CLINICAL NURSING

CONTRIBUTORS

Margaret A. Colliton, D.Sc.N.
Private Practice, New Haven, Connecticut,
and Administrator of Wellspring, an intermediate
psychiatric treatment facility

Carole A. LaFleur, R.N., M.S.N.
Chief, Advanced Clinical Practice and Director of Special Services
Visiting Nurse Association of Metropolitan Detroit
Detroit, Michigan

Kathlene F. Monahan, R.N., M.S.N.
Associate Professor of Nursing, College of Nursing,
Wayne State University, Detroit, Michigan

Rita H. O'Neil, R.N., M.S.
Associate Professor of Nursing, College of Nursing
Southeastern Massachusetts University
North Dartmouth, Massachusetts

Elizabeth Ford Pitorak, R.N., M.S.N.
Clinical Nursing Specialist
Frances Payne Bolton School of Nursing,
Case Western Reserve University, Cleveland, Ohio

Gloria J. Smokvina, R.N., Ph.D.
Associate Professor of Nursing,
Purdue University Calumet
Hammond, Indiana

Jean Stallwood-Hess, R.N., M.S.N.
Associate Professor of Nursing, College of Nursing
Wayne State University, Detroit, Michigan

Norma Peters Thomas, R.N., M.S.
Visiting Lecturer, College of Nursing
Southeastern Massachusetts University, North Dartmouth, Massachusetts

Gayle A. Traver, R.N., M.S.N.
Associate Professor of Nursing, College of Nursing,
Assistant Professor of Medicine, College of Medicine
University of Arizona, Tucson, Arizona

Jean A. Werner-Beland, R.N., M.N., F.A.A.N.
Associate Professor of Nursing, College of Nursing
Wayne State University, Detroit, Michigan

Judith A. Wood, R.N., M.S.N.,
Assistant Professor of Medical-Surgical Nursing,
Frances Payne Bolton School of Nursing
Case Western Reserve University, Cleveland, Ohio

CLINICAL NURSING

Pathophysiological and Psychosocial Approaches

Fourth Edition

Irene L. Beland R.N., M.S.
Emeritus Professor of Nursing, College of Nursing, Wayne State University, Detroit, Michigan

Joyce Y. Passos, R.N., Ph.D.
Dean, College of Nursing, Southeastern Massachusetts University, North Dartmouth, Massachusetts

Macmillan Publishing Co., Inc.
New York

Collier Macmillan Publishers
London

Printed in the United States of America

Macmillan Publishing Co., Inc.
866 Third Avenue, New York, New York 10022

Collier Macmillan Canada, Ltd.

Library of Congress Cataloging in Publication Data

Beland, Irene L
Clinical Nursing.

Includes bibliograhies and index.
1. Nursing. I. Passos, Joyce Y., joint author.
II. Title. [DNLM: 1. Nursing. 2. Nursing care.
3. Nurse—Patient relations. WY 100 B426c]
RT41.B34 1981 610.73 80–27131
ISBN 0–02–307890–1

Printing: 1 2 3 4 5 6 7 8 Year: 1 2 3 4 5 6 7 8

PREFACE

Development of content in the first edition was shaped by presentation of a number of concepts developed by a group of faculty of Wayne State University College of Nursing.

1. Adaptation is basic to survival.
   a. The human organism is flexible and permits adaptations at all levels of activity (physiological, psychological, social).
   b. As an organism increases in complexity, specialized structures are required to facilitate adaptive functions.
   c. In health, physiological and psychological changes are regulated within limits.
   d. Some of the effects observed in disease result from the utilization of adaptive mechanisms.
   e. In disease, adaptation may be deficient, excessive, disorganized, or initiated by inappropriate stimuli.
   f. The physiological and psychological changes occurring in disease have a cause or causes, and within limits, some of them serve a useful purpose.
2. Heredity and environment interact to create individual potentials and differences.
3. Patient needs determine patient care.
4. Organization facilitates the utilization of resources to meet human needs.
5. Optimum health is a desirable goal.
6. The value of an observation depends on the integrity and detachment with which it is made and on its specificity.
7. Perceptions of reality vary with the perceiver.
8. The interaction of multiple factors determines the outcome of a situation.
9. Progress from disease toward health involves an increase in the capacity of the patient to cope with stress. During illness and recovery, the patient's needs shift from dependence, to independence, to interdependence.
10. Manifestations of disease and behavior during illness result from:
    a. An attempt on the part of the organism to adapt to or to compensate for disturbed function.
    b. The mobilization of defense mechanisms.
    c. The effect of injury on cells comprising a tissue or organ.
    d. The meaning that a disease and its treatment has for a person.
11. What a person does when he is ill depends on

what he believes to be the cause of his illness and how he thinks it should be treated.

12. Therapy in disease includes one or more of the following: neutralizing the cause, encouraging compensatory mechanisms, and providing rest to the diseased organ so that healing can take place.
13. Respect for the rights and dignity of man is fundamental in a democratic society. This is just as essential to the sick as to the well.
14. Mutual trust is basic to the establishment of constructive nurse-patient relationships.
15. Acceptance of the patient involves considering the meaning of his behavior and recognizing that it has a cause and serves a purpose. It does not require the nurse to compromise personal values.
16. The behavior of a person is affected by and affects all persons and events with which he is involved.
17. Rehabilitation is a continuous process which begins with the first contact with the patient.
18. The patient has a right to participate in plans concerning his welfare.
19. The nurse has a responsibility to assist the patient and his family to utilize his resources constructively.
20. Nurses have an obligation to explore interests and aptitudes with the patient to increase his skills in living.
21. Nursing procedures can be used to facilitate communication.
22. There are limits to what can be accomplished by medical science.
23. Birth, growth, health, disease, and death are all phenomena of life.

These concepts have remained fundamental to all subsequent editions, including the fourth edition.

The objectives and approach of the fourth edition are similar to those of previous editions. The fourth edition is still intended for the nursing student, with substantial background in humanities, and in the natural and social sciences, who is studying nursing of the sick individual for the first time. Although nurses play many roles, this book emphasizes the central function of nurses in ministering to and acting in behalf of the individual. The approach that is used has been developed in the teaching of medical–surgical nursing over a period of many years. An attempt has been made to organize a vast quantity of material into a meaningful whole and to present the person who is ill as a total individual, not as a sick arm, leg, or heart. To further this objective the content of one chapter is related to and built upon earlier chapters and anticipates the content of later ones. Content is selected from the biological, physical, and social sciences. Emphasis is on normal as well as pathological physiology. Throughout the text the relationship of the function of one part to that of other parts of the body has been stressed. Since alteration in the function of one part is likely to affect other functions, including psychological and emotional functioning, these relationships are included. Further, an attempt has been made to organize all aspects of a function so that the interrelationships of different bodily functions are shown. As an example, one vital function is the maintenance of nutrition. All elements entering into the nutritional status from those affecting food supply and the ingestion, digestion, and absorption of food, to its utilization by cells, are presented. Through this approach, it is hoped that the student will have a broader base from which to evaluate the needs of each individual. A conscientious effort has been made to show how a variety of elements such as age, hereditary background, cultural background, state of nutrition, causative agent or agents, and the organs affected influence the effects of illness and the behavior manifested by the person and his nursing requirements.

No attempt has been made to include a wide variety of procedures. For the most part, procedures are included for the purpose of illustrating or emphasizing a point or points. Although the nurse does have a responsibility for using machines properly and for knowing whether or not they are operating properly, little attention has been given to the operation and care of machines employed in the treatment of disease. When directions provided by the manufacturer are inadequate, technicians should be available to instruct in the use and care of complicated machines.

Major organizational changes have been made to highlight the concept of *adaptation*, which is central to this edition as it has been to all previous editions. Other benefits of the major reorganization are that material should be easier to locate, and smaller chapters should facilitate student learning. Content is presented in three sections, comprised of 52 chapters which are organized into nine units.

Section One, consisting of eight chapters organized into two units, provides historical and contemporary perspectives on health and illness, including emphasis on the stress-adaptation model which is presented from a variety of perspectives.

Section Two, consisting of 21 chapters organized into four units, presents factors which influence dynamic equilibrium. The first set of factors (Unit III) are the internal and external environmental agents capable of producing injury; these injurious agents are considered stressors. The second set of factors (Unit IV) are the regulatory and control mechanisms with which we are endowed to sense and respond to stressors in such a way that essential life processes are protected. The third set of factors (Unit VI) are the nature and interrelatedness of essential life processes which must be regulated and maintained to assure the person's survival, growth and development. Unit V elaborates the nurse's role in supporting the individual's mechanisms of response to potential and actual injury.

Section Three, consisting of 23 chapters organized into three units, presents nursing management of clinical problems associated with (1) psychosocial aspects of illness and injury (Unit VII), (2) alterations in regulatory and response mechanisms (Unit VIII), and (3) alterations in essential life processes (Unit IX).

The authors express appreciation to all their students and faculty colleagues whose questions and suggestions have shaped this and previous editions. We especially thank all those who have contributed to, used, and shared their evaluations of previous editions.

Special thanks are given to B. Wallace Hood, Jr., Executive Editor of Macmillan Publishing Co., Inc., for his initiation and unstinting support of the major reorganization; to Sandra P. Young, for invaluable secretarial assistance in preparing the manuscript; and to Benjamin A. Passos, M.D., without whose encouragement, consultation, and innumerable services this edition would not have been completed.

Finally, the authors are grateful for the cooperation, assistance, and patience of Ellen Rope and other members of the staff of Macmillan Publishing Co., Inc., during the preparation and production of this edition.

I. L. B.
J. Y. P.

CONTENTS

Section ONE Historical and Contemporary Perspectives on Health and Illness

Section TWO Factors Influencing Dynamic Equilibrium

SECTION ONE

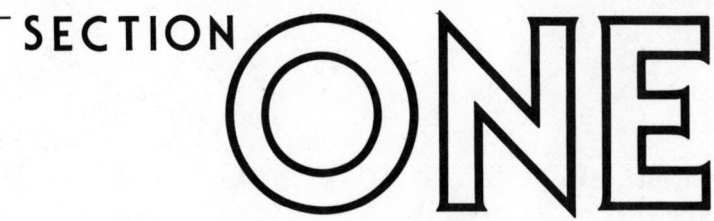

Historical and Contemporary Perspectives on Health and Illness

UNIT I

The Health-Illness Spectrum

Health of mind and body is so fundamental to the good life that if we believe men have any personal rights at all as human beings, then they have an absolute moral right to such a measure of good health as society and society alone is able to give them.

ARISTOTLE

INTRODUCTION

Although health and illness are often viewed as separate entities, they are not. All aspects of life, which begins with conception and ends in death, are interrelated. The theoretical framework for this and later chapters is that in health people are able to adapt successfully to their environment. In illness their adaptive capacity is limited in some way. In the words of Dubos (1965, p. xvii), "the states of health or disease are the expressions of the success or failure experienced by the organism in its efforts to respond adaptively to environmental challenges." Later he says that

> Human life is thus the outcome of the interplay between three separate classes of determinants, namely: the lasting and universal characteristics of man's nature, which are inscribed in his flesh and bone; the ephemeral conditions which man encounters at a given moment: and last but not least, man's ability to choose between alternatives and to decide upon a course of action *(Dubos, 1965, pp. xviii–ix).*

Dunn (1959) emphasizes the relationship of health and disease by saying that "it is essential to shift from considering sickness and wellness as a dichotomy toward thinking of disease and health as a graduated scale." What Dunn calls high-level wellness is at one end of the scale, whereas death is at the other. Pellegrino (1971) expresses a similar view: "it is better to think of each person as being located on a continuous spectrum extending from obvious disease through the absence of discernible disease to a state of optimum functioning in all spheres." He further states that no individual is entirely free from some physical, emotional, or social distress that impairs satisfaction in life or the ability to function optimally. The position of a person on the continuum depends on the interaction of all the influencing factors.

Not everyone agrees that disease is inevitable. There is some scientific basis for the hope that eventually the diseases now prevalent can be controlled. It is expected of health professionals in contemporary society that they be prepared and willing to address human needs related to *both* care of the sick and maintenance of health. Those expectations can be expressed as objectives for the health professions.

Objectives for the Health Professions

With the exception of 1 and 3, the following objectives are stated in terms of *PREVENTION,* which is the key concept in contemporary professional nursing (Beland & Passos, 1973):

1. The promotion of health
2. *Prevention* of the onset of illness or disease or the maintenance of health
3. Restoration of the sick person to health (cure)
4. *Prevention* of the extension of injury consequent to illness or disease
5. *Prevention* of complications of disease and/or its medical treatment
6. *Prevention* of avoidable deleterious dependence as a consequence of disease and/or its medical treatment
7. *Prevention* of death as an avoidable consequence of disease, injury, or medical treatment
8. *Prevention* of avoidable suffering in the presence of incurable or irreversible disease

From an examination of past and present-day health problems, a foundation can be laid for thinking of what nurses can contribute to the achievement of each of these objectives. Because in subsequent units, these objectives will be considered in detail in relation to specific nursing problems, only an overview will be given in this unit.

References Cited

Beland, I. L., and Passos, J. Y. "The Current Status of Baccalaureate Education." In Faye G. Abdellah et al., *New Directions in Patient-Centered Nursing.* New York: Macmillan Publishing Co., Inc., 1973, p. 259.

Dubos, R. "Health and Creative Adaptation." *Human Nature,* 1:2–10, 1978.

Dubos, R. *Man Adapting.* New Haven: Yale University Press, 1965, pp. xvii and xii–xix.

Dunn, H. "High-Level Wellness for Man and Society." *Am. J. Public Health,* 49 (1959), 787.

Pellegrino, E. D. "Medicine Looks at Health Maintenance—Health Maintenance: An idea in search of an organization." In Warren Perry and Joseph E. Necharch, eds. *Proceedings of an Institute on Health Maintenance: Challenge for the Allied Health Professions.* Buffalo, N.Y.: School of Health Related Professions, 1971, p. 14.

1

Historical Perspectives on Disease Causation

All theories have a life history. They start tentatively, grow piecemeal, and slowly become mature. Then they can successfully handle new facts and also have considerable predictive value. But sooner or later a discrepancy appears between fact and theory. Then the theory will become modified, perhaps will entirely disintegrate, to be succeeded by something new.

KING, 1963

To provide a background for understanding how knowledge, social beliefs and customs, and other circumstances affect health care the following areas will be considered: (1) theories to explain disease causation from early recorded history to the present, (2) changes in threats to health and health practices as knowledge increased, and (3) the evolution of legislation and social structures to promote health and to prevent injury and disease. Some ideas have been present throughout recorded history and most advances are built on past accomplishments. As an example, history records in different forms humankind's desire to live indefinitely. This desire persists today, despite evidence that the maximum life span for each species is predetermined (Hayflick, 1968). What has been accomplished is an increase in the number of persons who approach the maximum by decreasing the mortality rate among infants, young children, and those in middle age. Rosenfeld (1973) summarizes a variety of studies of factors influencing the rate of aging. One interesting finding has been that within species, individuals with a lower body temperature live longer than those individuals with higher temperatures.

Theories of Disease Causation

Throughout the course of history human beings have tried to explain their relationship to their environment and to each other. They have also tried to explain the significant events in life, including the nature of disease, its causes, prevention, and treatment. In the process theories and practices have been developed that were and are based on preceived cause–effect relationships. These attempts to define disease, its prevention, and its treatment have influenced the development of cultures throughout the world. These theories were related to the level of knowledge as well as to the social circumstances of the time. Even today some health practices are based on empirical rather than scientific knowledge. Effective preventive measures were introduced before the cause of infectious disease was known. Before the time of Christ, the Romans had developed a public water supply and a sewage disposal system. The latter continues in use to the present time. Smallpox was prevented by vaccination long before its cause was known. Although written records are incomplete, surgical skills were highly developed in ancient times.

To emphasize the point that people still act on empirical knowledge, twentieth-century examples follow. In Kurdistan in 1958, bubonic plague was still endemic. The plague season began in September and lasted until May. When the villagers noted an increase in the rat population in September, they moved from the village to the center of a field. Although the villagers did not know that fleas transmit plague from the sick rats to humans, the move from the village to the field was successful because it removed the people from the habitat of the sick rats and the vehicle of transmission of the plague, the flea. Plague was controlled not because the people understood how plague is transmitted, but because the increase in the rat population was regarded as an omen of an impending epidemic of a deadly disease (Gascar, 1958).

Moreover, action based on empirical knowledge is not limited to unsophisticated peoples. The use of many drugs is based on an observed cause–effect relationship rather than on knowledge of their effect on cellular activity. An ancient Chinese practice that is causing considerable interest, acupuncture, had its origin in the observation that soldiers hit in certain areas suffered no pain. Why it is effective in preventing and relieving some types of pain is unknown.

Some theories of disease causation date back to the beginning of humankind. Others are of recent origin; none has been entirely relegated to the past. Some of the important theories are as follows:

1. Disease is caused by the evil influence of supernatural powers.
2. Disease is punishment for sin and the result of the wrath of an essentially righteous god.
3. Disease is part of the natural order and can be explained on a rational basis.
4. Disease is caused by the epidemic constitution of the atmosphere, miasmic influences, and filth.
5. Disease is caused by a germ.
6. Many diseases require not only a necessary condition (a microbe or other agent) but also a sufficient cause.
7. Disease results from the interaction of multiple factors.
8. Disease results from a disturbance in the adaptive capacity of the individual.
9. Disease is due to a failure to live properly—either as a result of the person's own or society's failure.

Numbers 1 through 5 are discussed in this chapter and 6 through 9 are discussed in Chapter 2. There are many more theories of disease causation. Some, such as the germ theory, have withstood the test of time. Others, such as focal infection as a cause of disease—for example, arthritis due to an infection in tonsils or teeth—have not. In some instances healthy teeth were extracted without alleviating the arthritis.

The Malign Influence of Supernatural Powers

The first, or demonic, theory, though probably the oldest theory of the causation of disease, has not been entirely eliminated. Usually this theory is expressed in one of three ways. Living persons (witches) have the power to cause disease in other living persons (witches were believed to have an evil influence because of supernatural powers). This power is exercised in different ways: The witch casts a spell on someone whom she or he dislikes, or an individual has some power such as the evil eye. Even today one may hear an expression of the belief that one person is able to harm others by supernatural powers. Sam Thrill says, "You had better stay away from me; I always bring other people bad luck."

A second form of the demonic theory is that disease is caused by the spirits of the disembodied dead. This idea is the basis for some of the burial rites practiced by primitive peoples. It is not unknown today, however.

A third expression of the demonic theory is that disease results from superhuman abilities of inanimate objects. Stones, trees, animals, and natural events are ascribed special qualities that enable them to act in a malevolent fashion (Winslow, 1943, p. 34).

When a demon is held to be responsible for disease, prevention and treatment are directed toward the demon rather than the person who is sick. The principal methods employed are exorcism, evasion, and sacrificial propitiation. The individual who is possessed of a devil is beaten or given a vile-tasting medicine. Trephining (making a hole in the skull) was originally performed to provide an avenue of escape for the demon who had taken over the body of the sick person. Evasion, or avoiding the demon, is achieved by rituals that are prescribed to prevent contact between the potential victim and the evil spirit. The people of Kurdistan, by moving from the village to the field, were practicing a form of evasion. Sacrifices are made to appease the god who is believed to cause the epidemic. The sacrifice is really a bribe. The person makes the sacrifice not to atone for wrongdoing but to avoid harm from an evil spirit.

Punishment for Sin

A second theory of disease causation is that the wrath of an essentially righteous god decrees disease as a punishment for sin. Winslow (1943) states that this concept of disease causation reached its height among Semitic peoples and is best expressed in the Old Testament. This belief, however, was not limited to the Hebrews. The Hindus believed the epidemic of plague (1896–1897) was a punishment imposed on them by their god Siva. "Sin-caused" disease was treated by sacrifices of atonement to the offended god. Earlier modes of treatment, such as magical practices to appease demons, were condemned in this era. The theory of disease as a punishment for sin introduced a new concept, as it is based on a universal law.

The Hebrews also gave cleanliness a spiritual value. Early humans had practiced bathing for reasons of comfort. Other ancients such as the Egyptians required those entering temples to be clean, but the Hebrews had the most clearly formalized rules of hygiene institutionalized in their religion. Their hygienic laws are spelled out in the Book of Leviticus. They include practices relating to food, personal hygiene, clothing, diseases, and environmental sanitation. Without these laws there is doubt that the Jews would have been able to escape from Egypt. In fact, the Bible is replete with illustrations indicating the status of medicine of the time.

Part of the Natural Order

The first known reference to the idea that events in the universe can be explained on a rational basis appeared in the sixth century B.C. in the writings of the Ionic Greeks. Again in the words of Winslow (1943), "The Hebrews gave us a universe of moral law; but the Greeks clearly visualized for the first time in human history a universe of natural law." Thus the Greeks introduced a new way of thinking about disease. They stressed observation as a tool for learning about disease and advocated looking at the patient rather than assuming that his or her disease was something imposed from without by another being.

The Epidemic Constitution of the Atmosphere, Miasmic Influences, and Filth

In the period between Hippocrates and Pasteur, emphasis was on epidemic constitution of the atmosphere, miasmic influences.[1] According to this theory, disease is propagated by (1) the air, (2) diseased persons, and (3) goods transported from infected places. One or more of these agents was employed to explain epidemics at different times and places. For example, when plague was destroying much of the population of the world, the cause of the pandemic was believed to be a malign conjunction of planets over the Indian Ocean. They produced "corrupt vapors, raised by and disseminated through the air by the blasts of the heavy and turbid southerly winds" (Winslow, 1943, p. 182). References to atmospheric conditions as factors in the cause of disease are not unknown at the present time. Natural disasters, inasmuch as they disrupt measures taken to protect water and food supplies, can be sources of epidemic disease. What the individuals do at the time, however, depends on what they believe to be the source of illness. If they believe that the cause of the illness is borne on a "turbid southerly wind," nothing much can be done to avoid disease. If, however, they believe that when water and sewage pipes are broken, human feces containing pathogens may contaminate the drinking water, measures such as boiling the water or adding chlorine are likely to be accepted as necessary.

Because miasmic influences were held to be particularly dangerous at night, houses were often tightly sealed during the hours of darkness to prevent disease. To prevent the spread of disease from a sick person to the community, the sick person and his or her family were confined in the house. It was thought that if the house was sealed, disease-producing air would be prevented from escaping into the atmosphere. This also prevented contact of the sick person, objects used in his or her care, and the members of the family with members of the community. Because it usually increased the degree of contact among family members, sealing the house practically ensured that every family member would contract the disease.

[1] Miasmic influences means air poisoned or polluted by vapors rising from swamps, marshy grounds, and putrid or decaying matter and filth.

The Middle Ages, Including the Eighteenth Century

In Europe in the Middle Ages, epidemics of plague, syphilis, and cholera killed vast numbers of people. In the famous London plague of 1665, 68,596 Londoners died. Such a terrifying event called for drastic action. Consequently, it is not surprising that, besides sealing the family and person dying from plague into the house, dogs and cats were killed, as they were believed to be the source of the disease. Because of lack of knowledge of plague or its mode of transmission, flea-infested rats were allowed to run free.

By the end of the eighteenth century, plague, which had been a major threat to the populations of Europe for 400 years, was no longer a serious problem. It had been recognized as being contagious and measures appropriate to its eradication were undertaken. Plague has not been eradicated, however, as its incidence has been rising in the Republic of Vietnam and was high in 1968. Plague has also recently been reported in the United States.

Some of the practices introduced in the Middle Ages have been continued into this century. Thus in the recent past persons who were ill with certain infectious diseases, as well as their human and animal contacts, were confined for the longest usual incubation period. Although current practices vary somewhat in different legal jurisdictions and with different diseases, restriction of movement is usually limited to those sick with the disease. The movement of susceptible contacts may be limited during the longest usual incubation period. If, by the end of the incubation period, the contacts are well, restriction on their movement is lifted. Such practices as placarding the house have been discontinued.

Although serious pandemics occurred in the Middle Ages, they have not been confined to this period in history. References are made in the Old Testament to ancient pestilences sent by God to punish people for having sinned. The last great pandemic occurred during World War I, when influenza spread to all corners of the earth. More people died as a result of influenza than from battle injuries. In the United States few people escaped, and because of the rapidity with which influenza spreads, entire families were ill at the same time.

Why were plague, cholera, and typhoid common? The theory that epidemic diseases were caused by the constitution of the air, miasmic influences, and filth may appear to be strange. Considering, however, the state of knowledge and the conditions under which people lived, the theory was reasonable. It is difficult, if not impossible, for the modern-day middle- or upper-class American to imagine the conditions of filth under which people lived. People living in cities were crowded together. Provisions for safe water and food supplies, as well as for the sanitary disposal of human wastes, were limited and exceedingly primitive.[2]

Facilities for bathing and for maintaining general cleanliness were lacking. Furthermore, similar conditions still exist in many parts of the world. While traveling, the writer observed people using the same ditch as a source of water for drinking and cooking, for washing clothes, and for disposal of excreta. Overcrowding and limited provisions for personal and community hygiene are not unknown in some sections of the United States.

[2] For an account of the sanitary conditions in England and other parts of the world, Winslow (1943, pp. 236–66) is highly recommended.

The Nineteenth Century

Although measures instituted to control the spread of disease during each pandemic depended on the state of knowledge and the prevailing theories of disease causation, they were not limited to past knowledge. For knowledge was added to by those who made accurate observations from which valid inferences were drawn. As an example, in 1854 John Snow proved that cholera was spread by contaminated water and contact with the cholera victim despite the fact that the cholera vibrio was not identified for another 27 years. His conclusions were based on detailed observation of the habits of those who did and did not develop cholera.

The Sanitary Movement

Another significant advance derived from the observation that disease and filth were associated; the great sanitary movement developed first in England and shortly thereafter in America. By the beginning of the nineteenth century, the modern public health movement had been born. The leaders of this movement were lay people and social reformers, among them John Howard (eighteenth century) and Edwin Chadwick (early nineteenth century). Neither was a physician. John Howard was a sheriff who found appalling the conditions in the jails for which he was responsible. The sanitary procedures that he instituted appear to be elementary. At the time they were put into effect, however, they were most progressive. Walls were to be whitewashed each year. The walls were to be washed and cells ventilated regularly. Hot and cold water was to be made available to the prisoners for bathing. Clean clothes were also to be lent to prisoners, if necessary. Unfortunately, conditions in jails continue to be unsatisfactory.

Chadwick, who was a social reformer, studied living conditions in the slums of London. His studies led to administrative reform and to laws relating to conditions affecting the health of the poor. His report, *Conditions of the Labouring Population of Great Britain,* was published in 1842. It served as the basis for the sanitary reform that spread over the civilized world. In the early years of industrialization in England, living conditions were indescribably bad. One source of information is the novels of Charles Dickens. He not only wrote about the horrible social evils of the time but lent powerful support to the social reformers. In the United States, Shattuck (1948) made a similar contribution.

Shortly after Chadwick's report was published, another event contributed to knowledge of the practical importance of cleanliness to health and recovery from disease. Florence Nightingale went to Turkey where the Crimean War was in progress (1853–1856). Aided by thirty-seven assistants, she was able to reduce the death rate of soldiers hospitalized in Scutari from 42 to 2 per cent. Miss Nightingale had knowledge neither of germs nor of antibiotics. Previous to her appearance, cholera and dysentery ran rampant among the men who were hospitalized. She and her assistants used soap, water, clean linen, and humane care, with the result that she accomplished more than the entire British Medical Department in saving the lives of British soldiers.

Though Miss Nightingale was the first to reduce the death rate among soldiers by reducing the incidence of infection, she was not the first to note the disastrous effects of infections among soldiers. An early Greek historian, Thucydides, wrote, "Appalling too was the rapidity with which men caught the infection, dying like sheep if they attended one another; and this was the principal cause of mortality."

Not too long after the close of the Crimean War, the American Civil War (1861–1865) was fought. As in the Crimean War, infectious diseases were responsible for a high mortality rate. Dysentery, typhoid fever, and tetanus killed more than the wounds of battle. Approximately 300,000 men died, and two thirds of them died from disease.

The Germ Theory of Disease

At the time Miss Nightingale was saving lives in Scutari by instituting hygienic and humane care, Pasteur was disproving the theory of spontaneous generation and developing the germ theory of disease. As is usually true when new ideas are proposed or discoveries are made, Pasteur was not solely responsible for either accomplishment, as the theory of spontaneous generation had been questioned earlier. What is important, however, is that, as a result of the work of Pasteur, the idea was accepted that living beings, no matter how small, had their origin not from dead or decaying matter, but from other similar beings. Translated into the germ theory of disease, a specific microorganism is a necessary condition in the development of each infectious disease. Anthrax does not develop unless the anthrax bacillus is present. The natural culmination of the germ theory of disease was Koch's postulates. They are a set of criteria that can be utilized to prove that a specific microorganism does or does not cause a specific disease.

Without improvements in the power and precision of the microscope many of the discoveries supporting the germ theory could not have been made. It might be added that without the technological developments of the nineteenth and twentieth centuries much less would be known about the cause, prevention, effects, and treatment of a great number of diseases. In the period following the discoveries of Pasteur and Koch, the attention of scientists was on identifying the specific agents responsible for disease. The sanitary movement, which was introduced by the social reformers, now had a scientific basis.

The germ theory, along with related accomplishments, encouraged the hope that for each disease a specific causative agent could and would be identified. With knowledge of the cause, specific preventive and curative measures would follow; in some instances, this has happened. For example, although diphtheria has probably existed in epidemic form since the earliest times, it was not until 1826 that a French physician, Bretonneau de Tours, placed the clinical diagnosis of diphtheria on fairly firm ground. The diphtheria bacillus, or Klebs–Löffler bacillus, was seen and described by Klebs in 1883 and established as the cause of diphtheria by Löffler in 1884. From his observations of patients and animals with the disease. Löffler postulated that the bacillus secreted a diffusible toxin that was responsible for many of the effects of the disease. After this theory was proved by other investigators, the toxin was used to stimulate animals (the horse) to produce antitoxin. The antitoxin was found to provide passive immunity against diphtheria and, when administered early in the course of the disease, to hasten recovery and prevent serious complications.

Unfortunately, the relationship between cause, prevention, and cure does not fall so neatly into place with many infectious diseases. An effective preventive measure was available for smallpox before its cause was known. There are as yet no specific methods available for its treatment. In the twentieth century vaccines have been developed that are effective in the prevention of a number of other diseases, including poliomyelitis, tetanus, measles, and whooping cough. There is no method available to modify the course of poliomyelitis or whooping cough. Both must run their course. Conversely, for some infectious diseases for which there is no specific preventive measure, there are effective chemotherapeutic or antibiotic agents; pneumococcal pneumonia is an example.

Some of the changes in laws and attitudes that had their beginnings in the nineteenth century include sanitary and housing codes, laws to protect the quality of food, the supply of water, and the work and home environment. Later, as workers organized to promote and protect their rights, hours of work were shortened. Conditions under which women and children could work were defined. The right of the worker to a living wage was established. With machines, the workers were not only able to increase production of goods, but by sharing in the rewards of increased production the workers were able to improve their standard of living and health status. Members of groups such as fraternal organizations joined together to provide for insurance for their families in the event of death. Later, commercial insurance companies were formed for this purpose and the types of insurance were expanded to cover other kinds of human disaster.

Only a few of the accomplishments of the nineteenth century have been reviewed. As one reads about them, one cannot help but be impressed with their significance to health. In the first half of the century foundation for a sanitary revolution was laid. In the second half the scientific basis for sanitation was discovered and the germ theory of causation of infectious disease was shown to be valid.

The germ theory was not only important to the control of infectious diseases, it was also equally important to the development of modern surgery. During the twentieth century surgical techniques have been developed to the point where almost all organs are subject to surgical intervention, including the successful transplantation of some organs from one person to another.

The Twentieth Century

The twentieth century is marked by two worlds: that part in which the problems created by lack of sanitation, unsuitable and overcrowded housing, inadequate food and medical care predominate, and that part in which these problems have been minimized. Unfortunately, many more people live in the underdeveloped areas of the world than in industrialized countries. Even in highly developed countries not all of the conditions believed to be prerequisite to good health are equally available to all segments of the population. Further, industrialization, or as it is commonly called, progress, has brought with it threats to health. As an example, the Aswan Dam was built to increase food production in Egypt. It has had the unfortunate effect of providing an environment favorable to the multiplication of the snail, which the schistosoma requires for part of its life cycle. As a result, the incidence of schistosomiasis, a very serious disease, is increasing greatly. Air pollution in industrialized countries is believed to be a factor in the incidence of the chronic degenerative diseases of middle and old age.

Even where knowledge and resources are sufficient to control infectious disease, it has not been eliminated. In fact, some such as the venereal diseases are increasing. Furthermore, wherever infectious diseases are brought under control, the average length of life has increased and the incidence of the diseases common to middle and later life has risen. A significant point is that these latter diseases are not new; what is new is their relative frequency. It may be possible to delay the onset and progress of these diseases or even to eliminate them. Thomas (1972) proposes that the major diseases eventually will be brought under control. Should this happen, each individual will live out a life span as programmed in his or her cells, as stated earlier.

What remains to be done? Despite increases in knowledge and skills, much remains to be done. A high quality of health care is not equally available to all people. Much is yet to be learned about the prevention, causes, and treatment of a number of important diseases. Even when knowledge is available, people do not always use it. Why not? One problem is the development of habits and practices conducive to health as well as the control of the external environment. In many diseases the individual's behavior is as important as or more important than the causative agent(s).

Among the many other questions to be answered are the following: How can priorities be changed so that keeping an individual well is considered as challenging as curing him or her of a catastrophic illness? What kinds of facilities, services, support, and personnel are required to make health maintenance a reality? To what extent does regular health surveillance make a difference in the health of people?

Other questions that require answers include the following: Why do cells respond in self-destructive ways to harmless substances? Why do they fail to respond in appropriate ways to their own regulators, and what actually happens in cells in the prepathogenic period of chronic degenerative diseases? Although there is some information about the biochemistry of aging, much remains to be learned. There are many other questions that require answers before the prevention of chronic disease is established on a sound basis. Is aging inevitable or is it a disease and therefore subject to control (Rosenfeld, 1973)? Equally significant is the problem of how to implement knowledge so that it is used [by professionals as well as the public].

Some Accomplishments in the Field of Medicine

It is outside the scope of this chapter to recount all the accomplishments in the field of medicine in the twentieth century. It is also well to remember that as in other fields of knowledge, the present is dependent upon the past. Thus the control of infectious disease has been a continuation and development of knowledge gained in the nineteenth century. Developments in surgery depend upon methods to prevent infection, to produce anesthesia, and to control bleeding (see chapter 50). Medical therapies were extended by the discovery of new drugs as well as by refinements in the use of those already known.

The use of instruments in the diagnosis of disease has been greatly expanded. The first instrument generally used in diagnosis was the stethoscope, which was introduced in 1816 by Laennec (Reiser, 1979). Stephen Hales, an English minister, is credited with making the first measurements of arterial blood pressure in 1733, by inserting a glass rod into the femoral artery of a horse. The present sphygmomanometer was introduced at the end of the nineteenth century. Today arterial blood pressure can be measured and recorded electronically. The sophistication of present-day diagnostic instruments is illustrated by computed axial tomography ("cat scanning") [Abrams & McNeil, 1978]. With each advance some problems are solved and others are created. For example, questions arise when a diagnostic instrument is very expensive. Does its use justify the expense? Does every hospital need one? If the answer is no, which hospitals do need one? There are other questions as well.

As another example, in the treatment of chronic renal failure, there is the question of which patients will be selected for renal transplants or be provided with kidney machines. Involved is a limited supply of kidneys for transplantation and the high cost of either procedure. Thus ethical as well as financial questions are involved.

Another problem created by the advances in medicine is that because some diseases have appeared to be cured miraculously people have come to expect cures for all diseases. People find it difficult to believe that there are no quick and easy answers to diseases such as cancer and heart disease. There is also a common belief that any problem can be solved by the spending of enough money. Thus in 1977, $160 billion was spent on health care. Unrealistic expectations are encouraged by news stories, and concern about medical competence is aroused by stories of unnecessary surgery and malpractice (Abelson, 1978).

No attempt has been made here to summarize all the advances and problems created and still remaining in health and sickness care. Much has been accomplished, and with each accomplishment one is reminded that much more needs to be done.

References Cited

Abelson, P. "A View of Health Research and Care." *Science,* **200** (1978), 43–44.

Abrams, H. L. and McNeil, B. J. "Medical Implications of Computed Tomography ("Cat Scanning"). *N. Engl. J. Med.,* 298 (1978), 255–61.

Gascar, P. "Died of Plague: Ramsara's Daughter, 14 Years." *World Health,* 11 (1958), 12.

Hayflick, L. "Human Cells and Aging." *Sci. Am.,* 218 (1968), 32–37.

King, L. S. *The Growth of Medical Thought.* Chicago: University of Chicago Press, 1963, p. 232.

Reiser, S. J. "The Medical Influence of the Stethoscope." *Sci. Am.,* 240 (1979), 148–56.

Rosenfeld, A. "The Longevity Seekers." *Sat. Rev. Sci.,* 1 (1973), 46–51.

Shattuck, L. *Report of the Sanitary Commission of Massachusetts, 1850.* Cambridge, Mass.: Harvard University Press, 1948.

Thomas, L. "Guessing and Knowing: Reflections of the Science and Technology of Medicine." *Sat. Rev. Sci.,* 55 (1972), 52–57.

Winslow, C. E. A. *The Conquest of Epidemic Disease.* Princeton, N.J.: Princeton University Press, 1943.

General References

Alcott, L. M. *Hospital Sketches.* Ed. by B. Z. Jones. Cambridge, Mass.: Harvard University Press, 1960.

Bowers, J. Z. and Purcell, E. G., eds. *Advances in American Medicine.* New York: Josiah Macy, Jr., Foundation, 1976.

Defoe, D. *The Plague in London,* London: George Bell & Sons, 1889.

Duffy, J. *Epidemics of Colonial America.* Baton Rouge: Louisiana State University Press, 1953.

Garrison, F. H. *History of Medicine,* 4th ed. Philadelphia: W. B. Saunders Company, 1929.

Stent, G. S. Prematurity and Uniqueness in Scientific Discovery. *Sci. Am.,* 227:84–93, Dec. 1972.

2

The Nature and Scope of Disease

In America the passion for physical well-being . . . is general.
ALEXIS DE TOCQUEVILLE, 1835

The Nature of Disease

This chapter will consider the nature of disease and some of the factors that influence the cause, prevention, treatment, and cure of disease. Whenever considering disease, however, the nurse should keep uppermost in mind and actions Besson's (1967) injunction that professionals deal "more with people and less with patients . . . more with the human conditions, and less with formalin fixed pathology . . . more with the sociocultural hazards than with the biological ones . . . more with a continuum of care, less with the episode of sickness." No one approach to the care of people, sick or well, should be excluded. At one time one is more important than another. Humans are at the same time biological, sociocultural, and psychological beings.

DEFINITION OF DISEASE

In contrast to health, disease is a state in which the individual is no longer in equilibrium with the forces in the external and internal environment (see Figure 2-1). Francis (1960) expresses this concept of disease in the following statement: "disease is a reaction to a stress which extends beyond the bounds of individual reserve and adaptability." Engle (1960) defines *disease* as "failures or disturbances in the growth, development, functions, and adjustments of the organism as a whole or of any of its systems." Engle (1960, p. 469) also emphasizes the importance of defining disease as a natural phenomenon.

To clarify differences between a state of health and a state of disease, the essential features of each are summarized in Table 2-1.

Etiologic Agents

In the preceding section disease has been defined and some of the factors influencing the capacity of the organism to respond to disturbances in its environment in ways that prevent disequilibrium have been considered. However, success in preventing disequilibrium depends not only on the capacity of the individual to react appropriately but also on the nature of the agent eliciting the response and on the interaction of both elements. Moreover, neither health nor disease results from a single factor. Rather both health and disease are the consequence of the interaction of many factors within the host and its environment—physical, biological, psychological, and social (see Figure 2-1).

Engel (1960, pp. 478–83) states that agents or conditions placing strain on the adaptive capacity of the individual are of four general types: (1) agents causing injury by their physical and chemical properties, (2) physical and chemical agents required for cellular

Figure 2-1. Simplified illustration of factors influencing health equilibrium. (Reproduced with permission of The Blakiston Division, McGraw-Hill Book Company, Inc., from *Preventive Medicine for the Doctor in His Community,* 3rd ed., 1965, p. 49, by Hugh R. Leavell and E. Gurney Clark.)

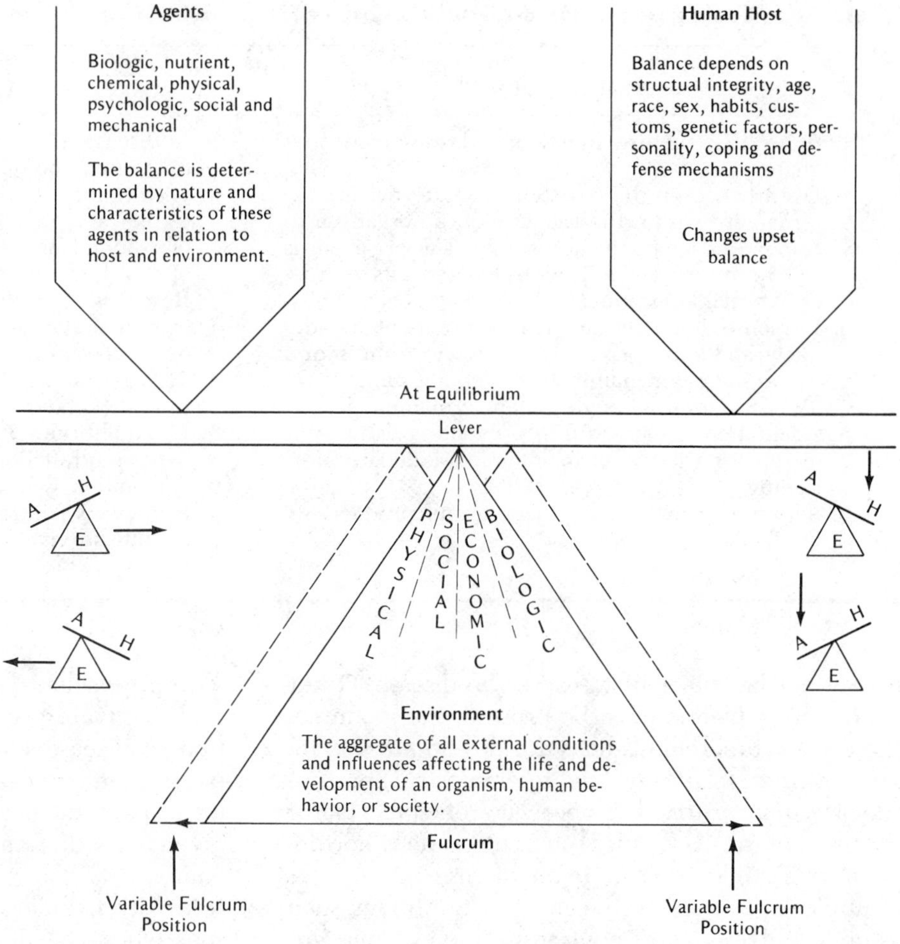

processes that result in injury when they are supplied in insufficient quantities,[1] (3) living agents, including microorganisms and parasites, and (4) psychological stress.

The disease-producing power of a pathogenic agent depends on the following: (1) its nature and characteristics, (2) its ability to maintain life and potency, (3) its ability to gain entrance and to establish itself in the host, (4) its source and reservoirs, and (5) vehicles and conditions for its dissemination. These factors are of importance in diseases caused by physical or chemical agents as well as those caused by living organisms. Knowledge of these factors contributes to the prevention, control, and treatment of disease, as well as to the identification of a disease-producing agent and its removal from the environment or the reduction of its effects. The application of the preceding to physical, chemical, and biological agents is made in Unit III. In addition to the preceding, certain other factors influence whether or not pathogenic agents are able to cause injury. Highly virulent microorganisms may overwhelm the host before there is an opportunity to mobilize defenses. A chemical agent may be so concentrated that many cells are injured and death is inevitable. A physical injury may be so violent that all vital processes are immediately and completely depressed. For example, a head-on collision in an automobile may result in the sudden death of all its occupants. A single exposure of a susceptible individual to the influenza virus is usually sufficient to cause disease.

The Concept of Not Only a Necessary Condition but a Sufficient Cause

Some agents do not cause disease on a single exposure and sometimes do not result in disease after repeated exposures. Not only do some etiologic agents require repeated exposures over a period of time, but the development of a particular disease may depend on the combined effect of several factors. These observations have led to the concept of the necessary and sufficient cause (Rogers, 1962). According to this concept, some diseases do not develop in the absence of a specific agent. This agent is necessary to the development of the disease, but by itself

[1] Some required substances can also cause injury when they are ingested in excessive quantities.

TABLE 2-1. *Comparison of the Essential Features of Health and Disease*

What is Health?	What is Disease?
1. In health, structure, function, and reserve are adequate.	1. In disease, structure, function, or reserve is inadequate (may be one or all).
2. Disturbances in the environment (internal and external) are within the capacity of the organism to respond or adapt to successfully. The organism is able to cope successfully with changes in its internal or external environment.	2. Disturbances in the environment (internal and external) are outside the capacity of the organism to respond or adapt to successfully. At the time of death, all adaptive powers are lost.
3. Responses to disturbances in environment are adequate and appropriate. They protect from injury.	3. Responses to disturbances in the environment are inadequate, excessive, or inappropriate. They may be sources of injury.
4. As a result of a dynamic state of equilibrium, stability of the internal environment is maintained.	4. There is failure to maintain stability within limits; that is, function is outside limits.
5. Adaptation is successful in preventing damage or in repairing it and in maintaining adequate functioning.	5. Disequilibrium in one area may lead to disturbances in function in other areas.
6. Survival, growth, reproduction, and productivity are facilitated.	6. Adaptation is unsuccessful in some respects; that is, there is failure of adaptation at some level, including survival.

it may not be sufficient to cause the disease. Other contributing factors must be present. For example, the disease tuberculosis does not develop in the absence of the *Mycobacterium tuberculosis.* Therefore the *Mycobacterium* is a necessary etiologic factor in tuberculosis. As a rule, tuberculosis does not develop on a single exposure to the disease but requires multiple exposures. Moreover, other conditions, such as undernutrition, are required to provide sufficient cause for the development of tuberculosis. In epidemiologic terms, tuberculosis requires both a necessary and a sufficient cause for disease to occur.

Multiple Factors in Disease Causation

In many of the chronic degenerative diseases the necessary condition for their development is not known, if such a factor exists. They appear to be the result of multiple factors, some of which have their origin in the individual and others in the external environment. Before disease develops, the sum total of all the factors must be sufficient to damage the cellular machinery and cause disease. Because chronic degenerative diseases require months or years to develop, it is difficult to assess the degree to which each factor is responsible.

Not all the factors contributing to the development of chronic disease are necessarily of a physical or chemical nature, nor are they of extrinsic origin. Apparently, genetic constitution predisposes an individual to some diseases and protects him or her from others. Psychological and social stresses can also impose strain on the capacity of the individual to cope with physical and chemical agents. Therefore when multiple factors appear to be involved in the causation of disease, the extent to which each factor—physical, chemical, genetic, microbiologic, physiologic, psychological, and social—is responsible in a given individual varies. When these and other factors combine so that the total effect is sufficient to interfere with cellular processes, disease results. In persons whose genetic constitutions predisposes them to a given disease, less in the way of other factors is required than in individuals who are not so predisposed. Conversely, an individual who is not predisposed to a given disease can develop it, if one or more other etiologic factors are sufficiently intense.

Methods of Studying Disease

Natural History of Disease

Another way to view disease (or health) is to examine its natural history. The term *natural history* is defined as the course taken by disease from beginning to end—that is, (1) the factors in the initiation of the disease, (2) the possible course of the disease to cure or to death, and (3) how environmental and genetic factors modify the course (Van Peenen, 1966).

It can be seen in Figure 2-2 that the development of a disease takes place in two periods. During the first, the prepathogenic period, the host, agent, and environment interact to produce a stimulus. It is dur-

Figure 2-2. Diagram showing the application of preventive medicine. (Reproduced with permission of The Blakiston Division, McGraw-Hill Book Company, Inc., from *Preventive Medicine for the Doctor in His Community,* 3rd ed., 1965, p. 27, by Hugh R. Leavell and E. Gurney Clark.)

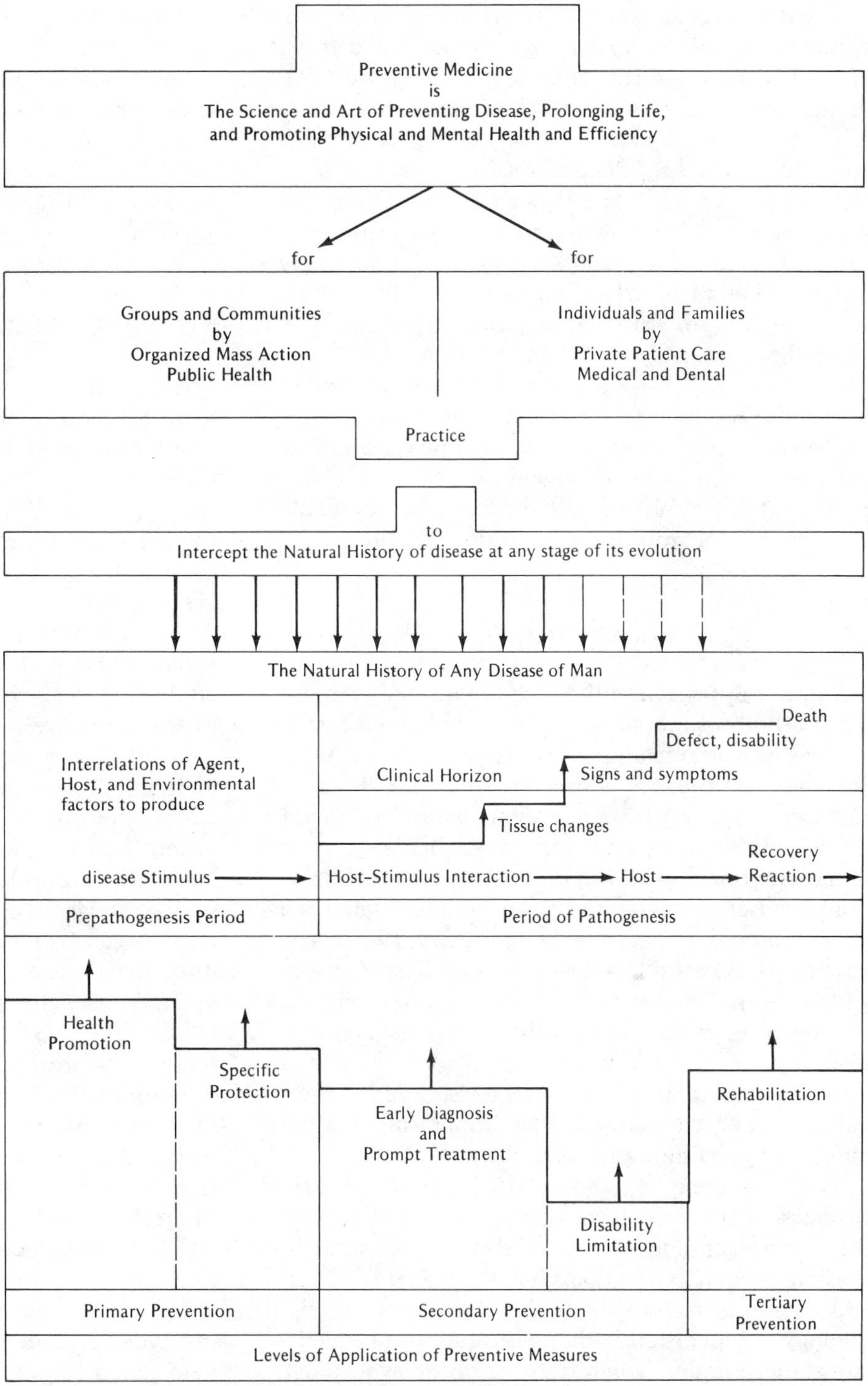

ing the prepathogenic period that measures should be instituted to prevent a disease or delay its onset. During the second, the pathogenic period, disease develops. It is during this period that the clinical manifestations become evident. Depending on the balance among the host, agent, and environment, the individual may fully recover, may be partially or completely disabled, or may die.

Study the Disease Characteristics

A disease may be studied by focusing attention on its characteristic features. It is described in terms of (1) causative or etiologic agents; (2) mechanisms by which the causative agent produces its effect, such as pathophysiology, psychopathology, sociopathology; (3) the nature of its onset—sudden or gradual;

(4) the characteristic signs and symptoms; (5) the predicted outcome or prognosis; (6) the preventive measures; and (7) the therapeutic measures. Although individuals who are sick are unique in many respects, diseases and patterns of response to diseases are not. They occur in classes or groups having common characteristics. Many persons may have the same disease. The cause and manifestations of a disease as well as the methods by which it is effectively prevented and treated are similar in individuals who have the disease. For example, measles is caused by a specific virus. Although manifestations vary in degree of severity, they are similar in all individuals who contract measles. Measles is effectively prevented by one attack of the disease or by vaccination. Treatment of the person who has measles is nonspecific inasmuch as no curative measures are available to shorten or modify the severity of the illness.

Study the Epidemiology

Another approach to the study of disease is to use the methods of epidemiology. The term *epidemiology* has its origin in and relates to its use in identifying the community factors in epidemic diseases. *Epidemiology* may be defined very simply as "medical detection." The same general methods are used in the identification of the person or persons responsible for a crime. A more comprehensive definition of *epidemiology* is given by Frost (Maxcy, 1941): "the science which considers the occurrence, distribution, and types of diseases of mankind, in distinct epochs of time, at varying points on the earth's surface, and secondly, will render an account of the relations of these diseases to inherent characteristics of the individual and to the external conditions surrounding him and determining his manner of life."

As the science of epidemiology has developed, workers in the field have come to appreciate that the same techniques and questions are useful in studying such noninfectious diseases as mental illness and atherosclerosis. Paul (1966) states that "epidemiology is concerned with measurements of the circumstances under which diseases occur, where diseases tend to flourish, and where they do not. . . . Epidemiology deals with circumstances involving more than one person, a group of people upon whom something has been thrust. . . ." The group may be small or large.

In the epidemiologic approach to disease not only the sick but also the well are studied. Answers are sought to such questions as the following: Who is sick? Who is well? What are the characteristics of those who are sick? Of the well? What are the etiologic agents? What are the characteristics of each causative agent? What are the factors in the environment bringing the susceptible host and the etiologic agent or agents together? The aswers to these questions serve as the basis for other questions. Which of the factors that have been identified as contributing to the development of the disease can be controlled? How can this control be most effectively applied?

Study the Sick Person

A fourth approach to the study of disease is to focus attention not on the disease per se but on the person who is ill. In this approach some of the questions that arise include the following: How has this disease come about? What effect does it have on the cells, tissues, and organs? Why did this particular person develop this particular illness at this time? What social and economic factors are involved? What purpose if any, does this illness serve the person? What purposes do the changes, physiologic and psychological, serve in the adjustment of the individual to the causative factors in the illness?

To illustrate, suppose a group of people become ill. Using the first approach, the study of the causative agent, the disease is described as having a sudden onset; the cause is *Staphylococcus aureus,* which releases an enterotoxin; the enterotoxin induces acute gastroenteritis; the signs and symptoms associated with the gastroenteritis include severe nausea, vomiting, diarrhea, and prostration. In most persons who are affected, the symptoms last only a few hours. Of the 100 persons who developed symptoms, 98 recovered promptly. Two died. Using the second, or epidemiologic approach, the persons who became ill were of all age groups above the age of 2 years. About 2 hours previous to the onset of symptoms they had all eaten ham at a community supper. Those who ate roast beef did not become ill. No one else in the community suffered the same symptoms. Further investigation revealed that the day was very hot and that the ham was sliced and was not refrigerated after it was cooked. The woman who sliced the ham had an infected finger. Both of the persons who died were elderly men.

In the third approach to the study of disease, attention is centered on each sick individual. The responses of each person are subject to investigation and evaluation. For example, both Marie Skinny and her date, John Robust, ate ham. Marie was only mildly sick, whereas John was severely ill. Marie convalesced slowly, whereas John recovered promptly. Elderly Mr. Claro died, whereas equally elderly Mrs. Claro suffered only a few minor symptoms. Questions arising include the following: Why should John, who was sicker than Marie, recover more promptly than Marie? Why did Mr. Claro die and his wife recover? Some answers to these and other questions are easy to obtain. Others require extensive knowledge of the individual, his or her capacity for response, and what has happened to the individual throughout his or her lifetime.

Inherent in each individual is the tendency to recover. The mechanisms involved are not well understood. However, this tendency makes the evaluation of therapeutic intervention difficult. This is particularly true when a chronic disease goes into a temporary or permanent remission. When a person regains apparent health, questions remain. To what extent did the treatment affect recovery? Were its effects positive, negative, or neutral? That is, did the treatment facilitate recovery, interfere with it, or have no effect at all?

Because of insufficient knowledge, some questions cannot be answered at this time. The fact that John was sicker than Marie may or may not be completely explained by the fact that she ate sparingly of the ham whereas John ate not only his serving but the remaining portion of Marie's. Certainly it does not explain why her recovery was prolonged. That Mr. Claro died may be explained in part by the fact that he had a diseased heart, but other factors may well have been of importance.

All of these approaches to the study of disease and its effects are important. Knowledge of the causes and manifestations of a particular disease is necessary to recognize illness caused by it and to introduce measures to limit its effects. The epidemiologic approach aims at the identification of those elements within or without the individual that are subject to control and the institution of measures to protect the population from harmful agents. As a result of study of incidents such as the community supper cited here, laws governing the handling of food have been enacted. Educational programs have been instituted to inform people of the procedures that are necessary for their protection. The fact that food poisoning continues to occur when conditions combine not only to introduce the *Staphylococcus aureus* but to favor its multiplication introduces the human factor. This brings the discussion to a summary of the third factor in the study of disease, that is, the individual. In the United States information is widely disseminated about the conditions favoring food poisoning. Why, then, should food be handled in such a manner that food poisoning occurs? The answers here are to be found in individual human beings. Each human being is an important factor in when, how, and why he or she becomes ill.

The incident of the community supper also serves to emphasize another concept that has been receiving increased emphasis in the literature. That is, any situation, including illness and recovery from illness, depends on the interaction of multiple factors. When the factors placing strain on individuals are within their adaptive capacity, they remain well. When they exceed the individuals' adaptive capacity, illness results. The nature of the illness, the degree of the individuals' illness, and the speed with which they recover can also involve multiple factors.

Prevention of Disease

All except the first objective of the health professions listed at the beginning of Unit I are concerned with prevention, that is, forestalling the occurrence of disease or injury or of some of its effects by prior action. With the exception of the first "prevention objective" all relate to the prevention of some effect or outcome of illness.

Hilbert (1977) defines prevention as including such activities as health education, adequate housing, good nutrition, and an environment that is physically and emotionally safe. He classifies preventive activities under three headings.

1. Certain government activities in which the public is largely passive. Activities include purification of water, sewage disposal, food sanitation, regulation regarding the safety and efficacy of drugs, and occupational safety. This group of activities would also include building codes, automobile design including seatbelts, control of air pollution, the disposal of dangerous chemicals including nuclear wastes, and many other activities that are designed to protect the health and lives of people.
2. So-called health care given to people by health professionals. These activities include many of the procedures included in a routine health examination, such as blood pressure measurement, the Pap smear, and urine and blood analysis. The findings may be used to counsel patients and/or to advise treatment of existing disease. At this time patients may be immunized against communicable diseases. Within this group of preventive activities is the reporting of diseases such as gonorrhea and syphilis as required by law.
3. Taking an active and continuing role as an individual. This category of activities include minimizing risk-taking behavior, as discussed in relation to the health habits survey, as well as taking responsibility for obtaining required immunizations, carrying out the regimens prescribed for the prevention and control of diseases such as obe-

sity, diabetes, and heart disease. The problem with this group of activities is to motivate the individual to do what is needed for the protection of health.

Stages in Prevention

Conditions in industrialized countries are quite different from those of the past. Progress in disease prevention was made in three stages. In the first stage the environment was rendered safe and the individual was protected from harmful influences in the environment. In this period applications of knowledge of bacteriology and immunology were made. Sanitation of food and water supplies and immunization against smallpox, diphtheria, and other infectious diseases were important contributions of the first stage to the health of the public.

In the second stage some diseases were brought under control by the introduction of new drugs and vaccines. Drugs have made a significant contribution to the control of such diseases as tuberculosis, syphilis, gonorrhea, and pneumonia. Hope that such diseases as tuberculosis and syphilis would be eradicated by the so-called wonder drugs has been replaced by the sobering knowledge that even today good control of an infectious disease depends on the constant application of all the available knowledge. Drugs have not proved to be the complete answer to the control of disease. Moreover, the value of an agent in the control or cure of an infectious disease is sometimes difficult to evaluate. To illustrate, the death rate for diphtheria, pneumonia, and tuberculosis had all dropped before modern methods of prevention and treatment were known.

The challenge of the third and present era of prevention is the prevention of noninfectious diseases. These are the diseases that have their highest incidence in maturity and the later years of life.

Levels of Prevention

Primary Prevention

Specific and identifiable measures are taken to forestall disease or injury. Examples include immunization against acute infectious disease and the development of habits that lessen the chances of being injured. Sanitary sewage disposal and clean air and water prevent disease by modifying the environment.

Secondary Prevention

Measures are taken to limit or stop the progress of an already established disease or injury, to prevent complications and sequelae, and to limit disability (see Figure 2-2).

That complete cure of disease is not always possible is well known. In some conditions, such as acute poliomyelitis, recovery from the acute infection may be complete, but there may be some degree of residual disability. In others, such as cerebrovascular accident, the patient may recover with or without disability, but the primary disease, atherosclerosis, remains. In these patients complete restoration to the preillness state may be impossible, but the effects of the disease may be modified so that disability is minimized. The limitation of disability is often a challenge. Its achievement depends on the evaluation and use of the patient's strengths and assets, psychological as well as physical, and a program of education and work whereby the patient learns to use all available resources constructively. Accomplishment requires that both the nurse and the patient be aware of, accept, and work toward realistic goals.

Tertiary Prevention

Measures are taken to maintain an incurably ill person at his or her optimum level of activity and to forestall unnecessary suffering.

Objectives of Preventive Activities

All levels of prevention involve one or more of the following:

1. Prevention of infectious diseases by specific measures and sanitary social procedures
2. Protection from exposure to harmful physical agents
3. Prevention or correction of dietary deficiencies and excesses
4. Development of habits and attitudes that favor a healthy state

The development of a viable program of prevention depends on community acceptance and support. It also depends on the state of knowledge, the resources available to procure necessary supplies and equipment, and persons possessing the imagination, knowledge, and skills required to utilize current knowledge and techniques. For example, one of the deciding factors in whether a community can have a sanitary water supply and a safe method of disposing of its wastes is whether or not it has or is willing to spend the money to build and to equip suitable facilities. Moreover, money is required to provide the necessary staff with a variety of knowledges and skills to operate and maintain them so that they can accomplish their purpose. Furthermore, the population must accept the need for these facilities and know how to use them. Use of a particular preventive measure depends in part on the knowledge of the group or individual that the measure is available and effective. The group must also accept a particular procedure as being necessary and desirable. Whether a facility or change in behavior will be adopted by a group of people depends on the degree to which its performance takes into account local customs, habits, and beliefs.

To illustrate, in a mountainous region the population had no sanitary facilities whatsoever. A young physician under the sponsorship of a foundation developed a community center to provide for some of the basic needs of the people. Among the services included were prenatal and postnatal and well-baby clinics. A part of these clinics was a pit privy where women were sent to collect urine specimens. Through this procedure they were taught to use it. Out in the community this physician promoted a factory to build pit privies. Some 35 people were employed by it. As the result of the work of one man who had some financial support, a community need had been identified and a practical solution selected. This involved not only providing equipment but helping people learn how to use it. In the process work was provided for some members of the community. This solution to the problem of sanitary waste disposal was the best that the community could support at that time.

Knowledge

Prevention is based on knowledge—knowledge of potential threats, risks, who is at risk, and measures of control. This knowledge may be empirical, based on observed cause–effect relationships, or the result of sophisticated scientific work. Every individual, in any geographic area, is at risk. Some of this risk is common to the general population. Some factors, such as age, life style, and occupation, either make an individual more vulnerable or modify the kinds of threats in the environment. Technology that has made possible the control of some environmental hazards has brought with it others.

Potential Threats

Despite past accomplishments, water and food continue to be sources of disease. With rising populations in sprawling urban areas sewage disposal plants may be inadequate to the task or housing may be built in advance of adequate disposal systems. In addition, water may contain high levels of nitrogen from runoff from barnyards, fields, and even city lawns. Long-lived pesticides and herbicides as well as industrial chemicals add other types of pollutants (see Chapter 12).

Similar to water, food can be the bearer of old and new threats to health. Bacteria and pesticide and herbicide residues are all too common. Food preservatives may at once lengthen the life span of food and be an agent of disease. Food value may be reduced by the addition of fillers. Overrefining removes essential elements. Snack foods, such as potato chips and carbonated beverages, may replace foods essential to nutrition.

In industrialized societies air is polluted by dusts, fumes, gases, and such materials as lead, nitrogen oxides, radioactive substances, and carbon monoxide. Unless air pollution is heavy, people may not be aware of it, and special equipment and techniques are required to identify the types and amounts of pollutants.

Heavy pollution resulting from both coal smoke and automobile exhaust gases is readily detected by the general population, which has suffered from its effects. Impetus was given to the study of air pollution by the London and Donora air disasters. According to Thomas (1959), urban air pollution stems from two sources. One, the London type, is primarily coal smoke, which contains appreciable amounts of sulfur dioxide combined with a more or less dense fog. The other, the Los Angeles type, is primarily automobile exhaust gases. It contains none of the components of the London smog. The irritating and damaging compounds result from the action of sunshine on the substances contained in exhaust gas. Many cities have to cope to some degree with both types of air pollution.

It is important to establish who is at risk, so that efforts can be concentrated where they will be most effective. Clean air, water, and food are important to the health of all segments of the population. Immunization against childhood infectious diseases is most important to young and school-age children. Lead poisoning is a threat to children from 1 to 5 years old living in deteriorated housing or where there is a high concentration of automobile exhaust gas (see Chapter 12).

Industrial workers are at risk as a result of their occupations. It is true that much has been done to create and enforce standards contributing to health and safety in factories and in other places of employment. Machinery is constructed with the safety of the worker in mind, and the worker is provided with clothing that is designed for protection from the hazards of the particular job. In addition, educational programs are conducted to teach employees how to work safely and what to do in the event that a fellow worker is injured. Campaigns are conducted to increase their interest and pride in their safety record. Workers' compensation laws and various types of insurance protect the health of employees by establishing and enforcing safety standards. Insurance also provides a means of support for employees and their families in the event of injury incurred while they are at work. Equally important to those who are permanently disabled is provision for their continued support.

Despite the accomplishments, people continue to be exposed to carcinogenic (cancer-producing) agents, such as asbestos and uranium. Beryllium poisoning and mine disasters still occur. According to one estimate, 100,000 deaths result each year from occupational diseases. Some industrial hazards also threaten those who live near factories and foundries. Wildlife, including fish, has been threatened by industrial wastes. Multiple factors enter into the solution of these similar problems, involving as they do the jobs of workers, economics, technological development, and a host of other considerations.

In some instances multiple factors place some individuals at risk. Deaths from automobile accidents continue to rise. Three factors are involved—the driver, the automobile, and the highway. In half or more of the fatal accidents, the use of alcohol is involved. Risk-taking behavior, such as excessive speed or cutting in and out of traffic, makes its contribution to the toll. Many agree that uniform traffic regulations would remove one traffic hazard. Yet every state continues to have its own. Why?

Besides knowledge of the population at risk, prevention may require knowledge of attitudes, values, and habits. No matter how well conceived a plan is, it will not be effective unless it is accepted and used by the population for whom it is intended. As an example, there are more effective ways of preventing dental caries than the fluoridation of water, but none of the other methods work in the population as a whole. As another example, Towle (1960) reported a study of the administration of vaccines by injection to a group of people living in India. In the early part of the study most of the candidates for immunization were men. After making this observation, the investigators placed a screen in such a position that the women could be hidden from the view of men. Following this adjustment the number of women seeking immunization did not differ materially from the number of men. Success in implementing the immunization program was dependent on making a significant observation, and then asking the question. "Why?" A plan was then made based on the local habits, customs, and beliefs of the people.

Many city, state, and even federal laws have been enacted for the purpose of protecting the general public from agents causing injury and disease. Examples include laws or regulations to control traffic, housing and building construction, water supplies, food handling, the preparation and serving of food in restaurants, and sewage disposal. Pure food and drug laws protect the quality of food and drugs (Goodman & Gilman, 1975). Other laws are discussed in Chapter 4.

The Nurse in Prevention

In exercising responsibilities in prevention the nurse has a number of functions:

1. The nurse gathers data in order to identify persons at risk and potential environmental hazards.
2. The nurse initiates preventive measures.
3. The nurse enlists the cooperation of the patient, family, and other professionals by the use of interpersonal counseling and teaching skills.
4. The nurse by word and deed supports community activities directed toward maintaining or improving health standards.

Objectives 3 Through 8: Care of the Sick (see p. 4)

A prominent feature of our health care system is the care of the sick. Sooner or later in the life of every individual, sickness becomes a reality. Depending on the nature of the causative agent or agents and capacity to respond, the individual may be mildly or seriously ill; recover promptly or experience a lingering illness; die suddenly or slowly; recover spontaneously without, or even in spite of, treatment or die despite excellent and intensive therapy.

In the American culture there is a tendency to equate recovery from illness with success and chronicity or death with failure. When a patient recovers, nurses as well as doctors take credit for the patient's success. Moreover, patients, nurses, and doctors frequently expect not only that patients should get well but that they should recover quickly and pleasantly. When they do not recover or they die, the nurse and/or physician feels that he or she must have failed in some respect.

Restoration to Health: Cure

The accomplishment of the third objective depends on two factors—the availability of a method of treatment and the capacity of the sick person to respond appropriately. The tendency toward recovery may be so great that the patient gets well with no treatment or despite meddlesome or harmful treatment. One aspect of an appropriate response to treatment is the desire of the patient to recover. A seriously ill or frail patient may be saved by specific and energetic therapy combined with the strong desire to recover.

Approaches to Therapy

One approach to the cure of disease is to attempt to eradicate the disease-producing agent. Elimination of the etiologic agent may be accomplished by administering a chemical or physical agent capable of reaching and destroying it or the diseased tissue without affecting healthy tissue. Examples include the use of antibiotic and chemotherapeutic agents to eradicate microorganisms and the use of x-ray, radioactive isotopes, or chemotherapeutic agents in the treatment of malignant neoplasms. Surgery is effective in eradicating disease by correcting structural defects or by removing diseased tissues.

Cure may also be effected by supplying a substance normally produced in the body, such as the thyroid hormone or an antibody such as antitoxin. An example of specific antiserum is diphtheria antitoxin, which is successful in the treatment of diphtheria. In patients who respond to substances that are not usually harmful, relief may be effected by limiting the contact of the patient with the harmful agent or by counteracting abnormal response. The person with hay fever can prevent or lessen the severity of an attack by eliminating from the environment substances to which he or she has a sensitivity. The severity of the reaction may also be lessened by taking an antihistamine or epinephrine.

When a disease is the result of the lack of a substance required in the body economy, cure may be effected by increasing the supply of the substance that is deficient. For example, scurvy is cured by adding ascorbic acid to the diet. Sometimes the physiologic disturbance occurring as a result of disease is so severe that the body is unable to restore balance or overcome the disease without aid. In these instances, needed materials are supplied to support body responses or defenses. For example, the temperature of the body may rise to a level that, if continued, will produce cellular damage. Temperature-lowering procedures such as the use of a hypothermia blanket or antipyretic drugs may be administered to reduce the temperature until such time as effective body controls are reestablished. Further, the prevention of unneccessary disability depends on the intelligent nursing of the patient during the acute phase of illness. Months of therapy may be required to correct the effects not of disease or injury but of inadequate care.

During the period of rehabilitation of the patient, nursing contributes to the progress of the patient in many ways. The patient is helped by an attitude of realistic optimism. The patient can be encouraged to try, even when these efforts are faltering. The nurse may find it difficult to decide when the patient should try to act and when the nurse should do things for, or help, the patient. In sympathy for the patient the nurse may forget that struggle is essential to growth or become impatient when the patient is discouraged or depressed. The chicken that escapes from the egg shell does so because it struggles. The chicken that does not struggle dies. The patient is helped in the struggle when the nurse gives recognition to his or her effort and difficulty. Recognizing successes and helping the patient to accept failures also contribute to emotional support. For some patients a source of irritation may act as a stimulus. For example, elderly Mrs. Elm was irascible and depressed following a stroke. Her nurse noted that she was a perfectionist who was greatly irritated by a crooked window shade or picture. Each day the nurse, unobtrusively but purposefully, pulled a window shade out of line. This seemingly minor action strengthened Mrs. Elm's feeling that nothing would be done properly if she was not there, and she began to make an effort to recover. The nurse was successful in helping Mrs. Elm because she was able to motivate her toward recovery. She concentrated on identifying what Mrs. Elm needed and not on her failure to conform to her own expectations of how a patient should respond. Judgment is required on the part of the nurse to assess the ability of the patient to perform so that he or she is not pushed beyond capacity. Both thought and experience are required to learn when to wait and when and how to encourage the patient to continue trying. Physical and emotional readiness are both important factors in rehabilitation.

The family of the patient is also important to rehabilitation. Family members can be a help or a hindrance, depending on their relationship with the patient and on their understanding and acceptance of the program planned. The nurse can help them to accept what can be and is being done for the patient. They, too, need support to watch a patient struggle.

They are more likely to be cooperative when they understand the plan of care and the what, how, and why of their contribution.

As a result of increased interest in rehabilitation, patients who have disorders associated with serious degrees of limitation of function are living more active lives than ever before in history. They are self-supporting, drive cars, go to ball games and dances, take vacation trips, marry, rear families, and carry on lives that are as active as those of persons not physically handicapped.

Incurable or Irreversible Disease

Not all persons who have an incurable or irreversible disease are in the terminal (end) phase of illness. A number of incurable diseases are compatible with a long and happy life. Further, even those who have life-threatening disease, such as metastatic cancer or heart disease, may live more or less active lives for extended periods of time and even die from some other type of illness. The objective in caring for incurably ill persons is to maintain them at their optimal level of function. If this objective is achieved, unnecessary suffering is prevented. The focus of care should be on what can be done rather than on what cannot be done.[2] See Chapter 34 for a detailed discussion of care of the terminally ill person.

[2] For an extensive discussion of death and dying see Virginia Henderson and Gladys Nite, *Principles and Practice of Nursing*, 6th Ed. New York: Macmillan, 1978, pp. 1929–2007.

References Cited

Besson, G. "The Health–Illness Spectrum." *Am. J. Pub. Health*, **57** (1967), 1904.

Engel, G. L. "A Unified Concept of Health and Disease." *Pers. Biol. Med.*, 3 (1960), 459.

Francis, T., Jr. "Research in Preventive Medicine." *JAMA*, **172** (1960), 994.

Goodman, L. S., and Gilman, A., eds. *The Pharmacological Basis of Therapeutics*, 5th ed. New York: Macmillan Publishing Co., Inc., 1975, p. 42.

Henderson, V., and Nite, G. *Principles and Practice of Nursing*, 6th ed. New York: Macmillan Publishing Co., Inc., 1978, pp. 1929–2000.

Hilbert, M. S. "Prevention." *Am. J. Pub. Health*, **67** (1977), 353–56.

Maxcy, K. F., ed. *Papers of Wade Hampton Frost, M.D.* New York: The Commonwealth Fund, 1941, p. 494.

Paul, J. R. *Clinical Epidemiology*, rev. ed. Chicago: University of Chicago Press, 1966, p. 4.

Rogers, E. S. "Man, Ecology, and the Control of Disease." *Pub. Health Rep.*, **77** (1962), 756.

Thomas, M. D. "New Understanding from Current Atmospheric Pollution Research." *Am. J. Pub. Health*, **49** (1959), 664–65.

Towle, R. L. "New Horizon in Mass Inoculation." *Publ. Health Rep.*, **75** (1960), 471–76.

Van Peenen, H. J. *Essentials of Pathology*. Chicago: Year Book Medical Publishers, Inc., 1966, p. 22.

General References

Fabrega, H. "The Scientific Usefulness of the Idea of Illness." *Persp. Biol. Med.*, **22** (Summer 1979), 545–58.

Hart, N. A. and Keidel, G. C. "The Suicidal Adolescent." *Am. J. Nurs.*, **79** (1979), 80–84.

Hover, J., and Juelsgaard, N. "The Sick Role Reconceptualized." *Nurs. Forum*, **17** (1978), 406–15.

Langer, W. L. "The Prevention of Smallpox before Jenner." *Sci. Am.*, **234** (1976), 112–17.

Major, R. H. *Disease and Destiny*. New York: Appleton-Century-Crofts, 1936.

Motulsky, A. G. "Biased Ascertainment and Natural History of Diseases." *N. Engl. J. Med.*, **298** (1978), 196–97.

Sackett, D. L. "Patients and Therapies: Getting the Two Together." *N. Engl. J. Med.*, **298** (1978), 278–79.

Sigerist, H. E. *Civilization and Disease*. Chicago: University of Chicago Press, 1943.

Simpson, R. R. *Shakespeare and Medicine*. Edinburgh: E. & S. Livingstone Ltd., 1959.

3

Factors Influencing Health and Levels of Wellness

According to the great equation, Medical Care equals Health. But the Great Equation is wrong. More available medical care does not equal better health. The best estimates are that the medical system (doctors, drugs, hospitals) affects about 10 per cent of the usual indices for measuring health: whether you live at all (infant mortality), how well you live (days lost due to sickness), how long you live (adult mortality). The remaining 90 per cent are determined by factors over which doctors have little or no control, from individual life style (smoking, exercise, worry), to social conditions (income, eating habits, physiological inheritance), to the physical environment (air and water quality). Most of the bad things that happen to people are at present beyond the reach of medicine.

AARON WILDAVSKY

Wildavsky, Aaron *"Doing Better and Feeling Worse:* The Political Pathology of Health Policy" *Daedalus,* 106:405 (Spring) 1977

The Maintenance of Health

Assisting people to promote their health is the first objective of members of the health professions. Beyond general agreement that health is more than a lack of disease, definitions of health do not go very far toward establishing the specific nature of health.[1] Undoubtedly there are many reasons for this. Most people who feel well and are able to carry out their social roles believe themselves to be healthy. A disease may be well established or even far advanced before a person has signs and symptoms indicating illness. As an example, a person with essential hypertension may feel well until a serious complication develops, such as a stroke or heart attack.

DEFINITIONS OF HEALTH

The definitions that follow reflect the lack of a clear conceptualization of the nature of health.

Perkins (1938) defines *health* as "a state of relative equilibrium of body form and function which results from its successful dynamic adjustment to forces tending to disturb it. It is not a passive interplay between the body substance and forces impinging on it, but an active response of body forces working toward readjustment." Francis (1960) extends the concept of adequate structure and function by adding *adequate reserve.* With the addition of the term *adequate reserve* to the definition, an individual can be presumed to be in a state of health as long as

[1] The World Health Organization's definition of *health:* "the state of complete physical, mental, and social well-being and not merely the absence of disease or infirmity."

he or she is able to adapt to changes in the environment in such a manner that structure, function, and reserve capacity are preserved. In fact, an individual is likely to appear to be healthy as long as his or her reserve capacity is sufficient to carry on usual activities.

Besson (1967) includes the environment in his definition of health and changes the emphasis. He states,

> Optimal health is not a condition of an individual, but a state of interaction between self and environment. It is a ceaseless struggle between a basically hostile environment and a series of defenses we are endowed with and which we add to when necessary. The homeostatic balance of forces is our goal and this may be accomplished by decreasing the threat of the environment or by raising the capability of the host to defend himself.

Sargent (1972) emphasizes adaptability in his definition when he states, "Health must be defined and measured in terms of adaptive capacity toward environmental circumstances and hazards.—When adaptability fails, he is ill."

"True health is closer to the Greek idea of health as harmony between the varied components of man's organism and his life situation. It is a positive concept and one which is even consistent with the existence of some anatomical defect or disability" (Goldsmith, 1972).

Dubos (1978) states that, "For human beings, health transcends biological fitness. It is primarily a measure of each person's ability to do and become what he wants to become. Good health implies an individual's success in functioning within his particular set of values, and as such is extremely relative." He goes on to emphasize that health reflects a person's success in adapting to environmental challenges. Dubos (1978) emphasizes that health is a creative adaptive process that requires conscious choices and participation by the individual in selecting a mode of life. In other words, according to this concept, each person, not the physician, has the major responsibility for his or her own health.

Despite some differences in emphasis, these authors emphasize that the healthy individual is one who is able to adapt to a changing environment. Through appropriate changes in behavior, the healthy behave in ways that promote the survival of the species as well as their own well-being and self-fulfillment. As stated in Chapter 4, the health care system is really a sickness care system. If the goal to promote health is to be accomplished, some health workers must shift their emphasis from death and disease to health and its fulfillment (Galdston, 1954). Chapter 4 describes some current efforts to strengthen the prevention and promotion emphasis in health care delivery systems.

Health Status Indicators

In the past, when acute infectious diseases were the common cause of illness and death, it was relatively easy to distinguish between the sick and the well. Chronic diseases are different, for they develop insidiously and the person who is chronically ill may consider him or herself to be well until the disease is far advanced. Moreover, a number of illnesses may be present at one time, either developing more or less independently or with one a sequelae of another. As an example, a person may have cancer and heart disease. In another person, disease of the blood vessels may develop as in long-standing diabetes mellitus. In fact, about 85 per cent of the chronically ill are ambulatory and many are unaware that they are ill. Because there is difficulty in defining valid and reliable measures of health, health is inferred from such indices as life expectancy, mortality rates, including infant mortality, morbidity, and disability rates. These are measures of the quantity of life and the loss of health, not of health per se.

Purposes

According to Bickner (1970) health status indicators serve three general purposes: public information, administration, and medical science. Health professionals use health status indicators to inform the general public and legislators in matters of health and the need to support research and health care. For administrators, health status indicators provide information for the selection of priorities, planning, management, and decision making. Medical science uses them in determining priorities and in selecting areas for research.

Criteria

According to Sullivan (1966), a health index for the purpose of measuring trends in the health level of the United States population should meet two criteria: "1) It should show changes over time in significant aspects of the health of the living as well as in mortality. 2) It should be subject to analysis into components which provide a useful description of health problems underlying index values." As Sullivan states, "death is a well-defined event, more difficult to decide is, what else can and should be measured."

Types

Life Expectancy Rates

Improvement in life expectancy rates is among the most frequently quoted of health status indicators. The validity of life expectancy rates depends on the availability and accuracy of written records. People's memories tend to be inaccurate and very old people tend to exaggerate their ages.

Life expectancy rates vary over the world, reflecting as they do sociocultural, economic, and political characteristics of each country or community.

In the United States, if the 1975 mortality rates continue to prevail during the lifetime of those born that year, three quarters can expect to reach their sixty-fifth birthday, over half their seventy-fifth, and one quarter their eighty-fifth *(Health in the United States, 1976–1977)*. Within the age group over 65, the proportion between the ages 65 and 74 is decreasing, and those 75 years or older is increasing. However, most of the gain in life expectancy continues to be in the early years of life as a result of a continuing decline in infant mortality. Some of the increase in life expectancy since 1970 is due to a decrease in the mortality from ischemic heart disease, cerebrovascular disease, and accidents. Although the nonwhite population has a shorter life expectancy than the white population, they have made greater gains than whites. Presently, white females have the best record of longevity, with nonwhite females being second. The smallest gains have been made by white males.

Increased longevity is reflected in the fact that in 1900 only one person in twenty-five lived to be 65 years of age. Today one in nine lives 65 years or longer with the result that there are now more than 23 million Americans 65 years of age or older. The prediction is that the proportion of those over 65 to those under 65 will soon increase to one in five. Further, this increase in the elderly population is not limited to the United States, but is a worldwide phenomenon.

Because the amount of illness and disability increases with age, the increase in the number of those over 65 has many implications for society as well as for the members of the health professions. The following are among the questions to be answered: What kind of facilities and services are needed to maintain the health of this segment of the population? How can those needing care during illness and its consequences be identified and served?

As stated previously, there is abundant evidence that socioeconomic conditions affect health and longevity. Those with the lowest income have the shortest life expectancy; those with the highest income have the longest life expectancy. Professional men and businessmen listed in the 1950–1951 *Who's Who in America* have lived longer than men in the general population. College graduates live longer than noncollege graduates. Clergymen, teachers, and lawyers live longer than the average. This advantage continues to be reported as a series of studies reported in the *Statistical Bulletin* (Metropolitan Life Insurance Company, 1968, 1971) show that cabinet officers, congressmen, and Supreme Court justices, in that order, have lower death rates than men in the general population. The mortality ratio varies from 91 per cent for cabinet officers to 71 per cent for Supreme Court justices. Judges and attorneys listed in *Who's Who in America* also have a lower death rate than their contemporaries. National Health Survey (Linder, 1966) statistics confirm clearly and in quantitative terms the generally accepted idea that there is a positive relation between poor health and low income. People with incomes of $2,000 per year had more days of disability than those in the next higher bracket, for example.

Antonovsky (1967) reviews a large number of life expectancy studies. These studies show that over the course of history, whatever index is used and the number of classes considered, the lowest class has the poorest life expectancy. Furthermore, the class differences are greatest in young and middle adulthood and tend to disappear after age 65.

A similar effect can be noted in different segments of the American population. Despite improvement over this century, nonwhite Americans still have a shorter life span than white Americans. In 1900–1902 the newborn nonwhite male could expect to live about 32.5 years, and the females 35.0 years. In 1967 the nonwhite male had a life expectancy at birth of 61.1 years and the female of 68.2 years (Metropolitan Life Insurance Company, 1970).

In an attempt to answer the question of why the poor have a lower level of health than the affluent, Pratt (1971) studied three different socioeconomic groups. Among her findings was a positive relationship between the level of health practices and the level of health. Those with good health practices tended to have good health, whereas those with poor health practices tended to have more health problems. However, the health status of the affluent with poor health practices tended to be better than that of their poorer counterparts. Another finding of interest to nurses was that although both groups tended to use medical services during illness, those in the lower socioeconomic group used fewer preventive and medical specialist services than the more affluent group. Though women in the higher socioeconomic group had more general health knowledge than women in the lower group, neither group was very knowledgeable. Further, there was little relationship between the level of general knowledge and the level of health practices. To be used, information needs to be specific. Replication and extension of Pratt's study by nurses might lead to some useful changes in nursing practice. Other questions to be answered include the following: What other factors have a direct bearing on health? What methods of instruction are effective and ineffective with varying socioeconomic and age groups? How can preventive services be made available to the poor? What can be done to encourage their use? Many other questions will occur to the individual who wishes to add to knowledge of why the poor are less healthy than the more affluent.

General Mortality

Although mortality statistics have been widely used as an index of health status, they were of much more value when acute infectious diseases were the leading cause of death (see Figure 3-1). They are useful inasmuch as they are available and provide data for comparing causes of death among nations, between areas of a country, and from one year or period to the next. Mortality statistics have a number of limitations as health status indicators. When chronic diseases are the cause of mortality, a number of diseases may be present in the same individual. Which one or ones were responsible for death? Further, autopsies are performed on less than one half of those who die. Without an autopsy, the diagnosis of the cause of death can be incorrect. At best, mortality statistics tell the cause of death. They do not provide information about the quality of the life of the person who died or what effect the disease had on the person's life. Despite their disadvantages, mortality statistics are used to make decisions about where money and effort should be concentrated in the study and treatment of disease.

Because they continue to be emphasized, nurses should be familiar with the leading causes of death and with the changes that have occurred in this century. (See Figure 3-1 which demonstrates clearly the changing pattern.)

Because the causes of death vary with age and

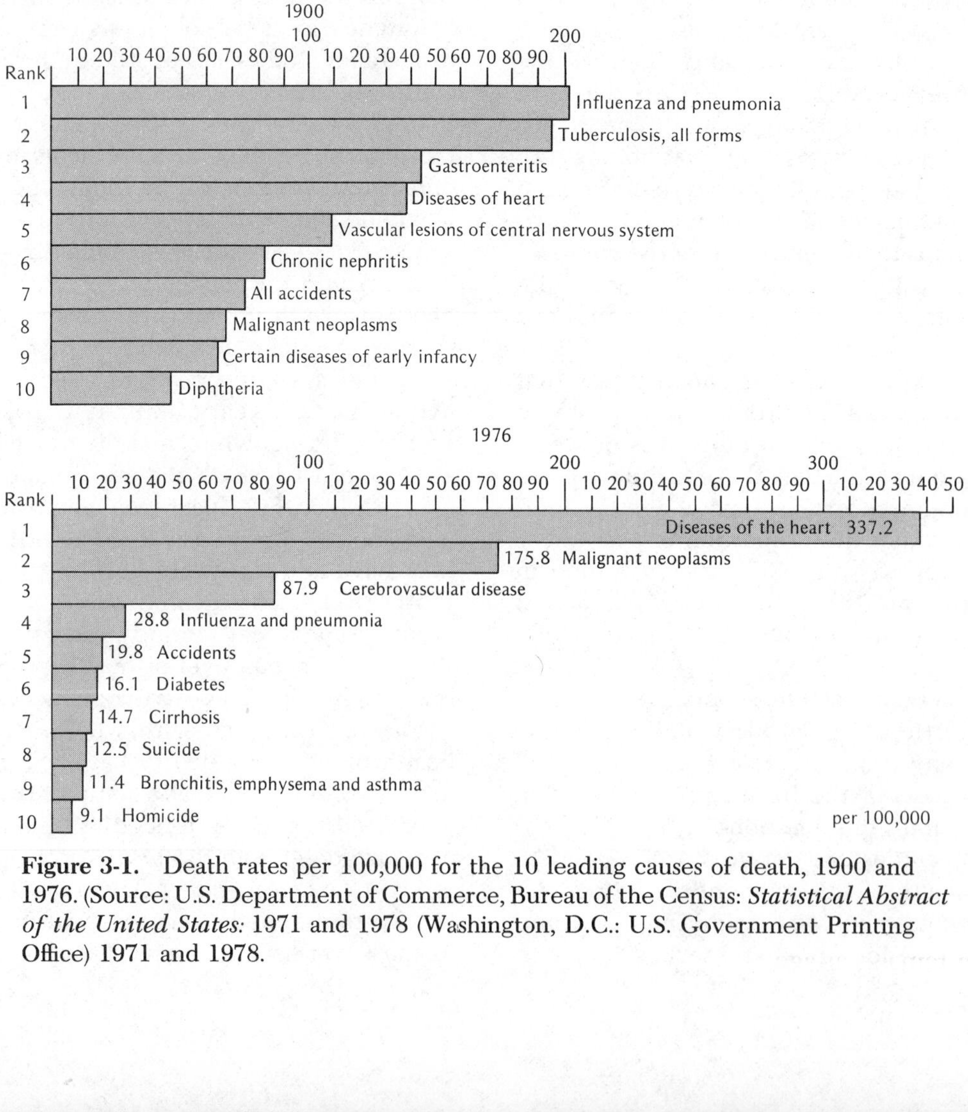

Figure 3-1. Death rates per 100,000 for the 10 leading causes of death, 1900 and 1976. (Source: U.S. Department of Commerce, Bureau of the Census: *Statistical Abstract of the United States:* 1971 and 1978 (Washington, D.C.: U.S. Government Printing Office) 1971 and 1978.

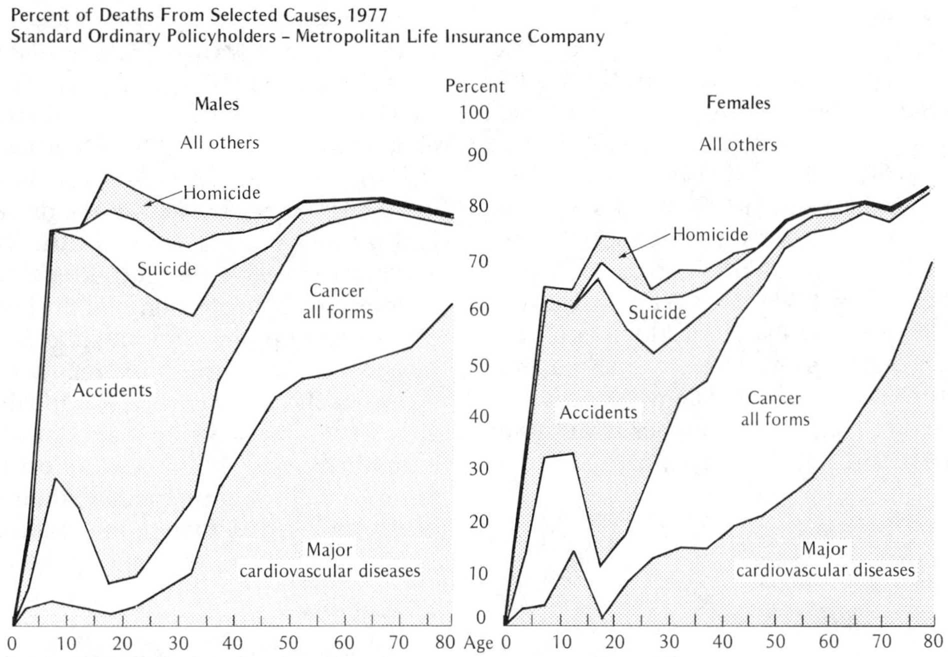

Figure 3-2. Percent of deaths from specified causes by sex and age, 1977. [From *Stat. Bull. Metropol. Life Ins. Co. 59*:14 (July–Sept.) 1978.]

sex, other information is needed (see Figure 3-2). Although the data in Figure 3-2 are derived from individuals with enough income to own ordinary life insurance, the pattern is similar to that of the entire population.

In both sexes, accidents are the first cause of death between 1 and 30 years. In males accidents continue in first place until age 35. The importance of accidents as a cause of death and disability is emphasized by the fact that over 100,000 deaths from automobile and home injury accidents expected in 1977 (Hilbert, 1977). In the 15- to 30-year age range, homicide and suicide in both sexes take a significant number of lives. This includes the young adult who is attending college. Because of the stigma associated with suicide, some deaths resulting from it may be reported as accidental. A significant number of suicides occur in children under 10 years of age.

In both sexes, following birth there is a sharp rise in the incidence of cancer, with a peak at about 10 years of age. The incidence then drops and in males causes less than 10 per cent of deaths between the ages of 18 and 40. The incidence then rises and between the ages of 40 and 70, cancer causes about 20 per cent of the deaths in males. In females the percentage of deaths from cancer is higher than in males in most age groups.

Although cardiovascular—renal disease is the first cause of death, it is not until age 35 for males and age 60 for females that it achieves this position. It causes about 65 per cent of the deaths in males and 70 per cent in females at age 80.

Other diseases among the first ten causes of death include diabetes mellitus; influenza and pneumonia, the only acute infectious diseases; cirrhosis of the liver; and arteriosclerosis. The increasing incidence of cirrhosis of the liver as well as of homicide and automobile accident deaths undoubtedly reflects the increasing abuse of alcohol (see Figure 3-2).

In fact, there is evidence that alcohol is a direct or contributing cause of death in a substantial number of persons. The true number is not known because of underreporting. Further, by themselves mortality rates do not provide other significant information, because they are averages of the population as a whole. Such factors as socioeconomic status, occupation, education, place of residence, nutritional status, and personal habits are all factors in longevity. In general, those in the highest socioeconomic groups with the most education live longer than those in the lower socioeconomic groups. Thus, on the average, lawyers live longer than clerks or day laborers. In fact, mortality statistics were more useful when infectious diseases were the main causes of death than they are today.

Among the questions to be pondered are the following: From the point of view of society, which of these causes of mortality are most significant? Why? If only a limited number of dollars is available for research into disease causation and prevention, for what should it be spent? Why? Where is the money spent? Why? Why do children kill themselves? How can the incidence of death from violence in 15- through 24-year-old males be reduced?

Infant Mortality

The infant mortality rate, which is an accepted index of health, is decreasing throughout the world. In the United States, the infant death rate has declined more than 50 per cent in the last 30 years. In 1946 it was 33.8 per 1,000 live births, in 1969–1971 it had fallen to 20.0 and in 1977 to 14.0. Within the United States there are wide differences in the reported rates. As an example, in 1976 they ranged from a low of 11.0 per 1,000 live births in Hawaii to a high of 25.3 in the District of Columbia (*Vital Statistics Report,* 1979, p. 7). Despite marked improvement in the mortality among nonwhite infants, their death rates are considerably higher than those of white babies. In 1975, the mortality rate for nonwhite infants was 22.9 per 1,000 live births. For white infants, it was 14.4 deaths per 1,000 live births (see Figure 3-3) (*Forward Plan for Health,* 1976). By October 1978, the infant mortality rate had declined to 13.7 per 1,000 live births (*Vital Statistics Report,* 1979).

Among the reasons cited for the reduction in infant mortality are (1) greater availability of medical and health services for mothers and babies, (2) better socioeconomic conditions, and (3) changes in the childbearing population. In spite of this decrease in mortality, one of the very real concerns is the increase in the number of teenage and even younger girls who now become pregnant. Because of their immaturity as well as their failure to seek medical supervision during pregnancy, they and their babies are at a higher risk than their sisters in their twenties.

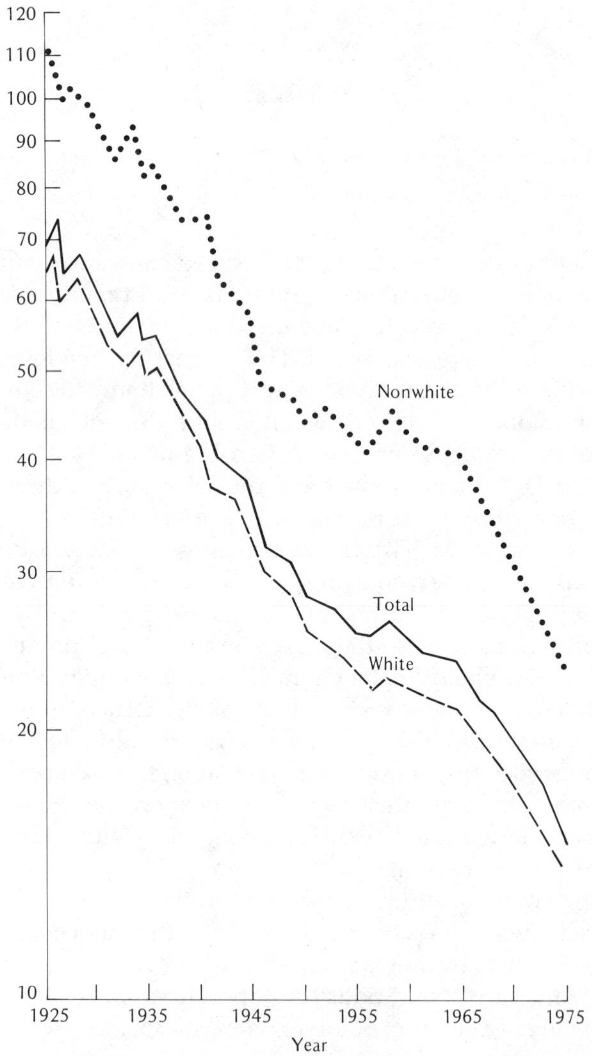

Figure 3-3. Infant mortality rates by color: United States, 1925–75. (*Forward Plan for Health,* U.S. Department of Health, Education, and Welfare, Public Health Service, 1976.)

Disability

Disease affects not only the quantity of life, but its quality. Unless death is sudden, the sick person experiences a period of partial or complete inability to function physically, mentally, socially, and economically. The degree of impairment may vary from not feeling well to complete incapacity and may last from a few hours to many years.

Although some diseases and injuries are more disabling than others, the person involved also makes a great difference. As an example, one person goes to bed at the first sign of a cold; another tries to work despite evidence of pneumonia. One person expects to feel unwell some of the time and pays little or no attention to minor or even major signs

Age	Restricted activity	Bed disability	Work loss[1]
	Disability days per person per year		
Under 6 years . .	12.1	4.7	. . .
6–16 years	10.5	4.3	. . .
17–24 years . . .	12.3	5.1	4.6
25–34 years . . .	14.5	5.5	5.1
35–44 years . . .	17.0	6.2	5.2
45–54 years . . .	21.1	7.7	5.5
55–64 years . . .	28.0	9.3	6.1
65–74 years . . .	34.0	10.3	3.5
75 years . . . . . . and over	46.2	17.4	8.9

[1] Currently employed persons 17 years of age and over.

NOTE: The rate for school-loss days per person per year for school-age children 6–16 years of age in 1975 was 5.1 days.

Figure 3-4. Disability days per person per year, by type of disability and age: United States, 1975. (*Disability Days,* United States 1975, Series 10, Number 118. Publication No. (PHS) 78–1546. U.S. Department of Health, Education, and Welfare, p. 4, June 1978.)

Karla Wise
Class of 87
FSC

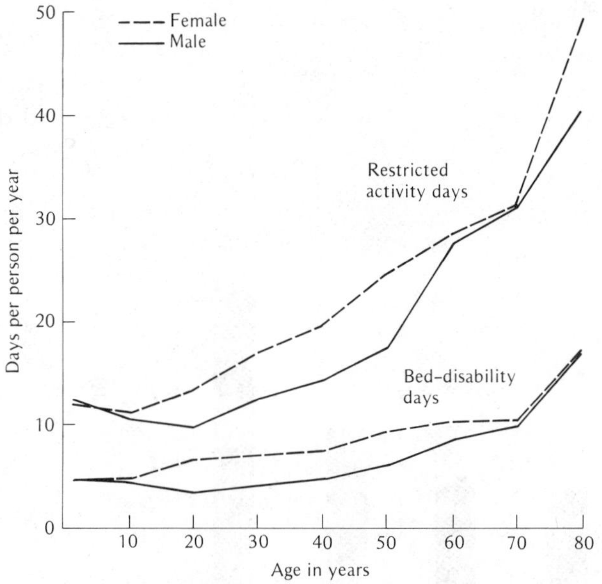

Figure 3-5. Disability days by type of disability, age and sex. (*Disability Days,* United States, 1975, Series 10, Number 118. Publication No. (PHS) 78–1546. U.S. Department of Health, Education, and Welfare, p. 4, June 1978.)

and symptoms; another person expects to feel well all of the time and seeks treatment for any discomfort. Other factors influencing the amount of disability are age, the amount of schooling, income, and occupation. The incidence of disability increases with age. Recovery from acute disabling conditions takes longer after 65 years of age. The more years of formal schooling and the higher the income, the fewer days of disability experienced (see Figures 3-4 and 3-5).

Indices of Disability

Among the indices used to determine the trend of disability in the United States by the National Center for Health Statistics of the United States Public Health Service are work-loss, restricted-activity, and bed-disability days. These data were obtained by household interviews and other types of surveys (see Figures 3-6 and 3-7).

Causes of Disability

Respiratory conditions cause more lost work days than any other acute conditions, including injuries and digestive system disorders. Injuries are responsible for a significant number of work-loss days among workers.

Among the chronic disorders, heart disease is the most common cause of disability; almost as many people are disabled by arthritis and rheumatism. Other frequent causes of disability are mental and nervous conditions, asthma and hay fever, hypertension without heart involvement, conditions of the genitourinary and digestive system, visual impairments, impariments of the musculoskeletal systems, diabetes, varicose veins, peptic ulcers, and partial or complete paralysis. Some of these disorders, such as arthritis and rheumatism, are responsible for years of human misery as well as loss of productivity (see Figure 3-8).

Data obtained by the Health Interview Survey (Bauer, 1972) from persons with incomes under $5,000 indicated that low-income persons are in poorer health than those with higher incomes. A number of studies cited in this report show that low-income persons have less access to medical care and the quality and range of services is much less than is available to those with higher incomes.[2] At the

Table D: Disability days per person per year, by race, type of disability day, and sex: United States, 1975

Type of disability day and sex	Race	
	White	Black
Restricted activity	Disability day per person per year	
Both sexes	17.5	21.4
Male	15.4	17.7
Female	19.4	24.7
Bed disability		
Both sexes	6.2	9.2
Male	5.2	7.4
Female	7.2	10.8
Work loss[1]		
Both sexes	5.0	7.4
Male	4.7	7.3
Female	5.4	7.4
School loss[1]		
Both sexes	5.2	4.8
Male	4.8	4.7
Female	5.6	5.0

[1] Currently employed persons 17 years of age and over.
[2] Persons 6–16 years of age.

Figure 3-6. Disability days by race, type of disability, and sex: United States, 1975. (*Disability Days,* United States, 1975, Series 10, Number 118. Publication No. (PHS) 78–1546. U.S. Department of Health, Education, and Welfare, p. 4, June 1978.)

[2] This disparity in health care for low- and high-income persons is not new; it has existed since Greco-Roman times.

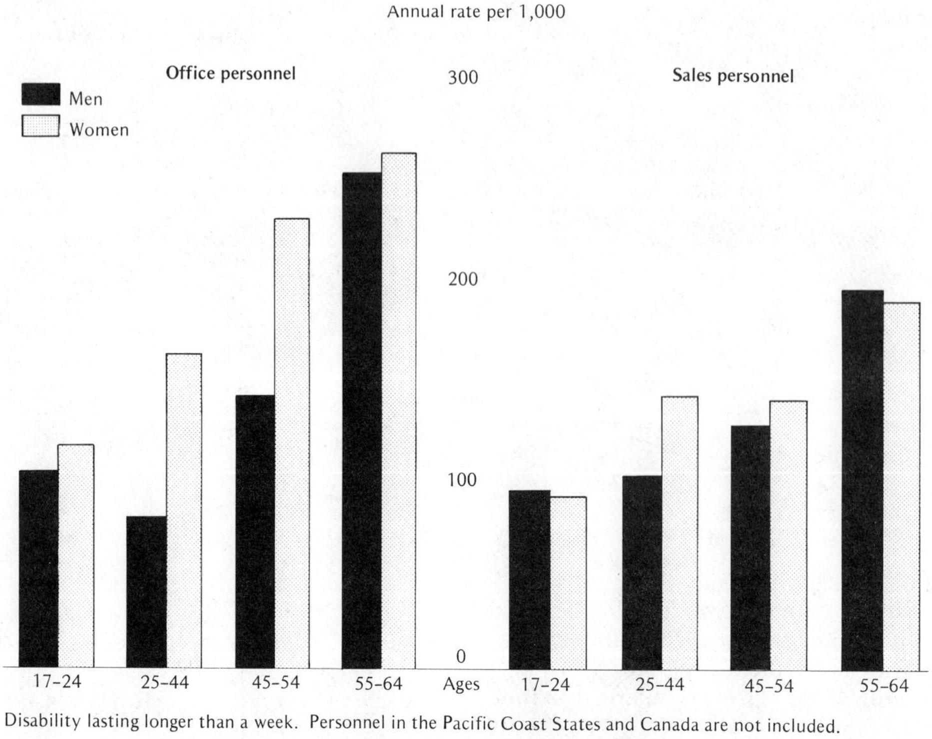

Figure 3-7. Incidence of Disability—1976: Personnel of the Metropolitan Life Insurance Company, by sex and type of position. (Metropolitan Life *Stat. Bulletin,* July–August, 1977, *58,* p. 12.)

same time those with incomes under $5,000 were found to have more limitation of activity, more disability, and more hospitalizations than the total population.

In both males and females the amount and degree of disability, restricted activity, and bed disability is inversely related to income. That is, the lower the income the more disability, and the higher the income the less the amount of disability. Without more data, the cause and effect relationship cannot be established. That is, to what extent does disability result in less income and to what extent does low income result in a greater incidence of disability? (See Figures 3-9 and 3-10). Both factors may be involved. Race is also a factor in the amount and degree of disability, as blacks have more disability than whites. The question here is: To what extent is the higher incidence of disability in blacks due to the fact that their average income is less than that of whites?

In a study of the leading causes of disability in 1976 among office and sales personnel made by the Metropolitan Life Insurance Company (1977), it was concluded that (1) the amount of disability increases with age, and (2) older employees were disabled more often than younger employees, (3) women had the highest incidence of disability, (4) in all age groups the disability rate at ages 55 to 64, was more than double than that at age 25, (5) there was wide seasonal variation with the highest incidence occurring during the winter and the lowest rates in the summer, (6) the rate fluctuated more for women than for men, and (7) the causes of disability differed with age and occupation. (See Figure 3-11 for details.) In other words, this study supported the findings of earlier studies.

Another approach to disability is to predict the length of a disability-free life. To do this, the National Center for Health Statistics (Sullivan, 1971) combined morbidity and mortality statistics. From this, they arrived at a formula for predicting the expectation of a disability-free life. The expectation for a disability-free lifetime was about 65 years in the United States in the mid-1960s compared to the conventional life expectancy of about 70 years (see Figure 3-12). The expected lifetime duration of disability was about 5 years. About 2 years of disability can be expected to occur before 65 years of age and 3 years after. Expectation of a life free of disability is about 68 years. Expectation of bed disability is about 2 years, 1 year of which occurs after 65 years of age. Males have less bed disability than females. Differences between whites and nonwhites are not great.

The so-called health status indicators are really indices of loss of health. Perhaps in the future, mea-

Figure 3-8. Metropolitan Life Insurance Company: Leading Causes of Disability, 1976. *Stat. Bulletin,* July–August, 1977, *58,* 11.

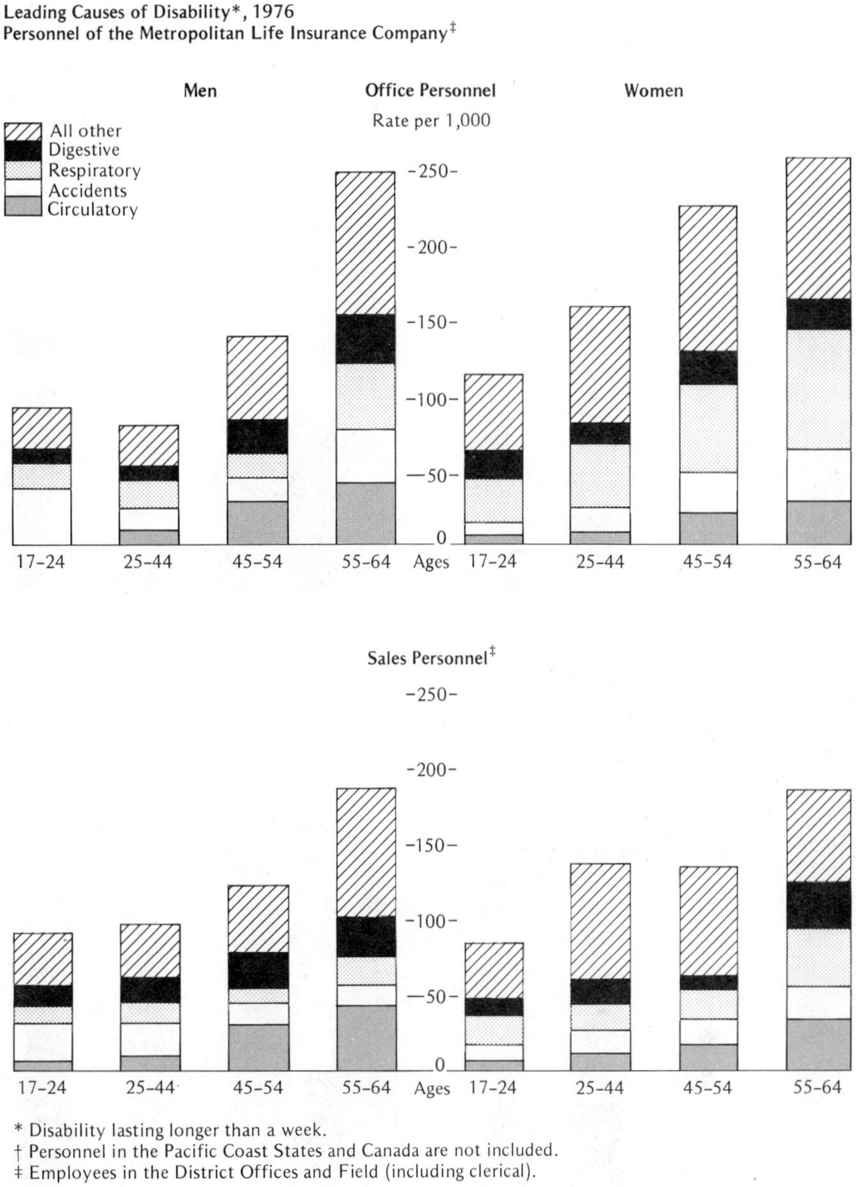

sures will be developed that can in fact be used to measure the state of health. As an example, it may eventually be possible to measure the degree to which an individual's activities are in tune with physiologic rhythms. (See the discussion of circadian rhythms and homeostasis in Chapter 6.)

Risk Factors

An indirect approach to the study of health is to identify those practices or events that promote health or place it at risk. When evaluating these studies, it must be remembered that health results from many interacting factors, some of which are subject to control by the individual or the community. Others, at least in our present state of knowledge, are not. It must also be remembered that the desire for simple and understandable explanations of complex problems is common (Thomas, 1978).

Among the studies of the influence of health practices on health status are those of Belloc and Breslow (1972). In this study, questionnaires were sent to about 7,000 adults over 45 years of age asking each about certain health habits. Five years later the death certificates of the 371 persons who had died were compared with the answers they gave to the questions. There were more deaths among heavy drinkers and smokers than among those who did not drink or smoke. Other conditions or habits having a greater incidence among those who died than among those who lived were not eating breakfast, snacking, getting too little or too much sleep, and

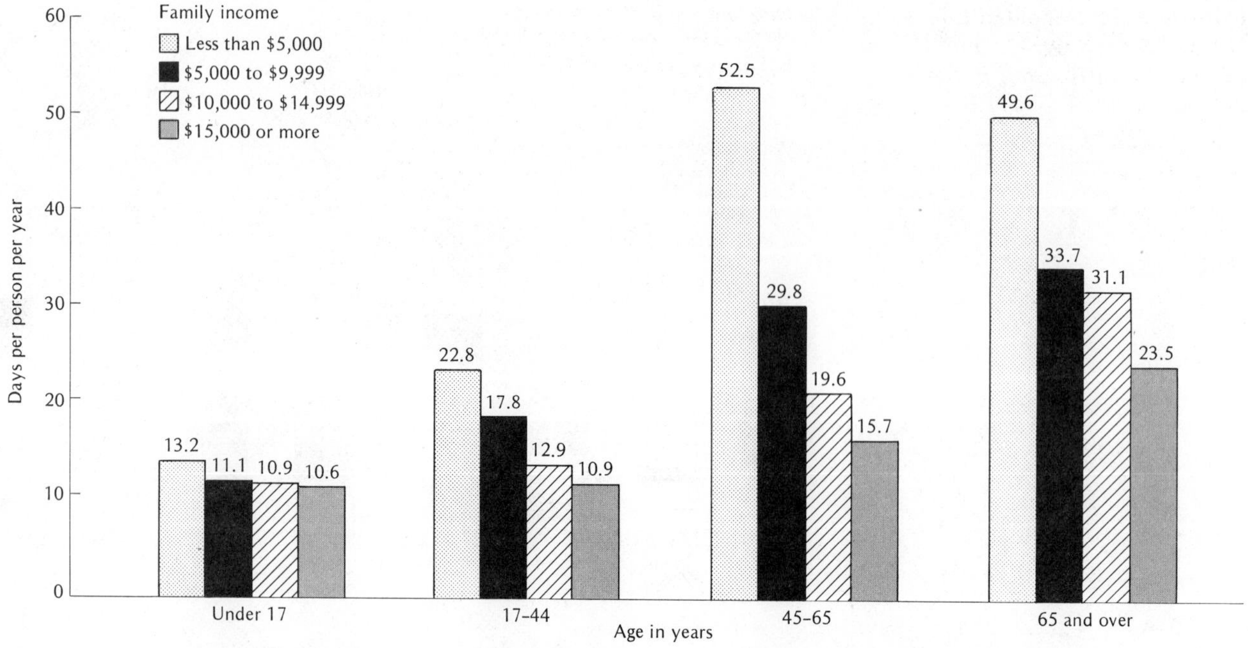

Figure 3-9. Number of restricted-activity days per person per year, by family income and age: United States, 1975. (*Disability Days,* U.S. Department of Health, Education, and Welfare, National Center for Health Statistics, June 1978, p. 19.)

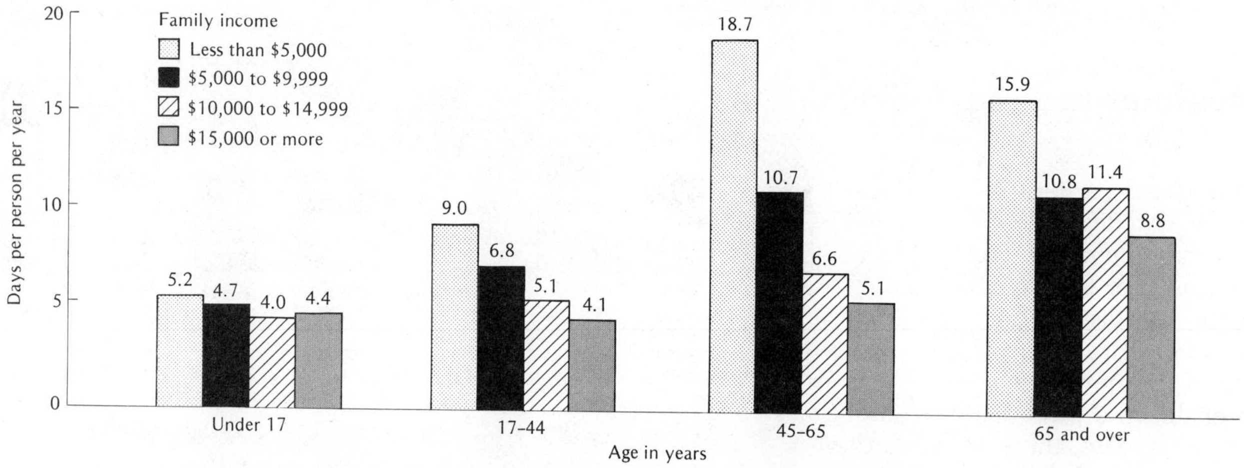

Figure 3-10. Number of bed-disability days per person per year, by family income and age: United States, 1975. (*Disability Days,* U.S. Department of Health, Education, and Welfare, National Center for Health Statistics, June 1978, p. 19.)

failure to exercise regularly. Further, Breslow (1978) reported that at every age from 20 to 70, persons who followed all seven health habits[3] were in better health than those who practiced only a few of these habits. In fact, those who practiced all seven were in better health than those who practiced five, and so on. The average health status of those 70 years of age who practiced all seven good health practices was about the same as that of those 35 to 44 years old who reported three or fewer. The results were similar for all age groups studied.

Thomas (1978) points out that the state of health of those studied was not known at the time the study was initiated. It is possible that those who did not practice the health measures were unable to do so. Further, the fact that smoking and excessive use of alcohol have a detrimental effect is well documented. The extent to which the other practices influence life expectancy is not known.

[3] That is, eating moderately, eating regularly, eating breakfast, exercising regularly, sleeping 7 to 8 hours, *not* smoking, and drinking moderately, if at all.

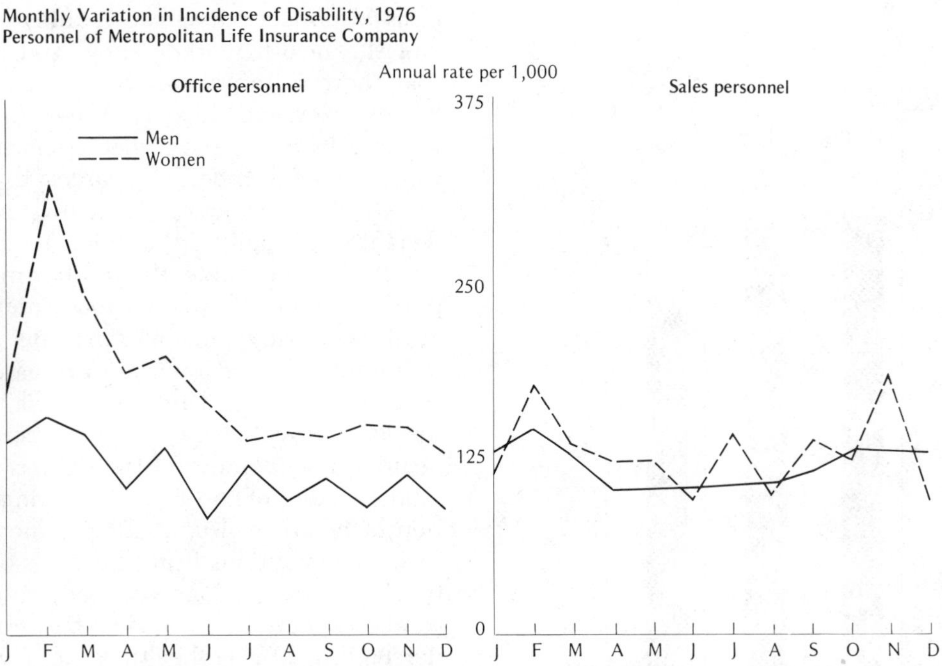

Disability lasting long than a week. Claims classified according to month of initial payment. Personnel in the Pacific Coast States and Canada are not included.

Figure 3-11. Monthly variation in incidence of disability, 1976: Personnel of Metropolitan Life Insurance Company, by sex and type of position. (Metropolitan Life *Stat. Bulletin,* July–August, 1977, *58,* p. 12.)

Measures to Promote Health

As stated earlier, the promotion of health is accepted as a desirable objective. However, very little is known about how to measure health or even how to achieve or maintain it. In much of the literature, little or no distinction is made between the promotion of health and the primary prevention of disease. Although knowledge and techniques are available to enable the physician to identify and categorize various disease, there is little information and few techniques to help distinguish among and classify different degrees of health.

For want of more definitive knowledge, conditions contributing to healthful living will be considered as facilitating the accomplishment of the objective "to promote health" and the measures more directly related to the prevention of specific diseases as facilitating the accomplishment of the objective "to prevent disease or disability from disease." The discerning reader will note that there is overlapping between the two.

The Commission on Chronic Illness (1957) lists the following as among the most important components of healthful living:

Nutrition—adequate, safe, and well-distributed food supplies as well as appropriate levels of personal nutrition.

Mental hygiene—beginning at an early age, it is important that the individual develop an equanimity in the face of the natural and inevitable frustrations of living; appreciation of the values of family life; acceptance of oneself and one's limitations.

Adequate housing—including proper safeguards against accidents for persons of all ages, and particular safeguards for children and for the aged and handicapped.

Moderate and well-balanced personal habits—restraints in use of alcohol and tobacco, sufficient rest and an appropriate amount of exercise, careful attention to personal hygiene.

A useful and productive role in society.

General education and education specifically for health.

A safe and healthful working environment.

Recreation, including access to recreational opportunities and facilities on the one hand, and proper balancing of recreational activities against satisfying work on the other.

A sense of personal security, related to such things as access to health services; legalized provisions for minimum wages and some sort of job security; provision for income maintenance during illness or following retirement.

To this list may be added another concept—a system of values that serves as a guide to action. Beginning at an early age, the individual should be helped to develop a sense of purpose in life, that is, who and why he or she is and where he or she is going. The individual's goals should be based on a whole-

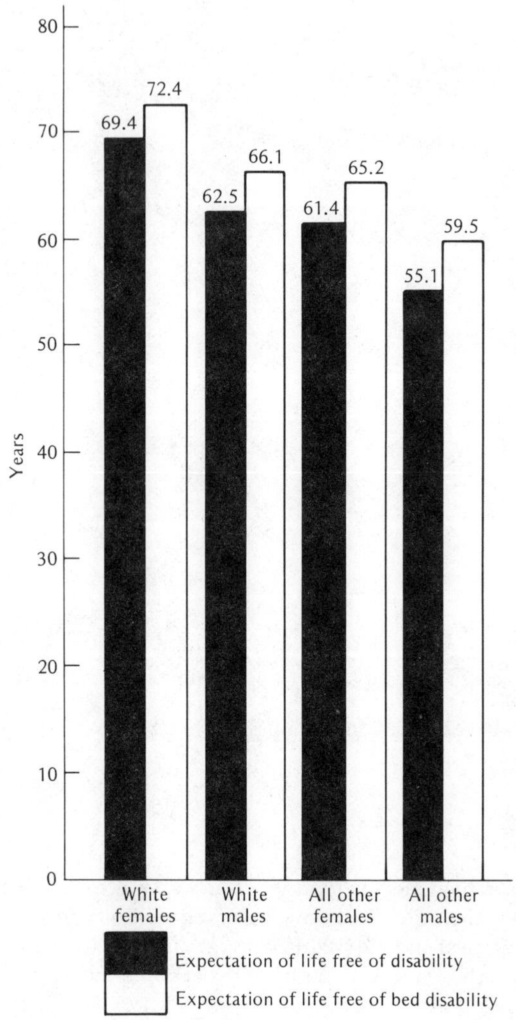

Figure 3-12. Approximate expectations of life free of disability and life free of bed disability for whites and other persons by sex, United States, mid-1960s. [Reproduced from *HSMHA Health Rep.*, *86*:350 (Apr.) 1971. "A Single Index of Mortality and Morbidity." Daniel F. Sullivan.]

some appreciation of the rights and dignity of others.

The promotion of health is both an individual and a social responsibility. Whenever a large group of people live in a limited area, regulations are necessary to protect the general welfare. The individual has a responsibility to cooperate in protecting not only one's own personal rights but also those of others.

One of the best-known and -organized efforts in the field of health promotion is the well-baby clinic. The baby is examined regularly and the mother is given guidance in care. Data are available by which the growth and development of the child can be measured. This information is useful in reassuring the mother that her baby is developing normally; in turn it may contribute to the mother's being more relaxed in the care of her baby. It may also be the basis for unnecessary anxiety, unless both the mother and the health worker know and accept the fact that there is much variation in the rate at which babies grow and develop. When the development of the baby is in some respect abnormal, the mother can be aided in modifying care so that health is promoted. For example, the baby may be gaining weight too rapidly. In addition to recognizing that obesity is undesirable, the mother may require support to modify the baby's food intake. Attendance at the well-baby clinic also provides an opportunity to immunize the baby against diseases such as measles, poliomyelitis, and diphtheria. Thus through services provided to the baby and mother, the healthy development of the baby is promoted.

Knowledge of the factors assisting in the promotion of health will undoubtedly increase in the future. Contributions from the fields of biochemistry, biophysics, psychology, sociology, and anthropology can be expected to provide a basis for a greater understanding of what health is and how it is measured and promoted than is now available. Among the questions being explored by social scientists are how to impart information about health so that it is effective, how to change attitudes, and how to improve communication between and among various groups.

As with other members of society, nurses have a personal responsibility to promote their own health. As society expects the contributions of an individual to be commensurate with education and opportunities, nurses have more responsibility than the ordinary citizen to promote their own health. As professional nurses they also work with individuals and groups to help them raise their standards of health. Nurses also have a responsibility as citizens to promote community projects, such as improved housing and slum clearance, that contribute to the general health and welfare of the entire community.

Some of the hazards to health in an urban, industrialized society were referred to in Chapter 1. They will be discussed in detail in Unit III, as well as in later chapters. Related conditions—economic status, education, and general standard of living—also affect the health of the population.

Other Ways of Looking at Health Problems

There are other ways of looking at the health problems that affect the practice of nursing. One is to examine some of the problems that arise out of illness and disability. These include some of the measurable costs of illness and disability to the community and to the individual. Hospitals, health departments, clinics, and all the services for the prevention and treatment of illness are costly and, according to most predictions, are becoming more so. The individual wage earner who is ill often suffers complete or partial loss of income. He or she may have to go into debt to pay for care or to care for the needs of his or her family. When the homemaker is ill and especially when there are children, a substitute mother may have to be employed. This may place a considerable financial burden on the family.

There are other losses that are more difficult to measure than the direct costs of the illness. These include the loss of productivity of a worker and sometimes of those who depend on the worker's service or the product that he or she produces for their work. Who can place a monetary value on the loss of the homemaker from the home or the teacher from the classroom? Few substitute mothers or teachers can pick up where their predecessor left off and carry on fully. The adverse effects from the death or disability of a parent on growing children include the gamut from insufficient food and clothing to effects of emotional deprivation and premature cessation of schooling. These things do not always happen, but they can and do occur. For example, Mrs. Alphonse, the 35-year-old mother of ten children, has severe, crippling rheumatoid arthritis. The children range in age from a few months to 12 years. During the last year and a half, Mrs. Alphonse has been in the hospital most of the time. The children have been cared for by grandparents filling in for a series of housekeepers, most of whom leave after a few weeks. Though the children have not been neglected physically, who can predict the effect of the absence of the mother from the home and exposure to a continuing state of anxiety about the mother and the costs of her care?

In addition to the problems created for children by death or disability of a parent, other members of the family are also affected. The average age of widows is 56. Among the problems that widows have to, or are likely to have to, face are adjusting to single living, coping with real or feared inadequacy of income to meet their needs and those of dependent children, and remaining in or changing their living arrangements. Older widows with little or no family, few friends, and no interests outside their families may have little incentive to continue living. The purpose and meaning of their lives may be gone. The older, friendless widow is often lonely. Unless she has or can find a way to support herself emotionally and financially, she may have to depend on her children or the community for both types of support.

Nurses cannot solve all the economic and social problems arising out of illness, but they can be helpful to patients by being aware that they exist. They may also assist by helping the patient to explore his or her resources and those in the community. With their special knowledge of the problems created by sickness, nurses should be able to give constructive leadership to the community in its efforts to solve some of the problems arising as a result of illness.

Summary

In summary, the role of the nurse in the maintenance of health and prevention of illness and conditions leading to illness includes

1. Knowledge required for the recognition of conditions or situations that are favorable or unfavorable to health
2. Skill in instituting preventive measures and in supporting community efforts to institute these measures
3. Recognition and use of the fact that disease prevention requires three general approaches: (a) maintenance of a healthy environment, (b) involvement of each individual in health maintenance, and (c) selection of methods of health protection that are acceptable and practical
4. Knowledge required to identify the symptoms and signs indicating health or illness. This knowledge is essential in the nurse's role as a case finder.
5. Knowledge required to make judgments as to the urgency of the need of the patient for attention: Does the patient require the immediate attention of a physician? Should he or she be subject to careful observation? Can the patient's needs be met at this particular time by the practice of nursing?
6. Knowledge required to make judgments as to the appropriate course of action: To whom should the patient and the problem be referred?
7. Confidence to press for action when the condition of the patient appears to require it
8. Knowledge of and competence in the practice of nursing (See Chapter 8 for the steps in problem solving.)

References Cited

Antonovsky, A. "Social Class, Life Expectancy and Overall Mortality." *Milbank Mem. Fund Q.*, **45** (1967), 31–73.
Bauer, M. L. *Health Characteristics of Low-Income Per-*

sons. DHEW Publication No. HSM 73–1500, Vital and Health Statistics series 10, No. 74. Washington, D.C.: U.S. Government Printing Office, 1972, pp. 1–2.

Belloc, N. B., and Breslow, L. "Relationship of Physical Health Status and Health Practices." *Preventive Medicine,* **1** (1972), 409–21.

Besson, G. "The Health-Illness Spectrum." *Am. J. Pub. Health,* **57** (1967), 1904.

Bickner, R. E. "Measurement and Indices of Health." In *Outcomes Conference I-II: Methodology of Identifying, Measuring and Evaluating Outcomes of Health Service Programs, Systems and Subsystems* Ed. by Carl E. Hopkins. Rockville, Md.: National Center for Health Services and Development, Health Services and Mental Health Administration, 1970, pp. 133–49.

Breslow, L. "Prospects for Improving Health Through Reducing Risk Factors," *Preventive Medicine,* **7** (1978), 449–58.

Commission on Chronic Illness. *Chronic Illness in the United States,* Vol. I. *Prevention of Chronic Illness.* Cambridge, Mass.: Harvard University Press, 1957, pp. 9–10.

Dubos, R. "Health and Creative Adaptation." *Human Nature,* **1** (1978), 2–10.

Forward Plan for Health, Washington, D.C.: U.S. Department of Health, Education, and Welfare, Public Health Service, 1976.

Francis, T., Jr. "Research in Preventive Medicine." *JAMA,* **172** (1960), 994.

Galdston, I. *The Meaning of Social Medicine.* Cambridge, Mass.: Harvard University Press, 1954, p. 32.

Goldsmith, S. B. "Status of Health Status Indicators." *HSHMA Health Rep.,* **87** (1972), 219.

Health in the United States, 1976–1977. U.S. Department of Health, Education, and Welfare. DHEW Publication No. HRA 77–1232. Washington, D.C.: U.S. Government Printing Office, 1977, p. 8.

Hilbert, M. S. "Prevention." *Am. J. Pub. Health,* **67** (1977), 353–56.

Linder, F. E. "The Health of the American People." *Am. Sci.,* **214** (1966), 28.

Metropolitan Life Insurance Company. *Stat. Bull.,* **49** (1968), 3.

Metropolitan Life Insurance Company. *Stat. Bull.,* **51** (1970), 5–8.

Metropolitan Life Insurance Company. *Stat. Bull.,* **52** (1971), 3–4.

Metropolitan Life Insurance Company. *Stat. Bull.,* **58** (1977), 12.

Perkins, W. H. *Cause and Prevention of Disease.* Philadelphia: Lea & Febiger, 1938, p. 21.

Pratt, L. "The Relationship of Socioeconomic Status to Health." *Am. J. Pub. Health,* **61** (1971), 281–91.

Sargent, F., II. "Man-Environment-Problems for Public Health." *Am. J. Pub. Health,* **62** (1972), 631.

Sullivan, D. F. "A Single Index of Mortality and Morbidity." *HSMHA Health Rep.* **86** (1971), 347–54.

Sullivan, D. F. "Conceptual Problems in Developing an Index of Health." In *Vital and Health Statistics,* U.S. Department of Health, Education, and Welfare, Washington, D.C.: U.S. Government Printing Office, 1966.

Thomas, L. "Notes of a Biology-Watcher on Magic in Medicine." *N. Engl. J. Med.* **299** (1978), 461–63.

Vital Statistics Report, Washington, D.C.: U.S. Government Printing Office, Jan. 1979.

General References

Anderson, F. "Preventive Aspects of Geriatric Medicine." *Postgrad. Med.,* **48** (1972), 157–61.

Anderson, G. et al. "Gypsy Culture and Health Care." *Am. J. Nurs.,* **73** (1973), 282–85.

Aschmann, H. "The Persistent Guajero." *Natural History,* **84** (1975), 28–37.

"Births, Marriages, Divorces, and Deaths for November, 1978." *Monthly Vital Statistics Report, Provisional Statistics,* **27** (Jan. 31, 1979), 4.

Cheraskin, E., and Ringsdorf, W. M. "Predictive Medicine III. An Ecologic Approach." *J. Amer. Geriatr. Soc.,* **19** (1971), 505–10.

Glittenberg, J. "Adapting Health Care to a Cultural Setting." *Am. J. Nurs.,* **74** (1974), 2218–21.

Hilleboe, H. E. "Modern Concepts of Prevention in Community Health." *Am. J. Pub. Health,* **61** (1971), 1000–6.

Lerner, M. "Social Differences in Physical Health." In *Poverty and Health* Ed. by John Kosa, Aaron Antonovsky, and Irving K. Zola. Cambridge, Mass.: Harvard University Press, 1969, pp. 69–112.

Leventhal, H. "Fear Appeals and Persuasion: The Differentiation of a Motivational Construct." *Am. J. Pub. Health,* **61** (1971), 1208–24.

Lewis, C. E., and Lewis, M. A. "The Potential Impact of Sexual Equality on Health." *N. Engl. J. Med.,* **297** (1977), 863–68.

Maslach, C. "Burnout." *Human Behav.* **5** (1976), 16–22.

Saward, E., and Sorensen, A. "The Current Emphasis on Preventive Medicine." *Science,* **200** (1978), 889–94.

Schuman, L. M. "Approaches to Primary Prevention of Disease." *Pub. Health Rep.,* **85** (1970), 1–9.

Thomas, L. "Biomedical Science and Human Health: The Long-Range Prospect." *Daedalus,* **106** (1977), 163–71.

Westoff, C. F. "Marriage and Fertility in the Developed Countries." *Sci. Am.,* **239** (1978), 31–37.

4

Contemporary Health Care Systems and Legislation

The basic issue facing government today is how to provide or pay for quality care at an affordable price. Quality care can be defined as exactly what the person needs—no more, no less. The old adage, "The right patient in the right bed, at the right time and at the right cost," is appropriate. Over-care of a patient is administratively wasteful and may even be detrimental to the patient's overall well-being. Under-care is hazardous to his or her health. In order to achieve a goal of quality care at an affordable price, it is essential to balance patient needs and actual services provided (outcomes) with costs.

FAYE G. ABDELLAH

Abdellah, Faye G. *Health Care in the 1980's Who provides? Who Plans? Who Pays?* New York: National League For Nursing. Publication No. 52–1755, 1979

Contemporary Health Care Systems

An adequate discussion of the health–illness system in the United States is outside the scope of this book. Major problems in the financing and delivery of health care will be considered briefly, as will some of the health-related legislation. Basic information relating to health and illness, facilities and services for providing care, and methods of financing it are summarized in Table 4-1. For those interested in further information, references are included at the end of the chapter.

Unfortunately, it often takes time for authorities to agree to use the same terminology for the same phenomena. Notable examples were seen in Chapter 3, in discussion of health and wellness, which are difficult to define clearly. In Figures 4-1 and 4-2, different terminology is used to refer to essentially the same states. Figure 4-1 is a health status scale, the focus of which is the major forms of available health service. Table 4-1 indicates the focus of major forms of health service. The important services of home, nursing home, and hospice care have been added to Figure 4-1, because of their growing importance in the two decades since Rogers (1960) developed the health status scale showing the focus of major forms of health service.

DEFINITIONS

System. "A system is a set of elements that are actively interrelated and that operate in some sense as a bounded unit" (Baker, 1971).

Primary care.[1] "The term Primary Care has two dimensions: (a) a person's first contact in any given episode of illness with the health care system that leads to a decision of what must be done to help resolve his problems; and (b) the responsibility for

[1] The definitions of primary, acute, and long-term care are taken from a report of the Secretary's Committee to Study Extended Roles for Nurses. *Extending the Scope of Nursing Practice* (Washington, D.C.: Department of Health, Education, and Welfare, 1971), pp. 8–12.

TABLE 4-1 ***Basic Information Relating State of Health, Facilities and Types of Service, and Financing of Health Care***

State of Health	Facilities and Types of Service*	Financing*
Optimum health, well	Research into factors in health maintenance Research into the mechanisms of disease Private medical practice Group medical practice Health maintenance organizations Nursing clinics Well-being clinics (for elderly) Well-baby clinics Family health clinics Schools, health education Community clinics Neighborhood health centers	Individuals Foundations Government agencies Universities—private and public supported Private insurance plans A. Types 1. Blue Cross, Blue Shield 2. Comercial 3. Independent plans such as H.I.P. and Kaiser Permanente (fee for enrolling in the plan, capitation system)
Less than optimum health, worried well, early illness	Many of the above, plus Free clinics Emergency rooms Outpatient clinics Home care	B. Kinds of insurance provided 1. Sickness 2. Disability 3. Income protection, including sick leave
Overt illness, including disability	As above, plus Hospitals Extended-care facilities Hospices	Medicare
Approaching death	Nursing homes	Medicaid

* The availability of each of the above depends on various factors.

the continuum of care, i.e., maintenance of health, evaluation and management of symptoms, and appropriate referrals."

Acute care. "Acute care consists of those services that treat the acute phase of illness or disability and has as its purpose the restoration of normal life processes and functions."

Long-term care. "Long-term care consists of those services designed to provide symptomatic treatment, maintenance and rehabilitative services for patients of all age groups in a variety of health care settings."

TYPES

In Figure 4-2 Garfield (1970) suggests an organization for a delivery system. The focus in Figure 4-2 is the point at which the person enters the system. Unlike the present system, which is focused on the sick, this proposal recognizes that the well also require attention. In this figure he uses the term *well* rather than *optimum health.* Further, he also recognizes that the worried well, that is, healthy persons who for some reason are concerned about their health status, have a legitimate need for care. Possibly some lonely people who visit physicians regularly fall into this category. Depending upon the state of the individual, a person enters the system through the Health-Testing and Referral Service or goes directly to the Health-Care Center or the Sick-Care Center. This system recognizes that well people have legitimate health care needs and require services that are different from those for sick people. Some of these needs are outlined. Garfield also indicates the relative responsibilities of physicians and others in different parts of the system. Both Figures 4-1 and 4-2 indicate that a given individual may move from one part of the system to the other, depending on his or her state of health. Further, both are one system because the various components are interrelated and connected. Nurses must continue to explore the question of what responsibility they can appropriately assume in each part of a system such as that suggested in Figure 4-2.

Figure 4-3 illustrates another concept of a health care system, developed in the planning of the Wayne State University–Health Care Institute. The focus in this system is on the patient. Entry into the system may be by way of referral from community agencies

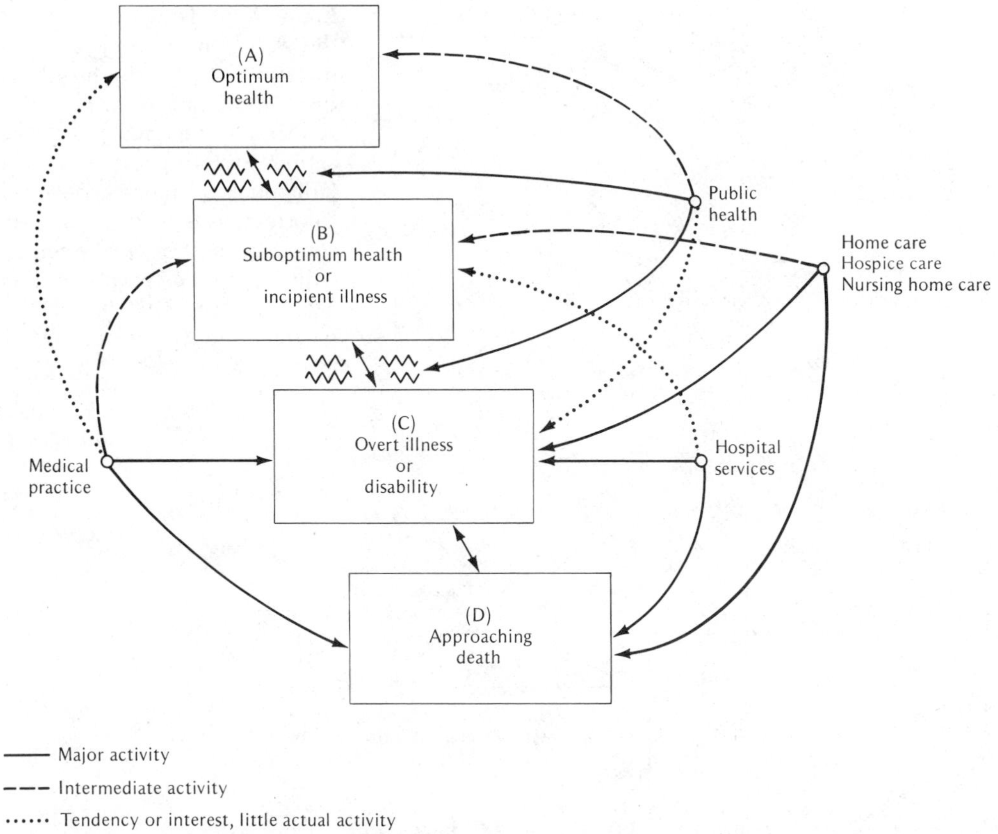

Figure 4-1. Health status scale showing focus of major forms of health service. *Solid line,* major activity; *dashed line,* intermediate activity; *dotted line,* tendency or interest, little actual activity. (Adapted with permission of Macmillan Publishing Co., Inc., from *Human Ecology and Health,* Fig. 24, p. 176, by Edward S. Rogers. Copyright © Edward S. Rogers, 1960.)

or a private physician who requests either primary care, specialty care service, or consumer services such as child care. Depending upon the needs of the person seeking health or sickness care, the person is referred to the appropriate service as listed in column III of Figure 4-3.

Provision of services of Figure 4-3

Again depending upon his or her needs, the person is referred for follow-up to the appropriate agency or service as listed in column IV. Once in the system, the person has a variety of services available, which continue through follow-up. The overall goal is to provide comprehensive care to each person entering the system. Which of the services is used depends upon the needs and desires of each individual entering the system. This figure includes the major types of facilities as well as names of the different personnel required to provide a complete range of services to patients. The plan also provides for the interdisciplinary instruction of health service professionals.

These figures do not refer to the environment, nor should they be expected to. This subject will be dealt with in Chapter 6, as well as in other chapters.

Problems in Meeting Health Care Needs

PRIORITIES

As stated earlier, the focus of the current health care system is primarily on sickness care. Strictly speaking, it is not a system, because the care provided is neither comprehensive nor continuous. Emphasis has rewarded the study of disease. Further funds for study of fundamental biological questions as well as the prevention and treatment of various diseases too often depend on political expediency. It is easier to get money for the dramatic than for the ordinary. Thus great sums of money have been

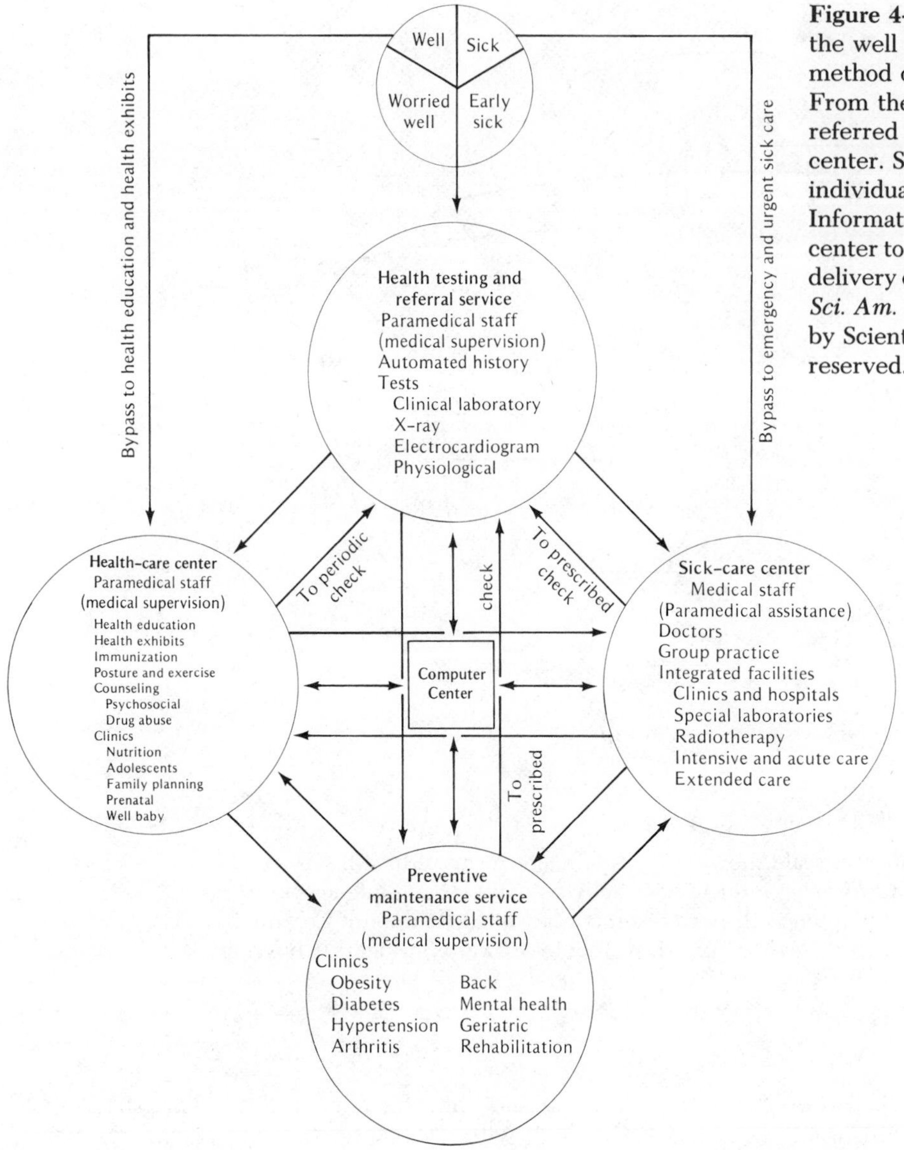

Figure 4-2. New delivery system, separates the well from the sick. Establishes a new method of entry, the health-testing service. From the point of entry the individual is referred to the appropriate health or sick-care center. System provides for the movement of individuals from one type of center to another. Information is readily transferred from one center to another via the computer. (From The delivery of medical care, by Sidney R. Garfield, *Sci. Am.* (Apr.) 1970, p. 22. Copyright © 1970 by Scientific American, Inc. All rights reserved.)

and are being spent on developing a mechanical heart, which even if it is perfected will benefit relatively few. Comparatively little money is being spent to study the basic mechanisms in the development of arteriosclerosis. Discontinuing the Framingham study is a classic example (Kannel, 1970). Were this knowledge available and applied, a number of important diseases could be prevented.

Costs

A second problem is the rapidly escalating cost of medical care resulting from inflation and the use of highly sophisticated technology. During the first half of the century, much of the nursing of hospitalized patients was provided by students. Nonstudent employees were poorly paid in comparison to other workers. In effect, care of the sick was subsidized by nursing and other students and the paid employees. Another factor in the high cost of medical care is the failure to prevent disease as well as to detect and treat early illness. When a crisis occurs, treatment may require specialized personnel and sophisticated machines. When illness is catastrophic or requires long-term treatment, costs escalate to the point where middle-class persons as well as those with limited incomes may be bankrupted. A significant force in the escalation of costs has been the infusion of millions of dollars from the federal government into the purchase of hospital and medical insurance. Finally, the increasing number of malpractice suits is leading physicians to overuse diagnostic tests.

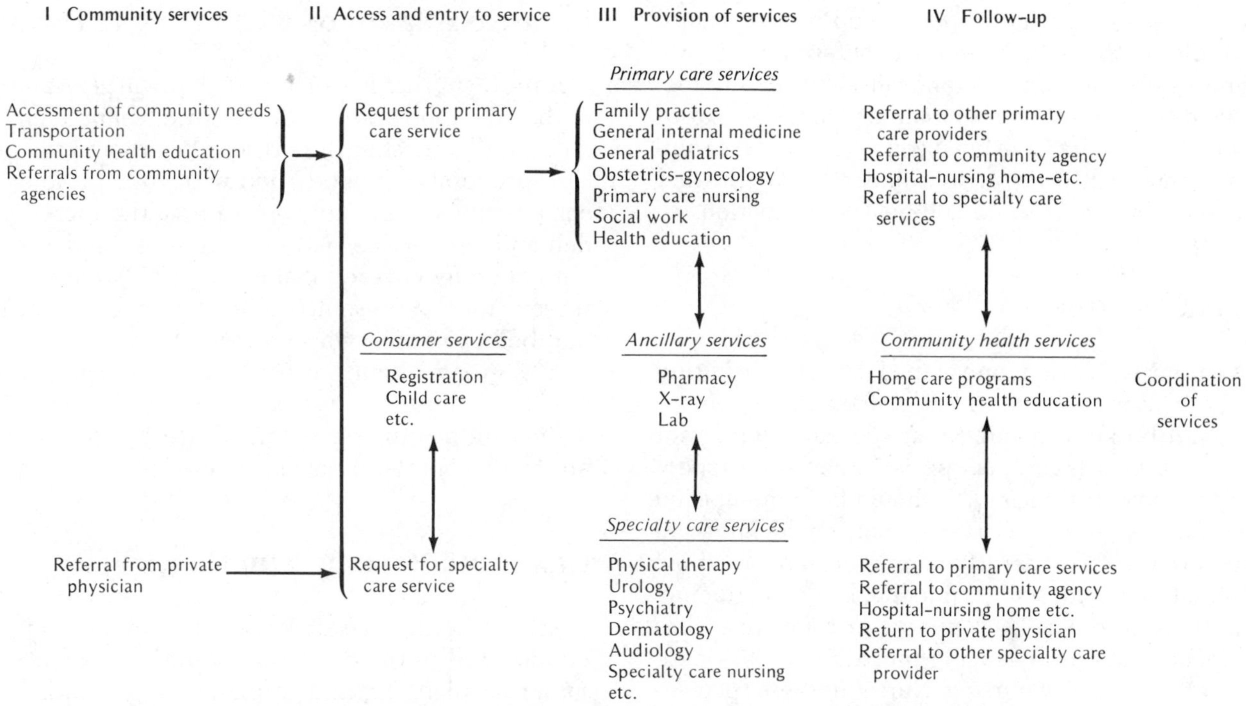

Figure 4-3. Patient Entry to the WSU/HCI Health Care System.

Another factor contributing to the high costs of medical care is that the delivery system is inefficient and uneconomic. As an example, hospitals have been overused because other types of agencies, such as home care, have failed to be used or developed. In some areas, there is an excess of hospital beds. Attention is now being directed toward improving this situation. In one area, a group of hospitals plan together so that the services required by their community are provided and unnecessary duplication is avoided. Laboratory and x-ray as well as support services such as central laundries may be shared. In one Wisconsin community, two hospitals have jointly employed one nurse to help the nursing staff in each hospital develop an in-service program. This and other examples of cooperation will undoubtedly help to reduce the cost and improve the quality of health care.

Availability

A third problem is the availability of health and sickness care. Part of this problem stems from an apparent or real lack of personnel. There is some question as to the extent of the shortage of physicians and other health personnel. There is no doubt but what there are too few physicians in some areas. Rural areas that once supported as many as three physicians may no longer have any. Ghetto areas in large cities may have to depend on city hospital outpatient clinics and emergency rooms. To receive care people may have to wait in line for hours. Were the truth acknowledged, many in the working and middle classes are also dependent upon hospital emergency rooms when prompt medical attention is required. Depending upon the location of the hospital and the area that it serves, these people may also have to wait for intolerably long periods of time. In addition to the shortage of physicians in general, there is a critical problem of geographic and specialty maldistribution. Many have migrated to suburban areas; too few have specialized in general practice and internal medicine and too many in specialized areas. Approaches to this problem include increasing the number of graduates from medical school and providing financial and other incentives to encourage young physicians to practice in areas of greatest need. One result has been an increase in the number of physicians specializing in family practice. Another solution has been to import graduates of foreign medical schools. In some large cities 50 per cent or more of the intern and resident staffs come from other countries.

A number of approaches have been made to increase the quantity of health care available. Money has also been allocated to increase the numbers of nurses graduating from nursing schools as well as to prepare them and others such as medics from the armed services to assume responsibility for routine procedures formerly performed by physicians. In addition there has been a proliferation of programs to prepare persons for limited but highly specialized activities such as pulmonary care. The extent to which numbers have been considered to be a solution to the health care crisis is illustrated by the fact that there are now some 200 health occupations.

Specialization

As indicated earlier, one of the factors contributing to the present situation is specialization. However, it should be kept in mind that specialization is not unique to health care, as specialization is an aspect of a technological society. It should be remembered that at one time a learned person could know all that was known. Presently no one person can know all about one field, such as nursing, law, or medicine. Examples of specialization, and in some instances subspecialization, in nursing include coronary care and cardiac surgery nursing. Nurses in these specialities learn a great deal about the needs of patients who have a particular type of illness. They are able to anticipate possible problems, to interpret changes in cardiac status, and to initiate measures that may be life saving. They have the kind of authority and competence that comes from having sound knowledge and experience. All the above are desirable. However, like other specialists, they can forget that a person is more than a heart (or any other organ). As an example, Mr. Sams, who suffered a severe myocardial infarction, was placed in an intensive coronary care unit. All the modern equipment was applied so that his status could be evaluated continuously. Despite receiving what was thought to be excellent care, he suffered because nurses and physicians talked about him. They seldom talked to or with him. He was frightened by what was said and by the concentration on machines and the intensity with which they were observed. Although specialization is not of itself responsible for depersonalization, each person must keep in focus the fact that it is a person, not an organ, that is receiving care.

Fragmentation

Another problem that has developed as the number of specialized health occupations have increased in the fragmentation of patient care. How can the many activities required in the care of some patients be coordinated so that the patients receive what is required without being exhausted or feeling like the patches on a quilt? Who is best prepared to do the coordination? Is it the nurse?

Decisions Based on Insufficient Data

A problem that has received all too little attention is that decisions are made on insufficient data. As an example, most of the present health and sickness care proposals are concerned with cost. Little or no consideration is being given to how the increase in demand for service will be met when and if costs are generally covered (Schwartz, 1972). One of the reasons for the present health care crises is that the number of people who are able to pay for health care is greater than the present system can accommodate. Attention must be given to the method of delivering health and sickness care if the system is not to be completely overwhelmed.

Changing Role of The Consumer

As in other aspects of society, consideration is being devoted to the decision-making role of the consumer in planning and implementing health care. The resolution of this question involves the attitude that consumers do in fact have a significant role, and it involves the identification of areas where the consumer has the knowledge and competence to make judgments. As implied above, increasing emphasis is being placed upon the role and responsibility of each person for the maintenance of his or her health. Individuals require knowledge of the effects of their life style on their health and life. They need to know the alternatives so that they can make an informed choice. Each person's situation must be considered if a reasonable plan is to be initiated. It should be remembered that most people select the alternative that is easiest for them. Knowledge of and by itself does not necessarily lead to a change in behavior. Many elements must be considered, such as education level, cultural background, socioeconomic status, occupation, as well as what a particular practice means to a person (Milio, 1976).

Legitimacy of consumer involvement in decision making has been acknowledged in comprehensive health planning legislation. As in other human services, providers of service must keep in mind that health service is for people, not for the providers.

One approach to the involvement of consumers in health care has been the development of health centers to meet the health needs of the people of a neighborhood. Residents of the community have an active part in planning and carrying out the program. These centers provide a variety of services to the community, such as the identification and referral of sick or probably sick for medical attention, instruction in normal nutrition or diabetic care, supervision of pregnant women, well-baby care, day care for preschool children, and activity centers for all age groups from the young to the aged. The effectiveness of these centers has been increased by involvement of people living in the area in the planning and conduct of the centers. One nurse with the assistance of persons recruited from the neighborhood provides a variety of health and social services to a group of people who might otherwise be neglected (Milio, 1967). Appropriate medical and social services must be available for referral. When the clientele of these centers is poor, financial support is a major problem.

Accountability

Accountability is a recurring theme in this book. Any person in any profession is held accountable to others in the profession for the quality of service that he or she renders. A good bit of attention has been paid to this type of accountability. The professional also has another kind of accountability, that is, accountability to society. As an example, Mary Claro visits elderly Mr. Bush and finds him living on bread and tea. She explores the situation and learns that Mr. Bush is spending $75 of his monthly income of $95 for rent. As a result of Miss Claro's actions, Mr. Bush receives adequate food. If Miss Claro stops at this point, she is fulfilling her responsibility to Mr. Bush. She has not, however, met her responsibility to society, that is, to initiate, support, and contribute to programs to prevent near starvation among the aged.

Lag Between Discovery and Application

One further problem will be mentioned: the lag between discovery of knowledge and its application. The reasons for this lag are varied. They range from sloth, greed, resistance to change, ignorance, and lack of money, to honest disagreement.

An example of a disease whose prevention lagged behind the knowledge of its prevention is typhoid fever. The history of the control of typhoid fever can be traced through changes in its importance as a cause of death. In 1905 typhoid fever caused more deaths than any other infectious disease. Moreover, the death rate was higher than it needed to be, as the rate was much higher in the United States than in Europe. Although typhoid fever decreased steadily as a cause of death after 1900, not until 1919 was there a sharp drop in its incidence. In some parts of the world it continues to be a significant cause of morbidity and mortality.

Health and Sickness Care Agencies

Table 4-1 lists some of the different types of agencies designed to provide for health maintenance and care of the sick. Not all the agencies listed will be discussed. There has been a proliferation in not only the types of health occupations but also in the number and types of agencies. With all the shortcomings of health and sickness care, it should be remembered that modern medicine is less than 50 years old, having begun with the discovery that the sulfonamides had a bacteriostatic effect. People and institutions are having difficulty keeping up with a world in which new knowledge is doubling every 7 to 8 years. The fact that expectations exceed the capacity to deliver is a reality.

Classification

Agencies may be classified according to their controlling body, the source of their support, or the type of service that they render. When classified according to their source of support, they are official or voluntary. Official agencies are controlled by some branch of the government—national, state, or local. Voluntary agencies are of two general types, nonprofit and proprietary. As the term implies, *voluntary* agencies are sponsored by some organization such as a religious body or a group of public-spirited citizens. They are supported by their users and by contributions of services by other persons. When income is insufficient to cover costs, additional funds are donated by individuals or groups such as the United Community Fund, a religious group, or private citizens.

In the Midwest and Far West United States, some hospitals under the aegis of local governments are financed on a basis similar to that of voluntary hospitals. Their major support comes from their users; minimal support is received from taxation.

Proprietary agencies are operated for the profit of their owners. To make a profit there is the possibility that either cost to the patient is high or the standard of services suffers. To date many nursing homes are proprietary. A hope for the future is that they will be integrated into the nonprofit health care system.

In addition to the classification of hospitals by ownership or type of controlling body, they may be classified by the type of patients treated. Thus they may be general or specialized. General hospitals provide care for people with a variety of medical problems.

Specialized hospitals limit their clientele to some group or type of patient or problem.

Just as hospitals may be sponsored by the government or by voluntary agencies, so may public health agencies. Although voluntary agencies carry out other activities, their major function is to provide nursing care for patients who are sick at home.

Hospitals

Prior to the twentieth century, with the exception of the indigent, most persons who were ill were cared for at home. There were few nurses and most of the care during sickness was given by physicians and members of the patient's family. In the past 50 years the number of hospital beds has quadrupled. After World War II, the number of beds in federal hospitals increased sharply. After 1950 the most marked increase was in hospitals providing short-term care. Among the reasons for the increase is that hospitals are no longer looked on as places to go to die. Rather they are expected to give sophisticated diagnostic and therapeutic care, thereby restoring the patient to the best possible state of health.

There is increasing emphasis on the development of facilities and services. Thus there is a trend toward building medical complexes that provide services for people in all stages of the health–sickness and disability continuum. There are facilities for diagnosis, treatment, care during critical stages of illness, convalescent care, and, as needed, rehabilitative and/or long-term care. An indispensable aspect is an arrangement whereby patients can move from one facility to another as their condition dictates.

Within the hospital itself, patients may be assigned to different areas, depending on the type and degree of illness. For example, a patient may be admitted to a diagnostic unit and later transferred to the operating room for a surgical procedure. From there the patient goes to a recovery room or to an intensive-care unit. With the concentration of patients having particular needs in a localized area, specialized equipment can be readily available and nursing personnel can develop a high degree of competence. This plan has some possible disadvantages. Unless provisions are made for continuing care, the patient may be transferred from one area of the hospital to another much as from one foreign country to another. What appears to the patient to be an abrupt change in expectations may increase his or her anxiety and sense of depersonalization. With adequate planning and followthrough, the patient does not have to experience these feelings. Certainly a real effort should be made to interpret a move from an intensive-care unit to a convalescent-care unit as a major step in progress from sickness to health. Provision should also be made for the personnel in the intensive-care unit to follow the progress of the patient.

Another possible danger in assigning patients to units on the basis of stage of diagnosis or degree of illness is that patients who appear to be less acutely ill or convalescent will be neglected. Care may be limited to meeting physical needs, the administration of medicines and treatments, and the performance of diagnostic tests. The period in which a patient is undergoing diagnosis is often characterized by anxiety. Perhaps the most important statement to be made at this point is that the priority of needs differs with different degrees of illness but that all sick people have needs. These needs should be identified and plans made to satisfy them.

Increasingly, hospitals are providing care for individuals who do not have a family physician or who become sick when the physician is not available. There is also an increasing trend for hospitals to serve as the hub or nucleus for a wide spectrum of ambulatory services.

Community Clinics

There is also a trend toward taking health centers to people rather than requiring people to go to distant centers. This has resulted in the development of neighborhood health centers, community clinics, and free clinics. Free clinics have developed in response to the need of individuals who do not fit into or feel comfortable in the traditional health and sickness care facilities.

Home Care

Another trend stimulated by the cost of medical and hospital care is movement toward caring for less acutely ill patients in their homes. Home care, as it is called, is a boon to the person who requires one or more professional services but does not require all the facilities of a hospital for the acutely ill. In many communities chronically ill persons can receive the care they require at home. Home care may be sponsored by hospitals or community agencies such as visiting nurse associations. To illustrate, Mrs. Albert, aged 35, has a chronic neurologic disorder, multiple sclerosis. She has four young children ranging in age from 1 to 14 years. Though she required hospitalization at the onset of her illness, she is able to spend most of her time at home. In addition to medical supervision, she is visited daily by a visiting nurse, who supervises her activity and exercise. A physical therapist visits her once a week to evaluate the effect of her activity program. The nurse has taught Mr. Albert to administer a preparation of the adrenocorticotropic hormone by intramuscular injection. The nurse consulted the agency dietitian about how to help Mrs. Albert plan a low-fat diet. An occupational therapist is available but has not been consulted, because Mrs. Albert is kept busy supervising the children and the household. Because the Visiting Nurse Service also provides household aides, one is assigned to assist Mrs. Albert. Because the number of services and amount of care required by Mrs. Albert are great, even home care is expensive, though less so than hospital care. One of the values of home care that cannot be measured in terms of money is that Mrs. Albert fulfills within the limits of her ability her role as wife and mother. For many persons home care may not play as vital a role, but it does make it possible for the person to live a more nearly normal life.

There is also a trend toward caring for patients in the terminal stages of illness at home and toward keeping the patient active as long as is practical. To do this, the family must be emotionally and physically able to care for the patient at home. The willingness of the family to have the patient at home is perhaps the most important factor in determining whether the patient can be cared for there. Mrs. Lottie Gamely is a good example of how a seriously disabled person may be cared for at home. Despite being bedridden and unable to turn in bed without help, she remained at home until the week before her death. During her last months she maintained her role as mother to her two children, aged 8 and 10. Before they left for school in the morning she checked them in the same manner as do healthy mothers. She saw to it that they performed their household chores and did their homework. She comforted them and she disciplined them. Household help was required. Medical and nursing care was available and provided.

Besides remaining useful, the patient's needs are often easier to meet at home than they are in the hospital. Food prepared at home is more palatable than hospital food. Visiting by friends and relatives is easier. The schedule and timing of the activities of the day are likely to be familiar. Medical and nursing supervision is necessary to the success of home care. They are required not only for the patient's safety but so that the strain on the family is not excessive. There is always the possibility that the patient will be neglected or become a sickroom tyrant. Neither is desired or desirable. It is also essential to be able to transfer the patient to the hospital when necessary.

Hospital personnel, including physicians, tend to minimize the problems faced by the chronically ill patient after discharge from the hospital. The result is that not all patients who require assistance at home are referred to the Visiting Nurse Service or other community agencies for guidance. The amount and type of assistance needed vary. Not all patients require as much help as Mrs. Albert or Mrs. Gamely; some require more. Further, no single type of service will meet the needs of all persons or even the same person at different times of life.

Hospice Care

About 30 years ago a British physician, Dr. Cicely Saunders, proposed and implemented the concept that the terminally ill have a right to die in a homelike setting as free of pain as possible. Today she heads a hospice, St. Christopher's in London, which serves as a model for hospices throughout the world. Presently there are about 75 hospices in operation in the United States and at least 150 in the planning stage (*Changing Times*, 1979).

Objectives

Unlike the objectives of a hospital, which are to cure or control a disease and to rehabilitate, the objective of the hospice is to prevent and relieve suffering of the patient and family and/or significant others. In other words, these persons have an unfavorable prognosis and the course of *their* disease is predicted to be in its final stages. Most persons entering hospices are in the last stages of cancer, although those with other diseases may also be admitted. At this point, emphasis is on the *quality* not the quantity of life. Everyone involved recognizes that the course of the disease is not likely to change but that much can be done to ease the suffering of the patient and family. Care of the family continues not only through the course of the patient's illness but beyond.

General Guidelines

The care must be under the supervision of a licensed physician in cooperation with a responsible family member 24 hours a day and 7 days a week. This does not mean that the patient is not involved in making decisions about care for as long as possible. Where does the patient receive care? When feasible, the patient should be cared for at home. In the experience of Hospice, Inc., in New Haven, Connecticut, a home care-based facility, 70 per cent of their patients are able to die in their own homes (Abdellah, 1979). In those instances where a patient's needs and desires are too demanding or specialized, the patient may be hospitalized or admitted to an inpatient facility. Points that must be considered when deciding where the patient will receive care are: Is the family willing and able physically and emotionally to care for the patient at home? Can an environment be maintained that is conducive to the patient's and the family's well-being? When the patient is cared for at home, the family needs instruction in managing symptoms, including pain, as well as basic nursing care, diet, medications, and exercise. Family members require emotional support while the patient is dying and during bereavement. Meeting the needs of the patient and the family requires a team of physicians, nurses, mental health workers, chaplains, social workers, and volunteers. When necessary to relieve pain, special therapies such as surgery, x-ray, or chemotherapy may be used.

An inpatient facility should be available and used when the patient's needs make it desirable. This facility should be homelike and open to the family 24 hours a day. There should be a comfortable sitting room where patient and family can meet in private.

It is well to remember that a hospice is neither a hospital nor a nursing home. It is an organization for caring for those persons who have received definitive treatment and whose disease is no longer responding to therapeutic measures and for whom no further therapy is to be given. Cure is no longer likely. The purpose of the hospice is to make it possible for the person in the last stages of disease to die in as homelike a situation as possible with the relief of pain and suffering. Maintenance of the *quality* of the dying patient's life is the goal. Much can be done to accomplish this goal. Whether or not a special facility is available, the hospice concept can be practiced. Certainly it is easier with an organization. For example, following therapy for cancer, Martha Black's disease no longer responded to treatment. She spent her last days in the hospital. Her wish to have her care given by her husband was granted. Her pain and suffering were kept at a minimum. Most important to Mr. and Mrs. Black was that they were able to share her last few days.

Systems of Payment for Medical Care

According to Terris (1978), there are three basic systems of payment for medical care: public assistance, health insurance, and national health service. Presently in the United States, there are two: health insurance and public assistance. Terris does not include the continued direct payment for the full cost of care. Despite more than 50 years of effort, Congress has not passed a National Health Plan. With each new Congress, bills that are introduced fail to pass.

Health Insurance

Of all the problems facing the health and sickness care system none is receiving more attention than its cost. One approach to the solution of high costs to the individual has been the development of insurance plans. Most of the plans have been one of three types: insurance to protect against an acute disabling illness, insurance to pay the cost of a major or catastrophic illness, and insurance to prevent the loss of income during illness. Benefits are often limited to a stated period of hospitalization and exclude certain diseases.

Insurance plans may be privately or government sponsored. Privately-sponsored plans may be nonprofit or profit making. The best known nonprofit plan is Blue Cross (hospital insurance) and Blue Shield (doctor insurance). Both Blue Cross and Blue Shield are fee-for-service plans. Some commercial plans have a very low or zero margin of profit.

In many of these plans, the hospital or physician is paid for service rendered. The hospital is paid when a patient is hospitalized, the physician when a service such as an appendectomy or an electrocardiogram is performed.

Health Maintenance Organizations (HMOs)

A second method of payment is through a health maintenance organization (HMO). This is a system for providing comprehensive and quality health care for a prepaid sum of money. The physician or organization receives the same amount of money whether clients are sick or well. Though many HMOs offer a full range of services, emphasis is upon ambulatory rather than hospital care. Originally it was hoped that quality care could be provided at less cost than the fee-for-service plan. However, in a study reported by the Metropolitan Life Insurance Company of an HMO in St. Louis (April–June 1978), total costs were about the same as in a fee-for-service plan. However, less was spent on in-hospital care and more on ambulatory and preventive care than in the fee for service. The latter is considered to be the better use of money.

The concept of prepaid group practice has been in existence for about 40 years. Included in the successful early plans were the Health Insurance Plan of Greater New York (HIP) and the Kaiser plans on the West Coast. Despite the success of a few plans, growth has been slow. As of February 1978, there were only 51 "qualified" HMOs, with an enrollment of about 4 million.

One of the early problems with HMOs was that laws governing their formation were inflexible and required excessive services. In 1976 amendments to the legislation increased flexibility and thereby made it possible to develop more competitive plans.[2] Financing of HMOs may be by insurance, such as Blue Cross-Blue Shield, or by direct payment by an employing agency or an individual.

Another type of insurance that helps to ease the financial burden of illness is income insurance. It may be purchased or provided by paid sick leave. An employed individual is allowed a set number of days each year when he or she may be absent from work without the loss of wages or salary. In some situations sick leave is cumulative. With the increase in the incidence of long-term illness, insurance covering extended periods of illness and providing income is of great importance. Many persons between the ages of 18 and 65 do not have this type of insurance available to them at costs they can afford to pay.

Health-Related Legislation

Health legislation is far from new, for as long as there has been organized government, there have been rules or laws governing human activities that were believed to protect our well-being. Among the oldest laws are those related to sanitation and food safety. During this century, laws having implications to health have continued to be enacted. Many city, state, and even federal laws have been enacted for the purpose of protecting the general public from agents causing injury and disease. Examples include laws or regulations to control traffic, housing and building construction, water supplies, food handling, the preparation and serving of food in restaurants, and sewage disposal. Pure food and drug laws protect the quality of food and drugs. As an example the 91st Congress passed over 20 health-related laws (Abdellah, 1973).

Important as health legislation is, space does not permit detailed coverage. Thus this discussion will be limited to a few laws that are based on the general principle that health is a right.

Workers' Compensation

The first workers' compensation law was enacted in 1910. It covered injuries caused by accidents. Later amendments included programs to protect the worker from diseases resulting from health hazards.

Social Security Act of 1935[3]

As a result of the Depression that began in 1929, the fact that industrial workers were not always able to protect themselves against unemployment was recognized. In 1935 the Social Security Act was passed. It had three provisions based on the principle that society has an obligation to provide for the security of its people. The first provision was for unemployment compensation to be handled by the states. The second was establishment of an annuity that was to be paid at age 65 or on retirement of its members. This provision combines some of the features of private insurance with the responsibility of society to provide for those in need. The third provided for special categories of needy persons, including the aged, the blind, the crippled and disabled, and dependent children. In this law the government assumed responsibility for helping people provide for the future. In the intervening years the number of persons covered and the benefits have been increased.

Medicare

In 1965 the Social Security Act was further amended to provide specified health services to those 65 years of age or older as a right through the application of social insurance principles. The purpose of Medicare is to protect the aged against the high cost of medical and hospital care. However, the cost of Medicare is pegged to hospital costs,

[2] For an extensive summary of health-related legislation, see Henderson, Virginia, and Nite, Gladys. *Principles and Practice of Nursing*, 6th ed. New York: Macmillan Publishing Co., Inc., 1978.

[3] Information about who qualifies for health insurance for the aged may be obtained from the Superintendent of Documents, U.S. Government Printing Office, Washington, D.C. 20402.

which have been rising. Because of increased deductible and increasing cost, Medicare pays for less and less of the cost of medical care.

Medicaid

At the same time as the Medicare law was enacted, under Title XIX monies were made available on a matching basis to states for various categories of needy people. When the two social security amendments of 1965 took full effect, about 25 per cent of the population was covered.

The principal effect of Medicare and to a lesser extent Medicaid has been to reduce the financial barriers to medical care. Because of exclusions and deductibles, Medicare pays less than half the costs of medical care for the aged. Those who can afford it carry some type of supplementary insurance, such as Blue Cross and Blue Shield–65 insurance. Further raises in the deductible that must be met before an individual is eligible for Medicare increases the barrier for those that need it the most. Those unable to pay for the additional cost of care are likely to neglect evidence of illness until it causes a crisis. Evidence that having means to pay for medical care increases its use is borne out by the fact that during the first 5 years of Medicare, use accelerated each year.

Whatever the reasons, studies (West, 1971) indicate that a high proportion of Medicare payments are spent on a relatively few persons. Twenty per cent of those covered received no covered medical care. In 1970 just under 50 per cent used sufficient services to be eligible for reimbursement. There were 7.5 per cent who were reimbursed $2,000 or more and who accounted for 39 per cent of the funds spent. About 20 per cent are hospitalized each year.

In 1972 the 92nd Congress set a precedent by extending Medicare to cover one catastrophic illness, kidney disease. Beginning July 1, 1973, persons requiring hemodialysis and/or kidney transplant who are under 65 and covered by Social Security will be covered by Medicare. Further, those who have been covered by Social Security and have been disabled for two or more years will also become eligible for Medicare.

Title XIX or Medicaid was intended to aid the states in providing medical care to needy people under 65 years of age, not only for persons on welfare, but for those whose incomes were insufficient to bear the cost of sickness. In actual practice in most states, it has been limited to persons on welfare (Gorman, 1971). According to some, the financing of the health and sickness care for many of the poor is worse than it was before Medicaid.

Goal of Past and Present Insurance Plans

Most insurance plans have had as their stated goal the reduction of the cost of medical care to people. Most are fee for service, that is, service is required if providers are to have an income. Some critics of current plans say that the real goal is the support of the providers of care. As emphasized earlier, plans have generally been crisis oriented. Relatively few of these programs provide for health maintenance or even for ambulatory care. Despite some exceptions, most insurance plans require hospitalization for full coverage. Insurance plans such as Medicare and especially Medicaid have failed because they have created a demand that cannot be met by present personnel and facilities. There is no incentive for prevention.

Professional Standards Review Organization (PSRO)

Concern for the quality of medical care led to the 1972 amendment of the Social Security Act. It resulted in the creation of the Professional Standards Review Organization (PSRO). The purpose of this organization was to formulate explicit criteria, norms, and standards to be met in the medical care of Medicaid and Medicare recipients and eventually of all recipients of medical care. In order to facilitate the achievement of the purpose of this amendment, the country was to be divided into areas (states or parts of states), and coordinated by the National Council with the Department of Health, Education, and Welfare (HEW) at the top of an apex.

Evaluation of the extent to which the criteria and norms are met is performed by a coordinator (usually a nurse). It includes an assessment of such factors as whether or not (1) the admission of a patient was justified, (2) the length of stay was appropriate, and (3) the care prescribed conformed to the standards and criteria of the PSRO (Donabedian, 1978).

National Health Planning and Resources Development Act of 1974 (HSA)

In an attempt to provide for equal access to quality health care and at the same time control the inflationary rise in health care costs, Congress passed Public Law 93–641. The act states the following purpose: "To Amend the Public Health Service Act to assure the development of a national health policy and of effective state and area health planning and resources development programs, and for other purposes." In order to achieve the intent of this law, the nation was divided into areas. As an example, seven counties in southeastern Michigan were formed into the Comprehensive Health Planning Council of Southeast Michigan. Further, the achievement of the goals of this law requires an effective partnership between the public and private sectors of the community. Community participation in the health care decision-making process was accepted as essential.

The scope of activities encompassed by P.L. 93–641 is demonstrated by the national priorities for improving the health care system. They include the following:

1. Primary care for medically underserved
2. Multiinstitutional systems for coordination or consolidation of services
3. Multiinstitutional arrangements for sharing support services
4. Prevention of disease
5. Development of medical group practices
6. Improvements in quality services
7. Provision of various levels of care
8. Training and increased utilization of physician assistants and nurse clinicians
9. Uniform cost accounting, simplified reimbursement, and utilization reporting system
10. Health education

These priorities for which plans are to be made are indeed impressive. However, the question must be asked "Is health planning working?" The answer, according to Bachman (1979), is "Not yet." As an example, much of the effort of the Comprehensive Health Planning Council of Southeast Michigan has been devoted to determining the number of hospital beds required in the area and setting limits on the expansion of hospitals.

The reasons for the inability to answer this question affirmatively are many. There is little agreement on what constitutes health. Most definitions are general and difficult to define in specific terms (see Chapter 3). Health status indicators are at a rudimentary level. Little is known about how and to what extent health care services actually contribute to health. Knowledge by itself is not sufficient to motivate people to avoid or discontinue practices hazardous to health (Chapter 3). One of the most serious weaknesses of health planning at this time is that cost-benefits on human life are not acceptable either politically or publicly. Yet, as a society, we will have to come to a resolution of what the need for health care as defined by professionals is and what we can afford.

In the words of Bachman (1979),

> There are no easy formulas for objective social determinations of need, nor are there likely soon to be any. Planning is not a simple, value-free, quantitative endeavor that involves gathering all the data on institutional health services delivery and plugging them mechanistically into expert calculations to determine what we need. Rather, through planning, we must decide how much health care is enough. Planning, in other words, is as much or more a political activity than a scientific one.

Lewis (1977) makes the above point when he says, "Although advances in medicine depend on the generation of new knowledge, changes in the health-care system depend on alterations in social and political values."

Despite the problems in implementing the National Health Planning and Resources Development Act, it is the structure through which all plans for changing, adding to, or developing new structures and agencies have to pass. Guidelines will be refined and need will be defined in realistic terms.

Other Legislation

Food and Drug Acts

A law going back to the early twentieth century is the Harrison Narcotic Act of 1914, which regulates the importation, manufacture, sale, dispensing or prescribing, and use of cocaine and opium and all their derivatives. The new synthetic preparations known to cause addiction are also included. Although the Harrison Act was intended to be regulatory, it is administered as if it were criminal or prohibitory in nature. In a discussion of the need for the reassessment of the problem of drug addiction, Murtagh (1963) made a plea for changes that would make it possible to treat the drug addict as a medical rather than a legal problem. Although the intent of the Harrison Act is to protect society, it has also created problems in relation to drug addiction. Drug-related problems led to passage of the Comprehensive Drug Abuse Prevention and Control Act of 1970. To protect the public health from unscrupulous drug manufacturers, the Federal Food, Drug and Cosmetic Acts were passed first in 1906 and revised in 1938, 1962, and 1967.

Among other laws passed by the 89th Congress, some were amendments of previous laws and some were new, such as the Cigarette Labeling Law. These laws have as their general purposes: (1) protection from health hazards in the environment, (2) making health facilities and services available to people, and (3) increasing the knowledge and skill of health service personnel. At each congressional session other laws, including antipollution acts and car safety, have been enacted.

The National Health Survey

Not only has Congress been interested in legislation protecting public safety, but it has been interested in determining the health status of the people. In 1956, Congress established the National Health Survey and charged it with collecting the facts about national health problems and the level and extent of medical care. To gather data, two types of activities were initiated: the health interview survey and the health examination survey. The purpose of the health interview survey is to measure the social dimensions of health. The health examination survey collects "precise physiological and diagnostic data by means of comprehensive clinical examinations with objective measurements and tests" (Linder, 1966). In the beginning, representative samples of adults ages 18 to 79 were examined. In the second part of the study 7,000 children aged 6 to 11 were examined. In addition to the above, data were also collected from health facilities (Linder, 1966).

Although no attempt will be made to summarize all the data gathered in this study, a few will be cited. In 1964, civilian nonhospitalized persons experienced more than 3 billion days of disability because of injury or illness. About 2 million people in the United States know that they have diabetes. A substantially larger number have symptoms generally attributed to diabetes but have not been so diagnosed. From this study information was obtained about the relationship of economic status to health and illness (see Chapter 3).

The Future

In planning for the future, several problems must be kept in perspective. Not only is medical care expensive and poorly distributed, but it is primarily sickness oriented. According to some authorities at least 25 per cent of the population is medically indigent. As stated earlier, a catastrophic illness can bankrupt a middle-class family. One solution that has been under consideration for at least 50 years is national health insurance.

Other health-related issues that have been and will continue to be of concern to all levels of government include (1) drug and narcotic use, (2) mental illness, (3) population control, (4) nutrition, (5) housing, (6) pollution control, (7) highway safety, (8) infectious disease control, (9) use of tobacco, and (10) alcoholism. Another issue that will have to be faced is how people's expectations of a health care system can be modified or met.

Despite the tendency on the part of Americans to believe that the solution to any problem is money, authorities warn that money alone will not solve the health care crisis. In fact, it will only make the situation worse. If the crisis is to be solved, the delivery system as well as the method of financing requires change. Some of the changes being suggested are not new. In fact they were made as much as 35 years ago. These changes are not likely to come about easily, involving as they do politics, powerful vested interests, sincere beliefs, lack of organization of consumers, and many other factors.

A question that must be answered is whether or not one large system of health and sickness care can meet the needs of everyone. Possibly a number of plans should be developed so that the consumer has an opportunity to select the kind of plan that best suits him or her. Though much has been made of the importance of the individual being able to choose a physician, doubts are expressed as to whether or not this is now a fact.

At this point all that can be said is that sooner or later there will be extensions of health care insurance. It is now known that improvement in health services involves more than removal of financial barriers. Burns (1966) emphasizes some of the principles that are basic to any system of health care:

1. Availability of appropriate health services to all people. In the discussion of this point, Burns (1966) makes a plea for giving children wherever they live priority in health care.
2. Attention should be given to high-quality medical services.
3. There should be an orderly organization of health services. What this principle means is that all services from the promotion of health and the prevention of disease to rehabilitation should be provided. Unnecessary duplication of services should be avoided.
4. Finally, attention should be given to economy in the use of health services.

To this list should be added the necessity to identify and correct those conditions that lead to ill health and premature death. Services must be provided in a manner acceptable to the recipients.

Burns (1971) summarizes the important issues as "the characteristics of an efficient and socially acceptable health services delivery system and the nature of the organizational structures, financial arrangements and administrative systems most likely to bring it into effect."

The first step in enactment of a health care program is the belief that health care is a right, not a concession. Without this belief and the actions that stem from it, people will not have the benefit of alternative forms of health care to complement the sickness care that is now the primary focus of medicine and most health agencies. Further, large segments of the population will receive care primarily in crisis situations, which call for the expenditure of large sums of money and involve considerable suffering.

References Cited

Abdellah, F. G. et al. *System of Delivery of Health Services.* New York: Macmillan Publishing Co., Inc., 1973, pp. 538–39.

Abdellah, F. G. "Preparing for the Health Care Issues of the 1980's." In *Health Care in the 1980's, Who Provides? Who Plans? Who Pays?* Pub. No. 52-1755. New York: National League for Nursing, 1979, pp. 8–10.

Bachman, L. "Health Planning—The Next Step." *Partnership for Health* (Comprehensive Health Planning Council of Southeastern Michigan), 7 (1979), 10–11.

Baker, F. "General Systems Theory, Research, and Medical Care." In *Systems and Medical Care,* Ed. by A. Sheldon et al. Cambridge, Mass.: The M.I.T. Press, 1971, p. 5.

"A Better Way for Dying." *Changing Times,* 33 (1979), 22.

Burns, E. M. "Policy Decisions Facing the United States in Financing and Organizing Health Care." *Pub. Health Rep.,* **81** (1966), 676.

Burns, E. M. "A Critical Review of National Health Insurance Proposals." *HSMHA Health Rep.,* **86** (1971), 120.

Donabedian, A. "The Quality of Medical Care." *Science,* **200** (1978), 856–63.

Garfield, S. R. "The Delivery of Medical Care." *Sci. Am.,* **222** (1970), 15–23.

Gorman, M. "The Impact of National Health Insurance on the Delivery of Health Care." *Am. J. Publ. Health,* **61** (1971), 962–71.

Henderson, V., and Nite, G. *Principles and Practice of Nursing,* 6th ed. New York: Macmillan Publishing Co., Inc., 1978.

Kannel, W. B. "The Framingham Study and Chronic Disease Prevention." *Hosp. Pract.,* **5** (1970), 78–87, 92–94.

Lewis, C. E. "Health-Services Research and Innovations in Health-Care Delivery." *N. Engl. J. Med.,* **297** (1977), 423–27.

Linder, F. E. "The Health of the American People." *Sci. Am.,* **214** (1966), 24.

Metropolitan Life Insurance Company. "Health Maintenance Organizations." *Stat. Bull.* **59** (April–June 1978), 56.

Milio, N. "A Framework for Prevention: Changing Health-Damaging to Health-Generalizing Life Patterns." *Am. J. Pub. Health,* **66** (1976), 435.

Milio, N. "Project in a Negro Ghetto." *Am. J. Nurs.,* **67** (1967), 1006–09.

Murtagh, J. M. "Dilemma for Drug Addicts." *America,* **108** (1963) 740–42.

Rogers, E. S. *Human Ecology and Health.* New York: Macmillan Publishing Co., Inc., 1960, Fig. 24, p. 176.

Schwartz, W. B. "Policy Analysis, Politics and the Problems of Health Care." *N. Engl. J. Med.,* **286** (1972), 1057–58.

Terris, M. "The Three World Systems of Medical Care: Trends and Prospects." *Am. J. Publ Health,* **68** (1978), 1125.

West, H. "Five Years of Medicare—A Statistical Review." *Soc. Sec. Bull.,* **34** (1971), 17–27.

General References

Abernathy, W. J. "Regional Planning of Primary Health Care Services." *Medical Care,* **10** (1972), 380–94.

Alcott, L. M. "Chapter 1. Projecting the Economic Cost of Illness: Introduction." *Pub. Health Rep.,* **93** (1978), 500–07.

Ball, B. M. "National Health Insurance: Comments on Selected Issues." *Science,* **200** (1978), 864–70.

Bates, L. E. "Health Maintenance Organizations, a Prototype: New York." *Hospitals,* **45** (1971), 59–60.

Burns, E. M. "Health Insurance: Not If, or When, but What Kind?" *Am. J. Pub. Health,* **61** (1971), 2164–75.

Callahan, E. B. "Extending Hospital Services into the Home." *Am. J. Nurs.,* **61** (1961), 59–62.

Falk, I. S. "National Health Insurance for the United States." *Pub. Health Rep.,* **92** (1977), 399–406.

Frank, K. D. "Government Support of Nursing-Home Care." *N. Engl. J. Med.,* **287** (1972), 538–45.

Hamburg, D., and Brown, S. S. "The Science Base and Social Context of Health Maintenance: An Overview." *Science,* **200** (1978), 847–49.

Isaacs, M. "Toward a National Health Policy: A Realistic View." *Am. J. Nurs.,* **78** (1978), 848–51.

Kramer, M. "The Consumer's Influence on Health Care." *Nurs. Outlook,* **20** (1972), 574–78.

Leininger, M. "An Open Health Care System Model." *Nurs. Outlook,* **21** (1973), 171–75.

Lister, J. L. "Access to Primary Care. The Paradox of Medical Care—Prospect for Change." *N. Engl. J. Med.,* **300** (1979), 1474–76.

Loewenstein, R. "Early Effects of Medicare on Health Care of the Aged." *Soc. Sec. Bull,* **34** (1971), 3–20.

Mauksch, I. C. "On National Health Insurance." *Am. J. Nurs.,* **78** (1978), 1323–27.
Mechanic, D. "Approaches to Controlling the Costs of Medical Care: Short-Range and Long-Range Alternatives." *N. Engl. J. Med.,* **298** (1978), 310–18.
Paige, R. L., and Looney, J. F. "Hospice Care for the Adult." *Am. J. Nurs.,* **77** (1977), 1812–15.
Perrin, E. C., and Goodman, H C. "Telephone Management of Acute Pediatric Illnesses." *N. Engl. J. Med.,* **298** (1978), 130–35.
Pluckhan, M. L. "Professional Territoriality, A Problem Affecting the Delivery of Health Care." *Nurs. Forum,* **11** (1972), 300–10.
Robinson, D. "Primary Medical Practice in the United Kingdom and the United States." *N. Engl. J. Med.,* **297** (1977), 188–93.
Sargent, E. G. "Evolution of a Home Care Plan." *Am. J. Nurs.,* **61** (1961), 88–91.
Schwartz, D. "Nursing Needs of Chronically Ill Ambulatory Patients." *Nurs. Res.,* **9** (1960), 185–88.
Trager, B. "Home Health Services and Health Insurance." *Med. Care,* **9** (1971), 89–98.

UNIT II

Concepts Basic to the Theory and Practice of Nursing

The trick, Fletcher, is that we are trying to overcome our limitations in order, patiently. We don't tackle flying through rock until a little later in the program.
BACH, 1970

INTRODUCTION

The explosion of information in health-related fields makes it impossible for this, or indeed any, textbook to present exhaustive coverage of content relevant to its topic. The growth rate of scientific fields has been measured by the number of years required for the literature in the field to double. Menard (1971) suggestes that a "normal field" doubles in 15 years, a very "slow field" may double in 45 years, a very "fast field" may double in 5 years. Many of the fields from which nursing draws facts and concepts relevant to understanding and modifying human behavior are fast fields; nursing itself appears to have moved from a slow to a normal field since mid-century. Obviously, the student of nursing will be unable to garner all, or even most, of the facts and concepts relevant to nursing in one textbook, or in one educational program, or in one lifetime. Our goal is to present sufficient facts to support generalizations or concepts in order to provide a base for effective thinking about patient problems. But ultimately it is our values that determine our behavior; and facts and concepts are needed to inform our values.

Beliefs Underlying the Selection of Content

Certain beliefs underlie the selection of content for this book.

1. *Every person is an individual human being with dignity and rights.* A person does not, or should not, lose dignity and rights as an individual because he or she is sick or well, old or young, clean or unclean, rich or poor, criminal or law-abiding.
2. *Every person has physiological, psychological, social, and spiritual needs that must be met in order to survive, grow, and be productive.* The healthy person is able to meet needs through his or her own efforts. When ill, an individual requires assistance in meeting one or more needs. Because of lack of specialized knowledge and skills, the person may also require assistance to maintain an optimum state of health.
3. *The practice of professional nursing requires a specialized body of knowledge.* This body of knowledge consists of facts, concepts, principles, and theories, and is derived from the humanities and the biological, physical, and behavioral sciences. It is neccessary to the understanding of (1) the needs of people; (2) the importance of the ability to adapt physiologically, emotionally, and socially to changes in the environment; (3) the results of failure to adapt; and (4) the role of the nurse as a helping professional.
4. *Professional nursing has a real contribution to make in the promotion of health, in the prevention of disease, and in the care of those who are sick, those who will be cured, and those for whom cure is unlikely and/or for whom this is the last illness.* The phrase "to give nursing care" has real meaning when it expresses the attitude of the nurse in expressing concern for the patient's welfare. The nurse does this freely and without the expectation of the reward of the patient's gratitude. Nor will the patient always accept what the nurse has to offer in ways that she or he expects. In fact, the patient may reject the nurse's efforts. Rejection by the patient of the nurse's service should not result in the rejection by the nurse of the person served. In other words, care is given unconditionally. The nurse expresses concern for the patient both by doing and by the manner of doing.
5. *Nursing is a profession whose practitioners, by virtue of their intellectual capacity, education, and moral outlook, are capable of the exercise of intellectual and moral judgments at a high level of responsibility.* Despite the fact that nursing, as it is practiced today, is not always on a professional level, increasing numbers of nurses exhibit critical professional characteristics: professional competence, an understanding of society, ethical behavior, and scholarly concern.

References Cited

Bach, R. *Jonathan Livingston Seagull.* New York: Macmillan Publishing Co., Inc., 1970, p. 86.

Menard, H. W. *Science: Growth and Change.* Cambridge, Mass.: Harvard University Press, 1971.

5

Clinical Nursing—A Systems Approach

The field covered by general systems theory is a vast intellectual, conceptual, technical area that is as yet loosely circumscribed. The applications of general systems theory range from abstract mathematical equations that attempt to define a particular system to awesome, complex, self-regulating machines. In some of the disciplines for which systems theory is relevant, the immediate problems include questions and issues on the nature of man and society, pollution, overpopulation, and criminality.

RIZZO

Rizzo, Nicholas D.: "General Systems Theory: Its Impact in Health Fields" in: Werley, Harriet H., Zuzich, Ann, Zajkowski, Myron and Zagornik, A. Dawn, Eds. *Health Research: The Systems Approach.* New York: Springer Publishing Company, 1976, p. 15.

Clinical Nursing—Origin and Definition of Terms

Clinical nursing is a term widely used to describe the functions and responsibilities of a nurse engaged in providing direct services to people, as opposed to the nurse whose functions and responsibilities relate to management, administration, education, or research. The origin of the word *clinical* is the Latin *clinicus,* meaning a bedridden person, which has become more broadly defined as having to do with the observation and treatment of disease in patients, as distinguished from experimental or laboratory study of disease. The designation of persons as patients also originates from a Latin term, *pati,* meaning to suffer. In common usage, a patient is one who is receiving medical care to alleviate some form of suffering, i.e., services from a physician intended to diagnose, treat, or prevent disease. Feinstein (1967) describes the clinician in medicine as a practitioner who "provides treatment to the sufferer, accepting responsibility for the life entrusted to him by the patient or family, and planning the strategy and executing the tactics of therapeutic care." The clinician in nursing as much as, and in some instances more than, medicine renders services designed to prevent or alleviate suffering, whatever its cause. Whenever the person served has potential or known disease, whether or not the disease is the cause of suffering, nursing practice is partially within the jurisdiction of medicine, and the person served by nursing is appropriately referred to as a patient.

This book, *Clinical Nursing,* is about the nursing of persons whose problems are associated with pathophysiology.[1] The derangement of function that characterizes the illness of the person may be central, peripheral, or unrelated to the problems with which nursing is assisting the patient, but because people respond as an integrated whole to changes in their internal and external environment, identification of the nature and probable cause of a patient's problem requires that the nurse have extensive knowledge of both pathophysiologic and psychosocial phenomena. Whatever its nature, illness is the consequence of the interaction of multiple factors—the susceptible host, the etiologic agent(s), and the

[1] *Pathophysiology* is the study of mechanisms by which disease occurs in living organisms, the responses of the body to the disease process, and the effects of these pathophysiologic mechanisms on normal function (Groër & Shekleton, 1979). The term usually refers to alteration in function as distinguished from structural defects.

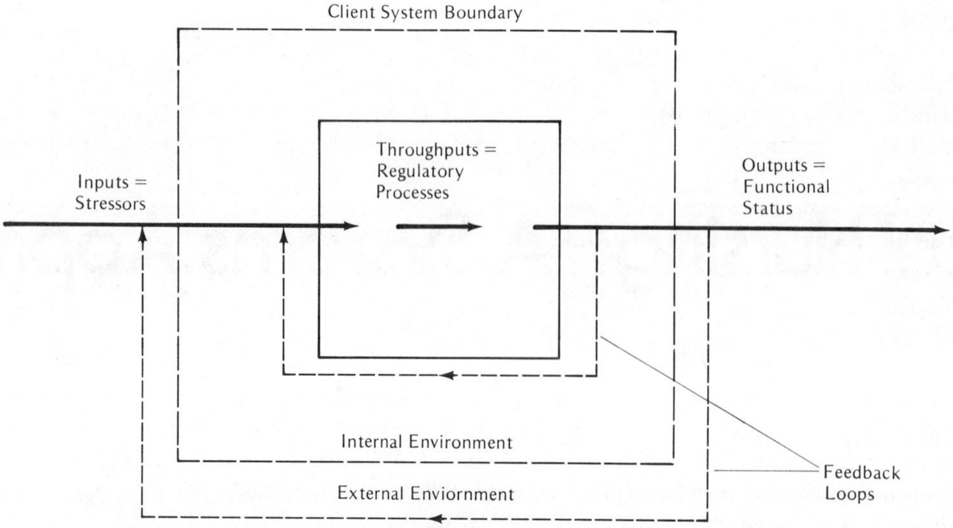

Figure 5-1. Basic elements of an open system.

environment. Disturbances at any level of organization—biochemical, cellular, systemic, psychological, interpersonal, or social—are likely to result in disturbances at other levels. For example, Mr. Quick is angry with his wife. Not only does he feel and look angry, but he also manifests his anger by changes in behavior. On the biochemical and physiologic levels, secretion of catecholamines increases. Among the changes occurring are increases in the amounts of blood glucose and cholesterol. His muscles contract, he loses his appetite, and his blood vessels constrict. On the interpersonal level, he shouts at his wife, is sharp with his son, and is rude to the neighbor next door. He gets into his car and backs out of the driveway, narrowly missing a 2-year-old child playing in the street. In other words, Mr. Quick is angry as a whole individual, and he manifests his anger as a unit, not as a part. The situation in which he is an actor is operating as a total "system," as a set of elements that are actively interrelated and that operate in some sense as a bounded unit. Elements of the system include Mr. Quick, his wife, his neighbor, the availability of a car, the presence of the 2-year-old child, and the unidentified events that elicited the anger.

Because the individual's ability to adapt can be directly affected by conditions that, on superficial consideration, seem very far removed from the immediate situation, seeking for probable causes of a patient's present situation from the universe of possibilities can be overwhelming unless one imposes some structure on the search. The systems approach is one method of imposing such structure, by identifying components of a complex whole and determining the relationships among the components.

General Systems Theory

Although there has been a proliferation of "systems theories," which differ greatly in their concepts and definitions of basic terms, all have a common goal: to organize the findings in some or all of the sciences of life and behavior into a single conceptual structure (Miller, 1978, p. 1). Concepts basic to Miller's general living systems theory are *space, time, matter, energy,* and *information,* because living systems exist in space and consist of matter and energy organized by information over time (Miller, 1978, p. 9). All levels of systems, from cosmic to microscopic,[2] are *open systems,* composed of "subsystems which process inputs, throughputs, and outputs of various forms of matter, energy, and information" (Miller, p. 1). The processes of critical subsystems are essential for life; some subsystems process matter or energy, some process information, and some process all three. Von Bertalanffy (1968, p. 39) describes an *open system* as one that maintains itself in a continuous inflow and outflow, a building up and breaking down of components, never—while alive—being in a state of chemical and thermodynamic equilibrium, but maintained instead in a so-called steady state.

This approach to describing, explaining, and predicting the behavior of open systems in terms of their wholeness, as a function of the interrelationship

[2] Miller identifies seven hierarchical levels: cell, organ, organism, group, organization, society, and supranational. Each higher level system is made up of the lower level system(s), i.e., the subsystems of each level in the hierarchy consist of all the systems that fall below it in the hierarchy (1968, p. 25).

of their component parts, is uniquely adaptable to the holistic approach to the care of people which has been the hallmark of modern nursing. Dubos (1979) affirmed the necessity for a holistic approach when he observed that "reducing the normal and pathological processes of life to the phenomena of molecular biology is simply not sufficient if we are to understand the human condition in health and disease."

In their various roles, nurses provide care to individuals, families, nonfamily groups, and communities; these consumers of nursing are sometimes referred to as nursing's client systems. Figure 5-1 displays basic elements of any open system, applied to the clients served by nursing. This textbook focuses on the individual as the client system, but the model is equally applicable to nursing practice with families, nonfamily groups, and communities. As shown in Figure 5-1, the general systems' terms *input, throughput,* and *output* are equated with the following terms used by nurses to describe the client system:

General Systems Term		Nursing Term		Definition of Nursing Usage
INPUT	=	STRESSOR	=	any physical, biological, chemical, psychological or sociocultural agent or event which challenges and activates the regulatory processes of the client system; the agent/event is potentially injurious if the response of regulatory processes are not successful in maintaining or restoring the system's steady state
THROUGHPUT	=	REGULATORY PROCESSES	=	physiological, psychological, sociocultural, political mechanisms of the client system, which operate to keep the system in the steady state, in the presence of constant challenges from the internal and external environment
OUTPUT	=	FUNCTIONAL STATUS	=	the extent to which the client system is able to perform health-related activities unaided

Every system but the smallest has subsystems, every system but the largest has suprasystems, and the boundary of each unit is determined by the objectives, or performance characteristics, of that unit (Churchman, 1968, p. 29). The boundary of a unit may shift to include fewer or more components, as the objectives or performance characteristics of the unit change. For example, a body system may constitute a whole system level of concern to the nurse, or it may be viewed as a subsystem component of a larger regulatory mechanism. To illustrate, if the objective or characteristic performance of the unit is to provide oxygen from the external environment to the blood and to remove carbon dioxide from the blood to the external environment, then the system boundary need include only the respiratory system. However, if the objective of the unit is to regulate respiration, this function is not complete until oxygen is combined in the cell with hydrogen to form water or with a compound containing a carbon to form carbon dioxide. The boundary of the system for regulation of respiration must include provisions for breathing, diffusion of gases, transport of gases to and from cells, oxidation–reduction reactions in cells, and regulation of all the preceding components of respiration; within this unit the respiratory system becomes a subsystem. If the objective of the unit is to set a world record in the 100-yard dash, then the system boundary must include all components of the whole individual who has this aspiration; within this unit the regulation of respiration becomes a subsystem. If the objective of the unit is to clean up the atmosphere by means of the Environmental Protection Agency programs, then the individual who aspires to set a world record in the 100-yard dash becomes a subsystem of that social unit.

Five System Levels of Analysis

In professional fields, particularly those regulated by certification or licensure of practitioners, the system boundary derives from the nature of the service provided to, or expected by, the society. As previously indicated, the client system boundary of concern in this textbook is the individual person whose problems, or altered functional status, are associated with pathophysiology; because of that association, the person is frequently referred to as *the patient.* Obtaining information about the patient as an open system is the first critical step in clinical nursing. Figure 5-2 illustrates five system levels of concern to the nurse in selecting relevant information to guide person-oriented nursing care. The circles are purposely not concentric, as it is only those components of the sub- and suprasystems that directly impinge upon the person as a functional unit, or system, about which the nurse must have information. The five system levels and their components can be defined as follows:

1. *The individual person,* as the pivotal system: his or her perceptions, habits, resources, liabilities, goals, and so on.
2. *The microsystems,* as subsystems of the individual: biochemical; cellular; organ; traditional body systems, such as pulmonary–cardiovascular, reticuloendothelial, musculoskeletal, and so on.
3. *The proximal suprasystem,* as the system that operates closest to, and has the greatest influence on, the individual's well-being in his or her usual surroundings: family, significant others, employment status, housing, and so on.
4. *The intermediate suprasystem,* as the system that operates closest to, and has the greatest influence on, the individual's well-being when transplanted from his or her usual surroundings to a health care agency: institutional policies and practices of the agency, staff members and practices within the unit of the agency where the individual is receiving care, and so on.
5. *The distal suprasystem,* as the system within which social institutions are developed, controlled, and coordinated: characteristics of the community from which the individual comes and/or to which he or she will return, such as the work community, the residential community, the religious community, the political system, and so on.

To illustrate the use of the five-level systems model as a guide to assessment, information related to an understanding of an individual's nutritional status is presented according to four of the five system levels and some of their component parts, or subsystems. The intermediate suprasystem has been omitted, because it is the source of information that is very specific to the setting in which the patient is encountered. See Figure 5-3 for system levels of information related to nutritional status.

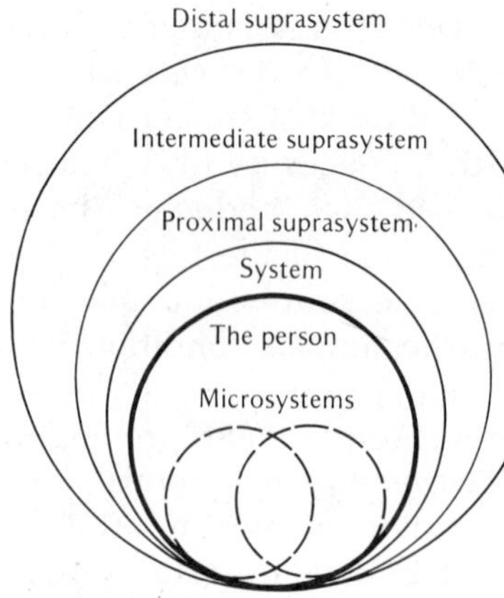

Figure 5-2. System levels of concern to the nurse in selecting relevant information for person-oriented nursing care.

Decision Making about Health as a Function of the Client System

One of the most significant functions of the patient system is to make health-related decisions. The nurse acts as a "regulatory process," through the use of teaching and counseling skills, to help the individual formulate all possible alternatives available in the present situation and to weigh the anticipated positive and negative consequences of each alternative to the individual and to others who are important to him or her. The ultimate choice among alternatives will reveal the most cherished values of which the individual may not have been aware prior to having been faced with the present situation and with this approach to making decisions. The nurse's work is not done when the decision has been made; very often, the greatest need for comfort, support, and reaffirmation comes when the individual is experiencing the aftermath of the decision (Janis & Mann, 1977). This phenomenon is common with persons who have made the decision to stop drinking, smoking, overeating, or to leave an abusive spouse or a stressful job.

Figure 5-3. System levels of information related to nutritional status. (This figure is modified from a model developed by Associate Professor Ann Marie Hedquist, R.D., a faculty member of the College of Nursing, Southeastern Massachusetts University, for use in teaching a systems approach to human nutrition. The idea for Hedquist's model was stimulated by the following article: Howard Brody. The systems view of man: Implications for medicine, science, and ethics. *Persp. Biol. Med.* 17:71–92, Autumn 1973.)

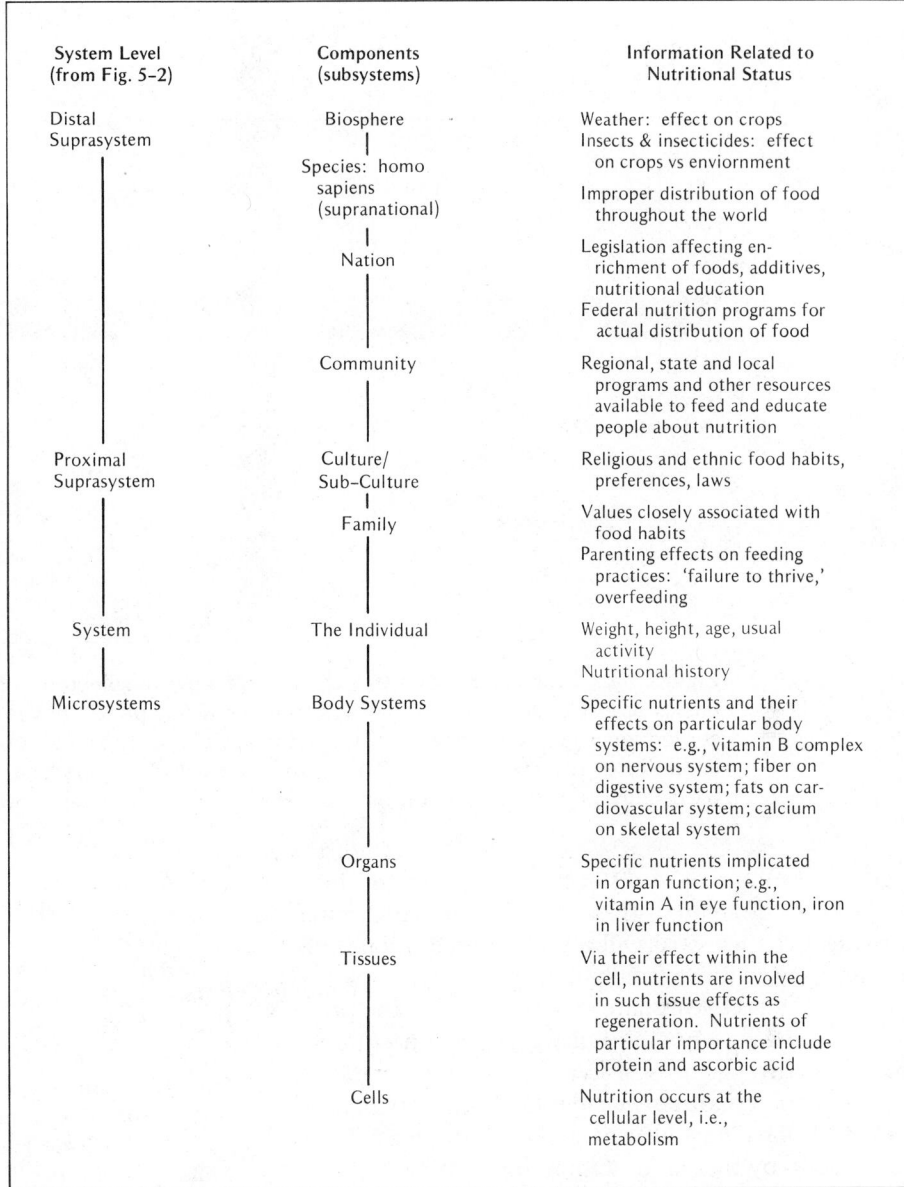

System Level (from Fig. 5-2)	Components (subsystems)	Information Related to Nutritional Status
Distal Suprasystem	Biosphere	Weather: effect on crops Insects & insecticides: effect on crops vs enviornment
	Species: homo sapiens (supranational)	Improper distribution of food throughout the world
	Nation	Legislation affecting enrichment of foods, additives, nutritional education Federal nutrition programs for actual distribution of food
	Community	Regional, state and local programs and other resources available to feed and educate people about nutrition
Proximal Suprasystem	Culture/ Sub-Culture	Religious and ethnic food habits, preferences, laws
	Family	Values closely associated with food habits Parenting effects on feeding practices: 'failure to thrive,' overfeeding
System	The Individual	Weight, height, age, usual activity Nutritional history
Microsystems	Body Systems	Specific nutrients and their effects on particular body systems: e.g., vitamin B complex on nervous system; fiber on digestive system; fats on cardiovascular system; calcium on skeletal system
	Organs	Specific nutrients implicated in organ function; e.g., vitamin A in eye function, iron in liver function
	Tissues	Via their effect within the cell, nutrients are involved in such tissue effects as regeneration. Nutrients of particular importance include protein and ascorbic acid
	Cells	Nutrition occurs at the cellular level, i.e., metabolism

An Adaptation Framework for Viewing Consequences of Selected Behavior Patterns

Many of the health problems represented in our nation's morbidity and mortality statistics are at least partially, if not primarily, the result of behavior patterns either deliberately or unconsciously selected by the victims: heart disease, cancer, accidental injuries, alcoholic cirrhosis of the liver. The only approach to reducing or eliminating some of our most debilitating and chronic diseases is to help people develop alternative patterns of eating, drinking, exercising, and dealing with the pressures of life.

There are two types of effects of any selected, habitual behavior; one effect is immediate and the other is delayed. The immediate effect is an internal one, the way it makes one feel at that moment; this effect can be considered the comfort dimension. The delayed effect is an external one, the alterations which occur over time in one's structure and self-help ability; this effect can be considered the functional dimension. A behavior such as overeating, which may be both adaptive and functional in its early stages, soon may lead to obesity; this condition may still be adaptive, in relation to how the individual feels while eating, but it tends to be dysfunctional in relation to its effects over time on mobility, energy, grooming, and self-concept. If overeating continues, it becomes maladaptive, the effects becoming

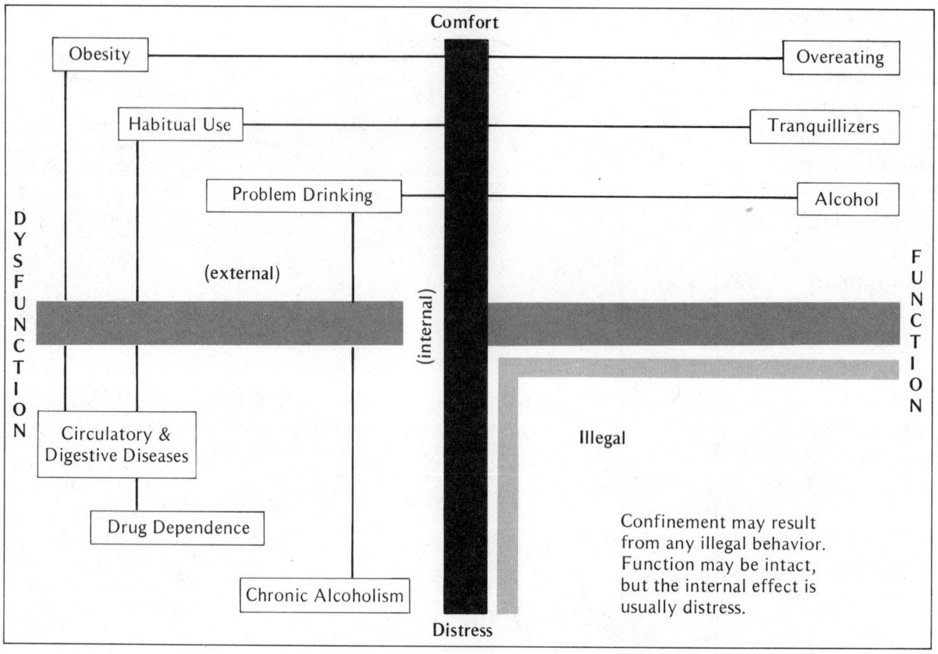

Figure 5-4. Framework for viewing consequences of selected behavior patterns. (J. Passos & E. Chandler developed this framework for plotting the comfort-functional consequences of clients' habitual behaviors, as a first step in identifying assets and liabilities of any client system. The framework was developed for use in the baccalaureate nursing program at Boston State College, Boston, Massachusetts, 1976.)

both dysfunctional *and* uncomfortable, as the individual may develop distressing digestive and circulatory disturbances that will require increasing modification in activities of daily living.

Nurses need to estimate and help reduce the probability of dysfunction and distress as a consequence of unhealthy patterns of living. The framework for viewing the adaptive/maladaptive consequences of selected behavior patterns shown in Figure 5-4 was developed by the junior author and a colleague. The framework is intended to assist the nurse in predicting the consequences of the patient's present habits, based on patient data gathered from all system levels.

Although it would be impossible to include information from all system levels in the discussion of every topic in the book, repeated emphasis is placed on the relationship of events in sub- and suprasystems, and the ways in which these affect, and are affected by, the individual as an open system.

References Cited

Churchman, C. W. *The Systems Approach.* New York: Dell Publishing Co., Inc., 1968, p. 29.

Dubos, R. Preface. In *Ways of Health: Holistic Approaches to Ancient and Contemporary Medicine.* Ed. by D. S. Sobel. New York: Harcourt Brace Jovanovich, Inc., 1979, p. xiii.

Feinstein, A. R. *Clinical Judgment.* Baltimore: The Williams & Wilkins Company, 1967, p. 21.

Groër, M. E., and Shekleton, M. E. *Basic Pathophysiology.* St. Louis: The C. V. Mosby Company, 1979, p. 3.

Janis, I. L., and Mann, L. *Decision Making: A Psychological Analysis of Conflict, Choice, and Commitment.* New York: The Free Press, 1977.

Miller, J. G. *Living Systems.* New York: McGraw-Hill Book Company, 1978.

Von Bertalanffy, L. *General Systems Theory.* New York: George Braziller, Inc., 1968.

General References

Abdellah, F. G., Beland, I. L., Martin, A., and Matheney, R. V. *New Directions in Patient-Centered Nursing.* New York: Macmillan Publishing Co., Inc., 1973.

Becknell, E. P., and Smith, D. M. *System of Nursing Practice.* Philadelphia: F. A. Davis Co., 1975.

Brodt, D. E. "A Synergistic Theory of Nursing." *Am. J. Nurs.*, **69** (Aug. 1969), 1674–76.

Putt, A. M. *General Systems Theory Applied to Nursing.* Boston: Little, Brown and Company, 1978.

Rubin, A. "A Theory of Clinical Nursing." *Nurs. Res.*, **17** (May–June 1968), 210–12.

6

Man-Environment Concept: Homeostasis and Adaptation

"The living being is an agency of such sort that each disturbing influence induces by itself the calling forth of compensatory activity to neutralize or repair the disturbance. The higher in the scale of living beings, the more numerous, the more perfect and the more complicated do these regulatory agencies become. They tend to free the organism completely from the unfavorable influences and changes occurring in the environment."

LÉON FREDERICQ, 1885

Quoted in: Cannon, Walter B., *The Wisdom of the Body.* New York: W. W. Norton & Company, Inc., 1932, p. 21.

Man-Environment Concept

The process of living involves the interplay of an organism and its environment. This interplay or interrelationship is known as an *ecological system.*

Ecology. Biologists define *ecology* as "the study of the interaction of organisms with their environment." Sociologists add to this definition "the relationship of human groups to their material resources and the consequent social and cultural patterns."

Environment. That which surrounds a thing or organism. Banks (1971) states, "Environment should be considered as the total economic, physical, natural, social and cultural complex within which man lives."

All organisms modify their environment and are modified by it. They remove materials from it for their use, and add products of their activities to it. In other words, there is a give and take between the organism and the environment. When the amount of energy and material taken from the environment is returned in about the same amounts, the system is said to be in a state of equilibrium. When more is taken than returned, there is a state of disequilibrium. Humans differ from other organisms by the rate and extent of the changes that they make. There are societies, such as those of the Navahos in the United States and the Zulus in Africa, that emphasize living in balance with nature; the result of this emphasis is that little is taken from the environment. The environment that the parent bequeaths to the child is little changed from that which the parent inherited from his or her parents.

In modern industrialized societies, however, people are taking more from the environment than they are returning to it, thus creating a state of disequilibrium. Even when humans and their environment are in a state of equilibrium, the nature of the interrelation shifts because both the natural environment and humankind are continuously changing. Some of these changes occur in a regular pattern; others do not. As examples, temperature and light intensity change during each 24-hour period and, for much of the world, from season to season. Atmospheric pressure, as well as other climatic conditions such as humidity, varies, but in a less predictable pattern.

Sargent (1972) summarizes these interrelationships as follows:

There is an inexorable bond uniting living organisms with their environment. This bond is complex, for it encompasses not only relationships among organisms but also between organisms and their physical-chemical surroundings. In the biotic realm, for example, we find that animals depend upon plants. Plants capture solar energy and store it in plant nutrients. To fulfill their nutrient requirements, certain animals eat plants. These herbivores are in turn eaten by carnivores. In the physical realm, we find that plants, for example, depend upon solar radiation and atmospheric carbon dioxide and water to accomplish the photosynthetic production of nutrients. At the same time all living organisms, plants and animals, depend upon atmospheric oxygen to provide for the release of energy from these same nutrients.

Environmental Conditions

External Environment

Conditions or circumstances in the external environment can be classified as life-supporting and as hazardous. Among the agents essential to survival are air, water, nutrients, and shelter. Other agents favoring survival include people and a variety of other living organisms, from microorganisms to highly complicated multicellular organisms of both plant and animal origin. Even essential agents may be harmful when exposure is excessive or unbalanced. Those required in minute amounts, such as copper, are deadly poisons in larger amounts. As an example, oxygen is required for survival. However, continued high concentrations of oxygen damage the respiratory membranes and can cause blindness in newborn babies.

Temperatures of about 68°F (21°C) are essential to comfort, but unprotected exposure to low or high temperatures causes cell injury and death. Ultraviolet light converts certain chemicals in the skin to vitamin D, but excessive exposure causes burns. Sound in controlled amounts adds variety, but in excess it leads to fatigue and hearing loss. People may by their actions improve the environment and make it a more fit place to live, or they may damage it by their actions. A major concern is how to protect both humankind and nature. People, including nurses, also form part of each individual's environment. Like other agents, people may be beneficial, neutral, or harmful. In Unit III some of the hazards in the environment and their effects will be considered in detail.

Management of the environment is possibly the nurse's most nearly independent function. Florence Nightingale (1860, p. 5) recognized the significance of the natural environment in the care of the sick when she wrote

> the thing which strikes the experienced observer most forcibly is this, that symptoms or suffering generally considered to be inevitable and incident to the disease are very often not symptoms of disease at all, but of something quite different—of the want of fresh air, or of light, or of warmth, or of quiet, or of cleanliness, or of punctuality and care in the administration of diet, of each or all of these.

To this should be added the people—nurses, physicians, paramedical personnel, family, friends, and others—who enter and leave the environment of the patient in the course of a day. Constructive management of all the elements in the environment of the patient so that his or her safety and well-being are protected is a considerable and too often neglected task. (See Unit VII for a discussion of the psychosocial aspects of patient care.)

Internal Environment

The environment that has been discussed is that which lies outside the body and is in contact with the skin and mucous membranes. In the following section the internal environment or the fluid surrounding cells and carrying materials to and from them will be considered. Similar to the dependence of health on relative stability within the external environment, health is also dependent on the maintenance of relative stability of the physical and chemical characteristics of the fluid comprising the internal environment.

Survival of the cell and maintenance of its function are dependent on conditions in the cell's immediate fluid environment. It is from this environment that the cell obtains a continued supply of nutrients and into which it discharges its products, some of which are necessary to physiologic functioning, and some of which are wastes. For all cells, this immediate environment is a pool of water in which a variety of substances such as sodium chloride and glucose are dissolved. For unicellular organisms, such as the amoeba, the fluid environment is a pond or puddle of water. For humans and other large multicellular organisms, blood, lymph, and interstitial fluid form the immediate environment of the cells. These fluids are known as the internal environment. The fluids composing the internal environment not only serve individual cells as such but are the medium by which all body cells are united to and affected by the activities of all other cells within the entire organism (see Chapter 27).

Historical Development of the Concept of the Internal Environment

Hippocrates, and later Galen, taught that humans are composed of four humours. They were healthy when these humours were in correct balance; disease was the result of imbalance. (See Chapter 1, theories of disease causation, number 6.) This doctrine is based on the concept that the universe is composed of four elements: fire, water, earth, and air. As part of the universe, humans were seen as composed of the four humours that corresponded to the four elements of the earth: blood (fire), phlegm (earth), yellow bile (air), and black bile (water). This theory was expanded by later physicians. They believed that when one humour dominated the others, it determined the physical and emotional characteristics of a person. Terms derived from this concept are still used to describe the behavioral characteristics of people. Thus a jolly, optimistic person, inclined to be fat, is said to be sanguine; one who is slow-moving and not easily aroused is described as phlegmatic; one who is easily angered or quick-tempered is choleric; and one who is depressed, peevish, or solitary is melancholic.

This theory of body fluids was not challenged until 1858, when *Cellular Pathology* was published by Virchow. As a result of this work, the cell was recognized as the important entity in health and disease. In 1878 Claude Bernard introduced the concept that cells live in the fluid that bathes them. This fluid—blood, lymph, and tissue fluid—he called the *milieu intérieur.* He believed that all vital activities have but one objective, the maintenance of the stability of the *milieu intérieur.*

Homeostasis

Cannon (1939) further elaborated and extended the scope of the work of Bernard. Like Bernard, he considered the stability of the internal environment its most important feature. He emphasized that although the blood and other fluids were constantly absorbing materials from the external environment and from the cells, the composition of these fluids was maintained in a stable condition. In describing his concept of how the stability of the internal environment was maintained, Cannon (1939, p. 24) states, "The coordinated physiological processes which maintain most of the steady states in the organism are so complex and so peculiar to living beings—involving, as they may, the brain and nerves, the heart, lungs, kidneys and spleen, all working cooperatively—that I have suggested a special designation for these states, homeostasis."[1] He elaborated further that the term does not imply stagnation but rather variation within limits. These variations occur in a predictable manner. For example, body temperature varies from 1 to 2°F each 24 hours. In persons who sleep at night, it is lowest in the night and highest in the late afternoon and early evening. Thus the limits that are maintained vary from one part of the day to another in a regular fashion. Further, in health the upper and lower limits are regulated in such a manner that these limits are maintained. Conditions are maintained within limits as long as the individual is capable of making appropriate adaptations to change.

[1] Some authorities object to the term *homeostasis,* as it implies a static rather than dynamic state, and prefer the term *homeokinesis.* However, *homeostasis* is generally used in physiologic and medical literature.

Maintenance of Homeostasis

The maintenance of homeostasis depends on a variety of elements. Substances required by cells must be available in adequate quantity. Material supplies include water, oxygen, and a variety of nutrients, including sources of calories, tissue-building materials, electrolytes, and regulators not synthesized or present in the body. The intake, storage, and elimination of excesses of supply are regulated so that the level of each substance is maintained within well-defined limits. It is not surprising that a large number of structures and regulatory functions are involved in maintaining homeostasis.

Structures Supporting Homeostasis

Because of their size and complexity, multicellular organisms require specialized structures to supply cells with needed materials, to remove the waste products of metabolism, and to maintain the stability of the internal environment. The healthy organism is capable of responding to disturbances in such a manner that damage is prevented or repaired. The kinds of structures that fulfill this function include the following:

1. Structures where required substances are absorbed from the external environment and, when necessary, modified so that they can enter the internal environment. For example, oxygen is absorbed into the blood unchanged. The air from which oxygen is taken, however, requires conditioning. Nutrients usually require reduction to simpler forms before they can be absorbed, and provision for elimination of indigestible substances is also necessary. Materials enter or leave the external environment through semipermeable membranes that separate the internal from the external environment. These semipermeable

membranes act to protect the internal environment from too rapid change or from the entrance of potentially harmful or nonusable particles.
2. Structures such as the heart and blood vessels that transport materials from points of entry to cells and from cells to points of elimination or exit.
3. Structures that store or eliminate excesses of intake and by-products of metabolism. For example, glucose is stored as glycogen in the liver and muscles; much of the excess is stored as fat. Excess sodium is normally excreted in the urine.
4. Structures that make movement in the external environment possible. They enable the individual to seek food and water, to alter the environment to suit his or her needs, to overcome or avoid danger, and to find a mate.
5. Structures that reproduce themselves—to replace worn-out cells, to repair injury, or to produce a new organism.
6. Structures that protect the organism from injury.
7. Finally, structures that regulate and integrate the activities of all individual cells and aggregates of cells so that the organism functions as a whole.

Conditions of Homeostasis

Conditions that must be maintained within limits include osmolality, blood pressure, level of glucose in the blood, cation–anion balance and concentration, hydrogen ion concentration, and body temperature. Conditions in the external environment must be within the limits to which people can adapt. For example, one's capacity to adapt to extremes of temperature, high altitude, water and food supply, and physical trauma is limited. However, people are able to live in some hostile environments by adapting them to their needs.

Control Systems

Similar to other systems, a homeostatic control system is a collection of interconnected elements functioning to achieve a goal, in this instance the relative constancy of physical and chemical characteristics of the internal environment. As in other regulatory systems, those concerned with homeostasis have (1) sensors stimulated by specific disturbances in the environment, (2) structures to communicate information to a (3) center or centers that receive and evaluate it and initiate messages, and (4) structures to convey these messages to appropriate (5) effector cells (muscle or gland cells). Upon stimulation, the effector cells act to correct the disturbance.

Specifically, homeostasis is regulated by the autonomic nervous system and the endocrine system. Although the autonomic nervous system is largely involuntary, it must be remembered that all parts of the nervous system have interconnections. Thus the autonomic nervous system receives messages not only from sensors in the internal environment but also from the cerebral cortex, which receives messages from both the internal and external environments.

Hormonal Regulation

In addition to nervous control of homeostatic mechanisms, hormones also play an important role. Their production is directly or indirectly subject to control by the hypothalamus. In some cases the action of a hormone enhances the action of the nervous system. For example, epinephrine and norepinephrine support the action of the sympathetic nervous system.

The adrenal steroids have many and varied physiologic effects. They play a role in the regulation of water and electrolyte balance as well as in carbohydrate, protein, fat, and purine metabolism. They are essential to survival. In their absence, the individual is unable to cope with even moderate changes in activity and environmental temperature or with mild illness or psychologic stress. To quote Haynes and Larner (1975), "The adrenal cortex is the organ, *par excellence,* of homeostasis, being importantly responsible for the relative freedom that higher organisms exhibit in a constantly changing environment." In the absence of the adrenal steroids survival is possible only in a rigidly controlled environment. [See Chapters 15, 18, and 22 for a more complete discussion of adrenal steroids.]

Other hormones, such as insulin, thyroxine, parathormone, and antidiuretic hormone, also function in homeostasis. Insulin is necessary for the utilization of glucose and directly or indirectly for the metabolism of fat and protein. Thyroxine regulates the rate of cellular metabolism and parathormone the level of calcium in the blood. The antidiuretic hormone participates in homeostatic regulation of water by increasing the rate at which water is reabsorbed by the renal tubules. No mention has been made of the role of the adenohypophysis in governing its so-called target glands or of its function in growth. The purpose has not been to review in detail all the structures that function in the control of homeostasis but rather to indicate the complex nature of its regulation.

Feedback Mechanisms

A living organism is an open system, that is, it is continuously exchanging materials and energy with

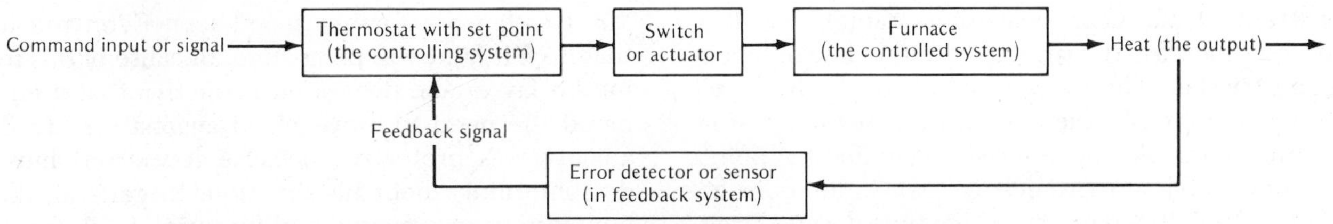

Figure 6-1. Components of a negative feedback control system represented by a room thermostat. (From *Physiology: A Regulatory Systems Approach,* by F. L. Strand, Macmillan Publishing Company, Inc., New York, 1978, Fig. 1-4, p. 6. Used with permission of Macmillan Publishing Company, Inc.)

its environment. This exchange is so regulated that, in health, physical and chemical characteristics are kept relatively constant.

Most physiologic activities are regulated by negative feedbacks, that is, a change in one direction is counteracted or opposed by a change in the opposite direction. In other words, the reaction to change is negative to the stimulus. In contrast, change in a positive feedback system causes more of the same. As an example, in a negative feedback system, ingestion of glucose causes a rise in the level of glucose in the blood. The rise acts as a stimulus to the blood glucose–lowering mechanism, and the blood glucose falls. In a positive feedback system, ingestion of glucose causes the blood glucose to rise even when it is elevated above normal. Clearly, a negative feedback system is self-correcting. A positive feedback system is self-perpetuating. Most homeostatic mechanisms are regulated by a closed-loop (continuous-circuit) negative feedback system. See Figure 6-1 for components of a negative feedback system represented by a room thermostat. (See Unit V for discussion of the body's defense mechanisms.)

The organism's capacity to meet its physiologic needs results from the fact that the cells, tissues, organs, and systems, as well as the entire organism, can respond to disturbances in the environment in such a manner that injury is prevented or damage is corrected.

Four Features of Homeostasis

To summarize and to clarify the concepts of homeostasis, the four features of homeostasis as outlined by Cannon (1939, pp. 299–300) will be stated and then applied to one condition of homeostasis, the maintenance of blood pressure. The characteristic features of homeostasis are as follows:

1. Maintenance of constancy in an open system continually subjected to disturbance requires some mechanism to prevent change.
2. The maintenance of a steady state requires that any tendency to change is automatically met by increased effectiveness of mechanisms to resist change.
3. Regulation of any homeostatic condition may require one or more mechanisms acting at the same time or successively.
4. Homeostasis does not happen by chance but is the result of organized self-government.

These postulates are illustrated by citing the instance of Mr. Brave. Mr. Brave was awakened at night by pain in his upper abdomen and a feeling of nausea. Shortly after awakening, he vomited what he and his wife described as a bowlful of bright red blood. Both were frightened. Mrs. Brave called the family physician, who suggested that Mr. Brave be taken to the hospital. When he was admitted to the hospital his blood pressure was 120/76. This was his usual blood pressure and is well within the normal range. Let us suppose that he had lost 450 ml of blood and examine the maintenance of arterial blood pressure as a homeostatic function.

Arterial blood pressure is one factor in maintaining tissue perfusion. It is dependent on agencies acting to elevate it, balanced against those acting to lower it. Arterial blood pressure depends on the relationship of the blood volume to the capacity (capacitance) of the chamber (blood vessels) that holds it and the force with which the blood is driven into the arteries. The viscosity of the blood is also a factor in that a viscid fluid offers more resistance to being moved than does a thin or watery one. All these factors can be altered so that blood pressure is raised, lowered, or maintained. In terms of Cannon's *first postulate,* the loss of blood tends to disturb the relationship between the volume of blood and the size of the chamber in which it is contained. Because Mr. Brave is able to maintain his blood pressure within normal limits, there must be some mechanism operating to counteract the effect of blood loss.

The *second postulate* suggests further that as blood continues to be lost and the tendency for the blood pressure to fall is increased the mechanisms elevating blood pressure must become increasingly active.

For example, the heart beats more rapidly and the arterioles increase the resistance to the flow of blood by constriction. The heart responds to the increase in resistance by contracting with greater force. For the time being, blood pressure is maintained. A point of considerable importance is that some persons maintain their blood pressure for a time despite large losses of blood, only to have it fall suddenly to a dangerously low level. This emphasizes the necessity for acting on the knowledge that, although individuals differ in their capacity to adapt, there are limits to this capacity. No single measure of the status of a patient should be considered to be infallible or apart from other evidence.

The *third postulate* that there must be a number of agencies acting together or successively to regulate a homeostatic condition. Review of physiology reveals that the heart and blood vessels are no exception. They are regulated by the autonomic nervous system and by hormones as well as by other chemicals, such as angiotensin, the activity of which depends on a substance secreted by the kidney. Blood volume is also regulated by a number of mechanisms. All of these will be discussed in detail later in connection with shock and hypertension. A number of factors interact to prevent the fall of Mr. Brave's blood pressure.

The *fourth postulate* states that the changes following disturbances in homeostasis do not happen by accident but that disturbances in physiologic processes call forth specific responses. This implies that there are receptors stimulated by change, and when these receptors are stimulated, a set of reactions is initiated to correct the disturbance. To illustrate by analogy, in any city in which the services are organized to meet the needs of the community, a call to the fire department brings forth fire fighters and fire-fighting equipment. Unless the fire is a big one or is in a critical area, the amount of equipment delivered is likely to be limited. It may or may not bring the police. In the instance of Mr. Brave, the stimulus initiating changes in his behavior was the loss of blood and what the loss of blood meant to him. Receptors sensitive to the level of the blood volume initiated impulses that resulted in the activation of mechanisms to maintain or to prevent the fall in his blood pressure. Thus Mr. Brave was protected from the harmful effects of blood loss.

By now it should be clear that Mr. Brave was able to maintain his blood pressure because of multiple agencies acting to overcome the blood pressure–lowering effects of blood loss. In addition to those cited, other mechanisms served either to reduce blood loss or to protect him from its effects. Contraction of blood vessels at the site of bleeding, combined with the tendency of the blood to clot, served to protect Mr. Brave from further blood loss. Even the fact that he felt faint was protective. Because of this feeling he lay down, decreased his activity, and eliminated the need to move blood against gravity. His anxiety was protective because it spurred him to do something about his situation. In general, then, homeostasis was maintained because Mr. Brave was able to regulate supplies and processes in such a way that excesses were eliminated and deficits corrected.

Nursing Functions

As indicated, in health the needs of the cells are met automatically by the integrated and coordinated activity of all the cells, including those in specialized facilities. In illness the capacity of the individual to cope with disturbances in the environment in such a manner that his or her needs are satisfied is reduced. In patients with medical–surgical diagnoses, the incapacity frequently lies in an inability to meet one or more physiologic needs. Many of the activities of the nurse in the care of these patients are directed toward (1) gathering information about the nature of the external and internal environment of the patients, (2) modifying the external environment so the adaptations the patients are required to make are within their capacity, (3) supporting the efforts of the patients to adapt or to respond, and (4) providing them with the materials required to maintain the constancy of their internal environment.

Circadian Rhythms

In discussing homeostasis, the point was made that through regulation, the physical and chemical characteristics of body fluids are maintained in a relatively stable state. Earlier the point was made that humans and environment change in relation to each other. In nature this regular recurrence of certain events—starting at one point, moving in a predictable pattern, and returning to the starting point—has long been observed. Tides rise and fall, day follows night, summer follows spring. Some cycles recur each 24 hours, others at shorter or longer intervals.

It has been established that all forms of life from one-celled to multicellular organisms demonstrate rhythmic variations every 24 hours. In other words, at all levels of organization rhythmic activity is characteristic of life. It further appears that this rhythmic activity involves at least two factors: (1) an endogenous, clocklike mechanism controlling each rhythm and (2) environmental (exogenous) cues that influence the cyclic variations.

Despite the importance of other biological rhythms, those that have been most extensively studied are circadian rhythm, that is, those recurring approximately each 24 hours. The exact length of each cycle is usually a bit shorter or longer than 24 hours.

Definitions

Cycle. A cycle may be defined as a single complete execution of periodically repeated phenomena.

Phase. Phase is the term used to indicate the time relationship of the peaks and troughs of the cycle to the external environment. A biological clock is said to be in phase when peaks and troughs occur at the expected time. In other words, the cycle is synchronized. It is out of phase or desynchronized when the crest or trough occurs at an unusual time. To illustrate, the temperature crest occurs late in the afternoon or early evening. Body temperature is out of phase when the crest occurs at a different time.

Amplitude. Amplitude may be defined as the extent or range of the change in the cycle each day. In some people the amplitude or range of change of body temperature is greater than in others.

Circadian rhythms. Circadian rhythms are those that complete a cycle each day—*circa* (around) and *dia* (day). However, they are not precisely 24 hours in length. They differ in length not only between species, but among individuals of the same species. Each person marches to his or her own drummer.

Infradian rhythms. Infradian rhythms have longer, slower cycles than circadian rhythms.

Ultradian rhythms. Ultradian rhythms have shorter and faster rhythms than circadian rhythms.

Dysrythmia. Dysrythmia is a condition in which an organism (animal or human being) is out of phase with the environment.

Desynchronization. Desynchronization is a condition in which rhythms are out of phase with each other.

Environmental Cues

As stated previously, an internal clock influenced by changes in the external environment regulates each rhythm. Among the environmental cues appearing to influence the period, timing, and amplitude of cyclic variations are alternation of (1) day and night, (2) heat and cold, (3) silence and sound, (4) hours of work and leisure, and (5) other activities

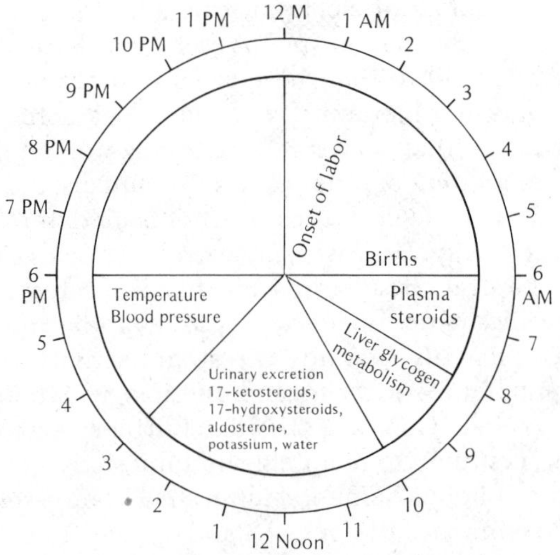

Figure 6-2. Physiologic crests in biological clock (for persons who sleep from 11 P.M. to 8 A.M.).

of daily life. Though other terms have been used, these environmental factors are called synchronizers, that is, the "clock or calendar time givers." In other words, physiologic rhythms are timed in relation to recurring events in the environment. They serve very much as clocks serve to determine daily activities. It must be emphasized, however, that physiologic rhythms are not entirely dependent upon synchronizers as physiologic rhythms continue in their absence. (See Figures 6-2 and 6-3 for crests and troughs of physiologic rhythms.)

Biological Clocks

The mechanisms for measuring time in the body are known as biological clocks. Similar to a manmade

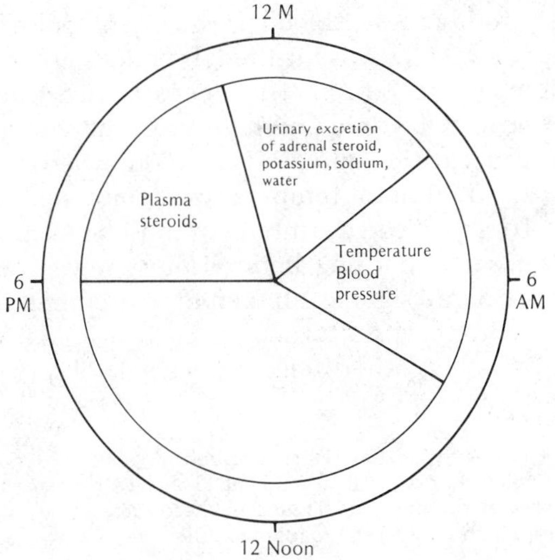

Figure 6-3. Physiologic troughs in biological clock (for persons who sleep from 11 P.M. to 8 A.M.).

clock, a biological clock must be able to communicate time information and to reset itself. At this time, scientists believe that there are a number of clocks arranged in a hierarchy, with one clock acting as a pacemaker that serves to synchronize or integrate the functioning of other clocks. In humans, the location of the biological clocks has not been determined with certainty. However, in several mammals a dominate central circadian pacemaker is located in the suprachiasmatic nucleus of the hypothalamus. It drives the daily rhythms in rest and activity as well as some neuroendocrine and physiological functions (Wehr and Goodwin, 1978). Further, biological clocks continue to maintain rhythmic activity in the absence of environmental input. In a number of vertebrate animals, the pineal gland appears to be associated with a biological clock, which communicates time information through its output of melatonin (Binkley, 1979). However, there must be other biological clocks, as animals that do not have pineal glands exhibit circadian rhythms.

Functions Exhibiting Periodicity

Of the many physiologic activities showing periodicity in humans and animals, only a few will be considered. These are (1) body temperature, (2) blood pressure, (3) pulse, (4) urine formation, (5) blood plasma and urinary corticosteroids, (6) sleep–activity, (7) cell division, (8) skin reactions to histamine, and (9) resistance–susceptibility cycles. These particular cycles have been studied and this knowledge has relevance to the prevention of disease and the restoration of health.

Body Temperature, Blood Pressure, Pulse

Body temperature, blood pressure, and pulse have similar cycles.[2] Levels for these functions are lowest at night in the person who sleeps at night and is active in the daytime and highest in the late afternoon and early evening.[3] Thus if knowledge of a patient's minimum temperature, pulse, or blood pressure is desired, measurement must be made during the early morning hours. Conversely, if maximum levels are significant, then measurements must be made in the late afternoon or early evening. With these as well as other functions, a single observation provides information only about the state of a function at the time the observation is made. Valid inferences generally require repeated observations.

The timing of screening examinations for hypertension is of particular importance. It is possible for a person to have a normal blood pressure in the morning and a high blood pressure in the afternoon. If this is the case, then screening examinations for hypertension should be performed in the afternoon. A true picture of the state of an individual's blood pressure depends upon 3- to 4-hour monitoring day and night. Because nurses functioning in primary care will be increasingly involved in separating the well from the early sick, nurses might initiate studies to determine the best time of day to screen day, afternoon, and night workers for early hypertension.

[2] The cycles for all functions described are those observed in people who sleep at night from about 11 P.M. to 7 A.M. and who are active in the daytime. Timing of these same cycles will be different for those who are adapted to other sleep–activity schedules.

[3] In some individuals temperature rises to its crest more rapidly than it does in others.

Urine Formation

Urine output of water, potassium, sodium, and other constituents is also cyclical. It is greatest in the late morning and early afternoon and least between 11 P.M. and 3 A.M. This pattern continues despite the intake of fluid before retiring and allows for a period of sleep uninterrupted by having to empty the bladder. If this pattern holds for the sick person, should some decrease in hourly urine output be expected between the hours of 11 P.M. and 3 A.M.? Might not individuals be more susceptible to overloading the cardiovascular system with fluid at night than at other times of the day? It would seem that nurses should study urine output in patients as well as the effect that intravenous solutions have on the output at different times of the day. Studies could also be made of the relationship of the excretion of potassium and other elements to the time of day. If there is in fact a significant difference, how does this difference change the timing and pattern of administering fluids to patients?

Blood Plasma and Adrenal Steroids

Adrenal steroids are not secreted in uniform amounts over a 24-hour period. The rate of secretion is highest in early morning and lowest between 11 P.M. and 3 A.M. Some time after the plasma adrenal steroid crest or trough is reached, urinary excretion of 17-ketosteroids and 17-hydroxysteroids rises or falls. (See Figures 6-1 and 6-2.)

A number of physiologic and pathologic events coincide with either the crest or trough of adrenal secretion. Eosinophil levels rise during the trough and fall during the crest of adrenal steroid secretion. Conversely, some of the neutrophils rise to a maximum during the day and fall to a minimum at night. Other elements in the blood such as gamma globulin also show a circadian rhythm. Asthmatic attacks are most common when plasma steroids are low and skin sensitivity to histamine is greatest. Short-acting barbiturates delay the increase in adrenal steroids. Does this effect help to explain distortions of mood and impairment in performance ability experienced by some people who have taken barbiturates to induce sleep?

Sleep–Activity Cycles

Every 24 hours, living beings alternate periods of activity with sleep. Some animals are nocturnal (active at night and sleeping by day). Others are active by day and sleep at night. In addition, there is evidence that mental and physical performance varies from one time of day to another. Some are at their best early in the day (morning people), whereas others are "afternoon or night people." Despite the significance of knowing when a given person is at his or her best, there is as yet no means of mapping each person's hourly physical or mental performance rhythm. One interesting point about the sleep and activity cycle is that it serves as a synchronizer for many physiologic functions.

In the human body there appears to be two clocks regulating sleep. One governs dreaming (REM—rapid eye movements sleep). This clock also controls the daily rise and fall in body temperature. There are also slight rises in the heart rate and blood pressure. The other clock regulates the nondreaming part of sleep. When a person's usual pattern of sleep activity is disrupted, either by rapid travel across time zones or by changes in working hours, he or she experiences symptoms of dysrythmia to some degree. These effects may be aggravated by a lack of sleep either from failure to go to sleep or from early rising. Sleep disturbances can be minimized by either going to bed earlier for a few nights before traveling east or later when flying west. Not only does sleep form a part of the daily sleep–activity rhythm, but it occurs in predictable cycles.

Cell Division

Not unexpectedly, cells have been found to divide at different rates at different times of the day. Further, the time at which some cancer cells divide differs from that of healthy cells of the same tissue. In studies on mice, it has been possible to determine these time differences. Cytotoxic (agents harmful to cells) drugs can then be given when the malignant cells are most susceptible and healthy cells less susceptible. Dosage of drugs that kill the animal if given when healthy cells are most susceptible are well tolerated during periods of relative cellular inactivity. The desired effect, death of the cancer cells, is achieved.

Resistance and Susceptibility

Studies made on humans and animals indicate that there are regularly recurring times each 24 hours when resistance and susceptibility to infection or responsiveness to drugs is greatest. Wongwiwat (1972) found that mice inoculated intraperitoneally with type I pneumococci during the dark period survived longer than those inoculated during the light period. It appears from this as well as other studies that the time of exposure to pathogenic microorganisms is a factor in determining whether or not one develops an infection as well as whether one lives or dies.

The fact that death most frequently occurs in the early morning hours may be related to one or more biological rhythms.

Disruption of Biological Rhythms

As discussed earlier, biological rhythms are synchronized with conditions in the environment. Therefore anything that disturbs this relationship suddenly will cause desynchronization. As an example, until very recently people were born, lived, and died in the same place. When they did move, travel was slow and they were able to adapt to new temporal relationships as they moved. Today with jet planes it is possible to be in New York in the morning and in Honolulu or London 8 hours later. In this interval as many as six time zones may have been crossed. Biological rhythms that were synchronized in New York are no longer in harmony with the environment. In other words, the person is dysrhythmic, for no longer are his or her biological clocks functioning in harmony with the environment. The person becomes desynchronized because his or her pacemaker clock and other clocks are not functioning in harmony with each other. Evidence of desynchronization of the elements in the hierarchy include disturbances in the person's thinking and learning ability, physical distress, depression, and anxiety. Desynchronization continues for at least 2 weeks, as not all rhythms return to normal at the same rate.

Other rhythms are also disturbed and take varying periods of time to be resynchronized. As an example, potassium metabolism only takes about a day. Temperature rhythms take from a week to 10 days or more. By the time or even before adaptation is accomplished, the traveler may be off again.

Most of the early studies of biological rhythms in humans have been made on travelers. There are, however, others who are exposed to changes that may result in desynchronization. This includes those who work rotating shifts or highly irregular hours. Because it may take 2 weeks or longer for some cycles to become synchronized, frequent changes in shifts may have a detrimental effect on health. There is evidence that some individuals never adapt and should not choose occupations requiring changes in shift. There is also evidence that daily and weekly shift changes are detrimental and should be eliminated whenever possible. Studies of the effects of shift rotation on circadian rhythms of workers including nurses continue to be made. Questions under investigation include: How does change of shift affect the ability of nurses (others) to function and to experience satisfaction? What is the optimum length of time for an individual to work a given shift?

Hospitalization

A change that may be responsible for desynchronization is hospitalization. For some individuals, timing of activities may be disrupted more than for others. Mealtimes as well as hours of sleep may be considerably different for the hospitalized patient from those to which he or she is accustomed.

Besides changes in schedules, other elements such as bedrest may contribute to desynchronization of circadian rhythms in sick people. Winget (1972) found that both heart rate (up) and body temperature (down) rhythms were affected during and for at least 10 days after discontinuing bedrest. Felton (1979) cites a study of the effects of bedrest of 5 or more days on renin secretion. It has been shown that the pattern of secretion of renin, a substance secreted into the blood by the kidney, is disrupted in individuals on extended bedrest. Renin activates a powerful vasoconstrictor, angiotensin. In health, the secretion of renin is at a minimum at midnight and gradually increases thereafter. As a consequence of the kidney's failure to secrete renin in a normal pattern, the blood vessels of the person who had been on prolonged bedrest do not contract appropriately when the person assumes the upright position. This possibility should be anticipated, and the patient should be assisted to rise slowly. The patient should be encouraged to sit on the side of the bed, swinging his or her legs, and then be supported to a standing position. (See Chapter 50 for preambulation leg exercises.)

If the effects of a drug as well as its effectiveness vary with the time it is administered in relation to the phase of circadian rhythms, should the dosage and the time of administration of some drugs be varied according to the crest and trough of one or more rhythms? For example, should adrenal hormones be administered so that their maximum absorption more clearly matches that of normal secretion? Even when data are gathered about personal habits, this information may not be used. Might not nurses institute studies to determine the extent to which patients' bodily rhythms are desynchronized as well as methods to prevent desynchronization?

There is evidence that desynchronization is a factor in manic-depressive illness. In this illness not only is more melatonin secreted than normal, but the peak occurs earlier than normal and decreases before daylight. In normal people the peak occurs just before dawn and ends abruptly at dawn. A hypothesis suggested by Wehr and Goodwin (1978) is that the clocks regulating different brain chemicals get out of synchronization so that two powerful chemicals that should counterbalance each other rise and fall together.

From this brief presentation, application of knowledge about circadian rhythms and the careful collection of data may result in improved methods of promoting and restoring health.

Adaptation

Another factor in the ability to maintain health is the capacity to adapt. Adaptation is another expression of humans' and other living beings' interaction with their environment. The definition of the concept *adaptation* varies with the orientation of the person who defines it. Thus biologists define adaptation as the structural and functional changes that make a species better suited to a particular environment. The anthropologist adds the dimension of changing the environment in such a manner that it is better suited to human needs. This is accomplished mainly by cultural means. In this discussion the classical definition is modified to include individuals as well as groups and temporary as well as permanent changes. Therefore, adaptation is defined as the temporary or permanent changes in structure, function, behavior, or culture that enable an individual or group to survive in a particular environment.

It must be remembered that adaptation involves a response that favors survival in a particular environment. It differs from tolerance inasmuch as it is a positive response whereas tolerance is accomplished by the loss of function. As an example, adaptation of hearing implies that acuity is improved. Tolerance implies that hearing is diminished or lost as a result of overexposure to a loud noise, such as rock music or the clang of noisy machinery.

Environment as a Factor in Adaptation

It should be noted that environmental conditions may favor the survival of certain individuals and the disappearance of others. For example, in England in rural areas a species of moth is commonly found to be light-colored. In industrial areas the dark variety predominate, as they blend into the soot-blackened branches and trunks of trees, whereas the light-colored variety are easily identified by birds and eaten. In rural areas the situation is reversed. Thus environment is a significant factor in which variety of moths (or of other species) disappears and which continues to live and reproduce its kind.

Mechanisms of Adaptation

Adaptation occurs at all levels of organization. In unicellular organisms the cell carries on all life processes. In multicellular organisms, some cells specialize, and with specialization, some of the capacity of these cells to adapt is lost. For example, the growth potential of nerve and muscle cells is so small that it is of little practical significance. Cellular specialization, however, is to the overall advantage of the individual. It makes the individual better able to find food and water, escape enemies, and modify the environment so that it meets his or her needs. All cells retain one common characteristic—they carry on the biochemical activities essential to metabolism. Although all cells are capable of adapting to changes in the supply of food, those with a high rate of metabolism are quickly injured by marked deprivation.

In addition to being able to adapt the rate of metabolism to the supply of nutrients, some cells can respond to a change in the environment by undergoing cell division. For example, following a small injury to the skin or mucous membrane, epithelial cells multiply and repair the damage. More extensive breaks are repaired by fibrous connective tissue. Squamous epithelium may replace other types of epithelial tissues when they are subjected to irritating substances over a period of time.

Among plants and nonhuman animals, genetic mutation is the principal mechanism for making long-term adaptations.

There are numerous examples of successful structural and functional adaptations in nature. Birds, adapted to living in the desert, conserve water by excreting solid urine. Certain sea birds have developed salt-excreting glands that enable them to drink seawater. Despite having kidneys that are less efficient in removing salt than human kidneys, they are able to maintain the concentration of salt in their extracellular fluid at about the same level. Humans, having no comparable structure, are unable to use seawater. When they drink it, they dehydrate themselves by using their body water to eliminate the excess salt into their urine. The dehydration is further increased by the diarrhea that results from the high concentration of magnesium in the seawater (Schmidt-Nielson, 1959).

At times the capacity of certain organisms to adapt has been a disadvantage to humans. For example, the fact that mosquitos have developed resistance to DDT and other insecticides enables them to survive and makes the eradication of malaria difficult. A similar case is *Staphylococcus aureus,* of which strains resistant to penicillin have come to predominate. For a brief time, infections caused by this organism were brought under rapid control, but the capacity of the *Staphylococcus* to adapt has enabled it to survive. Not all species, however, have been successful in adapting to change. The mammoth dinosaurs are extinct because they were unable to adapt to changes from a tropical to a temperate climate or, what appears to be more likely, to a reduction in the amount of food available.

Human Adaptation

Humans also adapt to climate, geography, physical activity, and disease. These adaptations may be temporary or permanent. They may also involve genetic mutation or the development of a potential characteristic. Thus climate may influence which genetic characteristics survive or predominate. As examples, body build appears to be influenced by climate and by the type of activities in which the individual customarily engages. The short, stocky frame of the Eskimos and the layer of fat under their skin serve to prevent heat loss. In tropical Africa, natives have a long, thin trunk that facilitates the loss of heat from core tissues.

Populations living at high altitudes make several adaptations that enable them to maintain the supply of oxygen to their cells. Among these adaptations are an increase in the size of the chest cavity and a secondary polycythemia, that is, an elevated erythrocyte count and volume of hemoglobin. At very high altitudes the values from hemoglobin and erythrocytes may be double that found in individuals living at or near sea level. Despite the low atmospheric pressure, people who are adapted to a high altitude carry on the same activities as those living at or near sea level. These activities include doing the most strenuous types of physical work. Given time, most healthy individuals can become adapted to high altitudes.

Humans as well as nonhuman animals adapt to some pathogenic microorganisms by developing an immunity to them. For some microorganisms, such as the virus causing smallpox, humans have been able to develop a vaccine that causes their bodies to produce antibodies that protect them from the disease. Others, either because they have diminished in virulence or because humans have developed some resistance to them, do not cause as much damage as they once did.

Temporary Adaptations

Some adaptations may be temporary. An example of a temporary protective biological adaptation is the capacity to tan the skin. Tanning on exposure to the sunlight offers some protection to the deeper layers of the skin. Persons whose skin does not tan run the risk of sunburn on each exposure to the sun. The fact that the races that developed in the tropics have dark skins whereas those in northern countries have fair skins is believed to represent a more permanent type of adaptation of the skin to environmental conditions.

Structures have a reserve capacity that enables them to increase their size and ability to do work. The stimulus may be either physiologic or pathologic. As examples, the heavy muscles of the manual laborer or the professional wrestler illustrate an adaptation to activities requiring muscular activity. Enlargement of the myocardium in essential hypertension is another illustration of biological adaptation to increased work.

As suggested earlier, polycythemia may be primary or secondary. The secondary type develops in response to a deficient supply of oxygen to the tissues, as occurs at high altitudes or in conditions in which arterial and venous blood are mixed. Primary polycythemia occurs when the bone marrow fails to respond appropriately to its regulators. The effects in both instances are the same, a rise in the number of erythrocytes and in the volume of hemoglobin.

One of the factors that has enabled humans to adapt so that they are able to survive in widely differing environments has been the development of cultures. Through the process of developing a culture, the rules by which members live are defined. These rules are the "thou shalts" and "thou shalt nots." In stable cultures, the rules by which people live are generally accepted, understood, and adhered to (see Chapter 31).

Mutual Adaptation

Another type of adaptation might be called mutual adaptation. In mutual adaptation, two species live together well enough that both survive. Numerous examples can be cited in nature, but we cite only one. When a population is first exposed to a new microorganism, the effects are often disasterous. However, after passing through many generations, the surviving population and the microorganism adapt to each other in such a manner that both survive. Our mouths and gastrointestinal tracts are teeming with microorganisms with which we live in harmony. Some diseases such as tuberculosis and syphilis are less deadly in long-exposed populations than in the newly exposed.

Disease as an Adaptation

It is interesting to note that occasionally an abnormality serves as an asset in a particular environment. Sickle-cell anemia is one such condition. For some reason it confers, or is associated with, some characteristic that increases resistance to malaria. In malarious areas of Africa, sickle-cell anemia is advantageous to the individual because it increases the chances of survival. In nonmalarious areas, such as the United States, it has no survival value. It is possible that some of the responses observed in a number of diseases and following injury have adaptive value, that is, favor survival. Kluger (1978) has suggested that moderate fever may be one such response.

As will be considered later, some believe that diabetes mellitus favored survival in a feast or famine society. A number of other diseases such as essential hypertension may once have favored survival. Because of a changed environment, they are now viewed by some as diseases of adaptation.

Adaptation to Food

A universal adaptation, that is, one that is common to all groups of people, is to the type of food available in an area. Whatever plant or animal is most abundant is utilized as the principal food. In some areas of the world, one or possibly two plants serve as the basic foods: potatoes, rice, and wheat. In others the principal food is corn, a fruit, or meat. The manner in which food is prepared reflects its abundance or scarcity and the means that are available to prepare it. Meat may be added to vegetables or sauces for flavor or to make a little meat go a long way. Because people take their food habits with them wherever they go, they may continue to select and to prepare foods in a certain way despite changes in environment or in the availability of specific foods. In fact, changes in food habits are made only with difficulty. A common observation is that persons migrating from one area of the world to another adopt a new language but continue to cling to old food habits.

In general, humans have the capacity to adapt to a wider range of conditions than do other species. Not only can they learn, but they can profit from learning and communicate learning to others. Humans are able to modify their external environment to their needs, as well as to foresee future needs and to make plans to meet them. Though many species are restricted geographically to a limited area, humans can roam the earth or live out their life span in the place where they were born. In either situation they alter their environment to suit their needs. Humans' capacity to adapt the environment to their needs increased greatly when they began to build shelters, make clothing and fire, cultivate plants, and domesticate animals as sources of food and power. In modern times the adaptations of the environment have been further increased by the achievement of a high degree of refinement and efficiency in industrial and agricultural methods and tools.

Factors Influencing the Capacity to Adapt

Among the factors influencing the adaptive capacity of an individual are genetic constitution, the extent to which needs have been met in the past, level of learning, anatomic integrity, and emotional state.

Genetic Constitution

Genetic constitution, or heredity, determines the potential and the limits for the growth and development of both structure and functions in the individual. Through influencing the biochemical activities of cells, genes affect the capacity of the organism to adapt to changes imposed on it from within or from without. The effects of genes range from the activity of enzyme systems in cells to body build and the pigmentation of the skin. Some abnormalities are transmitted by genes and are incompatible with life. Some are evident at birth; some appear early in life; and others do not make their appearance until late in life. An abnormality may be seriously handicapping or produce little or no disability. As stated earlier, a defective gene may be advantageous in certain environments.

Needs

The adaptive potential is determined by heredity. Whether or not the individual achieves his or her potential depends on a variety of factors. Very important is the extent to which the individual's physiologic as well as psychological needs have been met in the past, most particularly in early life. An inadequate intake of high-quality proteins in infancy and early childhood predisposes to liver disease and may impair intellectual capacity. A child who is seriously deprived of love is susceptible to failure to develop emotionally.

Anatomic Integrity

Anatomic integrity affects the capacity to adapt. As examples, the individual who has been brain-injured may be less able to cope with emotional and physical stress than a healthy person. A child with a defective intraventricular septum may not achieve full mental or physical growth. Neither will he or she be able to be as active as a healthy child. Depending on the nature of the environment, an individual achieves or fails to achieve intellectual and physical potential.

Learning and Experience

How well individuals achieve their adaptive potential also depends on how they have learned to satisfy their needs and to react to stressors as well as to conditions to which they have been exposed. Further, level of learning influences the flexibility of individuals. In general, educated persons are more adaptable than noneducated ones. Experiences along the way may predispose the individual to health or to disease later in life. For example, repeated streptococcal infections may predispose a person to rheumatic fever and the rheumatic fever to a reduction in the capacity of the heart to adapt. As a result of the effects of repeated illness, as well as of the attitudes of parents and others during periods of illness or health, the person may come to prefer illness to health. Schooling may be interrupted and the individual's incentive to learn impaired.

Age

Adaptability is generally greatest in youth and young middle life and least at the extremes of life. In infants and young children, the capacity to adapt is limited by the fact that not all organs and systems are fully mature. At birth the kidneys, nervous system, and immunologic systems are not fully developed. For example, the kidney is not able to concentrate urine as efficiently in the young infant as during youth and adult life. As a consequence of the immaturity of the nervous system and lack of experience, the infant is unable to evaluate the external environment and to modify it in terms of his or her needs. As a result of immaturity, the infant, and to a lesser extent the child, depends on others for safety and welfare.

In the later years of life, adaptive capacity declines. Not all the factors in this process are fully understood. One seems to be a lessening of the reserve capacity of vital organs and with it the inability to cope with rapidly increasing loads such as a rapid increase in blood volume during an intravenous infusion or blood transfusion. Aging persons should also be protected from a sudden increase in muscular activity, as muscle activity increases the amount of blood being returned to the heart. Infections such as pneumonia may not be accompanied by the usual signs and symptoms. Temperature may be only slightly elevated or within normal limits. Therefore, when there is evidence that an elderly person is ill, other signs and symptoms should be considered significant despite a normal or near-normal temperature. The aged are often able to cope with one stressor, even a serious one such as major surgery, but are seriously threatened by multiple stressors such as surgery complicated by massive blood loss or infection.

Characteristic Features of Adaptation

Whatever the power of the individual to adapt, adaptation is characterized by a number of features.

Involvement of Entire Organism

As stated previously, one feature is that adaptation involves the entire organism. Mr. Brave illustrates this concept. He awakened with a feeling of nausea and vomited a large amount of bright red blood. After he vomited, he saw the blood and was frightened. He called his wife, who called his physician, who asked him to go to the hospital—which is a social response to medical knowledge and equipment. Mr. Brave's fear or anxiety was so great that he did not delay putting himself under the care of his physician. But it was not so great the he was immobilized. His body was also reacting. His sympathoadrenal medullary system constricted his peripheral blood vessels. He looked pale and felt cold, dizzy, and faint. He lay on the bed until the ambulance arrived. His heart and respiratory rates increased. Although the picture is not complete, enough has been presented to emphasize the point that Mr. Brave reacted as a whole individual.

Time

A second feature of adaptation is related to time. Given time, an organism is able to adapt to a greater degree of change than it can when it is called on to adapt suddenly. In the instance of Mr. Brave, had he lost small amounts of blood over a period of time, he would have been able to tolerate a lower hemoglobin level than when he lost blood rapidly. With a slow loss of blood, he would probably have tolerated a hemoglobin of 4 g (25 per cent) or less without exhibiting manifestations of marked circulatory distress at rest. In contrast, with a rapid loss of blood, a hemoglobin of 50 per cent is accompanied by manifestations indicative of a serious impairment in the blood supply to vital tissues. There are a number of explanations for the differences in behavior of an individual following the slow and rapid loss of blood. In contrast to a rapid loss of blood, with a slow loss blood volume is not diminished and the tissues have time to adapt to a decrease in oxygen supply. With a sufficient decrease in the oxygen, signs and symptoms of circulatory distress appear. They include palpitation, rapid heart rate, shortness of breath, and possibly dizziness. Depending on the extent to which the hemoglobin level is diminished, these manifestations may appear with activity and disappear with rest or be present much of the time.

Each individual is called upon to respond not only to body changes but also to changes in the environment and in his or her relationship to it. When these changes occur slowly and are not too great in number, the individual may have little difficulty in adapting to them. When, however, many changes occur in a relatively short period of time, one's capacity to adapt may be threatened. Both the number of changes and the rate of change are factors in their effect. Toffler (1970) points out that a characteristic feature of modern technological cultures is change—he calls the result of rapid and multiple changes "future shock." The effects are similar to the culture shock that occurs when one travels to a new and different culture. In both states the unprepared individual enters a strange or foreign culture. Toffler (1970) says,

> Culture shock is what happens when a traveler finds himself in a place where yes may mean no, where a "fixed price" is negotiable, where to be kept waiting in an outer office is no cause for insult, where laughter may signify anger. It is what happens when the familiar psychological cues that help an individual to function in society are replaced by new ones that are strange and incomprehensible. . . . The culture shock phenomenon accounts for much of the bewilderment, frustration, and disorientation that plagues Americans in their dealings with other societies. It causes a breakdown in communication, a misreading of reality, an inability to cope. Yet culture shock is relatively mild in comparison with the much more serious malady, future shock. Future shock is the dizzying disorientation brought on by the premature arrival of the

future. It may well be the most important disease of tomorrow.

Toffler also makes another distinction between culture and future shock. Persons who are in culture shock know that they can go home again, home to the familiar, where they know what to expect and where they and their associates share common values. With future shock there is no home to go to.

Flexibility

A third feature of adaptation is that the more flexible the organism is in its capacity to adapt, the greater is its capacity to survive. If, for example, the only mechanism available to adapt to the loss of blood was to constrict blood vessels, people would be much more vulnerable and much less able to survive injuries involving blood loss than they are. Flexibility is as significant in psychological and social adaptation as it is in physiologic responses.

An illustration of the adaptation to available materials and climate is observed in the building of houses. Among the materials used are snow, wood, cement, cinders, sand, clay, aluminum, steel, and skins of animals. Houses vary in size from one room to 100 or more. Depending on climate and availability of fuel, they may be airy or almost airtight. Their shapes are varied. In fact, any adequate description of the varieties of ways in which humans have adapted materials to their need for shelter would be impossible to list in this volume.

Energy

A fourth feature of adaptation is that the organism generally, though not always, uses the mechanism that is most economical of energy. The fact that adaptation also requires energy should not be overlooked. Adaptation is usually integrative in character and is usually the best that the organism can do at a given time. In illness there is always some decrease in the capacity of a person to adapt. The sick person is not at his or her best, and allowance should be made for the inability to cope with the environment and the resultant frustration of needs.

Adequacy

A fifth feature is that the adaptive response may be adequate to the situation or it may be deficient, excessive, or inappropriate. To illustrate, following a meal, the blood sugar rises. In the healthy individual, as the blood sugar rises, insulin is secreted and glucose is removed from the blood by the liver and converted to glycogen. Some glucose may be temporarily stored in the muscles and areolar connective tissues. Approximately 2 hours after a meal, the level of sugar in the blood drops to, or slightly below the fasting level. As the level of glucose in the blood drops, mechanisms responsible for its fall are counteracted and the level of glucose in the blood rises to the normal range for the fasting blood glucose. (One of Cannon's characteristics of homeostatic mechanism.) An elevation in the level of glucose that is sustained above the upper limits of normal is usually caused by a relative or absolute lack of insulin.

To sum up, adaptation enables living organisms to respond to changes in their environment in such a manner that injury is prevented or damage is repaired. Although all living organisms possess the power of adaptation, not only species, but also individuals of the same species vary in their capacity to adapt. As with other characteristics, there is a

Figure 6-4. Nursing intervention in the field of interacting forces to promote adaptation. (Modified from Hopps, H. C.: *Principles of Pathology,* 2nd ed. New York, Appleton-Century-Crofts, 1964, p. 5.)

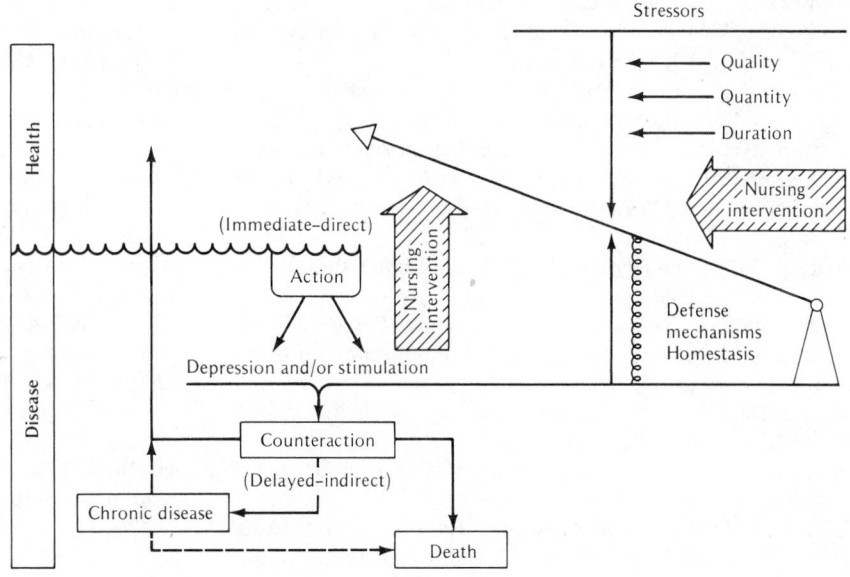

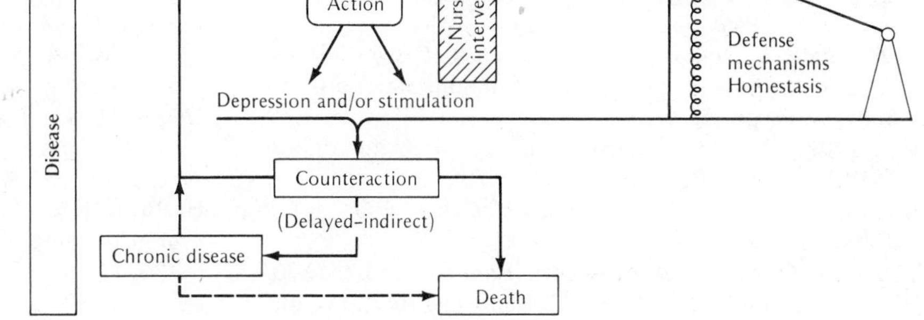

range to the capacity to adapt. When this range is exceeded, health or even life is threatened.

Nurse's Responsibilities in Promoting Adaptation

The nurse has several responsibilities, which include (1) to assess the adaptive capacity of the individual, (2) to modify the environment to the patient so that he or she is protected from excessive demands, and (3) to assist the patient in utilizing adaptive capacities to the patient's benefit.

To accomplish the goal of promoting adaptation, nursing intervenes at either of two points in the field of interacting forces of the life space of the client system. Intervention aims either at preventing stressors from impinging on the patient, thus conserving adaptive resources, or at maintaining, supplementing, or substituting for defense mechanisms which are inadequate to deal with unavoidable stressors. Location of nursing intervention in the field of forces across the health-illness spectrum is illustrated in Figure 6-4.

References Cited

Banks, O. H. "Comprehensive Health Planning in Relation to Environment Problems." *Am. J. Pub. Health*, **61** (1973), 1971.

Binkley, S. "A Time-Keeping Enzyme in the Pineal Gland." *Sci. Am.*, **240** (1979), 66–71.

Cannon, W. B. *The Wisdom of the Body*, rev. and enlarged ed. New York: W. W. Norton & Company, Inc. 1939, p. 24.

Felton, G. "Biological Rhythm Research: Application to Nursing." *News and Views: J. Detroit District Nurses Assoc.*, Fall 1978 and Winter 1979.

Haynes, R. C., and Larner, J. "Adreno-corticotropic Hormone: Adreno-corticotropic Steroids and Their Synthetic Analogs." In *The Pharmacological Basis of Therapeutics*, 5th ed. Ed. by Louis Goodman and Alfred Gilman. New York: Macmillan Publishing Co., Inc., 1975, p. 1478.

Kluger, M. J. "The Evolution and Adaptive Value of Fever." *Amer. Sci.*, **66** (1978), 38–43.

Nightingale, F. *Notes on Nursing: What It Is and What It Is Not*, rev. and enlarged ed. London: Harrison and Sons, 1860, pp. 5, 85, 92.

Sargent, F., II. "Man–Environment—Problems for Public Health." *Am. J. Pub. Health*, **62** (1972), 631.

Schmidt-Nielsen, K. "Salt Glands." *Sci. Am.*, **200** (1959), 109–16.

Toffler, A. *Future Shock*. New York: Random House, 1970.

Wehr, T. A., and Goodwin, F. K. "Biological Rhythms and Affective Illness." *Weekly Psychiatry Update Series*. Princeton, N.J.: BioMedia Inc., 1978, Lesson 28, Vol. 2.

Winget, C. M. et al. "Circadian Rhythm Asynchronism in Man During Hypokinesis." *Appl. Physiol.*, **33** (1972), 640–43.

Wongwiwat, M. et al. "Circadian Rhythms of Resistance of Mice to Acute Pneumococcal Infection." *Infect. Immun.*, **5**: 4 (1972), 442–48.

General References

Adams, M. S. "Genetic Consequences of Cultural Adaptation." *Med. Clin. North Am.*, **53** (1969), 977–89.

Baker, P. T. "Human Adaptation to High Altitude." *Science*, **163** (1969), 1149–56.

Buchsbaum, M. S. "The Chemistry of Brain Clocks." *Psychol. Today*, **8** (1979), 124.

Burnet, F. M. "The Implications of Global Homeostasis." *Impact of Science on Society*, **22** (1972), 305–14.

Burnside, I. M. "You Cope, of Course." *Am. J. Nurs.*, **71** (1971), 2354–57.

Busse, E. W. "Biologic and Sociologic Changes Affecting Adaptation in Mid and Late Life." *Ann. Intern. Med.*, **75** (1971), 115–20.

Chekov, quoted in Trilling, L. *The Experience of Literature*. Garden City, N.Y.: Doubleday & Company, Inc., 1967, 5501.

Coelho, G. V. et al. *Coping and Adaptation: A Behavioral Sciences Bibliography*, Public Health Services Publication No. 2087. Chevy Chase, Md.: National Institute of Mental Health, 1970.

Cohen, Y. A., ed. *Man in Adaptation: The Cultural Present*. Chicago: Aldine Publishing Company, 1974.

Edelstein, R. R. "The Time Factor in Relation to Illness as a Fertile Nuring Research Area: Review of the Literature." *Nurs. Res.*, **21** (1972), 72–76.

Felton, G. "Effect of Time Cycle Change on Blood Pressure and Temperature in Young Women." *Nurs. Res.*, **19** (1970), 48–58.

Felton, G. "Rhythmic Correlates of Shift Work." In *Communicating Nursing Research*. Vol. 6. Collaboration and Competition. Ed. by M. V. Batey. Boulder, Colo.: Western Interstate Commission for Higher Education, 1973, pp. 73–89.

Frisancho, A. "Functional Adaptation to High Altitude Hypoxia." *Science*, **187** (1975), 313–19.

Goosen, G. M., and Bush, A. "Adaptation: A Feedback Process." *ANS Advances in Nursing Science*, **1** (1979), 51–65.

Hagen, T. C., Lawrence, A. M., and Kirsteins, L. "Autoregulation of Growth Hormone Secretion in Normal Subjects." *Metabolism*, **21** (1972), 603–10.

Hastings, J. W. "The Biology of Circadian Rhythms from Man to Micro-Organism." *N. Engl. J. Med.*, **282** (1970), 435–41.

Jacobs, B. B., and Uphoff, D. E. "Immunological Modification: A Basic Survival Mechanism." *Science,* **185** (1974), 582–87.

Johnsgard, P. A. "Quail Music." *Natural History,* **83** (1974), 34–39.

Jones, P. S. "An Adaptation Model for Nursing Practice." *Am. J. Nurs.,* **78** (1968), 1900–06.

Lenfant, C. et al. "Adaptation to High Altitude." *N. Engl. J. Med.,* **284** (1971), 1298–1309.

Lewontin, R. C. "Adaptation." *Sci. Amer.,* **239** (1978), 213–30.

Luce, G. G. *Biological Rhythms in Human and Animal Physiology.* New York: Dover Publications, Inc., 1971.

Luce, G. G. *Biological Rhythms in Psychiatry and Medicine.* Chevy Chase, Md.: National Institute of Mental Health, 1970.

Natalini, J. J. "The Human Body as a Biological Clock." *Amer. J. Nurs.,* **77** (1977), 1130–32.

Rabkin, J. G., and Struening, E. L. "Life Events, Stress and Illness." *Science,* **194** (1976), 1013–20.

Reres, M. "Coping with Stress in Nursing." *Amer. Nurse,* 1977, p. 4.

Roy, Sister C. *Introduction to Nursing: An Adaptation Model.* Englewood Cliffs, N.J.: Prentice-Hall, Inc., 1976.

Selye, H. "Homeostasis and Heterostasis." *Perspect. Biol. Med.,* **16** (1973), 441–45.

Soodak, H., and Iberall, A. "Homeokinetics: A Physical Science for Complex Systems." *Science,* **201** (1978), 578–82.

Tom, C. V., and Lanuza, D. M. "Biological Rhythms." *Nurs. Clin. North Am.,* **11** (1976), 569–638.

7

Human Needs—The Basis of Nursing

The cause of every need of a living being is also the cause of the satisfaction of the need.

PFLÜGER, 1877
Quoted in: Cannon, Walter B., *The Wisdom of the Body.* New York: W. W. Norton & Company, Inc., 1932, p. 21.

Definitions of Need

The nursing care of each patient should be based on individual needs. Briefly stated, patient needs determine patient care. But what is a "need"? Definitions of patient need have varied greatly in sophistication and utility. An early oversimplification defined patient need as "what the patient wants as opposed to what is good for him" (Anderson, 1957). A more complex and potentially more useful definition of need was formulated by Murray (1938) and paraphrased by King (1962) as follows:

> a concept that stands for a force of some nature in the brain region, an organizing force that affects thinking, knowing, perceiving in such a way as to change an existing, unsatisfying situation in certain directions. Each need is accompanied by a particular feeling or emotion, and even though sometimes weak or momentary, it usually persists and gives rise to overt behavior or fantasy, which may change the external circumstances sufficiently to appease or satisfy the organism and still the need.

Needs must be satisfied if the organism is to carry on one or more of the activities of life. These activities may be classified as (1) use of food and oxygen with the release of energy, (2) response to the environment, (3) growth, (4) reproduction, and (5) productivity. Needs may arise from, or be met at, any of the levels of organization of the human being—biochemical, cellular, systemic, psychological, interpersonal, and social.

According to Gordon (1961–1962), four basic phenomena of the nervous system make it possible for humans to adapt, to survive, and to satisfy their needs in an ever-changing environment. They are pain, hunger, fear, and rage.

Frequently in nursing literature the problem of a patient toward which nursing care is directed will be referred to as the patient's *nursing need.* In their study of the elderly ambulatory patient, Schwartz, Henley, and Zeitz (1964) presumed that a nursing need existed "when an unsolved health problem was identified, which nursing attention seemed likely to solve, to improve, to modify, or to evaluate with profit to the patient" (p. 192). With the increasing emphasis on the necessity of interdisciplinary approaches to patient care, the common core of observations essential to effective professional activity render the notion of nursing need ineffectual. When the patient has needs that cannot be met unaided, we suggest that those unmet needs be referred to as *patient problems,* some of which will be addressed by nursing, some by medical and other health team members, and some by collaborative efforts of several team members.

Classification of Needs

Patient needs have been classified in a variety of ways, with most of the schemes drawing heavily on Maslow's (1954) hierarchy of human needs: physiologic, safety, belongingness and love, and esteem needs; self-actualization; and the need to know and to understand. In this section needs will be considered in five broad categories. They are the (1) physiologic, (2) safety, (3) psychological, (4) social, and (5) spiritual needs. In the following chapters the basis for understanding each of the needs of the patient will be discussed in some detail. As the various needs are discussed, the fact that a human being functions as a whole should not be lost from sight. A disturbance in the capacity of an individual to meet one or more needs affects the whole person, not just a part. Moreover, a disturbance in the capacity of the individual to meet one need may interfere with the ability to meet other needs. Except in the terminal stages of an illness, however, the patient can be expected to be able to meet some of his or her needs without the aid of others.

Requirements of health care regulatory agencies that there be documentation of the nature and outcomes of all care provided by practitioners in the health care field have increased attention to finding ways in which to determine the extent to which patients' needs have been met. This has led to a variety of classification schemes. The most notable of these in nursing is the grassroots effort to order a taxonomy, or classification, of nursing diagnoses, an effort being coordinated by the National Group for Classification of Nursing Diagnoses, based at the St. Louis University School of Nursing (Gebbie & Lavin, 1974; Gordon, 1976). The approach to classification is to group patient problems according to the type of human need which individuals or families are unable to meet unaided when faced with health-related difficulties. Because of the similarity of the major emerging categories of diagnoses to the alterations approach of subsequent chapters in this book, further elaboration on specific diagnostic categories will be dealt with in appropriate chapters.

Roberts (1978) focuses on eleven major behaviors common to hospitalized patients, which constitute patient problems best described through the integrating mechanisms of the systems model. These behaviors are also commonly encountered by nurses practicing in settings other than hospitals, and they overlap substantially with emerging categories of nursing diagnoses: anxiety, pain, sensory deprivation, stress, powerlessness, loss, hopelessness, hostility and anger, loneliness, altered body image, and maladaptations to available space and territory.

Daubert (1979) has described a five-level patient classification system, in use by the Visiting Nurse Association of New Haven, which is based on patients' rehabilitation potential. Each level has an identified ultimate program objective and a set of subobjectives that become the outcome criteria to judge the extent to which patient needs have been met, presumably as a result of services rendered. The description and program objective of each level or patient group in the classification appears in Table 7-1.

Patient Needs Determine Patient Care

For nursing care to be based on the needs of the patient, it is obvious that the nurse must be able to identify what they are. The nurse must have an understanding of what is meant by the term *need*, as well as of which needs take priority. Moreover, to understand how needs are affected by illness and how to assist the patient in meeting needs, some knowledge of the mechanisms used for defense and protection against changes in the environment is necessary. Knowledge of the mechanisms utilized to limit and to repair injury or disturbance is also essential. Finally, assessment of the success of the patient in meeting his or her own needs depends on knowledge of the behavior that indicates success or failure.

All living beings have needs. On the cellular level they are similar for all organisms. Humans differ from other living beings in their psychological, social, and spiritual needs. The needs common to all species are sometimes referred to as basic or survival needs. These are the requirements that must be met to maintain life. Basic needs are prepotent, or take precedence, over others. However, it is important to remember that one of the ways in which humans differ from other living beings is in their ability to override domination by basic needs through the exercise of free will. An example of this is the individual who voluntarily subjects him or herself to a prolonged hunger strike to bring attention to a social issue. Another example is a report by returning American prisoners of the Vietnam War. Four men living in a room 8 feet square and eating a diet of thin cabbage and rice soup for several years, creatively maintained morale by sharing memorized portions of the Bible with one another. Prisoners

TABLE 7-1. ***Description and Objectives of Five Patient Groups in a VNA Patient Classification System***

GROUP I	Patients with acute, nonchronic, episodic-type disease or disability who will return to preillness level of functioning
Objective:	Complete elimination of the existing health problem or need for which the patient was admitted to VNA
GROUP II	Patients with chronic disease(s) or disabilities who are experiencing an acute episode of illness but have the potential for returning to preepisodic level of functioning
Objective:	Management of chronic health problem(s) by patient/family without ongoing VNA services
GROUP III	Patients with chronic disease(s) or disabilities who, even though a return to preillness level of functioning is not possible, will have the potential for increasing their level of functioning and will eventually function without VNA services
Objective:	Rehabilitation of the patient to maximum level of physical, emotional, and social functioning without continued VNA services
GROUP IV	Patients with chronic disease(s) or disabilities who cannot be maintained at home without ongoing VNA services
Objective:	Maintenance of a chronically-ill patient at home to his or her maximum level of functioning with ongoing VNA services
GROUP V	Patients with an end-stage illness
Objective:	Maintenance of the patient in comfort and dignity during the end stage of illness

Adapted with permission of the American Journal of Nursing Company, from Daubert, E. A., "Patient classification system and outcome criteria." *Nurs. Outlook,* 27 (July 1979), 450–54.

in other cells benefited by Bible passages tapped in Morse code and whispered under doors. Spiritual values were chosen to dominate basic needs (Hitt, 1973). (See Chapter 32.)

Another way to state the concept that basic needs are prepotent over others is that needs are organized in a hierarchy, with lower needs demanding satisfaction first. They must be satisfied before other needs are manifested and given attention. For example, physiologic needs must be met to some degree before psychological needs can be expressed. Even among the basic needs some are more urgent than others. Some physiologic needs, such as the need for oxygen, take precedence over the need for food or water. Knowledge of the fact that some needs are more important to survival than others has implications for the practice of nursing. For example, the patient who is acutely short of oxygen is unlikely to be interested in food, much less in conversation or other intellectual activities. Even more significant, this person's survival may well depend on correction of the oxygen deficit. Most students have at some time tried to study when they were cold, hungry, or angry and found that they were unsuccessful until they put on a sweater, had something to eat, or recovered from their anger.

Material relating to all needs will be integrated throughout. There are, however, a few general points that bear emphasis at this time. The first group relates to safety, and the second group relates to optimizing patient behavior through manipulation of environmental factors.

In regard to safety, there are three important dimensions: one relates to the patient, another to the unsafe act, and a third to the responsibilities of those caring for the patient. Safety as related to the patient has two aspects: (1) a real danger or threat to the patient's welfare and (2) the patient's feeling of safety or danger. Threats to the safety of the patient may have their origin in either the internal or external environment. As an example, the life of the patient is threatened by any condition that deprives the patient of some substance required by his or her cells or by failure to remove excesses of supply or products of metabolism. The life of the patient may also be endangered by conditions in the external environment, such as extremes in temperature or radioactive substances or rays. What the person regards as being unsafe depends on past experience and the unknown elements in the situation. A patient who interprets symptoms as indicating the presence of a disease such as cancer is likely to be frightened during the period of diagnosis. Another patient feels unsafe when his or her light is not answered promptly. The patient wonders whether or not help can be depended upon if it is really needed.

Accident prevention in all settings is a primary responsibility of the nurse. In health care facilities, particularly in hospitals, the potential for accidents poses a real threat to the patient's welfare. All accidents have their origin in an unsafe act. Knowledge of certain facts about unsafe acts contributes to their control. Few unsafe acts result in injury and still fewer result in death. The person who is responsible for an accident is not always the one who is injured. Sometimes the relationship between the unsafe act and the accident is not immediate or direct. Moreover, an accident may result from a series of unsafe acts. This point is illustrated by the instance of the man who was killed by an iron bar falling from an open window. The first unsafe act was the construction of a building with windows opening directly over the street. The second was the use of an iron bar to prop a window open. The third was failure to remove the bar from the window sill preparatory to opening the window. When the effect of an unsafe act is delayed, the identification of who is responsible may be difficult, if not impossible.

The control of accidents depends on knowledge of the potential dangers and of the human factors entering into the performance of unsafe acts. Accident prevention takes planning, preparation, and instruction so that people may learn what the dangers are and develop the attitude that accidents can and should be prevented. Their prevention is the responsibility of everyone.

The second group of points relates to the impact of environmental factors on patient behavior. Consideration of the physical environment will be included in later chapters, as appropriate to selected topics. Emphasis here is on selected effects of the people with whom the patient interacts in the intermediate suprasystem.

In every type of health care agency, the number and variety of "allied health personnel" has proliferated at an alarming rate. Most of these workers are described as technicians, whose training varies in length and adequacy as widely as the specialized tasks they are prepared to perform. Gribbin (1973) described several tragic consequences of the acts of poorly trained and supervised technicians, including the death of a 23-year-old man who had had successful brain surgery for a head injury sustained while playing touch football; while the young man was in the recovery room, an inhalation technician inserted a tube too far, it slid into one of the bronchi, and the patient died of complications caused by oxygen deprivation. The professional nurse is responsible for assessing not only the needs of the patient, but also the nature and quality of the resources available in the setting to meet those needs. When actions of other persons in the setting result in distress or danger to the patient, the nurse has an obligation to know where, how, and to whom to proceed within the organization as the advocate of patient welfare.

The professional nurse must understand and be prepared to support or modify the reciprocal influence of the behavior of patient and personnel. When nurses and other health workers hold stereotyped role expectations for themselves and patients, the deviant behavior of patients who are unable or unwilling to comply often results in personnel labeling the patients as uncooperative, belligerent, or even as mentally ill. Davidites (1971) found, in her experience as a psychiatric nurse working with the staff on a medical unit, that patients were expected to be cooperative, cheerful, submissive, and nonquestioning about their illnesses, but that not all patients whose behavior deviated from those expectations were considered "problems." Only those patients whose behavior interfered with a nurse's ability to function according to the nurse's role expectations were brought up for discussion. Davidites reported a dramatic success in modifying "deviant behavior" of a problem patient, not by intervening directly with the patient, but by effecting a change in the attitude and approach of health team members to the patient, which subsequently made the so-called deviant behavior unnecessary. This approach to modifying behavior by altering factors in the environment to which patients appear to be responding is based on operant theory (Skinner, 1938), which proposes that behavior is governed by its consequences, that is, behavior that is rewarded, or positively reinforced, will increase, whereas behavior that is not rewarded (either by negative reinforcement or by withholding reinforcement) will decrease or disappear. Nurses and other health case workers are constantly rewarding or punishing patients for their behavior, but seldom with a conscious and therapeutic purpose. In an exploratory study of patients in an extended care facility, Mikulic (1971) found that only 25 per cent of appropriately independent patient behaviors were positively reinforced by nursing staff, whereas for 75 per cent of independent behaviors reinforcement was either negative or withheld. However, over 88 per cent of inappropriately dependent patient behaviors were positively reinforced by nursing staff, and reinforcement was withheld for only about 12 per cent of dependent behaviors; no dependent behaviors were negatively reinforced.

Mikulic's study used operant theory as a way to describe alarming events in a naturally occurring nursing situation; she did not attempt to use operant conditioning as an approach to modifying patient behavior. However, operant conditioning has been used successfully as an approach to modifying not only psychological, but also physiologic, behavior of patients. Weiss and Engel (1971) reported success in reducing premature ventricular contractions (a type of irregular rhythm of the heart), and Grosicki (1968) accomplished a dramatic reduction of episodes of incontinence by using techniques of operant conditioning. Despite some rather dramatic results from use of these approaches to behavior modification, the nurse must realize and accept the responsibility first to understand the factors that affect the satisfaction and frustration of human needs in general, and of his or her patient in particular, before attempting to design nursing measures to modify behavior.

Capacity to Tolerate Frustration of Needs

The capacity of the individual to tolerate frustration of one or more needs depends on a number of factors.

Adequacy of Structures and Processes

The adequacy of an individual's structures and processes for meeting needs and adapting to change is exemplified by the brain-damaged individual, such as one who has had a stroke, who may have very little tolerance for frustration. The individual becomes excited or upset when faced with minor difficulties. A general anesthetic reduces the ability of the person to adapt the caliber of blood vessels to changes in position. The child who is born with a defect in the structure of the heart may be unable to meet the need of tissues for oxygen during exercise. In general the individual can tolerate the frustration of a need better if the condition that is responsible develops slowly rather than rapidly. Time allows the organism an opportunity to adapt to the change both by altering its requirements and by initiating mechanisms that increase the effectiveness with which it utilizes its supplies. The capacity to tolerate frustration, particularly of psychological needs, depends also on the degree to which the need has been met in the past, especially in early life. Because illness involves the failure to meet one or more needs, the capacity of the sick person to tolerate frustration of needs is often limited. For example, the patient who is in the period immediately following a major operation is unable to anticipate and adapt to changes in the environment. Changes such as a move from the stretcher to the bed, or loud noises, may be followed by a fall in blood pressure. Until the patient fully recovers from the anesthetic, he or she must be protected from falling out of bed. Until the patient is up and about, procedures to maintain airway patency are required. Until the alimentary canal can tolerate them, food and fluids must be administered parenterally.

As has been previously implied, the capacity of an individual to meet needs depends on processes and mechanisms that in health are regulated so that their action is appropriate, effective, and constructive. Structures and processes are required for the regulation of intake, distribution, use, storage, output, and elimination of excesses of supply or of waste products resulting from activity. Not only are individual processes regulated so that a need is met, but each process is regulated so that it is integrated into the activities of the total individual. In humans many structures and functions may be involved in satisfying one need. To illustrate, the physiological need for water involves structures and processes through which a deficit of water is recognized and is translated into the sensation of thirst. Further, coordinated activity is required to obtain, drink, and absorb water into the blood stream. Many more processes are involved in the distribution of water to the cells, in its temporary storage, and in the elimination of an excess by the kidney.

Availability of Supplies or Materials

All living things are open systems, provided with the structures and processes necessary to obtain from the environment the resources and raw materials needed for growth and development. Lack of adequate resources will produce alterations in function, and ultimately the death of the individual. For example, the requirement for oxygen cannot be met unless there is oxygen in the atmosphere. The need to be loved and to give love cannot be met unless love is available.

Adequacy of Coordination of Activities of Participants in Care

The individual's care cannot be said to be comprehensive, and will rarely be effective, without close coordination of the contributions of the many specialized professionals and technicians, and family and friends, who presently participate in providing care for the individual. For example, to meet the food requirements of a patient, persons from a number of disciplines combine their efforts to make the proper food available to the patient. The physician prescribes the diet. The dietitian translates the prescription into food and is responsible for its preparation and serving. When patients require formal dietary instruction, this is frequently the responsibility of the dietitian. The nurse prepares patients for their meals and feeds them, when necessary. She or he answers patients' questions about their nutritional needs or diet, or refers them to the physician or dietitian. The nutritional needs of many patients are met by each individual nurse, physician, and dietitian performing his or her functions. When problems arise, however, their solution may depend on the combined efforts of the nurse, dietitian, physician, patient, and even the members of the family.

To illustrate, Mary Ellen Cliff was a young woman with a diagnosis of rheumatoid arthritis. She ate very little and consequently was weak, lacking in energy, thin, and frail looking. She was cared for at home by her mother and a visiting nurse who visited her twice a week. In the course of her visits the nurse learned that Mary Ellen ate poorly. She discussed this problem with Mary Ellen's physician, who said that her weakness and lack of energy were directly related to inadequate food intake. He prescribed a high-calorie diet and said that he would again talk to Mary Ellen about the importance of eating. To evaluate Mary Ellen's food pattern, the nurse asked her to keep a record of her food intake for three days. The nurse gave Mary Ellen and her mother instructions about how to make the study and told how the information was to be used. As a result of the study, the nurse's previous suspicion that Mrs. Cliff was an indifferent and unimaginative cook was borne out. Part of the problem stemmed from poorly prepared and unattractively served food. The nurse arranged for a consultation with the agency dietitian. The dietitian talked with the physician, and then she planned a diet that included foods Mary Ellen liked and that if eaten would be adequate to her needs. She also suggested that the nurse take some recipes with her that Mrs. Cliff might try to use. Mary Ellen was encouraged to try to eat even when she did not feel like it. After six months of continued effort Mary Ellen had gained 10 pounds and her appetite had improved considerably. She was able to be out of bed and was beginning to think about seeking employment. Mrs. Cliff's cooking, though not in the gourmet class, was much improved. In this particular instance the nurse carried much of the responsibility for the instruction and the management of the patient and her mother. The solution of the problem, however, depended on the cooperative efforts of the members of several disciplines.

Patient Rights

The consumer movement in health care delivery may be a strong ally for nursing in bringing about what ought to be in health care. Kibrick (1973) observed that "consumers are making two separate sets of demands on the health care delivery system: one, the curing of illness—the doctor's role; the other, 'total patient care,' including preventive care, coping with illness, and the eventual restoration of health—the nurse's potential role." An example of the demands of consumers can be seen in the report of a group of women on proceedings of a 1969 conference on "Women and Their Bodies" (A Woman's View of Health Care, 1973). The women contend that the first and most important task of the individual is to gain control of his or her own life and destiny, and that this effort begins with gaining control of one's own body. When one is a consumer of health or medical care, the source of power to control one's body is knowledge. The women recommend that the consumer must insist on enough information to negotiate the system instead of allowing the system to negotiate them. The right of the patient to information as a basis for informed consent to treatment is one of several considerations in the twelve-point Patients' Bill of Rights (AHA, 1973) approved, distributed, and promoted by the American Hospital Association in 1973. The medical literature is also beginning to legitimatize the concept of patients' rights. Chiles (1967) elaborated four rights of patients: (1) the right to privacy, (2) the right to pain, (3) the right to truth, and (4) the right to die. He includes under the right to privacy the right to keep one's own counsel. The patient should not be expected to expose him or herself emotionally any more than to be exposed physically. The environment should be such that the patient feels accepted and respected.

In discussing the right to pain, Chiles does not mean that the patient should be subjected to unnecessary or cruel pain. Rather, pain should be accepted as a warning and a plea that the patient be taken seriously. Whatever its cause, pain indicates that something is wrong and that the patient is suffering. Chiles is of the opinion that patients who want the truth should have it. If persons were certain that they could have the truth when they want it, at least some of them would be saved needless worry. Those with serious illness would then have someone to share their suffering.

Nursing has formally endorsed the concept of patients' rights for three decades. The Code for Nurses (ANA Committee on Ethical, Legal and Professional Standards, 1968), a guide to the ethical principles that should govern the practice, conduct, and relationships of the nurse, was adopted by the American Nurses' Association (ANA) in 1950, and revised in 1960 and 1968. Three of the ten standards of the Code speak directly to patients' rights:

Standard 1. The nurse provides services with respect for the dignity of man, unrestricted by considerations of nationality, race, creed, color, or status.

Standard 2. The nurse safeguards the individual's right to privacy by judiciously protecting information of a confidential nature, sharing only that information relevant to his care.

Standard 4. The nurse acts to safeguard the patient when his care and safety are affected by incompetent, unethical, or illegal conduct of any person.

In 1979, the National League for Nursing (NLN) issued a position paper on the responsibility of nurses to uphold patients' rights in their own practice and to make their influence felt indirectly when the practice of other health team members appears to be in violation of patients' rights. The NLN position emphasizes the patient's right to privacy; to humane and unprejudiced treatment; to information about every aspect of care, from the names and preparation of those caring for him or her to the cost of the care and services provided; to refuse observation and treatment; to have access to all records concerning her or his care; and to be fully informed about rights in all health care settings.

Historically, access to health care has been considered a privilege rather than a right. A concomitant of that conviction has been that one of the expectations of the patient role, by both the care givers and the patient, has been that the patient surrender control over space, interactions, and decision making. References to patient rights, such as those that appear in professional codes, have had no legal sanction until recently. In May 1979, Massachusetts became the third state, following Colorado and New York, to enact a Patients' Bill of Rights (Patients' Bill of Rights Now Law, 1979). It protects every patient or resident in any facility licensed or subject to licensing in Massachusetts by the Department of Public Health. Each person must receive written notice of these rights on admission to the facility. Any person who feels his or her rights as defined have been violated may bring a civil action against the facility. The provisions of the law are very similar to, but more specific than, the NLN position on patients' rights, and the law contains numerous references to specific rights the physician must guarantee to the patient in a facility.

The growing emphasis on patients' rights is part of the consumer protection movement that has arisen as a reaction at least in part to the dominance achieved by professions in American society. Bayles (1978), in arguing against the autonomy of professions except as a means to be used in particular cases, claims that the professions have constituted in American aristocracy whose theoretical foundations are no sounder than those of previous aristocracies. He insists, as does the patients' rights movement, that decisions about ends should be made by clients, provided that those ends are legally permissible. Another source of the movement to return the patient to the central position of control in health care arises from disillusionment of the public with the fallibility of medical technology. Knowles (1977) admonished the public that the next major advances in the health of the American people must be determined by what the individual is willing to do for him or herself and for society at large. "If he is willing to follow reasonable rules for healthy living, he can extend his life and enhance his own and the nation's productivity. . . . He can either remain the problem or become the solution to it; beneficent government cannot." Advocates of holistic and humanistic health care would place this personal responsibility of the consumer at the center of control of the health care system (Holden, 1978). The emphasis on the rights and responsibilities of the consumer is consistent with prevailing definitions of the goals of nursing, but overselling the benefits of self-responsibility may lead to yet another cycle of unrealistic consumer expectations. Shapiro (1979) urges that we be conservative in our expectations of benefits to be derived from success in helping individuals assume responsibility for their own health:

> No matter how purely we eat and drink, no matter how carefully we guard the air we breathe, no matter how much we become involved with our doctors and they with us, the mortality rate will still be 100 per cent. Not all diseases and decay are self-induced. The process of living wears us down as much as we wear ourselves down. Somehow the rhetoric of the be-responsible movement suggests that we can postpone and even reverse this inevitable process of decay. Ironically, we have come full circle to the notion of omnipotence in health care, only this time around it is not the physician who is omnipotent but the patient.

Patients have the right to expect that the nurse will help them to determine not only what they expect and desire as the outcome of their care but also to assess what it is realistic to expect. This quality of collaboration with the patient is the essence of the ethical practice of nursing, which requires a partnership with the patient, based on trust, in which the dignity of the individual and his or her right to understand and contribute to the plan of care are recognized. What competencies and considerations are required for this ethical nursing practice?

Personalization of Care

Basic to the treatment of each patient as an individual is respect for the patient as a person. This respect is demonstrated in many ways. The treatment of each patient with the same courtesy that one expects from one's associates goes a long way toward establishing the fact that the patient is an individual. This courtesy should be extended to the patient's family and friends. They have a right to be concerned about the patient and his or her welfare as well as to have a role to play in the patient's recovery. An effort should be made to allow the family to express their feelings and to interpret their behavior in the light of its meanings. The effect of their behavior on the patient should also be evaluated. When some change is necessary, explanations should be in terms of the needs of the patient and recognition should be given to the interest of the family in the welfare of the patient.

If the nurse accepts the responsibility for the welfare of the patient, she or he will intervene when the quality or quantity of visiting is likely to be detrimental to patient interests. An exaggerated, but true, example of the abdication by the nurse of the responsibility to protect the patient from harm is illustrated by the following anecdote. Mary Lively, age 17, was hospitalized on Friday night. She had been in an automobile accident and had two crushed lumbar vertebrae and some superficial scalp wounds. On the following Sunday she and her roommate had 84 visitors. When Mary's mother visited her in the evening, she found Mary in a state of near collapse. When Mrs. Lively complained, she was told that it was the responsibility of the family to regulate visitors. Though she had visited Mary in the morning, she had not been in the hospital at the time when most of the visitors arrived. She had asked that a sign be placed on the door indicating that not more than two visitors be admitted at a time. The visitors cooperated. They lined up and entered the room two at a time until the room was full. The conclusion that the nurse in this situation had lost sight of her responsibility to protect the patient and that she failed to exercise reasonable judgment is an understatement. Moreover, patients other than those immediately involved must have suffered.

One's name is a unique characteristic of each person. Therefore a way to show respect for an individual is to call him or her by name and title. Despite a trend toward informality, an adult should be called by the surname preceded by the appropriate title, that is, Mr., Mrs., or Ms. Unless there is a specific and identified reason, an adult should not be addressed by first name. Certainly first names should not be used to indicate that the social or economic status of the patient is less than that of the care givers. Calling an elderly person "Grandma" or "Grandpa" may express affection, but it may also be interpreted by the patient to indicate a lack of respect for the individual and his or her potential. Some elderly persons bitterly resent being called "Grandpa" or "Grandma" by anyone except their grandchildren. A patient who is addressed by first name or who is nameless does not always express resentment openly, but this does not mean that no resentment is felt.

Americans do not often understand it, but in most societies using one's first name—without the intermediate process of a seasoning relationship—seems rude and even disruptive. To people of many cultural backgrounds, the "relentless familiarity" of our tendency to be on a first-name basis with people from all walks of life has a cheap ring (Morrow, 1977). Only after the nurse has developed a working relationship with the patient and family will she or he be able to evaluate whether the patient would feel more comfortable with a less formal form of address.

Respect for individuals is expressed by nurses when they greet patients when entering their presence and include them in any conversation carried on in their presence. Other courtesies too often neglected include asking the permission of patients when it is necessary to interrupt their activities or care. Patients' care should not be interrupted unless it is absolutely necessary. Respect for patients as individuals also includes sensitivity to their feelings. This is expressed when nurses try to modify their behavior so that the patients know that their feelings are appreciated. Nurses try to avoid being excessively cheerful in the presence of downcast or depressed patients. On the other hand, they also avoid being depressed themselves.

Respect is evidenced when the patient's suggestions, opinions, and concerns are treated with courtesy and thoughtfulness. It is also evidenced when the nurse protects the patient from unnecessary embarrassment by protecting modesty and by helping in preparations for the visit of the physician or family.

Respect for the patient is demonstrated by creating an environment in which the patient is able to express feelings and by interpreting behavior as an expression of an unmet need or needs and then acting appropriately. Sometimes a patient who feels depersonalized is demanding and aggressive. He or she fights to be recognized as a human being. The patient may relax when certain that the nursing staff can be depended on to meet his or her needs as an individual.

Nurses are likely to find individualization of each patient's care easier if they have some awareness of their own values as well as biases and prejudices. No one is completely free of prejudice. When an individual knows his or her values, biases, and prejudices, he or she may be able to limit or maximize their effect on the care provided for the patient. An example of limiting the negative effects of prejudice is seen in the case of Mrs. Laura, a public health nurse, who took pride in being unprejudiced. One day as she was thinking about how unsuccessful she had been with the Hill family, she thought, "How could anyone be successful with those hillbillies?" As she talked about her experience later, she said she was shocked to learn that she too had prejudices and thought of people not as individuals but as stereotypes. After she recognized what she had been feeling, she was better able to manage her feelings and as a result to enlist the cooperation of Mrs. Hill.

Three situations involving the need to individualize care of a patient will be presented. In the first situation, failure to meet an obvious or overt need of the patient contributed to the patient's feeling of depersonalization and to failure of the nursing personnel to experience satisfaction. In the second situation, the nurse recognized and met a covert need of a patient. The last illustrates why it is impossible to individualize care by rule.

The first patient, Mrs. Devoted Family, had undergone major surgery several days previous to the incident cited. Following her operation, both she and her family expressed openly and volubly their concern about her progress. One of her less serious complaints, from the point of view of the personnel, was that her feet were cold. Though she complained to everyone who participated in her care, nothing was done to relieve her discomfort. Her family took their mother's discomfort seriously and bought her a lovely white wool shawl, which they placed over her feet. A few days later the shawl was discarded with the bed linen. Naturally, Mrs. Family and her children were upset. The nursing staff responded by saying that they had no responsibility for the personal belongings of the patient; nothing could be done to recover the shawl. In this instance the simple procedure of placing a bath blanket over Mrs. Family's feet might have been sufficient to relieve her discomfort. Mrs. Family might well have had her feelings of importance enhanced had the nurse placed a blanket over her feet in such a manner that the patient knew that the nurse wanted her to be comfortable. Moreover, the manner of the nurse might also have suggested that if the blanket did not accomplish the objective there were other things that she could and would do. She could give Mrs. Family a hot-water bottle (if her condition permitted) or ask her daughter to bring her some bed or ankle socks. In any event the patient's feeling of depersonalization might have been reduced by any one of several simple acts. As it was, both the patient and her family felt that Mrs. Family was neglected. She had suffered a double injury—cold feet and a lack of appropriate action to correct her discomfort as well as the loss of a valued possession. These feelings were strengthened by the loss of the shawl and failure of the nursing staff to appear to make any effort to retrieve it. The nursing staff was also deprived because they failed to achieve any sense of satisfaction in the care of Mrs. Family.

The next patient is Mr. Johnson. In the care of Mr. Johnson the nurse recognized and responded to a need that the patient was unable to express directly. Mr. Johnson was a middle-aged, obese man with a diagnosis of far advanced carcinoma of the lung. He was allowed bathroom privileges and permitted to sit in a chair as he desired. Patients who were up and about were expected to take their own sponge baths. Showers and bathtubs were not available. One busy morning just before noon his nurse stopped to check with Mr. Johnson to see whether or not he had taken his bath. In response to her inquiry he said, "I did the best I could." The nurse might have said, "I'll make your bed, or send the aide in to do it." She, however, interpreted Mr. Johnson's statement as saying, "I was not able to take a very good bath and I'd like to be given one." She thought a moment about his reply and realized that although he was up and about even a small amount of exertion caused Mr. Johnson to be short of breath. She got a basin of warm water and *gave* him a bath. As she was bathing him, he lay back against his pillows, sighed, and relaxed, saying, "This is the first bath that I've had since I came here."

The third patient is Mrs. Willow, a young middle-aged woman who some months earlier had had a radical mastectomy for cancer of the breast. The cancer has since metastasized to her spine and now impinged on her spinal cord. She was unable to control the movements of her lower extremities. Slight movement or jarring of her body resulted in muscular spasms accompanied by severe pain. Mrs. Willow was in the hospital for the purpose of determining the amount of a curarizing drug that would control the muscular spasms without paralyzing the muscles of respiration. After spending 3 days in a ten-bed ward, she was moved to a double room and was placed in the bed next to the door. She spent her days sitting in bed and guarding herself each time someone came into the room. Her general expression was that of a frightened fawn. In this instance the head nurse at the daily nursing care conference talked with the group about Mrs. Willow. Together they worked out ways to protect Mrs. Willow from avoidable suffering. A sign was placed on the door to warn those who were entering to avoid jarring her bed. The dietary aide was asked to call a nurse when Mrs. Willow's tray was ready rather than to deliver it to the room. As soon as the patient in the bed away from the door was discharged, Mrs. Willow's bed was moved. A special procedure was planned with Mrs. Willow so that her bed linen could be changed without causing her unnecessary discomfort. Other procedures were also modified. Information about Mrs. Willow's special needs and techniques for meeting those needs were communicated to all staff members by written entries on the nursing kardex and on the progress notes of her record.

Though there was no possibility of cure for either Mr. Johnson or Mrs. Willow, both these patients benefited from thoughtful and creative nursing. In both these instances, the nurses also experienced satisfaction, inasmuch as they concentrated on and were able to improve the situation of the patient. In the care of these patients, nurses demonstrated their concern for the welfare of the patient largely through physical care, and they exercised judgment within the realm of nursing. In neither instance was the amount of time involved great. In fact, time was probably saved in the care of Mrs. Willow.

Preparation of Patients for What to Expect

The patient needs and is entitled to an explanation of the care given, which prepares the patient not only for what to expect but also for what is expected of her or him. Wertham (1952), a psychiatrist, commented on his own experience as a patient: "Medical and surgical patients need psychological advice about how they should act, what their experiences mean; they need psychological preparation for what to expect; they need guidance, so that they can make the best of their possibilities."

Not all patients need or want the same informational preparation. Based on responses of 139 medical–surgical patients and their nurses to the importance of 60 information items, Dodge (1972) concluded that patients want specific information about their condition, and nurses think it is more important for patients to know what to expect in care.

A sound principle to guide the nurse in deciding what information is necessary for preparing any patient for what to expect is to inform the patient about those aspects of his or her condition and care that require some changes in behavior. A patient frequently requires information about such hospital routines as when meals are served and medicines administered, when friends may visit or telephone, and how to call the nurse. He or she needs to know the extent of, and reasons for, limitations on freedom to move about. In addition, the patient needs to have some idea about how he or she will feel during subsequent events in treatment and care. Johnson (1972) contends that much of the discomfort or distress experienced by patients in the course of their experience with medical and nursing care derives from inadequate or erroneous information about the sensory component of the experience. She is conducting a number of laboratory and field studies to test her hypothesis that a discrepancy between expectations about sensations and experience during a threatening event results in distress (Johnson, 1975).

To prepare patients to participate in and benefit from their care requires a broad spectrum of skills, but perhaps the most critical skill to the nurse's success is *communication.* Most people who are ill, or who have submitted themselves for examination or treatment by health care professionals are experiencing some degree of anxiety. In assessing and intervening to help an anxious person, the nurse must enable the person to reveal the nature and source of distress if she or he is to be successful in helping to improve the patient's ability to cope with the situation. The nurse who can approach the patient with appropriate self-disclosure communication will usually be more effective in helping the person cope than will the nurse whose communication is more impersonal. This predicted outcome derives from two related propositions:

1. As anxiety levels tend to increase, levels of self-disclosure tend to decrease.
2. Self-disclosure behavior in one person encourages the other to self-disclose, thereby reducing anxiety in both persons (Johnson, 1979).

In a study of the effects of anxiety on disclosure between seventy nurses and sixty-eight patients in medical–surgical, psychiatric, and critical care units, Johnson (1979) found evidence to support the first proposition, that anxiety responses to stress decrease levels of self-disclosure. However, to the detriment of the patients, there was low reciprocal self-disclosure between nurses and patients. The nurse who has little or no information about what the patient is experiencing has a critical deficiency in the data base needed to provide effective care.

Preparing children for what to expect in their care presents special problems, due in part to their fears and their inability to verbalize them. Miller (1979) reviewed, from a developmental perspective, all published research on children's fears. Findings suggest that children's fears change with age in a way that may parallel cognitive and perceptual development, with fears becoming better articulated, more varied, and more realistic as children move from age 1 to 12 years. An indispensable part of the data base for nursing care—particularly for children, but also for adolescents and adults—is description of the patient's fears. From that data will come guidance for structuring the patient's perceptions of threatening events in such a way that distress and anxiety can be decreased and coping ability increased.

Because of the effects of high levels of anxiety on the ability to attend and to learn, anxious patients frequently need to have instructions repeated a number of times. Because the patient often has questions about his or her illness and the plan of therapy, the nurse will find it helpful to know what information the physician has given the patient. Even when the physician has given the patient a careful explanation of the disease and of what is required in its treatment, the patient may have failed to comprehend what was said. When the nurse knows what the patient has been told, she or he can answer the patient's questions or refer them to the physician with the expectation that tension will be relieved rather than increased.

Part of preparing the patient for what to expect is to determine what the patient expects and wants to know. Patients are frequently subjected to unnecessary anxiety unless time has been taken to determine what their expectations are. To illustrate, Mrs. Fox, who had had heart surgery 2 weeks previously, was found lying on a cart in the hall outside the room where cardiac catheterizations were performed. The nurse who stopped to greet her learned that she had "been waiting for hours," and that she expected "to be stabbed in the back" without benefit of anesthesia. However, the catheter was to be introduced through an arm vein, and if someone had taken the time to determine her understanding of the procedure and to correct her misinformation, she might have been relieved of unnecessary suffering. Moreover, she might have been less apprehensive if someone had stayed with her.

Determination of what the patient expects and wants to know helps to prevent giving information that suggests problems or difficulties that were not anticipated. Wertham (1952) made this point in regard to his own situation. A surgeon made the comment to him that phlebitis seldom affects the arms. Previous to this time the possibility that his arms might be involved had not occurred to him, and it became a source of worry. He found himself trying to detect pain first in one arm and then in the other.

Participation of Patient as Partner in Care

Patients are helped to be partners in their own care when they are prepared for what to expect and for what is expected of them. When they are able to help themselves by such activities as exercising, deep breathing, and coughing, they know that they have a part in recovery. Moreover, appraisal of how long a painful procedure will take and comments indicating progress help to keep the patients informed about how long they have to continue to brace themselves. Further, both types of comments assure patients that the person who is performing the procedure is aware of their needs. They are then better able to follow instructions relative to their part in the procedure.

A patient is often asked to assume responsibility for aspects of his or her own care. When this is done, the patient should be encouraged to take this responsibility because it furthers recovery. Too often patients gain the impression that they are asked to bathe themselves or ambulate because the nurses are too busy or do not want to care for them rather than because activity is part of their therapeutic regimen.

At other times patients wish to retain certain responsibilities or privileges. These are sometimes denied them without adequate thought being given to the reason for the refusal or to the value that the responsibility has to them. To illustrate, Mrs. Lottie Gamely had disseminated cancer of the breast which had metastasized to the cervical spine. She was in more or less constant pain and was very fearful lest any activity increase it. Her husband brought her some tablets of Empirin[1] compound, which she planned to take as needed. In the course of giving her care, the nurse discovered the Empirin in her

[1] Trade name for tablets containing phenacetin, 0.15 g (gr. 2½); acetylsalicylic acid, 0.23 g (gr. 3½); and caffeine 30 mg (gr. ½).

bedside table. Before removing the medication, she talked with Mrs. Gamely's physician. The decision was made to leave the drug at the bedside because it gave Mrs. Gamely the feeling that she had some control over her pain.[2] The possibility of any harm resulting was negligible. Later this patient expressed her feeling that she was a partner in her care. This was revealed when the nurse told Mrs. Gamely that she was going on vacation and that she had enjoyed working with her. Mrs. Gamely responded by saying, "I've enjoyed working with you, too."

The satisfaction of the wish of the patient to be considered a partner in care depends on the belief that each individual, sick or well, has a right to participate in plans concerning his or her welfare. The nurse has a responsibility to provide the individual with the information needed in order to consider the alternatives, to carry out a decision after it is made, or to change his or her mind. Sometimes a patient is pressed to make decisions that he or she is unable or unprepared to make. If the patient feels censured or blamed for failing to make the "right" decision, he or she may be unable to change the decision. Physicians and nurses sometimes forget that a patient may be asked to adjust to or make a decision about a procedure that may affect the entire course of life and to do it quickly. Human beings tend to react to change with anxiety. Excessive anxiety makes the objective evaluation of the situation by the patient difficult, if not impossible.

In the practice of nursing, the nurse will see persons whose diseases require prompt action and yet who refuse treatment. The nurse's first obligation is to try to determine the extent to which the person understands the nature and purpose of the proposed treatment and its significance to his or her health and survival. If the individual reveals misconceptions, either about the severity of the condition or about the nature and purpose of the medical treatment, the nurse then works collaboratively with the physician to clarify the patient's understanding. However, if the refusal to accept treatment derives from concerns that have priority for the individual over health, or even survival, then the nurse is responsible to identify the nature of the need which is preeminent, to respond to that need if possible, or to help the individual mobilize appropriate resources to address the need. In addition, the nurse works collaboratively with the physician to gain the person's cooperation with whatever medical therapy will provide comfort and palliation.

[2] In increasing numbers of health care institutions, selected patients assume responsibility for taking their own medications.

References Cited

"AHA adopts Patients' Bill of Rights." *Am. J. Nurs.*, **73** (March 1973), 418.

Anderson, L. C. "The Nurse and Research." *Milt. Med.*, **121** (1957), 308–11.

Bayles, M. D. "Against Professional Autonomy." *Nat. Forum*, **58** (Summer 1978), 23–26.

Chiles, R. E. "The Rights of Patients." *N. Engl. J. Med.*, **277** (24 Aug. 1967), 409–11.

Committee on Ethical, Legal and Professional Standards. *The Code for Nurses*, Kansas City, Mo.: American Nurses Assoc., 1968.

Daubert, E. A. "Patient Classification System and Outcome Criteria." *Nurs. Outlook*, **27** (July 1979), 450–454.

Davidites, R. M. "A Social Systems Approach to Deviant Behavior." *Am. J. Nurs.*, **71** (Aug. 1971), 1588–89.

Dodge, J. S. "What Patients Should Be Told: Patients' and Nurses' Beliefs." *Am. J. Nurs.*, **72** (Oct. 1972), 1852–54.

Gebbie, K., and Lavin, M. A. "Classifying Nursing Diagnoses." *Am. J. Nurs.*, **44** (Feb. 1974), 250–53.

Gordon, G. "To Live or Not to Live with Your Job." *Nurs. Forum*, **1** (Winter 1961–1962), 38.

Gordon, M. "Nursing Diagnosis and the Diagnostic Process." *Am. J. Nurs.* **76** (Aug. 1976), 1298–1300.

Gribbin, A. "The Medical Misfits." *The National Observer*, 21 April 1973.

Grosicki, J. P. "Effect of Operant Conditioning on Modification of Incontinence in Neuropsychiatric Geriatric Patients." *Nurs. Res.*, **17**:4 (July–Aug. 1968), 304–11.

Hitt, R. "The POW Story: Seven Years of Prison and Prayer." *Eternity*, June 1973, p. 48.

Holden, C. "Holistic Health Concepts Gaining Momentum. *Science*, **200** (2 June 1978), 1029.

Johnson, J. E. "Effects of Structuring Patients' Expectations on Their Reactions to Threatening Events." *Nurs. Res.*, **21** (Nov.–Dec. 1972), 499–504.

Johnson, J. E., et al. "Altering Children's Distress Behavior during Orthopedic Cast Removal." *Nurs. Res.*, **24** (Nov.–Dec. 1975), 404–10.

Johnson, M. N. "Anxiety/Stress and the Effects on Disclosure between Nurses and Patients." *Advances in Nurs. Sci.*, **1** (July 1979), 1–20.

Kibrick, A. "Nursing '73: Time for New Leadership." *Nurs. Outlook*, **21** (April 1973), 227.

King, S. H. *Perceptions of Illness and Medical Practice.* New York: Russell Sage Foundation, 1962, p. 43.

Knowles, J. H. "Responsibility for Health." *Science*, **198** (16 Dec. 1977), 1103.

Maslow, A. H. *Motivation and Personality.* New York: Harper & Row, Publishers, 1954.

Mikulic, M. A. "Reinforcement of Independent and Dependent Patient Behaviors by Nursing Personnel: An Exploratory Study." *Nurs. Res.*, **20** (March–April 1971), 162–65.

Miller, S. R. "Children's Fears: A Review of the Literature with Implications for Nursing Research and Practice. *Nurs. Res.*, **28** (July–Aug. 1979), 217–23.

Morrow, L. "A Nation without Last Names." *Time,* 11 July 1977, p. 43.

Murray, H. A. *Explorations in Personality.* New York: Oxford University Press, 1938, pp. 123–24.

"Patient's Bill of Rights Now Law." *The Mass. Nurse,* **48** (July 1979), 1–2.

Roberts, S. L. *Behavioral Concepts and Nursing throughout the Life Span.* Englewood Cliffs, N.J.: Prentice-Hall, Inc., 1978.

Schwartz, D. et al. *The Elderly Ambulatory Patient: Nursing and Psychosocial Needs.* New York: Macmillan Publishing Co., Inc., 1964.

Shapiro, J. "The Psychology of Responsibility." *N. Engl. J. Med.,* **301** (26 July 1979), 211–12.

Skinner, B. F. *Behavior of Organisms.* New York: Appleton-Century Company, 1938.

Weiss, T., and Engel, B. T. "Operant Conditioning of Heart Rate in Patients with Premature Ventricular Contractions." *Psychosom. Med.,* **33**:4 (July–Aug. 1971), 301–20.

Wertham, F. "A Psychosomatic Study of Myself. In *When Doctors Are Patients.* Ed. by M. Pinner and B. Miller. New York: W. W. Norton & Company, Inc., 1952, p. 115.

"A Woman's View of Health Care." *The Sunday News Magazine,* (Detroit, Mich.), 29 April 1973.

General References

Abdellah, F. G., Beland, I. L., Martin, A., and Matheney, R. V. *New Directions in Patient-Centered Nursing.* New York: Macmillan Publishing Co., Inc., 1973.

Anthony, W. A., and Carkhuff, R. R. *The Art of Health Care: A Handbook of Psychological First Aid Skills.* Amherst, Mass.: Human Resources Development Press, Inc., 1976.

Smith, D. W. "Patienthood and Its Threat to Privacy." *Am. J. Nurs.,* **69** (March 1969), 508–13.

Sutterley, D., and Donnelly, G. *Perspectives in Human Development: Nursing throughout the Life Cycle,* 2nd ed. Philadelphia: J. B. Lippincott Company, 1980.

Veatch, R. M. *Case Studies in Medical Ethics.* Cambridge, Mass.: Harvard University Press, 1977.

8

The Nurse, the Nursing Process, and Its Documentation

Greek scientists in their century or two of life remade the universe. They leaped to the truth by an intuition, they saw a whole made up of related parts, and with the sweep of their vision the old world of hodgepodge and magic fell away and a world of order took its place. They could only begin the detailed investigation of the parts, but, ever since, Science has by an infinite labor confirmed their intuition of the whole. Greek artists found a disorganized world of human beings, a complex mass made up of units unrelated and disordered, and they too had an intuition of parts all belonging to a whole. They saw what is permanently important in a man and unites him to the rest.

EDITH HAMILTON
Hamilton, Edith: *The Greek Way* New York: W. W. Norton & Company, Inc., 1942, p. 336

Definitions of Nursing by the Profession

During our transition from an agrarian to a scientific–humanistic society, the dominant functions of nursing have been modified as an inevitable consequence of changes in the social, economic, political, educational, and scientific–technological milieu in which the consumer and practitioner of nursing meet. As functions change and proliferate, consensus among nurses on the essence of nursing has continued to elude us. The elusiveness of a sound and lasting definition of nursing as a practice discipline is undoubtedly due in large part to the fact that there has been more theorizing than data gathering about nursing practice. Positions taken in this century on the nature and contribution of nursing have resulted more often from deductive than from inductive reasoning, as evidenced by Henderson's (1972) review of published studies in nursing from 1900 through 1959. Review of the years 1957 to 1959 revealed less than a dozen studies concerned with characterizing patients' needs for nursing care. Only one study was addressed to the processes by which the nurse identifies nursing problems, (Abdellah, 1957), and none sought relationships between care provided and changes in patterns of patients' needs or responses. Fortunately, much progress has been made in both the quality and quantity of patient-care studies conducted by nurses within the decade of the 1970s, due largely to the increased number of well-prepared nurses who are functioning in the field of clinical nursing.

However, the attempt to define nursing goes back well beyond the turn of the century, for over 100 years ago Florence Nightingale (1860, p. 2) wrote that nursing signified "little more than the administration of medicines and the application of poultices." She continued by saying that it ought to signify the proper use of fresh air, warmth, cleanliness, and quiet and the proper selection and administration of diet—all at the least expense of vital power to the patient. Moreover, Miss Nightingale (1860,

p. 4) did not limit nursing to the care of the sick, for she wrote, "The same laws of health, or of nursing, for they are in reality the same, obtain among the well as among the sick."

The relatively stable essence of nursing is captured in one of the most widely quoted definitions of nursing, by Henderson (1978, p. 34).

> The unique function of nurses is to help people, sick or well, in the performance of those activities contributing to health or its recovery (or to a peaceful death) that they would perform unaided if they had the necessary strength, will or knowledge. It is likewise the function of nurses to help people gain independence as rapidly as possible.

Henderson (1964, p. 63) proposed fourteen activities contributing to health with which nursing is responsible for assisting the individual, and suggested that existing or potential loss of the power to control or perform those activities signals the existence of a nursing problem. A time dimension has been introduced into the definition of nursing by Rubin (1968), who states that "enabling another to achieve control of function appropriate in time and space may well be a succinct description of *nursing*," and by Orlando (1972, p. 8), who contends that "nursing is historically rooted in an immediate responsiveness to individuals assumed to be suffering helplessness in immediate situations." Orlando believes that the fundamental task of professional nursing in patient care is to give sufficient attention to the patient's reactions in the immediate experiences to help him or her avoid, or obtain relief or diminution of helplessness suffered or anticipated.

The nursing literature of the last decade or so has produced a plethora of expository pronouncements on the nature, philosophy, and science of nursing. From these has emerged a recurrent theme that *nursing is a service to help people adapt at an optimal level of function within their own goal systems.*

Necessary Personal Attributes

Somewhat paradoxically, there have been many fewer changes in definitions of the essence of nursing throughout the last century than there have been in stipulations of the personal attributes presumed to be necessary to function effectively as a nurse. Florence Nightingale's requirements for a nurse seem, in this era of emphasis on assertiveness and power-brokering in nursing, strangely incongruous with her visionary emphasis on health promotion as the essence of nursing. She required that a nurse be:

1. Chaste, in the sense of the Sermon on the Mount
2. Sober, in spirit as well as in drink
3. Honest
4. Truthful
5. Trustworthy to carry out directions intelligently and perfectly
6. Punctual to a second
7. Quiet yet quick; quick without hurry; gentle without slowness; discreet without self-importance
8. Cheerful, hopeful
9. Cleanly to the point of exquisiteness
10. Thinking of the patient and not of herself (Seymer, 1954)

Another dramatic illustration of the change in stipulated attributes is the relationship of the nurse to the physician. In 1907, Isabel Hampton Robb required "implicit obedience and loyalty to the physician" (Robb, 1907). This attribute can be a liability for current practice. In the decade of the 1970s, nurses have been held responsible in court for failure to report physicians' mistakes. Stanley (1979, p. 27) proposes that each nurse is ethically and legally responsible to "report any concern about medical practice to the person involved, and then to administrative personnel if the situation is serious. Make sure any behavior you observe is documented, and take the problem outside the hospital if there is no response to your first steps."

Functions as Measured by Licensing Examination

Behaving accountably not only in one's own practice but also in relation to the performance of other practitioners involves a high degree of risk taking by the nurse, which must rest solidly on a strong self-concept and a rich and current fund of knowledge. These characteristics are difficult to measure, and there has long been concern within the nursing profession about the extent to which the national State Board Test Pool Examination (SBTPE) constitutes a valid measure of the critical performance requirements for safe and effective nursing practice. In 1971, the Council of State Boards of Nursing authorized the National League for Nursing to conduct a study to examine the validity of the SBTPE. The criterion test was to be developed from behaviors identified by content analysis of over 13,000 critical incidents of nursing behaviors collected from 2,795 nurses at all levels of experience and responsibility in five clinical specialties: medical–surgical, maternal–newborn, pediatric, community health, and psychiatric nursing. Participants from 67 health care agencies in all 4 geographic regions of the country contributed descriptions of incidents in which there

TABLE 8-1. ***Ten Areas of Behavior Identified as Critical Requirements for Safe–Effective Nursing Practice****

I. Exercises professional prerogatives based on clinical judgment
II. Promotes patient's ability to cope with immediate, long-range, or potential health-related change
III. Helps maintain patient comfort and normal body functions
IV. Takes precautionary and preventive measures in giving patient care
V. Checks, compares, verifies, monitors, and follows up medication and treatment processes
VI. Interprets symptom complex and intervenes appropriately
VII. Responds to emergencies
VIII. Obtains, records, and exchanges information on behalf of the patient
IX. Utilizes patient care planning
X. Teaches and supervises other staff

* Subcategories and examples of these behavioral categories are reported in Jacobs, A. M., Fivars, G., Edwards, D. S., and Fitzpatrick, R., *Critical Requirements for Safe-Effective Nursing Practice,* Kansas City, Mo.: American Nurses' Association, 1978.

had been a "near miss" in relation to the comfort, safety, or well-being of patients, clients, or families. The 10 areas of behavior in the resultant category structure of Critical Requirements for Safe-Effective Nursing Practice appear in Table 8-1. See Appendix A for the complete category structure of Critical Requirements for Safe-Effective Nursing Practice.

STANDARDS OF NURSING PRACTICE

The official definition of nursing by the profession is the result of pooling expert opinion, and it is contained in the generic Standards of Nursing Practice first drafted by the Congress for Nursing Practice of the American Nurses' Association in 1971 (Congress for Nursing Practice, 1973; 1975). The generic standards apply to nursing practice in any setting; elaboration for practice with distinct populations is found in the sets of standards subsequently formulated by the various divisions on practice of the American Nurses' Association. Each standard is supported by a rationale and by assessment factors, which are to be used in determining achievement of the standard. The generic Standards of Nursing Practice appear in Table 8-2.

TABLE 8-2. ***Generic Standards of Nursing Practice (Council for Nursing Practice, 1973)***

Standard I

The Collection of Data about the Health Status of the Client/Patient Is Systematic and Continuous. The Data Are Accessible, Communicated, and Recorded.

Rationale: Comprehensive care requires complete and ongoing collection of data about the client/patient to determine the nursing care needs of the client/patient. All health status data about the client/patient must be available for all members of the health care team.

Assessment Factors:

1. Health status data include:
   —Growth and development
   —Biophysical status
   —Emotional status
   —Cultural, religious, socioeconomic background
   —Performance of activities of daily living
   —Patterns of coping
   —Interaction patterns
   —Client's/patient's perception of and satisfaction with his health status
   —Environment (physical, social, emotional, ecological)
   —Available and accessible human and material resources
2. Data are collected from:
   —Client/patient, family, significant others
   —Health care personnel
   —Individuals within the immediate environment and/or the community

Continued . . . .

Table 8-2 *(Continued)*

3. Data are obtained by:
   —Interview
   —Examination
   —Observation
   —Reading records, reports, etc.
4. There is a format for the collection of data which:
   —Provides for a systematic collection of data
   —Facilitates the completeness of data collection
5. Continuous collection of data is evident by:
   —Frequent updating
   —Recording of changes in health status
6. The data are:
   —Accessible on the client/patient records
   —Retrievable from record-keeping systems
   —Confidential when appropriate

Standard II
Nursing Diagnoses Are Derived from Health Status Data.

Rationale: The health status of the client/patient is the basis for determining the nursing care needs. The data are analyzed and compared to norms when possible.

Assessment Factors:
1. The client's/patient's health status is compared to the norm in order to determine if there is a deviation from the norm and the degree and direction of deviation.
2. The client's/patient's capabilities and limitations are identified.
3. The nursing diagnoses are related to and congruent with the diagnoses of all other professionals caring for the client/patient.

Standard III
The Plan of Nursing Care Includes Goals Derived from the Nursing Diagnoses.

Rationale: The determination of the results to be achieved is an essential part of planning care.

Assessment Factors:
1. Goals are mutually set with the client/patient and pertinent others:
   —They are congruent with other planned therapies.
   —They are stated in realistic and measurable terms.
   —They are assigned a time period for achievement.
2. Goals are established to maximize functional capabilities and are congruent with:
   —Growth and development
   —Biophysical status
   —Behavioral patterns
   —Human and material resources

Standard IV
The Plan of Nursing Care Includes Priorities and the Prescribed Nursing Approaches or Measures to Achieve the Goals Derived from the Nursing Diagnoses.

Rationale: Nursing actions are planned to promote, maintain and restore the client's/patient's well-being.

Assessment Factors:
1. Physiological measures are planned to manage (prevent or control) specific patient problems and are related to the nursing diagnoses and goals of care, e.g. ADL, use of self-help devices, etc.
2. Psychosocial measures are specific to the client's/patient's nursing care problem and to the nursing care goals, e.g. techniques to control aggression, motivation.
3. Teaching-learning principles are incorporated into the plan of care and objectives for learning stated in behavioral terms, e.g. specification of content for learner's level, reinforcement, readiness, etc.
4. Approaches are planned to provide for a therapeutic environment:
   —Physical environmental factors are used to influence the therapeutic environment, e.g. control of noise, control of temperature, etc.
   —Psychosocial measures are used to structure the environment for therapeutic ends, e.g. paternal participation in all phases of the maternity experience.
   —Group behaviors are used to structure interaction and influence the therapeutic environment, e.g. conformity, ethos, territorial rights, locomotion, etc.

Continued . . . .

TABLE 8-2 *(Continued)*

5. Approaches are specified for orientation of the client/patient to:
   —New roles and relationships
   —Relevant health (human and material) resources.
   —Modifications in plan of nursing care
   —Relationship of modifications in nursing care plan to the total care plan
6. The plan of nursing care includes the utilization of available and appropriate resources:
   —Human resources—other health personnel
   —Material resources
   —Community
7. The plan includes an ordered sequence of nursing actions.
8. Nursing approaches are planned on the basis of current scientific knowledge.

Standard V
Nursing Actions Provide for Client/Patient Participation in Health Promotion, Maintenance and Restoration.

Rationale: The client/patient and family are continually involved in nursing care.

Assessment Factors:
1. The client/patient and family are kept informed about:
   —Current health status
   —Changes in health status
   —Total health care plan
   —Nursing care plan
   —Roles of health care personnel
   —Health care resources
2. The client/patient and family are provided with the information needed to make decisions and choices about:
   —Promoting, maintaining and restoring health
   —Seeking and utilizing appropriate health care personnel
   —Maintaining and using health care resources

Standard VI
Nursing Actions Assist the Client/Patient to Maximize His Health Capabilities.

Rationale: Nursing actions are designed to promote, maintain and restore health.

Assessment Factors:
1. Nursing actions:
   —Are consistent with the plan of care.
   —Are based on scientific principles.
   —Are individualized to the specific situation.
   —Are used to provide a safe and therapeutic environment.
   —Employ teaching-learning opportunities for the client/patient.
   —Include utilization of appropriate resources.
2. Nursing actions are directed by the client's/patient's physical, physiological, psychological and social behavior associated with:
   —Ingestion of food, fluid and nutrients
   —Elimination of body wastes and excesses in fluid
   —Locomotion and exercise
   —Regulatory mechanisms—body heat, metabolism
   —Relating to others
   —Self-actualization

Standard VII
The Client's/Patient's Progress or Lack of Progress toward Goal Achievement Is Determined by the Client/Patient and Nurse.

Rationale: The quality of nursing care depends upon comprehensive and intelligent determination of nursing's impact upon the health status of the client/patient. The client/patient is an essential part of this determination.

Assessment Factors:
1. Current data about the client/patient are used to measure his progress toward goal achievement.
2. Nursing actions are analyzed for their effectiveness in the goal achievement of the client/patient.
3. The client/patient evaluates nursing actions and goal achievement.

Continued . . . .

Table 8-2 *(Continued)*

4. Provision is made for nursing follow-up of a particular client/patient to determine the long-term effects of nursing care.

Standard VIII

The Client's/Patient's Progress or Lack of Progress toward Goal Achievement Directs Reassessment, Reordering of Priorities, New Goal Setting and Revision of the Plan of Nursing Care.

Rationale: The nursing process remains the same, but the input of new information may dictate new or revised approaches.

Assessment Factors:

1. Reassessment is directed by goal achievement or lack of goal achievement.
2. New priorities and goals are determined and additional nursing approaches are prescribed appropriately.
3. New nursing actions are accurately and appropriately initiated.

Used with permission of the American Nurses' Association, from *Standards of Nursing Practice,* Kansas City, Mo.: American Nurses' Association, 1973, by the Congress for Nursing Practice, Pub. No. NP-41 180M 12/73.

Educational Preparation for Entry into Nursing Practice

Despite the growing consensus on the characteristics of and requirements for the practice of professional nursing, debate has raged for decades about what constitutes appropriate minimal educational preparation for entry into nursing practice. The debate about distinctions between levels of nursing education and practice intensified in the wake of the 1978 American Nurses' Association Convention, which passed a resolution that the baccalaureate degree should be the minimum preparation for entry into professional nursing practice by 1985 (ANA Convention '78, 1978, p. 1232). With few exceptions, proponents of both sides of the debate rest their positions on a very limited data base. Absence of patient data in support of arguments for or against proliferation of levels of preparation for nurses has fostered dissension within nursing and has added to confusion about nursing in public forums. Despite their confusion, consumers are amazingly consistent in what they expect from nursing.

Definitions of Nursing by the Consumer

What Patients Want from Nursing

In 1957, Abdellah and Levine (1957) reported a study conducted to determine what patients want from nursing. Their findings indicated that a patient wants

1. To be treated as an individual, that is, he wants his care to be personalized rather than depersonalized
2. An explanation of his care
3. To be considered as a partner in his care
4. To have his behavior as a sick person accepted as a part of his illness
5. To be treated with thoughtfulness, kindness, and firmness

The importance to patient welfare of personalized caring from nursing has been more often heralded than provided by nurses. Norris (1973) contends that "if there is any group of people who do not feel cared for by nurses or other health professionals, it is the American public—sick or well." She claims that the notion that nursing is patient-centered is a delusion that overlooks the fact that the needs of physicians, demands of the system or bureaucracy, secretarial duties, supervision of innumerable personnel, and urgent needs of many patients all take precedence over consideration of and concern for individual patients. This conflict between multiple demands of the work situation and nursing's professed commitment to personalized caring constitutes a persistent dilemma for practicing nurses.

Murphy (1979), a nurse ethicist, has described the present century as a dark period in the history of nursing ethics. She attributes the deterioration in the nurse–patient relationship to the effect of the social forces of technology and the bureaucratization of health care institutions. In her research on the moral reasoning of nurses, Murphy has found three basic models of the nurse-patient relationship exhibited by nurses faced with moral conflict arising between responding to human needs and adhering to the commands of authority: (1) the bureaucratic model; (2) the physician-advocate model; and (3) the patient-advocate model. Murphy's findings indicate that a significant number of nurses are not oriented toward the rights and claims of patients when ethical conflicts must be faced.

Serious and sustained efforts must be made in both preprofessional and continuing education programs to develop and evaluate the ability of nurses to engage in moral reasoning and to act in ethical conflicts as the patient advocate.

In the 15 years following Abdellah and Levine's study, expectations of nursing by consumers appear to have been adversely affected, perhaps by encounters with the realities described by Norris. In 1972, White (1972) reported on a study, done in three metropolitan hospitals, of the opinions of 100 nurses and 300 of their assigned patients. Each respondent was asked to rate 50 nursing activities on a scale of extreme to no importance. Patients and nurses agreed on the extreme importance of carrying out physicians' orders and the slight importance of preparation for discharge. Patients attributed greater importance than nurses to physical care, and nurses attributed greater importance than patients to psychosocial aspects of care. Nursing activities classified by White as psychosocial aspects of care included items addressed to the personalized caring which Abdellah and Levine's subjects wanted from nursing. A possible explanation for the findings in White's study is that patients responded in terms of the way the world is, whereas nurses responded in terms of the way the world ought to be.

In 1979, a survey of 1,000 adult consumers matched to the U.S. census was conducted to determine how nurses rate with the public (Lee, 1979(a)). Results indicated that nurses seem to be held in "heartwarming esteem" by the public, but an esteem founded on nursing's long-standing aura of absolute dependability and concern rather than on the public's clear recognition of nurses' expertise. "What the public appears to *value* most is the traditional 'dedicated handmaiden'; four out of five people still adhere to the traditional view, and two-thirds of the respondents regard nurses as doctors' assistants" (Lee, 1979 (a), p. 25). This opinion is shared by three out of four physicians in a national sample of over 500 physicians surveyed to determine how they rate nurses (Lee, 1979 (b)); 75 per cent regard nurses as their assistants, and nothing more, although they respect nurses and highly value nursing's contribution to the well-being of patients.

Public Image of Nurses' Expanded Role

The one exception to the public's traditional image of nursing is the growing awareness and support of "expanded role" nursing. Sixty per cent of respondents believe that nurses should perform some procedures now done mainly by physicians; but their justification was to cut health care costs (Lee, 1979 (a), p. 37). The vast majority of both the physicians and consumers surveyed agreed that nurses should spend more time with patients; it would appear that at least in defining nursing as a personal and direct service, the profession, the public, and physicians agree.

Children's Perceptions of Nursing

Apparently children's perceptions of nursing are somewhat closer to the profession's definition of nursing than are the perceptions of adults. Children's images of nurses were inferred from a survey of 134 children from 8 to 11 years of age, who were asked four questions: What do nurses do? What do you like/dislike about nurses? Would you want to be a nurse? (Robinson, 1979). A slim majority of the children perceived the nurse as devoted to helping people, as opposed to focusing on tasks.

Nursing Role	Percentage of Respondents
People helper	58
Task-oriented worker	51
Doctor's helper	34
Mother figure/caretaker	15
Giver of treats	10
Authority figure	1.5

The growing number of nurses engaged in expanded roles and independent nursing practice are a potential catalyst to change consumer expectations of nursing, provided that those nurses retain a strong commitment to nursing. In a study of the image of nursing, Benton (1979) interviewed eighteen master's prepared psychiatric/mental health nurses, six of whom were engaged in independent nursing practice; four of the six independent nurse practitioners declined to identify themselves as nurses to their clients. Benton commented on the grave implications of such marginal commitment:

> In essence, we have a circular situation in which the public and stereotyped image of nursing remains unattractive to many potential candidates, yet the nurses who function in nontraditional and possibly more appealing and challenging roles are not visible enough *as nurses* to change the public image of nursing. (Benton, 1979, p. 392)

In the final analysis, the legal definition of nursing is the official statement expressed in the Nurse Practice Act of each state. Both the consumer and the nurse contribute to this legal definition.

Some Roles of the Nurse in Patient Care

In responding appropriately to what patients require and desire from nursing, a nurse plays many roles. Sociologists suggest that the actions taken by nurses in the care of patients can be classified under two roles. One, the therapeutic or instrumental role, includes all those actions directed toward the prevention and treatment of disease. The other is the expressive role or mother-substitute role. It includes all those activities directed toward creating an environment in which the patient feels comforted, accepted, protected, cared for, and supported. The emphasis in the performance of the expressive role is not on cure, but on care. Johnson and Martin (1958) and Schulman (1958) emphasize that the physical care of the patient is an important vehicle for communicating to the patient the concern of the nurse for his or her welfare. Physical care is made professional by the manner in which it is provided and by the degree to which the nurse identifies and meets other needs of the patient. Nurses too often fail to respect the importance of physical care to the patient, both to his or her immediate welfare and as a means of establishing a helping relationship.

The critical significance of physical contact in establishing a helping relationship with a person who is physically ill derives from the association between space and interpersonal relationship. Hall (1966), based on his study of the distance used between people in interaction with each other, identified four personal distance zones that reflect how those interacting feel about each other: intimate zone, 0 to 1½ feet; personal zone, 1½ to 4 feet; social zone, 4 to 12 feet; and public zone, 12 to 25 feet. The nurse must breach the boundary of the intimate zone to obtain information about the patient's physical status and to minister to physical needs. In interviews with adult patients on acute medical and surgical units to obtain their recollections of and reactions to touch and closeness with nurses, Durr (1971) found that 62 per cent of the patients reported that nurses spent the most time within the intimate zone, especially when they were very ill. More important, patients believed that this was the appropriate area for nurses to occupy. Obviously, skillful use of the hands by nurses is necessary not only to monitor and apply medical therapy to patients' bodily functions and to ensure that their physical needs are met, but also to communicate the nurse's respect and compassion for the individual.

The Context of Role Relationships

Both space and time are critical ingredients in judging the appropriateness of the context within which the nurse works to fulfill both the therapeutic-instrument and the expressive roles with the patient. Cultures view the importance of context, and thus the use of space and time, very differently. Hall (Friedman, 1979) proposes that the cultures of the world can be placed on a continuum, based on the amount of communication contained in the nonverbal context compared with the amount in the verbal message. Some cultures, like our own, are low-context, which means that they tend to put more emphasis on the verbal message and less on the context. In a low-context culture, you "get down to business" very quickly. In a high-context culture, it takes considerably longer to get to the business at hand, because people have developed a need to know more about you before a relationship can develop. The source of most of the really important information is nonverbal communication.

Nonverbal Communication in Role Performance

Fully 65 per cent of all communication between people is nonverbal (Kundu, 1976). *Nonverbal communication* is the sum of all the body language and environmental manipulations that are used in the process of communication; the nonverbal element is by far the most important, as it conveys the feelings and attitudes of both speaker and listener in the exchange. Because of the importance of nonverbal communication to the nurse's ability to fulfill the various roles in patient care, it requires elaboration here. Communication is discussed more fully in later chapters dealing with the psychosocial aspects of patient care. The following characteristics of nonverbal communication will help the nurse to interpret and use body language more effectively in developing the nurse–patient relationship.

1. Nonverbal communication communicates information *only* about what is happening at the time the communicators are together.
2. Nonverbal communication usually gives information about the kind of relationship the communicators have.
3. Nonverbal communication can only send information in certain ways, because of the limited nature of expression a body has; the only way in which gestures and

expressions can be modified is by altering their magnitude.
4. There are no fixed meanings for individual nonverbal signals as there are for words. (Kundu, 1976)

The first obligation of the nurse who wishes to improve effectiveness as a nonverbal communicator is to develop awareness of what body language she or he customarily uses to express feelings and attitudes, so that the nurse may use this mode of communication deliberately to hasten the development of the relationship with the patient.

Therapeutic Touch

Relevant to both the therapeutic and expressive roles of the nurse is the increasing attention being given to the practice and scientific basis of therapeutic touch, which is described as energy transfer to support an individual's coping abilities by the laying on of hands by the nurse. Boguslawski (1979) states three concepts basic to understanding the healing process inherent in therapeutic touch as a nursing intervention:

1. The individual is an energy field;
2. The individual and the environment are continually, simultaneously, and mutually exchanging energy with each other; and
3. Universal order is a force innate in all energy fields.

The benefit of human contact to maintaining an optimal level of functioning is central to the practices of those who use what is called the holistic approach to health care. The East-West Academy of Healing Arts has formalized this belief in its prescription that "four hugs a day is the minimum of energy contact that everyone needs to maintain a sense of vitality and aliveness" (McCarty, 1979).

However valid the four-hugs-a-day regimen may be, not all patients—or nurses—are ready for that much structure in the touching aspect of their relationship. Some people feel uncomfortable when touched. If we were deprived of touch early in life, we are apt to be awkward later in life in relationships in which touch is used or expected (Goodykoontz, 1979). Ujhely (1979) gives wise counsel on the use of touch by the nurse:

> Obviously, there are no clear-cut answers about when to touch. We should be guided by our own philosophy about the purpose and meaning of another person's suffering, as well as our goals for that person's development. A second component is our attitude toward suffering, our tolerance of it, and our philosophy concerning its validity.

The Expressive Role

That aspect of the therapeutic role of the nurse which has as its goal the prevention and cure of disease will be discussed in detail in later chapters. Inasmuch as all patients experience the manner in which they are nursed, the expressive role of the nurse will be considered further here. Johnson and Martin (1958) state that the objective of the expressive role is the relief of tension in the group. The group is composed of the physician, nurse, and patient. Though they do not so state, the group actually consists of all those who have some relationship to the patient, including the members of the family and friends. They further state that, in any social system, certain problems must be solved if the system is to maintain itself. That is, it must move forward toward the accomplishment of a common goal and it must maintain internal equilibrium. They explain by stating that "relationships between the social system members must be harmonious and integrated and each member must feel good both within himself and toward other group members." They emphasize the importance of the nurse in this role by suggesting that it is here that the nurse is the expert and as such should give leadership. Nurses stand as intermediaries between the patient and the physician and what the physician does for and to the patient. If this view is accepted, nurses also stand between the patient and the other persons who participate in his or her care. To fulfill this role, they must know what the common goal or objective is and give leadership to those working toward its achievement. They lead by utilizing their skills in such a manner that each person feels "good within himself and toward other members of the group." Johnson and Martin emphasize that the physical care of the patient is important because it gives the nurse an opportunity to reduce the tension of the patient and to promote good feeling.

Schulman (1958) compares the feeling that the nurse should have for the patient with the feeling of a mother for her child. The early phase of the mother–child relationship is largely physical and marked by tenderness and compassion. The mother tends her child and stands between the child and harm. She comforts the child and soothes hurts. As the child grows and develops in ability to care for him or herself, she encourages independence. The mother gives of herself and of her material resources to meet the child's needs, because it is her child.

Johnson and Martin (p. 376) state that the expressive role of the nurse can be carried too far and that the needs and wants of a patient can be so gratified that he or she prefers sickness to health. As in other situations, multiple factors contribute to the preference of the patient for sickness to health. The nurse should not necessarily assume responsibility for the patient's behavior but, along with other data, the nurse must be willing and able to examine her or his own behavior to be sure that it is not contributing to the situation. The nurse shares with the physician the responsibility for recognizing the signs indicating that the patient is finding the secondary gains of illness preferable to the healthy state and for providing the necessary help to move the patient toward recovery.

A second problem in the practice of the expressive role concerns nurses. They must have and convey to the patient a very real concern for his or her welfare and at the same time develop themselves the ability to evaluate objectively both the patient's behavior and the effect of their own behavior on the patient. They may find that in one instance they were too supporting and in another they withdrew their support too soon, or were too permissive or too limiting. Nurses may also find that they felt so strongly with the patient that they were unable to give him or her the necessary support to consider the alternatives or to do what had to be done. Psychologists emphasize that the more the person is concerned with self, the less he or she is able to be concerned with others. Nurses contribute to the welfare of the patient when they not only are able to communicate to the patient their interest in and concern for his or her welfare, but also maintain enough objectivity to evaluate his or her needs and act in the manner that is best suited to meet them.

Through the skillful practice of the expressive role, the nurse helps to create an environment of trust essential to the comfort and well-being of the patient. The confidence of the patient is built on being accepted as an individual and on the confidence of the nurse to be able to meet his or her needs. It is facilitated by the way care is provided, by its timing, and by attention to details of care, especially those that are important to the patient. It is strengthened by keeping promises and by keeping the patient informed about the status of those that take time to fulfill. For example, Mr. Samuel was promised a high-low bed. When the nurse called the storeroom, she learned that one would not be available for several hours. She relayed this information to Mr. Samuel. Later, when it had not arrived at the expected time, she called the storeroom and then told Mr. Samuel that the bed was on its way. The fact that the nurse kept Mr. Samuel informed helped to develop his confidence that she was concerned with his welfare.

The nurse may not always be able to fulfill all the expectations of the patient, or always be responsible for the fact that they are not met. The nurse is responsible for trying to determine what they are and for considering them in the patient's care. Most persons who are sick enough to require medical and nursing care suffer some degree of anxiety. When they are hospitalized, the environment is strange and frightening. Sick persons should not be expected to be at their best. Despite their illness, they remain human beings and should be treated with courtesy and thoughtfulness. Interest in them as persons, concern for their welfare, kindness, and a desire to be helpful should all contribute to their confidence that their needs will be met.

This section has considered the nature of professional nursing as a human service. The following section presents the concept of the nursing process.

The Nursing Process—Its Properties and Purposes

Although the outward and visible signs of nursing are what the nurse does for, with, or in behalf of a patient, the nurse's actions are based on a series of intellectual processes that are not directly visible. Together these intellectual activities and nursing actions are called the *nursing process*. Essentially, the nursing process is a systematic method of problem solving applied to nursing situations, and based on the scientific process. The foundation for the scientific process was laid by philosophers such as Sir Francis Bacon and Sir Isaac Newton. It was further developed and refined by the great scientists who followed them. The general rules followed by the scientist are (1) observed and choose facts, (2) form a hypothesis that links the facts together, and (3) carry out a sufficient number of experiments to prove or disprove this hypothesis. These three general rules have been further defined and clarified to include the activities involved in the nursing process.

Before one can solve a problem, the problem must first be correctly identified. Johnson (D. M. Johnson, 1961) describes three phases of the problem-solving process: the preparation phase, when one is engaged in identifying the problem; the production phase, when one turns out possible solutions; and the judgment phase, when one selects a particular solution, then subsequently criticizes or evaluates it. All three phases are instances of causal thinking, which requires the substitution of verbal symbols for perceptions of reality. The right words may not automatically produce the right actions, and it is possible to arrive at the right action via intuition or experience, but the right words are an essential part of the process of causal thinking; and causal thinking is essential for the identification of the possible reasons for and significance of a patient's behavior. Those who do not use words and symbols easily will have difficulty with the causal thinking required for problem identification and problem solving. Weed (1968) insists it is the capacity to formulate and pursue a problem that distinguishes a good clinician.

Nursing Diagnosis

An explicit statement of the presenting problem is an essential element of the problem-solving process. When the problem-solving process is used in a patient-centered approach to nursing practice, the explicit statement of the patient's presenting problem to be addressed by nursing constitutes the *patient's problem,* or—as previously described—the *nursing diagnosis.* The problem may be an unmet need or difficulty the patient is actually experiencing at the moment, or one for which the total situation puts him or her at some degree of risk in the future.

Nursing Process as Problem Solving

There has been an almost infinite variety of definitions of the properties of nursing process as a problem-solving approach to patient care in recent years. Any definition incorporating consideration of the three general rules cited earlier, which guide the use of scientific process, is probably a usable definition; however, each nurse must have a definition that has meaning for and gives direction to her or his own nursing practice. The definition of nursing process developed by the authors and clinical nursing colleagues consists of three basic processes—observation, inference, and action—used to accomplish the steps in each of four components of the nursing process. The relationships among basic processes, steps, and components are illustrated in Figure 8-1. The four components and their respective steps are given in Table 8-3.

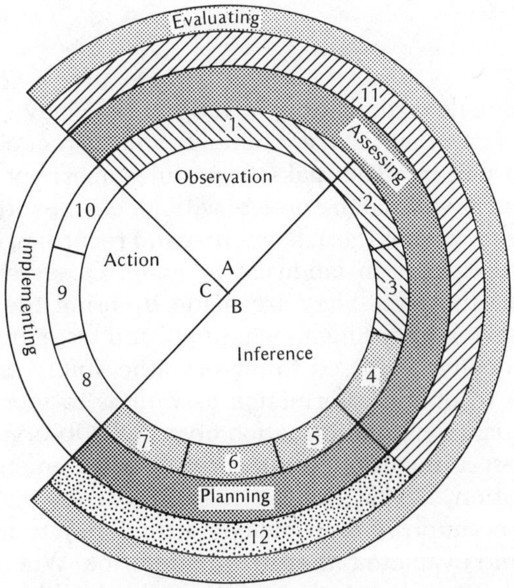

Figure 8-1. A conceptual model of the nursing process. *Central segments A, B,* and *C* represent the basic processes used in planning, providing and evaluating nursing care. The numerals represent the twelve steps to be accomplished by each of the three central processes, within the four components of the nursing process. The *outer circle* represents *evaluation as re-assessment and re-planning,* the fourth component of the nursing process.

Purposes of Nursing Process

The purposes of the nursing process are to meet the general objectives toward which the nursing care of all patients is directed. Again, these may be defined in various ways, any one of which is acceptable, but each nurse must have in mind a clear notion of what the purposes of the nursing care are. The following objectives constitute our beliefs about the purposes of the nursing process:

1. To personalize the care of each patient.
2. To ascertain, support, and maintain the patient's capacity for meeting his or her physiologic, psychological, social, and spiritual needs as well as recognizing strengths and limitations.
3. To protect the patient from the threats to safety, comfort, and well-being.
4. To support, comfort, and sustain the patient and to ease his or her suffering during all phases of illness.
5. To assist in the restoration of the patient to the fullest capacity of which he or she is capable.
6. To consider the patient's family members and friends as persons who have a legitimate interest and a role to play in the patient's well-being.
7. To assist the patient and the patient's family in planning for required care.

In pursuit of the general objectives elaborated here, there must be a complementarity between the type of problems presented by patients and the goal the nurse pursues in an effort to help the patient meet an otherwise unmet need (i.e., patient problem).

There is a parallelism between classes of patient problems (or nursing diagnoses) and classes of nursing goals. For example, if a patient with advanced cancer is on a drug that suppresses the immune sys-

TABLE 8-3. ***Components of the Nursing Process***

Components	Steps*
Assessing	1. *Collect data.* This is a systematic gathering of information about the subjective and objective state of the patient and the situation, using the interview to gather subjective data, and the observational skills of inspection, palpation, percussion, and auscultation to gather objective data.
	2. *Analyze data.* This is a methodical examination and separation of collected information into relevant categories.
	3. *Interpret data.* This is the identification of strengths and limitations of the individual, and determination of the presence, nature, and priority of patient problems.
Planning	4. *Specify the patient problem* to which nursing care will be directed. This is the formulation of the nursing diagnosis, as a succinct statement of the unmet need with which patient requires assistance from nursing.
	5. *Identify goals (or objectives).* This is the formulation of a statement of the behavior which is expected to result from planned action.
	6. *Consider alternative approaches.* In view of the nature and probable source of the patient's unmet needs, what actions or approaches are most likely to achieve the stated goal of terminal behavior of the patient?
	7. *Select one approach from alternatives.* The approach both consistent with the stated goal and feasible in the setting in terms of available resources is selected.
Implementing	8. *Communicate plan to all persons affected.* Use written and verbal communication as appropriate.
	9. *Coordinate plan with other therapeutic plans.* Dovetail the purposes, techniques, and timing of the plan for nursing with the medical, physical therapy, nutritional, and so on, plans of care.
	10. *Carry out the plan.*
Evaluating	11. *Reassess the patient and the situation.* This step consists of repeated measures of the same dimensions addressed in steps 1 through 4, to determine what, if any, progress has been made toward stated goals.
	12. *Appropriately modify the plan.* This step consists of repeating steps 4 through 7, in light of new assessment.

* Numbered steps correspond with numbers in Figure 8-1.

tem (i.e., the system that defends the body against injury from biological or chemical agents), then one of the goals of the nursing care is to protect the patient from exposure to persons with colds, any known low-grade infections, or carriers of any infectious diseases. The data required to identify the patient problem must include some description of *situational context* to which the individual's behavior appears to be a response, and the goal for the care *must be negotiated with the individual, family, and other significant participants in care.*

Two Basic Processes in Nursing

The action process of nursing will be discussed in subsequent sections as appropriate to selected topics. General aspects of the two remaining processes will be discussed briefly here.

Observation

Throughout the history of modern nursing the value of observation has been recognized. Florence Nightingale wrote (1860, p. 160), "For it may safely be said, not that the habit of ready and correct observation will by itself make us useful nurses, but that without it we shall be useless with all our devotion."

Observation is the act of noting and recording facts or occurrences in language or code. Observations involve the real. They are made by using the five senses: sight, hearing, touch, smell, and taste. Instruments can be utilized to increase the ability of the senses to obtain information as well as to measure and quantify the information obtained. Observation is a description, not an interpretation, judgment, or evaluation. Certain difficulties enter into the making of observations. These include a tendency to interpret and evaluate rather than to describe. When the word of others has to be taken, the likelihood of error is increased. There are limits to the ability of any person to observe accurately, remember, and report. Past experiences influence what an observer "sees," for what is seen depends in part on what is in the environment and in part on what the observer is. There is always the possibility of overlooking or underestimating significant clues as well as misinterpreting or overestimating their importance. As an experiment, note the ways in which different people describe and interpret a similar incident or statement.

Skill in observation can be increased by systematic and regular practice. This practice can be done in any setting from an aquarium to a zoo. Group practice followed by a comparison of notes is useful in improving observational skills.

In reports or records of observations, what has been noted should be described as carefully and specifically as possible. When describing what a patient says, use the exact words as far as is possible. Judge what is recorded by the following concept: *The value of an observation depends on the integrity and detachment with which it is made and on its specificity.*

In gathering and recording information about each subjective and objective symptom of the patient, the nurse should obtain measures of the seven variables suggested by Morgan and Engel (1969, p. 35) as mandatory dimensions to explore in symptom analysis:

1. *Location:* Where is the symptom located?
2. *Quality:* What is it like?
3. *Quantity:* How intense is it?
4. *Chronology:* When did the symptom begin and what course has it followed?
5. *Setting:* Under what circumstances does it take place?
6. *Aggravating and alleviating factors:* What makes it worse or better?
7. *Associated manifestations:* What other symptoms or phenomena are associated with it?

Subjective data gathering. Nursing process ideally begins with purposeful conversation with the patient and with members of the family and others knowledgeable and concerned about him or her. Purposeful conversation initiated by the nurse is *interviewing.* The goals of the initial interview are to begin building a personal relationship and to determine how the patient interprets the situation, what the patient's expectations are for him or herself and for others, past health history, and the pattern of activities of daily living. Skill in both verbal and nonverbal communication is essential to successful interviewing. Above all, the nurse must remember that the interview can rarely be completed, in terms of meeting its stated goals, in one session. This is particularly true if the patient comes from a high-context culture, which requires staging of the goals over time.

Bootay (1978, p. 50) offers ten rules to promote a satisfying and productive interview. Those rules appear in Table 8-4. Purposeful conversation as a therapeutic nursing tool is discussed in Chapter 19 and Unit VII.

Objective data gathering. Much attention has been devoted in recent years to extending the observational skills of nurses by formalizing their use of inspection, palpation, percussion and auscultation in the physical examination of the patient (Bates, 1974 & 1979; Sana & Judge, 1975; Murray & Zentner, 1975; Gillies & Alyn, 1976; Sauvé & Pecherer, 1977; Sherman & Fields, 1978). The organizing schema used by most authorities is the traditional patient history and review of body systems format used by physicians to facilitate communication between

TABLE 8-4. *Ten Rules about Interviewing*

1. Know what an interview is for and how it fits into the nursing process. See yourself as an interviewer when you ask questions, not just a nurse doing busy work.
2. Explain the interview in a way that will help the patient understand how it benefits him. Suggest that you establish a cooperative relationship.
3. Schedule the interview for a time convenient for both you and the patient.
4. Keep the environment as free from distractions as possible, and try to make the patient physically and emotionally comfortable.
5. Encourage the patient to communicate more expressively by asking open-ended questions, keeping related events in time sequence, and referring back to questions already answered. Never rush. Give him plenty of time to answer each question.
6. Use your common sense and sensitivity. Show your personal concern for the patient. Reach out and touch him.
7. Keep your questions centered on the patient's problems. Remember, you have to use the information you gather to write a care plan.
8. Don't insist the patient tell you more than he's comfortable telling you. Never imply that he won't receive adequate care from health-team members if he doesn't cooperate.
9. Look on interviewing as an ongoing process. Make every encounter with the patient a meaningful one.
10. Conclude your interview by identifying the patient's needs and share your plans about meeting those needs with him. Give him the opportunity to correct any misconceptions.

Used with permission of Intermed Communications, Inc., from "Interviewing Your Patient: How to Get the Most from Your Questions," in *Documenting Patient Care Responsibly,* © 1978, p. 50, by L. S. Bootay.

Back of the Card

Assessment Framework

The following is a framework for systematic, comprehensive assessment based on Maslow's heirarchy of needs. Dr. Abraham Maslow purports that man's behavior is motivated by "basic needs" common to all people. The behavior which expresses the most dominant need will be influenced by the culture, education, experience, and opportunities available to the person.

Putting the needs into a heirarchy suggests that some are more basic to life than others; however, there is a vital interrelatedness among them, eg. loss of one's self-esteem can influence one's appetite and therefore nutritional status.

Using the framework as a mental screen during patient assessment ensures total or comprehensive assessment. Significant patient data obtained during initial assessment should be recorded in all areas of human need to provide base line information. Without base line information, change in a patient's status or performance cannot be determined. Strengths and limitations, and the associated patient problems are inferred from analysis of patient data. Particular strengths can be very important in helping patients with the need areas that have deficiencies, eg. knowing that the patient can well afford dietetic foods can facilitate planning a diet for a diabetic or someone with malnutrition.

Front of the Card

Assessment Framework

For each area the current status and influencing factors are identified.

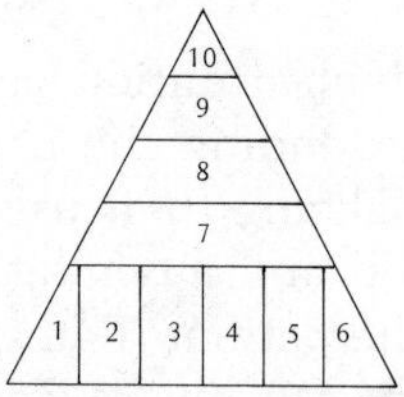

1. Respiration
2. Nutrition
3. Elimination
4. Rest and activity
5. Protective mechanisms
6. Sexuality
7. Security
8. Love and belonging
9. Self-esteem
10. Self-actualization

1. Rate, depth, color, Hbg, cough, change with activity, smoker, partial pressure, circulatory status, etc.
2. Meal pattern, likes and dislikes, wt., ht., cultural or religious connotation, etc.
3. Pattern, past difficulties, remedies, etc.
4. Pattern, facilitators and rituals, limitations, etc.
5. Skin, reflexes, bony structure, musculature, immunity, white blood cell count, pain and temperature responses, allergies, etc.
6. Maturity, femininity, masculinity, marital status, cultural significance, etc.
7. Economic and educational status, insurance, employment, feelings about hospitalization, religion, dependency, defense mechanisms, etc.
8. Family, significant others, pets, clubs, etc.
9. Achievement, recognition from others, ambition, etc.
10. Fulfillment, what one feels good about, peace of mind, etc.

Figure 8-2. Assessment framework based on Maslow's hierarchy of needs: a pocket guide (Passos & Janzen, 1974).

nurse and physician about the person who is to receive care. The traditional format is frequently modified, usually by addition of perceptual and patterns of living variables, by nurse practitioners engaged in delivery of primary care. The reader is referred to the authors cited above for further information on extended assessment skills necessary for the nurse who is functioning either as the initial assessor of the patient or in an expanded role. Acquisition of those skills necessary to gather both subjective and objective data necessary to plan and evaluate care occurs appropriately in the fundamental skills portion of the first course in nursing; this text does not deal systematically with those very important psychomotor skills. However, the type of data needed to assess patients with various alterations is presented with each chapter that focuses on alterations.

Maslow's Hierarchy of Human Needs: An Assessment Framework

In an effort to find a guide to patient assessment that would be comprehensive, human-needs oriented, concise, and available for use by the nurse involved in the care of the sick, the junior author and a colleague developed the Assessment Framework shown in Figure 8-2 (Passos & Janzen, 1974). The narrative describes Maslow's hierarchy of human needs, on which assessment is to be based, and it is printed on the back of a 3 by 5 file card. On the front of the card is the ten-category pyramid of human needs, with suggested types of information that will assist the nurse in determining whether or not the patient requires assistance to meet his or her needs in each area. The card is plasticized and is to be carried in the nurse's pocket for easy access as a mental screen during assessment activities. At the end of this chapter, following the section on documentation of care, is a suggested format for recording the data base; the format follows the pocket assessment framework.

Other Assessment Guides

In recent years a number of guides have been suggested to help nurses systematize the gathering and interpretation of data needed to plan and evaluate patient care. These guides and the data-gathering process to which they refer have been called by such various terms as nursing history; health appraisal; nursing or admission interview; and guide to the assessment of patient or nursing needs and patient or nursing problems. Whatever the terms, all refer to a variety of organized sets of questions or topics that direct the information-gathering efforts of the nurse as a first step in developing a plan of care for the patient. Mayers (1972) has identified a number of beneficial effects of this initial information-gathering process: (1) it begins the nurse–patient relationship, (2) it begins patient involvement, (3) it begins the nurse's commitment, (4) it saves time and energy of both patient and nurse, and (5) it allows the nurse and patient to reach an agreement on the purposes and conditions of their association for a specified period of time.

To collect the information required to make a nursing diagnosis, knowledge and skill in the field of interpersonal relationships, as well as in the observation and interpretation of the signs and symptoms indicating deviations from normal functioning and behavior, are essential. Not all the desired information is available for every patient, nor is it always necessary. Some of it may be obtained from the patient's hospital chart and medical history or from the family or physician. Moreover, continuous assessment is essential. As the patient recovers or fails his or her needs change. As a consequence, nursing care requirements also change.

After the data are collected, they should be analyzed and the problems that can be met through the practice of nursing identified. Problems outside the province of nursing or that are shared with other disciplines should be referred to the appropriate persons.

Inference

The term *inference* can be defined quite simply as a conclusion arrived at by reasoning from a fact or facts that are known. Hammond (1966) defines an inductive inference as the process of reasoning from a specific fact or facts to the general case. Kelly (1966) defines clinical inference as "making a judgment about the state of the patient and/or the nursing needs of the patient." Depending on a variety of factors, inferences may be perfect or imperfect, theoretical or empirical, and statistical or intuitive. Hammond (1966, p. 28) states that "Nearly all of our actions are based upon imperfect inductive inferences based on uncertain, probabilistic information. . . . our inferences are normally 'uncertainty-geared.' " He further states that many inferences made by nurses about the state of the patient are empirical and intuitive rather than theoretical or statistical.[1] The nurse is faced with the problem of correctly inferring the state of the patient from uncertain and incomplete data. Though the nurse lacks theoretical knowledge, she or he is expected to make judgments on the medical state of the patient. This requires thinking not only like a nurse but like a physician. The studies of Hammond and his associates indicate that the inferential tasks of the nurse are highly complex. Further, the nurse often needs far more knowledge than is generally appreciated.

An example of the type of clinical inference made by a nurse is evidenced when she or he tries to predict or foretell the possible outcomes of the patient's problems as well as of the efforts made to solve or relieve those problems, based on the observations made and classified during the assessment. Some predictions will be reasonably accurate, whereas others may be less so. For example, a patient who has had an appendectomy and is up and about and eating well can be expected to recover. The nurse can predict with some assurance that if the patient who has had a stroke or has been burned is kept in good alignment, he or she is less likely to develop contractures than one who is not. The patient who knows medication will be given promptly if pain occurs generally requires less medication than the one who is uncertain. An example of a more complex inferential task is seen in the case of Mrs. David, who has had a pituitary tumor removed. Shortly after the operation she regains consciousness and appears to be recovering as expected. She complains of thirst and voids from 500 to 700 ml of urine every 1 to 2 hours. What do these observations mean? Certainly the fact that Mrs. David knows who and where she is are favorable signs. What does the fact that she says she is thirsty and voids 500 to 700 ml of urine

[1] Empirical inference—one based on past experience. Theoretical inference—one based on knowledge. Intuitive inference—the knowing of something without conscious learning. Statistical inference—relationship established by mathematical treatment of data.

every 1 to 2 hours mean? Unless the nurse knows that these signs accompany a deficiency of the antidiuretic hormone, a real possibility is that this patient may die as a result of excessive loss of water from the blood.

The Hypothesis

Many of the nurse's interpretations or conclusions about the meaning of assessment data constitute hypotheses. A *hypothesis* is a tentative proposition[2] suggested as an explanation of some phenomenon or as a solution to a problem (Ary et al., 1972). The use of hypotheses enables us to use both induction, with its emphasis on observation, and deduction, with its emphasis on reason, thus uniting experience and reason to produce a powerful tool to seek new knowledge. Hypotheses present only a *suggested* explanation of or solution to a problem; support or rejection depends upon results obtained by testing them in the real world of patient care. Feinstein (1967) contends that the clinician in every aspect of the management of patient problems is conducting a clinical experiment. For example, several hypotheses might be suggested to explain Mrs. David's large urine output. One is that she was overhydrated during the surgical procedure. Another is that she has diabetes insipidus. A better guess is that the trauma incurred during the operation resulted in swelling with pressure on the tissues surrounding the neurohypophysis. As pressure increased, release of the antidiuretic hormone decreased—a condition that is readily treated when recognized.

To clarify and summarize, two further examples are presented. Mrs. Smart is lying quietly in bed. Her hair is neat and she has polish on her fingernails. On her bedside table is a picture of a little boy. These are observations or facts. What inferences can be made from these facts? Are there enough facts to conclude that the little boy is her son? He may not be; he may be her nephew or grandson or the child of a friend. What are her feelings toward him? What other *facts* must be known before these questions can be answered? This point should be emphasized: through observations the *facts* in a situation are determined. These facts have value inasmuch as they are accurately and clearly described.

Sometimes the data available are inadequate to explain the event: then an educated guess, or hypothesis, may be made. For example, a man whose blood pressure is 90/60 arrived in a hospital emergency room following an automobile collision. There is a large wound in his right arm from which he has been bleeding. Though his normal blood pressure is not known, from the known facts the inference that he is in shock is reasonable. What is fact and what is assumed to be fact should be kept clearly in mind. As new evidence is uncovered, new or different interpretations may be required.

Based on the data collected and their meaning, the nurse makes one or more decisions. Stated simply, she or he determines what the patient's nursing needs are. In the case of Mrs. David, the nurse notes the disparity between the patient's intake and output. She also knows that if output continues to exceed intake the patient will soon be in serious trouble. The nurse has a number of alternatives. She can continue to observe the patient and see if the condition corrects itself. She can encourage Mrs. David to drink as much fluid as she can. She can report her observation to the physician. Because the nurse knows that after surgery performed in the region of the neurohypophysis increased urine output and marked thirst indicate a decreased release of ADH, she decides to report her observations to the physician.

After the nurse has decided what the patient's unmet needs are, she or he translates them into nursing objectives and establishes priorities. As part of the decision-making process, the nurse considers the patient's wants and wishes as well as her or his own interpretation of what the patient's needs are. For example, Mrs. Giat is unconscious. Among her unmet needs are such requirements as maintaining a clear airway, preventing skin breakdown, maintaining fluid intake, and maintaining good body alignment. The nurse states the needs as objectives and decides which takes first priority, second, and so on. Actually all are important.

For each objective, the nurse must consider what approaches can be used to achieve it. After the possibilities have been identified, the nurse selects the one or ones that appear to be most feasible.

At this point the nurse is or should be ready to continue through the rest of the nursing process. The remaining steps should be clear as stated in Table 8-3. From the preceding discussion it should be evident that sound nursing practice is based on a high level of intellectual activity.

Documentation of Patient Care

The decade of the seventies has been characterized by many commentators as the decade of accountability. The health care industry has been a prime target of social reformers and government regulatory agencies, and all providers of health service have increasingly been held accountable for describing and justifying their services. Although the primary stimulus to this movement seems to have been cost containment, nursing has benefited in other ways. One of the prime benefits to nursing

[2] A *proposition* is a statement in which the predicate affirms something about the subject.

of the increasingly stringent requirements for documentation of care provided has been to help nurses make explicit their contribution to patient care.

Since World War II, the records written by nurses, particularly in the care of the sick, had degenerated to a series of notations confirming that prescribed medical therapy had been carried out, with a sprinkling of comments on patients' responses to medical therapy. Even in agencies where patients received excellent assistance from nurses in coping with illness and with the struggle to regain control and self-sufficiency, the nursing contribution was usually not retrievable from the written record; all too often, nurses themselves could not identify their explicit contribution to patient care.

The Problem-Oriented Approach (POR)

As pressures have mounted to improve documentation of care, the problem-oriented approach to the medical record (POMR) (Weed, 1968) has gained increasing acceptance by both physicians and many other health professionals. Weed's concept of the problem oriented medical record as a way to logically organize information about a patient around the patient's problems is an explicit application of the scientific method to patient management. The POMR is an informational system, used as a tool by professionals engaged in the process of problem solving with and for patients. The system has four basic components: the data base, problem list, plan, and progress notes. SOAP a form for recording progress notes which is a central technique of Weed's POMR, is an acronym for the order of classes of information to be recorded:

Recorded Information	Component of POMR
*S*ubjective data, obtained by interview	Data base
*O*bjective data, obtained by physical examination skills (inspection, palpation, percussion, auscultation), laboratory and other diagnostic tests	Data base
*A*ssessment	Problem list
*P*lan	Plan/orders/approach
Monitoring of patient's progress by recording appropriate SOAP for each active problem on the original problem list	Progress notes

Many nurses quickly saw the applicability of the POMR and its SOAP format to the nursing process. In adapting the SOAP format to the nursing process, some nurses have extended the format to "SOAP-IER" notes:

*S*ubjective data
*O*bjective data
*A*ssessment
*P*lan
*I*mplementation of plan
*E*valuation of the implemented plan
*R*evision of the plan if it was ineffective, or if problem has been resolved (Vasey, 1978)

Although it may be useful for nurses to describe elements of *I*mplementation (see Steps 8, 9, and 10 in Table 8-3), the addition of *E*valuation and *R*evision of the plan are probably redundant, since evaluation is the purpose, process, and product of the SOAP recording in the progress notes (see Steps 11 and 12 in Table 8-3).

The following format for documenting nursing care provides a way for organizing and recording the data base, the problem list, the plan of care, and the progress notes. Areas of need (ID) to be assessed derive from Maslow's hierarchy of needs, as illustrated on the pocket assessment framework in Figure 8-2. In each of the ten areas of need, provision is made to separate subjective from objective data to facilitate comparisons of perception with objective measures related to the area of need. The format for documenting nursing care provides inadequate detail to serve as a guide to the specific measures that must be made of innumerable variables relevant to each area of need. See Appendix B for a Guide for Assessing the Needs of the Patient, which is offered to assist the nurse in identifying what data to collect.

We believe there is a common core of historical and physical appraisal data needed by both medicine and nursing to identify patient problems, formulate goals, and develop the plan of care. There are increasing opportunities for the nurse to conduct the initial appraisal of the patient's health status. The suggested format is intended to present the results of the nurse's findings in a manner which not only will support the plan of nursing care, but also will optimize communication and collaboration with the patient's physician, should the patient need medical care.

In this chapter nursing as a profession and the broad role of the nurse have been reviewed. Because the writers believe that nursing has the responsibility for assisting the patient to meet needs that he or she is unable to meet alone, a concept of need was explored in Chapter 7. Because nursing is a complex activity, the nursing process has been outlined and discussed. A nursing guide for collecting data about patients has been outlined, and a format proposed for documentation of care.

Proposed Format for Documentation: Comprehensive Data Base, Problem List, Plan, and Progress Notes for Documenting Nursing Care[3]

I. Assessment

A. Vital Statistics

Name: (Initials only)		*Setting:*
Marital Status:	S M Sep W D (circle)	*Religion:*
Age	*Sex:* M F (circle)	*Race:*
Nationality:		*Occupation:*
Level of Responsiveness:		*Source/ Reliability of History:*

B. Patient's Description of Present Illness (Chief Complaint—Major Concern) This section begins with the patient's statement of problem, and the patient's own words are recorded as the chief complaint/major concern.

C. Medical Diagnoses and Prescriptions (All medical orders that will require preparation of or adaptation by the patient). *LIST.*

D. Areas of Need: (Maslow's Heirarchy) Record measures of variables relevant to each area of need. Include both significant normal and abnormal findings.

1. Respiration
S 0

2. Nutrition
S 0

3. Elimination
S 0

4. Rest and activity
S 0

5. Protection
S 0

6. Sexuality
S 0

7. Security
S 0

8. Love and belonging
S 0

9. Self-esteem
S 0

10. Self-actualization
S 0

E. This section consists of your *Summary and Analysis* of data recorded in Sections A–D.

Strengths *Limitations*

F. This section is your *Interpretation* of the problems or needs suggested by the data analysis.

Nursing diagnosis(es)—problem list
Number nature and probable cause of patient problems

II. Plan

A. Goals, stated as expected/accepted patient behaviors

B. Actions

III. Progress Notes (includes evaluation as reassessment, with emphasis on progress toward goals).

Date *Note*

[3] This format is modified from a form developed by the following graduate faculty in the department of Medical–Surgical Nursing, College of Nursing, Wayne State University, Detroit, Mich.: Mary Delaney-Naumoff, Barbara Jones, Kathlene Monaban, Jean Stallwood-Hess, Dawn Zagornik, Erica Janzen, and Joyce Passos.

References Cited

Abdellah, F. G. "Methods of Identifying Covert Aspects of Nursing Problems." *Nurs. Res.*, **6** (June 1957), 4–23.

Abdellah, F. G., and Levine, E. "What Patients Say about Their Nursing Care." *Hospitals,* **31** (1 Nov. 1957), 44.

ANA Convention '78. *Amer. J. Nurs.*, **78** (July 1978), 1231–46.

Ary, D. et al. *Introduction to Research in Education,* New York: Holt, Rinehart and Winston, 1972, pp. 71–72.

Bates, B. *A Guide to Physical Examination.* Philadelphia: J. B. Lippincott Company, 1974; 2nd ed., 1979.

Benton, D. W. "You Want to Be a *What?*" *Nurs. Outlook,* **27** (June 1979), 388–93.

Boguslawski, M. "The Use of Therapeutic Touch in Nursing." *J. Cont. Ed. in Nurs.,* **10** (July–Aug. 1979), 9–13.

Bootay, L. S. "Interviewing Your Patient: How to Get the Most from Your Questions." In *Documenting Patient Care Responsibly.* Ed. by J. Robinson. Horsham, Pa.: Intermed Communications, Inc., 1978, p. 50.

Congress for Nursing Practice. *Standards of Nursing Practice.* Kansas City, Mo.: American Nurses' Assoc., 1973, Pub. No. NP-41 180M 12/73.

Congress for Nursing Practice. *A Plan for Implementation of the Standards of Nursing Practice.* Kansas City, Mo.: American Nurses' Assoc., 1975, Pub. No. NP-51 7M 11/75.

Durr, C. A. "Hands that Help . . . But How?" *Nurs. Forum,* **10**:4 (1971), 397.

Feinstein, A. R. *Clinical Judgment.* Baltimore: The Williams & Wilkins Company, 1967, p. 21.

Friedman, Kenneth (interview of E. T. Hall). "Learning the Arabs' Silent Language." *Psychol. Today,* **13** (Aug. 1979), 45–54.

Gillies, D. A., and Alyn, I. B. *Patient Assessment and Management by the Nurse Practitioner.* Philadelphia: W. B. Saunders Company, 1976.

Goodykoontz, L. "Touch: Attitudes and Practice." *Nurs. Forum,* **18**:1 (1979), 4–17.

Hall, E. T. *The Hidden Dimension.* Garden City, N.Y.: Doubleday & Company, Inc., 1966, p. 108.

Hammond, K. R. "Clinical Inference in Nursing: II. A Psychologist's Viewpoint." *Nurs. Res.,* **15** (Winter 1966), 27.

Henderson, V. "The Nature of Nursing." *Am. J. Nurs.,* **64** (Aug. 1964), 63–67.

Henderson, V. *Nursing Studies Index.* Vol. IV-I. Philadelphia: J. B. Lippincott Company, 1963, 1966, 1970, 1972.

Henderson, V., and Nite, G. *Principles and Practice of Nursing,* 6th ed. New York: Macmillan Publishing Co., Inc., 1978.

Jacobs, A. M., Fivars, G., Edwards, D. S., and Fitzpatrick, R. *Critical Requirements for Safe/Effective Nursing Practice.* Kansas City, Mo.: American Nurses' Assoc., 1978, Pub. No. B-41 1.5M 5/78.

Johnson, D. M. *Psychology: A Problem-Solving Approach.* New York: Harper & Row, Publishers, 1961, p. 252.

Johnson, M. M., and Martin, H. W. "A Sociological Analysis of the Nurse Role." *Am. J. Nurs.,* **58** (March 1958), 374.

Kelly, K. "Clinical Inference in Nursing: I. A Nurse's Viewpoint." *Nurs. Res.,* **15** (Winter 1966), 24.

Kundu, M. R. "Visual Literacy: Teaching Non-Verbal Communication through Television." *Ed. Technol.,* Aug. 1976, pp. 31–33.

Lee, A. A. "How Nurses Rate with M.D.'s. *RN,* **42** (July 1979[b]), 21–30.

Lee, A. A. "How Nurses Rate with the Public." *RN,* **42** (June 1979[a]), 25–39.

Malasanos, L., Moss, M., and Stoltenberg-Allen, K. *Health Assessment.* Saint Louis: The C. V. Mosby Company, 1977.

Maslow, A. H. *Motivation and Personality.* New York: Harper & Row, Publishers, 1954.

Mayers, M. G. *A Systematic Approach to the Nursing Care Plan.* New York: Appleton-Century-Crofts, 1972, pp. 230–32.

McCarty, P. "Energy: Tapping the Body's Natural Resource." *Amer. Nurse,* **11**:8 (20 June 1979), 13.

Morgan, W. L., and Engel, G. L. *The Clinical Approach to the Patient.* Philadelphia: W. B. Saunders Company, 1969, p. 35.

Murphy, C. P. "Ethical Aspects of Decision Making in Nursing." In *Political, Social and Educational Forces on Nursing: Impact of Social Forces.* New York: National League for Nursing, 1979, pp. 17–25, Pub. No. 15–1774.

Murray, R., and Zentner, J. *Nursing Assessment and Health Promotion through the Life Span.* Englewood Cliffs, N.J.: Prentice-Hall, Inc., 1975.

Nightingale, F. *Notes on Nursing: What It Is, and What It Is Not,* rev. and enlarged ed. London: Harrison and Sons, 1860.

Norris, C. M. "Delusions that Trap Nurses." *Nurs. Outlook,* **21** (Jan. 1973), 18–21.

Nursing's Role in Patient's Rights. New York: National League for Nursing, 1979, Pub. No. 11–1671.

Orlando, I. J. *The Discipline and Teaching of Nursing Process.* New York: G. P. Putnam's Sons, 1972.

Passos, J. Y., and Janzen, E. "Assessment Framework Based on Maslow's Hierarchy of Human Needs." Unpublished pocket guide for use in workshops on nursing process, Detroit, Mich.: Wayne State University College of Nursing, 1974.

Robb, I. H. *Educational Standards for Nurses.* Cleveland, Ohio: E. C. Koeckert, 1907, p. 21.

Robinson, C. "An (Unabashed) Assessment of Nurses by Their Most Demanding Patients." *RN,* **42** (June 1979), 35.

Robinson, J., ed. *Documenting Patient Care Responsibly.* Horsham, Pa.: Intermed Communications, Inc., 1978.

Rubin, R. "Body Image and Self-Esteem." *Nurs. Outlook,* **16** (June 1968), 23.

Sana, J. M., and Judge, R. D. *Physical Appraisal Methods in Nursing Practice.* Boston: Little, Brown and Company, 1975.

Sauvé, M. J., and Pecherer, A. *Concepts and Skills in Physical Assessment.* Philadelphia: W. B. Saunders Company, 1977.

Schulman, S. "Basic Functional Roles in Nursing: Mother Surrogate and Healer." *Patients, Physicians and Illness.* Ed. by E. Gartley Jaco. New York: The Free Press, 1958, pp. 528–37.

Seymer, L. R. *Selected Writings of Florence Nightingale.* New York: Macmillan Publishing Co., Inc., 1954, pp. 351–52.

Sherman, J. L., and Fields, S. K. *Guide to Patient Evaluation,* 3rd ed. Garden City, N.Y.: Medical Examination Publishing Co., Inc., 1978.

Stanley, L. "Dangerous Doctors: What to Do When the M.D. Is Wrong." *RN,* **42** (March 1979), 22–30, p. 27.

Ujhely, G. B. "Touch: Reflections and Perceptions." *Nurs. Forum,* **18** (1979), 18–32.

Vasey, E. K. "Documenting Patient Care: How the System Works." In *Documenting Patient Care Responsibly.* Ed. by J. Robinson. Horsham, Pa.: Intermed Communications, Inc., 1978, pp. 25–33.

Weed, L. L. "Medical Records that Guide and Teach." *N. Engl. J. Med.,* **278** (21 March 1968), 652–55.

White, M. B. "Importance of Selected Nursing Activities." *Nurs. Res.,* **21** (Jan.–Feb. 1972), 4–14.

General References

Anthony, W. A., and Carkhuff, R. R. *The Art of Health Care: A Handbook of Psychological First Aid Skills.* Amherst, Mass.: Human Resources Development Press, Inc., 1976.

Archer, C. O., and Swearinger, D. "Application of Benjamin Franklin's Decision-Making Model to the Clinical Setting." *Nurs. Forum,* **16**:4 (1977), 319–28.

Becknell, E. P., and Smith, D. M. *System of Nursing Practice.* Philadelphia: F. A. Davis Company, 1975.

Berggren, H. J., and Zagornik, A. D. "Teaching Nursing Process to Beginning Students." *Nurs. Outlook,* **16** (July 1968), 32–35.

Berni, R., and Readey, H. *Problem-Oriented Medical Record Implementation: Allied Health Peer Review.* Saint Louis: The C. V. Mosby Company, 1974.

Burgess, A. W. *Nursing: Levels of Health Intervention.* Englewood Cliffs, N.J.: Prentice-Hall, Inc., 1978.

Campbell, C. *Nursing Diagnosis and Intervention in Nursing Practice.* New York: John Wiley & Sons, Inc., 1978.

"Communicating with Patients—A Seven Article Series." *Am. J. Nurs.,* **79** (June 1979), 1074–84.

Curran, W. J. "The Sarkewicz Decision." *N. Engl. J. Med.,* **298** (2 March 1978), 499–500.

"Ethical Dilemmas in Nursing—A Special Supplement." *Am. J. Nurs.,* **77** (May 1977), 845–76.

Gordon, M. "Nursing Diagnosis and the Diagnostic Process." *Am. J. Nurs.,* **76** (Aug. 1976), 1298–1300.

Gorry, A. G. et al. "The Diagnostic Importance of the Normal Finding." *N. Engl. J. Med.,* **298** (2 March 1978), 486–89.

Johnson, D. E. "Professional Practice and Specialization in Nursing." *Image,* **1** (1968), 2–7.

Komorita, N. I. "Nursing Diagnosis." *Am. J. Nurs.,* **63** (Dec. 1963), 83–86.

Langham, P. "Open Forum: On Teaching Ethics to Nurses." *Nurs. Forum,* **16**:3,4 (1977), 220–49.

Lash, A. A. "A Re-Examination of Nursing Diagnosis." *Nurs. Forum,* **17**:4 (1978), 332–43.

LeBow, M. D. *Behavior Modification: A Significant Method in Nursing Practice.* Englewood Cliffs, N.J.: Prentice-Hall, Inc., 1973.

Marriner, A. *The Nursing Process.* Saint Louis: The C. V. Mosby Company, 1975.

McPhetridge, L. M. "Nursing History: One Means to Personalize Care." *Am. J. Nurs.,* **68** (Jan. 1968), 68–75.

Parker, J. C., and Rubin, L. J. *Process as Content: Curriculum Design and the Application of Knowledge.* Chicago: Rand McNally & Company, 1966.

Passos, J. Y. "Accountability: The Long Road Back to Professional Practice." *J. New York Nurs. Assoc.,* **7** (Dec. 1976), 27–38.

"The Role of a Nurse in 1887." *Nurs. Forum,* **10**:1 (1971), 31.

Shoemaker, J. "How Nursing Diagnosis Helps Focus Your Care." *Nurs. 79,* **42** (Aug. 1979), 55–61.

Verhonick, P. J. "Clinical Investigations in Nursing." *Nurs. Forum,* **10**:1 (1971), 80–88.

Walter, J. B., Pardee, G. P., and Molbo, D. M. *Dynamics of Problem-Oriented Approaches: Patient Care and Documentation.* Philadelphia: J. B. Lippincott Company, 1976.

Wiedenbach, E. *Clinical Nursing: A Helping Art.* New York: Springer Verlag New York, Inc., 1964.

Wollowick, A. "Will the Nursing Profession Become Extinct?" *Nurs. Forum,* **9** (1970), 408–13.

SECTION TWO

Factors Influencing Dynamic Equilibrium

UNIT III

Nature and Cellular Effects of Injurious Agents

The environment of the industrialized society is not only beclouded by products from the combustion of fuel, but it is also increasingly burdened by vast numbers of new chemicals of ambiguous potential used in medicine, agriculture, food processing, the cosmetic industry, and in vermin control. In addition, other products such as detergents, bleaches, and cleansing fluids—some highly toxic—are an essential part of the contemporary human environment.

(SMILLIE & KILBOURNE, 1963)

In Chapter 2, the various etiologic agents were classified as those causing direct injury to cells (biological, physical, and chemical agents) and those inducing their effect indirectly through the mental apparatus (psychological injuring agents). This unit is concerned with the nature and effects of selected biological, physical, and chemical agents, particularly the effects on cellular function and structure, and the implications for the practice of nursing.

Potential injurious agents have their origin in either the external or internal environment of the individual. Many of the harmful agents in the external and possibly in the internal environment are of human making. Moreover, they are of increasing variety and potency. Some of the noxious agents in the environment are not new. They are an augmentation of preexisting natural hazards. For example, ever since lightning ignited a tinder-dry prairie or forest, humankind has been exposed to smoke. When they learned to use fire for their own purposes, they increased the intensity of exposure by inhaling smoke from a campfire or a poorly constructed fireplace. Inventions such as the furnace and steam and diesel engines have increased the quantity of smoke spewed into the atmosphere. Though many cities have accomplished miracles in controlling the pollution of the air with smoke, much remains to be done. Whatever the quantity of smoke in the air, many persons expose their respiratory tissues more or less continually during their waking hours to tobacco smoke. The harmful effects of this practice are well documented.

The nurse is responsible for helping individuals to understand and, when possible, to avoid and/or eliminate harmful agents from their environment. When it is not possible to eliminate or avoid harmful environmental agents, the nurse works to help people protect themselves in ways that prevent or minimize injury. When injury is sustained, the nurse supports those mechanisms which are activated to limit or repair injury.

To fulfill these responsibilities, the nurse must understand the characteristics of cell injury and of the agents that commonly produce cell injury. The purpose of this unit is to promote understanding of those characteristics, as a basis for prevention and treatment of cellular injury.

Reference Cited

Smillie, W. G., and Kilbourne, E. D. *Preventive Medicine and Public Health*, 3rd ed. New York: Macmillan Publishing Co., Inc., 1963, p. 275.

General References

Groër, M. E., and Shekleton, M. E. *Basic Pathophysiology: A Conceptual Approach*. St. Louis: The C. V. Mosby Company, 1979.

Guyton, A. C. *Textbook of Medical Physiology*, 5th ed. Philadelphia: W. B. Saunders Company, 1976.

LaVia, M. F., and Hill, R. B., Jr. *Principles of Pathobiology*, 2nd ed. New York: Oxford University Press, 1975.

Biological Agents

Amantadine: Adjunct to Flu Vaccine." *Science News*, **116** (3 Nov. 1979), 311.

Fiddes, J. C. "The Nucleotide Sequence of a Viral DNA." *Sci. Am.*, **237** (Dec. 1977), 54–67.

Fox, J. P., Hall, C. E., and Elveback, L. R. *Epidemiology: Man and Disease*. New York: Macmillan Publishing Co., Inc., 1970.

Gallucci, B. B., and Reheis, C. "Infection, Nutrition and the Compromised Patient." *Infection Control, Topics in Clinical Nursing* (E. Larson, ed.), 1:2 (July 1979), 27–28.

Kaplan, M., and Webster, R. G. "The Epidemiology of Influenza. *Sci. Am.*, **237** (Dec. 1977), 88–106.

Marx, J. L. "Viral Messenger Structure: Some Surprising New Developments." *Science*, **197** (26 Aug. 1977), 853–5, 923.

Mazia, D. "The Cell Cycle." *Sci. Am.*, **230**:55–64 (Jan. 1974), 61–62.

McNeill, W. H. *Plaques and Peoples*. New York: Anchor Press, 1977.

Meyer, K. F. "The Ecology of Psittacosis and Ornithosis." *Medicine*, **21** (May 1942), 175–76.

Miller, J. A. "Hot Bug for Energy." *Sci. News*, **116** (3 Nov. 1979), 317.

Schiff, E. R., and Chiproot, R. "Chronic Hepatitis: Guidelines for Diagnosis and Management." *Hosp. Med.*, **14** (Sept. 1978), 59–75.

Schoenbaum, S. C. "Vaccination for Influenza–Any Alternatives?" *N. Engl. J. Med.*, **298** (16 March 1978), 621–22.

Thompson, M. *The Cry and the Covenant*. Garden City, N.Y.: Doubleday & Company, Inc., 1949.

Chemical Agents

Alcohol

Burkhalter, P. K. *Nursing Care of the Alcoholic and Drug Abuser*. New York: McGraw-Hill Book Company, 1975.

Clarren, S. K., and Smith, D. W. "The Fetal Alcohol Syndrome." *N. Engl. J. Med.*, **298** (11 May 1978), 1063–67.

Gibbins, R. J. et al. *Research Advances in Alcohol and Drug Problems*. New York: John Wiley & Sons, vol 1, 1974; vol. 2, 1975.

Isselbacher, K. J. "Metabolic and Hepatic Effects of Alcohol." *N. Engl. J. Med.*, **296** (17 March 1977), 612–16.

Drugs

Govoni, L. E., and Hayes, J. E. *Drugs and Nursing Implications*, 3rd ed. New York: Appleton-Century-Crofts, 1978.

Hansten, P. D. *Drug Interactions*. Philadelphia: Lea & Febiger, 1975.

Physicians' Desk Reference, 33rd ed. Oradell, N.J.: Medical Economics Co., 1979.

9

Cell Injury—Ischemia

Virchow dominated German medicine for fifty years, established the cellular theory of diseases, and influenced world-wide medical progress.

POOLE

Gray Poole, Doctors Who Saved Lives *New York: Dodd, Mead & Company, 1966, p. 59.*

Characteristics of Cell Injury

Causes of Cell Injury

Agents that cause direct injury may be classified as biological, physical, and chemical. They also can be classified according to the manner in which they cause injury, that is, as an agent, situation, or condition that:

1. Deprives the cell of something it requires such as oxygen, calories, vitamins. (See Unit VI.)
2. Cripples the cell machinery by
   a. The lack of a necessary enzyme due to a genetic defect. (See Chapter 14.)
   b. The toxic effect of an endogenous or exogenous chemical or bacterial poison on an enzyme or enzyme system.
   c. The effect of physical agents such as heat, cold, or radioactive materials on enzymes or enzyme systems.
3. Alters the nature of proteins within cells through physical or chemical systems.
4. Produces antigen–antibody responses. (See Chapter 24.)

Nature of Cell Injury

As with the response of the entire organism to an injuring agent, individual cells may be healthy, adapted to the injuring agent, injured, or dead. Degrees of injury may be so slight that the cell is able to repair itself while maintaining its function and structural integrity, or so great that it dies immediately with or without appreciable structural change. The significance to the nurse of the nature and severity of cell injury is related to the way in which injury alters the primary functions of the individual as an open system. The primary functions include: (1) reproduction, (2) environmental exchange, (3) internal transport, (4) internal communication, and (5) adjustment to the external environment. The participation of each of the ten organ systems in maintaining the primary functions is shown in Figure 9-1.

In sudden and overwhelming injuries there may be less structural change than in those that are of long standing. Knowledge of this fact is utilized when tissue is prepared for microscopic examination. It is quickly frozen or otherwise treated so that structural changes are minimized. The structure of the tissue and cells must be preserved for the comparison between it and so-called normal cells to be mean-

Organ System	Primary Functions: Reproduction	Environmental Exchange	Internal Transport	Internal Communication	Adjustment to Environment
Circulatory	S	P	P	P	S
Integument	S	P	S	S	P[1]
Skeletal	S	S	S	S	P
Excretory	P[2]	P	S	S	S
Respiratory	S	P	S	S	S
Digestive	S	P	S	S	S
Nervous	S	S	S	P	P
Endocrine	P	S	S	P	P
Reproductive	P	NE	NE	NE	NE
Muscular	S	S	P	S	P

KEY: P = primary role; S = supportive role; NE = nonessential

[1] In its censory capacity.

[2] Since reproductive systems commonly utilize excretory ducts.

Figure 9-1. Participation of the ten organ systems in the primary functions of multicellular organisms. (Used with permission of Macmillan Publishing Company, Inc., from *Biology,* 2nd ed., 1979, p. 194, by J. F. Case.)

ingful. Further, a number of different agents have similar effects on cell structure.

Because of its function as a major organ of detoxification, the liver's cells are damaged by a variety of chemicals. By the time enough damage occurs to impair liver function, the changes in liver structure are characteristic of injury and tissue responses to it, but not of any particular toxic substance. (Chapter 44.)

Sequence of Events

Knowledge of the sequence of events in cell injury is incomplete. However, it is known that the first effects of injuring agents are on the molecular and biochemical elements in the cell, with the result that most types of cell injury affect the ability of the cell to (1) produce the energy required to support metabolic processes, (2) synthesize proteins, (3) maintain homeostatic conditions within the cell, and (4) reproduce.

Factors Affecting the Degree of Cell Injury

Two general factors affect the degree of cell injury: the potency of the injuring agent and the susceptibility of the cell and/or individual to injury.

Potency of the Agent: Quality, Quantity, and Duration of Exposure

The potency of the injuring agent is influenced by its nature, concentration, and in some instances the length of the exposure. As examples, cyanide is a highly toxic chemical that in minute amounts wrecks cell machinery. Substances such as asbestos, coal dust, and silica require excessive and/or prolonged exposure to be harmful. The effect of deprivation of nutrients depends not only on the degree, but on whether or not the deficiency is of a single substance or is a balanced deficiency of several nutrients. Generalized undernutrition is better tolerated than a diet adequate in calories but lacking in protein or one vitamin such as thiamine.

Susceptibility of the Host

In many instances the individual (or cell) is a factor in the degree of injury sustained after exposure. A critical factor can be the stage of growth and development, that is, the age of the individual. For example, the drug thalidomide was supposed to be a mild and relatively safe sedative. It was safe when administered to adults, unless the adult happened to be a prospective mother who was in the early stages of pregnancy. Even then the drug appeared to be safe for the mother, but an unusual number of infants born of mothers who had taken thalidomide during the first 6 weeks of pregnancy were born with a deformity called phocomelia (seal limb). Although the reason for the susceptibility of the embryo to thalidomide is not known, the drug arrests and deranges the development of the embryo exposed to it. It is generally thought that drugs that produce fetal deformities exert their action at the time the affected part is undergoing differentiation. Some infants were only slightly deformed, whereas others were born with multiple anomalies, including serious deformities of all four extremities and of the viscera (Taussig, 1962). The nature and extent of deformity depend on the time of differentiation in the embryo in relation to the ingestion of the drug and its action. The differences between the effects of thalidomide on the adult and embryo serve to emphasize that the susceptibility of the individual can be a factor in the effect of a chemical agent. In this instance, immaturity was the critical factor. In other instances, it may be something else, such as blood supply to a part or body temperature.

Responses to Injury

Many injuries are so minor that cell damage or even cell death passes unnoticed. In more extensive but sublethal injuries cells respond to damage by alterations in their normal biological mechanisms. When sublethal injuries are prolonged, cells are able to adapt to the presence of abnormal stimuli by new or altered steady states. Examples of altered steady states include altered growth and development, atrophy, hypertrophy, hyperplasia, metaplasia, and neoplasia. As a consequence of some types of prolonged injury, normal as well as abnormal substances accumulate within cells, thus causing further interference with normal biologic mechanisms.

Changes in Growth and Development

One of the responses to cell injury is some alteration in the cell's growth and development. Basically, the growth and development of a cell is dependent on (1) the capacity of the cell to proliferate and differentiate, (2) its supply of nutrients, and (3) the degree to which its activity is stimulated. In the process of development, some types of cells, such as those of connective and epithelial tissues, retain their capacity to proliferate (multiply) and differentiate (breed true). Others, such as nerve and muscle cells, sacrifice these properties as they specialize. The manner in which cells of different types respond to abnormal conditions is influenced by inherent cell functions. A stimulus, normal or abnormal, can depress or increase a cell function, but it cannot make a cell take on a new function.

Responses to Deprivation

The effects of deprivation on growth and development of cells depend on multiple factors. In general, however, when cells are deprived of an essential nutrient or stimulation, they lose substance. The cell, like larger functioning units in the body, is capable of adapting to a decrease in the supply of nutrients or to a decrease in the functional demands made on it by decreasing its substance. As with other homeostatic mechanisms there are limits to adaptation. When the degree of deprivation is too great, the cell dies. The scientific term for the loss of substance, and with it a decrease in the size and functional capacity of a cell, tissue, or organ, is *atrophy.* Some authorities include a decrease in the number of cells in a tissue in the definition of atrophy. For example, as a muscle atrophies it loses strength or becomes weak. In some instances atrophy can be prevented or reversed if conditions leading to it are corrected soon enough. For instance, muscle atrophy that accompanies insufficient exercise can be reversed and the muscle can be restored to its former strength by exercise.

Atrophy

Atrophy has many causes, not all of which are abnormal. Atrophy is involutional when some tissue or organ diminishes in size as a result of the normal aging process; to maintain its youthful structure would be abnormal. For example, at the time of menopause, sexual organs, including the breasts of women, diminish in size. In old age all organs undergo some decrease in size. As a result elderly persons are not quite as tall as they were in their youth and they do not weigh as much. Shock (1962) quotes a study made in Canada that illustrates the decline in weight from middle to old age. Men who weighed 167 lb at ages 35 to 40 showed a decline in average weight to 155 lb at 65 years or older. They weighed 12 lb less at 65 than they did at 35 or 40 years of age. In a study made on a group of men in the United States, men who averaged 168 lb at ages 65 to 69 weighed, on the average, 148 lb at the ages 90 to 94; that is, they lost approximately 20 lb during this period. Not only does the total body weight decrease, but individual organs decrease in weight after middle age. Shock indicates that the average weight of the brain at autopsy drops from 1,375 g (3.03 lb) to 1,232 g (2.72 lb) between the ages of 30 and 90. Mrs. Sabin illustrates these changes very well. At 95 years of age she weighs only 145 pounds. Her highest weight was 215 pounds. She has lost about 2 inches in height. Her skin is loose and wrinkled, her hair thin and sparse. With her loss of tissue she has lost strength. She is no longer as energetic as she was in her youth. She spends her days in her rocking chair.

Pathologic Atrophy

Pathologic atrophy classified according to its etiology is (1) disuse, (2) deficient blood supply or ischemic, (3) pressure, (4) neurogenic, (5) endocrine, or (6) generalized atrophy.

DISUSE ATROPHY is one of the forms commonly seen by the nurse. In some instances, disuse atrophy can be prevented or limited by the practice of nursing. In disuse atrophy there is a wasting of tissue, especially that of the muscle and bone. The development and maintenance of the size, strength, and composition of muscle and bone are influenced by the amount of strain placed on them. This is supported by the principle that, in nature, parts develop in proportion to the stresses and strains placed on them. In a tree the trunk is larger and stronger than the branches. The branches proximal to the trunk are larger in diameter than those distal to it. Patients may lose weight and strength from want of exercise. Inactivity and immobilization lead to muscle and bone atrophy. The results of the demineralization of the bone are known as osteoporosis and can be seen on x-ray. Sometimes the decalcification of the bone may proceed at such a rapid rate that calculi are formed in the urine. The weakness experienced by the patient who has been on bedrest is caused in part by generalized atrophy.

A striking example of disuse atrophy can be observed by comparing the size of a limb that has been encased in a cast with that of its free mate. (See Figure 9-3 for the effect of casting on muscle strength.) To minimize disuse atrophy, unless there is some contraindication, bed patients should be encouraged to exercise. All patients should have arms and legs put through the normal range of motion each day. This can be done as they are bathed. The nurse should use reasonable judgment. Motion should not be forced beyond the normal range nor should it cause pain. Patients who are able should be taught to do exercises such as wriggling their toes, moving the legs up and down in bed, and doing muscle-setting exercises. When the patients' condition permits, activities such as boosting or raising themselves up in bed, reaching, and turning help to maintain muscle strength. For patients who are paralyzed or who are unable to get out of bed, strain on muscles and bones may be increased by the use of the standing board. The circoelectric bed makes this procedure easy to perform.

ISCHEMIC ATROPHY is also commonly seen in care of the sick. When the blood supply to tissue is deficient, the tissue adapts by undergoing atrophy. This will be further expanded in the following discussion of pressure atrophy.

PRESSURE ATROPHY. Although pressure may have other effects, it predisposes to atrophy by causing ischemia. There are many examples of pressure causing atrophy by reducing the blood supply. For example, hydrocephalus is a condition in which cerebrospinal fluid accumulates within the ventricles and stretches the brain cortex. This causes pressure on blood vessels and diminishes their capacity to carry blood. Brain cell nutrition is thereby reduced, and atrophy ensues. Another example is the atrophy of glandular structures such as the kidney or liver following obstruction of a ureter or the common bile duct. As a result of the blocking of the duct, urine accumulates in the ureter or bile in the bile ducts, distends the ducts, and causes back pressure. The distended ducts press on blood vessels and reduce the blood supply to the affected organ. If ischemia is marked, and if it is allowed to continue, the functioning cells may die. With a decrease in the number of parenchymal[1] cells, there is a decrease in the functional capacity of the organ. With stagnation of bile or urine, growth of bacteria is favored. Thus, atrophic injury resulting from stagnation and ischemia is extended by injury to the organ resulting from infection.

NEUROGENIC ATROPHY. Loss of normal stimulation of tissues is accompanied by atrophy. When a muscle loses its motor nerve supply, it wastes or atrophies. For example, in anterior poliomyelitis, destruction of the motor horn cells in the spinal cord deprives muscles of normal stimulation and the muscles become flaccid or limp. Muscles permanently deprived of their motor nerve supply eventually degenerate. Injuries to sensory nerves may have a similar effect.

ENDOCRINE ATROPHY. Secretion by some endocrine glands is under the control of the anterior hypophysis (pituitary). The relationship of the anterior pituitary to its target glands is essentially that of a system of negative feedbacks. The anterior pituitary produces a number of tropic (stimulating) hormones, each of which stimulates a specific endocrine gland. The gland so stimulated increases the secretion of its hormone. As the level of the hormone from the target gland rises, the secretion of the tropic hormone is depressed. The glands known to be under the control of the anterior pituitary are the adrenal cortex, the thyroid, and the gonads. The tropic hormones are ACTH (adrenocorticotropic), TSH (thyrotropic), and GSH (gonadotropic). Some of the hormones secreted by the anterior pituitary, notably ACTH, have effects other than stimulation of target glands. The preceding is an oversimplified description of the relationship of the anterior pituitary gland to its target glands. The brain and liver both play a part in the system. Atrophy of its target glands may result from failure of the anterior pituitary to

[1] *Parenchymal* cells are those that constitute the essential parts of an organ that are concerned with its function, in contradistinction to the cells that constitute the supporting framework of the organ.

produce its tropic hormones. Because of the negative feedback relationship of the anterior pituitary with its target glands, atrophy of a target gland can also be produced by the administration of large doses of its hormones. To illustrate, atrophy of the adrenal cortex has been observed when large dosages of cortisone or hydrocortisone have been administered over a period of time. When thyroxine is administered in the absence of a thyroid deficiency, the thyroid gland adapts by decreasing its secretion of thyroxine.

GENERALIZED ATROPHY is caused by a variety of conditions. It is most frequently associated with a lack of calories or a serious debilitating disease. An infrequent cause is destruction of the anterior pituitary gland following childbirth.

In a broad sense, atrophy occurs when stimulation or nutrition falls below that required to maintain the optimum number, size, and strength of the cells. The factors initiating atrophy may be physiological or pathological. As an adaptive mechanism atrophy permits cells to survive unfavorable conditions.

The Nurse

The nurse through the practice of nursing can help to prevent atrophy by encouraging and assisting the patient to exercise, by preventing and relieving pressure, and by assisting the patient in maintaining food intake.

Responses to Increased Nutrition and Activity and to an Unfavorable Environment

Just as cells adapt to lessened nutrition or strain by decreasing in size or number, they can respond to an increase in nutrition and activity by an increase in size and/or in number of cells. The term *hypertrophy* is used to indicate an enlargement in the volume of parenchymal tissue. *Hyperplasia* denotes an increase in the number of cells. Whether cells undergo hypertrophy or hyperplasia depends in part on whether or not they are able to regenerate or reproduce themselves. Highly specialized cells, such as nerve cells, skeletal and cardiac muscle cells, and, to a lesser extent, smooth muscle cells, do not proliferate, and they therefore respond to stimuli for increased function by hypertrophy.

Both hypertrophy and hyperplasia are adaptive and they are beneficial when they enable the cell (organ) to meet increased demands for function. Furthermore, both are organized processes. Possibly hypertrophy occurs because the capacity of the cell for anabolism is greater than it generally uses. With a higher rate of anabolism there is an increase in the storage of materials in the cell and the cell becomes larger. In terms of function, hypertrophy increases the capacity of the cell to do work.

Hypertrophy

There are many examples of hypertrophy. The bulging muscles of the wrestler or the weight lifter are examples of hypertrophy of skeletal muscles in response to increased work. Figures 9-2 and 9-3 show the relationship of strength to muscular hypertrophy and atrophy. The same adaptation may be observed in the person who has lost the function of the lower extremities and uses his or her arm and shoulder muscles as legs. Hypertrophy also enables the myocardium to move the blood against an increase in resistance such as is produced by stenosis of a heart valve, coarctation of the aorta, or arteriolar constriction in essential hypertension. These disorders are examples of adaptations to a pathologic process enabling the organism to survive. Unfortunately, the capacity of the individual to nourish the increase in muscle tissue may not keep pace with the increase in size. Eventually the muscle becomes ischemic and fails.

Smooth muscle also undergoes hypertrophy when its work is increased. For example, hyperplasia of the prostate gland obstructs the urethra, causing increased resistance to the flow of urine. The smooth muscle of the urinary bladder wall responds by increasing the size of the muscle fibers. For a time this results in a sufficient increase in force to move the urine through the narrowed urethra. In time, the bladder wall may reach several times its normal thickness. Although capacity to undergo hypertrophy is adaptive, in this instance the stimulus is patho-

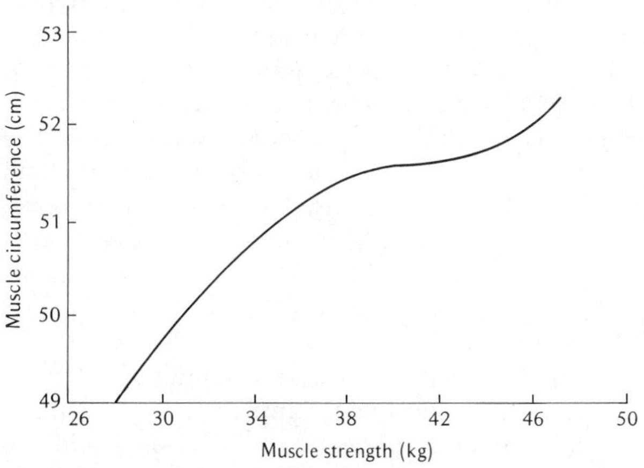

Figure 9-2. Increase in the strength of muscle with hypertrophy. The increase in total muscle circumference is due to an increase in individual muscle fiber size as a result of isometric training. (Used with permission of Macmillan Publishing Company, Inc., from *Physiology: A Regulatory Systems Approach,* 1978, p. 501, by F. L. Strand.)

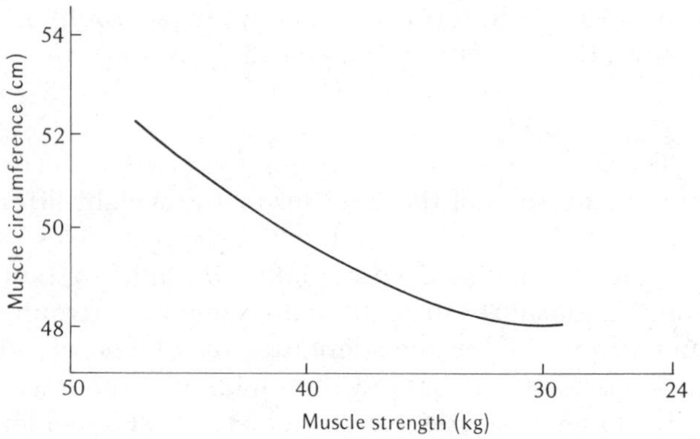

Figure 9-3. Decrease in the strength of muscle with atrophy. The decrease in the total muscle circumference is due to a decrease in individual muscle fiber size following prolonged immobilization in a plaster cast. (Used with permission of Macmillan Publishing Company, Inc., from *Physiology: A Regulatory Systems Approach,* 1978, p. 501, by F. L. Strand.)

logic. Hypertrophy of the pyloric muscle, with a narrowing or stenosis of the outlet of the stomach, occurs in infants of 2 to 3 weeks of age. The infant manifests projectile vomiting, rapid loss of weight, and constipation or obstipation.

Hypertrophy can be expected to develop in any muscle called on to increase its work over that it normally does. Hypertrophy is adaptive when it enables the organ to perform a greater amount of work. It is maladaptive when it narrows the lumen of a tube.

The extent to which any organ or tissue can respond to a stimulus for an increase in function is limited. A factor in this limitation is the ability to increase the blood supply in proportion to the increase in the amount of tissue. To illustrate, hypertrophy of the myocardium is limited by the capacity of the coronary arteries to provide a supply of blood adequate to its needs. The increase in bulk demands an increased supply of nutrients. Moreover, as the heart muscle enlarges, it causes pressure on the small vessels and thereby decreases circulation. The consequence is an ischemic heart muscle and, eventually, failure.

Hyperplasia

Hyperplasia, which involves the multiplication of cells, is a somewhat more complex process than hypertrophy. In hyperplasia two cells are derived from one cell. Hyperplasia is physiologic. It occurs only in response to a need, the process is organized, and it is terminated when the need is met. Daughter cells are similar to those from which they derive, which means that they are differentiated. Hyperplasia is possible because cells have a built-in capacity to grow and to multiply. The capacity of the bone marrow, the lymphoid tissue, and the reticuloendothelial tissue to undergo hyperplasia enables the organism to cope with infection, restore blood cells after blood loss or abnormal destruction of blood cells, and adapt to living at high altitudes. Hyperplasia of an organ around or adjacent to a tubular structure may interfere with its drainage. As an example, hyperplasia of the prostate gland (benign prostatic *hypertrophy*) blocks the urethra, as the prostate enlarges, and interferes with emptying the urinary bladder.

Hyperplasia and hypertrophy may occur together. Following the removal of one kidney, the other one enlarges. The enlargement is caused by an increase in both the size of the tubules and the number of cells lining them.

In summary, hypertrophy and hyperplasia are adaptive responses to an increase in stimulation, which may be either pathologic or physiologic. As a consequence of these responses, an organ or part can increase the amount of work it performs. Without this adaptive capacity, life would be greatly shortened by many diseases and would not be possible in some environments.

Metaplasia

Besides being able to adapt to environmental conditions by increasing the size and/or number of cells, some types of cells are able to adapt by a process known as *metaplasia.* In metaplasia one type of tissue is changed to another. Metaplasia involves two factors. The tissue must contain incompletely differentiated cells that have the potential for maturing into different types of cells, and the environment must be unfavorable to the type of cell normally found in the tissue. For example, the different types of epithelial tissues have their origin in a common cell, the basal cell. When conditions are unfavorable to a given type of epithelial tissue, it is transformed to a type better suited to the particular environmental conditions. Squamous cell epithelium usually replaces other types. Conditions predisposing to epithelial cell metaplasia include chronic irritation by physical and chemical agents, certain vitamin deficiencies, and direct exposure of a mucous membrane to the external environment. For example, the mucous membrane in the trachea undergoes a transformation to squamous cell epithelium following a tracheostomy. The capacity to undergo metaplasia enables the cell or tissue to survive unfavorable conditions.

Neoplasia

Whereas metaplasia is a process whereby a healthy cell adapts by differentiating into another type of healthy cell, *neoplasia* is a process in which adaption results in an abnormal cell. Cell proliferation continues without regard to the needs of the body, and cell differentiation also departs from the normal. Depending on the nature of the neoplasm, cells may be similar to those of the parent cell (differentiated) or be so different (undifferentiated) that the cells from which they originated are difficult if not impossible to determine. These latter cells are said to be anaplastic. (See Chapter 51.)

Failure to Grow and Develop: Agenesis

The failure of an organ or tissue to develop in the embryo is known as agenesis. Literally translated, *agenesis* means "without beginning." Occasionally an individual is born with only one of a pair of organs such as the kidney. This individual may very well live a normal life span. However, when neither kidney develops, life after birth is shortened to a few days or weeks. When the organ is one that is essential to life, death occurs at or before birth.

Aplasia

Aplasia is a condition in which there is defective development or absence of a part. A lesser degree of aplasia, in that some tissue is present, in hypoplasia. In *hypoplasia,* the amount of tissue is insufficient to meet the functional requirements of the body. For example, as a consequence of failure to develop or as a result of exposure to toxic agents, the bone marrow may be aplastic or hypoplastic. A child may be born with aplastic or hypoplastic bone marrow. He or she may develop a disease or be exposed to an environmental condition causing partial or complete destruction of the bone marrow. There are many agents capable fo injuring bone marrow. Among them are x-rays and radioactive materials and bone marrow poisons such as benzene. Evidence of an aplastic or hypoplastic bone marrow can be obtained from low blood cell counts and from biopsy of the bone marrow. As a consequence of hypoplasia, the individual not only is unable to adapt to conditions requiring an increase in the number of blood cells but may not be able to manufacture enough cells to meet ordinary needs. The person whose bone marrow is aplastic can do neither.

The normal cell has the capacity to adapt to increased or decreased supply of materials or stimulation by increasing its size and strength (hypertrophy) or by decreasing its size and strength (atrophy). The integrity of the structure is further protected by the capacity of some cells to proliferate (multiply) and to undergo *hyperplasia.* Certain cells are able to protect themselves by differentiating into a type of cell better suited to the environmental conditions to which they are exposed. Failure of cells to proliferate whether because of a low growth potential or a deficiency or absence of tissue robs the individual of an important means of defense against injury.

Degeneration

In addition to failures to grow and mature, previously healthy cell activities may deteriorate or degenerate. In the various forms of degeneration, different substances accumulate within the cells. In some types the name is descriptive of the substance accumulating within the cell. In others it is descriptive of the appearance of the cell. Thus in fatty degeneration, fat accumulates within the cell. In cloudy swelling, changes take place that, as the name suggests, cause the cell to appear cloudy instead of clear. When a degenerative process is terminated during the phase in which chemical activity is altered, it may be reversed and the cell restored to normal. This presupposes that the changes do not overwhelm the cellular enzymes, especially those in sensitive tissues, beyond the point of recovery. After structural changes occur, the cell goes on to necrosis or death. When there are blood vessels, blood cells, and connective tissues in the area of the necrotic cells, they respond with inflammation.

Infiltration

Healthy cells may also be damaged by being overloaded with metabolites; the resulting condition is known as an infiltration. In infiltration the cell is damaged. Despite many possible disturbances in intermediary metabolism, the most common are those involving fat, glucose, amyloid, and calcium. Disturbances in the metabolism of glucose are discussed in Chapters 44 and 52. Disturbances in the metabolism of fat are usually of one of two types. One or both types may be present in a tissue at one time. Although the mechanisms by which they affect tissue are different, they are both known as fatty infiltration. In the first type adipose tissue cells undergo hyperplasia. They infiltrate tissues of organs where they are not normally present. In the other, fat particles enter (infiltrate) cells and displace cellular elements. Severe obesity is an example of the first type. Adipose tissue cells undergo hyperplasia and infiltrate tissues in which they are not normally found, such as the heart muscle. They do not enter the muscle cells, but they lie between muscle fibers. They neither cause cellular degeneration nor provoke an inflammatory response. Because of their number, they occupy space and interfere mechanically with function.

Adipose tissue may also fill space left by the atrophy of the parenchyma of organs. Replacement of parenchymatous tissue by adipose tissue sometimes follows normal involution of organs, such as the thymus at puberty. It is also associated with pathology. Atrophy of muscle, especially when it results from a loss of the nerve supply to the muscle, may be accompanied by an increase in adipose tissue. When this happens, the affected extremity may maintain its normal size, despite the loss of muscle tissue. With the loss of muscle, the function of the extremity is lost.

In the other type of fatty infiltration, lipids enter the cells of the organ and displace its normal elements. Cells may be so overdistended by fat that they rupture. One organ in which this type of fatty infiltration occurs is the liver. Though fatty infiltration of the liver may develop rapidly, it usually develops slowly. In the United States, the most common cause is chronic alcoholism. In parts of the world where the supply of high-quality proteins is deficient and malnutrition is made more severe by diarrhea, a disease called kwashiorkor is common among young children. One of its striking features is fatty degeneration of the liver. (See Chapter 44.)

Ingestion of poisons, such as phosphorus, is followed by the rapid development of fatty degeneration. Though the liver is perhaps the most common site of fatty degeneration, other organs such as the heart muscle may be affected. Fatty degeneration of the heart is a serious complication of diphtheria and of marked and long-standing anemia, particularly pernicious anemia. Phosphorus poisoning has become infrequent, because phosphorus is no longer used in matches. Diptheria is easily prevented by immunization. Patients with pernicious anemia can be protected by adequate treatment. In the latter two conditions, the nurse contributes through participating in public and individual education and by assisting with the required procedures.

Despite the importance of disorders characterized by fatty infiltration of vital organs, the disease with the highest incidence in which disordered metabolism of lipids is strongly implicated is atherosclerosis. The effects of this disorder will be considered in Chapters 42 and 43.

Amyloid Degeneration

In infections such as empyema, tertiary syphilis, and tuberculosis, a starchlike substance known as amyloid is deposited in the cells of the body. The organs most likely to be affected are the kidneys, spleen, liver, and adrenal glands. As with fatty degeneration, amyloid degeneration usually develops slowly and does not cause acute cellular degeneration or stimulate an acute inflammatory response. It does result in atrophy of the cell, probably as a result of interference with cellular nutrition. Symptoms resulting from the failure of function depend on the extent of damage to the affected organs. Though a number of organs may be involved, death is usually from renal failure.

Cell Death

In those conditions in which cellular injury is sufficiently great or prolonged, death of the cell occurs. Throughout the course of life, body cells die and are replaced. For example, epithelial cells of the skin and mucous membranes, as well as blood cells, mature, live out their life span, and die. However, when a group of cells die not as a result of aging but from some injury, the condition is known as *necrosis.* It usually results from a lack of oxygen. Terms such as *gangrene* and *infarction* also imply death of cells but have more specific meanings.

Gangrene

Gangrene is the term ordinarily used to indicate the death of a large section of an organ, an entire organ or part (such as a portion of the bowel, the appendix, or gallbladder), or an extremity such as a hand or leg.

Gangrene may be classified as wet or dry. Wet gangrene develops in those conditions in which there is fluid in the tissue. It occurs in disorders in which there is an obstruction of the venous return from a tissue or an organ. In dry gangrene, death of tissue results from obstruction of the arterial circulation. As a consequence the tissue becomes dehydrated and shriveled. It is blackened and mummified in appearance. The area of dead tissue is usually clearly demarcated from the living tissue by a red zone of granulation tissue.

Infarct

Infarct is the term used to indicate a localized area of necrosis resulting when the blood supply to an area falls below the level required for cells to survive. Infarction results from the obstruction of an artery at a point where both the main blood supply and the collateral circulation are blocked. It also occurs when the tissue requirements are raised above the capacity of the diseased vessels to deliver blood. Although an infarction may occur in any tissue, those that require a large supply of blood and/or have a poor collateral circulation are particularly vulnerable. Organs in which infarctions are commonly found are the brain, heart, kidney, and lung.

The consequences of an infarction depend on its location and extent. A large infarct in a vital organ such as the heart, lung, or brain may be responsible for sudden death. When the infarcted area is small enough for the function of the organ to be maintained, it is healed by fibrous tissue substitution, that is, by the formation of scar tissue. Residual effects will depend on its size and location. The reserve capacity of the organ will, however, be reduced in proportion to the amount of loss of parenchymal tissue.

Ischemia

In the preceding section some of the possible effects of cell injury were considered. Because alteration in blood supply is so frequently associated with cell injury, whatever the causative agent, effects of depriving cells of their blood supply are discussed here in detail. Figure 9-4 summarizes the temporal sequence of cellular events that occur in ischemic injury.

Ischemia is a condition in which the quantity or quality of blood delivered to the tissues is insufficient to supply their needs for oxygen and nutrients under varying degrees of activity. At one extreme, sufficient oxygen is delivered to meet ordinary but not unusual needs. At the other, barely enough blood is supplied to maintain life even at complete rest.

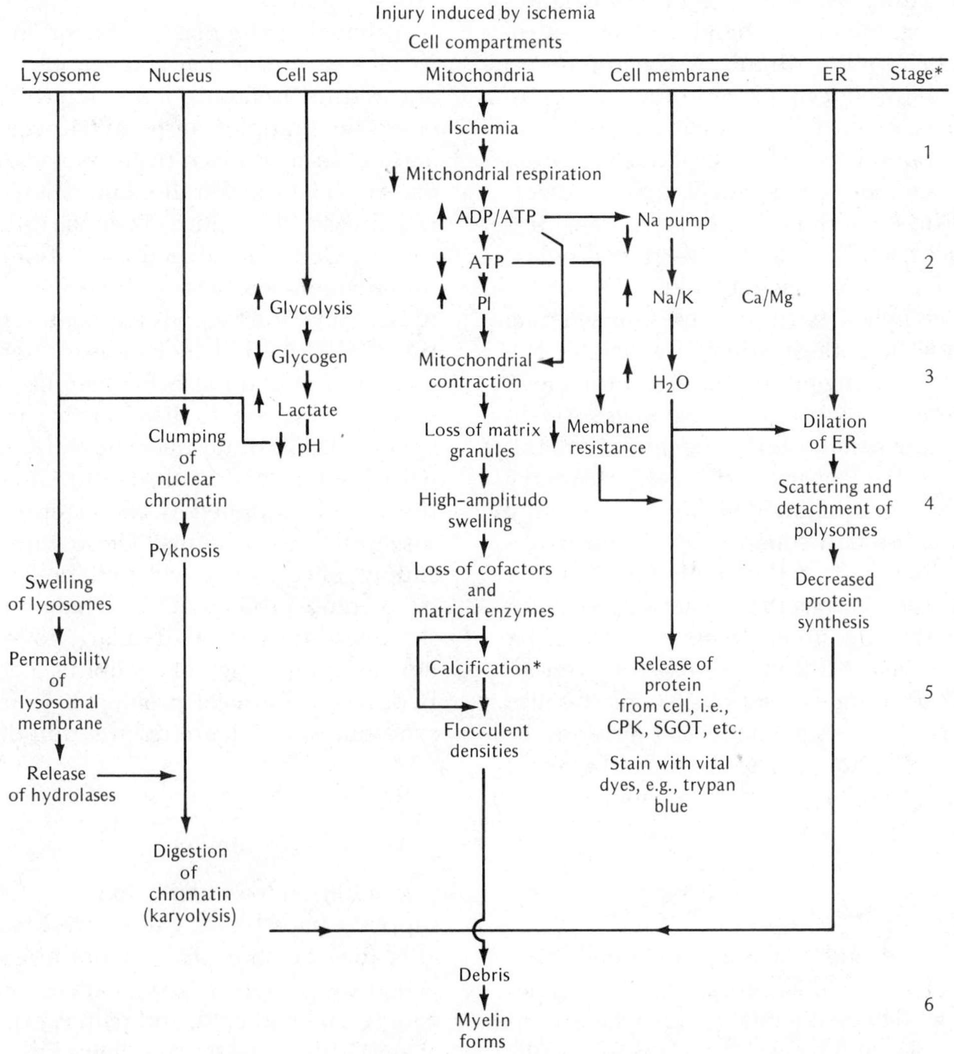

*Calcification does not generally occur in the centers of infarcts unless reflow of blood is permitted.
*Numbers at the right correspond to the temporal sequence of events.

Figure 9-4. Flow sheet of sequential events that occur in ischemic injury. (Used with permission of Universities Associated for Research and Education in Pathology, Inc., from *Cell Injury,* 1974, by D. Scarpelli and B. F. Trump.)

Causes

Ischemia may be generalized or limited to a small area of tissue. Generalized ischemia results from (1) the failure of the heart as a pump; (2) a lack in the quantity or quality of the blood; (3) generalized and excessive resistance of arterioles to the flow of blood; (4) excessive dilatation of veins, which increases their capacity to hold blood and thereby reduces the amount of blood returned to the heart; and (5) failure of the lungs to oxygenate blood. In all these conditions cell nutrition suffers.

Localized ischemia can be of intrinsic or extrinsic origin. The most common intrinsic causes of ischemia are arterial occlusion and interference with the venous return, which will be discussed in Chapters 42 and 43. A less usual cause of ischemia is Raynaud's disease. Arteries supplying the hands and/or feet respond to cold or to other stimuli by constricting so greatly that no blood can pass through them to the tissue. Consequently, the involved areas are blanched and painful. Because the attack is brief, tissue necrosis seldom occurs. Small areas of ulceration of the skin sometimes do develop. The frequency of attacks can be reduced by preventing exposure to inciting agents, such as cold.

Among the common extrinsic causes of ischemia are prolonged sitting; the resting of a part of the body, particularly a bony prominence, against a firm surface; and constricting casts and bandages. Swelling of tissues, as the result of either edema[2] or inflammation, reduces the capacity of vessels to carry blood. The effects of swelling develop more rapidly in solid tissues or those surrounded by a nonexpansible wall, such as a cast or the skull. Any increase in tension in tissues lessens the capacity of veins to remove blood from the area. Unless corrected, the swelling that results leads to a decrease or even an interruption of arterial blood supply. Neoplasms also cause ischemia by pressing on either arteries or veins. Changes in the function or structure of arteries and/or veins are frequent causes of ischemia.

Effects

Although marked and prolonged ischemia leads to the death of cells, cells differ greatly in their capacity to tolerate it. The suddenness with which ischemia develops also influences the outcome. Cells maintaining a high metabolic rate, such as those in the brain, tolerate ischemia poorly. Cells adapt to slowly developing ischemia by reducing their metabolic rate and cellular substance; that is, they atrophy. This adaptation is successful *only* as long as the tissue nutrition is maintained at a level high enough to sustain the life of the cells and the cells are not stimulated to function beyond this point. Tissues rendered ischemic by one cause have a smaller tolerance for other ischemia-inducing conditions than do normal tissues. For example, Mr. Brown, who has occlusive vascular disease in the arteries in his legs, is more susceptible to the effects of pressure on his heels than is his roommate, who has healthy arteries. When death of cells does occur, continuity of structure may be maintained by the formation of scar tissue. With the loss of parenchymatous cells, the reserve capacity of the organ is reduced and with it the capacity to adapt to changes in the environment.

Although ischemia is a factor in many illnesses, its effects on the skin and muscle will be discussed at this time. Ischemia of the skin results from a single cause or multiple causes. Whatever the etiology, it acts to cause localized tissue anoxia. As stated earlier, external pressure on the skin, edema, occlusive arterial disease, and failure of venous return are common causes. Generalized undernutrition, particularly of protein and ascorbic acid, increases the susceptibility to ischemia. For reasons not completely understood, tissues deprived of their sensory nerve supply have increased susceptibility to ischemia. Because the sensory nerve supply to the tissue is part of the warning system, its loss diminishes the capacity of the individual to detect and evaluate threats of injury to the tissue. Cells supplied by end arteries are particularly susceptible to ischemia. Those with a double blood supply or a well-developed collateral circulation have some protection. The ischemic effect on the skin and muscle, particularly over bony prominences, is formation of decubitus ulcers, or bedsores. Bedsores are a major problem associated with disuse syndromes, which are discussed in detail in Chapter 45.

Arterial Obstruction

In addition to ischemia in which tissues are undersupplied with blood, the entire blood supply to an area may be shut off by acute arterial obstruction. When the venous return is adequate, the tissue becomes pale and cold, and pain is experienced in the area. Tissue breakdown follows unless the condition is rapidly corrected.

Muscle Ischemia

Ischemia of muscle is frequently the result of a partial or complete occlusion of an artery. The most marked manifestation in acute ischemia is pain. Al-

[2] *Edema* is a condition in which the interstitial (between tissue) spaces or serous cavities retain an abnormal amount of fluid.

though a lack of oxygen to the tissues may be responsible for the pain, just why pain occurs is not completely clear. There is, however, no doubt about the reality of pain. When occlusion is complete, the pain continues for a day or two and then subsides. When the ischemia is relative rather than absolute, the pain is initiated by any condition increasing the need of the muscle for oxygen or food. This can be physical exercise, such as walking or running, or it can be an emotional state, such as anger or fear. The pain is relieved by rest. The ease with which the pain is precipitated depends on a number of factors, one being the degree to which the circulation to the tissue is compromised. When the pain occurs in an extremity, it is referred to as claudication. When the myocardium is involved, the condition is known as angina pectoris. The basis for the pain is the same in both instances. Arteries supplying the muscle of the heart or the extremities are unable to adapt the supply of blood to the requirement of the tissues for nutrition.

The responsibilities of the nurse in the care of patients with the occlusion of arteries supplying various organs will be considered in Chapter 42. However, these patients have a reduction in their capacity to adapt the supply of blood to the needs of the ischemic tissue. With impaired blood supply the tissue is susceptible to necrosis. Therefore, the tissue should be protected from conditions that increase its nutritional requirements, such as heat or exercise. When possible, measures to increase the flow of blood are instituted.

Venous Obstruction

Because venous pressure is relatively low in comparison to arterial pressure, veins are more easily obstructed than are arteries. When the venous return is obstructed, blood is delivered to the tissue but is not removed. As previously stated, in arterial obstruction the problem is one of supply. In venous obstruction, it is one of pickup and return. In venous obstruction or insufficiency, the blood remains in the tissue longer than is usual. The hemoglobin loses its oxygen, the quantity of reduced hemoglobin in the area is increased, and the tissue takes on a bluish tinge, or is cyanotic. In lightly pigmented skin, the bluish tinge is directly visible; in heavily pigmented skin, the hue is more gray. The increase in filtration pressure that accompanies venous obstruction increases the amount of fluid in the interstitial space and causes swelling (edema). This further obstructs the venous return and interferes with lymphatic drainage. A vicious circle is initiated. As the venous pressure rises, filtration pressure also rises, which further adds to imbalance between the quantity of fluid leaving the vascular system and returning to it; as more fluid enters the interstitial space and less fluid returns to the intravascular space, swelling increases. Eventually, tissue fluid pressure may equal the filtration pressure, and the blood flow to the area ceases. Venous stasis plus the diminishing arterial circulation to the tissues favors bacterial growth. With the growth of bacteria, tissues are liquefied and putrefaction occurs. As the products of bacterial growth and the necrotic tissue are absorbed, the patient becomes toxic. Inflammation with its signs and symptoms develops in the area adjacent to the necrotic tissue. Tissues in a confined space are particularly susceptible to venous obstruction.

Signs and symptoms indicating obstruction to the venous return are swelling, coldness, cyanosis/grayness or pallor, numbness and tingling, and failure to be able to move exposed fingers or toes. The numbness and tingling and the inability to move are caused by pressure on sensory and motor nerves. Unless the pressure is relieved promptly, irreversible nerve damage is likely.

Venous obstruction is commonly caused by a condition that interferes with venous return and at the same time allows arterial blood to enter. The tight-fitting cast or bandage is a good example. Another is the abdominal hernia. A loop of intestine is trapped in a hernial ring. This leads to obstruction of the venous return and, unless treated promptly, to gangrene of the trapped bowel. Surgery is usually required to reduce the hernia (removal of the bowel from the ring). When an extremity is in a cast or bandage, excessive swelling can often be prevented by elevating the limb, thus allowing gravity to facilitate return of the interstitial fluid to the intravascular space.

While reading the next four chapters on the injurious effects of selected biological, physical, and chemical agents, it should be remembered that a variety of dissimilar agents have similar effects on cells.

References Cited

Shock, N. W. "The Physiology of Aging." *Sci. Am.*, **206** (Jan. 1962), 108.

Taussig, H. B. "The Thalidomide Syndrome." *Sci. Am.*, **207** (Aug. 1962), 29–35.

10

Biological Agents

Another giant step for mankind—world eradication of smallpox.

WORLD HEALTH ORGANIZATION
OCTOBER 1979

Mechanisms of Cell Injury

Humans represent only one form of animal life in the global ecosystem, and in the natural order other forms of life threaten its existence, from large predatory carnivores to the smallest microscopic parasites. Humans consider these parasites to be enemies, as they consider a man-eating tiger, though both are as much a part of nature as humans. In fact, probably the great majority of microorganisms are either highly beneficial or of no consequence to humankind. Relatively few are harmful or disease-producing. However, those few potentially disease-producing biological agents are among the common causes of cell damage and death. It is not known how they act. Suggested possibilities of the action of bacterial endo- and exotoxins include (1) injury to cell membranes, (2) impairment of protein synthesis, (3) interference with cell respiration, or (4) inducement of immunologic alterations. Viruses enter a cell where, according to a considerable body of evidence, the viral DNA or RNA becomes incorporated into the genome or the messenger RNA system and thereby alters the homeostatic control of the cell. A question for which answers are incomplete is why some viruses (cytocidal) destroy cells, whereas others (oncogenic) stimulate cell growth. A partial answer is that the cytocidal viruses usually proliferate and mature in the host cell, after which they burst out of the cell thereby destroying it. Oncogenic viruses do not usually mature within the cell. Is the cause of cell death by the cytocidal viruses merely the explosion of the cell or is some other factor responsible?

Dramatic advances in biomedical technology have greatly increased research on biologic agents. An example of the rapidly expanding knowledge about biological injuring agents began in the 1950s with the identification of the Epstein-Barr virus as belonging to the herpes group of viruses on the basis of its double-strand DNA structure. Subsequent investigation has demonstrated that the Epstein-Barr virus is perhaps the most common of all the viruses that infect people, known to cause infectious mononucleosis and suspected of causing two types of cancer: Burkitt's lymphoma and nasopharyngeal carcinoma (Henle, 1979).

PATHOGENS

Disease-producing organisms are called *pathogens,* and when they enter the human body and start to multiply, they have initiated an infection. If this process results in manifest disease, it is called an infectious disease. This is a parasitic process because the pathogen is getting its nourishment from the host's substance. An infectious disease can be de-

This chapter has been revised by Jean Stallwood-Hess, R.N., M.S.N., Associate Professor, College of Nursing, Wayne State University, Detroit, Michigan.

scribed as "no more and no less than part of that eternal struggle in which every living organism strives to convert all the available foodstuff in its universe into living organisms of its own species" (Burnet & White, 1972). When trying to control infections, it is essential to remember that many infections occur without any evidence of pathology, and that these "silent" infections may be more important in the spread of the pathogen to other individuals than are the ones producing signs and symptoms.

General Characteristics of Infectious Diseases

Although infectious diseases have a number of similar characteristics, they are also very different from one another. One characteristic common to all is that *a pathogenic microorganism is a necessary factor to the development of disease.* The microorganism may be a virus, rickettsia, bacterium, yeast, mold, protozoan, or other parasite. The microbe is capable of being transmitted from one host, usually another human being but possibly a lower animal species, to another susceptible host. The infectious disease may occur with great frequency if the pathogen is readily transmissible, such as influenza virus during an epidemic, or it may occur infrequently and only under special conditions, as encephalitis. It may be self-limiting, that is, run a relatively predictable course and be self-terminating; or it may have no natural termination point but continue indefinitely. It may result in a more or less permanent immunity or be characterized by repeated attacks. The infectious process may be relatively mild or cause great destruction, death, or permanent disability. Different microorganisms have a predilection for specific organs or tissues of the body for reasons not completely understood but in part determined by their fastidious growth requirements. The period of time required by different microorganisms to establish themselves in the body and induce disease varies from hours to many months or even years.

The pathogenic microorganism is a necessary factor in the development of an infectious disease, but it may or may not be sufficient. It is now known that other equally significant factors influence the *susceptibility of the host.* For instance, susceptibility to some infectious diseases can be lessened by vaccines and other immunizing agents. Other organisms that are usually considered to be part of the natural microflora harmless to humans can produce serious disease if the normal defense mechanisms of the body are drastically altered.

Infectious Diseases and Present-Day Control Efforts

Definitions

The following short list of definitions of words frequently used in relation to infectious diseases will clarify their meaning as they are used throughout this chapter.

Carrier. An apparently well person in whom pathogenic microorganisms live and multiply without apparent ill effect, and can be disseminated to others.

Communicable disease. An illness caused by a specific infectious agent or its toxic products that is transmitted directly or indirectly from an infected person or animal to a susceptible host.

Contamination. The presence of pathogenic microorganisms on a body or inanimate objects. The term *contamination* is often used to indicate the possibility rather than the known presence of microorganisms.

Endemic. A disease or infectious agent that is continuously present in a community, or the usual amount of the disease.

Epidemic. A temporary and significant increase in the incidence of a disease above what is normally expected at a given time.

Infection. The entry and multiplication of an infectious agent in the body of humans or animals. Infection is *not* synonymous with infectious disease; the result may be inapparent or manifest.

Nosocomial infection. An infection or infectious disease arising within the hospital or other institution.

Pandemic. A worldwide epidemic.

Sporadic. The occasional occurrence of a disease, at a low level of incidence.

The Great Killers

Throughout the course of history five infectious diseases—plague, smallpox, cholera, typhus, and yellow fever—have been the great killers. Today they are still on the list of the six internationally quarantinable diseases, with louse-borne relapsing fever. None of them are believed to be major threats to the United States currently. However, modern air travel makes possible the importation of any of them, at any time, as long as pockets of disease remain anywhere in the world.

Modern medical science and technology would like to be able to eradicate the great killers. In a practical sense this is difficult, so efforts are aimed at control. *Eradication* means literally the "rooting out" of a disease. This may be possible on a national scale, but the optimistic goal in the United States in the first quarter of this century to eradicate *tuberculosis* has not been achieved yet, a half century later. On a global scale, efforts are being made to eradicate *malaria.*

The World Health Organization (WHO) as of October 26, 1979, has officially declared the world free of *smallpox.* Conquering this disease, which has been the world's worst pestilence at least since the time of the Egyptian pharaohs, is one of humanity's great, genuine triumphs (*Science News,* November 3, 1979). Credit for the success of the WHO eradication program is given, among other things, to an improved vaccine of assured potency and the use of the jet injector gun, which makes it possible to vaccinate up to 1,000 people an hour. Eradication was nearly accomplished 4 years ago, but some cases were reported in Bangladesh, India, Ethiopia, and Nepal.

The World Health Organization will shortly recommend that member countries stop all vaccinations against smallpox, and travelers will need smallpox certificates no longer. Halfden Mahler, director general of WHO, says these events will save the world community $1 billion, which can now be utilized to solve other health problems (*Science News,* November 3, 1979).

However, as long as smallpox virus remains viable in laboratories around the world, threat of the disease remains, as evidenced by a recently diagnosed case in a laboratory worker in London in 1973 and two deaths in visitors of another patient on the same ward (Center for Disease Control, April 7, 1973). In 1978, smallpox virus escaped from a laboratory at the University Medical School in Birmingham, England, infecting a female photographer working on another floor of the building. As she lay dying, her mother developed smallpox. The laboratory director committed suicide (Detroit Free Press, 1979). These examples illustrate the tenuous use of the term *eradication.*

Malaria is the other major disease against which a WHO eradication program has been launched. The disease remains endemic in many parts of the world, including Africa, Central and South America, and Southeast Asia. In Liberia about 37 per cent of hospital patients are suffering from malaria, and this is thought to be the general pattern in Africa. The eradication program is aimed at mosquito elimination, for not only is the mosquito the vector for the malarial parasite, it requires the mosquito for part of its life cycle. Malarious areas have been sprayed with insecticides such as DDT (dichlorodiphenyltrichloroethane). Unfortunately, some mosquitoes have become resistant to DDT, thus greatly complicating the problem of eradication, and the current controversy about the long-range health effects of human exposure to DDT adds another complication. Eradication efforts are combined with preventive chemotherapy in many areas and groups, such as our military personnel going into malarious areas. In Tanzania and Uganda some residents are protected by replacing ordinary table salt with salt containing a controlled amount of chloroquine (Around the World, 1969). However, malarial parasites are developing resistance to the synthetic drugs of choice for prevention and treatment.

Control, or the reduction to relatively low levels of incidence, is the more practical approach taken toward other serious infectious diseases. *Yellow fever* is still endemic in several areas of the world, including Central and northern South America. Epidemics occur in Africa; for example, one occurred in Angola in 1971. The jungle cycle of the disease involving tree-top monkeys and their mosquitoes that exists in the Americas make a vaccination program for people in high-risk occupations more appropriate for control than a mosquito eradication program. There were 797 confirmed cases of *plague* reported to WHO in 1971 and many more unconfirmed cases, the majority in the Republic of South Vietnam. Many varieties of rodents act as lower vertebrate hosts for the plague bacillus, and it would be virtually impossible to eradicate them, so efforts are exerted to prevent infected rodents from coming in contact with humans.

Cholera is once more a dominant global public health problem and has been termed pandemic. The cases reported in 1970 numbered 46,500, and more than three times this number occurred the following year. The cases reported from Africa increased nearly six times in 1971 over the preceding year, and there was a major outbreak in India among the refugees in West Bengal. Cholera presents a great threat to any area with poor standards of sanitation. In 1978, there were 74,632 reported cases of cholera. *Louse-borne typhus* and *louse-borne relapsing fever* remain as infectious disease problems in very limited areas today (Center for Disease Control, July 6, 1979).

The incidence of *poliomyelitis* is increasing in all parts of the world that do not have vaccination programs. In addition, children in tropical countries have poor sero-conversion rates in response to live virus poliomyelitis vaccine as compared to children in temperate climates. The pandemic status of *gonorrhea* is substantiated by the fact that marked and continued increases in infections are being reported from all over the world. The trend for *syphilis* is more varied, but this is a great health problem in a country such as Ethiopia, which lacks the facilities and the personnel to apply the usual control measure of contact tracing.

Many areas of the world have large disease burdens caused by tissue-inhabiting nematodes, such as *schistosomiasis* and *onchocerciasis. Filariasis* is estimated to affect 250 million people; it is becoming worse in the developing countries, where the influx of people to urban centers is creating peripheral slum areas lacking sanitation, which provide more breeding places for the mosquito vector. These parasitic diseases are sometimes referred to as the "cancers" of developing nations (Schultz, 1977, p. 259).

Among the infectious diseases having a high morbidity rate in the United States are some of the acute infectious diseases of childhood (such as *mumps* and *chickenpox*), acute infections of the respiratory system (the *common cold, influenza, pneumonia*), and acute infections involving the gastrointestinal system. Other more serious infectious diseases include *viral hepatitis, syphilis, gonorrhea, tuberculosis, staphylococcal infections*, and infections caused by normal inhabitants of the alimentary canal. There is always the possibility that citizens returning from Southeast Asia may reintroduce diseases that are not now usually problems in this country. They include *malaria, dengue, plague, helminthic infections*, and *Japanese B encephalitis virus infections*, among others.

The most probable source of forty-seven cases of *plasmodium vivax malaria* that occurred among needle-sharing users of intravenous heroin in Bakersfield, California, during the six-month period beginning November 1970 was a recent Vietnam returnee (Friedman et al., 1973, pp. 302–7). Also, increased incidents of malaria including some deaths in 1978 were attributed to returning American tourists.

In addition to control efforts directed against these more frequent infections, there is a great need to maintain vigilance to be sure that major diseases of the past do not reappear. Diphtheria was responsible for an outbreak in Texas in 1967–1969 (Stewart, 1970, pp. 949–54) and in Seattle in 1972–1973. There was an epidemic of poliomyelitis in a private school in Connecticut in 1972 (Center for Disease Control, October 28, 1972). Typhoid fever spread through a farm labor camp in Florida in 1973 (Center for Disease Control, March 3, 1973). Despite the fact that measles vaccine has been available for several years, measles has not been eradicated in the United States. Such experiences with preventable infectious diseases usually stem from one or two main sources—*susceptible groups that are not being reached by vaccination programs* or *pockets of susceptibles who hold personal beliefs against vaccination.* The typhoid outbreak illustrates another means by which infectious diseases occur, a breakdown in well chlorination.

Status of the United States in Control of the Great Killers

What is the status of the United States in respect to the diseases that are, or have been, the big killers? The louse-borne fevers and cholera are no longer believed to represent major threats, though there has been an increased incidence of cholera in certain parts of the world. This belief is based on the premise that an introduction of these diseases is unlikely, and, if it did occur, it could be contained rapidly before it could spread in an American city (Reeves, 1972, pp. 251–59). Smallpox vaccine is no longer included in the armamentarium of immunizing substances recommended for every infant.

Yellow fever, despite its endemic persistence in Central and South America, is not considered an epidemic threat because of knowledge about vector control and the existence of a satisfactory vaccine. Plague is endemic in the wild rodent population in the western states, but routine surveillance of urban rat populations in the affected area, it is hoped, will prevent their becoming a major source of infection for humans. The few cases that have occurred in recent years have been associated with rural exposure.

The purpose of presenting this brief survey of some of the more important potentially epidemic infectious diseases in the world of today is to emphasize that although some infectious diseases are under control, others continue to be a real threat.

Discoveries Involving the Incidence of Certain Infectious Diseases

In the nineteenth and twentieth centuries, a variety of discoveries have contributed to the reduction in the incidence of infectious disease, although in some instances the problem of prevention and control has increased. Included among the more important discoveries are the following:

1. Sanitary measures can effectively control the spread of enteric bacterial diseases.
2. A microorganism is a necessary factor in the etiology of infectious diseases.
3. Techniques have been developed to identify many but not all microbes.

4. Immunity to some diseases can be induced
   a. By injecting antibodies specific for the disease (temporary or passive immunity).
   b. By introducing antigenic substances (active artificially acquired immunity).
   c. By having the disease (active acquired immunity).
5. Some diseases can be cured by antimicrobial agents. For example, penicillin cures syphilis.
6. Some diseases are transmitted by an insect vector, and in some instances the microbe also spends part of its life cycle in the insect.
7. Measures to eliminate insect and animal vectors have been discovered and used.
8. Improvement in living standards, including nutrition and housing, has enhanced resistance or decreased exposure to some infectious diseases.
9. Some microorganisms have developed resistance not only to one but to a number of antimicrobial agents.
10. Some pathogenic microorganisms inhabit healthy carriers and can be disseminated to susceptible persons and cause disease.
11. Some airborne diseases are spread by droplets and others by droplet nuclei.

All of the preceding are of significance in any program of prevention and control of infectious disease.

Man and Microorganism: the Concept of Ecological Equilibrium

Despite a large body of knowledge about microbial agents, how they reach their potential hosts, and the influence of resulting infections on the human body, many questions remain to be answered. Among some of the more intriguing questions to be answered are the following: Why was the incidence of some infectious diseases decreasing before the advent of antimicrobial agents? Precisely what are the mechanisms involved in the recovery from viral infections? How can we explain the entire phenomenon of humoral immunity? What is the role of cell-mediated immunity, both in the pathogenesis of infections and in the defense against infections? What is the role of such infectious agents as slow viruses in the development of chronic disease, e.g., cancer? How do infectious agents trigger autoimmune disease, such as glomerulonephritis following a streptococcal infection? Though the answers to these questions are still far from complete, enough is known to be able to say with confidence that the development of infectious disease depends on the state of equilibrium that exists between the host, the etiologic agent or agents, and the factors in the environment that bring the agent and host together or influence their interaction.

Types of Host–Agent Relationships

There are three types of relationships that may exist between a host and its microorganisms. These are *symbiosis*, *commensalism*, and *parasitism*.

Symbiosis

Before a healthy baby enters the birth canal, he or she is free of microorganisms. Beginning with the birth process and continuing throughout the person's lifetime a relationship with a variety of microorganisms is acquired and developed. Depending on the host and microbe, their relationship varies all the way from one of mutual benefit to the production of serious disease in humans. *The state in which a host and microbe live in a mutually beneficial relationship is known as symbiosis.* In a symbiotic association, both partners derive advantages from their complementariness, usually nutritional, and often require each other's presence for their complete development. For example, microorganisms living in the alimentary canal obtain their nutrients from its contents. In return they synthesize certain essential nutritional elements, such as enzymes and vitamins, to supplement the dietary intake. Both human and microbe profit from the arrangement. There is growing evidence that bacteria in the intestinal tract have a beneficial effect on the strucutre of the mucosa, and in some poorly understood way, increase resistance to some infections.

Commensalism

A second type or relationship between the host and the microorganisms is called commensalism. *The microorganisms are dependent on the host, but under normal conditions they neither injure nor benefit it.* The microorganisms of this intermediate range of the normal or indigenous microbiota generally have been classed as commensals. Though these organisms are considered harmless, it is becoming more and more difficult to differentiate them from pathogens. The fact that true pathogens can achieve a state of equilibrium with the host is demonstrated by the healthy carrier. Microorganisms that ordinarily persist in the body without causing any obvious harm (the commensals) are responsible for the microbial diseases most common today when the infected person is under physiologic stress. Disease is the result of a disturbance in the ecological equilibrium.

Parasitism

In a parasitic relationship *one organism derives significant benefit from the other at the expense of the host.* In the instances in which the commensals cause disease, they become parasitic. Of the organisms living in a parasitic relationship with the host, some are able to live independently of the host as well as with it. These are known as the *facultative parasites. Staphylococci* and *Streptococci* are examples. Other microorganisms are dependent on the host for survival and for propagation. They are known as *obligatory parasites. Treponema pallidum* is one example. It dies very quickly after leaving the body; however, it can be propagated in an experimental animal, the rabbit.

Ecological Equilibrium Disturbed

The relationship existing between humans and microbes is an excellent example of the concept that adaptation is basic to survival. As a result of adaptations, both humans and microorganisms exist in a state of ecological equilibrium. Anything tending to disturb the equilibrium in favor of humans (the host) leads to a reduction in the incidence of disease. Any disturbance in the state of equilibrium favoring the microorganisms increases the incidence of disease. This relationship and the results of disturbing the balance are the same as illustrated in the diagram of the health–illness spectrum in Chapter 3. Survival of the microbe depends on its maintaining and reproaching itself without destroying the host. Wisely, but not too well, microorganisms have been successful in doing this. For example, when a group of people is exposed to microorganism for the first time, both the attack and mortality rates are high. When the group has lived with the same microorganism for a long time, both the attack and the mortality rates tend to be low. The late Theobold Smith summarized this point in a much-quoted statement, "Whenever you find a parasite that has affected a given host over a long period of time, you will find that the infection does not interfere with the survival of the host and is of low virulence." Examples abound of the fatal outcome of the exposure of a group of people to a new (to them) pathogenic organism. Simpson (1954, pp. 679–87) has pointed out that the Europeans were able to conquer America by "waging unpremeditated and unrecognized biologic warfare." His thesis was that smallpox, tuberculosis, and similar infections killed far more Amerindians that swords and rifles ever did. Records show that entire tribes were killed by smallpox.

The results of the adaptation of humans to their microbes, and vice versa, are illustrated by the effects of tuberculosis among successive generations of Indians after they moved onto the Qu Appelle Valley Reservation in the 1800s. In the first and second generations many individuals experienced acute generalized forms of the disease, and the death rate was high. Extensive glandular involvement, a sign of high susceptibility, affected up to 30 per cent of school-age children. By the third generation, though the disease was still epidemic, it showed a tendency to localize in the lung, and glandular involvement had fallen to 7 per cent. In the fourth generation, glandular evidence of tuberculosis occurred in less than 1 per cent of schoolchildren (Ferguson, 1955).

Although not as well documented, a similar process of adaptation can be traced for syphilis. Although this disease had probably existed at an epidemic level earlier, it reached epidemic proportions in western Europe in the late 1490s and, according to historic reports, ravaged many countries. Apparently the spirochete was extraordinarily virulent, because reports describe a very severe disease, frequently fatal in the second stage, so that most people considered it a new and unknown entity. The disease became much milder by the middle of the next century and acquired gradually the venereal mode of transmission that is common today. Currently more than half the infected people either have a spontaneous cure or develop no later symptoms related to the infection.

These adaptations may be due to a change in the virulence of the organism, the resistance of the host, or both, but it is now a relatively mild disease in its early stages, showing that some degree of equilibrium between agent and host has been reached. It seems fairly certain that such factors as stress, nutritional state, and weather conditions alter the susceptibility of the host. Although host factors were known to play a part in the infectious process, in the past emphasis has been placed on the number and virulence of germs as the significant factor. With the use of immunosuppressive and cytotoxic drugs in organ transplants and in the treatment of cancer, it has been learned that almost any microbe can cause disease if the defensive physiologic responses are sufficiently depressed. Thus coliforms, diphtheroids, yeasts, and other organisms that are usually nonpathogenic cause endogenous infections. To reemphasize this point, a microorganism is a necessary factor in the development of an infectious disease. Whether it is sufficient to cause disease depends on the relationship of host, microorganism, and environment. To express the relationship of host and microorganism, Stewart (1968) rewrote Theobald Smith's equation:

$$\text{Severity of disease} = \frac{\text{number} \times \text{virulence of organisms}}{\text{susceptibility of host}}$$

The relationship of the three elements—host, agent, and environment (refer again to Chapter 2)—during health is that of equilibrium. When a change in any one element occurs, the balance is lost. Examples of the four possible changes diagrammed in Chapter 2 are well known for infectious diseases. An extremely rainy season, providing many breeding places, can increase the mosquito population and thus greatly increase the risk of the host acquiring an infectious agent (of malaria or encephalitis) transmitted by that insect. A change in weather conditions, such as a cold storm front moving into an area, can increase the congregation of people indoors and facilitate the transmission of common cold agents. A lax attitude in a community toward childhood immunizations will increase the number of susceptibles and thus the incidence of measles or poliomyelitis, among other diseases. A mutation in an influenza virus can easily circumvent the immunity acquired from previous infections and produce an epidemic.

Humans have for centuries been able to alter their external environment and adapt it to their needs. To some extent they have influenced the infections that attack them in this way. Now they are able to alter their internal environment as well, and the unsatisfactory side effects of this are just being realized. Through the use of antimicrobial agents, irradiation, and corticosteroid drugs humans are able to change the internal environment and therefore the nature of the normal flora of their bodies.

In the gastrointestinal tract many microorganisms live in a state of equilibrium not only with their host but with each other. Apparently, when this equilibrium is not disturbed, the growth of some species tends to suppress that of others. Exactly how this is accomplished is only beginning to be understood. When the balance among the microorganisms is disturbed, some species may grow and multiply in excess and may therefore cause disease. For example, the tetracycline antibiotics inhibit the growth and multiplication of the gram-negative bacteria forming part of the normal flora of the intestinal feces. Tetracycline-resistant organisms including yeasts, fecal streptococci, *Proteus*, and *Pseudomonas* are allowed to flourish, and sometimes they produce clinical disease and death. In the nasopharynx, alpha streptococci are commensals. Located in other parts of the body, such as the heart valves, they are pathogens.

The occurrence of infection is also influenced by the fact that some true pathogenic organisms survive long periods of time in human tissues, occasionally for an entire lifetime. Sometimes the agents cause no sign of illness in the individual, as in a carrier of *Salmonella typhosa* or *paratyphi*, but are excreted either regularly or intermittently and are a source of infection to others. Other agents persist in a latent state and when conditions are right emerge as overt disease in the individual and again are transmissible to others. A familiar example is herpes simplex virus infection. After the host is first infected, the virus persists in a latent state and the characteristic lesions, cold sores, appear only under certain conditions such as a febrile illness or exposure to strong sunlight. Infection with the tubercle bacilli does not usually manifest itself as overt disease, for the body is able to restrict multiplication of the bacilli, and its occurrence can be detected only by a positive reaction to a skin test. However, the bacilli persist in a latent state for several years until some disturbance in the environment upsets the equilibrium and disease develops. This disturbance is probably a combination of factors, including lowered nutritional status, stress, increased susceptibility related to increased age, and so on. This ability to remain viable but latent for many years is thought to help explain the marked shift in incidence of tuberculosis from young people to those past middle age that has occurred in this country. Many other organisms have this capacity to assume a protective state, but the phenomenon is not clearly understood. It is an adaptation that enables microorganisms to survive.

Evidence is accumulating of another phenomenon of the ecological equilibrium between humans and their microorganisms known as "slow virus infections" (Marx, 1973). These are manifest as a group of persistent degenerative diseases especially of the central nervous system, believed to be caused by both known and unidentified viruses. Conventional measles virus has been isolated from the brains of patients suffering from subacute sclerosing panencephalitis (SSPE) (Jabbour, 1969; Youmans, 1975). The average time interval between the measles infection and the development of SSPE was 6 years. It is suggested that either immunologic immaturity or a defective immune system allows the suppression of the measles virus rather than its total elimination. There is speculation that multiple sclerosis may have a similar etiology. In each of these examples a change in the ecological equilibrium has favored the agent to the disadvantage of the host. Successful prevention and control of infectious diseases result when equilibrium is maintained or tipped in favor of the host.

Essential Interactions for Development of Infections

As stated previously, three factors are involved in the development of an infection or an infectious disease: host, microbe, and environment.

Host Susceptibility

Susceptibility is usually thought of as those conditions making an individual more liable to a condition or disease. Conversely, resistance decreases the individual's liability. These terms refer to the risk level the person has of acquiring a certain disease.

Host resistance to a number of important infectious diseases can be increased by vaccines and other immunizing agents. The nurse should keep informed about which diseases can be prevented and the schedule required to maintain immunity to each (See Henderson and Nite, 1978, for excellent table on immunization schedules, p. 2043). The nurse as well as the physician has a responsibility to determine the immune status of individuals under their care. This responsibility is not limited to nurses employed in well-baby clinics and schools but applies to all nurses. The best form of treatment of any disease is prevention. However, it is also important for the nurse to know that the duration of immunity acquired in this way has varying periods of effectiveness, that no vaccine necessarily is effective for every individual, and that a large dose of infecting organisms may be able to overcome immunity.

Other factors in host susceptibility are heredity, state of nutrition, hormonal balance, age, sex, the integrity of the host's defense mechanisms, and presence of other diseases. Susceptibility to disease also depends on the past experience of the individual with a given microorganism or its antigenic components.

Heredity

A possible genetic influence on susceptibility or resistance is difficult to discern because it is almost impossible to eliminate environmental factors. Studies with laboratory animals have yielded more exact information than has come from studies of human disease. Susceptible or resistant strains of animals have been developed by inbreeding, but to specific agents, not to all infections. A genetic resistance has been shown to a leukemia virus and to tuberculosis in different strains of mice. A study of tuberculosis in twins indicates the possibility of a genetic factor in human tuberculosis (Kallman & Reisner, 1943). When one of a pair of heterozygous twins develops tuberculosis, the chances of the other twin having it are one in three. In homozygous twins the chances are three out of four.

The contribution of the immune response or inflammatory reaction to overall lowered host resistance is vividly demonstrated in individuals being studied with congenital deficiencies or inborn errors of metabolism. In children with severe congenital humoral immune deficiencies, there are numerous recurrent severe bacterial infections such as otitis media, pneumonia, septicemia, pyoderma, and gastroenteritis. They also may fail to thrive and have chronic diarrhea and malabsorption problems. Cell-mediated deficiencies in children may also produce failure to thrive and proneness to severe viral, fungal (candida), and bacterial infections such as tuberculosis and pseudomonas. An injection of BCG (bacillus Calmette-Guérin) vaccine or a smallpox vaccination may be fatal in these children (Allen, 1976).

A severe and usually fatal neutropenia characterizes some congenital diseases. Chronic granulomatous disease and Chédiak–Higaski syndrome produce defective white blood cells which fail to destroy phagocytized bacteria. There are tendencies to recurrent bacterial infections in skin, lungs, and perianal tissue in affected persons (Allen, 1976).

Nutritional Status

There is an association between nutritional status and the incidence and severity of infections. Writing on interactions of nutrition and infection, Scrimshaw and Behar (1969) noted that malnutrition of any severity acted synergistically with infections by most classes of bacteria, especially the pyogenic pathogens. Occasionally antagonistic effects occurred, especially with some viruses and protozoal infections. In the synergistic interaction, malnutrition lowers host resistance to infection and infectious disease exaggerates an existing deficient nutritional state. Measles, which we know as a mild disease, causes high mortality rates among children who are malnourished, as in Guatemala and parts of Africa. The exact mechanisms of how malnutrition aggravates infection are slowly being identified. Antibodies are similar in nature to proteins, and it is to be expected that severe depletion of body proteins would reduce the synthesis of antibodies. Studies in laboratory animals have shown that nutritional deficiencies interfere with antibody formation and with leukocyte response and activity. However, as Scrimshaw cautioned, nothing is known about which if any of these mechanisms are involved if the nutritional deficiency is subclinical. Limited observations on children with congenital deficiencies of the humoral immune system show that host resistance dependent on cellular immunity might be enhanced in some forms of malnutrition (Jose et al., 1971).

Nurses working in areas of the world where serious malnutrition exists need to consider special problems in regard to infectious diseases and malnutrition. The ordinary communicable diseases are usually accompanied by a reduced appetite and a resulting altered diet, frequently liquids lacking needed food elements. This, plus decreased protein absorption, can add insult to an already poor nutritional status. Antibody formation is depressed by malnutrition; therefore serologic response to artificial immunizing agents is poorer than usual. Poliomyelitis, for example, can occur in a recently immunized child. These problems are not necessarily limited to developing countries but may also be found to some extent in sections of this country where economic conditions are very poor.

Hormonal Balance

Hormones secreted by the endocrine glands have an influence on host resistance and response to infection. The incidence of paralytic poliomyelitis was higher in pregnant women than in women comparable in every way except for pregnancy. The explanation was thought to be the hormonal changes existing during the pregnancy. Cortisone and its related analogues diminish resistance to tuberculosis, probably by suppressing the inflammatory response. The use of corticosteroids in the treatment of a variety of diseases contributes to the increase in infections caused by microbes of the normal flora. In addition, these preparations can depress antibody formation and suppress interferon production. Persons whose adrenal cortices hypersecrete the glucocorticoids also have an increased susceptibility to infection.

Age

With increasing age, an individual develops protection against many infectious diseases because of immunity acquired either as the result of natural infection or artificial immunization. This masks in part the fact that our ability to deal effectively with infection in the absence of specific immunity tends to decrease with age. The opportunity for exposure also confuses the picture, which for the common communicable diseases steadily decreases from shortly after individuals enter school until they become parents in their own right. Severity of infectious disease varies with age. The greatest incidence of deaths from common infectious diseases such as measles and whooping cough is highest in young children, but infectious hepatitis is rarely severe enough to produce jaundice in this age group. The highest incidence of deaths during an influenza epidemic is usually in the elderly, and though underlying conditions account for some of the excess, there seems to be a greater susceptibility to the infection itself.

Burnet and White have summarized the relationship of humans and infectious disease as the "five ages of man" (1972). Age one is represented by the infant who needs both the protection of maternal antibody and a carefully controlled environment because of its high susceptibility. Age two is the child who is easily infected, but is able to deal satisfactorily with most infections and build life-long immunity against many. Age three is the young adult who is less easily infected and deals rapidly with local infections, but is likely to be overwhelmed by too vigorous a reaction to general infections if he or she has no immunity. During later adulthood, age four, the individual is usually free from anything but minor illness. In old age, age five, there is an increasing susceptibility to infection.

Sex

Incidence of some infectious diseases varies according to sex, as does severity. Women report a higher number of respiratory infections, but the death rate for men is higher. Presenting symptoms of gonorrhea are frequently much milder in females than in males. Males over 10 years have a higher incidence of toxoplasmosis than females. Many other examples could be given. Some of the differences are probably related as much or more to opportunities for exposure than to true differences in susceptibility. Other reasons may include hormonal or hereditary sex-linked explanations.

Washburn et al. (1965) proposed a genetic origin for sex-related differences in susceptibility. Based on a study of hospital charts and autopsy records, a significant sex difference, unfavorable to males, was found in the incidence of bacterial meningitis at all ages and of septicemia among newborn infants and children. These investigators speculated that the female's greater resistance to infection came from her heterozygosity of genes on the X chromosome, which are now known to control immunoglobulin synthesis and thymic function. Later investigators have agreed with this hypothesis.

Many other factors appear to influence susceptibility to infection. For many of these, the belief that they do is based more on observation than on clear understanding of why they do.

Host Defenses and Routes of Spread

In the following outline the characteristics of the host that provide some protection as he or she enters into the development of an infectious disease are summarized. The routes of spread after an infectious agent has penetrated the first line of defense of the host are also included.

1. Characteristics of host defense mechanisms
   a. Anatomic and physiologic barriers to the entrance of microorganisms (discussed in Unit V)
      (1) Intact skin and mucous membranes
      (2) Structures and functions that protect the entrances to the respiratory and gastrointestinal tract
      (3) Character of secretions and body fluids
         (a) pH (acid pH inhibits bacterial growth)
         (b) Lysozyme produced by leukocytes found in tears, saliva, and other body fluids; lyses bacteria and is bactericidal
         (c) Properidin system
         (d) Bactericidins
         (e) Agglutinins
         (f) Opsonins
         (g) Interferon
      (4) Anatomic barriers within the tissues
         (a) Continuous matrix
         (b) Fibrin barrier
   b. Cell-mediated responses (discussed in Unit V)
      (1) Microphages (neutrophils—highly mobile, quickly responding somewhat vulnerable)
      (2) Macrophages
   c. Humoral-mediated responses (discussed in Unit V)
      (1) Antitoxin—directly neutralize toxins
      (2) Antibacterial or antiviral antibodies combine with a specific substance at the surface of a virus or bacterium and produce a new surface about which leukocytes can spread and more easily ingest the microorganism
   d. Inflammatory response (discussed in Chapter 25)
   e. Other host factors
      (1) Heredity (genetic)
      (2) Age
      (3) Sex
      (4) Nutritional state
      (5) Hormonal balance
      (6) Inhibition of virulent strains by normal flora
2. Routes of spread after a microbe has penetrated the first line of defense
   a. Intercellular spaces—direct extension to contiguous tissues
   b. Lymphatics
      (1) Arrest at lymph node
      (2) Spreads from the lymph node through lymphatics to blood stream
   c. Blood stream
   d. Ingested by macrophages but not destroyed—carried to other parts of the body
   e. Spillage or escape from a hollow organ
      (1) Direct extension
      (2) Perforation of the hollow organ

Etiologic Agent

The Pathogenic Microorganism

Pathogenic microorganisms have certain properties that are important to disease causation. Some of these properties are common for all such organisms, such as the ability to cause infection. In general, as the infecting dose increases so does the chance of disease. Other properties vary greatly between species of microorganisms and even within species. Some characteristics are intrinsic to the organisms, including morphology, growth requirements, viability, resistance to physical or chemical substances, antigenic character, and host range. Other properties relate to the behavior of the parasites in their hosts, such as infectivity, pathogenicity, and virulence. Some of the characteristics of microorganisms influencing their ability to survive and establish themselves have been selected for discussion with specific examples. These include (1) morphology; (2) growth requirements; (3) resistance to physical or chemical agents; (4) infectivity, pathogenicity, virulence; and (5) toxin production.

Morphology

The morphology of microorganisms (size, shape, structure) influences their ability to survive and to establish themselves. Many bacteria form capsules that offer some protection against the body defenses. In some instances, as, for example, the pneumococcus, the microbe is dependent on its capsule for its pathogenicity. The protein coat of the virus not only protects the nucleic acid core but has a special affinity for complementary receptors on the surface of susceptible cells. Some bacteria, such as those causing botulism and tetanus, are spore formers and in this form are unusually resistant to heat, drying, and chemicals.

Growth Requirements

In general the principles of biochemistry are the same for all living organisms, and many microorganisms pathogenic for humans grow best under circumstances similar to the human internal environment. Some have very fastidious growth requirements. For example, those of the spirochete of syphilis are such that they have not been grown in vitro in a laboratory. For the particular requirements of a specific microorganism, refer to a textbook of microbiology.

Pathogenic organisms in general are parasites in that they have lost the ability to synthesize some amino acids and vitamins that they require. Some need oxygen, others can exist only in an anaerobic environment. Reproduction is largely a matter of growth and division. Most bacteria have a wide range of temperature tolerance.

An interesting example of extreme temperature tolerance is a newly discovered genus of bacteria, *Thermoanaerofacter ethanolicus,* which has three distinctive characteristics: (1) survivability at high temperatures (172°F, 78°C); (2) growth without air; and (3) the ability to produce alcohol (ethanol). Research indicates that newly discovered bacteria may someday supply alcohol for commercial use (*Science News,* November 3, 1979, p. 317). Some humans may even try to permanently infect themselves with this organism to produce an internal "still."

Unlike bacteria, viruses have no metabolism and are capable of reproducing only within living cells. Like bacteria, viruses which are relatively harmless abound. Other groups of pathogenic microorganisms, such as protozoa and rickettsia, have some special requirements also.

Resistance to Physical and Chemical Agents

The use of a variety of physical and chemical agents to control pathogenic microorganisms and the ways in which these act is not within the scope of this chapter. In earlier times they were used to remove or destroy pathogens before they had an opportunity to enter the body, but it was believed that little could be done to destroy the majority of them once they had produced disease. The introduction of antibiotic drugs in the 1930s changed this belief and led to the expectation that bacterial illnesses at least could be effectively treated. It must be remembered that because of their intracellular characteristics, most viruses are protected against antimicrobial drugs. There has been substantive progress in developing chemicals that can be effectively used in treating selected viral diseases, such as *Vidarabine* for herpes simplex encephalitis; *Idoxuridine* for viral keratitis; and amantadine hydrochloride for type A influenza (*Science News,* November 3, 1979, p. 311).

One of the more serious problems in the treatment of bacterial infections today is that despite a high degree of effectiveness when first introduced, most antimicrobial drugs lose their effectiveness against certain infectious agents after a period of use. Why should a once-effective agent become ineffective? For example, why should penicillin, which was once highly effective against *Staphylococcus aureus,* become ineffective? There are two major mechanisms: (1) as susceptible strains are killed, resistant strains multiply without competition and predominate; (2) bacterial drug resistance develops as the result of either mutation or the transfer of genetic material from resistant to sensitive organisms.

Changes in the resistance of bacteria to drugs can be the result of mutation. Although spontaneous mutation probably does not occur very often in nature, it seems possible that in a medical situation opportunities would exist to increase the likelihood of an error in the reconstruction of the DNA molecule when cell division takes place. Exposure to irradiation or certain chemicals could be precipitators.

Interest in genetic transfer of bacterial drug resistance was stimulated by the report from Japan in 1959 of a resistance (R) factor in the cytoplasm of some bacteria capable of transferring resistance to multiple drugs simultaneously. This mechanism operates mainly among the gram-negative organisms, either of the same or different strains. During a process called conjugation, the transfer takes place. It occurs in a few moments. The bowel is a good location for this. The genetic transfer confers drug resistance, sometimes to as many as six drugs or more. The other mechanism for genetic transfer of drug resistance is phage transfer. Phage is the name given to the small viruses parasitic on bacteria. When a phage starts an infection in a susceptible organism it carries with it DNA that has the genetic code for resistance. It is thought that resistance to only one or two drugs is conferred at one time. Bacterial drug resistance may occur in a single step over one or two days, or it may be gradual. Interestingly, the use of antibiotics in livestock feeds may contribute to increasing drug resistance among disease-causing bacteria (More Feed Additives, 1979).

From the clinical point of view, bacterial drug resistance is important for several reasons. It drastically reduces the antibiotics suitable for treating infections. It severely handicaps treatment when resistance has developed to the main drug effective on a specific organism, such as chloramphenicol for *Salmonella typhi.* Many of the organisms developing drug resistance cause serious diseases. Bacteria which have developed resistance to multiple drugs and are capable of passing R factor to other organisms include shigella (dysentery), *Pseudomonas aeruginosa* (purulent infections), those causing plague, cholera, and most responsible for urinary tract infections. The R factor mechanism does not appear to exist in gram-positive organisms such as streptococcus or staphylococcus. Further, the infecting organism does not need to be resistant at the time it enters the body, as it can be rapidly infected by R factors from bacteria normally found in the large intestine.

Infectivity, Pathogenicity, Virulence

These characteristics of microorganisms relate specifically to their action within the host. An understanding of these properties is necessary in order to understand the complete spectrum of the infectious process and is helpful in the establishment of effective control programs. *Infectivity* is the capacity of microorganisms to enter the tissues of the host, lodge, and multiply. In ordinary observations, the measure of infectivity is how much overt disease occurs in susceptible people following exposure to the agent. With laboratory support to detect subclinical infections, it is possible to get a much more accurate estimate of the infectivity of the microorganism. *Pathogenicity* refers to the capacity of a microorganism to produce disease once it has established an infection, a measure of the number of infections that actually result in disease. The organisms that produce disease are therefore called pathogens. *Virulence* applies to the severity of the disease produced. Therefore the organisms that produce severe, rapidly developing disease are often termed highly virulent. There is a tendency to use the three terms interchangeably, but each has a distinct meaning of its own and indicates a specific aspect of the interaction between host and agent.

Each of these three characteristics has a wide range of variation, between species of microorganisms, strains of the same species, and human hosts. Many of the factors that determine conditions in the human host have already been discussed. Some of the factors operating on the agent, other than inherent genetic character, include the site where it gains entrance to the host, the rapidity and extent to which it multiplies in the host, how much tissue damage it causes, and whether or not it produces a toxin. A high level of infectivity probably makes it easier for an agent to perpetuate the species. It is difficult to get a direct measure of the level of infectivity of an agent in humans. A measure was obtained for polio viruses in studies on the development of natural immunity to these agents in Louisiana. When polio virus was introduced into families, more than 90 per cent of the naturally susceptible children became infected, on the basis of antibody formation (Gelfand et al., 1959).

The range of pathogenicity is from completely inapparent infections, as happens at least 75 per cent of the time when polio virus is transmitted, to overt illness every time a susceptible host is exposed to the agent, as with measles. An illness that is almost always very mild, such as the common cold, is caused by agents with low virulence, but other infections where death is a frequent outcome, as with rabies virus, are said to be caused by highly virulent agents. It should be obvious that no agent ranks at the same spot on the scale for all three of these characteristics. Measles virus has high infectivity and pathogenicity but very low virulence.

The antigenicity of a microorganism, or its ability to induce specific immunity, was classed as an intrinsic characteristic, but it is also host related. The mechanisms of the immune system are presented in detail in Chapter 24. An infection with some organisms is followed by durable life-long immunity against subsequent disease with the same organisms. Other infections confer little or no immunity. Some of the reasons for these differences lie in the intrinsic properties of the agents; others are probably related to the immune system of the host.

Microorganisms vary greatly in their power to invade and disseminate themselves throughout the body. At one end of the scale are the noninvasive toxin producers, such as the organisms of tetanus and botulism, and at the other end of the scale are the highly invasive organisms of plague and anthrax. Most microorganisms that have any degree of invasiveness have some sort of capsule or protective covering. The capsule appears to protect the microorganism against the defense mechanisms of the host. Without its capsule, the pathogen is quickly destroyed by phagocytes. Even viruses have a protein coat or "capsule" surrounding the central core of nucleic acid. The protein capsule attaches itself to the cell, but only the nucleic acid enters. After the virus multiplies within the cell, the cell must build protein to surround the nucleic acid before the cell releases the virus.

Toxin Production

As indicated earlier, pathogenic microorganisms may be present in the tissues without causing manifestations of disease. For clinical evidence of disease to appear, the organism must not only establish itself in the host but multiply in sufficient numbers to overcome host resistance and to induce tissue response. Whether or not the microbe is successful in causing disease depends on the relationship of its infectivity, pathogenicity, and numbers to the nonspecific and specific resistance of the host. After the microorganism becomes adapted to a susceptible host, it may then induce local and systemic effects, by one or more mechanisms.

Some bacteria, such as the diphtheria bacillus, secrete water-soluble *toxins* that are distributed by the blood to all regions of the body. These *exotoxins* are responsible for the systemic manifestations of disease in diphtheria, botulism, tetanus, and gas gangrene. They are highly specific, as each exotoxin acts as an antigen stimulating the body to produce a specific antitoxin (an antibody) that neutralizes that specific toxin.

The exotoxin not only stimulates the antibody-producing mechanism of a victim of a disease, but it can be used to stimulate an animal, such as a sheep or a horse, to produce antitoxin. Serum obtained from such a treated animal contains the specific antibody or antitoxin, and can be used to confer passive immunity, that is, to neutralize toxin in the blood of an infected human host. To protect a person who has a disease caused by an exotoxin-forming microbe, the antitoxin must be given early, for after a toxin has combined with cellular constituents, antitoxin is of little or no benefit. Persons with a disease such as diphtheria or tetanus must receive antitoxin at once if they are to benefit. Nurses acting as case finders may be responsible for getting patients under medical care. In an epidemic of diphtheria in one large city, a school nurse was credited with recognizing the possibility that the children who were sick had diphtheria. When her suspicions were verified, sick children were treated with antitoxin and measures were undertaken to prevent the spread of the disease to others by immunizing schoolchildren and other contacts. A modified toxin (toxoid) can also be used to stimulate the production of antitoxin by the individual. The toxin may be converted to toxoid by a chemical such as formalin.

Although the general manifestations occurring in tetanus, diphtheria, and botulism differ, as do the local effects of the organisms involved, the specific exotoxins produced in each of these diseases cause injury to the nervous system. The exotoxin of diphtheria also injures the myocardium. Each of the exotoxins varies in degree of toxicity; however, exotoxins are among the most highly poisonous substances known.

Diphtheria bacilli can produce toxin when they are latently infected by a bacterial virus. In typical disease, the organisms lodge in the throat and remain in that area. The toxin produced spreads rapidly through the body and produces the generalized symptoms of acute illness. The invaded site in the throat ulcerates, and a membrane grows over this area that may extend through the glottis into the larynx and tracheobronchial tree, where it can cause death by suffocation.

Other organisms producing toxin belong to the genus *Clostridia* and among other diseases produce tetanus, botulism, and gas gangrene. They are spore formers and either completely or nearly completely anaerobic. *C. botulinum,* the agent of botulism, usually does not cause injury by the growth of microorganisms in the alimentary canal or in the tissues but by the actual ingestion of an exotoxin produced by the microorganisms growing in bland vegetables or fish canned at temperatures insufficient to kill the spores. There is no local growth of organisms to cause injury. This is the most lethal toxin known and acts to block transmission of impulses on certain nerve fibers. Fortunately it can be destroyed easily by boiling such vegetables as home-canned corn, beans, or peas for five minutes before they are eaten. Commercially canned vegetables are rarely sources of botulism because they are subjected to high temperatures during the process of canning. It is helpful to know botulism can occur in babies fed raw honey.

Tetanus is produced by the toxin of *C. tetani.* The organism itself remains localized at the site of entry and must have necrotic tissue in order to grow. *C. tetani* is very common and has been known to cause disease after small or insignificant wounds have healed. All accidentally incurred wounds should be thoroughly cleansed and attention paid to the immunity status of the patient. Persons who have been previously immunized for tetanus are given a booster dose. Tetanus toxoid has been demonstrated to be an effective immunizing antigen, but it takes time to produce immunity. When the immunity status is unknown or there has been no previous immunization procedure, the administration of tetanus antitoxin must be considered. Because this material is contained in horse serum, individuals who are to receive it should be tested for sensitivity to the foreign protein previous to its administration. Otherwise severe hypersensitivity reactions or even tetanus may develop. Tetanus neonatorum can be a serious problem in areas of the world where sanitation is poor and contamination of the unhealed umbilicus can occur.

Several species of clostridia have been encountered in gas gangrene, *C. perfringens (welchii)* most frequently, following a traumatic injury. The organisms proliferate, producing a cellulitis and a toxin. The usual incubation period is from 1 to 4 days, though the range is from 6 hours to 6 weeks. The onset of gas gangrene is often heralded by severe pain in the affected part and a sweetish, foul odor. Bubbles of gas may be seen in the drainage from the wound. Because the disease progresses rapidly, the area around the wound should be inspected regularly. Though this is usually done by the physician, the nurse should be alert to such signs and symptoms as pain in the injured part and the characteristic odor, both of which indicate the possible development of gas gangrene. The physician should be notified promptly, as the life or limb of a patient literally depends on the promptness with which treatment is instituted. As yet there is no effective way to protect individuals by either active or passive immunization. Protection depends primarily on thorough cleansing and debridement of the wound.

In addition to exotoxins, bacteria also form substances known as endotoxins. Endotoxins differ from exotoxins in that they are not liberated in appreciable amounts during the life of the bacterial cell, but they are released as the cell degenerates. Endotoxins also differ in that they are not specific to a given organism. They appear to be a fairly homogeneous group of substances that probably cause injury by a similar chemical process. Among the physiologic changes endotoxins cause are severe shock and fever. The implications to nursing of both these conditions are discussed elsewhere.

Many microorganisms have the power to invade healthy tissues. Not all the factors that enable microorganisms to do this and to disseminate themselves throughout the body are known. Bacteria form nontoxic substances that facilitate their spread, which vary from species to species. They play a role in the infectious process by protecting microorganisms from the defense mechanisms of the body or by enabling them to spread throughout tissue. The nontoxic *polysaccharide capsule* of pneumococcus permits it to be invasive by inhibiting phagocytosis. Many pathogenic staphylococci produce a substance called *coagulase.* Coagulase and certain factors in the blood serum interact to form fibrin clots in small blood vessels supplying the infected area. It is a factor in the formation of fibrin walls around areas of tissue infected by the staphylococcus. The fibrin wall serves to protect from the defenses of the body such as phagocytosis and from antistaphylococcal drugs, and thereby favors their persistence in tissues.

Hemolysins and *leukocidins,* also produced by pathogenic staphylococci, dissolve erythrocytes and leukocytes, respectively. *Streptokinase,* an extracellular enzyme, has the opposite effect of coagulase. It digests coagulated plasma and is thought to be an important factor in the spread of organisms such as hemolytic streptococci throughout the body. It has been used experimentally to digest blood clots formed in blood vessels in disease. *Clostridium welchii* produces *collagenase* and *lecithinase.* These substances dissolve collagen and lecithin and thereby facilitate the spread of the microorganisms throughout the tissue.

A group of enzymes, formed by certain bacteria including streptococci, are known as *hyaluronidases.* They act as spreading factors because they have the power to increase the permeability of tissues. Hyaluronidase is sometimes added to fluids administered subcutaneously to increase tissue permeability and, as a consequence, to increase the rate at which the fluid is absorbed, such as in a sprained joint.

To summarize, the following characteristics of bacteria or their products may enhance pathogenicity:

1. Polysaccharide capsule inhibits phagocytosis
2. Toxin production
   a. Exotoxin
   b. Endotoxin
3. Other substances
   a. Coagulase
   b. Streptokinase
   c. Collagenase
   d. Lecithinase
   e. Hyaluronidase
4. Other factors
   a. Number, virulence, and invasiveness are sufficient to overcome local body defenses. Reaches a tissue where it is able to establish itself, grow, and multiply.

Characteristics of Viruses

There are many varieties of viruses responsible for human, animal, and plant diseases, including a high percentage of acute illnesses among human beings. Currently it is estimated that about 200 viruses can produce the syndrome called the common cold. The majority of viral infections are "inapparent" or "subclinical," but any particular virus is capable of producing a wide spectrum of symptoms from a silent infection to a fatal illness. They cause minor illnesses and such serious diseases as smallpox, yellow fever, and hepatitis. In addition veterinary virologists are aware of several viral diseases in which months or years pass before overt disease appears (the best known is scrapie in sheep) and it is now believed the same process can occur in humans. Some viruses, such as that of herpes simplex, cause the recurrence of acute disease years after the first infection, and others can persist in humans for years after the original infection, causing no symptoms. They are known to cause some forms of cancer in animals, and the possibility that they are involved in some human cancers is being actively investigated.

Youmans (1975) mentions a new class of infectious agents, which resemble the classic virus but differ from them. They elicit no demonstrable immune response, withstand boiling and formaldehyde, and survive short periods of autoclaving. Because they have incubation periods of a year or more, viroids resemble slow viruses mentioned previously.

Much of the information about the relationship of the virus to the host has been obtained from the study of bacteriophages (viruses that attack bacteria). Phages are highly specific for the bacteria they attack, and this specificity is very helpful in identifying the precise strains of staphylococcus or of typhoid bacillus responsible for an outbreak. Another advance followed the discovery by Enders, Weller, and Robbins (1949) that poliomyelitis virus could be grown in mammalian cells in test tubes. *Today nearly all viruses can be grown in cell cultures.* Other developments that have contributed greatly to knowledge of viruses are electron microscopy and x-ray diffraction techniques.

Viruses cannot be regarded as true microorganisms, and in a strict sense they probably should not be considered living things (Chang, 1977, p. 2). In contrast to the cellular microorganisms, they contain only one type of nucleic acid (DNA or RNA). This nucleic acid core is surrounded by a protein coat that enables the virus to survive outside the cell, helps it penetrate susceptible cells, and contains the antigenic material. After a virus enters the cell, the protein dissolves. The nucleic acid takes over the metabolic machinery of the cell to reproduce itself and to direct synthesis of protein to coat the new nucleic acid molecules. If the cell dies, it undergoes lysis and the viruses are released. If the cell lives, viruses may be released one at a time. In either event, the new viruses are free to enter other cells, where they multiply. In virus diseases, signs and symptoms may be caused by the response of cells to the virus as well as to cell necrosis.

Viruses tend to be of small size. The unit of measurement used is the nanometer (nm), which is equal to one-millionth of a millimeter. The largest viruses (poxviruses) measure about 200 nm, influenza virus 100 to 120 nm and the smallest viruses, adeno-associated viruses, about 20 nms. They are considered "filterable" agents, because they will pass through a millipore filter of a 450-nm pore size that excludes bacteria.

Specific viruses prefer particular hosts and tissues, but in experimental situations they can be induced to grow in the tissues of other animals. One way to attenuate the virulence of a virus is by passage in an unnatural host. As an example, when the smallpox virus is passed through a calf it is attenuated, but it retains sufficient antigenicity to induce immunity to smallpox for a period of 3 or 4 years.

The capacity of viruses to alter their character in nature has great practical significance. Influenza provides a good example. Influenza virus type A has caused several pandemics and many more localized epidemics, and is always present in large population centers. Differences in the incidence and severity of the disease are caused in part by the number of susceptible individuals and their degree of susceptibility; in part they are due to changes in antigens or a mutation of the virus. Pandemic occurrence of influenza is the result of major changes in the antigens, which occurred recently in the pandemic of Asian influenza in 1957 and the Hong Kong outbreak in 1968, and an outbreak of type A influenza in January 1978. The epidemics of influenza every few years are associated with minor changes in the antigenic composition called *antigenic drift.*

An interesting discovery that may have some implications in the prevention and treatment of viral diseases was made by Isaacs about 21 years ago—that some virus-infected cells produce a protein, which he called *interferon.* This protein substance acts only on cells. When released, it protects susceptible cells from invasion and stimulates the production of a second antiviral protein that inhibits the translation of viral nucleic acid by susceptible cells. Some viruses stimulate interferon production better than others. Interferons are specific to an animal species and are harmless to that animal. Progress continues to be made in synthesizing interferon in the laboratory. However, it will be some time before production of interferon on a commercial basis will be possible. Another approach would be to stimulate production by the individual, either by an infection with an attenuated virus or by a nonviral inducer (Fenner and White, 1970).

Viruses are classified in a number of ways: according to type of nucleic acid in the core (RNA or DNA); according to their biologic, chemical, and physical properties; or according to the way they are transmitted and enter the body, as respiratory viruses, enteric viruses, or arborviruses. For more detailed information on virus classification, see Hoeprich (1977).

Once viruses have reached susceptible cells, they can produce localized effects, generalized effects, or both. Those that penetrate cells of the respiratory tract can cause localized symptoms of a head cold or may penetrate to deeper parts and produce such diseases as influenza and pneumonia. Viruses that infect the intestinal tract must be able to survive the acid in the gastric juice and the bile. Arborviruses, transmitted by the bite of an arthropod, generally cause systemic infections. In generalized viral infections, once the virus has entered the body it selects a site for multiplication. This establishes viremia, the widespread dissemination of the virus in the body. Sites frequently selected are the skin, central nervous system, heart, liver, and certain glands.

Cellular responses induced by viruses are of two types and can occur alone or in combination. Tissues invaded by a virus may undergo hyperplasia. A familiar example is the common wart. This ability to induce hyperplasia in tissues supports the possibility that viruses may play a role in initiating some types of human neoplasms as they do in some plants and animals. Hyperplasia may be followed by necrosis of cells. The lesions formed in smallpox are characterized by hyperplasia followed by necrosis. Necrosis can occur alone. The lesions in the anterior horn cells in poliomyelitis are characterized by necrosis. In infection caused by viruses, damage to and rearrangement of chromosomes have been noted.

Most viruses are capable of inducing immunity. For some virus diseases, vaccines have been prepared that are successful in establishing active artificial immunity. The oldest is the vaccine for smallpox. The diseases in which the virus travels through the blood stream to cause disease are the ones in which antibodies are most successful in preventing a second attack. Also, when a specific virus is frequently present in a community, individuals have the opportunity to have repeated subclinical infections that help boost the level of immunity. Disease syndromes in which a variety of viruses appear to be involved, such as the common cold, probably will never be entirely preventable by immunization. Possibly this is not undesirable. Scientists have discovered that for a time after one virus infection an animal is not susceptible to infection by another. This is thought to be partly due to interferon synthesis, but other mechanisms are probably also at work.

Physical and Chemical Characteristics of Viruses

Some of the physical and chemical characteristics of viruses have practical implications in the practice of nursing. Most viruses are destroyed by heating to 60°C (140°F) *for 30 minutes.* An important exception is the virus of serum hepatitis. It is able to withstand heating to 60°C *for 4 hours.* Because it is highly infectious, as little as 0.01 ml of plasma can carry enough virus to cause disease or to contaminate a batch of pooled plasma. Persons without a history of hepatitis may be carriers of the virus. The virus of infectious hepatitis, although less resistant to heat, may also be transmitted in blood plasma. For this reason authorities generally recommend that needles, syringes, pipettes, and other articles contaminated by blood be sterilized by autoclave for 15 minutes. Because of the possibility of transmitting infectious and serum hepatitis, as well as for economic reasons, many agencies use disposable syringes, needles, and other equipment.

To prevent self-infection, the nurse should avoid needle pricks after drawing blood or giving injections. In the event that the nurse is pricked by a needle, the supervisor should be notified, so that arrangements can be made for preventive therapy, such as immune globulin.

The viruses of hepatitis are known to be present in the feces, blood, and urine. From the available evidence, nasopharyngeal secretions probably do not contain virus. Because the likelihood of spreading disease is increased by overcrowding and contaminated food and water, preventive measures should be directed toward relieving overcrowding and the sanitary disposal of feces.

The virus of infectious hepatitis also withstands residual chlorine of 1 part per million. This resistance is of significance, as the virus leaves the body in the feces and is ingested from food and water. In large cities the water supply is usually safe. The swimming pool in the back yard can be a source of infection unless care is taken to keep it clean and to disinfect the water. Poorly constructed and overcrowded camp sites are also hazardous. Some epidemics of hepatitis have had their origin in oysters and clams obtained from contaminated water and eaten raw.

To prevent the spread of infectious hepatitis, the patient should be isolated until the jaundice subsides, and a gown be worn over the uniform. As for any infectious disease, provision should be made for the sanitary disposal of contaminated articles and body discharges. Gloves are also recommended for persons having direct contact with the patient or contaminated articles. Everyone who enters the room should wash his or her hands on leaving. If possible, such patients should have their own toilet.

In the care of the patient with a virus infection, the nurse has two general responsibilities. One of these is to meet the needs of the patient for nursing care. The other is to prevent the spread of the disease. The same principles apply to the spread of virus infections as to those caused by true microorganisms. The fact that viruses are relatively resistant to conditions in the external environment should be taken into account when planning an effective method for preventing their spread. The only viruses that consistently leave the body in feces are enteroviruses, but adenoviruses frequently do also. As for viruses spread from the respiratory tract, a properly worn mask on the person who has a cold should be reasonably effective in preventing its transmission to others. For most practical purposes this is not feasible in everyday life. In special situations in hospital, isolation procedures may specify that the nurse wear a mask during close patient contact.

The Environment

Besides a pathogenic microorganism and a susceptible host, conditions in the environment must facilitate interaction if an infectious disease is to develop. As an example of the environment facilitating host and agent interaction, bilharziasis has increased in incidence as a result of vast systems of irrigation constructed to improve living standards. Some authorities say that it is the most common and important parasitic disease in humans as it affects the young and causes a high degree of disability. Conditions required for the propagation of the snail in which the *Schistosoma* (a flatworm) spends part of its life cycle are provided by the environment. The eggs of the organism are voided or defecated into the water by infected persons. They hatch and the larvae enter a suitable fresh-water snail. After a period of time, free-swimming larvae leave the snail. They pierce the skin of a person wading, working, or swimming in the water. From the site of entry they are carried by the blood to the liver, where they mature. The essential point here is that customs and habits, i.e., discharging human excreta wherever convenient and the provision of suitable conditions for the propagation of a pathogenic microorganism, provide the conditions in the environment required to transmit the disease. The practices of working, wading, and swimming provide the final conditions necessary to spread the disease. Control of bilharziasis could be effected by the sanitary disposal of urine and feces.

Various conditions in the environment facilitate or prevent the transmission of a pathogenic microorganism to humans. They include such factors as customs, changes in values and mores, climate, geography, sanitary procedures, housing, neighborhoods, and the adequacy of health facilities. For those diseases to which immunity can be developed, the proportion of susceptibles to nonsusceptibles is a significant factor in the control of spread.

The Transmission of Infectious Diseases

The Reservoir Mechanism

In the preceding sections, three essential interactions for development of infection—the susceptible host, the pathogenic microorganism, and the environment—were explored. Following, the elements involved in transmitting the organism from its source to a susceptible host will be considered.

In order for a pathogenic microorganism to survive, it must have a suitable shelter in which to propagate its species and from which progeny can be disseminated before being overcome by the defenses of the host. The place where such shelter is provided is frequently termed a reservoir, be it the tissues of people, animals, or insects or even human wastes and food and water contaminated by them. In a strict sense, a reservoir is a storage receptacle and the term implies inactivity. It seems more accurate to use the term *reservoir mechanism* to describe the total process of bringing the infectious agent in contact with new susceptible hosts, because a continuing chain of transmission is required to perpetuate any microbial species.

This concept of a reservoir mechanism for microbial species perpetuation includes human hosts who shelter pathogenic microorganisms and from whom the microorganisms can be disseminated. These hosts can be apparently well, in the prodromal stages of illness, or mildly or seriously ill. The apparently well person whose mucous membranes or secretions are found to contain pathogenic microorganisms is called a carrier. The reasons that some individuals become healthy carriers are not well understood. Diseases in which carriers serve as disseminators include typhoid fever, diphtheria, and infections caused by staphylococci and streptococci. After recovery from typhoid fever the individual's biliary tract can continue to act as a reservoir source for typhoid bacilli. Virulent diphtheria bacilli, staphylococci, or streptococci can be found on the mucosa of persons who have not experienced an apparent infection. This healthy carrier state can be of either short or long duration and may be constant or intermittent.

Persons who are ill with an infectious disease can also disseminate pathogenic microorganisms. The number available for dissemination does not necessarily correspond with the stage or degree of illness. For example, the most infectious stage of measles is the prodromal stage, that is, before the rash appears and when the eyes and nose are weepy. The peak period of infectious hepatitis A precedes the onset of icterus (jaundice). Mumps virus can be transmitted up to 6 days before any glandular swelling appears. Polio viruses can be excreted in the feces for weeks after recovery of the host. The degree of illness apparently does not govern the transmission of microorganisms, as is well illustrated by poliomyelitis. Probably over 90 per cent of infections are inapparent, somewhere between 4 and 8 per cent abortive, and not more than 2 per cent develop into typical paralytic disease. No matter what the host's response to the polio virus infection he or she can be the source of a highly virulent illness in a susceptible contact. Terms such as *inapparent infection, missed cases,* and *abortive cases* are used to describe the situation in which an individual apparently reacted to pathogenic organisms without experiencing the "normal" manifestations of the disease.

In addition to people, animals or insects may be involved in the reservoir mechanism. Diseases of animals to which human beings are susceptible are known as *zoonoses.* The list includes rabies, tularemia, and psittacosis. In some parts of the world the zoonoses are of much more significance than in the United States. As a group, they are important not only because they are animal diseases that are transmissible to humans under normal conditions, but because they add to the problem of disease control. Possibly the best-known example of a disease where an insect is involved in the reservoir mechanism is malaria. It is essential that the plasmodium spend some time in the mosquito to complete part of its developmental cycle before it can be pathogenic to humans.

Portal of Exit from Host

For the infectious process to succeed, a microorganism must have a mode of escape from the host, or "portal of exit," as part of the reservoir mechanism. These escape routes include the respiratory, gastrointestinal, and urinary tracts, open lesions of the skin, and occasionally blood itself. In some instances escape of the microorganism depends on some other living organism, such as a biting insect. In others they are excreted directly by the infected host.

One of the most common natural avenues of escape for microorganisms is the respiratory tract. Agents growing on or in respiratory membranes can be found in saliva an mucous secretions. Very few are liberated during quiet breathing, but talking, coughing, and sneezing eject large numbers of particles in various sizes. Larger droplets settle to the ground rapidly, within 1 or 2 minutes, where they become incorporated in dust. The smaller ejected droplets evaporate almost instantly, leaving a droplet nucleus that contains any organism originally present in the droplet. They are so light that they remain suspended in air currents and are carried wherever the air goes.

Most of the pathogenic microorganisms discharged from the gastrointestinal tract are expelled with the feces. In addition to the normal flora of the intestinal tract, which under certain circumstances can cause disease, feces can contain truly pathogenic organisms. It is the common mode of transmission for the etiologic agents of typhoid fever, cholera, and amoebic dysentery, and frequently for several viral diseases such as Coxsackie virus infections. This is significant because it has been estimated that 50 to 60 per cent, dry weight, fecal material consists of bacteria and other microorganisms. Worms or their eggs may also be contained in the feces and, when ingested by another, cause disease. The control of infectious diseases of the gastrointestinal tract has been accomplished largely by providing sanitary facilities for the discharge of feces and by controlling water and food supplies. The same facilities also serve to prevent the dissemination of microorganisms contained in urine. Open lesions serve as a route of escape either by direct contact or by contact with its discharge.

Vehicle of Transmission

Once a microorganism has escaped from an infected person, it must have a means of transportation to a susceptible host. The simplest mode of transmission is direct transfer by close personal contact. The organism may be passed directly by touching, kissing, or sexual contact. The venereal diseases are called that because they are usually transmitted sexually, by direct contact with the lesion or the secretions. Infectious mononucleosis is called the "kissing disease" by those who believe it is transmitted by saliva. Organisms can also be passed by the direct propulsion of small droplets or droplet nuclei that settle on or very near mucous membranes of the mouth, nose, or the conjunctiva. For example, Mary Sue arises in the morning with the "sniffles," which she interprets as a cold. After she goes to school she sneezes part of the day, spraying droplets of nasal and pharyngeal secretions in all directions. Children in the room inhale the droplets or droplet nuclei, and within a few days several of her classmates have colds.

Microorganisms may also be passed indirectly from one person to another by means of air currents, contaminated dust, hands, water, food, or objects. To be transmitted indirectly, microorganisms must be able to survive for at least a time outside the body. Organisms such as the *Treponema pallidum* and the gonococcus are fragile and survive for only brief periods outside the body. They are therefore unlikely to be transmitted by indirect contact. In contrast, tubercle bacilli are capable of living for extended periods of time outside the host and may be transmitted indirectly.

Indirect transmission of microorganisms by food or water is properly termed *vehicle transmission.* Organisms that can utilize the nutrients of the food substance for their own growth and reproduction, such as bacteria, are often responsible for a sharp outbreak of an infectious disease. An example of this is the traditional one of an epidemic of staphylococcal food poisoning following a church supper where some article of food was contaminated by the person preparing it and then not properly stored until the time it was served. Other organisms, such as viruses, not capable of multiplying while in a vehicle but of retaining their infectivity, are also transmitted this way. There have been outbreaks of disease due to food contaminated with hepatitis virus. Vector-borne transmission of microorganisms can also occur. Some vectors play a mechanical role in transferring, merely providing a ride for the pathogen on their contaminated feet or legs and then wiping it off on exposed food or human skin. The pathogen may get scratched in as a reaction to the sting of a fly bite. Other vectors, usually arthropods, play a truly biologic role, in that the agent must infect the vector and multiply within it before transmission can occur. Plague and St. Louis encephalitis are transmitted by biologic vectors.

Portal of Entry

Besides requiring a portal of exit from the host and a vehicle for transmission, microorganisms must be able to find a portal of entry into the new host. To be effective, a portal of enty must provide the pathogen with ready access to a tissue where it can lodge and multiply. The same structures, that is, the respiratory tract, mouth, skin, and mucous membranes, that are sites for the escape of microorganisms are also portals for their entry into the new host. Organisms of most respiratory diseases can lodge and multiply only in the membranes of the upper respiratory tract. Many intestinal infections are caused by agents that, because of certain intrinsic properties, can survive the trip through the stomach. However, before a microorganism can cause disease, it must get past the defenses that guard each of these structures. (Refer to Chapter 24 and 25.) Even when the microorganism makes its way past these defenses, the specific resistance of the individual may be sufficient to overcome the microorganism so that disease does not occur.

Factors affecting the susceptibility of the host to any type of illness have been considered. One critical characteristic is the degree to which the individual is or is not immune to the pathogenic microorganism. Immunity is seldom absolute. Whether or not disease results from exposure to pathogenic microorganisms depends on the interaction of the host and the microorganism.

In summary, the infectious disease process has been presented as a reservoir mechanism providing a continuing chain of transmission from an infected to a susceptible host. The essential factors in this process are summarized in Table 10-1.

Table 10-1. *Infectious Disease Process*

Reservoir Mechanism	Essential Factors
1. A causative or etiologic agent (a necessary factor)	Bacteria Fungi Protozoa Rickettsiae Viruses
2. An infected host	Human beings Animals and insects
3. A portal of exit	Respiratory tract—sputum, droplets, droplet nuclei Alimentary canal—feces, saliva Genital tract—secretions, open lesions Urinary tract—urine Skin lesions—drainage Blood
4. A mode of transmission	Direct: Personal contact—secretions, open lesions Indirect: Vehicles—air, dust, food, water, blood, fingers Vectors—insects, arthropods, animals
5. A portal of entry	Respiratory tract, mouth, broken skin or mucous membrane
6. A susceptible host	

The Stages of Illness

The course of an infectious disease is usually divided into three stages. The first, or *incubation,* period is the time that elapses between the entrance of the microorganism into the body and the appearance of clinical signs and symptoms. In terms of the microorganism, the incubation period is the time it takes to adapt to the host and achieve a rate of multiplication sufficient to cause evidence of disease. The length of the incubation period is different for each acute communicable disease but is constant for any one disease. As examples, the incubation period for measles is 10 to 14 days and not longer than 21 days. In meningococcus meningitis, it varies from 2 to 21 days. In those diseases in which not only a specific microorganism but other factors play a dominant role in their development, the length of the incubation period may be difficult to determine. For example, from the time of the primary tubercular infection to the development of progressive pulmonary disease, years may elapse, because other factors in the host determine the actual development of disease. A similar situation exists for the infectious diseases caused by agents that can assume a latent state in the body. The first infection with the virus of herpes simplex is thought to take place early in life and may or may not cause overt illness. The typical lesion of a cold sore reappears over the lifetime when other conditions in the host are right.

The second stage is the *period of illness.* As with the incubation period, in general the length of the period of illness is predictable for a given disease but varies from one type to another. A self-limiting disease may run its course in a few hours or extend for a few weeks at most. The old saying "If a cold is treated it lasts 2 weeks and if it is not treated it lasts 14 days" applies here. Most of the acute communicable diseases are of relatively short duration. Some, such as tuberculosis, may continue to be active for years or months. Of course, the existence and effectiveness of chemotherapy must be kept in mind. As yet there is no specific drug with which to treat the common cold, but the course of tuberculosis can frequently be altered drastically. As in noninfectious diseases, the degree and severity of illness vary from one individual to another. Some individuals have antibodies in their blood indicating that they must have reacted to a given microorganism, but they have no knowledge of ever having had the disease. Nevertheless, these antibodies can protect them from a severe form of the disease. Other individuals experience mild attacks, whereas in still others the course of the disease is so rapid and so severe that the patient becomes ill and dies within a few hours. When the course of a disease is unusually rapid and the manifestations are unusually severe and uncontrollable, it is said to be fulminating. (The term fulminating can be applied to any disease in which the manifestations are unusually severe and which progress in a short time to death.) For example, John Harvey felt fine yesterday. This morning he awakened with a shaking chill, feeling very ill. He had a fever that continued to rise. Despite intensive therapy, he died less than 24 hours after the onset of his illness. He was diagnosed as having fulminating pneumococcal pneumonia, type III. At the onset of his illness he was not a weakened old man but healthy and robust. Despite the possibility of an infectious disease being fulminating, the tendency toward recovery is strong in most acute communicable diseases.

The onset of the period of illness of some acute communicable diseases is usually marked by a prodromal period. During this period the individual has early manifestations of the impending illness but does not have the specific signs and symptoms. One of the problems in the control of diseases such as measles is that the prodromal symptoms are similar to those of a common cold. This morning when Mary Sue went to school with "just a cold," she might well have been in the prodromal phase of measles or another acute communicable disease.

Following the onset of illness, the individual experiences a period in which the specific manifestations of the particular illness are evident and he or she is sick. Depending on the nature of the disease and the person who is ill, he or she may go into the third stage of the infectious illness, which is the *period of convalescence,* and may recover completely; develop complications such as measles encephalitis; recover with permanent sequellae, such as the residual paralyzed limb due to poliomyelitis; or die.

Characteristic Signs and Symptoms in Acute Infectious Disease

During the period of illness most patients have fever. The fever may be constant, intermittent, or remittent. A fever is said to be constant when the amount of variation is less than 2°. It is remittent when it varies more than 2° but does not drop to normal. The type of fever, the degree of elevation, and the length of time it persists are reasonably characteristic for each disease. For example, in untreated pneumococcal pneumonia following a shaking chill, the temperature rises rapidly. It can be expected to remain elevated to from 38.8°C (102°F) to 40°C (104°F) for 5 to 9 days. The fever then falls rapidly, that is, *by crisis,* to below normal. Unless the patient develops a complication, the temperature does not again rise above normal, and from that point on the patient recovers rapidly. When the temperature does not fall within the expected period of time, or if it rises above normal after the crisis, a complication such as lung abscess or empyema is suspected. Accurate determination and recording of the temperature are important in assessing the progress of the patient toward recovery. Although some deviation from the expected pattern does not always indicate that the patient is developing complications, it may.

Along with fever, the patient can be expected to have an elevation in pulse and respiratory rates. Other signs and symptoms are more or less characteristic for each disease. The illness is terminated when the body's defense mechanisms are sufficient to overcome the causative agent. For example, in diphtheria, recovery occurs when sufficient antibodies are formed to neutralize the exotoxin. With the neutralization of the exotoxin, the phagocytes are then able to overcome the diphtheria bacilli.

In some infectious diseases, notably typhoid fever, which is becoming much less of a threat to the general public, but still a risk to laboratory workers, the patient may appear to be recovering only to have a recurrence of symptoms. Usually the course of the second illness is not as severe, nor does it last as long as the original attack. Recurrence of infection in patients treated by antimicrobial agents also happens. Apparently the antimicrobial drug suppresses but does not kill the microbe. The recurrence is caused by the multiplication of the microorganism following the termination of drug therapy.

Not all infectious diseases are self-limiting. The period of illness in some diseases, such as tuberculosis, may depend as much or more on conditions within the person who is ill as it does on the virulence and invasiveness of the microorganism.

During *convalescence,* which follows the period of illness, the patient returns to health. Its length will depend on how long the patient has been ill as well as on how well his or her general condition was maintained during the illness. Some illnesses are more debilitating than others. For example, though the period of illness from influenza may not be unduly long, patients often complain of being weak and easily fatigued for weeks. In the past when patients with typhoid fever were starved, convalescence was delayed until their nutritional status was improved. Attention to nutrition during the period of illness as well as in the period of convalescence is important.

The requirements of the patient who has an infectious disease should be evaluated in the same manner as the requirements of persons with other illnesses. Particular attention should be paid to the person who is isolated. Many, but not all, patients who are isolated feel rejected by nursing and medical personnel. Because drainage from an ulcer on her leg contained virulent staphylococci, Mrs. Brown was placed on isolation precautions. Because no single rooms were available, the curtains were drawn about her bed. At 11 A.M. a nurse opened the curtains to speak to Mrs. Brown. Her breakfast tray was still sitting on her bedside table and her bed was in complete disarray. When the nurse spoke to Mrs. Brown, she burst into tears. As she sobbed, she spoke of her feelings of desolation at being deserted. "You would think that I had leprosy or something. What do I have that makes everyone afraid and avoid me? It must be awfully bad."

Not all patients who are isolated, however, feel neglected. Mrs. Solo, who was also screened from other patients in a large ward, thanked the nurse for making it possible for her to have privacy. The differences in the responses of the two patients was due to differences in their perception of a similar situation.

The nurse, too, should examine how she or he feels about the particular illness. It is not uncommon for nurses to express fear of diseases such as tuberculosis or syphilis. Nurses should also know how they feel about people who have these diseases. Although one cannot always completely change one's feelings, they are easier to control when one knows what they are. Some fears arise from ignorance of the manner by which specific infectious diseases are spread and from not knowing what can be done to prevent their spread.

The role of the nurse in meeting the psychological needs of patients will be discussed in Unit VII. During the period when the patient is acutely ill, attention should be directed toward conserving the patient's energy, providing comfort, relieving symptoms associated with fever, and maintaining fluid intake and, if possible, intake of food. Rest should be provided and unnecessary stimulation avoided. Because fever activates the herpes virus, cold sores on the lips and face of the patient may cause discomfort. Camphor ice or some type of bland or mildly stimulating ointment, prescribed by the physician, should be applied as necessary. Unless the patient breathes through his or her mouth, it will remain clean and moist if fluid intake is adequate, and the patient should be given whatever assistance is required to maintain this fluid intake. Mouth care is important to the comfort of the patient even when the mouth appears to be clean. During illness and convalescence, the patient should be protected from unnecessary exposure to other infectious agents.

During convalescence the needs of the patient will not be particularly different from those of the patient undergoing a surgical procedure or some other illness. Some patients, especially those having had typhoid fever or diphtheria, may continue to discharge virulent bacteria. Precautions designed to protect others may therefore have to be continued during or after the period of convalescence.

The Prevention and Control of Infectious Diseases

Epidemiologists are concerned with three kinds of prevention, which can be used as models for infection prevention and control.

1. *Primary Prevention:* general health promotion, reducing exposure, altering susceptibility, providing specific protective measures—that is, preventing the disease before it starts.
2. *Secondary Prevention:* early detection and treatment of infection.
3. *Tertiary Prevention:* alleviation of disability and restoration to effective functioning (Larson, 1979).

As has been stated, control of infections and the diseases they cause consists basically of determining where and how the chain of transmission can be broken successfully. It is important to control infections, because the individual with a subclinical infection can be a source of serious disease for susceptible contacts. Therefore, accurate detecting and diagnosing are essential. Burnet and White (1972) consider there are "three basic approaches available to public health authorities. They are, first, preventing the entry of the parasite by quarantine measures; secondly, breaking the chain of transmission by what can be broadly called environmental sanitation; and thirdly, protection of the susceptible individual by immunization or chemoprophylaxis." These three basic approaches may be considered as *primary prevention.*

Preventing Entry of the Parasite

A country that is free of any particular infectious disease does not want to have that disease imported by visitors or citizens returning from an infected country. The historic approach to the problem has been the institution of quarantine regulations, or the limitation of freedom of movement of persons or animals exposed to the communicable disease for the longest incubation period of the disease. This procedure hopefully would prevent contact with susceptible people or animals. The practice dates from the fourteenth century, when the port of Venice tried to protect itself from pandemic plague by making ships from infected ports wait 40 days before entering. The procedures have been changed repeatedly over the years, and now quarantine is rarely used. As said earlier in the chapter, only six human diseases are now on the international quarantine list, but this has been revised since smallpox is eradicated.

Quarantine was used in the community when the patient with a communicable disease and all members of the family were restricted to their premises under penalty of law. A placard was nailed on the outside of the house to warn others not to enter. Sometimes the wage earner was allowed to leave, but could not return to the home until the end of the prescribed period of quarantine. The effectiveness of this practice was always questionable, and it has been replaced by isolation of the patient.

International control of animal diseases poses still more of a problem. This includes both human and economic dangers. The possibility of importation was well demonstrated in 1930 when outbreaks of psittacosis occurred in several countries following shipments of parrots from South America (Meyer, 1942). Part of the campaign to eradicate foot and mouth disease in cattle in this country was to forbid shipment of animals into the United States from Mexico. Brucellosis was eradicated state by state, and as each state achieved the goal, it banned shipments of animals from states still having the disease.

Break the Chain of Transmission

Efforts to control an infectious disease may be aimed at any factor in the disease-producing process. Various characteristics of the etiologic agent must be considered in order to determine whether or not it is a good target for control activities. These have been discussed in some detail. In addition, in a number of infectious diseases the identification of the causative organism is essential both to the proper treatment of the patient and to the protection of noninfected individuals. For example, a diagnosis of tuberculosis carries with it the possibility that long-term treatment will be required and the possibility that others have been or will be infected. The tubercle bacillus may be found in the sputum, gastric washings, or urine. Verification may require that one or more of the above be injected into a guinea pig. In many bacterial infections, such as staphylococcal infections, it is increasingly important to determine the range of antibiotic resistance of the agent in order to institute successful therapy. In general, the causative agent for bacterial infections can be identified and this knowledge helps in establishing a diagnosis, as well as in control. Virus identification is too time-consuming to be of any help to the patient as a rule, but can be important from the standpoint of control.

The nurse frequently is responsible for collecting body discharges to be examined for pathogenic microorganisms. The inside of the container to be used for the specimen should be sterile at the time the collection is made. The discharges and containers should be handled in such a way that the outside of the container is kept clean. The nurse should protect her or his hands from contact with potentially contaminated material. Finally, the nurse's hands should be thoroughly washed after the collection procedure has been completed.

Infected human hosts may be isolated during the period of illness and for as long as they shed pathogenic organisms. One reason, though not the only one, for treating patients who have tuberculosis in hospitals is to remove them from the community, where they may be a source of infection to others. Since the introduction of antimicrobial agents, the length of hospitalization has been shortened, and often eliminated. Patients must continue treatment for varying periods of time on an outpatient basis. Therapy of the patient who has tuberculosis has three aims. One is eradication or at least suppression of the organism. The second is prevention of the transmission of the infection. The third is helping the patient learn a way of life that will enable him or her to live in healthful coexistence with the *Mycobacterium tuberculosis.* Even before the days of antituberculosis drugs, the tubercular process was arrested in many patients by a program of rest—both mental and physical, a nutritious diet, and attention to individual factors in each patient. The atmosphere in the sanitarium was calm and unhurried. Because the individual patient is a key factor in recovery, he or she must be taught early the nature of the disease and what the patient's part is in recovery and in maintaining health. Patients also learn how to protect others. The program of therapy serves to assist patients not only to arrest the tubercular process, but to learn a way of life that will enable them to keep their disease under control.

Surgical therapy has made a contribution to controlling tuberculosis. Some surgical procedures result in temporary or permanent collapse of the affected area in the lung. In either event the purpose is to assist the body in healing diseased tissue. When the disease process is localized in one organ or part of an organ, the diseased tissue may be removed surgically. For example, when tuberculosis involves one kidney and not the other, the diseased kidney is usually removed. In pulmonary tuberculosis, a lung may be partially or entirely removed. In some instances, portions of both lungs may be excised. Eradication of the source of infection by surgical removal of the infected tissue is not limited to tuberculosis, as persons who are typhoid carriers can sometimes be cured by cholecystectomy.

The most important measures available to control tuberculosis are the antimicrobial drugs. Although Goodman and Gilman (1975) list a number of drugs, they state that the primary ones used singly or in combination are isoniazid, ethambutol, rifampin, and streptomycin. When a single drug is considered sufficient, the compound employed is isoniazid. When antitubercular drugs were first introduced, the hope was entertained that humankind now would have a means of effectively and easily eradicating tuberculosis. Despite the fact that the original expectations have not been realized, the mortality rate and to a lesser extent the morbidity rate continue to fall in the United States. But the disease remains a major threat to health in most developing countries. Further, in Great Britain, drug-resistant tuberculosis is increasing despite a decrease in morbidity and mortality rates. Although it is possible to cure tuberculosis, cure is not certain. Therefore regular follow-up is essential to discover reactivated disease process.

Case finding is important but is not an end in itself. It is done so that patients who have tuberculosis can be identified and brought under treatment. The initiation of prompt and effective treatment, not only with antimicrobial drugs but with measures designed to improve the resistance of the host to tuberculosis, is imperative. The earlier the disease is discovered, the easier it is to prevent damage.

Antibacterials are also useful in the eradication of other infectious diseases. Among diseases treated with success are syphilis, gonorrhea, and bacillary infections such as those caused by the pneumococcus, meningococcus, and hemolytic streptococcus.

Animals also act as sources of infection for humans, and this danger may be reduced or eradicated by killing diseased animals. For example, in the past, bovine tuberculosis was a problem in dairy cattle partly for this reason. After methods for the identification of tuberculous cattle were developed, programs were instituted to identify and to destroy diseased animals. Farmers were somewhat resistant to this program because they saw it as an economic problem. They did not find it easy to accept as a fact that healthy-looking cows were diseased and must be sold for a price far below their value as producers of milk. The program has, however, been effective in eradicating bovine tuberculosis among cattle and therefore among humans. When the reservoir of disease is in one or more species of wild animals, the problem of eradication is difficult.

For control measures directed against the actual mechanism of transport from the source of infection to a susceptible host, community efforts are highly important as well as personal actions. For most diseases spread by the air-borne route, where the causative microorganisms are expelled in nasal secretions and saliva, care on the part of the infected host to try to contain such secretions is about the only control possible, other than protection of susceptible hosts by immunization. Diseases spread by personal contact, such as gonorrhea and syphilis, can only be controlled by knowledge and abstinence until adequate antimicrobial treatment has been secured. Other mechanisms of transmission are largely controlled by community action. Sewage services for the disinfection and disposal of human wastes do much to break the fecal–oral route, although hand washing is valuable. As people concentrate in an area in larger and larger numbers, the problem of protecting them from their own excreta increases. This has been solved in the developed countries but still is a major problem for countries currently becoming industrialized. Such activities as the filtration and chlorination of water supplies, the pasteurization of milk, the supervision and inspection of food and food handlers, all help prevent the spread of food-borne disease. Destruction of insect vectors blocks this path of transmission. Eradication of the *Anopheles* mosquito, for example, eliminates the biological vector of malaria.

Reduce the Number of Susceptible People

The third method by which the chain of transmission can be broken is to reduce the number of persons in the community who are susceptible to the disease. This may be done by administering antibodies (passive immunity) or by stimulating the person to form antibodies by administering a vaccine or other immunizing agent. (See Chapter 24.) Sometimes antibodies are administered to persons sick with a disease in order to modify the course of the disease. Examples of this include specific antitoxins for diphtheria or tetanus, and gamma globulin for infectious hepatitis. Whether or not the person develops an active immunity as a result of the infection depends on the time the antiserum is administered in relation to the onset of the disease, as well as other factors. The immunization procedures that are most effective are those most nearly like the natural process. Immunizations for poliomyelitis, mumps, and measles, in which living but attenuated viruses are administered, and for tetanus and diphtheria, in which attenuated toxin is injected, are very successful. Killed organisms are not usually as effective as live ones, in that the duration of the resulting immunity is thought not to be so long-lived. Many problems must be solved before a vaccine can be produced and administered to human beings. The most important test that a vaccine must pass is that of safety. Although there is no such thing as absolute safety, the element of risk should be far below the natural risk involved, both in the severity of side effects caused by the vaccine and in the risk of actually acquiring disease.

Influenza vaccine presents special problems. It is useful in preventing the rapid spread of influenza through the community when the strain responsible for the current epidemic is identified in time to allow for the production of the vaccine. But influenza virus is noted for its antigenic shifts, with new mutant strains appearing periodically, and with little if any homologous antigenic components of previous strains. The major pandemics of influenza have been caused by such new strains of virus because no one has any immunity to them.

Influenza immunization is, therefore, valuable only if the antigenicity of the vaccine matches that of the virus involved in a given epidemic. As mentioned previously, amantadine hydrochloride, one of the few antiviral drugs on the market is useful in preventing type A influenza, particularly in institutional settings.

Skin tests, available for the identification of persons who have or have not reacted to specific antigens, are of two types. They are epitomized by the Schick test for immunity against diphtheria, and the tuberculin test for tubercular infection. In the Schick test a minute quantity of weak diphtheria toxin is injected intradermally, usually on the anterior surface of the forearm. Persons lacking neutralizing antitoxin develop, within 24 to 72 hours, a swollen reddened lesion at the site of the injection, indicating that the injected toxin has damaged skin cells and the individual is susceptible to diphtheria. Those who do not react to the toxin have sufficient antibodies to neutralize it. If diphtheria bacilli enter the throat, there is a good chance they will not be able to establish an infection and excrete toxin. If they do, the resulting disease will be mild.

In contrast, for tuberculosis, antigenic protein material, tuberculin, is injected intradermally to demonstrate the presence or absence of a tubercular infection by determining whether or not there is a delayed hypersensitivity reaction to the injected foreign protein. If lymphocytes have been sensitized by exposure to the tubercle bacillus, they will have antibodylike receptors on their surface, will be immobilized by the injected toxin, and will liberate substances that injure local capillaries. Thus a reddened, indurated area at the site of the test after

48 to 72 hours indicates a positive reaction, proof that the person at some time has had a tubercular infection. Two sources of material are available for tuberculin testing. One is an extract of the tubercle bacillus, called old tuberculin or simply OT. The other is a purified protein derivative, or PPD, prepared by growing the bacilli on special synthetic media. The material may be injected into the skin (Mantoux), scratched into the skin (Von Pirquet), applied as a patch test (Vollmer), or pressed in with a special many-pronged device (Heaf). The primary use of tuberculin testing in the community today is to find new infections or new cases. A positive test does not indicate whether or not the person presently has active tuberculosis, so those who have positive tuberculin skin tests then have a chest x-ray. Once hypersensitivity has developed, it usually persists for life. Isoniazid given as a prophylactic for 1 year is recommended for all tuberculin-positive children and for young adults with positive skin tests of less than 2 years duration (Bader, July, 1979, p. 10).

Authorities in public health point out that the control of an infectious disease does not depend on the eradication of the infectious agent or the immunization of all who are susceptible. They do not underestimate the desirability of this goal, but they are aware of the difficulty of attaining total eradication or immunization. The spread of a contagious disease can be fairly effectively controlled provided a sufficient proportion of the population is immune to it. This is called *herd immunity*—the indirect protection existing for the susceptible because many of the people around the person are less susceptible to infection and therefore less likely to transmit pathogenic organisms to him or her. In the past there has been much discussion about what percentage of people needed to be immunized in order to prevent an epidemic of measles or rubella. Today the more important question is whether the vaccine prevents infection, or merely disease. If the vaccinated person is able to get infected and then shed the agent, there is the possibility that he or she could be a source of disease for susceptible contacts. It has been shown, on the basis of rises in antibody levels occurring in people vaccinated against such diseases as influenza and measles, that they were reinfected following exposure to a naturally occurring virus. It is not as easy to prove that they have actually transmitted the infection, but the possibility exists.

A marked increase in the incidence of measles has occurred in this country in the last few years, although the overall number of cases and deaths since 1912 has greatly declined. Even in a country where the great majority of children have been immunized, pockets may exist where, for cultural or socioeconomic reasons, many susceptibles live and mini-epidemics do occur.

Diagnosis

The diagnosis of infectious disease is based on three types of findings, not all of which are present in every instance. The first and most definitive diagnostic finding is the *identification of the etiologic agent.* Sometimes this is not necessary because the manifestations of the illness presented by the patient are so specific. The *symptoms of disease* presented by the patient are the second diagnostic aid to the physician. Third is the *identification of specific types of serologic and/or immunologic response* to the microorganisms.

The importance of identification of the causative organism has already been mentioned. Although many of the manifestations of infectious diseases are similar from one disease to another, for many the patterns of signs and symptoms are fairly characteristic for each disease. Frequently there are one or two effects that are pathognomonic of a particular disease. For example, a physician once said that an experienced nurse helped him arrive at a diagnosis of measles because she recognized the characteristic brassy cough. A highly elevated temperature in an apparently healthy child, which falls when the rash appears, is typical of roseola infantum. When the patient is at least moderately ill and there are other patients in the community with the same infectious disease, the problem of diagnosis may be relatively easy. When the manifestations presented by the patient are not very marked and there are few other sick persons, the problem of diagnosis may be more difficult. This may be complicated by diseases that now occur infrequently. The modern-day physician may never have heard the peculiar labored breathing that his or her grandparents would have recognized immediately as typical of diphtheria.

The third group of findings that are of diagnostic value are the serologic and/or immunologic responses of the infected individual. These are based on the fact that specific immunochemical changes take place in the blood or cells that can be determined by appropriate procedures. The tuberculin-test reaction is one example. If a blood sample is drawn early in the course of an infectious illness, and another 3 or 4 weeks later, they can be tested against a battery of viral antigens. A fourfold or greater rise in antibody level against a certain virus indicates that this was probably the etiologic agent. As stated earlier, this procedure usually takes too long actually to aid in the treatment of the patient but may aid in retrospective confirmation of the diagnosis.

To a limited extent with viral infections, but more frequently with bacterial infections, it must be remembered that similar reactive changes can be temporarily induced by a number of other agents. Thus a false-positive reaction to the less specific tests for syphilis may be caused by such disorders as infectious mononucleosis, malaria, and viral pneumonia. A long-term disease, lupus erythematosus, is frequently accompanied by a positive serologic test for syphilis, despite the absence of a true syphilitic infection. A false-positive tuberculin test may be produced by an infection with atypical mycobacteria.

Skin-sensitizing antibodies are also formed in response to certain other microorganisms. For example, the pathologic changes that occur in blastomycosis are often similar to those of tuberculosis. A patient may be found on x-ray to have pathology suggesting tuberculosis and yet have a negative tuberculin test and no tubercle bacilli in sputum or gastric washings. Injection of antigenic material into the patient's skin from the organism causing blastomycosis may reveal sensitization to it.

In summary, infectious diseases in humans are the result of the interrelationships of factors about the biological agent (organism) the host (humans), and the environment common to agent and host. Any successful nursing plan to prevent or control the spread of infectious disease must appropriately answer the questions, Who protects from whom? Why? From what? and How?

References Cited

Allen, J. *Infection and the Compromised Host.* Baltimore: The Williams & Wilkins Company, 1976.

"Around the World: Salt Against Malaria," *World Health* (March, 1969), 34.

Bader, M. "Infection Control: Immunization." In E. Larson (Ed.), *Infection Control, Topics in Clinical Nursing,* **1**(2) (July 1979), 7–21.

Burnet, M., and White, D. O. *Natural History of Infectious Disease,* 4th ed. London: Cambridge University Press, 1972.

Center for Disease Control. *Morbidity and Mortality Weekly Reports,* April 7, 1973; July 6, 1979; Oct. 28, 1972; March 3, 1973.

Center for Disease Control. "Reported Measles Cases and Deaths per 100,000 Population in the United States for the Years 1912–1974." *Mobidity & Mortality Weekly Report Supplement, Summary,* 1974.

Chang, R. S. "Attributes of Microorganisms." In *Infectious Diseases.* Ed. by P. D. Hoeprich. New York: Harper & Row, Publishers, 1977, pp. 2–12.

Detroit Free Press, Nov. 13, 1979.

Enders, J. F., Weller, T. H., and Robbins, F. C. "Cultivation of the Lansing Strain of Poliomyelitis Virus in Cultures of Various Human Embryonic Tissues." *Science,* **109** (Jan. 1949), 85–87.

Fenner, F. J., and White, D. O. *Medical Virology.* New York: Academic Press, Inc., 1970, p. 119.

Ferguson, R. G. *Studies in Tuberculosis.* Toronto: Toronto University Press, 1955, pp. 6–9, 37–38.

Friedman, C. T. H. et al. "A Malaria Epidemic among Heroin Users." *Am. J. Tropical Med. Hygiene,* **22** (May 1973), 302–7.

Gelfand, H. M., LeBlanc, L., Potash, L., and Fox, J. P. "Studies on the Development of Natural Immunity to Poliomyelitis in Louisiana. IV. Natural Infections with Polioviruses Following Immunization with a Formalin-Inactivated Vaccine." *Am. J. Hygiene,* **70** (1959), 320.

Goodman, L., and Gilman, A. *The Pharmacological Basis of Therapeutics,* 5th ed. New York: Macmillan Publishing Co., Inc., 1975, p. 1214.

Henderson, V., and Nite, G. *Principles and Practice of Nursing,* 6th ed. New York: Macmillan Publishing Co., Inc., 1978, pp. 886–905, 1705–69, 2043.

Henle, W. et al. "The Epstein-Barr Virus." *Sci. Am.,* **241** (July 1979), 48–59.

Hoeprich, R. O., ed. *Infectious Diseases,* 2nd ed. New York: Harper & Row, Publishers, 1977.

Jabbour, J. T. et al. "Subacute Sclerosing Panencepholitis. A Multidisciplinary Study of Eight Cases." *JAMA,* **207** (24 March 1969), 2248–54.

Jose, D. G., Cooper, W. C., and Good, R. A. "How Protein Deficiency Enhances Cellular Immunity." *JAMA,* **218** (29 Nov. 1971), 1428–29.

Kallman, F. J., and Reisner, D. "Twin Studies on the Significance of Genetic Factors in Tuberculosis." *Am. Rev. Tuberculosis,* **47** (1943), 549–74.

Larson, E. "Hands: The Healers and Killers." In *Infection Control, Topics in Clinical Nursing.* Ed. by E. Larson. **1**:2 (July 1979), 59–65.

Marx, J. L. "Slow Viruses: Role in Persistent Disease." *Science,* **180** (29 June 1973), 1351–54.

"More Feed Additives." *Science News,* **116,** 197 (Sept. 22, 1979).

Meyer, K. F. "The Ecology of Psittacosis and Ornithosis." *Medicine,* **21**:175–76 (May) 1942.

"No More Smallpox." *Science News,* **116** (3 Nov. 1979), 310.

Reeves, W. C. "Can the War to Contain Infectious Diseases Be Lost?" *Am. J. Tropical Med. Hygiene,* **21** (May 1972), 251–59.

Schultz, M. G. et al. "Current Concepts in Parasitology." *N. Engl. J. Med.,* **297**:23 (8 Dec. 1977), 1259–64. p. 1259.

Scrimshaw, N. S. and Behar, M. "Malnutrition," in E. D. Kilbourne and W. G. Smillie, eds., *Human Ecology and Public Health,* 4th ed. New York: Macmillan Publishing Co., Inc., 1969, pp. 284–307.

Simpson, H. N. "The Impact of Disease on American History." *N. Engl. J. Med.,* **250** (22 April 1954), 679–87.

Stewart, G. T. "Limitations of the Germ Theory." *Lancet,* **1** (18 May 1968), 1079.

Stewart, J. C. "Analysis of the Diphtheria Outbreak in Austin, Texas, 1967–1969." *Pub. Health Rep.,* **85** (Nov. 1970), 949–54.

Washburn, T. C., Medearis, D. M., and Childs, B. "Sex Differences in Susceptibility to Infections." *Pediatrics,* **35** (Jan. 1965), 57–64.

Youmans, G., Paterson, P., and Sommers, H. *The Biologic and Clinical Basis of Infectious Diseases.* Philadelphia: W. B. Saunders Company, 1975.

11

Physical Agents

In the age of technology which now surrounds us, and which boasts of its triumphs over nature, one thing is ever more apparent to the anthropologist—the student of man. We have not really conquered nature because we have not conquered ourselves. It is modern man, Homo sapiens, *"the wise" as he styles himself, who is now the secret nightmare of man. It is his own long shadow that falls across his restless nights and that follows soundlessly after the pacing feet of statesmen.*

EISELEY

Loren Eiseley, "An Evolutionist Looks at Modern Man" in *Adventures of the Mind."* Richard Thruelsen and John Kobler, Editors. New York: Alfred A. Knopf. 1959, p. 3.

Overview

Although microorganisms are probably the most common type of stressor to challenge our body's defense mechanisms, physical agents are among the most common factors contributing to ischemia and ultimately to cellular necrosis. Physical agents include trauma, extremes of temperature, electricity, gravity, and radioactive rays.

The effects of traumatic injury are further elaborated in Unit V and in Chapters 47 and 50, which address problems associated with surgical trauma. Problems associated with extremes of temperature sufficient to cause cell injury are discussed in Chapter 37, and Chapter 51 presents in detail the consequences of the cytotoxic agents used in treatment of malignant tumors. Emphasis in this chapter is on the nature and effects of radiation.

Trauma

Although the term *trauma* is used to denote any type of agent producing emotional or physical shock, it is used here to indicate a physical force. Trauma is capable of causing all degrees of tissue injury from relatively minor abrasions to lethal disruption of the continuity of critical organs and tissues.

Abrasions

Abrasions are lesions resulting from the scraping of epithelial cells from the skin or mucous membrane by friction. They are produced by pulling or pushing the area over a rough surface. The skinned knee of the child who falls on a sidewalk is an example. Abrasions of the skin can be caused by pulling a sheet from underneath a patient without lifting or turning him or her or by pulling (dragging) a patient over the sheets. Obese or heavy comatose patients who are difficult to move and turn are most likely to suffer from this treatment. Besides causing unnecessary discomfort, an abrasion robs the patient of one primary barrier to infection, that is, intact skin. In the care of the patient, attention should be given to the protection of the skin and mucous membranes from ill-advised friction, by rolling or lifting or lubrication of tubes. These procedures also protect underlying tissues from injury by the shearing force.

Contusion or Bruise

Crushing injury to deeper layers of tissue is termed a *contusion* or *bruise*. Contusions are caused by the application of force to tissue, thereby injuring the underlying structures. Contusion frequently results from striking a part of the body against a hard object such as a table or chair. In a contusion there may be extensive damage to soft tissues, including blood vessels, with subsequent bleeding into the tissues. The surface layer of skin or mucous membrane may or may not be ruptured. Particularly in debilitated patients, a bruised area may serve as the site favorable to the growth of pathogenic bacteria. Free blood in the tissues provides food for their growth, and swelling interferes with the body's ability to increase the number of leukocytes in the area. In all individuals, blood escaping into the soft tissue acts as a foreign body and induces an inflammatory response. Pain on pressure or movement of the tissue is usual.

Contusion of the Brain

In traumatic injuries involving the skull, the brain may be contused or bruised. Contusions of the brain occur even in the absence of skull fractures. In infants brain hemorrhage is the most common cause of accidental death. It may result from vigorous "burping" or repeated, relatively mild shaking (Caffey, 1972). The bleeding may create further injury by increasing intracranial pressure. Sometimes the volume of blood escaping from the blood vessels is insufficient to cause a significant increase in intracranial pressure, but the clot that forms attracts and holds water. Venous bleeding is likely to increase intracranial pressure more slowly than does arterial bleeding. Bleeding into the space between the dura and the skull also takes time to increase intracranial pressure. (See Chapter 36.) Days or weeks may elapse after the injury before signs of increased intracranial pressure are seen.

An injury unique to the brain is the so-called contrecoup, in which the bruise occurs at a site other than at the point at which the skull suffers trauma. A contrecoup injury is most likely to occur when the body has been in motion at the moment of injury and the head is brought to an abrupt stop by the injuring force. As an example, a contrecoup injury may occur when the head strikes the windshield in an automobile accident. The same type of injury may result from a fall. The course of events in the development of a contrecoup injury can be simulated by taking a full pail of water and walking rapidly—a sudden stop will cause the water to splash. Emergency-room nurses, as well as those caring for patients who have suffered head injuries, should be alert to the possibility that the brain has been bruised despite absence of obvious injury to the scalp or skull. Identification of the site of injury depends on careful observation of the signs and symptoms presented by the patient. Changes in level of consciousness and of vital signs should be reported without delay. Because the brain is susceptible to edema after it is shaken (concussion) or bruised, the patient should be encouraged to lie quietly, and care should be taken to protect the head from jarring or sudden movements.

Lacerations

Lacerations, injuries in which there is a disruption of the continuity of surface-layer tissue, also result from trauma. Depending on the instrument causing the laceration, the resulting wound may be superficial or extend deep into the tissues. Puncture wounds such as those caused by a nail or other similar instrument and those in which tissue is crushed and devitalized offer conditions favorable to the growth of *Clostridium perfringens (welchii)* and *Clostridium tetani.* Lacerations not only disrupt natural defenses but may be accompanied by contusions and bleeding. Attention should be paid to minimizing the contamination of the wound and, if necessary, to controlling bleeding.

Prevalent Extrinsic Agents

Although this section is looking at trauma as one type of injuring agent, it should be pointed out that two extrinsic agents are largely responsible for the great increase in serious and fatal traumatic injuries in our society: (1) the automobile, driven in an unsafe manner primarily by persons under the influence of alcohol and drugs, and (2) the increased availability and use of handguns (Rushforth et al., 1977).

To summarize, trauma injures tissue by removing

surface cells; by crushing tissues, including blood vessels; and by disrupting the continuity of tissue. The terms used to indicate the type of injury resulting from trauma are, respectively, *abrasion, contusion,* and *laceration.* Trauma predisposes to further ill effects by disrupting the body's first line of defense against microorganisms: the intact skin and mucous membranes. By devitalizing tissues it renders them liable to infection by one or more types of clostridia. Prevention of infections by these organisms can usually be accomplished by passive and active immunization against *Clostridium tetani* and by thorough cleansing and debridement of the wound.

Extremes of Temperature

Hypothermia

A second physical agent causing cellular (tissue) injury is a low temperature, or cold. Healthy cells can survive the gradual reduction of temperature to 20°C (68°F). Esophageal temperatures below 78°F are associated with an extremely poor prognosis. When tissue is actually frozen, further injury is caused by the formation of ice crystals. Hypothermia is accompanied by metabolic acidosis and physiological hypotension. Exposure to moist cold over a long period of time damages capillary endothelium and increases its permeability. As fluid leaks into the tissues, the erythrocytes are concentrated in the capillaries with the result that they tend to pack in clumps and obstruct the flow of blood, thus causing ischemia. When these changes occur in the feet, the condition is known as immersion or trenchfoot. This condition can be a problem to hunters and campers. It can be prevented by a boot developed in Iceland during the Korean War.

Hyperthermia

Humans tolerate a greater degree of lowering than of raising tissue temperatures, as the range of temperature compatible with cell survival varies from 30° to 45°C (88° to 114°F). A body temperature over 42.5°C (108.5°F) is tolerated for only a short time. Two factors, length of exposure and degree of temperature elevation, are significant factors in the degree of injury. As examples, exposure of the skin to temperatures below 45°C (114°F) for 20 minutes causes only minimal injury. Temperatures of 60°C (140°F) and above for as little as a minute cause full-thickness burns.

Effects of Raising Tissue Temperatures

The earliest change in cells in which the temperature is compatible with life is an increase in the metabolic rate of about 7 per cent for each degree of temperature elevation.[1] When the temperature of tissues rises above a critical level, cell proteins are denatured, critical enzyme systems are inactivated, and the affected cells die. See Chapter 37 for discussion of cause, effect, and care of patients with hypothermia and hyperthermia.

Thermal Burns

In thermal burns, heat is applied directly or indirectly as radiant energy to the skin. Damage is not limited to the skin as the constituents of blood and blood vessels may also be affected. In minor burns the changes in the skin and other organs are minimal. In major burns the entire body is affected (see Chapter 49).

Classification

Over the course of history a variety of classifications have been employed to express the extent of tissue damage resulting from burns. The most recent classification is simply (1) partial-thickness injury to the skin and (2) full-thickness injury to the skin. The older classification identifies burns by degrees of injury: first-degree burns—erythema; second-degree burns—death of the epidermis, with the appendages of the epidermis remaining viable in the dermis; third-degree burns—death not only of the epidermis, but of its appendages in the dermis; and fourth-degree burns—charring or carbonification of the skin. First- and second-degree burns are partial-thickness burns. Third- and fourth-degree burns are full-thickness burns. The seriousness of a thermal burn depends not only on the depth of the burn but also on its extent.

Burn Prevention and Control

Burn prevention and control are based on three types of information: (1) incidence of burns, (2) who is burned, and (3) what causes burns.

Incidence and Who Is Affected

Each year at least 2 million persons are burned seriously enough to require medical attention or to

[1] This is a biologic example of a chemical principle that the speed of a chemical reaction is directly proportional to the temperature.

restrict their activity for a day or more. Of these about 100,000 require hospitalization and from 9,000 to 12,000 die. In addition to causing loss of life and human suffering, fires destroy about $3 billion worth of property.[2] Burns are second only to transport accidents as a cause of death among children 1 to 4 years of age. They are the second cause of accidental death among 5- to 14-year-olds and among those over 40 years of age. In the past more boys have been burned than girls, but more girls died than boys, because of the kinds of clothing they wore. As the styles and fabrics used in both boys and girls clothing become similar, this distinction may vanish. In a study made in six counties in southeastern Missouri the incidence of burns was higher among nonwhites than among whites and among those living in cities than those in rural areas (Garner & Love, 1969).

Causes

In the Missouri study (Garner & Love, 1969, p. 28) the leading sources of burn injuries were in this order: stove, grease, hot water, hot iron, space heater, matches, exhaust pipe, campfire or bonfire, hot drink, gas vapors, and others. Sixty-one per cent of the fatal burns occurred in a building fire and over 21 per cent were caused by explosions. Over one half of the minor injuries were due to contact with a hot object and about 26 per cent were due to steam, hot liquid, and grease. *More than half the burns occurred in the living room and kitchen.*

Unsafe acts leading to burning include careless smoking; explosions from the reckless handling of volatile fluids such as alcohol, benzine, and gasoline; drying clothing too close to an open fire or heater; and defective stoves, heaters, and wiring. The improper or excessive storage of flammable materials provides fuel. Pans placed on a stove with handles extending over the edge result in scalding when pulled by a child or caught in loose clothing. All these as well as other unsafe acts result in burns ranging from minor to fatal injuries.

Burn Prevention Program

In the Missouri Burn Injury Prevention project the burn death rate in the project area was reduced by 43 per cent. The first step in this program was to gather epidemiological data. The next step was the development of a community action program based on the following premises about the readiness of each individual to learn safety behaviors:

a. Safety matters are salient.
b. Belief that he is susceptible.
c. Belief that it would have serious consequences for him or his family.
d. Belief that recommended control measures will be effective.

One area in which progress has been made is in the development of flame-resistant materials for use in children's clothing and furnishings for homes, hospitals, airplanes, and other areas where fire is likely or difficult to contain. Legislation has been enacted to further the development and use of fire-resistant fabrics. Much remains to be done, particularly in the enforcement of existing statutes. Public education is needed so that the public will (1) support the stronger legislation and enforcement of laws requiring the use of fire-resistant fabrics, (2) support research to develop fire/heat resistant fabrics, and (3) practice fire prevention. As in other areas, prevention of burns is everyone's business.

Electrical Injury

For an electrical injury to occur, some part of the body must complete the circuit between two conductors. The path taken is generally the most direct between the two contact points. Harmful effects depend on the kind of current, the path taken by the current, the duration of the flow, and the amount of current.

In the past the usual sources of electrical injury were lightning, fallen or broken high tension lines, or damaged electrical cords or outlets. Hazards to persons undergoing diagnosis or medical treatment have been greatly increased by the use of electrically powered machines. These range from commonly used electric beds, heating pads, and suction pumps to respirators and hemodialysis machines. These machines make care easier and more efficient. Without a source of power such as electricity, some diagnostic and therapeutic measures could not be performed. Risks in their use can be minimized by persons who understand the basic principles of electricity and who know what the dangers are and how to minimize them (Sovie & Fruehan, 1972).

Electricity causes cellular injury in a variety of ways. It produces cellular necrosis by direct coagulation of proteins and by changes in the polarity of cells, which result in an increase in their permeability. Furthermore, resistance to the passage of the electric current through a tissue produces heat that has the same effect on tissue as heat from any other source. The effect of controlled amounts of electric current on the tissue depends on whether the cur-

[2] Deaths from explosions are included in some figures.

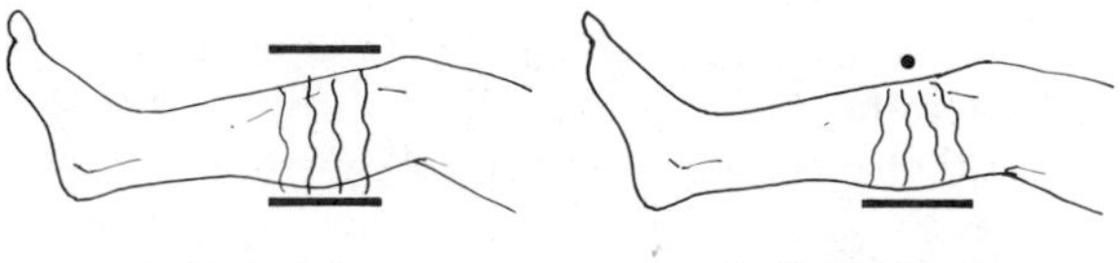

A. To heal tissue B. To destroy tissue

Figure 11-1. Diffuse and concentrated distribution of electric current passing through tissue in diathermy.

rent is widely diffused through the tissue or is concentrated at a narrow point. When the current is diffused, the tissue is warmed. When it is concentrated, tissue is destroyed at the point of concentration. In either instance a high-frequency alternating current is passed through the tissue from one electrode to another (see Figure 11-1). One source of burns is a metal intrauterine device. Before a woman is treated over the abdomen or pelvis with shortwave diathermy, such a device must be removed.

Death from exposure to an electric current is usually caused by its effects on the heart and brain tissue. Exposure of the heart to 110-volt electric current alternating at 60 cycles per second induces ventricular fibrillation, because one of the stimuli is bound to come at the end of the refractory period when the heart is most susceptible to fibrillation. In contrast, an electric current may be used to stop ventricular fibrillation or to initiate contraction in a heart that has stopped beating.

Gravity

The final physical injuring agent to be considered is *gravity*. Human evolution has taken place on the surface of the earth, under the influence of the constant and pervasive force of gravity.[3]

In health, our regulatory processes operate optimally under the amount of force created by gravity at sea level. As modern technology takes us deeper into the earth, our bodies become heavier, that is, they sustain greater force; as we travel further into space, away from the earth's surface, our bodies weigh less, that is, they sustain less force. Space flight research has demonstrated that changes in gravitational force can produce marked alterations in both biologic function and structure, such as net body mass, bone mineralization, mass of body musculature, distribution of body fluids, cardiovascular function, mineral and nitrogen balance, and vestibular function (Page, 1977). When change in gravitational force is great in either quantity or duration, serious cell injury or death may result from failure of adaptation to the altered environmental pressure.

[3] *Gravity* is the accelerating tendency of bodies toward the center of the earth or toward the center of other heavenly bodies such as the moon. This tendency is the force with which all bodies in the universe attract one another. The force is proportional to the product of the masses of the objects and inversely proportional to the square of the distance between them.

Newton's laws of motion, which deal with inertia, momentum, and action and reaction, explain the behavior of matter within gravitational force (Flitter, 1972).

Radiation

Although radiation is another form of physical energy capable of injuring cells, some forms of radiation are essential to the biological processes of living things (see Table 11-1). Rays may be classified as those that can be seen, light rays; those that can be felt, heat rays; and those that cannot be detected by any of the five senses. All may be classified by their length. In nature infrared light and ultraviolet rays are required for specific biological activities. Appropriately controlled microwaves and waves causing ionization are useful. In sufficient dosages, with the possible exception of light rays,[4] all are capable of causing serious damage to living things. In Table 11-1, the length in Angstroms, sources, mode of exposure, penetrating power, and biological and injurious effects of and protection against the various types of rays have been summarized.

Definitions

The following discussion of radiation will be facilitated by definition of some of the terms used.

Atom. An electrically neutral basic unit of matter resembling a miniature solar system, with its nucleus made up of protons and neutrons surrounded by enough revolving electrons to balance electrically the protons in the nucleus. The hydrogen atom, with one proton and one electron (and therefore no neutron), serves as a basis for determining the atomic number and weight of other atoms (Routh, 1953, p. 28).
See Figure 11-2 for an illustration of atomic structure and chemical reactions possible because of atomic structure.

Proton. A positively charged particle of mass 1 within the nucleus of the atom, which may be considered

[4] Light rays, as LASER beams, are being used to destroy abnormal cells, but the light rays are in a state greatly amplified from their natural form. (LASER is the acronym for *l*ight *a*mplification by *s*timulated *e*mission of *r*adiation.)

a hydrogen atom minus its one electron (Routh, 1953, p. 27).

Electron. A negatively charged particle whose mass equals 1/1,837 of the mass of the hydrogen atom, which revolves in orbit around the nucleus of the atom (Routh, 1953, p. 27).

Neutron. An uncharged or electrically neutral particle of mass 1, found in nuclei of atoms.

Atomic number. That number which equals the number of revolving electrons of the atom. Because the atom must be electrically neutral, the atomic number also equals the number of protons in the nucleus (Routh, 1953, p. 30).

Atomic weight. That number which equals the sum of the total number of protons and neutrons in the nucleus of the atom (Routh, 1953, p. 30).

Radiation. The process by which the nucleus of an unstable particle emits particles and/or energy in the process of decay to a more stable element (DiSaia et al., 1975, p. 24).

Ionization. The process whereby one atom permanently donates the electron(s) of its outer valence shell to another atom that completes its valence shell by accepting the electron(s). The electrically charged particles that result from the transfer of electron(s) are called *ions.* The donor atom becomes positively charged; the recipient atom becomes negatively charged. See Figure 11-3 for an illustration of the process of ionization.

Ionizing radiation. Radiation capable of causing ionization, even of air; the physical force whose characteristic ability is to transfer its energy to matter by separating orbital electrons from their atoms and thus forming physical ion pairs (Danforth, 1977, p. 1092).

Photon. A discrete quantity of energy of visible light, or any other electromagnetic radiation; waves or particles without mass (Blakiston's, 1972, p. 1184; DiSaia et al., 1975, p. 24).

Positron. An elementary particle having the mass of an electron but carrying a unit of positive charge; highly unstable, dissipates as radiation as soon as it encounters an electron, which is annihilated with it (Blakiston's, 1972, p. 1227).

Alpha rays. Positively charged helium atoms. An alpha particle is the nucleus of the helium atom minus the pair of planetary electrons, consisting of two protons and two neutrons with a positive charge of two units (Routh, 1953, p. 43).

Beta rays (beta particles). Streams of electrons or positrons traveling at the speed of light. (Routh, 1953, p. 45).

Gamma rays. Photons; electromagnetic radiation emitted from within an excited nucleus; can be considered as either waves or particles without mass (DiSaia et al., 1975, p. 24).

X-rays. Photons; electromagnetic radiation similar to gamma rays, but originating outside the atomic nucleus (DiSaia, et al., 1975, p. 24).

Radioactive isotopes. Those isotopes in which the nucleus undergoes spontaneous disintegration with the production of new elements and three types of rays—alpha, beta, and gamma rays. Some radioactive elements such as radium occur in nature; others are produced artificially. In the process of degeneration, a radioactive isotope may form another radioactive isotope or it may decompose immediately to a stable atom.

Half-life. The period of time it takes one half of the atoms of a radioactive element to disintegrate or to become stable. The rate of disintegration of a radioactive element depends only on its atomic structure; changes in temperature or pressure or chemical combination or any other measurable conditions have no effect on the length of its half-life. The half-life of different elements varies from a few seconds to several billion years.

Angstrom unit (A.U.). A unit of length equal to 10^8 centimeters (1/100 millionth of a centimeter); used to measure wavelengths of visible light, x rays, and radium radiation (Blakiston's, 1972, p. 91). See Figure 11-4 for an illustration of measurement at the microscopic level.

Dyne. The amount of force which, when acting continuously on a mass of 1 gm for 1 second, will accelerate the mass 1 cm per sec (Blakiston's, 1972, p. 471).

Erg. A unit of work, representing the work done in moving a body against the force of 1 dyne through a distance of 1 cm (Blakiston's, 1972, p. 521).

Roentgen *(r).* The unit of measurement of radiations, based upon ionization produced in air; 1 r = the amount of radiation that will liberate 1 electrostatic unit of electricity per cubic centimeter of air under standard conditions of temperature and pressure. One r corresponds to the dissipation, in air, of about 83 ergs per gm (Danforth, 1971, p. 1062).

Radiation absorbed dose (rad). The unit of measurement of radiation absorbed, in material other than air, which is independent of the energy of the radiation and of the absorbing material. Dissipation of energy when material other than air is exposed to ionization depends upon (1) the effective atomic number and (2) the quality of the radiation involved. One rad = the amount of ionizing radiation that transfers 100 ergs per gm to the absorbing material (Danforth, 1971, p. 1062).

Electron volt (ev). The energy of motion acquired by an electron accelerated through a potential difference of 1 volt.

TABLE 11-1. *Characteristics of Radiation**

Type of Radiation	Length	Sources of Particles or Rays (waves)	Mode of Exposure	Penetrating Power	Biological Effects	Protection Against	Injurious Effects
Infrared—heat rays	7,000 to 500,000 A	Solar energy; heated objects	Contact with skin or other tissues	1 to 10 mm	Can be felt; heats tissues that absorb it; moderate exposure causes a transient erythema of the skin	Clothing; shelter; shading; avoiding contact with flame and heated objects	Thermal burns
Visible light	3,900 to 7,700 A	Sunlight	Contact with skin; focused on retina		Vision		Little if any at ordinary intensities
Ultraviolet	2,000 to 3,900 A	Sunlight; artificial ultraviolet light—sunlamp	Contact with skin and other tissues	Little	Photochemical processes such as photosynthesis in green plants; vitamin D from precursors in irradiated skin; kills bacteria and viruses	Limited length of exposure; clothing; shelter; shading	Sunburn, a photochemical reaction; senile degenerative changes accelerated; farmer's or sailor's skin; hyperkeratosis and carcinoma of the skin more frequent in exposed than nonexposed areas
Electromagnetic waves as microwaves & short waves	1 mm to 1 m	Electrical energy converted to microwaves	Through skin and mucous membranes Inadequately insulated and improperly used microwave ovens and careless use of radar	Penetrates deeply	Insufficient energy to produce ionization; heats the tissue as it penetrates—molecules bounce back and forth causing friction	Shielding by insulation	Degenerative lesion in heart, kidney, and other organs in experimental animals; cataracts and testicular atrophy
Alpha particles	0.1 A	Helium atom, doubly ionized	Ingestion; inhalation; through breaks in the skin; introduction into a body cavity or tissue in diagnosis or treatment	Minimal—completely absorbed or stopped by a few centimeters of air or a thin piece of paper	Either ionizes cell constituents directly and makes them unstable *or* ionizes water in the cell and forms products such as ionized hydrogen or hydroxyl radicals; these products	Very easily absorbed; distance; shielding; rubber gloves; filtration mask; protective clothing	Because of limited penetrating power, alpha particles are essentially harmless unless inhaled or ingested

					react with other cell constituents to ionize them		
Beta particles (negatrons)	0.1 A	Electron particles of small mass carry a negative charge; radioactive nuclei emitted by ^{131}I, ^{198}Au, ^{226}Ra	As above	Only a few millimeters of tissue at most; 2 mm thickness of brass; 1 mm of lead	As above	Easily absorbed; as above; copper and aluminum filters	Local tissue injury at site of application including tissues to which beta particles are applied in the interior of the body; when ingested or inhaled in sufficient quantities causes injury as listed below
Gamma rays	1 to 0.1 A	1. Roentgen rays or x rays produced by bombarding a metallic target with high-speed electrons; no charge 2. X rays originating in the nuclei of atoms, e.g., ^{198}Au, ^{226}Ra; a range of charges	As above, plus exposure to rays in the environment; scatter x rays from diagnostic or therapeutic x rays	Great; can traverse, that is, pass through, the entire body	As above	Penetrates several inches of metal; lead is commonly used for shielding; concrete	1. Prompt effects a. Hematopoietic system b. Gastrointestinal system c. Nervous system 2. Delayed effects a. Genetic aberrations b. Induction of malignant neoplasms c. Reduction in the life span d. Other effects such as (1) sterility, (2) cataracts
Neutrons or neutron rays; uncharged particles; electrons; deuterons	0.1 A	Cyclotron and from the so-called atomic pile; atom bomb (nuclear fission and transmutation)	1. Explosion of atom bomb 2. Working with neutrons 3. During therapy	Passes; in general, very penetrating		Very penetrating—concrete slows down	See gamma rays
Protons	0.1 A	Positively charged hydrogen nuclei					

* Information in this table was synthesized by I. L. Beland from cited and easily accessible references and from personal knowledge.

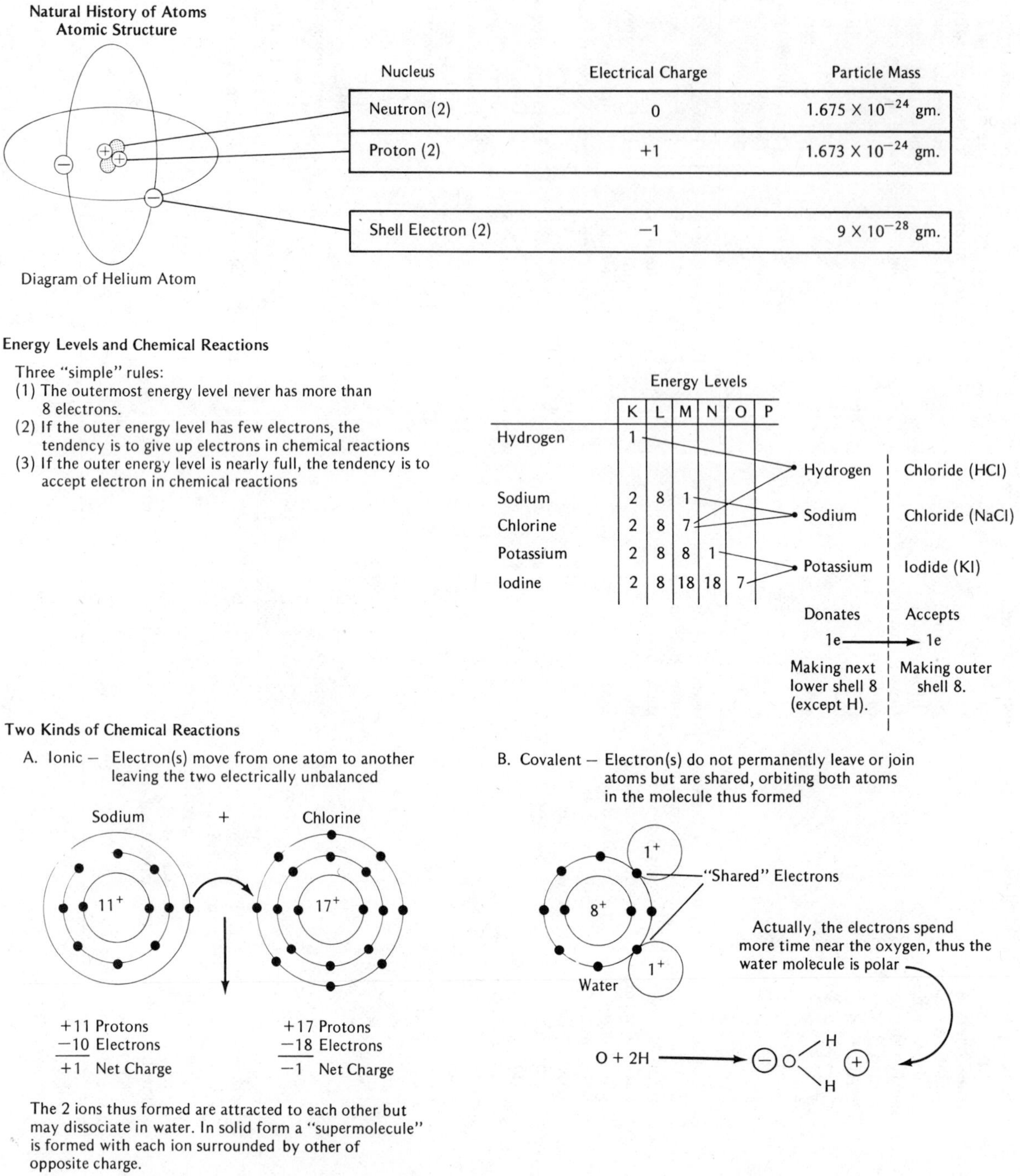
Natural History of Atoms
Atomic Structure
Nucleus
Electrical Charge
Particle Mass
Neutron (2)
0
1.675 X 10^{-24} gm.
Proton (2)
+1
1.673 X 10^{-24} gm.
Shell Electron (2)
−1
9 X 10^{-28} gm.
Diagram of Helium Atom
Energy Levels and Chemical Reactions
Three "simple" rules:
(1) The outermost energy level never has more than 8 electrons.
(2) If the outer energy level has few electrons, the tendency is to give up electrons in chemical reactions
(3) If the outer energy level is nearly full, the tendency is to accept electron in chemical reactions
Energy Levels
K L M N O P
Hydrogen 1
Sodium 2 8 1
Chlorine 2 8 7
Potassium 2 8 8 1
Iodine 2 8 18 18 7
Hydrogen
Chloride (HCl)
Sodium
Chloride (NaCl)
Potassium
Iodide (KI)
Donates
Accepts
1e
1e
Making next lower shell 8 (except H).
Making outer shell 8.
Two Kinds of Chemical Reactions
A. Ionic — Electron(s) move from one atom to another leaving the two electrically unbalanced
Sodium
+
Chlorine
11$^+$
17$^+$
+11 Protons
−10 Electrons
+1 Net Charge
+17 Protons
−18 Electrons
−1 Net Charge
The 2 ions thus formed are attracted to each other but may dissociate in water. In solid form a "supermolecule" is formed with each ion surrounded by other of opposite charge.
B. Covalent — Electron(s) do not permanently leave or join atoms but are shared, orbiting both atoms in the molecule thus formed
1$^+$
8$^+$
1$^+$
"Shared" Electrons
Water
Actually, the electrons spend more time near the oxygen, thus the water molecule is polar
O + 2H
H
H

Figure 11-2. Atomic structure and chemical reactions. (Used with permission of Macmillan Publishing Company, Inc., from *Biology,* 2nd ed., 1979, p. 84, by J. F. Case.)

Kiloelectron volt (kev). The equivalent of 1,000 ev.

Millielectron volt (mev). The equivalent of 1 million ev.

Roentgen-equivalent-man (rem). The dose unit equal to *any* type of ionizing radiation that produces, in humans, the same biologic effect as 1 r of x-rays or gamma rays; i.e., dose in rems = dose in rads × RBE (relative biologic effectiveness) of the radiation in question (Rhein, 1976, p. 35).

Infrared Waves

Depending on their length, infrared waves can penetrate the skin from 1 to 10 millimeters where they may produce heat and with it a transient erythema. With excessive exposure, edema, blistering, and necrosis of the skin characteristic of heat burns are produced. The most serious injury caused by infrared rays is heat coagulation of the retina. Like

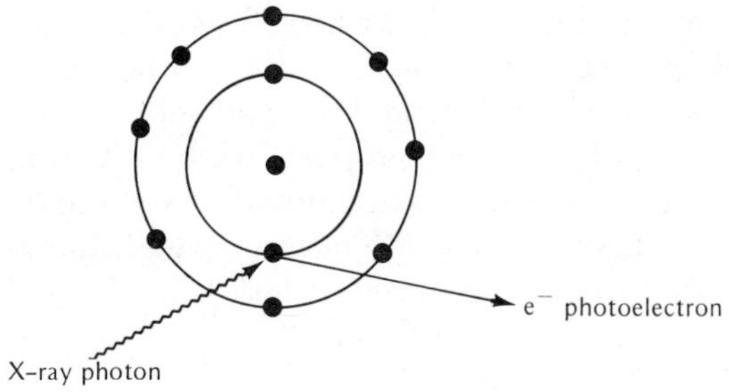

Figure 11-3. Ionization is a process by which orbital electrons are ejected. A low-energy x-ray photon which is a "packet" of x-ray energy "hits" an atom and interacts with an orbital electron, transferring its energy to electron and knocking it out of orbit. This produces a photoelectron, which can cause further ionization, and leaves behind a charged atom, or ion. (Used with permission of The C. V. Mosby Company from *Basic Pathophysiology: A Conceptual Approach,* 1979, p. 171, by M. E. Gröer & M. E. Shekleton.)

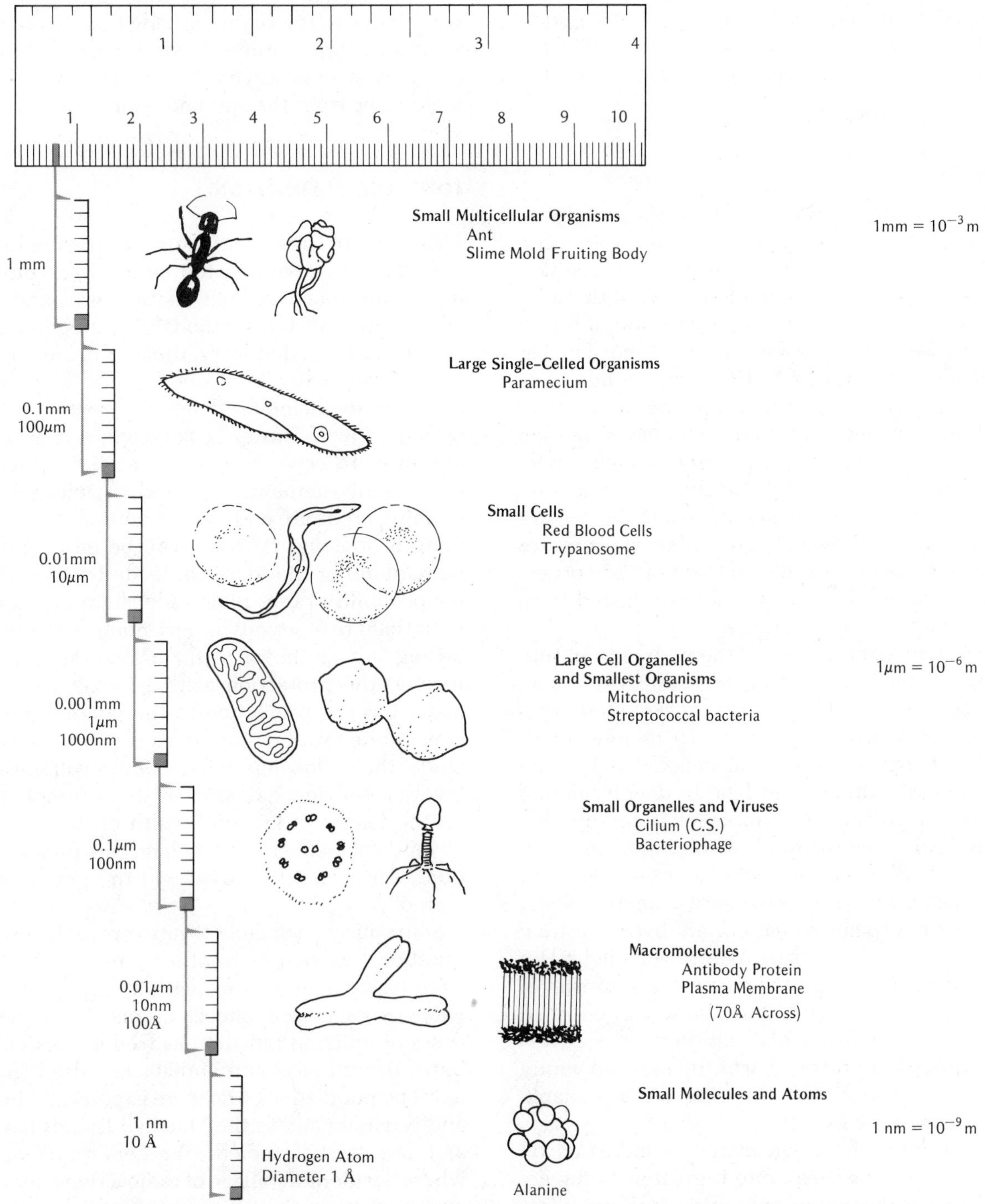

Figure 11-4. Measurement at the microscopic level. (Used with permission of Macmillan Publishing Company, Inc., from *Biology,* 2nd ed., 1979, p. 36, by J. F. Case.)

light rays, infrared rays can be refracted and focused on the retina. Excessive exposure can be caused by staring directly at the sun during an eclipse. Because of a lack of light rays, the pupil of the eye remains open and the infrared rays concentrate on the retina. The fovea is the usual site of injury, with the result that fine vision is impaired or lost.

Ultraviolet Rays (Waves)

Ultraviolet rays lie just beyond the violet end of the visible spectrum. As can be noted in Table 11–1, ultraviolet rays have beneficial as well as injurious effects.

Sunburn

Sunburn is a complex process that can be induced by exposure to the sun's ultraviolet rays or to ultraviolet light (lamp). On sufficient exposure of the skin to sun's rays, there is a sensation of warmth and a transient reddening of the skin due to the infrared rays. Because ultraviolet-ray injury to the skin has a latent period of from 2 to 12 hours, an individual may incur a serious burn before being aware of it. These burns range from a mild erythema of the skin through second-degree burns. Fever and leukocytosis are not common unless the burns are severe. However, the cornea and conjunctiva of the eye are very sensitive to ultraviolet light and short exposures may produce keratitis (inflammation of the cornea) and conjunctivitis. The eyes can be protected from ultraviolet light by dark glasses.

Persons who tan can protect themselves from sunburn by gradually increasing exposure to the sun. Tolerance is built up by starting with a limited exposure and extending the time by 10 minutes or so each day. Despite the general belief that tanning of the skin is conducive to health, deeply tanned skin is damaged skin. A number of factors modify the length of exposure to ultraviolet light that can be tolerated. Blondes and redheads are much more sensitive to ultraviolet rays than are brunettes. Some people, for unexplained reasons, are hypersensitive and cannot tolerate exposure to ultraviolet light. Hypersensitivity (photosensitivity) is a characteristic of a rare disease, porphyria. It is also a side effect of the phenothiazine group of drugs. Protective covering is required to prevent burns. Infants and young children are susceptible to burning and are unable to protect themselves.

Concentration of ultraviolet rays is increased by reflection. Therefore, exposure is greater during activities such as boating or swimming. Because ultraviolet rays pass through clouds, sunburn is possible on cloudy days. Though the shade from trees provides some protection against sunburn, protection is only partial. Exposed areas are therefore liable to sunburn even when a person is shaded by a tree.

Prolonged or extended overexposure of the skin to the rays of the sun intensifies the rate at which it ages. It also predisposes to carcinoma of the skin. The incidence of carcinoma of the skin is higher among those living in tropical climates than those living in temperate or arctic regions. It is also higher among farmers and sailors than among those who work indoors. It is higher among those who tan their skins for social reasons. Great grandma's sunbonnet and long sleeves served a useful purpose; they protected her from the sun and cancer of the skin.

Ionizing Radiation

Because of the extensive use of ionizing radiation, as well as its awesome potentialities, everyone should have some knowledge of its nature, uses, and dangers and of some of the methods of protection from its effects. Since its discovery, the uses of ionizing radiation have greatly increased. It was first used primarily in medicine for diagnosis, treatment, and research. Now, industry is developing it as a source of power. Its capacity as an agent of destruction has been amply demonstrated and is well known. Depending on its use and the precautions taken in handling it, ionizing radiation can be either a boon to humankind or the source of its destruction. The latter possibility raises philosophical and ethical questions that are of serious import. Some of the problems arising out of the peaceful uses of atomic energy include the protection of those who work with it, as well as the protection of the general population from atomic wastes. Questions requiring answers include the following: What effects will raising the level of ionizing radiation in the atmosphere have on the length of life and health of the people now alive? What effects will it have on future generations? How can it be used and the population protected?

Some answers or clues to answers to the preceding questions, as well as to others, are being obtained from experimental work with a variety of animals. Knowledge of the effects of massive generalized doses of ionizing radiation as well as those of small, but repeated, doses on humans are also being studied. The populations who were exposed at Hiroshima and Nagasaki and in the Marshall Islands have been and are being studied. Workers in laboratories, where accidental spillage of radioactive materials has occurred, have also been subjected to intensive and extensive study. Knowledge of the local effects of small, but repeated exposure to ionizing radiation has been obtained from a variety of sources. Physicians who pioneered the use of x rays and radium developed cancers on exposed areas. They also had a higher incidence of leukemia than do present-day radiologists.

Knowledge has also been obtained from the effects radiation has had on industrial workers. For example, girls were employed to paint the dials of watches with radium salts. In the process, they moistened the brushes that they used by placing them in their mouths. Radium and thorium contained in the paint were absorbed and stored in the bones of the girls. Eventually they developed cancer of the nasal sinuses and osteogenic sarcoma. This tragedy had one positive aspect. Useful information was gained about the long-term effects of low-level exposures to internal emitters of radiation.

Sources

Despite the tendency to think of ionizing radiation as something new, it has existed since the beginning of time. Sources of natural radiation include cosmic rays and the crust of the earth. Exposure is greater at high than at low altitudes and in regions containing uranium and thorium deposits. Although the extent to which the general population is exposed differs, everyone is and always has been exposed to radioactivity. The largest source of exposure to ionizing radiation is the natural background, for which there are no practical methods of limiting exposure. The next largest source of exposure in the United States is medical uses of ionizing radiation, particularly for diagnostic tests, and especially chest x-rays (Eason & Brooks, 1972). This source is elaborated on later in the discussion of medical uses of ionizing radiation.

Effects

All radioactive material, whether in the form of electromagnetic rays (gamma rays) or particles such as the alpha or beta particles or neutrons, has the same effect on tissues. Delario (1953) stated that all radiations directly or indirectly produce their tissue effect through ionization. Regardless of its source, *all ionizing radiation acts by a single mechanism that evokes an identical tissue change,* that is, DEGENERATION. If the effect on the tissue is marked, cells undergo necrosis. Although the effect on cells is the same, the power of various rays and particles to produce that effect differs, because of differences in their penetration of tissues or other materials. A curious fact is that the less they are able to penetrate, the more ion pairs they produce in the tissues through which they pass. Alpha particles, which have the least penetrating power, produce more ion pairs than do either beta particles or gamma rays. However, because gamma rays and neutrons have the greatest penetrating power, they are by far the most damaging type of radiation. Because alpha particles are filtered by air or a single sheet of paper, they are unlikely to have an opportunity to come in contact with much tissue. Likewise, the extent of damage caused by beta particles is limited by their poor power of penetration. They cause superficial injuries when tissues are exposed to them. Furthermore, beta particles may cause serious injury when they are ingested or inhaled in large quantities as after an atomic explosion. Likewise they can affect tissues in the interior of the body when they are introduced by a cut or injection. Unlike alpha and beta particles, gamma rays and neutrons can traverse the entire body. (See Table 11-1 for a review of the various types of radiation.)

Sensitivity

Despite differing degrees of sensitivity, all living things are sensitive to the injuring effect of ionizing radiation. An early misconception was that it injured animals, particularly humans, but had little if any effect on plants. To test the validity of this belief, Woodwell (1963) studied the effects of ionizing radiation on plants. From these studies, he learned not only that plants are sensitive to ionizing radiation of an intensity sufficient to injure human beings, but that different plants have different degrees of sensitivity. For example, pine trees are more sensitive than oak trees and weeds are highly resistant. Moreover, when a forest is destroyed by ionizing radiation, it upsets the ecological system in the forest. As an illustration, white oak trees were more sensitive to irradiation than some of the insects living on them. Therefore, though not all trees were killed by radioactivity, those remaining died because they were stripped of their leaves by the proportionately larger number of insects. There were many other similar imbalances. One implication of these studies relates to the disposal of atomic wastes. All forms of life are liable to destruction in any area exposed to sufficient radioactivity to injure humans.

All cells are equally damaged by ionizing radiation, but dividing cells are more susceptible than resting cells. Nondividing cells are frequently able to repair the radiation-induced damage, whereas cell division prevents such repair and often multiplies radiation injury. Many of the radiated cells will not die until they try to divide, and this may occur sometimes as long as several months or years after exposure to radiation. The expression of effects of exposure to ionizing radiation may be classified as (1) more or less immediate somatic effects, (2) delayed somatic effects, and (3) genetic effects. The genetic effects are not manifested in the exposed individual, but cause genetic mutations that may appear in future generations (Plant, 1969).

A tragic example of delayed somatic effects has been seen in recent years in the dramatic increase in cancer of the thyroid. From the early 1920s until the early 1950s, when x-ray therapy was first suspected as a cause of thyroid cancer, more than a million people—mostly children and adolescents—had received head and neck radiation for such benign conditions as enlarged tonsils and adenoids, mastoiditis, and skin conditions such as acne and eczema (Guimond & Wilson, 1979).

Not only do tissues vary in their sensitivity to ionizing radiation, but the degree to which any tissue is sensitive can be altered to some extent. Any condition, such as hyperthyroidism or fever, which elevates the metabolic rate increases tissue sensitivity. The reverse is also true. A decrease in metabolism is accompanied by a decrease in sensitivity. Sensitivity is also related to the degree of cellular differentiation and to the ability of the tissue to reproduce. The more highly differentiated a cell or tissue, the more resistant it is to the effects of radiation. The greater the capacity of the tissue to proliferate, the less its resistance is to the effects of radiation. This fact helps to explain the sensitivity of bone marrow and germ cells to irradiation. Cells undergoing reproduction are particularly sensitive when they are in the prophase of mitosis. Immature cells are more sensitive to irradiation than are mature cells.

Factors Determining the Effect of Ionizing Radiation

Intracellular organization is arranged in a hierarchy with relatively few DNA molecules at the top acting as a storehouse of information and director of activities. DNA communicates its messages by way of RNA. (See Chapter 6, Part A.) When a cell is exposed to the radioactive particle or ray, molecules are hit at random. Because the number of DNA–RNA complexes are relatively few compared to other types of molecules, their chances of being hit are also less. The extent of cell damage depends on the damage to the DNA–RNA system and the number of other molecules affected. With little or no damage to DNA–RNA and few other molecules injured, the cell may repair itself. A change in the DNA structure results in a change in messages and an alteration in the type or types of proteins synthesized. Destruction of DNA and/or widespread destruction of molecules causes cell death.

Factors that must be taken into consideration when evaluating the possible total effects of radiation include the likelihood of injury to the tissues exposed, the function of these tissues, and the period of time over which the radiation is absorbed. The effects of a single large dose may be quite different from those resulting from small repeated exposures applied over a period of time. The effects of irradiation also are modified by the size of the area exposed.

Effects of Total Body Irradiation

According to Warren (1961), irradiation of the entire body with massive doses, such as occurred in Hiroshima and Nagasaki, results in unconsciousness, and death occurs shortly after exposure.[5] Unless the person who receives a dose of total body irradiation is so heavily irradiated that he or she dies from damage to the brain or is burned or struck by flying debris, the person may not be immediately aware of the fact that injury has occurred. Depending on the seriousness of the injury, symptoms may appear in a few minutes or be delayed for 8 to 10 days. The early symptoms may last for a brief period and then return sometime between the fifth and twentieth days. The effect is similar to that of skin reactions following local applications of irradiation.

Early symptoms are nausea, vomiting, and diarrhea. Increased capillary and cell permeability throughout the body leads to a progressive loss of fluid and electrolytes with the development of shock. Death occurs in a few days. Bleeding into the skin and mucous membranes occurs. It is evidenced by petechiae and ecchymoses of the skin as well as frank bleeding from the mouth and gastrointestinal tract. One of the factors in the bleeding is a depression in the level of circulating thrombocytes. The leukocytes also disappear from the blood, and this decreases the resistance of the person to infection. Because of their longer life span, erythrocytes do not disappear as rapidly as do the other blood cells. Ulcerations in the gastrointestinal tract provide portals of entry for bacteria. With the decrease in resistance, infection follows. Weakness and fever are a consequence of the infection and the malnutrition that result from the nausea and vomiting. In patients who survive, fever and weakness may persist for months. During the period of recovery, patients should be protected from infection and all forms of stress, including physical exertion.

Because it is assumed that after any exposure there is some permanent injury, radiation injury may be cumulative over the life span.

[5] Other serious injuries incurred as the result of an atomic explosion are blast injuries, flash and thermal burns, and trauma from falling debris.

Other effects result from less intense exposures to ionizing radiation. They may follow its use in therapy as well as exposure to peaceful and warlike applications of nuclear energy. Some of the effects, such as the induction of malignant neoplasms, the reduction in the life span, and genetic aberrations, may take months, years, or generations to make their appearance. They may result from single or multiple exposures.

The effects of total body irradiation can be summarized as

1. Prompt effects (within a few days or weeks)
   a. None—exposure of entire body to less than 200 rads or superficial injury from exposure to alpha or beta particles
   b. Hematopoietic form (200 to 400 or 500 rads)
      (1) Lymphopenia.
      (2) Leukopenia
      (3) Anemia
      (4) Loss of immune response
   c. Gastrointestinal form (400 or 500 to 1,000 rads)
      (1) Nausea, vomiting
      (2) Diarrhea
      (3) Ulceration and infection
   d. Central nervous system form (greater than 1,000 rads)
2. Delayed effects (months or years)
   a. Genetic abberations
   b. Induction of malignant neoplasms
   c. Reduction in life span
   d. Other effects
      (1) Sterility
      (2) Cataracts

Figure 11-5 shows the relationship, in adult rats, between dose and survival time following a single total-body exposure to x rays.

In those who have received a lethal dose of irradiation, no treatment is known that is effective in preventing death or in restoring the person to health. Those who have lesser exposures benefit from blood transfusions, antibiotics, protection from infection, maintenance of nutrition and of water and electrolyte balance, and emotional support. Because of widespread knowledge of the possible harmful effects of ionizing radiation, emotional support is essential.

Medical Uses of Ionizing Radiation

The use of ionizing radiation for diagnosis and treatment has been one of the major advances in medical science in the twentieth century. Radiology and nuclear medicine are the two medical specialties that use ionizing radiation in diagnosis and treatment

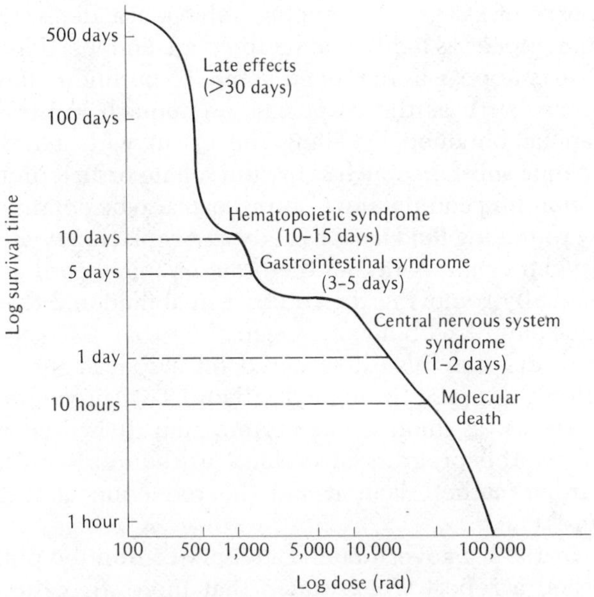

Figure 11-5. Relationship between dose and survival time for adult rats following a single total-body exposure of x-rays. Radiation damage produces many alterations, leading to breakdown of steady state. (Used with permission of Prentice-Hall, Inc., from *Radiation Biology*, 1968, pp. 222, by A. P. Casarett.)

of disease. *Radiology* uses *x-rays* to obtain information about body *structures; nuclear medicine* applies radioactive tracers that emit *gamma rays* to measure and alter substances involved in all types of *metabolic processes* (Wagner & North, 1976). Diagnostic use of radioactive tracers evolved from perfection of the automatic rectilinear scanner,[6] first developed by Cassen in 1951, which moves over the area of interest, mapping the distribution of the tracer and providing information about the nature, speed, and location of physiologic and biochemical processes (Wagner & North, 1976).

Diagnosis

X-RAYS. The most common form of ionizing radiation employed in medicine is the x-ray. Though x-rays are utilized in therapy, they have their most frequent use in diagnosis. According to the FDA Bureau of Radiological Health, about 130 million Americans undergo diagnostic x-rays yearly. X rays, like light rays, sensitize photographic plate on contact. Because they penetrate body tissues in inverse proportion to the density of the tissues, dense tissues filter out a higher proportion of the x rays than do less dense ones. Therefore when a body containing tissues of varying densities is placed between the

[6] The CAT scanner is presently the most popular piece of equipment for this purpose. (CAT is the acronym for Computerized Axial Tomography.)

source of x-rays and a photographic plate, dense tissues appear as light areas on the plate and less dense tissues appear as darkened areas. To outline hollow organs such as the esophagus or stomach, contrast can be obtained by filling the organ with a radiopaque substance such as barium sulfate or an iodine-containing compound. Contrast can also be obtained by removing fluid from a cavity and replacing it with oxygen or air. X-rays of the brain or spinal cord are made by removing the cerebrospinal fluid and then replacing it with air or oxygen.

X-rays may also be focused on a special screen after they pass through the body. This procedure is known as fluoroscopic examination. It is used to follow the progress of certain procedures such as cardiac catheterization and the reduction of fractures.

In 1972, a governmental advisory committee published a report which stated that there *are* cancer risks from low doses of ionizing radiation in the range delivered in diagnostic x-ray procedures. It had previously been taken for granted that genetic risks from exposure at those levels were greater than somatic risks (Rhein, 1976, p. 30). The caution generated in the wake of the 1972 report is attributable to the stature of the group who authored the report: the National Academy of Sciences–National Research Council Advisory Committee on the Biological Effects of Ionizing Radiations.

In determining whether the advantages of radiologic examination outweigh the benefits to an individual patient, the physician—with the informed consent of the patient—is still the final judge. In 1971, the American College of Radiology, with the cooperation of the American Medical Association and the assistance of the Food and Drug Administration's Bureau of Radiological Health, stated a position which has not been overruled to date: "In almost every medical situation, when a physician feels there is a reasonable expectation that radiological examination will benefit the health of an individual, radiation hazard is not a contraindication" (Rhein, 1976, p. 30).

Unlike exposure to natural sources of irradiation, exposure to ionizing radiation during its use in diagnosis and treatment can be minimized. Most of the radiation exposure from its medical uses comes from diagnostic x-rays. Under federal guidelines dangers in the use of nuclear radiation have been minimized. These dangers have not been as well controlled in the use of x-radiation, but both federal and state governments are giving leadership in the control of x-ray devices (Johnson, 1972). When well-designed and maintained equipment is used by competent x-ray professionals and technicians, diagnostic radiation provides information without undue risk to the patient. In the hands of the untrained or the unscrupulous, there are few forces available that can cause more harm and human misery. The physician who has special training has credentials that can be presented, if necessary, to the patient. Should the patient have any doubt about the competence of a physician, he or she should inquire at the local medical society and/or health department for information. The nurse as a citizen and as a health educator has a responsibility for educating the public about the uses and abuses of x-radiation. The nurse should have at least enough knowledge to appreciate its dangers and benefits and should have some basis for self-protection and for aiding others to protect themselves.

GAMMA RAYS. Gamma-emitting radioactive isotopes are also used in diagnosis. An isotope such as iodine 131 (^{131}I) is administered orally or intravenously. Though it is largely a beta emitter, enough gamma rays are formed to penetrate the overlying tissues and be counted by a radiation-sensitive instrument located outside the body or be converted into a series of dots on film or paper. When the latter procedure is used, it is called a scan, as a brain scan or thyroid scan. These tests are based on the fact that stable and radioactive isotopes behave in the body in a similar manner. As an example, thyroid tissue removes iodine from the blood and concentrates it within itself. ^{131}I is useful in determining the activity of the thyroid gland as well as in locating distant metastasis in thyroid cancer. In some of the scanning tests patients should be prepared to remain in a fixed position. Following the administration of an isotope, body fluids or secretions may be examined in a similar manner. Urine may be checked to determine the rate of excretion of ^{131}I.

In addition to the widespread use of ^{131}I to evaluate thyroid function, there is a growing array of other radioactive isotopes in common use to evaluate the functions of the cardiovascular system, the liver, the gut, and the kidney. Table 11-2 presents some of the commonly used isotopes and the diagnostic purposes for which they are used.

Because procedures for the preparation of patients for diagnostic tests vary from one institution to another, directions will not be detailed here. Each nurse is responsible for determining what is required for each patient and ascertaining that the patient understand what is being done and what is expected of him or her. Printed directions are of help, especially for patients who are undergoing diagnosis on an outpatient basis.

Before leaving the discussion of the use of radioactive isotopes for medical diagnosis, it should be mentioned that dramatic progress has been made in developing ultrasound as a tool which may be equally

TABLE 11-2. ***Name, Symbol, and Diagnostic Purpose of Some Radioactive Isotopes in Common Use****

Name	Symbol	Diagnostic Purpose
Sodium chromate	^{52}Cr	To determine red cell mass
Sodium iodide	^{131}I or ^{125}I	To determine plasma volume
Sodium Potassium	^{24}Na ^{42}K	To determine circulation time
Gold	^{198}Au	To distinguish liver abscesses from hepatitis
Krypton	^{85}Kr	To determine cerebral blood flow
Xenon	^{133}Xe	To determine blood flow in leg muscles and coronary arteries
Cobalt	^{60}Co– or ^{58}Co-labeled cyancobalamin	To determine intestinal absorption in pernicious anemia
Iron	^{55}Fe and ^{59}Fe	To determine use and storage of iron
Technitium-99m	^{99m}Tc	To visualize liver, spleen, bone marrow; for brain and thyroid scanning; plus other uses

* Information taken from R. P. Walton & J. A. Richardson, "Pharmacology." In *Rypins' Medical Licensure Examinations,* 12th ed. Ed. by A. W. Wright, Philadelphia: J. B. Lippincott Company, 1975, pp. 555–653, see pages 636–637.

effective and less hazardous to patients and personnel than present radiation sources.

Ultrasound is a method of examining the interior of the body painlessly and with a minimum of risk and expense. Although the technique was tried in the 1940s, the electronic technology was not sufficiently perfected until ultrasound was used for radar and sonar. Pulses of ultra-high-frequency (UHF) sound waves send back echoes from tissues of varying density; from the echoes, pictorial images of the organs can be constructed. Since the early 1960s, millions of patients have been examined by ultrasonic techiques with no reported adverse effects (Devey & Wells, 1978). There are no unpleasant sensations and no elaborate preparations of the patient for diagnostic examination by ultrasound. The nurse should make it her or his business to observe the equipment and procedure to be used with the patients in order to provide specific informational preparation to the patient.

Therapy

Many of the same sources and methods of application can be used in therapy as well as in diagnosis. Among the previously mentioned isotopes used for diagnostic purposes (see Table 11-2), both sodium iodide (^{131}I) and cobalt (^{60}Co) are also used in radiation therapy. In addition, sodium phosphate (^{32}P) is used to treat polycthemia and boron (^{10}B) to treat brain tumors (Walton & Richardson, 1975, pp. 635–36).

The energy and penetrating power of ionizing radiation increase as the photon wavelength decreases. Thus, differences in the physical characteristics of the radiation used are of great importance. The clinically important changes occur with radiation generated in the range of 400 to 800 kev. Above this energy, the advantages are reduced absorption of radiation in bone, less damage to the skin at the portal of entry, better tolerance of the vasculoconnective tissue, greater radiation at the depth relative to the surface dose, and reduced lateral scatter of radiation in the tissues (DiSaia et al., 1977, p. 1096). See Table 11-3 for the amount and source of voltage of various modes of external radiation.

The reduced skin effect of supervoltage radiation as compared with orthovoltage radiation is based on the physical fact that, with higher energy radiation, forward scattering is greater and lateral scattering less in the absorber. With supervoltage radiation, the

TABLE 11-3. ***Amount and Source of Voltage of Modalities of External Radiation****

Modality	Voltage	Source
Low voltage (superficial)	85–150 kev	x-ray
Medium voltage (orthovoltage)	180–400 kev	x-ray
Supervoltage	500 kev–8 mev	x-ray ^{60}Co ^{147}Cs ^{226}Ra
Megavoltage	Above supervoltage energy	Betatron Synchrotron Linear accelerator

* DiSaia, P. J., Nolan, J. F., & Arneson, A. N. "Radiation Therapy in Gynecology." In *Obstetrics and Gynecology,* 3rd ed. Ed. by D. N. Danforth. Hagerstown, Md.: Harper & Row, Publishers, 1977, chap. 54, p. 1096.

maximum ionization occurs below the level of the epidermis. As photons and resultant electrons become more energetic, they travel a greater distance into absorbing material. Therefore, the percentage of radiation at any specific depth, compared with the surface dose, increases as the energy increases (DiSaia et al., 1977, p. 1097). When selecting the source of radiation to be used in the treatment of a given patient, the **radiotherapist** considers many factors including the location of the tissue to be treated, the tolerance of adjacent tissues, and the rays or particles available for use. Whatever source of radiation is selected will operate on the *inverse square law:* "The intensity of radiation from a point source varies inversely as the square of the distance from the source" (DiSaia et al., 1975, p. 24).

To illustrate the operation of the inverse square law, the dose rate at a distance of 2 cm from a source is one fourth the dose from that same source at a distance of 1 cm; at 3 cm the dose rate is one ninth of the dose rate at 1 cm. Therapy may be administered externally through the skin and tissues over the organ, applied directly to the organ, or administered internally.

Some isotopes can be temporarily or permanently implanted. At one time the only available isotope for implantation was radium or its emanation, radon 222, which is a gas. Among those now available are cobalt 60, cesium 137, iridium 192, tantalum 182, gold 198, and iodine 125, (Kendall, 1967). Whether the seeds or applicators are temporarily or permanently implanted depends on the half-life of the isotope and the organ being treated. In providing and assigning others to provide nursing care to patients with an isotope implant, the nurse is guided by the inverse square law in identifying the distance zone around the patient within which direct care activities must be carried out dextrously and quickly, for the control of exposure of the nursing staff. Care should be taken to involve the patient in developing the schedule and sequence of nursing activities and ensuring understanding of the necessity for staff to place distance between themselves and the patient. Extra effort should be exerted to maintain forms of communication that do not require the nurse to be in the intimate zone, to prevent the patient from experiencing unnecessary levels of isolation and the perception of rejection.

In the timing of therapy with ionizing radiation, the physician must consider whether surgery is a part of the treatment, because ionizing radiation delays wound healing. When it is used before surgical therapy, time must be allowed for the tissue to recover. Following surgery, treatment must be delayed to allow time for healing to take place.

Effects on the Skin

Ionizing radiation, whether applied as rays or particles, has a local as well as a general or systemic effect. Evidence of the local effect is presented by changes in the skin through which the radiation passes. Although modern methods of treatment lessen the number of patients having marked skin reactions, the application of radiation through the skin to neoplasms is always accompanied by some changes in the skin. The physician is responsible for preparing the patient and family to expect reddening and possibly some desquamation of the skin. The fact that the nurse knows that this is expected and takes it as a matter of course is supporting to the patient. Any expression of surprise may lead to doubts as to whether the treatment is being properly applied or is producing the expected effect. Furthermore, the changes in the skin should be spoken of as a reaction rather than as a burn. The term *burn* may suggest carelessness, which the term *reaction* does not. Because the reaction is temporary, the use of this word is also reassuring. The use of correct terminology helps to protect the patient from unnecessary stress.

In 24 to 48 hours after a large dose of radiation, the skin develops an active erythema that disappears in a few days. A week or so later the erythema reappears. This time it develops gradually but increases in intensity until it resembles a severe sunburn. Blistering edema and desquamation may take place. In severe reactions the area may be very painful and continue to be painful for about a month. Examination of the skin and underlying tissue reveals degeneration of cells in the epidermis. Small blood vessels, especially the arterioles, also undergo degeneration. Some of the vessels are thrombosed. Capillary permeability is increased, and the tissue is hyperemic. In 6 or 8 weeks the skin begins to regenerate. The appendages of the skin, such as the hair follicles and the sweat glands, do not regenerate. The resulting skin is thin and pigmented. The underlying tissue has a poor blood supply. When the injury is severe, skin atrophy, dryness, telangiectasis (dilated veins), and hyperkeratosis are common. Deep ulcers that heal poorly may form.

Skin Care

When the method used to administer radioactive rays or substances is such that damage to the skin is minimal, special care of the skin may not be required. If there is an obvious reaction, the skin requires special care. The tissue is susceptible to pressure, trauma, and infection. Gentleness is essential. Because the skin is fragile, washing should either be omitted or be limited to the use of clear water. Oily substances should not be placed on the skin unless specifically ordered by the physician. Oil prevents the evaporation of perspiration and predisposes to maceration of the skin by keeping it moist. The skin should be protected from the effects of pressure from bed coverings or clothing by the use of bed cradles and lightweight, loose clothing.

Outpatients should be directed to wear loose clothing. No corsets, girdles, or garter belts should be worn by patients being treated over the trunk. Tape should not be placed on the skin in treated areas. With the exception of cornstarch, powders should not be applied to the skin exposed to irradiation during the period of therapy. Many commercially prepared powders contain zinc. The radioactive rays or particles ionize zinc or other ionizable substances. These ions produce further injury of the skin.

If the skin breaks down, it must be treated aseptically. Patients treated on an outpatient basis should be warned against exposure of the treated areas to the rays of the sun, as they increase the damage to the skin. The patient should also be instructed not to remove marks placed on the skin by the physician because they serve as guides to treatment. Nurses should assume responsibility for making certain that patients understand the instructions given by the physician. Repetition is necessary to learning for those who are under severe stress.

The reactions of mucous membranes are similar to those of the skin. Erythema occurs first. When the reaction is severe, it may be followed by the formation of a tough adherent grayish-white membrane. Some disturbance in function is to be expected. When the mouth is irradiated, secretion by the salivary glands may be depressed or the glands destroyed. Soreness makes it difficult for the patient to eat. A mouthwash of lidocaine (Xylocaine) applied before each meal increases comfort while eating. Mucous membranes react more quickly than the skin, but the reaction does not last long and the mucous membranes of the mouth heal fairly rapidly.

Irradiation of the pharynx results in dysphagia, which may be relieved (if the physician agrees) by gargling with aspirin. Irradiation of the esophagus causes dysphagia and soreness in the chest. Patients who have heavy pelvic irradiation may develop an extremely painful proctitis.

Systemic Effects

As stated earlier, patients who are treated with ionizing radiation may have systemic as well as local reactions during treatment. Depression of the bone marrow is accompanied by leukopenia, anemia, and thrombocytopenia. One type of systemic reaction is sometimes referred to as irradiation sickness. A number of factors contribute to its development. They include the location and intensity of the treatment and the emotional state of the patient. Treatments over the abdominal organs are more likely to be accompanied by systemic reactions than are those over other parts of the body. The symptoms presented by the patient include anorexia, nausea, vomiting, and diarrhea. These symptoms are seldom of serious import, but they add to the discomfort of the patient. There are a number of theories about the cause of the symptoms in radiation sickness. Some authorities believe the symptoms are caused by the effect of ionizing radiation on the bone marrow, lymph nodes, and gastrointestinal mucosa. Others believe that emotional factors are primarily responsible. Those who support the latter view point out that patients have many fears, some of which are aroused by the treatment itself and the meanings that it has. This theory is supported by the large number of agents used in the treatment of radiation sickness. The specific value of any of them is doubtful and their value may lie in the enthusiastic attitude of the physician and the confidence of the patient in the physician. Figure 11-6 shows the complex pathophysiologic interactions that underlie the symptoms in acute radiation syndrome.

Whatever the cause of the symptoms, patients are usually very miserable. They have difficulty in eating and are often worried by this fact. They lose food and fluids through vomiting and diarrhea. When these symptoms are severe, they can lead to dehydration and electrolyte imbalance. Intravenous fluids may be necessary to restore hydration and electrolytes. Compazine, an antinausea drug, may be pre-

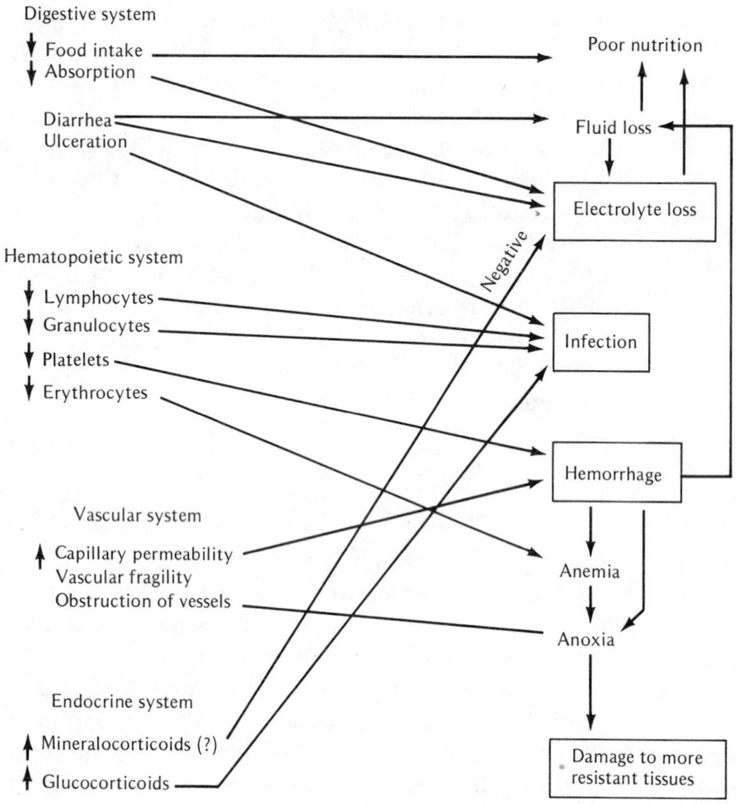

Figure 11-6. Pathophysiologic interactions in acute radiation syndrome. (Used with permission of Prentice-Hall, Inc., from *Radiation Biology,* 1968, p. 223, by A. P. Casarett.)

scribed. For some patients the food intake may be increased by adjusting the times at which meals are served. The patient who is treated early in the morning may be able to eat in the late afternoon or early evening. Food likes and dislikes should be given special consideration. This is no time to try to reform the food habits of the patient. A bottle of "Coke" or ginger ale may not meet all nutritional requirements but either provides glucose and water. Adjustments made in the timing, or in the foods served, also help to convey to the patient the concern for his or her welfare. The objectives toward which the patient's care should be directed include the following: to minimize the undesirable effects of ionizing radiation and to provide the patient with support and comfort. For further suggestions about nursing actions in the care of patients with nausea and vomiting, see Chapter 44.

The nurse should also take into account the method by which radiation therapy is being applied. When external radiation therapy is used, the patient should be prepared to be placed in a room alone. The patient should know that there is a small window in the room through which he or she can be seen at all times and that there is an intercommunication system that will enable communication with the person responsible for treatment. In the care of patients in whom an applicator containing a radioactive element, such as radium or its salt radon, or cobalt 60, is placed directly in the organ, the nurse has additional responsibilities and objectives. They include the following: (1) to care for the patient in such a manner that the applicator stays in place; (2) to prevent the loss of the radioactive element, usually radium; (3) to notify the physician who is to remove the applicator at the proper time; and (4) to protect the personnel (and others) from the harmful effects of radiation.

To illustrate the accomplishment of the objectives stated, the care of Mrs. Erie, who was treated for cancer of the cervix by the implantation of radium, will be presented. Mrs. Erie was prepared psychologically and physiologically for the treatment. She knew what to expect and what was expected of her. Measures were instituted the day before the procedure was to be done to cleanse her intestinal tract and vagina. She was taken to the operating room for the actual insertion of radium. Radon, with a half-life of less than 4 days might have been used. On her return she was to lie quietly and to avoid unnecessary movement in order to keep the applicator in the position in which it was placed. An indwelling catheter had also been inserted, so that she would not have to use the bedpan for urination.

Mrs. Erie's physician had explained to her why she needed to lie still. Because she was a very conscientious person, she scarcely moved. As anyone who has tried knows, lying in one position is very tiring. Mrs. Erie's back ached and she was generally uncomfortable. To reduce the backache, the nurse slipped her hand under the small of Mrs. Erie's back. She helped her move her legs and encouraged her to move her arms. She answered Mrs. Erie's light promptly and visited her frequently. The nurse performed those tasks for Mrs. Erie that Mrs. Erie could not do for herself. One of the objectives that the nurse considered very important was to make what was for Mrs. Erie a trying time less difficult. To protect herself, the nurse maintained a distance of at least a yard between herself and the patient when she was not actually giving care.

In addition to providing care for the patient, the nurse has a responsibility to prevent the loss of radium. The specific procedures in the prevention of the loss of radium vary from institution to institution and with the part of the body into which it is placed. However, there should be a regular system for informing all who care for the patient that the patient is under treatment. There should also be a system for saving and checking dressings after they are removed and before they are discarded. If the applicator containing the radium escapes the cavity in which it was placed, it should not be replaced, but the physician should be notified immediately. If the radium is applied in an area where it may be dislodged by movement, the patient must remain quiet until it has been removed.

Depending on the site of implantation, a patient may or may not need special treatment after the removal of the applicator. In this instance, Mrs. Erie had a profuse vaginal discharge for which her physician prescribed mild antiseptic douches.

Some of the instructions to the patient have been presented. Outpatients who are undergoing therapy should be impressed with the importance of keeping their appointments. It is understandable that the patient may be reluctant to return when beginning to recover from the effects of the previous treatment.

The patient or family may fear that the patient is radioactive. The only time a patient is a possible source of danger is when a therapeutic dose of ionizing radiation has been given, either by implantation or other internal means. As indicated earlier, the danger lasts only as long as the applicator is in the body or until the half-life of the isotope has elapsed. Even during this period no one needs to be concerned if two principles are obeyed: (1) the time spent with the patient is limited and (2) a distance from him or her is maintained.

Latent Effects

Two latent effects that are particular hazards to the person who handles and works with radioactive materials are radiation-induced cancer of the skin and leukemia. Physicians who pioneered the use of x-ray and radium developed carcinoma of the skin of the hands. In some instances the neoplastic changes occurred fairly early. In others it was delayed for years. Leukemia was once twice as frequent among physicians as in the general population. Now that more stringent precautions are taken to prevent exposure, the incidence of leukemia among physicians does not differ greatly from its incidence in other persons. Employed by those who know and respect its dangers as well as its uses, it can be controlled and utilized to benefit humanity. In the hands of the ignorant or careless it may be a lethal weapon both for the user and for the victims. Protection from the hazards of radiation is important both for those who work with it and for patients. As stated previously, standards have been set for the protection of both workers and patients from the harmful effects of radioactivity. Some of these have been put into law.

Guides to Protection

The following principles, if acted upon, serve as guides to protection. Nurses are responsible for protecting patients and their relatives as well as themselves and their assistants. Ionizing radiation may injure tissue without producing immediate effects. When the degree of injury is small, the effects may not be evident for weeks, or even months or years. Its effects are cumulative. Some tissues are more sensitive than others. Because of the sensitivity of the gonads to radiation, special precautions should be taken to protect them in both patients and personnel. The effects on the gonads include the possibility of mutations of germ cells and of sterility.

Effective protective measures are based on shielding, distance, and time or length of exposure. The measures that are necessary depend on whether the source emits rays or particles. Because rays have the greatest power of penetration, lead-impregnated walls or materials are required for protection. Most radioactive isotopes are primarily beta emitters. To affect deeper tissues they must be taken into the body by ingestion or inhalation or be introduced by injection. Otherwise, their effect is primarily on the skin. Knowledge of what happens to the isotope in the body as well as its half-life is also important. For example, radium salts or strontium 90 are stored in bone. Because both have a long half-life, they may initiate changes that result in cancer of the bone or in leukemia. Last, the quantity of radiation to which the individual is exposed can be determined. This is of particular importance to personnel employed in radiotherapy or who care for patients receiving radioisotope therapy. Badges containing material sensitive to radioactivity are worn and examined at regular intervals. They serve to remind personnel of hidden danger. Should they indicate excessive exposure, procedures can be initiated to find the cause and to limit the exposure of the individual who has been exposed excessively. Some authorities believe that every person should have an available record of all radiation exposure. This type of record is especially important for persons working in the field.

Nurses who are responsible for the care of patients receiving ionizing radiation need to be concerned for their own protection only when patients are receiving treatment with radium or radioactive isotopes. As stated earlier, the principal source of harm from beta-emitting particles is from ingestion or inhalation of these materials. Protection is afforded by distance, shielding, the length of exposure, and checking. Provided the nurse is conscientious about carrying out appropriate protective measures, there is no need to worry about being harmed.

For nurses who do not work in x-ray departments or in radioisotope laboratories, the usual sources of contact with ionizing radiation are limited to (1) radioactive isotopes that are to be administered to or implanted into a patient and (2) the patient who is being treated, and (3) his or her excretions. In the handling of radioactive materials, protection is afforded by shielding and distance. They are transported in lead containers with long handles, which enable the person to keep the container at a distance. If the material is to be ingested, the patient removes the glass from the lead container and drinks the "cocktail" previously prepared in the isotope laboratory. After the glass is emptied, it is rinsed by the patient and replaced in the container. Radium is also transported in a lead-covered case and kept at a distance by a long handle.

In the care of patients receiving internal therapy with radioisotopes, the nurse is protected by limiting the time spent in close contact with the patient and by the way in which equipment is handled. Bed linens or other materials subject to contamination are handled without shaking so that a minimum of dust is raised. Thorough hand washing and keeping the nails short and clean are important.

Because some of the isotopes such as ^{131}I are excreted in the urine and feces, the nurse should check to determine whether urine or feces should be collected and saved for the duration of the half-life of the isotope. Contamination of linen, the floor, or equipment should be checked by the radiation department. They should also supervise the cleaning of the floor, should it be contaminated. The patient should either be confined to bed or be in a private room. In working with radioactive materials, the nurse should remember that an unsafe act may endanger not only herself or himself but many other persons. Finally, relatives and visitors of patients should be instructed so that they can visit safely and comfortably.

Many points relative to protection have previously been made but will be repeated for the sake of emphasis. Protection should take into account the length of the half-life of the isotope, the size of the dosage administered to the patient, and the route of excretion. To illustrate, the effective half-life of ^{131}I is 6 days. When it is administered as a tracer dose, the amount given is very small. It is excreted in the urine. No precautions need be observed in the care of the patients, but the urine should be saved in special bottles for checking. Because the drug is given by mouth, breakfast is limited to toast and coffee, and other food is withheld for 3 hours to allow time for the absorption of iodine. The study also requires that the patient should not have been receiving an iodine-containing drug within the past 2 weeks. Because the patient who is treated with ^{131}I receives a larger quantity of the isotope, precautions should be observed in care. The precautions include the wearing of rubber gloves when giving direct care and the protection of the mattress and pillows with rubber covering. Linens used by the patient should be saved and checked. The urine of the patient should be saved and sent to the laboratory for checking. Should any be spilled, the radiological laboratory should be called to superintend the cleaning up.

The rules for the handling of patients receiving radioactive isotopes are usually made by the radiologist and/or the health physicist. They are applied by those who care for patients. The measures required are simple, but they will be ineffective unless they are strictly followed. It is a common observation that persons are likely to be very careful when they first work in a new project and to become careless later. Certainly knowledge of how to protect oneself should make the nurse more comfortable in the care of patients and, in turn, improve the quality of the care of the patient. In caring for a patient who is undergoing radiation therapy, the nurse should work quickly without seeming hurried. An attempt should be made to reduce the patient's feeling of isolation by frequent short visits. Diversional therapy such as reading, radio, television, or handiwork may be helpful to those patients who feel well enough to enjoy them.

Cytotoxic Agents

In addition to radioactive isotopes, a number of chemicals are used in medicine as cytotoxic agents. They include (1) alkylating agents, (2) antimetabolites, (3) plant alkaloids and antibiotics, (4) hormones, and (5) miscellaneous agents. Although the specific manner in which these agents act is different, they all cause death of cells. As with ionizing radiation, the most rapidly dividing cells appear to be the most sensitive. These include the cells found in the bone marrow, mucous membranes of the gastrointestinal tract, skin, and hair follicles. Because of their effects, these drugs are used in the study of cellular processes and in the treatment of certain types of malignant neoplasms. Possible toxic effects include (1) stomatitis; (2) nausea, vomiting, and diarrhea; (3) loss of hair; and (4) the suppression of the bone marrow. When a patient is treated with large doses of one of these drugs, he or she becomes highly susceptible to infection. To protect the patient, reverse isolation procedures may be instituted or the patient may be placed in a Life Island Isolator. Measures used in the care of patients undergoing radiation therapy are also applicable to patients undergoing chemotherapy. For information about cytotoxic drugs, see Goodman and Gilman (1975, ch. 62). There is voluminous specialized literature on cancer chemotherapy, which is further detailed in Chapter 39.

References Cited

Blakiston's Gould Medical Dictionary, 3rd ed. New York: McGraw-Hill Book Company, 1972.

Caffey, J. "On the Theory and Practice of Shaking Infants." *Am. J. Dis. Child,* **124** (Aug. 1972), 161–69.

Danforth, D. N., ed. *Textbook of Obstetrics and Gynecology,* 2nd ed. New York: Harper & Row, Publishers, 1971; 3rd ed., 1977.

Delario, A. J. *Roentgen, Radium, and Radioisotopes Therapy.* Philadelphia: Lea & Febiger, 1953, p. 61.

Devey, G. B., and Wells, P. N. T. "Ultrasound in Medical Diagnosis." *Sci. Am.,* **238** (May 1978), 98–112.

DiSaia, P. J. et al. *Synopsis of Gynecologic Oncology.* New York: John Wiley & Sons, 1975.

DiSaia, P. J., Nolan, J. F., and Arneson, A. N. "Radiation Therapy in Gynecology." In *Obstetrics and Gynecology,* 3rd ed. Ed. by D. N. Danforth, Hagerstown, Md.: Harper & Row, Publishers, 1977, pp. 1092–107.

Eason, C. F., and Brooks, B. G. "Should Medical Radiation Exposure Be Recorded?" *Am. J. Pub. Health,* **62** (Sept. 1972), 1189.

Flitter, H. H. *An Introduction to Physics in Nursing,* 6th ed. St. Louis: The C. V. Mosby Company, 1972, p. 46.

Garner, L. M., and Love, D. M. *A Community Action Approach for Prevention of Burn Injuries.* Washington, D. C.: U.S. Government Printing Office, 1969.

Goodman, L. S., and Gilman, A. *The Pharmacological Basis of Therapeutics,* 5th ed. New York: Macmillan Publishing Co., Inc., 1975.

Guimond, J. H., and Wilson, S. G. "Postirradiation Thyroid Disorders." *Am. J. Nurs.,* **79** (July 1979), 1256–58.

Johnson, P. C. "Benefits and Risks in Nuclear Medicine." *Am. J. Pub. Health,* **62** (Dec. 1972), 1571.

Kendall, E. B. "Care of Patients Treated with Sealed Sources of Radioisotopes." *Nurs. Clin. North Am.,* **2** (March 1967), 98.

Page, N. "Weightlessness: A Matter of Gravity." *N. Engl. J. Med.,* **297**(7 July 1977), 32–36.

Plant, R. "The Dangerous Atom." *World Health,* (Jan. 1969), p. 15.

Rhein, R. W. "X-rays: How Much Is Too Much?" *Med. World News,* **17** (27 Dec. 1976), 30–36.

Routh, J. I. *20th Century Chemistry,* Philadelphia: W. B. Saunders Company, 1953.

Rushforth, N. B. et al. "Violent Death in a Metropolitan County." *N. Engl. J. Med.,* **297** (8 Sept. 1977), 531–38.

Sovie, M. D., and Fruehan, C. T. "Protecting the Patient from Electrical Hazards." *Nurs. Clin. North Am.,* **7** (Sept. 1972), 469–80.

Wagner, H. N., Jr., and North, W. "What Is Nuclear Medicine All About?" *Dis. A Month,* **23** (Nov. 1976), pp. 6–7.

Walton, R. P., and Richardson, J. A. "Pharmacology." In *Rypins' Medical Licensure Examinations,* 12th ed. Ed. by A. W. Wright. Philadelphia: J. B. Lippincott Company, 1975, pp. 555–653.

Warren, S. *The Pathology of Ionizing Radiation,* Springfield, Ill.: Charles C Thomas, Publisher, 1961, p. 3.

Woodwell, G. M. "The Ecological Effects of Radiation." *Sci. Am.,* **208** (June 1963), 40–49.

12

Chemical Poisons of Extrinsic Origin

The sedge is wither'd from the lake,
And no birds sing.
KEATS

Overview

A variety of chemical agents injure or destroy tissues and cells. Their effects may be direct or indirect. They may occur naturally or be manmade. According to the Public Health Service, a new and potentially toxic chemical is introduced into industry every 20 seconds.

The environmental costs of industrialization and technologic development in the second half of the twentieth century are creating an increasingly hostile and risk-laden environment, with innumerable new sources of chemical injury to us all. Communities, nations, and international forums lack the tools, and in many instances the will, to decide or even to distinguish between what is possible and what is desirable. Examples are legion of conflict between the advantages of using a new technology and the effect of that technology on both the quality and quantity of life of people affected. Examples come from the current events of our time: growing opposition to nuclear power plants; resistance of many people who live near international airports to the use of the supersonic jets with their horrendous noise pollution; and persistent opposition by local communities targeted for location of industrial chemical waste dumps. Most of us want the benefits of new technologies, but we prefer that someone else pay the cost in quality of life and health.

Comar (1977) proposes three principles to clarify decision making about use of technologic options:

1. In every environmental and health assessment, the risk or effect (biological and economic) of a given action should be weighed against the risk or effect of not taking that action.
2. All risks or effects should be expressed in terms of the changes that would be produced in our existing state of well-being.
3. In all estimates of risks or effects, there should be a clear statement of the uncertainties that pertain to the assessment to be used in decision making.

These principles constitute a framework for cost-benefit analysis. However, efforts to apply cost-benefit analysis to technologic manipulations of the environment frequently are ineffective because of the inadequacy of our quantitative knowledge of relevant ecological and social factors (Westman, 1977).

The following discussion focuses on known chemical poisons in our environment, some of which we have been exposed to for centuries and others which are new by-products of our technology. For example, cyanide is a highly effective poison, because it blocks the action of the respiratory enzymes in the cell. As the result of this action, cells are unable to release the energy from nutrients required for their activities. Death from cyanide poisoning is certain and occurs in a matter of minutes. The only method of prevention is to avoid the inhalation or ingestion of chemicals containing cyanide.

Certain chemicals coagulate cellular proteins. Examples include phenol and formaldehyde.

Carbon Monoxide

Carbon monoxide is a powerful poison, causing its effect indirectly and possibly directly. The fact that hemoglobin has 300 times more affinity for carbon monoxide than for oxygen has long been known. Carbon monoxide reduces the amount of hemoglobin available to carry oxygen, thereby depriving cells of it. Rhodes (1971) reported that carbon monoxide also inhibits oxygen use in mammalian cells. Not only is the cell deprived of oxygen, but it cannot use all that is delivered. Tissues having the greatest need for oxygen such as the brain and heart are likely to be injured first by severe or prolonged carbon monoxide poisoning. Sources of dangerous amounts of carbon monoxide include defective heating devices, automobile exhaust gases, particularly from defective automobiles in slow-moving traffic or operating in a closed garage, and possibly cigarette smoking. Any of the preceding situations is aggravated by inadequate ventilation. Protection is afforded by adequate venting of stoves and automobiles and ventilation of areas where carbon monoxide is produced. Treatment is based on the law of mass action; that is, the rate of a chemical reaction is proportional to the concentration of each reacting substance. In other words, patients are treated with high concentrations of oxygen. With a large number of oxygen molecules competing for reduced hemoglobin molecules, the chances of forming oxyhemoglobin are increased. (See Chapter 39 for details of oxygen administration.)

Fat Solvents

A group of toxic chemicals employed in industry and in the home are the fat solvents, which have their effect in fatty tissues. Benzene, because of its affinity for bone marrow, causes death relatively quickly. Other fat solvents such as chloroform or carbon tetrachloride are concentrated in the liver, kidney, and brain and produce tissue necrosis in the affected organs. Because fat solvents are volatile and are used in the dry-cleaning industry, special precautions are necessary to protect workers. Protection of patrons from the danger of fat solvents was one of the problems that had to be solved before "do-it-yourself" dry-cleaning establishments could be made relatively safe. Precautions should also be taken by those who use these agents at home. Directions on containers should be followed explicitly. One way to limit the quantity inhaled is to work out of doors. Dry-cleaning fluids should be stored out of reach of children, and bottles of "spot remover" should be stored away from medicines and food. Had Mr. Curly and his wife followed this rule, he might have been spared a long hospitalization and permanent renal injury. One night he awakened with indigestion. He went to the medicine cupboard and drank what he thought was a popular remedy for indigestion. Instead it was dry-cleaning agent. As a result of the toxic effect of the solution and delay in treatment, Mr. Curly experienced gastroenteritis, injury to the liver, and permanent and serious injury to his kidneys.

Another source of chemical poisons is bacterial toxins and enzymes. (See Chapter 10.)

Heavy Metals

Another group of toxic chemicals are the heavy metals such as mercury, arsenic, and lead. Heavy metals have toxic effects on enzyme systems. Although mercury harms cells in other parts of the body, death is usually from its effect on the kidney. Small quantities of mercury in the form of organic compounds are used as diuretics, because they inhibit enzyme systems concerned with the reabsorption of sodium ions and fixed anions. Toxic dosages of mercury salts cause necrosis of the renal tubules and result in failure of kidney function.

The effects of arsenic are widespread: it damages the brain, heart, bone marrow, and kidneys. One of the interesting points about arsenic is that in times past, it was the favorite agent in fact and fiction to eliminate one's enemies (Kesselring, 1947). Arsenic is an ingredient in insecticides, rat poisons, and crabgrass killers. Children should be protected from the danger of accidental poisoning by proper handling and storage of supplies of arsenic-containing compounds and by the substitution of less toxic agents.

Lead Poisoning

Although the problem of lead poisoning, plumbism, is far from new, it is greater in industrialized societies than in nonindustrialized societies of the past and present. In addition to the lead-polluted air inhaled by everyone, certain segments of the population are at even greater risk. They are (1) young children who chew leaded paint chips, (2) workers in certain industries where exposure is not adequately controlled, (3) persons who drink quantities of lead-contaminated moonshine whiskey, and (4) those who eat or drink from improperly lead-glazed pottery.

Despite the importance of knowing the extent to which levels of lead in the blood of the general population are harmful, there is even a more urgent need to prevent lead poisoning in young children. In this group it causes serious illness, mental retardation, and death. In addition to damaging the brain and peripheral nerves, lead injures other organs such as the kidney. Fielding and Russo (1977, p. 944) identify the innumerable and ubiquitous sources of lead poisoning of children:

> Although new paint for household use will soon contain less than 0.06 per cent lead, thousands of houses have paint that contains well over 1 per cent. Many of these surfaces are flaking and peeling. Those that are not often chalk and contribute to lead in dust. Air-borne lead of small particle size is readily absorbed through the lung; large particles fall out into dust and are swallowed by children. The largest contribution to lead in the atmosphere is automobile emissions. Foodstuffs contribute a substantial amount of lead to the daily intake, much of which is added to the food during processing. Water may be a source in areas where the mineral content is low, the water acidic, and old leaded pipes still in place. Newsprint and some ceramic tableware may contain lead. Decorative decals and glazes on the exterior of some glasses contain considerable amounts of lead. This lead, leachable by dilute acids, can also flake off the glass, and represents a potential hazard for some children.

Knowledge of how lead causes its toxic effects is incomplete. However, its effects on metabolism have been studied in detail. Like other heavy metals, it inhibits the activity of enzymes. In the case of lead the affected enzyme systems are those that are dependent on the presence of free sulfhydryl groups for their activity. Lead makes the sulfhydryl groups unavailable to the enzymes that require them. One of the results of the inhibitory effect of lead on the sulfhydryl-dependent enzymes is a disturbance in the synthesis of heme (the iron-containing portion of the hemoglobin molecule). Heme is also an essential part of other respiratory pigments, the cytochromes, which play essential parts in energy metabolism (Chisolm, 1971). The effects on the blood are first seen as a shortened life span of the red blood cells. Later there is an anemia characterized by a decrease in the number of red cells, with each cell carrying less than the normal complement of hemoglobin.

Lead poisoning is a preventable disease. Prevention lies in eliminating the sources of exposure. For young children this means removing lead-contaminated paint and plaster or covering it with paneling. Neither painting the surface with a water-based paint nor covering it with wallpaper is adequate.

Because preventive measures have not been uniformly applied, what is often the first step in the prevention of acute and chronic lead poisoning is the identification and treatment of children whose bodies—blood, soft tissues, and bone—carry excessive quantities of lead. Currently large cities such as Detroit, under the auspices of their health departments, conduct lead detection centers where children of ages 1 to 5 may have their blood tested for lead without cost. Children with high blood levels are treated and the source of the lead is eliminated. Treatment is of little permanent value unless lead is removed from the environment.

Nurses have an important role to play in the prevention of lead poisoning as well as the identification of already affected children. In their home visits they should look for evidence of peeling paint. When there is such, the paint should be checked for lead. Sick, anemic-looking children particularly in the 1- to 5-year age group should arouse the nurse's suspicion that lead poisoning is a possibility. Mothers living in areas where lead poisoning is endemic should be encouraged to take their young children to lead detection clinics. The earlier the disease is discovered and treated, the better the child's chance of escaping serious injury. For a more complete discussion of the action of heavy metals, see Goodman and Gilman (1975, pp. 912–45).

Insecticides, Rodent, and Weed Killers

An important group of man-made noxious chemicals include insecticides and rodent and weed killers. Each year there are more of these chemicals available. Synthetic organic pesticide production is increasing at a rate of about 15 per cent per year. Between 1963 and 1969 herbicide sales rose 271 per cent (U.S. DHEW, 1969). The use of chemicals to control insects and rodents is not new. Some of the old preparations such as the inorganic preparations containing lead, mercury, and arsenic are highly toxic to humans. This is not to say that they have been without value, for both the old and new chemicals have contributed to the control of diseases such as malaria and yellow fever and to increasing the food supply. According to one estimate, previous to 1945 the loss of crops and stored commodities to pests was at least 10 per cent. Despite their usefulness in controlling pests and weeds, all such chemicals are potentially harmful to humans and/or the environment.

Unlike the older insecticides, the newer ones are synthetic organic compounds. Each class has its uses and dangers. The organochlorines (DDT is the best-known example, but it is no longer available to the general population) are highly effective in killing certain groups of insects. Although they are less toxic to humans than the organophosphates, they are chemically stable and have been found in the soil 10 years after their use. Further, once-susceptible insects become resistant to its effects.

The organophosphates have a wide range of effectiveness. They are biodegradable and do not persist in the environment. Although they are less damaging to the environment than the organochlorines, they are more hazardous for humans. They inhibit the enzyme cholinesterase, thus preventing the destruction of acetylcholine. Serious symptoms, and even death, can follow when a critical level of enzyme inhibition is reached.

It is outside the scope of this chapter to present a comprehensive view of a great number of chemical agents. New ones are continually being added. They are prepared in the form of dusts, sprays, and aerosols. About 350 million pounds of pesticides are used each year in the United States. Because of the large quantity used, there has been an increase in the level of certain toxic compounds in the environment. Pesticides have on occasion caused the widespread destruction of wildlife. Acute insecticide poisoning is responsible for about 150 deaths a year. About half the deaths are among children. In the state of California alone as many as 1100 instances of acute insecticide poisoning have occurred among agricultural workers in a single year. Aerosol preparations carry with them an additional danger, as the containers can explode if damaged or heated. Because these chemicals are relatively new, there has been little or no time to evaluate their long-term effects on human health. Depending on the form in which they are employed, these chemical agents may be inhaled, ingested, or absorbed through the skin. Some general safety precautions include:

1. Act on the principle that despite differences in degree of toxicity, all are potentially dangerous.
2. When selecting, ask the question, "How does the benefit compare to the risk?"
3. Use the least toxic chemical that will be effective. In some instances, other methods are adequate. For example, tabacco worms can be manually removed from tomato plants.
4. Do not use more than necessary.
5. Use granular preparations rather than dusts and liquid sprays.
6. Follow the instructions on the container.
7. Place insecticide containers where they are out of the reach of children.
8. Do not store or use toxic chemicals around food.

Nitrogen Fertilizers

In the area around Limbow, U.S.A., many of the wells have been rendered unfit for use by either human beings or animals by chemicals containing nitrogen. Over a period of years commercial fertilizers containing large quantities of nitrogen have been employed in enriching the soil. Because nitrogenous compounds are highly soluble, each rain carries them further into the subsoil. Eventually the nitrogenous chemicals reach the water supplying the wells. Although the high nitrogen content of drinking water does not appear to harm mature animals, it causes a serious illness in immature animals, including human infants.

Food Additives

Another possible hazard about which there is little information is the chemicals added to food to preserve it or to improve its palatability or appearance. These chemicals may be added when the food is processed or during the growing stage. As a simple example, coloring is used to create pink ice cream or green lime sherbet.

Industrial Poisons

Some of the hazards associated with the exposure of the population of cities and industrial areas to pollution of the air was presented in Chapter 6. Water in some areas is also rendered unfit for human use and dangerous to fish by detergents and industrial wastes. In industry, a variety of chemicals are potential sources of danger against which workers require protection. Chemicals to which industrial workers are exposed include arsenic, thallium, beryllium, aliphatic hydrocarbons, nickel, chromium, asbestos, and benzol. Although a number of sources

Place of interview________________ Date ________
Name of interviewer________________________
Patient's name____________________________
Ethnic group________________ Age____ Sex________
Birthplace________________ Occupation________
Last grade attended________________________

1. For what reason did you come to this agency?
2. What do you most want help with at the present time?

Drinking History

3. How old were you when you started drinking alcohol regulary?
4. How long have you had problems with alcohol?
5. How often do you drink alcoholic beverages?
6. What kinds of alcoholic beverages do you drink?
7. How much of each alcoholic beverage do you drink?
*8. When did you have your last drink?
*9. When did you start your last drinking bout?
*10. What have you been drinking during this last drinking episode?
*11. How much alcohol did you consume each day during your last drinking episode?
*12. Has your drinking created problems for you in any of the following areas?
with spouse________ on the job________
with family________ with children________
with friends________ ________
13. Have you ever been injured because of drinking? Yes____ No____ in fights____ auto accident____ accidental fall____ other ________
14. Have you ever been arrested because of drinking? Yes____No____ On what charge:
DWI______ drunk in public______ fights______ other (specify)______
15. Have you ever been in prison or jail because of drinking? Yes____No____
16. What previous treatments have you had for alcohol problems?
Date Place
________ ________
________ ________

Symptoms Related to Gastrointestinal System

*17. What have you been eating during this most recent drinking bout?
*18. What is your usual eating pattern?
(a) When not drinking:
(b) When drinking:
19. Have you had recent changes in appetite?
20. Have you had any recent weight changes?
21. Are you on a special diet?
22. What fluids do you drink other than alcohol?
Kind of fluid and amount per day.
regular coffee____ tea____ water____
decaffeinated coffee____ juices____ milk____
23. Do you have frequent irritation of your mouth and throat?
24. Are you having pain in your stomach?
25. Are you bothered by heartburn or gas?
*26. Are you nauseated?
*27. Are you vomiting or having dry heaves?
*28. Have you ever vomited blood? If yes, when?
*29. Have you ever had stomach ulcers or other stomach problems?
30. How frequently and for what reason do you use aspirin?
31. What medications do you use to relieve stomach pain?
32. Are you having pain in your abdomen?
33. Are you having diarrhea or constipation?
34. Do you have hemorrhoids?
35. Have you had bleeding from your bowels?
36. Have you noted a change in the color of your stool?
clay colored____ black____ bright red____
37. What problems have you had in the past with your bowels?
38. What medications do you use to relieve abdominal or bowel pains?
39. Have you ever had problems with your pancreas?
*40. Has you skin or the white of your eyes ever turned yellow?
*41. Have you ever had problems with your liver?
*42. Do you have diabetes? If yes, what medication do you take?

Symptoms Relating to Neurological System

43. Have you noticed any change in the amount of alcohol it takes to get the effect you desire? If yes, describe the change.
*44. What reactions occur when you stop drinking?
tremors________ d.t.'s________
seizures________ other________
hear or see things______ ________
*45. Have you ever taken Dilantin or any other drug for seizures?
46. Have you ever experienced a period of time you don't remember when drinking?
47. Have you experienced tingling, pain, or numbness in hands or feet?
48. Have you experienced muscle pain in your legs or arms?
*49. Are you experiencing any difficulty in keeping your balance?
*50. Are you experiencing any difficulty with your vision?
*51. Do you have problems with your sleep? If yes, describe.
52. How many hours do you usually sleep?________
when sober________
when drinking________
53. Do you feel rested after a night's sleep?
54. What do you do when you are unable to sleep?
55. Have you noticed any recent changes in your sex life? If yes, describe.

Symptoms Relating to Cardiovascular and Pulmonary System

*56. Do you have heart trouble? If yes, describe.
*57. Do you have swelling of the hands and feet?
*58. Do you have shortness of breath?
*59. Do you have chest pain?
*60 Are you taking any medication for heart disease?
61. Have you had pneumonia?
62. Have you ever had tuberculosis? If yes, are you taking any medication for it?

*Indicates questions providing important information for a quick survey of intoxicated patients.

OVER . . . . .

Figure 12-1. A nursing history tool for use with patients with alcohol problems. (Used with permission of American Journal of Nursing Co., from Assessing alcoholic patients, *Am. J. Nurs.* 76:785–789, May 1976, pp. 787–788, by E. Heinemann & N. Estes.)

63. Do you have frequent infections? (e.g., colds, flu, boils, sores that don't heal quickly).
64. Do you have a chronic cough? If yes, describe.
65. Have you ever coughed up blood or phlegm?
66. Describe any other lung problems you have had.
67. Do you smoke? If yes, how many packs a day?

Psychosocial Status

68. What is your marital status?
69. With whom do you live?
70. Does this person have alcoholism or use alcohol regularly?
    Yes____ No____
71. To whom do you feel close?
72. Do your neighbors, relatives, and/or friends use alcohol regularly? Yes____ No____
73. How many children do you have?
74. How often do you see your children?
75. Describe the place you live.
    type of residence (i.e., house, apartment, room, etc.)
    cooking facilities
    number of stairs
    availability and type of transportation
76. Have you had mental or emotional problems?
    depression________ suicidal attempt________
    nervousness (anxiety)____ other________
    loneliness________ ________
77. Are you currently involved in a counseling program?
*78. Are you currently taking medication for emotional problems? If yes, describe.
79. Are you actively affiliated with a religious group?
80. What is your current employment status?
81. Do you have some special job skills?
82. If employed, how does this period of treatment affect your employment?
83. If unemployed, what is your current source of income?
84. What hobbies or special interests do you have?
85. How do you spend a typical day at home?

Drug Taking Other Than Alcohol

*86. What drugs do you take that you haven't mentioned?
    prescribed drugs ________
    over-the-counter drugs ________
    drugs obtained on the street ________
*87. What is your usual manner of taking drugs?
    as directed ________
    more than directed ________
    less than directed ________
*88. Are you allergic to any drugs?

Final Questions

89. What are your ideas for managing your drinking when you leave this agency?
90. Are there any further comments you would like to make?
91. Are there any questions you would like to ask?

Write a summary of the nursing history interview.

1. Describe your overall impressions of the client (mood, attitude, intelligence, ability to relate, social skills, general physical and emotional health, level of orientation, reliability of information given).
2. List all the problems identified in order of priority.
3. Suggest a plan of action for each problem identified.

of injury to cells have been cited, there are others and the number will undoubtedly be increased in the future. Because many chemicals are stable (they do not deteriorate into harmless compounds) and highly toxic, increasing attention is being devoted to regulating their use and to devising ways of protecting workers from unnecessary exposure to them.

Hazards of Abuse of Self-Selected Substances

No discussion of noxious chemicals is complete without mention of the heavy toll on the nation's health of the abuse of tobacco, alcohol, and drugs. One of the tragic aspects of substance abuse is that it injures not only the individual who elects to use the substance but, in the case of the pregnant woman, sometimes also does irreversible damage to the unborn child.

In 1976, the total cost of medical care and lost earnings attributable to smoking and alcohol abuse was estimated at $59.9 billion—about 25 per cent of the nation's total economic cost of illness in that year (Luce & Schweitzer, 1978).

Tobacco

Over the last two decades increasing attention has been devoted to the question of the relationship of cigarette smoking to the genesis of disease. Hammond (1962) reported that not only was the incidence of cancer of the lung higher among cigarette smokers, but the total death rate from all causes among this group was far higher than among nonsmokers. He states that this finding is the most significant of all. Though the death rate is lowest among nonsmokers, those who stop smoking have a longer life expectancy than those who continue to smoke. There is also an adverse relationship between the number of cigarettes smoked and life expectancy. The more cigarettes smoked, the shorter the life span.

In January 1964, the Surgeon General of the United States released a report based on a long series of major research projects establishing smoking as a significant health hazard. More recent reports support earlier findings. In 1968 the Public Health Service published the following statement (U.S. DHEW, 1968):

1. Cigarette smokers have substantially higher rates of death and disability than their nonsmoking counterparts

in the population. This means that cigarette smokers tend to die at earlier ages and experience more days of disability than comparable nonsmokers.

2. A substantial portion of earlier deaths and excess disability would not have occurred if those affected had never smoked.

3. If it were not for cigarette smoking, practically none of the earlier deaths from lung cancer would have occurred; nor a substantial portion of the earlier deaths from chronic bronchopulmonary diseases (commonly diagnosed as chronic bronchitis or pulmonary emphysema or both); nor a portion of the earlier deaths of cardiovascular origin. Excess disability from chronic pulmonary and cardiovascular diseases would also be less.

4. Cessation or appreciable reduction of cigarette smoking could delay or avert a substantial portion of deaths which occur from lung cancer, a substantial portion of the earlier deaths and excess disability from chronic bronchopulmonary diseases, and a portion of the earlier deaths and excess disability of cardiovascular origin.

The elimination of smoking involves not only the changing of the attitudes and behavior of smokers but also the economics of tobacco growers, manufacturers, advertisers, and others.

ALCOHOLS

Ethyl alcohol

Although the effects of the long-term excessive use of ethyl alcohol are not within the scope of this chapter, alcoholism is an increasing problem in the United States. In fact, it is the leading cause of drug abuse; and due to its effect in producing alcoholic cirrhosis of the liver, it has finally appeared in the top ten causes of death in the United States (see Chapter 3). There are well over 9 million alcoholics in the United States, although statistics are unreliable because of the large number who are not diagnosed. Many alcoholics begin to use alcohol before their teenage years and are chronic alcoholics before they reach the end of adolescence. Alcoholism is not a new problem, nor is it one that is unique to industrialized societies. Be that as it may, prevention of alcoholism and treatment of alcoholics are current urgent needs. A critical facet of identifying victims of alcoholism early in their disease is obtaining a good history in four major problem areas (Heinemann & Estes, 1976): (1) drinking history; (2) symptoms related to damage-prone systems; (3) psychosocial status; and (4) use of other drugs. Figure 12–1 presents a nursing history tool for use with patients with alcohol problems.

It has been conclusively demonstrated that heavy drinking during pregnancy increases the risk to the offspring (Ouellette et al., 1977). The types of injury that may be sustained by the unborn child of the chronic alcoholic mother include craniofacial, limb, and cardiovascular defects associated with prenatal onset growth deficiency and delay in development. During the first trimester, the period when organs are forming, the fetus is most vulnerable to developing structural abnormalities as a result of cell injury due to alcohol (Luke, 1977).

Methyl alcohol

Methyl alcohol commonly called wood alcohol, is a highly toxic substance that produces its effect indirectly. It is converted first to formaldehyde and then to formic acid. Methyl alcohol is thought to become toxic through conversion to formaldehyde. Formic acid itself is nearly innocuous. Acidosis results from the inhibition of aerobic metabolism (in particular the enzyme lactic dehydrogenase) with accumulation of organic acids, especially lactic acid. In nonlethal doses, methyl alcohol causes blindness by injuring the retina. During Prohibition, poisoning from methyl or wood alcohol was not uncommon. Whenever the number of illegal stills in operation increases, there is an increase in the number of persons poisoned by wood or methyl alcohol. Ethyl alcohol takes smaller amounts to induce inebriation.

DRUGS

Drugs are chemicals that when administered in appropriate amounts are expected to be beneficial. For some, the margin between the effective therapeutic dose and the toxic dose may be wide. For others, the margin may be very small. At one time, it was believed that there was a threshold of exposure to certain physical and chemical agents below which no harmful effects occurred. Scientists, therefore, tried to establish safe levels of exposure. It is now known that some agents have delayed effects that may be manifested months or years after the initial exposure to the substance. As a consequence, the concept of safe level of exposure has been replaced by the "permissible dose." Basically, permissible dose means that the possibility that exposure to a particular agent will cause harm is slight. At times it means that the risks involved are less than the possible benefits. At times the condition of a person alters the quantity of the drug that he or she can tolerate. For example, acetylsalicylic acid (aspirin) is a drug found in every medicine chest—and possibly in almost every purse. Few people are aware of the toxic potentialities of aspirin. Yet when a child

TABLE 12-1. ***Signs and Symptoms Associated with Poisoning by Specific Drugs and Chemicals****

Acetaminophen: anorexia, nausea, vomiting, delayed onset of symptoms, jaundice, hypoglycemia, encephalopathy and hepatic failure

Alcohol: depressed sensorium, odor on breath

Amphetamines: toxic psychosis, hyperthermia, flushing, increased blood pressure, dilated pupils, hallucinations, seizures, tachycardia

Antifreeze: metabolic acidosis, hypocalcemia, renal failure

Arsenic: garlicky breath, vomiting, profuse diarrhea

Barbiturates: tense vesicular skin lesions, coma, nystagmus, drowsiness, ataxia, slurred speech

Boric acid: lobster red skin, blue green diarrhea, severe acidosis, convulsions, coma

Bromide: pigmentation, dementia, acne, psychosis, hyperchloremia

Caffeine: vomiting, extreme miosis, visual disturbance, glycosuria, acetonuria, salivation, muscle twitching

Carbon Monoxide: red skin color, coal gas odor, bullae, cyanotic

Cocaine: perforated nasal septum, dilated pupils, psychosis, delusions, tachycardia

Cyanide: bitter almond odor on breath, convulsions, coma, abnormal EKG

Diazepam: euphorogenic (sometimes), progressive central nervous system depression

Digitalis: visual disturbances, delirium, abnormal EKG, nausea

Disulfiram: flushing, pulsating headache, circulatory collapse, acrid breath odor

Ethchlorvynol: deep coma, pungent aromatic odor, lowered pulse and blood pressure, pink gastric aspirate

Fluoride: decreased serum potassium and magnesium, tetany

Gasoline: distinctive odor, choking, pulmonary infiltrates

Glutethimide: dilated pupils, coma, prolonged respiratory depression, laryngeal spasms

Heroin: coma, decreased blood pressure, respiration, and pulse, miosis, needle marks

Hydrocarbons: pulmonary edema, lipid pneumonia, tinnitus, convulsions, ventricular fibrillation

Iron: diarrhea, coma, bloody vomiting, radiopaque on x-ray, hypotension

Isopropyl Alcohol: severe gastritis, acetonemia with normogylcemia

Lead: severe abdominal pain, increased blood pressure, milky vomitus, convulsions, muscle weakness, metallic taste, anorexia, encephalopathy

LSD: hallucinations, dilated pupils, bleeding disorder, confusion, agitation

Mercury: stomatis, gingivitis, colitis, nephrotic syndrome

Methadone: miosis, coma, lowered pulse, blood pressure and respiration; transient response to narcotic antagonist

Methaqualone: increased reflexes, tonic clonic spasms

Methyl alcohol: alcoholic patient, hyperventilation, decreased vision

Mushrooms: nausea, vomiting, delayed liver and renal failure

Organophosphate: miotic pupils, cramps, bronchorrhea, salivation, lacrimation, urination, defecation

Paraquat: oropharnyx burning, headache, vomiting, diarrhea, acute renal failure, pleural effusion

Phencyclidine: muscle twitching, prolonged psychosis, mild increase in blood pressure and pulse, nystagmus, altering state of consciousness

Tricyclic antidepressants: ileus, supraventricular arrhythmia, convulsion, respond to physostigmine, radiopaque on x-ray

Phenothiazines: postural hypotension, hypothermia, miosis, tremor, radiopaque on x-ray of abdomen, increased QT interval on EKG

Salicylates: hyperventilation, vomiting, fever, bleeding, acidosis

Strychnine: stiff neck, status epilepticus

Scopolamine: tachycardia, decreased secretions, urinary retention, dilated pupil, hallucination, confusion, dry skin

* Used with permission of Health Sciences Media and Research Services, Inc., from Tong, T. G., "Incidence and Clinical Signs of Poisoning and Toxic Overdose," *Nurse Practitioner*, **2** (Nov.–Dec. 1976), 35–36, p. 36.

TABLE 12-2. *Treatment of Specific Drug and Chemical Overdoses of Relatively Frequent Occurrence**

Agent/Drug	Special Problems	Treatment
Narcotics, propoxyphene, pentazocine, diphenoxylate	Opiate overdosed patients classically present with pinpoint pupils (unless anoxic), areflexie, respiratory depression. Begin cardiopulmonary resuscitation if needed and protect airway and vital functions. Severe abstinence symptoms may be experienced by the opiate dependent user during recovery from the acute overdose or may be precipitated by narcotic antagonists. The symptoms can be adequately managed with supportive care alone.	Any comatose patient with small pupils, bradycardia, hypotension, and depressed respiration should be given a narcotic antagonist. Naloxone is clearly the drug of choice and will reverse all symptoms of the overdose. Commonly used narcotics, such as heroin, have a relatively short elimination half-life: methadone has a much longer half-life and therefore repeated administration of the antagonist over 24 to 36 hours may be necessary.
Organophosphate Insecticides	Poisoning can occur from ingestion and from absorption through the skin. Five important physical signs are characteristic: salivation, lacrimation, urination, defecation and constriction of the pupils. Response to large amounts of atropine confirms the diagnosis.	Pralidoxime can be used in organophosphate but not carbamate poisoning. Thorough decontamination must be carried out.
Tricyclic Antidepressants	Cardiovascular effects are most serious. Supraventricular tachyarrhythmias, quinidine-like myocardial toxicity are seen. Other serious symptoms include; ileus, hypotherma, and convulsions.	Because of protein binding and large tissue distribution, forced diuresis and dialysis are not effective in removing the drug. Monitor EKG and vital signs for at least 48 hours. Physostigmine is an antidote for central nervous system and atropinic cardiac toxicities. In severe overdoses with tachyarrhythmias and heart block, cardiac pacing should be used before physostigmine or antiarrhythmics, e.g., lidocaine or phenytoin are given.
Phenothiazines	The number of cases is increasing among children and adults. There are three common clinical syndromes: hypotension, arrhythmias and atropmism. Other effects include quinidine-like effects on EKG, dystonic reactions, hypothermia, seizures and ileus. Although common to find dilated pupils in most, constricted pupils may be seen in more severely poisoned patients. The phenothiazines are radiopaque.	Dystonic reactions are seen occasionally and diphenhydramine 50 mg (IV) is given for these reactions.
Sedative-hypnotics	Central nervous system depression, coma, hypotension, hypoxia, respiratory and cardiac failure are seen. Withdrawal with hyper-irritability and more serious seizures can occur 16–24 hours following discontinued use. Simultaneous ingestion with other depressants (alcohol) is common. The nonbarbiturate sedative hypnotics, e.g., chloral hydrate, glutethimide, ethchlorvynol, meprobamate etc. may be much more toxic with longer duration of coma in the overdose circumstance. In the acute sedative-hypnotic overdose, prolonged absence (24 hours) of brain activity and function may be reversible and have a favorable outcome.	Treatment is supportive. For the number of overdoses involving barbiturates, there is a remarkably high recovery rate. Respiratory assistance, hydration, management of hypotension and maintaining adequate urine output are important treatment considerations. Do not use respiratory stimulants to arouse overdosed patients from coma. If physical dependence to sedative-hypnotic drugs is established in an acute overdose patient, treatment for withdrawal should be closely supervised, preferably in a hospital setting.

Alcohol	Severe hypoglycemia may occur in children following ingestion of large quantities. Varying degrees of intoxicated behavioral changes and central nervous system depression are seen.	Convulsions associated with hypoglycemia are seen and can be treated with diazepam and glucose. Treatment is supportive. Children need careful evaluation for neurologic and metabolic abnormalities.
Aspirin	In acute overdose, peak salicylate levels may not occur until at least 6 hours after ingestion. Consider severity on basis of blood salicylic acid level and interval between ingestion and measurement. Avoid metabolic acidosis since this will enhance salicylate distribution to the brain. Hyperventilation, tinnitus, fever, acidosis, hypoglycemia are seen in the aspirin overdose.	Alkalinization of urine to promote elimination of the salicylates. Administration of potassium and fluids can facilitate attempts at alkalinization of the urine. Removal of aspirin by emesis has been successful even 10 hours after ingestion. Activated charcoal is a useful adjunct to treatment of aspirin overdose.
Hydrocarbons/ Petroleum distillates	Vomiting and diarrhea are often experienced. Central nervous system depression can occur. Aspiration pneumonitis is a serious complication. Chemical pneumonitis has occurred even after intraveneous injection of hydrocarbon material (lighter fluid).	Emesis before central nervous depression occurs followed by cathartics may provide some protection against absorption and major toxicities (hepatic, etc.). Lavage is reserved for patient with absent gag reflex, coma or convulsions, and must be preceded by intubation with a cuffed endotracheal tube. Steroid use in these circumstances is controversial. Treatment is supportive.
Corrosives	Concentrated solutions of caustic material can cause burns of the esophagus that characteristically progress from inflammatory phase to necrosis and constriction. Source: liquid and crystalline corrosives. Clinitest® tablets, household bleaches (some), electric dishwasher soaps.	Immediate treatment is dilution with copious amounts of water. Emesis and lavage should be avoided. Olive oil, vinegar, juices, should not be given. Esophagoscopy should be performed. Corticosteroids should be given if burns are found and patient should be evaluated for surgical follow-up.
"Street drugs" LSD PCP Amphetamine Cocaine	Illicit drug overdoses and "bad trips" seldom ever involve a "pure" agent.	Treatment is primarily supportive, reduction of sensory stimulation, reassurance and "talking down." Restraints tend to increase anxiety. Where the patient is extremely hyperactive, diazepam (0.1 mg/kg-10 mg) is preferred since chloropromazine may produce synergistic hypotension (seen with MDA, STP DMI, etc.) and also can potentiate seizure activity by lowering threshold. Particularly where phencyclidine (PCP) has been taken, reducing sensory stimulations is often helpful. Marked suicidal depression may follow an amphetamine episode. In chronic abuse, withdrawal from amphetamine is relatively safe, unlike withdrawal from barbiturates and other sedatives.
Methanol	Ingestion (usually as a substitute for ethanol) is highly toxic and can cause blindness. There may be a 6- to 30-hour symptom-free period followed by severe abdominal pain and muscle weakness. Hyperventilation, profound metabolic acidosis are seen.	Methanol levels greater than 50mg% in the blood is an indication for hemodialysis.
Ethylene glycol (antifreeze)	Metabolism to oxalic acid produces renal damage with significant renal tubular necrosis and failure. Ethanol can inhibit this reaction. Examine urine for oxalate crystals.	Renal status must be evaluated and hemodialysis should begin in severe poisonings (marked acidosis, electrolyte abnormalities, renal failure).

Continued . . . .

Table 12-2. *(Cont.)*

Agent/Drug	Special Problems	Treatment
Household products	Cleaning agents, bleaches, solvents and cosmetics constitute the largest group of potential toxins found in the home. Many of the products are relatively non toxic in the amounts usually ingested. Adhesives, ballpoint pen inks, bubble bath, soap, chalk, crayons, lipsticks, eye makeup, perfumes, deodorants, incense, pencil, shampoo, putty, non-lead-containing paints, shoe polish, vitamins without iron generally produce insignificant toxicity unless ingested in large doses.	All soaps and detergents can cause gastrointestinal irritation, other toxic manifestations range from none (bar soaps) to severe mucous membrane damage, hypocalcemia (electric dishwasher detergents). Treatment of the severe toxicities should include immediate dilution and supportive care. Many liquid general purpose cleaners and polishes contain petroleum distillates and ingestion should be treated as hydrocarbon ingestion. Ammonia causes toxicity by exposure to its vapors (which can be decontaminated) or by ingestion (which should be treated as a corrosive ingestion). Bleaches are generally only moderately toxic and will not cause esophageal burns or strictures. Sodium perborate is highly toxic and management requires removal, support of vital functions and control of seizures (if they occur). Effects from common household solvents such as acetone are similar to ethanol when ingested except for more central nervous system depression. Treatment is supportive care, decontamination and minimizing further absorption.

* Used with permission of Health Sciences Media and Research Services, Inc., from Tong, T. G., "Treatment of Poisoning and Toxic Overdose," *Nurse Practitioner,* **2** (Jan.–Feb. 1977), 29–43, pp. 30–31.

finds a bottle of a hundred or so aspirin tablets and eats them, the acetylsalicylic acid can cause fatal acidosis. Occasionally an individual is so sensitive to aspirin that one 5-grain tablet can cause serious effects or even death. A laxative taken to treat a digestive upset may cause the perforation of an inflamed appendix. The concept that certain drugs are safe and that within limits all drugs are safe is being replaced by the concept that safety is a relative matter. Furthermore, safety cannot always be judged by the immediate effects of a drug.

We presently have an epidemic in our country of self-administration of over-the-counter and illicit drugs. Reference will be made in a later section to the most frequent causes of poisoning and how to treat victims. But here, emphasis is given again to the injury done to unborn children of pregnant women taking drugs. The human fetus exposed to the effect of drugs taken by the mother may develop behavioral birth defects as well as physical deformities. The most firmly established human behavioral *teratogens* [1] are drugs that also cause physical deformities: alcohol, thalidomide, anticonvulsant drugs (hydantoin or trimethadione). Other drugs which are suspected of producing behavioral birth defects are narcotics, including methadone and heroin, and the synthetic sex hormones (Kolata, 1978). Researchers are looking for subtle and common defects in behavior, such as shorter attention span, lower intelligence or hyperactivity.

Alcohol–drug Interactions

In addition to the cell injury that can be produced by alcohol taken in excess on a regular basis, even occasional or moderate drinkers who are taking some medication subject themselves to a high risk of tissue damage. Of the 100 most frequently prescribed drugs, more than half contain at least one ingredient known to interact adversely with alcohol. Most adverse effects due to alcohol–drug interactions are accidental, but the medical toll is high, including an estimated 2500 deaths a year and 47,000 emergency room admissions a year (Secretary of HEW, 1978). The drugs that most frequently have altered therapeutic and/or adverse effects when taken with alcohol include not only sedatives, hypnotics, narcotics, antidepressants, and tranquilizers but also marihuana and other psychoactive substances, as well as certain antihistamines, analgesics, anticoagulants, and antiinfective agents (Alcohol–Drug Interactions, 1979).

[1] A *teratogen* is any agent which causes abnormal development in an embryo.

Recognition and Treatment of Poisoning

Symptoms of poisoning from chemicals of extrinsic origin are often confusing and sometimes misleading, because of the frequent mixtures of multiple drugs and chemicals involved. Table 12–1 presents signs and symptoms associated with poisoning by specific drugs and chemicals (Tong, 1976).

Four poisons must be diagnosed immediately so that the appropriate antidote can be given: (1) organophosphates; (2) methanol; (3) cyanide; and (4) the opiates. Each of these substances has a specific antidote which must be given promptly to be effective (Tong, 1977). In general, overzealous or inappropriate use of an antidote may complicate the initial injury and result in additional poisoning. Careful use of drugs and therapeutic measures for supportive treatment are likely to be more beneficial than an antidote in the majority of poisoning cases. Table 12–2 describes treatment of specific drug and chemical overdoses which occur with relative frequency (Tong, 1977).

References Cited

"Alcohol–Drug Interactions." *FDA Drug Bull.*, **9** (June 1979), 10–12.

Chisolm, J. J., Jr. "Lead Poisoning." *Sci. Am.*, **224** (Feb. 1971), 17.

Comar, C., "Environmental Assessment: A Pragmatic View." *Science,* **198** 567 (Nov. 1977).

Fielding, J. E., and Russo, P. K. "Exposure to Lead: Sources and Effects." *N. Engl. J. Med.*, **297** (27, Oct. 1977), 943–44.

Goodman, L. S., and Gilman, A. *The Pharmacological Basis of Therapeutics,* 5th ed., New York: Macmillan Publishing Co., Inc., 1975.

Hammond, E. C. "The Effects of Smoking." *Sci. Am.*, **207** (July 1962), 42.

Heinemann, E., and Estes, N. "Assessing Alcoholic Patients." *Am. J. Nurs.*, **76** (May 1976), 785–89.

Kesselring, J. "Arsenic and Old Lace." In *Best Plays of the Modern American Theatre,* 2nd series. Ed. by John Grassner. New York: Crown Publishers, Inc., 1947, pp. 459–510.

Kolata, G. B. "Behavioral Teratology: Birth Defects of the Mind." *Science,* **202** (17 Nov. 1978), 732–34.

Luce, B. R., and Schweitzer, S. O. "Smoking and Alcohol Abuse: A Comparison of Their Economic Consequences." *N. Engl. J. Med.*, **298** (9 Mar. 1978), 569–71.

Luke, B. "Maternal Alcoholism and the Fetal Alcohol Syndrome." *Am. J. Nurs.*, **77** (Dec. 1977), 1924–26.

Ouellette, E. M. et al. "Adverse Effects on Offspring of

Maternal Alcohol Abuse during Pregnancy." *N. Engl J. Med.*, **297** (8 Sept. 1977), 528–30.

Rhodes, M. L. "Dangers of Exposure to Carbon Monoxide." *HSMHA Health Rep.*, **86** (Oct. 1971), 888–89.

Secretary of Health, Education, and Welfare. *Third Special Report to the U.S. Congress on Alcohol and Health.* Technical Support Document: HEW, PHS, ADAMAHA, NIAAA, June 1978.

Tong, T. G. "Poisoning and Its Treatment. Part 1: Incidence and Clinical Signs of Poisoning and Toxic Overdose." *Nurse Practitioner,* **2** (Nov.–Dec. 1976), 35–36.

Tong, T. G. "Poisoning and Its Treatment. Part 2: Treatment of Poisoning and Toxic Overdose." *Nurse Practitioner,* **2** (Jan.–Feb. 1977), 29–43.

U.S. Department of Health, Education, and Welfare. *Report of the Secretary's Commission on Pesticides and Their Relationship to Environmental Health,* Washington, D.C.: U.S. Government Printing Office, 1969, p. 46.

U.S. Department of Health, Education, and Welfare. *The Health Consequences of Smoking.* Washington, D.C.: U.S. Government Printing Office, 1968, pp. 3–4.

Westman, W. E. "How Much Are Nature's Services Worth?" *Science,* **197** (2 Sept. 1977), 960–64.

13

Physical and Chemical Agents of Intrinsic Origin

Science is nothing else than the search to discover unity in the wild variety of nature—or more exactly, in the variety of our experience.

J. BRONOWSKI
Science And Human Values, 2nd Ed. New York: Harper & Row, Publishers, Incorporated, 1965, Revised ed., p. 16.

Overview

In the preceding discussion, some of the agents found in the external environment having deleterious effects on the structure and functions of cells have been presented. Cellular injury may also be caused by physical or chemical agents of intrinsic origin. It may result from the abnormal distribution or concentration of one or more body constituents or from the failure of one or more steps in the utilization of substances within the cell. The latter is usually caused by the lack of one or more enzymes or by some condition interfering with their action. As a consequence, substances that are necessary to the body economy or that are the product of a step in metabolism accumulate within or around the cells. Chemically inert substances may act as foreign bodies and provoke an inflammatory response. In addition, chemically active substances may also alter chemical and physical conditions within the cell and have an adverse effect on the activity of cellular enzymes. The effects of the accumulation of normal or abnormal products within or around cells can be summarized as follows: (1) As they accumulate they occupy space, thereby encroaching on normal cellular constituents. (2) They alter the physical and chemical conditions in and around the cell, thereby interfering with the activity of enzymes. Some of these conditions are reversible when detected early. If they are allowed to progress, they lead to death of parenchymal cells and all that their loss implies.

Disturbances in Calcium and Phosphorus Metabolism

Like other body constituents, calcium and phosphorus are subject to disturbances in their metabolism. Normally they exist in the blood plasma in a concentration very close to saturation. About one half of the plasma calcium is in an ionized form and the other half is bound to protein and is therefore in a colloidal form. The latter serves as a reserve supply that can be added to or subtracted from as needed. Phosphorus also exists in the plasma in differing states. These include the phospholipids and ester lipids and inorganic phosphorus in the form of mono- and dibasic phosphate ions. There is a reciprocal relationship between the levels of calcium and phosphate ions in the blood. When the level of one is raised, that of the other is depressed. The product of their levels must be kept below a certain point or precipitation of calcium occurs.

Because of their reciprocal relationship, anything that affects the level of one also affects the level of the other. Their levels in the plasma, however, represent a balance between intake and output. Absorption of calcium from the gastrointestinal tract is increased by vitamin D_2, or calciferol. Calciferol also increases the excretion of phosphates in the urine. Although authorities are not in complete agreement as to the action of parathormone, it is believed to regulate the excretion of phosphates by the kidney and absorption of calcium from the gut and bone. When the level of phosphates in the plasma falls, the calcium level rises. The source of the calcium is absorption either from the gastrointestinal tract or from the bone. The bone serves as an important reserve supply of both calcium and phosphorus.

Abnormal Calcification

Abnormal calcification may take place when tissue is diseased or in certain types of disturbances of calcium and phosphorus metabolism. There are many conditions in which calcification of diseased tissues occurs. Although calcium may be laid down in injured cells, it is more commonly deposited between cells. Occasionally bone is formed at the site of its deposit. The ultimate effect depends on the tissues involved and the effect of the calcification on the functioning of involved or related organs. For example, calcification of fibrous tissue in an old tubercle or thrombus is an expected reaction of the body to a particular type of injury. It is also regarded as beneficial rather than harmful. Calcification of the medial layer of middle-sized arteries results in so-called pipestem arteries. This type of calcification is relatively harmless. In contrast, calcification of the pericardium, which sometimes follows tuberculosis or pneumococcal pericarditis, causes constrictive pericarditis. The firm wall formed around the heart limits its ability to dilate and therefore to fill during diastole. Calcification of the heart valves following the healing of rheumatic fever contributes to their rigidity and deformity and their failure to open or close properly.

Disturbances in calcium metabolism leading to hypercalcemia can result in metastatic calcification, that is, the calcification of distant organs. The disorders most frequently responsible are hyperparathyroidism, excessive intake of calciferol, and primary disease of the bone associated with excessive decalcification. The structures that are most commonly sites of calcification are the gastric mucosa, the renal tubules, and the alveolar walls of the lungs. As stated earlier, calcium is in the blood in a nearly saturated solution. Any condition that raises its level or decreases its solubility favors calcium precipitation. Calcium is more soluble in an acid than in an alkaline solution. Therefore, in the presence of hypercalcemia, precipitation of calcium is most likely in tissues where acid and alkaline conditions follow each other. As examples, in the stomach, following secretion the cells secreting hydrochloric acid are left with an excess of hydroxyl ions and are therefore relatively alkaline. In the kidney tubule, cells are in an alkaline state after the excretion of acid phosphate. The effect on the patient depends on which organ is calcified.

In nursing, knowledge that excessive intake of vitamin D may result in pathology should serve as a basis for instructing parents and patients to limit the dosage of vitamin D to that prescribed by the physician. This is the instance where some is good, but more is definitely not better.

Lithiasis

Another pathological condition resulting from the precipitation of calcium and phosphorus and sometimes other blood constituents is the formation of concretions or stones. The terms used to indicate their formation or presence are *lithiasis* and *calculi.* Stones are formed in hollow organs and their ducts, primarily in the biliary and urinary tracts. Though their composition varies, they are generally composed of calcium, phosphorus, and organic matter. The formation of stones depends on two factors: (1) a focus, usually of organic materials, and (2) a soluble substance that is a crystalloid in solution that precipitates on the organic particles such as bacteria, epithelial cells, or tissue debris. The substance that precipitates depends on the constituents of the fluid in the hollow organ or duct. For example, calculi formed in the gallbladder may be composed of cholesterol, calcium, or bilirubin or a mixture of two or more of these substances. Those formed in the urinary tract are most likely to be a mixture of calcium oxalate and phosphate.

The effects of lithiasis depend on such factors as the size of the stones and the structure in which they are located. Small stones generally cause more trouble than large stones, because the small stone is more likely to move into a duct and cause obstruction and muscle spasm. Muscle spasm is accompanied by severe cramping pain, which is referred to as colic. The patient with a stone in the common bile duct accompanied by pain is said to have biliary colic. The patient with a stone in the ureter has renal colic. In both instances, the pain is thought to be caused by the muscle spasm induced by obstruction and stretching of the tube. The pain, which is often accompanied by some degree of shock, is severe, often exquisitely so.

If the stone remains in the duct, it also causes obstruction. The consequences of the obstruction depend, in part, on its location. An obstruction in the cystic duct from the gallbladder may cause pressure on the blood supply of the duct and be followed by gangrene of the gallbladder and spillage of bile into the peritoneal cavity. Obstruction of the common bile duct or a ureter interferes with the drainage of the liver or the kidney, respectively. This leads to pressure and stasis and, if unrelieved, to infection and eventually to the atrophy or necrosis of the affected organ. Other effects will depend on the function of the organ.

Methods of Therapy

At this time there is no known method of dissolving calculi that are already formed. Because fat in the stomach initiates a reflex that initiates contraction of the gallbladder, patients who are subject to biliary colic are advised to restrict their intake of fat. The nurse can assist patients by helping them to learn what foods to include or reject from their diet. For patients who have, or who are predisposed to, renal calculi, teaching them to maintain an adequate or even a high fluid intake may help to keep the urine diluted and thus prevent the formation of stones. When a patient is admitted in acute colic, measures should be taken to relieve the pain as rapidly as possible. This usually involves the injection of an analgesic such as morphine or Demerol Hydrochloride[1] and an antispasmodic such as atropine, scopolamine,[2] and/or papaverine. The decision of which drug or drugs to be used is the responsibility of the physician. The nurse is responsible for making the needs of the patient known to the physician and for instituting prescribed therapy as soon as possible.

Body Fluids

Another source of injury to cells is the patient's own secretions and body fluids. As stated earlier, blood escaping from blood vessels causes damage by occupying space, by irritation, and by increasing the number of osmotically active particles in the area. There is usually an inflammatory response in tissues into which there has been bleeding. Interstitial fluid or lymph, when it accumulates in excessive quantities, interferes with tissue nutrition because it occupies space.

Digestive juices are also capable of causing cell injury when they escape from the gastrointestinal tract or when the balance between the resistance of the mucous membrane lining the tract and the digesting action of the secretion is upset. Gastric, pancreatic, and intestinal juices contain protein-splitting enzymes. When they come in direct contact with cells, these enzymes break down the protein constituents of cells into polypeptides or amino acids and thereby disrupt the structure of cells. The digesting action of the various secretions is modified by their pH. In health, gastric juice is acid, and secretions in the intestine are alkaline. A prolonged or marked lowering of the pH of the gastric juice is a frequent finding in peptic ulcers. Although ulceration may occur anywhere along the alimentary canal, the stomach, the proximal portion of the duodenum, and the large intestine are the most common sites. Ulcerative disease of the large bowel is often disabling. Not all the factors responsible for ulceration along the alimentary canal are understood. In many instances multiple factors probably interact to disturb the balance between the digesting action of the juices in the stomach or intestines and the efficiency with which the mechanisms for the protection of the mucous lining act. The results of this failure are disruption of cell structure and the formation of sores opening to the surface of the mucous lining of the alimentary canal. The size and depth of the ulcers vary with the location, acuteness of the condition, and other factors.

Specific therapy of ulceration along the gastrointestinal tract is directed toward providing conditions favorable to healing. To the extent to which the ulceration is related to the patient's way of life, healing and continued good health may also depend on the identification and control of predisposing factors. Thus Mrs. Johns, who has an active duodenal ulcer, is admitted to the hospital for treatment. She is thereby removed from her usual environment. In addition, a therapeutic regimen is instituted to accomplish two general objectives. One is to decrease the motor and secretory activity of the alimentary canal and the other is to decrease the digesting power of the gastric juice. As soon as Mrs. Johns is well enough, a program of instruction is begun that will help her learn to manage her life and disease so that the possibility of future ulcerations is decreased. The problems associated with the therapy of the patient with peptic ulcer are described more fully in Chapter 46.

Digestive juices also have a destructive action on cell proteins of structures outside the alimentary canal. Pancreatic enzymes, when activated by a reflux of bile into the duct of Wirsung, digest the pancreas. This serious condition may be induced by obstruction of the ampulla of Vater by biliary calculi or by scar tissue. Fistulae, especially those from the small intestine, usually heal with great difficulty.

[1] Trade name for meperidine hydrochloride.
[2] Also known as hyoscine hydrobromide, B.P.

Sometimes they are of great size. Healing is facilitated by preventing digestive enzymes from coming in contact with body tissues. This is not easy.

An abnormal opening such as an ileostomy or colostomy allows the intestinal contents to escape onto the abdominal wall. Unless appropriate measures are instituted, breakdown of the skin is inevitable. The situation is more acute when the feces are fluid than when they are solid, as the watery state brings the enzymes in contact with the skin. The proper application of an ileostomy or colostomy bag reduces this possibility to a great extent. Other measures are discussed elsewhere.

Continued exposure of the skin to urine predisposes to its breakdown. The skin does not tolerate being wet over long periods of time as this predisposes the skin to maceration and lessens its resistance to destructive agents. In addition, with standing, urea contained in urine is decomposed by bacteria to ammonia, a highly irritating substance. When urine escapes onto the skin, prevention of irritation depends on the conscientious use of measures designed to prevent urine from coming in contact with the skin or to remove it by washing the exposed areas of the skin with soap and water and changing the bed linen promptly.

Adaptation as a Source of Injury

Earlier the capacity to adapt structure and function was discussed as a means of the survival of the individual or species. It can also be the cause of disease or injury. Among the first to make the relationship between adaptive responses and the etiology of disease was Claude Bernard. He proposed that disease could result when a response was faulty in degree or magnitude or when in correcting one defect other responses were initiated that resulted in injury. As an illustration, direct injury to cells causes an inflammation. When the inflammatory response is excessive, swelling may impede the flow of blood and tissue nutrition may be so greatly impaired that cells die from a lack of nutrients and oxygen. When a sufficient number of parenchymal cells are killed, scar tissue proliferates and as it matures it shortens. Tissues may be deprived of their blood supply and tubular organs obstructed. As a consequence of the inflammatory process and scar tissue formation, more harm may be done to the involved organ than the initial injury caused.

As another example, hypoxia is a stimulus to the formation of erythrocytes. Possibly, in some instances, the disease polycythemia vera is initiated by hypoxia. The capacity to increase the number of circulating erythrocytes at high altitudes and in certain congenital defects of the heart is homeostatic. In the absence of an appropriate stimulus and when the number of cells formed is excessive and continued, the condition is maladaptive.

Another concept of the relationship of adaption to disease causation was introduced by Selye, who proposed that the organism undergoes certain stereotyped general and local adaptive reactions to injury irrespective of its cause. To the extent to which these responses are appropriate in kind and degree, they assist the sick person in coping with the injury and its effects. Although Selye classified the phases of the adaptive response to illness under different names, they have come to be called the stage of injury or the alarm reaction, the "catabolic" phase and the "anabolic" phase. (See Unit V for a discussion of the response of the body to injury.)

Selye, *(1956)* further suggested that certain diseases are "diseases of adaptation." According to Selye, these diseases are not the result of some external agent such as a microbe, but they result from the inability of the body to cope with injury by appropriate adaptive responses. These diseases may involve the body tissues or the structures regulating the metabolic responses to injury. Thus in addition to the body tissues, the nervous system, the anterior hypophysis, or the adrenal cortex may be involved. Disturbances in adaptation may be manifested during any stage of the body's metabolic response to injury. Thus disturbances in adaptation occur during the stage of the "alarm reaction." Evidence of shock is not at all uncommon among individuals who have experienced severe injury of various types. In certain acute fulminating infections, such as an infection caused by the meningococci, the alarm reaction may be profound. On examination the adrenal cortex is found to be destroyed by hemorrhage into the cortices of both glands.

Disorders of adaptation may also occur during the other stages of the "adaptive" syndrome. Thus there are disorders of adaptation during the catabolic phase of the general adaptation syndrome. Lesions similar to, but not identical with, those induced by the injection of large doses of aldosterone into animals are observed in a great variety of human diseases. These include disseminated lupus erythematosus, diffuse collagen diseases, dermatomyositis, psoriasis, acute and chronic nephritis, ulcerative colitis, as well as a number of allergic states such as asthma and allergic rhinitis and certain psychiatric states.

Similarly, disorders may result from failure of adaptation during the anabolic response to injury. Many patients, particularly those with wasting diseases, go through the early stages of illness satisfactorily only to falter in the anabolic (restoration-of-body-tissue) stage. The malnourished and seriously burned or injured patient may have a prolonged anabolic phase. Ill health in chronic illnesses, such as rheumatic fever or arthritis, may also be prolonged by failure to adapt during the anabolic phase of illness.

A number of diseases such as sickle-cell anemia and diabetes mellitus, once had survival value for the human species. One view of neoplasia is that neoplastic change enables cells to survive injury. Hypertension is also classified by some as a disorder of adaptation.

From the work of Selye and other investigators, there are now known to be changes occurring in the body that represent the body's reaction to injury. Inasmuch as they are appropriate in kind and degree, they facilitate survival and recovery. When they are excessive, inappropriate, or inadequate, they can be sources of disease.

Immune Responses

Immune responses may also be the source of injury. These responses involve the mechanisms through which cells distinguish self from nonself. Disorders of immunity usually involve a defect in the immunologic system leading to: (1) its failure to respond to threats such as bacteria or viruses, (2) a response to harmless substances, and (3) inability to distinguish self from nonself, causing injury to its own tissues. (See Chapter 24.)

Aging as a Cause of Cell Injury

Earlier in the chapter evidence of atrophy associated with aging was presented. The biologic mechanisms underlying the aging process are of much interest, though they are incompletely understood. It is not known if aging is controlled and progresses in a fashion similar to growth and development from the embryo to maturity. On the basis of a number of different types of observations, longevity is believed to have a genetic basis. At conception each individual is programmed to live a long or short time for his or her species. There is a truism, "if one wishes to live a long life, he should select long-lived grandparents." There is also laboratory evidence to support the theory that potential life span is genetically determined. Hayflick (1970) as well as other scientists have shown that in tissue culture, healthy cells divide for a predictable number of generations. Then mitotic activity ceases and the cells undergo degeneration and die.

Many of the current theories of biologic aging involve altered protein metabolism. According to Barrows (1971), during senescence the efficiency with which DNA messages are transcribed and translated becomes reduced by use, with the result that certain proteins are synthesized at reduced rates or imperfectly. These proteins regulate certain body functions, including adaptation to stress.

The extent to which environmental factors influence aging is not known. However, in experimental animals such as the rotifer, the rate at which aging occurs can be altered by changing environmental conditions. Barrows (1971, p.8) states that the life span of the rotifer can be altered by underfeeding and by environmental temperature. These conditions did not alter the program for the organism's total life span, but they alter the rate at which specific events occur. In other words, they change the rate at which information is transmitted.

Among environmental conditions that may affect the rate of aging and cause cell injury are (1) infections, (2) immune responses, (3) failure to remove harmful waste products, (4) extrinsic poisoning, and (5) radiation damage. Among questions that have been raised are the following: Is the overfed child, like the overfed rotifer, likely to have a shorter life span than a less well-fed sibling? Is the fact that children are larger than their parents an advantage or disadvantage? As answers are found for these and other questions, child feeding and other practices may be altered to favor living out the potential life span.

Iatrogenic Disease

The term *iatrogenic* has its origin from *iatros*, "physician"; *iasthai*, "to cure or heal"; and *genesis*, "the beginning or origin." Therefore iatrogenic disease is defined as disease having its origin in treatment of disease. Accordingly, bedsores are iatrogenic when they are associated with immobilization prescribed in treatment of disease. Phocomelia induced by thalidomide is iatrogenic, as is aplasia of the bone marrow following therapy with cytoplastic drug. A single catheterization can, through injuring the mucosa of the urethra or bladder or by introducing microorganisms, result in cystitis. Illness induced by a misinterpretation of a careless remark is also a source of iatrogenic illness that can be as incapacitating as some of the structural injuries induced by physical and chemical agents. From the preceding examples, it can be seen that iatrogenic disease is a common event. It can occur in any situation in which disease is being treated.

With the increased legitimate use of prescription drugs, there is an inevitable concurrent increased risk of drug-induced iatrogenic disease. All newly marked drugs should be routinely evaluated through compulsory registration and follow-up studies of the earliest users (Jick, 1977). Risk–benefit information should be presented to the patient in seeking his or her consent to be treated with any prescription drug. Nurses have a responsibility to be alert to evidence indicating adverse effects of a treatment. They also have a responsibility to observe safety precautions as indicated.

Control Measures

General measures used in the control of potentially harmful agents do not differ in principle from those used in the control of microorganisms. Furthermore, living agents cause disease by their chemical and physical effects. Toxins formed by bacteria are poisonous chemicals. Control measures are based on information about sources of noxious agents, their vehicles for transmission, the forms in which they are harmful, and portals of entry as well as how they reach susceptible cells.

Summary

In this chapter some of the causes and effects of injury to cells have been presented. Emphasis has been on the nature of the responses to injury rather than on the agents causing the injury. Agents leading to cellular injury may have their origin in the external or the internal environment or originate within the cell itself. Injury to the cell may result from a deficiency of, or an excess of, or imbalance among substances required by the cell or substances useful to the organism in its activities. Cellular injuries may be induced by agents interfering with machinery of the cell for utilizing nutrients or by alteration of the nature of the proteins within the cell including its membrane. Within limits, cells are capable of adapting to unfavorable conditions. They do this by undergoing atrophy or hypertrophy or hyperplasia or by altering their character. Furthermore, cells repair the changes induced by injury, provided the structure of the cell itself is not altered.

In relation to tissue injury, the nurse has a responsibility to prevent injury, and to forestall conditions leading to further injury. The responsibilities of the nurse encompass a variety of activities ranging from public education to the direct care of the sick. Public education includes activities such as teaching how to protect children from accidental poisoning and what to do should poisoning occur or be suspected. It includes teaching how to make the living and working environment safe. Workers should know what the hazards are in their place of work, what the employer is doing to protect them, and what they need to do to protect themselves. They should be informed about the laws protecting their safety and make sure that employers and workers alike comply with them. Some of the activities in the care of the sick to prevent injury or to protect already injured tissues have been indicated. More will be included in later chapters.

Survival of the patient who has suffered cellular injury often depends on the protection of damaged tissues until healing has taken place. Although the physician plans the therapeutic regimen, the nurse is frequently responsible for its effectiveness. The nurse makes many of the observations that are used to evaluate the response of the patient to disease and treatment and helps to interpret both preventive and therapeutic measures to the patient and family.

References Cited

Barrows, C. H. "The Challenge—Mechanisms of Biological Aging." *Gerontologist,* **11** (Spring 1971), 10.

Hayflick, L. "Aging under Glass." *Exp. Gerontol.,* **5** (Dec. 1970), 293.

Jick, H. "The Discovery of Drug-Induced Illness." *N. Engl. J. Med.,* **296** (3 March, 1977), 481–85.

Selye, H. *The Stress of Life.* New York: McGraw-Hill Book Company, 1956, p. 128.

UNIT IV

Regulatory and Control Mechanisms

Living things, including people, go to a considerable amount of trouble to stay alive. Some of the work and effort involved in staying alive is expended at the level of consciousness, but fortunately much of it is carried on automatically under the direction of the two great communication systems of the body—the nervous system and the endocrine system. In any multicellular organism which consists of cooperative clusters of highly differentiated cells there are systems of signals and mechanisms for the transmission of messages from one part of the organism to another.

TEPPERMAN, 1973

General Aspects of Regulation

The three preceding units have detailed the delicate balance between physical, chemical, and biological agents in the human environment and the circumstances under which they may produce cellular injury. Emphasis has been placed on the difficulty of predicting whether human response to these agents will result in remaining healthy or becoming ill. A major factor influencing that outcome is the capability of the individual's information-processing system to detect the agent and to mobilize and integrate appropriate responses.

The mechanisms regulating and integrating physiologic and psychological processes are only beginning to be understood. This should not be surprising, as regulation takes place on many levels and is highly complex. The general function of regulation is to enable the organism to modify its behavior so that it adapts to its environment and/or adapts the environment to its needs. Most adaptive behavior is of one of the following types: (1) the defensive escape and avoidance reactions that serve to protect the organism from injury; (2) the reactions concerned with providing materials for energy, for the maintenance of protoplasm, and for growth; and (3) the responses required for the perpetuation of the species. In a broad sense, all these reactions contribute to the maintenance of intracellular as well as extracellular homeostasis. Any disturbance in homeostasis acts as a stimulus that initiates activity resulting in its restoration.

Adaptations to the environment involve all aspects of function, from those taking place within individual cells to the integrated functioning of the organism as a whole. Within the cell, literally thousands of different biochemical reactions occur simultaneously. They are regulated so that controlled amounts of energy are released and the structure and function of the cell are maintained within limits. This is accomplished despite differences in the supply of nutrients and the demands placed on the cell by the organism.

Governance of the body, which is a society of cells, dictates that some cells will reproduce and others will not. Among those that do not reproduce at all are cells of tissues that perform special services for the society, such as cells of the nervous and muscular systems. Among those cells that do reproduce, production is either modulated to compensate for continual loss of old cells, in such tissues as skin, epithelial linings, and the blood-forming system, or initiated as a bodily response to external stimuli, as in the healing of wounds and immunity reactions. Only in malignant cancer do individual cells defy governance of the organism and repeat the growth cycle in response to private impulses (Mazia, 1974).

Metabolic activities are regulated so that anabolism and catabolism are kept equal. If equilibrium is disturbed, adjustments are made to restore balance. Proteins are synthesized to maintain the protoplasm of the cell. The growth potential of the cell is controlled so that cells grow and divide only in response to specific stimuli. It is increasingly evident that the cell membrane is a major factor in regulation of cellular activities.

Growth ceases when the need of the organism has been met. The physical and chemical structure of the cell is maintained. Despite the fact that each individual originates from a single cell formed by the union of two germ cells, genetic activity is so regulated that cells differentiate into different types of tissues, some of which have highly specialized functions. Intracellular regulation is probably as complicated as the regulation of the whole individual. Adaptations of multicellular organisms depend on structures and physiologic processes whereby messages are communicated from one area of the body to another. Activities in which the entire organism participates to a greater or lesser degree include those involved in the maintenance of physiologic and psychological homeostasis, locomotion, sensation, and psychic processes. All these activities depend on the function of individual cells, tissues, organs, and systems, but no part of the organism functions independently of other parts. There is an amazing unity of biological control at all levels of organization. Through regulation, structure and function of the parts are maintained within limits, so that the needs of the entire organism are met. Priority is usually given to basic needs. When the basic needs are met more or less automatically, attention can be devoted to higher needs.

Regulatory agencies are of two general types—chemical and *neurochemical, or neurohumoral.* Formerly, the regulation of intracellular activities was thought to be entirely chemical. Recent findings support the belief that the nervous system probably also participates. Chemical regulators within the cell include genes, enzymes, and vitamins. Products of metabolism, such as carbon dioxide, also influence the activity of the cells; consequently, they are regulatory. Two types of agencies are involved in the communication of messages from one part of the body to another. The older and more primitive type is the hormones; the other is the nervous system.

To reiterate, regulation enables the organism to maintain the function of cells, tissues, organs, and systems within the central range described as normal. Regulatory mechanisms prevent the excessive excursions of function that are incompatible with the safety and survival of the individual. They do this despite changes in the internal or external environment. A change in the internal or external environment acts as a stimulus that sets into motion a change or series of changes that correct the effects of disturbance or remove the individual from it.

References Cited

Mazia, D. "The Cell Cycle." *Sci. Am.*, **230** (Jan. 1974), 55–64, pp. 61–62.

Tepperman, J. *Metabolic and Endocrine Physiology,* 3rd ed. Chicago: Year Book Medical Publishers, Inc., 1973, p. 1.

14

Chemical Regulation of Intracellular Activities

Man masters nature not by force but by understanding. That is why science has succeeded where magic failed: because it has looked for no spell to cast on nature.

J. BRONOWSKI

Jacob Bronowski quoted in Ebison, Maurice: *The Harvest of a Quiet Eye.* Bristol and London: The Institute of Physics, 1977.

This chapter provides a brief summary of the roles of the cell membrane, genes, chromosomes, and enzymes in the regulation of intracellular activities.

The Cell Membrane and the Cell

The study of cell membranes is presently one of the most active fields in biology. It has been well established that the cell membrane is an active participant in the regulation of intracellular activities. The cell membrane is not a wall or a skin or a sieve. It is an active and responsive part of the cell; it decides what is inside and what is outside and what the outside does to the inside. Cell membranes have "faces" that enables cells to recognize and influence one another. The membranes are also communication systems. Things outside a cell do not necessarily act on the cell interior by passing through the membrane; they may simply change the membrane in some way that causes the membrane, in turn, to make changes in the cell interior (Mazia, 1974, p. 63). Among the many phenomena in which the cell membrane is now believed to be involved, are the following:

1. The distribution of ions and solutes between the cell and its environment
2. The rate at which substances enter or leave the cell and consequently the regulation of cellular metabolism
3. Bioelectric potentials
4. Immunochemical reactions
5. Cell recognition, the way in which cells recognize foreign bodies or cells (Strand, 1978, p. 13).

Proliferation of Cells

Not all cells replace themselves; some, such as neurons and oocytes are part of the genetic endowment at birth. Others replace themselves rapidly, such as those that constitute the skin and mucous membranes. For these cells that replace themselves, the cell cycle has four phases. The duration of each of the four phases of the typical cell cycle is remarkably similar for individual cells of the same kind, as well as for cells of different kinds: (1) The first and longest phase is the initial growth phase (G), lasting about eight hours. (2) The second phase (S) begins when the cell begins to synthesize DNA, the genetic material of the chromosomes, and associated proteins. Chromosome replication requires about 6 hours. (3)

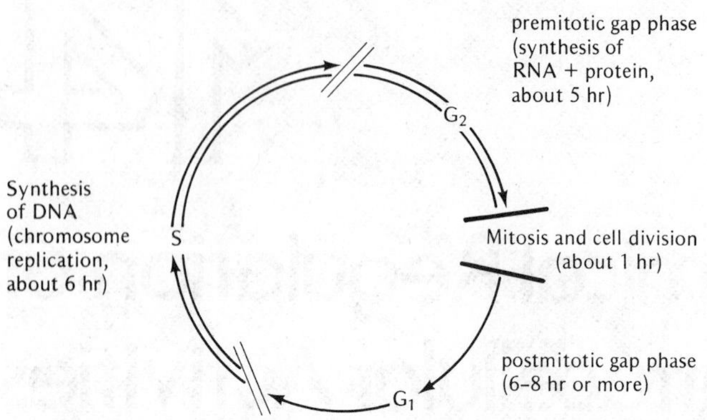

Figure 14-1. The four phases of the cell cycle for a typical mammalian cell. (Used with permission of Macmillan Publishing Company, Inc., from *Physiology: A regulatory systems approach,* 1978, by F. L. Strand, Fig. 2-22, page 20.)

The third phase (G2) begins when the replication of chromosomes is terminated. During the G2 phase of continued growth, the cell becomes twice its original size, which requires about 5 hours. (4) The fourth phase (M) is the period of mitosis and cell division, lasting about 1 hour, and terminating with the production of identical daughter cells that begin the cycle all over again (Mazia, 1974, pp. 56–57). This process of mitosis is illustrated in Figure 14-1.

The Transmission of Hereditary Information

DNA

Modern genetics can be traced back to the work of Mendel. In 1866 Mendel published his work in which he demonstrated that certain characteristics of peas are transmitted in an orderly and predictable pattern from parent to progeny. Despite the accuracy of his observations, Mendel did not know how or by what means hereditary characteristics were transmitted. In 1869, Miescher isolated a substance from the nucleus of the cell that he called nuclein; today this nuclein is called DNA. He knew that it contained nitrogen and phosphorus, but he had no idea about what it was or how it functioned. The specific question "What are genes and how do they act?" has been asked for about 50 years. Since approximately 1913 it has been known that genes—the individual units of heredity—are strung along chromosomes, which are threadlike structures in the nucleus of the cell. In 1953 James D. Watson and Francis H. C. Crick first described the information-

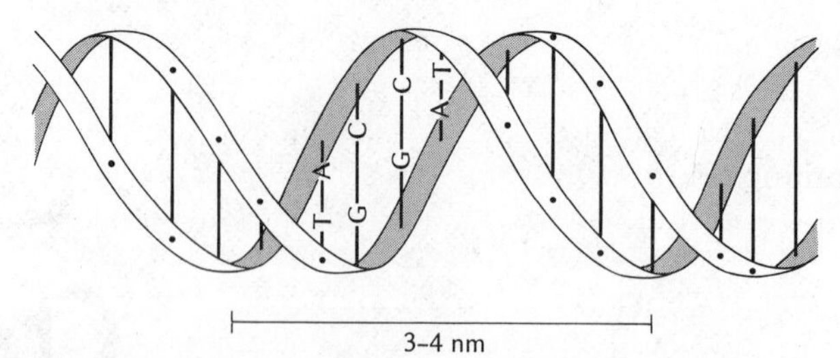

Figure 14-2. The twisted helix of the DNA molecule as suggested by Watson and Crick in 1953. The chains are joined by hydrogen bonding between the base pairs. A = adenine, C = cytosine, G = guanine, and T = thymine. (Used with permission of Macmillan Publishing Co., Inc., from *Physiology: A regulatory systems approach,* 1978, by F. L. Strand, p. 39, Fig. 3-14.)

giving part of the cell as a giant molecule of deoxyribonucleic acid, or, as it is commonly called, DNA (Watson & Crick, 1953).

From studies made over the past few years DNA has been demonstrated to be present in the nuclei of all cells. Small amounts have been found in mitochondria. It is the chemical control system that governs heredity. Not only does it transmit information from one generation to the next, but it directs all the processes within the cell. Although most of the DNA remains in the nucleus of the cell, it regulates the activities of all its parts. It has the capacity to divide into two parts in such a way that each new part is an exact copy of the original.

The DNA molecule is a double helix that is sometimes described as a coiled ladder or spiral staircase (see Figure 14-2). A single helix is composed of four kinds of nucleotides (Crick, 1962). Each nucleotide is connected to the next by a phosphate bridge between the deoxyribose sugars.[1] These alternating units of deoxyribose and phosphate form the backbone of the DNA molecule. The nucleotide bases of one helix are hydrogen-bonded to those of a second helix and may be thought of as forming the rungs in a ladder. Adenine is normally bound to thymine and cytosine to guanine. Although the bases are attached at regular intervals, their order is not regular. It is the sequence of the bases that is believed to carry the genetic message. More specifically, the order in which the bases are attached to the backbone of the nucleic acid determines the sequence of the amino acids in the proteins. They therefore code whether the protein that is synthesized is that of a human, mouse, or tree. In an individual the sequence and arrangement of the amino acids within the DNA

[1] Nucleotides are formed from a combination of a purine or pyrimidine base with a sugar and phosphoric acid. In DNA, the sugar is deoxyribose. The four bases in the DNA molecule are the purines, *adenine* and *guanine,* and the pyrimidines, *cytosine* and *thymine.*

molecule determine whether the protein synthesized is muscle or insulin or whether either is formed at all. Proteins contain most or all of the 20 common amino acids. Each amino acid is directed to its proper place in the protein chain by the sequence of bases in the DNA molecule. When the fact that a typical protein molecule contains approximately 200 subunits linked together in a specific sequence is considered, the possibilities for mistakes in sequence would appear to be large.

DNA, which is present in the nucleus as well as the mitochondria of all cells, normally transfers information by three mechanisms: duplication, transcription, and translation. These mechanisms are illustrated in Figure 14-3. DNA can also transfer information in a few species of bacteria, and possibly in other species, by a process of transformation (Tomasz, 1969).

Duplication. A process whereby DNA provides exact copies of itself for transmission from one generation to the next. The language and the alphabet are the same in the copy as in the original (Spiegelman, 1964).

Transcription. A process whereby a copy is made of the original. The copy resembles but is not the same as the original. The language is the same, but the alphabet differs slightly. The copy that is called RNA is located in the nucleus and in the cytoplasm. It is of two types, messenger or template RNA and transfer RNA. RNA has two main functions. It carries the genetic information from the nucleus to the ribosomes and acts as the pattern or template for the synthesis of polypeptides. DNA directs the formation of mRNA. The sugar in the RNA molecule is ribose instead of deoxyribose and uracil is substituted for thymine (Spiegelman, 1964).

Translation. A process whereby one language is rendered into another. In this instance the 4-element language of RNA is translated into the 20-element language of the proteins (Spiegelman, 1964).

Transformation. A process whereby DNA penetrates a cell and becomes incorporated into the genetic apparatus of the cell. Transformation has been demonstrated in only a few species of bacteria. The significance of transformation may extend beyond bacteria, however, because viruses enter cells of higher plants and animals, as well. Although genetic combination of viral DNA with cellular DNA has been hypothesized, until recently support has been lacking. Dulbecco and his associates report evidence that a fragment of viral DNA attaches itself at one or multiple sites to the cell's own DNA and becomes a part of the genetic message that is duplicated each time the cell divides. Furthermore, it prevents the cell from responding to normal controls, thus changing it into a cancer cell (Science, Nov. 1968).

Further support for the possibility that viral DNA induces some forms of cancer comes from studies of DNA isolated from mitochondria. Although its function is not known, small amounts of DNA are

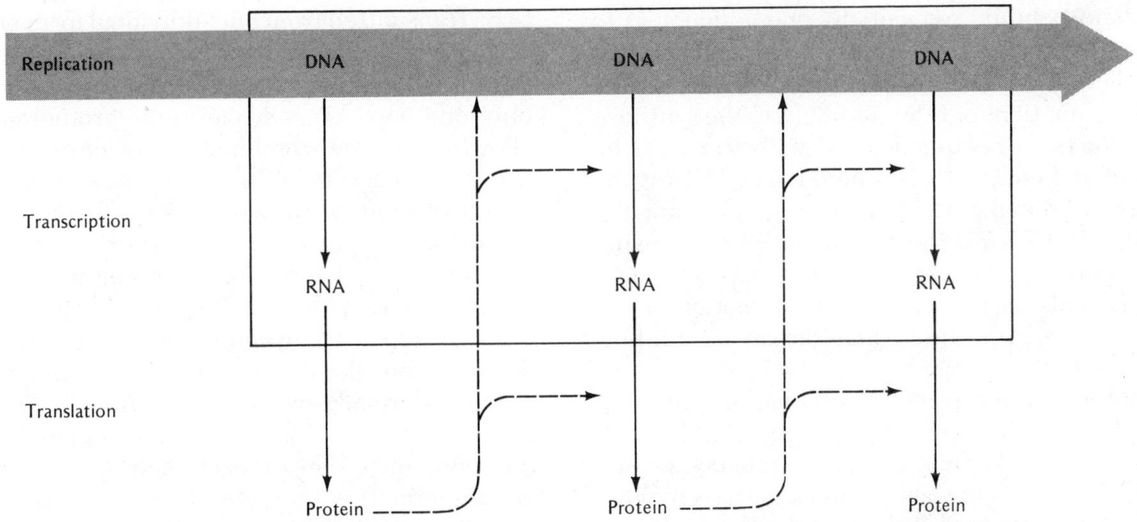

Figure 14-3. The central concept of molecular biology. DNA supplies information for its own reproduction (replication) and for production of RNA (transcription), which in turn supplies information for protein synthesis (translation). Dotted lines indicate that protein synthesis leads directly or indirectly to all materials necessary for further cycles of replication, transcription, and translation. (Used with permission of Macmillan Publishing Company, Inc., from *Biology*, 2nd ed., by J. F. Case, p. 112, Fig. 8-2.)

found in the mitochondria. The first DNA to be studied came from the laboratory strain of human cells called HeLa cells. Later, three patients with leukemia were found to have similar chains of mitochondrial DNA in their leukocytes (Science, Jan. 1968).

RNA

Because DNA is localized in the nucleus of the cell, some means is required to transfer its instructions to sites of synthesis in the cytoplasm. Ribonucleic acid (RNA) is required for this purpose. Brachet (1961) states that DNA directs the formation of RNA, and RNA, which is present in both the nucleus and the cytoplasm, acts as an intermediary arranging the amino acids in the proper sequence in the synthesis of protein. There are actually three kinds of RNA. The first is messenger, or template, RNA. It specifies the sequence of amino acids in the protein to be synthesized. The second RNA, transfer RNA, transports the amino acids to the proper sites on messenger RNA. The third type is ribosomal RNA, which in conjunction with specific proteins forms the ribosomes. According to Nirenberg (1963), for each of the twenty naturally occurring amino acids there is a specific enzyme; each cell contains a specific enzyme that functions to attach a specific amino acid to its particular transfer RNA.

In the synthesis of a polypeptide chain or protein, mRNA attaches itself in the cytoplasm to groups of ribosomes called polysomes. The ribosomes move along the mRNA, reading the base code, removing one amino acid from one of the twenty transfer RNAs, and bonding sequentially one amino acid to the next by peptide linkage until the chain is complete. Three nucleotide bases code for one amino acid. The functions of DNA and RNA in the synthesis of protein have been compared with those of the architect and contractor or builder. The DNA is the architect who makes the blueprints or plans for the building. The RNA is the contractor who, following the directions of the architect, constructs a building of bricks and mortar. The size and function of the building depend on the original directions and how they have been executed.

Nirenberg (1963, p. 80) states that the number of proteins required by a typical cell to perform its functions is not known, but it is probably several hundred. Most, if not all, proteins act as enzymes to direct the hundreds of chemical reactions going on continuously within each cell. As a consequence of the lack of or the presence of an abnormal protein or enzyme, there may be a failure in one or more chemical reactions in the cell that can result in the synthesis of an abnormal substance or the failure to use one or more metabolites.

Chromosomes

Chromosomes are giant molecules consisting of protein, deoxyribonucleic acid, and a small amount of ribonucleic acid (Crick, 1954). Each human adult cell contains forty-six chromosomes. There are twenty-two homologous pairs, called autosomes, and two sex chromosomes. Females have two X chromosomes and males one X and one Y. To prevent the doubling of chromosomes in each germ cell, or gamete, the diploid number is reduced to a haploid number of chromosomes by a process known as meiosis. Each gamete contains either an X or a Y chromosome. The ovum normally contains one X chromosome. The sperm may contain an X or a Y chromosome. The sex of the individual depends on whether the sperm fertilizing the egg carries an X or a Y (sex) chromosome. Although the X chromosome carries many genes other than those determining sex, the Y chromosome carries little other genetic material.

The genetic information carried on chromosomes is transmitted to daughter cells under two different sets of circumstances. One of these occurs whenever a somatic cell (i.e., a nongerm cell) divides. This process, called *mitosis,* functions to transmit identical copies of each gene to each daughter cell, thus maintaining a uniform genetic makeup in all cells of a single organism (see Figure 14-4). The other set of circumstances prevails when genetic information is to be transmitted from one individual to an offspring. This process, called *meiosis,* functions to produce germ cells (i.e., eggs or spermatozoa) that possess only one copy of each parental chromosome, thus allowing for new combinations of chromosomes to occur when egg and sperm cells fuse during fertilization (Goldstein & Brown, 1977, p. 314).

During the process of meiosis, the forty-six chromosomes of an immature germ cell arrange themselves in twenty-three pairs at the center of the nucleus, each pair being composed of one chromosome derived from the mother and its homologous chromosome derived from the father. At a specified point in the meiotic process, the two partner chromosomes separate, only one of each pair going into each daughter cell, or gamete. Thus, meiosis produces gametes with a reduction in the number of chromosomes from forty-six to twenty-three, each gamete having received one chromosome from each of the twenty-three pairs. The assortment of the chromosomes within each pair is random, so that each germ

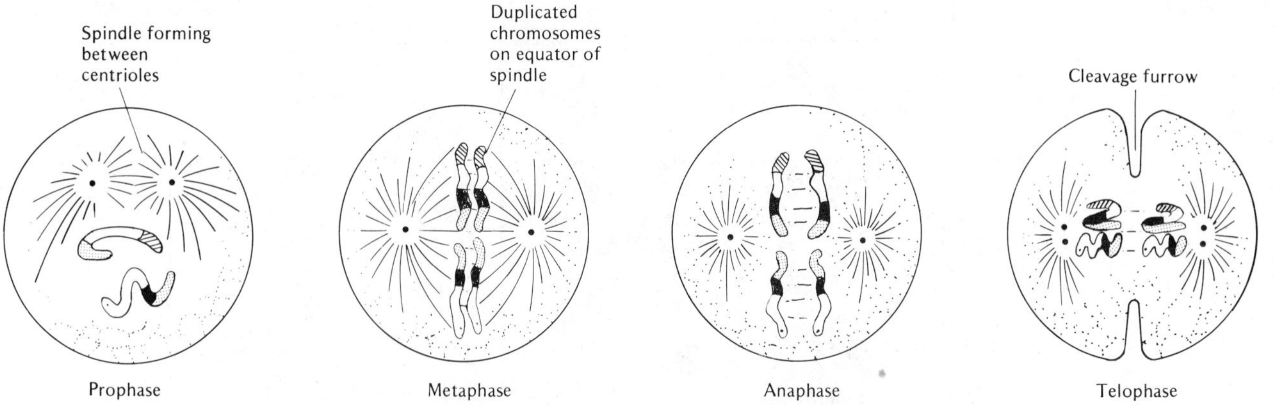

Figure 14-4. Mitosis in an animal cell, showing the duplication of the DNA of the chromosomes and its subsequent equal distribution to each of the daughter cells. (Used with permission of Macmillan Publishing Company, Inc., from *Physiology: A regulatory systems approach,* 1978, by F. L. Strand, Fig. 2-23, p. 21.)

cell receives a different combination of maternal and paternal chromosomes. During the process of fertilization, the fusion of egg and sperm cells, each of which has twenty-three chromosomes, results ultimately in an individual with forty-six chromosomes (Goldstein & Brown, 1977).

GENES

More than one third of the proteins (and hence genes) in each human being exist in a form that differs from the one present in the majority of the population. This remarkable degree of genetic variability, or polymorphism, among normal people accounts for much of the naturally occurring variation in body traits such as height, intelligence, and blood pressure. Moreover, these genetic differences produce marked variations in the ability of individuals to handle every environmental challenge, including those that produce disease. Thus, every human disease can be considered to occur as a result of an interaction between a given individuals's genetic makeup and the environment. In certain diseases, however, the genetic component is so overwhelming that it expresses itself in a predictable manner without a requirement for extraordinary environmental challenges. Such diseases are termed *genetic disorders* (Goldstein & Brown, 1977, p. 313).

After Gregor Mendel established the principle of genetic transmission, Johannsen, in 1909, introduced the word *gene* to denote a unit of heredity. A structural gene is now defined, operationally, as a functional unit of inheritance situated on a chromosome and responsible for the synthesis of a specific polypeptide. It has been estimated that there are probably at least 10,000 genes in humans. Since the number of well-documented examples of genetic variability is of the order of 1000, it is apparent that despite the acceleration in discovery of new genetic entities 90 per cent of the human genome remains to be discovered (Bearn, 1979, p. 31).

Molecular Basis of Gene Expression

All hereditary information is transmitted from parent to offspring through the inheritance of specific molecules of deoxyribonucleic acid (DNA). DNA is a linear polymer composed of purine and pyrimidine bases whose sequence ultimately determines the sequence of amino acids in every protein molecule made by the body. The four types of bases in DNA are arranged in groups of three, each group forming a code word, or codon, that signifies a particular amino acid. A *gene* represents the total sequence of bases in DNA that specifies the amino acid sequence of a single polypeptide chain of a protein molecule (Goldstein & Brown, 1977, p. 313). The genetic code is displayed in Table 14-1.

The genome is the total of all the genes in the cell. Each gene directs the synthesis of a polypeptide chain. When it is considered as the smallest unit of genetic material directing the synthesis of a specific polypeptide, it is sometimes called a *cistron.* Each gene is derived from a preexisting gene. Genes are self-reproducing inasmuch as they copy themselves when they divide. Each gene has a specific position, or locus, on a chromosome. The gene occupying the same relative position on a corresponding chromosome is known as an allelomorph, or *allele.* Although a gene usually stays on the same chromosome, it may exchange with its allele by a process known as crossing over. Crossing over makes the recombination of genes possible. Chromosomes can also break

Table 14-1. *The Genetic Code**

UUU	Phe	UCU	Ser	UAU	Tyr	UGU	Cys
UUC	Phe	UCC	Ser	UAC	Tyr	UGC	Cys
UUA	Leu	UCA	Ser	UAA	STOP	UCA	STOP
UUG	Leu	UCG	Ser	UAG	STOP	UGG	Trp
CUU	Leu	CCU	Pro	CAU	His	CGU	Arg
CUC	Leu	CCC	Pro	CAC	His	CGC	Arg
CUA	Leu	CCA	Pro	CAA	Gln	CGA	Arg
CUG	Leu	CCG	Pro	CAG	Gln	CGG	Arg
AUU	Ile	ACU	Thr	AAU	Asn	AGU	Ser
AUC	Ile	ACC	Thr	AAC	Asn	AGC	Ser
AUA	Ile	ACA	Thr	AAA	Lys	AGA	Arg
AUG	Met	ACG	Thr	AAG	Lys	AGG	Arg
GUU	Val	GCU	Ala	GAU	Asp	GGU	Gly
GUC	Val	GCC	Ala	GAC	Asp	GGC	Gly
GUA	Val	GCA	Ala	GAA	Glu	GGA	Gly
GUG	Val	GCG	Ala	GAG	Glu	GGG	Gly

* The specific triplet of bases (codon) will determine the amino acid synthesized. The nonsense codes, which do not code for any amino acid, are shown in boxes. (Used with permission of Macmillan Publishing Co., Inc., from Strand, F. L., *Physiology: A Regulatory Systems Approach*, 1978, p. 40, Table 3-3.)

and recombine. Damage to a chromosome can occur and be repaired.

If both genes of a pair influence a given trait in the same way, the individual is said to be homozygous for that characteristic. If one member influences a character differently from the other, the individual is said to be heterozygous. For example, if both genes influence growth in such a way that tallness results, then the individual is said to be homozygous for tallness. If, however, one gene is for tallness and the other is for shortness, then the individual is heterozygous for height. The trait exerting its influence over the other one is said to be dominant. The one that is hidden is recessive. Thus, if the person is heterozygous for height and at maturity is tall, tallness is dominant over shortness. Dominance may or may not be complete. For example, sickle-cell anemia is a disorder in which a defective gene produces an abnormal form of hemoglobin. The person who has one normal gene and one sickle-cell gene synthesizes two kinds of hemoglobin, one normal, or hemoglobin A, and the other abnormal, or hemoglobin S. Through the use of appropriate methods, both types can be identified. Whether the person evidences sickle-cell disease depends on the proportion of normal to abnormal hemoglobin. Only a slight excess of abnormal to normal hemoglobin is sufficient to cause sickle-cell disease. Persons who have some abnormal hemoglobin but who do not have sickle-cell disease are known as carriers. Although they do not have the disease, they can transmit the tendency to their offspring. The gene for sickle-cell anemia illustrates a point made earlier; that is, genes direct the synthesis of proteins, and the specific character of a protein depends on the instructions relayed to the ribosomes by a specific gene. Sickle-cell hemoglobin differs from normal hemoglobin in only one respect; the amino acid valine is substituted for glutamic acid at a specific point in the hemoglobin molecule. Hemoglobin S, when deoxygenated, tends to form crystalloid aggregates that cause distortion of the erythrocytes.

Linkage

When genes for different traits are carried by the same chromosome, this condition is known as *linkage.* Linkage is the basis for certain hereditary disorders associated with sex. The X chromosome carries genes for traits other than those that affect sex differentiation. Because the Y chromosome carries little genetic material, some of the genes on the X chromosome may not be matched by a corresponding gene on the Y chromosome. If the unopposed gene is defective, its effect will be evident in the individual. As a consequence of linkage, the genes for sex-linked diseases such as hemophilia pass from father to daughter. Because the daughter has two X chromosomes, the defective gene is opposed by a normal allele and the daughter carries the trait for, but does not develop, the disease. The affected father's sons are free from the defective gene because they get their Y chromosomes from him and their X chromosomes from their mother. The sons of the carrier mother run a 50:50 chance of receiving a defective gene and her daughters have the same chance of becoming carriers. A famous example of a female carrier of a sex-linked disease is Queen Victoria. Several of her great-grandsons were hemophiliacs because her granddaughters were carriers of the gene for hemophilia.

Mutation

A gene may change in character, or mutate. Mutations may be spontaneous or induced by radiation or chemicals. Plant and animal experiments have demonstrated that the higher the dose of irradiation, the larger the number of mutations produced. Moreover there is no minimum dosage of irradiation below which mutations do not occur. A wide variety of chemicals have been shown to induce mutations in experimental animals, but very little is known about their effects in humans.

Although mutations are generally harmful, they do not have to be. Mutant strains that are resistant to specific diseases or that are more productive than old strains have been developed in plants and animals. As examples, turkeys with broad breasts and a high proportion of white meat, and alfalfa that is resistant to drought have been developed through selective breeding. In humans, desirable mutations are less likely to be noticed than undesirable ones and may therefore be overlooked.

Another point is that a gene may favor survival under one circumstance and be detrimental under another. As examples, carriers of the sickle-cell trait are more resistant to malaria than persons who are not so endowed. Because hypoxia increases the tendency toward red cells sickling, a sickle-cell carrier is at a disadvantage at high altitudes.

Neel (1962) calls the gene (genes) for diabetes mellitus the "thrifty gene" and postulates that at one time it may have favored survival. Growth is accelerated and, in the female diabetic child, the menarche is early. Thus a girl's chances of reproducing during her short life span are improved. Furthermore, the tendency of diabetics toward obesity may have protected them during periods of famine.

In some instances when a gene no longer endows individuals with a selective advantage, its frequency may decrease. As an example, in certain parts of Africa about 4 per cent of the population has sickle-cell anemia and as high as one in three are carriers. In the United States, the frequency of the gene is falling in each generation. In 1973 it was estimated that about 8 per cent of American blacks possess the sickle-cell trait (Cooper & Bunn, 1977).

From the discussion of the sickle-cell gene, it would appear reasonable to conclude that recessive genes will eventually disappear. In fact, in small isolated populations either dominant or recessive genes can be increased in frequency. In large randomly mating populations, however, dominants do not increase at the expense of the recessives. In other words, the relative proportion of different genotypes remains unchanged.

Summary

Despite a lack of knowledge of the mechanisms for the control of genes, in differentiated cells they must be regulated. Almost all cells contain the same genes (genomes), yet these cells behave differently one from another. As an example, muscle cells and nerve cells are presumed to have the same genes, but they differ both in structure and function. Although smooth muscle and striated muscle have some common characteristics, they differ in some respects. Apparently some genes are active and others are inactive. Why this is so is being explored, but there are no certain answers (Britten & Davidson, 1969).

Although there are still many unanswered questions in genetics, knowledge has been greatly expanded since the discovery of DNA. Basic to reading the literature is an understanding of the vocabulary and of the processes of meiosis and mitosis.

Enzymes

Enzymes are proteins that are synthesized under the direction of the genes. Once synthesized, enzymes are regulated in several ways. An enzyme may be synthesized in an inactive form, called a *zymogen,* which must be enzymatically or otherwise converted into an active form. This stratagem is useful if an enzyme, for example, a protease, might do damage at the site of synthesis and must be kept in the inactive zymogen form until it reaches the proper site for its action.

In another type of regulation, an enzyme may have two forms, one more active than the other, and be switched back and forth between the two by other enzymes in accordance with the requirements of the cell. Glycogen phosphorylase, the enzyme that breaks down glycogen (the storage carbohydrate of animal cells) into glucose-1-phosphate, is a well-known example. The most active form of the enzyme is a four-peptide chain subunit. This is broken down into less active two-chain subunits by one enzyme and reconstituted into the four-chain more active form by another (Case, 1979, p. 139).

Finally, there is a large group of regulatory enzymes that are affected by *modulator molecules* that may be their own substrates or substrates of related reactions. These enzymes have been named allosteric enzymes by J. Monod, J. P. Changeux, and F. Jacob, who first proposed their mechanism of action. The name allosteric was given because it means "another structure," reflecting the idea that the enzyme changes its activity by means of changes in its structure. Allosteric enzyme molecules possess at least two critical sites. One is the enzymatic site where the reaction the enzyme mediates takes place. A different site, the allosteric site, allows the modulator molecule to bind in a reversible way. This binding of the modulator with the enzyme serves to influence the properties of the enzymatic site, perhaps by a change in the shape of that part of the molecule. Very commonly the allosteric enzyme is the first in a series of related reactions, so that changes in its level of activity may control the entire sequence. Alternatively, allosteric enzymes may occur at branch points in complex reaction systems, so as to control the flow of molecules among the various possible alternative routes. Modulator molecules may either increase or decrease the level of activity of the enzymes on which they act (Case, 1979, p. 140).

Enzymes within cells are organized into teams that function as organic catalysts in biochemical reactions. Like inorganic catalysts, they do not initiate, but they enter into, intermediate stages of chemical reactions. They affect the speed of chemical reactions without themselves appearing in the final product. Organic catalysts have the advantage of being effective at lower temperatures than inorganic catalysts. During a chemical reaction in which catalysts are involved, they combine momentarily with the substance whose reaction they are speeding. In the absence of enzymes or other catalytic agents, the rate at which many chemical reactions occur at body temperature is so slow that life could not exist. The actions of most enzymes are specific; that is, they act on a single substance or a closely related group of substances. Some enzymes are concentrated in a particular type of tissue. For example, among the enzymes found in the cells of the lung are those that catalyze the conversion of the bicarbonate ion to carbon dioxide. Enzymes in the kidney catalyze the reabsorption of glucose and the excretion of urea. The synthesis of enzymes is common to all living cells. Some of the products of bacteria, such as exotoxins, may be enzymes. One factor in bacterial resistance to penicillin is that bacteria synthesize an enzyme, pencillinase, that destroys penicillin. Frieden (1959) quotes the biochemist Ernest Borek as follows: "We live because we have enzymes. Everything we do—walking, thinking, reading these lines—is done with some enzymic process." And in the words of Frieden himself, "Life is essentially a system of cooperating enzyme reactions."

Only a few of the many thousands of biochemical reactions catalyzed by enzymes in human beings are illustrated by the following reactions: (1) the hydrolysis of foods in the alimentary canal; (2) the movement of substances across cell and other membranes; (3) the transformation of carbohydrate, fat, and protein into energy; (4) the synthesis and storage of glycogen and fat; (5) the synthesis of proteins; (6) the synthesis and degradation of hormones; (7) the formation of a blood clot; and (8) the digestion of tissue and other debris associated with inflammation. The preceding list of body processes in which enzymes are involved is in no sense complete, for all biochemical processes in the body require the presence of enzymes. Anything interfering with the activity of one or more enzyme systems can be expected to have widespread effects.

References Cited

Bearn, A. G. "Introduction: Genetic Principles." In *Cecil Textbook of Medicine,* 15th ed. Ed. by P. B. Beeson et al. Philadelphia: W. B. Saunders Company, 1979, pp. 31–34.

Brachet, J. "The Living Cell." *Sci. Am.,* **205** (Sept. 1961), 52.

Britten, R. J., and Davidson, E. H. " Gene Regulation for Higher Cells: A Theory." *Science,* **165** (25 July 1969), 349.

Case, J. F. *Biology,* 2nd ed. New York: Macmillan Publishing Co., Inc., 1979.

Cooper, R. A., and Bunn, H. F. "Hemolytic Anemias and Hemoglobinopathies." In *Harrison's Principles of Internal Medicine,* 8th ed. Ed. by G. W. Thorn et al. New York: McGraw-Hill Book Company, 1977, pp. 1674–97, 1689.

Crick, F. H. C. "The Genetic Code." *Sci. Am.,* **207** (Oct. 1962), 66–74.

Crick, F. H. C. "The Structure of the Hereditary Material." *Sci. Am.,* **191** (Oct. 1954), 54.

Frieden, E. "The Enzyme-Substrate Complex." *Sci. Am.,* **201** (Aug. 1959), 125.

Goldstein, J. L., and Brown, M. S. "Genetic Aspects of Human Disease." In *Harrison's Principles of Internal*

Medicine, 8th ed. Ed. by G. W. Thorn et al. New York: McGraw-Hill Book Company, 1977, pp. 313–29.

Mazia, D. "The Cell Cycle." *Sci. Am.,* **230** (Jan. 1974), 55–64.

Needleman, P., and Kaley, G. "Cardiac and Coronary Prostaglandin Synthesis and Function." *N. Engl. J. Med.,* **298** (18 May 1978), 1122–28.

Neel, J. V. "Diabetes Mellitus: A 'Thrifty' Genotype Rendered Detrimental by 'Progress' ? " *Am. J. Hum. Genet.,* **14** (Dec. 1962), 355.

Nirenberg, M. W. "The Genetic Code: II." *Sci. Am.,* **208** (March 1963), 83.

"Science and the Citizen: Interlocked DNA," *Sci. Am.,* **218:**46–51 (Jan.) 1968.

"Science and the Citizen: Subversive DNA," *Sci. Am.,* **219:**56 (Nov.) 1968.

Spiegelman, S. "Hybrid Nucleic Acids." *Sci. Am.,* **210** (May 1964), 48.

Strand, F. L. *Physiology: A Regulatory Systems Approach.* New York: Macmillan Publishing Co., Inc., 1978.

Tomasz, A. "Cellular Factors in Genetic Transformation." *Sci. Am.,* **220** (Jan. 1969), 38–44.

Watson, J. D., and Crick, F. H. C. "Molecular Structure of Nucleic Acids: A Structure for Deoxyribose Nucleic Acid." *Nature,* **17**(25 April 1953), 737–38.

General References

Arber, W. "Promotion and Limitation of Genetic Exchange." *Science,* **205** (27 July 1979), 361–65.

Caplan, A. I., and Ordahl, C. P. "Irreversible Gene Repression Model for Control of Development." *Science,* **201** (14 July 1978), 120–30.

Crow, J. F. "Genes that Violate Mendel's Rules." *Sci. Am.,* **240** (Feb. 1979), 134–46.

Hayflick, L. "The Cell Biology of Human Aging." *Sci. Am.,* **242** (Jan. 1980), 58–65.

Hinkle, P. C., and McCarty, R. E. "How Cells Make ATP." *Sci. Am.,* **238** (March 1978), 104–23.

Kolata, G. B. "Polypeptide Hormones: What Are They Doing in Cells?" *Science,* **201** (8 Sept. 1978), 895–97.

Lazarides, E., and Revel, J. P. "The Molecular Basis of Cell Movement." *Sci. Am.,* **240** (May 1979), 100–13.

Libassi, P. T. "Two for the Cellular Seesaw: A Balanced View of Biochemistry." *The Sciences,* Dec. 1974, pp. 15–20.

Lodish, H. F., and Rothman, J. E. "The Assembly of Cell Membranes." *Sci. Am.,* **240** (Jan. 1979), 48–63.

Marx, J. L. "Brain Peptides: Is Substance P a Transmitter of Pain Signals?" *Science,* **205** (31 Aug. 1979), 886–89.

Marx, J. L. "Gene Structure: More Surprising Developments." *Science,* **199** (3 Feb. 1978), 517–18.

Marx, J. L. "Gene Transfer in Mammalian Cells: Mediated by Chromosomes," *Science,* **197** (8 July 1977), 146–48.

Marx, J. L. "Interferon (II): Learning About How It Works." *Science,* **204** (22 June 1979), 1293–95.

Marx, J. L. "Newly Made Proteins Zip through the Cell." *Science,* **207** (11 Jan. 1980), 164–67.

Staehelin, L. A., and Hull, B. E. "Junctions Between Living Cells." *Sci. Am.,* **238** (May 1978), 140–52.

Ulmer, D. D. "Trace Elements." *N. Engl. J. Med.,* **297** (11 Aug. 1977), 318–20.

Wolpert, L. "Pattern Formation in Biological Development." *Sci. Am.,* **239** (Oct. 1978), 154–64.

DNA

Abelson, P. H. "Recombinant DNA." *Science,* **197** (19 Aug. 1977), 721.

Baxter, J. D. "Recombinant DNA and Medical Progress." *Hosp. Prac.,* **15** (Feb. 1980), 57–67.

Bennett, W., and Gurin, J. "Science that Frightens Scientists." *Atlantic Monthly,* **239:**2 (Feb. 1977), 43-62.

Cooke, R. "MIT Scientific Team Finds New Form of DNA." *The Boston Globe,* 7 Dec. 1979.

Genes and Chromosomes

Khorana, H. G. "Total Synthesis of a Gene." *Science,* **203** (16 Feb. 1979), 614–25.

Lucchesi, J. C. "Gene Dosage Compensation and the Evolution of Sex Chromosomes." *Science,* **202** (17 Nov. 1978), 711–16.

Ronn, A. M. "Laser Chemistry." *Sci. Am.,* **240** (May 1979), 114–28.

Enzymes

Binkley, S. "A Timekeeping Enzyme in the Pineal Gland." *Sci. Am.,* **240** (April 1979), 66–71.

Guillemin, R. "Peptides in the Brain: The New Endocrinology of the Neuron." *Science,* **202** (27 Oct. 1978), 390–402.

15

Chemical Regulation by Hormones

The Race is not to the swift, nor the battle to the strong.

ECCLESIASTES 9:11

Communication Mechanisms

In large multicellular organisms, the activities of cells and the structures of which they are a part must be integrated and coordinated so that each accomplishes its functions and has its needs met. Basic elements in a regulatory mechanism are (1) receptors or sensors sensitive to changes in the environment—gain, loss, or expenditure; (2) a means of communicating information (structural or humoral); (3) centers for the reception and interpretation of messages from the receptors; (4) centers for the initiation of messages as well as for the detection and correction of errors; and (5) a means of communication to effector or target cells which receive and respond to the message.

There are two agencies for communicating information from one part of the body to another—the nervous and endocrine systems. In the past these systems were considered independently of each other. Because of the many interrelations between them, a specialty in neuroendocrinology has developed. Directly or indirectly, secretion of most, if not all, hormones is under the control of the nervous system. Conversely, the level of most hormones directly or indirectly affects the functioning of the central nervous system.

There are many overlapping functions between the nervous and endocrine systems. The adrenal medulla is part of the sympathetic nervous system, and its products, epinephrine and norepinephrine, are also secreted by other portions of the system. Tepperman (1973) compares the two systems to a wireless communication system (endocrine) and a telegraph system (nervous system). Endocrine glands form chemical substances that are distributed by the blood to all parts of the body. They have their effect on target or specialized cells that are especially responsive to them.

Hormones

A common definition of *hormones* is chemical regulators synthesized by specialized organs, the endocrine glands. Hormones are distinguished from other chemicals in that they:

1. Are produced by a specialized gland or by a localized group of cells and are secreted directly into the blood stream
2. Exert their effects on distant parts of the body, not where they are locally produced
3. Act upon their target cells by regulating the rates of specific metabolic reactions; this is accomplished through the regulation of appropriate enzyme activity
4. Are required—because they are not utilized to provide energy—in very small amounts and may be excitatory or inhibitory in their effect, depending on their concentration and the physiological

state of the responding tissue (Strand, 1978, p. 161).

Hormones are carried by the blood and other body fluids to the cells of the body. Specific structures on which they have a marked effect are called target tissues, or organs. Despite seeming specificity, the action of hormones is not limited to their target organs; rather they all probably have widespread effects. The actions of hormones influence the rate not only of energy metabolism, but of mineral metabolism, as well as the growth and development of the organism.

Tissue Hormone

Although some scientists define hormones as chemicals secreted by specialized cells and delivered to distant sites by the extracellular fluids, others include in the definition chemicals having their effect in the tissues where they are released. As an example, the kidney is able to regulate its own blood flow. One of the chemicals involved in its regulation is the renin–angiotensin system. Angiotensin is a hormone formed in the blood in response to renin, which is formed in the juxtaglomerular apparatus in the kidney. Although angiotensin can elevate the systemic blood pressure, it is not believed to reach sufficient levels to do so very frequently. Its principal effect is on the blood vessels within the kidney itself, probably on the efferent arterioles (Berman & Vertes, 1973).

In addition to its influence on blood flow through the kidney, the renin–angiotensin system may also stimulate the release of aldosterone by the adrenal cortex. (See Chapter 27.) A reninlike substance has been isolated from the pregnant uterus. It is believed to regulate blood flow through the placenta.

Classification of Hormones by Chemical Structure

Classified according to their chemical structure, they are *steroids, proteins and polypeptides,* and *amines.* The sex hormones and the adrenocortical hormones are steroids. They are secreted by glands having their origin in the mesenchymal zone in the embryo. There are some overlapping functions of adrenocortical and sex hormones. As an example, women patients receiving or secreting large quantities of adrenocortical hormones undergo masculinizing changes.

Hormones from the adenohypophysis, pancreas, and parathyroid are proteins or large polypeptides. Those secreted by the thyroid, adrenal medulla, and neurohypophysis are amines. Although most naturally occurring hormones are more effective when administered parenterally, proteins and polypeptides must be administered by injection; otherwise they are destroyed by digestion.

Action of Hormones

The mechanism(s) by which hormones act is largely unknown. However, there is some support for each of four theories that have been proposed to explain their actions: (1) they regulate the activity of enzymes, (2) they act on membranes, (3) they alter the activity of genes, and (4) they bring about the release of ions or other small molecules within cells.

Control of Enzyme Activity

The first and oldest theory is that hormones control the action of enzymes. This theory was proposed after the discovery was made that vitamins enter the cell and act as coenzymes. A hormone may enhance or inhibit the action of an enzyme or the order in which enzymes act. Some hormones have been shown to interact with specific enzymes in the test tube, but thus far this action has not been demonstrated in living organisms.

Action on Membranes

There is evidence that hormones do act on membranes. As an example, insulin does increase the quantity of glucose entering muscle and fat cells, but this is not unique, for exercise and hypoxia have a similar effect. Whether or not the mechanism of action is the same is not known.

Action of Genes

A third theory proposed to explain some of the actions of hormones is that they alter the activity of genes. One factor in achieving maturity is that genetic information comes into play in the correct order and at the proper time. Karlson (1963) stated that, because hormones reach all the tissues, they may well act as timing devices for the development of peripheral organs.

Davidson (1965) cited evidence supporting the hypothesis that hormones regulate the activity of genes. This hypothesis may explain some of the puzzling features of hormone activity, such as the time lag between the administration of some hormones and the appearance of their effects. As an illustration, within 10 to 15 minutes after the administration of thyroxine, new messenger RNA is synthesized and within an hour synthesis of all classes of RNA has been stimulated. Within 10 hours, RNA–DNA polymerase has been increased. This is followed later by a general increase in protein synthesis.

Mechanisms of Hormone Action

Hormones direct cellular metabolism, usually through their influence on selected enzyme-catalyzed reactions and by their influence on the transport of solutes across membranes. This brings the necessary substrates into the cell for the enzymes to work on and accelerates the removal of the end products from the cell and into the circulation (Strand, 1978, p. 174).

Through Second Messenger—Cyclic AMP

One basic mechanism of action of hormones is believed to be action through second messenger—cyclic AMP. Sutherland and his associates (1968) introduced a concept of hormone action that they call the "second messenger concept," the first messenger being hormone. According to this concept, as a result of the action of the hormone at or near the cell membrane, a second messenger, a chemical known as cyclic 3′ 5′-AMP (adenosine monophosphate) is released within the cell where it mediates a variety of hormonal responses. There may well be other second messengers that react with one or many proteins and enzymes.

Sutherland et al. (1965) have demonstrated that epinephrine acts by causing liver cells to release cyclic 3′ 5′-AMP, which in turn causes glycogen to be converted to glucose. Other hormones believed to act in a similar manner are ACTH on the adrenal cortex and vasopressin on the kidney. The end products of the reaction are different in the three target organs. In the liver, glucose is released; in the adrenal cortex, glucocorticoids are released; and in the kidney there is a change in the permeability to water.

On the Genome

Unlike hormones that utilize cyclic AMP as a mediator (most polypeptide and amino acid derivatives), steroid hormones enter the cell, where they may enter the *nucleus* directly or bind with intracellular protein receptors in the soluble part of the *cytoplasm.* The formation of the hormone-receptor complex apparently facilitates the entry of the hormone into the nucleus, where it reacts with DNA. This leads to changes in protein synthesis in the cytoplasm of the cell, appropriate to the biochemical organization of that specific cell. For example, testosterone entering a muscle cell will, through its action on the DNA of the genome, influence protein synthesis on the ribosomes to increase muscle protein. Progesterone will influence the growth of the cells lining the uterus. The specificity of the action of a hormone requires first that a cell have the requisite receptors in the plasma membrane or cytoplasm and also the necessary biochemical machinery to respond to the changes thus initiated (Strand, 1978, p. 178). A model for steroid hormone action on the target cell is presented in Figure 15-1.

As more is learned about the regulation of intracellular homeostasis, the action(s) of various hormones will be clarified. To date, efforts have tended to be concentrated on finding a single action for each hormone. It may be that a hormone has more than one fundamental action in a given cell. It may also be that it acts differently from one cell to another.

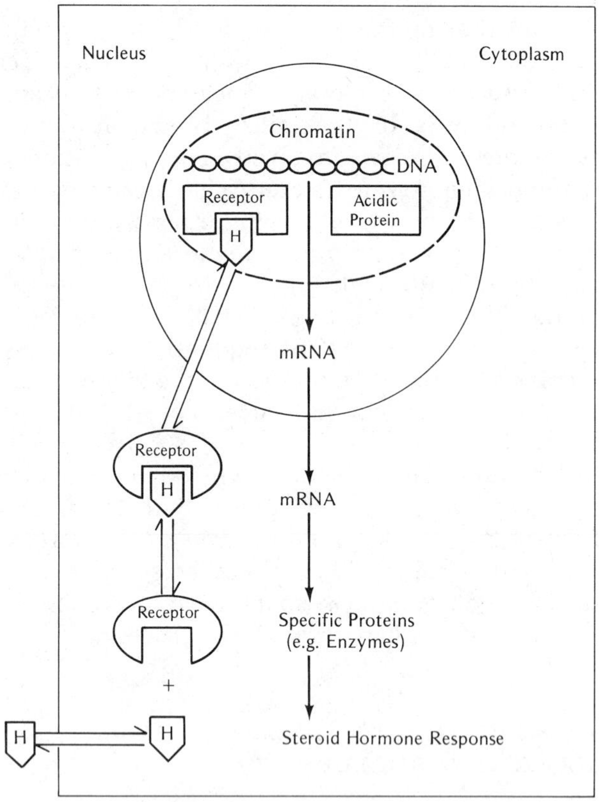

Figure 15-1. Model for Steroid Hormone Action on the Target Cell. The sequence of events shown has been verified to some extent for the following steroid hormones: estradiol, testosterone, progesterone, cortisol and analogues and aldosterone. The pentagon designated H represents the steroid hormone molecule. The cytosol receptor protein is designated receptor; change in shape signifies an apparent change in protein conformation or dimerization. mRNA denotes messenger RNA. (Used with permission of the Massachusetts Medical Society from "Thyroid Hormone Action at the Cell Level," *N. Engl. J. Med.* 300: (18 Jan. 1979), 117–22, by K. Sterling, Fig. 1, p. 119.)

Permissive Actions

Certain hormones have what is referred to as a permissive action. They condition the animal to adapt to or respond to the environment. In other words, they affect the manner in which the organism responds under a given set of circumstances. To illustrate, the adrenocortical hormones are essential for the organism to respond to any form of stress, be it physical, chemical, or emotional. In other words, a minimum level of adrenocortical hormones is required for adequate cell and tissue functioning. In the human being, the thyroid hormones sensitize the individual to epinephrine. The patient who is hyperthyroid is hypersensitive to epinephrine. A therapeutic dose of epinephrine may induce ventricular fibrillation in such a person. Hypothyroidism increases the sensitivity of the nervous system to depressant drugs such as codeine, morphine, and meperidine. A single dose of any depressant drug may result in profound depression of the nervous system. The actions of other hormones are also determined by conditions in the body. In hyperthyroidism, the possibility of liver injury can be reduced by an adequate intake of the vitamin thiamine.

Broad Functions

Hormones may also be classed as those essential to life and those required for normal growth and development. For example, the adrenocortical hormones are necessary to life. The same is true for insulin. Although the thyroid hormones are required for normal growth and development and for healthy physical and mental functioning, their absence does not result in the death of the individual.

Some Generalizations about Hormones

Some hormones act on all or most cells, whereas others have more limited effects. It may be that there are receptor sites in cells that are specific for particular hormones. Thus all cells are believed to respond to thyroxine and the growth hormone. Insulin is required by muscle and fat cells to utilize normal amounts of glucose, whereas nerve and brain cells do not require it. Some of the releasing hormones act only on their target glands. As an example, the thyrotropic hormone causes the thyroid gland to release its hormones.

Some hormones, such as the steroids and thyroxine, have specific carrier proteins. It is not known whether the polypeptides do.

The half-life[1] of hormones varies. For some it is only a few minutes; for others it is a matter of days. Epinephrine has a short half-life, and thyroxine's is long. When hormones are used in therapy, one factor determining the frequency with which they are administered is their half-life.

Hormones are not believed to initiate functions. They alter the rate of reactions, usually by enhancing them, but in some instances by limiting them. Thus the cells metabolize glucose in the absence of insulin. In the presence of insulin, the rate at which glucose is removed from the blood and metabolized by cells is accelerated.

Another characteristic of hormones is that none is secreted at a precisely uniform rate. Some hormones, such as the adrenal steroids, are secreted according to a daily (diurnal) rhythm. Others, such as the gonadotropins and the female sex hormones, maintain a cyclical rhythm. Still others, such as insulin, are secreted in response to the level of a constituent in the blood. Some, such as insulin, are secreted somewhat in excess of the quantity required. As a consequence, after the blood glucose is raised, its level in the blood may drop slightly lower than it was before glucose was ingested. It then returns to normal.

Hormones are effective in relatively small amounts. The effective dose of triiodothyronine and aldosterone is in the microgram range. Because of the minute quantities of hormones found in the plasma, direct measurement is difficult.

Hormones are continuously lost from the body either by excretion or by metabolic inactivation, and they must be replaced. Inactivation occurs in the target organ or liver. Excretion is by the kidney. Effects of hypersecretion may therefore be caused by oversecretion by a particular gland or by failure of a mechanism by which a particular hormone is inactivated. For example, aldosterone is inactivated by the liver. One of the factors in edema in diseases in which there is functional failure of the liver may be an elevation in the level of aldosterone.

For some hormones a latent period exists between their administration and the time effects become apparent. In the case of epinephrine or insulin, the length of the latent period is relatively short. Thyroxine, on the other hand, has a long latent period, taking from 8 to 14 days to act. After absorption, thyroxine immediately combines in the blood with a plasma protein from which it is slowly released to the cells. This accounts for the long half-life of thyroxine.

For reasons that are not understood, individuals

[1] The half-life of hormones is the time required for the substances to lose one half of their activity through biological processes.

tend to be hypersensitive to hormones that they lack. The patient who is hypothyroid requires a smaller dosage of thyroxine to cause symptoms of hyperthyroidism than the one who is euthyroid.[2] Persons with the growth-onset type of diabetes mellitus are very sensitive to exogenous insulin.

There are a number of other generalizations that may be made about hormones. Each hormone has widespread effects on the organism. Few, if any, functions are exclusively dependent for regulation on one hormone. Most functions are dependent on a number of hormones in adequate balance and sequence. Several hormones may act at the same time or in a series. A hormone may oppose or supplement the action of another. For example, insulin lowers blood sugar; the adrenal glucocorticoids, epinephrine and glucagon, oppose the action of insulin by elevating it. The growth and thyroid hormones have synergistic effects on growth. Some hormones have overlapping actions. Oxytocin and vasopressin have long been known to have some common pharmacologic properties. This is also true of the mineralo- and glucocorticoids secreted by the cortex of the adrenal gland. Their actions are quantitatively, but not qualitatively, different. Because hormones do not initiate functions, but only modify them, other elements may be responsible for disturbances in functions regulated by particular hormones. To illustrate, growth depends not only on adequate secretion of thyroid and growth hormones, but also on the genetic background and nutrition of the individual. A serious or prolonged illness at a critical period in the life of a child may also stunt growth. Although thyroid hormones regulate the rate of energy metabolism, other factors contribute to it. This is demonstrated by the fact that, in the absence of the thyroid gland, the basal metabolic rate[3] falls about 35 per cent. Expressed in the usual terms for reporting, the metabolic rate of an individual without a thyroid gland is about −35. Other factors are responsible for the remaining 65 per cent of the metabolic rate.

In health, the level of each hormone is maintained within physiologic limits, as well as in a state of equilibrium with other hormones, by at least two types of regulatory mechanisms. One type is a negative feedback relationship between the regulator and the target gland. (In negative feedback, there is a regulatory relationship between two factors or elements in which the increase in one results in an increase in the activity of the second, but the increase in the activity of the second results in a decrease in the activity of the first. See also Chapter 5 for negative feedback systems.) In the other type, no feedback relationship between two glands has been demonstrated. Rather, stimulation or depression of secretion results from the level of a component of the blood such as glucose, water, or the sodium cation. An example of a negative feedback is the relationship of the anterior pituitary to the adrenal cortex. The level of production of the adrenal glucocorticoids is increased by adrenocorticotropin (ACTH) from the anterior pituitary. As the concentration of the glucocorticoids rises, the secretion of ACTH is depressed. As the level of the glucocorticoids falls, the secretion of ACTH rises. Superficially, the preceding relationship is true. It is now known that the release of ACTH and other tropic hormones requires the intervention of the releasing factor from the hypothalamus. Where no feedback mechanism is known to exist, the rate of hormone production is presumed to be controlled by some mechanism at the site of the formation of the hormone. This may be nervous, chemical, or physical in origin.

The relationship between the nervous system and the secretion of hormones is central to an understanding of the functions of the endocrine system. Little doubt exists at the present time that the release of a number of hormones is under the control of the nervous system. Regulatory mechanisms can be viewed as parts of one system, organized in a hierarchy with the nervous system as the head. In some instances the exact means by which the nervous system controls the secretion of hormones is not clear. In others the relationship of the chemical regulator to its neural counterpart is so intimate that they appear to be part of the same mechanism. For instance, the relationship between the sympathetic nervous system and the adrenal medulla, which has been described earlier, is so close that some authorities speak of them as the sympathoadrenal system. There is an embryologic, anatomic, and functional basis for this hypothesis.

The neurohypophysis (posterior pituitary) is generally described as an anatomic and functional extension of the nervous system. Like the adrenal medulla, the neurohypophysis originates from embryonic structures in common with the nervous system. There are also clearly defined nerve pathways between nuclei (groups of cells) in the hypothalamus and the neurohypophysis. The hormones released by the posterior pituitary, vasopressin and oxytocin, are believed to be synthesized in nuclei in the hypothalamus, after which they travel down to the gland, where they are released on stimulation.

The hypothalamus stands in a key position between the nervous and endocrine systems. Either

[2] *Euthyroidism* is the condition in which the thyroid gland is functioning normally, its secretion being of proper amount and constitution.

[3] See Chapter 20 for detailed discussion of the procedure and significance of results for basal metabolic rate assessment.

directly or indirectly the hypothalamus serves as a center for the exchange of messages between higher centers in the nervous system and endocrine glands. The hypothalamus receives and relays messages from the higher centers to the appropriate endocrine gland. It also sends messages to the higher centers apprising them of conditions within the organism.

Processes Regulated by Hormones

As implied earlier, hormones participate in the regulation and integration of all important body activities. The functions in which hormones play a significant role are summarized as follows:

1. Hormones are important to reproduction and all the activities related to it.
2. Hormones are essential to growth and to structural and biochemical differentiation.
3. Hormones participate in the regulation of intra- and extracellular homeostasis (Tepperman, 1973, p. 4).

The variety of metabolic (biochemical) reactions regulated by hormones include (1) energy metabolism—that is, the rate of oxidation–reduction reactions in the mitochondria in the cytoplasm of cells; (2) calcium–phosphorus balance between body fluids and bony structures; (3) water balance; (4) electrolyte balance; and (5) metabolism of carbohydrates, proteins, and fats and the rate of transport of materials across cell membranes. Not only are these reactions regulated in relation to supply, but they also are regulated in relation to conditions in the internal and external environments. Furthermore, hormones not only modify the rate of body functions in health, but they also integrate many responses of the organism to injury or threats of injury. They also modify the course of some diseases. For instance, some breast cancers appear to be dependent on ovarian and adrenocortical hormones for their growth. In hormone-dependent cancers of the breast, regression of the growth may follow removal of the ovaries and adrenal glands. In contrast, the growth of some malignant neoplasms is inhibited by the adrenocortical hormones. Some children with acute leukemia improve for a time when they are treated with adrenocortical steroids.

Summary

To summarize, hormones are essential for the communication of information from one area of the body to another. They are produced by the glands comprising the endocrine system. Each gland in the system is an individual organ. There exists, however, among the endocrine glands a complicated relationship and a complex, yet unified working together toward a common goal—the maintenance of homeostasis, to ensure the survival and reproduction of the individual.

The Endocrine Glands[4]

Anterior Pituitary (Adenohypophysis)

The anterior pituitary in humans is a small structure, about the size of a pea, and it is located along with the neurohypophysis just below the center of the brain in the sella turcica. The function of the anterior pituitary (hypophysis) is controlled by the secretion of releasing and inhibitory factors (hormones) from special neurons in the hypothalamus; these hypothalamic factors, or hormones, reach the anterior pituitary by way of the hypothalamic–hypophyseal portal vessels (Guyton, 1976, p. 993). For each anterior pituitary hormone, there is a corresponding hypothalamic releasing or inhibitory factor. (See Table 15-1.) Despite its small size, the anterior pituitary secretes at least seven important hormones. These hormones control growth, sexual development, reproduction, and adrenocortical and thyroid activity.

The hormones secreted by the anterior pituitary induce their effect in two ways. They affect tissues directly, and they regulate the output of hormones of other glands, such as the adrenal cortex, thyroid, and gonads (ovaries and testes).

Because of the difficulty of discussing the tropic hormones without also including the hormones secreted by their target glands, they will be considered with the gland that they stimulate. The general relationship of the hypothalamus, the anterior tropic hormones, and the target glands is illustrated in Figure 15-2.

The Growth Hormone

Secretion of the growth hormone is regulated by the hypothalamus. Somatotropin-releasing factor is thought to be formed in the paraventricular nuclei and delivered to the anterior pituitary via the hy-

[4] Contributions to this section of the chapter were made by Judith Landry Valone, R.N., M.S.N., Ob-Gyn Clinical Specialist, Brookline, Massachusetts.

TABLE 15-1 *Some Anterior Pituitary Hormones and Corresponding Hypothalamic Factors*

Hormones Secreted by Anterior Pituitary (Hypophysis)	Some Corresponding Hypothalamic Factors (Hormones)
Growth hormone (GH)	Growth hormone releasing factor (GRF) (also called somatotropin-releasing factor)
Adrenocorticotropin (ACTH)	Corticotropin-releasing factor (CRF)
Gonadotropins:	
Follicle-stimulating hormone (FSH)	Follicle-stimulating hormone-releasing factor (FRF)
Luteinizing hormone (LH)	Luteinizing hormone-releasing factor (LRF)
Thyroid-stimulating hormone (TSH)	Thyroid-stimulating releasing factor (TRF)
Prolactin (PRL)	Prolactin inhibitory factor (PIF)
Melanocyte-stimulating hormone (MSH)	

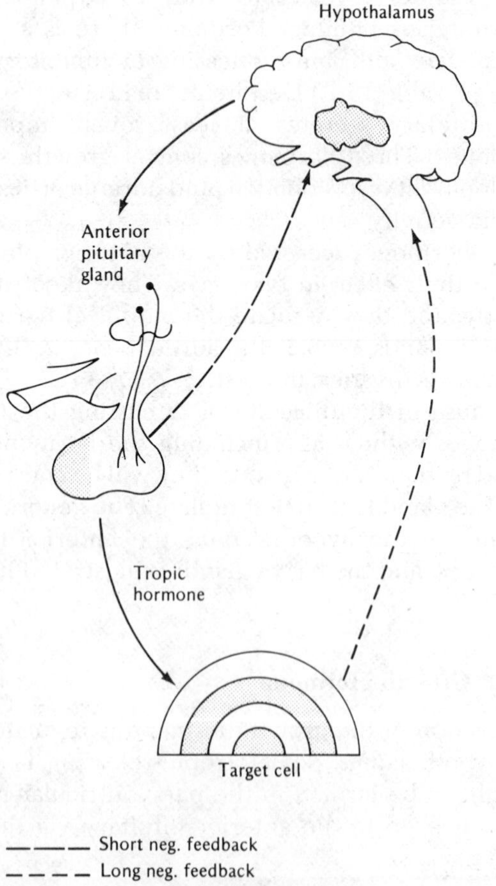

Figure 15-2. Feedback relationships among the hypothalamus, the anterior pituitary gland, and the target cell. (After a drawing by Leola Hogan.)

pothalamic–hypophyseal portal vessels. Not all the factors influencing its release are known, but there is now convincing evidence that most, if not all, of the effects of the factors are mediated by neural mechanisms. Among the factors that have been shown to control secretion of GH are fasting; exercise; onset of sleep; arginine infusion; alterations in protein intake; changes in blood glucose levels; and the administration of glucagon, vasopressin, L-dopa, and estrogens (Martin, 1973). The corticosteroids lessen its release.

The human growth hormone has three metabolic effects: (1) anabolic, (2) lipolytic, and (3) diabetogenic. In its anabolic effect it stimulates the rate of growth, particularly of muscles and epiphyseal cartilages. It stimulates all aspects of protein metabolism. These effects are evident when there is a plentiful supply of nutrients and insulin is present. Absence of the growth hormone before maturity is accompanied by a marked slowing of the rate of growth. Factors other than the lack of the growth hormone also contribute to failure to grow.

The lipolytic and diabetogenic effects of the growth hormone are similar to those seen in starvation. Among these are an increase in the mobilization of free fatty acids, an increase in fat in the liver, loss of body fat, ketonemia, decreased peripheral utilization of glucose, and resistance to insulin.

From animal experiments and the observation of patients with disorders of growth hormone secretion, the interdependence of hormones becomes clearer.

Among the hormones interacting metabolically with the growth hormone are insulin, adrenal glucocorticoids, thyroid hormones, and glucagon. Diabetes mellitus in pancreatectomized animals is mild if the animal is also hypophysectomized. Growth retardation is frequently observed in children receiving large doses of the adrenal glucocorticoids. In animals that are hypothyroid and lack the growth hormone, both hormones must be replaced for growth to proceed normally.

Hypersecretion

Hypersecretion of the growth hormone in an immature animal leads to overgrowth of the skeleton, or *giantism*. Hypersecretion after growth has ceased leads to a condition known as *acromegaly*. A characteristic feature in acromegaly is an enlargement of flat bones, such as those of the hands, feet, and head. The lower jaw enlarges and the face takes on a coarse appearance. There is also an enlargement of all viscera except the brain. Acromegaly may be accompanied by symptoms of hyperthyroidism and of diabetes mellitus. Many patients can be cured by irradiation of the pituitary gland. The skeletal changes are permanent, however.

Posterior Pituitary (Neurohypophysis)

Modern theory postulates that antidiuretic hormone (ADH) or vasopressin and oxytocin are synthesized by the neurons of the supraoptic and paraventricular nuclei. They are stored in and released by the neurohypophysis. The principal effect of ADH is to increase reabsorption of water by the renal tubules. In massive hemorrhage, ADH has a blood pressure–raising effect. The stimulus to secretion is an increase in the osmolality of the blood.

The disorder with which the hypofunction of the neurohypophysis is most commonly associated is diabetes insipidus. The characteristic effect is a large volume of urine of low specific gravity. There may be as many as 15 to 28 liters of urine per day, and its specific gravity ranges from 1.001 to 1.005. With this large loss of water, hypovolemia with dry skin and intense thirst occur. The polyuria is not lessened by depriving the patient of water, nor is the specific gravity of the urine increased. Polydipsia is secondary to the polyuria. Thirst may be so intense that, unless continually supplied with water, the patient will drink whatever fluid is available including, in extreme cases, his or her own urine.

When the cause of polyuria and polydipsia is in doubt, the patient may be deprived of water for a period of time. When water is withheld, the patient should be closely observed for signs indicating the development of hypovolemia. Changes in the rate and volume of the pulse as well as any decrease in the blood pressure should be reported immediately. Because polyuria and polydipsia may have psychogenic causes, the patient should also be observed to determine whether or not he or she has access to water and other fluids.

The treatment of diabetes insipidus has two aspects. When a pituitary lesion is responsible, it is corrected. Until this is done and in those persons who have a permanent loss of function, replacement therapy with ADH is indicated. This usually is required throughout the life of the individual. The antidiuretic hormone may be administered by subcutaneous or intramuscular injection or by nasal insufflation. In the latter, a solution containing pituitary hormones is sprayed deeply into each nostril to obviate the need for injections. The presence of upper respiratory infection or rhinitis will markedly decrease the absorption of the drug. When replacement is in the form of vasopressin tannate in oil, it is administered intramuscularly. It is best given at night to prevent polyuria and thus to help the patient experience a good night's sleep. The patient (or nurse) should be instructed to warm the vial of vasopressin tannate and to shake it repeatedly and thoroughly, until the powder is distributed as a slightly cloudy suspension, because the active material has a tendency to precipitate out of the oil.

Disorders arising from hyperfunction of the neurohypophysis have not been described. Although hypersecretion of the neurohypophysis can occur, when it does it is an appropriate or inappropriate response to injury or threat thereof. Secretion returns to normal when the crisis is past. As an example, some authorities ascribe the retention of water after major surgery or a serious injury to an increase in the secretion of the antidiuretic hormone. A factor in edema in heart failure may be the inappropriate secretion of the antidiuretic hormone. Neither of the preceding can in any sense be considered to be caused by a disordered function of the neurohypophysis.

In addition to disorders caused by abnormal secretion, tumors of the pituitary gland are occasionally responsible for pressure on related structures. The usual cause is an adenoma (tumor originating in gland cells). The most serious effect of enlargement of the pituitary gland is blindness as a result of pressure on the optic chiasm. The optic chiasm is formed by the fibers of the optic nerves that pass over the pituitary gland on their way to the visual areas in the occipital lobes of the brain. Fibers from the retina on the lateral side travel to the same side of the brain. Those on the inner, or nasal, side of the retina cross and go to the opposite side of the brain. As the lesion enlarges, pressure on the optic tracts leads to the loss of one or more fields of vision and eventually to complete blindness. Because of the proximity of the floor of the brain, there may be disturbances in vegetative functions. Depending on the nature of the lesion, removal may be by irradiation or by surgical means. Irradiation is used when at all possible, because of the difficulties involved in exposing the area.

The Adrenal Gland

The adrenal gland consists of two parts, the medulla and the cortex.

The Adrenal Medulla

The medulla arises along with the sympathetic nervous system from the neural crest. It secretes two hormones, epinephrine and norepinephrine. The latter is also released at the nerve ending of the sympathetic nervous system. Both hormones are secreted continuously in small amounts. The adrenal medulla, along with the sympathetic nervous system, appears to regulate functions enabling the organism to adapt to emergency situations. It responds readily to stimulation by the sympathetic nervous system in a wide variety of conditions, with the result that a message borne by a preganglionic fiber of the sympathetic nervous system is converted to a bloodborne one. The release of the hormones epinephrine and norepinephrine by the adrenal medulla contributes to the widespread reaction following activation of the sympathetic nervous system. As emphasized previously, the action of the sympathetic nervous system and that of hormones secreted by the adrenal medulla are similar. Emergency conditions activating the sympathoadrenal system include hemorrhage, hypoglycemia, hypoxia, pain, strenuous exercise, fear, and anger, as well as various pharmacologic agents. (See Chapter 22.)

The physiologic effects of the two hormones are different. Norepinephrine acts primarily on the alpha receptors. It increases both diastolic and systolic blood pressure by increasing the peripheral resistance. Epinephrine acts on both the alpha and beta receptors. Its actions are principally inhibitory and metabolic. It increases the contractility and excitability of the heart muscle, thereby increasing cardiac output. It facilitates the flow of blood to the muscles, brain, and viscera and increases the basal metabolic rate. It enhances the blood sugar by stimulating the conversion of glycogen to glucose by the liver and by decreasing the uptake of glucose by muscle. It inhibits smooth muscle contraction. The adrenal medulla is not necessary to maintain life but contributes to the ability of the organism to cope with stress.

Hormones of the Adrenal Cortex

Adrenocortical hormones are classified into three groups according to their major effects:

1. Glucocorticoids
2. Mineralocorticoids
3. Adrenal androgens

Glucocorticoids include cortisone; corticosterone; and hydrocortisone, also known as cortisol and compound F. In humans, the principal glucocorticoid is hydrocortisone (Guyton, 1976, p. 1024).

The major mineralocorticoid is aldosterone. Others, 11-deoxycorticosterone and 18-hydroxy-11-deoxycorticosterone, are much less important than aldosterone. The mineralocorticoids, as their name implies, regulate

1. Extracellular fluid volume through a direct effect on the reabsorption of the sodium cation by the renal tubule, and
2. The renal tubular excretion of potassium

All adrenal steroids affect sodium retention and potassium and chloride excretion to some degree. (See Chapter 27.) All these hormones have their origin in a common chemical, cholesterol. A lack, or a decreased activity, of an enzyme calatyzing one hormone results in increased formation of the others.

Effects of Glucocorticoids

The glucocorticoids such as cortisone and hydrocortisone have a number of effects that are not exhibited to any degree by the mineralocorticoids. These include the following:

1. They have a significant effect on body water—its distribution and excretion.
2. They enhance protein catabolism and inhibit protein synthesis and amino acid uptake.
3. They antagonize the action of insulin.
4. They affect the metabolism of glucose.
   a. They increase the synthesis of glucose by the liver (gluconeogenesis). The source of glucose is mobilization of amino acids from peripheral supporting structures such as bone, skin, muscle, and connective tissue. Amino acids are deaminized in the liver and converted to glycogen. The glycogen is converted to glucose, which is released into the blood, thereby elevating the level of blood glucose.
5. Glucocorticoids influence the defense mecha-

nisms in the body. High concentrations act to suppress inflammation, inhibit the formation of scar tissue, and impair cellular-mediated immunity.

They are also believed to have a significant role in adaptation to many kinds of stresses, such as traumatic injuries (surgical or accidental), burns, severe infections, and other similar challenges to the organism. The mechanisms by which the adrenocortical hormones participate in these complex events have not been elucidated. Other hormonal, neural, and nutritional factors also influence the response of the individual to injury. Current and future studies will undoubtedly contribute to an understanding of all the factors involved in the response of an individual to stress. Although some animals can be maintained on aldosterone, humans require hydrocortisone or corticosterone for their survival.

6. The secretion of ACTH is regulated by the hypothalamus. The level of hydrocortisone in the blood, the presence of stress-inducing factors and the sleep-wake cycle regulate the production of corticotropin-releasing factor (CRF) from the hypothalamus, which regulates the release of ACTH from the pituitary.
7. The glucocorticoids appear to play a permissive role in metabolism. Many cells appear to respond to other influences such as neural or hormonal stimulation only when there is a certain basic level of adrenocortical hormones.
8. The glucocorticoids influence (directly or indirectly) emotional status. In adrenal insufficiency, patients are often depressed and anxious. By adequate replacement therapy, these effects are ameliorated. The long-term administration of large dosages of adrenal steroids in the therapy of patients with rheumatoid arthritis may result in euphoria (an unrealistic optimism or cheerfulness) or even in a frankly psychotic state in persons who are predisposed to this condition.

Influences on Hormonal Secretions

The secretion of cortisol (hydrocortisone) fluctuates regularly according to a circadian rhythm. The highest levels are noted in the morning between 4 and 6 o'clock. The lowest levels are found in the evening. The secretion of cortisol and adrenal androgen is controlled by ACTH, secreted by the anterior pituitary gland. ACTH also exhibits a diurnal rhythm.

A decrease in the level of cortisol, or the presence of certain stressors such as pyrogens, surgery, hypoglycemia, exercise, or severe emotional trauma, result in an increased release of ACTH in response to the hypothalamic release of corticotropin-releasing factor (CRF). The presence of cortisol decreases the responsiveness of the anterior pituitary to CRF stimulation, thereby maintaining blood cortisol concentration within a certain range by a negative feedback mechanism. As the level of adrenocortical hormones rises, the production of ACTH by the anterior pituitary declines. Many environmental, chemical, and psychological factors influence the release of ACTH. Although ACTH may have some effect on the secretion of aldosterone, it appears to be regulated by the concentration of sodium and potassium in the body fluids. After the removal of the pituitary gland, secretion of aldosterone is maintained. In some instances, it is increased over prehypophysectomy levels.

Summary

To recapitulate, adrenocortical hormones have widespread effects on the metabolism of protein, carbohydrates, lipids, and the electrolytes sodium, potassium, and calcium. They also affect and are affected by hormones elaborated by other glands. They are essential to survival.

The Thyroid Gland

The thyroid gland synthesizes two hormones, thyroxine (T_4) and triiodothyronine (T_3) from the amino acid tyrosine and iodine. Thyroxine (T_4) is produced exclusively by the thyroid gland whereas T_3 is produced by the conversion of T_4 to T_3 in peripheral tissue. In normal subjects the ratio of T_4 to T_3 is about 10 to 1 (Larsen, 1975). This ratio is altered by the presence of hyperthyroidism. The effects of thyroxine (T_4) and triiodothyronine (T_3) are similar. They differ inasmuch as triiodothyronine is three to five times more potent than thyroxine. Its action is more rapid but less sustained than that of thyroxine. Thyroxine has a long latent period and a prolonged action. It takes about 8 to 10 days for it to cause its maximum effect and the effect lasts for 5 to 6 weeks.

Regulation of Thyroid Secretion

The thyrotropic hormone (TSH) secreted by the anterior pituitary regulates thyroid activity. TSH and the thyroid gland are in a negative feedback relationship with each other. As do other hormones secreted by the anterior pituitary, the hypothalamus secretes a thyrotropic releasing factor (TRF) that can increase the output of TSH. Thus changes in environmental conditions such as heat, cold, and emotional stress can alter thyroid activity. As with any function regulated by a negative feedback mechanism, the organism is protected from either hypo- or hyperactivity.

The person is protected not only from endogenous hormone, but from exogenous hormone. Thus the euthyroid person who ingests thyroid hormone is, within limits, protected against thyroid excess. As the level of ingested thyroid hormone rises, the individual's own production of thyroid hormone falls.

In addition to the regulatory effects of the thyrotropic hormone, the synthesis and release of the thyroid hormones are dependent upon the entry of iodine into the thyroid, normal pathways of iodine metabolism within the thyroid, and the concurrent synthesis of protein thyroglobulin (Thorn et al., 1977).

Actions of the Thyroid Hormones

Although it is possible to describe many of the effects of the thyroid hormones as well as the consequences of a lack or excess, where and how they act are not known. The following hypotheses are among the suggested mechanisms of action. (1) Thyroid hormone may act via nuclear transcription, similar to models of steroid hormone action, penetrating the plasma membrane and binding to specific cytosal receptors, which then enter the nucleus of the cell and increase the transcription of the genetic message to form more messenger RNA (mRNA). (2) Free hormone, existing in equilibrium with T_3 bound to specific cytosal receptors, binds to receptors in the nucleus and mitochondria of the cell, increasing the formation of mRNA, thereby directing protein synthesis. (3) Last, the demonstrated stimulation of the transport of sodium across the plasma membrane, resulting in the increase in oxygen consumption by the cell, may be a primary action of thyroid hormone or may be a major effect of the hormone on the cell (Sternig, 1979).

The thyroid hormones affect the rate of metabolism of proteins, lipids, and carbohydrates, as well as of water, minerals, and vitamins. In physiologic amounts, the thyroid hormones promote protein synthesis and fat breakdown. In hyperthyroidism the increased secretion of thyroid hormones is reflected by an increase in the loss of nitrogen in the urine and by a lowering in the level of cholesterol (a lipid) in the blood. In hypothyroidism the concentration of cholesterol in the blood rises. Thyroid hormones also have an influence on calcium metabolism, for osteoporosis frequently accompanies severe hyperthyroidism.

The thyroid hormones are essential to the normal physical and mental growth and development of the child. A child who is born without functioning thyroid tissue or who develops this condition soon after birth fails to develop either physically or mentally. The child's development is dependent upon the promptness with which the deficiency is detected and treatment initiated. Maturation of the skeleton and other body structures is delayed. Mental development is also retarded. Hypothyroidism in a child results in a characteristic type of dwarfism known as *cretinism.* Normal growth is dependent upon the presence of the growth hormone as well. In older children and adults hypothyroidism is evidenced by physical and mental slowing. These effects can, however, be reversed by the ingestion of adequate amounts of thyroid hormones.

Parathyroid Function

Among the regulators of the stability of the composition of the internal environment is the parathyroid hormone. In humans, there are usually four parathyroid glands, lying behind the thyroid gland, which secrete the parathyroid hormone, *parathormone.*

The first biologically active extracts of the parathyroid were prepared by Collip in 1925, but the complete structure of the hormone was not determined until 1970 (Habener & Potts, 1978). Now that the hormone has been obtained in pure form, physiologists and biochemists are able to study its mode of action.

Prior to the purification of parathyroid hormone, there was a considerable body of knowledge about the effects of the hormone. This knowledge was obtained by observing the consequences of disease or by removing the parathyroid glands and by administering crude extracts containing the hormone to animals. The parathyroid hormone regulates the level of calcium and phosphate ions in the body fluids so that their product is maintained at a constant level. Calcium and phosphate ions are regulated so that when the level of one or the other rises, the other falls. A rise in the level of calcium ions in the blood, therefore, is accompanied by an increase in the excretion of the phosphate ions in the urine. Conversely, a rise in the level of the phosphate ions results in an increase in the excretion of the calcium ions.

Unlike the thyroid hormones and certain other hormones, the secretion of the parathyroid hormone is not under the control of the anterior pituitary gland. Secretion is regulated by the concentration of calcium in body fluids. By a fall in the level of calcium in the blood, secretion is increased. Conversely, as the level of calcium rises, secretion of the hormone is decreased.

To maintain the extracellular concentration of calcium within physiologic limits, parathyroid hormone acts on the bones, the kidney, and on absorption from the gut. It increases the activity of bone-destroying cells, or osteoclasts, with the result that calcium is released from the bone to be utilized elsewhere. The hormone also acts to increase the excretion of phosphate in the urine. Both actions are essential to the homeostasis of calcium and phosphate ions. During periods of increased calcium need, such as growth, pregnancy, and lactation, or the intake of a diet low in calcium, parathyroid hormone, in conjunction with vitamin D, responds to increased demand by increasing the efficiency of calcium absorption from the gut.

In brief, then, the level of calcium ions in extracellular fluid, as well as their relationship to phosphate ions, is regulated by the parathyroid hormones. Parathyroid hormone increases the rate of release of calcium from the bones, the excretion of phosphate by the kidney, and the reabsorption of calcium by the kidney and absorption from the alimentary canal. This complicated regulating mechanism provides for both rapid and slow responses to changes in the level of the parathyroid hormone. The kidneys and the gastrointestinal tract are sensitive and respond rapidly to small changes in its level. Bone, on the other hand, is much less sensitive and responds slowly.

As in other homeostatic conditions, the concentration of calcium in body fluids is maintained by several regulatory agencies. The parathyroid hormone appears to regulate body processes so that the relationship of calcium to phosphate ions is maintained at a constant level. The level of calcium ions in body fluids is also maintained constant. Vitamin D supplements the action of the parathyroid hormone in maintaining the constancy of calcium ions in the body fluids. In climates and cultures where people are scantily clad, ingestion of vitamin D is unnecessary, because the skin manufactures vitamin D when it is exposed to sunlight. When most of the skin surface is covered with clothing, the addition of vitamin D from exogenous sources is necessary.

Functions of Calcium and Phosphate Ions

Calcium and phosphate ions are important in the formation of new bone. The source of these ions for the newly forming bone is the extracellular fluid of the body. These ions are considered to be in simple equilibrium with the new bone; that is, calcium and phosphate ions move into and out of the bone depending on their level in the body fluids. When the level of vitamin D falls, the level of calcium and phosphate falls. These minerals are therefore unavailable for deposit in the collagen of the newly forming bone. As a consequence the bones stop growing and bend out of shape. The resulting disorder is known as rickets.

Other functions that are dependent on the level and ratio of calcium to phosphate include (1) the normal transmission of nerve impulses, (2) the contraction of muscles, and (3) the coagulation of blood. When the level of calcium and phosphate in body fluids falls below a critical level, the irritability of nerve and muscle fibers increases. The patient suffers from tetany, which is characterized by painful muscle spasms. An outstanding feature of the condition is carpopedal spasm. The muscles of the hands and feet contract powerfully and painfully. The hands assume a characteristic position. Spasms of the muscles of the face can be precipitated by tapping over the facial nerve. This is known as Chvostek's sign. Tetany can be relieved by the intravenous injection of calcium gluconate.

The action of digitalis is enchanced by calcium. The size of the dose and the rate of administration of calcium to a patient who is digitalized should be less than in those who have not been digitalized. Patients who have been digitalized and who are given calcium should be observed for evidence of digitalis toxicity.

Besides the parathyroid hormone and vitamin D, other hormones also play a role in the regulation of the calcium–phosphate balance. These include calcitonin, the sex and adrenocortical steroids, the growth hormone from the anterior pituitary, insulin, and the thyroid hormone.

The level of calcium and phosphate ions in body fluids depends not only on the integrity of the regulatory mechanisms, but also on the adequacy of the supply of calcium in the diet and the health of the gastrointestinal tract, the bones, and the kidney.

Female Reproduction

The purpose of the female reproductive system is the cyclic preparation of an ovum capable of being fertilized and the preparation of the body for conception and gestation should fertilization occur. This cyclic activity, frequently referred to as the menstrual cycle but more appropriately called the female sexual cycle, is dependent upon an intact hypothalamic-pituitary-ovarian axis. The reproductive system, then, becomes an area appropriately studied within the context of its endocrinologic function.

The female sexual cycle is dependent upon the interaction of three specific levels of hormones: hypothalamic-releasing hormones, pituitary gonadotropin, and ovarian hormones (see Figure 15-3).

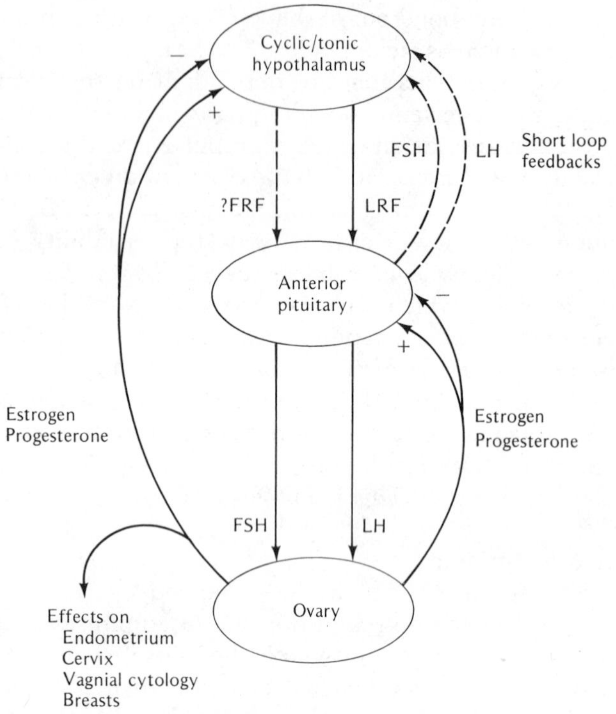

Figure 15-3. Diagramatic representation of the hypothalamic-pituitary-ovarian axis. (FRF, follicle-stimulating hormone releasing factor; LRF, luteinizing hormone releasing factor) [Used with permission of Harper & Row, Publishers, from "Evaluation of Anovulatory Cycles and Induction of Ovulation," *Clin. Obs. & Gyn.* 22 (1):145–67, Mar. 1979, by M. L. Taymor, Fig. 1, p. 146.]

The Tonic and Cyclic Centers

The sequential nature of the menstrual cycle results from a delicate balance in the neuroendocrine control mechanisms constituted by stimuli from the cerebral cortex mediated by nerve fibers in the hypothalamus that liberate substances into the capillary plexus of the median eminence.[5] These substances or releasing factors are carried via the venous portal system between the hypothalamus and the adenohypophysis or anterior lobe of the pituitary, where the releasing hormones exert neurohormonal control. Two types of hypothalamic control centers, tonic and cyclic, are believed to be responsible for the hypothalamic regulation of the anterior pituitary (Taymor, 1979). In response to LH–RH the anterior pituitary secretes gonadotropins, follicle-stimulating hormone (FSH) and luteinizing-hormone (LH). Both of these are small glycoproteins, which exert their effects on the ovary in the female and in the testis in the male. FSH and LH initiate their response on the cell membrane after binding to specific membrane receptors. Hormone-induced responses are mediated by cyclic adenosine monophosphate (cAMP) (Hsueh, 1978). Cyclic AMP has been shown to be the second messenger for many hormones, including membrane-related gonadotropin-induced release, induced by LH–RH, and steroidogenesis induced by LH and FSH (Sutherland, 1972; Marsh, 1976). See the discussion of cAMP under mechanisms of action of hormones earlier in this chapter.

The reciprocal relations of the hypothalamus, pituitary, ovary and endometrium are shown in Figure 15-3. The major influence of the two gonadotropins is upon the ova-containing follicles which respond by secreting predominantly estrogens, by increasing cell numbers, and ultimately producing follicular fluid, which results in the mature graafian follicle. The rise in blood estrogen from the follicle triggers LH release. The mature follicle may then react to the sudden surge of LH by rupture and expulsion of the egg at the time of ovulation. The ruptured follicle develops into a corpus luteum which produces progesterone and estrogen during its limited life span.

The cyclic center responds to sex steroid feedback and sets the rhythm for the menstrual cycle. The ovarian steroids affect the growth and development of both primary and secondary sexual characteristics (see Table 15-2). In the normal male or in the female with a disorder affecting the cyclic center such as polycystic ovarian disease, only the tonic center activity is in evidence. This tonic discharge of releasing factors is reflected in a tonic rather than a cyclic release of gonadotropins.

The Female Sexual Cycle

An understanding of the nature and sequence of events in different phases of the female sexual cycle is necessary in order not only to study the mechanisms of endocrinologic control, but also to understand and manage abnormalities of the menstrual cycle.

The female sexual, or menstrual, cycle is a sequence of morphological changes in the female reproductive system, particularly in the endometrium that in the absence of fertilization culminates in an episode of uterine bleeding called the menstrual period or menstruation. The bleeding phase or menstruation thus is the periodic discharge of blood and of disintegrating uterine mucosa that has been built up for the reception of a fertilized ovum but has not been utilized. The term menstruation characterizes a regular or normal menstrual cycle and cannot properly be applied to anovulatory or dysfunctional

[5] Luteinizing hormone–releasing hormone (LH–RH) is carried from the hypothalamus directly to the anterior pituitary via long and short portal vessels.

TABLE 15-2 *Biologic Effects of Estrogen and Progesterone on Primary and Secondary Sex Characteristics*

Structure	Effect of Estrogen	Effect of Progesterone*
Vagina	—increase in size —change of vaginal mucosa to multilayer structure more resistant to trauma and infection	—alteration of vaginal epithelium resulting in desquamation of superficial cells, decrease in thickness of lining and infiltration with leukocytes
Cervix	—growth in size and vascularity —development of mucous glands —secretion of cervical mucus	—change in amount, electrolyte-content, and physical-chemical characteristics of cervical mucus
Uterus	—marked proliferation of endometrium and development of glands —hypertrophy of myometrium and alteration of myometrial irritability	—promotion of secretory changes in endometrium in preparation for implantation —decrease in contractibility of myometrium preventing expulsion of ovum
Fallopian tubes	—development of mucosal lining and musculature —enhanced activity of ciliated and secretory cells to promote movement of fertilized ovum	—promotion of secretory changes in mucosal lining for nutrition of fertilized ovum —decreased contractibility of smooth muscle
Breast	—fat deposition —development of stromal tissue —growth of extensive ductile system	—development of lobules and alveoli in preparation for lactation
Skeleton	—increased osteoblastic activity —retention of calcium and phosphate in matrix of bone —early uniting of the epiphyses with shafts of long bones	
Skin	—development of soft, smooth texture —increase in thickness of skin —increase in pigmentation, particularly of scars and the areolar of breasts	
Electrolyte balance	—sodium and H_2O retention by kidney tubules	—H_2O and electrolyte loss by ability to antagonize effects of aldosterone at renal tubule†
Metabolism and fat deposition	—increased metabolic rate —increased deposition of fat in subcutaneous tissues, especially marked in thighs and buttocks	—mild catabolic effect on body protein —nitrogen excretion

* On estrogen-primed substrate.
† Compensatory secretion of aldosterone believed to occur, leading to H_2O retention.

bleeding, or to the discharge of blood during pregnancy or to bleeding caused by the presence of neoplasms or other abnormalities. Thus, the menstrual cycle is a repetitious phenomenon for the purpose of preparing the endometrium for the reception and nidation (embedding) of the egg in the event that the egg is fertilized. The menstrual cycle is the interval between the onset of one period and the onset

TABLE 15-3 *Histology of the menstrual cycle**

Day of Cycle	Ovary	Endometrial Phase	Endometrial Histology
1 to 4	Degenerating corpus luteum	Menstrual	Infiltration of leukocytes, degeneration and breakdown of endometrium, hemorrhage and sloughing of endometrium
5 to 12	Developing follicle … Mature follicle	Proliferative (estrogen)	Regeneration of endometrium from basalis; glands rounded, regular, with piled-up cells; mitoses; stromal cells elongated and spindly with scanty cytoplasm
13 to 15	Ovulation		
16 to 28	Corpus luteum	Secretory (estrogen + progesterone)	Glandular epithelium lines up in single layer; subnuclear vacuolization, followed soon by peripheral vacuolization of glandular epithelium with basal nuclei; glands tortuous, saw-toothed; stroma edematous in early stages; later, stromal cells swollen, rounded, finally decidua-like; congestion of blood vessels and infiltration of polymorphonuclears and lymphocytes in final stages

* Used with permission of The C. V. Mosby Company from *Synopsis of Pathology*, 9th ed., by W. A. D. Anderson & T. M. Scotti, Table 22-2, p. 939.

of the next. Its average length is 16 to 30 days. The *proliferative* or *follicular phase* begins with the first day of menstrual bleeding and continues until ovulation occurs. The *secretory* or *luteal phase* begins with the formation of the corpus luteum and ends with the cessation of its endocrinologic function. A summary of the events in the menstrual cycle is presented in Table 15-3.

Control of the Female Sexual Cycle

It is probable that the full complement of eggs (estimated as at least 150,000 in the two ovaries) is present at birth and that no further formation of eggs occurs after birth. If this is true, the implication is that some of the eggs must lie dormant within the ovary for 40 years or more before they complete their maturation in the current ovulatory cycle or degenerate. Of this large number of eggs, only about 400 may be successfully ovulated during the sexual life of the woman; the rest degenerate. It is also important to understand that the eggs present in the postnatal ovary are primary oocytes, that is, they have already entered upon the maturation cycle and are arrested in the prophase of the first maturation division. All subsequent divisions of these cells are by reduction division (meiosis) (Danforth, 1977, p. 88).

A group of primary oocytes begins to mature at the beginning of each menstrual cycle under the influence of pituitary gonadotropins, probably chiefly follicle-stimulating hormone (FSH), but also luteinizing hormone (LH), during the follicular phase which lasts about 14 days. The sudden release of a high level of pituitary LH into the blood stream causes rupture of usually only one follicle with the formation of a single corpus luteum that has a life span of about 12 to 13 days. The number of maturing follicles in any cycle is constant (Lipschutz's law of follicular constancy), and if one ovary is removed the number of maturing follicles in the remaining ovary is approximately doubled (Danforth, 1977, p. 89). The follicles not ovulated all regress in a process called *atresia* (Danforth, 1977, p. 90). The explaination as to why only one follicle ruptures and how that one is selected are at present complete mysteries (Erickson, 1978). It is postulated that one follicle begins to outgrow the remaining follicles, thereby producing more estrogen and progesterone and creating a hormonal milieu less susceptible to falling levels of FSH and LH. The cycle is then regulated each month with an average total duration of 28 days for both the follicular, corpora lutea (luteal) and regression phases. When the corpus luteum regresses and its hormones are withdrawn, endometrial shedding (menstruation) occurs.

The process of ovulation is a sequence of structural and biochemical changes resulting in the rupture of the mature follicle and the expulsion of the follicular fluid, including the ovum, outward into the abdomen. The endocrinologic control of ovulation appears to depend upon a mechanism of biphasic or positive feedback (Naftalin & Tolis, 1978). High levels of circulating estrogens are thought to trigger the outpouring of gonadotropin-releasing hormone (GnRH) from the hypothalamus, which causes the resultant surge of LH from the anterior pituitary. The LH surge is necessary for ovulation to occur (Speroff et al., 1978, p. 55).

The luteal or secretory phase of the cycle begins with the process of luteinization of the remaining cells of the ruptured follicle to form the *corpus luteum.* The corpus luteum, a transitory gland, is formed in and from the cellular structures of the follicle that has ovulated. The basic function of the corpus luteum is to elaborate two hormones, estrogen and progesterone. These two hormones prepare the endometrium for implantation of a fertilized ovum and aid in the maintenance of the pregnancy for approximately 8 weeks. Unless conception occurs, the life span of the corpus luteum is approximately 14 days. If pregnancy does not ensue, the corpus luteum undergoes certain changes, which lead to the phenomenon of menstruation (Brewer, 1967, p. 63), at which time the levels of estrogen and progesterone fall sharply, leading to an increase in circulating gonadotropins and the beginning of another follicular phase.

The cyclic occurrence of the menses, the expulsion from the uterus of desquamated tissue and blood, results from the rapid involution of endometrium which occurs at the end of the luteal or secretory phase. The loss of hormonal stimulation and the resultant vasospasm lead to necrosis, separation, and expulsion of the uterine contents. Hormonal control of the female sexual cycle is illustrated in Figure 15-4.

Puberty and Menarche

Puberty refers to the transitional developmental phase between childhood and full maturity. One of

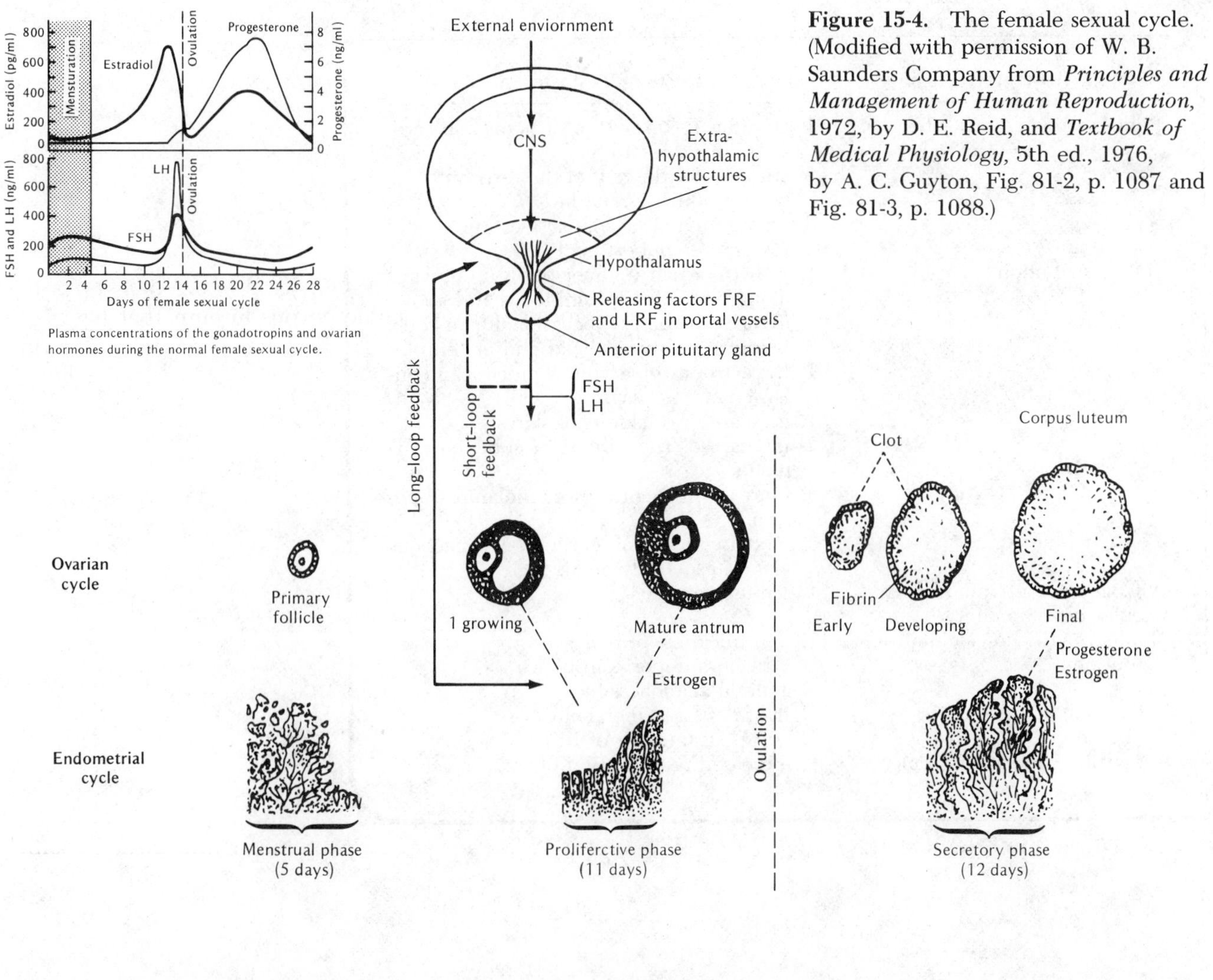

Figure 15-4. The female sexual cycle. (Modified with permission of W. B. Saunders Company from *Principles and Management of Human Reproduction,* 1972, by D. E. Reid, and *Textbook of Medical Physiology,* 5th ed., 1976, by A. C. Guyton, Fig. 81-2, p. 1087 and Fig. 81-3, p. 1088.)

the manifestations of this phase, but only one of many, is the appearance of the first menstrual period to which the term *menarche* is applied. Novak (1975) stresses the distinction because the mistake is often made of referring to the occurrence of the first menstrual period as the age of puberty. At puberty, activation of the hypothalamus results in the production and release of follicle-stimulating releasing hormone (FSRH) and luteinizing hormone releasing hormone (LHRH) as the first step in sexual maturation. A third factor, prolactin or luteotrophic hormone inhibiting hormone (PIH) whose action is inhibitory rather than stimulatory, is also present in the hypothalamus and is released at this time. Thus, the hypothalamic controlling mechanisms are stimulatory for pituitary FSH and LH and they are inhibitory for prolactin (lactogenic hormone).

Anovulatory Cycle

Menstruation may occur without ovulation and a large proportion of such anovulatory cycles are noted in young adolescents and in women approaching the menopause. Such cycles are relatively uncommon during active reproductive life (Novak, 1975). Cyclic menstrual bleeding that is not preceded by ovulation and corpus luteum formation is caused by an imbalance in the normal cyclic reciprocity in the hypothalamic-pituitary-gonadal axis. The ovaries produce estrogen but no progesterone because the ovarian cycle is incomplete. Therefore, the progesterone-deprived endometrium has a proliferative pattern throughout the entire anovulatory cycle (Willson, 1975).

Control of Male Reproduction

Male reproduction is dependent, as is the female sexual cycle, upon the interaction of three specific levels of hormones: hypothalamic-releasing hormones, pituitary gonadotropins, and androgen pro-

TABLE 15-4 *Biologic Effects of Testosterone on Primary and Secondary Sex Characteristics**

Structure(s)	Effects of Testosterone
Penis, scrotum, and testes	1. stimulus for growth of a penis and scrotum during fetal life 2. stimulus for descent of the testis into the scrotum during fetal life 3. enlargement of penis, scrotum, and testes after puberty
Hair distribution	1. growth of hair (1) over pubis (2) upward along linea alba to umbilicus and above (3) face (4) chest (5) occasionally on back. 2. baldness on top of head and at temples
Voice	1. hypertrophy of laryngeal mucosa and enlargement of larynx
Skin	1. increase in thickness of skin 2. increase of ruggedness of subcutaneous tissue 3. increase in quantities of melanin deposition 4. increase in rate of secretion of sebaceous glands, especially of the face
Nitrogen retention and muscular development	1. ↑ musculature
Bone growth and calcium retention	1. ↑ in thickness of bones 2. ↑ calcium deposits in bones 3. general anabolic effect
Basal metabolism	1. ↑ rate of basal metabolism
Red blood cells	1. 20% ↑ in number of RBCs
Electrolyte and H_2O balance	1. increased reabsorption of sodium

* Based on Guyton, 1976, pp. 1079–81.

duction by the testis. As in the female, luteinizing hormone–releasing hormone (LH–RH) is carried from the hypothalamus to the anterior pituitary via long and short portal vessels. In response to LH–RH, the anterior pituitary secretes gonadotropins, follicle-stimulating hormone (FSH) and luteinizing hormone (LH). Follicle-stimulating hormone, in the male, is responsible for the growth and maturation of the testicular tubules at puberty and for the stimulation of spermatogenesis. Luteinizing hormone (LH) stimulates the interstitial cells of the testis to produce testosterone. Function of the testis is dependent upon both FSH and LH, since spermatogenesis cannot proceed without testosterone.

A negative feedback relationship between the production of LH and the level of testosterone has been demonstrated. The failure of spermatogenesis is associated with a marked elevation in the amount of FSH produced by the anterior pituitary; however, the mechanism of regulation is not known. An inhibiting hormone, sometimes called inhibin, at the presence of estrogen secreted by the testis may play a role in the regulation of FSH production and spermatogenesis.

Testosterone, produced by the interstitial or Leydig cells, is responsible for the development of primary and secondary sexual characteristics. See Table 15-4 for the biologic effects of testosterone on primary and secondary sexual characteristics.

References Cited

Anderson, W. A. D., and Scotti, T. M. *Synopsis of Pathology,* 9th ed. St. Louis: The C. V. Mosby Company, 1976, pp. 938–40.

Berman, L. B., and Vertes, V. "The Pathophysiology of Renin." *Clin. Symp.,* **25**:5 (1973).

Brewer, J. I., and DeCosta, E. J. *Textbook of Gynecology,* 4th ed. Baltimore: The Williams & Wilkins Company, 1967.

Danforth, D. N., ed. *Obstetrics and Gynecology,* 3rd ed. Hagerstown, Md.: Harper & Row, Publishers, 1977.

Davidson, E. H. "Hormones and Genes." *Sci. Am.,* **212** (June 1965), 36.

Erickson, G. F. "Normal Ovarian Function." *Clin. Obstet. & Gynecol.,* **21** (March 1978), 31–52.

Guyton, A. C. *Textbook of Medical Physiology,* 5th ed. Philadelphia: W. B. Saunders Company, 1976.

Habener, J. F., and Potts, J. T. "Biosynthesis of Parathyroid Hormone (First of two parts)." *N. Engl. J. Med.,* **299** (Sept. 14, 1978), 580–85.

Hsueh, A. J. W. "Current Developments in the Mechanism of Action of Reproductive Hormones." *Clin. Obstet. & Gynecol.,* **21** (March 1978), 53–66.

Karlson, P. "New Concepts on the Mode of Action of Hormones." *Perspect. Biol. Med.,* **6** (Winter 1963), 208.

Larsen, P. R. "Thyroidal Triiodothyronine and Thyroxine in Graves' Disease: Correlation with Presurgical Treatment, Thyroid Status and Iodine Content." *J. Clin. Endocrin. & Metab.,* **41** (1975), 1098–104.

Marsh, J. M. "The Role of Cyclic AMP in Gonadol Steroidogenesis." *Biol. Reprod.,* **14** (1976), 30.

Martin, J. B. "Neural Regulation of Growth Hormone Secretion." *N. Engl. J. Med.,* **288** (28 June 1973), 1384–93.

Naftalin, F., and Tolis, G. "Neuroendocrine Regulation of the Menstrual Cycle." *Clin. Obstet. & Gynecol.,* **21** (March 1978), 17–29.

Novak, E. R. et al. *Novak's Textbook of Gynecology,* 9th ed. Baltimore: The Williams & Wilkins Company, 1975, pp. 90–93.

Reid, D. E. et al. *Principles and Management of Human Reproduction.* Philadelphia: W. B. Saunders Company, 1972.

Speroff, L. et al. *Clinical Gynecologic Endocrinology and Infertility,* 2nd ed. Baltimore: The Williams & Wilkins Company, 1978.

Sternig, K. "Thyroid Hormone Action at the Cellular Level (First of two parts)." *N. Engl. J. Med.,* **300** (18 Jan. 1979), 117–23.

Strand, F. L. *Physiology: A Regulatory Systems Approach.* New York: Macmillan Publishing Co., Inc., 1978.

Sutherland, E. W. "Studies on the Mechanism of Hormone Action." *Science,* **177** (1972), 401.

Sutherland, E. W. et al. "The Action of Epinephrine and the Role of Adenyl Cyclase System in Hormone Action." *Recent Prog. Horm. Res.,* **21** (1965), 628–29.

Sutherland, E. W. et al. "Some Aspects of the Biological Role of Adenosine 3', 5' Monophosphate (Cyclic AMP)." *Circulation,* **37** (Feb. 1968), 300.

Taymor, M. D. "Evaluation of Anovulatory Cycles and Induction of Ovulation." *Clin. Obstet. & Gynecol.,* **22** (March 1979), 145–67.

Tepperman, J. *Metabolic and Endocrine Physiology,* 3rd ed. Chicago: Year Book Medical Publishers, Inc., 1973.

Thorn, G. W. et al., eds. *Harrison's Principles of Internal Medicine,* 7th ed. New York: McGraw-Hill Book Company, 1977.

Willson, J. R. et al. *Obstetrics and Gynecology,* 5th ed. St. Louis: The C. V. Mosby Co., 1975, p. 69.

General References

Crews, D. "The Hormonal Control of Behavior in a Lizard." *Sci. Am.,* **241** (Aug. 1979), 180–87.

Frohman, L. A. "Neurotransmitters as Regulators of Endocrine Function." *Hosp. Practice,* **10**:4 (April 1975), 54–67.

Jarrett, L., and McDonald, J. M. "Hormone Receptors: From Basic Research to Clinical Applications." *Arch. Pathol. & Lab. Med.,* **101** (March 1977), 156–58.
Schally, A. V. "Aspects of Hypothalamic Regulation of the Pituitary Gland." *Science,* **202** (6 Oct. 1978), 18–28.

Thyroid

Burrow, G. N. "Hyperthyroidism during Pregnancy." *N. Eng. J. Med.,* **298** (19 Jan. 1978), 150–53.
Guimond, J. H., and Wilson, S. G. "Postirradiation Thyroid Disorders." *Am. J. Nurs.,* **79** (July 1979), 1256–58.
Oppenheimer, J. H. "Thyroid Hormone Action at the Cellular Level." *Science,* **203** (9 March 1979), 971–79.
Sterling, K. "Thyroid Hormone Action at the Cell Level." *N. Eng. J. Med.,* **300** (18 Jan. 1979), 117–22, pt. 1. (25 Jan. 1979), 173–76, pt. 2.

Parathyroid

Habener, J. F., and Potts, J. T. "Biosynthesis of Parathyroid Hormone. *N. Engl. J. Med.,* **299** (21 Sept. 1978), 635–44.

Gonads

Dietz, J. "Endocrine Cure for Impotent Men Reported." *The Boston Globe,* 18 Feb. 1980.
Frantz, A. G. "Prolactin." *N. Engl. J. Med.,* **298** (26 Jan. 1978), 201–7.
Tolis, G. "Prolactin: Physiology and Pathology." *Hosp. Practice,* **15** (Feb. 1980), 85–95.
Wilson, J. D. "Sex Hormones and Sexual Behavior." *N. Engl. J. Med.,* **300** (31 May 1979), 1269–70.

16

The Nature and Organization of Neural Regulation

These three scientists, Dale, Loewi and Cannon, working in England, Germany and America, were Prometheans in the full sense of the word. They were opening up a new world, revealing new concepts, enormously enriching our knowledge of the physical basis of behavior and, ultimately, of the chemistry of the mind. The concept of the brain as a complex computer entirely electrical in its workings was shown to be a gross oversimplification. The nervous system was far more complex than any computer man could even conceive. In addition to the myriad pulses passing along the nerve fibers, whose flow Sherrington compared to a cosmic dance, there were a host of chemical processes, substances generated with flashlike suddenness in infinitesimal amounts, produced, destroyed, regenerated, destroyed again. The whole nervous system was a seething mass of chemical reactions and any interference with those reactions could halt the working of the whole machine.

DE ROPP

Robert S. De Ropp: *The New Prometheans.* Delacorte Press/Seymour Lawrence, 1972, p. 176–77.

Overview—Governing Principles

Any complex multicellular organism requires means by which its activities can be controlled. Organisms with highly elaborate differentiated systems demand means for relating these to one another, for adjusting to varying demands. Previous chapters of this unit have discussed various regulatory systems that facilitate these adjustments. As research frontiers on regulatory processes expand, there appears to be less justification for separating the contribution of neural and endocrine function. For example, there is evidence that not only do neurohypophyseal hormones modify endocrine function but that pituitary hormones may be transported directly to the brain to modify brain function (Bergland & Page, 1979).

The nervous system, which will be the concern of this section, stands in position to integrate, direct, and control all the regulatory systems. With a mature and functionally perfect nervous system, the bodily life of the organism goes on smoothly, meeting exquisitely, in the environment to which it is suited, its needs as an individual. When there are defects in the nervous system, the organism may be handicapped only slightly and able to compensate quite satisfactorily, or, as is the case in any complex organization with a highly elaborate administrative system when departments are absent or ineffective, chaos can result.

The history of the nervous system reaches far back in evolution; and the basic patterns of the simpler forms of animal life have been used, built upon, and elaborated until it is hard to see in the healthy adult the simple beginnings of so complicated a structure. By returning to the early life of the embryo and following the first weeks of its development, it may be seen that certain principles of growth will hold as well for the nervous system within the body as for the body as a whole. The following governing principles are basic to understanding the nervous system. They will be stated here and subsequently referred to or applied in discussion.

1. *Growth proceeds in a cephalocaudal direction.*
2. *The more important an organ or system is to the economy of the body as a whole, the more provisions there are for protecting its structure and blood supply.*
3. *The more highly specialized a tissue, the less able it is to survive severe and sudden deficits in supply.*
4. *After destruction of nerve cells, those remaining are unable to replace those that are lost.*
5. *Within the nervous system there is a hierarchy of control. No single part functions separately from other parts.*
6. *The nervous system imposes regulation and control not only on organs and systems of the body but also on itself.*
7. *In general, higher centers inhibit lower, and phylogenetically newer parts inhibit older.*
8. *The later in embryonic life a part of the nervous system develops, the more susceptible it is to injury.*

Embryonic Development

The earliest aggregation of cells that will shortly be delegated to undertake the elaboration of the nervous system is seen first at the anterior dorsal part of the embryo. As development proceeds, it is at the cephalic end that evaginations and foldings that indicate the primitive brain occur. The simpler cord, growing caudally, retains for some time an appearance reminiscent of the nervous system of segmented animals such as worms, the nerves growing out from it seeming to pursue the primitive muscles that develop earlier (Principle 1).

Organization of the Central Nervous System

Mechanisms for Protection

Because the central nervous system is the system responsible for the control and regulation of all others, the economy of the body dictates that it be well protected (Principle 2). This protection is provided by shielding of brain and cord by (1) bony structures, (2) membranous coverings of brain and cord by meninges, (3) shock-absorbing qualities of the cerebrospinal fluid (CSF), (4) chemical protection by the blood–brain barrier, and (5) nutritional guarantees of a rich blood supply.

Bony Structures

Although the bony protector lies outside the nervous system, its structure needs to be appreciated nevertheless, because a break in the integrity of the protectors may constitute a threat to the nervous system they guard. For example, a compound fracture of the skull may be serious not so much on its own account as for the hazard of brain injury or infection it presents to the contents within.

The human nervous system is well protected. The brain, after the period of rapid growth in infancy is over, is enclosed in a relatively *rigid cranium of bone* that is shaped by its inner tables to conform to and support the friable tissues that lie within the several fossae of the skull. In like manner, the spinal cord is guarded by a *chain of vertebrae,* rigid in themselves but held into a flexible tunnel for the cord by means of the *heavy cartilaginous disks* between their bodies and by powerful *tendinous and muscle attachments.* The safety of parts of the cord is enhanced by additional fixation offered by the *shoulder and sacral girdles,* although the thoracic section of the cord does not profit from such an additional shield.

Membranous Coverings

Within the skull and vertebral column are three membranous coverings, *the meninges.* The outermost, the *dura mater,* is a heavy, relatively nonelastic tissue that forms a cloaklike covering for brain and cord and is reflected at these points to form deep folds: one, the *falx,* between the two cerebral hemispheres; the second, the *tentorium,* between the cerebral hemispheres and the cerebellum; and third, between the lobes of the cerebellum, the *falx cerebelli.* Like that of the skull, the protection offered by the dura is mechanical, and the partition erected by the falx tends to cut down on the transmission of pressure, or force, from hemisphere to hemisphere. The tentorium affords a comparable shield between the forebrain and the more vital structures of the midbrain and medulla below.

The second meningis, or *arachnoid,* is thin and made up of a delicate, fibrous, weblike tissue that both separates it from and joins it to the *pia mater,* the third membrane. Filling this mesh is the cerebrospinal fluid, which eventually will be returned

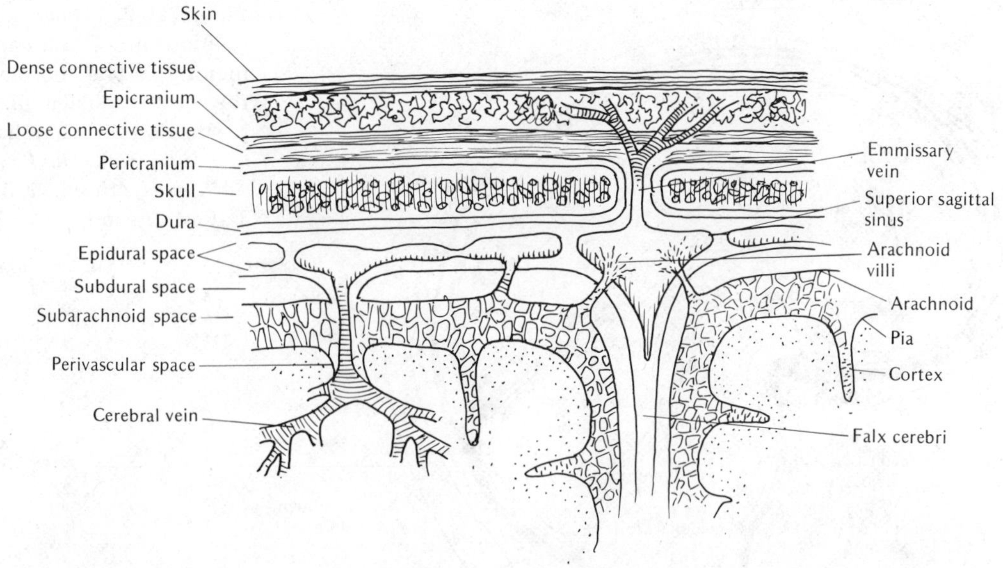

Figure 16-1. Diagrammatic coronal section through the head, including the layers of the scalp and the superficial cerebral cortex. This shows the emissary veins and the relations of the arachnoid villi to the dural sinuses. (Adapted with permission of the McGraw-Hill Book Company from *A Functional Approach to Neuroanatomy,* by E. L. House and B. Pansky. Copyright © McGraw-Hill Book Company, Inc., 1965, Fig. 44, p. 68.)

to the blood by way of specialized structures of the arachnoid called villi, granulations, or the pacchionian bodies. (See Figure 16-1.)

The pia mater is also a thin membrane but tougher than the arachnoid, its connective tissue fibers being thoroughly interwoven. The pia is closely applied to the nervous system, helping to hold the very soft substance of brain in form and shape. In so doing, it follows the gyri and sulci and cuffs the blood vessels penetrating the surface of the brain. The thick mat of blood vessels that are integral parts of the choroid plexuses is borne by the pia. Together they extend into the ventricles. This rich blood supply, and the action by which the pia seems to resist invasion by microorganisms, a matter that will subsequently be discussed briefly, as well as its apparently purely mechanical function of support, qualify the pia as a protector of the central nervous system. The pia and arachnoid together are referred to as the *leptomeninges.*

Cerebrospinal Fluid

The *cerebrospinal fluid* found circulating in the subarachnoid space has its origin largely in the choroid plexuses in the ventricles of the brain. These are fluid-filled cavities that serve as another means for absorbing shock. The ventricular system is rather like a short series of little lakes, spring-fed, that are connected to one another by canals of varying width to reach a marsh that spreads wide to cover the brain and eventually drains, by way of the arachnoid granulations, into the great channels of the dural sinuses. Thus the brain floats on a fluid cushion; and because the specific gravities of the brain and cerebrospinal fluid are about the same, a blow to the head moves all the cranial contents together so that contortion is at a minimum. (See Figure 16-2.)

In the analogy, the "springs" are the choroid plexuses, which are little clusters of blood vessels covered by the pia mater and a single layer of cuboidal epithelial cells, the whole rather resembling a raspberry, that project into the lateral, third, and fourth ventricles. Cerebrospinal fluid is extravasated from them continuously at a rate estimated to be about 840 ml per day. (Guyton, 1976, p. 415). Nothing is found in cerebrospinal fluid that is not found in blood, but the concentrations are quite different, which implies that the fluid is a choroid secretion rather than a filtrate. (See Table 16-1.)

The secreted fluid passes from the lateral ventricles through their foramina (of Monro) into the third ventricle, where continuation of the choroid plexus contributes to the volume that passes through the aqueduct of Sylvius into the fourth ventricle where still more fluid is formed. In the fourth ventricle are two foramina (of Luschka) placed laterally and one (of Magendie) in the midline that permit passage of fluid into the *cisterna magna* and out into the subarachnoid spaces, the "marsh" over the brain. Only a small amount of cerebrospinal fluid is required to float the spinal cord and *cauda equina,*

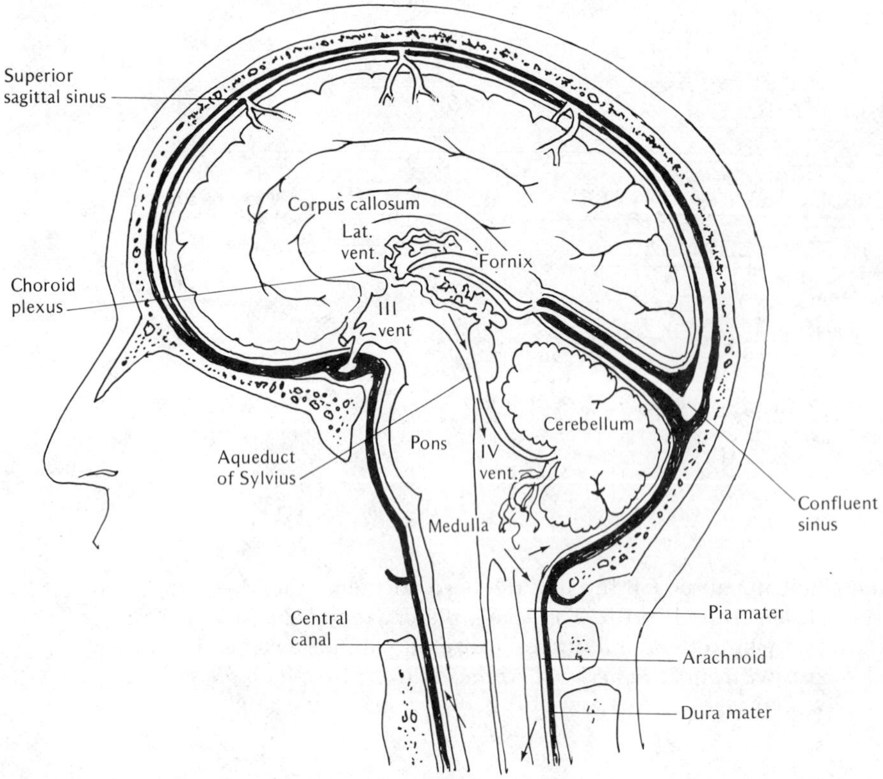

Figure 16-2. Diagram showing relationship of brain and cord to meninges. The choroid plexus forms the cerebrospinal fluid. (Modified with permission of Macmillan Publishing Co., Inc., from *The Principal Nervous Pathways*, 4th ed., 1952, by Andrew T. Rasmussen.)

that cluster of spinal nerves that supplies the lower part of the body and that was seemingly left to drag behind by the uneven rate of growth, in early life, of cord and spinal column. It is this slender column of fluid in the lumbar spinal subarachnoid space that the physician taps to determine the present chemical or bacteriological composition of the patient's cerebrospinal fluid or to determine the intracranial pressure.

The arachnoid granulations protrude through the venous walls and permit easy return to the blood of water and electrolytes as well as small protein molecules, for the osmotic gradient favors this. The amounts of fluid secreted and absorbed daily are normally the same, which is some five to six times the total volume of the entire cerebrospinal cavity (Guyton, 1976, p. 415). Circulation is maintained because

Table 16-1

Average	Blood Plasma	Cerebro-spinal Fluid
Protein, mg per 100 ml	7,500	20
Na, mEq per liter	137	141
Cl, mEq per liter	101	124
K, mEq per liter	4.9	3.3
Glucose, mg per 100 ml	92	61

the pressure in the capillaries at the point of secretion is greater than in the area of absorption.

Blood–Brain Barrier

The fourth protector of the nervous system is determined more by inference than by vision: This is the *blood–cerebrospinal fluid barrier* and *blood–brain barrier*. Under normal circumstances, not all substances that circulate freely in the blood stream and pass into interstitial spaces of the body cells will pass into the cerebrospinal fluid or brain parenchyma. These barriers are highly permeable to water, carbon dioxide, and oxygen, slightly permeable to the electrolytes, such as sodium, chloride, and potassium, and almost totally impermeable to substances such as arsenic, sulfur, and gold.

The cause of the low permeability of the barriers is the fact that endothelial cells of the capillaries are joined to each other by so-called tight junctions; that is, the membranes of the adjacent endothelial cells are almost fused with each other rather than having split-pores between them, as is the case in most other capillaries of the body. However, in addition to the tight junctions, the capillaries are also surrounded by glial "feet" that abut the outsides of the capillaries, which some physiologists have suggested decrease the permeability of the capillaries (Guyton, 1976, p. 418).

The barriers tend to protect the central nervous

system from being affected by many agents that are potentially harmful. The presence of the barriers is important to appreciate in drug therapy. When a drug is prescribed to treat an infection in the nervous system—meningococcic meningitis, for example—it is necessary to use one that penetrates the barriers such as sulfadiazine; many other forms of sulfa do not, and would be ineffective.

Blood Supply of the Brain

The tissue of the nervous system, which will be discussed subsequently, is the most specialized of any tissue of the body and as such demands and receives a rich blood supply. The brain alone receives about 700 ml per minute (14 per cent of total resting cardiac output) (Guyton, 1976, p. 251). This is provided both by the carotid arteries, which enter at the base of the skull and divide to form the middle and anterior cerebral arteries, and by the two vertebral arteries, which branch off the subclavian artery and enter through the foramen magnum to form the basilar artery. These great vessels deliver to the brain blood that has only recently left the heart and is rich in oxygen and nutrients. Both the carotid and vertebral arteries variously coalesce, branch, and subdivide to assure excellent blood supply to all areas, the smallest arteries eventually forming capillaries from which veins arise that return to the subarachnoid spaces, and finally to the dural sinuses through which the brain is drained at last into the internal jugular veins that return to the superior vena cava.

A test frequently performed in the course of a diagnostic spinal tap illustrates some points discussed in the foregoing paragraphs. With a manometer attached to a lumbar-puncture needle inserted into the spinal canal, the cerebrospinal fluid will be noted to oscillate in direct relation to both the patient's pulse and respiration. If pressure is then applied to the patient's neck over the jugular veins, there will be a prompt rise in the column of cerebrospinal fluid in the manometer. Partial occlusion occasioned by jugular-vein compression has temporarily interfered with blood leaving the cranium, but the arterial inflow continues. This increases the volume of the intracranial blood and hence increases the intracranial pressure, which is reflected at once in the height of the fluid column in the manometer.

Cerebral Metabolism

Brain tissue demands a continuous supply of oxygen and glucose to meet its large energy requirements. In the absence of oxygen, cerebral function can be supported for only 10 seconds before symptoms result. The brain can survive for only 1 to 1½ hours in the absence of glucose, before symptoms of hypoglycemia appear. (Principle 3: The more specialized a tissue, the less able it is to survive severe and sudden deficits in supply.)

Neural Structure

Although nerve cells have certain features in common and are quite unlike cells of other tissues—muscle, bone, and blood, for instance—these nerve cells vary greatly from one another, for they are well adapted in form to the special activities they carry on. In discussing a "typical nerve cell," one needs to understand that many nerve cells will be structurally quite different in appearance from the "typical" one used for illustration.

A nerve cell and all that is contained within it together with the processes of the cell are termed a *neuron,* the structural unit of nerve tissue. The processes that convey impulses to the cell are termed *dendrites* and are referred to as *afferent processes* (*ad* meaning "to," *ferre* meaning "to bring"). Those that convey impulses away from the cell for delivery to a muscle or gland or to the dendrites of another nerve cell are *axons* and are referred to as *efferent processes* (*ex* meaning "from"). When an axon of one cell delivers its message to the dendrites of another, the point of transfer is a *synapse* (*syn* meaning "together," *aptein* meaning "clasp"). The surface membrane of neurons and their synaptic connections are the essence of the remarkable process that establishes the integration of the nervous system (Stevens, 1979). It is believed that the synapse offers some resistance to passage of nerve impulses and that the frequency with which impulses are sent along a pathway may influence this resistance so that it is reduced, a factor that may well be a part of perfecting manual or mental skills. Certain drugs, of which strychnine is an example, act at the synapse to speed up or delay transmission. The nerve impulse is generated by the flow of sodium and potassium ions through molecular channels embedded in the nerve membrane (Keynes, 1979).

Inside the nerve cell will be found all the activities of any cell, with the exception of those having to do with cell division and replication. Because nerve cells cannot replace themselves, there will be no centrosome and no mitotic activities to be seen. (Principle 4: After destruction of nerve cells, those remaining are unable to replace those that are lost.) *Nissl bodies,* seen only in nerve cells, appear as heavily stained granules scattered plentifully about in healthy nerve cells. They are nucleoprotein in nature, are concentrations of RNA, and respond promptly to illness of the cell by breaking up and largely disappearing, a situation referred to as *chromolysis.* This is a reversible process, and if the cell recovers, the Nissl substance returns as before. Mitochondria are very numerous, as would be expected in a type of cell with vigorous metabolism.

The description of nerve fibers that follows applies both to afferent and efferent fibers of the peripheral nerves and to efferent fibers within the central nervous system. The only difference that needs to be mentioned is that nerve fibers within the central nervous system lack a *neurolemma* (sheath of Schwann), the outer cellular sheath of the peripheral nerve that permits successful regrowth after destruction of the fiber within, a privilege not accorded to nerve fibers lying within the central axis. Nerve fibers are simple in structure, being tubes of plasma, containing elongated protein molecules (Stevens, 1979).

The *myelin* coat that covers many fibers serves to insulate the fiber and speed conduction along it. Myelinization is the work of the cell of the neurolemma sheath, the Schwann cell, and may involve the neuron itself as well (Stevens, 1979). The process begins in fetal life and continues actively until the individual is about 2 years old and, to a lesser extent, into adolescence. The developing *structure,* with the appearance of myelin, can be seen to correlate with

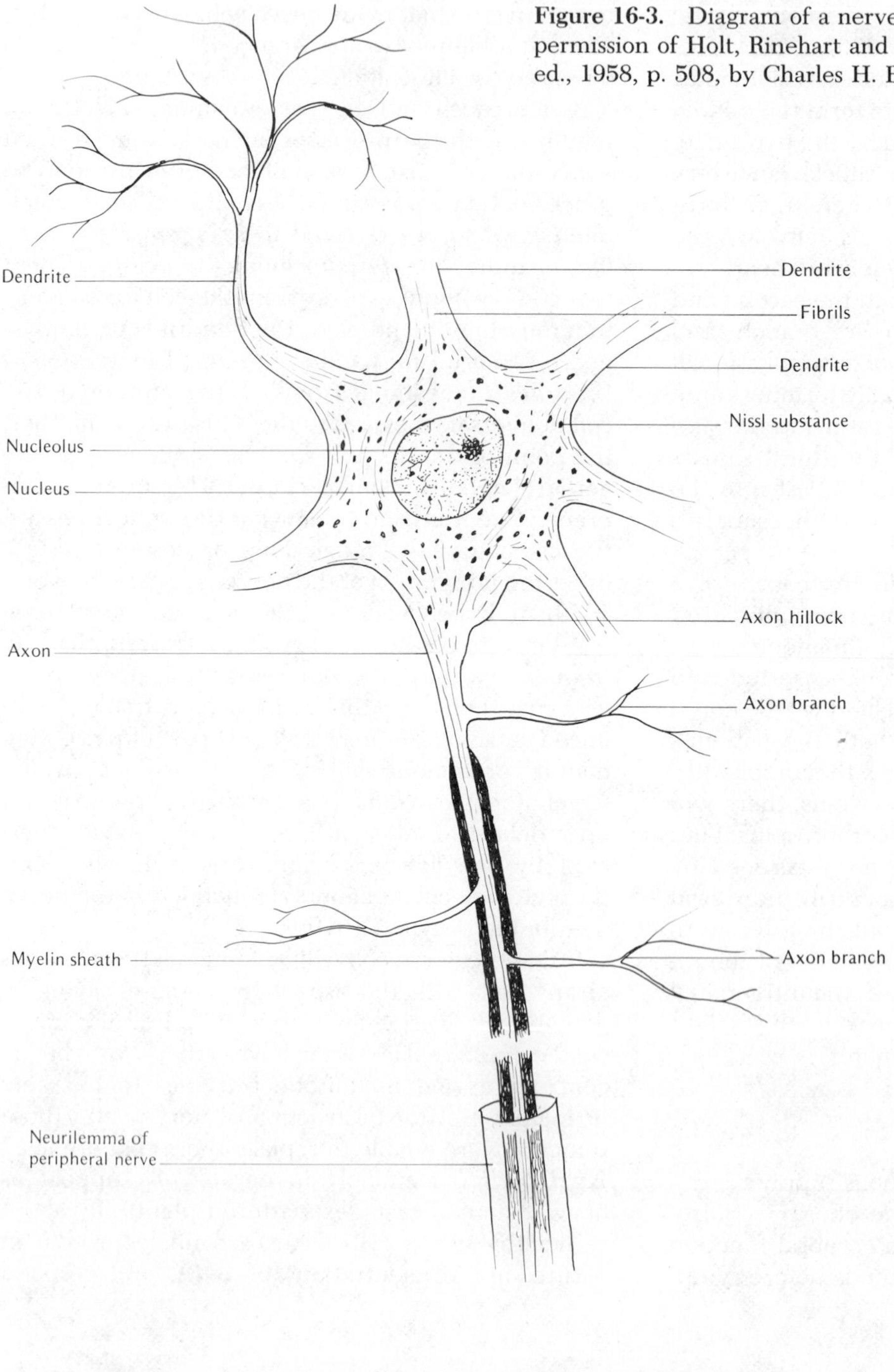

Figure 16-3. Diagram of a nerve cell with processes. (Adapted with permission of Holt, Rinehart and Winston from *The Living Body,* 4th ed., 1958, p. 508, by Charles H. Best and Norman B. Taylor.)

the control of *function* in the maturing organism; for example, it is useless to expect conscious control of bowel and bladder by a child before the age of about 2 years, when myelinization has proceeded to a point where this is possible. It is myelin that names the *white matter* of the nervous system, for nerve cells, or *gray matter,* have no glittering fatty covering to reflect light.

Inside the central nervous system where nerves are without a neurolemma, the process of myelinization depends on certain of the *neuroglial cells.* The neuroglial cells are accessory to the cells of the nervous system and may be likened to connective tissue cells in the body as a whole, in that they support both structure and functions of other tissues. These cells are of several types, *astrocytes, oligocytes,* and *microcytes.* Unlike nerve cells, they are possessed of centrosomes and are capable of reproducing themselves. More than half of intracranial neoplasms are tumors of the neuroglia.

Figures 16-3 and 16-4 show that the nerve fiber itself emerges naked from the cell but, as it proceeds, is very soon wrapped in myelin and covered over by a thin neurolemma. The myelin sheath, however, is broken at short intervals, and the neurolemma appears to be nipped in at this point. Each interruption is termed a *node of Ranvier.* The continuity of the nerve fiber and that of the neurolemma remain; only that of the myelin is broken. Because myelin acts to insulate the contained fiber, nerve fibers that conduct rapidly and for which discreteness of function is important, as, for instance, that of discriminating touch, are heavily insulated by myelin. The neurolemma of each node of Ranvier has a single flattened cell that is vital to the repair of a damaged fiber, a process that, when comprehended, will make clear some points of importance for the care of patients who have suffered damage to peripheral nerves.

Peripheral Nerve Injury

When rapidly growing, skinny Sarah stumbles up the back steps, she trips, falls, and knocks over a milk bottle. As she and the bottle tumble down the steps, the bottle breaks and Sarah cuts her forearm deeply on a fragment of the heavy glass bottle. In addition to incising skin, blood vessels, and muscle, Sarah severs the radial nerve, which is a *mixed peripheral* nerve that supplies a part of her hand. It is a *peripheral* nerve because it lies outside the central nervous system and supplies peripheral areas, and it is *mixed* because it contains, bound up in its structure, many nerve fibers with and without myelin, each with a neurolemma, some of which carry information from Sarah's hand to her spinal cord and brain (afferent fibers) and some of which, the axons of cells located in her spinal cord (efferent

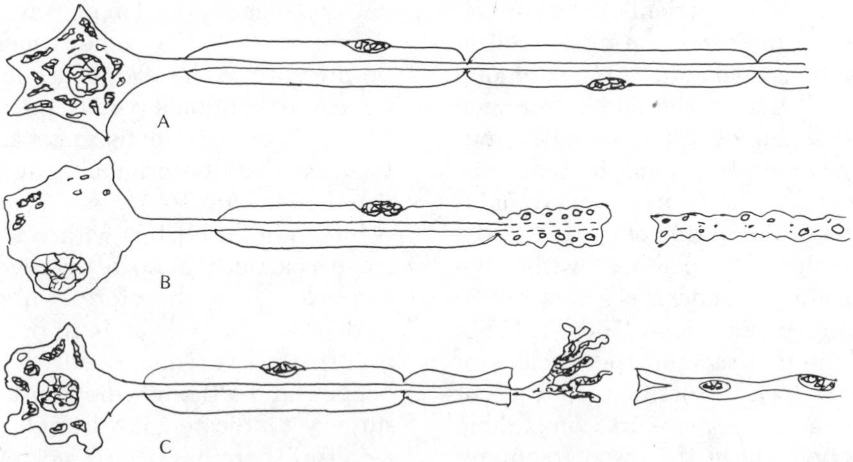

Figure 16-4. Diagram of nerve regeneration. *A.* A normal neuron with its axon enclosed in myelin and a neurolemma sheath. Two nodes are shown. *B.* A neuron two or three days after section of the axon. Retrograde degeneration back to first node proximal to cut; swelling and chromolysis of the cell body, with displacement of the nucleus. Wallerian degeneration in the distal stump; the axon disintegrates, the myelin breaks down into droplets, and only the neurolemma survives. *C.* Beginning of regeneration. The axon sprouts into profuse branches. The cell body reverts toward normal. If a branch of the axon reaches the surviving neurolemma sheath of the distal stump, it will grow down it and restore functional continuity. (Adapted with permission of the J. B. Lippincott Company from *Textbook of Neuroanatomy,* 2nd ed., 1969, Fig. 4-11, p. 50, by H. Chandler Elliott.)

fibers), are responsible for delivering directions for action to the muscles and glands of her hand. The mixed nerve is like a telephone cable in some respects, containing many insulated wires, each with assigned work to perform.

In such an injury, the patient cannot feel anything in the parts once supplied by the now severed nerve: the area supplied is *anesthetic*, or without feeling. The afferent fibers are cut. She cannot move the parts either, and, very shortly, the muscles will begin to atrophy. If an appropriate electric current is supplied, there will be a failure to respond to galvanic current although there continues to be a response to faradic current: the so-called *reaction of degeneration*. This paresis of the parts must follow the break in continuity of the efferent fibers. The muscles are present but they have now lost their innervation: they are *denervated* and cannot act.

Sarah has excellent surgical care, no infection, and good health. Her well-repaired wound heals cleanly. She is careful to follow the directions given her to protect the partly anesthetic hand from thermal or mechanical injury and, a few months later, notes curious prickly sensations, pain, and tingling in her hand. These abnormal sensations, or *paresthesias*, continue to herald the fact that nerve repair is progressing, and eventually Sarah may regain much of what she lost when the radial nerve was severed by the fragment of glass.

The process of reinnervation of the partly denervated hand can be understood by following what goes on in a single fiber of the patient's radial nerve. This fiber originates as the axon of a motor cell in the anterior horn of the spinal cord. It is a very long fiber and was cut well toward the end. After such an injury, the distal fragment of the axon becomes swollen, the myelin disintegrates, and both are disposed of by phagocytosis. The neurolemma remains and survives. On the proximal side of the cut nerve as well there are changes. The cell body within the cord may demonstrate profound shock because of the damage to its process far away. The Nissl substance undergoes chromolysis, and the nucleus of the cell itself loses its central position. At the cut end of the axon, degeneration occurs comparable to that which is happening in the distal fragment, but this proceeds only as far as the next node of Ranvier. In a few days' time, when the cell has recovered its normal healthy state and the injured fiber fragments have been carried away, new little nerve fibrils begin to emerge from the node. They wave about seeming to seek guidance and a path. There are many of them, but it is obvious that only a few will find the waiting neurolemma of the distal stump that is essential both to guiding them to the muscles they should supply and also to provision of myelin needed for efficient performance.

Many of the new fibrils find no way and eventually disappear. If the break between proximal and distal fragments is great, more than a few millimeters, the regenerating fibrils will not find the distal neurolemma at all and, although they will continue to grow for some time, will ball themselves up in a little matted tumor, or *neuroma*, that can be a source of pain. The hand will, of course, remain without innervation and the part will be useless.

The most favorable outcome possible from a peripheral nerve injury such as the one described is not by any means the commonest and depends on circumstances only partly subject to control. At the time of the injury great care must be taken to prevent overvigorous application of a tourniquet. Blood lost can be replaced if it is necessary to do so—a little free bleeding is an effective douche to wash the damaged parts—but compression of the nerve higher up with resulting hypoxia to the entire arm from a tight tourniquet will seriously insult already damaged tissues.

Sarah's mother took a smoothly ironed linen guest towel, laid Sarah's forearm on it, and bandaged the whole forearm from wrist to elbow very firmly with a strip torn from an old sheet, before driving her to the hospital. The towel was reasonably clean, having been ironed and stored in a linen drawer probably free of pathogenic bacteria. Firm pressure exerted over the length of the forearm checks but does not stop bleeding and in no way interferes with arterial supply. The emergency treatment provides gentle pressure to the bleeding points locally and does not cause additional pain to the patient and thereby increased demand on her mechanisms for adaptation to stress that the original trauma has already activated. (See Unit V.)

Infection cured but with resultant scarring may leave a barrier that no newly regenerating axon fibril can cross. It is, therefore, important for everyone to do everything possible to prevent infection from occurring. Everyone needs to be one's brother's keeper; and although the gentlest and most skillful surgery is indicated, it will not bring the best possible results if there has been a lack of respect by anyone for bacteria, for the vulnerability of injured tissue, or for the person of the injured patient.

The third principle given at the beginning of the chapter stated that the more highly specialized a tissue, the less likely it is to survive deficits in supply. A neuron, nerve cell and fiber, has been described, and the effects of injury discussed. Although all nerve tissue is specialized, the specialization varies in degree. We have seen in the foregoing that even the most homogeneous part of the neuron, the fiber, suffers actual dissolution at its point of injury for a measurable distance toward its cell (up to the next node of Ranvier), and that the sensitive cell itself, though many inches away, reflects the shock when serious injury to the fiber is sustained. However, recovery of the shocked cell is prompt, as is the cell's immediate attention to repair its fiber. But this regeneration is not a simple process even in the fiber. It is one that demands no interference with the prescribed sequence and is possible only in the peripheral nerves.

Destruction of Myelin

There are progressive diseases of the nervous system that are known as demyelinating diseases. Of these, *multiple sclerosis* (MS) is the most prevalent. The nurse will see slow, hesitant, inaccurate activity in patients with multiple sclerosis manifested in speech as well as in gross and other fine motor skills. This inadequacy demonstrates the loss of the rapid discrete conduction that their previously well-insulated nerve fibers had accorded them.

Multiple sclerosis may prove to be an autoimmune disease. The myelin sheath is attacked and destroyed, probably by the body's own immune defenses mobilized as a result of a much earlier viral infection. Many investigators believe the causative agent is the measles (rubeola) virus. Obviously, not all people exposed to measles develop MS; evidence suggests that those who do develop MS have a specific immune response gene that renders them susceptible following a viral infection (Maugh, 1977).

Symptoms arise from the altered function of affected myelinated nerves. Patches of destroyed myelin are replaced by scar tissue that interrupts and distorts transmission of impulses. The most common symptoms include numbness, loss of coordination, hand tremors, loss of balance, speech difficulties, and paralysis.

If the viral etiology is proven, it may be possible to eradicate new cases of MS within the next 10 years by immunization. However, present knowledge of causes brings no new hope of cure to MS victims, who now number 500,000 in the United States alone (Maugh, 1977). There is no known cure for MS, for which the peak incidence occurs at age 30, with predominance in women. The disease creates obvious obstacles to achievement of the developmental tasks of young adulthood and the middle years—namely, intimacy and solidarity (young adult) and generativity (middle years). In addition to helping the patient and family accept and safely adapt to the patient's progressive loss of self-help ability, nursing care must be directed toward preventing isolation and self-absorption, which characterize failure of development in the age-group affected by MS. (See Unit VII for approaches to caring for patients with developmental crises.)

The Functional Unit of the Nervous System

As the neuron is the unit of nerve structure, the *reflex arc* is the unit of function. Because nervous structures exist to direct, control, and integrate all parts of the organism, discussion of the reflex arc involves end organs and nerves as well as neurons. In the broadest sense, these are a structure to receive a stimulus and one to react to a stimulus, which may be referred to simply as *receptor* and *effector* end organs. Thus, in simplest form, one may see the reflex arc illustrated when the patellar tendon, the receptor end organ, is stretched by a sharp blow on it, and the leg, the effector end organ, extends in response. This reaction implies the presence of an afferent nerve to convey the impulse to the spinal cord, intact synapses within the cord, and an efferent nerve to take the message for contraction out to the muscles of the leg. All parts of the circuit are needed. Any break in the circuit results in loss of the reflex. Each reflex, whenever elicited, is invariably repeated in the same pattern. It represents a pathway that has become useful to the animal over generations and, as it were, brooks no interference with its habits. A little thought will recall many familiar reflexes: the blink of the eye in response to threat, withdrawal of the finger from a flame, and so on. In the case of peripheral nerve transection described previously, both afferent and efferent fibers were cut by the injury, so the hand was neither aware of the injury nor able to move to react. In poliomyelitis, however, the reflex will be lost because the motor cell in the spinal cord is destroyed by disease; and although the message from the struck tendon can be conveyed to the cord, there is no longer a motor cell within to activate an impulse to be conveyed out to the muscle of the leg.

This cell in the anterior horn of the spinal cord has many dendrites. All directions for the control of motion that are coming down from the brain by way of the descending tracts will eventually end at the synapses on these dendrites. This cell with its processes is therefore called the *lower motor neuron.* The axons that proceed from it to form the spinal and then peripheral nerves are called the *final common path.* In other words, all motion, consciously planned or not, must in the end be effected through these large motor cells and be carried out through these axons, a pathway that, though it may begin as far away as the cortex of the brain, is the last segment in the road on the way to the effector end organ (muscle or gland), and is common for all travelers. The name is a good one; it is the final pathway, to be used by all.

The simple cord reflex used to illustrate a reflex arc requires no planning on the part of individuals, but ordinarily they are aware that it has occurred. They may see it; they may be aware of the coldness or heat of the instrument that struck the knee; they may even inhibit the reflex by an elaborate play of higher activities on these simple ones that have not actually required any involvement of their brain at all.

THE SPINAL CORD

Because this chapter is concerned with the over all administrative system of the body, it is necessary to understand more than the last and simplest unit of action, to appreciate the main channels of communication, some of the lower and higher administrative branches, and how they influence one another. The discussion has referred already to the spinal cord and structures within it, the motor cells with their many dendrites around which axons synapse, bringing impulses from the brain above. Much of the cord is devoted to conveying information up and down its length and also to delivering some of the messages at appropriate stops along the way. The remainder of the cord is concerned with its relations to the periphery of the body. Structurally, the cord reflects these functions. Only slightly larger in diameter than a pencil, it is somewhat elliptical in shape with some increase in size at the thoracic and sacral enlargements. Neatly suspended in the spinal foramina of the vertebrae, two roots emerge on each side, one dorsal and one ventral, and pass through foramina in each vertebra. These roots presently join, and from this point on belong to the peripheral nervous system, which has just been discussed briefly in considering the reflex arc.

Looked at in cross section, the cord shows a central, H-shaped portion made up of cells, or gray matter, lying with a heavy border of fiber masses, or white matter. Many of the cells are those of neurons that are responsible for intercommunication within the cord: these are connectors that constitute a large part of the bulk of nervous tissue and are termed *internuncial* neurons. The white matter or nerve fibers of the cord tend to be grouped according to function; each group of fibers that is fairly discrete is called a *tract* and has a name. The form of the name usually indicates the direction of the tract, the point of origin being stated first and the destination second. Thus the *spinocerebellar tract* names a group of nerve fibers that conveys from the spinal cord to the cerebellum, which may be required to act on this knowledge, information about the state of contraction of muscles. A tract, then, represents a group of nerve fibers all of which have the same function.

Ascending Tracts

The first neuron implicated in conveying a sensation to the brain is the neuron whose cell is located in a small swelling in the dorsal root just outside the spinal cord, called the posterior or *dorsal root ganglion* (see Figure 16-5). The processes of this cell extend in two directions; the shorter one extends centrally to enter the cord in the dorsal part and the other extends to the periphery to end in muscle, in skin, or around a hair follicle. This process extending to the periphery should be recognized as a single afferent unit in the cable of the peripheral nerve. It will terminate in one or another of a specialized nerve ending, peculiarly adapted to its place and function. Fibers that carry pain are naked and end in little brushes that cover a considerable surface, a square centimeter (Elliott, 1963, p. 118), and may overlap one another, whereas touch, for which the animal requires far more discrimination than for

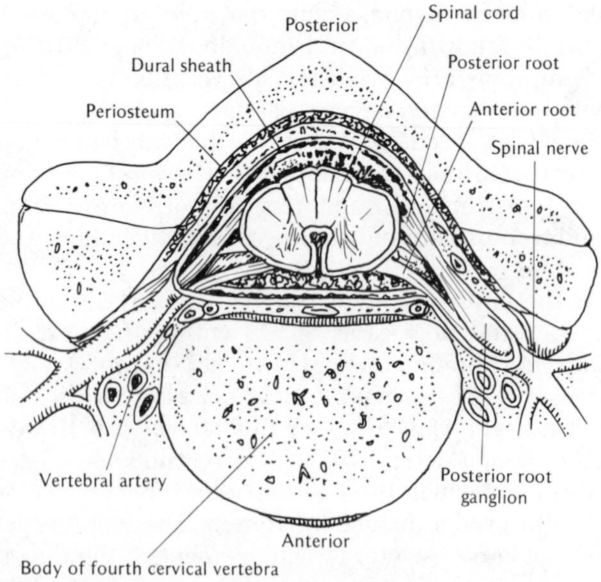

Figure 16-5. Cross section of vertebral column at the level of the fourth cervical vertebra, showing spinal cord in position. (Adapted with permission of the J. B. Lippincott Company from *Basic Physiology and Anatomy*, 1964, Fig. 136, p. 203, by Ellen E. Chaffee and Ester M. Greisheimer.)

pain, is provided with a myelinated fiber and three kinds of specialized endings. Cold, heat, pressure—each is represented by its own ending adapted to meet the need (see Figure 16-6). Each specialized ending, on stimulation, sends the message along the sensory nerve fiber to the cell in the dorsal root ganglion whence it proceeds into the dorsomesial part of the cord. If this sensation is one of pain or temperature, the fiber, on entering the cord, ascends a segment or two and ends on the dendrites of a second neuron that immediately *decussates* (crosses over to the other side), to travel in the *spinothalamic* tract in the lateral part of the spinal cord to the thalamus (see Figure 16-7).

The *proprioceptive* pathway accounts for the conveyance of those sensations that are peculiarly one's own, within oneself (*proprio* meaning "own"). These are the muscle–tendon–joint sensations and vibration. It is by means of these columns that one is aware of one's position in space. It is not, for example, necessary to look at one's foot to know where it is and whether or not the knee is bent. These fibers enter the cord by way of the dorsal root and sweep upward into the great wedge-shaped columns that occupy the whole dorsum of the cord. These columns are variously named, and the student should recognize *dorsal* or *posterior columns, fasciculus gracilis* and *fasciculus cuneatus,* and *dorsal fasciculus* as terms that indicate these tracts that proceed without decussation to the medulla, where the fibers end on secondary neurons. These fibers decussate at once and proceed as the *medial lemniscus* to the thalamus.

Reference has been made previously to the spinocerebellar tract, another afferent pathway of the spinal cord, but this one goes to the cerebellum. This tract lies at the periphery of the cord in two distinct divisions. The fibers conduct with great rapidity and are heavily myelineated. They ascend for a considerable way before they synapse with secondary neurons that are scattered along in the dorsal columns. Because the cerebellum is responsible for rapid adjustments of posture, it requires quick and accurate information. The spinocerebellar tract keeps the cerebellum continously informed on the state of contraction of muscles and of any change in tension. A disease that is not commonly seen today, tertiary syphilis, may result in degeneration of the dorsal columns which, it will be recalled, convey also part of touch as well as proprioception and vibration. Patients with this disease suffer many disabilities, of which loss of position sense, *ataxia* (without order), and awkward, faulty coordination (cerebellar adjustment) are conspicuous. This condition is called *tabes dorsalis* (*tabes* meaning "decay," *dorsalis* meaning "of the back").

Figure 16-6. Specialized nerve endings. (Adapted with permission of Macmillan Publishing Co., Inc., from *Anatomy and Physiology,* 14th ed., 1961, Fig. 169, p. 202, by Diana Clifford Kimber, Carolyn E. Gray, Caroline E. Stackpole, and Lutie C. Leavell.)

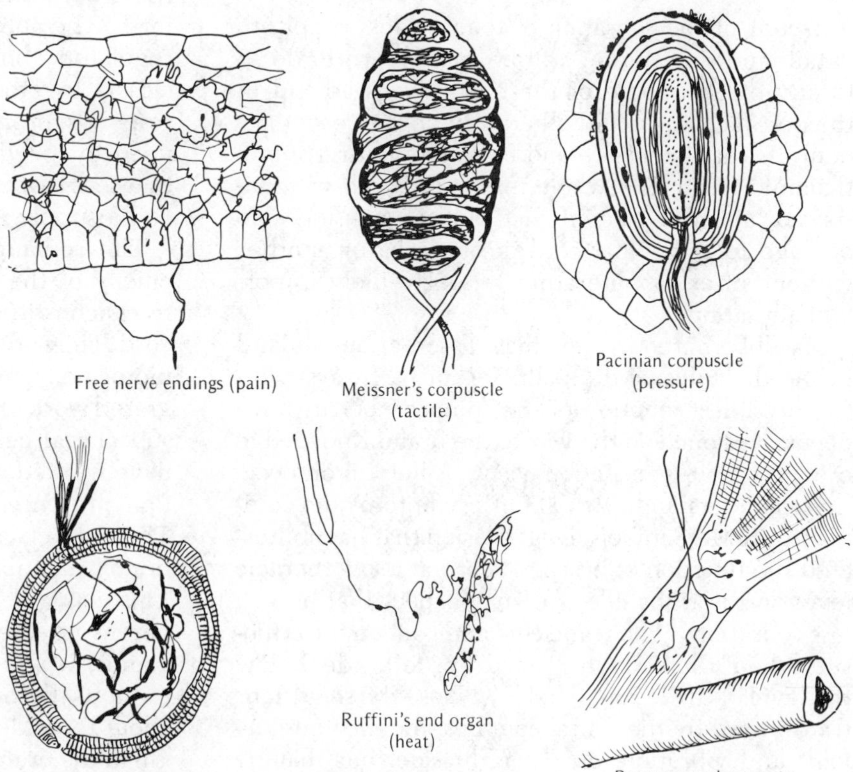

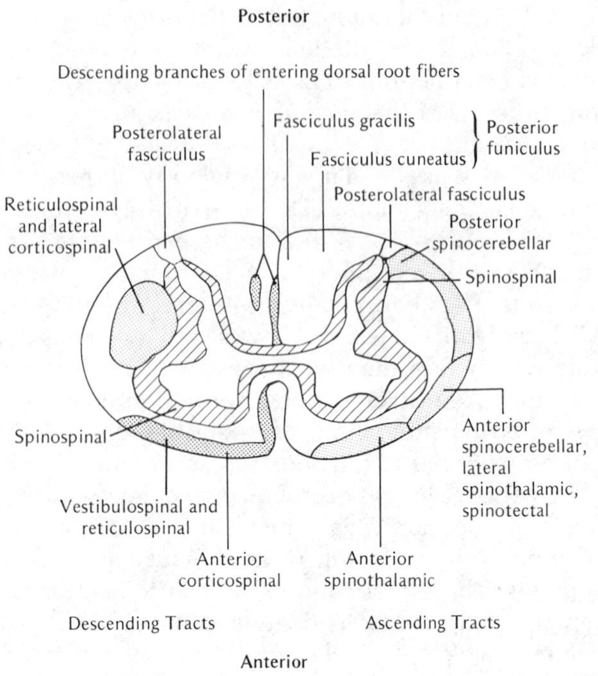

Figure 16-7. The main tracts of the spinal cord. Afferent, ascending tracts on the right side; efferent, descending tracts on the left. It must be remembered, however, that both ascending and descending fibers are present on each side. (Adapted with permission of the W. B. Saunders Company from *Fundamentals of Neurology,* 5th ed., 1968, Fig. 134, p. 246, by Ernest Gardner.)

Ascent of the sensation of touch is less simple to detail, and no attempt will be made here to do so to any extent. Some of the touch axons ascend in the dorsal columns and others end on the secondary neurons that decussate and form the ventral spinothalamic tract. The whole inflow of touch is widespread, an arrangement that permits considerable damage to the spinal cord in one area or another without utterly obliterating this extremely important sensation.

It will be noted by now that (1) sensations all land in the thalamus, and (2) all afferent pathways, with the possible exception of the spinocerebellar, have decussated once on the way to the brain. Knowledge of where that decussation occurs is helpful on occasion to understanding a patient's symptoms and complaints. If Mr. Samuelson has a lesion that has obliterated the function of his spinal cord at a low thoracic level on the right side, one may expect that he will lose sensations of heat and cold and pain on the opposite side of the body, his "good," or left, side, below the level of the lesion; that he will lose the sensations transmitted by the dorsal columns, muscle–tendon–joint and vibration, on the right side; but that he will retain some awareness of touch, however defective, on both sides. The nurse who is aware of the patient's sensory deficit will recognize the hazards involved in mechanical or thermal damage to Mr. Samuelson's legs and also to his peace of mind if he notes the defective perception in his "good," left leg.

Up to this point we have considered these structures in the spinal cord—the afferent pathways and the neurons that convey messages within the cord—and we have mentioned the large motor cells of the anterior horn of spinal cord gray matter that form, with their processes, the *lower motor neuron* and whose axons are the *final common path.* A third cell found in the *thoracolumbar* part of the cord belongs to the efferent system of the *sympathetic nervous system.* The axons of these cells emerge from the anterior, or motor, root of the cord along with those of the anterior horn cell, and most of them have a synapse with dendrites of cells in the sympathetic chain lying paravertebrally outside. The cells of the *parasympathetic nervous system,* or *craniosacral* division of the autonomic nervous system, are quite differently placed. The cells of the cranial division are found in the brain stem and those of the sacral division in the sacral cord, in two compact masses and some scattered cells. (See Chapter 18 for further discussion of the autonomic nervous system.) Hormones are chemicals, and chemicals act diffusely; even chemicals that act quickly may not be at hand at the right moment unless there is something authoritative that reacts quickly to call them forth. The autonomic nervous system and the other regulators, hormones, enzymes, and so on, work closely together, but it is the nervous system that responds promptly when, for instance, there is a need to speed up the heart in an emergency, and that sees to it that epinephrine is produced promptly and a supply maintained.

The remaining parts of the spinal cord consist chiefly of the descending or efferent tracts. These tracts constitute the rest of the white matter of the cord. They are concerned with bringing to the lower motor neuron the results of the concerted and integrated work of the higher centers: the cortex, various subcortical cell masses, and the cerebellum, which have worked and planned together on the information presented to them by the afferent pathways. These tracts are now bringing the result of the brain's planning to deliver to the anterior horn cell. This cell will send it out by way of the peripheral nerves to the final performers, the muscles and glands. It will be simpler, because the student has by now the outlines of the circuit traced, to learn about these descending tracts from their sites of origin in the brain. Therefore discussion of the descending tracts will be included in Chapter 17 with brain function.

References Cited

Bergland, R. M., and Page, R. B. "Pituitary-Brain Vascular Relations: A New Paradigm." *Science,* **204** (6 April 1979), 18–24.

Elliott, H. C. *Textbook of Neuroanatomy.* Philadelphia: J. B. Lippincott Company, 1963.

Guyton, A. C. *Textbook of Medical Physiology,* 5th ed. Philadelphia: W. B. Saunders Company, 1976.

Keynes, R. D. "Ion Channels in the Nerve-Cell Membrane." *Sci. Am.,* **240** (March 1979), 126–35.

Maugh, T. H., III. "Multiple Sclerosis: Genetic Link, Viruses Suspected." *Science,* **195** (18 Feb. 1977), 667–69.

Stevens, C. F. "The Neuron." *Sci. Am.,* **241** (Sept. 1979), 54–65.

General References

Bannister, R. *Brain's Clinical Neurology,* 4th ed. New York: Oxford University Press, 1973.

Clark, R. G. *Manter and Gatz's Essentials of Clinical Neuroanatomy and Neurophysiology,* 5th ed. Philadelphia: F. A. Davis Company, 1975.

Gardner, E. *Fundamentals of Neurology,* 5th ed. Philadelphia: J. B. Lippincott Company, 1968.

Kurland, L. T., Kurtzke, J. F., and Goldberg, I. D. *Epidemiology of Neurologic and Sense Organ Disorders,* Cambridge, Mass.: Harvard University Press, 1973.

Matzke, H. A., and Foltz, F. M. *Synopsis of Neuroanatomy,* 2nd ed. New York: Oxford University Press, 1972.

Truex, R. C., and Carpenter, M. B. *Human Neuroanatomy,* 6th ed. Baltimore: The Williams & Wilkins Company, 1969.

17

Integration of Neural Regulation—Brain Function

No one knows what he can do til he tries

MAXIM 786, PUBLILIUS SYRUS

Overview of the Brain

It is now time to reexamine the cranial cavity to discuss the brain, which is itself responsible for originating much of what is carried out by the cord and peripheral nerves as well as all that goes on in respect to the special senses, vision, hearing, and so on, and everything that we think of as "brains," such as higher thought, emotion, learning, and memory.

Learning and memory are neural functions of great consequence for the nurse in dealing with any patient problem for which teaching is an appropriate part of nursing management. Although progress is slow in unlocking the secrets of the mechanisms by which we learn and remember, it is now generally believed that learning and memory would not be possible in any form without the existence of a particular group of previously nonfunctional synapses that "open" only as the result of a specific unconditional stimulus from the environment. As yet there is not sufficient evidence to support a biochemical theory of learning, which contends that the critical physiologic event in learning is the very first activation of a previously nonfunctional synapse. Most researchers believe that protein synthesis is a crucial factor in the process. Edelman, an immunologist, suggests that mechanisms similar to those that enable immunologically active cells to recognize foreign material may also play a role in the brain's own memory system (Stoler, 1974). It has also been shown that memory, a necessary ingredient of learning, depends upon emotional arousal, and that the arousal state of an individual is regulated through those neurons that use catecholamines as transmitters (Huttunen, 1973). These findings are another link in the chain of evidence for unitary regulation of autonomic and central nervous system functions; for the indivisibility of mind, body, and emotions. The nurse who would help a patient to learn must reach him or her through feeling as well as reason.

The profound influence exerted on learning by the quality of interpersonal communication is presently acknowledged though poorly understood. Many studies have demonstrated that the power of expectation alone can influence the behavior of others (Rosenthal, 1973). Nurses use this powerful tool to support and motivate patients when helping them to formulate realistic goals and showing by patient and persistent assistance that they fully expect the patients to achieve those goals. The "Head Start" programs of the late 1960s for preschool-age children were an effort to promote childhood development through increasing environmental stimuli. Although the results with the Head Start children were inconclusive, there is experimental evidence that animals placed in an enriched or impoverished environment exhibit measurable changes in brain anatomy and chemistry (Rosenzweig et al., 1972).

As the brain developed in higher animals from the simple linear structure seen in worms, and tended to concentrate at the anterior end of the animal, it bent back upon itself, and, in higher mammals and humans, developed and enormously enlarged certain parts, notably the cerebral hemispheres. These great hemispheres, that bubble over and obscure almost all else seen by the casual viewer, cover up the evidence that remains of the curves and bends in the structure of the brain, which is finally crammed into a space and maintained at a weight (1,400 gm) that a human can support and still not be top-heavy. Study of the brain's development in the embryo does demonstrate these changes, and even in the cut adult brain one can easily note that the lower parts, *medulla oblongata,* or *bulb,* and *midbrain,* are in direct linear continuity with the cord and are smaller and less complicated in physical form than are other much larger, evolutionarily newer, parts. These newer parts, some of the cerebellum, and the cerebral hemispheres show, even on gross examination, much greater bulk than bulb and midbrain, and reveal an enormous surface area that has been achieved by wrinkling and folding of the surface layers. Even a cursory view of the cut brain should demonstrate two other points that are helpful in looking at the structural basis for control and integration of function from a developmental point of view and that recall principles stated in the beginning of the chapter. (Principle 5: Within the nervous system there is a hierarchy of control. No single part functions separately from other parts. Principle 6: The nervous system imposes regulation and control not only on organs and systems of the body but also on itself. Principle 7: In general, higher centers inhibit lower centers and phylogenetically newer parts of the brain inhibit older or lower centers.)

On examination of the brain, two things are striking: (1) Heavy bands of white matter are evident running between parts recognizable as gray matter, and (2) although it is obvious that the surface of cerebrum and cerebellum is gray matter, that is, made up of nerve cells, there are a good many other masses of cells lying embedded in white matter paired up along the central axis. These clumps of gray matter, literally covered up, and to an extent metaphorically as well, by the cerebral hemispheres, are referred to as *nuclei.*[1] They were present and more completely dominant in simpler animals before the cerebral cortex developed and overwhelmed them. We shall make frequent reference to these cell masses from now on, for although in humans they are by no means at the top of the hierarchy of control, they are of great importance to them, and when any of these structures are damaged directly or thrown out of kilter by being poorly informed, integrated performance is handicapped. Studies of integrated performance have demonstrated that an individual can continue to function normally after the two hemispheres of the healthy brain have been split or disconnected from each other. However, disease localized in only one of the hemispheres creates predictable difficulties because of specialized functions of each hemisphere. It is well established that the left hemisphere dominates language ability. Ornstein (1973) suggests that the left hemisphere is the logician and the right hemisphere the artist. Anatomical asymmetries normally found between the cerebral hemispheres may help to explain the range of human talents, recovery from acquired disorders of language function (such as the loss of speech—*aphasia*—which sometimes accompanies stroke), some dementing illnesses of middle life, and certain childhood learning disabilities (Galaburda et al., 1978).

What one sees, hears, smells, tastes, or feels must involve anatomically many parts if it is to be physiologically useful. One must not simply see or hear the car coming round the corner but retreat to the curb to avoid being struck, an act that utilizes many nervous connections from the instant the eye or ear perceives the threat until the muscles of trunk and leg effect the life-saving backward steps. This activity involves sense organs, the cerebral cortex, the cerebellum and subcortical cell masses, reticular formation in the brain stem, and efferent tracts in the cord. All these will be considered in their turn. Before going further it may be well to review, restate somewhat differently, and add a bit.

Above the cord, the relatively simple form of an H-shaped mass of cells surrounded by fiber tracts becomes modified. Centrally, from bulb to thalamus, there is the reticular formation, a loose-appearing network of cells and nerve fibers in which some quite discrete cell masses are seen. From the bulb to the *pons* (bridge) the pairs of cranial nerves branch off; the cells of these nerves form nuclei that are embedded in pairs along the way (see Figure 17-1). Still larger masses of cells are to be found as one moves upward, and all are surrounded by the great masses of white matter, tracts carrying their messages from one area to another, connecting, projecting, and associating the work of their cells. The greatest bulk of white matter will be found in the cerebral hemispheres, and there, too, are the greatest number of nerve cells, spread in the thin wrinkled layers of the *cerebral cortex* (*cortex* meaning "bark"). It is these millions of cells that initiate; and it is their fibers, their axons and dendrites (some so short that they run only between cells of the cortex itself and some so long that they pass all the way to the spinal cord), that make possible those activities that are most characteristically human—complex thinking, memory, judgment, and highly developed learning

[1] This use of the word *nuclei* may confuse the student. The term as used in this paragraph, and as used considerably in the text that follows, means a group of nerve cells and does not refer to the central structure of a single cell. Examples: (1)The *red nucleus* (group of cells) is in the midbrain. (2) The two major divisions of a cell are the *nucleus* (the central organizing part of a single cell) and the *cytoplasm.*

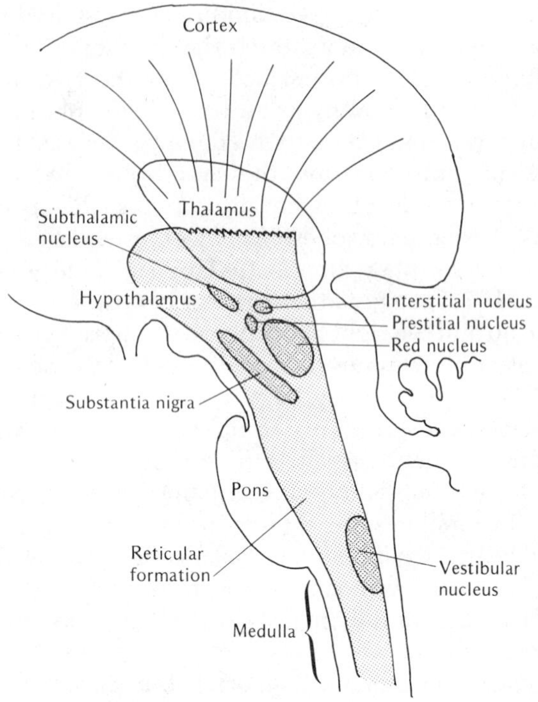

Figure 17-1. The reticular formation and its relationship to adjacent structures of the brain stem and cerebrum. (Adapted with permission of the W. B. Saunders Company from *Textbook of Medical Physiology,* 5th ed., 1976, Fig. 52-1, p. 695, by Arthur Guyton.)

skills. These cells are at the top of the hierarchy: they are newest in evolutionary and embryologic development. Although the most human, they are least vital in a biological sense and the most intolerant of hypoglycemia and anoxia. (Principle 8: The later in embryonic life that a part of the nervous system develops, the more susceptible it is to injury.)

Looking at the nervous system from a developmental point of view and at the cerebral hemispheres as latecomers, one will realize that biologic control and integration must have been possible for the organism before the cerebrum was there. The structures involved, which are both dominated by the cerebrum in humans and yet important to the integrity of cerebral function, are the vestibular nuclei belonging to the eighth cranial nerve, thalamus, cerebellum, basal ganglia, reticular formation, and a number of cell masses enclosed within it.

Reticular Formation

Some of these cell masses, or nuclei, just referred to, seem in the course of evolution to have condensed from a more diffuse-appearing substance, made up of scattered cells and fibers, that extends along the central axis from the bulb through the pons to the posterior part of the hypothalamus and into the ventral thalamus. This diffuse nerve cell—fiber system is called the *reticular formation* (*reticulum* meaning "net"). The reticular formation has become a subject of intense interest to neurophysiologists relatively recently. Although there is still much to be learned about this interesting area, certain contributions of the reticular formation at different levels throughout its length have nevertheless been determined.

Functionally the reticular formation of the brain stem corresponds to the internuncial neurons of the spinal cord, neurons that work like the U.S. Senate page boys, taking information from one committee of the legislature to another, committees that will facilitate or inhibit action. In this formation, a vast number of reflex connections are made: all those for the cranial nerves and many others, some of which will be noted in discussion of the basal ganglia. Stimulation of parts of the reticular formation excites muscle activity, whereas stimulation of other parts inhibits it—a sort of brake-and-throttle action.

An important part of the life of any animal is sleep; and for animals that must respond quickly to the advent of danger or the presence of approaching prey, a ready change to alertness is as vital. The anterior part of the reticular formation alerts the whole cerebrum. This is accomplished by connections to the hypothalamus, to the thalamus, and thence to both the cortex and basal ganglia. The brain, thus made alert, is quickly cleared for action whether this be for the sleeping cat to waken and run across the lawn and leap into the grape arbor to escape the collie dog, or to develop a strategy and adjust its entire muscular system in order to catch a field mouse in the meadow in the evening.

In disease, the effect of this reticular activating system on the cortex as a whole can be illustrated by two examples. In an attack of *grand mal* epilepsy, it can be shown electrically that this part of the reticular formation is excessively stimulated. An electroencephalogram will demonstrate that the entire cerebral cortex is experiencing extreme neuronal activity during the convulsion (Guyton, 1976, p. 737). On the other hand, when this area is destroyed, either by disease or by mutilation, of which encephalitis and gunshot wounds are examples, the patient presents the appearance of being asleep and cannot be wakened.

In subsequent chapters the student will become familiar with the neurophysiology of respiration (respiratory center) and with factors that affect arterial pressure (vasomotor center). These are parts of the reticular formation. The needs of the body for more or less pulmonary ventilation are mediated through connections in the reticular formation, as are other homeostatic mechanisms; so are the sympathetic and parasympathetic control of the heart and vascular system, and relays from the hypothalamus for control of temperature and other affairs of metabolism.

Thalamus

Anatomically, the *thalamus* lies above the brain stem and beneath the cortex, seeming to push up against the floor of the lateral ventricles. It is bounded on its sides and below by the fibers of the internal capsule that are wedged between the thalamus and basal ganglia. Although the most primitive part of the thalamus has no connections to the cortex because it developed in simple animals that had none, the rest of the thalamus is organized into large nuclei, cells onto which specific sensory tracts discharge and from which the information they bear is sent on to the cortex to be associated with different information coming from other thalamic sources, and is appreciated, integrated and acted on. The cerebral cortex, in turn, reports to the thalamus. The trip by the sensations to the cortex and back seems by some means to have modified and refined the traveler, for the thalamus itself has a sort of coarse, undisciplined, conscious awareness that can be demonstrated when the cortex of an animal is removed. The creature reacts excessively: the decorticated cat will spit and snarl in response to a stimulus at which a normal cat would simply rise, stretch, and walk away. The cat with the mutilated nervous system has no means by which to evaluate the stimulus: if it is of a noxious nature, no matter how minor, the cat "gives it all he has" in response. The normal cat, on the other hand, has all the integrating mechanisms intact and, evaluating the minor nature of the annoyance as just that, the cat simply moves away and conserves energy for a real emergency.

Absence of the cortex results in dementia with impaired memory, speech, judgment, and insight and *intensity of affect* (an emotional response out or relation to the stimulus). This intensity of affect is caused by loss of the disciplining effect of the intact cortex on the thalamus and is an illustration of Principle 7: Higher centers inhibit lower and phylogenetically newer parts inhibit older. Pleasure centers of the brain previously believed to be located in the thalamus are now seen as belonging to a system of pathways that appears to play a role in learning and memory, a complex referred to as the brain-reward system. The boundaries of the brain-reward system have been extended deep into the brainstem and far forward into the cortex of the frontal lobe of the cerebrum. All the reward systems do, however, have pathways through the medial forebrain bundle, suggesting that this region of the hypothalamus may be described as the relay station through which the brain-reward pathways course (Routtenberg, 1978).

Psychoactive drugs that *enhance transmission* at dopamine (DA) and norepinephrine (NE) synapses tend to *potentiate* self-stimulation or initiation behaviors and to enhance learning and memory; psychoactive drugs that *block transmission* at DA and NE synapses tend to *inhibit* self-stimulation or initia-

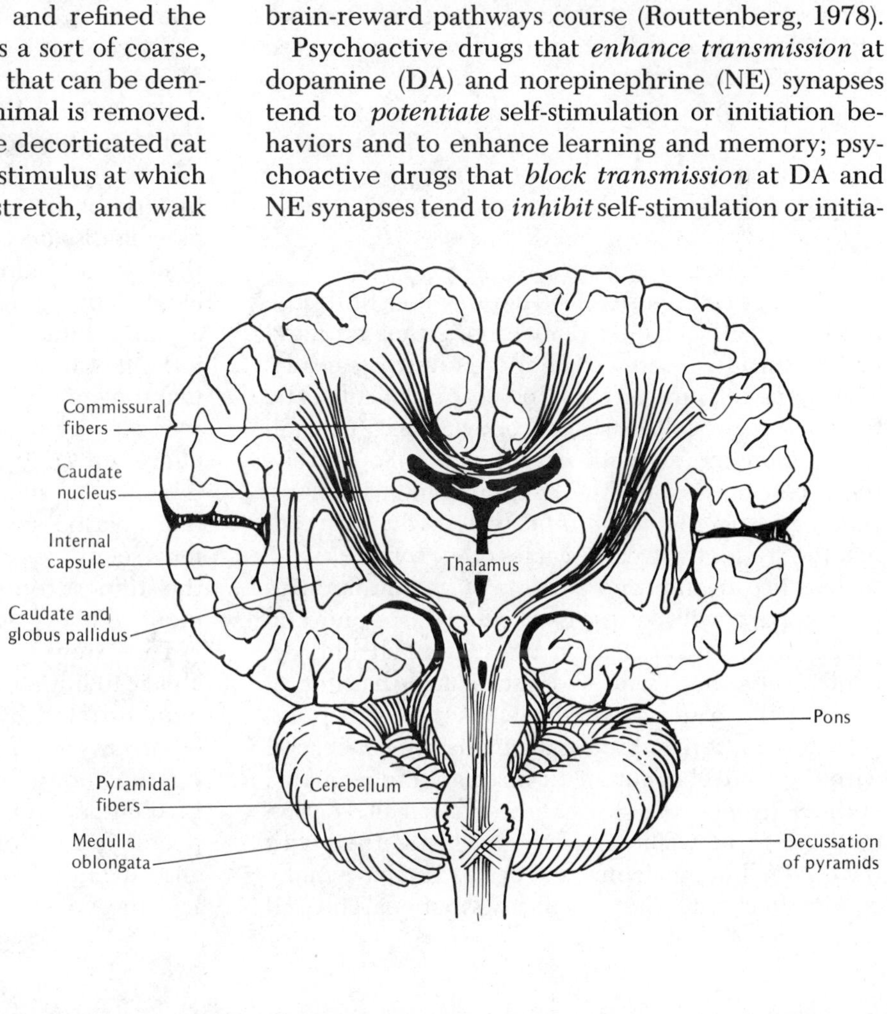

Figure 17-2. Vertical transverse section through the brain. (Adapted with permission of Holt, Rinehart and Winston from *The Living Body*, 4th ed., 1958, Fig. 12-16, p. 538, by Charles H. Best and Norman B. Taylor.)

tion behaviors and to impair learning and memory (Routtenberg, 1978).

Intensive investigation is being done to identify possible biochemical factors that contribute to affective disorders, especially to depression, one of our major health problems. Present evidence indicates that depressed patients have a functional deficit of norepinephrine in the brain. It is now taken for granted that the affective tone of the mind that determines our moods and attitudes depends especially on the balance of the neurotransmitters; the cause–effect relationship is not clear. Many drugs, such as lithium, being used to treat depressive states exert their effect on the metabolic processes of the catecholamines rather than on any discrete region of the brain (Maas, 1973).

The thalamus has connections to all the subcortical cell masses that have been mentioned, the hypothalamus, basal ganglia, red nucleus, and so on, and to the cerebellum. It is a most important correlation center that must have its material in order before presenting it to the cortex and that must then take an active part—as an intermediary to be kept informed—in order that no details of the performance that is ordered by the cortex, on the basis of information received, should go astray.

Although the thalamus is to be thought of chiefly as sensory, the basal ganglia, also large cell masses situated nearby, are parts of the motor system (see Figure 17-2).

Basal Ganglia

The large cell masses or nuclei that constitute the basal ganglia lie slightly caudal to the thalamus and on the outside of the wedge of the internal capsule. The nomenclature of these bodies is difficult. The term *corpus striatum* (striped body) can be used almost synonymously with *basal ganglia.* Separately, these cell masses are the *caudate* (tailed) nucleus, *putamen,* and *globus pallidus* (pale body). In reading, the student will come across other terms as well, such as *neostriatum* and *paleostriatum.* In this chapter the parts will be discussed simply as a unit and called the basal ganglia, but the student should recognize the other terms and also realize that not all parts of the basal ganglia have identical functions.

In general terms, the basal ganglia are concerned with the control of automatic associated movements of the body (e.g., the swing of the arms in alternation to the legs in walking). They work together with the cerebellum, thalamus, and cortex and have many connections with the reticular formation. The red nucleus in the reticular formation of the midbrain is the origin of a main efferent descending tract, the *rubrospinal,* which carries directions for control to the lower motor neuron and thence to muscles or glands.

Some of the motor tracts originating in the brainstem are short and completely contained within the brain itself (e.g., for eye movements), whereas others run in close proximity to the voluntary motor tract, the pyramidal, whose origin is cortical. All these tracts decussate and therefore exert control on the side of the body opposite their origin. The student can easily determine their origins and destinations simply by their names: reticulospinal, reticulobulbar, and so on. Their great responsibility for the perfection of motor control can be grasped best by observing the problems of those who have disease in any of the nuclei from which they rise.

When there is injury or disease referable to the basal ganglia and nearby nuclei in the reticular formation, the individual is greatly handicapped. Depending on the part involved, the individual not only loses automatic associated control but also is beset with a variety of nuisance movements that plague him or her, and also by alteration in muscle tone, a rigidity that makes every move more difficult. The student can easily learn to recognize these aberrations.

Athetosis is a writhing, wormlike squirminess. In *chorea* there are contractions of muscles occurring without control, so that the sequence of movement is interrupted and the patient accomplishes nothing effectively, for he or she is repeatedly thrown off by jerks of interrupted patterns. The *tremor* of basal ganglia disease is most obvious in the hands, which tend to be held pointing medially, fingers rather close, moving against the thumb in what is called a "pill-rolling" tremor. *Hemiballismus* is a violent jerking of large parts of the body. Like other abnormal movements of basal ganglia disease, hemiballismus may be provoked or made worse by voluntary efforts for controlled movement on the part of the patient. The rigidity seen in damage to basal ganglia is of a plastic type. When quite at ease, the individual may seem free of it, but on effort or with anxiety, the stiffness returns to resist the smooth accomplishment of every act.

The extent to which one is disabled by loss of the ability to initiate or control movement is graphically demonstrated by the increasing number of victims of *Parkinson's disease,* which is characterized by disturbance in muscle tone and bodily posture, and by involuntary movement. Approximately 1.5 million people in the United States have Parkinson's disease, and this number is growing as life spans lengthen. It is the nation's third most disabling disease and is considered the most common neurological disorder of the aging. Patients, predominantly men, usually experience the first symptoms when they reach their sixties (Fishbach, 1978).

As nothing has yet been discovered to cure or completely arrest the disease, treatment is symptomatic, and includes physical therapy, supportive psychological services, and drug therapy. In addition to Parkinson's disease, some types of cerebral palsy are diseases wherein the basal ganglia are affected.

Vestibular Nuclei

That portion of the eighth cranial nerve that comes from the vestibular, or labyrinthine, portion of the ear and is concerned with informing the brain of the position and change of direction of the head in order that appropriate adjustments can be made to maintain equilibrium is called the vestibular portion of the eighth, or auditory, nerve. It has four nuclei in an irregular line along the floor of the fourth ventricle at the level of the caudal portion of the pons and upper portion of the medulla oblongata. As the vestibular fibers coming from the peripheral sense organ, the ear, enter the central nervous system, they bifurcate. Some of the branches go to a fifth vestibular nucleus in that part of the cerebellum that is phylogenetically the oldest, having arisen in animals (fishes) whose most important problem in coordination is maintaining appropriate swimming position. (You will recall noting that the dying goldfish keeps losing this position and slips over onto its side.) The other branches go to one or another of the four pairs of vestibular nuclei more centrally located. The bulk of the fibers of secondary neurons collects to form a tract, the vestibulospinal, that descends in the cord and ends on cells many of which control extensor muscles of the limbs.[2]

The whole vestibular apparatus, from ear to brainstem to cerebellar nuclei to efferent cell in the cord, helps to keep the animal on an even keel. When the horse is galloping round the ring, its legs on the inside must take up more sharply or it will topple on the curving track. The horse's vestibular apparatus contributes to maintaining perfection of gait even though this demands continuous adjustment because of the constant curve of the riding ring.

[2] When the brainstem is cut across just above these nuclei, the decerebrated animal goes into a state of *extensor rigidity.* This state may be seen in human beings when, through disease, the brainstem and cord are functionally cut off from control of higher parts, as with any large intracerebral mass that compresses the upper brainstem. This is called in humans *decerebrate rigidity.* (See Principles 6 and 7.)

Cerebellum

The cerebellum is the largest division of the brain after the cerebral hemispheres. Situated posterior to the central axis, it is connected by three large masses of white matter, the cerebellar peduncles, to the pons, midbrain, and medulla oblongata. The cerebellar cortex consists of two layers whose cells are provided with an enormous number of processes. The Purkinje cell, which is the effector cell, has so extensive a provision of branching dendrites that it looks like a microscopic Japanese barberry bush. The cellular structure and arrangement of the cerebellar cortex are such that incoming stimuli will excite a wide cortical area (see Figure 17-3).

The cerebellum has evolved with the increasing complexity of the animal, as has the rest of the brain, and several divisions can be recognized that are correlated with phylogenetic age. We have spoken of one, the most primitive, that is simply an outgrowth of the vestibular system, but shall here, as was done in the case of the basal ganglia, discuss briefly the function of the cerebellum, not in parts, but as a whole.

In reviewing the material to this point the student will recall that

1. The afferent tracts to the cerebellum report to it the existing state of contraction of muscles and changes in tension; that the fibers are heavily myelinated and conduct with great rapidity.
2. The basal ganglia, concerned with control of associated movement and acting on information received from thalamus and cortex, report to midbrain centers.
3. The reflex connections of the cranial nerves, vestibular included, whose nuclei are in bulb and pons, take place in the reticular formation.
4. There are connections of these structures to thalamus and cerebral cortex.

It must, then, be evident, with mention of the large peduncles of white matter that bind the cerebellum to all these structures by way of their connections to the brainstem, that the cerebellum works with them all, and this is the case. Its work is in association with others, not independent. There is, for example, no tract running from cerebellum to cord. In its function the cerebellum illustrates especially well the second parts of the fourth and the

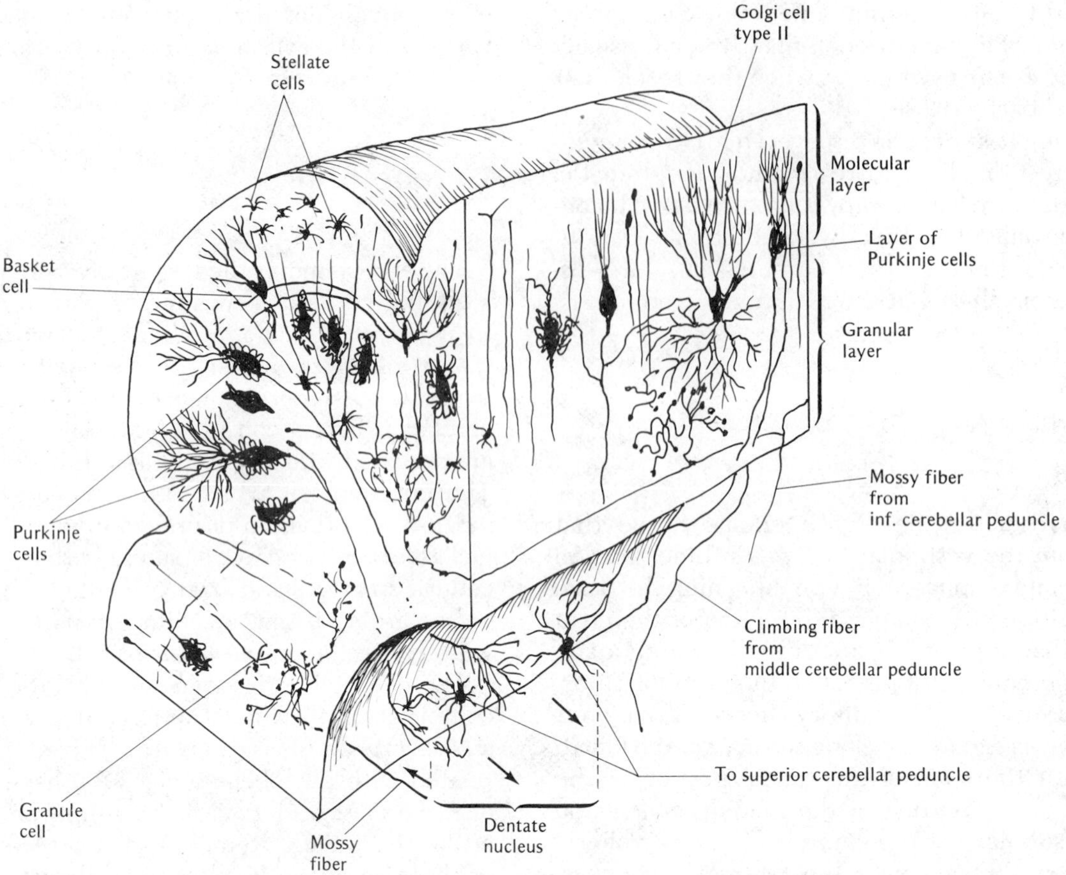

Figure 17-3. Cerebellar cortex drawn in three dimensions to show geometry of location of Purjinke cells, Golgi cells, granule, basket and stellate cells, with terminals of climbing and mossy fibers. (Adapted with permission of The Williams & Wilkins Co. from *Best and Taylor's Physiological Basis of Medical Practice,* 9th ed., 1973, Fig. 9.38, Sec. 9, p. 45, by John R. Brobeck.)

fifth principles. (No single part of the nervous system functions separately from other parts. The nervous system imposes regulation and control not only on organs and systems of the body but also on itself.)

Cerebellar Function

Specifically, the cerebellum accepts on many dendrites the motor impulses discharged from the various centers we have just reviewed and spreads them widely in the cerebellar cortex. Although these incoming impulses, which represent a plan for action to be undertaken, have already been organized to some extent, they need a final revision with correction of errors. This is the work of the cerebellum. If more impulses for a given movement have been initiated than will be required, the cerebellum can arrange to have them cut down; if too great speed has been undertaken, this will be inhibited by instructions to the motor cortex to excite antagonist muscles and inhibit agonists. The revisionist activities of the cerebellum are accompanied by very efficient and extremely rapid feedback mechanisms that Guyton, terming them servomechanisms, compares to the control system of an automatic pilot in an airplane (see Figure 17-4).

When the cerebellum is diseased and this servomechanism breaks down, the individual no longer is able unconsciously to make the necessary corrections. He or she does not predict very well how a sequence of planned motions will come out, and the faster the motions, the worse the results. A common test of this is to ask the patient to rotate the forearm and hand rapidly. It is a simple thing to do with an intact cerebellum, but results in a futile jumble of uncoordinated moves when there is cerebellar disease. This inability to perform rapidly coordinated movements is called *adiadochokinesia.* Taking demands rapidly coordinated sequential movements. When these cannot be effected, speech may become nearly unintelligible. Some syllables are too loud or too soft, held too long or not long enough, and the patient is said to have *dysarthria.* Cerebellar disease

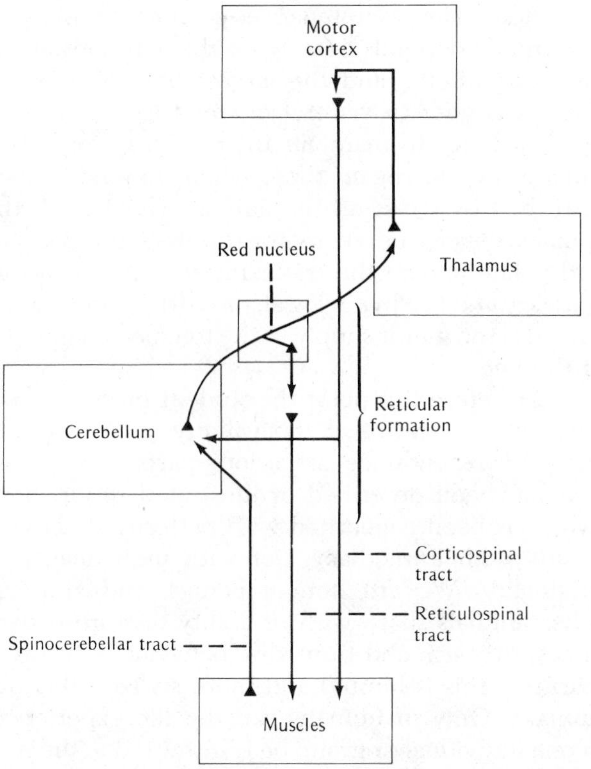

Figure 17-4. Pathways of cerebellar "error" control of voluntary movements. (Adapted with permission of the W. B. Saunders Company from *Textbook of Medical Physiology*, 5th ed., 1976, Fig. 53-13, p. 721, by Arthur Guyton.)

results also in *dysmetria*, a faulty ability to measure. The individual over- or undershoots the mark when reaching for something. *Asynergia* is also a problem for the patient with defective cerebellar function. The student will recognize the meaning from remembering its use in pharmacology. Synergistic drugs work together effectively to enhance one another; but the cerebellar patient's activity is asynergic—nothing works together. Hypotonia, tremor, nystagmus, and ataxia may all be noted in disease of the cerebellum. The patient, being competent intellectually, will make conscious attempts to compensate for errors that the previously intact cerebellum would not have permitted. Some efforts are more successful than others. The patient can make an ataxic gait safer by walking with his or her legs far apart, thrusting the pelvis forward, and holding onto the furniture. No amount of intelligence, conscious planning, or years of experience in the act will enable the patient now to perform neatly an act such as cracking and emptying a soft-boiled egg.

Signs of cerebellar injury, disease, or surgery derive from interference with one or both of the following:

1. The fine tuning function of the cerebellum in relation to voluntary movement of skeletal muscles
2. The proximity of cranial nerves IX through XII, which originate near the cerebellum

The patient may experience difficulty with gait *(ataxia)*,[3] speech, and eye movements *(nystagmus)*, in addition to difficulty with swallowing, tasting, salivating, and regulating heart rate; with respiration and gastrointestinal function; and with moving shoulders and head (Wheeler, 1977).

This is, perhaps, a good place to stop and illustrate in a small way a basic reason for a professional nurse's having some understanding of the nervous system. One learns that, ordinarily, a patient should be permitted to undertake independently or with assistance all the activities of daily living that are possible. This is better for morale than having them done for the patient. It may help him or her to recover. Like all generalizations, this one must be accepted with wariness, and the knowledge that generalizations have their exceptions. The nurse who understands the basis for the awkwardness of a cerebellar patient knows that the patient will be nothing but worse off for the attempt to open his or her own eggs, being left frustrated, humiliated, and hungry. The nurse will see that this and similar little services are performed for the patient.

Great imagination, skill, and patience are required of both the nurse and patient to safely maximize the patient's self-help ability in sitting, standing, walking, eating, and restoring normal bowel movement patterns, as well as in remaining oriented, hopeful, and convinced of his or her own worth, despite usually profound alteration in body image.

Cranial Nerves

Previously the statement was made and has since been referred to that the reflex connections for cranial nerves were centered in the reticular formation; little, however, has yet been said about the cranial nerves themselves other than the vestibular portion and nuclei of the eighth, and a statement that the nuclei of the cranial nerves are paired along either side of the center, in bulb and pons. There are several points by which it is interesting to compare cranial with peripheral nerves. (1) They are specialized,

[3] *Ataxia* occurs only during voluntary movements, particularly fine movements involving more than one joint, and is characterized by errors in the speed, range, force, and timing of purposive movements (Wheeler, 1977, p. 264).

in that some are sensory, some motor. Although some have both a sensory and a motor component, these have their own nuclei and are quite discrete. (2) Their fibers are without neurolemma and cannot regenerate. They seem in some respects rather more like tracts than nerves. The cranial nerves are very frequently referred to by number instead of name in speaking and in designation on the patient's chart. It is convenient to know the names that belong to the roman numerals, but some persons find the task of learning them difficult. There is a mnemonic that has helped students for generations to learn the names.[4] A brief discussion of arrangement may also help, especially if the student will keep in mind the arrangement of features in the head of an animal such as a dog. The sense organ right out in front in animals is the snout; so the *olfactory* nerve is the most anterior, number I. Eyes come next; so *ocular* is II, large nerves whose fibers cross at the optic chiasm above the pituitary and proceed as *optic tracts* to the visual cortex. These two cranial nerves are sensory. But eyes need to be moved; and III, *oculomotor,* IV, *trochlear,* and VI, *abducens,* provide this control. III includes parasympathetic fibers to constrict the pupil of the eye. Eyes are set in a face that is both above and below them; the Vth nerve, *trigeminal,* emerges between IV and VI. This great nerve, with three branches, is sensory (pain, temperature, touch, proprioception) to face and scalp and motor to muscles of mastication. The slender VIIth nerve, the facial, supplies motion to the muscles of expression of the face and taste to the anterior two thirds of the tongue. It pursues a circuitous route intracranially and fans out to supply a large area extracranially, and not infrequently is damaged either centrally or peripherally. Sadly collapsed muscles of the face result. Ears are double organs set to deal with hearing and to assist with balancing. Cranial nerve VIII has two divisions, auditory and vestibular, each coming from the appropriate portion of the ear. Not much below the ears, the throat begins where one finds IX, the glossopharyngeal (tongue–pharynx), which is largely sensory, supplying taste to the posterior third of the tongue and feeling to the upper pharynx. X is the vagus, the main outflow for the cranial division of the parasympathetic fraction of the autonomic nervous system. It is sensory to auricle, pharynx, larynx, and viscera of chest and abdomen, and motor to pharynx, larynx, base of tongue, and autonomic ganglia of chest and abdomen. The maintenance of homeostasis (see Chapter 6) depends heavily on the activities of the parasympathetic, and the largest bulk of fibers of the vagus goes to visceral organs that are assisted by its activity to maintain their normal vegetative functions or to regain these when they have been disturbed by stress on the animal. The XIth is the spinal accessory nerve, motor supply to the pharynx and palate and to the trapezius and sternomastoid muscles, and the hypoglossal, or XIIth cranial nerve, provides the motor supply to the tongue and muscles of the neck.

Long before this point the student must have become clearly aware of the validity of Principle 5, the interdependence of various parts. Everything that has been described or illustrated so far, however, has been concerned with patterns of activity, mostly with immediacy, not with individuality or originality. We are human beings, and although other animals share with us ability to store experiences, to learn, and to modify behavior in terms of learning, this is limited and more stylized than for humans. Only in humans can the life experiences of one individual or group be transmitted to the next generations so that they can be appreciated and used. However great the genius of an individual, even of a true innovator, in a sense, the works produced are never completely his or her own creation. Human heritage, the effects on consciousness of work and techniques of artists who preceded the individual, have been received and integrated. Although what he or she builds, paints, or composes may seem to be quite unlike anything that has been done before, the unique product of the creative genius of one person, it could not have been built or painted so had other artists not left their buildings, paintings, musical scores, and poetry.

In this respect, the oriole's nest hanging in perfect level and balance from the elm branch is different. We admire it and say, "It is a work of art." But the beautiful structure perfectly adapted to the needs of orioles would not satisfy all definitions of a "work of art" for, exquisite as it is, the nest of one is like that of another, like that of the parent, and of the next generation. The characteristics the nest has are those of the bird's species or class, not of itself as an individual builder; one oriole's nest will provoke neither more nor less admiration from us than that of another.

With these last notes on structure and function of the nervous system we have reached the top of the ascent from the cord and peripheral nerves and shall remain at this height long enough to gain a view, though cursory, of the activities of the human cerebral cortex. Then, with a quick descent on the motor tracts, the circuit will be completed.

[4]
On	*Old*	*Olympus'*	*Topmost*	*Top*
olfactory	optic	oculomotor	trochlear	trigeminal
A	*Finn*	*And*	*German*	*Viewed*
abducens	facial	auditory	glossopharyngeal	vagus
Some	*Hops*			
spinal accessory	hypoglossal			

The Cerebral Cortex and its Function

The activities of the cerebral cortex are intimately and inextricably tied to the thalamus. The connections in both directions, thalamus to cortex and cortex to thalamus, are innumerable, constituting most elaborate feedback situations whereby impressions arriving at the thalamus by way of afferent pathways are relayed to appropriate parts of the cortex for analysis. Because analysis may demonstrate the need of appreciation from other parts of the cortex before final actions are taken, this factor may require another trip to the thalamus and relay by still other neurons to different parts of the cortex. These corticothalamic relays may have both immediate and long-lasting effects, relatively simple and quite complex. The sensory stimulus may cause a *motor response,* and the total experience may provoke new thoughts and also be stored in *memory,* perhaps to be useful in the future, three results differing from each other considerably but all necessary for humans.

The student who wishes to learn any considerable amount of what is known today of the functions of the cerebral cortex is referred to a contemporary medical or neurophysiology text. The knowledge is incomplete at best, and the following text is but an overall summary. Structurally, the cortex is a very thin, layered structure, the thickest part not more than 4 mm. The area is enormous, however. If one could flatten out its convoluted surface, it would cover more than 2 square yards. Considering the size of a single cell, this surface, even though only a few millimeters deep, provides a large acreage for a human being to manage and direct the work of the body, to think, plan, act rationally or not, communicate with others, and develop cultural and ethical behavior. This thin sheet of cells shows, histologically, six layers. Seen in microscopic section, the cell processes form a veritable mat, providing communication with cells in all layers, passing to more distant areas in the same or opposite hemispheres, or being themselves parts of the afferent and efferent systems to the brain and cord below.

Sensorimotor Function

The cerebral cortex looks quite homogeneous, yet certainly there are parts that are specialized in function. Considerable areas seem not to have a single function but only to reinforce by presenting wider areas for association. Figure 17-5 shows broad areas

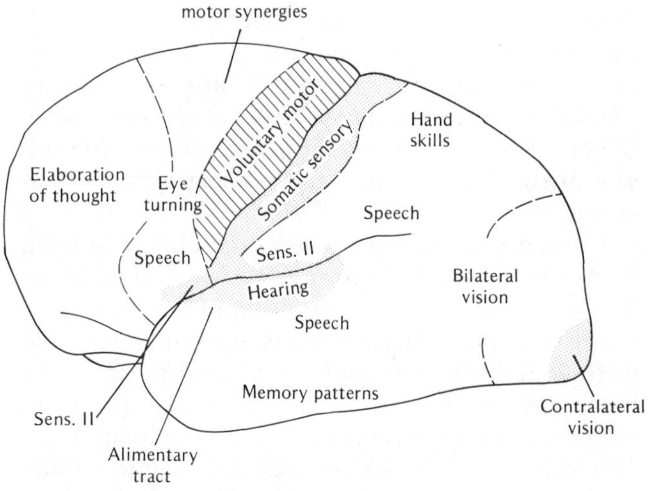

Figure 17-5. Functional areas of the human cerebral cortex as determined by electrical stimulation of the cortex during neurosurgical operations and by neurologic examinations of patients with destroyed cortical regions. (Adapted with permission of Macmillan Publishing Co., Inc., from *The Cerebral Cortex of Man,* 1950, Fig. 117, p. 221, by Wilder Penfield and Theodore Rasmussen.)

of cortical localization. One of the most interesting of these for human beings is the surface of the temporal lobe at the angular gyrus. This small region bears responsibility for interpreting sensory experience from whatever source. Complex and elaborate memories are stored here (Guyton, 1976, p. 656), and any damage to the area has serious effect on intellectual competence. Even though the entire visual and auditory apparatus from eye and ear to visual and auditory cortex may be intact, if there is loss of the interpretive area no proper use can be made of the sensory experience; it will not be integrated with previous experiences and so is valueless. For example, on walking toward a railroad crossing the individual might see the flashing red light and hear the noise of the approaching train but even though, before damage occurred, the meaning of this sight and sound was clear to the person and his or her behavior appropriate in terms of the correct interpretation and recollection, now the individual walks on, for the signals are meaningless and have no value anymore.

This experience (memory)–sensation–interpretation–reaction cycle is of paramount importance to the nurse in understanding and easing a person's perception of and response to illness. In health, about 90 per cent of our informational input comes to us through vision; for the sighted, vision completely dominates, and even shapes the meaning of, touch (Rock & Harris, 1967). Illness is frequently associated with some degree of impairment of visual acuity. When caring for the blind and/or sick individual, the nurse must consider ways to supplement the critical visual sense with sound and touch. The meaning and use of touch in patient care are receiving increased attention by nurse researchers and practitioners. (See Unit II and references for further discussion of the consequences and nursing management of sensory deprivation.)

The most anterior parts of the cerebrum in front of the motor areas are termed the prefrontal lobes. There are connections from these to the hypothalamus that evoke responses associated with anger and distress and other responses mediated by the autonomic nervous system. For the most part, however, the prefrontal lobes seem to have a disciplinary function to perform. Without specialized function themselves, they provide a considerable area for reinforcement. In their presence, the individual has the means to work at complicated problems, resist distraction, deal with abstract thought, and weigh the relative merits of one line of behavior against another. If they are cut off from their influence on the rest of the brain, individuals are unable to discipline themselves to any of these complex activities. They are incapable of abstract reasoning, although they can follow concrete patterns of behavior. They may perform correctly the arithmetical tasks involved but be unable to solve a problem that presents no interesting challenge to them, for they are too easily distracted to grasp its import. Social behavior may be quite unorthodox and unsatisfactory to others, for the individuals respond directly to impulses without evaluation of consequences. This apparent isolation of the braking, inhibiting, or disciplinary effect of the frontal lobes is sometimes one of the unfortunate consequences of encephalitis, an inflammation of the brain.

Human beings can talk; it is their most important means of communication. They read and write and use symbols to express themselves by these means. These activities are very complicated, utilizing many areas of the cortex, some highly specialized. These are sometimes selectively destroyed by hemorrhage, tumor, or disease, and the patient may have any of the following resultant disabilities: being unable to form words although knowing what he or she wants to say *(motor aphasia);* being unable to comprehend by word or gesture what is said to him or her *(sensory aphasia);* one variety of sensory aphasia is an inability to attach meaning to words heard *(auditory agnosia,* or *word deafness);* and there may be a similar problem with words read *(visual agnosia,* or *word blindness).*

It is common knowledge that in right-handed persons the left hemisphere has ascendency over the right after early childhood. Motor speech for these persons is largely handled by the appropriate area—low in the premotor cortex—of the left hemisphere. One of the frequent and most trying disabilities of those who suffer a cerebral accident or *stroke* resulting in damage to this hemisphere is not the weakness of arm and leg so much as the maddening inability to express, in words, the thought that the mind can formulate. The student has probably noted that, in right-handed persons, the stroke that occurs in the right hemisphere does not have this unhappy result.

Mention of these difficulties with communication brings us at last to the parts of the cortex concerned with the control of motion and appreciation of sensations. There are large areas of the surface of the brain that, when stimulated, will result in movement of one or another group of muscles. These must all be included under the term *motor cortex,* although some parts considerably overlap areas that are sensory (see Figure 17-6). The cortical region right around the central sulcus is purely motor. The number of cells that are present and responsible for initiating voluntary control of a part relate to fineness of control expected of that part; thus there are more cells in the cortical area concerned with voluntary control of the fingers that can be trained to operate with great dexterity than in the region devoted to control of the muscles of the thigh, where voluntary control of muscles to any great degree is unnecessary.

Figure 17-5 demonstrates the considerable surface devoted to sensory functions, the special senses, and body sensations. Although, for example, the primary auditory cortex recognizes sounds, and bilateral ablation of this area of cortex will result in deafness, the sounds are not analyzed into useful forms until

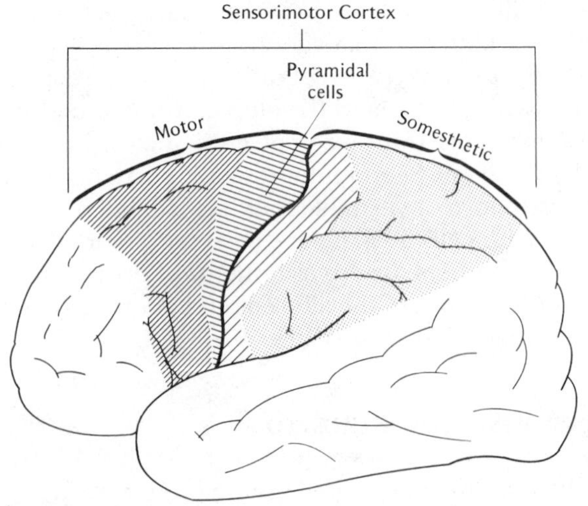

Figure 17-6. Relationship of the motor cortex to the somesthetic cortex. (Used with permission of the W. B. Saunders Company from *Textbook of Medical Physiology,* 5th ed., 1976, Figure 53-1, p. 710, by Arthur Guyton.)

they have undergone switchbacks to the brainstem and again to the cerebrum where, in the angular gyrus of the temporal lobe, they are correctly interpreted, having been correlated with other experiences, and can be intelligently acted on. For example, the auditory motor cortex is stimulated by the train whistle, the sound coming to it from the eighth nerve by way of the thalamus. Switchback to the reticular formation results in alerting the necessary cortical areas so that when the angular gyrus and other parts of the cortex put everything together, the person will note the flashing red lights and stop the car. (Sound was used here as an example. A like process occurs with other sensations.)

A curious example of sensory defect is not uncommonly seen in children who have cerebral palsy with spastic hemiplegia of a type wherein there is cortical damage that includes the somatosensory areas just posterior to the central sulcus. These children have an *astereognosis,* an inability to identify a familiar object by the feel and form in the affected hand. With eyes closed they will accept a key and say that it is cold and that is has weight, but until they open their eyes they cannot identify the key. Such damage can occur later in life but then it is not such a handicap as it is to the child, who is such an active learner.

Motor Function

Under discussion of the cerebellum and cell masses in the brainstem something was said about the coordination of unconscious muscle activity and automatic associated motion and the efferent tracts that arise from these nuclei. With this brief discussion of the cerebral cortex, there has been mention of voluntary control. It is evident that these systems work together. The motor systems of the brain are very complex and, as yet, by no means completely understood or worked out. In a very general way the *pyramidal,* or *corticospinal,* system is largely concerned with the control of voluntary motion, and those pathways that have to do with the coordination of unconscious adjustments and with the control of automatic associated movements are termed *extrapyramidal* or *extracorticospinal* (*extra* meaning "outside of"). A perfectly executed "voluntary" act implicates not only the pyramidal and extrapyramidal but sensory systems as well.

In humans, control of voluntary motor activity is usually achieved by the second year of life. Most infants can accurately reach for an object by the age of 6 months, can sit erect by 8 months, can crawl by 10 months, can stand by 12 months, and can walk steadily by 15 months. With only slight variation in timing, the sequence of these events is rarely altered. Current research suggests that cognitive, or hypothesis-forming, development also begins about the age of 9 months (Kagan, 1972).

It will help to remember that the human's ability to move is regulated by three highly interdependent motor systems: (1) the pyramidal tract, responsible for *initiation* of voluntary movements, whose efferent fibers arise in the motor strip of the cerebral cortex and terminate on the lower motor neurons; (2) the cerebellar system, responsible for *coordination* of movements, which comprises the afferent and efferent fibers of the cerebellum and associated nuclei; and (3) the extrapyramidal system, responsible for the *maintenance of posture,* which consists of a number of paired nuclei and associated pathways.

Injury to or lesions of these systems tend to produce the following results: (1) injury to the pyramidal results in paralysis of voluntary movement; (2) cerebellar injury causes tremors on movement, incoordination, dyssynergia, and ataxia; and (3) extrapyramidal injury results in abnormal position and postural reflexes, usually present at rest (Klawans, 1970).

Motor-neuron diseases are due to primary abnormalities of anterior-horn cells and motor cranial nerve nuclei. Clinical features are attributable to degeneration of motor nuclei at the spinal and/or brainstem levels, usually with involvement of the Betz cells of the cortex and demyelination of the corticobulbar and corticospinal (pyramidal) tracts; manifestations include muscle wasting, weakness, and involuntary contraction or twitching of groups of muscles (Bobowick & Brody, 1973). Although multiple factors can contribute to impairments in a person's ability to move, the leading cause of major deficits in locomotion is stroke. The American Neurological Association estimates that 55 per cent of the 2.5 million stroke survivors in the United States each year are left with sufficient disability to require special care, and 15 per cent are so totally disabled that institutionalization is necessary. The most economical and effective approach is to prevent stroke, by controlling those high-risk factors found to predispose to stroke: severe hypertension, obesity, elevated hematocrit levels, and EKG abnormalities (Staving off stroke, 1974). (See Chapter 50 for restorative care.)

Loss of mobility has profound effects not only on the function of all body systems, which seem designed to operate most effectively in support of a physically active person, but also on one's concept of self as a worthwhile person. Patients with some degree of sudden onset paralysis resulting from causes such as curable infections or traumatic injury usually have the opportunity to work through new ways of adapting, and often live long, happy, and productive lives despite their paralysis (see Chapters

34 and 50). But a patient whose mobility is eroded bit by bit, by a progressive degenerative disease such as *amyotrophic lateral sclerosis,*[5] no sooner adapts to one level of impairment than his or her function deteriorates further. The patient with a fatal progressive degenerative disease presents a profound challenge to the nurse: not only must physical and psychological care strike the delicate balance between necessary dependence and independence, but also the nurse must convey to patient and family that the patient is valued and his or her life is significant, despite deterioration of self-sufficiency (Boyle & Ciuca, 1976).

Another major cause of locomotion deficits is the degeneration of neurologic function as a consequence of aging. High accident rates among the aged are attributable to progressive atherosclerosis, which affects cerebral, cerebellar proprioceptive, and cardiac function to produce weakness, incoordination, general dysfunction of homeostatic mechanisms, and impaired hearing, vision, and gait. In persons over 64 years of age, accidents are the seventh most common cause of death (Rodstein, 1973).

To demonstrate the highly complex and largely automatic nature of so-called voluntary movement, the student is asked here to sit in a chair from a standing position while paying the most alert attention possible to all that goes on. Although the student will not note everything, he or she will nevertheless realize that the strictly voluntary, consciously willed part of the act is only a small fraction and that the sensory awareness of one's initial position and the shifts that were made while neatly lowering oneself to the chair were coordinated and adjusted with an exactness impossible had they depended on conscious planning alone.

The voluntary part of the controlled act of sitting down originated in cells of the motor cortex just anterior to the central sulcus. There are large cells there, the cells of Betz, whose heavy axons form a conspicuous fraction of the pyramidal tract. But the entire sensory motor cortex contributes to this tract whose fibers gather together first in the *internal capsule.* (The internal capsule is a massive band of white matter that contains the bulk of all fibers running to and from the cortex. It forms a sharp angle and appears to be squeezed in between thalamus and basal ganglia.) The fibers of the descending pyramidal tract give off collaterals to basal ganglia, reticular formation and nuclei therein, and indirectly to the cerebellum, as they continue through the pons to the medulla oblongata. Here they appear on the surface, and, as they continue caudally, most of the fibers decussate. The few that do not are found in the ventral part of the spinal cord, but the major number that decussate form the lateral *pyramidal tracts* that occupy a considerable fraction of the lateral white matter of the cord, running just anterior to the important extrapyramidal tract, the rubrospinal. As the text indicates, these two systems, pyramidal and extrapyramidal, are repeatedly in communication with each other through brainstem nuclei. The term *extrapyramidal* is not a good one; the interplay is too close. As is the case with all efferent tracts, the termination is on the lower motor neuron (anterior motor neuron in the spinal cord). It is the anterior horn cell there that will send the impulse to muscle or gland along the final common path. Interference with the tract at any point or with the cortical cells from which it arises will necessarily result in some measure of weakness and inadequacy of voluntary control, especially in fine discriminative movements.

The origin of the pyramidal tract is higher than that of the extrapyramidal pathways, and Principle 7 reminds us that higher centers tend to inhibit lower. When a patient has damage to the pyramidal pathway, these inhibiting forces are released and one sees activity that the wholly intact nervous system has under disciplined control after babyhood. There is constantly increased muscle tone, spasticity, with increased tendon reflexes and a marked tendency to develop contractures, absence of surface reflexes (abdominal and cremasteric), and the Babinski reflex is present (upturning of the big toe and fanning of the others when the plantar surface of the foot is gently stimulated). Any number of pathologic states in the nervous system will in some way encroach on the pyramidal tract so that testing for its integrity by eliciting abdominal reflexes and a normal plantar response (clenching of the toes and withdrawal on plantar stimulation) are commonly part of any general physical examination. If the person's responses to these are normal and there are no obvious signs of central nervous system disease, the physician will often assume that no further neurologic testing is necessary.

Nurses may observe the signs of involvement of the pyramidal tract in the course of daily care of a patient after a cerebrovascular accident, or stroke. The abnormal reflex responses are demonstrated in the course of the bath, and the others will be noted during range-of-motion exercises.

[5] *Amyotrophic lateral sclerosis* (ALS) is a fatal disease characterized by progressive degeneration of the anterior horn cells of the spinal cord, the motor nuclei of the lower cranial nerves, and the corticobulbar and corticospinal tracts. It occurs usually in men between the ages of 40 and 70, has no known cause, and the only treatment is supportive. There are no paresthesias or apparent sensory changes, and no loss of mental acuity due to the disease. Death is eventually caused by aspiration, pneumonia, and respiratory failure. See Boyle & Ciuca (1976) for a sensitive case study of one man's final weeks with ALS.

The brain controls every organ system in the body. When electrical activity of one part of the brain is modified, changes occur in almost every other area. However, there is reason to be optimistic that one day persons with lesions of some part of their motor system will again be able to control their own movements. Research is in progress to apply operant conditioning techniques to turning on and off the electrical activity of the brain as a whole, or specifically selected parts, in the hope that such techniques may help to control such disorders as Parkinson's disease, and even may be successful in controlling movement of artificial limbs.

By perfectly performing the act of sitting down in the chair, we have involved nearly everything that has been discussed in this section on the nervous system. An effort has been made to increase the student's knowledge of the nervous system beyond that gained in the basic course in anatomy and physiology and so to provide a basis for understanding difficulties patients may have that relate to involvement of the nervous system. Then it is easier to observe intelligently, to analyze the patient's needs for nursing care more specifically, and thereafter to meet them wisely. The central nervous system is not a thing apart even though shut up in a bony box. It is nourished by the same blood supply and suffers insults from many of the same agents that injure the rest of the body. Whatever types of patients being cared for, the nurse will inevitably find some with complications involving the nervous system. Often it is the nurse who is present when these signs first manifest themselves, and the professional nurse should be prepared to recognize their import. Before the nurse is prepared to plan care for patients whose problems have a neurologic component or origin, she or he must consider the functions of the autonomic nervous system and its relationship to the central nervous system. Chapter 18 discusses autonomic control mechanisms and their participation in protection and response of the individual faced with threatening events.

References Cited

Bobowick, A. R., and Brody, J. A. "Epidemiology of Motor-Neuron Diseases." *N. Engl. J. Med.*, **288** (17 May 1973), 1047–55.

Boyle, M. A., and Ciuca, R. L. "Amyotrophic Lateral Sclerosis." *Am. J. Nurs.* **76** (1976) 66–68.

Fischbach, F. T. "Easing Adjustments to Parkinson's Disease." *Am J. Nurs.*, **78** (Jan. 1978), 66–69.

Galaburda, A. M. et al. "Right-Left Asymmetries in the Brain." *Science,* **199** (24 Feb. 1978), 852–56.

Guyton, A. C. *Textbook of Medical Physiology,* 5th ed. Philadelphia: W. B. Saunders Company, 1976.

Huttunen, M. O. "General Model for the Molecular Events in Synapses during Learning." *Perspect. Biol. Med.*, **17** (Autumn 1973), 103–8.

Kagan, J. "Do Infants Think?" *Sci. Am.*, **226** (March 1972), 74–82.

Klawans, H. L., Jr., and Cohen, M. M. "Diseases of the Extrapyramidal System." *DM,* (Jan. 1970), p. 4.

Maas, J. W. "The Biology of Depression: Where We Stand." *Med. World News* (Psychiatry Issue), (1973), pp. 69–70.

Ornstein, R. E. "Right and Left Thinking." *Psychol. Today,* **6** (May 1973), 87–92.

Rock, I., and Harris, C. "Vision and Touch." *Sci. Am.*, **216** (May 1967), 96–104.

Rodstein, M. "Accidents: Epidemiology and Prevention." *Med. World News* (Special Volume on Geriatrics), (1973), pp. 28–31.

Rosenthal, R. "The Pygmalion Effect Lives." *Psychol. Today,* **7** (Sept. 1973), 56–64.

Rosenzweig, M. R. et al. "Brain Changes in Response to Experience." *Sci. Am.*, **226** (Feb. 1972), 22–29.

Routtenberg, A. "The Reward System of the Brain." *Sci. Am.*, **239** (Nov. 1978), 154–64.

Stoler, P. "Exploring the Frontiers of the Mind." *Time,* **103** (14 Jan. 1974), 50–59.

"Staving Off Stroke." *Med. World News,* **15** (8 Feb. 1974), 47–53.

Wheeler, P. "Care of a Patient with a Cerebellar Tumor." *Am. J. Nurs,* **77** (Feb. 1977), 263–66.

General References

Barbizet, J. *Human Memory and Its Pathology,* San Francisco: W. H. Freeman and Company, Publishers, 1970.

Cannon, W. B. *Bodily Changes in Pain, Hunger, Fear and Rage,* Newton Centre, Mass.: Charles T. Branford Co., 1929.

Eccles, J. C. *The Understanding of the Brain.* New York: McGraw-Hill Book Company, 1973.

Hamburg, D. A., Pribram, K. H., and Strunkard, A. J. eds. *Perception and Its Disorders.* Baltimore: The Williams & Wilkins Company, 1970.

Held, R. H., and Richards, W., eds., *Perception: Mechanisms and Models—Readings from Scientific American.* San Francisco: W. H. Freeman and Company, Publishers, 1972.

Langworthy, O. R. *The Sensory Control of Posture and Movement.* Baltimore: The Williams & Wilkins Company, 1970.

Teyler, T. J., ed. *Altered States of Awareness: Readings from Scientific American.* San Francisco: W. H. Freeman and Company, Publishers, 1972.

Thompson, R. F., ed. *Physiological Psychology: Readings*

from Scientific American. San Francisco: W. H. Freeman and Company, Publishers, 1971.

General Neurologic Function

Cabanac, M. "Physiological Role of Pleasure." *Science,* **173** (17 Sept. 1971), 1103–07.

Fine, W. "Cerebral Symptomology in Old Age." *Nurs. Mirror,* **132** (30 April 1971), 37–39.

Gardner, M. A. "Responsiveness as a Measure of Consciousness." *Am. J. Nurs.,* **68** (May 1968), 1034–38.

Geschwind, N. "Specializations of the Human Brain." *Sci. Am.,* **241** (Sept. 1979), 180–201.

Hess, W. R., and Fischer, H. "Brain and Consciousness: A Discussion of the Brain." *Perspect. Biol. Med.,* **17** (Autumn 1973), 109–18.

Iversen. L. L. "The Chemistry of the Brain." *Sci. Am.,* **241** (Sept. 1979), 134–49.

Johnson, L. C. "Are Stages of Sleep Related to Waking Behavior?" *Am. Scientist,* **61** (May–June 1973), 326–38.

Kolata, G. B. "Sex Hormones and Brain Development." *Science,* **205** (7 Sept. 1979), 985–87.

National Dairy Council. "Malnutrition, Learning and Behavior." *Dairy Council Digest,* **44** (Nov.–Dec. 1973), 31–34.

Nauta, W. J. H., and Feirtag, M. "The Organization of the Brain." *Sci. Am.,* **241** (Sept. 1979), 88–111.

Penfield, W. "The Mechanism of Memory. Reported by Morris Fishbein." *Med. World News,* **10** (4 April 1969), 56.

Sensory Function

Barnett, K. "A Survey of the Current Utilization of Touch by Health Team Personnel with Hospitalized Patients." *Int. J. Nurs. Stud.,* **9** (Nov. 1972), 195–208.

Barnett, K. "A Theoretical Construct of the Concepts of Touch as They Relate to Nursing." *Nurs. Res.,* **21** (March–April 1972), 102–10.

DeThomasco, M. T. "Touch Power and the Screen of Loneliness." *Perspect. Psychiatr. Care,* **9** (14 July 1971), 112–18.

Dominian, J. "The Psychological Significance of Touch." *Nurs. Times,* **67** (22 July 1971), 896–98.

Motor Function

Ahlquist, R. P. "Adrenergic Receptors: A Personal and Practical View." *Perspect. Biol. Med.,* **17** (Autumn 1973), 119–22.

Eisler, T. "Parkinsonism—New Drugs and New Approaches." *Dis.-a-Month,* **25** (March 1979), no. 6.

Erb, E. "Improving Speech in Parkinson's Disease." *Am. J. Nurs.,* **73** (Nov. 1973), 1910–11.

Evarts, E. V. "Brain Mechanisms of Movement." *Sci. Am.,* **241** (Sept. 1979), 164–79.

Greenblatt, D. J., and Shader, R. I. "Anticholinergics." *N. Engl. J. Med.,* **288** (7 June 1973), 1215–19.

18

Autonomic Control Mechanisms

The development of even a simple nervous system such as the autonomic system is clearly a complicated business. Nevertheless, neurobiologists have made a good deal of progress in identifying the influences regulating autonomic development. They do not have all the answers, but they think they are on the right track.

JEAN L. MARX
Jean L. Marx: "New Information About the Development of the Autonomic Nervous System," *Science 206*:437 (26 October) 1979.

The Autonomic Nervous System

Functions

The function of the autonomic nervous system (ANS) is visceral control, because its fibers (1) transmit information to the spinal cord and brain from the viscera, and (2) provide a significant part of the motor control of all cardiac and smooth muscle, of exocrine glands, and possibly of certain endocrine glands. In some organs and systems, such as the digestive tract, the ANS shares the control of function with intrinsic and extrinsic hormonal mechanisms. As indicated previously, hormonal and autonomic controls are alike in that both appear to be "involuntary," operating without the person's having to be aware of their activity. But they are highly interdependent, and both are under the influence of the central nervous system.[1] The intimacy of the relationship between the autonomic and central nervous systems is illustrated in Figure 18-1, which shows the distribution of autonomic fibers and their connections with the central nervous system.

The ANS is responsible for the internal adjustments necessary to maintain the stability of the internal environment described by Cannon as *homeostasis* (see Chapter 6 and Unit V). Through its various activities the autonomic system contributes to the maintenance of the constancy of composisition of the fluid environment of the body's cells: it serves to combat forces, acting within or without, which tend to cause variations in this environment. Regulation of the composition of the body fluids and their temperature, quantity, and distribution is effected through the actions of the autonomic nerves upon circulatory, respiratory, excretory, and glandular organs (Brobeck, 1973, p. 59).

Relationship of Sympathetic and Parasympathetic Fibers

Most of the effector organs of the ANS are supplied with sympathetic and parasympathetic fibers, their effects being delicately balanced against each other.

[1] For an excellent discussion and diagram of the way in which various negative feedback systems operate to establish regulations of physiologic processes, see "Control Systems That Establish Regulations," in *Best & Taylor's Physiological Basis of Medical Practice,* 9th ed., by J. R. Brobeck (Baltimore: The Williams & Wilkins Company, 1973), sec. 9, pp. 121–36.

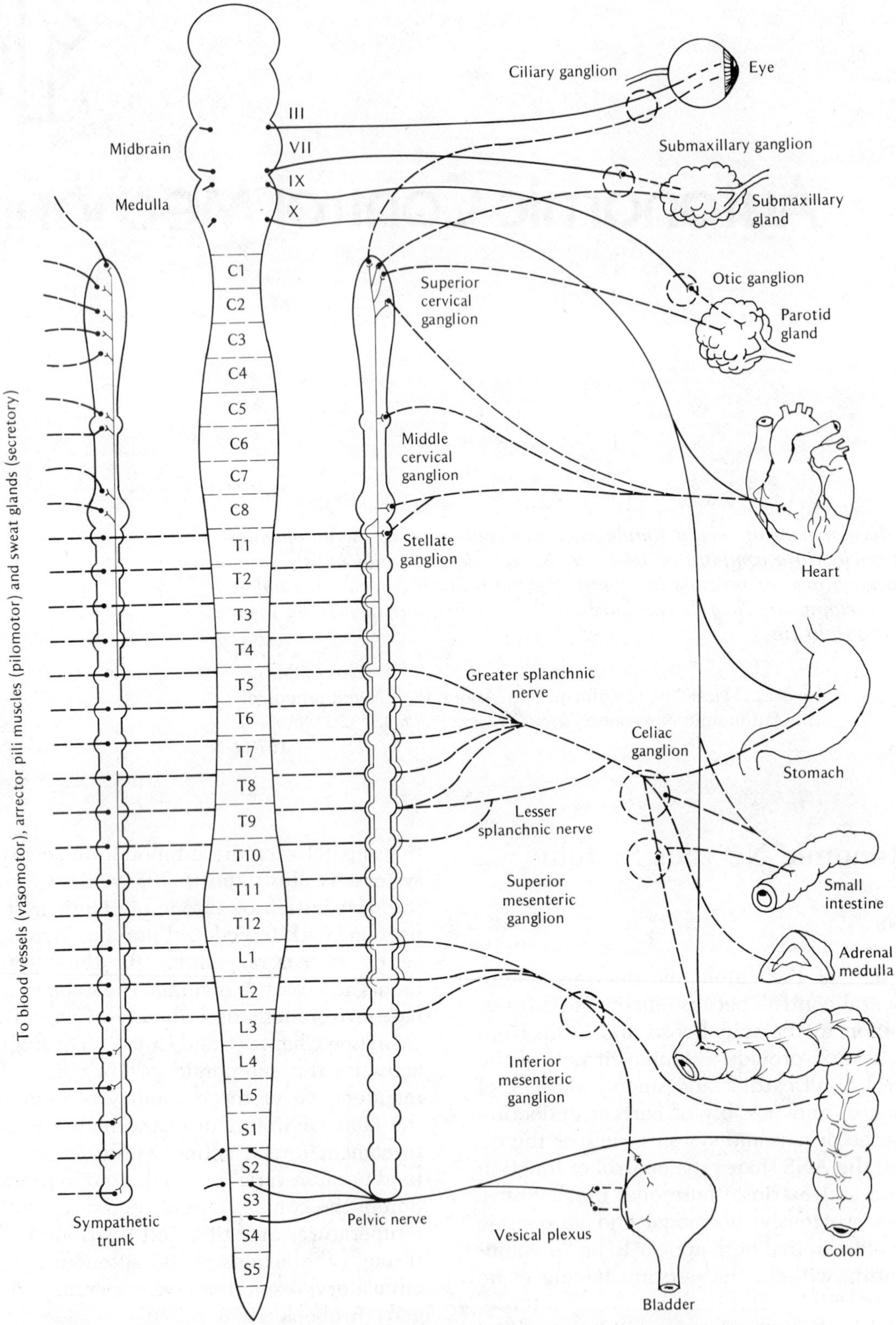

Figure 18-1. Connections of autonomic or visceromotor system. Craniosacral components are in *dashed lines;* thoracolumbar connections are in *solid lines.* Course of postganglionic fibers is shown by *dotted lines.* (Adapted with permission of The Williams & Wilkins Co. from *Bailey's Textbook of Histology,* 16th ed., 1971, Fig. 9-4, p. 233, by W. M. Copenhaver, R. P. Bunge, and M. B. Bunge.)

Interruption of the effects of one type of fibers generally results in the effects of the other type becoming more prominent. To illustrate, heart action is slowed by stimulating the vagus (a parasympathetic nerve) but accelerated by stimulation of sympathetic fibers. Following interruption of the vagus nerve, cardiac rate increases (Brobeck, 1973).

Although the postganglionic fibers of the visceral system have cell bodies located outside the brain and cord, the cell bodies and dendrites of the preganglionic fibers are in the hypothalamus, brainstem, and spinal cord. One functional difference between the somatic and visceral systems is that the somatic system acts more rapidly than the visceral.

Control of Autonomic Functions

Until recently, the hypothalamus was said to be the level of highest control of autonomic functions, containing "head ganglia" for sympathetic and parasympathetic divisions. Subsequent findings suggest that there are no discrete centers for autonomic control in the hypothalamus, although its lateral regions tend to excite and its medial region tends to inhibit whatever control system is being investigated. It has also been demonstrated that autonomic responses can be evoked by stimulation of certain regions of the cerebral cortex, the cerebellum, and the limbic system (a central region believed to be responsible for emotional experience) (Brobeck, 1973). Many of the manifestations associated with a stress response are due to the fact that, in addition to participating in regulation of the autonomic nervous system, the hypothalamus also participates in regulation of endocrine glands, body weight, and fluid and electrolyte balance. All visceral as well as somatic sensory and motor functions are subject to fundamental regulation not only by the hypothalamus, but also by the reticular formation.

With the exception of the smooth muscle of the blood vessels, the muscle of the hair follicles, and the sweat glands, all visceral organs are innervated by both sympathetic and parasympathetic systems. Although the sweat glands are supplied by the sympathetic nervous system, they are cholinergic; that is, acetylcholine is released at the effector cell rather than norepinephrine (see Figure 18-2). The sympathetic and parasympathetic systems function so that visceral activity is regulated and the needs of the organism are met under differing conditions. Because the sympathoadrenal system stimulates an organ under some circumstances and depresses it under others, some authorities postulate two different types of receptor substance in the effector cells—the alpha and the beta receptor substance. Although the sympathoadrenal system is continuously active, it acts most intensely during stress and emergency situations. Many of the signs and symptoms observed in patients who are under acute stress are caused by sympathoadrenal activity. As examples, many of the signs and symptoms observed in early shock or hypoglycemia are caused by sympathoadrenal activity.

To reiterate the few generalizations made about the autonomic nervous system, under emergency conditions the sympathoadrenal system regulates those activities in which energy stores are utilized with the result that the individual is prepared for flight, fight, or freeze. Conversely, the parasympathetic nervous system regulates activities associated with conservation and restoration of energy stores. As stated earlier, the functions of the two systems are integrated and are not antagonistic to each other. It was once believed that the sympathoadrenal system always acted as a unit when the individual was in danger. It is now known, however, that a part can be activated independently of other parts. Thus it can regulate nonemergency functions such as body temperatures (Hemingway & Price, 1968).

Figure 18-2. Peripheral structure of the sympathetic and parasympathetic divisions of the autonomic nervous system.

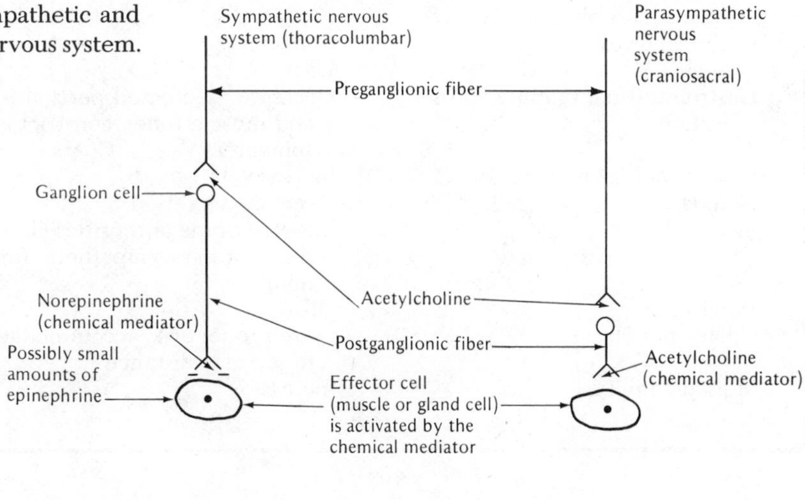

The parasympathetic nervous system consists of the third, seventh, ninth, and tenth cranial nerves and branches of the second, third, and fourth sacral nerves. There are no interconnections among the fibers forming these nerves. In the parasympathetic system, the ganglia lie in, or very close to, the organ that they stimulate with the result that preganglionic fibers are long and postganglionic fibers very short. There are very few connections among ganglia. The chemical mediator between the preganglionic fiber and the ganglion and the postganglionic fiber and the effector cell is acetylcholine (see Figure 18-2). Evidence suggests that the addicting properties and withdrawal symptoms of heroin and morphine may be related to their effect on acetylcholine (How Heroin May Hang on in Body, 1972).

The preganglionic fibers of the sympathoadrenal system originate from cells in the thoracolumbar portions of the spinal cord. The preganglionic fibers branch in the vertebral ganglia (cells lying peripheral to the spinal cord). Some are parallel to the cord, and others are located in the abdominal cavity or near an organ. Depending on their location, these ganglia are known as vertebral, collateral, or terminal. The preganglionic fibers of the sympathoadrenal system branch widely and often synapse with cells located in more than one ganglion. Some of the branches synapse with ganglionic cells, whereas others pass through the ganglia to higher or lower vertebral ganglia or to collateral ganglia. Preganglionic fibers are generally relatively short and postganglionic fibers are long. One exception is the fibers supplying the adrenal medulla, as it is supplied with preganglionic fibers. Stimulation of the sympathetic nervous system results in stimulation of the adrenal medulla.

Some of the effects of activation of the two divisions of the autonomic nervous system are summarized in Table 18-1. For a more detailed discussion of the autonomic nervous system, see Guyton (1976, pp. 768–81).

Nature and Effects of Chemical Mediators

Another relationship exists between the sympathetic nervous system and the adrenal medulla. The chemical mediator between the sympathetic postganglionic fiber and the effector cell—muscle or gland—is norepinephrine. Epinephrine and small amounts of norepinephrine are secreted by the adrenal medulla. Both these chemicals augment and prolong the action of the sympathetic nervous system. Synthesis of norepinephrine begins in the axoplasm of the terminal nerve endings of adrenergic nerve fibers but is completed inside the vesicles. The basic steps are the following (Guyton, 1976, p. 771):

1. $\text{Tyrosine} \xrightarrow{hydroxylation} \text{DOPA}$
2. $\text{DOPA} \xrightarrow{decarboxylation} \text{dopamine}$

Table 18-1 *Selected Actions Resulting from Activation of the Sympathetic and Parasympathetic Divisions of the Autonomic Nervous System*

Site of Effector Cells	Activation of Sympathetic Division (Thoracolumbar) Tends To	Activation of Parasympathetic Division (Craniosacral) Tends To
Heart	Increase rate and output	Decrease rate and output
Coronary arteries	Dilate	
Blood vessels in nose, salivary glands, and pharynx	Constrict	Dilate
Cutaneous vessels	Constrict	
Bronchi	Dilate	Constrict
Gastrointestinal motility and secretion	Decrease (decreased peristalsis and muscle tone); constrict sphincters	Increase; relax sphincters
Glycogenolysis by liver	Increase	
Glands	Decrease secretion	Increase secretion
Sweat glands	Increase (some authorities classify this as a parasympathetic function)	
Pupil of eye	Dilate	Constrict
Ciliary muscles	Lessen tone; eyes accommodated to see at a distance	Contract ciliary muscles; eyes accommodated to see near objects
Mental activity	Increase	

3. Transport of dopamine into the vesicles
4. Dopamine $\xrightarrow{hydroxylation}$ norepinephrine
   In the adrenal medulla this reaction goes still one step further to form epinephrine as follows:
5. Norepinephrine $\xrightarrow{methylation}$ epinephrine

As in the parasympathetic nervous system, the chemical mediator between the preganglionic fiber and the ganglion cells is acetylcholine.

Current research on embryological development of the cells which become principal neurons of the autonomic nervous system suggests that the development of cholinergic mechanisms takes precedence and that adrenergic neurons may develop only when cholinergic sites have been occupied (Bunge et al., 1978). Catecholamines have both local and far-reaching effects; they influence metabolic processes through the sympathetic nerves and the adrenal medulla. Norepinephrine influences metabolism in the innervated tissue in the immediate vicinity of release, whereas epinephrine when released from the adrenal medulla into the circulation affects cells throughout the body (Landsberg & Young, 1978). This mechanism of communication is analogous to communication in the endocrine system and provides further support for understanding neuroendocrine function as a unitary regulatory process. In both the nervous and endocrine systems, chemical messengers (respectively hormones and neurotransmitters) are released from one cell, travel through the extracellular medium and bind to receptors on the surface of a second cell to modify its activity. The intracellular effects of many hormones and neurotransmitters appear to be mediated by the same substance, the second-messenger cyclic AMP (Nathanson & Greengard, 1977).

It appears that catecholamine systems, specifically norepinephrine and dopamine, play a fundamental role in mediating the interaction between the individual and the environment and that abnormalities in function of these neurotransmitters may be linked to behavioral pathology of such disorders as Parkinson's disease, the schizophrenias and possibly other affective disorders (Antelman & Caggiula, 1977).

Though anatomically the sweat glands belong to the sympathetic nervous system, their innervation is cholinergic; that is, the chemical mediator for the postganglionic fibers supplying sweat glands is acetylcholine. Depending on their orientation, some authorities classify the nerve supply to the sweat glands as parasympathetic, whereas others consider them to be controlled by the sympathetic nervous system.

One effect of increased sympathoadrenal activity deserving emphasis is that the seriously ill or injured patient is often unusually alert. Whereas a high degree of alertness is protective in a hostile environment, it may be an unnecessary source of stress to the patient who is under professional care. In fact, the climate surrounding the patient ought to be such that the patient can trust others to be responsible for his or her care. Conversations in the vicinity of the patient should take into account the possibility that the patient is overly alert. Nothing should be said that is likely to increase anxiety. A useful rule is not to talk in the presence of the patient without including him or her in the conversation. Furthermore, noise, jarring, and other forms of unnecessary stimulation should be avoided, as the patient is likely to be unusually sensitive to them.

TABLE 18-2 *Comparison of Effects of Stimulating Alpha and Beta Receptors*

Alpha Receptor	Beta Receptor
Vasoconstriction	Vasodilatation in muscles
Dilatation of pupil	
Increased heart rate	Increased strength of heart contraction
Relaxation of intestine	Relaxation of uterine muscle
Conversion of glycogen to glucose	Bronchial relaxation

As stated earlier, differences in behavior resulting from stimulation of the sympathoadrenal system are explained by proposing two different types of receptor substances. Some authorities suggest that norepinephrine affects only effector cells containing alpha receptors. Epinephrine affects both (see Table 18-2).

Interference with Nerve Impulse Transmission

Sympathectomy by surgical or chemical means is employed in the therapy of diseases of blood vessels in which vascular spasm is believed to be a factor. It is most commonly used in the treatment of essential hypertension, severe Raynaud's disease, and occlusive arterial disease involving the extremities. In surgical sympathectomy, a few to many pre- or postganglionic fibers of vertebral sympathetic ganglia are interrupted and a section of the fiber is removed. The number and location of the fibers to be excised depend on the disorder under treatment. Preganglionic fibers to collateral or terminal sympathetic ganglia may also be interrupted. In splanchnicectomy the preganglionic fibers to the celiac ganglia, the superior and inferior mesenteric plexuses, may be severed and removed. Instead of surgical interruption and excision of sympathetic fibers, a similar effect may be obtained by chemical means. There are a number of drugs that inactivate the autonomic nervous system by blocking the transmission of impulses through autonomic ganglia (ganglionic blocking agents). These drugs act by reducing the number of impulses reaching blood vessels and thereby reducing vascular tone and blood pressure. To evaluate the effectiveness of blocking agents, the blood pressure should be taken in the lying, sitting, and standing positions. One undesirable effect of extensive surgical and chemical sympathectomies is that they limit the capacity to adapt the diameter of the blood vessels to changes in position. Blood pressure falls when the affected person assumes the upright position after having been in the recumbent position. The patient should therefore be instructed to assume the upright position slowly. When postural hypotension is severe, excessive pooling of blood in the legs may be prevented by wrapping them from instep to groin with elastic bandages. (See Chapter 52 for preambulation exercises to minimize postural hypotension.)

Clinical Illustrations

Myasthenia Gravis

The classic illustration of disease which involves interference with transmission of impulses across the myoneural junction is *myasthenia gravis.* The clinical and physiologic manifestations of myasthenia gravis are attributable to a reduction in the number of acetylcholine receptors at neuromuscular junctions. This results in a decrease of the "safety margin" of neuromuscular transmission, with frequent transmission failure. The receptor deficit is due to an autoimmune attack directed specifically against the acetylcholine receptors. In most patients, antibodies to acetylcholine receptor are present, and there is evidence that they have a pathogenetic role in the disease. The mechanism of antibody action may involve acceleration of the rate of degradation and blocking of the receptors (Drachman, 1978).

Modern treatment of myasthenia gravis is successful in returning most patients to productive lives. Anticholinesterase agents[2] improve neuromuscular transmission but do not correct the basic receptor defect. Thymectomy and adrenal corticosteroids apparently interfere with the autoimmune reaction. As more is learned about the immune mechanisms in the disease, specific methods of immunotherapy may be devised to correct the abnormalities in individual patients (Drachman, 1978).

Fortunately, myasthenia gravis is relatively rare; in 1974, it was estimated that about 50,000 persons in the United States were known to have the disease (Carini & Owens, 1974, p. 207). The muscular weakness and easy fatigability characteristic of the disease most frequently affect the facial, oculomotor (causing pathognomonic drooping of the eyelids), laryngeal, pharyngeal, and respiratory muscles.

Major nursing responsibilities include teaching drug effects and adminstration; helping the patient and family to plan physical activity to coincide with peak action of anticholinesterase drugs and to design an adequate sleep, rest, and activity schedule for hospital and home; and being prepared to deal effectively with impending respiratory arrest if respiratory muscles should fail. See Chapter 40 for nursing in ventilatory crisis.

Huntington's Chorea

A more devastating example of pathology related to neurotransmitter abnormalities is seen in *Huntington's chorea,* a disease characterized by bizarre choreiform (irregular, involuntary, twisting, writhing) movements, speech disturbances, and mental deterioration that gradually lead to dementia. Huntington's chorea is an hereditary disease transmitted via an autosomal dominant gene by both sexes, with each child having a 50 per cent chance of inheriting the disease. People have been known to live 30 years following onset of the earliest symptoms, which are usually indicative of impaired concentration and reasoning (Stipe, 1979). The disease is progressive and incurable but not fatal; death usually results from the secondary complications of heart failure, aspiration, or pneumonia.

The defective gene appears to orchestrate imbalance in three neurotransmitters: an excess of dopamine, an excitatory neurotransmitter, in relation to levels of acetylcholine and gamma aminobutyric acid (GABA), an inhibitory neurotransmitter. Drug therapy is aimed at restoring balance among these three neurotransmitters and thus lessening choreiform movements. Dopamine antagonists such as haloperidol and chlorpromazine (Thorazine) may partially control involuntary movements, but the patient progressively requires more assistance with self-care to ensure safety and comfort, and family and staff progressively need help to accept and pro-

[2] During acute attacks of myasthenia gravis, the anticholinesterase agent of choice is parenteral neostigmine; for long-term management, oral neostigmine, pyridostigmine (Mestinon bromide), or ambemonium (Mytelase Chloride) is usually the drug of choice (Adams, 1977).

tect the patient as his or her mental and emotional status become more labile.

Further discussion of ANS function in defending against and responding to bodily injury, and the nurse's role in helping the patient with a sympathoadrenal response, is presented in Unit V.

Summary—Neural Regulation

Stimulus, receptor, arousal system, integrator, and effector—if any are absent or weak, the response is lacking or inappropriate. The nurse whose care is based on thorough initial and ongoing assessment of the person's total behavior, including neurologic function, is in a position to enhance or weaken the force of the circuit.

References Cited

Adams, R. D. "Myasthenia Gravis and Episodic Muscular Weakness." In *Harrison's Principles of Internal Medicine,* 8th ed. Ed. by G. W. Thorn et al. New York: McGraw-Hill Book Company, 1977, p. 1998.

Antelman, S. M., and Caggiula, A. R. "Norepinephrine–Dopamine Interactions and Behavior." *Science,* **195** (18 Feb. 1977), 646–54.

Brobeck, J. R., ed. *Best & Taylor's Physiological Basis of Medical Practice.* 9th ed. Baltimore: The Williams & Wilkins Company, 1973.

Bunge, R. et al. "Nature and Nurture in Development of the Autonomic Neuron." *Science,* **199** (31 March 1978), 1409–16.

Carini, E., and Owens, G. *Neurological and Neurosurgical Nursing.* St. Louis: The C. V. Mosby Company, 1974.

Drachman, D. B. "Myasthenia Gravis." *N. Engl. J. Med.,* **298** (26 Jan. 1978), 186–92.

Guyton, A. C. *Textbook of Medical Physiology,* 5th ed. Philadelphia: W. B. Saunders Company, 1976.

Hemingway, A., and Price, W. M. "The Autonomic Nervous System and Regulation of Body Temperature." *Anesthesiology,* **29,** 694 (July–Aug. 1968).

"How Heroin May Hang on in the Body." *Med. World News,* **13** (28 April 1972), 17–18.

Landsberg, L., and Young, J. B. "Fasting, Feeding and Regulation of the Sympathetic Nervous System." *N. Engl. J. Med.,* **298** (8 June 1978), 1295–1301.

Nathanson, J. A., and Greengard, P. "Second Messengers in the Brain." *Sci. Am.,* **237** (Aug. 1977), 108–19.

Stipe, J. et al. "Huntington's Disease." *Am. J. Nurs.,* **79** (Aug. 1979), 1428–33.

UNIT V

Supporting Mechanisms of Response to Potential and Actual Injury

As the essence of things must always remain unknown, we can learn only relations, and phenomena are merely the result of relations.

CLAUDE BERNARD

Overview of Defenses Against and Responses to Injury

More times than we are aware of, our automatically regulated defenses prevent us from sustaining cellular injury by preventing contact of an injuring agent: as many more times, we are unaware of the repair of injured cells when the agent does succeed in making contact. But even when an individual is aware of the injury, and of the response of his or her body to the injury, the individual is not necessarily considered to be experiencing illness.

Illness exists when (1) the individual recognizes some difference, discomfort, or dysfunction within himself, or (2) society recognizes and labels some discomfort, dysfunction, or deviance in an individual or group. The standard or norm against which the individual and/or society measures the health–illness axis is highly unstable, and often situationally determined (Chafetz, 1972).

Whatever the interpretation assigned to an individual's responses to injury, there are certain regularities or patterns of response traceable to activation of the human defense mechanisms.

Three Types of Defense Mechanisms to Protect Homeostasis

There are basically three types of defense mechanisms to protect a human being's internal environment from external injuring agents:

1. The first line of defense consists of the *mechanical and chemical properties* of the skin, mucous membranes, and other tissues in contact with the outside environment. Special weapons of the skin include keratin and the sweat and sebaceous

glands. Mucous membranes protect by ciliary action and their bactericidal power. Some tissues have specialized secretions, such as saliva, tears, earwax; respiratory membranes have mucus and cilia; tonsils and tracheal lymph nodes protect the oropharynx; and the lungs are further protected by the detergent properties of alveolar fluid.
2. The second line of defense is *cellular* and is based on localized tissue reactions, the most important of which is phagocytosis.
3. The third line of defense is *humoral,* activated when the injuring agent is not deterred by other defenses, and penetrates the tissues, invading the blood (Timiras, 1972).

Some understanding of the physiologic mechanisms by which the organism responds to injury is essential to planning and meeting the needs of sick patients. During the early stages of an acute illness or following a serious injury, the energy and the resources of the patient are concentrated on survival.

Nursing Objectives in the Care of the Acutely Ill

1. To prevent further injury
2. To ascertain the degree and extent of injury as a basis for modifying nursing care
3. To support the patient and modify the environment and nursing care so that he or she can use energy to recover (survive)
4. To observe the reactions of the patient so that care can be altered as patient needs change and that, inasmuch as is possible, complications can be prevented
5. To provide the patient with materials and services required during the various phases of illness
6. As the patient recovers, to shift responsibility to the patient for meeting his or her own needs.

How the Body Protects Itself Against Injury

Although emphasis is on the response of the organism after it is injured, a brief discussion of protective structures and functions follows.

First Line of Defense: Mechanical and Chemical Properties of Contact Tissues

Body structure is protective. Bony cages shelter vital organs such as the brain, heart, and lungs. The eye is recessed in the skull and is further guarded by the nose and the outward jutting of the brow. Injury great enough to disrupt the continuity of bones is almost always accompanied by injury to underlying or surrounding structures.

Barriers against the entrance of foreign matter into the body include sensory receptors that are stimulated by conditions in the external environment, the intact skin and mucous membranes, mechanisms for conditioning air as it passes through the respiratory tract and for the removal of particles that do reach the alveoli, and mechanisms for the rejection of irritating substances from the gastrointestinal tract. The hydrogen ion concentration of secretions in the stomach, mouth, and vagina offers some protection against microorganisms. The presence of enzymes such as lysozyme injures the cell wall and causes the bacteria to lyse, mainly because of environmental conditions. Because secretions by glands in these organs are stimulated by irritation, there is an increased volume of fluid to dilute and wash away noxious agents.

Reflexes such as coughing, sneezing, vomiting, dodging, and blinking initiate activities enabling the individual to remove or avoid harmful agents. Often protection involves a number of mechanisms. For example, a particle of dust gains access to the cornea of the eye where it stimulates sensitive nerve endings in the cornea. Exquisitely severe pain demands relief, and the person suffering it is prompted to initiate measures for the removal of the foreign body. Simultaneously the lacrimal glands secrete tears that dilute the foreign material (when this is possible) and wash it away by flooding. Blinking of the eyelids distributes the tears over the eyeballs and tends to prevent the entrance of new particles. A person in whom the cornea and sclera are insensitive to pain or who cannot secrete tears lacks a primary defense mechanism. To prevent irreparable injury to the affected eye, this person must institute a regular schedule of procedures that substitute for the ones that have been lost. Because the person does not suffer pain when a foreign body enters the eye, he or she must develop the habit of inspecting the sclera for redness several times a day. The person should also consciously blink the eyes at regular intervals, and may have to bathe the eyes with saline solution. The person should try to identify sources of injury and then utilize appropriate measures for protection against them. For example, on windy days or when there is the possibility of exposure to dust, he or she should wear goggle-type glasses.

Second Line of Defense: Cellular Reactions

As discussed in Unit III, cells can alter their size and strength in response to increased or decreased stimulation (hypertrophy–atrophy). Some can adapt to a change in the environment by undergoing metaplasia. The organs of most persons are capable of doing more work than they are ordinarily called on to do.

Even when the first lines of defense are penetrated, in some instances the body is able to destroy or localize an injuring agent. As an example, a cut in the skin allows pathogenic microbes to enter. The germs may be destroyed by local defense mechanisms before they are able to multiply. If they do multiply, they may never leave the site of entry because the body's localizing mechanisms are effective. One of the barriers to spread is hyaluronic acid, an intracellular cement of gellike consistency. It is permeable to small particles such as water and electrolytes but less permeable to large particles such as bacteria, protein molecules, and cells. Other localizing factors will be discussed later.

Third Line of Defense: Humoral Reactions

Assuming that injurious agents get beyond the second line of defense, they may be destroyed or inactivated by reticuloendothelial cells in the lymph nodes, the spleen, or liver or destroyed by phagocytic cells in the blood. The body is further protected by the ability of the liver and kidneys to excrete bacteria and certain chemicals into the bile or urine. Depending on the effectiveness of the body's defense mechanisms, injuring agents may be eliminated without appearing to cause harm, may be localized to the site of injury, or may escape to be destroyed or eliminated at more distant sites or may cause overt injury.

Responses to Limit and Repair Cellular Injury

Despite protective structures and the capacity to respond to the environment so that injury is prevented, injury to cells does occur. When cells are injured, survival depends on the capacity of the organism to react in such a manner that the injury to cells is limited and damage is repaired. As with other homeostatic mechanisms, there are limits to the capacity of any individual to withstand injury. The damage to the total organism or to a vital structure may be so great that death occurs immediately. At the other end of the scale, because human beings are thinking, learning, remembering, and feeling organisms, they sometimes respond to symbols of danger when no real threat exists. Responses to imaginary danger may be as incapacitating as responses to tissue injury.

In injury or illness of a serious nature, not only the cells in and around the site of injury but those throughout the entire organism participate in the response. Many of the manifestations observed in illness arise from the local and general responses of the organism to cell damage. They are initiated by a noxious agent sufficiently potent to cause direct injury to cells or to alert the mental apparatus to the possibility of serious danger. Similar to other homeostatic mechanisms, responses to injury may be excessive or deficient in degree or they may be inappropriate to the stimulus. As will be emphasized later, a response may be the cause of injury.

The stimulus initiating one or more of the responses to injury may be damaging to cell structure or a symbol implying danger to the individual. To illustrate, fire, by raising the environmental temperature above that tolerated by the tissue, injures the tissue. Cells in the burned area are affected by the products released by injured or killed cells and respond in ways that are protective. The pain associated with even a small burn acts as a stimulus for responses involving the entire organism. When more than a limited area of tissue is burned, the individual can be expected to respond on all levels of organization, from the biochemical level to the highest integrative centers in the brain. Some of these same reactions can be elicited by a situation in which fire is perceived as being a source of danger. Seeing a flame where none should be elicits behavior similar to that in which actual burning has occurred. Even a fire siren may alarm an individual who has recently experienced a severe burn.

Many of the responses occurring during illness are to injury or danger rather than to the specific agent. They are therefore nonspecific or stereotyped rather than specific responses. Though there are modifying factors, the magnitude of reaction is usually in proportion to the extent of the danger or injury. There are also patterns of response that can be attributed to particular etiological agents. For example, during the prodromal stage of the acute infectious diseases of childhood, the child is ill but the nature of the illness may be unclear for several days. Unless the child develops a rash or some other feature of a specific disease, the illness will be attributed to a cold or a virus. Antibodies specific to the causative agent may be isolated from the child's blood. The final outcome in any illness depends on two general factors: the nature and extent of the injury and the appropriateness and adequacy of the response of the individual.

Humans have a remarkable capacity to respond to changes in their internal and external environment in such a manner that function is maintained within physiologic and psychological limits. As long as disturbances do not exceed the adaptive capacity of the individual, energy is available for growth and reproduction and to alter conditions in the external environment. When conditions in the environment are such that the survival of the organism is threatened, energy is utilized to escape from, or to overcome, the injuring agent and to make necessary repairs.

A special case of threatening environmental conditions is the experience of hospitalization. Whatever the nature of the events perceived as threatening by the patient, he or she is often unable to (and sometimes unwilling to risk) escape from, or to confront the cause of, the distress. Volicer (1973) found that the event related to hospitalization which was assigned the highest stress value by 216 adults was the possibility of loss of function of the senses, such as eyesight and hearing.

Finally, through the use of the intellect, humans evaluate and modify their environment so that they protect themselves against many potential dangers. Through the enactment and enforcement of laws, they regulate their own behavior and that of others so that all are protected from disease and injury.

In general, the magnitude of a response to injury varies with the extent of the injury. Some agents inflict more damage and provoke a greater reaction than others, and injuries to certain body structures are accompanied by a greater response than are others. The characteristics of the person who is ill also influence his or her response. Persons who are at the extremes of age usually respond less vigorously than do children and young adults. The response of persons in middle life is not as vigorous as that of young adults, but it is greater than that of the elderly. There are exceptions. Mrs. Malone, aged 96, is one. She experienced and recovered from pneumonia. At the height of her illness, she had a fever of 102°F. It is not uncommon for persons of advanced age to have little or no elevation in temperature in disorders commonly causing fever in younger persons. Males usually respond more vigorously than females, but the fact that vigorous young men respond actively does not mean that they have a higher recovery rate from serious illness than women do. In fact, there is some evidence that the reverse is true. As might be expected, the well-nourished react more actively than the poorly nourished and vigorous, healthy persons more than debilitated or sickly ones. In general, the vigor of homeostatic responses to illness or injury is greater in those with a good adaptive capacity and less in those whose adaptive capacity is deficient.

As stated earlier, the ultimate goal of the homeostatic responses to injury or to dangers perceived as sources of injury is survival. The attainment of this goal involves escaping from, or overcoming, noxious agents and repairing disturbances or damage that results. At the time the individual is threatened with, or suffers, severe injury or illness, a whole series of integrated reactions are initiated involving the neuromuscular, neuroendocrine, circulatory, respiratory, and reticuloendothelial systems. Structures and functions not immediately useful to survival are suppressed. The significance of the preceding to nursing will be indicated as the various responses are discussed.

Supporting Mechanisms of Response to Actual or Potential Injury

In this unit, mechanisms by which the organism responds to injury are presented. Inasmuch as these responses are appropriate and adequate, the survival of the organism is facilitated.

Though the role of the nurse is indicated throughout each chapter, objectives of care may be summarized as follows: (1) To control, or to teach the patient to control, agents causing injury of the tissue. This includes many activities: the prevention of fires and automobile accidents, the protection of an allergic person from the antigen or antigens to which he or she is susceptible, the maintenance of asepsis in the operating room and cleanliness in the areas where patients reside, and the prevention of sunburn. (2) To provide the necessary conditions for the tissue response to be adequate to the needs of the situation. This too involves a variety of activities ranging from those that have to do with supporting the arterial or venous circulation to providing the necessary nutritional elements. Although points are illustrated in many instances by relating the content to events occurring in patients treated by surgical therapy, all persons who are ill undergo similar responses. They may be less obvious and are sometimes of a lesser degree. All illness, however, of whatever degree is compounded of injury and the response of the individual to the injury. The responses to injury detailed in this unit are summarized in tabular format in Appendix D.

References Cited

Chafetz, M. E. "Definition of Illness: When Is a Person a Patient?" *Med. Insight*, 4 (May 1972), 60–66.

Timiras, P. S. *Developmental Physiology and Aging*. New York: Macmillan Publishing Co., Inc., 1972, pp. 224–45.

Volicer, B. J. "Perceived Stress Levels of Events Associated with the Experience of Hospitalization." *Nurs. Res.*, 22 (Nov.–Dec. 1973), 491–97.

19

Psychological Responses*

No one is so accursed by fate,
No one so utterly desolate,
But some heart, though unknown,
Responds unto his own.

Endymion [1842]. Stanza 8
LONGFELLOW
In Bartlett's Familiar Quotations by John Bartlett. Thirteenth and Centennial Edition 1955, Boston: Little, Brown and Company, p. 521a.

In the discussion of the psychological aspects of illness, the following points will be considered: (1) the concept of homeostasis, (2) a definition of psychological stress, (3) some purposes served by intellectual responses to illness, (4) the differences in definition of the sick role as a source of psychological stress, (5) the emotional reactions of a person who recognizes he or she is ill, and (6) the emotional reactions of significant others to illness.

Emotional Homeostasis

Although the concept of homeostasis was introduced by Cannon (1939) to explain the constancy of internal physiological environment of cells in the body, psychologists have adapted the concept to encompass the emotional state. Thus used, *homeostasis* refers to a general condition of psychological integration (Kallmann, 1959).

> Homeostasis is the ensemble of regulations that maintain variables constant and direct the organism toward a goal, and are performed by feedback mechanisms, that is, the result of the reaction is monitored back to the "receptor" side so that the system is held stable or is led toward a target or a goal (von Bertalanffy, 1974, p. 1160).

As with physiologic homeostasis, emotional homeostasis depends on having certain needs fulfilled. Whereas the supplies required to satisfy physiologic needs are materials such as oxygen or water, those required to meet psychological needs are nonmaterial, though they may be represented, symbolically, by material objects. Psychological needs are the conditions, situations, actions, or effects of action that the individual perceives, experiences, and represents in his or her mind as having meaning. Depending on the situation and its meaning, the person may feel safe and protected, esteemed by others and self, and loved. Conversely, in other situations the individual may feel threatened, unsafe, unesteemed, endangered, and unloved. The satisfaction of psychological needs depends on the person having structures that function in such a manner that he or she is able to perceive and evaluate anything that impinges on his or her being. Psychological homeo-

* This chapter revised by Jean A. Werner-Beland, M.N., R.N., Associate Professor of Nursing, Wayne State University, College of Nursing, Detroit, Michigan.

stasis implies, as does physiologic homeostasis, the presence of processes or mechanisms that regulate, maintain, or restore emotional or psychological stability in a changing environment.

Agents that endanger psychological homeostasis may have their origin in either the internal or external environment of the individual. They are similar to agents that threaten physiologic homeostasis in that they may result from an excess or deficit of supply. They differ from agents that threaten physiologic homeostasis in that the individual responds not only to the agent itself but to what it symbolizes. Consequently, fear and anxiety can be engendered by harmless things. The individual feels and behaves in the presence of the symbol as if in the presence of the thing it represents to him or her. As a consequence of this phenomenon, much of what a person fears is learned.

To illustrate, Mrs. Simon is afraid of dying. Despite her knowledge that her illness is minor and not considered to threaten her life, she has all the signs and symptoms of being terrified. She has no understanding of why she is reacting in this way. Her fear does not diminish when she is given logical and reasonable explanations. Illness of any sort symbolizes total destruction to Mrs. Simon, and she responds to the symbolic meaning of illness rather than to the reality of the situation.

As in physiologic homeostasis, individuals differ in their capacity to adapt. Many factors contribute to this difference. Some of these may be inborn, others may be learned, and still others may result from disease. For example, the capacity of the brain-injured child or adult to adapt to frustration is less than that of the non-brain–injured person. This must be recognized and the environment adapted so that expectations are kept within the person's ability to function. Though the capacity to tolerate psychological stress differs from one individual to another, all people have a limit. As stated earlier, there are many factors in illness that contribute to the disruption of psychological homeostasis, with the end result an increase in psychological stress.

Psychological Stress

As a basis for the discussion of the causes of psychological stress, Engel's definition of stress is quoted: "Psychological stress refers to all processes, whether originating in the external environment or within the person, which impose a demand or requirement upon the organism, the resolution or handling of which necessitates work or activity of the mental apparatus before any other system is involved or activated" (1960, p. 480).

It is difficult to determine which situations or conditions requiring adaptation will actually be stressful to the individual's adaptive capacity. Stress is likely to occur because the adaptive capacity of the individual is limited or because the condition to which the individual is required to adapt is extreme. In other words, because adaptation is a learned process, the person's previously learned methods of adaptation may not be adequate to deal initially with a situation, and stress results. Psychological stresses place strain on the adaptive capacity of the organism by acting on the brain and mental apparatus (Engel, 1960). Although other agents that place strain on the adaptive capacity of the organism may produce psychological stress, this action is secondary. Their primary effect is on biochemical processes, cells, organs, or system. Psychological stress may also, and often does, involve structures other than the mental apparatus, but is primary effect is on the mental apparatus. Whatever the cause of the disturbance, agents that act as stimuli result in the initiation of mechanisms of response that serve to reduce or relieve the discomfort. In general these mechanisms enable the individual to attack or to withdraw from the danger or to play dead (possum).

From the previous statements one can assume that adaptation is not a static condition. We have mentioned the individual's need to strive for emotional homeostasis, which requires continuing use of adaptive processes. It also would be well to mention *heterostasis*, or the concept that deals with the tendency of the organism to seek imbalance or new stimuli, which, in turn, lead to new levels of adaptation (Sargent and Mayman, 1959). The latter concept is important in health care because it clearly implies that an individual can acquire new learning from a state of imbalance such as illness or disability. The positive or negative quality of this learning often depends on the kind of assistance the patient receives from health professionals and others in the course of the illness.

During illness the individual may lose or be threatened with the loss of something that has value. He or she is almost certain to suffer painful procedures or to fear such a possibility. The fear is often increased by the fact that the patient does not know what to expect and therefore fears the worst. In the process of growing up, the individual learns to master drives so that needs can be met in keeping with reality. Sometimes the manner in which the individual regards his or her drives is a source of conflict. During illness these conflicts may be intensified. Whatever the specific source of psychological stress in illness, it leads to unpleasant feelings such as anxiety, anger, helplessness, hopelessness, guilt, shame, and disgust. To counteract these feelings and to restore emotional homeostasis, psychological defense mechanisms that have been relatively effective in the past will be initiated. When *defense mechanisms* such as *rationalization, projection, sublimation, displacement,* or *denial* are ineffective or inadequate to restore emotional homeostasis, physiologic and/or behavioral changes follow.

Some Causes of Psychological Stress

What actually will be disturbing to any patient during illness and how he or she will react are highly individual matters. There are, however, some causes of psychological stress that occur frequently enough that they should be considered when each patient's needs are assessed. Engel classifies the causes of psychological stress as (1) the loss of something that is of value to the person, (2) injury or threat of injury to the body, and (3) the frustration of drives. These, obviously, are interrelated. Contained within Engel's list of causes are other elements such as the altered concept of self, failure of the intellect to resolve the illness, threats to economic security, confusion in the definition of the sick role, and fears that needs will not be adequately met.

Threats to Self-Concept

The first of these subelements, self-concept, includes all the ideas, conscious and unconscious feelings, beliefs, and attitudes that persons have about themselves and their possessions. In their concept of themselves they attempt to answer the questions "Where am I?" "What am I?" "Who am I?" Among the many things that persons may or may not value about themselves are their body image or picture of themselves; their feeling of being intact or whole; their role and status in their family, community, and job; their adequacy and acceptability as a marriage partner; their success and sense of fulfillment; and their hope that tomorrow will be better than today. They may value family, home, state, and country. Other values that may be threatened during illness include the way in which they regard financial, physical, or emotional dependence and independence; how they feel about relinquishing control over events that relate to their welfare; as well as the way in which they ordinarily relate to other people.

Because they threaten the self-concept of the individual in some way, certain types of disease are more likely to cause psychological stress than others. These include those that cause disfigurement, especially of the face, or the loss of a part that is easily identified, such as an extremity. Diseases or treatments that threaten the organs of reproduction are also sources of anxiety. Some diseases such as venereal diseases are regarded as bringing disgrace on the person and family. In some groups tuberculosis and cancer are also perceived as a cause for shame. Mental illness and mental retardation fall into the same category. Other diseases such as heart disease or cancer are associated in the minds of many people with death. In addition cancer is generally equated with an extended and painful illness.

Failure of the Intellect to Resolve Illness

Failure of the intellect to resolve illness and all its consequences is also a source of psychological stress for many persons. In illness each individual reacts closely to the way he or she does in other crises in life—at least initially. Reactions are often complex, involving both intellect and emotions. Through the use of their intelligence, human beings are often able to foresee the consequences of their actions and to plan to avert injury or correct the damage that has been done. Inasmuch as they are able to acquire knowledge and to grasp and identify the significant factors in their situation and to use their capacity to reason and think, to modify their behavior, or to adapt the environment to meet their needs, intelligence is useful to humans. However, what if intelligence fails? What if illness imposes such overwhelming changes on the physical functioning of the person that intelligence fails in every way except to tell the person that this time reason cannot get him or her out of this mess? Anxiety increases, and various defensive maneuvers are called into action to protect the individual from experiencing the full impact of what has happened.

How well a person uses intelligence depends on numerous factors, including educational background and emotional state. Hence a highly intelligent and well-educated person (not excluding physicians or nurses) may act irrationally as well as rationally in a personal crisis such as illness. Intelligence is useful to the individual only as long as he or she can remain objective, identify the nature of the threat, and plan protection or elimination of the threat. It fails inasmuch as the knowledge on which decisions are based is inadequate, inaccurate, or not applicable, or the person's emotional state is such that he or she is unable to use this knowledge. The theories of crisis intervention take these points into account. The significance of crisis intervention is in helping an individual utilize intelligence to do problem solving in relation to the immediate critical situation in his or her life. If the person in crisis receives appropriate help—that is, help that allows the person to think through the problem and come to some conclusions about acceptable solutions or alternatives—the experience can lead to new, more mature levels of adaptation.

This does not imply that education and intelligence are of no importance when a person is ill. However, the point that intelligence is not synonymous with years of schooling is worth making. Some people who are intelligent but who have had little opportunity to go to school are well educated. Because of the tendency to equate schooling with education and with intelligence, quite intelligent but unschooled people may be treated as if they were not capable of understanding or of participating in plans for their care.

When a patient's level of education is similar to that of the people responsible for care, communication is facilitated. They are more likely to have similar vocabularies and values than when their backgrounds differ widely. When there are differences in background, the degree of success with which the needs of patients are met depends on the extent to which these differences are taken into account.

Differences in Perception of the Sick Role

Another source of psychological stress to the patient, family, and those who provide care is the difference in their respective concepts about the appropriate role and behavior of each other in illness. The role of the sick person in the American culture has been studied and defined by sociologists. Parsons (1958) defines illness as a "socially institutionalized role-type" characterized in the American culture by some incapacity to carry on the normally expected role and tasks. He summarizes the American culture view of illness as follows:

1. The person is exempted from role obligations.
2. He or she is not held responsible for being ill.
3. This state is held to be legitimate, if the person accepts the need for help and cooperates with those who help him or her.

The meaning of each of these will be clarified later in this chapter.

To understand how a patient arrives at his or her particular version of the sick role, it is necessary to review certain psychological developmental facts (Linn, 1977, p. 364). In infancy did the person receive sensitive, loving care when ill? If so, there probably will be less panic later in life when the same person becomes ill. On the other hand, it is speculated that if care given during infancy came from a cold, unresponsive, withdrawn source, when this person becomes ill as an adult he or she will exhibit panic or excessive displays of discomfort (both physical and psychological) when ill (Linn, 1977).

Conflict, with its accompanying psychological stress, arises between the patient and the people providing health care when differences in interpretation of their respective roles arise. If the patient is interpreting his or her role in one way and the nurse is interpreting the patient's role differently, there is little or no communication taking place between them. Each has a set of values to which the other is expected to conform, but when conformity does not take place power struggles frequently occur. The patient will start behaving in ways that are intended to maintain his or her role image, and the nurse probably will react in a similar manner.

In general, when there is an increase in nonconformity, there is a counterincrease in rigidity. Thus if a nurse does not conform to the patient's stereotype of "nurse," the patient may become more rigid and determined in an effort to make sure that the nurse does conform. For example, if the patient's stereotype is that all nurses are crabby, he or she may unconsciously behave in such a way that the nurse will eventually get angry. Then the patient has reinforcement for his or her view. These situations work both ways. In an instance where a patient is not able to accept the need for help and continues to be uncooperative with those who provide help the patient is demeaned, treated with suspicion, or discharged as a hopeless case. What may be operating in the latter example is that the patient and nurse are defining *help* in different ways and neither is able to communicate this difference to the other. Anxiety usually increases on both sides. After all, the nurse is taught that nurses are supposed to be helpful. Failing in this, she or he becomes anxious. The patients, at some level, must want help or they would cease being patients. Failing to get the assistance they think would be useful to them, they too get anxious. The breech between the helper and the one seeking help usually widens unless someone, usually the nurse, can stop and make a conscious effort to look at what is getting in the way of satisfactory and satisfying care.

Similar struggles frequently occur between the patient and family, between the patient and the community, or between the patient and the hospital culture. The patient begins to sense pressure to conform to a stereotype that comes from a group and not just from an individual. Finding that behaving in accordance with personal feelings and standards gains nothing, the patient may gradually fall into the system's stereotype of what patients should be in order to get needed attention. The writer recently observed a situation where one norm of ward culture was to yell. The patients who yelled the loudest received the most favorable attention from the nursing staff. This usually made new patients and new staff members very uneasy, especially if they came from backgrounds where people spoke quietly, said what they meant, and were listened to. The new patient, for example, would expect that when he turned on his call light a nurse would respond, he would tell her what he wanted, and then she would take some appropriate action. However, this did not happen. Finally, even the most mild-mannered patients recognized that in this culture sick people were expected to yell. If you did not yell, apparently you were not considered to be sick enough to need attention.

The nurse does not have to search very far for examples of strained nurse–patient relationships that occur when a patient violates one of Parsons's norms for illness. Let us look at the one that says that a patient is not held responsible for his or her illness. What happens if a person is hospitalized because of self-inflicted wounds or because of blatant disregard for measures that might have maintained health? What usually happens is that the staff will either help the patient deny responsibility for the illness, or treat the patient with contempt, or both. Another aspect of this norm is that the patient may be relieved of responsibility for the illness, but he or she is almost always judged as being responsible for personal behavior. There is a tendency in the American culture to evaluate the expression of emotion in terms of good (desirable) or bad (undesirable). Thus anger, or the expression of anger, is bad, and people who express anger are treated as if they were bad. This view neglects the fact that emotions are the substance of life. They give it color and meaning. Emotions are useful when they are directed toward socially acceptable goals. Their usefulness is impaired when they are inappropriate to the situation or excessive or deficient in degree. Anger, when properly controlled and directed toward the accomplishment of goals, may serve as a spur to the correction of an injustice. When it is uncontrolled, or excessive in amount, it may be destructive. What is appropriate is in the eye of the beholder. For example, what the nurse may think is appropriate behavior for a patient in a given situation may not be what the patient feels is appropriate. When their views differ widely, conflict may result.

Regression is another part of illness that frequently leads to confusion in the definition of the sick role. Holmes and Werner write that "Not only is regression a necessary concomitant of an illness, but also it always accompanies and is fostered by hospitalization" (1966, p. 66). In other words, return to a less mature level of behavior is observable in any illness—even the common cold. Linn (1977) writes that "The sick role in adult life is regularly associated with the phenomenon of regression" (p. 3). People may become more dependent, insist that they be taken care of, become short-tempered, and engage in a variety of behaviors that were not common to their personality when they were well. In addition, the very nature of health care demands that a patient give up certain independent functions and rely instead on the judgment of those individuals from whom help is sought. Conflict arises because the limits of the sick role and the helper role are difficult to define. There are double messages going from patient to staff and vice versa. The nurses may make it clear that patients must submit to all types of care and at the same time expect patients to behave as mature adults. Patients frequently behave as if they expect to be treated as mature, capable adults and at the same time insist that their "patient status" give them the right to have even the most unreasonable demands met.

The point was made previously that illness involves relinquishing, to a greater or lesser degree, the ability of the person to control events in relation to himself or herself. This is not only related to actual need imposed by the physical inability to perform certain functions but again is related to the way we define the sick role. According to our perceptions, the person is exempted from role obligations of making decisions. Furthermore, because the patient is not held responsible for being ill, he or she is treated as if unable to assume responsibility for anything. The patient is told when to go to bed, when to get out of bed, when and what can be eaten, and when to bathe. The patient may be asked to perform procedures that he or she does not feel able to do. For example, Mrs. Mel had a hysterectomy following several days of severe hemorrhage. On the day after surgery the nurse entered the room and said, "Now it is time for you to get up." Mrs. Mel asked, "How can I get up? I have all these tubes and I feel too weak." She had three tubes, one into her stomach, one into her urinary bladder, and another connected to a needle in a vein in her left arm. "Doctor's orders," said the nurse. "All patients get up the day after surgery. Just turn on your side and swing your feet over the edge of the bed and raise up as you do so." Mrs. Mel got up because she felt she was helpless to alter the situation. She also felt that the nurse was harsh and unfeeling. Mrs. Mel's feeling that she was called on to perform activities for which she was unprepared and without adequate physical and emotional support is all too common. The nurse could have assisted the patient better by acknowledging her question and her concern and by explaining why it was necessary for her to be out of bed so soon after surgery. Some expression from the nurse that indicated that she appreciated how Mrs. Mel felt and that she would help her might have reduced Mrs. Mel's fear.

In conclusion, there are at least three very important variables that affect the role definition of the sick. One that has not been dealt with in any systematic way is the source(s) and *availability of funding for treatment.* Under some insurance plans, an individual with an emotional disturbance can receive treatment in a psychiatric unit of a general hospital for *X* number of days. As long as the insurance coverage is continued, the person is viewed as being sick. When the limit of the insurance coverage is reached, the patient frequently is discharged whether or not the condition has actually undergone a change for the better. The discharge is justified on the basis that the patient is now ready for discontinuance of treatment or is treatable as an outpatient. It would be interesting to study how many treatments and procedures are withheld from patients who do not have the necessary finances. The physically disabled often have the terms of their patient role defined by the Division of Vocational Rehabilitation when this is the source of funding for their care. As mentioned previously, even the title of the agency draws attention to the fact that rehabilitation efforts are vocational. Little money goes into dealing with the psychological aspects of rehabilitation or toward rehabilitation in relation to readjusting to family, social, or sex roles. Spitzer, Swanson, and Lehr (1969) refer to the family as an *audience which helps determine the careers of psychiatric patients.* This is our second variable, and the concept has meaning for the physically ill individual as well, and can be expanded to include work associates and significant others as part of the audience. Continuing observations of the reactions of these significant others to the illness of one of its members should give the nurse a clearer picture of some of the elements operating in the way the patient engages in care, as well as some of the factors that will be operating in the care and health maintenance of the patient once he or she leaves the hospital. The third variable, the *meaning that illness has to the individual,* is also critical in identifying how a person formulates the sick role. This latter concept will be dealt with in some detail elsewhere in this chapter.

Other Sources of Stress to the Individual

There are many ways in which the performance of various aspects of patient care can be a source of psychological stress and unnecessary anxiety. Such instances occur because we are more oriented to the necessity for completing tasks than we are to the fact that we are caring for a person who has not abdicated his or her entire sense of self-responsibility. Because we fail to take the psychological needs of the patient into account, the following omissions in care often occur:

1. Failure to prepare the patient for what to expect and when to expect it
2. Failure to provide consistency in care
3. Lack of skill in handling the patient or the equipment—including awkwardness, roughness, uncertainty about how to proceed, and failure to give necessary emotional and physical support
4. Lack of needed supplies
5. Changing the performance of a procedure without explanation
6. Failure to observe the patient's modesty patterns by omitting such things as adequate covering and screening while performing procedures
7. Making thoughtless or careless remarks in the presence of the patient that suggest dangers that may or may not exist.

Diagnostic and therapeutic procedures that are performed by as many strangers as there are procedures are sources of anxiety to patients. There is always the possibility that the patient knows or believes that a procedure may be harmful or painful as well as helpful. No list of situations in which the performance of a procedure may add to the patient's anxiety will ever by complete. However, awareness of some common ways in which anxiety is prevented or provoked should be helpful when planning patient care. To illustrate, Mrs. Taylor was to have a urea clearance test on Tuesday. On Monday the physician told her about the test and that she would be moved to the treatment room for it. Later the nurse found Mrs. Taylor weeping. As the nurse attempted to comfort Mrs. Taylor, she learned that the patient called the treatment room the "death room." This belief had its origin in the fact that the artificial kidney was in this room and that some of the patients who went into the room died. The nurse reported Mrs. Taylor's feeling to the physician, who replied, "That is the reason that she looked so forlorn when I told her about the test." He arranged to perform the procedure in Mrs. Taylor's room and, of course, talked with her about the change of plans. In this example it was possible to change a physical aspect of a procedure and therefore reduce the threat to the patient. This may not always be true. When it is not, the nurse can still be helpful to the patient by recognizing his or her feelings, by trying to understand the source of the anxiety, and by planning alternatives that might alleviate it.

The cost to the patient and family because of pain and suffering, or the fear of pain and suffering, is a real part of any illness. Here nurses can do much through the use of appropriate measures to relieve and prevent unnecessary pain.

Although the psychological cost of pain and suffering is great, the actual expense of illness is also a source of anxiety to patients and their families. Here, too, patients are by cultural definition exempted from their role obligations but only to a degree. They are not exempted from the obligation of paying for their care or other debts. Direct costs are of great concern to those whose incomes are limited and who do not have hospital and medical insurance. This is especially true of people who have always been able to meet their financial obligations. Since the advent of Medicare, the burden of the cost of medical care for the elderly has been greatly reduced. However, care for this age group is still a costly matter. The costs of hospitalization and medical care are also the expenses that are the most obvious to the nurse. Patients may have insurance that pays their medical expenses and still be extremely concerned because illness is accompanied by loss of income, the inability to meet other obligations such as mortgage payment, or additional burdens such as payments for child care. Even relatively short illnesses may make serious demands on a limited income. Other costs of illness include the demands made on family members to visit the sick or to provide for care if he or she is not hospitalized. Sometimes this means the expense of traveling long distances, of shifting home responsibilities to meet the patient's needs, and so forth.

The nurse is not responsible for the cost of illness, but she or he should be aware that it may be a problem for the patient. Nurses can attempt to find out the nature of the patient's concern and alert the physician to the fact that the patient is worried. Depending on the nature of the situation, the problem may be referred to a social worker or a community agency. In communities where home-care plans are available, some patients may be able to receive the care they need at home. From the patient's point of view this may be more satisfactory as well as less expensive. Patients are not always aware of available community services. The nurse should be aware of community resources, so that she or he can bring these to the attention of the patient and family.

Illustrations of the Relationship between Defined Sick Role and Psychological Stress

To illustrate how differences in definition of the sick role may produce psychological stress, six patients will be presented.

First there is Mr. Tompkins, admitted to ward X. By the very act of admission to the hospital he was separated from his responsibilities as a husband, father, and executive. Hospitalization also established the fact that he was incapable of carrying on his normal role activities. Correct sickroom behavior for Mr. Tompkins and his visitors was interpreted to mean the avoidance of talking about his business or the problems that his son was having in school. In fact, visitors were expected to "cheer him up." Anyone who violated this code was immediately labeled as harmful to his welfare. His employer assured him that he was not being held responsible for his illness by providing him with sick leave and medical and hospital insurance and the assurance that his job would be waiting for him when he recovered. His coworkers took up a collection for flowers and sent him cards to indicate their support and concern.

The diagnosis—peptic ulcer—afforded Mr. Tompkins a certain amount of status in the community. It was assumed to indicate that he was hard-working and successful. Therefore he was allowed to be hospitalized without the loss of status. He could refuse to do certain things commonly expected of persons in his social or employment group. He could even refer to his ulcer with modest pride because it was considered, by some, to be one of the badges of success.

Mr. Tompkins was accepted as a sick person capable of being helped. He recognized that he was ill and placed himself in the hands of professional people. He was considered cooperative or uncooperative to the degree to which he did or did not question care, follow orders, and the like. If he was "cooperative" he won favor for himself, the title of "good patient," and the approval of the personnel concerned with his care. To the degree that he questioned his treatment and did not follow orders and suggestions he was labeled "uncooperative." The intensity of his behavior earned him the titles "demanding, unreasonable, stubborn, impossible, and neurotic." Under these circumstances he was held responsible for his behavior and care was withheld or was given in a way that was intended to remind Mr. Tompkins of his role as a patient. This tactic seldom succeeds in doing anything except make the patient feel misunderstood. The patient often continues to exhibit the offending behavior or may increase the intensity of his efforts in order to be recognized as an individual. The staff, failing to recognize the defensive nature of Mr. Tompkins's behavior, accomplishes little by resorting to maneuvers that deprive him of care he needs until he acts in accordance with some mystical model for "good patient."

Next there is Mr. Helm, who was hospitalized following an acute myocardial infarction. His illness constituted a serious threat to his self-concept. He always had taken great pride in the fact that he was strong and healthy. He had boasted to his friends that he never lost a day of work because of illness. He always perceived being sick as a sign of weakness. The onset of the myocardial infarction was accompanied by severe substernal pain. Mr. Helm felt frightened, angry, and helpless. He tried to tell himself that the pain would go away—that it was probably indigestion. When the pain became very severe, he called his doctor.

After his admission to the hospital, Mr. Helm made many demands on the nursing staff for attention. When he turned on his light, he expected it to be answered immediately. Through his behavior he indicated that he wanted what he wanted when he wanted it. His behavior demonstrated his need to feel that he had some control over his situation. Though he vented his angry feelings on the nursing staff and his wife, he did not feel safe in attacking his physician. He covered his angry feelings by telling the doctor stories and making light of the situation. As Mr. Helm began to improve, and the physician was able to reassure him that his heart was healing, he began to press for changes in his medical regimen and in the management of the nursing unit. In fact, he did this to some extent from the beginning by refusing to use a commode and insisting that he use the bathroom. Part of his reaction to illness was to deny its severity and also to deny the change from his role as a well person to that of a sick person.

It was evident that Mr. Helm's behavior did not conform to what is usually expected. If others did not recognize the true meaning of Mr. Helm's behavior they might have thought that Mr. Helm did not like them. Feeling that they have been rejected by the patient might make it difficult for others to attend to his needs. Conversely, if they were able to accept Mr. Helm as a sick man whose behavior was in keeping with his effort to cope with a critical situation in his life, they might have been able to identify his needs and provide a therapeutic environment for him. Even when the nurse recognizes that a patient's behavior has a cause and serves a purpose, acceptance of the patient who violates the "rules" may not be easy. Knowledge of possible sources of conflict should facilitate their identification and serve as a basis for making appropriate adjustments in the patient's environment.

In the room next to Mr. Helm was Mr. Quinn. He, too, was in the hospital for the treatment of a myocardial infarction. At the onset of the pain under his sternum, Mr. Quinn also felt helpless and frightened. In contrast to Mr. Helm, however, he was described as a good patient because he conformed to the cultural definition of a sick person. After consulting his physician, Mr. Quinn went to the hospital, where he cooperated with the prescribed care. That is, he followed orders exactly. He lay quietly, permitting himself to be fed and bathed. He seldom asked for anything and, when he did, he was both patient and polite. Instead of reacting with anger, he responded to his fears and feelings of helplessness by withdrawing from interactions. He became dependent on others for his care and allowed his dependency without murmur. Although nursing care provided well for his physical needs, his psychological needs were in danger of being overlooked. Mr. Quinn was worried not so much about whether he would die but about his ability to return to his job as a riveter in an automobile plant and about what would happen to his wife and five children if he were not able to work. He always had been able to provide for his family. He had hoped to send his sons to college. Because Mr. Quinn was quiet and undemanding, there was also danger of his being left alone for long periods of time. Elements in establishing a therapeutic environment for Mr. Quinn included instituting a pattern of regular visits and trying to establish a nurse–patient relationship in which he felt comfortable expressing his concerns.

Each of the next two patients had an above-the-knee leg amputation. Though the surgical procedure was similar for both patients, their emotional reactions were quite different.

The first patient was Mrs. Oeski, an elderly Polish woman. She seemed to have little concern about the loss of her leg per se. She was, however, very fearful that she would no longer be able to go up and down stairs. This was serious, for though her home had a "company" kitchen and dining room on the first floor, these were seldom used. The kitchen that was used for everyday living was in the basement. Her concept of herself as a homemaker appeared to be more important than that of her physical self. She worked hard to learn to use her prosthesis so that she would be able to walk up and down stairs. Her family were also interested in what they could do to make it possible for her to go up and down stairs. Because of Mrs. Oeski's personal resources and goals and the support given her by her family, she was able to be rehabilitated to the point where she could continue her homemaking role. The fact that she was highly motivated toward a goal was very helpful to her.

Down the corridor from Mrs. Oeski was Mr. Young. His amputation followed an accident in which a basket of ingots fell on his right leg and crushed it. For days afterward he lay with his face to the wall and refused to eat, be bathed, or perform any activity that was considered necessary to his welfare. Though he guarded against anyone seeing him weep, the nurses were sure that he did. He lacked interest in his children and in events that had interested him previously. His general appearance was that of a dejected, depressed person. It was assumed that he was mourning the loss of his leg.

If nurses who provide care for Mr. Young recognize that grief reactions frequently follow the loss of a part or a function of the body, they also must understand that each person views the body as part of his or her identity and self-image. To some people their body represents almost their total self-image and is of extreme importance to them. Others may have their identity anchored in other aspects of their being such as their intellect, and although their body is important to them, it may not be as significantly important as it is for others. These factors have a bearing on the magnitude of the grieving that is present. The more importance the body has to identity, the greater the grief reaction and vice versa. However, everyone can be expected to grieve to some extent.

In Mr. Young's case the nurses recognized that the behavior, although symptomatic of grief, violated two tenets of the accepted sick role in the American culture. Mr. Young did not cooperate with those responsible for his care nor did he make an effort to recover. His crying, although appropriate to his grief, is considered inappropriate for a man in this culture. The nurses who provided Mr. Young's care were able to accept his behavior as having meaning and were able to provide an environment in which he was able to express his grief and examine his feelings. With this help he was able to move forward and began making plans for his rehabilitation.

Mary Belle Smith represents another manifestation of role confusion resulting from illness. She had rheumatic fever at ages three and seven followed by mitral stenosis. As a consequence, she spent little time in school and was overprotected by her family. At age 23 she had a mitral commissurotomy, which, according to the surgeon, was a success. Mary Belle, however, continued to behave like an invalid and resisted all efforts at rehabilitation. Her self-concept remained unaltered and she continued to cope with life in the only way she knew. She only knew how to relate to others as an invalid and continued to do so. Mary Belle's reaction is not unique. It is representative of a more deeply seated psychological problem than some of the acute reactions to crisis cited in the previous examples. Therefore, Mary Belle will have greater difficulty changing her self-concept and may require professional psychiatric help to do so. Kaplan (1956), in a study of patients having cardiac surgery, found that some did not recover despite the correction of their physical disability. In some instances the patient continued to be a cardiac invalid; in others he or she developed other disabilities. According to Kaplan, the patient who uses heart disease as a means of adapting psychologically to problems in life is less likely to be benefited by surgery than one who does not. This reaction is not unique to patients with heart disease. Studies of patients with diseases such as asthma, arthritis, and duodenal ulcer favor a similar conclusion.

Sometimes people make self-derogatory remarks in an attempt to get others to reaffirm their role perception and give reassurance that they really are acceptable. At times the person wants to be assured that what happened was interpreted in a favorable light. For example, Mrs. Terry had a hysterectomy. As she passed through the stage of excitement in her recovery from a general anesthetic, she cried, screamed, and thrashed about in bed. She was aware of her behavior but was unable to control it. Later, when the effects of the anesthetic had diminished, she said to the nurse, "I behaved very badly when I was under the ancsthetic, didn't I?" The nurse replied, "You certainly did." Mrs. Terry burst into tears. She had not wanted to have fears confirmed. What she wanted was to be reassured that her behavior was not unusual. Had the nurse stopped to examine the intent of Mrs. Terry's question, she could have responded in such a way that Mrs. Terry might have been relieved.

Through the examination of the manner in which some patients reacted to illness, a few of the causes of psychological stress related to role definition have been reviewed. Another way to learn about the psychological needs of patients during illness is to examine the reactions of patients during the different stages of illness. These are the stage of onset, the stage of accepted illness, and the stage of convalescence. Some attention will be given to the ways in which patients are expected to react and how these expectations may affect the care they receive.

Emotional Reactions of the Person Who Is Ill

The significant principle is that anxiety alerts the person to danger. The amount of anxiety provoked in any illness depends on the meaning the illness has to the individual. When the person recognizes that the illness does not respond to home remedies or that he or she cannot explain its cause or effects satisfactorily, anxiety may act as a stimulus for seeking attention. In contrast, the person may be so anxious that he or she denies the illness and attempts to avoid its symptoms. The individual is too busy to see the doctor, the doctor is too busy to see him or her, or there is an important meeting coming up, and so on. This denial may be so complete that the person cannot recognize that he or she is ill even though it may be obvious to family and associates. Denial in some degree is a common psychological defense against anxiety, and the degree of the denial usually serves as a clue to the degree of anxiety with which the individual is struggling.

Acceptance of illness requires that the individual place himself or herself in the hands of others. To do this the person must return to earlier modes of behaving, or regress. Inasmuch as he or she is able to allow this, the individual will be able to follow orders and allow others to attend to personal, emotional, and physical needs.

According to Barker et al. (1953), if the patient can tolerate being dependent on others, he or she regresses to a more childlike state that is characterized by the following four features:

1. Patients become self-centered. They see events and people in relation to themselves and existing for their benefit. They become demanding and less able to wait to have needs and wants satisfied. Where they were once considerate of the needs of others, they now are concerned only with their own. Perrine (1971) refers to this as the "period of protest." He also identifies openness and honest evaluation of one's condition as an important need of the patient during this period. But many patients are, as Perrine described himself, afraid to ask direct questions because they do not want to know the answers, but at the same time they do want the information. The result is that the patient remains "trapped in ignorance and fear" unless someone intervenes. Perrine writes that it is during this period that he remembers with gratitude the people who continued to support him even while he was resisting. One of the criteria by which a patient may be judged as recovering from and or adapting to the limitations imposed by illness is evidence of less self-centeredness. On the other hand, it is quite possible that the patient may go through periods of despair and detachment before being emotionally ready to accept the illness as a part of life that may or may not have lasting physical as well as psychological implications.
2. Patients interests become circumscribed; that is, they are interested in what is happening to them at the present time. Things that were of interest to them before they became ill may be of little concern now. For example, when a patient was well he was an avid baseball fan, but when he is ill he will not even watch the World Series games on television.
3. Patients are dependent emotionally on those who care for them. They often personalize the actions of those who care for them as being a direct indication of their acceptance or rejection of them. When a new nurse is assigned to their care, they may interpret this to mean that the nurse who cared for them previously dislikes them. In addition, their feelings may be ambivalent—one minute they feel one way and the next minute they feel the opposite. Nurses should learn to recognize this shift in tone. Once recognized, the patients' expression of feelings can be more easily dealt with as part of their total illness.
4. Patients become preoccupied with their bodily functions. They are concerned with what they eat or do no eat, with whether the food is suitable for an invalid, with their bowel functions, with the amount of time they sleep, and so on.

Recognition of the value and characteristics of regression in illness should be helpful to the nurse in understanding the patient and his or her behavior. It is stated in *Social Interaction and Patient Care* (Lederer, 1965, p. 162) that "It is conceivable that through social and emotional regression the sick person re-distributes his energies to facilitate the healing process or possibly that the regressive integration is in itself an essential factor in the healing process." Regression helps the patient because it makes it possible for him or her to depend on others to do many things that, when well, the patient could and would do for himself or herself. This includes activities that are of a personal nature. As the patient was growing up and became able to care for personal needs, this was accepted as evidence of maturation. Therefore activities such as bathing, feeding, enemas, and catheterizations have psychological significance that surpasses the actual procedure. Often these activities are not acceptable to the patient because they demand that control be relinquished over some of the first, and most basic, functions that were mastered in life. When a patient is able to allow others to care for him or her, however, the energy thus conserved can be redirected toward the process of getting well.

As his or her condition improves the patient is expected to resume self-responsibility. In general, the belief is held that the sooner the patient can resume normal activities, the more rapid the recovery will be. However, the patient needs to understand that these activities are as much a part of the plan of therapy as are medications and diet. Patients too often interpret being asked to bathe themselves as the nurses' shifting some of their work on the patients because they are too busy or unwilling to help. Very often the nurses reinforce this feeling because they feel guilty about letting the patients care for themselves or do not understand why this activity is important to the patients' recovery. The patients need to know that nurses are standing by to help if and when they require help.

The person with an illness or disability frequently feels angry. The anger is often associated with the feeling that being ill or hurt is an injustice. The person may be angry at what has happened to him or her, angry at being helpless, and so forth. What is even more difficult is that the person does not know where to direct this anger or, in some instances does not even know why the anger exists—only that it does. Because he or she cannot shout at the walls and gain satisfaction in the expression of anger, the patient frequently displaces anger onto people in the environment because they are real and will react. The patient may express anger at those who care for him or her, including friends, family, nurses, and other health workers. If the nurse recognizes that the patient's behavior is part of the reaction to illness and knows that it serves a purpose, then she or he is better able to help the patient explore or examine the situation without becoming upset or hurt. Families frequently require some support in order to develop understanding of the situation. There is some evidence to support the observation that patients who are able to express their hostility during illness make more rapid recoveries than those who do not.

Some patients turn their anger inward and become depressed. Some degree of depression is probably associated with any serious illness and indeed may be a necessary stage in recovery. Inasmuch as depression enables the patient to withdraw and conserve energy, it is protective. When it gets in the way of any movement toward health, depression is considered to be destructive. Sutherland (1952) found that patients who had radical mastectomies almost always evidenced some depression during their first few days at home. In families where the patients' depression and increased dependency were accepted, patients made more rapid recovery than those whose families did not accept this behavior.

The depression that accompanies the loss of a part or of an ability that has been important to the patient may be an expression of grief, as was seen in the case of Mr. Young. Acceptance by the nursing staff of the fact that a patient not only does but has the right to mourn the loss of part of himself or herself and may need help in expressing grief is fundamental to an adequate plan of care. The nurse may think that the patient should be glad to be rid of a gangrenous leg, but the patient views the situation differently. Because the leg was part of the patient's body, part of his or her self-concept or image, opportunities for the expression of sorrow in an understanding and accepting environment may lessen the need for feelings of self-pity or self-chastisement. People often find it easier to do what they have to do when they feel that others are trying to understand their point of view.

When illness is a serious threat to the individual's integrity, he or she is likely to become confused. Confusion may cover up other feelings such as anxiety, anger, or the fear of being dependent. Confusion makes people feel less responsbile for their other feelings because these are hidden under the blanket of the confusion. For example, Mrs. Wilson found her husband dead in bed beside her. She went next door for help but could not remember going or how she got there. She kept repeating, "What did I do? How did I get to your house? I can't remember, I'm so confused. I do not know what to do." The thing she stated as being most helpful to her was that, after confirming the fact that her husband was dead, the neighbors assumed responsibility for calling the doctor, the relatives, and so on. They took the necessary responsibility and appeared to have the situation under control. Sometimes confusion is not as evident as in the instance of Mrs. Wilson. Confusion may show only when the patient is called on to remember or to learn. It is likely, however, that it is more common than is generally appreciated. This is one reason instructions and explanations given to patients need to be repeated, sometimes over and over. Nurses should not be surprised when patients forget or distort instructions given to them by themselves or physicians. Confusion tends to limit the person's perception of reality in many situations.

As implied, patients may adapt to illness by attack or withdrawal. Each method has its advantages and disadvantages and implications for nursing. During illness the patient needs energy to recover. The patient who adapts by attack should be protected from circumstances that increase the feeling that he or she has to use aggressive behavior to have needs met. This is often difficult for nursing personnel (and others), because sick people are expected to follow orders and appreciate the care that is offered them. When the patient demands attention and does not seem to appreciate the efforts made in his or her behalf, the nurses may feel frustrated and ineffectual. If the nurse understands that the use of aggressive behavior is the patient's attempt at adapting to illness, the nurse should feel less responsible for the behavior. She or he might then find it easier to understand the patient's motivation, plan care to assure the patient that needed care will be given, and assist him or her in looking at other ways of getting needs met without having to use attack.

The patient who withdraws during illness is also

trying to adapt. Withdrawal serves the positive purpose of conserving energy, but the patient does not gain insight into what the illness means personally or what he or she needs to do differently in order to adapt in a healthier way. The withdrawn patient is likely to be considered a "good patient" unless he or she becomes overly dependent on those who provide care. The problems in care derive from the ability of those who provide care to accept the patient in the regressed state and also to prevent the withdrawal from going too far. This means that those who care for the patient must recognize when the patient no longer needs to conserve energy and can assume responsibility for meeting some of his or her own needs and for making decision. This transition may take considerable time, especially when the patient has been seriously ill. It also requires skillful assessment on the part of the staff and consistent messages about expectations so that the patient is not being asked to assume responsibility one minute and being told he or she cannot the next.

During the stage of convalescence the patient is exptected to progress from illness to physical and emotional health. He or she must give up dependent and self-centered behavior and fend for himself or herself again. Lederer (1965) states that there are many similarities between the dynamics of adolescence and illness. During the stages of illness the patient goes from dependence to independence and finally to interdependence. Some patients find it difficult to give up being the center of attention and to assume responsibility for themselves again. When patients have been able to enjoy the legitimate claim to dependency that illness affords, and which they may deny themselves when well, they may go through a rather difficult dependent–independent struggle on the road to recovery.

Recovery may also be delayed if illness provides more satisfactions than does health. The many factors that contribute to the development of a preference for illness to health will not be discussed in detail. They are, however, defined as the secondary gains of illness. For some reason illness provides more security and satisfaction than health for certain people. Mary Belle, who continued to be an invalid despite correction of her cardiac disability, was one example. There are techniques that may reduce the likelihood of this happening. The first is to encourage patients to assume responsibility by including them in the decision-making process concerning their care. As this is done the patients should understand that, as they assume responsibility, they help themselves recover and that assistance is available if and when they require it. When and how to help patients requires judgment so that they are not assisted unnecessarily and thus robbed of the feeling of accomplishment. Nor, on the other hand, should they be pushed beyond their capacity to perform. The nurse must be able to stand by and wait as the patient struggles, but she or he must also be alert enough to restructure the patient's learning experience when the struggle seems insurmountable and the same goal can be reached in another way. Through grappling with the problem and experiencing some successes as well as being able to look at the things that cause frustration, the patient gains the strength to progress toward recovery.

A few practices that are useful in helping patients with long-term illnesses keep before them the objective of returning to the community and an active life are restricting visitors as little as possible, permitting overnight leaves from the hospital, encouraging family and friends to take patients to community events, having patients wear their own clothing when at all possible, encouraging self-expression and participation in activities that are of interest in the hospital, and moving the patient to home care as soon as the situation permits. During hospitalization a patient can be assisted to use time constructively by reviewing the home situation and thinking ahead about the kinds of physical adaptations that will help the patient live as normally as possible. If the house has stairs and the patient is in a wheel chair, what needs to be done so he or she can move about and not be confined to one area? Who, in the community, is available to help the patient maintain outside contacts at home? What other professional assistance such as physical therapy and occupational therapy is available to help the patient learn useful diversional or self-maintaining activities? These are some of the questions nurses need to ask themselves when planning patient care. There are many social agencies and social clubs whose aim is to help people help themselves. The patient should be familiarized with some of the available resources so he or she does not begin to feel that posthospitalization offers nothing but isolation and frustration. In addition to planning for physical needs, the patient should be helped to look at how the nondisabled respond to the disabled and how he or she anticipates reacting in situations where others are either oversolicitous or studiously ignore his or her limitations.

Emotional Reactions of Others to an Individual's Illness

It is difficult to categorize the responses of others to the illness of a significant individual. As mentioned throughout this chapter, the responses of individuals to illness—whether this be the patient, family, or significant others, including care givers—are determined by social, cultural, psychological, economic, and family factors. In close relationship such as husband–wife or parent–child, illness in one of the members usually triggers a response in the other that can be examined within the framework of grieving. The more serious the illness, and the greater the threat it poses to the security of others, the more intense their reactions might be expected to be. Delaney-Naumoff (1980) gives a brief glimpse at the response of a man who had a serious myocardial infarction. The entire family, including the patient, seemed to have been on an upward social spiral when the breadwinner became ill. Economics and social position seemed to play a major role in the way the patient and his family responded. Everything was invested in a growing business that left little cash reserve to cover an event such as a serious illness. When the family's income producer became ill, the family became increasingly concerned about its social position and continued economic well-being. These had been priority issues before the advent of illness and they continued to be priority issues. These people were caught in a sudden disaster, but one cannot expect their attitudes and values to change in as short a time as it takes to have a coronary. I am sure many parallels to this example can be found in the clinical area of nursing practice. A wife who enjoyed a dependent relationship with her husband when he was well might react intensely to threatened alterations in this relationship if her husband becomes ill. A husband who has avoided anything that is traditionally accepted as "woman's work" may find himself in considerable conflict if his wife becomes ill and he has to assume the bulk of household and parenting tasks. Each situation has to be evaluated on its own merits, taking into account preillness adaptation and coping patterns, role relationships, cultural and social stereotypes or misconceptions about the type of illness problem that has occurred, and so on. French and Schwartz (1976) give an example of an elderly man whose adult sons and daughter thought their father's terminal carcinoma of the bladder was "contagious." Although all were attentive to most of the father's needs, his bladder and catheter care were neglected because his children feared the contagion. No amount of health teaching seemed to convince them otherwise. Although the exact source of this erroneous believe was not identified, the fact remained that it created a problem in health care that the nurse had to deal with even though she did not fully understand the basis for the belief. In nursing we strive to identify causal factors and to plan care based upon that understanding. However, this case example points out that sometimes care must be given when the only awareness the nurse has is that a problem exists or has been created by certain behavioral responses of the patient or his or her significant others.

References Cited

Barker, R. G., Wright, B. A., and Conick, M. R. *Adjustment to Physical Handicap and Illness: A Survey of the Social Psychology of Physique and Disability,* (rev. ed.) New York: Social Sciences Research Council, 1953.

Cannon, W. B. *The Wisdom of the Body.* New York: W. W. Norton & Company, Inc., 1939.

Delaney-Naumoff, M. "Loss of Heart." In *Grief Responses to Long-term Illness and Disability.* Ed. by J. Werner-Beland, Reston, Va.: Reston Publishing Co., Inc., 1980.

Engel, G. L. "A Unique Concept of Health and Disease." *Perspect. in Biol. Med.,* 3 (Summer 1960), 480.

French, J., and Schwartz, D. R. "Terminal Care at Home in Two Cultures." In *Transcultural Nursing: A Book of Readings.* Ed. by P. J. Brink. Englewood Cliffs, N.J.: Prentice-Hall, Inc., 1976.

Holmes, M. J., and Werner, J. A. *Psychiatric Nursing in a Therapeutic Community.* New York: Macmillan Publishing Co., Inc., 1966.

Kallmann, F. J. "The Genetics of Mental Illness." In *The American Handbook of Psychiatry.* Ed. by S. Arieti. Basic Books, Inc., Publishers, 1959.

Kaplan, S. M. "Psychological Aspects of Cardiac Disease." *Psychosom. Med.,* **118** (May–June 1956), 221–33.

Lederer, H. D. "How the Sick View Their World." In *Social Interaction and Patient Care.* Ed. by J. K. Skipper, Jr., and R. C. Leonard. Philadelphia: J. B. Lippincott Company, 1965.

Linn, Louis, "Basic Principles of Management in Psychosomatic Medicine." In *Psychosomatic Medicine: Its Clinical Application.* Ed. by E. D. Wittkower and H. Warnes. Hagerstown, Md.: Harper & Row, Publishers, 1977.

Parsons, T. "Definitions of Health and Illness in Light of American Values and Social Structure." In *Patients, Physicians and Illness.* Ed. by E. G. Jaco. New York: The Free Press, 1958.

Perrine, G. "Needs Met and Unmet." *Am. J. Nurs.,* **71:** 11, (1971), 2128–29.

Sargent, H. D., and Mayman, M. "Clinical Psychology." In *American Handbook of Psychiatry,* Vol. 2. Ed. by S. Arieti. New York: Basic Books, Inc., Publishers, 1959.

Spitzer, S. P., Swanson, R. M., and Lehr, R. "Audience Reactions and Careers of Psychiatric Patients." *Family Process,* **2** (1969), 159–81.

Sutherland, A. "The Psychological Impact of Cancer Surgery." *Pub. Health Rep.,* **67** (1952), 1139–43.

von Bertalanffy, L. "General System Theory and Psychiatry." In *American Handbook of Psychiatry,* 2nd ed., Vol. 1. Ed. by S. Arieti. New York: Basic Books, Inc., Publishers, 1974.

General References

Busse, E. W., and Pfeiffer, E., eds. *Behavior and Adaptation in Late Life.* Boston: Little, Brown and Company, 1969.

May, R. *Power and Innocence: A Search for the Sources of Violence.* New York: W. W. Norton & Company, Inc., 1972.

Selye, H. *Stress.* Montreal, Can.: Acta Inc., Medical Publishers, 1950.

Selye, H. *The Story of the Adaptation Syndrome.* Montreal, Can.: Acta Inc., Medical Publishers, 1952.

Selye, H. *The Stress of Life.* New York: McGraw-Hill Book Company, 1956.

20

Thermal Response

The ability to maintain a stable body temperature over a range of environmental temperatures and of metabolic activity permits predictable response of the receptor, integrating and effector mechanisms of the body. The homeotherm is thus free, within broad limits, to determine his own activities rather than have them determined for him by environmental conditions.

BELDING, 1967

Overview

Environmental temperatures influence the growth and development of both individuals and nations. Advances in technology in the highly developed nations have minimized the retarding effects of hot and cold climates on the growth and development of their children, but in underdeveloped countries these environmental stresses continue to have a direct and often deleterious effect (Harrison & Cleeg, 1969).

The ability of the individual to perceive and respond appropriately to temperature changes in the internal and external environment is critical to his or her comfort, safety, and survival. In the self-sufficient individual, many aspects of temperature regulation are accomplished instinctively or subconsciously, under the surveillance of an effective neuroendocrine system. However, illness is frequently associated with alteration in internal body temperature and with impairment in the individual's ability to make necessary modifications in the temperature of the external environment.

Mandatory aspects of nursing assessment include determination of body temperature and of the internal and external factors that appear to be influencing it. Nursing care is then directed toward (1) supporting those factors that contribute to a safe and effective level of body temperature, and toward (2) eliminating or minimizing those factors that interfere with maintaining an optimal level of body temperature.

When accurately determined, the measurement of body temperature assists both the physician and nurse to make a number of inferences about the state of the patient as well as the nature of his or her illness. Ensuring the accuracy of temperature readings of patients is primarily the responsibility of the nurse.

Temperature Regulation and Variation

As one of the critical homeostatic conditions of human beings, body temperature is regulated by a numer of interrelated negative feedback systems. Not all animals have the human capability to regulate body temperature in the presence of changes in temperature of the external environment. Depending on their ability to regulate their temperatures, animals are classified as homeothermic (warm-blooded) or poikilothermic (cold-blooded). Homeothermic animals maintain their body temperatures within limits, whereas poikilothermic animals do not.

Although this classification is generally useful, it is not completely accurate, because hibernating animals are homeothermic when they are active and poikilothermic during periods of hibernation. Their body temperature is subject to homeostatic control when they are active and is determined by the temperature of the environment when they are hibernating. In humans, factors that interfere with the production or loss of body heat may result in the individual's becoming poikilothermic (Heller et al., 1978). Examples of such factors include lesions of the hypothalamus and low cervical cord injuries.

Two major characteristics indicate that humans are a tropical homeotherm: (1) their critical body temperature is higher than that of most other animals and (2) they have a well-developed capacity to sweat, being able to produce up to 1 liter per hour for several hours, with a heat loss as high as 600 kcal per hour. Their success in adapting to temperate and frigid climates is largely a result of their use of intelligence to manipulate external environmental conditions (Belding, 1967, pp. 481–510.

Unlike some substances required by the body, heat is both necessary for and a product of cellular activity. All bodily processes are affected by temperature. Within the limits of the tissue tolerance, biochemical reactions within cells are accelerated by increasing body temperature and slowed by decreasing body temperature. With increased body temperatures, oxyhemoglobin is dissociated more rapidly than at normal temperatures, the heart rate is increased, and wound healing is accelerated. The purpose of temperature-regulating mechanisms is to prevent injurious effects of extremes of temperature on body cells. There is recent speculation that some metabolic cycles which appear futile, insofar as they seem to produce only heat, may provide a unique and rapid mechanism to accelerate metabolic pathways in times of urgent need (Cahill, 1980).

As indicated in Chapter 9, injury to cells is brought about by (1) depriving cells of required materials, (2) crippling cellular machinery by interfering with the action of enzymes that enable the cell to use materials, and (3) altering the nature of intracellular proteins.

Temperature Measurement Scales

Before introducing specific values of normal and altered thermal states, it is necessary to consider current temperature measurement scales. The two most widely used scales for measuring body temperature are the centigrade (C) and Fahrenheit (F) scales. The centigrade scale, generally employed in laboratories and scientific work, is consistent with the 100-unit divisions of the metric system. The 0°C point marks the temperature of melting ice, or the freezing point of water; the 100°C point marks the temperature at which water boils at sea level. Therefore one unit, or 1°C, represents 0.01 the amount of heat required to change melting ice to boiling water. In support of the effort to adopt the centigrade scale as a universal system for measuring and reporting temperature, most of the values in this discussion are reported in degrees centigrade. Rules for the conversion of degrees centigrade to Fahrenheit are based on the fact that $1°F = \frac{5}{9}°C$.

Rules to convert degrees centigrade to Fahrenheit:

A. When degree C is:	To find degree F, you:
1. Above 0°C	Multiply by 9, divide by 5, add 32.
2. Between 0°C and −17.8°C	Multiply by 9, divide by 5, subtract from 32.
3. Below −17.8°C	Multiply by 9, divide by 5, subtract 32.

The following conversion rules are as accurate as, and perhaps simpler to remember than, those above (Routh, 1953).

B. To convert degrees C to degrees F, add 40, multiply by $\frac{9}{5}$, and subtract 40 from the result.

C. To convert degrees F to degrees C, add 40, multiply by $\frac{5}{9}$, and subtract 40 from the result.

Example: Convert 98.6°F to degrees C.

$$98.6°F + 40 = 138.6$$
$$138.6 \times \frac{5}{9} = 693 \div 9 = 77.0$$
$$77.0 - 40 = 37.0°C$$

The *U.S. Pharmacopeia* suggests the following conversion formulae which are slightly less accurate, but quicker.

$$C \text{ to } F = (\tfrac{9}{5} \times C) + 32 = F$$
$$F \text{ to } C = (F - 32) \times \tfrac{5}{9} = C$$

Normal Body Temperature

Although humans are homeothermic, the temperature of their tissues varies from one part of the body to another. There is no one body temperature, but rather a series of gradients, from the "hottest" organ, the liver [normally about 38°C (100°F)] to the "coldest" organ, the uncovered skin [normally 5.5° to 8.3°C (10° to 15°F) cooler]. Authorities agree that the temperature of the core tissues, the nervous system, and the organs in the abdominal and thoracic cavity is regulated. Whether the temperature of the peripheral tissues is regulated is not known.

HEAT PRODUCTION: METABOLISM AND BODY TEMPERATURE

Body temperature may be considered a reliable indicator of metabolic activity. Metabolic activity, which is the total of all chemical reactions in all cells, is expressed in terms of the rate of heat liberation during chemical reactions. Basal metabolic rate (BMR), which measures the liters of oxygen used in the resting state per unit of time, is an indirect measure of energy released during chemical reactions in the cells. The energy equivalent of oxygen, which is the quantity of oxygen liberated per liter of oxygen used in the body, averages about 4.8 kcal (Guyton, 1976, p. 953). Any factors that affect metabolic rate affect heat production, and therefore will have a direct effect on body temperature.

Factors that Decrease Metabolic Rate

Factors that decrease metabolic rate, and thus lower body temperature, include the following:

1. *Tropical climate.*
2. *Sleep.* BMR drops 1 to 15 per cent, as a result of decreased muscle tone and decreased activity of the sympathetic nervous system.
3. *Malnutrition.* BMR may drop as much as 20 to 30 per cent, because of scarcity of nutrients necessary for cell metabolism.

Factors that Increase Metabolic Rate

Factors that increase metabolic rate, and thus raise body temperature, include the following:

1. *Cold climate.* Exposure to a cold environment increases our rate of metabolic heat production, which then maintains our internal body temperature at an optimal level. A clothed individual maintains an internal body temperature of about 37°C (98.6°F). The ambient, or environmental, temperature which favors heat loss passively down a temperature gradient, to maintain the optimal internal temperature 37°C, is about 22°C (71.6°F) [Heller et al., 1978].
2. *Exercise.* The major source of body heat is contraction of skeletal muscles. During exercise, rectal temperature normally rises as high as 40°C (104°F). There is evidence that during exercise there is elevation of the thermal point at which the heat-dissipating mechanisms are activated (Ganong, 1973, p. 169). Shivering is a rapid, involuntary contraction of muscles that occurs as a body response to a sudden drop in core temperatures or a sudden elevation of the lower level of the "thermostat" in hypothalamic centers. When the "thermostat" is raised by chemical agents, the sudden onset of shivering is called a "chill."
3. *Specific dynamic action of food.* The effect of protein on metabolic rate is greater than that of carbohydrates or fat, but ingestion of any food is always followed by increased metabolic rate. The fate of food energy in heat production is as follows: (a) about 60 per cent becomes heat during formation of adenosine triphosphate (ATP); (b) about 15 per cent becomes heat when energy is transferred from ATP to the functional systems of cells; and (c) of the 25 per cent of energy that finally reaches functional systems of cells, the major proportion also becomes heat.
4. *Epinephrine and norepinephrine.* Stimulation of the sympathetic nervous system may increase metabolic rate as much as 25 per cent. Increase develops rapidly but is short-lived. Norepinephrine is the trigger for a unique mechanism of heat production in the infant; the metabolism of brown fat. Brown fat has a unique metabolic device for oxidizing fatty acids and turning the resulting chemical energy mainly into heat. The rate of heat production is controlled by release of norepinephrine from sympathetic nerves, which directly innervate the brown fat (Strand, 1978, p. 382). See Figure 20-1 for the distribution for brown fat in infants.
5. *Thyroid hormone.* Increased production may raise metabolic rate as much as 100 per cent. Increase develops slowly, but is prolonged.
6. *Growth hormone.* Increased levels may raise metabolic rate as much as 15 to 20 per cent. This partially explains the higher body temperature of the young person.
7. *Male sex hormone.* Except in infancy, males have a metabolic rate 10 to 15 per cent higher than that of females.
8. *Female sex hormones.* During the proliferative phase of the menstrual cycle, body temperature is low. At the time of ovulation the temperature often falls and then rises. During the period that follows, the temperature remains up and then falls just prior to the onset of menstruation. Fluctuations in body temperature may be used as a

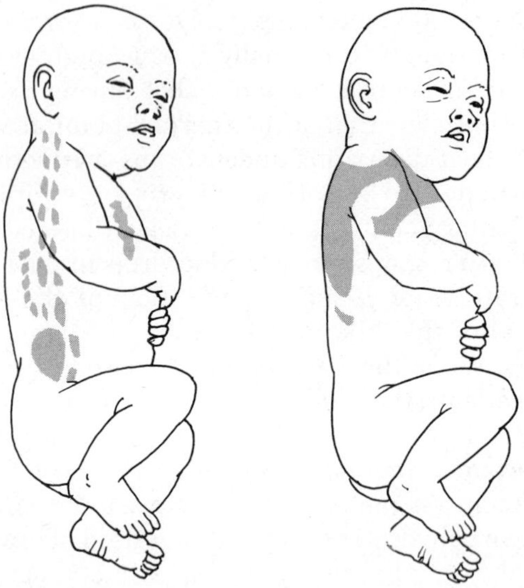

Figure 20-1. Brown fat is deposited in young infants between the shoulder blades, along the spine, behind the breastbone, and around the neck. (Used with permission of Macmillan Publishing Company, Inc., from *Physiology*, 1978, by F. L. Strand, Fig. 21-5, p. 382.)

basis for determining the so-called safe period in family planning.

9. *Age.* Metabolic rate of the newborn is almost twice that of persons in their sixth and seventh decades of life.
10. *Emotion.* Increased metabolic rate that accompanies emotional states is probably due to the interacting effects of nervous system stimulation, hormonal secretion, and muscle contraction. Cassidy (1976) found that healthy female subjects (18 to 25 years of age) had a wider temperature range on days when they had to make more adjustment than usual to life events.
11. *Fever.* An abnormal elevation in body temperature from any cause increases metabolic rate. The rate of all chemical reactions increases approximately 13 per cent for every 1°C rise in body temperature (7 per cent for each 1°F of elevation). See the discussion of fever later in this chapter.
12. *Time of day.* The normal human core temperature undergoes a regular diurnal fluctuation of 0.5° to 0.7°C, with the highest levels reached in the evening and the lowest levels about 6:00 A.M. (Ganong, 1973, p. 169).

Cyclic Temperature Changes

A daily temperature rhythm has been noted for most people, but the high and low points over a 24-hour period vary for each individual. There is some correlation between the high point and the time of greatest efficiency and activity. Early risers appear to have their high point in the morning but reach their lowest temperature later in the day. Those who are sluggish and dazed in the mornings record their lowest temperature at this time, and there is an elevated temperature later in the day, or even at night, when they feel most active and enterprising (Strand, 1978, p. 380).

Attempts to change the cycle in individuals have met with dubious success, but the correlation between temperature and activity remains. Subjects who were able to reverse their habits of work and sleep also changed their temperature cycles. Those who were unable to make the change successfully did not make the physiological temperature adjustment (Strand, 1978, p. 381). See Figure 20-2 for comparison of the temperature and sleep cycles of one individual who succeeded and one who failed to adapt to a change in pattern of activity and sleep.

The preceding factors that increase heat production by increasing metabolism constitute only one of two ways to increase body temperature. A second set of factors that increase body temperature includes those that prevent heat loss or that introduce heat from the external environment. Factors that lessen heat loss include peripheral vasoconstriction, dehydration, edema, or still or moist air. Introduction of heat from the external environment is accomplished by topical applications of heat and by ingestion of hot foods and liquids.

Heat Loss

Body temperature is maintained by balancing heat production and heat loss. Moving from the previous discussion of heat production to the other side of the balance, heat is lost by (1) radiation, (2) convection, (3) conduction, and (4) evaporation.

Mechanisms of Heat Loss

Radiation is defined as the transfer of heat by means of waves. These waves are like radio waves in all respects except length. Radiation differs from other means of transferring heat inasmuch as it does not need a medium to pass through space. *Convection* can be defined simply as the movement of heat from one site to another by currents of air or fluid. As air warms it tends to expand; it becomes less dense and therefore rises. As it rises cooler air takes its place. It in turn warms, expands, and rises and is replaced by cooler air. Heat exchange by radiation and convection is influenced by air temperature and humidity, skin temperature, and the amount of body surface area exposed for transfer of heat (Belding, 1967, p. 482). In *conduction,* heat is transferred from

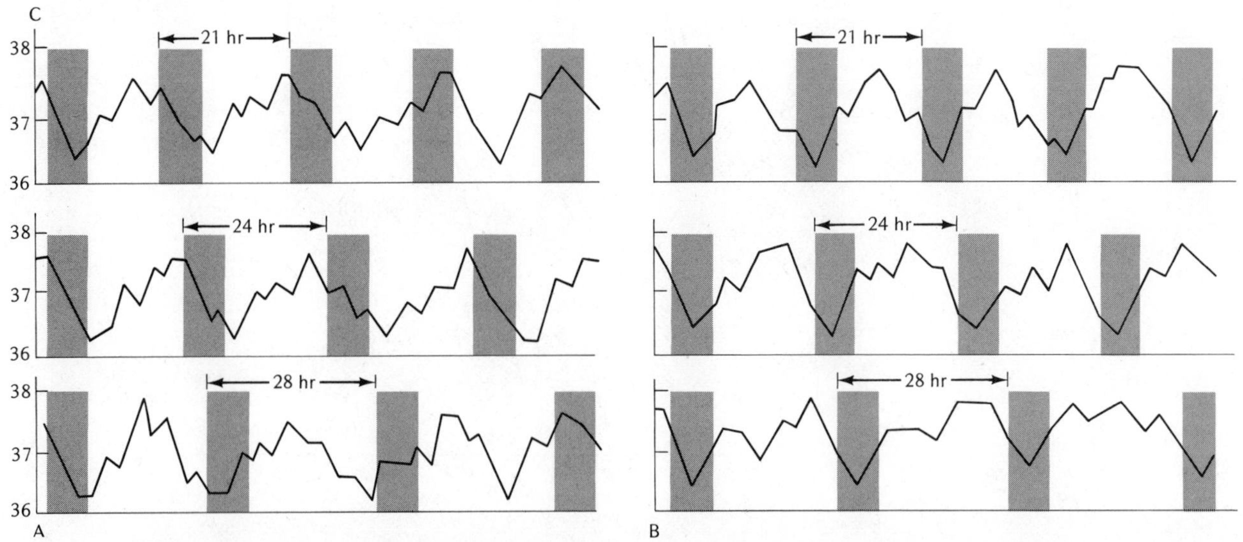

Figure 20-2. Correlation of body temperature with differences in sleep cycles. (A) This individual maintained the 24-hr temperature cycle despite alterations in the sleep cycle from a 20- to a 28-hr day. (B) Temperature cycles in this subject followed the changes in the length of the day, probably indicating an ability to perform more efficiently under these varying circumstances than subject A. (Used with permission of Macmillan Publishing Company, Inc., from *Physiology*, 1978, by F. L. Strand, p. 381, Fig. 21-3.)

one molecule to adjacent ones. A good example of conduction is the transfer of heat from a metal coffee pot to its handle. The wall of the pot is heated by the hot water and the heat is transferred directly to adjacent metal in the handle. This movement of heat can be observed by holding the handle and feeling it warm. Skin conduction is the first line of defense for thermal regulation. It is accomplished by adjustment of blood flow through the skin, with direct effect on skin temperature and heat transfer by radiation and convection (Belding, 1967, p. 489). *Evaporation* is a process whereby water is converted to steam. A significant site for evaporative loss is the lungs. The amount of heat lost through the lungs with breathing is proportional to the ventilatory volume and the difference in water vapor pressure between inspired and expired air (Belding, 1967, p. 483).

Heat loss through the skin is primarily by radiation, convection, and evaporation.

Functions of the Skin in Control of Heat Loss

Human skin is constructed in ways that permit control of heat loss. Three structures found in skin influence heat loss.

1. *Hair* impedes radiative heat loss by forming an insulating layer of still air just above the skin surface in animals that have a significant coat. The effectiveness of this insulating air coat can be varied by raising or lowering the air-entrapping hairs by means of tiny muscles attached to the base of each hair. Birds accomplish the same thing by ruffling their feathers. Humans retain a vestige of this mechanism in the "goose bumps" which appear when one feels cold (Case, 1979, p. 387).
2. *Blood vessels* lying in the skin are an element of its heat-controlling equipment. Expanded to their greatest diameter, they carry much more blood near to the surface than when they are contracted. Expanded, they exert a cooling influence because the large quantity of warm blood that flows through the skin loses heat rapidly by radiation. When these vessels are constricted, the effect is to prevent heat loss (Case, 1979, p. 387).
3. *The skin's complement of glands* is an element of its heat-controlling equipment. Sebaceous glands secrete a fatty material onto the base of hairs and play no role in temperature regulation. However, sweat glands are very effective cooling devices. Humans have sweat glands everywhere in the skin. When our sweat glands are operating maximally, they secrete as much as 10 to 15 liters of sweat per day—roughly half the water in the body. Thermal energy is used to evaporate all that water from the skin. At the usual temperature of the body surface, about 580 kcal are used up to evaporate a liter of sweat. Sweating, particularly in dry air, is thus an extremely effective cooling mechanism (Case, 1979, p. 387). See Figure 20-3 for diagrammatic representation of thermoregulatory structures of the skin.

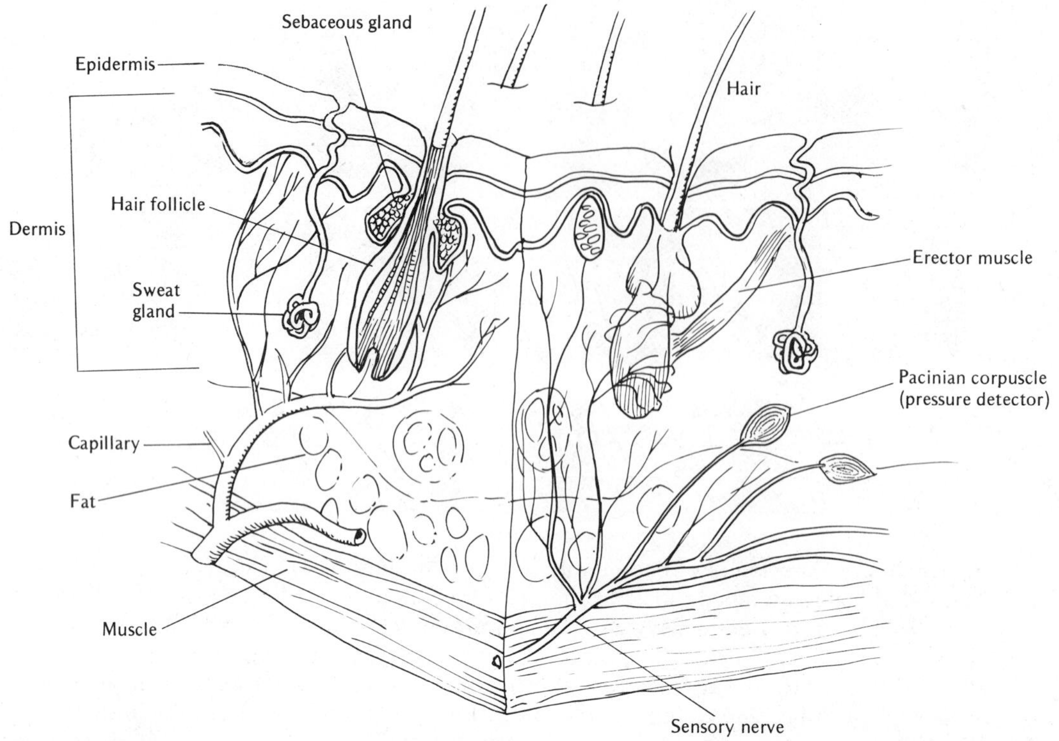

Figure 20-3. The skin is a multipurpose organ active in physical protection, thermoregulation and information gathering. (Used with permission of Macmillan Publishing Company, Inc., from *Biology,* 2nd ed., 1979, by J. F. Case, p. 386, Fig. 19-11.)

Other Avenues of Heat Loss

Some heat is lost in the urine, feces, and expired air. In the deeper tissues and the muscles, blood absorbs the heat produced in the tissue and transports it to the skin, where it is transferred to the external environment, thereby cooling the blood. The transfer of heat from the tissue to the blood and from the blood to the tissue illustrates one of the laws of thermodynamics; that is, energy travels from an area of greater energy to an area of lesser energy; that is, heat moves from the warmer to the cooler tissues.

Heat is not necessarily always lost to the external environment. In the extremities heat may be transferred from the arteries to the cooler blood in the veins by a countercurrent heat transfer mechanism. See Figure 20-4 for illustration of the operation of countercurrent heat transfer in the upper extremity, exposed to low atmospheric temperature.

Other Factors Influencing Heat Loss

Heat loss may be facilitated by increasing the circulation of blood through the skin, by increasing the amount of skin exposed to the environment, and by increasing the capacity of the air surrounding the body to take on heat or moisture. Body structure also affects the rate at which heat is lost. The apron of fat, the omentum, that hangs in front of the abdominal organs protects them from the loss of heat. A layer of fat under the skin insulates the deeper tissues and reduces heat loss. As stated previously, the layer of fat under the skin of the Eskimo plus his short, stocky frame is a type of adaptation to a cold climate, as fat acts as insulating material. However, in a tropical climate obesity is not necessarily a significant barrier to heat loss, because the dermal vascular bed is mostly external to adipose tissue. However, more energy is required for the overweight person to do work in a hot environment, and this places an added strain on the cardiovascular system (Belding, 1967, pp. 499–500). In tropical regions of Africa, adaptation has been in the direction of a long, lean trunk.

Clothing decreases heat loss because it is a poor conductor of heat and it traps air, which is also a poor conductor. Because air is trapped in the spaces between fibers, loosely woven woolens are effective in preventing heat loss under certain conditions (when the air is still). In windy climates, close-woven or impervious materials may be more effective than heavy ones, because the body heat is trapped and prevented from dissipation by the wind. Still air limits heat loss, whereas moving air promotes heat loss by replacing the warm, moist layer of air that sur-

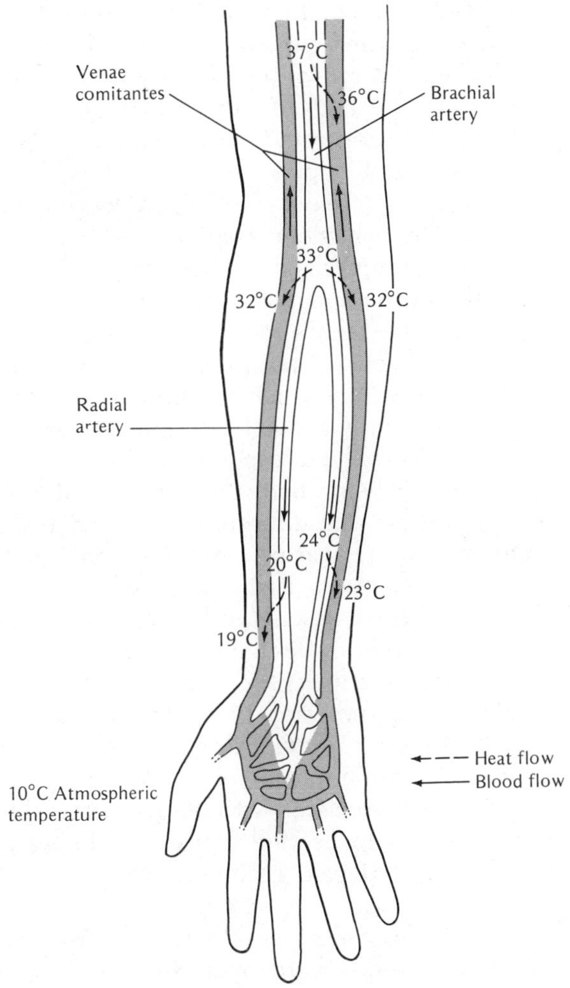

Figure 20-4. When atmospheric temperature is low, warm blood leaving the arm arteries loses heat to the chilled blood returning from the hand through the veins. Thus warmed venous blood is returned to the body. Heat loss is further minimized by vasoconstriction of surface blood vessels. (Used with permission of Macmillan Publishing Company, Inc., from *Physiology,* 1978, by F. L. Strand, p. 383, Fig. 21-6.)

rounds the body with a layer of cooler, drier air. Therefore an electric fan increases comfort on a hot day, and the wind increases the danger of frostbite on a cold one. Chilling is therefore related not only to the temperature but to the movement of air. Thus a "windbreaker" coat may offer more protection from the cold on a windy day than a heavier, "warmer" coat. In caring for the sick, the nurse should keep in mind that clothing serves as a barrier against heat transfer, both into and out of the body, by reducing radiation, convection, and conduction. Therefore the *hyper*thermic patient being cooled should be covered only enough to prevent embarrassment to him or her, whereas the *hypo*thermic patient being warmed should have fabric in contact with all possible surfaces

Atmospheric Humidity and Temperature

The extent to which the air is saturated with moisture is also a factor in heat loss. One of the ways in which heat is transferred from the skin to the external environment is through the evaporation of the water secreted by the sweat glands in the form of perspiration. The sweating mechanism responds to elevation of skin temperatures above normal values. Within limits, sufficient sweat will be produced to maintain thermal balance, but the capacity to sweat appears to fall with length of exposure to elevated temperatures. Effectiveness of sweat for cooling depends upon its evaporation. After days or weeks of habituation to hot environments, there is a 1° to 2°C downward shift in the skin temperature at which sweat glands are activated, with resulting decreased circulatory strain. In infants, the sweating mechanism begins to function about the eighteenth day of life. Prior to that time infants are very vulnerable to upward changes in temperature, primarily because of poorly developed mechanisms for heat loss.

Conversion of a liquid to a vapor requires energy in the form of heat to overcome the cohesion of molecules. Water requires more heat to vaporize than any other liquid. This property is called the latent heat of vaporization, because the heat remains in the steam until it forms water and releases the heat. There is a limit to the amount of water vapor that the air can hold before it becomes saturated. This amount varies with the temperature. The lower the temperature, the lower the absolute amount of water the air will hold before it is saturated. This is demonstrated in hot weather when the humidity is relatively high. During the night and in the early morning when the temperature is low, the capacity of the air to hold moisture is reduced, and although it remains saturated, or nearly so, some of the air vapor is precipitated as dew. As the humidity falls, the grass dries slowly or quickly, depending on the degree of saturation of the air and whether or not there is a wind. For example, this morning the temperature was 63°F and the humidity was 93 per cent. At noon the temperature was 85°F and the humidity was 63 per cent. The absolute amount of moisture in the air is as great as or greater at noon than it was earlier in the day. The amount that the air is capable of holding has been increased by the increase in temperature.

Another factor in comfort is the relationship of the humidity to the temperature. This is expressed as the comfort index. As the humidity rises in relation to the temperature, comfort declines. Cooling systems are designed differently for use in hot moist and hot dry climates. In hot moist climates an essential feature of a cooling system is a device to remove moisture as well as heat. In fact, unless the temperature is extreme, comfort can be greatly increased by the removal of excessive moisture, despite little or no decrease in temperature. In hot dry climates cooling may be effected by increasing evaporation. Rather than removing moisture, it is added as air is circulated. The windows may be open to supply fresh dry air. Temperature in the room falls because of the heat used in evaporation. Persons driving through a hot dry region sometimes utilize a similar device to cool their cars. They hang wet towels in the car. Cooling is effected by evaporation. The dripping water bags hung on the fenders of cars driven through the desert are based on the same principle.

In addition to its high latent heat of vaporization, water has other properties that facilitate heat loss and therefore help to protect the tissues from overheating. They include its high specific heat and its high conductivity. Specific heat is defined as the amount of heat required to raise the temperature of 1 g of water 1°C. Water has a specific heat of 1, which is the highest of all liquids. All others have a specific heat of less than 1. Defined in terms of numbers, 1 g of water absorbs 1 kcal of heat in rising 1°C. As a consequence, body fluids are capable of absorbing relatively large amounts of heat with little change in temperature.

Regulation of Body Temperature

Although body temperature is regulated, the temperature of the external environment affects the ease with which this is accomplished. Heat loss may be facilitated by cooling the environment, by removing moisture or dehumidifying room air, by warming and humidifying inspired air, by changing body position to increase amount of body surface exposed, by removing clothing, by increasing air currents, and by applying fluids that are cooler than the body to the skin. Conversely, heat loss may be diminished by changing body position to decrease amount of body surface exposed, increasing the environmental temperature, by adding moisture or humidifying it, by covering the body, by reducing air currents, and by immersing the body in warm water.

Control System

Similar to other bodily processes, the temperature of the body is subject to nervous and hormonal control.

Despite a lack of knowledge of the number of circuits involved in the nervous control of body temperature, it behaves as if it were a closed-loop negative feedback system. Information is fed into the hypothalamus by the temperature of the blood circulating through it and/or by sensory receptors in other parts of the body. In the hypothalamus the information is interpreted and converted (transduced) into neural impulses that initiate behavior that increases or decreases rates of heat loss and heat production. The behavioral responses to thermal information are summarized in Table 20-1.

Thermal information about the environment is picked up by the body's temperature sensors. The body has two types of temperature sense organs: (1) warmth receptors, which respond maximally to temperatures slightly above body temperature, and (2) cold receptors, which respond maximally to temperatures slightly below body temperature. Mapping experiments show that discrete cold-sensitive spots outnumber discrete warmth-sensitive spots in the skin. Warmth receptors discharge between 20° and 45°C, with maximal discharge between 37.5° and 40°C, and cessation of discharge above 45°C. Cold receptors discharge between 10° and 41°C, with maximal discharge between 15° and 20°C; paradoxically, cold receptors resume discharge above 45°C in conjunction with discharge of pain receptors. The sensation of heat associated with temperatures above 45°C is believed to be due to this combined discharge of cold and pain receptors (Ganong, 1973, p. 76).

Information from peripheral temperature receptors is transmitted inward over the lateral spinothalamic tract of the spinal cord, which carries impulses of pain and temperature to the thalamus, where automatic responses are integrated and initiated. Fine discrimination and initiation of voluntary responses occur only if and when messages reach the cerebral cortex.

Satinoff (1978) has proposed modification of the currently accepted view that the hypothalamus is the sole integrator of body temperature. He describes the hypothalamus as the most important among many integrators, in that it coordinates the activity of other intregrating mechanisms at lower levels of the neuroaxis. Satinoff's model proposes there are as many integrators as there are thermoregulatory responses; each level of neural integration is facilitated or inhibited by levels above and below. Satinoff proposes that the purpose of such a complicated arrangement is to achieve finer and finer control over body temperature.

Control of temperature regulation is exerted through the autonomic nervous system and through endocrine activity. The sympathetic system is activated by cold stimuli and reduces heat dissipation by reducing blood flow through the skin and decreasing sweat production. In addition, heat production

TABLE 20-1 *Behavioral Responses to Thermal Information**

Thermoregulatory Mechanisms	Activated By
A. Those that increase or prevent decrease in body temperature:	
1. By stimulating heat production	Cold
Shivering	
Hunger	
Increased voluntary activity	
Increased endocrine activity	
2. By decreasing heat loss	Cold
Cutaneous vasoconstriction	
Curling up the body	
"Goose flesh" (horripilation)	
B. Those that decrease or prevent increase in body temperature:	
1. By increasing heat loss	Heat
Cutaneous vasodilation	
Sweating	
Increased rate of respiration—panting	
Stretching out the body	
2. By decreasing heat production	Heat
Anorexia	
Apathy and inertia	
Decreased endocrine activity	

* Information in this table is based on Timiras, P. S., *Developmental Physiology and Aging.* New York: Macmillan Publishing Co., Inc., 1972, p. 213.

is increased through increased adrenaline release and by activation of the thyroid gland, when cold exposure is prolonged. When a person is exposed to heat stimuli, cooling mechanisms of vasodilatation and sweating are activated through the parasympathetic nervous system (Case, 1979). See Figure 20-5 for a model of the body temperature control system.

The hypothalamus appears to function as a central thermoreceptive area, integrating sensory information from three sources: (1) thermal receptors located in the periphery, (2) thermal-sensitive cells in the hypothalamus, and (3) "core" receptors located in deep body tissues. The anterior hypothalamus is associated with mechanisms responsible for heat loss, that is, for those reflex responses activated by warmth; regions of the posterior hypothalamus are associated with heat production mechanisms, that is, those reflex responses activated by cold (Plum, 1979). Injury to the region of the anterior hypothalamus results in elevation of body temperature; injury to the region of the posterior hypothalamus results in abnormally low body temperature. Stimulation of the area increasing heat production results in inhibition of the area facilitating heat loss. There is some evidence indicating that there are heat-regulating centers in the spinal cord. The principal centers are, however, in the hypothalamus and nearby preoptic nuclei. Messages from the hypothalamus are conveyed to the surface of the body by the sympathetic, or thoracolumbar, division of the autonomic nervous system. It innervates both the sweat glands and the peripheral blood vessels. Although the postganglionic fibers supplying the sweat glands are cholinergic, they respond to stimulation of the sympathetic nervous system. According to Hemingway and Price (1968), nonshivering heat production in the cold-adapted individual is controlled or influenced by the sympathetic nervous system.

Age-related factors significantly influence temperature regulation. In the infant who has established the ability to sweat, heat loss exceeds capacity to produce heat. Although the infant responds to cold by shivering and by increasing his or her metabolic rate, the losses are too great to maintain heat balance. Because he or she lacks subcutaneous fat and has a relatively larger body surface, the premature infant has more difficulty in maintaining a stable body temperature than the full-term infant (Silverman & Parke, 1965).

In infants and children the temperature response in illness is often greater than in adults. They have a higher metabolic rate; therefore there is more heat to eliminate. Normally they have a larger proportion of their body water in the interstitial fluid space, and their kidneys do not concentrate urine as effectively as do those of adults.

In contrast to the child and younger adult, who

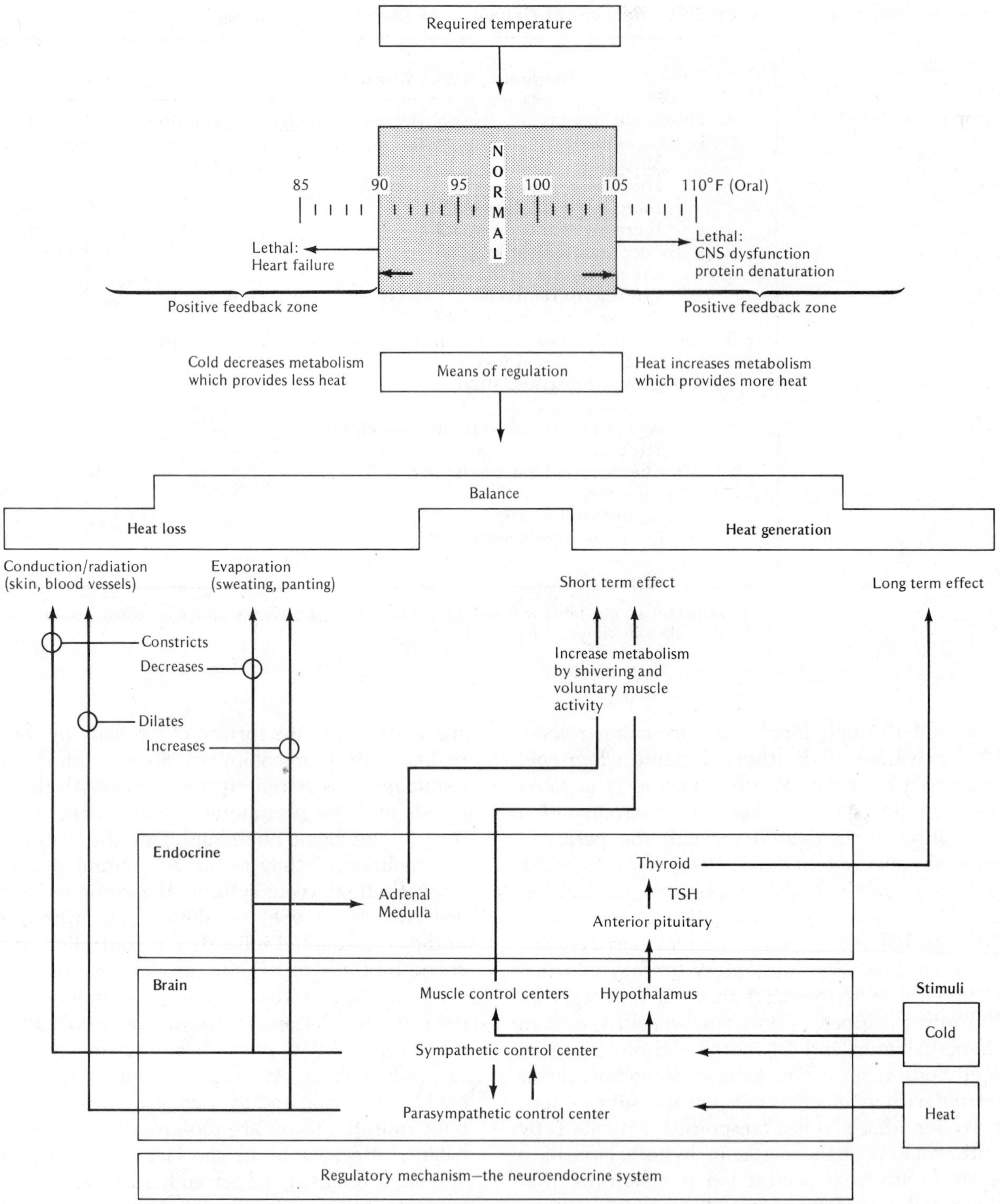

Figure 20-5. The body temperature control system. (Used with permission of Macmillan Publishing Company, Inc., from *Biology*, 2nd ed., 1979, by J. F. Case, p. 389, Fig. 19-14.)

respond to a variety of etiologic agents by developing a fever, elderly and debilitated persons may have little or even no elevation of temperature when ill. Therefore absence of a fever should not lead the nurse to discount other evidence that the elderly person is ill. Failure to develop a fever under circumstances when it is usual is generally a poor prognostic sign.

Range of Body Temperature

Vertebrates, including humans, function most efficiently within a narrow range of body temperatures. The upper limit for survival is about 45°C (113°F), when proteins begin to denature and become inactivated; the lower limit is slightly below 0°C (32°F), when intracellular water begins to form ice crystals that rupture and kill cells (Heller et al., 1978). Temperature-regulating mechanisms, if effective, maintain body temperature within the upper and lower limits compatible with survival. Figure 20-5 shows the temperature range within which negative feedback operates effectively to maintain temperature within limits compatible with life. As with many other pathological states, when temperature exceeds the limits beyond which control mechanisms can no longer maintain homeostasis, control changes to positive feedback mechanisms, which are frequently irreversible (see Figure 20-5). Although survival is possible with body temperatures in the range of 30 to 45°C (88° to 115°F), upper-limit temperatures in excess of 42.5°C (108.5°F) can be tolerated for only *brief* periods. Tolerance to lower-limit temperatures is very variable, depending on moisture and rate of cooling. The most efficient temperature regulation occurs between 34° and 41°C (93° to 105.8°F). Except in persons who have a brain lesion, heat stroke, overwhelming sepsis, or dehydration, or who are moribund, temperatures seldom rise above 41°C.

Adaptation to Extremes in Temperature

Within limits humans are capable of adapting to extremes in temperature. Most individuals have an excess of sweat glands, not all of which function at the same time. Persons born in tropical climates have more sweat glands functioning at one time than those who are born in temperate climates, but they do not have visible drops of sweat. Given time, a nonadapted but healthy person adapts physiologically to elevated environmental temperatures. Evidence that adaptation to heat occurs is that the first hot days of summer are more uncomfortable than later hot days. Changes taking place during adaptation to heat include increased salt conservation, probably caused by increased aldosterone secretion, and a small decrease in metabolic rate. The ability to retain salt takes longer to develop than the other changes. The pulse rate, which is increased in the beginning, returns to normal levels. Flushing of the skin because of vasodilatation decreases as adaptation develops. Edema of the hands and the feet is common until adaptation occurs and the individual may have many signs and symptoms similar to those observed during illness. Some people, especially those with a limited cardiac reserve, have a limited capacity to adapt to heat. This is evidenced by an increase in pulse rate. Also, in the adaptive process the tendency to conserve salt may aggravate previous salt and water retention and place an added strain on a limited cardiac reserve.

Persons who are elderly or who have a cardiac disorder should be encouraged to reduce physical activity during hot weather. This is most important at its onset. Because of impaired function of the cardiovascular and pulmonary systems, they are unable to deliver promptly to the skin an increased volume of oxygenated blood. Other measures reducing the burden on the heart and the thermoregulatory systems include the wearing of lightweight clothing and use of electric fans and air conditioning. It is also important for the person to maintain fluid intake without exceeding excretory capacity. When sweating is profuse, it is often difficult to replace the fluid loss by voluntary drinking. When air conditioning is not available, patients who are in congestive heart failure are sometimes placed in oxygen tents in hot weather. Although the increase in oxygen supply may be beneficial, the air conditioning reduces the demands made on the circulatory system to facilitate the loss of heat. When the patient is removed from the tent, he or she may be called on to adapt both to a reduction in environmental oxygen and to an increase in the temperature of the surroundings. Consequently, the tent may be removed gradually. When this is done, it is well to take it off during the cooler parts of the day and to replace it when it is hot.

Summary of Regulation

To summarize the physiology of temperature regulation, temperature is one of the conditions that is homeostatically controlled by the nervous, hormonal, and circulatory systems. The heat-regulating centers in the nervous system regulate body temperature primarily by increasing or decreasing the diameter of blood vessels in the skin and by shivering. The hormonal system influences heat production and salt retention, which in turn increase water retention and in this way aid in the transfer of heat from the interior of the body to the external environment. The temperature known to be regulated is that of the deeper, or core, tissues of the body. Body temperature varies with such factors as activity, emotion, environmental conditions, and the time of day. Body temperatures can be elevated by procedures interfering with heat loss, such as hot baths, hot weather, and strenuous muscular exercise. Children are likely to respond with greater swings in temperature than adults. Elderly people often respond less actively than younger persons.

One of the most common findings in disease is some disturbance in temperature regulation. Although temperatures below the lower range of normal do occur, the most common change is an elevation above the upper limits of normal. Because some people normally maintain a temperature somewhat higher than average, the upper limit of normal is difficult to define exactly. However, for persons resting quietly in bed, an oral temperature of 37.5°C (99.5°F) is usually accepted as the upper limit of normal. The condition in which the body temperature is elevated above normal in disease is called fever.

Measuring Body Temperature

The purpose of measuring body temperature is to estimate as accurately as possible the temperature of the interior of the body. Whether or not the temperature recorded by the thermometer accurately reflects the temperature of the body depends on the care with which the procedure is performed and the accuracy of the thermometer. The thermometer should be placed in an area of the body that contains large blood vessels and that is protected insofar as possible from outside influences. The most accurate determinations of body temperature are made by readings taken at the tympanic (ear drum) membrane. This location is of little practical value, due to technical problems. Since minute changes in body temperature are less important than ease and comfort of measurement, readings are usually taken orally, rectally, and occasionally in the axillary fossa (Strand, 1978, p. 380).

Whatever site is used, the thermometer should be kept in place long enough to register the true temperature. When a mercury thermometer is used, care should be taken to shake the mercury down before the thermometer is reused. Despite their importance to the safety of the patient, certain basic techniques related to taking measurements of body temperature are not discussed here. It is important to be certain that (1) the thermometer is clean when it is inserted and (2) the thermometer is introduced in such a manner that it does not damage body tissue.

Not only do the temperatures of various parts of the body differ, but the temperatures at the same site vary from one time of the day to another. As previously indicated, internal body temperature rises and falls with clocklike regularity, in the course of a day, with the rhythm depending on neither muscular activity nor food intake (Luce, 1971). The lowest temperature is reached sometime between 3 and 6 A.M. Then it begins to rise until it reaches its highest point between 7 and 10 P.M. When temperatures are taken once a day, the time selected should reflect the peak temperature. For most moderately well patients a temperature reading taken about 7 P.M. is most satisfactory. When a patient's temperature rises rapidly, readings may need to be made every 10 to 15 minutes in order to determine the peak temperature as well as to protect the patient should his or her temperature rise excessively. Sims (1965) suggests that temperatures taken at 7 A.M. and 7 P.M. will provide knowledge of the peak and trough, and that a 6-hour schedule beginning about 7 A.M. will provide sufficient information about the temperature of most patients.

Sites Used for Temperature Determination

Although the tympanic membrane and other sites have been used for experimental studies, the sites commonly used are the mouth, rectum, and axilla. Authorities differ as to the range of normal for each of these sites. Despite the assumption that the rectum most accurately reflects core body temperatures, some authorities believe that equally or more accurate temperature readings may be made in the mouth or axilla.

From the studies made by Nichols and her associates (1966), factors influencing the accuracy of temperature readings included the reliability of the thermometers and the time they were left in place. Of fifty-two oral thermometers tested for reliability, thirty-five were accurate at 95.4°F. At 105.8°F only five were accurate. Of fifty-two rectal thermometers tested, only sixteen were accurate at 95.4°F and three at 105.8°F.

The ease and accuracy of taking measurements of body temperature of persons in acute and long-term care facilities is being advanced by the widespread use of electronic probes. New models of the probe are pliable plastic, with a highly accurate thermistor embedded in the tip. The probe can usually be cleaned with soap and water, alcohol, Zephiran Chloride, or any other sterilizing agent, or a plastic probe sheath can be applied for use with each individual, and then disposed. The reading of the body temperature is recorded on the dial of a separate case which contains the power source. Without the plastic sheath, a stable reading may be recorded within as little as 30 seconds. However, as with any electronic equipment, the electronic thermometer requires regular maintenance to remain accurate. The same explanations and care should be given to the patient, regardless of the type of measuring instrument being used to record the body temperature.

Findings from studies of the time required to obtain accurate oral measurements of body temperature do not agree on the minimum time required; recommendations vary from 4 minutes (Soo, 1973) to 11 minutes (Nichols & Kucha, 1973) to reach the maximum reading. Pending further studies, the nurse might use the following placement times recommended by Nichols et al., (1966) as a guide to obtain reasonably accurate readings; oral, 7 minutes; axillary, 10 minutes; and rectal, 2 minutes. The only procedure to ensure that the thermometer has reached the maximum reading is to remove the thermometer from the selected site at the recommended time, make a reading, replace the thermometer for about a minute, and repeat the reading. If the recorded temperature has not changed, you probably have the maximum reading; if the temperature reading has changed, repeat the cycle until you obtain two consecutive identical readings.

Except in infants and young children, the oral cavity is the most common site used for measuring body temperature. Findings from investigations of the effect of oral temperature readings of a variety of preceding oral events support the belief that cold fluids produce significant changes, but evidence on the effect of smoking was conflicting (Woodman et al., 1967; Verhonick & Werley, 1963).

Kintzel (1966) could not support the assumption that the administration of oxygen by either nasal catheter or tent had a significant effect on oral temperature readings. In fact, she suggests that by changing from oral to rectal thermometers at the time oxygen therapy is instituted a greater error may be introduced than if oral temperatures are continued. On the basis of her findings, Kintzel recommends that no change be made in the site used for temperature determination when oxygen therapy is prescribed.

General Nursing Objectives Related to Temperature Regulation

Knowledge of temperature regulation has a bearing on meeting the needs of all patients as well as those with fevers. One general objective in the nursing of patients is *to protect the patient from conditions that place strain on the adaptive capacity* of the individual. Certainly temperatures outside the range of comfort increase metabolism and, as a result, the activity of all tissues and organs. Although the effect of small or moderate changes in environmental temperature may be of no consequence as far as the heat-regulating center is concerned, they may place serious strain on the heart or blood vessels. In heart disease or shock, they may well have serious consequences. Methods that can be used to protect the patient from the consequences of high environmental temperatures have already been suggested. Patients should also be protected from chilling by adequate bed covering and warm clothing. Covered hot-water bottles to the feet, with attention to their temperature, bed socks, bed jackets, and sweaters help to protect patients from chilling. People, especially the elderly, who are accustomed to wearing their underwear in bed should be permitted to continue the practice when at all possible. Screens in front of open windows or doors may reduce drafts, which some patients find chilling. When bathing patients, especially during those times of the year when the environmental temperature is low, care should be taken that the bath water is warm and that the person is kept covered and the skin is thoroughly dried.

The second objective is *to make observations* not only *of the body temperature* readings, but also of *any other signs and symptoms indicating deviations from health or response to disease and/or its treatment.* The prompt reporting and recording of clearly described observations of patient responses are crucial to the identification of patient problems and to joint planning and evaluation of patient care by the nurse and physician.

References Cited

Belding, H. S. "Resistance to Heat in Man and Other Homeothermic Animals." In *Thermobiology.* Ed. by A. H. Rose. New York: Academic Press, Inc., 1967, p. 479.

Cahill, G. F., Jr. "Metabolic Memory." *N. Engl. J. Med.*, **302** (14 Feb. 1980), 396–97.

Case, J. F. *Biology*, 2nd ed. New York: Macmillan Publishing Co., Inc., 1979, pp. 385–90.

Cassidy, C. A. "The Relationship between Life Changes, Physical Symptoms, and Body Temperature Range: Temperature Changes Related to Adjustments to Life Events." *Image*, **8**:2 (June 1976), 30–35.

Ganong, W. F. *Review of Medical Physiology*, 6th ed. Los Altos: Lange Medical Publications, 1973.

Guyton, A. C. *Textbook of Medical Physiology*, 5th ed. Philadelphia: W. B. Saunders Company, 1976.

Harrison, G. A., and Cleeg, E. J. "Environmental Factors Influencing Mammalian Growth." In *Physiology and Pathology of Adaptation Mechanisms.* Ed. by E. Bajusz. New York: Pergamon Press, Inc., 1969, p. 84.

Heller, H. C. et al. "The Thermostat of Vertebrate Animals." *Sci. Am.*, **239** (Aug. 1978), 102–13.

Hemingway, A., and Price, W. M. "The Autonomic Nervous System and Regulation of Body Temperature." *Anesthesiology,* **29** (July–Aug. 1968), 693.

Kintzel, K. C. "A Comparative Study of Oral and Rectal Temperatures in Patients Receiving Two Forms of Oxygen Therapy." In *ANA Clinical Sessions.* New York: Appleton-Century-Crofts, 1966, p. 102.

Luce, G. G. *Biological Rhythms in Human and Animal Physiology.* New York: Dover Publications, Inc., 1971, pp. 44–45.

Nichols, G. A. et al. "Oral, Axillary, and Rectal Temperature Determinations and Relationships." *Nurs. Res.,* **15** (Fall 1966), 308.

Nichols, G. A., and Kucha, D. H. "Taking Adult Temperatures: Oral Measurements." *Nurs. Res.,* **22** (Jan.–Feb. 1973), 93.

Plum, F. "The Hypothalamus and Neurologic Disorders: Heat Regulation." In *Cecil Textbook of Medicine,* 15th ed. Philadelphia: W. B. Saunders Company, 1979, pp. 715–19.

Routh, J. I. *20th Century Chemistry.* Phildelphia: W. B. Saunders Company, 1953, p. 19.

Satinoff, E. "Neural Organization and Evolution of Thermal Regulation in Mammals." *Science,* **201** (7 July 1978), 16–22.

Silverman, W. A., and Parke, P. C. "Keep Him Warm." *Am. J. Nurs.,* **65** (Oct. 1965), 81.

Sims, R. S. "Temperature Recording in a Teaching Hospital." *Lancet,* **2** (11 Sept. 1965), 535–36.

Soo, B. "Temperatures and Their Accuracy." *Nurs. Res.,* **22** (Jan.–Feb. 1973), 93.

Strand, F. L. *Physiology: A Regulatory Systems Approach.* New York: Macmillan Publishing Co., Inc., 1978, pp. 380–86.

Verhonick, P. J., and Werley, H. H. "Experimentation in Nursing Practice in the Army." *Nurs. Outlook,* **11** (March 1963), 205.

Woodman, E. A. et al. "Sources of Unrealiability in Oral Temperatures." *Nurs. Res.,* **16** (Summer 1967), 276–79.

General References

Abbey, J. C. et al. "How Long Is That Thermometer Accurate?" *Am. J. Nurs.* **78** (Aug. 1978) 1375–76.

Adolph, E. F. et al. *Physiology in Man in the Desert.* New York: Interscience Publishers, Inc., 1947.

Baker, M. A. "A Brain-Cooling system in Mammals." *Sci. Am.,* **240** (May 1979), 130–39.

Barnett, S. A., and Mount, L. E. "Resistance to Cold in Mammals." In *Thermobiology.* Ed. by A. H. Rose. New York: Academic Press, Inc., 1967, pp. 411–77.

Benzinger, T. H. "The Human Thermostat." *Sci. Am.,* **204** (Jan. 1961), 134–47.

Christensen, H. N., and Cellarius, R. A. *Introduction to Bioenergetics: Thermodynamics for the Biologist.* Philadelphia: W. B. Saunders Company, 1972.

Felton, G. "Effect of Time Cycle Change on Blood Pressure and Temperature in Young Women." *Nurs. Res.,* **19** (Jan.–Feb. 1970), 48–58.

Folk, G. E., Jr. *Introduction to Environmental Physiology.* Philadelphia: Lea & Febiger, 1966, p. 92.

Goldsmith, R. "Use of Clothing Records to Demonstrate Acclimatization to Cold in Man." *J. Appl. Physiol.,* **15** (Sept. 1960), 776–80.

"Guaging a Safe 'Time-out' for Stopped Hearts." *Med. World News,* **14** (26 Jan. 1973), 62E.

Lutz, L., and Perlstein, P. H. "Temperature Control in Newborn Babies." *Nurs. Clin. North Am.,* **6** (March 1971), 15–23.

Matzke, H. A., and Foltz, F. M. *Synopsis of Neuroanatomy,* 2nd ed. New York: Oxford University Press, 1972, p. 24.

Netter, F. H. *The Ciba Collection of Medical Illustrations: Vol. I—The Nervous System.* New York: Ciba Corporation, 1962, pp. 160–61.

Nichols, G. A., and Verhonick, P. J. "Time and Temperature." *Am. J. Nurs.,* **67** (Nov. 1967), 2304–06.

Purintum, L. R., and Bishop, B. E. "How Accurate Are Clinical Thermometers?" *Am. J. Nurs.,* **69** (Jan. 1969), 99–100.

Torrance, J. T. "Temperature Readings in Premature Infants." *Nurs. Res.,* **17** (July–Aug. 1968), 312–20.

Verhonick, P. J., and Nichols, G. A. "Temperature Measurement in Nursing Practice and Research." *Can. Nurse,* **64** (June 1968), 41–43.

Walker, V. H., and Selminoff, E. D. "A Note on the Accurancy of the Temperature, Pulse and Respiration Procedure." *Nurs. Res.,* **14** (Winter 1965), 72–76.

21

Neuromuscular Responses

Self-movement is one of the most obvious properties of animals, including men. At first it was regarded as a property of living things alone. Then men made machines which moved themselves, and in the seventeenth century philosophers began to explain animals as machines. Descartes thought that a muscle shortened because it was blown out by "animal spirits" pumped down the nerves from the brain.

VANNEVARR BUSH
Vannevar Bush in Caryl P. Haskins

Essential Structures and Processes

One of the primary and earliest responses to threat of or actual injury is the alteration of position in space. There are, obviously, many other types of stimuli that result in movement. At the very minimum, this response depends on a receptor connected by nerve cells and fibers to an effector. Receptors contain cells sensitive to changes in the internal or external environment. The retina of the eye contains receptor cells sensitive to light. Effector cells are capable of some overt activity. These cells are of two general types, muscle and gland cells. Between the receptor and effector cells are afferent (sensory) nerve fibers that convey messages from the receptor cells to centers, groups of cells, in the spinal cord and brain where "decisions" are made (see Chapters 16 and 17). From the centers, messages are sent by way of efferent pathways to a few or to many effector cells. Alteration of position in space requires not only intact neuromuscular units but also a metabolic response adequate to supply the necessary muscular energy. The direct source of energy for a muscle's activity is adenosine triphosphate (ATP); the release of energy from the splitting of ATP into adenosine diphosphate (ADP) and phosphoric acid is what powers muscle contractions. The ATP must be continuously resynthesized from its products as soon as it is broken down. The energy needed for the recombination of ADP and phosphoric acid into ATP is supplied by another energy-yielding reaction in the cells: the splitting of creatine phosphate, which must also be resynthesized continuously. The two ultimate sources of energy for the resynthesis of the phosphagens are combustion of food and glycolysis (see Chapter 29). In summary, the muscular energy system consists of five reactions, three of which yield energy and two of which absorb energy (Margaria, 1972). This energy system operates not only to power the muscles for movement, but also to provide fuel to power cellular activity in response to injury that was not avoided by movement. (See metabolic responses to injury, Appendix D, and Chapter 29.) Joints must be functional so that areas of the body can be moved, and the bones must be sufficiently rigid to be moved by the muscles.

Three Ways to Respond to Danger

Response to danger or to injury by alteration of position in space may be manifested in one or more of three ways. One is to *flee* or run away. A second is to remain and *fight* the enemy. A third is to become immobile or *freeze*, by contracting opposing sets of muscles. Each type of reaction is appropriate in different situations. On awakening, Mr. All notes that his apartment is on fire and that the blaze is sufficiently large that fighting it is out of the question; to try is to court disaster. Immobility is even more inappropriate. To flee as quickly as possible is the only reasonable course of action. Under other circumstances, such as in the presence of a lion or a poisonous reptile, immobility is the only response likely to be successful.

Frequently the manner in which the individual reacts is entirely automatic. Sometimes a person is able to control the impulse to act and to make a conscious decision as to the most appropriate course of action. An illustration of more or less automatic behavior occurred when Mr. All, who had taken his son John with him as he left his burning apartment, found that John had returned to get his clothing. Although Mr. All had to go through flames, he returned to the apartment. Despite suffering painful burns, he was able to rescue his son and to protect him from the fire. He had no recollection of his actions or of what had happened to him. Had his reaction not been more or less automatic, he probably would not have been able to save his son.

The following item taken from the news illustrates the type of situation in which survival results from making a conscious decision. A young woman was trapped in a walk-in freezer. Despite feelings of panic, she remembered that freezing could be delayed by continued movement. To maintain her self-control and to keep herself moving, she concentrated on counting the cans of food stored in the refrigerator. Fortunately, her mother missed her before she suffered serious injury. She survived because she was able to act intelligently and to modify her behavior appropriately. One factor that was very helpful to her was the certainty that her mother would miss her soon enough so that she would be rescued in time.

Sustained Muscular Contraction—Contemporary Response to Feelings of Aggression

Despite the value of "flight, fight, and freeze" to the past survival of the human species, the number of situations in which they now serve a useful purpose is quite limited. In fact, fight and flight are both modes of behavior that are disapproved of in the American culture. Persons who fight in public are censured or jailed for disturbing the peace. Those who openly flee are called cowards. This leaves only one mode of behavior, that is, immobility in circumstances eliciting a fight-or-flight response. Some persons are in a state of constant muscular contraction. They behave as if they are in a continuous state of danger. Persons who have a large number of muscles contracted are likely to appear tense or strained. In some persons, contraction may be limited to a group of muscles such as those of the back or neck. Sustained muscular contraction, even in the absence of motion, requires the expenditure of energy, and it results in fatigue and muscular pain. In some instances it may predispose to disease.

Persons free of disease or pain who experience prolonged muscular contraction frequently are responding to feelings of hostility or aggression. Fromm (1973) distinguishes two different kinds of aggression in humans: (1) *benign* aggression, which is biologically adaptive, serves the suvival of the individual and the species, and ceases when the threat has ceased, and (2) *malignant* aggression, which is not biologically adaptive and is often destructive and cruel. Aggressiveness and rage, extreme forms of response to threatening events,[1] are judged by many to be modern people's greatest problem, because of the violence and destruction that can result when aggressive behavior is harnessed with advanced technology. Factors that influence aggressive behavior include heredity, hormones, stimulation of the reticular activating system, and learning through past experience. Technology now exists to control aggressiveness by surgical, chemical, and electrical manipulations of the nervous system, but the serious ethical issues raised by the spector of such controls have not been resolved. The use of tranquilizers that tend to reduce hostility is the only widespread practice aimed at modifying this response pattern. Laboratory studies of the aggressive and avoidance behavior of animals placed in stressful conditions, and the consequent degree of gastrointestinal ulceration, found that (1) when coping behavior was followed by persistence of the stressful stimulus, ulceration was aggravated; (2) when coping behavior was followed by stimuli not associated with the stressful stimulus, no ulceration was found; and (3) when animals could avoid and escape the stressor, they showed increased levels of brain norepinephrine, whereas helpless animals showed decreased norepi-

[1] Physiologic events that accompany these emotional responses are similar to those shown in Appendix D.

nephrine. Weiss (1973) suggests a causal sequence, from "helplessness" to behavioral depression dependent on changes in brain norepinephrine, with perpetuation of a vicious cycle; inability to cope alters neural biochemistry, which further accentuates depression, increasing inability to cope, which further alters neural biochemistry, and so on.

In caring for the person responding to a stressful condition, the nurse attempts to break this cycle by modifying the environment or the patient's perception of the situation, in such a way that his or her distress and/or sense of helplessness are reduced.

Muscular Tension in Illness

In illness, sustained muscular contraction is a not uncommon source of suffering. Headache is one of the most common complaints of people who are ill. One of the factors in its development may be spasm of the head and neck muscles. Backache, another frequent discomfort, results from sustained contraction of back muscles. (See discussion of common types of pain, Chapter 36.) Many other aches and pains of illness result from the effects of muscle tension. In a number of diseases, and following injury, a characteristic feature is increased muscular tension or even muscular spasm. For example, the person whose thyroid hypersecretes is in a continuous state of increased muscular tension. A small sudden noise initiates a startle reflex out of proportion to the stimulus. Disorders in which muscle spasm is a factor in pain include acute poliomyelitis, fractures, rheumatoid arthritis, peritonitis, biliary or renal colic, and menstrual cramps.

Prevention and Treatment Measures

Measures used in prevention and treatment of muscular tension vary. They are usually directed toward one or more of the following objectives: (1) to lessen the degree of muscular spasm, (2) to relieve the pain, and (3) to remove the cause. Measures that relieve muscle spasm are likely to relieve the pain associated with it. For example, the application of moist or dry heat over an area of a painful muscle is a well-known practice in folk medicine. In acute poliomyelitis, muscle spasm and pain may be relieved by the application of moist heat. In rheumatoid arthritis, use of salicylates with or without the applicatoin of heat will often afford relief. A number of muscle-relaxing drugs are also available. Diathermy may be employed to relieve pain by the application of heat. (See Chapter 11 for explanation.)

Under some circumstances, muscle spasm can be relieved by the application of traction, that is, by the application of a force opposing muscle contraction. After a period of time the muscle becomes fatigued and relaxes. As an example, traction is frequently employed in the treatment of fractures (broken bones) in which the ends of the bones are displaced. Traction is applied to lessen muscle spasm by fatiguing muscles. As the muscles relax, the two ends of the bone return to their normal position with the two parts of the bone in normal alignment and the ends of the bone just touching each other. Should the traction be removed, the muscles again contract and displace the fracture. When traction is utilized in the treatment of a fracture, everyone, including the patient and members of the family, should understand why it must be continuously applied. They should also know what conditions must be met for it to be effective. Under no circumstances should it be removed or lessened without a prescription of the physician. Traction may also be prescribed in the treatment of muscle spasm associated with pressure on nerve roots. For example, it is used to relax the muscles of the back in low-back pain or to relax the muscles of the neck when pain is caused by pressure on nerves supplying spastic muscles. When a patient is placed in traction, the nurse should know why the traction is applied and whether it may or may not be released.[2]

When pain results from the spasm of muscles in ducts or tubular structures such as a ureter or the common bile ducts, an analgesic or muscle-relaxing drug may be required to relieve pain. Thus morphine or one of its substitutes with or without a smooth-muscle relaxant such as papaverine is administered to relieve the pain.

Because muscle tension frequently accompanies illness and its treatment, the nurse should develop the habit of looking for evidence indicating its presence as well as for conditions that predispose to its development. The nurse should also develop skill in the performance of nursing measures that prevent and/or relieve muscle tension. Most of these are not difficult and require little complicated equipment. They do require a conviction on the part of the nurse that they are important to the welfare of the patient. One of the most important aspects is attention to the position and body alignment of the patient, not only when in bed but when up and about and sitting in a chair. Weak and flaccid muscles should be supported and protected from overstretching. When supports are required, they should support, rather than be held in place by, the patient. They should extend along the length of the part and they should be adjusted so that strain is not placed on another

[2] See the references for descriptions of the types of traction and methods of application.

structure. For example, when a sling is applied to support an arm, it should extend the entire length of the forearm. It is not enough to support the arm at the wrist.

One of the most frequent causes of discomfort in the patient confined to bed is back pain. It can often be prevented by use of a firm mattress or by the simple procedure of placing a board under the mattress. Frequent changes in position also aid in the prevention of prolonged strain on back and other muscles. When a patient is required to lie on his or her back continuously, a support under the lumbar curve of the back may prevent stretching of back muscles. A properly placed footboard and a cradle to prevent bed covering from weighing on weakened extremities are other measures that protect muscles from spasm or overstretching.

No matter how comfortable a position is at the start, it becomes less so as time elapses. There should therefore be a regular schedule for changing the position of weak and helpless patients. At the time their position is changed, the arms and legs should be put through the normal range of motion. Exercise not only promotes muscular relaxation by relieving strain on muscles used by the patient to maintain the position, but it acts as a stimulus to relaxation. A well-given backrub will further contribute to muscular relaxation. Any attention to the comfort of the patient should facilitate relaxation. It is difficult to relax when one has to look at a bright light, listen to a noise, or be too cold or too warm and not be able to correct the situation. The nurse should be alert to possible sources of irritation and take appropriate steps to prevent or eliminate them from the environment of the patient.

Because the psychological and social climate of the patient has an effect on physiologic status, these too may be the source of muscular tension. There are many sources of muscular tension in the course of an illness, and no effort will be made to enumerate them all. The nurse should develop the habit of looking for evidence of it. When patients look relaxed and comfortable, they probably are. When they appear to be tense or in poor position, they are likely to be uncomfortable. The nurse should also be alert to conditions in the environment of the patient—physical, psychological, or social—that are likely to induce tension, and should then act to correct them.

The following illustrations represent two relatively common nursing problems whose solutions are not very complicated. The first is Mr. All, who was introduced earlier. For the first 2 or 3 days after he was burned he paid little attention to his surroundings and showed no concern for anyone but himself. About the third day he began to ask about his son John, who was hospitalized after the fire. Despite everyone's effort to reassure him that John was not badly injured and would soon be discharged from the hospital, he was obviously worried. Arrangements were made for John to visit him. When he saw that John's burns were really of a minor nature, he was much relieved. This one visit did what verbal reassurance could not do; it convinced Mr. All that John was alive and would completely recover from his injury.

About a week or 10 days after Mr. All was burned, skin grafts were applied to his upper arms and neck, and he was instructed to lie still for 3 days as any movement might disrupt the contact between the skin graft and the underlying tissue. Because Mr. All understood and accepted the importance of remaining immobile to the success of skin grafting, he concentrated on lying quietly. Although he maintained the desired position, he experienced considerable muscular tension. Because the nurse knew that Mr. All was to lie in the same position for 3 days, she checked his mattress to be sure that it was firm and provided adequate support for him. To encourage Mr. All to relax, his back was rubbed at 2-hour intervals by inserting a hand between the mattress and the lumbar region of his back, and he was assisted in performing leg exercises. He was encouraged to wiggle his toes and to flex and extend his foot at the ankle. The nurse made a real effort to anticipate his needs and to visit him frequently. Because he was in a large ward, she encouraged ambulatory patients to stop briefly to see if he needed anything. As is frequently true when the arms are immobilized, one of his greatest sources of discomfort was an itching nose. When the nurse observed him wiggling his nose, she offered to scratch it for him. During the period immediately following skin grafting, the objective given precedence in Mr. All's nursing care was to minimize the sources of physiologic and phychological stress so that he could use his energy for recovery. His environment and nursing care were planned to meet this objective. Even so, he experienced discomfort. Despite the inability of the nurse to eliminate all of Mr. All's discomforts, she was able to minimize them and to make the experience more tolerable.

The second patient is Mrs. Carney, who had a radical amputation of the left breast. Her left arm was to be elevated in order to prevent swelling of the hand and arm. The positioning of the arm under circumstances such as Mrs. Carney's is based on the fact that water runs downhill. Therefore, distal parts should be higher than proximal parts. In terms of the particular structures, the hand should be higher than the elbow and the elbow higher than the shoulder. Unnecessary muscle tension can and should be prevented by arranging and balancing supporting apparatus, including pillows, so that it will support Mrs. Carney's arm. Briefly stated, supports should support.

The capacity to alter their position in space has been one of the significant factors in the survival of humans. It has enabled them to overcome danger, to find or produce food, to find mates, and to alter their environment so that it is better suited to their needs. In illness, the neuromuscular system reacts to the implied as well as to the real injury. Inasmuch as this response is appropriate, it contributes to survival. Even when muscle tension is appropriate, it adds to the fatigue and pain of illness. When the response is inappropriate or excessive, it increases the suffering of the patient, and it may be a factor in the development of undesired complications or sequelae.

The Nurse's Role in Helping the Person with a Neuromuscular Response

The nurse can help to lessen the severity of the neuromuscular response and its attendant discomforts by

1. Removing noxious stimuli from the external environment that the person, if able, would eliminate or remove. Some examples include bright lights, loud or sudden noises, overheated or underheated surroundings, inadequate ventilation, dripping faucets, blaring radio or television sets, overtalkative people, untidy surroundings.
2. Giving attention to the position of the person and changing the position regularly.
3. Providing for a comfortable bed.
4. Relieving muscle tension by putting extremities through the normal range of motion and rubbing the back.
5. Performing therapeutic procedures to relieve muscular spasm such as warm, moist packs; administering prescribed pain-relieving medications and supervising traction.
6. Preparing the person for what to expect and what is expected of him or her.
7. Identifying the implications that the illness has to the person and, if indicated, using appropriate resources to relieve him or her.
8. Modifying care of the person in relation to the severity, extent, and phase of the illness. This implies accepting the person and his or her behavior.

References Cited

Fromm, E. *The Anatomy of Human Destructiveness.* New York: Holt, Rinehart and Winston, 1973.

Margaria, R. "The Sources of Muscular Energy." *Sci. Am.,* **226** (March 1972), 84–91.

Weiss, J. M. "Psychological Factors in Stress and Disease." *Sci. Am.,* **226** (June 1973), 104–13.

General References

Brunner, N. A. *Orthopedic Nursing, A Programmed Aproach.* 2nd ed. St. Louis: The C. V. Mosby Company, 1975.

Chapman, C. B., ed. *Physiology of Muscular Exercise.* New York: American Heart Association, 1967.

Frohlich, E. D., ed. *Pathophysiology: Altered Regulatory Mechanisms in Disease.* Philadelphia: J. B. Lippincott Company, 1972.

Larson, C. A. and Gold, M. *Orthopedic Nursing,* 8th ed. St. Louis: The C. V. Mosby Company, 1974.

22

Sympathoadrenal Medullary Responses

The General Functions of the Autonomic System. *The diffuse influence of sympatho-adrenal activity allows, in structures where that activity is continuous and moderate, a widespread increase or decrease of function. Thus augmented activity of the sympatho-adrenal system may evoke extensive changes, as in dilating the pupils, accelerating the pulse, and contracting the blood vessels of the splanchnic area. Reduction of activity, on the other hand, permits these widely scattered organs to resume their former state or to become less affected.*

CANNON, WALTER B. and ROSENBLUETH, ARTURO. *Autonomic Neuro-Effector Systems.* New York: The Macmillan Company, 1937, pp. 8–9.

Sympathoadrenal Medullary Functions in Response to Stressful Events

Actions of the sympathetic divisions of the autonomic nervous system (ANS), together with the medulla of the adrenal gland, are directed toward strengthening fight-or-flight defenses against such environmental dangers as extremes of temperature, deprivation of water, or physical attack. Sympathetic effects involve the expenditure of energy, whereas parasympathetic effects appear to be concerned with acts of conservation and restoration. Examples of conservation brought about by the parasympathetic division include slowing of the heart, contraction of the pupil of the eye to protect it from intense light, and digestive processes that replenish energy stores of the body.

Any factor that impairs appropriate sympathoadrenal medullary response will interfere with liberation of epinephrine in response to an emergency or other stressful event, with the result that the individual will be unable to (1) perform hard physical work, (2) mobilize sugar from the liver on demand, (3) increase circulating red blood cells during excitement or exercise, and (4) conserve body heat in cold environments (Brobeck, 1973). The problems faced by a person with inadequate sympathoadrenal response are illustrated by the person in adrenal crisis, who is unable to adapt to even minor stresses. (Adrenal and thyroid dysfunctions are discussed in Chapter 35.) Although it has been demonstrated that the sympathetic division of the ANS is not essential to survival, the person with severe or prolonged impairment of the sympathoadrenal response must live under very controlled physical and emotional conditions if he or she is to remain in good health.

Participation of the sympathoadrenal response in the total response of an individual to injury is shown in Phase I of the table in Appendix D.

The Nurse's Role in Helping the Person with a Sympathoadrenal Response

The activity of the sympathoadrenal system can be expected to be increased in any person who suffers an injury or illness threatening survival. The nurse can help to support or appropriately modify the magnitude of the sympathoadrenal response by

1. Establishing severity of injury and degree of illness
2. Observing for signs and symptoms of increased sympathoadrenal activity, especially as evidenced by function of the nervous, cardiovascular, pulmonary, and renal systems
3. Looking for possible physical or emotional causes of increased sympathoadrenal activity, and acting on the basis of the cause(s) that appear most reasonable
4. Deft handling of the person's body
5. Allowing and encouraging dependency, including the surrender of the sense of obligation to make decisions

Assessment of Sympathoadrenal Response to Injury

Major surgery, severe burns, overwhelming infection, frightening sounds or sights, myocardial infarction, pain, and many other conditions stimulate the activity of the sympathetic nervous system. Many of the early symptoms that follow trauma are evidence of activation of the sympathoadrenal response to injury. The nurse who is the first or only person at the scene of an accident, or whose position requires initial screening of patients, must estimate the severity of injuries as the first step toward obtaining proper medical care. The trauma index (Emergency Handbook, 1973), shown in Figure 22-1 which was developed and tested at the University of Kansas Medical Center, provides a quick and reliable guide to estimation of the severity of injuries. The following criteria were used to select items to be included in the rating system: (1) data are obtainable without patient cooperation; (2) data are obtainable with little or no equipment; and (3) data are obtainable by paramedical personnel. The observer makes a quick but thorough assessment of the five patient characteristics listed in the left-hand column: the body region injured; the type of injury; and the cardiovascular, central nervous system, and respiratory status. He or she then selects one of the four descriptions that best fits the patient's situation, in each of the five areas, and writes in the blank boxes to the right of each row the number equivalent of the descriptions selected. Total score can range from 0 to 30 points, and scores within three ranges have been found to predict the following consequences: (1) rating of 0 to 7—usually lacerations, abrasions, contusions, or minor fractures, rarely requiring hospital admission; (2) rating of 8 to 18—variety of lesions, but confined to a single organ system, with admission

	One point	Three points	Four points	Six points	
Region	Skin or extremities	Back	Chest or abdomen	Head or neck	
Type of injury	Laceration or contusion	Stab wound	Blunt	Missile	
CV status	External hemorrhage	BP < 100 P > 100	BP < 80 P > 140	Absent pulses	
CNS status	Drowsy	Stupor	Motor or sensory loss	Coma	
Respiratory status	Chest pain	Dyspnea or hemoptysis	Evidence of aspiration	Apnea or cyanosis	
				Total	

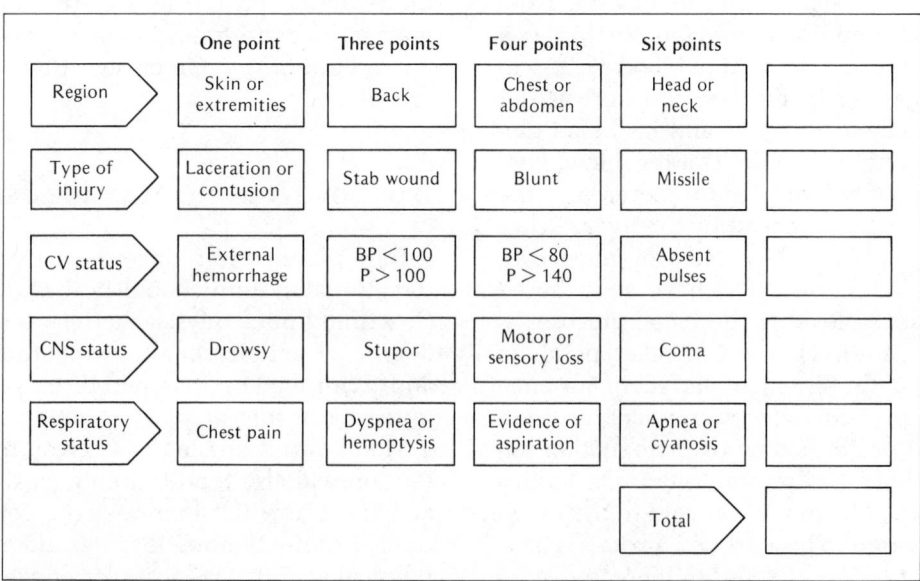

Figure 22-1. A trauma index to rate the severity of injuries. [Adapted with permission of Fischer-Murray, Inc., from "Fast Score for Medical Trauma" by John R. Kirkpatrick. *Emergency Medicine,* 4:93 (Oct.) 1972.]

to the hospital usually required, and injuries rarely fatal; and (3) rating over 18—severe, multiple injuries requiring intensive therapy, usually requiring admission to ICU, with a death rate approaching 50 per cent.

Regardless of the practice setting, the nurse cannot avoid encountering persons whose situation produces in them some evidence of activation of the sympathoadrenal response. Most, if not all, persons have experienced symptoms resulting from stimulation of the sympathetic nervous system. Mr. Brave (bleeding peptic ulcer), Mr. All (burned), and Mrs. Carney (amputation of breast) all had symptoms and signs indicating stimulation of the sympathetic nervous system. Both Mr. Brave and Mrs. Carney perspired profusely. All these patients had an increase in pulse rate. Mr. Brave complained that his heart pounded (palpitation). All breathed at a rapid rate. Though both Mr. Brave and Mrs. Carney lost blood, neither had an appreciable drop in blood pressure. Despite a loss of considerable volume of fluid into the burned area, and possibly in other tissue, Mr. All's blood pressure was maintained within normal limits. All three patients had some depression in gastrointestinal activity. In Mrs. Carney, diminished gastrointestinal activity was of short duration. In common with other patients who are seriously burned, Mr. All was predisposed to acute gastric dilatation. Consequently oral fluids were withheld for 2 days. When oral fluids were first prescribed, he was given 30 ml per hour for 4 hours. Because he did not complain of feelings of fullness, or of nausea, he was rapidly promoted to a full fluid and food intake.

Some degree of hyperglycemia may result from increased sympathoadrenal activty. On the third day after Mr. All was burned, his fasting blood sugar was 180 mg per 100 ml of blood. Because he was not known to have diabetes mellitus and his blood glucose returned to physiologic limits after a few days, the elevation probably indicated an increase in the release of glucose from glycogen by the liver. Other factors, including increased secretion of glucocorticoids by the adrenal cortex, may have contributed to the increase in the level of the blood glucose.

Mr. Brave had some evidence of so-called paralytic ileus. His abdomen was distended and silent (absence of peristalsis). To prevent overdistention of his stomach, his physician prescribed nasogastric suction until peristaltic activity was reestablished. On admission to the hospital, Mr. Brave was cold to the touch and pale; he appeared to be alert and anxious. These manifestations can all be ascribed to increased sympathoadrenal activity. Probably most patients have some increase in activity of the sympathoadrenal system at some stage of their illness. Even when illness is relatively minor, uncertainty about its causes or outcome may be a sufficiently potent stimulus to bring this about. When diagnostic or therapeutic procedures are perceived as indicating the possibility of a serious disease, or inducing pain, the likelihood of sympathoadrenal stimulation is further increased.

When a patient exhibits signs and symptoms indicative of increased sympathoadrenal activity, the nurse should seek answers to the following questions. Do the manifestations presented by the patient indicate that the illness is becoming more severe or that the patient is developing a complication? Are they the result of some physical or emotional stress associated with the illness or the patient's personal life? Is there something in the environment of the patient that probably explains their presence? Has the patient undergone, what is for him or her, an unusual degree of activity? Are the symptoms and signs transitory or do they persist? As an illustration, suppose that Mr. Brave has an increase in his pulse and respiratory rate. Because he has a history of hemorrhage, he may be bleeding. Depending on other circumstances the nurse will look for additional evidence that he is bleeding or will modify his care in some way. Perhaps a visitor has stayed too long or Mr. Brave is anxious because his wife, whom he expected at 2, has not arrived by 5 o'clock. If Mr. Brave is out of bed for the first time after several days of bedrest, the nurse will assist him to bed. She may then allow him to rest for a short period of time and then recheck his pulse and respiration. If indicated, she will take his blood pressure. Whatever the stimulus is, Mr. Brave is responding to it by increasing his circulatory and respiratory rates. Appropriate action on the part of the nurse depends on taking into consideration the possible causes and acting in light of the one or ones that appear most reasonable.

Basis of Nursing Management

Care planned to reduce the activity of the sympathoadrenal system should be based on two factors: (1) within limits, physical activity tends to lessen the degree of activity of the sympathoadrenal system, and (2) implied or imagined threats can act as stimuli initiating or augmenting its action.

Much of the nursing care given to relieve muscle tension will also tend to minimize sympathoadrenal activity. Care that increases the comfort of the patient promotes muscle relaxation. Within limits, physical activity has a similar effect. One of the values of early ambulation is that it decreases the intensity of the sympathoadrenal response. Patients whose condition allows them to get out of bed and to walk soon after injury or major surgical procedures usually have less pain and an earlier return of gastrointestinal activity than do those who are confined to bed for longer periods of time.

Not only does the sympathoadrenal system participate in the response of the individual to present and actual dangers to survival, but it is activated by fear or anxiety initiated by implied or imagined threats to well-being. When the nurse is successful in developing a trusting relationship with the patient, she or he can lessen the opportunities for the patient to imagine or magnify dangers in the situation (see Chapter 31).

The seriously ill patient who is fighting for life should not be required to make decisions or to be responsible for meeting his or her own needs. The patient is allowed and encouraged to be sick. He or she should be bathed, moved, turned, and assisted out of bed, as the condition demands, and should be held responsible neither for deciding when care is required nor for carrying it out. When giving care, the nurse should exercise judgment about its timing. When caring for a very ill patient, his or her welfare may demand that certain aspects of care be omitted or be given at a particular time. With some sick patients the nurse may have to say firmly and kindly, "I have come to give you a bath. You look miserable and the bath will help you to feel better," or "It is time for you to be turned to your other side or to get up." As the patient recovers, responsibility is shifted as he or she is able to assume it.

A person who has been seriously injured may not be able to face responsibility for, or the consequences of, that injury, and may build elaborate rationalizations to explain or justify himself or herself (Aronson, 1973). Once the person's survival is assured, and physiologic homeostasis is reestablished, the priority goal of care frequently becomes that of helping the person examine, acknowledge, and build on the consequences of the traumatic event. Confronting the person with the unreasonableness or unreality of his or her position or explanation is *not* appropriate while the person is still in the onset or shock phase of stress response. At that time, all the patient's energy is required to repair cellular damage.

Summary

One of the factors in the survival of humans has been their capacity to respond to threats of, or actual, injury by attacking or removing themselves from danger. Many of the processes involved in these responses are under the control of the sympathoadrenal system. Because the sympathoadrenal system can be activated by any change in the external or internal environment that is perceived to be a threat to survival, most serious illnesses are accompanied by increased sympathoadrenal activity. Trauma, including surgical therapy, is a stimulus to increased sympathoadrenal activity. The effect on the patient is a decrease in those activities not immediately essential to survival and an increase in those that are. Thus the individual is more alert, pupils are dilated, and he or she has increased muscle tension as well as an increase in heart and respiratory rate, increased sweating, and a rise in blood sugar. Activities not immediately essential to survival are depressed. Thus the alimentary canal is less active or may be temporarily paralyzed. Many of the discomforts and problems accompanying illness are caused by alterations in the activity of the autonomic nervous system. They should therefore be anticipated and dealt with by appropriate measures.

References Cited

Aronson, E. "The Rationalizing Animal." *Psychol. Today,* **6** (May 1973), 46–52.

Brobeck, J. R. "Neural Control Systems." In *Best & Taylor's Physiological Basis of Medical Practice,* 9th ed. Baltimore: The Williams and Wilkins Company, 1973, pp. 9–59.

Emergency Handbook for Rating Trauma. Nutley, N. J.: Roche Laboratories, Division of Hoffmann-LaRoche, Inc., 1973.

General References

Axelrod, J. "Noradrenaline: Fate and Control of Its Bio-Synthesis." *Science,* **173** (Aug. 13, 1971), 598–606.

Berkowitz, L. "The Case for Bottling Up Rage." *Psychol. Today,* **7** (July 1973), 24–31.

Brobeck, J. R., ed. *Best & Taylor's Physiological Basis of Medical Practice,* 9th ed. Baltimore: The Williams and Wilkins Company, 1973.

Busse, E. W. "Biologic and Sociologic Changes Affecting Adaptation in Mid and Late Life." *Ann. Intern. Med.,* **75** (July 1970), 115–20.

Di Cara, L. V. "Learning in the Autonomic Nervous System." *Sci. Am.,* **222** (Jan. 1970), 30–39.

Evarts, E. V. "Brain Mechanisms in Movement." *Sci. Am.,* **229** (July 1973), 96–103.

Frohlich, E. D., ed. *Pathophysiology: Altered Regulatory*

Mechanisms in Disease. Philadelphia: J. B. Lippincott Company, 1972.

Gentry, W. D., Musante, G. J., and Haney, T. "Anxiety and Urinary Sodium/Potassium as Stress Indicators on Admission to a Coronary-Care Unit." *Heart & Lung,* **2** (Nov.–Dec. 1973), 875–77.

Levine, S. "Stress and Behavior." *Sci. Am.,* **224** (Jan. 1971), 26–31.

Putt, A. M. "A Biofeedback Service by Nurses." *Am. J. Nurs.,* **79** (Jan. 1979), 88–89.

Selye, H. *Stress.* Montreal, Can.: Acta Inc., Medical Publishers, 1950.

Selye, H. *The Story of the Adaptation Syndrome.* Montreal, Can.: Acta Inc., Medical Publishers, 1952.

Selye, H. *The Stress of Life.* New York: McGraw-Hill Book Company, 1956.

Stephenson, C. A. "Stress in Critically Ill Patients." *Am. J. Nurs.,* **77** (Nov. 1977), 1806–09.

Sutterley, D. C., and Donnelly, G. F., eds. "Stress Management." *Topics in Clin. Nurs.,* **1**:1 (April 1979).

Wynn, V. "The Anabolic Steroids." *Practitioner,* **200** (April 1968), 509–18.

"Two Emergency Indexes to Tell Who Will Live." *Med. World News,* **14** (16 Nov. 1973), 89.

Wagner, M. M., ed. "Symposium on Emergency Nursing." *Nurs. Clin. North Am.,* **8** (Sept. 1973), 375–466.

White, K. M. "Evaluating the Trauma of Gunshot Wounds." *Am. J. Nurs.,* **77** (Oct. 1977), 1589–93.

23

Metabolic Responses

The concept that there is an integrated endocrine-metabolic sequence in convalescence, and one of survival value to the organism, places convalescence among those adaptive endocrine-metabolic sequences (of which pregnancy is another example) in which certain normal functions are compromised to achieve a specific survival objective.

FRANCIS D. MOORE

Francis D. Moore. *Metabolic Care of the Surgical Patient*, Philadelphia: W. B. Saunders Company, 1964, p. 27.

Role of Metabolic Processes in Response to Injury

In addition to muscular and visceral responses in illness that are largely regulated by the nervous system, there are also metabolic reactions to tissue injury. Even in these responses, the nervous system may participate in their initiation and regulation. Whereas muscular and visceral responses enable the organism to fight or flee its enemy, the metabolic responses have three objectives. They are (1) to maintain the stability of the organism during stress, (2) to repair damaged tissues, and (3) to restore the body to normal composition and activity. The care of the individual should therefore be planned to assist him or her in achieving these objectives.

Four Phases of Metabolic Response to Injury

The work of Moore (1959) and Selye (1946) are classic in metabolic responses to injury. Despite differences in terminology and emphasis, there are similarities between their findings.

Though there is overlapping between the various phases, Moore (1959) describes convalescence as taking place in four phases.

Phase I. Initial reaction to injury, lasts 2 to 4 days. The first phase serves three purposes: (1) the release of amino acids and electrolytes into the extracellular fluid, (2) maintenance of the extracellular fluid volume, and (3) conversion of body fat as sources of energy. During the first phase there is rapid catabolism of lean tissue and fat. For about 6 to 24 hours after major surgery or a severe injury, water and sodium chloride are retained in the body. Until the patient is eliminating water and salt at a normal rate, overloading is possible. The danger of overloading is greatest among patients with heart disease or who are elderly. In the period immediately following major surgery or injury, careful attention should be paid to the rate at which solutions are introduced intravenously, to the type of solution, and to the relation of intake to output. Nitrogen, potassium, and phosphates are lost in the urine. Clinically the patient is characterized by all the reactions to an acute injury. Hemorrhage, pain, and fear augment the reaction. The patient has tachycardia and a slight fever which persist for 2 or 3 days. Unless the patient is storing water, he or she loses weight as the result of tissue catabolism.

The changes in nitrogen metabolism that are a part of the stress response have been extensively studied. As a result of this response, lean tissues undergo catabolism and large amounts of nitrogen and potassium are lost in the urine. The catabolic response cannot be reversed and may be intensified by forced feeding. It can also be induced by the administration of cortisone or hydrocortisone.

In nondiabetic persons who have a healthy liver, marked changes in glucose metabolism are not usually evident during stress, whereas the person who is diabetic usually has an elevation in blood glucose unless measures are taken to prevent it. The adrenocortical hormones and insulin are physiologic antagonists. During stress the tolerance of the diabetic person for glucose is lessened. For a period following surgery, the diabetic patient requires more insulin than at other times. Following injury, considerable amounts of fats may be utilized as fuel. In patients who have diabetes mellitus, regular checking of the urine for glucose and acetone is therefore important.

In the first phase of the metabolic response to injury, the outpouring of adrenal steroids brings a marked suppression of many facets of the immunologic defense mechanism, producing a severe impairment in the ability of the patient to combat infection (Munster, 1973). When acute tubular necrosis of the kidney develops, there is suppression of both antibody production and cell-mediated lymphocyte function. In the lungs, both shock and overhydration affect the ability of pulmonary macrophages to deal with bacteria that have penetrated beyond the bronchial mucociliary barrier, thus predisposing to the very great threat of pneumonia. Reduction of portal blood flow has an adverse effect on the ability of the reticuloendothelial cells of the liver to remove such products as bacterial endotoxins.

Phase II. The turning point begins about the fourth day and continues for 2 or 3 days. Catabolism of tissue substance decreases, and preparations are made for anabolism. Clinically the patient appears improved. Appetite and spontaneous activity increase. He or she begins to be a bit less self-centered and more interested in the affairs of others, showing some concern for spouse, roommate, or the patient down the hall.

Phase III. Anabolic phase, characterized by protein synthesis, lasts 2 to 5 weeks. Anabolism begins 7 to 10 days after an extensive injury, to restore lean tissue to the person who has been injured. This phase involves the reconstruction of the lean tissues lost during the catabolic phase of illness. During this period, the person requires a generous dietary intake, and if it is not received, convalescence will be retarded as the patient will fail to gain the necessary weight, strength, and vigor. Wound healing continues normally, despite postoperative starvation (Perry, 1979). Progress through phase III depends, however, on an adequate intake of calories and protein. Unless adequate calories and protein are available during this period, the recovery of the patient may be seriously delayed. A patient may require between 2,000 and 3,000 calories per day. Progress means not only that wound healing occurs normally, but that the patient gains weight and strength. Attention must be paid to the food intake of patients following surgical treatment, severe trauma, burns, and severe infections. The glass of milk in the refrigerator for a between-meal or evening snack is important and contributes to recovery provided it is consumed by the patient. Further, because many surgical patients are discharged some time between the seventh and tenth days, attention should be given to preparing them so that they understand the importance of eating sufficient amounts and variety of food. Eating may not be a serious problem for those whose appetite is good, but in the elderly or chronically ill, a real effort may be required to assure adequate food intake. In the patient who has been seriously burned, losses of protein during phase I may have been very great. Infection of the burned areas may have aggravated that loss. For example, despite the fact that Mr. All ate quite well, his food intake was augmented by tube feeding to the point where his gastrointestinal tract was unable to tolerate food. Despite heroic efforts to maintain his caloric and protein intake, he lost 20 pounds during the first few weeks of his illness.

Phase IV. *Fat gain phase,* the final adjustment, lasts for several weeks or months. During this final phase, there is a return to full body weight and function. Fat deposits are restored, and the patient returns to work. During this phase the appetite of the patient may be very good. When the desired weight is reached, the patient may have to consciously limit food intake in order to prevent an excessive gain in weight.

Many of the extensive studies of metabolic responses of human beings to injury have been made on young men undergoing a surgical procedure, but some studies have been made on individuals who have suffered fractures or burns. There is no reason to suppose that patients who are seriously ill with nonsurgical diseases do not also have a metabolic reaction. Response to injury is believed to be universal, and many, though not all, authorities believe it to be homeostatic.

Knowledge of the systemic response to injury, disease, or surgical therapy is essential to determining the requirements of patients who have suffered injury or acute disease. Unless the reactions of the patient are understood, treatment may interfere with rather than support the responses that promote recovery.

Conditions Associated with the Intensity of a Metabolic Response

The intensity of a metabolic reaction varies with a number of conditions. For example, the catabolic response is greatest in well-nourished young males. A less intense response occurs in females, the elderly, and the poorly nourished of either sex. The degree and type of trauma also influence the reaction. Minor trauma induces a less intense response than major trauma. Following minor trauma, phase I is shorter. Phase II is scarcely noticeable, and the other two phases are passed through quickly. Burns and bone injury elicit a more vigorous response than can be predicted on the basis of the degree of injury. Extensive injury to soft tissues, including extensive surgery, also adds to the severity of the reaction. Infection is a potent activator of the metabolic response. Fever may also be a factor. There is evidence that a marked and prolonged metabolic response to injury predisposes to the development of decubiti. Among the seriously injured, tissue breakdown may occur in a matter of hours. Care that can ordinarily be counted on to prevent the development of decubiti may be ineffective. Under these circumstances they result not so much from neglect as from the vigor of the metabolic response of the patient. Because seriously injured patients are predisposed to decubiti, protective measures should be instituted immediately. Because tissue breakdown can be far advanced before external evidence such as reddening of the skin occurs, preventive care should not be delayed until signs appear (see Chapter 49).

The Nurse's Role in Helping the Person with a Metabolic Response

The metabolic response to injury can be intensified by apprehension and pain and by other factors such as chilling, fever, and infection. The nurse has a responsibility to provide an emotional and physical environment that reduces undesirable stimuli to a minimum. The nurse can help to support or appropriately modify the magnitude of the metabolic response and its attendant effects by

1. Observing for signs and symptoms of metabolic response, especially for evidence of adequate oxygenation and of water, electrolyte, and nitrogen balance
2. Minimizing circumstances which intensify the metabolic response, such as pain, apprehension, fatigue, chilling or fever, and infection
3. Protecting against overexertion, particularly in phases II and III

Bases of Nursing Management

Preoperative preparation of the patient for what to expect after operation, prompt relief of pain, gentleness in handling the patient, a quiet, nonstimulating environment, realistic expectations for and acceptance of the behavior of the patient—all should reduce the strain on the patient. The patient should be protected from too many stimuli from well-meaning friends and relatives, who stay too long or talk too much, who are too boisterous, or who come in too large numbers. The writer has seen patients newly operated on and seriously ill exhausted by too many visitors or by those who remained too long. Conversely, a relative or friend whose presence comforts or quiets the patient should have an opportunity to visit the patient or be encouraged to remain. When the necessity arises to lessen the number of visitors or the length of time that they stay, the interpretation should be in terms of the needs of the patient. The feelings of the visitor should be respected. The nurse may need to take initiative and use ingenuity in accomplishing the reduction in the number of visitors. When necessary, something can be arranged to do to or for the patient that requires the visitors to leave. The nurse may suggest to the visitors that cards and letters are greatly enjoyed. However, the regulation of visiting should be based on the needs and condition of the patient.

Occasionally the problem of no visitors to a patient arises. The patient may be far from home or have no surviving relatives or friends. Visits from the doctors and nurses are then especially welcome. If a volunteer service worker is available, she or he may be utilized to meet needs of the patient that are ordinarily met by the family. In addition to visiting the patient the worker may write letters for the patient, read, shop for minor necessities, and the like. Of course, what the volunteer does should be adapted to the requirements of the patient. A friendly and sympathetic person who sits quietly by the seriously ill patient's bed may make a significant contribution.

As a result of severe injury, major surgery, or serious illness, the person undergoes a variety of responses that are integrated by the neuroendocrine system. Among the changes are a series of metabolic responses by which the organism provides the materials for repair and restores itself to normal. These changes have been studied more extensively in animals and in patients who have been treated surgically than in patients with acute or chronic disease. The metabolic changes are characterized by a series of catabolic and anabolic changes that proceed through overlapping phases.

Apprehension, pain, and other circumstances associated with operative procedures intensify the response to injury. Through the intelligent practice of nursing, the emotional and physical climate of the patient can be controlled so that harmful stimuli are minimized. The nurse should give attention to those observations indicating the state of the water and electrolyte balance. As soon as patients are able to eat, food intake should be noted and attention given to those patients who eat poorly. Patients who suffered wasting diseases before surgical treatment require special attention to improve their nutritional status. Intelligent application of the knowledge of the changes taking place after injury can shorten the convalescence of the patient.

Just what initiates or ends the metabolic responses is not known at the present time. The metabolic changes following surgery or injury are assumed to be the result of homeostatic mechanisms that function to maintain the circulating fluid volume so that tissues may be supplied with nutrients and oxygen. The catabolic changes liberate both water and materials from which energy may be obtained to maintain body processes. The changes occurring in the later phases of the response to injury restore the body to preinjury condition.

Assistance with Locomotion

During each of the first three phases of response to injury, all patients require some assistance with locomotion. The need may range from total dependence on the nurse, as in the unconscious, paralyzed, or critically ill patient, to a need for minimal assistance with getting out of bed or ambulating. To meet the locomotion needs of patients, the nurse must use safe and effective body mechanics. Proper use of the body requires that the nurse remain physically fit and wear clothing that allows ease and comfort when one assumes correct work positions. Millen (1970) proposes that the following positions can be modified for use in all nursing techniques:

1. Broad base—feet apart, one foot forward for balance
2. Flex knees—flex hips
3. Keep back as straight as possible
4. Tighten abdominal and gluteal muscles
5. Set powerful leg muscles to
   a. *Push* (raising patient from bed, lifting object from floor, and so on)
   b. *Resist* (downward thrust of weight of patient being lowered to a chair, for example)

Selye's Theory of How the Body Responds to Injury

Selye proposes that the responses of the tissues during injury are the result of the reaction of sensitive tissues to an increase in secretions of the adrenopituitary axis. Much of the data on which this theory is based has been obtained by subjecting rats to varying types of physical, chemical, and psychological injury. From these studies, Selye postulated that no matter what agent was used to cause injury, certain nonspecific stereotyped reactions occur in the stressed organism. Like Cannon (1939), Selye believes that homeostatic responses may cause disturbances in the internal environment. He also postulates that certain diseases may result from prolonged overactivity of homeostatic mechanisms. These he calls the diseases of adaptation. He includes among the diseases of adaptation the collagen fiber diseases and degenerative vascular diseases (Selye, 1946, p. 127).

A decrease in "disease of adaptation" may be possible as a result of "learning" to control the autonomic nervous system through mastery of the "meditative state" as achieved by Yogis and other Far Eastern mystics. This dampening of nonproductive, inappropriate stress response in a technological age may be adaptive for coping with vicissitudes of the environment. Investigations in the 1950s and 1960s of the physiologic effects of meditation revealed as much as a 20 per cent reduction in metabolic rate; a predominance of alpha waves on electroencephalogram; increased skin resistance to electrical current consistent with low levels of anxiety; increased dilatation of peripheral blood vessels resulting from a decrease in production of norepinephrine; decreased serum lactate; and decreased heart rate (Wallace & Benson, 1972). The pattern of changes suggest that meditation generates an integrated response, or reflex, mediated by the CNS—a *hypo* metabolic counterpart to Cannon's "fight-or-flight."

The General Adaptation Syndrome

According to Selye (1946, pp. 119–20), increased endocrine secretion, particularly from the adrenopituitary axis, is responsible for the response of the organism to injury. This response may be general or local or both. In either instance it is nonspecific, because it may be elicited by any agent causing injury. The general response that Selye calls the "adaptation syndrome" takes place in three stages: (1) the alarm reaction, (2) the stage of resistance, and (3) the stage of exhaustion. The alarm reaction consists of two phases: (a) shock and (b) countershock. During the stage of shock and countershock the organism undergoes catabolic and other changes that result from the effects of the injury and response of the body to it. The "alarm reaction" as described by Selye is similar to phases I and II of the metabolic responses to injury as described by Moore. During countershock the organism is restored to its preinjury condition. In the stage of resistance the organism is adapted to the injuring agent. It can tolerate greater exposure to the injuring agent than can the nonadapted organism. Eventually, if the stress is continued, the animal loses its adaptation and goes into the stage of exhaustion. The stage of exhaustion is comparable to the shock of the earlier period.

Selye (1973) has more recently proposed the concept of *heterostasis,* to describe the unusual defense reactions which are mobilized in response to drug therapy to permit resistance to unusual aggression. The salient feature of heterostasis is not that substances foreign to the body are attacked, but that a new equilibrium between the body and an unusually high level of a potentially injurious agent is established. Heterostatic substances operate either by destroying the excess of the injuring agent (catatoxic action) or by making tissues tolerant to it (syntoxic action).

Whether or not the animal goes through all phases of the adaptation syndrome depends on its capacity to react as well as on the intensity and continuance of the injuring agent. Usually, when an injury is limited to a single insult and is within the adaptive capacity of the individual, recovery is complete. But any injury may be so severe that the vital processes of an individual are depressed to such an extent that death occurs immediately. Or the individual may die because his or her adaptive capacity is inadequate to cope with the injury. In contrast the individual may add to the damage by overreacting.

Fat embolism following multiple injuries may be an example of damaging consequences of the stress response. Some authorities believe that in addition to the release of fat from the marrow of fractured bones, the release of catecholamines that accompanies the stress response may mobilize fatty acids, altering the emulsion of fats in the blood stream. Symptoms of fat embolism usually appear within 24 to 72 hours following injury. The nurse should observe closely for and immediately report any sudden signs of tissue hypoxia; cyanosis (or slate-gray color, in the black patient); dyspnea or tachypnea; fever; change from alertness to confusion and/or agitation; changes in EKG tracings; and especially the appearance of the rash that typically distributes on the anterior chest, axilla, and soft palate mucosa and in the conjunctiva. Because shock is often a concurrent complication, the nurse can help prevent hypovolemia by closely watching fluid output and carefully maintaining fluid balance with prescribed fluids (del Bueno, 1973).

Selye believes that adrenocortical hormones not only affect the general responses of the organism but also modify the local response of tissue to injury. Further, the type of change in the tissues depends on whether the mineralocorticoids (aldosterone) or the glucocorticoids (cortisone) predominate. According to Selye, the mineralocorticoids are prophlogistic; that is, they stimulate the connective tissue to proliferate and enhance its inflammatory potential. In contrast, the glucocorticoids are anti-inflammatory or antiphlogistic. They inhibit proliferation of connective tissue and suppress the inflammatory process with the result that there is a reduction in the quantity of scar tissue formed in repair. Thus they may be prescribed in the treatment of rheumatic fever, rheumatoid arthritis, and other disorders in which an excessive or prolonged inflammatory response may lead to crippling scarring. Selye is of the opinion that the growth hormone from the anterior pituitary sensitizes the tissue to the mineralocorticoids. Other investigators do not agree that the changes in metabolism following tissue injury are caused solely by the action of the adrenocortical hormones.

Although the mechanisms of action of the adrenocortical hormones in response to injury are not known, these hormones are essential to the general response. Furthermore, cortisol and its analogues are used therapeutically to modify the local reaction of certain tissues to injury. (See Figure 23-1 for a diagram summarizing body responses to stress.)

Disorders of adaptation may occur at any phase of the "adaptation syndrome." As examples, rheumatic fever and rheumatoid arthritis occur during the catabolic phase. In other disorders the patient fails to progress into the anabolic phase. Patients in whom failure is most likely to occur are those with chronic debilitating conditions such as starvation, se-

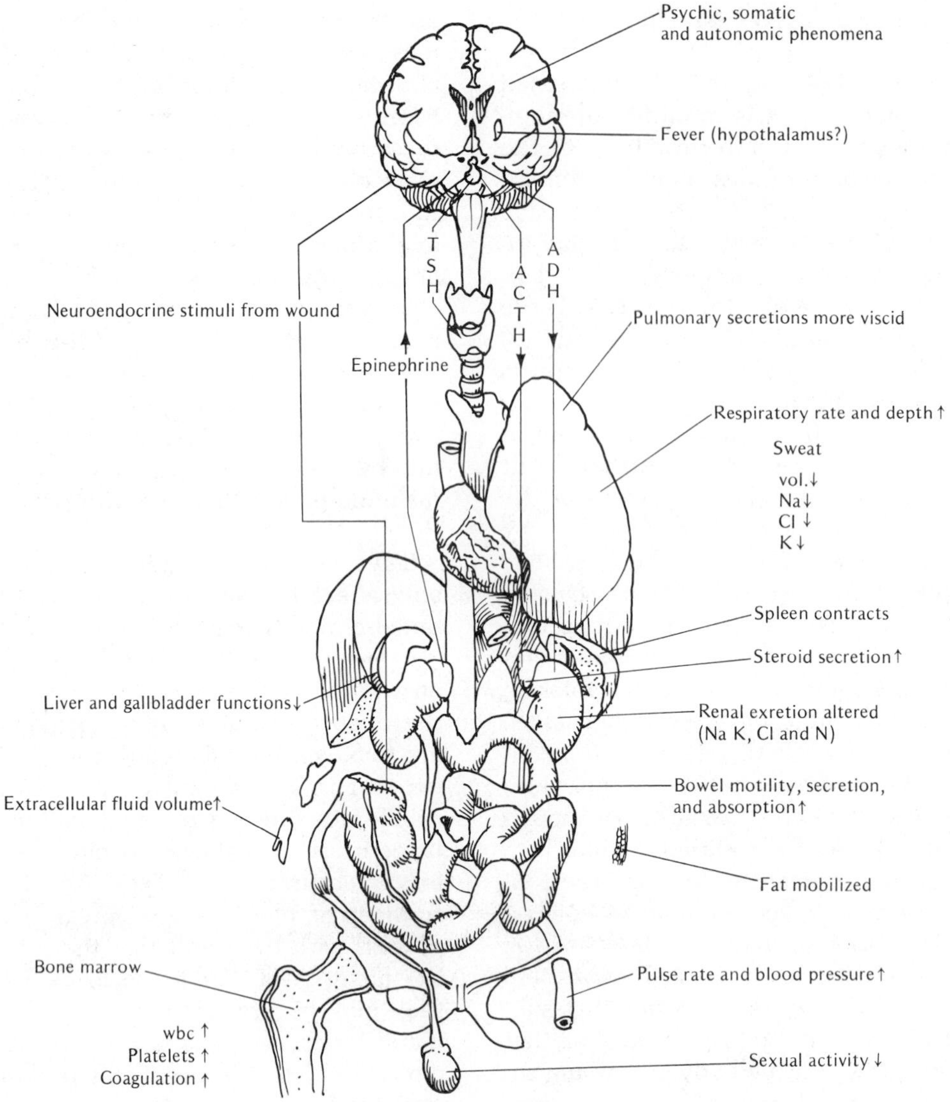

Figure 23-1. Reaction to stress. The first phase of surgical convalescence. Each system in the body participates in the total response to the stress of surgery, injury, or disease. Variations in response depend on the extent of surgery or injury and the severity of disease as well as the status of the patient prior to surgery or illness. In terms of metabolic responses, the chronically ill patient reacts to a lesser degree than does the previously well individual. Coordination of reactions to stress depends on the integrating roles of the nervous, circulatory, and endocrine systems. [After Hardy, courtesy of *Therapeutic Notes,* 67:203 (July–Aug.) 1960.]

vere burns, large draining wounds, hyperthyroidism, Cushing's syndrome, and many others.

References Cited

Cannon, W. B. *The Wisdom of the Body.* New York: W. W. Norton & Company, Inc., 1939, p. 22.

del Bueno, D. J. "Recognizing Fat Embolism in Patients with Multiple Injuries." *RN,* **36** (Jan. 1973), 48–55.

Millen, H. M. "Physically Fit for Nursing." *Am. J. Nurs.,* **70** (March 1970), 520–23.

Moore, F. D. *Metabolic Care of the Surgical Patient.* Philadelphia: W. B. Saunders Company, 1959, pp. 27–28.

Munster, A. M. "The Immunology of Injury." *Surg. Gynecol. Obstet.,* **137** (Oct. 1973), 666.

Perry, M. O. "Metabolic Response to Trauma." In *Principles of Surgery,* 3rd ed. Ed. by S. I. Schwartz et al. New York: McGraw-Hill Book Company, 1979, pp. 223–26.

Selye, H. "The General Adaptation Syndrome and the Diseases of Adaptation." *J. Clin. Endocrinol. Metab.,* **6** (Feb. 1946), 117–230.

Selye, H. "Homeostasis and Heterostasis." *Perspect. Biol. Med.,* **16** (1973), 441.

Wallace, R. K., and Benson, H. "The Physiology of Meditation." *Sci. Am.,* **226** (Feb. 1972), 84–90.

General References

Browse, N. L. *The Physiology and Pathology of Bed Rest.* Springfield, Ill.: Charles C Thomas, Publisher, 1965.

Busse, E. W. "Biologic and Sociologic Changes Affecting Adaptation in Mid and Late Life." *Ann. Intern. Med.,* **75** (July 1970), 115–20.

Frohlich, E. D., ed. *Pathophysiology: Altered Regulatory Mechanisms in Disease.* Philadelphia: J. B. Lippincott Company, 1972.

Hutchin, P. "Metabolic Response to Surgery." *Curr. Probl. in Surg.,* (April 1971).

Kaliner, M. A. "Extravascular Albumin." *N. Engl. J. Med.,* **301** (30 Aug. 1979), 497–99.

Pastan, I. "Cyclic AMP." *Sci. Am.,* **227** (Aug. 1972), 97–105.

Selye, H. *Stress.* Montreal, Can.: Acta Inc., Medical Publishers, 1950.

Selye, H. *The Story of the Adaptation Syndrome.* Montreal, Can.: Acta Inc., Medical Publishers, 1952.

Selye, H. *The Stress of Life.* New York: McGraw-Hill Book Company, 1956.

24

Immunologic Responses

A clue to rheumatoid arthritis

Rheumatoid arthritis is probably the most devastating of all forms of arthritis, causing excruciatingly painful joint inflammation, systemic disease and perhaps even death. Evidence to date suggests that rheumatoid arthritis is an autoimmune disease—that immune cells in the body (B cells) make antibodies that mistakenly attack the body's own tissues. The reason that B cells make autoantibodies may now have been found by Marius Teodorescu of the University of Illinois Medical Center in Chicago.

SCIENCE NEWS
Biomedicine: *Science News* 117:105 (Feb. 16) 1980.

Immunity

Whereas many of the responses to injury are nonspecific, most individuals also have, or are able to develop, resistance to specific microorganisms. The term *immunity* signifies a characteristic of the host that confers resistance to a specific agent. This characteristic is based on the ability of cells to distinguish "self" from "nonself" and to elaborate a specific agent that acts against foreign substances. The ability to recognize and to respond to foreign agents is certainly adaptive. It has contributed to survival of the species. Understandably enough, the first observations involving immune responses were made in relation to infectious diseases. Very early humans noted that after persons experienced and recovered from certain diseases they never had them again. Instances are reported in which material was taken from a smallpox lesion and inoculated into a susceptible host with the hope that he or she would have a mild case of the disease. In 1798 Jenner reported that persons inoculated with material from a cowpox lesion could be effectively protected from smallpox. Later workers in the field such as Pasteur, Koch, Metchnikoff, and Ehrlich added to the knowledge of immunity. From the time of Pasteur to the present, considerable effort has been devoted to developing vaccines against specific diseases. As emphasized in Chapter 10, a number of deadly and/or crippling diseases can now be prevented by vaccines and other immunizing agents.

Schwartz (1969) summarizes the developments in the field of immunology in the following:

> The control of disease by immunological means began in 1796, when Edward Jenner inoculated James Phipps with cowpox. Immunologic prophylaxis still flourishes, and the discovery that passive immunization prevents erythroblastosis is its latest triumph. Early in this century Clemens von Pirquet initiated another branch of immunology by establishing the principle that antibodies can be injurious. The central issues of clinical immunology, formulated in terms of these momentous discoveries, are the production of desired immunity and the elimination of undesired immune reactions. . . .

Recent developments stimulating the study of immunity include (1) the recognition of immunologic deficiency and its effects, (2) the overproduction of certain gamma globulins and of abnormal immunoglobulins (as an example, an abnormal protein is produced in myeloma, a malignant disorder of plasma cells), (3) the concept of autoimmune disease, and (4) the immunologic interference with organ transplants. Electron microscopy, fluorescent antibody techniques, immunoassay, and radioimmunoassay have made a considerable contribution to the understanding of the biochemical and physiologic aspects of immunity and immunopathology.

As knowledge of the immune response has increased, the field has been greatly expanded. It is now known that some of the responses involve many structures: the phagocytic system, the thymus, the lymphocytes, and the plasma cells and their secretory products, the immunoglobulins. Further, the immune response is not limited to microbes and homografts but can be elicited by a vast number and variety of agents. Similar to other body responses, immunologic responses may be appropriate in kind and degree. They may also be inadequate (hypo), excessive (hyper), or inappropriate to the stimulus.

Definitions

The following discussion of immunity will be facilitated by definition of some of the terms used.

Immunity. The state of being able to resist and/or overcome harmful agents or influences.
Active: Immunity acquired as a result of experience with an organism (usually specific and due to antibodies); also innate.
Passive: Immunity due to acquisition of maternal antibody or injection of antibody.
Adoptive: Immunity produced by the acquisition of immune lymphoid cells (DiSaia et al., 1975).

Immunology. The study of the immune response.

Immunogen. An antigen that incites specific immunity (DiSaia et al., 1975).

Adjuvant. A substance that when mixed with an antigen enhances its antigenicity (DiSaia et al., 1975).

Mitogen. A substance that stimulates mitosis and lymphocyte transformation; it may be associated with streptococci and some strains of staphylococci, as well as with protein of plant or animal sources.

Antigen (Ag). A substance that may be one of a variety of large molecules, many of them protein in nature, such as a part of a virus, bacterium, a foreign tissue cell, a fragment of a foreign tissue cell, or a polysaccharide. Lipids and nucleic acids are capable of becoming antigens after they combine with protein. With the exception of the erythrocytes and tissues sequestered from the blood stream, such as parts of the brain, the thyroid gland, and the lens of the eye, antigens stimulating the formation of antibodies are usually derived from other species or individuals. Antigen can react specifically with antibodies and under appropriate conditions can incite an individual to form specific antibodies.
Extrinsic: An antigen that is not a constituent of the cell.
Intrinsic: An antigen that is a constituent of the cell.
Occult: A self-antigen that does not reach antibody-forming tissues (DiSaia et al., 1975).

Isoantigen (alloantigen). An antigen that incites the formation of antibodies in genetically dissimilar members of the same species (DiSaia et al., 1975).

Hapten. An incomplete antigen. It requires another substance to become antigenic. It reacts with an antibody but does not by itself stimulate antibody formation.

Antibody (Ab). A humoral protein (commonly, if not always, a gamma globulin) that can be incited by an antigen or by a hapten combined with a carrier and that reacts specifically with the antigen or hapten. Some antibodies occur naturally without known antigen stimulation. Antibody can be detected by its ability to combine with an antigen. It is responsible for the recognition of foreign molecules or antigens (Edelman, 1973).

Isoantibody (alloantibody). An antibody produced by one individual that reacts specifically with an antigen present in another individual of the same species. The term *isoantibody* is commonly used in blood work and *alloantibody* in tissue transplantation work (DiSaia et al., 1975).

Immunoglobulins (Ig). Classes of globulins to which antibodies belong (DiSaia et al., 1975).

Histocompability. The degree to which cellular antigens are alike in two individuals of the same species. Histocompatibility is genetically determined. Histocompatibility Ags = transplantation Ags = HLA Ags.

Autograft (self-graft). Tissue transplanted from one part of the body to another. The tissue is accepted.

Isograft. Tissue transplanted from a donor of a highly inbred strain to a recipient of the same strain. Donor and recipient are genetically identical or nearly identical. The tissue is usually accepted.

Homograft (allograft). Tissue transplanted from one member of the same species to another (noninbred), as from one human to another. In the absence of immunosuppressive therapy, the tissue is rejected.

Heterograft (xenograft). Tissue transplanted from one species to another (e.g., goat to sheep). It is always rejected.

Normergy. A normal tissue response to a given substance.

Hypoergy. A deficient tissue response to a given substance.

Hyperergy. An exaggerated tissue response. In allergy the tissues hyperreact.

Allergen A substance (antigen or hapten) that incites hypersensitivity or allergy.

Allergy. A state of specific increased reactivity of tissues to repeated contacts with an antigen or hapten such as occurs in hay fever. The term is most commonly used to designate states of delayed sensitivity due to contact allergens and immediate sensitivities due to Prausnitz-Küstner antibodies (DiSaia et al., 1975).

Hypersensitivity. (used interchangeably with *allergy*). Delayed-type hypersensitivity is one in which the reaction is delayed for several hours and may last for days. The delayed type is mediated by immunologically competent cells. Immediate-type hypersensitivity is a wheal and flare reaction that begins immediately on contact with the allergen and disappears promptly. The immediate type is mediated by humoral antibodies.

Reagin (homocytotropic antibody). A skin-sensitizing antibody occurring in the skin of some persons who are allergic. These individuals have the immediate type of hypersensitivity. Reaction is characterized by a wheal and flare response about 20 minutes after the intradermal injection of antigen. IgE is important in forming reagin.

Atopy. An allergic disease of the wheal and erythema type in which there is usually a family history of allergic disease.

Bradykinin. A potent vasodilator that is released from the alpha-2-globulin fraction of the blood by proteolytic enzymes.

Histamine. A powerful vasodilator. Experimentally it has been demonstrated to produce asthmalike symptoms. It is a powerful stimulator of secretion of hydrochloric acid. It is found in mammalian tissues, especially mast cells. The breakdown of mast cells leads to liberation of histamine and serotonin.

Serotonin. A powerful smooth-muscle stimulator and vasoconstrictor. Serotonin is formed in the argentaffin cells of the gastrointestinal tract and is transported by the blood platelets. It is found in the brain and many other tissues.

Complement. A complex group of serum proteins, but not antibodies, which are responsible for immunologically-induced cell lysis (Edelman, 1973, p. 833). Complement acts to (1) increase capillary permeability, (2) cause neutrophil chemotaxis, (3) cause immune adherence of antigen–antibody complexes, (4) promote phagocytosis, and (5) cause damage to membranes of mammalian cells, bacteria, and viruses and possibly to basement membranes (Stroud, 1967).

Tolerance. A state in which the immunologic system does not react to a substance. Normally, an individual is tolerant of his or her own tissues.

Autoimmune disease. Any situation in which the autoimmune response, humoral or cellular, is responsible for tissue injury. The autoimmune response is represented by the appearance of antibodies in the human directed against self. These autoantibodies may reflect a normal response to tissue antigens which are separated anatomically from the immune system during fetal development and appear later as a consequence of tissue breakdown. Autoantibodies also may arise following abrogation of tolerance in a normal immune system by an exogenous antigen cross-reacting with self or because an abnormal immune system has lost the capacity to distinguish self. Autoantibodies do not necessarily indicate an autoimmune disease (Austen, 1977).

Structure and Function of the Immunologic System

There are some interesting parallels between the immune and nervous systems. They are unique among the organs of the body in their ability to respond adequately to an enormous variety of signals; both have cells that can both receive and transmit signals, and the signals can be either excitatory or inhibitory; both systems penetrate most other tissues, but seem to avoid each other;[1] and both systems "learn" from experience and build up a memory that is sustained by reinforcement but cannot be transmited to the next generation (Jerne, 1973).

The lymphocyte is the cell that stands at the center of the immune response. The essential initial step in the immune response is the contact of an antigen with receptors on the surface of lymphocytes derived from bone marrow (B-lymphocytes). This contact may be altered by interaction of the antigen with the macrophages or with lymphocytes derived from the thymus gland (T-lymphocytes). The contact alters the expression of the B-lymphocytes' genes, setting in motion a series of events, during which the cells divide and differentiate. The cell type evolves from one that is specialized to respond to an event in its environment to one that is uniquely adapted to the synthesis and secretion of antibody molecules (Lerner & Dixon, 1973). Children born without a thymus gland have normal amounts of im-

[1] The "blood–brain barrier" prevents lymphocytes from coming in contact with nerve cells.

munoglobulins, but they do not show hypersensitivity responses to various antigens. They either accept skin grafts from unrelated donors or reject them after a long delay.

The humoral system involves the immunoglobulins or circulating antibodies in the blood. Some authorities refer to this system as the gut-associated lymphoid-tissue system. The structures that may function in this way are the appendix and Peyer's patches. Others are not certain about the location of the tissue that plays a role similar to that of the thymus. These immunoglobulins are synthesized by fixed plasma cells in the lymph nodes and spleen and are secreted into the blood. Children with congenital agammaglobulinemia[2] lack plasma cells and humor antibodies, but they have normal cellular immunity (Science, 1969).

Both these systems are essential to combating a host of foreign substances, including not only microorganisms and homografts but a wide variety of other foreign agents.

In the words of Hall (1969), "in the absence of cell-mediated immune mechanisms the extravascular compartment, which means most of the body, has little in the way of an immunologically specific defense against bacteria and viruses in the early invasive stage of the disease process. For this reason, it seems proper to regard the evolution of cell-mediated immunity as an adaptive response to the major environmental threat, i.e., infectious disease." The rejection of homografts is, therefore, to be expected.

The thymus-dependent system reacts relatively quickly to microbes entering a tissue. Within 4 to 5 days after exposure, the lymphoid tissue produces large numbers of immunoblasts that pass into the affected tissue where they synthesize cellular antibodies. These antibodies help to limit the spread of infection from one cell to another. Immunoblasts may be of particular importance in the prevention of dissemination of virus and certain types of bacterial infection in tissues.

Hall (1969) discusses the relationship of cellular immunity to recovery from measles. Children with agammaglobulinemia recover from measles and develop immunity to them. In children treated with cortisone, the thymus-dependent system (cellular immunity) is eliminated. These children die from giant cell pneumonia and do not have a rash.

The thymus-independent system is slower acting and less accurate than the thymus-dependent system. It takes about 10 days after exposure to invasive organisms for humoral antibodies to reach peak levels in the blood. The lymphocyte in cellular ("T") and humoral ("B") immunity is illustrated in Figure 24-1.

The ability of tissues to react to antigenic agents by synthesizing antibodies and to distinguish between self and nonself has many applications in the field of medicine. On the positive side, the capacity of tissues to react to foreign substances by forming antibodies enables the individual to become immune to (protected against) a variety of infectious agents. On the negative side, it increases the hazards of blood transfusion, limits the extent to which tissues of one individual can be successfully transplanted to another, and is responsible for a number of diseases. As examples, because the body is able to form antibodies against the virus causing smallpox, immunity to smallpox can be developed. Before blood can

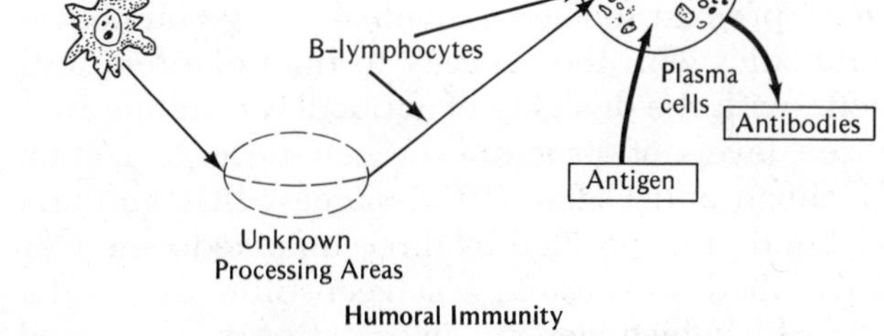

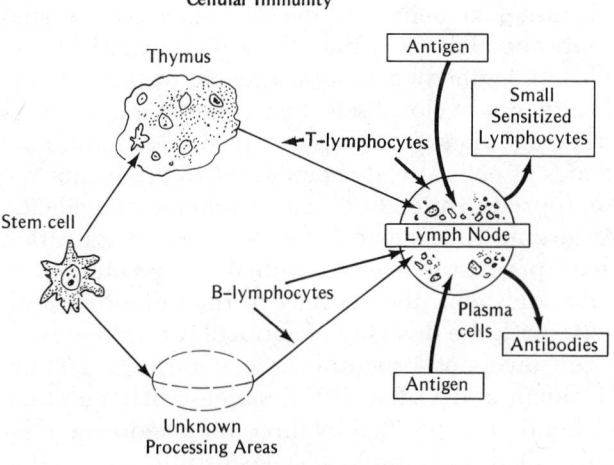

Figure 24-1. Formation of antibodies and sensitized lymphocytes by a lymph node in response to antigens. This figure also shows the origin of *thymic* ("T") and *bursal* ("B") lymphocytes that are responsible for the cellular and humoral immune processes of the lymph nodes. (Used with permission of the W. B. Saunders Company from *Textbook of Medical Physiology,* 5th ed., 1976, Fig. 7-1, p. 79, by Arthur C. Guyton.)

[2] Occasionally an individual is born who has congenital *agammaglobulinemia,* a disorder in which there is a failure in the synthesis of gamma globulin. It is probably caused by a defect in the formation of plasma cells. Agammaglobulinemia falls into three categories:

1. Primary congenital—sex-linked, recessive—male children
2. Primary acquired—no clear-cut hereditary basis and may appear in either sex at any time in life
3. Secondary—to neoplastic disease, e.g., Hodgkin's, other malignant lymphomas, multiple myeloma, and chronic lymphatic leukemia

Syndrome of primary agammaglobulinemia includes:

1. Recurrent pyogenic infections
2. Gastrointestinal symptoms (diarrhea; large, bulky, foul-smelling stools; and flat oral glucose tolerance curves)
3. Reticuloendothelial disorders
4. Arthritis and arthralgia

be safely transfused into an individual, the blood from the donor and the recipient must be matched to eliminate the possibility of the recipient's serum containing antibodies against the antigen in the donor's erythrocytes. Unless the donor is an identical twin or the recipient has agammaglobulinemia, or is treated with an immunosuppressive agent, the chances of tissue transplanted from one individual to another "taking" are negligible. The tissues of one individual are antigenic in another; that is, the tissues of the recipient recognize the transplanted tissue as "foreign" and form antibodies against it. This response is as normal as any response to a foreign antigen.

Immunoglobulins

The immunoglobulins are a heterogeneous group of plasma proteins with antibody activity. They vary in molecular weight from 140,000 to 1 million. Immunoglobulins (antibodies) are designated according to which one of the five types to which they belong; IgG, IgA, IgM, IgD and IgE. From the available evidence, antibodies appear to consist of two heavy (H) or long and two light (L) or short peptide chains joined by disulfide (—SS—) bonds. Immunoglobulins have two types of activity, antigenic and antibody. Their antigenic activity is used to distinguish one from the other. Both H and L chains probably contribute to the combining sites on the antibody molecule, but the H chain appears to have the most antibody activity. The L chain may contain the recognition site. The L chains are closely similar in all immunoglobulins, but the H chains serve to distinguish one class from the others (Gordon, 1974, pp. 34–48). Antibody activity is specific to the antigen. The theory of clonal selection suggests that molecular recognition of antigens occurs by selection among clones of cells already committed to producing the appropriate antibodies, each of different specificity. According to the clonal theory, it is necessary that there preexist in each individual a large number of antibodies with the capacity to bind different antigens, with the diversity of antibodies resulting from three levels of structural or genetic organization. Edelman and Galley (1973) suggest that immunoglobulins are specified by three unlinked gene clusters, called *translocons,* which constitute the mechanism by which genetic information is combined. According to this hypothesis the translocon is the basic unit of immunoglobulin evolution, different groups of immunoglobulin chains having arisen by duplication and various chromosomal rearrangements of a precursor gene cluster. Some authorities suggest that the first step in the formation of antibodies is the phagocytosis of antigen by the macrophages. They then transfer the information in a form of RNA or the antigen itself to the lymphocytes that synthesize antibodies. The fact that a mixture of leukocytes is more effective in antibody formation than lymphocytes alone supports this view.

Stages in the Development of Immunity

As previously emphasized, body structures and functions prevent many foreign agents from penetrating the body's surface. After a germ or other foreign substance gains access to the internal environment, the body is faced with three tasks: capture, recognition, and response (Janeway, 1968). *Capture,* which is *the first stage* of the specific response to bacteria, involves at least three processes: ingestion (phagocytosis), intracellular killing, and digestion of antigens. Although capture is the first stage of the specific response, it will be discussed later with phagocytosis.

The *second stage, recognition,* is poorly understood. After lymphocytes have contact with a foreign antigen, they are able to recognize it as being different from its host. This means that the lymphocyte has some means of distinguishing between host and foreign chemical configurations. On subsequent exposures to the antigen the lymphoid cells "remember" that they have had previous contact with a specific foreign agent. The latter is called *immunologic memory.* According to Janeway (1968), immunologic memory is clearly associated with the small lymphocyte. The second time the lymphocyte has contact with an antigen, it responds more quickly and to a greater degree than it did the first time.

Immunologists at the National Institute of Allergy and Infectious Diseases report that large doses of vitamin A given to experimental animals strongly stimulate the immune response, increasing the count of antibody-forming cells in the spleen to more than three times the level in untreated animals. In addition, vitamin A was found to prevent the well-known immunosuppression of conticosteroids. In patient care, vitamin A has been used successfully to reduce the incidence of stress ulcers among burned, traumatized, and postoperative patients (Vitamin A, 1973). (See Chapter 52 for more on etiology of stress ulcers.) *The third stage,* that is, *response,* will be considered later.

Allergy

Like other homeostatic mechanisms, the immunologic defense system can be a source of disease. Two abnormalities, agammaglobulinemia in which the individual is unable to form humoral antibodies against foreign materials and absence of the thymus, have been previously mentioned. Primary immune deficiency is a severe but, fortunately, rare problem. There are about twenty types, classified according to the part of immune function which is missing. Most immunodeficiencies are due to a deficit of antibodies, reflected in low immunoglobulin —G, —A, or —M levels. In about one fourth of patients, antibodies *and* cells are lacking (Stiehm, 1973). Many autoimmune diseases are far more common in the aged. Waning of immunologic responsiveness begins in early adult life, accelerating in old age. Immunologic inadequacies of the aged have been attributed to an intrinsic deficiency in the immunocompetent cell population (Gerber, 1973).

A far more frequent malady is allergy. The word *allergy* was introduced in 1907 by von Pirquet to describe altered reaction of tissues after repeated contact with microorganisms and antigenic agents such as foreign serums, tuberculin, and vaccine virus. Subsequently, the term *allergy* has come to include a large group of conditions in which the tissues or organs of a person respond on repeated contacts with a foreign material in a way that is different from the manner in which other members of the same species react. Allergy differs from beneficial immunologic reactions in that it does harm to body tissues. Crowle (1960) referred to allergy as an immunologic mistake. It is immunity gone wrong.

Although the preceding has been the classic view of allergy, allergic responses are now thought to be beneficial in supporting the host's responses to microbial antigens. As an example, granulocytes, macrophages, and serum proteins including antibodies and complement accumulate at the site of a localized allergic response to microbes. Some types of microbes, such as *Mycobacterium tuberculosis,* can multiply in "nonactivated" macrophages, whereas they are destroyed in "activated" ones. It is also possible that delayed-type reactions enhance antibody formation.

ANTIGENS

Antigens vary in their capacity to induce antibody formation from those that are seldom antigenic to those that almost always are. Horse serum induces hypersensitivity in a high percentage of instances on the first exposure to it. Poison ivy will eventually induce hypersensitivity, if exposure continues to be repeated. As indicated earlier, large molecules are more likely to be antigenic than small molecules. Chemically, antigens are usually proteins or polysaccharides, though they may be lipids or nucleic acids. According to one hypothesis, polysaccharides do not become antigenic until they attach themselves to a protein molecule. Lipids and nucleic acids must be attached to a protein molecule to be allergenic. A vast variety of substances are therefore potentially antigenic. Some of the more common ones are the plant pollens, animal danders, seafoods, berries, eggs, chocolate, and wheat. Foreign serums, tuberculin, and vaccine viruses as well as drugs such as penicillin, streptomycin sulfate, heavy metals, sulfonamides, iodides, and barbiturates are also common offenders. Antigens may be introduced in the body by injection, inhalation, ingestion, or contact with the skin.

Just as antigenic agents vary in potency, individuals vary in their capacity to become allergic or hypersensitive. Many of the common forms of allergy depend on a hereditary factor. What is inherited is not the allergic manifestation but the tendency to become allergic. For example, a parent has asthma; his or her child develops urticaria. Physical, chemical, and emotional factors also play a role in the development of allergy. They may be significant not only in inducing hypersensitivity but in prolonging a particular allergic response. Some persons appear to be hypersensitive to certain substances on their first contact with them. Others evidence great resistance to even common allergens. For example, some babies are unable to tolerate wheat or eggs from their first exposure to them. One theory advanced to explain this observation is that antigenic material is transferred from the mother to the fetus in utero.

In the more usual conception of allergy, the tissues most likely to become hypersensitive are those in contact with the external environment, that is, the skin and the respiratory and gastrointestinal tracts. Hall (1969) states that immunoblasts are commonly observed in the parenchyma of the alveoli and the interstitial tissue of the gut. When there is a high concentration of antibodies in the circulating blood, circulatory collapse may follow reexposure to the antigen. The tissues in which allergic responses are manifested are sometimes referred to as shock tissues. It is not known whether they have a greater tendency to become sensitized or whether they become sensitized because they have greater exposure to allergens.

Immunologic Disorders

Immunologic disorders can be classified in different ways, such as (1) the length of time elapsing between exposure to an antigen to which the individual has been sensitized and the development of an allergic response, and (2) according to the mechanism underlying the response. The first is the traditional classification: immediate and delayed response. The mechanisms for these two types of disorders are different. The immediate type is mediated by humoral antibodies, whereas the delayed type is mediated by immunologically competent cells. Further, the immediate type of hypersensitivity reactions may be either local or general. They may also be cytotropic (cell-stimulating) or cytolytic (cell-damaging) anaphylaxis.

Schwartz (1969) classifies harmful immunologic mechanisms as (1) anaphylaxis, (2) cytolysis, (3) injury by soluble antigen–antibody complexes, and (4) delayed hypersensitivity.

Immediate-Type Hypersensitivity: Cytotropic Type

It can be noted that the immediate type of hypersensitivity can be induced by several types of antigens. Either genetic plus environmental factors or previous sensitization with a foreign protein or drug predisposes to it. In those disorders in which genetic factors play a role, sensitivity is said to be natural and the resulting diseases are called atopic diseases. They include infantile eczema, which is often followed in later life by respiratory allergies; hay fever; allergic rhinitis; and asthma. Other atopic allergies include urticaria, gastrointestinal allergies, and in some instances migraine headaches. Although the tendency to atopic allergy is a characteristic of an individual throughout his or her lifetime, the antigens to which the individual is sensitive and the manifestations of the atopic state may change (Sherman, 1965).

In atopic individuals an antibody, which is variously called the homocytotropic skin-sensitizing or reaginic antibody, or simply reagin, or IgE (Austen, 1977, p. 392), mediates the wheal and flare reaction. In normal persons, it is present in millimicrogram amounts; in allergic individuals it is present in microgram amounts. IgE adheres to leukocytes and mast cells. An allergic reaction occurs when IgE bound to these cells comes in contact with the appropriate antigen.

Anaphylaxis

The most serious immediate-type hypersensitivity reaction is cytotropic *anaphylaxis.* Acute anaphylaxis is a true medical emergency requiring immediate treatment within seconds after the onset of symptoms, which may occur from seconds to hours after exposure to antigen. The most common agents which cause acute anaphylaxis include antibiotics, especially penicillin; aspirin; radiopaque contrast media; heterogenous serum; and stinging insects (Queng & McGovern, 1976, p. 33). Fundamental pathophysiological features of acute anaphylaxis are illustrated in Figure 24-2.

The symptoms of acute anaphylaxis arise from the organ systems which are targeted by the chemical mediators released in the antigen–antibody interaction: these shock organs are primarily the pulmonary system, including the upper respiratory tract, and the vascular system. Cutaneous and respiratory symptoms are the most frequent early manifestations of anaphylaxis; without prompt and effective treatment of immediate reactions, vascular collapse and death may occur within 15 minutes (Queng & McGovern, 1976).

Initial Symptoms

Diffuse erythema (redness of the skin); pruritus (itching); urticaria (eruption of itching wheals)

May be Accompanied by

Sneezing; rhinorrhea (discharge from nasal mucosa); cough; tightness in chest; wheezing

May be Followed by

Dyspnea; laryngeal stridor; hypoxia with cyanosis

May be Followed by Symptoms of Vascular Collapse, which May Also Occur Without Preceding Respiratory Distress

Faintness or syncope; pale and cold skin; hypotension; tachycardia; arrhythmia; and cardiac arrest

The specific manifestations of anaphylactic shock differ with each species.

Immediate treatment of anaphylaxis is the administration of aqueous epinephrine 1:1,000, 0.1 to 0.5 ml subcutaneously or intramuscularly; if the patient is in anaphylactic shock, aqueous epinephrine is administered slowly intravenously, 0.1 ml in 10 ml of normal saline. General measures are directed toward (1) establishing and maintaining the airway (see Chapter 40) and (2) restoring blood volume (see Chapters 45 and 52).

Physiologic Reactions

Although a cytotropic (cell-stimulating) reaction including atopy involves the entire body, it is usually

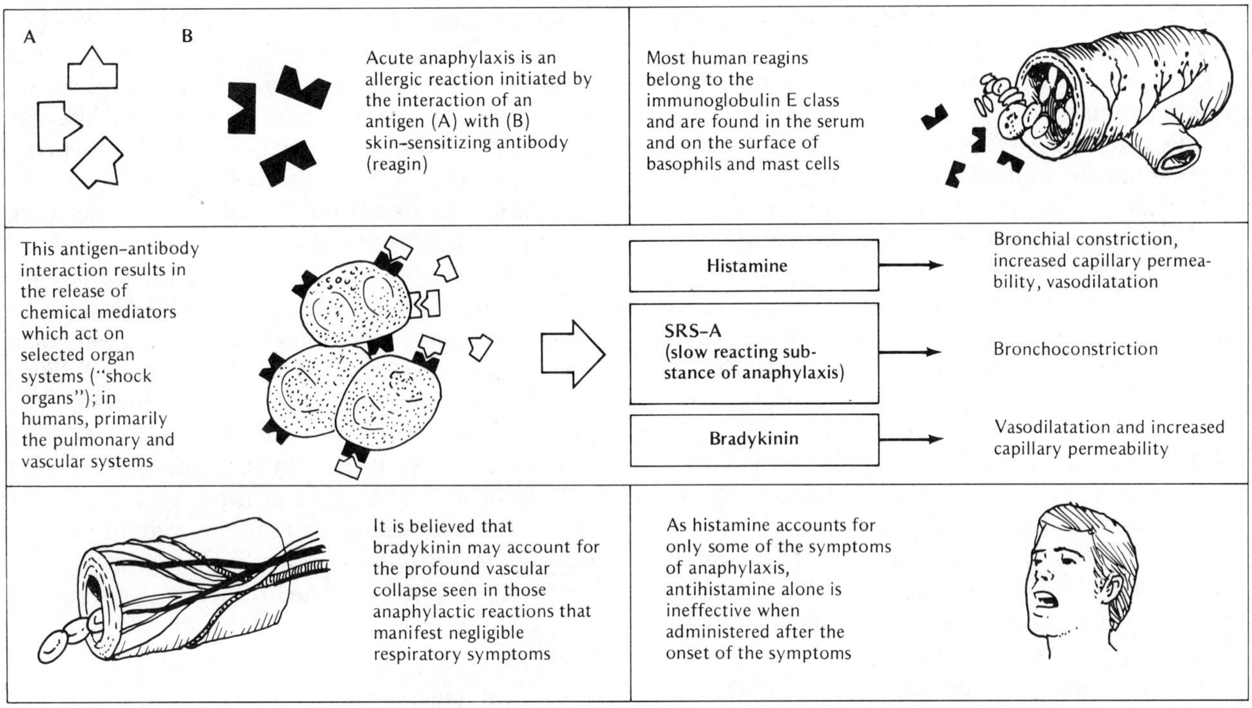

Figure 24-2. Fundamental pathophysiologic features of acute anaphylaxis. (Used with permission of Hospital Publications, Inc., from Acute anapylaxis. *Hosp. Med.* 12:31–43, Sept. 1976, p. 32, by J. T. Queng & J. P. McGovern.)

manifested by a specific or shock organ. Target organs are most frequently those that are in contact with the external environment. Interestingly enough, the lymphocytes and plasma cells are commonly observed in the alveolar parenchyma and the interstitium of the mucosa of the small intestine. Many of the manifestations of atopic disease occur in organs supplied by the autonomic nervous system.

Vascular Reactions

The characteristic vascular change is an increase in capillary permeability with loss of fluid into the interstitial spaces. The resulting edema may be noted as swelling of the face, eyelids, and lips. When edema of the larynx occurs, it may be an immediate threat to life as it impairs ventilation by obstructing the airway. When the blood vessels themselves are the shock or target organ, loss of fluid from the capillaries may be so great that blood volume is diminished sufficiently to cause a serious decrease in cardiac output and arterial blood pressure. When the capillaries are dilated, the skin is flushed or red. From the preceding it should be obvious that increased capillary permeability threatens the life of the individual by predisposing to laryngeal edema and loss of blood volume. Because the manifestations develop rapidly, the patient should be observed for flushing of the skin and any puffiness of the face, mouth, or eyelids. Any patient in whom these signs appear should be treated immediately. *Epinephrine should be immediately available to be administered in situations where systemic reactions are a possibility.*

Skin Reactions

When a small amount of antigen is injected into previously sensitized skin, a swelling with erythema or reddening occurs at the site. It is believed that the skin-sensitizing antibody sensitizes certain cells, particularly the mast cells and blood platelets. The capillaries dilate, causing local erythema. Then the arterioles dilate, causing the flare. The skin response is utilized in identifying hypersensitive individuals. As little as 0.1 ml of antigen diluted 1:10 is injected into the skin. Within a matter of minutes the reaction occurs. Knowledge that the individual is sensitized to the antigen may prevent a life-threatening experience.

The typical skin lesion is known as a wheal or hive. Hives, which may be single or multiple, are localized areas of swelling caused by increased capillary permeability. They are red, hot, and accompanied by intense itching. Although they can be seen on the skin, they may also occur in the gastrointestinal and tracheobronchial mucosa.

Itching, especially when generalized, is important not because it threatens the life of the individual but because it serves as a warning that a general systemic reaction is developing. When a patient has received a potentially antigenic drug such as penicillin, itching should be regarded as indicating the patient is developing a systemic response. The fact of itching should be immediately reported to the patient's physician. *In any situation in which a generalized hypersensitivity reaction is a possibility, epinephrine should be prepared and be immediately available.* Life-threatening allergic responses occur relatively infrequently. Therein lies a danger, for preparation may not have been made for this possibility.

Diagnostic Skin Tests

As previously stated, various body tissues may be sensitized to specific antigens. Because antibodies are frequently found in the skin, and it is conveniently located, the skin may be used (1) to identify individuals who are sensitized to horse serum or other antigens; (2) to check the effectiveness of certain immunization procedures, as the Schick test[3] for diphtheria; (3) to trace the distribution of a disease such as tuberculosis in the community; and (4) to establish the nature of the diagnosis as an example to distinguish between tuberculosis and histoplasmosis.

Skin tests may be performed by injecting a dilute solution of the desired antigen into the skin or by placing a small quantity of the solution on the skin and abrading or scratching it with a hypodermic needle. The scratch test is believed to be safer than intradermal injection because the rate of absorption of the antigen is slower. In the intradermal test, 0.1 to 0.2 ml of a given dilution of the antigen is injected into the skin. In patients known to be or suspected of being hypersensitive, the dilution should be appropriately large. The patient or a member of the family should be asked if he or she has had the particular type of injection previously and, if so, what the reaction to it was. Skin reactions, similar to other allergic responses, may be immediate or delayed. The immediate reaction occurs within a few minutes after the antigenic material is injected and lasts only a short time; the area should therefore be subject to continuous observation. With a positive reaction, the skin becomes red or flushed. Careful observation of the site where antigenic material is injected is important if an immediate response is to be detected. When the patient is to receive an antigenic agent such as tetanus antitoxin (horse serum), detection of a positive response may prevent the patient from developing a serious response or even be life saving. A person who is found to be sensitized to horse serum and who requires tetanus antitoxin can be temporarily immunized by small but increasing doses of antigenic material. The first dose may be no larger than the initial test dose. The safety of the patient depends on identifying the fact that he or she is sensitive and on rigid adherence to the schedule for increasing the dosage and for its timing.

The skin reaction in the delayed type of hypersensitivity takes several hours to appear. It may or may not have been preceded by the immediate type of reaction. The skin at the site of the injection is red, hot, and swollen. The swelling is firm. The lesion lasts longer than it does in the immediate reaction.

In some skin tests, such as the Schick test, reddening of the skin indicates that the individual has not developed antibodies against the antigen. Antibodies protect the skin from the antigen rather than sensitizing it.

[3] The Schick test is a skin test for susceptibility to *Corynebacterium diphtheriae* toxin, the antigen responsible for tissue injury in the infectious disease, diphtheria.

Smooth Muscle Reactions

In target organs containing smooth muscle, the musculature contracts. In humans, contraction of the musculature of the bronchi causes labored breathing characteristic of asthma. Increased contractions of the gastrointestinal musculature causes vomiting and diarrhea.

Mucous Membrane Reactions

Increased capillary permeability in the mucosa results in redness, swelling, weeping, and itching. Mucous glands hypersecrete mucus, thereby predisposing to obstruction of the tracheobronchial tree.

Some Atopic Allergies

There is a group of common human allergies, including nonseasonal vasomotor rhinitis, hay fever, infantile eczema, urticaria, and angioedema, as well as some migraine headaches and gastrointestinal disorders, having a number of features in common. They all appear to be based on *a common predisposing hereditary factor.* The characteristic lesion in the allergic tissues is the wheal or hive. In many instances, symptoms and signs appear promptly on exposure to the allergen. Injection of the offending allergen into the skin is followed by the immediate type of response.

There are some instances, however, in which individuals who are predisposed by heredity to become allergic do not develop signs and symptoms following exposure to an allergen for 12 to 24 hours. For example, Silas Cornflower has a positive family history for allergy, as his mother had urticaria when she ate strawberries or seafood. Injection of minute quantities of antigenic material from either strawberries or seafood results in a raised swollen area at the site of injection (wheal). Mr. Cornflower has asthma when he is exposed to dog dander, but his symptoms do not develop immediately on exposure. They are delayed for 12 to 24 hours after he is in close proximity to a dog. Skin tests do not show the immediate type of reaction. The mechanism in the delayed type of immunologic responses must be different from that in the immediate type. How it differs is not known.

Hay Fever

In hay fever (seasonal vasomotor rhinitis) and nonseasonal rhinitis the mucous membranes lining the nose, related structures, and conjunctiva are affected. The manifestations include tearing and redness of the eyes, burning of both the eyes and nasal mucosa, sneezing, watery discharge from the nose, and obstruction to the passage of air by congestion of the nasal mucosa. The severity of symptoms varies from mild to so severe that the patient cannot get sufficient rest. Seasonal and nonseasonal vasomotor rhinitis differ principally in the antigens to which the person is sensitive. They include pollens—ragweed is a common offender and is responsible for seasonal vasomotor rhinitis—house dust, animal danders, drugs, foods, and the products of infection. With the exception of ragweed, all the other materials cause nonseasonal vasomotor rhinitis. Besides causing varying amounts of discomfort, vasomotor rhinitis predisposes to allergic asthma.

Allergic Asthma

In allergic asthma, the basic lesion is the same as in other allergic responses of the immediate type, but the lesions occur in the bronchial tubes. Three factors are commonly considered to be responsible for allergic asthma: (1) the inhalation of allergens, causing seasonal or nonseasonal asthma; (2) infection of the respiratory tract, causing intermittent or chronic symptoms; and (3) a combination of the first two. The same antigens causing allergic rhinitis may also be responsible for allergic asthma. Because of the variety of factors involved in allergic asthma, it may be seasonal, nonseasonal, or chronic.

Because the bronchi are involved in allergic asthma, there are three responses contributing to the development of symptoms: (1) increased capillary permeability in the mucosa lining the bronchi, (2) spasm or contraction of bronchial musculature, and (3) increased secretion of mucus. All these changes contribute to the interference with breathing—the major manifestation in asthma. At the onset of an attack, the patient is likely to experience a feeling of suffocation, and his or her behavior may suggest a state of panic or acute anxiety. For example, Mrs. Pine, who had been hospitalized for the treatment of asthma, developed an acute attack. She turned on her light. Before the nurse had time to reach her room, she called out for the nurse to hurry. Mrs. Pine appeared to be frightened and she did not want to be left alone. The feelings of suffocation accompanying an attack of asthma probably always engender fear and anxiety and may prolong the attack, after it is under way. Whatever the cause, cell injury results in the release of histamine and serotonin. Any serious threat to oxygen supply and to the removal of carbon dioxide can be expected to have a similar effect.

Emotional factors may also trigger attacks of asthma. As an illustration, one morning Mrs. Pine thought that she had been given a drug to which she was allergic and she developed a full-blown attack of asthma. What had actually occurred was that a laboratory assistant had drawn blood. The attack had been triggered by a thought rather than a material substance. It was no less severe, however. She required the same treatment as any patient experiencing an acute attack of asthma. During the attack Mrs. Pine sat with her feet hanging over the edge of the bed. She was supporting herself with her hands and arms in a winglike position. This position enabled her to make maximum use of her accessory muscles of respiration. Because bronchi dilate with inspiration and are smaller with expiration, air is trapped in the lungs, causing them to be distended and the chest to be in a continuous state of expansion. Therefore the efforts of the patient are directed toward forcing air out of the lung during expiration. Expiration appears more labored than inspiration. Her (Mrs. Pine's) respirations were accompanied by a wheeze that was audible to her and to those who were nearby. Coughing was stimulated by an increase in the secretion of mucus. Therapy for an acute asthmatic attack is directed toward (1) depressing the allergic response, (2) dilating the bronchi, (3) decreasing the anxiety of the patient, and (4) correcting the conditions predisposing to asthma. When at all possible, someone should stay with the patient who is in an acute attack of asthma. When only one person is available, the most reasonable course of action is to prepare and administer the prescribed drug or drugs. *Some of the same drugs that are effective in treatment of anaphylactic shock are also useful in relieving an acute attack of asthma.* These drugs include *epinephrine, ephedrine sulfate,* or *hydrochloride, aminophyllin, U.S.P., B.P., isoproterenerol hydrochloride, and Tedral.*[4] In a very acute attack, epinephrine is usually administered.

Skin Reactions

Skin reactions characteristic of the immediate type of allergy include infantile eczema, erythematous rashes, exfoliative dermatitis, and hives.[5]

Urticaria or hives of the skin is most frequently associated with allergy to foods. Drugs may also be responsible.

Wheal and erythema reactions occurring along the gastrointestinal tract, combined with the contraction of smooth muscle, cause symptoms such as nausea, vomiting, and diarrhea. Gastrointestinal allergies are likely to be caused by ingestants such as seafood, wheat, or eggs.

Immediate-Type Hypersensitivity: Cytolytic Type

A second harmful immune mechanism of the immediate type is cytolysis. Whereas in the cytotropic reaction cells are stimulated by the antigen–antibody in cytolytic or cytotoxic reaction, sensitized cells are directly injured. According to Schwartz (1969), the offending immunoglobulin is almost always IgG. The antigen may be of either intrinsic or extrinsic origin. An example of an intrinsic antigen is the Rh factor in the erythrocyte. An extrinsic antigen is penicillin. Whatever the offending antigen, coating of the cell with IgG makes it susceptible to damage by macrophages and other mononuclear cells. A series of changes occur that lead to the damage of red blood cells. Examples of disorders caused by cytolytic reactions are the hemolysis of red cells following the transfusion of mismatched blood, erythroblastosis in the newborn, some types of hemolytic anemia, thrombocytopenia, leukopenia, and a type of anemia induced by penicillin.

[4] Trade name for compound containing theophylline, 0.13 g; ephedrine hydrochloride, 24 mg; and phenobarbital, 8 mg.

[5] A number of terms are used to describe blisters. Blebs, vesicles, and bullae all imply blisters. Bullae are large blisters.

The Arthus Reaction

Another example of a cytolytic reaction is the Arthus phenomenon. An individual sensitized by repeated injections of a specific antigen may eventually respond to the same antigen by a localized inflammatory response at the site of the injection. Within 12 to 24 hours a centralized area of necrosis appears. The reaction requires (1) large amounts of antigen in the tissues, and (2) circulating antibodies (IgG). In the presence of complement, soluble antigen–antibody complexes are deposited in the blood vessels. As a result of their irritating effect large numbers of polymorphonuclear leukocytes enter the area and phagocytosize the antibody–antigen complexes. Protein-digesting enzymes are released. Platelets accumulate and blood clots. The result is an area of hemorrhagic necrosis. Healing is by repair (Kunkel, 1979).

A response that appears to be similar in many respects to the Arthus reaction is also mediated by soluble antigen–antibody aggregates. Instead of occurring at the site of injected antigen, the reaction occurs at a distant site such as in the kidney. Schwartz (1969) states that insoluble aggregates of antigens and antibodies are formed when antibodies are mixed with appropriate antigens. When increasing amounts of antigens are added, however, some of the molecules of the aggregate are rearranged and form soluble complexes. Because of their size insoluble immune aggregates are rapidly removed by the reticuloendothelial system. Conversely, the soluble complexes are not easily removed from the blood and they penetrate the walls of blood vessels. Because they are highly vascular organs, the kidneys are frequent sites of injury. Soluble immune aggregates deposit in the basement membranes of the glomeruli and activate the complement system. In response polymorphonuclear leukocytes enter the area and ingest the deposits. Lysosomal granules in the cell burst and release lytic enzymes, which then injure the basement membrane of the glomerulus.

From the preceding discussion, it should be obvious that there are a number of systemic and local allergic responses of the immediate type. The nature of the manifestations depends on whether or not the response is systemic or localized to an organ or part. The organs in which the manifestations are most prominent are those in direct contact with the external environment: the skin, the airway, and the gastrointestinal tract. The bone marrow may, however, be a primary site of reaction as well. In *anaphylactic shock,* the blood vessels throughout the body are affected. Two factors that seem to influence the nature of the response are the rate and site of exposure to an antigen. As stated in the previous section, most of the manifestations are caused by increased capillary permeability and by contraction of smooth muscle. Vascular collapse and obstruction of the airway as a result of edema of the larynx are the two most serious threats to the life of an individual. No person should be treated with a foreign serum or other type of antigenic agent without first determining whether or not he or she has been treated with it at some earlier time. Patients receiving horse serum should be tested previous to its administration by the injection of horse serum intradermally (into the skin). A reddening or flare indicates that the patient has been sensitized to horse serum.

Delayed-Type Hypersensitivity

Another harmful immunologic response is delayed hypersensitivity. The classic example is the response of the tissues to the tubercle bacillus. A similar type of reaction occurs in other chronic infections as well as in contact dermatitis. Although signs and symptoms usually occur within minutes after exposure to an antigen in the immediate type of hypersensitivity, there are a few exceptions such as serum sickness. In general, however, signs and symptoms are slower to develop in the delayed type than in the immediate type. In the immediate type the antibody circulates in the blood; in the delayed type it is bound to cells. The first is known as humoral antibody and the latter as a high-affinity or avidity antibody. Antibodies in the serum can be identified in and transferred in the serum.[6] Cellular antibodies cannot be transferred in the serum but require lymphocytes to which antibodies are bound. This class of reactions which involve T-lymphocytes in delayed-type hypersensitivity is termed cellular immunity (see Figure 24-1).

Differences in the Lesions

Whereas the lesion in the immediate type of hypersensitivity usually develops within a few minutes and may disappear within a short time, the lesion of the delayed type of hypersensitivity reaction takes several hours to appear. It is similar inasmuch as the area is red, hot, and swollen. The swelling is firmer and lasts longer than it does in the immediate type of reaction. When the reaction is severe, tissue cells may be killed and cellular necrosis may be evident. The initial damage may result from the combination of the antigen and the antibody. Further injury may be caused by substances released by the necrotic cells. With cellular injury, tissues also respond by inflammation. This response will be discussed later in the chapter. The classical example of the delayed type of hypersensitivity is the response of the tissues to tuberculin. Anyone whose tissues have been sensitized to *Mycobacterium tuberculosis* and has had a Mantoux or similar test has experienced the delayed type of allergic skin reaction. When this reaction is marked, there is some degree of tissue necrosis.

[6] Transfer of humoral antibodies from an immunized to a susceptible individual provides passive immunity.

Allergies of the Delayed Type

Allergies of the delayed type include contact dermatitis, poison ivy, drug allergies, and allergies of infections such as tuberculosis. Changes occurring in the tissues in a variety of other infections such as syphilis are believed to be attributable to hypersensitivity reactions. Symptoms in conditions such as athlete's foot may be the result of delayed hypersensitivity to the fungus causing the disorder. Following the administration of heterologous serum and certain drugs, including penicillin, changes take place in blood vessels that are characteristic of a delayed type of allergic response. The pathological changes in the blood vessels resemble those of periarteritis nodosa.

One of the most common examples of delayed hypersensitivity is contact dermatitis. Because of the frequency with which it occurs and its increasing incidence, contact dermatitis will be discussed in some detail. As a result of repeated contacts with a wide variety of simple as well as complex antigenic agents, including detergents, the skin becomes sensitized to an antigen. The agents that initiate or prolong dermatitis are numerous. The signs of dermatitis appear in sensitized skin from 12 to 48 hours after exposure to the antigen. They include (1) erythema and swelling, (2) oozing and/or vesiculation, (3) crusting and sealing, (4) thickening and evidence of repeated excoriation (the results of scratching), and (5) hyperpigmentation, scratch papule formation, and lichenification. The first three groups of signs occur during the acute phase and the latter two during the chronic phase of the disorder. The eventual outcome depends on the early identification and elimination of the cause. When contact dermatitis is allowed to persist, secondary changes follow and tend to prolong it.

Autoimmune Disease

Until recently most antigens were believed to be foreign substances that were introduced into, or entered, the individual from the outside environment. Some individuals, for reasons that are poorly understood, appear to lose their ability to identify their own tissues as being of themselves, for they react to certain of their own tissues as they would to foreign antigens. Diseases in which the body may possibly form antibodies against its own tissues are called autoimmune diseases. Though this theory offers an attractive explanation for the changes occurring in certain diseases such as rheumatic fever, multiple sclerosis, lupus erythematosus, periarteritis nodosa, and rheumatoid arthritis, it is largely unproved. One disorder usually cited as being caused by an antoimmune reaction against thyroglobulin is Hashimoto's disease of the thyroid (Gordon, 1974, p. 200). A number of observations have been made that lend support to the theory that tissues can become antigenic and thus stimulate the formation of antibodies against themselves. In diseases such as rheumatic fever, the onset is frequently preceded by a streptococcal infection occurring approximately 2 to 3 weeks earlier. How the infection or the products of bacterial growth induce changes in tissue cells is now known. It has been shown that streptococcus and the myocardium possess a common antigen—a body response to the streptococcal infection is also a response against myocardial tissue. Antibodies are formed in response to this antigen; they combine with the antigen and injure tissue cells. The damaged cells release histamine and possibly serotonin, both of which cause secondary changes that are possibly more damaging than the initial injury. Further destruction of healthy tissues may result from the contraction of scar tissue formed to replace dead tissue. One of the puzzling things about these diseases is that after they are initiated there is no sure way known to stop their progress.

Interferon

Two types of *interferon* are a part of the immunological response. Type I (standard) interferon is produced by both lymphoid and nonlymphoid cells in response to viruses, polynucleotides, and endotoxins. Type II (immune) interferon is produced by sensitized lymphocytes in response to specific antigens, mitogens, or antigen–antibody complexes, and serves as a mediator of *cellular immunity* (Hooks et al., 1979). Immune interferon has been found in the serum of patients with a number of antoimmune diseases: systemic lupus erythematosus (SLE); rheumatoid arthritis (RA); scleroderma; and Sjögren's syndrome. It may be that the production of interferon contributes to immunologic abberations in autoimmune diseases and also protects the already compromised patient from viral infections (Hooks et al., 1979). An example of the protection provided by interferon has been demonstrated by its use with immunosuppressed renal transplant patients. Following a 6-week course of prophylactic interferon administered to postrenal transplant patients during a 2-year trial period, Cheesemen et al. (1979) observed a decreased incidence of viremia after transplantation.

Homotransplantation

One of the most publicized accomplishments of the last decade or so has been the ability to transplant whole organs from one person to another. Successful transplantation presents a variety of problems. One problem that has been solved for organs such as the kidney and the heart has been the development of techniques for removing an organ from one individual and placing it in another in such a manner that it is supplied with blood and is able to carry out its function. A second and less easily solved problem is obtaining a sufficient number of healthy and viable organs. In the case of the heart, a living heart must be obtained from a person who has died. Many complex legal and ethical problems have surfaced in relation to the life-or-death status of the donor of organs to be transplanted. A frequently cited basis for the definition of death are the criteria for neurological death developed in 1968 by a committee of doctors at Harvard University. See Chapter 33 for the Harvard criteria, with discussion of brain death.

The third problem, which will be discussed briefly, is created because tissues of one individual recognize those of another as being foreign. As a consequence, homografts are almost always rejected by the immunologic response of the recipient to the donor's antigens (Amos, 1977).

To achieve success in homograft transplantation, histocompatible tissues must be used or some method found to induce a state in which the immune system fails to response to foreign antigen or antigens.[7] Because identical twins are genetically

[7] The same specific histocompatibility antigens (HL-A) that determine whether an individual will accept or reject a homotransplanted organ appear to be associated with such diseases as Hodgkin's, systemic lupus erythematosus (SLE), chronic glomerulonephritis, childhood asthma, and infectious mononucleosis. ["HL-A Antigens and Disease," *Med. World News,* **12** (13 Aug. 1971), 51.]

similar, a kidney or skin transplanted from one can be expected to be accepted by the other.

Another natural type of tolerance was reported by Owens in 1945. In cattle twins, vascular anastomoses frequently develop in utero. As a result, each twin of the nonidentical pair may have two different types of red blood cells, his or her own and that of the twin. Each retains the two types of red blood cells throughout his or her life span. Experimentally, animals can be made tolerant to foreign antigens during embryonic life.

Homografts present the immune mechanism with the same challenge as any foreign protein be it a virus or bacterium in a cell. The difference is in degree and not in kind, as homotransplanted cells are less antigenic than other foreign proteins. Another difference is that bacteria and viruses release toxins that provoke acute inflammatory responses. Most authorities believe that the initial rejection of the homograft is caused by a delayed type of hypersensitivity. There is evidence, however, that humoral factors are eventually involved.

Following the transplantation of tissue, there is a more or less typical and predictable sequence of events. For a few days the transplanted tissue remains viable and its blood supply appears to be developing. In 10 days to 2 weeks or more the graft becomes intensely inflamed, undergoes necrosis, and dies. A second graft from the same donor is more rapidly rejected than the first. The accelerated reaction is known as a "second-set" reaction. The second-set reaction is specific to the original donor and can be induced by prior inoculation of cells from the donor.

To achieve success in homograft transplantation, two methods are combined to increase the likelihood of the recipient accepting the donor's tissues. First, a donor is selected whose tissues have a minimum number of antigenic differences from the recipient. The fewer the foreign antigens that the recipient has to respond to, the greater the chance of success. Second, the recipient is altered in such a manner that tolerance to the foreign antigen is induced. On the hypothesis that the lymphocyte is responsible for antibody formation, total body radiation may be used to destroy the lymphocytes. Irradiation must be administered before transplantation. If administered at the same time or after exposure to the antigen, radiation has little effect. Some of the drugs used in the treatment of leukemia such as 6-mercaptopurine and certain antibiotics are useful in suppressing immune responses. They may be used not only to eliminate the initial response but to maintain tolerance to foreign tissues. A third method has been used to deplete the body's store of lymphocytes by draining the thoracic duct. Under certain circumstances antibody synthesis may be inhibited by overloading with antigen. This technique is called immunologic paralysis.

Prevention of or minimizing the immune response depends on limiting the number of antigens to which the recipient is exposed combined with altering the capacity to respond. The latter depends on understanding the role that various body components play. This includes not only lymphocytes but macrophages and other elements. Moreover, despite the importance of preventing the initial rejection of transplanted tissue, methods must be used to maintain continuing tolerance to foreign tissue.

As knowledge of the specialized differentiation of lymphoid-cell populations and their characteristic surface antigens is acquired, the production of antiserums directed against cell lineages committed to allograft rejection or even against other cell types is to be expected. The immunosuppressive effectiveness of antilymphocyte globulin is related to its capacity to reduce the number of peripheral-blood thymus-derived cells.

Nonspecific immunosuppression increases the incidence of microbial invasion, and the treatment of infection in patients given immunosuppressive agents has become a demanding subspecialty for experts in infectious diseases (Russell & Cosimi, 1979).

Foremost among the goals of transplantation biologists is to produce a specific and long-lasting alteration of responses in the recipient that is confined to the antigens in the donor tissue. There is mounting evidence from experimental immunology that such alterations are feasible. The search for improved immunosuppressive agents that favor specific reduction of the recipient's responsiveness to donor antigens has yielded two possible treatments of interest: administration of the fungal metabolite cyclosporin A, and irradiation directed by suitable shielding toward lymphoid centers throughout the body—"total lymphatic irradiation" (Russell & Cosimi, 1979).

With methods such as total body irradiation and with immunosuppressive agents the individual's capacity to respond to microorganisms is lost. Methods must be used to protect him or her from exposure to exogenous microbes. Protection from one's own organisms is a more difficult problem. (See Chapter 10.) The rejection problem accompanying transplantation may ultimately be resolved by use of cultured tissue whose antigenicity is lost as a result of having been grown in a culture medium for a critical period of time prior to transplantation (Maugh II, 1973).

In the more distant future, human beings will certainly continue to require renewal of individual structures or cell types. Major advances, even beyond the free and successful use of transferred human tissues, may include the use of structures from other species than our own (xenografts), the use of nonliving artificial devices and the use of new tissues fabricated *in vitro* by the guided differentiation of cells from the patient or another suitable donor. Success with any of these approaches would free transplantation from the restrictions that must always apply when human tissues are used (Russell & Cosimi, 1979).

For those who wish to pursue this subject in more detail, references are included at the end of this chapter. Because much research is in progress, future reports will undoubtedly be enlightening.

The Nurse's Role in Helping the Person with an Immunologic Response

Because allergic responses, however they are manifested, are the result of an immunologic mechanism, preventive and therapeutic measures are based on similar principles and are directed toward the achievement of three objectives. The site of the response and the requirements of the individual patient influence the selection of specific preventive and therapeutic measures. These factors also influence the decision as to which objective takes priority at a given moment in time. The primary objectives are (1) to prevent or limit the exposure of the patient to antigens to which he or she may be, or is known to be, hypersensitive; (2) to relieve or mitigate the effects produced by a hypersensitivity reaction; (3) to increase the resistance of the patient to a specific antigen.

Objective 1. Prevention or Limitation of Exposure to Antigens

The accomplishment of the first objective depends on knowledge of what the common allergens are, what their sources are, how they are transported in the environment, and how they gain entrance into the organism. Actually, this is the very knowledge that forms the background for the prevention of the spread of infectious agents causing disease. Because not all persons are allergic to the common allergens, knowledge of the particular antigens to which the patient is hypersensitive is also useful. Some of the substances to which people are frequently hypersensitive have been previously mentioned. Hypersensitivity to horse serum is so common and so easily developed that all persons are presumed to be sensitive to it unless they are shown not to be by skin testing. The use of skin testing in the identification of substances to which individuals are hypersensitive has also been discussed. Although skin testing is of value, it also has limitations. A reddened area indicates that the patient has antibodies for that antigen in the skin but it does not necessarily mean that he or she will have an allergic response when exposed to it. Why this is true is not known. Neither does the absence of a reddened area necessarily mean that the person is not hypersensitive to a particular antigen. Some persons have a high degree of hypersensitivity to an antigen, despite the absence of a positive skin reaction.

Because skin tests do not necessarily give complete information about the antigens to which an individual is hypersensitive, other methods have to be used in their identification. Perhaps the most important of these is the observation of a cause–effect relationship between contact with an antigen and the development of an allergic reaction on the part of the patient. Patients are often aware of these relationships. For example, Mrs. Cornflower knows that each time she eats strawberries she develops hives. In some instances an individual such as Mrs. Cornflower knows that if she eats one strawberry she becomes deathly sick. Her cousin Frank is able to eat a small serving of strawberries three or four times during the summer, but he has hives if he eats them more frequently. Nurses can help in identifying antigens when they observe and report events that are coincident. For example, Mrs. Batelman was hospitalized for treatment of an acute attack of allergic asthma. Following her recovery, her physician decided to remove some nasal polyps obstructing her breathing. Nasal polyps are a common sequela in allergic rhinitis. As part of her preparation for polypectomy, Mrs. Batelman was given ephedrine. Shortly thereafter, she began to wheeze and to show signs of a developing asthmatic attack. Despite the impending attack of asthma, the surgeon removed the polyps and the ephedrine was continued. Each time Mrs. Batelman received ephedrine, wheezing and difficulty in breathing were intensified. The nurse observed the apparent cause–effect relationship between the ephedrine and the difficulty in breathing exhibited by Mrs. Batelman. She brought her observation to the attention of the physician, who discontinued the drug. Mrs. Batelman's breathing improved and other evidence of asthma also cleared rapidly. Despite the usefulness of ephedrine in relieving asthmatic attacks in most individuals, in the instance of Mrs. Batelman it acted to trigger its onset.

Cause–effect relationships are frequently more difficult to establish than in the illustration cited here. To collect data, the patient may be instructed to keep a diary or a record of activities, including what he or she eats, and to describe any abnormal responses. For example, Mrs. Bobbin learned from keeping a diary that she was allergic to an insecticide used to kill mosquitoes. She developed asthmatic symptoms each evening after an insecticide containing pyrethrum was sprayed just outside the porch where she sat in the evening.

When a food is suspected to be allergenic, a diary may be employed or the patient may be placed on an elimination diet. The elimination diet may be approached in different ways. The patient may be instructed to eliminate one food at a time and observe the response or to eliminate all commonly allergenic foods and then add them to the diet one at a time. Before adding a new food, the patient should note any response to the one just previously included in the diet. Occasionally all foods except those that are rarely antigenic may be removed from the diet and then the above procedure followed. The success of any type of elimination diet in discovering antigenic foods depends on the patient and/or the person who prepares the food understanding why the diet is prescribed and what is entailed in its preparation. It must be understood that it is the specific food and not its method of preparation that is important. The food must be eliminated in all forms. The following example has its origin in the days before electricity was supplied to every farmhouse. Mrs. Farwell brought her three-year-old son, Bobby, to University Clinic for the treatment of atopic eczema. In an attempt to identify the offending allergen, the physician prescribed a diet from which all forms of wheat were to be eliminated. Mrs. Farwell was duly instructed and appeared to be interested and cooperative. A week later she returned with Bobby. He was no better. The physician checked with Mrs. Farwell to determine whether she had carried out the instructions. He asked her if Bobby had had any bread. She replied, "No, none at all. I toasted every bit of it." Mrs. Farwell did not have a toaster and she did not usually toast bread unless a member of the family was ill. She believed that toast was more easily digested than untoasted bread and was therefore more suitable than bread for a sick person. The making of toast was a cultural response to illness.

Patients sometimes eliminate foods from their diet because they are, or believe that they are, allergic to them. Although the avoidance of one or two specific foods is not likely to cause malnutrition, the exclusion of many foods may, and this possibility increases in proportion to the number of foods eliminated. Occasionally an individual appears for medical attention who has eliminated almost all types of food from his or her diet. It is quite important that persons for whom elimination diets are prescribed understand that the diet is temporary.

Prevention of Acute Drug Reactions

Because of the possibility of an acute hypersensitivity developing after the use of drugs, certain precautions should be taken. Before any drug is administered, the patient should be asked whether there is any history of allergy in the patient or family and whether he or she recalls ever having been treated with the drug to be used. Because of the common practice of treating infections in cows with penicillin, milk may contain penicillin. Persons who drink milk may be sensitized to penicillin without ever having been treated with it. For reasons not well understood, drugs applied to the skin are more likely to induce sensitivity reactions than those ingested or injected. When there is reason to suspect that an individual may be allergic, he or she should be tested for skin-sensitizing antibodies. When a patient inquires about the nature of a drug being taken, the nurse should at least ascertain the reason for the question. In some hospitals, only the physician tells the patient what drugs have been prescribed. The practice of withholding information from a patient about the drugs administered is being questioned. Some physicians now request the pharmacist to indicate on the label of the container the generic or trade name of drugs prescribed for and taken by the patient. Should the patient state that he or she is allergic to a given drug, it should be withheld until the physician has been notified. Even drugs such as aspirin can, in the occasional individual, be highly antigenic. When agents such as heterologous serum are administered, the patient should be skin-tested before the serum is administered, and a syringe containing acqueous 1:1,000 epinephrine should be prepared so that it will be immediately available should symptoms develop. In all patient areas, the following emergency drugs and equipment should be immediately available (Queng & McGovern, 1976, p. 39):

Drugs

- Aqueous epinephrine 1:1,000, for SC or IM injection
- Parenteral preparations of:
  - Antihistamine
  - Aminophylline
  - Vasopressors
  - Corticosteroid
  - Intravenous fluids

Equipment

- Sphygmomanometer and stethoscope
- Syringes and needles—IV, IM, SC

IV adapter
Oropharyngeal airways
Laryngoscope and endotracheal tube
Tourniquets
Oxygen
Tracheostomy set

Despite the infrequency of anaphylactic reactions, they can cause death unless they are treated immediately. Patients who are treated as outpatients should remain at least one-half hour after the injection of any potentially antigenic agent.

The danger to the individual who receives an antigen to which he or she has been sensitized can be illustrated by Mrs. Johns, who had a serious reaction to penicillin. Fortunately for Mrs. Johns, she had not left her physician's office when she experienced systemic or anaphylactic shock. The reaction might have been prevented had either the physician who prescribed the penicillin or the nurse who administered it questioned her about her previous experience with penicillin. Failure to do so very nearly cost Mrs. Johns her life. Almost immediately following an injection of penicillin, she developed hives and had great difficulty in breathing; in a matter of a few minutes her blood pressure dropped sharply and she became unconscious. The physician injected epinephrine and applied artificial respiration. As soon as an ambulance could be obtained, she was taken to a hospital. When her condition improved, the doctor learned that she had had penicillin on two previous occasions. After the second injection she had had swelling, reddening, and itching at the site where it was injected. She had not remembered to tell her doctor of this. Unlike horse serum, skin tests to determine sensitivity to penicillin are unreliable. The only protection of the patient lies in regular questioning of each patient before therapy with penicillin is initiated.

Adaptation of the Environment

In addition to assisting in various ways with the identification of antigenic agents, the nurse is often responsible for the preparation of an environment that is as nearly free of antigenic agents as is possible. She or he may also be helpful to the patient in planning the home environment. Extremes should be avoided in adapting the home to the needs of the allergic person. The same general points apply whether the patient is in the hospital or at home. Frequently, stripping the bedroom of unnecessary dust-catching furniture and draperies is all this is required. Overstuffed furniture, draperies, pillows, mattresses with ordinary covering, and rugs serve as reservoirs for the accumulation of dust, and they should be removed or covered with an impervious material. Mattresses can now be purchased with plasticized coverings that prevent them from accumulating dust. They do not require further covering. The rest of the house may be furnished as desired. For older children and adults, airborne allergens are of considerable importance. House dust and pollens are common antigens. When furniture is purchased for the home, ease of cleaning should be kept in mind.

The patient can use a Dacron[8] pillow. Sponge rubber may be used, but in time it tends to take on dust, and some persons are allergic to rubber. Allergic patients often take their own pillows with them to the hospital. Despite the possibility of the patient's losing the pillow, he or she should be permitted to keep it and a concerted effort should be made to prevent its loss.

The air may be a source of dust and pollens. Hot-air systems without adequate filters circulate considerable dust. For persons who are allergic to dust, filters should be installed in systems circulating air. They require regular cleansing or replacement. Many persons who are sensitive to pollens can reduce exposure enough to keep themselves fairly comfortable by sleeping in an air-conditioned room. When this is not possible, a window fan combined with a paper or glass-wool filter will give some relief by reducing the pollen count and cooling the room. Keeping the windows closed also reduces the pollen count in the house. For patients who have severe hay fever or asthma, and who are able to afford it, a trip to an area in which the pollen count is low may be indicated. Before the advent of air conditioning, certain areas of the United States were havens for hay fever sufferers. Persons who are sensitive to fungi are advised to avoid damp climates. Damp basements can be dried by the use of dehumidifiers. Anyone who has worked in the emergency room of a large city hospital cannot escape being impressed by the number of patients who come in for treatment of asthma on a warm, moist summer evening. In fact, physicians and nurses can sometimes be heard to say, "This is an asthma night." Many persons who are allergic learn to identify substances and circumstances that activate their symptoms and can plan to avoid them.

Animal danders are another common cause of hypersensitivity. Hypersensitive persons should be advised against acquiring a dog or cat if they do not already have one. When there is a pet in the home, its effect can be tested by removing it for a month or so. If the condition of the patient is improved, the patient and family should be advised to give the pet away. Should there be no difference in the patient's condition, there is no reason to do so.

[8] Synthetic Fiber.

In the control of contact dermatitis, the same general principles hold. The first step is to identify the offending antigen or antigens and then to make a plan to avoid them. Because of the variety of contactants, this is not always as easy to do as to narrate. The importance of prompt action cannot be overestimated. Secondary changes including infection may cause more problems than the original dermatitis. Sometimes, as in the instance of a housewife who is allergic to detergents, protection merely involves wearing rubber gloves when using detergents or substituting soap for them. To avoid dermatitis, she may have to wear gloves every time she uses a detergent.

At other times the problem is more complicated. For example, streptomycin sulfate has been found to induce hypersensitivity in a high proportion of those who work with it either in its preparation in factories or in hospitals. This problem has been minimized because streptomycin is now supplied in disposable syringes. Rubber gloves should be worn by nurses and pharmacists when they handle it. Contact dermatitis can occur in persons who handle penicillin, but this does not occur as commonly as it does with streptomycin. The amount of either of these drugs required to cause a reaction in sensitive persons may be infinitesimal. In one hospital where nurses had become sensitized to streptomycin, it was necessary to assign them to units where patients did not receive streptomycin.

On occasion, a nurse may develop a sensitivity to other drugs. In the experience of the writer one nurse was so highly sensitive to morphine that she developed a dermatitis each time she prepared even a single dose of it. To continue in the practice of nursing she had to arrange to be relieved of any responsibility for administering morphine, or being near where the drug was prepared. In nurses who develop contact dermatitis, the problem of control is often difficult. Any measures that can be taken to prevent its development are well worth taking. When the possibility of exposure to a sensitizing agent exists, thorough washing with soap and water will serve to remove the agent and thereby reduce the intensity of the contact. For example, after exposure to poison ivy a shower should be taken as soon as possible. Although both soap and water should be generously applied, this should be accompanied by minimum rubbing of the skin as the antigen of poison ivy does not induce sensitivity unless it is rubbed into the skin.

Summary—Nursing for Objective 1

The first step in the accomplishment of the objective to limit to prevent the exposure of the patient to substances to which he or she is hypersensitive is to identify the offending agent or agents. In some instances this can be accomplished by skin tests. In others, the antigenic agents cannot be identified by skin tests but may be by establishing a cause and effect relationship. This requires a form of medical detective work. The patient and others, including the nurse, try to identify the conditions associated with the onset of symptoms; their relationship to the patient's allergic manifestations can be tested by eliminating possible antigens one at a time from the environment and observing the results. In instances in which there is doubt, a suspected antigen may be further tested by its reintroduction into the environment of the patient. After the causative agent is identified, the next step is to plan how contact with the agent can be reduced or eliminated. Points to be considered include the nature of the antigen, its source or reservoir, vehicles by which it is transmitted, and portals of entry. The degree of sensitivity of the person is also a factor. In the person who is highly sensitive to an antigen, all exposure may have to be prevented. In the person who is less sensitive, restrictions on exposure may be less stringent.

Objective 2. Relief or Mitigation of the Allergic Response

When an allergic patient experiences an acute response to an allergen, the symptoms may be such that she or he is incapacitated or survival is threatened. Then efforts to relieve or mitigate the allergic response take priority. The urgency of the situation depends on the type and acuteness of the reactions of the patient. Prompt and energetic treatment may be necessary to save the life of a patient in anaphylactic shock or in status asthmaticus. Protection from further exposure to foreign serum or to an antigenic drug and palliation of the symptoms may meet the major requirements of a patient with serum or drug sickness. The patient with hay fever (allergic rhinitis) may be miserable, but his or her life is not usually in danger.

Drugs have an important role in the prevention and relief of allergic responses of various types. One of the most generally useful drugs is epinephrine. It is believed to act directly on effector cells, stimulating some and inhibiting others. Because the action of epinephrine is similar to that of the sympathetic nervous system, it is said to be sympathomimetic. It antagonizes the effects of the parasympathetic nervous system (cholinergic), other cholinergic chemicals, and histamine. In disorders such as anaphylaxis and acute asthma it may be life saving. *Epinephrine should always be in readiness in situations where an anaphylactic response is a possibility.* Because of its powerful bronchial dilatory action, it is often effective in the relief of asthmatic attacks that are resistant to other drugs. It affords symptomatic relief in urticaria, serum sickness, hay fever, angioneurotic edema, and other similar allergic disorders. It may be administered by subcutaneous, intramuscular, or intravenous injection or by inhalation. The usual range of dosage for subcutaneous injection for adults is from 0.2 to 0.5 ml of a 1:1,000 aqueous solution. Despite the fact that epinephrine is dispensed in ampules containing 1 ml, a nurse should not give more than 0.5 ml without special instructions from the physician. Smaller dosages are indicated when the patient is receiving the drug for the first time. Patients with hyperthyroidism and hypertension are especially susceptible to the effects of epinephrine, and it is contraindicated in these conditions. In any patient, an overdosage of epinephrine predisposes the patient to ventricular fibrillation.

When epinephrine is administered by inhalation, the exact dosage is difficult to control. The delivery of epinephrine to the bronchi requires that the solution be converted to a fine mist. It also requires that the solution be at least 1 part epinephrine to 100 parts water. A positive pressure machine and nebulizer may be used. An atomizer or nebulizer should be made entirely of glass or plastic. When the patient uses a hand-operated atomizer considerable practice may be needed to coordinate squeezing of the bulb with inspiration. Proper coordination is necessary to deliver and distribute the drug through the tracheobronchial tree. Oxygen may be used in a nebulizer to convert the solution to a fine mist and distribute it to the desired area. Whether an atomizer, a mask, or a nebulizer is used, the drug is inhaled through the mouth. The patient should be cautioned against overusage, as it causes dryness of the throat and irritation of the tracheobronchial tree. Should irritation of the airway occur, the patient may have to discontinue inhalations for several days. The nurse should note the frequency with which patients inhale epinephrine, and if it seems excessive, caution the patient or bring the observation to the attention of the physician. Because swallowing epinephrine causes epigastric pain, the patient should be taught to wash his or her mouth after each administration. Sometimes the mucus that is expectorated is pink, due to changes in the color of the drug. Bleeding is not necessarily indicated.

Ephedrine may be used to relax the smooth muscle of the bronchi in asthma. It has an advantage over epinephrine because it can be administered orally. Theophylline, U.S.P., is also prescribed because it relaxes the smooth muscle in the tracheobronchial tree.

The antihistaminics are a group of drugs providing relief in a number of allergic disorders. Among those in which antihistaminics are most beneficial are hay fever, serum sickness, urticaria, drug reactions, and angioneurotic edema. These are all forms of allergy in which exudation is a significant factor. The antihistaminic drugs have two general effects believed to be important in the treatment of allergy. They are supposed to counteract the effect of histamine by displacing histamine from receptor sites in the cell. This effect is called the blocking action of the antihistaminic drugs. Some authorities question the validity of this concept of their action. The chemical structure of some antihistamines bears little superficial resemblance to histamine. Therapeutic dosages of these drugs cause some depression of the central nervous system; they have a sedative effect in some persons and in others they cause restlessness, insomnia, and nervousness.

Cortisone and ACTH have proved to be useful not only in the relief of symptoms in acute attacks of asthma, hay fever, allergic dermatitis, and drug reactions but also in the treatment of chronic states. In some patients the relief lasts only as long as the drug is administered, in others relief may continue for months or longer.

Itching is frequently referred to as a troublesome symptom of allergic dermatoses. Although itching does not threaten the life of the patient and is not always incapacitating, it can cause a good bit of discomfort and reduce the patient's efficiency. Since the introduction of antihistaminic drugs, itching is often easier to control than it was in the past. In the care of the patient, the nurse may add to his or her comfort by the prevention of overheating of the room, as sweating increases itching. A cool environmental temperature reduces itching, whereas a warm one increases it. When wet dressings are ordered, at least twenty layers of gauze or an equal thickness of turkish toweling should be used. Dressings should be applied loosely and kept well soaked. One of the frequently used solutions is aluminum subacetate, or Burrows' solution, a mild astringent. To prevent increasing the concentration of the solution, water should be used to remoisten dried dressings.[9] When the patient is able to moisten the dressings, he or she may be given some of the solution or water and a syringe to keep the dressings moist. Though a nonporous material should be placed under the dressing to protect the bed, it should not be wrapped around the dressing. Interference with evaporation decreases heat loss and predisposes to elevating the temperature of the involved area. Before selecting material to protect the

[9] When a solution is used repeatedly to moisten the same dressings, the concentration of the solution increases. Water evaporates but the solute does not and its concentration therefore rises.

bed, the nurse should ascertain whether or not the patient is allergic to the material to be used.

Because most of the injury to the skin in allergic conditions is caused by scratching, every effort should be made to prevent and relieve the itching. The fingernails should be cut short. Sometimes the patient gets some relief by scratching the bed. Few symptoms are more unpleasant than itching. A patient with a severe dermatitis is likely to be irritable, because of being uncomfortable and having difficulty in obtaining rest and sleep. Whenever lotions or salves are applied to the skin in dermatitis, the nurse should observe the skin for signs of increasing irritation, that is, redness, swelling, or vesiculation, as some patients develop a sensitivity to the chemicals used in therapy.

Because contact dermatitis is likely to be a recurring problem, the patient should be taught to identify and to avoid agents in the environment to which he or she is sensitive. The patient should also be encouraged to institute palliative measures as soon as the characteristic lesions on the skin are noted. Scratching is to be avoided, as it excoriates the skin and predisposes to more itching as well as to infection. For many persons, contact dermatitis is a long-term problem. As in many other chronic disorders, control depends on the willingness and ability of the patient to carry out the preventive and therapeutic program.

OBJECTIVE 3. INCREASED RESISTANCE TO A SPECIFIC ANTIGEN

To increase the resistance of the patient to a specific antigen, the patient may be given small but increasing doses of an antigen over a period of time. The procedure for raising the resistance of the patient to a specific antigen is known as *hyposensitization.* In addition to the hyposensitization of a patient to foreign proteins, as previously discussed, some patients with hay fever benefit from being treated with offending pollens. Therapy is usually started 2 or 3 months before the expected onset of symptoms. They may be continued at 4-week intervals throughout the year. The injected antigen stimulates the formation of what is known as the blocking antibody. The blocking antibody is distinct from the preexisting sensitizing antibody. Increased tolerance for the antigen appears to be caused by the blocking antibody.

Knowledge of how hyposensitization to an allergen benefits the allergic patient is incomplete. Decreased sensitivity may in part be attributable to blocking antibodies, which are IgG immunoglobulins. Blocking antibodies are incomplete antibodies with the power to combine with antigen. They lack the ability to form insoluble antigen–antibody complexes.

Because emotional factors may predispose to, precipitate, perpetuate, or contribute to the development of complications, their significance in each patient requires evaluation. When emotional factors are of importance, the patient may require assistance in learning to identify situations aggravating the disorder and either avoid them or modify reaction to them. For example, Mrs. Cornwall usually develops an asthmatic attack when she smells, or imagines she smells, cigar smoke. Because the physician believes that emotional factors are probably involved in precipitating and prolonging Mrs. Cornwall's asthmatic attacks, he explores this possibility with her.

Summary

The discussion thus far has dealt with the immunologic tissue responses of the body, factors that incite them, and methods of predicting and controlling them. The capacity of the organism to produce antibodies is one of its mechanisms of defense against foreign invaders. It arises out of the capacity of the cells of the body to distinguish self from nonself. Steps in the immune response are schematically presented in Figure 24-3. As with other mechanisms of defense, immunologic responses are useful when they are initiated in response to truly harmful agents and in the amounts required by the situation. They are harmful when they are initiated in response to harmless substances or when the response is deficient or excessive. There is some evidence to support the theory that many chronic diseases may result from immunologic responses. Recent studies of immune responses are adding greatly to understanding this very important defense mechanism. This is a new and exciting field in medicine.

In the care of patients with the diseases of allergy, nurses have an opportunity to assist in the identification of agents that act as antigens, they care for patients during acute phases of illness, and they help to prepare the patient to live with his or her disorder.

Phagocytosis

Phagocytosis is a process whereby certain cells capture and ingest bacteria and other large particles such as tissue fragments and sometimes destroy them. See Figure 24-4 for a schematic illustration of the three ways in which phagocytosis of foreign substances by polymorphonuclear leukocytes

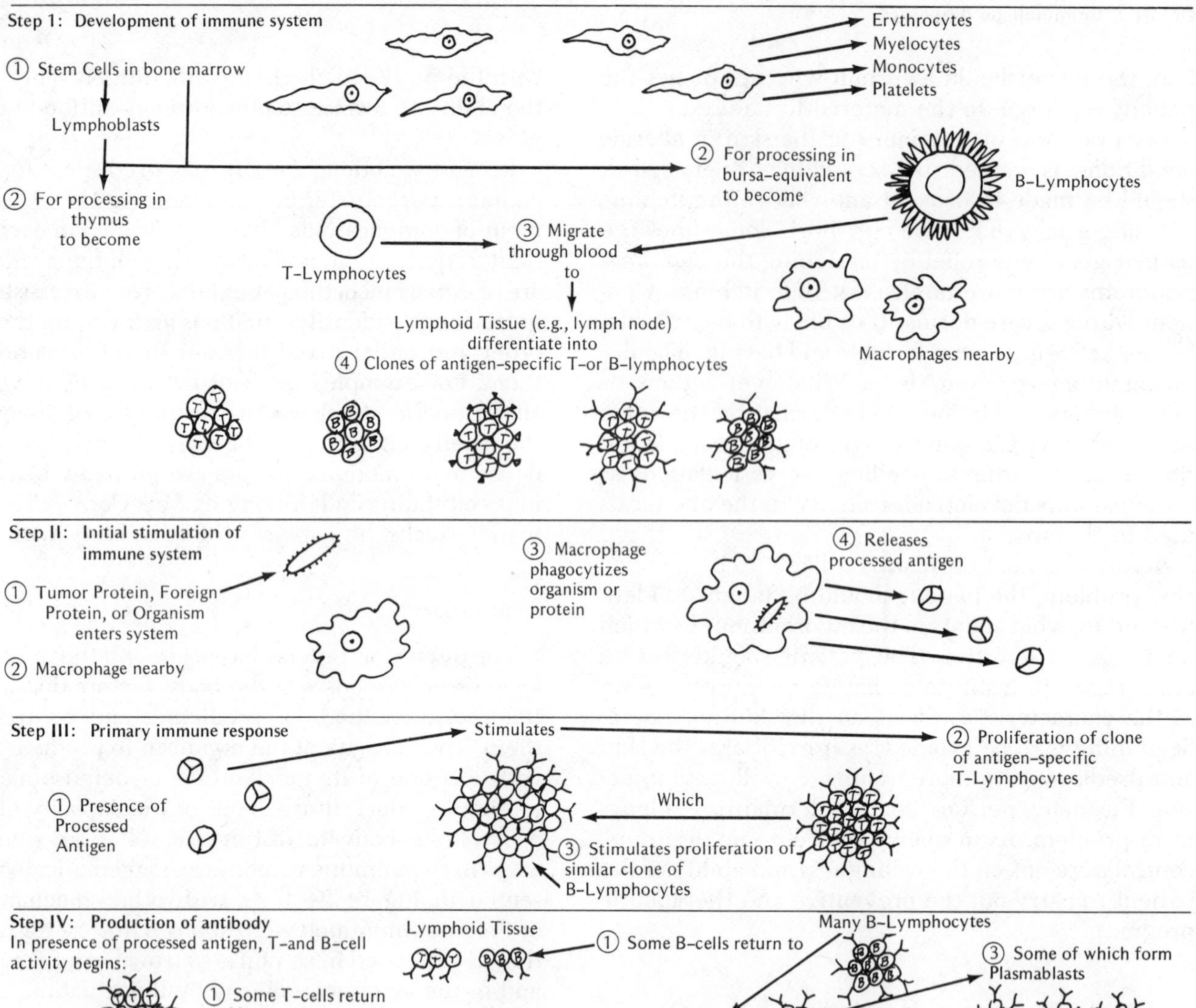

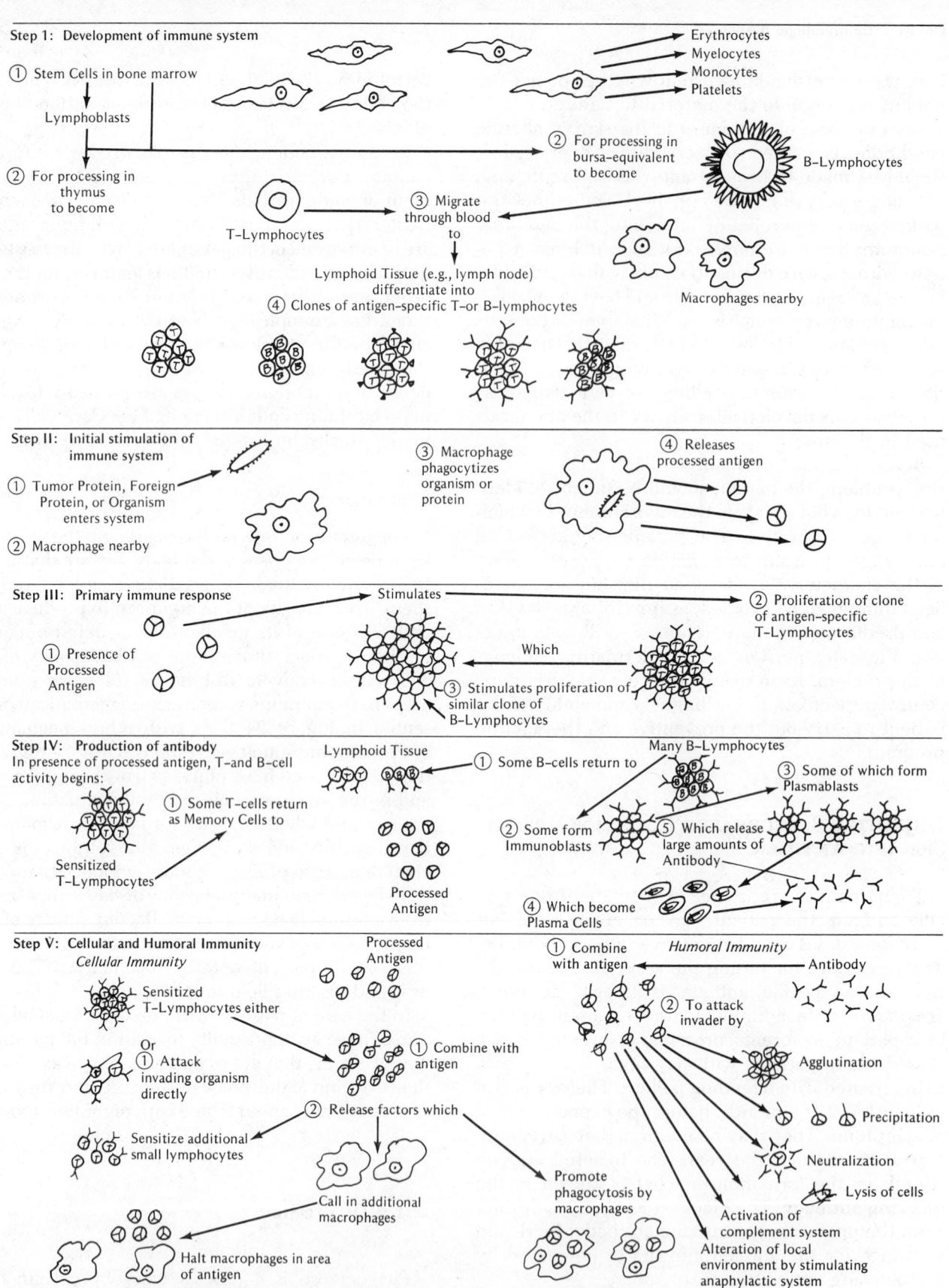

Figure 24-3. Steps in the immune response. (Adapted with permission of the American Journal of Nursing Company from The immune system: Its development and functions. *Am. J. Nurs.* 76:1614–18, Oct. 1976, by J. O. Nysather, A. E. Katz, & J. L. Lenth. Illustrated by F. Bozzo.)

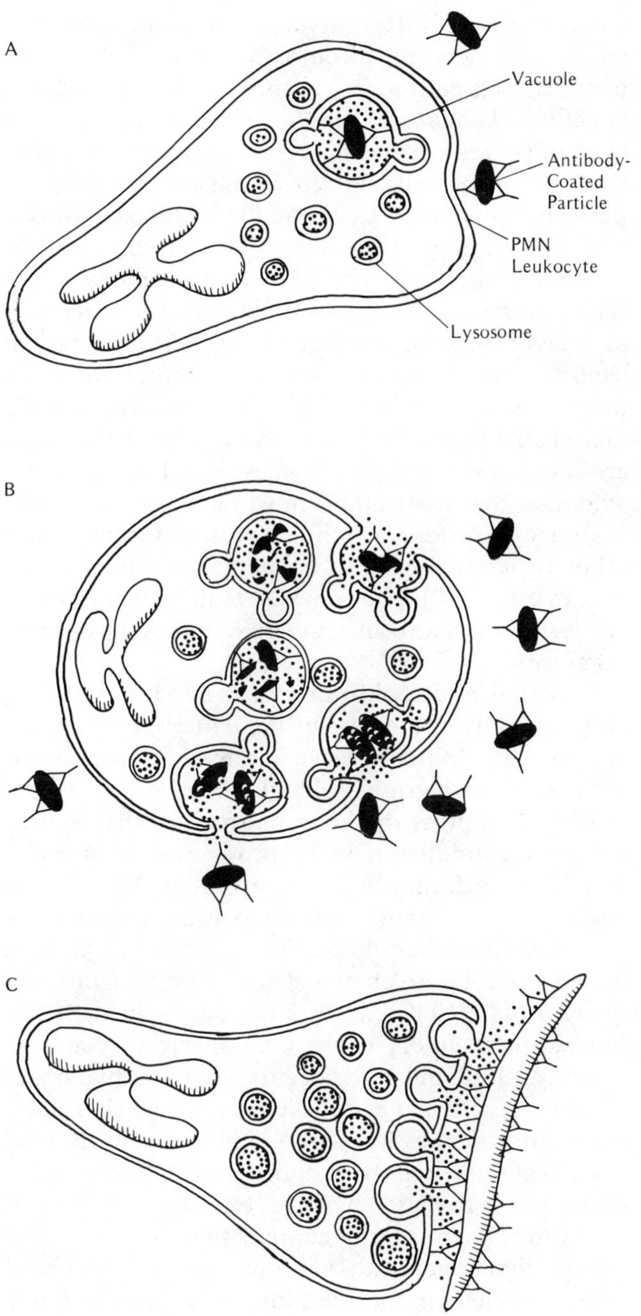

Figure 24-4. Phagocytosis of foreign substances by polymorphonuclear leukocytes (PMNs) can occur in three ways. Under "normal" conditions (i.e., a low particle-to-cell ratio) lysosomal enzymes are released into closed phagocytic vacuole (A). With high particle-to-cell ratio, release occurs before closure, with escape of enzymes into ambient area where they can damage tissues (B). Enzyme release also occurs when foreign body is too large for ingestion: PMN attaches to it and "bombards" it with enzymes (C). (Adapted with permission of Hospital Practice Publishing Co., Inc., from Leukocytes as secretory organs of inflammation. *Hosp. Practice* 13:53–62, Sept. 1978, Fig. 2, p. 55, by G. Weissmann.)

(PMNs) can occur. Some microbes escape from the phagocytes and may destroy them. Some survive and even multiply within the phagocyte. Sometimes the phagocyte acts as a vehicle to transport certain bacteria from one part of the body to another. For phagocytosis to occur, the particles must come in contact with the cell membranes. Globulin molecules called opsonins combine with particles and increase their likelihood of adhering to the phagocyte. After particles are ingested by the cells, lysosome granules within the cell break down and release digestive enzymes. This process of digestion requires the expenditure of energy. The utilization of glucose and oxygen goes up and the production of lactic acid rises. Attention to maintaining the nutritional state of the individual should help to support this extremely important defense mechanism.

Phagocytosis is one of the most important functions of white blood cells (leukocytes), which are the mobile units of the body's protective system. There are seven types of white blood cells (WBCs) normally found in the blood (Guyton, 1976, pp. 67–70).

Lymphocytes and plasma cells are critical to immunity, as discussed previously in this chapter; platelets activate the blood-clotting mechanism, and will be discussed in Chapter 42. Granulocytes (microphages), particularly the neutrophils, and monocytes (macrophages) are responsible for the important function of phagocytosis, and are further discussed here.

	Synonym or Precursor	Type of WBC
Phagocytic cells	Granulocyte = polymorphonuclear leukocyte = microcytic microphages	1. neutrophils 2. eosinophils 3. basophils
	Monocytes →	4. macrophages
		5. lymphocytes 6. plasma cells
	Megakaryocyte →	7. platelets

Macrophages

Phagocytic cells are classified according to size as macrophages and microphages, both of which are formed from the primitive reticuloendothelial stem cell, found in bone marrow, from which all blood cells are thought to arise. Macrophages are monocytic cells. They may be either fixed (stationary) or wandering. The fixed cells, tissue histiocytes, are permanently located in the interstitial tissues of the reticuloendothelial system. They are concentrated in the sinusoids of the liver (Kupffer's cells) and the spleen, the lung, the lymph nodes, and the blood vessels, particularly the veins. Apperly (1951) compared the fixed macrophages to the rural police, as they are scattered through the body at strategic points. They are highly phagocytic. They digest bacteria, foreign substances, worn-out red blood cells, and other cells, as well as remove certain dyes. They are also believed to form antibodies.

Macrophages are less numerous than the microphages but each cell has great phagocytic power. They are characteristic of chronic infection and the stage of resolution in acute infection. In chronic infection, macrophages fuse to form giant cells.

An interesting observation is that some species of bacteria, especially those causing chronic infections, may not only be transported by macrophages and multiply in them but may remain dormant for months or years. This may help to explain the development of immunity in diseases such as tularemia. The macrophage may also serve as a vehicle for the transport of some bacteria such as *M. tuberculosis.*

Microphages

Microphages are granulocytes also having their origin in the bone marrow. Of the three types of granulocytes, the neutrophils are the most abundant. They are much more numerous than the macrophages, but their phagocytic power is much less. During phagocytosis granulocytes can be seen to lose their granules. These granules contain phagocytin, a substance released into the phagocytic vacuoles, which contain bacteria. Following infection with certain types of bacteria or the death of tissue, a leukocytosis-promoting factor is released. This substance stimulates the bone marrow to release large numbers of microphages, particularly neutrophils. From a normal of 5,000 to 9,000 the number may rise as high as 20,000 to 30,000 cells per cubic mm of whole blood.

Neutrophils seem to be the body's first line of defense in combating infection and trauma. Neutrophils are thought to be drawn into the peripheral blood and toward the site of injury by products derived from necrotic tissue or bacteria. The process which impels cells to move from one area to another is called *chemotaxis.* All the granulocytes, as well as monocytes, are capable of active locomotion through vessel walls and through tissue. Neutrophils perform their protective function by phagocytosis—engulfment of particles and especially of bacteria. The neutrophils do not elaborate antibodies, but they transport enzymes which may be functional in phagocytosis. In phagocytizing certain types of bacteria, neutrophils require assistance of *opsonins,* the circulating antibodies which render the bacteria more liable to engulfment. Eosinophils and basophils are much less active in phagocytosis. There is some evidence that neutrophils must be present at a site of injury in order for lymphocytes, monocytes, and other reparative cells to be attracted subsequently (Widmann, 1973). The response to dead tissue is usually less than that to an acute infection by a pyogenic organism.

Although neutrophils are short-lived cells, living only, 3 or 4 days, the healthy bone marrow is capable of replacing them in large numbers. Some drugs, such as aminopyrine, sulfanilamide, and nitrogen mustards, depress the bone marrow, so that following their administration the production of granulocytes may be diminished or even absent. As discussed in Chapter 11, radioactive materials, including x-rays, have a similar effect. The capacity of the bone marrow to tolerate chemical and physical agents depressing its activity places a limitation on their use in treatment. Injury to the bone marrow by aminopyrine and sulfanilamide occurs when it is hypersensitive to a particular agent. Not all persons, therefore, experience depression of the bone marrow after ingestion of these agents. In contrast, nitrogen mustard and ionizing radiation have a cytotoxic effect on cells. The nitrogen mustards contain two or more alkyl groups that react with some of the constituents of cells. Radioactive materials injure the cells by ionizing substances within them. Though cells vary in sensitivity, all cells are injured when they receive a large enough dose of either type of agent.

When the number of neutrophils is markedly deficient, the condition is known as agranulocytosis. A better term would be *granulocytopenia.* Granulocytopenia is a serious disorder because the capacity of the person to protect himself or herself against microorganisms is impaired. Evidence of a loss of the capacity of tissues to protect themselves is seen as ulcerations in the mouth, pharynx, gastrointestinal tract, and vagina. When infection develops in the patient with agranulocytosis, the prognosis is very poor. Special precautions should be taken to protect these persons from infection.

Phagocytosis is not only an important mechanism of combating established disease, but it is important in preventing disease. In a healthy individual, the blood is highly efficient in destroying bacteria.

The effectiveness of phagocytosis is influenced by the structure of the tissues. Because dense tissues offer more opportunity for phagocytes to come in contact with bacteria or other foreign material than tissue spaces, phagocytosis is more efficient in them. Thus bacteria implanted in a solid tissue such as the gluteal muscle are more likely to be phagocytized than those placed in the peritoneal or pleural cavity.

As the frontiers of science illuminate more of the still dimly understood mechanisms of immunity, the nurse's role in supporting, or preventing a challenge to, the person's immunologic responses will undoubtedly expand.

References Cited

Amos, D. B. "Antigenicity and the Recognition of Foreignness." In *Davis-Christopher Textbook of Surgery,* 11th ed. Ed. by D. C. Sabiston. Philadelphia: W. B. Saunders Company, 1977, p. 464.

Apperly, F. L. *Patterns of Disease.* Philadelphia: J. B. Lippincott Company, 1951, p. 50.

Austen, K. F. "Introduction to Clinical Immunology." In *Harrison's Principles of Internal Medicine.* Ed. by G. W. Thorn et al. New York: McGraw-Hill Book Company, 1977, p. 386.

Cheesemen, S. H. et al. "Controlled Clinical Trial of Prophylactic Human-Leukocyte Interferon in Renal Transplantation." *N. Engl. J. Med.,* **300** (14 June 1979), 1345–49.

Crowle, A. J. "Delayed Hypersensitivity." *Sci. Am.,* **202** (April 1960), 129.

DiSaia, P. J. et al. *Synopsis of Gynecologic Oncology.* New York: John Wiley & Sons, Inc., 1975, pp. 328–33.

Edelman, G. M. "Antibody Structure and Molecular Immunology." *Science,* **180** (25 May 1973), 830–40.

Gerber, I. E. "Autoimmunity and the Aging Process." *Med. World News,* Special Issue on Geriatrics (1973), 16–19.

Gordon, B. L., II. *Essentials of Immunology,* 2nd ed. Philadelphia: F. A. Davis Company, 1974.

Guyton, A. C. *Textbook of Medical Physiology,* 5th ed. Philadelphia: W. B. Saunders Company, 1976.

Hall, J. G. "Effector Mechanisms in Immunity." *Lancet,* **1** (4 Jan. 1969), 27.

Hooks, J. J. et al. "Immune Interferon in the Circulation of Patients with Autoimmune Disease." *N. Engl. J. Med.,* **301** (5 July 1979), 5–8.

Janeway, C. A. "Progress in Immunology." *J. Pediat.,* **72** (June 1968), 886–87.

Jerne, N. K. "The Immune System." *Sci. Am.,* **229** (July 1973), 52–60.

Kunkel, H. G. "Introduction to Immune Disease." In *Cecil Textbook of Medicine,* 15th ed. Ed. by P. B. Beeson et al. Philadelphia: W. B. Saunders Company, 1979, p. 131.

Lerner, R. A. and Dixon, F. J. "The Human Lymphocyte as an Experimental Animal." *Sci. Am.,* **228** (June 1973), 82–91.

Maugh, T. H., II. "Tissue Cultures: Transplantation Without Immune Suppression. *Science,* **181** (7 Sept. 1973), 929–31.

Nysather, J. O. et al. "The Immune System: Its Development and Functions." *Am. J. Nurs.,* **76** (Oct. 1976), 1614–18.

Queng, J. T., and McGovern, J. P. "Acute Anaphylaxis." *Hosp. Med.,* **12** (Sept. 1976), 31–43.

Rose, N. R., Milgrom, F., and van Oss, C. J. *Principles of Immunology.* New York: Macmillan Publishing Co., Inc., 1973.

Russell, P. S., and Cosimi, A. B. "Transplantation." *N. Engl. J. Med.,* **301** (30 Aug. 1979), 470–79.

Schwartz, R. S. "Therapeutic Strategy in Clinical Immunology." *N. Engl. J. Med.,* **280** (13 Feb. 1969), 367–68.

"Science and the Citizen: Dual Immunology." *Sci. Am.,* **220** (Feb. 1969), 43.

Sherman, W. B. "Atopic Hypersensitivity." *Med. Clin. North Am.,* **49** (Nov. 1965), 1599.

Stiehm, E. R. "How to Spot the Child with Immunodeficiency." *Consultant,* **13** (Nov. 1973), 93–94.

Stroud, R. M. "Complement and Disease." *Postgrad. Med.,* **41** (April 1967), 387.

"Vitamin A May Enhance Immune Responses." *Med. World News,* **14** (14 Dec. 1973), 21.

Weissmann, G. "Leukocytes as Secretory Organs of Inflammation." *Hosp. Practice,* **13**:9 (Sept. 1978), 53–62.

Widmann, F. K. *Goodale's Clinical Interpretation of Laboratory Tests.* Philadelphia: F. A. Davis Company, 1973, p. 23.

General References

A Proposed Classification of Primary Immunologic Deficiencies." *Am. J. Med.,* **45** (Dec. 1968), 817–25.

Ammann, A. J., et al. "Thymus Transplantation: Permanent Reconstitution of Cellular Immunity." *N. Engl. J. Med.,* **289** (5 July 1973), 5–9.

Barnet, Sir M. *Self and Not-Self: Cellular Immunology.* New York: Cambridge University Press, 1969.

Benacerraf, B. "Suppressor T Cells and Suppressor Factor." *Hosp. Practice,* **13** (April 1978), 65–75.

Benacerraf, B., and McDevitt, H. O. "Histocompatibility—Linked Immune Response Genes." *Science,* **175** (21 Jan. 1972), 273–79.

Bretscher, P., and Cohn, M. "A Theory of Self–Nonself Discrimination." *Science,* **169** (11 Sept. 1970), 1042–49.

Bunting, F. W. "Immunity Against Infectious Diseases." *Nurs. Times,* **67** (27 May 1971), 634–36.

Code, C. F. "Reflections on Histamine, Gastric Secretion and the H_2 Receptor." *N. Engl. J. Med.,* **296** (23 June 1977), 1459–62.

Cohen, E. P. "On the Mechanism of Immunity—In Defense of Evolution." *Ann. Rev. Microbiol.*, **22** (1968), 283–304.

Craddock, C. G., Longmire, R., and McMillan, R. "Lymphocytes and the Immune Response." *N. Engl. J. Med.*, **285** (5 Aug. 1971), 324–30.

David, J. R. "Lymphocyte Mediators and Cellular Hypersensitivity." *N. Engl. J. Med.*, **288** (18 Jan. 1973), 143–49.

Dharan, M. "Immunoglobulin Abnormalities." *Am. J. Nurs.*, **76** (Oct. 1976), 1626–28.

Donley, D. L. "Nursing the Immunosuppressed Patient." *Am. J. Nurs.*, **76** (Oct. 1976), 1619–25.

Edelman, G. M. "The Structure and Function of Antibodies." *Sci. Am.*, **223** (Aug. 1970), 34–42.

Frohlich, E. D., ed. *Pathophysiology: Altered Regulatory Mechanisms in Disease.* Philadelphia: J. B. Lippincott Company, 1972.

Gewurz, H. "The Immunologic Role of Complement." *Hosp. Practice*, **2**:9 (Sept. 1967), 45–56.

Harkness, D. R. "Structure and Function of Immunoglobulins." *Postgrad. Med.*, **48** (Dec. 1970), 64–69.

"The Immunological Orchestra." *Lancet*, **1** (Jan. 27, 1968), 185–86.

Jacobs, S., and Cuatrecasas, P. "Cell Receptors in Disease." *N. Engl. J. Med.*, **297** (22 Dec. 1977), 1383–86.

Janeway, C. A. et al. *The Gamma Globulins.* Boston: Little, Brown and Company, 1967.

Lischner, H. W., and DiGeorge, A. M. "Role of Thymus in Humoral Immunity." *Lancet*, **2** (15 Nov. 1969), 1044–48.

Mackaness, G. B. "Cell-Mediated Immunity to Infection." *Hosp. Practice*, **5** (Sept. 1970), 73–77, 82–86.

Mayer, M. M. "The Complement System." *Sci. Am.*, **229** (Nov. 1973), 54–66.

Marx, J. L. "Interferon (I): On the Threshold of Clinical Application." *Science*, **204** (15 June 1979), 1183–86.

McIntyre, P. A. "Visualization of the Reticuloendothelial System." *Hosp. Practice*, **6** (July 1971), 77–80, 84–87.

Movat, H. Z. ed. *Inflammation, Immunity, and Hypersensitivity.* New York: Harper & Row, Publishers, Inc., 1971.

Müller-Eberhard, H. J. "Complement Abnormalities in Human Disease." *Hosp. Practice*, **13**:12 (Dec. 1978), 65–76.

Newhouse, M. et al. "Lung Defense Mechanisms." *N. Engl. J. Med.*, **295** (28 Oct. 1976), 990–98.

Notkins, A. L., and Koprowski, H. "How the Immune Response to a Virus Can Cause Disease." *Sci. Am.*, **228** (Jan. 1973), 22–31.

Parkman, R. et al. "Graft-Versus-Host Disease after Transfusions for Hemolysis in Newborns." *N. Engl. J. Med.*, **290** (14 Feb. 1974), 359–63.

Peterson, R. D. A. "Tissue Immunity and Tissue Typing." *Med. Clin. North Am.*, **54** (Jan. 1970), 43–58.

Plaut, A. G. "Microbial IgA Proteases." *N. Engl. J. Med.*, **298** (29 June 1978), 1459–63.

Prockop, D. J., and Guzman, N. A. "Collagen Diseases and the Biosynthesis of Collagen." *Hosp. Practice*, **12** (Dec. 1977), 61–68.

Rose, N. R., Milgrom, F., and van Oss, C. J. *Principles of Immunology.* New York: Macmillan Publishing Co., Inc., 1973.

Rosenburg, L. E., and Kidd, K. K. "HLA and Disease Susceptibility: A Primer." *N. Engl. J. Med.*, **297** (10 Nov. 1977), 1060–62.

Schatz, M., et al. "Immunologic Lung Disease." *N. Engl. J. Med.*, **300** (7 June 1979), 1310–20.

Siegal, F. P. "Suppressors in the Network of Immunity." *N. Engl. J. Med.*, **298** (12 Jan. 1978), 102–3.

Smith, D. W. "Survivors of Serious Illness." *Am. J. Nurs.*, **79** (March 1979), 440–46.

Vaisrub, S. "Nature's Experiment in Unnatural Aging." *JAMA*, **226** (24–31 Dec. 1973), 1565.

Walker, W. A., and Isselbacher, K. J. "Intestinal Antibodies." *N. Engl. J. Med.*, **297** (6 Oct. 1977), 767–72.

White, J. F. "Teaching Patients to Manage Systemic Lupus Erythematosus." *Nurs. 78*, **8**:9 (Sept. 1978), 26–34.

Wiener, A. S. "Histo-Compatibility, Immunodepression, and Immunologic Tolerance. *Med. Opinion Rev.*, **6** (March 1970), 70–75.

General References

Immunosuppression and Transplantation

Abouna, G. M. et al. "Massive Early Proteinuria Following Renal Homotransplantation." *JAMA*, **226** (5 Nov. 1973), 631–35.

Bach, F. H., and van Rood, J. J. "The Major Histocompatibility Complex—Genetics and Biology." *N. Engl. J. Med.*, **295** (1976), 806–813; 872–878; 927–936.

Barnard, C. N. "Heterotopic Versus Orthotopic Heart Transplantation." *Transplant Proc.*, **8** (1976), 15–19.

Batchelor, J. R., and Hackett, M. "HL-A Matching in Treatment of Burned Patients with Skin Allografts." *Lancet*, **2** (1970), 581–83.

Blumenstock, D. A. "Lung Transplantation Update." *Transplant Proc.*, **9** (1977), 1641–64.

Burke, J. F., May, J. W. Jr., Albright, N., et al. "Temporary Skin Transplantation and Immunosuppression for Extensive Burns." *N. Engl. J. Med.*, **290** (1974), 269–71.

Calne, R. Y. "Hepatic Transplantation." *Surg. Clin. North Am.*, **58** (1978), 321–33.

Calne, R. Y., Thiru, S., McMaster, P., et al. "Cyclosporin A in Patients Receiving Renal Allografts from Cadaver Donors." *Lancet*, **2** (1978), 1323–27.

Cantor, H., and Boyse, E. A. "Lymphocytes as Models for the Study of Mammalian Differentiation." *Immunol. Rev.*, **33** (1977), 105–24.

Cooper, K. D., Abrams, C. L., and Blagg, C. R. "The Potential of Cadaveric Kidneys for Transplantation." *Trans. Am. Soc. Artif. Intern. Organs*, **23** (1977), 416–20.

Cosimi, A. B., Burke, J. F., and Russell, P. S. "Transplantation of Skin." *Surg. Clin. North Am.*, **58** (1978), 435–51.

Cosimi, A. B., Delmonico, F. L., Burdick, J. F., et al. "Individualized Management of Immunosuppression According to Serial Monitoring of Immunocompetence." *Transplant Proc.*, **10** (1978), 647–50.

Dandavino, R., Trunet, P., Descamps, B., et al. "Prolonged Withdrawal of Azathioprine in Kidney Transplantation." *Transplant Proc.*, **10** (1978), 655–57.

Griepp, R. B. "A Decade of Human Heart Transplantation." *Transplant Proc.*, **11** (1977) 285–92.

Groczynski, R. M., Macrae, S., and Till, J. E. "Analysis of Mechanisms of Maintenance of Neonatally Induced Tolerance to Foreign Alloantigens." *Scand. J. Immunol.*, **7** (1978), 453–65.

Gunnarsson, R., Groth, C. G., Bottazzo, G. F., et al. "Islet Autoantibodies in Human Pancreatic Transplant Recipients." *Lancet*, **1** (1979), 926.

Hardy, J. D. "Surgical Management of Cushing's Syndrome with Emphasis on Adrenal Autotransplantation." *Ann. Surg.*, **188** (1978), 290–307.

"The HLA System." Ed. by W. F. Bodmen. *Br. Med. Bull.*, **34** (1978) 213–316.

Jamieson, S. M., Stinson, E. B., and Shumway, N. E. "Cardiac Transplantation in 150 Patients at Stanford University." *Br. Med. J.*, **1** (1979), 93–95.

Jonasson, O. "Transplantation of the Pancreas, 1978." *Transplant Proc.*, **11** (1979), 325–330.

Kaplan, S. R., and Calabresi, P. "Immunosuppressive Agents." *N. Engl. J. Med.*, **289** (6 Dec. 1973), 1234–36.

Lafferty, K. J., and Woolnough, J. "The Origin and Mechanism of the Allograft Reaction." *Immunol. Rev.*, **35** (1977), 231–62.

Langer, F., Gross, A. E., West, M., et al. "The Immunogenicity of Allograft Knee Joint Transplants." *Clin. Orthop.*, **132** (1978), 155–162.

Lernmark, A., Freedman, Z. R., Hofmann, C., et al., "Islet-Cell-Surface Antibodies in Juvenile Diabetes Mellitus." *N. Engl. J. Med.*, **299** (1978), 375–80.

Lower, R. R. "Is Heart Transplantation a Realistic Approach to Inoperable Heart Disease?" *Cardiovasc. Clin.*, **8** (1977), 319–22.

Moore, F. D., Burch, G. E., Harken, D. E., et al. "Cardiac and Other Organ Transplantation: In the Setting of Transplant Service as a National Effort." *JAMA*, **206** (1968), 2489–2500.

Powles, R. L., Barrett, A. J., Clink, H., et al. "Cyclosporin A for the Treatment of Graft-Versus-Host Disease in Man." *Lancet*, **2** (1978), 1327–31.

Reemtsma, K., Drusin, R., Edie, R., et al. "Cardiac Transplantation for Patients Requiring Mechanical Circulatory Support." *N. Engl. J. Med.*, **298** (1978), 670–71.

Rowley, D. A., Fitch, F. W., Stuart, F. B., Kohler, H., and Cosenza, H. "Specific Suppression of Immune Responses." *Science*, **181** (21 Sept. 1973), 1133–40.

Sade, R. M., Ballenger, J. F., Hohn, A. R., et al. "Cardiac Valve Replacement in Children: Comparison of Tissue with Mechanical Prosthesis." *J. Thorac. Cardiovasc. Surg.*, **78** (1979), 123–27.

Slavin, S., Reitz, B., Bieber, C. P., et al. "Transplantation Tolerance in Adult Rats Using Total Lymphatic Irradiation: Permanent Survival of Skin, Heart, and Marrow Allografts." *J. Exp. Med.*, **147** (1978), 700–7.

Starzl, T. E., Koep, L. J., Halgrimson, C. G., et al. "Liver Transplantation—1978." *Transplant Proc.*, **11** (1979), 240–46.

"Thank You for My Life." *Newsweek*, 16 Oct. 1972, pp. 72–73.

Thomas, F., Mendez-Picon, G., Thomas, J., et al. "Effect of Antilymphocyte–Globulin Potency on Survival of Cadaver Renal Transplant: Prospective Randomized Double-Blind Trial." *Lancet*, **2** (1977), 671–74.

Thompson, R., Knight, E., Ahmed, M., et al. "The Use of 'Fresh' Unstented Homograft Valves for Replacement of the Aortic Valve: Analysis of 6½ Years Experience." *Circulation*, **56** (1977), 837–40.

Wells, S. A., Jr., Stirman, J. A., Jr., Bolman, R. M., III, et al. "Transplantation of the Parathyroid Glands: Clinical and Experimental Results." *Surg. Clin. North Am.*, **59** (1978), 391–402.

Wood, C., Downing, B., McKenzie, I., et al. "Microvascular Transplantation of the Human Fallopian Tube." *Fertil. Steril.*, **29** (1978), 607–13.

Zinkernagel, R. M. "Major Transplantation Antigens in Host Responses to Infection." *Hosp. Practice*, **13** (July 1978), 83–92.

Allergic Responses

Bridgewater, S. C., and Voignier, R. R. "Allergies in Children." *Am. J. Nurs.*, **78** (April 1978), 613–21.

Cannon, P. J. "Antihistamines." *Practitioner*, **200** (Jan. 1968), 53–64.

Dave, V. K. "Contact Dermatitis." *Nurs. Times*, **67** (29 April 1971), 504–6.

Feinberg, S. M. "Allergies and Air Conditioning." *Am. J. Nurs.*, **66** (June 1966), 1333–36.

Hawkins, K. "Wet Dressings: Putting the Damper on Dermatitis." *Nurs. 78*, **8**:2 (Feb. 1978), 64–67.

Lockey, R. F., and Fox, R. W. "Allergic Emergencies." *Hosp. Med.*, **15** (June 1979), 64–78.

Saunders, N. A., and McFadden, E. R., Jr. "Asthma—An Update." *Dis.-a-Month*, **24**:11 (Aug. 1978).

Slavin, R. G. "Asthma in Adults. III. Occupational Asthma." *Hosp. Practice*, **13** (June 1978), 133–46.

Wanderer, A. A. "An 'Allergy' to Cold." *Hosp. Practice*, **14**:6 (June 1979), 136–37.

Wieczorek, R. R., and Horner-Rosner, B. "The Asthmatic Child: Preventing and Controlling Attacks. *Am. J. Nurs.*, **79** (Feb. 1979), 258–62.

25

Local Responses—Inflammation and Wound Healing

If the other person injures you, you may forget the injury; but if you injure him, you will always remember.

KAHLIL GIBRAN

Inflammation

To this point, the body defenses involving the body as a whole have been discussed. In addition to these responses, cells at the site of injury also react to injury in a characteristic and more or less stereotyped fashion. Similar to the more widespread responses, the local reactions to injury serve to limit the area of injury, to prepare the area for repair, and finally to replace the damaged tissue. Because inflammation is one of the most common responses of the body to injury, knowledge of the mechanisms involved in inflammation provides a basis for understanding the changes that occur in a wide variety of infectious and noninfectious diseases. Essentially the response of the tissue injured by an antigen–antibody reaction is one of inflammation. Even in those conditions in which inflammation is not considered to be an aspect of the disease, it may play a role. For example, in some patients who have cancer the body responds to the neoplastic cells (new growth cells) much as it does to a foreign body, with the result that surrounding tissues are inflamed.

Inflammation may be defined as *an active and aggressive response of tissue to injury.* It involves the blood vessels, fluid and cellular components of the blood, and surrounding connective tissue. It is a useful response because it serves to destroy or neutralize the injurious agent and to prepare the tissue for repair. Inflammation may cause harmful effects by virtue of its location or by an ineffective, excessive, or inappropriate response.

Progress in understanding the acute inflammatory process has been uneven and sometimes delayed by false steps and interpretations. In the first century, Celsus described the four cardinal signs of inflammation as rubor (redness), calor (heat), dolor (pain), and tumor (swelling). It was not until almost the end of the eighteenth century that John Hunter first established inflammation as a mechanism of defense. Cohnheim, a student of Virchow, recognized the part that blood vessels play in inflammation. He also described the margination and emigration of leukocytes. The part played by the leukocytes in phagocytosis was established by the Russian zoologist Metchnikoff when his study of inflammation was published in 1901. Though knowledge of the biochemical changes in the inflammatory process was, and still is, incomplete, the discoveries of Metchnikoff established an understanding of the fundamental nature of the process. With the development of electron microscopy and the rabbit's ear chamber, knowledge of the process has been further expanded.

CAUSES

Despite a tendency to think of inflammation as a response initiated primarily by microbes, it can be induced by any agent causing injury to tissue cells. Only a few of the possible causative agents will be discussed. Essentially they all act to injure tissue cells. The surrounding tissue then responds with inflammation. How the various types of agents injure cells was presented in Unit III. Physical agents that are common initiators of the inflammatory process are heat, cold, radiant rays including ultraviolet and infrared rays, radioactive rays, and trauma.

Chemical agents also act as irritants. They may be either extrinsic or intrinsic in origin or result from a combination of the two. Examples of extrinsic chemical irritants include strong acids and bases, insect bites, allergens, and the toxins manufactured by microorganisms. Chemical irritants of intrinsic origin are substances that are produced in the body. They may be normal substances, such as pancreatic juice that escapes from the gastrointestinal tract and comes in contact with tissues not protected from the digesting actions of its enzymes. Large areas of necrosis of the abdominal wall may occur in those who have the misfortune to have a fistulous tract from the small intestine to the surface of the body.

Perhaps the most common example of a body fluid that is "out of place" is blood. The body responds to blood that escapes into tissue from a break in a blood vessel as it does to a foreign body. Frequently soreness is the first sign of bleeding into a tissue. Soreness at the site of an intramuscular injection may result from the rupture of a small blood vessel during the insertion of a needle. Bruises caused by bumping furniture or other hard objects often pass unnoticed for a day or so and then come to attention because the area is painful.

Inflammation also develops in the tissue surrounding dead or necrotic tissue. In the degeneration of the dead tissue, products are formed that act as irritants. When the death of tissue is caused by the loss of its blood supply, the necrotic area may also serve as as site for the development of infection. The tissue, robbed of its blood supply, is no longer able to supply phagocytes to control microorganisms in the area. They are therefore able to establish themselves and grow and multiply in the tissue. For example, following infarction caused by the obstruction of a branch of the pulmonary artery by an embolus, Mr. Ash developed pneumonia. The original focus for the infection was in the infarcted tissue.

Products of metabolism may also act as irritants. They may be abnormal either in quantity or in kind or in the manner in which the body handles them. In gout, because of a defect in the metabolism of purines, uric acid crystals accumulate in the tissues about joints. The resulting inflammatory process is exceedingly painful. Because, according to folklore, gout is the result of high living, which it is not, persons who develop gout are often subjected to cruel jokes and ridicule.

Among other causes of inflammation are antigen–antibody reactions and neoplasms. From the preceding it is evident that a wide variety of agents can indeed initiate the inflammatory response.

Whatever the stimulus to inflammation, the characteristic physiologic events are believed to be mediated by one or more of the following chemicals elaborated by injured cells: histamine, 5-hydroxytryptamine (known also as 5-HT and serotonin), the kinins, slow-reacting substance in anaphylaxis (SRS-A), immunoglobulins, serum complement, and, most recently, prostaglandins.[1] Several investigators have hypothesized that prostaglandins participate in the regulation of inflammation by feedback inhibition, being inflammatory at low concentrations and antiinflammatory at higher concentrations (Prostaglandins, 1972).

Role of Blood Vessels

In the study of inflammation in the laboratory, immediately following the application of an irritant, blood vessels may be seen to constrict momentarily. Constriction is extremely transitory and is of no consequence. Following constriction, arterioles, then venules, and finally capillaries dilate, and more blood vessels come into view. Blood flows rapidly through the vessels and the tissue becomes bright red. This active increase in the flow of blood is known as hyperemia.

Associated with the greater blood flow is an increase in the filtration pressure of the blood and in the permeability of the capillaries with the result that a large volume of fluid, known as the inflammatory exudate, is moved into the interstitial space. In minor injuries, the increase in capillary permeability may be small so that little extra fluid escapes into the injured area. Neither is there an increase in the rate at which larger molecules in the blood plasma diffuse from the blood into the injured area. In more severe injuries, large molecules, most particularly proteins, escape into the inflammatory exudate in increased quantities. The effects of this loss of protein are not serious when the inflamed area is small. However, when the area is large, or when the loss continues over an extended period of time, the consequences may be serious. As an illustration, the patient who is burned may lose enormous quantities of proteins as well as of water and electrolytes into the burned area. Moreover, the absorption of chemicals released at the site of the burned or in-

[1] Prostaglandins are a group of hormonelike substances found in nearly all body tissues that participate in numerous processes in the human body. They are classified on the basis of their structure as E, F, A, or B (PGE_1, PGF, and so on).

jured tissue may increase the permeability of capillaries, throughout the body causing a generalized edema. Loss of fluid leads to a decrease in blood volume and concentration of the blood in the patient.

The extent to which fluid escapes into the tissue of the patient who has been burned can be illustrated by Mr. All. Examination of the intake and output record reveals that during the first 48 hours after he was burned the ratio of his fluid intake to output was 13,000 ml to 2,000 ml. Even when another 2,000 ml is added to his output to account for fluid lost by other avenues, he still lost at least 10 liters of fluid into the burned area. In addition to water, he lost protein and electrolytes. Human blister fluid contains about 4 g of protein per 100 ml of fluid. Because serum albumin is smaller in molecular size than the other blood proteins, a higher proportion of albumin is lost into the inflammatory exudate than of either globulin or fibrinogen.

The increase in filtration pressure plus the greater permeability of the capillaries upsets the balance between the quantity of fluid leaving the capillary and the quantity returning, in favor of the fluid escaping from the capillaries. The disequilibrium is further aggravated by the loss of protein from the blood plasma to the interstitial fluid. As protein is added to interstitial fluid, it increases its colloid osmotic pressure. When the quantity lost from the blood is large, the level of protein in the blood falls and with it the colloid osmotic pressure of the blood. The three factors contributing in varying degrees to the production of the inflammatory exudate may therefore be summarized as (1) the elevation of the filtration pressure of the blood, (2) the increased permeability of the capillaries, and (3) the increase in the colloid osmotic pressure of the tissue fluid in the area. The result is inflammatory edema. (See Chapter 11 for further discussion of edema.)

Dilatation

As is often true, it is easier to describe what happens than to explain why it happens. However, the current explanation is that on injury cells release a chemical or chemicals acting either directly or reflexly to dilate the blood vessels and to increase their permeability. Sir Thomas Lewis first described such a substance, which, because of its similarity to histamine, he called the H-substance. Menkin (1956) isolated a substance from the inflammatory exudate that he called *leukotaxine.*[2] It increases capillary permeability and in addition attracts leukocytes. Despite the ability of many chemicals to increase capillary permeability, convincing evidence that they are primarily responsible in inflammation is lacking.

Slowing of Blood Flow

During the early phase of the inflammatory reaction, the blood moves rapidly through the tissues. Later, depending on the severity of the injury, blood flow slows. The factors contributing to slowing include (1) the increased concentration of the blood in the capillaries that results from the loss of fluid into the inflamed area, (2) the increase in tissue fluid pressure that counteracts the increase in filtration pressure of the blood, and (3) possibly increased resistance to the flow of blood by the blood cells that adhere to the vascular endothelium.

With the slowing of the flow of blood, cells, especially the leukocytes, settle out of the main stream and line the vascular endothelium. This is known as the *pavementing of leukocytes.* Normally, the blood cells are carried in the axial stream with the leukocytes in the center and the smaller cells or erythrocytes surrounding them. The erythrocytes are separated from the vascular epithelium by a layer of plasma. In the inflammatory process, red cells tend to adhere together in clumps (blood sludge) that are larger than the leukocytes. They replace the leukocytes in the center of the stream. The leukocytes migrate peripherally, adhere to and enter the capillary wall, and pass between the endothelial cells by a process known as *emigration.* Because leukocytes accumulate in the injured area, they were believed to be attracted to the site by a process known as *chemotaxis.* Why they accumulate is questioned, as continuous observation shows that they move about at random.

Retardation of the blood flow may be so great that the blood moves forward only when the heart is contracting. This is one cause of a throbbing sensation. As long as some blood flow to the tissues is maintained, the process may be reversed and the tissues restored with little or no permanent harm. Blood flow, however, may be stopped by the formation of blood clots (thrombosis) in small vessels and by the pressure of inflammatory edema. Swelling caused by inflammatory edema is a particular hazard in tissues that have little space for distention, such as the brain or an extremity encased in a bandage or plaster cast. As the inflammatory edema increases, pressure on the small blood vessels increases, thereby decreasing their capacity to carry blood. The problem is aggravated by the fact that the venous return is restricted first, so that as blood continues to enter the tissue it adds to the swelling. Unless

[2] *Leukotaxine* is a cell-free nitrogenous material prepared from injured, acutely degenerating tissue and from inflammatory exudates.

the condition is corrected, tissue pressure eventually exceeds the arterial pressure and the blood flow to the tissue ceases. When an extremity is involved, swelling, pain, numbness and tingling, bluish discoloration of the skin, coldness, and inability to move the part are warning signs. When the brain is affected, signs of increasing intracranial pressure develop. (These are discussed in Chapter 36.) Proper elevation of the extremity encased in a cast will often support the venous return enough to prevent excessive swelling.

To illustrate, Mrs. Willow suffered a fractured tibia in a traffic accident. The fracture was reduced and the leg was encased in a cast. She was placed in a bed in which the mattress was slightly depressed at the foot of the bed. A nurse found her crying with pain and begging for a "shot." Instead of administering medication, the nurse examined Mrs. Willow's toes and found them to be cold and swollen. She could move her toes only with difficulty. The nurse then elevated Mrs. Willow's leg so that gravity aided the venous return.[3] She also told Mrs. Willow that she expected that her pain would be relieved shortly by the elevation of her foot and leg, but if it was not, she would call her physician and obtain a prescription for a pain-relieving medication. Should elevation fail to relieve the pain, the physician would also be apprised of this fact, as the cast might have to be cut to relieve the pressure. In about half an hour the nurse returned to see Mrs. Willow. She was comfortable and about to begin eating her breakfast. Her toes were warm and she could wiggle them.

Role of Cellular Elements

Neutrophils

The cells playing an active role in the acute inflammatory process have phagocytic action. Of these the neutrophils are most important in acute inflammation, as described previously. Both eosinophils and basophils transport significant amounts of histamine, the eosinophils carrying the larger portion. Despite their frequent temporal and spatial association with allergic responses, the role of eosinophils in the etiology or manifestations of allergic reactions is unclear, nor is it clear why eosinophils disappear promptly from the blood following injection of certain adrenal steroids (Widmann, 1973, p. 24). Function of basophils is not well understood, but they appear to play a role in heparin and histamine metabolism (Brobeck, 1973, pp. 4–62). The neutrophil plays an important role in inflammation, both when it is alive and after it dies. It is actively phagocytic when alive; that is, it ingests, kills, and digests microbes and their foreign material. After it dies it releases proteolytic enzymes that digest not only other dead cells and bacteria but itself. Thus neutrophils aid not only in overcoming the injurious agent but also in ridding the area of debris. The latter process is an essential step in the preparation of the tissue for healing. As neutrophils and macrophages are themselves destroyed as they phagocytize particulate matter, they release *endogenous pyrogen,* a substance which has a direct effect on the hypothalamic thermostat to increase its setting to febrile levels (Guyton, 1976, p. 966). Thus, the neutrophil contributes not only to the local reaction but to the total response of the individual.

[3] The nurse applied the second law of thermodynamics in which it is stated that energy runs downhill.

Macrophages

Both fixed and wandering macrophages have a number of important functions in inflammation. They act as scavengers. They phagocytize foreign bodies, cellular debris, and the more resistant organisms, such as *Mycobacterium tuberculosis* and fungi. They are called on to remove such substances as silica, talc, mineral oil, and sutures. They are essential to the reaction in tuberculosis as they form the epithelioid cells. They fuse to form giant cells, which are also found in the tubercle (the specific lesion of tuberculosis). They are necessary to the formation of fibrous connective tissue as they mature into fibroblasts.

Lymphocytes

The lymphocyte is the second most abundant leukocyte. It is smaller than the granulocyte and has a large nucleus with relatively little cytoplasm. It does not appear to be phagocytic to particulate matter.

As indicated in the discussion of immunity, lymphocytes play a role in immunologic responses. Small lymphocytes conditioned by the thymus recognize and are responsible for immunologic memory. Some authorities suggest that plasma cells originate from lymphocytes. It will be remembered that the plasma cells are the most active cells in the production of immunoglobulins.

Summarizing the role of leukocytes in the inflammation, leukocytes are essential to the inflammatory response. They function by phagocytosis (ingestion, killing, and digestion) of foreign bodies, bacteria, and the products of inflammation. Some of them form antibodies. Macrophages not only have a high phagocytic power, and form antibodies, but they contribute to the repair of the damage by maturing into fibroblasts and forming collagen. Without the power of phagocytosis the organism is at the mercy of any foreign invader. Not only do leukocytes increase in number in the injured area, but the number in the circulating blood is usually increased in all but minor injuries. The leukocyte count may reach 30,000 cells per cubic millimeter of blood[4] or rise even higher in severe systemic reactions to infection or tissue injury. In acute inflammation, the rise is usually in the neutrophils, particularly in the less mature forms. As neutrophils mature the nucleus undergoes segmentation; therefore the percentage of segmented cells drops when the number of neutrophils rises rapidly. In a few infections such as acute infectious mononucleosis and whooping cough, the lymphocyte count rises.

The number of leukocytes may also fall (leukopenia) in a number of infections. Infections in which this is true include typhoid fever, brucellosis, and malaria. As stated earlier, the count may be depressed in overwhelming infections or in any condition having a toxic effect on the bone marrow.

The reasons for leukocytosis are not known. It occurs not only in acute bacterial infections, such as pneumonia, but in conditions in which there is death of tissue, such as myocardial infarction and advanced malignant neoplasia. With leukocytosis there is often an associated increase in the sedimentation rate. The degree of increase in leukocyte count or sedimentation rate provides clues to the severity but not to the specific nature of the illness. Whether or not the level of the leukocytosis is in keeping with the apparent severity of illness is also significant. The obviously sick patient with a falling leukocyte count has a poor prognosis, for it indicates that the response of the patient is inadequate to the degree of illness.[5]

[4] Normal leukocyte (WBC) count is 4,000 to 11,000 cells per mm^3 of blood in the average adult (Widmann, 1973, p. 476).

[5] One of the most useful bits of objective data to include in initial and ongoing patient assessment is the report of hematologic examination of WBCs, including the differential count of (1) granulocytes, usually referred to as "polys," or PMNs, for polymorphonuclear leukocytes, and (2) lymphocytes; both are reported as a percentage of the total number of WBCs. Comparison of the patient's values with the range of normal, combined with close observation of the patient, provide a core of evidence for evaluating the inflammatory or immunologic response of the patient.

Differential WBC Count PMNs (Granulocytes)	Normal Range* (as % of WBCs)
Neutrophils	56.0
Eosinophils	2.7
Basophils	3.0
Lymphocytes	34.0

* Values as reported by Tilkian, S. M. et al. *Clinical Implications of Laboratory Tests,* 2nd ed. St. Louis: The C. V. Mosby Company, 1979, pp. 53–54.

Summary

In the preceding pages, the nature of the changes taking place in the blood vessels and in the blood cells occurring in inflammation have been considered. These changes have two purposes: (1) to destroy or localize the injuring agent and (2) to prepare the tissue for repair.

The dilatation and increased permeability of the blood vessels bring fluid to the area that contains antibodies and other substances to neutralize the toxins or to destroy the irritant. This fluid also dilutes the toxins and helps to restore homeostatic conditions by reducing the hydrogen ion concentration. It contains nutrients required for the release of energy and for the repair of cells. The leukocytes in the exudate phagocytose and destroy the irritant and the cellular debris.

Sequence of Events Following Tissue Injury

The early changes that have been discussed proceed somewhat as follows: The tissue is injured by an inflammant—heat, cold, radiant rays, chemicals, trauma, microorganisms, antigen–antibody reaction, or some combination thereof. Almost immediately the blood vessels in the area dilate and capillary permeability increases. The extent to which these changes take place depends on the severity of the injury. Blood flow increases and there is an outpouring of fluid containing protein and leukocytes. The polymorphonuclear leukocytes are concentrated around the irritant. When the inflammatory response is initiated by bacteria able to reproduce themselves, the bacteria may at first overcome the leukocytes. Leukocytes, however, are poured into the area and eventually they turn the tide in favor of the body. In the process, however, tissue cells, bacteria, and leukocytes are killed.

Abscess Formation

Fibrinogen that escapes from the blood is converted to fibrin.[6] It forms a meshwork in the area.

[6] The availability of fibrinogen as an element in the body's protective inflammatory response can be a source of injury when used inappropriately. Researchers at the immunopathology unit of Massachusetts General Hospital have identified at least two types of neoplastic cells that appear to use the body's own defense mechanisms as camouflage to evade detection and control. These cancer cells produce a protective gelatinous cocoon by extracting fibrinogen from blood vessels, which the tumor converts to the fibrin gel cocoon. As the tumor expands, it produces material to convert plasminogen into a very active enzyme which dissolves the fibrin closest to the tumor, thus creating space for growth. This process turns the body's own defense mechanisms to the advantage of the disease. Successful treatment may involve giving anticoagulants (see Chapter 42 for discussion of the self-sealing mechanism and coagulation) (Dvorak, 1979).

Antibodies are formed in increasing quantities and support the action of the phagocytes by neutralizing bacterial toxins. The wall of leukocytes surrounding the irritant deepens. The leukocytes are supported by a net formed of fibrin. The inner zone of leukocytes is composed of polymorphonuclear cells with lymphocytes, monocytes, and macrophages at the periphery. The area is bathed by a fluid rich in antibodies and nutrients. Obstruction of small blood and lymph vessels helps to block the spread of microorganisms. If the response is successful, the bacterial cells escaping from the area are phagocytosed in the blood and lymph. The central mass in the inflamed tissue is composed of dead cells and living and dead leukocytes and bacteria. These are digested. The entire zone of inflammation is called an abscess.

The abscess may rupture spontaneously or be opened. Drainage of the abscess to the outside facilitates healing by aiding in the removal of materials that would otherwise have to be digested and absorbed before healing can begin. Rupture of the abscess into a serous cavity, such as occurs in perforation of the appendix, leads to the dissemination of the contents of the abscess as well as those of the intestine into the peritoneal cavity, thus predisposing to localized or generalized peritonitis. Perforation with the development of peritonitis is one of the most serious complications in acute appendicitis. When leakage from the appendix is minimal, the body may be able to wall off the area with the formation of an appendiceal abscess.

Rupture of an abscess into the pleural space results in a condition called empyema, a disorder that is often resistant to treatment. Although the term *empyema,* when used by itself, usually refers to an accumulation of pus in the pleural cavity, it actually means a collection of pus in any natural body cavity. Therefore an accumulation of pus in the gallbladder is also empyema.

Understanding the nature of the walling-off process of inflammation is of importance in the practice of nursing. Premature or improper opening of an abscess may interfere with the mechanisms of the body for limiting spread of microorganisms and lead to their widespread dissemination. Manipulation of boils and pimples should be avoided until they have a well-defined area of pus in the center. Then they should be opened under surgical conditions. Care should be taken not to squeeze a pimple or a boil forcefully and the extruded pus should be prevented from coming in contact with the surrounding skin. Pus contains living bacteria and proteolytic enzymes that are able to digest both dead and living tissue. The combination of protein-digesting enzymes and viable bacteria predisposes to infection of the tissues with which they come in contact. Anyone changing dressings that cover draining wounds should protect himself or herself by using instruments to handle the dressings or by wearing gloves.

In addition to draining at the surface, an abscess may terminate in other ways. When an abscess is small or the injury to the tissue structure is minimal, the products of inflammation may be digested and absorbed into the circulation. This process is known as resolution. Following pneumonia, healing takes place by resolution. Enzymes released by the degenerating leukocytes digest and liquefy the material in the alveoli. Much of the exudate is removed by coughing. Following recovery from uncomplicated pneumococcal pneumonia there is no evidence of past disease. The lung is restored to its original condition and there is no evidence of scar tissue having been formed.

Still another way an abscess may terminate is for it to drain to the surface of the body through a sinus or tract. A sinus differs from a fistula in that a sinus is a tract draining an abscess, whereas a fistula is a tract between two hollow organs or between a hollow organ and the outside. An example of a sinus is a tract from a mediastinal abscess to a bronchus. An example of a fistula is a tract or passageway between the rectum and the vagina or from the colon through the abdominal wall to the outside.

Ulcer and Erosion Formation

Ulcers and erosions may also result from an inflammatory process. They are alike inasmuch as the surface layer of tissue, skin, or mucous membrane is lost. They differ in that an ulcer extends through the covering membrane, whereas an erosion involves only the covering membrane. Examples of ulcers include peptic ulcers and varicose ulcers. A common site of an erosion is the cervix uteri. In the formation of ulcers and erosions, the body mechanism for maintaining the integrity of tissue breaks down and the tissue destruction follows. In most people the tissue lining the stomach and duodenum is protected from the digesting action of gastric secretions. Any condition that upsets the balance between tissue resistance and protection from the digesting action of the gastric secretions so that digestion is favored predisposes to peptic ulcer formation. Varicose ulcers are essentially the result of inadequate tissue nutrition.

Factors Affecting the Outcome of the Inflammatory Response

The outcome of an inflammatory response depends on many factors including the agent responsible for injury to the tissues, the effectiveness of the individual's mechanisms of defense, and the specific tissues that are involved, as well as the nature and extent of the injury to the tissues. Factors influencing the capacity of an individual to respond to injury include age and general state of health and nutrition. When microorganisms are responsible, the body may or may not be able to localize them. Some bacteria are difficult to localize because they manufacture an enzyme, hyaluronidase, that destroys hyaluronic acid. Hyaluronic acid, a mucopolysaccharide, is a gel-like ground substance that acts as a cement substance between cells and to hold water in interstitial spaces. It is a component of synovial fluid, vitreous humor in the eye, and Wharton's jelly in the umbilical cord. It is also a constituent of the capsules of certain types of streptococci, pneumococci, and other microbes. Because *hyaluronidase* destroys the tissue hyaluronic acid and therefore allows greater spreading of materials in the tissue spaces, it is called *the spreading factor.* Production of hyaluronidase by such organisms as the staphylococcus and streptococcus enables them to break down the continuity of the tissue as well as the fibrin clots formed in the area of infection. When microorganisms are successful in disrupting barriers to their spread, they are then able to penetrate the surrounding tissue and cause cellulitis. With a breakdown of the local barriers to their spread, organisms may also enter the lymph and blood channels. Fibrin clots in the small venous and lymph channels may delay the entrance of bacteria into the general circulation. Lymph nodes in lymph channels also act as traps to remove and phagocytize microbes and other particles as well as to respond with acute inflammation (lymphadenitis). When bacteria enter and are circulated in the blood, the condition is known as bacteremia. When bacteria enter and multiply in the blood the condition is called septicemia. In some diseases, such as typhoid fever, bacteremia characteristically occurs in a particular phase of the illness. In others, such as pneumonia, the appearance of bacteremia is an unfavorable prognostic sign. Septicemia is always a serious and often fatal disorder. In either bacteremia or septicemia, microorganisms may be distributed through the body and set up sites of infection distant from the original infection.

Classification of Inflammation

Any condition that modifies the nature of the inflammatory response or is useful in identifying something about it can be used as a basis for classification. Inflammation may be classified according to (1) the causative or etiologic agent, (2) the characteristic type of exudate, (3) the location or site in which it occurs, and (4) the length of time the process has been in existence. Any classification of inflammation according to cause includes an endless variety of physical, chemical, and living agents. Some have their origin in the external environment and some in the internal environment of the individual.

Characteristic Types of Exudates

The character of the fluid exudate depends on the severity of the injury. In less severe injuries there may be very little exudate and what there is may differ very little in composition from normal interstitial fluid. As the severity of the injury increases, the damage to blood vessels increases and more components of the blood are found in the inflammatory exudate.

The inflammatory process may be classified according to the nature of the exudate. The exudate may be purulent, serous, serosanguineous, fibrinous, hemorrhagic, or catarrhal.

A *purulent exudate* is commonly known as pus. Although a number of other agents stimulate the production of a purulent exudate, it is most commonly associated with the so-called pyogenic bacteria. In these infections the exudate is rich in leukocytes. The purulent exudate or pus contains a large number of leukocytes, together with tissue debris and the products of digestion by proteolytic enzymes released by dead and dying leukocytes. The thick creamy pus found in the spinal fluid of the patient with meningococcic meningitis is an example of a purulent exudate associated with a pyogenic infection. Another more common example is the pus associated with staphylococcal infections of the hair follicle or a wound or the material occurring in the center of a pimple or boil (furuncle).

A *serous exudate,* which occurs in mild injuries, is a watery, low-protein fluid derived either from the blood or from the cells lining serous cavities and joint spaces. Perhaps the most common example of a serous exudate is the fluid found in the blisters or vesicles associated with second-degree burns. Mr. All had some blistering of his skin as a consequence of burns. These blisters contained a serous exudate. Another example of a serous exudate is the fluid that accumulates in the pleural cavity as a result of some types of pleurisy. This type of pleurisy is known as pleurisy with effusion. It is frequently caused by tuberculosis or by a malignant neoplasm in the lung.

Infections involving the peritoneum or the pericardium may likewise result in the production of a serous exudate. Pericarditis with effusion is likely to cause serious impairment in cardiac function. Relatively small amounts of fluid prevent the heart from dilating fully during diastole and interfere with the filling of the heart. This results in congestion of blood in the systemic venous circulation and reduces the quantity of blood available to circulate to the tissues.

In the more severe acute inflammatory processes, damage to capillaries may increase permeability to the extent that large molecules such as fibrinogen escape in the exudate. The fibrinogen is converted to fibrin and forms a sort of meshwork structure in the inflamed area. It also obstructs small lymph vessels and capillaries. These fibrin threads probably also function to prevent intravascular clotting, by removing thrombin from the blood, thus blocking the effect of thrombin on fibrinogen (Guyton, 1976, p. 106). The fibrin probably acts to delay the spread of microorganisms by providing a sort of maze through which bacteria must pass before they can escape into the surrounding tissue. This maze also increases the likelihood of the bacteria coming in contact with phagocytic cells. The fibrin network may contribute to the difficulty of removing all microorganisms from tissues even when the microorganisms are sensitive to antibiotics. The network acts to protect microorganisms by limiting their exposure to the therapeutic agents. Until the inflamed area is well walled off, it should be protected from trauma. A *fibrinous exudate* is characteristic of certain types of infections, such as pneumococcal pneumonia. The alveoli are filled with a fibrinous exudate containing large numbers of leukocytes. When the inflammatory process extends to the pleura, it causes the so-called fibrinous pleurisy. The fibrin on the surface of the pleura is sticky. Pain during breathing results from the pleural surfaces rubbing together. Though fibrinous pleurisy is an early finding in pneumonia, it also occurs in the absence of pneumonia.

Hemorrhagic Inflammation

In very severe inflammatory reactions, damage to the blood vessels may be so great that erythrocytes escape into the exudate. This may be observed as minute hemorrhages into the skin that are known as petechiae, which appear as small reddened areas in the skin. They are commonly found in subacute bacterial endocarditis. In fulminating infections the damage to blood vessels may be so great that bleeding into the subcutaneous tissues takes place. This gives the skin a dusky hue. The color of the skin is responsible for the black smallpox or meningitis of fact and legend.

Catarrhal Inflammation

Catarrhal inflammation occurs only in those tissues in which there are mucous glands—that is, in mucous membranes. The term is really a misnomer, but it continues to be used because of force of habit. The exudate from mucous membranes contains large amounts of mucinous material. It is one of the most frequent types of exudate because it is associated with inflammations of the respiratory tract. The clear mucinous exudate accompanying a common cold is an example. Mucous secretion may be increased by the exposure of the respiratory tract to chemical irritants such as those contained in smoke or smog.

Other Classifications

Inflammatory processes may also be classified according to the tissue or organ in which they are located. Students can recognize that the inflammatory process is involved when the suffix *itis* is added to the combining form indicating a tissue or organ. Inflammation of the trachea and bronchi, whatever the causative agent, is known as tracheobronchitis. The term *myositis* indicates that a muscle is inflamed. Myocarditis is used to indicate that the heart muscle is inflamed. Nephritis indicates that the site of inflammation is the kidney. None of these terms indicates the cause of the inflammatory process. The only information provided is that a particular organ is the site of an inflammatory process.

The inflammatory process may also be classified as to the length of time it has been in existence. This classification gives some clue as to the degree of activity of the process. Thus the terms *acute, subacute,* and *chronic* are used. Acute inflammations are those of recent origin and in which the process is active. The common cold is an example of a condition in which there is an acute inflammatory process. A recently incurred burn is another. An example of a condition that may go from the acute to the chronic stage is acute hemorrhagic nephritis. The kidney may recover fully following the acute phase of the disease or it may fail to do so and go into the subacute phase and finally into chronic nephritis.

Not all inflammatory processes are highly active at the beginning. Some inflammants are only mildly irritating and cause damage only by prolonged exposure. Such an irritant is silica. When it is inhaled into the lung, it sets up a simple inflammatory process in which the macrophage plays an important role. Because silica is indigestible, it cannot be destroyed by the macrophage. Macrophages, however, can wall it off by forming fibroblasts that mature into fibrous connective tissue. One particle of silica will not require a very large scar, but many particles do. Therefore to prevent serious scarring of the lung, workers who are exposed to silica dust require measures that reduce the chances of inhaling dust.

CAUSES OF SIGNS AND SYMPTOMS

The signs and symptoms in inflammation depend in part on the degree of response of the host, the nature of the inflammant, and the site of the injury. Mild irritants, including psychogenic stimuli triggered by a symbol of injury, may produce only a transient inflammation lasting only a few minutes or hours, whereas severe injury may last for days, weeks, or even months. The response may be limited to a small area or may involve the entire organism.

The cardinal signs of inflammation are increased *heat, redness, swelling, pain,* and *loss of function.* The rise in the temperature is caused mainly by an increase in blood supply, though there may also be some increase in the metabolic rate. With the increase in blood flow in the area, the temperature approaches that of the interior of the body. The increase in blood in the area is also responsible for the redness. Although the increased quantity of blood contributes to the swelling, swelling or inflammatory edema is mainly caused by the accumulation of the exudate in the tissue. Swelling causes pain because of pressure on sensory nerve endings. Some authorities believe that toxic metabolites are also a factor in pain.

Loss of function is partly caused by pain, as motion increases pain. Muscle spasm in the injured area also serves to splint or limit motion of the part. For example, following spillage of the contents of the gastrointestinal tract into the peritoneal cavity, the muscles of the abdominal wall contract and act as a physiologic splint. Even cuts involving skin over or near a joint induce some muscle spasm and a disinclination to move the joint because of the pain.

As a space-occupying mass, an area of inflammation may impinge on the circulation to an organ or obstruct a hollow organ or duct. For example, a localized area of inflammation of a structure within the cranial cavity may raise the intracranial pressure enough to deprive the entire brain of an adequate supply of blood. It may also cause pressure on the area of the brain where it is situated. An abscess in the mediastinum may interfere with swallowing by obstructing the esophagus from without. An abscess in the neck may obstruct the trachea by local pressure on it. In none of these examples does the inflammatory process directly involve the affected structures, but it causes its effects as a space-occupying mass.

In the description of inflammation thus far, emphasis has been on the local responses of tissues to injury. When only a relatively small number of cells are damaged, most, if not all, of the physiologic response is in the region of injury. When, however, the products of inflammation are absorbed into the blood stream in sufficient quantities, the whole organism becomes involved. Although the nature of the etiologic agent influences the severity and timing of the general physiologic manifestations, they are not unique to a single class. Therefore the manifestations of illness resulting from the escape of the products of inflammation into the general circulation can be observed in Mr. All (burns), Mr. Hoffer (myocardial infarct), and Mrs. Carney (radical mastectomy—major surgery), as well as Miss Mallow, who has pneumococcal pneumonia.

Generalized Signs and Symptoms

One important group of symptoms includes fever and the symptoms and signs that commonly accompany fever. (See Chapter 37.) The degree and character of fever vary with the causative agent. Following a major surgical procedure or an acute myocardial infarction, the temperature rises a degree or two and remains elevated for no more than 2 or 3 days. It should then return to normal and remain within the normal range. If it does not, or if the temperature rises higher than expected, this usually indicates that a complication is developing. Because the pattern of fever varies with each acute infectious disease, no attempt will be made to describe them here. The pulse and respiratory rate are usually, though not invariably, accelerated in proportion to the increase in temperature. Weakness and general malaise—a general feeling of unfitness—are common. Anorexia, or loss of appetite, is frequent; headache, backache, and generalized aching are not uncommon. Nausea may occur, with or without vomiting or diarrhea. Leukocytosis and an increase in the erythrocyte sedimentation rate occur in a wide variety of acute conditions—with and without infection. Some infections, such as pneumococcal pneumonia, may be preceded by a chill in adults or by a convulsion in infants and young children. In other conditions, such as advanced tuberculosis, subacute bacterial endocarditis, and malaria, chills, and fever may alternate with sweating (diaphoresis).

Weight loss may be marked if the inflammatory process (1) continues for more than a few days, (2) is severe, (3) is associated with fever, or (4) is associated with the loss of considerable quantities of tissue substance or nutrients. During fever, the metabolic rate is increased about 7 per cent for each degree of fever. With continued fever, the patient needs a substantial intake of calories to prevent weight loss. In long-continued inflammatory processes, particularly when associated with infection, the production of erythrocytes by the bone marrow may be depressed; normocytic anemia is a common finding in chronic infections.

Summary

Inflammation is one of a living organism's most important mechanisms of defense against injury. Inflammation is a defensive response to an injurious agent. It involves blood vessels; blood cells, particularly the leukocytes; tissue cells; the immunologic system; and cells of the reticuloendothelial system. It serves to neutralize, destroy, and limit the spread of inflammants and to prepare the tissues for repair.

The signs and symptoms accompanying the inflammatory process result from the response of the injured tissue and the person to injury as well as from the nature and severity of the injury. Inasmuch as the inflammatory process is a space-occupying mass, it may interfere with the function of organs. The signs and symptoms will depend on the extent to which function is disrupted. When sufficient products of the inflammatory process are absorbed, signs and symptoms indicate that the whole person is sick.

The Nurse's Role in Helping the Person with an Inflammatory Response

The specific therapy of any patient who has suffered cell injury and an accompanying inflammatory response will depend on such factors as the nature of the etiologic agent and the extent of the injury and its location, as well as on the adaptive capacity of the individual. In general, therapy will be directed toward (1) assisting the patient to overcome or eliminate the causative agent, (2) supporting the inflammatory response, and (3) providing substances required for the repair of the injured tissues. Attention is also given to the prevention of further injury so that the individual may be restored to health.

Six Principles to Guide Nursing Management

In planning the therapy of the patient, six principles serve as guides in the selection of specific measures.

PRINCIPLE ONE. *When appropriately used, rest favors healing.* How rest of an organ or part is achieved depends on its location and function. Both these factors—location and function of the affected part—are important in determining the degree of rest that it is possible to achieve. To illustrate, Mr. Carlos fractured his leg. Maintaining his leg at rest was relatively easy. It was placed in a cast or in traction with the two ends of the bone held in apposition. Mr. Carlos remained in bed until sufficient healing occurred. Even after he was out of bed he did not bear weight on his leg until healing was well underway or the leg was immobilized by a cast or brace. By way of contrast, despite the desirability of rest to the liver in the treatment of hepatitis, only relative rest can be secured. Mr. Devon,[7] who had a diagnosis of infectious hepatitis, was placed on a high-carbohydrate, high-protein, and low-fat diet. He was maintained at bedrest for several weeks in order to provide rest for the liver. Mr. Hoffer, immediately after suffering a myocardial infarction (heart attack), was also treated by bedrest, in order to reduce strain on the heart; he was fed, bathed, and—insofar as possible—protected from psychological and social stresses. Then his physical activity was gradually increased. Though bedrest is used less extensively than in the past, it is still believed to be an important form of treatment in infectious disease, in acute glomerulonephritis, and in acute rheumatic fever.

Bedrest is not without its hazards. As emphasized earlier, rest or lack of use of the body is accompanied by a loss of body substance and strength. Visceral and circulatory functions are depressed with the result that gastrointestinal function is disturbed and clotting of blood in vessels is favored. Respiratory excursions are lessened and this predisposes to atelectasis and pneumonia. (See Chapter 49 for discussion of the hazards of immobilization.) Despite these and other disadvantages, the indications for rest may be sufficiently great for the physician to prescribe it. When bedrest is prescribed, the nurse has the responsibility to select appropriate nursing measures so that physical and psychological rest are achieved.

PRINCIPLE TWO. *Survival depends on an adequate circulation of blood to and from the tissue.* The effectiveness of the inflammatory response as well as the life of the cells depends on (1) a continued supply of nutrients, leukocytes, antibodies, and other substances required by the tissue and (2) the removal of products of tissue metabolism as well as those of the inflammatory process. Heat in the form of dry or moist heat may be used to dilate the blood vessels. Because each tissue has a thermal death point, care should be taken to prevent burns. Moist heat is more dangerous than dry heat because it prevents evaporation. A temperature of from 40.5° to 46°C (105° to 115°F) is very hot. Exposure of the tissue to 85°C for as little as 10 seconds is sufficient to cause burning. With each degree that the temperature of tissue is raised, the metabolic rate goes up about 7 per cent. Patients with arterial diseases such as arteriosclerosis are sensitive to heat because they have a limited capacity to increase the delivery of nutrients to their tissues by dilating their arteries. Their ability

[7] In the treatment of hepatitis, restriction of activity is indicated during active phases, but prolonged bedrest following remission is unnecessary (Thorn et al., 1977, p. 1603).

to judge the temperature may also be defective. Should moist heat be applied to a patient with a diagnosis of arteriosclerosis, the temperature of the solution should be prescribed by the physician and should be checked with a thermometer. The dressings should be removed if the patient complains of pain and the physician should be notified. These patients should also be taught to check the temperature of bath water with a thermometer before stepping into the bathtub.

Heat is sometimes applied to extremities of patients in the form of a light cradle. Tissues can be protected by using a cradle in which the heat is controlled thermostatically. The temperature should not be allowed to go above 38°C (100.4°F) (Coffman, 1979); maximum vasodilatation can be expected between 30 and 34°C (between 86 and 95°F). When a cradle with a thermostatic control is not available, the patient can be afforded some measure of protection by using light bulbs of 25 watts or less. Despite great care, some patients have pain caused by muscle ischemia at environmental temperatures that are very little above ordinary room temperature. When this occurs, the heat should be discontinued and the physician notified.

Maintenance of the venous return is also important to the nutrition of tissues. In inflammation, distention of tissues by the inflammatory exudate causes pressure on veins, thereby interfering with the venous return. Elevation of an extremity is an important measure in promoting venous return. An elastic stocking or bandage is also useful in supporting the venous circulation. Should signs and symptoms that accompany impaired circulation occur in an extremity encased in a cast or bandage, measures to relieve the situation must be instituted promptly if tissue injury is to be prevented.

Care directed toward the maintenance of the circulation of inflamed tissue is important. Observation of the signs and symptoms indicating the status of the circulation in the tissue is imperative if indications that the circulation is failing are to be detected early and appropriate measures instituted in time.

PRINCIPLE THREE. *To provide the patient with specific assistance to overcome the causative agent.* This principle applies primarily to those conditions in which the causative agent propagates itself, or is a foreign body. At this time the main group of causative agents falling into the first category are microorganisms. There are two general, but specific, ways of attacking microorganisms or their products. One is to give the patient specific antibodies formed by an animal or another human being. The other is to administer a chemical that acts to weaken or to kill the microorganism. The use of specific therapy in the treatment of infectious disease is included in Chapter 38.

PRINCIPLE FOUR. *To modify the tissue response in inflammation so that tissue injury is prevented.* As in other body responses, the inflammatory reaction may be deficient or it may be excessive. In the first case, recovery may be threatened because the body is unable to overcome the irritant and prepare the tissue for repair. In the latter, the tissue is damaged by the excessive reaction. Agranulocytosis has been previously cited as an example of a condition in which the body response to injury may be inadequate. In individual patients in whom the inflammatory response is excessive, tissue damage may result. The control and effects of excessive swelling have been discussed. Necrotic areas are often repaired by fibrosis. Scar tissue may cause deformity of the affected tissue or organ. In disorders such as iritis, arthritis, and rheumatic fever, residual injury can sometimes be lessened by modifying the severity of the inflammatory response of the tissues. By limiting the exudative phase of the inflammatory response, tissue swelling is lessened. This contributes to the maintenance of the circulation to the tissues and therefore helps to prevent tissue necrosis. In the absence of tissue necrosis, fibrosis does not occur. To illustrate, in the treatment of iritis (inflammation of the iris of the eye) cortisone, hydrocortisone, or one of their synthetic analogues may be placed in the eye to reduce the severity of the inflammatory reaction and, as a consequence, the amount of scarring. Although authorities do not agree as to how the corticoids act, they reduce in some way the exudative response in inflammation. As a result, there is less tissue damage and a reduction in the amount of scar tissue formed in healing. Corticoids and salicylates are used in the treatment of arthritis and rheumatic fever for essentially the same reason. In the search for agent(s) responsible for transforming acute to chronic inflammation, which is characteristic of diseases such as arthritis, prostaglandins are receiving much attention. A major experimental treatment approach is to find compounds that effectively inhibit prostaglandin synthesis (Prostaglandins, 1972).

PRINCIPLE FIVE. *To allow healing to proceed by ensuring removal of the inflammatory debris, foreign bodies, blood clots, necrotic tissue, and the like.* In simple inflammations, the products of inflammation may be digested and absorbed into the blood stream. The blood vessels and tissue may be repaired leaving little or no evidence of the past inflammation. In pneumonia, the exudate in the lung may be coughed up and the tissue repaired without leaving any sign of the past infection. In boils, wound infections, empyema, and other similar infections, as well as those in which foreign bodies are present in the tissue, recovery may be hastened by the evacuation of pus, tissue debris, or foreign bodies. The removal of necrotic tissue and foreign bodies is called débridement; sometimes, as with a boil, this may need to be done only once. In other disorders, such as a serious wound infection, repeated opening of the wound may be required to facilitate drainage. Such wounds may be irrigated with isotonic saline or some other solution to remove debris and pus. When irrigation is done, enough force should be used to remove the purulent material. Care should be taken to prevent contamination of other areas of the skin of the patient and of the nurse.

PRINCIPLE SIX. *To institute procedures that help to support the patient in the reaction to his or her condition.* The support should be both emotional and physiologic, as one augments the other. No one is at his or her best when ill, and one should not be expected to be. Moore and his associates (Wilson, Moore, & Jepson, 1958) found that apprehension and fear before a surgical procedure were associated with a mild catabolic response. Attention to the needs of the patient and prompt relief of unnecessary pain should help to minimize suffering. Attention should be given to supplying the nutritional needs of each patient. There is evidence to indicate that in undernourished patients phagocytic ability is less than in those who are well nourished. Nutrients are necessary to the formation of antibodies and to the replacement of nutrients lost in the inflammatory exudate. Tissue substance lost as a result of the catabolic response to tissue injury must also be replaced by the food intake of the patient.

Water intake should be sufficient to replace that which is lost. Insensible perspiration may be increased by 1 liter or more in fever. Drenching diaphoresis may be responsible for the loss of 1 liter or more of water. A urine output of less than 1 liter usually indicates that the fluid intake of the patient is inadequate. This presupposes a normally functioning kidney.

Rest and reassurance may also be important ingredients in the care of the patient. The doctor usually orders the degree of activity that is allowed, but the nurse is the one who tries to modify the environment so that the patient is able to rest. Reassurance is discussed in Chapter 31.

Provided that the body is successful in removing, destroying, or neutralizing the injurious agent, the tissue goes on to repair the damage that has been done. Essentially the nature of repair is the same whether the continuity of the tissue is disrupted by a spontaneous process or by a carefully planned incision.

Wound Healing

Repair

The question of whether repair is the final stage of inflammation or is a separate response to injury is really of little importance. What is significant is that repair is a response to injury in which the body attempts to restore the injured tissue to normal. How this is accomplished depends on the severity and type of the injury as well as on the tissues that have been injured. There are three general ways in which repair may take place: healing by *recovery,* by *regeneration,* and by *replacement with scar tissue.* (See Figure 25-1 for schema of reparative processes.)

Recovery

In the discussion of possible outcomes of inflammation, the point was made that when injury to the tissue is minimal the products of inflammation are absorbed and the tissues are returned to their former condition. The restoration of tissue to its former state is known as *recovery.*

Regeneration

When the injury is more severe and cells are destroyed, repair may be accomplished by regeneration, a process in which cells are replaced by similar cells. Actually, regeneration of tissues such as the skin is a constant process. As the surface cells of the skin are shed, they are replaced by underlying cells, which are in turn replaced by cells at the base of the skin, each of which undergoes mitosis and divides into two cells. The process is carefully controlled, so that only as many cells are produced as are needed to replace those that are lost.

Regeneration of cells and tissues depends on two fundamental properties. One is the capacity of cells to proliferate or multiply. The other is the capacity of the organism to organize new cells into a functional pattern. Scientists have long been intrigued by the fact that animals, such as the salamander, are able to regenerate limbs following amputation. One of the factors in the regeneration of an organ is the ability of cells forming different types of tissue to regenerate at the same rate. In humans different types of tissue cells reproduce at different rates. The problem is complicated by the fact that fibrous connective tissue regenerates more rapidly and under less favorable circumstances than other types of tissues. Therefore even in tissues having the capacity

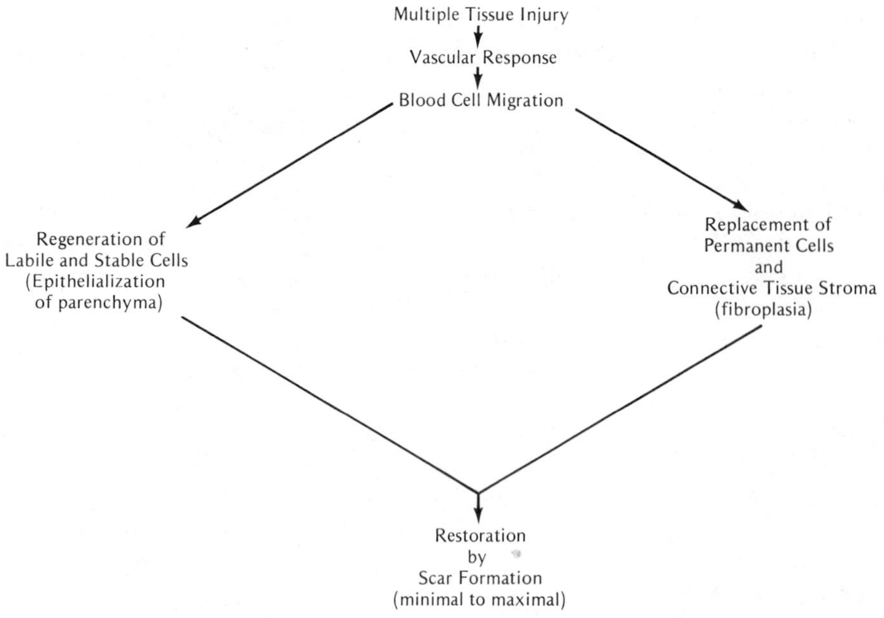

Figure 25-1. Schema of reparative processes. (Used with permission of W. B. Saunders Company from The nature of wound healing: Implications for nursing practice. *Nurs. Clin. N. Amer.* 14:667–82, Dec. 1979, p. 669, Fig. 2, by P. Bruno.)

to regenerate, healing may take place by scarring rather than by regeneration.

Not only are humans incapable of regenerating limbs, but the capacity of their tissues to regenerate varies. As stated previously, highly specialized cells such as those in nerve and muscle tissues are incapable of regeneration. Injuries are repaired by replacement with microglia (a connective tissue in the nervous system) and fibrous connective tissue. By way of contrast, tissues having their origin in the mesenchymal tissues (those that form the supporting structures for the parenchymal or functioning cells) have a great capacity for regeneration. Surface and glandular epithelium, bone, and lymphoid tissue are also able to regenerate adequately.

The capacity to produce an adequate number of differentiated cells is only one aspect of regeneration. Another is the capacity to organize these cells into functioning units with the necessary blood, lymph, and nerve supply. A good example of an organ in which the capacity to regenerate fails, not because cells do not proliferate but because the body is unable to properly organize them into functioning units, is the liver. The liver is susceptible to injury by a wide variety of agents: microorganisms; chemical poisons, such as chloroform or carbon tetrachloride; and undernutrition, as the liver is particularly susceptible to a lack of protein and of vitamin B in the diet. The liver fails to recover following injury not because liver cells do not have an adequate capacity to regenerate but because the body is unable to organize the cells around ducts. Despite the capacity to replace damaged liver cells, the resulting tissue is likely to be of little use. In a way, the liver is repaired much as a jerry-built house is constructed—a cell here and one there without thought as to where it should be placed to accomplish its function.

Replacement with Scar Tissue

The *third way* in which repair is achieved is by the *substitution of fibrous connective tissue for the injured tissue.* When fibrous connective tissue is used in repair, it serves as a patch to preserve or restore the continuity of the tissue. It does nothing more. Therefore when an injury to a vital organ is repaired by the substitution of fibrous connective tissue, the result is a decrease in the functional reserve in that organ. For example, a myocardial infarct heals by the formation of scar tissue. The extent to which the cardiac reserve is diminished will depend on the size of the scar. Following an attack of glomerulonephritis, scar tissue is formed to heal the kidney. The scarring may do more damage than the original disease process because as the scar tissue matures, it contracts and obstructs the flow of blood to the kidney. Functioning tissue dies as a consequence of loss of blood supply. In patients who die from the effects of glomerulonephritis, the kidney is frequently found to be a contracted mass consisting mostly of scar tissue.

The circumstances under which repair by the substitution of fibrous connective tissue occurs are (1) when conditions in the internal environment are unfavorable to mitosis, (2) when the quantity of tissue destroyed is too large for it to be replaced by regeneration of the cells in the area, (3) when highly specialized tissues have been destroyed, (4) when the rate at which parenchymal cells multiply is slow, and (5) when tissues are subjected to repeated injury.

As has been implied, healing by the formation of fibrous tissue serves a number of purposes. It restores the continuity of tissue after too great destruction of tissue. It walls off foreign bodies and disease processes such as tuberculosis. It reinforces weakened structures such as aneurysms of the aorta and other large arteries.[8] Fibrous connective tissue also plays an important role in the healing of thrombosis, infarctions, osteomyelitis, and nephritis as well as of many other conditions. When thrombi form in veins, fibrous tissue serves to hold the clot at the site of formation and to repair the damage. Following an infarction, scar tissue maintains tissue continuity.

Similar to other homeostatic mechanisms, tissue repair by the formation of scar tissue is beneficial when the process is initiated by an appropriate stimulus and is sufficient to correct the damage caused by injury. Likewise it may also be the source of harm. The principal harmful effects of scar tissue are (1) the unnecessary replacement of parenchymatous tissue, (2) interference with the function or drainage of an organ, or (3) the cutting off of the blood or nerve supply to an organ, and (4) the formation of an excessive quantity of scar tissue.

Certain of the characteristics of scar tissue account for some of its potentially harmful effects. It is composed largely of collagen. When a scar is subjected to slight or moderate stress, it tends to shorten or contract. When it is subjected to much stress, it tends to lengthen. Contraction of the scar does no harm when it is in the abdominal wall and the quantity of scar tissue is not excessive. However, when scar tissue is formed in or around an organ, it can be expected to interfere with the function of the organ as it matures, as sometimes happens in the healing of third-degree burns or in arthritis. In these patients, attention to maintaining the extremities in the appropriate position so that deformities caused by contractures can be prevented may be a lasting service to the patient.

Scar tissue located in areas where it is subjected to repeated strain may lengthen or extend. Sites that are subjected to considerable pressure include the wall of the heart and the arteries. Especially when an infarct in the wall of the heart is large or when the heart is subjected to repeated infarction and the quantity of scar tissue is large, the collagen fibers in the scar may be stretched by the pressure created as the heart contracts. Because they are not elastic, after they are lengthened they do not return to their former state. This results in a bulge or aneurysm. This bulge reduces the mechanical efficiency of the affected ventricle. Instead of only one area of relatively low pressure, that is, the artery, there are two, the artery and the distensible area in the wall of the heart. As the heart contracts, blood enters both the artery and the aneurysm. This increases the work of an already weakened heart.

Many of the general factors favoring tissue repair have already been indicated. They may be summarized as (1) a limited amount of injury and a high regenerative capacity of tissues, (2) an abundant supply of blood to the tissue as well as an adequate supply of protein and ascorbic acid, and finally (3) good health and youth. Regarding the last point, the most important practical difference between healing in the young and in the old is that the young tend to heal more rapidly than the old. The need for a good blood supply is obvious. Protein is necessary to supply the amino acids required for the formation of new tissue. Some authorities are inclined to interpret the metabolic response following injury as an adaptation by which the organism provides the tissues with the materials needed for healing. Because the metabolic response is greater in the young and healthy than in the old and feeble, perhaps this is one reason that they recover more quickly than do the old and feeble. Ascorbic acid, or vitamin C, is necessary for the formation of collagen—an essential element in fibrous tissue. The course of wound healing can be favorably influenced by adding to the wound otherwise deprived of them the following compounds: vitamin A, as well as C cited above; zinc; protein; and oxygen (Hunt, 1974). Evaluation of an ingredient found in a proprietary hemorrhoidal product, Preparation H, indicates that the substance is capable of stimulating wound oxygen consumption, epithelialization, and collagen synthesis (Goodson et al., 1976).

The presence of diseases such as uncontrolled diabetes mellitus or atherosclerosis delays repair. Though there is some disagreement among authorities about the effect of anemia on wound healing, it probably is not an important factor.

Local conditions in the injured tissue also have an effect on the healing. The exact nature of the stimulus to cellular proliferation is not known, but it is believed to be caused by a local factor or factors. As was emphasized in the discussion of inflammation, healing is delayed or prevented until the wound has been cleared of infection and any dead space has been obliterated. In the past, healing has been delayed by the introduction of foreign substances at the time the wound was made or treated. At various times throughout history, antiseptics and germicides

[8] An aneurysm is a bulge or outpouching in the wall of an artery. It usually results when the wall is weakened by a disease such as arteriosclerosis or symphilis. As it distends, the wall of the artery thins and is further weakened. Fibrous connective tissue strengthens the wall.

have been placed in wounds to destroy microorganisms. It is now known that any agent potent enough to kill bacteria also kills body cells. Furthermore, before healing can proceed normally, all foreign material must be removed. Because it acts as a foreign body when introduced into a wound, talc is no longer used to powder gloves. A form of treated cornstarch or Biosorb cream and powder have been substituted for it. Though it is much less likely than talc to produce a foreign-body reaction, cornstarch can and does. Therefore, it should be used as sparingly as possible in powdering the gloves. The outer surface of the gloves should be wiped or washed in sterile saline before the operation is started (Brooks, 1975).

The mechanism of injury also has a bearing on healing. A clean, incised wound free from infection is the most favorable to healing. Crushing wounds, fractures, especially those with much soft-tissue damage, and infection of wounds delay healing. They also are attended by the possibility of excessive scar tissue formation.

So that the reader may have some understanding of what is happening in a patient who is healing an area of injured tissue, the healing of a clean, incised wound will be briefly described. The process of healing all injuries is essentially the same. The principal difference between the healing of a clean, incised wound and an infected one, or one in which the tissue is subjected to long-standing injury, is in the quantity of scar tissue required to heal the defect. In a clean, incised wound only a small scar is required, which may form quickly; in other wounds, scarring may be extensive and delayed.

Preparatory to, and during, healing a number of things must be accomplished. The damaged cells and tissue debris must be removed. Bleeding must be stopped. The gap between the two severed edges of tissue must be bridged. The surgeon works carefully making the incision. Though a small clot of blood or fluid exudate is necessary to fill the defect between the two sides of the wound, a large clot delays healing. Therefore the surgeon carefully ligates (ties) the ends of each blood vessel as it is cut. Small vessels seal themselves by the formation of blood clots, which on retraction of the vessel form an effective plug in its end. The surgeon also facilitates healing by the careful approximation of like tissues to like tissues. As the surgeon completes this part in the healing of the wound, nature takes over.

Authorities usually describe healing as occurring in three phases. There is considerable overlapping among the various phases. They may all be going on at the same time in different parts of the wound. *The first phase,* which lasts from 3 to 5 days, is variously called the initial, the lag, the catabolic, and the inflammatory phase. These terms all have some virtue in that each describes some change or condition that is present in the tissues. The term *lag* has been used because the strength of the wound diminishes during this time. The term is, however, misleading because it implies that no changes are occurring in the tissue. This is not true, for exudation is increased and leukocytes accumulate in the area. Blood vessels dilate and the area becomes hyperemic. The fluid exudate and/or blood fills the space between the two edges of the wound and not only causes the edges of the wound to stick together but provides a meshlike framework for fibroblasts and budding capillaries. Materials essential to tissue repair accumulate. Fibroblasts appear and there is an increase in collagen. Without collagen, wound healing does not take place. Collagen does not form unless the proper materials and conditions are present. Capillary buds also begin to appear. Their formation coincides with the general catabolic response of the body as a whole. During this phase the patient looks and acts ill. Moore (1959) calls this the stage of injury or the adrenergic corticoid phase.

After 4 or 5 days the leukocytes begin to disappear from the wound. About this time the fibroblasts can be observed to be actively proliferating. During this phase collagen is formed and the newly formed tissue is highly vascular. Because of its appearance, the new tissue is called granulation tissue. As the collagen fibers mature, they tend to shorten or contract. Early in the process of wound healing, epithelial cells migrate and later proliferate to cover the wound surface. With large wounds the epithelial covering may be very thing and delicate. Care should be taken when the wound is dressed to protect these newly forming cells lest they be destroyed. In time, the scar, which was a bright pink, fades, because the blood vessels are squeezed out. The result is a mature scar, or a cicatrix. See Figure 25-2 for an illustration of healing of a superficial wound.

When a wound is infected, suppuration occurs and healing is delayed. At one time infection was so common that surgeons thought it was necessary to healing. The type of pus that was believed to favor healing was called laudable pus. When pus is present, the wound is said to heal by second intention. Healing is delayed and more granulation tissue is required to fill the defect than in the absence of infection. Occasionally, either because of the nature of the wound or because of its disruption, secondary closure is necessary. This is known as healing by third intention.

Currently, knowledge of the factors involved in wound healing is incomplete. Questions as to what initiates the process and what terminates it have not been answered. In experiments with rats, Selye has been able to prevent scar tissue formation by the

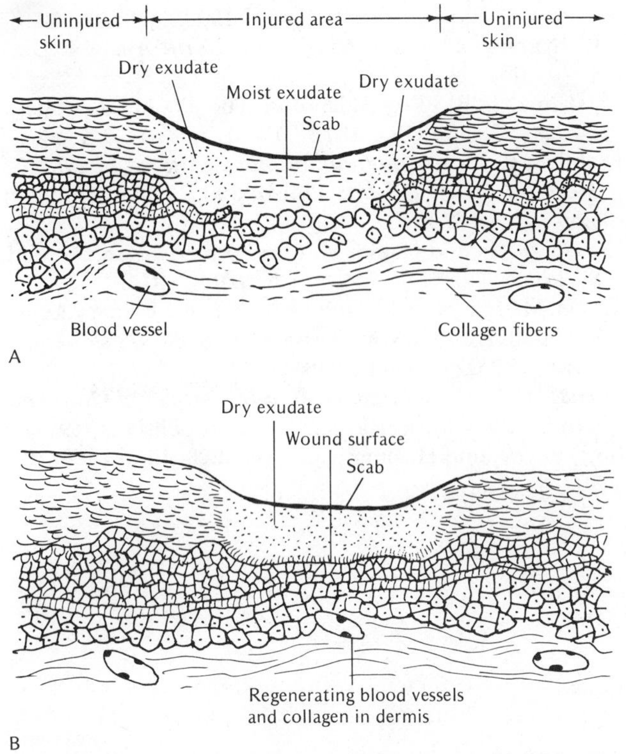

Figure 25-2. The healing of a superficial wound. (Used with permission of Macmillan Publishing Company, Inc., from *Physiology: A Regulatory Systems Approach,* 1978, by F. L. Strand, Fig. 19-12, p. 358.)

administration of cortisone and to augment its formation by administration of desoxycortisone. Exactly how cortisone, hydrocortisone, and related analogues act is not known. In rats the different adrenal cortical hormones depress or enhance the inflammatory response that follows tissue injury.

Earlier in this chapter the changes occurring in the tissue in response to injury were described. In Appendix D, changes that take place in the body as a whole and in the wound are summarized and correlated with the signs and symptoms that can be expected in the patient and his or her needs during each phase. The length of each phase varies with the extent of injury to the tissue as well as with the capacity of the individual to respond. The summary is based on the changes occurring in a patient who has a clean, incised wound such as is made in the performance of abdominal surgery. Changes are less marked in conditions in which the extent of injury to tissue is less and is more marked in those in which there is greater injury to the tissue.

During the twentieth century, techniques have been perfected and the knowledge of the changes that take place in the body as a whole, as well as in the wounded tissue, has increased. With expansion in the fields of physiology and biochemistry, clues are being uncovered that can be expected to lead to a knowledge of the factors that initiate the healing process, regulate its course, and terminate it. Interest is also centered on the biochemical changes that take place in the body as a whole following injury and during illness. The preceding discussion reemphasizes that the body acts as a unit. Biologically it gives priority to the injured tissue. As the understanding of these changes becomes more complete, care of the patient following injury can perhaps be planned to support body responses rather than to interfere with them. In other patients, such as those with glomerulonephritis or rheumatic fever, this knowledge may make it possible to limit the inflammatory response, including subsequent scarring, so that tissue structure and function may be preserved.

References Cited

Brobeck, J. R. "Neural Control Systems." In *Best & Taylor's Physiological Basis of Medical Practice,* 9th ed. Baltimore: The Williams & Wilkins Company, 1973, pp. 9–59.

Brooks, S. M. *Fundamentals of Operating Room Nursing.* St. Louis: The C. V. Mosby Company, 1975, p. 67.

Coffman, J. D. "Peripheral Vascular Diseases Due to Organic Arterial Obstruction." In *Cecil Textbook of Medicine,* 15th ed. Ed. by P. B. Beeson et al. Philadelphia: W. B. Saunders Company, 1979, p. 1301.

Dvorak, H. F., quoted in AP news release. "Tumors May Protect Selves in Cocoons, Researchers Find." *The Standard Times,* New Bedford, Mass., 6 Aug. 1979.

Goodson, W., et al. "Augmentation of Some Aspects of Wound Healing by a Skin Respiratory Factor." *J. Surg. Res.,* **21** (1976), 125–129.

Guyton, A. C. *Textbook of Medical Physiology,* 5th ed. Philadelphia: W. B. Saunders Company, 1976.

Hunt, T. K. "Diagnosis and Treatment of Wound Failure." *Adv. Surg.,* **8** (1974), 287.

Menkin, V. *Biochemical Mechanisms in Inflammation,* 2nd ed. Springfield, Ill.; Charles C. Thomas, Publisher, 1956, p. 11.

Moore, F. D. *Metabolic Care of the Surgical Patient.* Philadelphia: W. B. Saunders Company, 1959, pp. 27–28.

"Prostaglandins: Mediators of Inflammation?" *Science,* **177** (1 Sept. 1972), 780–81.

Thorn, G. W. et al. *Harrison's Principles of Internal Medicine,* 8th ed. New York: McGraw-Hill Book Company, 1977.

Tilkian, S. M. et al. *Clinical Implications of Laboratory Tests,* 2nd ed. St. Louis: The C. V. Mosby Company, 1979.

Widmann, F. K. *Goodale's Clinical Interpretation of Laboratory Tests,* Philadelphia: F. A. Davis Company, 1973, p. 23.

Wilson, G. M., Moore, F. D., and Jepson, R. P. "The Metabolic Disturbances Following Injury. In *Metabolic Disturbances in Clinical Medicine.* Ed. by G. A. Smart. Boston: Little, Brown and Company, 1958, p. 76.

General References

Babior, B. M. "Oxygen-Dependent Microbial Killing by Phagocytes. Part I." *N. Engl. J. Med.,* **298** (23 March 1978), 659–68. Part II. *N. Engl. J. Med.,* **298** (30 March 1978), 721–25.

Brunner, N. A. *Orthopedic Nursing, A Programmed Approach,* 2nd ed. St. Louis: The C. V. Mosby Company, 1975.

Bruno, P. "The Nature of Wound Healing: Implications for Nursing Practice. *Nurs. Clin. North Am.,* **14** (Dec. 1979), 667–82.

Di Palma, J. R. "Prostaglandins, The Potential Wonder Drugs." *RN,* **35** (Oct. 1972), 51–61.

Frohlich, E. D., ed., *Pathophysiology: Altered Regulatory Mechanisms in Disease.* Philadelphia: J. B. Lippincott Company, 1972.

Larson, C. A., and Gould, M. *Orthopedic Nursing,* 8th ed. St. Louis: The C. V. Mosby Company, 1974.

Mason, M., Matyk, P. M., and Doolan, S. A. "Urinary Ascorbic Acid Excretion in Postoperative Patients." *Am. J. Surg.,* **122** (Dec. 1971), 808–11.

Movat, H. Z. ed. *Inflammation, Immunity, and Hypersensitivity.* New York: Harper & Row, Publishers, 1971.

Ross, R. "Wound Healing." *Sci. Am.,* **220** (June 1969), 40–50.

UNIT VI

Regulation and Maintenance of Essential Life Processes

Unit VI focuses on those processes that are essential to the physical survival, growth, and development of the individual, by guaranteeing to all body cells an adequate supply of oxygen, water, and nutrients. The essential life processes are core subsystems of the individual as the focal system, and the regulatory and response mechanisms—discussed in Units IV and V, respectively—may be said to function at the interface of the individual's internal and external environments, in behalf of protecting the essential life processes. Unit III discussed common environmental agents (stressors) that are capable of producing cellular injury, and thereby capable of interfering with essential life processes.

Regulation of cellular events which make up the essential life processes is primarily automatic (i.e., continual function does not require awareness or volition on the part of the individual). However, the multiplicity of interconnections between central and autonomic nervous systems and the widespread effects of neurohormones make it inevitable that one's thoughts and emotions play a major role in determining the effectiveness with which the essential life processes function.

Although the nurse's role in helping persons with some of the most common alterations in essential life processes due to disuse, trauma, and disease is emphasized in Unit IX, some reference to nursing techniques and strategies appropriate to preventing and treating altered function accompanies explanation of related pathophysiology.

26

Exchange of O_2 and CO_2—Control of Ventilation*

A thing of beauty is a joy forever:
Its loveliness increases; it will never
Pass into nothingness; but still will keep
A bower quiet for us, and a sleep
Full of sweet dreams, and health, and quiet breathing.

John Keats, *Endymion*

Overview

Respiration in the broadest sense, refers to those processes contributing to cellular metabolic activities and the production of energy in the form of adenosine triphosphate (ATP). The production of energy requires oxygen, which reacts with simple sugars (CHO) and produces carbon dioxide and energy.

$$CHO + O_2 \longrightarrow CO_2 + H_2O + ATP$$

To maintain the production of energy, oxygen must be continually supplied and carbon dioxide eliminated from the cells and the system. Two physiologic systems are required to maintain this process of energy production at the cellular level. First, there must be a blood circulatory system, including the presence and function of hemoglobin. In other words, there must be a method of transporting the oxygen and carbon dioxide throughout the body. Second, there must be a ventilatory system that provides for the transport of oxygen and carbon dioxide between the body and the atmosphere. The ventilatory system is often referred to as the respiratory system, not including the broader biochemical definition of respiration previously stated. This more limited definition of respiration will be the one used in this chapter, with the emphasis of the chapter being placed on the transport of gases between the body and the atmosphere.

Other chapters will more thoroughly discuss the other phases or aspects of respiration, including the metabolic processes required for respiration at the cellular level. The sections within the present chapter are arranged according to a physiologic model. Four basic areas of lung function are discussed. These are: (1) lung mechanics or the forces and resistances to the movement of air in and out of the lung, (2) the exchange and transport of carbon dioxide and oxygen, (3) lung defense mechanisms, with emphasis on airway clearance, and (4) the control of respiration.

Each of these sections includes basic terminology, normal physiology, applied clinical physiology, and clinical examples. After these discussions there is a section devoted to special techniques used in respiratory care that have not been previously described. Now the reader is ready to integrate all of the preceding content in order to care for a patient. The last part of the chapter thus concentrates on nursing assessment and nursing intervention as exemplified in case studies. The case studies will also include discussions of specific pathology, its impact on physiologic function, and the total medical and nursing intervention required.

* This chapter has been revised by Gayle A. Traver, R.N., M.S.N., Associate Professor of Nursing, College of Nursing; Assistant Professor of Medicine, College of Medicine, University of Arizona.

The chapter has been arranged in this manner for a specific purpose. Many of the most common pulmonary diseases, such as emphysema, have no known cure or even specific therapy. Therefore the diseases are treated symptomatically. Even when specific therapy is known, the symptoms must be treated concurrently in order to ensure optimal patient response. Thus the nurse must be able to recognize symptoms and the physiologic basis for these symptoms in order to decide upon the appropriate nursing intervention. There is no "recipe" of nursing care for any diagnosis.

Much of the medical care of these patients is dependent upon knowledgeable and skilled nursing care. Treating an infection with an antibiotic is not successful if airway patency is not maintained. Ventilating a patient with a mechanical ventilator is not successful unless the patient receives good airway care and alert, knowledgeable anticipation and recognition of changes exhibited by the patient. In addition to participating and contributing to the medical care of the patient, the nurse can aid the patient and family by helping them to cope with the demands of the disease and its treatment. Therefore, a patient with a pulmonary disease must have knowledgeable and skilled nursing care at all times in order to ensure an adequate response to all aspects of the therapy.

Nursing care of the patient must not be "rote" activity but must be based on scientific theory. Only by understanding normal and abnormal physiology can the nurse understand why a problem has arisen or may arise and what effect the nursing care will have on it. Having a skill without knowing when to use it is detrimental to the patient. The nurse must have the knowledge to identify the problem, to identify the basis for that problem, and to identify the possible nursing intervention. The nurse must have the skills necessary to use the required intervention and, finally, must be able to evaluate both the therapeutic and the side effects of that intervention.

In summary, nursing care is basic to the care of the pulmonary patient. It is often the difference between successful and nonsuccessful treatment of the patient in the perception of both the provider and consumer.

Lung Mechanics

Lung mechanics refers to the forces and resistances to moving air in and out of the lungs. Although a complicated subject, the nurse must understand the basic concepts inherent in lung mechanics. It is this understanding that will aid the nurse in explaining the sensation of dyspnea to a patient, allow a more systematic approach to assessing the patient's respiratory pattern, and enable the nurse to have a scientific basis for nursing interventions aimed at improving ventilatory efficiency. Before discussing the physiologic principles basic to lung mechanics, it is important to realize that most *dyspnea,* the perceived sensation of difficulty in breathing, is not usually due to gas exchange abnormalities. Rather, dyspnea is most often more closely related to alteration in lung mechanics. In all instances, the patient's personal perception is an important component of dyspnea. Shortness of breath can be observed by others; dyspnea depends on the individual's perception of his or her breathing.

Inspiratory and Expiratory Forces

As a prerequisite to understanding some of the forces that influence the movement of air in and out of the lung, it must be remembered that the lung is enclosed in a bony cage, the thorax. The lung "wants" to return to its resting volume. This tendency is referred to as the elastic recoil of the lung. The resting volume is seen when the thorax is open during a surgical procedure; it is evident that the lung collapses and goes to a very small volume, although it does not become completely airless. Similarly, the chest wall wants to go to its resting volume. This volume, however, is larger than the resting volume of the lung alone. For example, if the patient has a complete pneumothorax of the left lung, observation of that patient will demonstrate that the thoracic cage on the left side is larger than on the right side. This situation arises because the thorax is no longer held to the smaller volume by the interplay between the lung and the thoracic wall. The result of the interaction of these two forces, the lung wanting to return to a smaller volume and the chest wall wanting to expand to a larger volume, is that a negative intrapleural pressure is created (negative being subatmospheric). The relationship between these two forces becomes equal and opposite at the end of a normal expiration with no pressure applied to the system. The volume left in the lung at this point of the respiratory cycle is defined as the functional residual capacity.

Inspiratory Muscles

If at the end of a normal expiration there is no pressure being applied to the system, then to increase the volume of the thorax requires that a certain amount of work and pressure be applied to the system. Therefore inspiration is an active act involving muscle contraction that will enlarge the bony thorax, creating a more negative pleural pressure, pulling the lung with it. The major muscles of inspiration are the diaphragm and the external intercostal muscles. The diaphragm is a large, domed muscle that forms the bottom of the thoracic cage and separates the thoracic cavity from the abdominal cavity. It is innervated by the phrenic nerve, which leaves the spinal cord at the level of the third to the fifth cervical vertebrae. As the diaphragm contracts, it increases the diameter of the thorax in a downward direction and also elevates the lower ribs. Concurrently, there is an increase in intra-abdominal pressure. On a maximal inspiration the diaphragm may move down as much as 10 cm. This action of the diaphragm is one that the nurse tries to encourage when teaching deep breathing.

By understanding the action of the diaphragm, there are also other observations that the nurse can make. First, of course, the patient's respiratory pattern can be observed, to see if it indicates effective use of the diaphragm or not. You can observe a slight bulging of the abdomen and a flaring of the lower ribs as the diaphragm descends on inspiration. It must be remembered that these observations alone do not ensure use of the diaphragm; such a conclusion would require fluoroscopy and actual observation of the movement of the diaphragm. If the lung is overinflated as in emphysema, the diaphragm is depressed and flattened even at the end of expiration. This situation results in mechanical inefficiency. Under such circumstances, contraction of the diaphragm causes an inward movement of the lower ribs rather than a flaring, and therefore can often be observed by the nurse. Such an observation would influence the nurse's approach to teaching breathing exercises to that patient.

In the care of the patient with an injury to the spinal cord, the nurse must recall that the phrenic innervation is derived from the third to fifth cervical level. Therefore, patients who have an injury below that level would be expected still to have diaphragmatic activity and adequate ventilation because the diaphragm accounts for more than 80 per cent of total ventilation. In those patients with an injury above the third to fifth cervical level there would be a loss of diaphragmatic activity, and mechanical ventilation would be required.

In considering innervation of the diaphragm, it must be remembered that the diaphragm consists of two leafs and receives innervation from both the left and the right phrenic nerves. Therefore, one leaf of the diaphragm can be paralyzed and the patient will still be able to maintain adequate ventilation. Such a situation may arise when a tumor of the lung involves the phrenic nerve on one or the other side. The diagnosis of a paralyzed diaphragm is made under fluoroscopy with visualization of the movement of the diaphragm. Simple observation of the patient's breathing during fluoroscopy will not always determine the presence or absence of a paralyzed diaphragm because the change in thoracic pressure may cause a movement of the diaphragm that appears to be normal. The test that is done to ascertain whether or not a diaphragm is paralyzed is called a "sniff" test. In this test the patient sniffs, which is a very rapid, quick inspiration. In the patient who has a paralyzed diaphragm there is a paradoxical movement of the paralyzed diaphragm, so that the leaf of the diaphragm with normal innervation will move downward but the paralyzed diaphragm will move upward during the sniff maneuver.

The other normal muscles of inspiration are the external intercostals. These muscles are innervated by nerves leaving the cord at the first through the eleventh thoracic segments. Their action is to elevate the anterior end of each rib, which then increases the anterior posterior diameter of the chest. The intercostals are not the major muscles of ventilation and account for only about 20 per cent of the ventilation of a normal individual. The effect of loss of the external intercostals is largely due to the loss of rigidity of the intercostal interspaces during inspiration. Because of this loss of rigidity and a certain "caving in" of the intercostal spaces, there is less room for volume expansion of the lung itself. The nurse must therefore be alert in observing whether a patient can use the intercostals effectively or not. It is also important to note that with lower cord injuries the intercostals would be lost before the diaphragm, as the nerves innervating the diaphragm leave the cord at a much higher level than do the nerves innervating the intercostal muscles. Should the patient not have use of the intercostal muscles, stress must be placed on developing a good diaphragmatic respiratory pattern.

There are other muscles that can be used to aid inspiration. These are called the accessory muscles and include the scalene, sternocleidomastoid, and many others. These muscles are not used in normal ventilation but are brought into play when ventilation must be increased markedly. Therefore the individual with a normal lung, should he or she be increasing ventilation, will use the accessory muscles. For patients with lung disease, these accessory muscles may be used during ventilation at rest because of the marked effort needed to expand the lung. The nurse should be careful to observe if a patient uses the accessory muscles at rest, at mild exercise, or only on strenuous exercise. Clinical observations also help the nurse to determine if the patient chronically uses the accessory muscles to aid respiration. These observations include hypertrophy of the neck muscles and callouses on the elbows indicating that the patient is frequently in the tripod posture (leaning on knees, table, or other object) in order to fix the muscles of the shoulder girdle. When these muscles are "fixed" they can be more effectively used to expand the chest rather than contraction simply resulting in shoulder movement. It should also be noted that upper limb exercise will often demand that the patient use these muscles for that activity rather than as respiratory muscles. Therefore, upper limb exercise is very difficult for patients who use their accessory muscles to breathe. Frequently the nurse can help to alleviate these problems. For example, it often helps to have the patient lean on an over-the-bed table, when washing his or her face, so that the shoulder girdle is fixed to aid respiration and the forearms can be used for the washing activity. Other upper limb activity should also be analyzed and adapted when appropriate. For example, vacuuming can be less of an impingement on the use of the respiratory muscles if the vacuum is pushed away with expiration and pulled toward the individual on inspiration. Thus the posturing and respiratory movements of the involved muscle groups are synchronized.

Expiratory Muscles

Expiration is usually a passive maneuver. The previous description of the interplay between the elastic recoil of the lung and the elastic recoil of the chest wall demonstrates that end expiration is at a resting point where the forces are negligible between the resting volumes of the lung and the chest wall. When expiration is carried below the normal resting volume or when expiration is extremely rapid and forced, the expiratory muscles will be brought into play to aid with the force and rate of expiration. The major expiratory muscle group is the abdominal musculature. The abdominal muscles are innervated from the lower thoracic vertebrae (sixth thoracic to first lumbar segments). As the abdominal muscles contract, they depress the lower ribs and flex the trunk. At the same time there is an increase in intra-abdominal pressure, which has an effect in moving the diaphragm upward. One of the best ways to picture how the abdominal muscles work in the forced expiratory maneuver is to consider one's posture and what happens when one coughs. An individual who coughs is usually in the upright position with the trunk flexed forward and feels the strain on the abdominal musculature. Those patients who have lost use of their abdominal musculature will have a great deal of difficulty in producing an effective cough due to inability to produce a forced expiration. The internal intercostal muscles are also expiratory muscles. These intercostals receive their innervation from T-1 to T-11, just as do the external intercostals. Their major action is to depress the ribs in a downward and inward motion and they also stiffen the intercostal space during the forced expiratory maneuver.

Resistances

In order to produce air flow and a change in lung volume, the muscle forces must overcome the elastic resistance of the lung and chest wall and the flow resistance produced by the airways. There are a variety of tests of lung function which have been developed to measure changes in volume, flows produced, resistance, and elastic properties of the lung and chest wall. Only selected tests of lung function will be discussed. These tests are used to help diagnose the physiologic basis of the patient's problem but, more important for the nurse, they can be used to plan appropriate nursing interventions. Examples of these applications to nursing care will be pointed out in the discussion of the various tests.

Measurement of Lung Volumes and Flow

Spirometry includes some very basic measurements of lung mechanics and is a common clinical test of the patient's lung function. Spirometry can be done at the bedside but is most often performed in a pulmonary function laboratory. During this study the patient breathes in and out of the spirometer and a tracing such as that depicted in Figure 26-1 is made of the amount of air that he or she is able to move during various maneuvers.

The following measurements are made in simple spirometry:

1. The inspiratory vital capacity (IVC). This is the maximal amount of air that can be inhaled after a maximal expiration.
2. Forced vital capacity (FVC). This is the maximal amount of air that can be forcefully exhaled after a maximal inspiration.
3. The forced expiratory volume in 1 second (FEV_1). This is a flow measurement, expressed as volume per unit time. The FEV_1 represents the maximal amount of air that can be exhaled in the first second of a forced vital capacity.
4. FEV_1/FVC. This ratio compares the amount of air that can be forcefully exhaled in 1 second to the total amount of air that can be forcefully ex-

haled after a maximal inspiration. The ratio should be greater than 70 per cent (see Figure 26-1).

5. Maximal voluntary ventilation (MVV). This measurement refers to the maximum amount of air that the patient can move in 1 minute by rapid deep breathing. The measurement is made over a 10- to 15- second period and then extrapolated for 1 minute. In the past, this measurement was referred to as maximum breathing capacity (MBC).
6. Tidal volume (V_T or TV). This is the amount of air moved in a normal breath.

Additional measurements of lung volumes may also be done, but these require more sophisticated techniques than simple spirometry. Such lung volumes include the following:

1. Total lung capacity (TLC). The total amount of air in the lung after a maximal inspiration.
2. Functional residual capacity (FRC). The amount of air left in the lung after a normal expiration. The functional residual capacity, or resting volume, is that lung volume when no inspiratory or expiratory forces are being applied.
3. Residual volume (RV). The amount of air left in the chest after a maximal expiration.

These measurements of mechanical lung function are used to aid in determining the diagnosis and plan of care for patients. From the results of spirometry, a physiologic diagnosis of an obstructive ventilatory defect or a restrictive ventilatory defect can be made. An obstructive defect is one which demonstrates slowed expiratory flows. The FEV_1 is decreased and the FEV_1/FVC is below 70 per cent. In an obstructive defect, the residual volume is usually increased because of the difficulty in getting air out of the lungs. A restrictive defect is one where flows are maintained but volume excursion is reduced. The vital capacity and FEV_1 are decreased, but the FEV_1 is decreased proportionately to the vital capacity so that the FEV_1/FVC ratio is normal, greater than 70 per cent. The residual volume and total lung capacity are both usually decreased. For the nurse, the results of these measurements can help to plan care. For example, a decreased vital capacity would indicate that the patient has difficulty in taking a deep breath. A decreased FEV_1 or decreased FEV_1/FVC ratio would indicate that the patient has difficulty generating rapid, forced expiratory flow rates. If the FEV_1 is below 500 cc the patient is usually short of breath at rest. If one remembers that the normal tidal volume is approximately 500 cc, and the FEV_1 for an adult male is 3 liters, it is evident that an FEV_1 of 500 cc denotes a great deal of limitation. At an FEV_1 of 800 to 1000 cc the patient may not be short of breath at rest, but any increase in ventilation (e.g., activities of daily living) will induce shortness of breath. Therefore the nurse can use the spirometry to help in planning care—that is, the nurse's expectation of the exercise tolerance of the patient and how activity should be planned.

Other Measurements of Mechanics

There are many more measurements that can be made of lung mechanics. It is not the purpose of this section to describe exactly how these measurements are made. But it is important that the nurse have a basic understanding of the meanings of these measurements and what implications they would have for the nurse who is caring for a patient.

Elastic Forces

Compliance is a measure of the distensibility of the lung. Compliance expresses the volume change of the lung per unit of pressure change. Compliance is often increased in such disease states as emphysema, where the lung distends more readily than does the normal lung; a greater volume change takes place for the same pressure change than would occur in the normal lung. In contrast, the patient with pul-

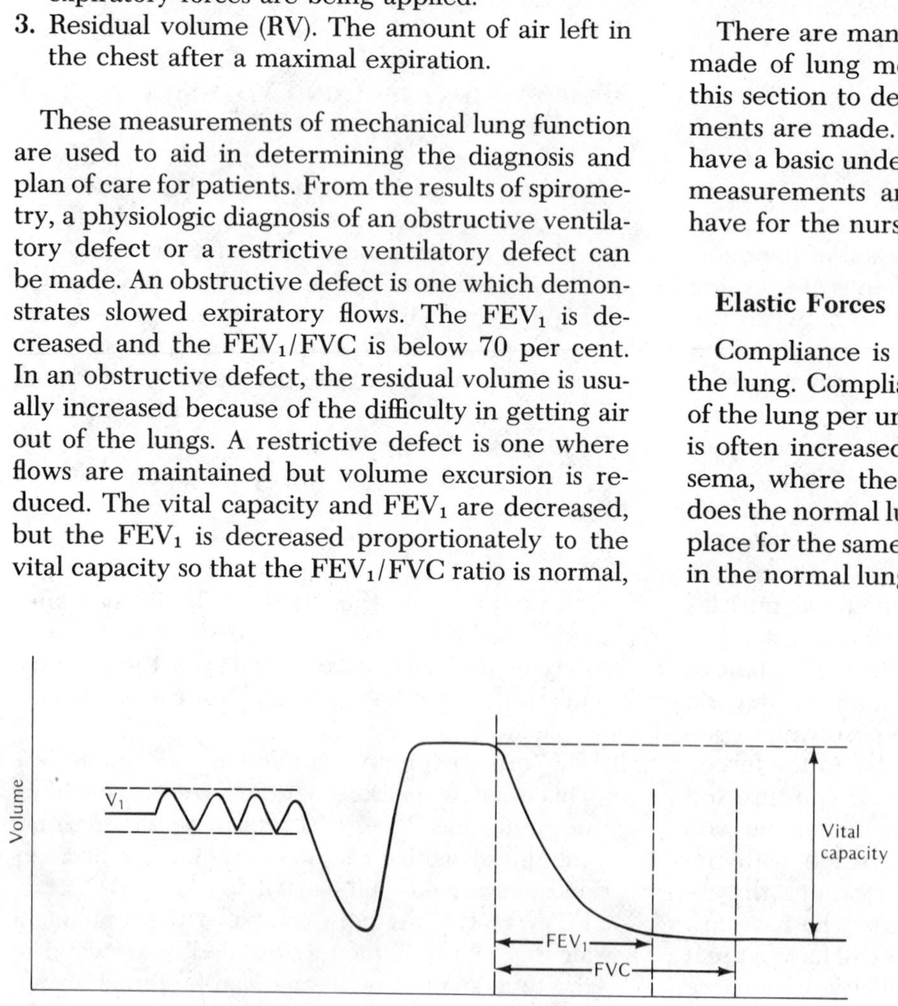

Figure 26-1. Spirogram.

monary interstitial or adult respiratory distress syndrome (ARDS) has what is called a "stiff lung" or decreased compliance. Therefore this patient produces a much smaller volume change for the same pressure change. Compliance is one measure of the elastic force that must be overcome to distend the lung. These elastic forces influence both inspiration and expiration. For example, let us compare the stretching of a tight spring to the stretching of a loose spring. The tight spring will be much harder to stretch than will the loose one. In other words, the tight spring is less compliant. On the other hand, the tight spring will have an increased elastic recoil; in other words, it will return to its original shape quickly when the extending force is removed. This picture of increased recoil is seen in the patient with a stiff lung or with fibrotic lung disease. The patient with emphysema has the combination of increased compliance and decreased elastic recoil. It takes less pressure change to get air into the lung. On exhalation, however, there is decreased elastic recoil and, therefore, the lung does not passively return to its original shape. Thus, the patient uses forced expiration to aid the return of the lung to a resting state.

These combinations of compliance and elastic recoil have implications for the nurse in teaching breathing exercises to the patient with emphysema. Because the increased compliance makes it easy for the patient to get air into the lungs, inhalation does not have to be stressed during breathing exercises. Exhalation, however, is difficult for this patient. Therefore the expiratory side of the respiratory cycle is stressed in teaching breathing exercises and the patient should be encouraged to use a slow respiratory cycle with a prolonged expiratory time to allow the lungs to come back to a resting volume. This slow respiratory rate will also decrease the work of breathing because it allows for a slow return to resting volume without extremely active use of the expiratory muscles, which would consume energy. The patient with fibrotic lung disease presents the opposite picture. Such a patient has low compliance and increased elastic recoil. This patient will tend to use a short inspiratory phase with a shallower breath than will the patient with emphysema. He or she will do this to decrease the work of breathing. To create a larger pressure change in order to inhale larger volumes would create more work for that patient. The patient with fibrotic lung disease also tends to have a rapid respiratory rate because the expiratory time is so short. Because the patient's lung has increased elastic recoil, it quickly springs back to its resting volume; therefore the expiratory phase takes place much more rapidly. Thus in this type of physiologic situation, it is more efficient for the patient to use a rapid rate than it is in the clinical picture demonstrated by the patient with emphysema.

Other factors must also be considered. One is the influence of surface tension and how it will affect the elastic recoil of the lung. The alveoli are frequently equated to bubbles. If we had two connecting bubbles of differing sizes, the smaller one would always empty into the larger because of the differences in surface tension and increased pressure in the smaller bubble. Yet in the lung this situation does not occur. In the lung, alveoli of different sizes will remain expanded; the smaller alveoli do not collapse and empty air into the larger alveoli. The explanation for this phenomenon is the presence of a lipoprotein material called surfactant. This material lines the alveolar surfaces and changes the surface tension of the alveoli. Surfactant is more active in small alveoli than in large alveoli. Therefore in the small alveoli, where surfactant is much more active, surface tension is reduced to a much greater extent. The result is that the pressures needed to ventilate the small and the large alveoli become more similar and therefore air will go to both spaces and not to just the large alveoli. There are some conditions where surface tension increases. The prime example is the hyaline membrane disease of the newborn. There are similar conditions in the adult, such as have been described in the adult respiratory distress syndrome, which affects surface active forces in the lung. Surface tension is also increased in the situation where the patient is unable periodically to sigh or deep-breathe. A sigh is a normal mechanism and appears to maintain the activity of surfactant. With a lack of such periodic deep breathing, as in pain, low-volume mechanical ventilation, and so on, alveolar collapse may occur. In any situation where the surface tension is increased, the elastic recoil in that area of the lung will be increased. Much greater pressures will be needed to expand the lung and the lung will tend to return to low lung volumes at end expiration.

Airway Resistance

Flow through the airways is dependent on the driving pressure and the resistance of the airways $\left(\dot{V}=\frac{P}{R}\right)$. One of the major determinants of resistance is the airway caliber. Therefore, as the airway lumen increases in diameter, resistance will decrease; as the diameter decreases, resistance is increased. It must be remembered that the airway diameter changes with both inspiration and expiration. Just as the lung expands during inspiration so do the airways. During expiration, on the other hand, the airways have a smaller diameter. In the same respect, the airway resistance will change at various lung volumes. Airway resistance will be less when at the top of the inspiratory vital capacity and will be greater when the lung is at low volumes such as residual volume. It has been noted in many situations that there is a discrepancy between the inspiratory vital capacity and the forced vital capacity. This finding has been explained by the fact that the forced expiration, by increasing the pleural pressure, creates a narrowing of the airway during the forced vital capacity, which results in obstruction of the airway. As the result of the obstruction, the patient cannot get as much air out of the lung as he or she was able to inhale during a slow, inspiratory, vital-capacity maneuver.

In disease states airway resistance is also affected. Many factors such as bronchospasm and bronchial secretions will increase resistance. In pure obstructive diseases the airway resistance is increased on expiration; in pure restrictive diseases it is normal at any absolute lung volume. If the resistance is abnormally increased, the patient must increase the driving pressure if flow is to be maintained. One way that this may be accomplished is to use an active, forced expiratory pattern. At the same time the forced expiratory pattern may lead to further narrowing of the airways in some patients, especially those with decreased elastic recoil. The airways are no longer "tethered" open by the recoil of the surrounding lung. These patients should therefore be taught to exhale slowly; it is more efficient to allow more time for expiration than to try to increase flow rates.

Nursing Applications

Many applications of the knowledge of lung mechanics have already been cited. Many relate to a knowledgeable assessment of the patient's respiratory pattern. Next, the decision whether or not that pattern needs to be modified has to be made. For examples we will examine two patients in greater detail: the first one is a postoperative patient who breathes too shallowly and at a normal-to-rapid rate, the second is a patient with an asthma attack who is breathing too rapidly. In the first instance, it is known that patients with upper abdominal or thoracic surgery have reduced lung volumes. If they do not periodically "sigh" (take a deep breath), small airways can collapse and atelectasis develop. To prevent occurrence and progression of these complications, the patient needs to deep breathe periodically. In the situation of the patient with asthma, an obstructive disease, the rapid forced respiratory rate causes greater airway collapse. As the patient gets less air out with each breath, the functional residual capacity increases and soon inspiratory excursion is limited. Both patients need to have their respiratory pattern modified but for different reasons.

The Postoperative Patient

For the postoperative patient with upper abdominal surgery, all lung volumes tend to be reduced. The reduction in vital capacity is frequently greater than 50 percent. Due to pain and other sequelae of the surgery, the diaphragm is in a higher-than-normal position. Initial efforts at deep breathing this patient are usually aimed at emphasizing an abdominal pattern. The patient is encouraged to breathe in slowly and deeply, allowing the abdomen to bulge, and then to exhale normally. Often placing the hands (nurse or patient) on the abdomen and instructing the patient to "push them away" aids in accentuating this motion. Many patients, however, are unable to perform this maneuver because of incisional pain. Instead, encouraging a lower thoracic pattern is often more effective. As mentioned earlier, lower rib movement also indicates diaphramatic excursion. Again it often helps to place the hands on the chest. (Allow the patient the opportunity to splint the abdominal incision with his or her hands, small pillow, towel or other means.) In attempts to modify the respiratory pattern of the postop patient, the hands are in constant contact with the chest wall or upper abdominal wall, depending on the pattern desired. The patient is encouraged "to push" the hands away on inspiration while on expiration the hands are used to compress the chest or abdomen. Since the postoperative patient has lung volumes that are too small, at the end of the maneuver he or she is always encouraged to inhale deeply, and is not left at the end of an expiration more forced than usual. In order to open "closed" airways or alveoli, it is also helpful to have the patient do a "yawn" maneuver or an inspiratory breath hold after inhaling as much air as possible. It has been found that many postoperative patients are better able to take a deep breath if they have a goal to reach and visual feedback their ability to reach that goal. There are several commercial devices available to help provide this feedback. The patient exhales normally and then inhales through the device which registers the volume inhaled and provides a signal to the patient if the preset volume has been accomplished. It should be remembered that these devices (i.e., incentive spirometry, tri-flow, and others) do not *make* the patient take a deep breath. They simply provide feedback which acts as a motivating force. Some patients profit from this type of feedback whereas others are capable of taking just as deep a breath without it.

The Asthmatic

The second example is that of the patient with asthma. This patient's major problem is airway obstruction. Emphasis in this situation is placed on exhalation. If the patient can exhale more slowly, the functional residual capacity will be decreased, allowing the patient to take a deeper breath. To simply encourage the patient to take a deep breath when the volume of air left after expiration is so much greater than normal is useless; there is no room left! At the same time, to tell a patient who is anxious and dyspneic to breath more slowly is also often foolhardy; if you feel like you're suffocating, you are not about to take slow deep breaths. In such cases the nurse should approach the patient calmly. Do not let your own anxiety increase the patient's fear and anxiety. Those emotions alone serve to increase the respiratory rate. Also it is usually best to approach the patient from the side. Approaching directly, face on, appears to impinge on the dyspneic patient's personal space and increase apprehension. Then, with the hands on either the upper abdomin or lower chest, exert pressure during exhalation, attempting to slightly lengthen each expiration. The hands should remain on the chest during inspiration, but the pressure should be released. The deep inhalation will follow spontaneously. The inspiratory maneuver is not stressed as in the previous patient. At the same time it is helpful to place one hand on the patient's shoulders, and rock the patient forward on expiration. This movement helps to increase intra-abdominal pressure and will help to push the diaphragm up. In both of these examples the patient's respiratory pattern needed to be modified. Because of different problems of lung mechanics, however, the approach was different in each case.

Gas Exchange

It must be remembered that gas exchange is not solely dependent upon the air moved in and out of the lungs. Rather, there must be movement of air in and out of the lungs and perfusion of the lung by the cardiovascular system. In addition, there must be a matching of this gas and blood. In other words, blood and air must be going to the same areas of the lung for effective gas exchange to take place. This exchange of oxygen and carbon dioxide is a dynamic process. Too many times people believe that as we breathe in, oxygen goes into the blood and as we breathe out carbon dioxide leaves the blood. Such a concept is erroneous. Perfusion of the lung is continuous, it does not stop and go with inspiration and expiration. Because blood is always circulating through the lung, there is a continuous exchange of gases across the alveolar capillary membrane. Second, all the air in the lung is not exchanged with each breath. This fact is evident when one realizes that in an adult male the total lung capacity is approximately 5 liters and the tidal volume is 500 cc. Rather, a balance is kept so that the alveolar gas composition remains relatively constant. The following sections will discuss gas exchange in terms of carbon dioxide and oxygen and will stress the nursing observations and nursing interventions required by patients who have various malfunctions of their gas exchange system.

Introduction to Blood Gases

A working knowledge of blood gases is a prerequisite in the care of the patient with pulmonary dysfunction. As recently as the early 1960s blood gas analysis was a research tool and was seldom used in the clinical management of the patient. Today, however, blood gas analysis is a common tool used to assess patient status in both the inpatient and outpatient settings. The uses of blood gas analysis are as follows:

1. To determine the need for oxygen therapy.
2. To monitor the response to oxygen therapy.
3. To determine acid–base status.
4. To evaluate operative risk, disability, and prognosis.

Blood gas analysis provides the following data:

Pa_{O_2} The partial pressure (P) of oxygen (O_2) in the arterial blood (a). Normal value at sea level is 85 to 95 mm Hg or torr. (Torr is equivalent to mm Hg.)

Pa_{CO_2} The partial pressure (P) of carbon dioxide (CO_2) in the arterial blood (a). Normal value is 36 to 44 mm Hg or torr.

pH The acidity or hydrogen ion concentration of the arterial blood. Normal value is 7.36 to 7.44.

Sa_{O_2} The per cent saturation of hemoglobin (S) with oxygen (O_2) in the arterial blood (a). Normal value at sea level is 95 to 98 per cent.

Partial Pressure

According to Dalton's law of partial pressures, in a mixture of gases each gas exerts its own pressure independently of all the others. The total pressure of the mixture of gases is equal to the sum of the pressures of the individual gases. For example, the total pressure of air at sea level is 760 mm Hg. The

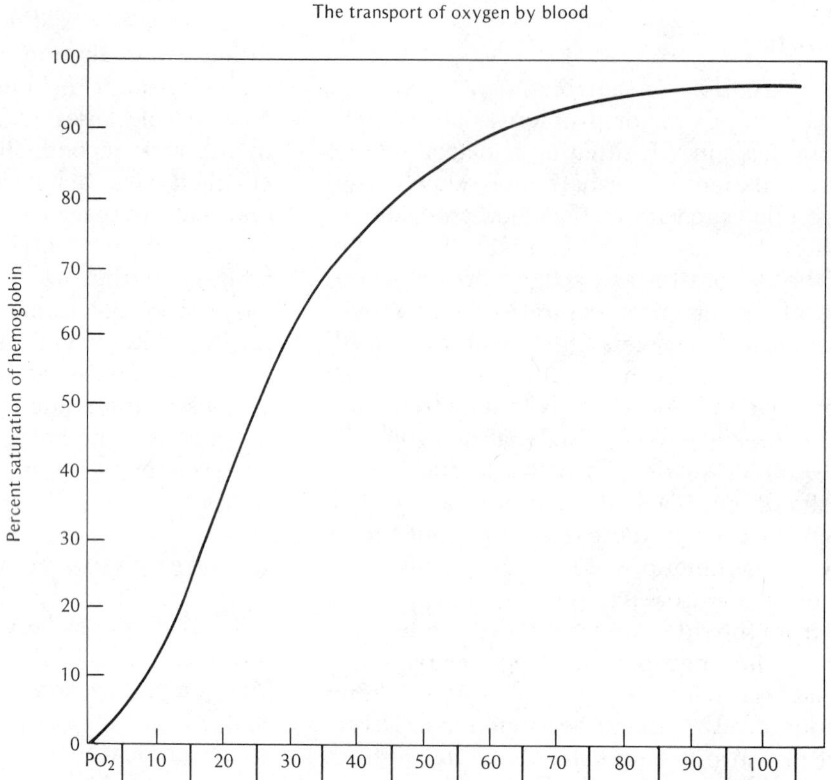

PO_2	10	20	30	40	50	60	70	80	90	100
A Whole blood O_2 cc O_2/100 ml blood	2.73	7.06	11.49	15.12	16.85	17.98	18.75	19.14	19.57	19.80
B Dissolved O_2 cc O_2/100 ml blood	0.03	0.06	0.09	0.12	0.15	0.18	0.21	0.24	0.27	0.30
C O_2 combined with Hb (A–B)	2.70	7.00	11.40	15.00	16.70	17.80	18.54	18.90	19.30	19.0
D % sat. of Hb $\frac{\text{Hb } O_2}{O_2 \text{ capacity}} \times 100$	13.5	35	57	75	83.5	89	92.7	94.5	96.5	97.5

Figure 26-2. Oxyhemoglobin dissociation curve. (From *Physiology of Respiration* by J. H. Comroe. Copyright © 1965 by Year Book Medical Publishers, Inc. Used by permission.)

composition of the air is approximately 21 per cent oxygen and 79 per cent nitrogen. The partial pressure of oxygen therefore would be 760 mm Hg × 21 per cent:

760	mm Hg (barometric pressure)
×0.21	oxygen fraction
159.6	mm Hg = the partial pressure of the inspired oxygen (PI_{O_2})

The partial pressure of the gas is thus dependent upon the total barometric pressure and the fraction of the specific gas present. At higher elevations, where the barometric pressure is less, the partial pressure of inspired oxygen in the air would be less even though the percentage would still be 21 per cent. The use of the *partial pressure* thus allows one to compare the quantity of a gas available in any mixture whereas the percentage allows one to know only what concentration of that gas is present, not the total quantity.

Measurement of Oxygen

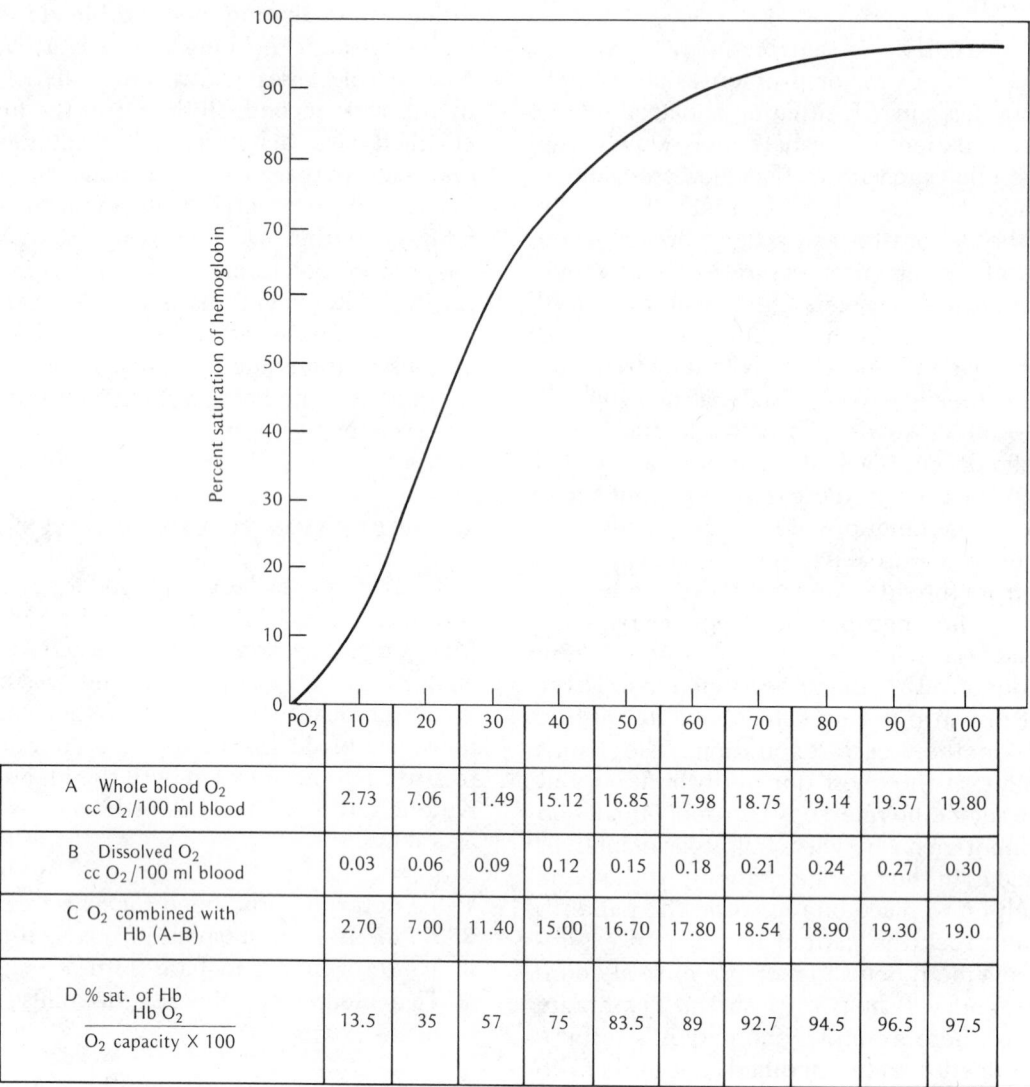

In the analysis of arterial blood, the measurement of Pa_{O_2} and the Sa_{O_2} is obtained. These two measurements represent the two ways in which oxygen is carried in the blood, dissolved (Pa_{O_2}), and in chemical combination with hemoglobin as oxyhemoglobin (Sa_{O_2}). At sea level a healthy individual with a normal amount of functioning hemoglobin would have an oxygen content of approximately 20 volumes per cent. In other words, every 100 ml of arterial blood contains 20 cc of oxygen. Of this 20 volumes per cent, most of the oxygen is carried in the form of oxyhemoglobin.

0.3	vol. per cent of dissolved oxygen
19.7	vol. per cent of oxygen combined with hemoglobin
20	vol. per cent—total oxygen content

Therefore normal functioning hemoglobin as well as the normal amount of hemoglobin is necessary for adequate oxygen transport.

It is important to understand that there is a relationship between the Pa_{O_2} and the Sa_{O_2}. The partial pressure acts as the driving force to the chemical combination of hemoglobin and oxygen. The relationship between the partial pressure and the oxygen saturation is demonstrated by the oxyhemoglobin dissociation curve, shown in Figure 26–2. The sigmoid shape of the curve shows that the oxygen content is protected so that even if the P_{O_2} drops from 100 mm Hg to 50 mm Hg, the saturation only falls to 80 per cent; the oxygen content is maintained at 16.8 volumes per cent, a change of only 3 volumes per cent assuming a normal amount of hemoglobin. Therefore when the P_{O_2} is greater than 50 mm Hg, large changes in the P_{O_2} result in relatively small changes in the saturation and content. Below a Pa_{O_2} of 50 mm Hg, the values fall on the steep part of the oxyhemoglobin dissociation curve. Therefore a change in the Pa_{O_2} from 50 to 25 mm Hg causes the saturation to fall to 50 per cent and the oxygen content to decrease greatly (oxygen content 10 volumes per cent).

Measurement of Carbon Dioxide

Carbon dioxide is the end product of all body metabolism and is also closely related to the body acid–base balance. The level of carbon dioxide found in the arterial blood is directly related to the metabolic rate of the body and inversely related to the ventilation. For this reason the adequacy of ventilation is defined by the arterial P_{CO_2}.

The total carbon dioxide content bears a nearly linear relationship to the Pa_{CO_2}. There are many ways of carrying carbon dioxide in our blood: dissolved, combined with water to form carbonic acid as bicarbonate, and in the form of carboamino compounds (CO_2 and protein). The CO_2 transport system is therefore not limited by the amount of hemoglobin present as in the oxygen transport system.

Measurement of pH and Acidity

Acidity is directly related to the hydrogen ion concentration (H^+). The greater the hydrogen ion concentration, the more acidic the substance. In the body the accumulation of carbon dioxide leads to an accumulation of hydrogen ions and an increased acidity, as follows:

$$CO_2 + H_2O \longleftrightarrow H_2CO_3 \longleftrightarrow H^+ + HCO_3^-$$

The pH is a convenient method of expressing the hydrogen ion concentration:

$$pH = -\log (H^+)$$

Because of the negative relationship between the hydrogen ion concentration and the pH, a low pH indicates a high hydrogen ion concentration and increased acidity. Also, the pH is a logarithmic expression of H^+ concentration so that small changes in the pH actually express large changes in H^+ concentration.

In the body acids and bases are kept in a delicate balance by a series of buffers. A buffer is a solution of a weak acid and its salt that prevents marked changes in hydrogen ion concentration. The major body buffer is the carbon dioxide/bicarbonate (HCO_3^-) system. The relationship of HCO_3^- and CO_2 to pH is as follows:

$$pH = pK + \log \frac{HA\ (salt)}{A\ (acid)} \quad or$$

$$pH = pK + \log \frac{HCO_3^-}{H_2CO_3}$$

This equation is called the Henderson–Hasselbach equation. The pK represents an equilibrium constant, which is 6.1 for the HCO_3^-/H_2CO_3 system. Because CO_2 is directly related to the amount of H_2CO_3 present, the equation is often simplified to an expression of the relationship of HCO_3^- to CO_2. When the pH is normal (7.4), the ratio of HCO_3^- to Co_2 is 20 to 1. As can be seen, any change in this ratio will lead to a change in the pH. As HCO_3^- increases, pH will increase; as CO_2 increases, pH will fall. The lung and kidney are the two major organs that maintain the 20:1 ratio.

Exchange and Transport of Carbon Dioxide

First, it is important to note that the ventilatory state is defined by the arterial P_{CO_2}. In other words, a patient should not be said to be hypoventilating unless the carbon dioxide is above normal, or hyperventilating unless the carbon dioxide is below normal. The terms *hyper-* or *hypoventilation,* thus, refer to alveolar ventilation, that amount of air that comes in contact with perfused alveoli. Alveolar ventilation (VA) is equal to the tidal volume (V_T) minus dead space (V_D) multiplied by respiratory rate. If the nurse wishes to describe the patient's breathing pattern, the appropriate words are *polypnea, tachypnea,* or *bradypnea.* As previously discussed, the level of carbon dioxide in the arterial blood is directly related to the metabolic rate of the body and inversely related to ventilation, thus making it a very close relationship between the P_{CO_2} and ventilation.

Hyperventilation

What, then, are the factors that may lead to the development of hypocapnia or what are the causes of hyperventilation? The most common is anxiety on the part of the patient. Another is increased ventilatory drive because of a central nervous system lesion. A third cause is mechanical overventilation. For example, a patient placed on a mechanical ventilator could be overventilated so that his or her P_{CO_2} is below normal. Another cause is the patient responding to a hypoxic or other drive to increase ventilation. If this drive is strong enough, the patient may become hypocapnic.

The effects of hyperventilation and a low P_{CO_2} are more related to the alkalosis which, ensues than to the P_{CO_2} itself. These changes are more evident in acute hyperventilation where the pH rises as the P_{CO_2} falls. In chronic hyperventilation the kidney compensates by excreting bicarbonate. Therefore there is less of a change in pH. In acute hyperventilation the patient often complains of feeling "lightheaded" and dizzy. He or she will have a sensation of tingling in fingertips and toes, and in cases of severe alkalosis, the patient may develop tetany. Some of the symptoms that the patient exhibits, such as the "lightheadedness," are due to the vasoconstrictor effect of the lowered P_{CO_2} and the change in cardiac return and therefore cardiac output caused by the high levels of thoracic pressure that often accompany the hyperventilation. The neuromuscular effects such as seen in tetany are due to the alkalosis, which causes a change in the resting membrane potential and makes the muscle much more responsive to stimuli.

In some cases the hyperventilation per se cannot be treated, for example, in central nervous system lesions. In other cases, such as anxiety, treatment involves working closely with the individual patient to try to decrease fears or the cause of anxiety. On a temporary basis the patient may be made to rebreathe his or her own expired carbon dioxide. This rebreathing can be accomplished by having the patient breathe in and out of a paper bag or by using a rebreathing tube; on a ventilator, deadspace may be added to the ventilator so that the patient rebreathes part of his or her own exhaled air with each breath, or the minute volume may be reduced (minute volume or $VE = RR \times V_T$).

In other cases where the hypocapnia is the result of increased drive to ventilation (acidemia, hypoxia, and so on), treatment is aimed at the underlying cause, because the hypocapnia is actually a compensatory mechanism.

Hypoventilation

Hypercapnia, an increased P_{CO_2}, is an anticipated problem in the care of many patients. Because of the many extreme metabolic effects of an acute change in P_{CO_2} and resulting acidemia, the nurse must be alert to the possibility of hypoventilation so that, if possible, its development can be prevented; if present it must be quickly diagnosed so that prompt treatment can be instituted.

Causes

There are four basic physiologic mechanisms which may lead to hypoventilation. Although they apply to all patients, they are especially important in the care of patients with underlying chronic lung disease. In persons with a previously normal lung there is a large reserve so that compensations for loss of some function is possible. In those with previous lung damage such compensation for a new insult to the lung is often not possible. Before proceeding to the mechanics of CO_2 retention it should be noted that chronic hypercapnia is not related to any single diagnosis. Rather it is seen in a variety of clinical situations: COPD, kyphoscoliosis, result of polio, and so on. At the same time not all of the patients who have one of these diagnoses have CO_2 retention. The mechanisms leading to carbon dioxide retention are as follows:

1. Reduced ventilatory drive. Because the excretion of carbon dioxide is dependent upon the patient's ventilation, anything that reduces his or her drive to breathe will, therefore, tend to increase the carbon dioxide levels. Included in this category clinically are the effects of sedation, narcotics, and anesthetic agents. This effect of oversedation may be seen in cases where the drug is self-administered (drug overdose) or where there is overuse of therapeutically ordered sedation. Some head injuries may also cause hypoventilation although hyperventilation is seen in many such cases. Many of the patients who exhibit chronic CO_2 retention have a reduced ventilatory drive; they no longer respond to an increased carbon dioxide level by increasing their ventilation. These patients then are extremely sensitive to the effects of sedation and narcotics.

2. Reduced ventilatory response. In this category the patient has a drive to breathe but is not able to respond to that drive. In other words, the patient cannot maintain ventilation. There are two subheadings within this mechanism. One includes those individuals who have an inability to move the thorax, such as those with neuromuscular diseases and deformities of the thorax. For example, a patient with a high spinal cord lesion has a drive to breathe but is unable to contract the diaphragm. Other less direct examples are patients who limit normal ventilation due to pain or fatigue. The second subheading is when involvement of the lung parenchyma and airways limits the ability of the lung itself to expand. An example is the patient with severe airways obstruction.
3. Increased dead-space ventilation. In this category there is an increased proportion of the inspired air that is in the trachea and airways but does not come in contact with the perfused alveoli. Patients with anxiety may increase anatomic dead-space ventilation by increasing the rate of respiration. As the rate increases, and if the total amount of air moved per minute (minute volume) remains the same, less air is available to the alveoli. For example, if Mr. A. takes one breath of 1,000 cc in a specified time and Mr. B takes four breaths of 250 cc in the same period of time, although the total number of air measured at the mouth would be the same, Mr. B is actually ventilating his alveoli much less than Mr. A. If we subtract the amount of dead-space per breath (in an adult male approximately 150 cc), Mr. A would have an alveolar ventilation of 850 cc and Mr. B would have an alveolar ventilation of only 400 cc. Patients may also have increased physiologic dead-space. In this situation air is reaching alveoli but there is no perfusion of those alveoli or the amount of blood flow is reduced in relation to the amount of air reaching that area. Such problems of increased alveolar dead-space ventilation are exhibited in patients with severe obstructive airway disease who have changes in pulmonary perfusion and in those patients who have a pulmonary embolus. Increasing dead space does not usually lead to carbon dioxide retention unless there is underlying chronic lung disease.
4. Increased carbon dioxide production. This problem is seen in states of increased metabolic rate, such as with exercise, hyperthyroidism, and infection. In patients with normal lungs the increase in carbon dioxide production does not usually lead to carbon dioxide retention. In patients with chronic carbon dioxide retention, however, increased carbon dioxide production is often reflected in an increased arterial P_{CO_2}. It should be re-emphasized that the presence of one of the factors discussed above does not mean the hypercapnia will be present. The nurse must be aware, however, that especially in extreme cases and in the presence of pre-existing chronic hypercapnia, the presence of any of these factors may lead to acute carbon dioxide retention. In any patient where one of four mechanisms pertains, it is important that the nurse observe the patient for the possibility of carbon dioxide retention. In the same respect, in those patients who have chronic carbon dioxide retention, it is part of the nurse's role to prohibit the development of these factors because she or he knows that they may well lead to additional acute carbon dioxide retention in that patient.

Effects

Chronic carbon dioxide retention with a compensated pH is usually well tolerated physiologically. Acute changes result in serious sequelae. Observation of the patient for the development of hypercapnia requires the nurse to know the physiologic effects of hypercapnia and those symptoms produced by the acidemia that accompanies an acute rise in carbon dioxide levels. Chronic hypercapnia alone with a compensated pH does not usually lead to any specific symptomatology. Therefore many of the symptoms of hypercapnia are actually symptoms of respiratory acidemia and the concurrent hypoxemia.

Because the changes in carbon dioxide, pH, and oxygen cause cerebral vasodilatation, the patient will often complain of a headache. The headache is often characterized as being an occipital throbbing headache that is worse when the patient awakens in the morning and does not appear to be affected by aspirin. The reason for the headache is that as the blood vessels in the central nervous system dilate, there is a resulting increase in cerebrospinal fluid pressure, which causes the headache. At the same time, there is the general elevation of cerebrospinal fluid pressure, and should a lumbar puncture be done for other reasons, it is not uncommon for the patient to exhibit an elevated pressure. In addition, the patient may exhibit papilledema and asterixis. Asterixis is usually noted first in the wrists and is demonstrated by having the patient hold his or her wrists in the extended position and observing the sudden flexion and withdrawal. This same "flapping" can be observed with other major muscle groups and is seen in the feet, tongue, and eyelids as well. General behavioral symptoms include drowsiness, tremors, confusion, and, if the CO_2 rise is large and acute resulting in a severe acidemia and hypoxemia, convulsions may occur. Should the nurse note a behavioral change in the patient, it is wise to investigate a possible physiologic mechanism for this behavioral change. For example, the patient may become "uncooperative" or "combative." These symptoms are not always derived from a psychological origin but sometimes from a physiologic change resulting from the lack of oxygen supply and inability to eliminate carbon dioxide from the central nervous system.

Hypercapnia, as stated, causes a decrease in the arterial oxygen tension. Whenever the arterial oxygen is increased, the level of carbon dioxide in the alveoli is also increased. Therefore there is less space left for oxygen and hence the arterial P_{O_2} will be decreased in an amount proportional to the rise in the P_{CO_2}. The symptoms related to the hypoxemia specifically will be discussed in the following section.

Blood gases, in addition to showing the change in P_{O_2}, will also show a change in the pH. As has been previously mentioned, there will be a fall in pH with a rise in the carbon dioxide level. In patients with chronic carbon dioxide retention, the pH change may be very slight, because of compensatory mechanisms of the kidney. This compensatory mechanism is demonstrated by an increase in the serum bicarbonate in the kidney's attempt to restore the 20:1 ratio of HCO_3^- to CO_2.

Hypercapnia and acidemia will also result in a low potassium level. As the serum becomes more acidotic and more hydrogen ions are available, the hydrogen ions enter the cell. In order to maintain electroneutrality, potassium leaves the cell. Initially a high serum potassium may be seen although total body potassium may be depleted. As the acidosis continues, low serum potassium levels may develop, indicating a severe deficit in the total body potassium. This hypokalemia may cause symptoms of muscle cramps and weakness. Severe cardiac arrhythmias may also occur.

A final symptom of carbon dioxide retention and acidosis is an additive effect to the pulmonary hypertension seen in hypoxemia. With a fall in pH and a concurrent hypoxemia, there is greater elevation of the pulmonary artery pressure than seen with hypoxemia alone. (See section on hypoxemia for further description.) In patients where this rise in pulmonary pressure puts an undue load on the right side of the heart, it is not uncommon for the nurse to observe signs of right-sided heart failure as a result of the increasing P_{CO_2} level. (See Chapter 44.)

Therapy

Dealing with carbon dioxide retention and its accompanying acidemia presents a need for very knowledgeable and aggressive nursing care. Specific treatment will vary, depending on whether the carbon dioxide retention and the ventilatory failure are chronic, acute, or chronic with superimposed acute ventilatory failure. In all cases, the hypoxemia is treated.

Chronic ventilatory failure is defined as the situation where the patient has a P_{CO_2} greater than 50 mm Hg but the pH is near normal. In other words, the body has been able to compensate for the pH change by retaining bicarbonate and the patient, therefore, does not show a severe pH change even though he or she may have severe carbon dioxide retention. Chronic ventilatory failure is seen in patients with chronic obstructive lung disease, primary idiopathic alveolar hypoventilation, kyphoscoliosis, and other such conditions. In such cases effort is not directed to lowering the carbon dioxide tension to the normal range. Rather, treatment emphasizes the prevention and early treatment of any acute exacerbation that would lead to a superimposed acute ventilatory failure. At the same time, the underlying disease is treated. The nurse must be alert to the fact that the patient does have chronic ventilatory failure. These patients may function quite well and not look like they are in any acute distress. However, all of the factors that would lead to carbon dioxide retention and that have been previously discussed could cause disastrous results in this type of patient. Therefore the nurse must be alert to teaching the patient to observe for respiratory infections or heart failure and must be very careful that within her or his own care regimen the nurse does not cause the patient to go into acute ventilatory failure (for example, by giving too much oxygen or requesting a sedation order).

The second type of ventilatory failure is acute ventilatory failure. In this situation, the P_{CO_2} is greater than 50 mm Hg and the pH shows an acidemia; there has not been compensation of the pH change. Acute ventilatory failure may be seen in some cases of drug overdose, acute trauma, severe pneumonia, and so on. If P_{CO_2} and pH changes are not severe (pH is still between 7.3 and 7.4, P_{CO_2} is close to 50 mm Hg), then treatment can often be aimed at the underlying cause of the ventilatory failure. In many cases, however, with the rapid change of P_{CO_2} and pH the patient becomes unresponsive and mechanical ventilation must be instituted. For specifics of the nursing care in such situations, the nurse is referred to the case studies and the special techniques of respiratory care.

The third general category of ventilatory failure is chronic ventilatory failure with superimposed acute ventilatory failure. Such an instance refers to the patient who has had chronic CO_2 retention and now has had an acute episode (such as might be precipitated by infection, sedation, and so on). The acute episode results in a sudden rise in the P_{CO_2}. The pH is not as low as would be expected with a pure acute ventilatory failure, but it is definitely out of the compensated range.

Within this last general category of mixed chronic and acute hypercapnia three types of therapy are possible. The one most commonly used today is referred to as the conservative approach to therapy. In this approach, therapy is aimed at the underlying cause. As the cause of the acute exacerbation is treated, the patient's P_{CO_2} and pH should return to the pre-exacerbation level. Treatment of this patient requires very knowledgeable and aggressive nursing care, for the patient must be kept awake and breathing so that the acidemia does not become more severe as the underlying cause of the failure is being treated. Therefore the nurse must frequently observe the patient. She or he must be very conscientious in having the patient deep breathe and cough and in maintaining a patent airway. The second mode of therapy involves the patient who is still alert but whose pH is falling to life-threatening levels (the pH is less than 7.2). In such cases some physicians recommend administering intravenous bicarbonate. The administration of bicarbonate will tend to reverse the pH change and return it to a more normal level, although acidemia will still be present. When the pH change is no longer life-threatening, time is gained to treat the underlying cause of the acute exacerbation in an effort to return the pH and P_{CO_2} to the patient's chronic level. If the patient is not alert or is not responding to the treatment of the underlying disease, this approach is not used. Some physicians are against using bicarbonate therapy unless there is a specific metabolic acidosis present; they feel that because bicarbonate adds to the CO_2 stores of the body, it can lead to further depression of ventilation. The third approach to therapy and one that is only seldom used is the institution of mechanical ventilation. When used, mechanical ventilation in this category of ventilatory failure is reserved for those patients with a reversible process who are unresponsive and therefore cannot be kept awake and breathing without the assistance of a ventilator. In such cases caution must be used so that the patient is not overventilated. Because this patient has chronic ventilatory failure and excess of bicarbonate on board in order to compensate the pH, it is dangerous to return him or her to a normal P_{CO_2} level. Instead, the patient must be ventilated to a point where the CO_2 is still elevated but the pH is within a normal range. Should the P_{CO_2} be lowered to a normal of 40 mm Hg, the pH may be extremely elevated and all the dangerous side effects of alkalemia will be encountered.

As can be seen, the type of therapy used depends very much on the philosophy of the physician, and the alert observation of the patient, and the nursing care capabilities in the situation. Therefore there is a great emphasis placed on the nursing care of the patient, not only nursing observation of the patient, but the nurse's active involvement in the type of therapy provided to that patient. In those situations where expert nursing care is not available, it is much more common to see more and more of these patients requiring mechanical ventilation. They require the ventilation because the nurse does not understand the physiology involved in the patient's condition and was not alert enough to observe him or her and to institute the proper nursing care. With expert nursing care, many of these patients survive these episodes of acute ventilatory failure extremely well.

The later section on special techniques used in respiratory care and the case study discussions will better exemplify the type of nursing care needed in individual situations. It must always be remembered that there is no recipe to the care of these individuals in acute ventilatory failure. *Ventilatory failure* is a physiologic term attributed to a variety of specific disease states. Therefore the nurse must be able to make astute observations and plan appropriate interventions for that patient depending on the interaction of his or her basic disease processes and the total effects and causes of the episode of acute ventilatory failure.

Exchange and Transport of Oxygen

One of the ultimate goals of gas exchange is to maintain adequate levels of oxygen at the tissue level. This exchange and delivery system depends on several things, including the following:

1. Ventilation of the lungs with air.
2. Perfusion of the lungs with blood.
3. The cardiac output.
4. The tissue demands for oxygen.
5. The carrying capacity of the blood (hemoglobin level).

If any part of the system is out of balance the patient would suffer the undesirable effects of tissue hypoxia. In order to assess the ability of the lungs to maintain the oxygen level of the arterial blood, the P_{O_2}, and the oxyhemoglobin saturation are measured as previously described. Hypoxemia is defined as levels of arterial P_{O_2} that are below normal (*Hypoxemia* refers specifically to low oxygen in the arterial blood whereas *hypoxia* refers to general or regional lack of tissue oxygen.) When the Pa_{O_2} is above normal levels, a state of hyperoxia is present.

The P_{O_2} provides information regarding the lungs'

ability to exchange oxygen, but the nurse must also be able to assess oxygen transport. An important factor is the oxygen content of the blood. As has been discussed, the results of blood gas analysis provide a P_{O_2} and Sa_{O_2}. The saturation measured is the saturation of the hemoglobin present; it does not tell you how much oxygen the hemoglobin should carry if the individual had a normal type and amount of hemoglobin. To illustrate, look at the following values for three patients.

	P_{O_2} (mm Hg)	Sa_{O_2} (%)	Hgb (g)	Oxygen Content (Vols %)
Patient A	80	95	15	19.3
Patient B	80	95	10	12.9
Patient C	33	61	15	12.4

Patients A and B have very acceptable numbers for Pa_{O_2} and Sa_{O_2}. Patient B, however, because his hemoglobin is very low has a very low total oxygen content. Regretfully, because his "numbers" look good, the fact that he is not delivering adequate amounts of oxygen to his tissues is frequently not recognized. Patient C, on the other hand, will be promptly recognized as having a low oxygen level. Yet the oxygen content of patient B is nearly the same as that of the patient with the very low P_{O_2}. Therefore the blood gas results must be analyzed in terms of the amount of hemoglobin present if a valid assessment of oxygen delivery is to be made. In addition to the ability to carry oxygen, assessment of the actual delivery of oxygen may also be done. This measurement is not a routine one except in intensive-care settings, as it requires the placement of a catheter in the pulmonary artery. Blood samples from the pulmonary artery allow measurement of the mixed venous oxygen tension ($P_{\bar{v}O_2}$) and mixed venous oxygen content. Abnormally low values ($P_{\bar{v}O_2}$ less than 40 mg and arteriovenous content difference greater than 6 volumes per cent) usually indicate a decreased cardiac output and inadequate delivery.

Hyperoxia

Although nurses are commonly aware of the problems of hypoxemia, they must also be aware of the problems of hyperoxia or an oxygen level above normal. The only way for the body to demonstrate an excess quantity of oxygen is to administer supplemental oxygen via an exogenous source. Such a situation is extremely common during artificial ventilation when special gas mixtures are administered via a mechanical ventilator. The saying that "if a little is good, a lot is better" is not true in the case of oxygen. Hyperoxia will have a variety of effects upon the pulmonary system. A few of these are as follows:

1. Hyperoxia may decrease ventilatory drive by decreasing the stimulation of the peripheral chemoreceptors. This situation is especially true in the patient with chronic carbon dioxide retention where the reduction of ventilatory drive can reach extremely hazardous levels.
2. Hyperoxia may also decrease surfactant production in the lung and impair the function of that surfactant. Because surfactant reduces surface tension in the alveoli, a lack of it can lead to atelectasis and an increase in the physiologic shunt (blood goes by unventilated alveoli). Therefore the result is that the oxygen therapy creates a problem that will cause a further problem of hypoxemia.
3. It has also been found that hyperoxia can decrease mucociliary clearance. Therefore in addition to affecting the distribution of gas in the lung, the hyperoxia will also decrease the effectiveness of the protective mechanisms of the lung.

The treatment for hyperoxia is basically to prevent its occurrence. Therefore the patient's blood gases should be carefully monitored during the administration of oxygen therapy so as not to produce hyperoxia and its resulting problems.

The effects of hyperoxia are most evident when the fraction of inspired oxygen (FI_{O_2}) is above 50 per cent. It has been stated that at inspired oxygen levels of 100 per cent, symptoms of oxygen toxicity occur within 12 hours, whereas at 60 per cent manifestations occur in several days (Senior, 1971). It has also been demonstrated that patients who received oxygen concentrations of 35 to 40 per cent for extended periods of time (years) on postmortem, demonstrate the results of oxygen toxicity in the lung parenchyma (Petty, Stanford, and Neff, 1971).

Although it is desirable not to administer oxygen at concentrations greater than 50 per cent in order to prevent these problems, if this level of inspired oxygen is required to supply oxygen adequately to the tissues, then that level must be administered. It has become common usage now in those patients who are demonstrating the need for very high inspired oxygen levels that the addition of a positive end expiratory pressure plateau is often helpful in decreasing the amount of oxygen required. Positive end expiratory pressure (PEEP) means that the patient exhales against a positive pressure and that airway pressures are never allowed to fall to atmospheric. When such therapy is initiated, it is often possible to decrease the inspired oxygen to less than 50 per cent and still maintain oxygenation of the patient. The specific therapeutic indications and physiologic applications of PEEP will be discussed in the section on special techniques.

Hypoxemia

Causes

Hypoxemia is a prominent problem in the care of the patient with pulmonary dysfunction. In order to recognize or anticipate this problem, the nurse must recognize the physiologic causes of arterial hypoxemia. First would be a low inspired oxygen tension. Because the arterial oxygen level depends on the inspired oxygen, any alteration in the inspired oxygen tension would change the arterial oxygen. The commonest cause of an abnormally low inspired oxygen tension (PI_{O_2}) is a decrease in the barometric pressure. For example, at elevations of 8,000 feet the normal Pa_{O_2} would fall to 60 to 70 mm Hg compared to the normal of 80 to 100 at sea level. It is therefore understandable that it would be dangerous for a person who had marginal oxygenation at sea level to undertake a trip to an area with a higher elevation.

The second cause of hypoxemia is hypoventilation. As previously discussed, hypoventilation results in an elevated alveolar P_{CO_2}. Because the amount of carbon dioxide present will affect the space left for oxygen in the alveolus, it is evident that an elevated carbon dioxide level will be accompanied by a lower-than-normal alveolar oxygen level. Therefore any state that results in an elevation of the carbon dioxide level will decrease the arterial P_{O_2}.

A third cause of hypoxemia is mismatching of ventilation and blood flow. Any situation which results in a reduction of the ratio of alveolar ventilation to capillary perfusion ($\dot{V}/\dot{Q}$) will lead to hypoxemia. The extreme of mismatching is a shunt, an absolute lack of ventilation with perfusion continuing. Thus a shunt means that there is an anatomic or physiologic alteration so that the blood travels through the lung without being exposed to ventilated alveoli. Therefore that blood will not have its oxygen level raised. It will still have the gas tension of venous blood. This venous blood is then mixed with normal arterialized (oxygenated) blood, the result being that the systemic circulation has a P_{O_2} that is below normal. The absolute value of the Pa_{O_2} will depend upon the ratio of venous to arterialized blood. There are some anatomic shunts found in the normal lung. These are the thebesian veins that empty into the aorta and some of the bronchial veins that anastomose directly with the pulmonary veins. The variance in the degree to which these normal shunts are present partially accounts for the range of normal arterial oxygen tension. The most common cause of abnormally high levels of anatomic shunts are pulmonary arteriovenous fistulas and congenital heart lesions; other pathologic conditions such as atelectasis or ARDS result in a shuntlike effect.

Most hypoxemia due to mismatching of ventilation and perfusion is due to areas of low $\dot{V}/\dot{Q}$. In such instances there may still be ventilation, but it is markedly reduced in comparison with the amount of perfusion. Some common clinical examples are bronchitis, emphysema, asthma, and interstitial fibrosis.

The usual blood gas picture is one of a low Pa_{O_2} and a low or normal Pa_{CO_2}. Blood that is not exposed to an adequately ventilated alveolus has a low P_{O_2} and high P_{CO_2}. In areas where the blood is exposed to normal alveoli, hyperventilation occurs in an attempt to compensate. Since CO_2 transport is not limited by hemoglobin, the CO_2 content of the blood in these hyperventilated areas can be markedly reduced. When the blood from areas of low $\dot{V}/\dot{Q}$ is mixed with the blood in contact with hyperventilated alveoli, the result is a low to normal P_{CO_2}. In the case of oxygen, such compensation is not possible. Since normal oxygen content depends on an oxyhemoglobin saturation of nearly 100 per cent, the blood in the hyperventilated areas does not have a significantly higher oxygen content; the hemoglobin cannot be supersaturated. Thus blood with a normal content is mixed with blood with a low content. The result is an arterial P_{O_2} which is lower than normal. Because of the mechanism by which the hypoxemia is produced, in cases of absolute shunt, oxygen therapy has little effect in raising the arterial P_{O_2}. The oxygen cannot reach the unventilated alveoli. In areas of low $\dot{V}/\dot{Q}$, the supplemental oxygen can reach the involved alveoli. So, even though they are underventilated, the P_{O_2} can be raised.

The fourth possible physiologic explanation of hypoxemia is a diffusion abnormality. In order for the blood to take up the oxygen, the oxygen must pass through the alveolar wall, into the capillary, through the plasma and red blood cells, and into the hemoglobin. This transfer is called diffusion and limitations of diffusion are sometimes referred to as alveolar capillary block. Physiologically, a diffusion block looks exactly like a ventilation perfusion abnormality, and careful studies have failed to prove that diffusion alone, under resting conditions, impairs gas transport.

The preceding discussion has summarized the various physiologic abnormalities that could lead to hypoxemia. As is evident, most clinical situations produce a situation that could potentially cause a problem in gas transport and hypoxemia. For example, any time a patient is placed in bed and does not take periodic deep breaths, there is the potential for the development of hypoxemia. By understanding the mechanisms of hypoxemia, the nurse can be alert to anticipating which patients may develop hypoxemia, and at the same time institute actions to prevent its occurrence. Similarly, if hypoxemia does develop the nurse should detect it as early as possible.

Effects

Clinically, the effects of hypoxemia are manifested by altered function of the end organs. Therefore the symptoms of hypoxemia are actually the physiologic effects of hypoxia. Because the oxygen stores of the body are only about 20 cc per kilogram and because the basal metabolic requirement is about 4 cc per kilogram per minute, the stored oxygen supply fails to support an adequate tissue oxygen tension in 2 to 4 minutes if the flow of oxygen to the tissues is blocked. If the lack of oxygen persists, the cells shift to anaerobic metabolic pathways and these changes can result in a metabolic acidosis and cell death. (Hypoxemia without carbon dioxide retention does not cause respiratory acidosis.) The system effects of hypoxemia can be described as follows:

1. *The central nervous system.* The central nervous system is particularly sensitive to hypoxemia because of its reliance on metabolism of simple sugars for energy production. The manifestations of hypoxemia include a decreased ability to concentrate, insomnia, headaches, and behavior that can range from restlessness to lethargy to coma. It is also not infrequent that Cheyne-Stokes' respirations may be observed, and finally EEG abnormalities will occur in the presence of hypoxemia. The degree to which many of these symptoms are exhibited by any specific patient will vary. Patients with chronic hypoxemia will not demonstrate these symptoms as would someone whose P_{O_2} fell acutely to the same level. On the other hand, it is interesting to note that recent studies have demonstrated an indication that scores on intelligence tests are elevated by the administration of oxygen to patients who have chronic hypoxemia (Krop et al., 1973). These effects of hypoxemia on the central nervous system are important to the nurse not only for early detection of signs of hypoxemia in terms of diagnostic criteria but also for how the nurse works with the patient who is chronically hypoxic. First, it is important to note that behavioral changes may often be related to physiologic dysfunction of the central nervous system and not just to the "uncooperativeness" of the patient. Therefore the nurse must be careful to determine whether or not the patient is being "uncooperative" or if this is in actuality a demonstration of the lack of oxygen supplied to the central nervous system. In the case of the patient who is hypoxemic the nurse must realize that the patient does indeed have a decreased ability to concentrate and that his or her comprehension may not be as good as when the patient is not hypoxemic. Therefore teaching sessions with the patient should be planned so as to last for only short periods of time and the materials presented in any session of teaching should be limited and very clearly explained with frequent repetition so that the patient is able to comprehend the material.
2. *Gastrointestinal system.* The manifestations of hypoxemia on the gastrointestinal system may include abnormal liver function and abdominal pain and, if there is severe hypoxemia, bowel infarction may occur.
3. *Genitourinary system.* Manifestations of hypoxemia on the genitourinary system include sodium retention with ensuing fluid retention. Hypoxemia appears to affect sodium retention in several ways. First of all, total urinary function may be decreased because of decreased glomerular filtration rate. Should the hypoxemia be severe enough to decrease cardiac function and therefore cardiac output, perfusion pressures will be further decreased. In addition, hypoxemia affects the function of both the distal and the proximal tubule so that sodium retention occurs. There may also be influences upon the secretions of hormones such as aldosterone that would affect sodium retention. Another effect of hypoxemia on the genitourinary system is that it is not uncommon for patients who are chronically hypoxic to have difficulty initiating or completing sexual intercourse. This problem is one of great concern to the patient and yet one that is very infrequently discussed.
4. *Cardiovascular system.* The manifestations of hypoxemia exhibited by the cardiovascular system are often some of the first symptoms to be detected clinically. There is an increase in cardiac output produced by an increase in the heart rate. Therefore it is not uncommon to see tachycardia in the presence of hypoxemia. With this increase in cardiac output, systolic hypertension may occur. As the hypoxemia continues to become more severe and the oxygen supply to the myocardium itself is inadequate, cardiac arrhythmias, angina, myocardial infarction, and heart failure may occur. Hypoxemia may also lead to the development of pulmonary hypertension, as there appears to

be an arteriolar constriction in the pulmonary vascular bed as a response to hypoxemia. In the peripheral circulation there will be some local vasoconstriction with an effort to shunt blood to vital organs where there will be a vasodilatation. In chronic hypoxemia, there is erythrocytosis with the development of polycythemia. This is called secondary polycythemia as it is the result of the response to the hypoxemia and is not a primary hematologic defect.

It should be noted that all the clinical manifestations of hypoxemia are quite vague and nonspecific. Not all of these symptoms will be exhibited in one patient, and therefore it is extremely difficult to diagnose hypoxemia and tissue hypoxia by one or two clinical symptoms. Hence the diagnosis of hypoxia must be made in view of the entire clinical setting, which would include an estimation of ventilation, cardiac output, and blood hemoglobin. It should also be noted that cyanosis was not mentioned as an outstanding symptom of hypoxemia. The detection of cyanosis is a very subjective observation and is also very unreliable. Cyanosis is present when there are 5 g of reduced hemoglobin per 100 ml blood (hemoglobin that is not carrying oxygen molecules). Therefore there must first be adequate hemoglobin present in order for the detection of cyanosis to be made. The patient who is anemic can be severely hypoxemic and also have a severe decrease in oxygen content because of the low hemoglobin level, yet he or she will not look cyanotic (because there is not 5 g of reduced hemoglobin). On the other hand, the patient who has a polycythemia with an elevated hematocrit and elevated hemoglobin level will tend to show cyanosis at an earlier point than would the normal individual. In addition, the visual detection of cyanosis is dependent upon the local circulation to the area. If there is poor capillary blood flow in the region where the observation of cyanosis is being made, it will not be detected even if there is reduced hemoglobin present. When one is observing for cyanosis it is recommended that the mucous membrane of the mouth and the tongue be observed. Too many times the observation is made in terms of the color of the nail beds. Often the patient is in such a position that the hands are in a dependent position, which leads to engorgement of those blood vessels. Therefore the cyanosis is due more to the circulatory disorder than to the amount of oxygen being supplied. Although the detection of cyanosis is still used clinically, the observer must remember that this is a subjective symptom and is also extremely unreliable. Therefore whenever there is a question as to the level of the patient's oxygenation, the arterial P_{O_2} should be measured.

Therapy

The treatment of hypoxemia is basically the administration of supplemental oxygen. It must be realized that even though oxygen therapy can be used to treat many types of hypoxia, it is not effective in all cases. For example, if the problem is low oxygen content resulting from a low hemoglobin level, the administration of oxygen alone will not correct that difficulty; the need is for an elevation of the hemoglobin to normal levels. In the same respect, should the tissue hypoxia be due to a decreased perfusion, administration of supplemental oxygen alone will not solve the problem and as previously mentioned in hypoxemia due to shunt, supplemental oxygen does not increase the alveolar P_{O_2} in the affected areas. In most cases, however, the administration of supplemental oxygen is extremely effective in correcting hypoxemia and its ensuing tissue hypoxia.

It must be remembered that oxygen is a drug and is given to treat a specific problem, the problem of hypoxemia. Because it is a drug, the oxygen should be given in very specific concentrations or at specific flow rates. In some cases administration of too much oxygen is potentially dangerous to the patient's well-being just as too little is dangerous. Therefore the oxygen must be given in a specific amount for the problem of hypoxemia. The response to the therapy is then monitored by way of arterial blood gases and the determination is made as to whether this amount of oxygen is sufficient or not.

The most common mode of oxygen supplementation is the use of the nasal cannula. Even at flows of 1 to 2 liters via the cannula, most patients have enough of a rise in arterial P_{O_2} to increase adequately oxygen delivery to the tissues. In some extreme cases, other modes of oxygen delivery are required, but again, it should be emphasized that the cannula is sufficient in the vast majority of cases. Because oxygen is administered to meet a specific need, it usually is required that the oxygen therapy be continuous. Only when the need for oxygen is intermittent should the administration of oxygen therapy be intermittent. For example, some patients may require oxygen supplementation only during exercise when there is an increased metabolic need for oxygen. Other patients may be able to maintain adequate oxygenation during the waking hours but at night with the problem of hypoventilation the arterial oxygen drops to more dangerous levels and supplemental oxygen is required. In other cases, however, it should be emphasized that oxygen therapy should be continuous. The use of intermittent oxygen, especially in the case of the patient with chronic carbon dioxide retention, can be potentially hazardous to the patient's well-being and is definitely not beneficial.

A variety of methods are available for the delivery of oxygen to the patient. These methods allow some flexibility in controlling the concentrations delivered; patient comfort is also a factor in selecting a method of delivering supplemental oxygen. For most oxygen therapy, adequate oxygen supplementation can be obtained through the use of a nasal cannula. The nasal cannula consists of dual prongs that are inserted into the nasal vestibule via both external nares. The inspired oxygen fraction that is ultimately delivered to the patient will be dependent upon the patient's minute volume, the patient's peak inspiratory flow rate, and the oxygen flow rate delivered through the equipment. The oxygen is delivered from the compressed gas source at a concentration of 100 per cent. Mixing then occurs in the pharynx, for as the patient inhales, the oxygen delivered is mixed with room air. Therefore as minute volume increases the actual oxygen fraction delivered to the patient will be less at a specified flow rate than it would be when the patient's minute volume was smaller. Studies on normal individuals have shown that the inspired oxygen at 2 liters per minute ranges from 23 to 28 per cent in nose breathers and from 22 to 48 per cent in mouth breathers. At 5 liters per minute the range is 32 to 47 per cent in nose breathers and to 33 to 63 per cent in mouth breathers (Waligora, 1970).

It is important to note that this method produces a higher concentration in mouth breathers than in nose breathers even though the oxygen flow is directed into the nose. The patient does not have to nose breathe. The major advantage of the cannula is, therefore, patient comfort and simplicity of use, and for these reasons it is currently the most common means of oxygen administration. The major disadvantage is the flow limitation, as most patients do not tolerate flows greater than 8 to 10 liters per minute.

The nasal catheter, which is a single tube inserted into the nasopharynx via the external nares, can also be used for the administration of nasal oxygen. It comes in a variety of sizes so that adjustment can be made for patient comfort. The inspired oxygen fraction that is delivered will vary, just as it does with the oxygen cannula. In normal subjects at a flow of 2 liters per minute, the inspired oxygen concentration ranges from 24 to 36 per cent in nose breathers and from 28 to 52 per cent in mouth breathers. At 5 liters per minute the range is 32 to 52 per cent in nose breathers and 34 to 63 per cent for mouth breathers (Waligora, 1970).

The major disadvantage of the nasal catheter is patient discomfort. It must be taped securely to prevent a change in its position, because if it should drift, it might stimulate a gag reflex or result in gastric insufflation. The catheter must also be changed every 6 to 8 hours in order to prevent mucous crusting. A final limitation that is similar to that of the oxygen cannula is that the patient usually does not tolerate flows greater than 8 to 10 liters per minute.

Oxygen masks may also be used to deliver oxygen supplementation. An oxygen mask should not, however, be used unless the flows required are greater than 6 liters per minute. With flows less than 6 liters per minute, there is carbon dioxide accumulation in the mask (added dead space) and the resulting inspired fraction delivered to the patient is less than would be expected. Therefore flows must be high enough to wash out most of the exhaled gas. Other disadvantages of the oxygen mask are patient discomfort, necessity to remove the mask for eating, drinking, expectorating, and the possibility of unintentional displacement of the mask by the patient's activity. The major advantage is that a mask will attain higher inspired oxygen concentrations than will the catheter or cannula and at high flows is usually better tolerated by the patient. A simple oxygen mask will deliver an inspired oxygen fraction equivalent to 40 to 65 per cent at 6 to 10 liters per minute of oxygen. The partial rebreathing mask that has a reservoir bag can attain an inspired oxygen fraction equivalent to 60 to 80 per cent at 6 to 10 liters per minute. When using the partial rebreathing mask care must be taken that flows are sufficient so that the reservoir meets the patient's inspiratory demands. Should the reservoir bag not meet the patient's inspiratory demands, there is a higher proportion of mixing with entrained room air and therefore the inspired oxygen fraction will be lower than expected. The nonbreathing mask has a reservoir bag and valves that regulate the direction of inspiratory and expiratory flows. The patient inhales from the reservoir bag and exhales through the side expiratory ports. With an adequate volume potential of the reservoir bag, high flows (up to flush) and a snugly fitting mask, an oxygen concentration of 95 per cent plus or minus 5 per cent can be delivered. The major advantage of this method is the high concentration of inspired oxygen that can be obtained. The disadvantages are the same as those for oxygen masks in general. In addition, there is a disadvantage of the mechanical limitations of the valve's reliability and the added resistance to the work of breathing.

The Venturi mask is an oxygen mask especially designed to deliver a specific inspired oxygen fraction regardless of the patient's minute volume and peak inspiratory flow rates. There are four concentration specific masks available so that there is a choice of inspired oxygen from 24 to 40 per cent. The mask operates on a Venturi principle so that it produces very high flow rates. There is a flow rate provided by the oxygen source itself plus the air added at the Venturi mix. This mask therefore has the advantage that a specific inspired oxygen concentration is delivered and that the dead-space effect is reduced because of the high flow rates. The disadvantages are the same as many of those of the other oxygen masks in that there is a need to remove the mask for eating, drinking, and expectoration. Condensation or deposition of foreign particles at the Venturi orifice could alter the oxygen concentration, but humidification of the oxygen source does not appear to alter the oxygen concentration.

Although supplemental oxygen treats the hypoxemia, the nurse must be alert to also treat the causative mechanism. For example, the patient is retaining secretions which leads to a problem of hypoxemia due to low $\dot{V}/\dot{Q}$. The nurse, by instituting airway care measures can affect the cause of the hypoxemia while ensuring adequate oxygenation by administering supplemental oxygen.

Lung Defense Mechanisms

Upper Airway

The upper airway (nose and mouth to the larynx) serves as the air-conditioning system for the respiratory tract as well as a passageway for the transport of gases (see Figure 26-3). Within its function as the air-conditioning system are included filtering, heating, and humidification of the inspired air. Filtering is most efficient when the inspired air passes through the nose rather than the mouth. As the air passes through the nose, flow is very turbulent as the passage is baffled by the turbinate bones. Particles that may be in the inspired air are thus more likely to impact and stick onto the mucus that lines the airway. During the air's passage through the upper airway, it is also heated to body temperature. This process occurs as the air is in close contact with the highly vascular mucous membrane. At the same time, the air is humidified to 100 per cent water vapor saturation at body temperature (remember that the warmer the air, the more water vapor it can hold). If the inspired air is not fully humidified during passage through the upper airway, water is extracted from the mucous lining in the lower airway. This process of extracting water from the mucous lining of the lower airway can lead to the inspissation of the mucus secreted in the lower airway. All these functions of the upper airway not only serve to protect the lower airway but also ensure that the inspired air has the properties that will enable the other defense mechanisms to be more effective.

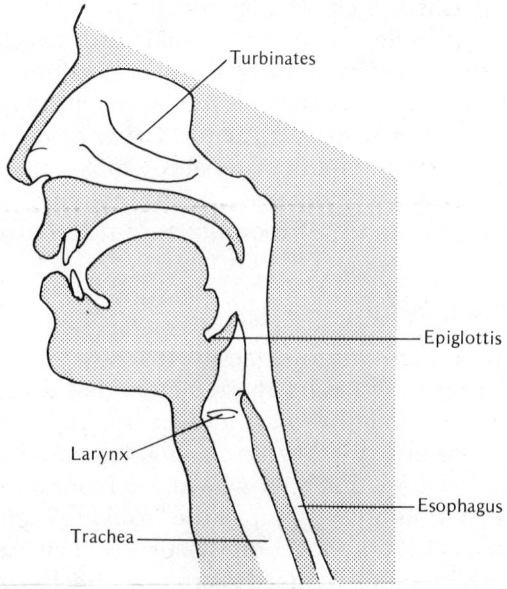

Figure 26-3. The upper airway.

Lower Airway

The basic defense mechanisms of the lower airway include (1) the mucociliary escalator system, (2) cough, and (3) macrophage clearance.

The Mucociliary Escalator System

The mucociliary escalator system requires a thin sheet of mucus and ciliary activity. The walls of the airways contain mucous glands that secrete a thin mucous coating that lines the airway down to the level of the respiratory bronchiole. In addition, the epithelium of the airway is ciliated. These cilia beat in a coordinated, rhythmic fashion toward the upper airway. As the inspired air passes down the airway, particles impact on the mucus and are entrapped. The layer of mucus is continually being moved by the ciliary action up the airway to the mouth, where the mucus with its trapped pollutants is swallowed. Everybody is continually clearing this mucus from the airway, although the amount raised to the upper airway at any one time is so small that it is not perceivable to the individual.

Cough

Cough is another important physiologic mechanism used to maintain a patent airway. The cough reflex is most easily stimulated in the larynx and at the carinae (points of airway bifurcation). An effective cough involves the following:

1. A deep breath. This maneuver produces dilation of airways so that air can pass distal to the secretions in addition to producing a large lung volume.
2. Closure of the glottis.
3. Active contraction of expiratory muscles. Active expiration against a closed glottis produces a high intrathoracic pressure (up to 100 cm water).
4. Sudden opening of the glottis. Because of the buildup of high intrathoracic pressures, opening of the glottis produces very high expulsive gas velocities.

In order for the airways to transmit a gas volume adequate for effective cough, they must have sufficient rigidity to prevent collapse. In diseases such as emphysema, the airways are "floppy" and may not remain open during the cough. In contrast, in pulmonary fibrosis (which produces a stiff lung), the volume available for expulsion may be insufficient in spite of competent airways.

Macrophage Clearance

The third defense mechanism is macrophage clearance. This system operates at the alveolar level and clears those particles that have not been removed from the airway by the other defense mechanisms. Small particles that reach the alveoli are engulfed or ingested by the alveolar macrophages and then cleared via the lymphatics and the mucociliary escalator system.

Factors Affecting Airway Clearance

A great many patients have some dysfunction of the defense mechanisms of the airways. If these mechanisms are not effective, the exchange of gas between the atmosphere and the alveoli will be inhibited with resulting hypoxemia and, in some patients, hypercapnia. First, the nurse must be able to recognize the factors that may affect the normal mechanisms of airway clearance. Only in this way can patient care problems be anticipated and treated effectively before they become so extreme that they produce gross limitations on gas exchange. A brief survey of these factors will be arranged into external and internal factors that affect the defense mechanism.

External Factors

Air pollution is one external factor that can affect the normal clearance of the airway. Air pollution includes industrial pollution and personal air pollution such as cigarette smoking. These inhaled irritants cause irritation of the airway, which can stimulate an increased production of mucus. At the same time, many of the pollutants also decrease ciliary activity. The resulting situation is one of increased mucus being present and decreased effectiveness of the airway in clearing the mucus.

Another factor that can affect the normal clearance mechanisms is low humidity of the inspired air, such as is seen in hot-air heating systems and the administration of compressed gases, such as oxygen and air. Even when the dry inspired air is inhaled through the nose and upper airway, it is frequently at such a low humidity before entering the airway that the upper airway is not successful in meeting its roles as the air-conditioning system. Thus water is extracted from the mucous lining of the lower airway and secretions become more viscid and less easily transported along the mucociliary escalator. The inhalation of dry air can also cause upper airway discomfort in the form of a sore throat. Low humidity of the inspired air becomes a special problem in those patients who are intubated, for the functions of the upper airway are bypassed. In such situations the air must be artificially heated to body temperature, be humidified to 100 per cent saturation at body temperature, and be as free as possible of foreign particles. In addition, intubation results in a less effective cough, because the glottis can no longer be closed to create the high intrathoracic pressures required for high expulsive flow rates.

A fourth external factor that affects the normal clearance of the airway is the use of drugs. There are many drugs, such as narcotics and sedatives, that will decrease the cough reflex. These same drugs may also inhibit the patient's spontaneous periodic deep breaths, which often stimulate the production of a cough reflex. The atropinelike drugs will decrease the water content of the secreted mucus in the airway and, thus, make it more difficult to move it along the mucociliary escalator. Other drugs, such as alcohol, components of tobacco smoke, and anesthetic gases, will decrease ciliary activity, again inhibiting clearance of secretions from the airway.

Internal Factors

There are also internal factors that will affect airway clearance. First are those factors that decrease the patient's ability to take a deep breath, such as, pain, neuromuscular diseases, and a decreased level of consciousness. Patients who do not periodically take deep breaths lose some of the "milking" activity that such action produces on the airway. This "milking" activity helps to move secretions mechanically up the airway. A deep breath is also necessary to produce an effective cough. There are also factors that decrease the individual's ability to generate high expiratory velocities as needed in cough. Examples of these factors would be the chronic obstructive lung diseases, muscle weakness, and pain. Infection is a third factor, for it will increase the mucus production of the patient and will put a greater burden on natural defense mechanisms. Next are those states that produce dehydration, with subsequent increase in the viscosity of the mucus produced. Such mucus is less easily transported and more difficult to remove by the cough mechanism. The last group of internal factors includes those conditions that would decrease macrophage activity at the alveolar level. Examples are patients who are immunologically suppressed as in cancer therapy and alcoholism.

Nursing Measures to Maintain Airway Patency

Because of the extreme importance of the maintenance of a patent airway, there are many implications for the initiation of therapeutic intervention in order to maintain function. This discussion will cover a great many methods of bronchial hygiene available to the nurse, but it is important to point out that not all of these techniques are required in each patient. In some patients bronchial hygiene simply requires increasing the fluid intake, in others bronchoscopy may be required. What is important to remember is that every program of bronchial hygiene must be individualized for the specific patient. In addition, not only do patients differ as to their needs for these respiratory therapy techniques, but the needs of any one individual patient may vary from day to day and even from hour to hour. Therefore this discussion of techniques will describe each of the techniques and not necessarily describe when it may be used. The discussions later in the chapter of actual patient care situations will bring into context the need for judgment as to when to use what technique and what signs and symptoms would be used to indicate the need for these types of therapy.

Humidification

The first implication is to prevent excessive drying of the mucous membrane by ensuring adequate humidification of therapeutic gases. Gases that come from a compressed source, such as wall or tanked oxygen and air, contain no water vapor. Therefore these gases must be at least partially humidified before they are administered to the patient. In the case of administering therapeutic oxygen through a nasal or oral device, a bubble humidifier is usually adequate. However, it must be remembered that this humidifier is only adequate when the upper airway is intact. The bubble humidifier provides approximately 20 per cent relative humidity and thus requires that the upper airway further humidify the air so that it is at 100 per cent humidity at body temperature when the air enters the lower airway. When the upper airway is bypassed, the inspired air or oxygen must be heated and humidified in order to ensure that the prerequisites are being met. A heated Cascade type of humidifier or a heated aerosol unit is used for this purpose.

Medications

A second therapeutic implication is to ensure the judicious use of narcotics and sedatives. It must be remembered that in the case of the patient who has pain, a narcotic may help in deep breathing and coughing. Yet overuse of such medication will actually decrease the patient's normal defense mechanisms for maintaining a patent airway. Therefore deep breathing and coughing should be done within a short period of time after the narcotic is given and the narcotic should not be used to such an extent that it prevents the patient from periodically taking a deep breath.

Deep Breathing and Coughing

Correctly teaching the patient how to deep breathe and cough is one of the most important roles of the nurse in maintaining the patient's patent airway. First, the nurse must remember to observe the patient for adequate chest expansion. A measurement of respiratory rate alone is not sufficient to determine the adequacy of the patient's ventilation. At times it may also be necessary actually to measure the volume of air the patient can exhale. An observation of chest expansion should show expansion of all diameters and not just a simple raising of the shoulders. When volumes are measured, a device such as the Wright respirometer can be used to measure the amount of air exhaled.

Methods of encouraging deep breathing have already been covered in the section on lung mechanics. The period of deep breathing may "milk" the airways encouraging the movement of secretion from smaller to larger airways. In addition the large inflations and deflations of the lung may mechanically stimulate a cough reflex.

In addition to ensuring that the patient can deep breathe effectively, the nurse must often teach him or her how to cough effectively. Many patients have a chronic cough and yet the cough maneuver is ineffective in raising secretions. There are several techniques used to teach patients to cough, and they will vary somewhat according to the physiologic problems that the patient exhibits. Remember that the tests of lung mechanics will help the nurse determine the approach to cough. For example, is the problem one of volume excursion or ability to generate high flows?

The cough techniques most widely used are the following:

1. Cascade cough.
2. End-expiratory cough.
3. "Huff" coughing.
4. Augmented cough.

These techniques may be used separately or in combination depending on the patient's problem.

The cascade cough is basically the normal cough or rather a series of coughs. Although patients are frequently taught to take a deep breath and then cough with one great, expulsive cough, seldom do we spontaneously cough in that manner. Rather, after one inhalation, we do a series of coughs, each with slightly less air in the lung. This maneuver makes the cough more effective over a greater part of the airways. If the cough was always performed at total lung capacity, it would only be effective in the trachea. By doing a series of coughs at successively lower lung volumes, coughing becomes effective out to the level of the segmental bronchi. It should be noted that in the normal healthy individual, coughing is only effective, meaning expectoration of mucus, to the level of segmental bronchi, certainly not to the alveolar level. Coughing may help to move mucus from smaller to larger airways, but such an effect has not been proven.

The end-expiratory cough is a maneuver especially effective in patients with bronchiectasis. It is also effective in patients with severe airway obstruction, and in other situations it can be used to stimulate a natural cough reflex. In the end-expiratory cough, the patient is usually instructed to do several deep breaths followed by slow, prolonged expirations. Then after two to three such maneuvers he or she is instructed to take a deep breath and breathe out slowly. After exhaling more than normally but still above residual volume, the patient should cough without inhaling first. This cough maneuver is the technique of choice in bronchiectasis (Macklem, 1973). In chronic obstructive lung disease, where a very forceful expiratory effort may lead to collapse of airways, this maneuver may facilitate the movement of secretions from smaller to larger airways. Then the end-expiratory cough can be followed by the cascade cough. The end-expiratory cough is also helpful in stimulating a cough reflex in the postoperative patient. Frequently it is easier for the patient with postoperative incisional pain to perform the end-expiratory cough than to cough at total lung capacity. Secretions can then be gradually moved up the airway and expectorated more easily. In the postoperative patient, the cough maneuver should always be followed by a deep inspiration.

The "huff" cough is another technique used to move secretions and to stimulate a natural cough. The "huff" cough is accomplished by having the patient take a deep breath and then do a series of short, forced expiratory maneuvers; the patient "huffs" on expiration. This technique is very similar to the cascade cough except that it is done with an open instead of closed glottis. The maneuver often stimulates a natural cough. If the patient has very "floppy" airways, this maneuver may lead to collapse of the airways and therefore not be beneficial. It may also be difficult for the postoperative patient because of incision discomfort from the rapid, repetitive forced expirations. In many patients, however, the increased expiratory flow rates move secretions to points in the airway where they stimulate a spontaneous cough.

A fourth approach to coughing is the augmented cough. This method is very helpful in patients who because of neuromuscular disease or fatigue are not able to generate maximal muscle contraction. Although postoperative patients or patients with chest trauma also have the problem of not being able to perform maximal expiratory muscle contraction, this technique is not used in such situations because of pain and possible trauma. In the augmented cough the nurse provides the muscle force that the patient is unable to generate. The cough may be augmented by chest or abdominal compression. Chest compression is also referred to as rib springing. This maneuver consists of having the patient take a deep breath or mechanically producing a deep breath. During the deep breath maneuver the hands are placed over the area of the thorax where there are retained secretions or on both sides of the lateral thorax if there is general weakness. At peak inspiration and just as the patient is going to begin to exhale, there is a forceful downward movement of the hands, forcing chest compression. This maneuver will produce rapid flow rates at peak expiration. The compression is then maintained and vibration is used throughout the rest of the expiratory maneuver. (The vibratory technique will be further described under postural drainage.) The other method of abdominal compression is helpful in patients who have loss or weakness of the abdominal muscles. As the patient inhales, the flat palm of the hand is placed at the upper abdomen below the xyphoid process. As the patient begins to exhale or, if possible, actively coughs, there is a sudden, abrupt pressure applied with the hand. The resulting increase in abdominal pressure (because of the reduction in size of the abdominal cavity) tends to force the diaphragm up and produce a higher expiratory flow rate than the patient would be able to produce spontaneously.

The methods described have assumed that the patient is capable of following instructions and generating a cough. For patients who are unable to follow instructions on how to cough, a spontaneous cough may often be stimulated by a stroking of the neck near the cricoid cartilage of the trachea. This maneuver will stimulate the natural cough reflex by irritation of the larynx and produce cough.

This discussion of means of teaching or stimulating effective cough in patients has ranged from the techniques that would be used in an outpatient setting or to any patient with chronic sputum retention to those patients who would be found in the intensive-care unit and who are in a more critical situation. Nursing judgment must be used to determine which technique would be most helpful in any given situation.

Aerosol Therapy

There are many patients who deep breathe and cough quite well; however, their secretions are so thick that they have difficulty moving them up the airway and expectorating them. There are several alternatives or methods of varying degrees of complexity that can be used in such a situation. The first is to ensure an adequate fluid intake. The oral fluid intake in itself can help to make secretions produced less viscid and therefore more easily expectorated. Another method is to add water particles directly to the airway through the administration of aerosol therapy. First, let us review just what aerosol therapy is. An aerosol by definition means that particles, not just water vapor, have been added to the inspired air. *Humidification* as discussed previously refers to the addition of water vapor or water in the gas form, whereas *aerosol* refers to water added in a particulate form. Therefore a bland (water or saline) aerosol can be used therapeutically in order to help liquefy secretions, or an aerosol may be used to administer particulate suspensions of medications, or an aerosol may be administered as a diagnostic tool—as a way of obtaining an induced sputum.

There are many disagreements about the therapeutic usefulness of bland aerosol therapy and it is important to discuss the pros and cons of such a type of therapy before discussing some of the actual techniques that can be used to deliver aerosol therapy.

Some clinicians argue that there is no evidence to support that the aerosol reaches the lower airway. As has already been discussed, the airway is anatomically constructed in such a way that inhaled particles will impact upon the mucous membrane so that entrance into the lower airway is inhibited. Just as this method is normally a "defense" mechanism of the airway, it will serve the same function during the administration of an aerosol. Therefore large particles tend to be filtered out of the air in the upper airway and only small particles will enter the lower airway. It has been estimated that, depending upon the type of generator used to produce the aerosol, only 10 to 20 per cent of the water particles inhaled will actually reach the lower airway (Wolfsdorf et al., 1969). Yet, at the same time, therapeutic results are observed in the patient. There are several factors that may account for this clinical finding. One is simply that even though the water particles are deposited in the upper airway, they are swallowed, and this in addition to the general fluid intake enhances fluid addition to the mucus produced. This amount would be miniscule, however. Second, methods that are presently used to detect the pattern of deposition may alter the properties of the water particles so that they may be deposited in different areas than in normal therapeutic use. It is known that particle deposition will be enhanced if the patient mouth breathes in that this respiratory pattern bypasses the baffling action of the turbinates in the nose and, second, that particle deposition in the lung is enhanced if the patient takes a slow deep breath with a short inspiratory hold at end inspiration (Wolfsdorf et al., 1969). It is unreasonable to assume that the patient will be able to deep breathe for the entire 20 to 30 minutes of the aerosol treatment; however, periodic deep breathing should be encouraged.

Aerosol therapy also causes side effects. First, inhalation of a water or saline aerosol may cause a decrease in the arterial oxygen tension. This is especially true in people with obstructive airway disease. The fall in the arterial P_{O_2} may be as much as 10 to 12 mm Hg, and although this may not be hazardous to persons with normal blood gases, it could be hazardous in those patients who have a borderline P_{O_2} (Pflug et al., 1970). Therefore it is important that the nurse make observations as to the patient's level of oxygenation during such therapy. A second side effect is that the aerosol will cause an increase in airway resistance (Pflug et al., 1970). Again, this is especially true in people with obstructive airway disease. The change in airway resistance by clinical observation appears to be related to the amount of water output produced by the aerosol generator. (The greater the water output, the greater the change in airway resistance.) This change in airway resistance causes some patients to wheeze, it increases the work of breathing, and generally increases the patient's complaint of discomfort. In the past, the nurse has often related this sensation of discomfort to a feeling of claustrophobia on the part of the patient, but it is important to realize that it is the physiologic side effects of the aerosol therapy that causes the patient's breathing to become more difficult. In addition to being related to the amount of water output, the change in airway resistance is also related to the type of solution aerosolized. An aerosol of normal physiologic saline produces a much greater increase in airway resistance than does an aerosol of water. The effect on airway resistance can often be eliminated by administration of an aerosolized bronchodilator prior to the water or saline aerosol.

When the aerosol is used to deliver moisture to the lower airways there are several types of aerosol generators available. The most common of these are the jet nebulizer, cold or heated, and the ultrasonic nebulizer. The jet nebulizer produces a smaller output than does the large model of the ultrasonic nebulizer and it also produces a larger particle size than does the ultrasonic nebulizer. The side effects of the aerosol produced by the jet nebulizer, however, are less than those of the ultrasonically produced aerosol.

The jet nebulizers may be run as either cold nebulizers or heated nebulizers. When a heating coil is added, the nebulizer will have a greater water output than it does when it is cold. In addition, many of the jet nebulizers are constructed so as to provide for an "air mix." (Room air is mixed with the compressed gas source.) As greater flow is added to these nebulizers, the water output is increased. In addition, because this greater flow is more likely to meet patient inspiratory demands, there is less mixing with the inspired air that would tend to evaporate some of the water particles. The ultrasonic nebulizer, because of its high water output, does not require heating, nor does it require additional air mix.

In the administration of aerosols, several other points should be remembered. First of all, there are a variety of ways by which the generator that produces the aerosol can be adapted to fit the patient's needs. The aerosol is always administered with the use of wide-bored tubing to help prevent the conglomeration and dropping out of water particles. The actual adaptation to the patient, however, is much more flexible. Examples are the aerosol mask, the tent, the face tent, in line with IPPB apparatus or with T-tubes or tracheostomy masks over artificial airways. Regardless of the specific method used, the nurse must ensure that the tubing does not become blocked with water and therefore stop gas flow through the tubing. (Water will collect in the dependent parts of the tubing, and it must be periodically emptied.) If the patient is receiving supplemental oxygen, oxygen must be continued during periods of aerosol therapy. (This is accomplished by continuing nasal oxygen or by driving the aerosol generator with an oxygen-enriched gas mixture.) If the therapeutic response desired of the aerosol therapy is the increased expectoration of secretions from the airway, it must be remembered that simply decreasing the viscosity of secretions will not necessarily enhance their movement up the mucociliary escalator. The patient must be taught to deep breathe and cough during the aerosol therapy in order to move secretions effectively from the lower airway.

In all aerosol therapy the patient must be closely observed for both therapeutic response and any side effects that may occur. By these observations the treatment can be adapted to the specific patient needs. It is foolhardy to aerosolize water to the patient's airway and at the same time increase the airway resistance to the level where the patient is less able to deep breathe and cough.

Postural Drainage

Postural drainage is another technique that can be used as a measure of bronchial hygiene. This technique consists of positioning the patient in such a way as to enhance gravity drainage from the lung. A complete segmental drainage of the lung will require 12 different positions, as shown in Figure 26-4. It is important to note that many patients do not require drainage of all areas of the lung. Many areas are able to drain quite well on their own, especially the upper lobe areas. Therefore the positions selected must be chosen according to the individual patient's needs. In addition, although Figure 26-4 depicts the various positions that are used, it is often found that these positions have to be slightly adapted according to patient needs. For example, various diseases will cause distortion of the anatomy of the lung. If a patient has a lung abscess that the nurse is attempting to drain by postural drainage, the formation of the abscess may have distorted the anatomy in such a way that a slightly different position from the one depicted for that specific segment may have to be used. In other situations the patient cannot tolerate the position that is advocated. For example, the extremely dyspneic patient may not be able to tolerate the head-down position, so that perhaps the best that can be accomplished is the prone or supine position, which at least is more efficient in draining secretions from the lower lobe than is the upright position. In other situations where the patient has an artificial airway, it is often impossible to get the patient in the prone position, and therefore drainage of the posterior segments is not feasible. A final consideration is the changes that may occur in cadiovas-

Upper Lobes

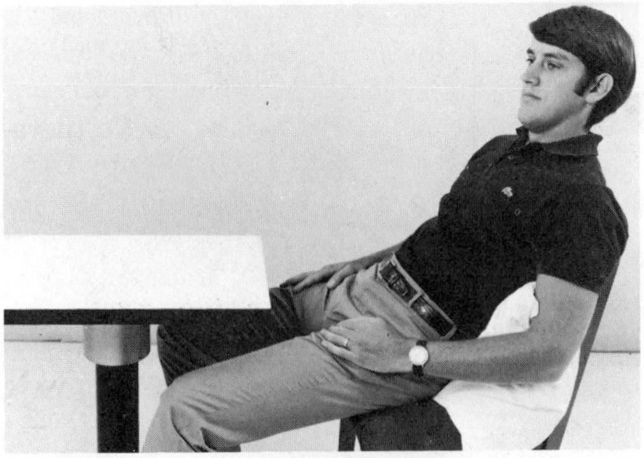

A. Left and right upper lobe—anterior apical segments. Sit in a chair leaning back against a pillow. Percuss and vibrate with hands at shoulders with fingers extending over collarbone in front. (Do both sides at same time.)

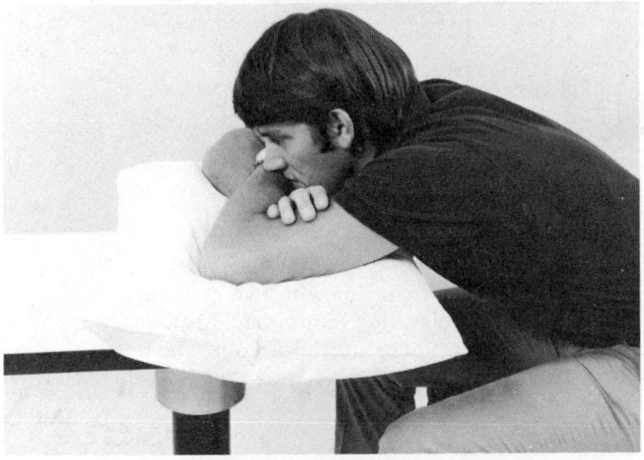

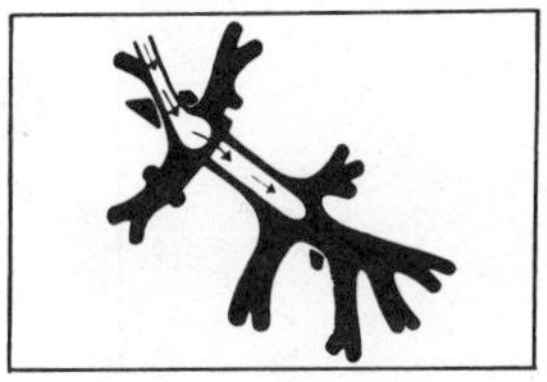

B. Left and right upper lobe—posterior apical segments. Sit in a chair leaning forward onto a pillow or table. Percuss and vibrate with hands at shoulders in back; fingers go a little over the shoulders. (Do both sides at same time.)

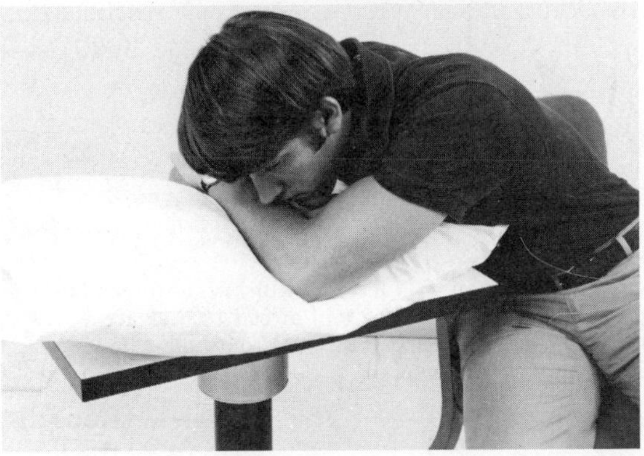

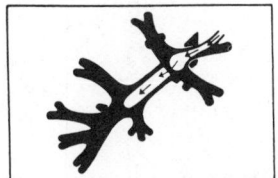

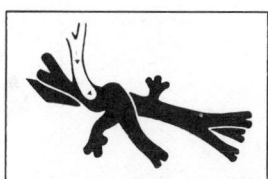

C. LUL—posterior segments. Sit sideways in a chair. Lean forward and to right side with arms folded on table. Percuss and vibrate over the left shoulder blade.

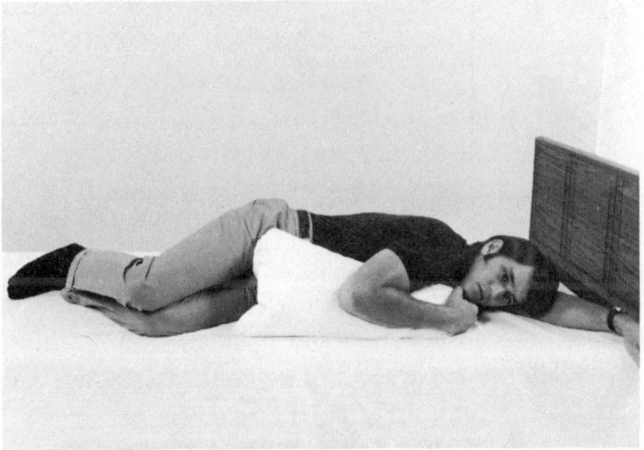

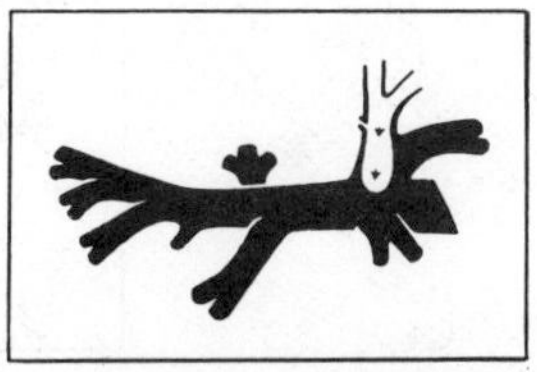

D. RUL—posterior segments. Lie on your left side. Put a pillow in front of you (from shoulders to hips) and roll slightly forward onto it (about one-fourth turn). The bed is flat. Percuss and vibrate over the right shoulder blade.

Figure 26-4. Postural drainage.

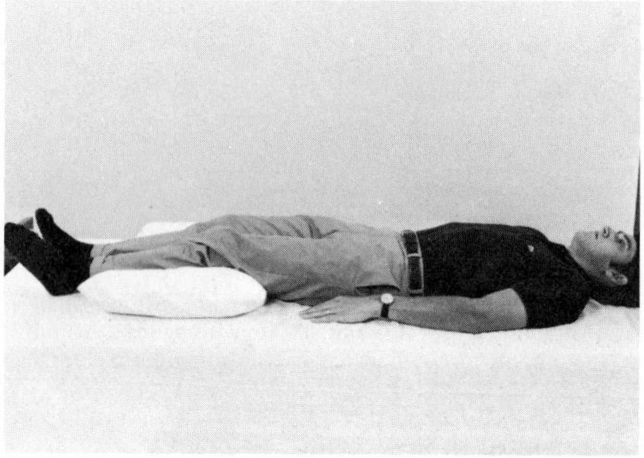

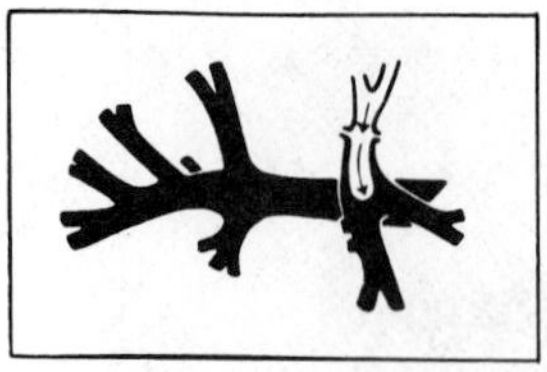

Upper lobes (continued)

E. Right and left anterior segments. Lie flat on back with a small pillow under your knees. Percuss and vibrate just below the collarbone. (Do both sides at the same time.)

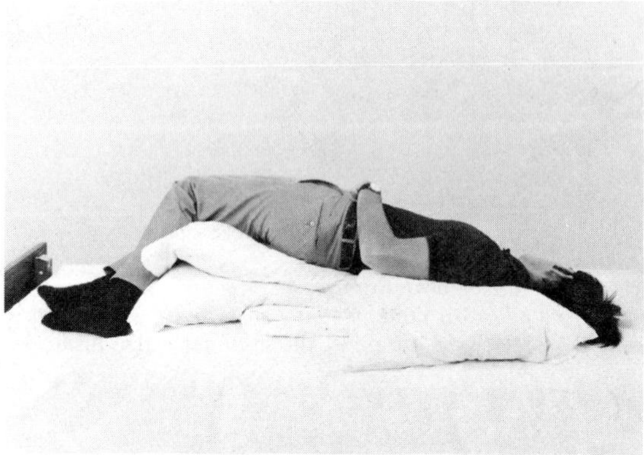

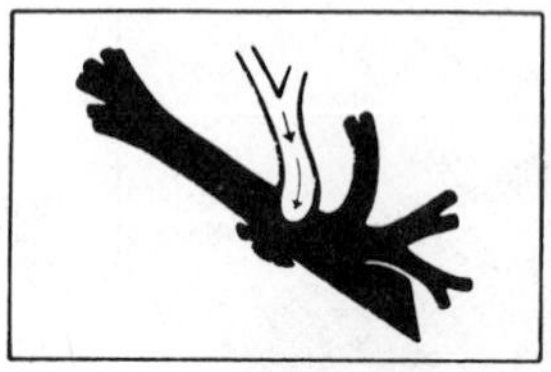

F. Lingula (LUL). Lie on your right side with two or three pillows under your hips (equivalent to elevating foot of bed 12"). Place a pillow behind your back and roll one-fourth turn onto the pillow. Percuss and vibrate over the left nipple.

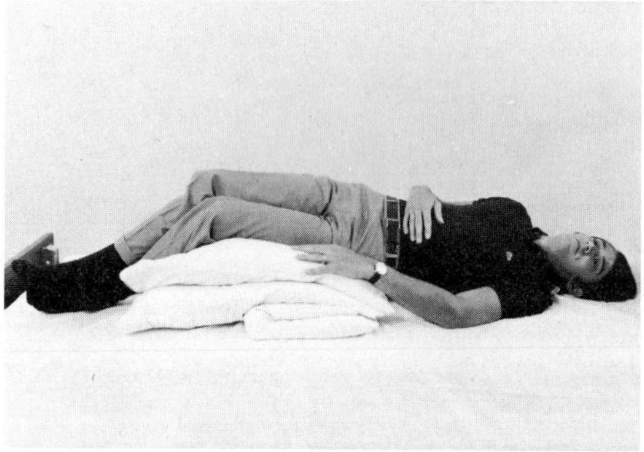

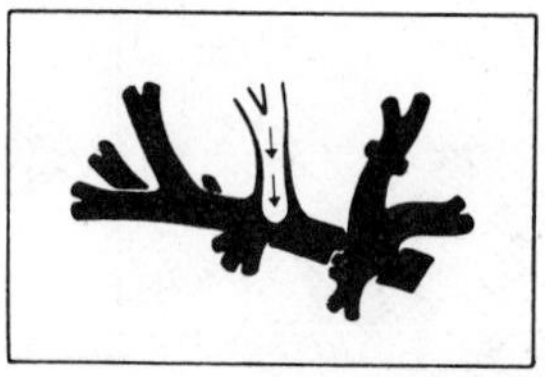

Middle lobe (right)

G. Middle lobe (right). Lie on your left side with two or three pillows under your hips (equivalent to elevating foot of bed 12"). Place a pillow behind your back and roll one-fourth turn onto the pillow. Percuss and vibrate over right nipple.

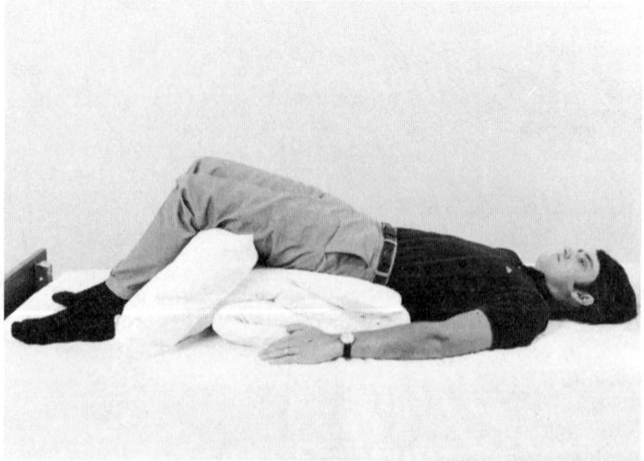

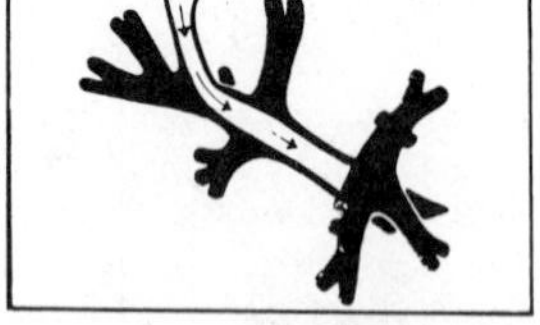

Lower lobes

H. Left and right anterior basal segment. Lie on back with three or four pillows under your hips (equivalent to elevating foot of bed (18-20"). Have knees flexed. Percuss and vibrate at lower ribs on both sides of front of chest.

Lower lobes
(continued)

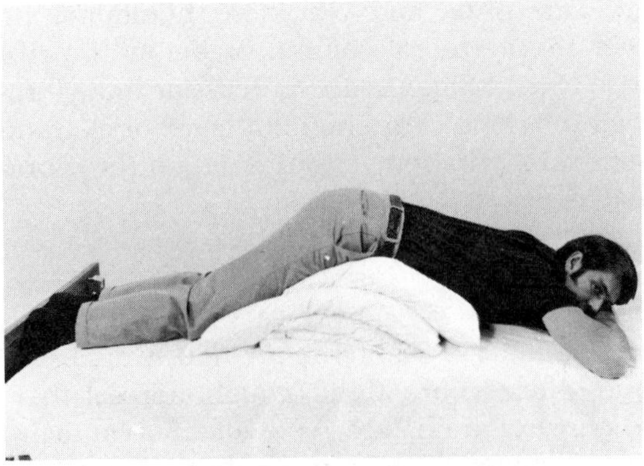
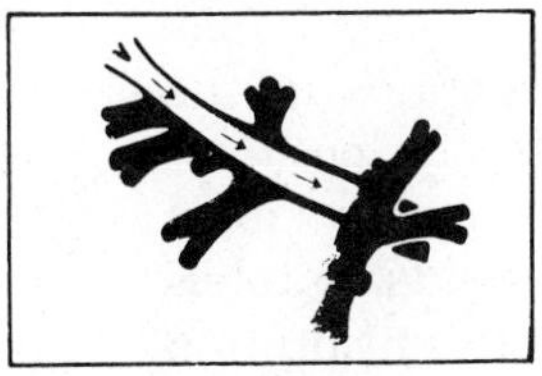

I. Left and right posterior basal segments. Lie on stomach with three or four pillows under your hips (equivalent to elevating foot of bed 18–20″). Percuss and vibrate at lower ribs on both sides of back of chest.

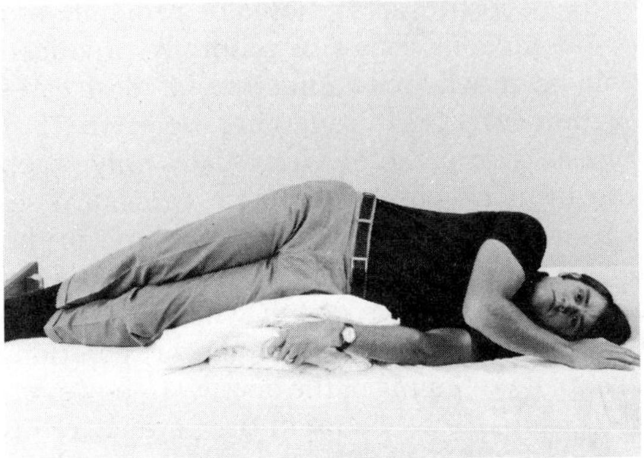
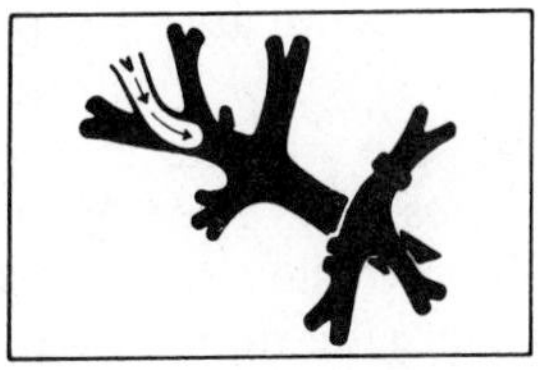

J. Right lateral basal segments. Lie on left side with three or four pillows under hips (equivalent to elevating foot of bed 18–20″). Percuss and vibrate at lower ribs on right side of chest.

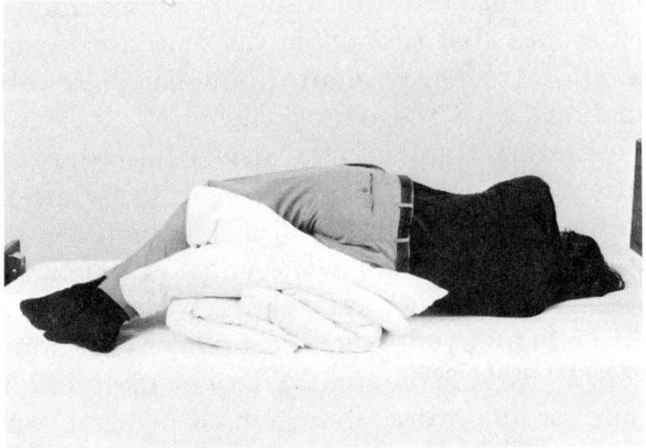
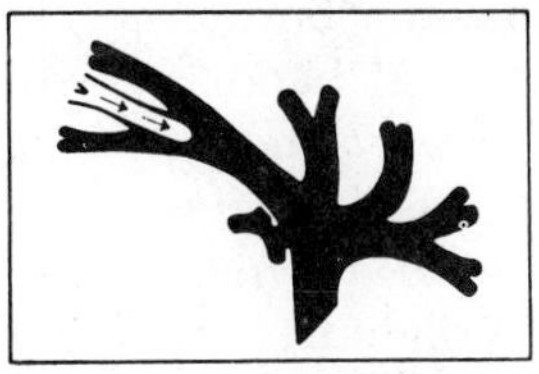

K. Left lateral basal segments. Lie on right side with three or four pillows under hips (equivalent to elevating foot of bed 18–20″). Percuss and vibrate at lower ribs on left side of chest.

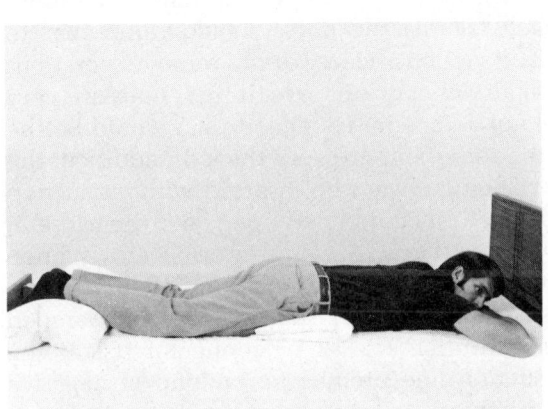
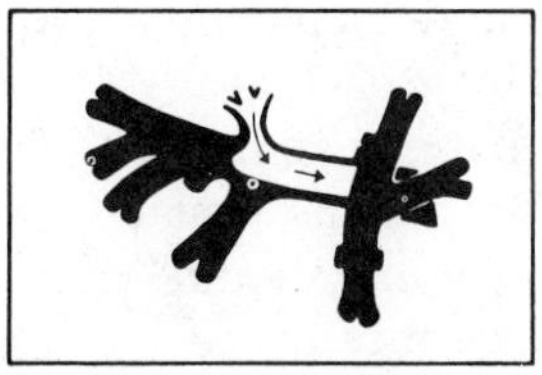

L. Superior segments. Lie flat on stomach with single pillow under stomach. Percuss and vibrate both sides at area between shoulder blade and lower ribs.

cular dynamics; for example, cardiac output may change and cerebral blood flow increases in the head-down position. For all patients, the positions used and the length of time in any one position must be individually determined. Most patients do tolerate postural drainage very well, and this institution of positioning is effective in increasing the removal of secretions from the lower airway.

If positioning alone is not successful, percussion and vibration may be added to the postural drainage. This technique is often said to be based on the "ketchup bottle" theory. In other words, if you turn the bottle upside down and the ketchup does not come out, you pound on it, which is percussion, and you shake it, which is vibration.

Percussion is a technique whereby the nurse's hand is placed in a stiffened, cupped position. The chest is then struck in a rhythmic fashion by flexing the wrist. The striking of the chest is actually done with the air pocket enclosed by the hand rather than by slapping. Percussion should produce a clopping type of sound, which has often been equated to the sound of a horse galloping. A slapping sound indicates that the technique is not being carried out correctly. The percussion is done for approximately 1 minute over the area of the chest that is being drained. After the area has been percussed, vibration is then carried out. For vibration the flat hand is placed over the area of the chest that is being drained. The patient is instructed to take a deep breath. On exhalation, the nurse tenses the arm muscles and from the shoulders, produces a slight tremor in the hands. At the same time, the chest is compressed, so that there is a simultaneous tremor and a downward compression of the chest. This pressure and tremor should be maintained until the patient has exhaled fully. After several vibrations, if the patient has not coughed spontaneously, he or she is instructed to cough voluntarily. Vibration is especially effective in moving secretions and should be repeated at least three or four times over each area of the chest being drained. If the patient is productive or if the nurse can "feel" secretions that have not yet been expectorated, vibration should be carried out several more times. The entire procedure of percussion and vibration is then repeated before placing the patient in another position. It is also helpful to have the patient return to a sitting posture after each position. Cough is usually more effective in this position, and therefore secretions that have been "moved" can often be expectorated when deep breathing and coughing is done in the sitting position. The forcefulness of both percussion and vibration must be modified to meet specific patient needs. In all situations it must be remembered that these techniques are always carried out on the rib cage. Percussion and vibration should not be done over the vertebral column or below the ribs at the base of the lung. Also the percussion and vibration should be done over one light layer of clothing to prevent skin irritation yet not dampen the vibration created.

Suctioning

In those patients in whom the previously discussed techniques of deep breathing, cough, aerosol therapy, and postural drainage are not effective in maintaining the patency of the airway, deep airway suctioning must be instituted. It should be remembered that the spontaneous cough or naturally produced cough will be much more effective in most cases than a suction catheter in removing secretions. For example, a suction catheter will usually only reach main-stem bronchi whereas a cough can move secretions from more distal points in the lung to the larger airways, where they can be expectorated. In addition, a good, effective cough will result in the expectoration of a far greater volume of secretions than will actual suctioning of the airway. If, however, the patient is unable to maintain the patency of his or her airways, then, of course, suctioning can be a life-saving measure. At the same time, the nurse must remember that suctioning does produce certain side effects. First, no matter how carefully the nurse suctions with the commonly used "whistle-tipped" catheters, trauma to the airway is produced. Observation of the airway via bronchoscopy after usual suctioning techniques will show many areas of trauma where the suction openings on the catheter have torn the mucosa (Sackner, Wanner, and Landa, 1972). This irritation of the airway by suctioning therefore disrupts the mucociliary blanket of the airway and produces irritation, which in itself can cause a greater production of secretions. To minimize such trauma the nurse should remember to use as little suction as necessary to remove secretions from the airway. For example, if secretions are very thin, less of a vacuum is needed than would be the case if the secretions are very thick. In addition, the catheter should always be inserted without suction being applied, should be left open, and the catheter should be withdrawn with intermittent suction rather than with continuous suction. The suction line attached to the catheter should never be clamped off in substitution for a "Y" connector. Clamping of the suction line produces a buildup of negative pressure behind the obstruction, so that when it is removed, the negative pressure is suddenly applied to the airway. Finally, the catheter should not be removed from the airway using an up-and-down motion. Instead it should be removed in one continuous movement. Research has led to the modification of suction catheters so that new designs produce less trauma than the older style catheters (Sackner et al., 1973).

Another side effect of which the nurse must be aware during suctioning is the production of hypoxemia. The introduction of a suction catheter produces additional obstruction to the airway as well as the removal of air from the airway. Therefore hypoxemia is the usual rather than the unusual occurrence during suctioning. To help alleviate the detrimental effects of hypoxemia to the patient, it is recommended that the patient be preoxygenated prior to the actual introduction of the suction catheter, that suctioning be for short intervals (no more than 15 to 20 seconds), and that oxygen be reinstituted immediately upon the completion of the suctioning technique. For patients receiving nasal oxygen, the oxygen should not be removed during suctioning.

A third consideration that always must be made when suctioning the lower airway is that the catheter is most likely to enter the right main-stem bronchus. It is very seldom that the catheter will enter into the left main-stem bronchus, and therefore adequate clearing of secretions from both sides of the lung is not ensured by suctioning techniques. Turning of the patient's head to the contralateral side or turning of the patient's head and hyperextending the neck does not ensure entrance of the catheter into the left main-stem bronchus (Haberman et al., 1973). This consistency of entrance into the right main-stem bronchus is due to the anatomy of the airway. The left main-stem bronchus is smaller in diameter than the right and leaves the carina at a sharper angle than does the right main-stem bronchus. Use of a curved bronchial catheter will help to ensure entrance into the left main-stem bronchus if this is a special problem in the care of the patient. These catheters have a stiffened angle on the distal end with a marker on the end that connects to the vacuum line (the marker allows the nurse to know in which direction the angled end of the catheter is pointing). When inserted to a level just above the carina, the catheter is turned so that the tip of the catheter points in the appropriate direction. Then, as the catheter is advanced, it is more likely to enter the left (or right) main-stem bronchus. Although the use of such a catheter may be highly successful, it requires that the person doing the suctioning be knowledgeable about the anatomy to be sure that the catheter tip is turned at the appropriate time.

The final area of consideration regarding suctioning that will be discussed is the prevention of the introduction of pathogens into the lower airway. Suctioning techniques must be as strictly clean as possible so that pathogens are not directly introduced into the lower airway. Such considerations become extremely important in those patients who are intubated, for they have already lost many of their normal defense mechanisms which would aid in the clearance of the airway. On the other hand, it must be remembered that it is virtually impossible to maintain a sterile suctioning technique. Any time nasotracheal suctioning is done, the catheter must be introduced through the upper airway, which is a grossly "dirty" area. As the catheter passes through the upper airway it is going to carry some organisms with it into the lower airway. Also, once a patient is intubated or tracheotomized it is ridiculous to believe that the end of that tube, which is exposed to the room environment, will remain sterile (meaning the complete absence of any organism). Therefore whenever the catheter is passed through such a tube it is likely that some organisms will be carried with the catheter. The purpose of suctioning techniques is therefore not to maintain a completely sterile technique but to maintain a strictly clean technique and to prevent the introduction of pathogens into the lower airway. The exact technique used will vary, but it is the principle that must be followed. It is, however, definitely recommended that a sterile, disposable catheter be used for every period of suctioning. A catheter should be used for one session of suctioning and then should be discarded. It is also recommended that a glove be worn on the hand that is manipulating the suction catheter. Although very strict handwashing techniques are often adequate, it is not uncommon for the nurse to have to touch something after hand washing. Therefore the glove that is put on immediately prior to entering the lower airway will prevent introduction of organisms that the nurse may be carrying on her or his hands from around the bedside. Solutions that are used to rinse the catheter should also be discarded after every use, for if they are exposed to room air, they will tend to grow organisms. One simple technique that has been very successful is the pouring of small amounts of the solution (sterile saline, sterile water, or tap water) into clean paper cups. The patient is then suctioned with a sterile disposable catheter with the nurse wearing a sterile disposable glove. After that session of suctioning, the glove, the catheter, the paper cup, and the remaining solution are discarded. The main source of the solution for the rinsing of the catheter may be kept in a large container, but it must be covered between uses and used only as a reservoir for the smaller containers.

Suctioning techniques vary according to whether the lower airway is being entered via an artificial passageway such as an endotracheal or nasotracheal tube or is being entered through the nasooropharynx. In the case of nasotracheal or orotracheal suctioning, the positioning of the patient in order to produce maximal opening of the airway is of prime importance. First, it is usually easier to pass the catheter through the nose, as this route produces a straighter drop into the trachea, whereas passage of the catheter through the oropharynx requires a greater curvature of the catheter to enter the anteriorly located trachea. Elevating the tip of the nose will also provide a straighter passage through the nose. The catheter should be very gently passed in a downward direction through the nose using a gentle rotation of the catheter in order to maneuver in between the various turbinates. Once the catheter is located in the posterior pharynx, the patient should be positioned much as for resuscitation. A pillow is placed behind the patient's back with the uppermost part of the pillow reaching only as high as the shoulders. (It is often easier to introduce the suction catheter with the patient in a semi-Fowler's position.) The head is then dropped back in such a way that the neck is hyperextended. Additional opening of the airway can be attained by a manipulation of the jaw whereby traction is applied to the lower jaw so that it is pulled up and out. The catheter has now been placed directly above the glottis and as the patient inhales, the catheter is quickly advanced and will usually enter the larynx.

Entrance into the larynx will usually produce a cough, which is evidence of entrance into the lower airway but is definitely not a reason for rapid removal of the catheter from the lower airway. Instead, the coughing helps to move more distal secretions to a point where they are accessible to the catheter. The catheter is then advanced as far as possible; in the adult male it can usually be advanced 22 inches, which is the entire length of the catheter, to attain an adequate depth of suctioning. Because one of the biggest problems in nasotracheal suctioning is ensuring the introduction of the catheter into the lower airway, it is important that with each passage of the catheter adequate airway clearance is attained. For this reason the following technique is helpful: The catheter is inserted into the lower airway and suction is applied during withdrawal. The catheter, however, is not completely withdrawn from the airway but is withdrawn only to a point between the carina and the larynx (a 22-inch catheter is withdrawn about 10 to 12 inches). The vacuum line is then removed from the catheter to prevent any further withdrawal of air and the patient is encouraged to deep breathe at this time. It should be remembered that for the patient who is on oxygen therapy, the oxygen is continued throughout this procedure. Oxygen administration by the nasal route may be continued or the oxygen line may be hooked directly to the suction catheter and the oxygen administered to the lower airway. After the patient has had several deep breaths, the suction line is again attached to the catheter and the catheter is reinserted to its full length and again withdrawn with intermittent suction to a point between the carina and the larynx. The procedure is repeated until secretions are no longer obtained during the suctioning. At that point the catheter is completely withdrawn from the airway, being sure that suction is intermittently applied during the complete withdrawal to remove secretions that have been moved higher into the trachea or into the upper airway. If the nurse encounters special difficulties in entering the trachea or in passing the catheter through the nares, it is often helpful to insert a nasopharyngeal tube. This is a small airway that is passed through the nose and terminates above the glottis. It ensures much easier access through the nares and the tube can often be directed above the glottis so that the catheter can be more easily passed into the trachea. In other situations, the nurse can often feel a certain anatomic deviation when passing a catheter and, although a semi-Fowler's position is generally recommended for the patient, in some patients a flat position or a side-lying position is often more expedient to facilitate the entrance of the catheter into the trachea.

For patients who have an endotracheal or tracheostomy tube inserted, it must be remembered that the introduction of the catheter produces a much more drastic increase in airway resistance than does the introduction of a catheter into a patient without such an artificial airway. Therefore in patients with artificial airways, the catheter is inserted once, without suction, and then withdrawn completely with intermittent suction. The patient is then either put back on the ventilator or allowed to breathe an oxygen-enriched mixture, whatever the situation warrants. For each session of suctioning, the catheter is completely withdrawn and is not left situated in the lower airway, as is done with nasotracheal suctioning. The latter technique is really not required in such situations because the artificial airway allows easy access to the lower airway. Adequate depth of insertion must be ensured just as with nasotracheal suctioning. With an oral or nasoendotracheal tube, the catheter can usually be inserted 18 to 22 inches in adult patients, with a tracheostomy tube 6 to 10 inches. If the catheter is not passed beyond the end of the artificial airway, secretions can accumulate at the end of the tube and cause complete airway obstruction.

If secretions are so thick that they are difficult to remove through the suction catheter, irrigation is often helpful. Five to 10 ml of sterile saline may be injected into the lower airway via the suction catheter or artificial airway (a syringe without a needle is used). This added liquid will often thin secretions sufficiently so that they can be removed. If irrigation alone is unsuccessful, then irrigation followed by deep breathing (done manually with a self-inflating bag) and then suctioning will frequently be effective. There are insufficient data to recommend that irrigation be considered an integral part of lower airway suctioning. The irrigating solution tends to remain in a bolus rather than dispensing and probably remains in the area of main-stem bronchi (Hanley et al., 1978).

Control of Ventilation

Central Regulatory Centers

The respiratory cycle requires a periodic contraction of the inspiratory muscles and then relaxation of those muscles to allow for expiration. This contraction and relaxation of the muscles occurs rhythmically and has a very definite pattern. The characteristics of the respiratory cycle are controlled by the respiratory centers of the central nervous system. It used to be thought that there was one specific area of the brain that controlled ventilation. It has now been found that this concept is incorrect; therefore it is preferable to speak of respiratory centers rather than of just one respiratory center. The areas of the central nervous system that do influence the respiratory cycle are found in the medulla and the pons. In addition, certain parts of the reticular formation of the brainstem are necessary to have normal periodic ventilatory movements. These respiratory centers are also influenced by the motor neurons in the spinal cord and nuclei of some of the cranial nerves. In addition to the input from these neural pathways, the central respiratory centers also receive input from the circulatory system. The respiratory centers therefore not only regulate the rhythm of the respiratory cycle but also serve as an integrator for the input from other stimuli. The neural impulses generated in the central respiratory centers are then transmitted to the motor neurons of the major thoracic respiratory muscles as well as to those of the sensory muscles.

It is evident that the brainstem, even when isolated from its other connections, demonstrates a rhythmic ventilatory activity that is automatic. Under normal conditions, however, the central nervous system respiratory centers are not isolated from the rest of the body. Therefore their effect is influenced by voluntary activity and feedback mechanisms. Voluntary activities that affect the rhythmicity of the respiratory center are exemplified by such actions as speech, swallowing, and breathholding. In these instances the cerebral cortex exerts a controlling effect on the respiratory centers in the brainstem. Feedback mechanisms that affect the rhythmicity of respiration are derived from a variety of ventilatory reflexes. The major categories of feedback mechanisms are the following (DeJours, 1966):

1. The mechanical conditions of the thoracic-pulmonary system, which influence the centers through appropriate receptive pathways.
2. The influence of humoral stimuli, including the partial pressures of oxygen, and carbon dioxide and the pH of the arterial blood and cerebrospinal fluid.

Mechanoreceptors

The pulmonary mechanoreceptors, which are innervated via the vagus, affect the rhythmic activity of the central respiratory centers. These receptors respond to the degree of lung inflation and are therefore often referred to as the stretch receptors. They are found in the walls of the small airways (terminal bronchioles). The greater the lung volume, the more the expiratory signals that are sent by the receptors to the central respiratory centers. Thus, an inspiration continues, more and more inhibitory or expiratory impulses are sent to the central nervous system. When these inhibitory impulses reach a certain level, the inspiratory centers at the central level decrease their activity and exhalation takes place. Then as lung volume decreases, the inhibitory signals also decrease and when a low point is reached, inspiration can again occur. Other receptors include those that respond to various irritants resulting in bronchoconstriction, those that respond to pulmonary interstitial edema with resulting tachypnea, and the baroreceptors that respond to changes in blood pressure. An increase in arterial blood pressure will cause hypoventilation or apnea by affecting the aortic and carotid sinus baroreceptors. Similarly, a decrease in arterial pressure will produce hyperventilation. It should be remembered that the baroreceptors have an inhibitory action; as they are stimulated (by an increase in pressure) they inhibit or decrease ventilation, just as they serve to decrease blood pressure.

Humoral Stimuli

The second major category of stimuli that affect respiration are the humoral stimuli.

One of the major humoral stimuli is carbon dioxide. An increase in arterial carbon dioxide tension will increase ventilation. This increase in ventilation is seen more dramatically as an increase in tidal volume; with added stimulation the rate of respiration also increases. A decrease in the level of arterial carbon dioxide will cause a decrease in alveolar ventilation. The carbon dioxide stimulus plays a role in both normal and abnormal ventilatory patterns. In normal respiration the major stimulus is the carbon dioxide effect on the central respiratory centers. In the abnormal situation where the arterial carbon dioxide level is chronically elevated, the effect of the carbon dioxide is more evident on the peripheral chemoreceptors. In this situation the central nervous system is depressed and therefore the prime stimulus is at the peripheral level. The peripheral chemoreceptors are located in the carotid and the aortic bodies. These receptors then have fibers that travel to the central nervous system and stimulate the respiratory system in that manner.

Hydrogen ions also act as a stimulus to ventilation. An increase in hydrogen ions (acidemia) will cause increased ventilation, whereas a decrease in hydrogen ions (alkalemia) will cause decreased ventilation. This effect of hydrogen ions on ventilation can be independent of the carbon dioxide level, for in metabolic acidosis hyperventilation will persist in spite of the existence of hypocapnia, which would normally decrease ventilation. Similarly, metabolic alkalosis can lead to a decrease in ventilation even with a coexisting hypercapnia.

Oxygen also acts as a ventilatory stimulus via a reflexogenic pathway; in other words, stimulation is at the peripheral level, which then influences the central nervous system. Although there is some controversy, it appears that the oxygen stimulus is the partial pressure of oxygen in the arterial blood rather than saturation. As the partial pressure of oxygen decreases it stimulates the aortic and carotid chemoreceptors and then reflexively increases the activity of the respiratory centers in the central nervous system. The central nervous system itself is depressed during severe hypoxemia because of the hypoxia of the respiratory center. This response of the peripheral chemoreceptors to the oxygen stimulus is one of the bases of oxygen therapy in the patient with chronic carbon dioxide retention. In patients who have chronic carbon dioxide retention, hypoxemia is also present. It is sometimes found that the response of the central nervous system to the carbon dioxide stimulus is depressed in such patients. Therefore ventilation is often maintained through the stimulus of hypoxemia. Administration of very high concentrations of oxygen to these patients could be dangerous. As the P_{o_2} is raised to normal levels, the stimulation of the peripheral chemoreceptors decreases and therefore ventilation could be depressed. For this reason oxygen is given at inspired concentrations sufficient to raise the oxygen content without raising the P_{o_2} to normal levels. In other words, a P_{o_2} in the range of 45 to 65 mm Hg is desirable in patients with carbon dioxide retention in that this level will maintain stimulation of the peripheral chemoreceptors but will at the same time ensure adequate oxygen content. This increase in the patrial pressure of oxygen in the arterial blood may have some effect on ventilation in that it is not infrequent that the P_{co_2} rises by about 5 mm Hg. However, it is usually possible to maintain stimulation of the respiratory center so that ventilation does not cease or become markedly depressed.

Epinephrine and norepinephrine also act as stimuli to ventilation. The injection of either of these substances will cause hyperventilation. The effect is usually self-limiting because of the development of hypocapnia and respiratory alkalosis as the result of the hyperventilation. These latter developments will then serve to depress ventilation and return it to a normal level. It is possible that this is one mechanism by which ventilation is increased during muscular exercise in that the blood concentrations of epinephrine and norepinephrine during exercise are very high.

There are many other stimuli that have been hypothesized to affect ventilation. The mechanisms and modes of action of these stimuli are not well known and will not be discussed in this area. Students with interest in this aspect of physiology of ventilation are referred to a physiology text.

One important clinical aspect of the regulation of ventilation is an explanation of periodic respiration. As we have seen, the chemical characteristics of the arterial blood—the P_{o_2}, P_{co_2}, and pH—will affect ventilation. Normally changes in these values are damped because of the relatively rapid circulation time and the buffering effect of the blood. In certain conditions, however, the ventilatory system may show oscillation. This will be especially true if the circulation time from the lungs to the respiratory center is increased. It is not uncommon in such a situation to have periodic respiration. Hypoxia may also result in a pattern of periodic ventilation because of the fact that simple, relatively normal activities, such as speaking or swallowing, may cause a drop in the P_{o_2}. A few seconds later, if this blood reaches the chemoreceptors, the low P_{o_2} then stimulates ventilation and a pattern of periodic ventilation may develop. Another cause of oscillation in the ventilatory pattern results from a change in respiratory center excitability. The latter is probably the cause of periodic respiration or Cheyne-Stokes' respirations[1] in patients who are sleeping. Such observations are especially evident at high altitudes for the patient who is hypoxic.

There are still many facts to be known about the control of ventilation. As more knowledge becomes available, it will probably be much easier to explain many of the observations that we presently make in patients. At the present time, however, it is important to understand that a variety of stimuli can affect ventilation and that these may in fact be the cause of an abnormal respiratory pattern.

References Cited

DeJours, P. *Respiration.* New York: Oxford University Press, 1966.

Haberman, P. B. et al. "Determinants of Successful Selective Tracheobronchial Suctioning." *N. Engl. J. Med.*, **289,** 20 (Nov. 1973), 1060–63.

Hanley et al. "What Happens To Intra-tracheal Saline Instillations?" *Am. Rev. Resp. Dis.* **117:** 4, Part 2 (Apr. 1978) 124.

Krop, H. D., et al. "Neuropsychologic Effects of Continuous Oxygen Therapy in Chronic Obstructive Pulmonary Disease." *Chest,* **64,** 3 (Sept. 1973), 317–22.

Macklem, P. "The Pathophysiology of Chronic Bronchitis and Emphysema." *Med. Clin. North Am.*, **57,** 3 (May 1973), 669–80.

Petty, T. L. et al. "Continuous Oxygen Therapy in Chronic Airway Obstruction." *Ann. Intern. Med.*, **75** (1971), 361–67.

Pflug, A. et al. "The effects of an Ultrasonic Aerosol on Pulmonary Mechanics and Arterial Blood Gases in Patients with Chronic Bronchitis." *Am. Rev. Respir. Dis.*, **101** (May 1970), 710.

Sackner, M. A., et al. "Pathogenesis and Prevention of Tracheobronchial Damage with Suction Procedures." *Chest,* **64,** 3 (Sept. 1973), 284–90.

Sackner, M. A. et al. "Applications of Broncho Fiberoscopy." *Chest,* **62** (Nov. 1972, Suppl.), 705–85.

Senior, R. M. et al. "Pulmonary Oxygen Toxicity." *JAMA,* **127** (Sept. 1971), 1373–77.

Waligora, Sister B. M. "The Effect of Nasal and Oral Breathing upon Nasopharyngeal Oxygen Concentrations." *Nurs. Res.*, **19** (Jan.–Feb. 1970), 75–78.

Wolfsdorf, J. et al. "Mist Therapy Reconsidered: An Evaluation of the Respiratory Deposition of Labelled Water Aerosols Produced by Jet and Ultrasonic Nebulizers." *Pediatrics,* **43** (May 1969), 799–808.

[1] Cheyne-Stokes' breathing is an irregular or cyclic type of arrhythmic breathing. The rate and depth of respiration increase to a maximum followed by a gradual decrease until there is a period of apnea lasting 10 to 20 seconds.

General References

O_2/CO_2 Exchange

Amborn, S. A. "Clinical Signs Associated with the Amount of Tracheobronchial Secretions." *Nurs. Res.*, **25,** 2 (1976), 121–26.

Andrewes, C. H. "The Viruses of the Common Cold." *Sci. Am.*, **203** (Dec. 1960), 88–102.

Bartlett, R. H. et al. "Respiratory Maneuvers to Prevent Postoperative Pulmonary Complications." *JAMA,* **224** (May 1973), 1017–21.

Betson, C. "Blood Gases." *Am. J. Nurs.*, **65,** 5 (May 1968), 1010–12.

Bluemle, M. L. "Tracheal Bacterial Count of Patients Following Suctioning." *Nurs. Res.*, **19** (March–April 1970), 116–21.

Brooks, W. "Replacing Ritual with Reason." *Am. J. Nurs.*, **69** (Nov. 1969), 2410–11.

Chester, E. et al. "Bronchodilator Therapy: Comparison of Acute Response to Three Methods of Administration." *Chest,* **62,** 4 (Oct. 1972), 394.

Cohen, S. "Blood-Gas and Acid-Base Concepts in Respiratory Care." *Am. J. Nurs.*, **76,** 6 (1976), 1–30.

Collart, M. E., and Brenneman, J. K. "Preventing Postoperative Atelectasis." *Am. J. Nurs.*, **71,** 10 (Oct. 1971), 1982–87.

Comroe, J. *Physiology of Respiration.* Chicago: Year Book Medical Publishers, 1965.

Dudley, D. L. *Psychophysiology of Respiration in Health and Disease.* New York: Appleton-Century-Crofts, 1969.

Fell, T., and Cheney, W. "Prevention of Hypoxia during Endotracheal Suction." *Ann. Surg.*, **174,** 1 (July 1971), 24–28.

Foss, G. "Postural Drainage." *Am. J. Nurs.*, **73,** 4 (April 1973), 666–70.

Goldsmith, J. R. "Health Effects of Air Pollution." *Basics of RD,* **4,** 2 (Nov. 1975).

Green, G. M. "Lung Defense Mechanisms." *Med. Clin. North Am.*, **57** (May 1973), 547.

Green, G. M. "In Defense of the Lung. J. Burns-Amberson Lecture." *Am. Rev. Respir. Dis.*, **102** (1970), 691–703.

Hedley-Whyte, J. et al. *Applied Physiology of Respiratory Care.* Boston: Little, Brown and Co., 1976.

Johanson, W. G., and Gould, K. G. "Lung Defense Mechanisms." *Basics of RD,* **6,** 2 (Nov. 1977).

Kearns, B. "Tracheostomy Suctioning Technique." *Can. Nurse,* **66** (Feb. 1970), 44–48.

Keyes, J. L. "Basic Mechanisms Involved in Acid-Base Homeostasis." *Heart and Lung,* **5,** 2 (March–April 1976), 239–46.

Keyes, J. L. "Blood-Gas Analysis and the assessment of Acid-Base Status." *Heart and Lung,* **5,** 2 (March–April 1976), 247–55.

Keyes, J. L. "Blood Gases and Blood-Gas Transport." *Heart and Lung,* **3,** 6 (Nov.–Dec. 1974), 945–54.

Kirmidi, B. et al. "Evaluation of Tracheobronchial Suction Technique." *J. Thorac. Cardiovasc. Surg.*, **59** (March 1970), 340–44.

Laws, A. K., and McIntyre, R. W. "Chest Physiotherapy." *Can. Anaesth. Soc. J.*, **16**, 6 (Nov. 1969), 487–93.

McFadden, E. R., and Lyons, H. A. "Arterial Blood Gas Tension in Asthma." *N. Engl. J. Med.*, **278** (9 May 1968), 1027–32.

Moody, L. "Asthma-Physiology and Patient Care." *Am. J. Nurs.*, **73** (July 1973), 1212–20.

Moody, L. E. "Primer for Pulmonary Hygiene." *Am. J. Nurs.*, **77**, 1 (Jan. 1977), 104–06.

Moody, L. E., and Martindale, C. L. "Effect of Pulmonary Hygiene Measures on Levels of Arterial Oxygen Saturation in Adults with Chronic Lung Disease." *Heart and Lung*, **7**, 2 (March–April 1978), 315–19.

Murray, J. F. "The Normal Lung." *The Basis for Diagnosis and Treatment of Pulmonary Disease.* Philadelphia: W. B. Saunders Co., 1976.

Naigow, D., and Powaser, M. M. "The Effect of Different Endotracheal Suction Procedures on Arterial Blood Gases in a Controlled Experimental Model." *Heart and Lung*, **6**, 5 (Sept.–Oct. 1977), 808–16.

Netter, F. H. *Respiratory System.* Summit, N.J.: CIBA Pharmaceutical Co., 1979.

Pace, W. R. *Pulmonary Physiology in Clinical Practice.* Philadelphia: F. A. Davis Co., 1970.

"Patient Assessment: Examination of the Chest and Lungs." *Am. J. Nurs.*, **76**, 9 (Sept. 1976), 1453.

Paulin, E. G., and Hornbein, T. F. "The Control of Breathing." *Basics of RD*, **7**, 2 (Nov. 1978).

Petty, T. L. et al. "Methods of Ambulatory Care." *Med. Clin. North Am.*, **57**, 3 (May 1973), 751–62.

Traver, G. "Assessment of Thorax and Lungs." *Am. J. Nurs.*, **73**, 3 (March 1973), 464–71.

Traver, G. "Respiratory Care: Roles of Allied Health Professionals." *Med. Clin. North Am.*, **57** (May 1973), 793–800.

Traver, G. A. et al. "Maximal Expiratory Flows Air Postural Drainage." *Am. Rev. Resp. Dis.*, **119**, 2 (Feb. 1979), 239–45.

Waldran, M. W. "Oxygen Transport." *Am. J. Nurs.*, **79**, 2 (Feb. 1979), 272–75.

Waligora, Sister B. M. "The Effect of Nasal and Oral Breathing upon Nasopharyngeal Oxygen Concentrations." *Nurs. Res.*, **19** (Jan.–Feb. 1970), 75–78.

Watts, N. "Improvement of Breathing Patterns." *Phys. Ther.*, **48**, 6 (1968), 563–76.

Weiler, Sister M. C. "Postoperative Patients Evaluate Preoperative Instruction." *Am. J. Nurs.*, **68**, 7 (July 1968), 1465–67.

West, J. B. "Causes of Carbon Dioxide Retention in Lung Disease." *N. Engl. J. Med.*, **284** (3 June, 1971), 1232–36.

Zuch, D. "Technic of Tracheo-Bronchial Toilet in the Conscious Patient." *Anaes.*, **6** (1951), 226–30.

A 70's Look at Asthma. Morris Plains, N.J.: Warner-Chilcott Laboratories, 1972.

27

Fluid and Electrolyte Balance

When they went ashore the animals that took up land life carried with them a part of the sea in their bodies, a heritage which they passed on to their children and which even today links each land animal with its origin in the ancient sea. Fish, amphibian, and reptile, warm-blooded bird and mammal—each of us carries in our veins a salty stream in which the elements sodium, potassium, and calcium are combined in almost the same proportions as in sea water. This is our inheritance from the day, untold millions of years ago, when a remote ancestor, having progressed from the one-celled to the many-celled stage, first developed a circulatory system in which the fluid was merely the water of the sea. In the same way, our lime-hardened skeletons are the heritage from the calcium-rich ocean of Cambrian time. Even the protoplasm that streams within each cell of our bodies has the chemical structure impressed upon all living matter when the first simple creatures were brought forth in the ancient sea. And as life itself began in the sea, so each of us begins his individual life in a miniature ocean within his mother's womb, and in the stages of his embryonic development repeats the steps by which his race evolved, from gill-breathing inhabitants of a water world to creatures able to live on land

CARSON, 1950

Overview

Just as a continuous supply of oxygen is necessary to life, maintenance of the composition and distribution of body fluids is also essential.

These fluids not only form the environment of the cells but also enter into their structure. In health, exchange between the internal and external environment is so regulated that (1) conditions favorable to the functioning of enzymes and hormones in cellular activities are preserved with the internal environment, (2) materials needed by the cells are supplied, and (3) products of metabolism are removed from the cells. As indicated in Unit IV, exchange between the internal and external environment is governed by both chemical and neural regulators. A major evolutionary event that contributed to the mobility and adaptability of humans was the development of the fast-acting autonomic nervous system, whose major function is to influence the flow of fluids in the internal environment by controlling smooth muscle action in the circulatory system.

In this chapter the discussion will be centered on (1) the constituents of the body fluids, (2) the function of each constituent, (3) the distribution and concentration of each constituent in the various fluid compartments, and (4) the effects of each on the volume, osmotic pressure, and hydrogen ion concentration in the body fluids. Most disturbances in fluid balance in the body are related to its volume, osmolality, and hydrogen ion concentration. Most illnesses, acute or chronic, are accompanied by some local or general disturbance in the body fluids. One of the factors in recovery is the ability of the individual to maintain or to restore the normal distribution and composition of body fluids. In order to anticipate and meet the needs of patients with understanding, the nurse requires some knowledge of the normal mechanisms for maintaining the constancy of the internal environment and the manner in which these mechanisms are disrupted in disease.

Body fluids are composed of water with electrolytes and nonelectrolytes suspended or dissolved in it. The types and concentrations of electrolytes in body fluids resemble those of seawater. According to one popular theory of the origin of life, the first living creatures developed in the sea. Those that were successful in making the adaptation to living on land took some of the sea with them in the form of extracellular fluid. Land animals, including humans, continue to surround their cells with fluids like those that were present in the primeval seas.

Undue loss of fluid is prevented by a watertight jacket—the skin. A special structure, the gastrointestinal tract, enables the organism to take from the external environment the materials required to replenish fluid constituents utilized by, or lost from, the body. The kidney, lung, and skin remove metabolic waste products and excesses in supply. All of these are regulated so that they function with remarkable accuracy in maintaining the composition and concentration of this fluid. The seas have no such means for protecting their composition and concentration. In the eons of their existence, water laden with minerals has been emptied into them by the rivers of the earth. Water is evaporated by the sun and wind with the result that minerals, especially salt, have become concentrated in the seawater.

Chemical Compounds in Solution

Understanding of the behavior of electrolytes in body fluids requires prior knowledge of atomic and subatomic particles as the basic units of matter. Three classes of chemical substances that make up matter are elements, compounds, and mixtures. The behavior of compounds in solution in body fluids is of central importance. A chemical compound is a molecule that consists of two or more elements that in turn are each made up of one or more atoms. Chemical compounds in solution may behave in one of two ways: (1) Their elements may remain intact, with no separation of atomic particles. These substances are called *nonelectrolytes*, examples of which are urea, glucose, and creatinine. (2) Their elements may break up *(dissociate)* into separate particles *(ions)* by the process of *ionization*. These substances are called *electrolytes*, examples of which are potassium chloride, magnesium sulfate, and sodium bicarbonate.

Terminology

Because mastery of terminology is essential to understanding of fluid and electrolyte balance, a number of terms will be defined and discussed.

Atom. An electrically neutral basic unit of matter resembling a miniature solar system, with its nucleus made up of protons and neutrons surrounded by enough revolving electrons to balance electrically the protons in the nucleus (Routh, 1953). The hydrogen atom, with one proton and one electron (and therefore no neutron), serves as a basis for determining the atomic number and weight of other atoms.

Proton. A positively charged particle of mass one within the nucleus of the atom, which may be considered a hydrogen atom minus its one electron (Routh, 1953).

Electron. A negatively charged particle whose mass equals 1/1,837 of the mass of the hydrogen atom, which revolves in orbit around the nucleus of the atom (Routh, 1953).

Neutron. An uncharged or electrically neutral particle of mass one.

Atomic number. That number which equals the number of revolving electrons of the atom. Because the atom must be electrically neutral, the atomic number also equals the number of protons in the nucleus (Routh, 1953).

Atomic weight. That number which equals the sum of the total number of protons and neutrons in the nucleus of the atom (Routh, 1953).

Ionization. The process whereby one atom permanently donates the electron(s) of its outer valence shell to another atom that completes its valence shell by accepting the electron(s). The electrically charged particles that result from the transfer of electron(s) are called *ions*. The donor atom becomes positively charged and will migrate, under the influence of an electric current, to the cathode (−) (negatively charged pole), thus being called a *cation*. The recipient atom becomes negatively charged and will migrate to the anode (+) (positively charged pole), thus being called an *anion*. For example, the hydrogen atom has one electron in its outer shell and the chloride atom has seven. The hydrogen atom, by giving up its electron, becomes a positively charged *cation* (H^+); the chloride atom fills its outer shell and becomes a negatively charged *anion* (Cl^-) (Pitts, 1963).

Valence. The measure of capacity of an atom or group of atoms (a radical) to combine with another atom or radical. The value for each atom or radical is determined by the number of electrons in the outer shell of the atom, with the single-electron hydrogen atom being the unit of comparison. *Negative valence* indicates the number of electrons an atom can take up; *positive valence* is the number of electrons an atom can give up.

Equivalent weight. A weight equal to the number of grams of an element that will chemically replace or react with 1 g (actually 1.008 g) of hydrogen or 8 g or parts of oxygen. The equivalent weight of an element is obtained by dividing its atomic weight by its valence. For example, the atomic weight of oxygen is 16. It has a valence of 2. Its equivalent weight is therefore 8. In forming water, 2 atoms (parts) of hydrogen combine with 1 atom (part) of oxygen. In terms of equivalent weights, 2.016 g of hydrogen combines with 16 g of oxygen to yield 18.016 g of water. To cite another example, 1 equivalent of potassium weighs 39.1 g. This is the amount of potassium that will combine with 8 g of oxygen. One equivalent of potassium (39.1 g) combines with 1 equivalent of chlorine, which weighs 35.5 g, to yield 74.6 g of potassium chloride.

Milliequivalent (mEq). The unit of measure of chemical activity of elements, equaling 0.001 of an equivalent weight. The number of milliequivalents per liter is determined by multiplying the milligrams per liter of the element by its valence and dividing by its atomic weight.

$$\text{mEq/L} = \frac{\text{mg/100 ml} \times 10 \times \text{valence}}{\text{atomic weight}}$$

Because the quantity of electrolytes found in a liter of body fluids is small, milliequivalents rather than equivalents are used to express the concentration of electrolytes in body fluids. Formerly, electrolytes in the blood were measured in milligrams per 100 ml of serum or plasma. The current trend is toward reporting them in milliequivalents per liter. The reason for this change is that the milliequivalent provides information about the number of anions or cations available to combine with cations and anions. To illustrate, the level of sodium cations in the blood serum ranges from 137 to 147 (average 142) mEq per liter. This means there are approximately 142 sodium cations available to combine with 142 anions. The average level of chloride ions in blood serum is 103 mEq per liter. Therefore, approximately 39 mEq of sodium are available to combine with other anions.

Electrolytes. Those substances that, when dissolved in water, are capable of carrying an electric current because they dissociate into electrically charged ions. Their chemical activity is measured in milliequivalents. The degree to which a dilute solution of a given electrolyte dissociates is constant, but it differs for each electrolyte. Strong electrolytes dissociate almost completely. They include most soluble salts and inorganic acids and bases.

Acids. Once defined as compounds yielding hydrogen ions, acids are now defined as *proton donors.* Though they exist in solution as H_3O^+ (hydronium ion), they are generally referred to as H^+.

Bases. Once defined as compounds yielding hydroxyl ions, bases are now defined as *proton acceptors.*

Buffer. A substance that protects a solution from changes in pH when an acid or base is added by acting to maintain the original hydrogen ion concentration of the solution. It is sometimes referred to as a chemical sponge. The buffering capacity of a solution is determined by the number of hydrogen ions it can take up or discharge per unit change of pH. The average adult has a total of about 1,000 mEq of total buffer bases, most of which are found in the tissue cells, with only a small part present in the blood (Wilson, 1973).

Buffer system is composed of a weak acid and a salt formed by neutralizing the weak acid with a strong base. A weak base and a salt formed by neutralizing the base with a strong acid functions similarly.

There are a number of buffer systems in the body. In blood the chief buffer systems are *oxyhemoglobin* and *reduced hemoglobin; bicarbonate* and *carbonic acid;* and *acid protein* and *B protein.* The bicarbonate–carbonic acid system is present in greatest concentration and is most important in maintaining the pH of blood and interstitial fluid (Wilson, 1973). In cells the main buffer systems are *sodium acid phosphate* and *bisodium phosphate,* and *acid protein* and *B protein.*

The body buffers acid far better than alkaline solutions, as might be expected in view of the fact that virtually all physiologic changes in the body such as those effected by exercise and fasting tend to cause an acidosis (Wilson, 1973).

Alkali reserve. A term used to refer to the sodium in the blood that is in combination with bicarbonate. It is called the alkali reserve because the sodium can combine with other anions. The term is really a misnomer.

Osmotic pressure. The force created by particles in solution that attracts water across a membrane that is fully permeable to water, but impermeable to the particles, ions, or molecules. The direction of flow of the water is always from the less concentrated toward the more concentrated solution. Flow continues until the solution on the two sides of the membrane is of equal concentration. An increase in the osmotic pressure of the fluid in one fluid compartment in the body results in the movement of water into that compartment.

Hydrostatic pressure. The force exerted by a fluid against the wall of the chamber in which it is contained. Literally, it means the pressure created by the standing weight of water. Applied to the blood, it includes not only the pressure created by the weight of blood against the wall of the capillary, but the force with which the blood is propelled.

Osmol. One gram molecular weight of a nonionized solute. One osmol of glucose is the molecular weight of the glucose expressed in grams. One gram molecular weight of sodium chloride yields two osmols because each molecule of sodium chloride breaks up into one sodium ion and one chloride ion.

Osmolality. The number of osmotically active particles per kilogram of water.

Osmolarity. The number of osmols per liter of solution.

Filtration. The separation of a liquid from a solid by passing the liquid through a semipermeable membrane. The force responsible is gravity or weight.

Diffusion. The distribution of one substance throughout another by the movement of molecules.

Hyponatremia. A condition characterized by too little sodium in the blood plasma.

Hypernatremia. A condition in which there is too much sodium in the blood plasma.

Hypokalemia. A condition in which there is too little potassium in the blood plasma.

Hyperkalemia. A condition in which there is too much potassium in the blood plasma.

Azotemia. A condition in which there is an excess of nitrogenous compounds in the blood plasma.

The Kidney

Because the kidney is essential to the maintenance of the internal environment, its functions are discussed here. The consequences of renal failure are considered in Chapter 41.

Renal Mechanisms to Regulate the Constancy of the Internal Environment

In health the kidney functions to maintain within limits (1) the volume of water in the extracellular fluid, (2) the concentration of electrolytes in extracellular fluid, (3) the osmolality of the extracellular fluid, and (4) the concentration of hydrogen ion in the extracellular fluid. The kidney is the site for the excretion of the wastes of metabolism, particularly those of protein catabolism. Under certain abnormal conditions, the kidney produces vasoexcitatory substances or their precursors. At the present time this is thought to revolve around the juxtaglomerular apparatus and the renin–angiotensin system; participation in regulation of calcium balance; and production of prostaglandins (Stein, 1979). The kidneys also secrete a substance (erythropoietin-stimulating factor) that influences the maturation of red blood cells.

Not only is the kidney a target organ of various hormones, but it also influences the metabolism of other organs and carries out its own endocrine functions, producing substances that regulate body processes that are carried out by other organs (Stein, 1979). Table 27-1 summarizes the hormones that affect renal function, and those affected and produced by the kidney.

Although the kidneys are frequently called organs of excretion, the above list of their functions indicates the inadequacy of this concept of renal function. The primary function of the kidneys is to regulate the volume and composition of the extracellular fluid; their excretory function is incidental to this regulatory function.

Blood Supply to the Kidney

Blood is supplied to the kidney by the renal arteries, which are branches of the abdominal aorta. Although renal mass accounts for only 0.5 per cent of body weight, the kidney receives 25 per cent of cardiac output and consumes 7 per cent of the body's total oxygen uptake, most of which is used for the metabolic processes of tubular transport (Epstein, 1979).[1] The renal circulation is actually a composite of several microcirculations, each with a specialized role. The glomerular circulation is specialized for filtration, the first step in urine formation; the cortical peritubular network is specialized for reabsorption of fluid and solutes; and the medullary circulation is specialized to facilitate concentration and dilution of urine (Brenner & Beeuwkes, 1978).

[1] More detailed discussions of the gross structure of the kidney may be found in most anatomy textbooks.

TABLE 27-1 *Hormones Affecting Renal Function and Those Affected and Produced by the Kidney.**

Hormones Affecting Renal Function

1. Renin-angiotensin-aldosterone (RAA) sequence
2. Antidiuretic hormone (ADH)
3. Prostaglandins
4. Adrenocortical hormones
5. Thyroid hormone
6. Parathyroid hormone
7. Kallikrein-kinin sequence

Hormones Produced By the Kidney

1. Renin—this inactive substance is not a true hormone (see Chap. 15), but is released from granules contained in the juxtaglomerular cells in response to one of the following developments:
   (a) reduced glomerular filtration rate (GFR)
   (b) reduced glomerular pressure
   (c) increased sympathetic stimulation of the kidneys (Guyton, 1976, p. 469).
2. 1,25-(OH_2)-D_3, also expressed as 1,25-dihydroxycholecalciferol
3. Prostaglandins

Hormones Affected By the Kidney

1. Insulin
2. Parathyroid hormone
3. RAA sequence
4. Adrenocortical hormones

* Information from Stein, J. H. "Hormones and the Kidney." *Hosp. Prac.,* **14**:91–95, 99–105 (July 1979), p. 92.

Unlike most capillaries, the glomerulus has an arteriole at its exit as well as its entrance (see Figure 27-1). The quantity of blood entering the glomerulus is regulated by the afferent arteriole. Dilation results in increased blood flow into the kidney and constriction results in a decrease. The efferent arteriole regulates the pressure of the blood in the glomerulus. With dilation, resistance to the outflow of blood from the glomerulus diminishes the glomerular filtration and pressure drops. With constriction, resistance to the flow of blood out of the glomerulus increases, resulting in an increased filtration pressure in the glomerulus. The vessels supplying the glomerular bed are short and have a wide lumen, allowing the glomerular capillary bed to act as a high-pressure system. This can be contrasted with the peritubular capillary bed, which is a low-pressure system. As a consequence of this arrangement, the kidney is able to closely adapt blood flow to its own and the body's needs.

The Nephron

The work of the kidney is performed by the nephron. In humans there are a million or more nephrons in each kidney. They are all basically similar in structure and each one is presumed to be grossly similar to all others in function. Nephrons are located in the cortex. Those situated near the periphery of the kidney are called cortical nephrons. Nephrons situated in the cortex adjacent to the medulla are called juxtamedullary nephrons. Classically, a nephron is described as consisting of a renal or malpighian corpuscle (glomerulus and Bowman's capsule), proximal convoluted tubule, loop of Henle, and a distal convoluted tubule. Finally, many nephrons empty into a collecting tubule. Although the glomeruli are found in the cortex, the proximal and distal renal tubules and especially the loop of Henle dip far down into the medulla of the kidney. (See Figure 27-1 for major characteristics of each portion of a juxtamedullary nephron.)

Filtration by the Glomeruli

Of the processes involved in the formation of urine, the first is filtration by the glomeruli. Filtration depends on the hydrostatic pressure created by the pumping action of the heart, the volume of blood circulating through the glomeruli, and the resistance offered by the afferent and efferent arterioles. The glomerular filtrate is an ultrafiltrate of the blood and as such it does not contain red cells or colloid materi-

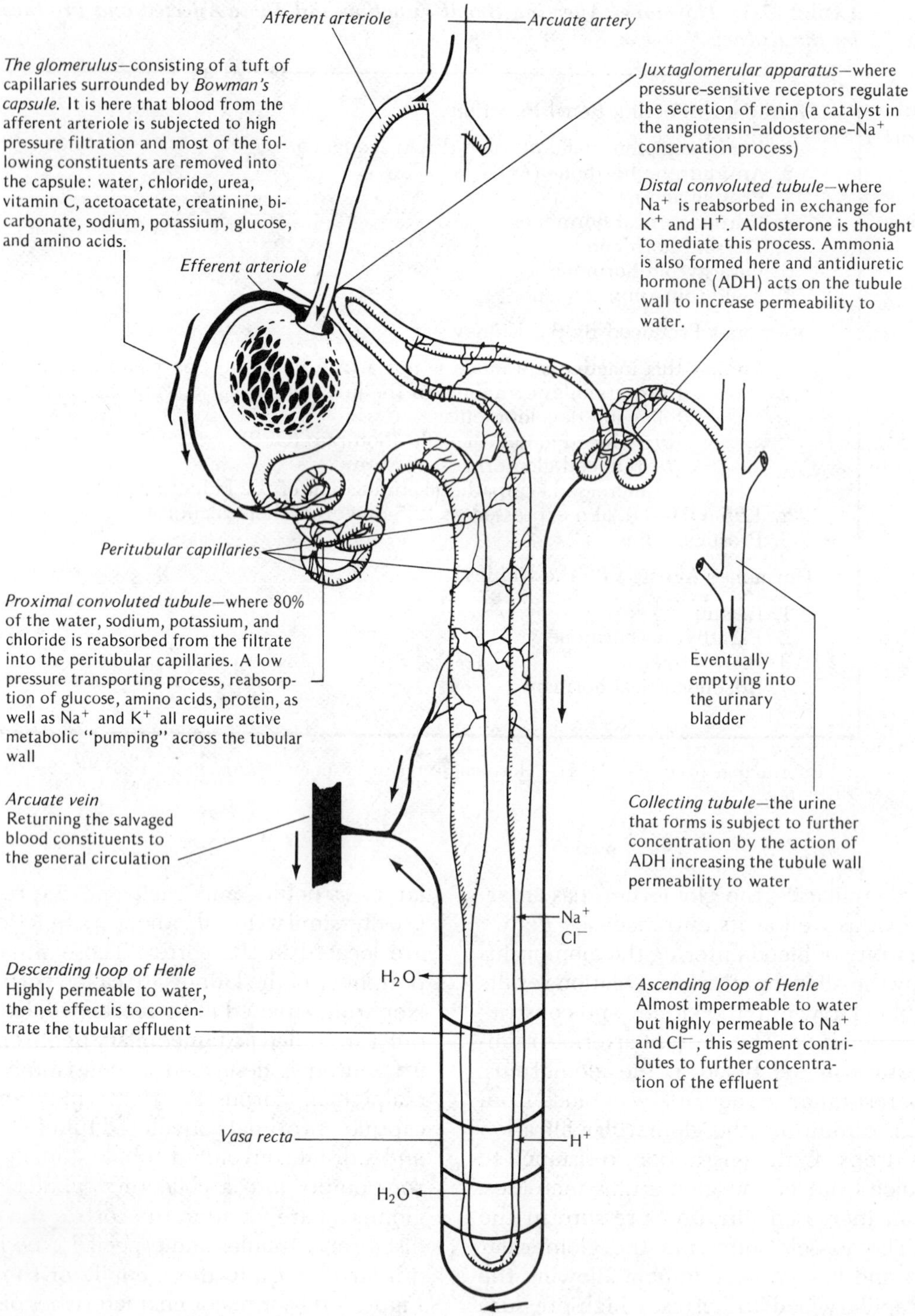
Afferent arteriole
Arcuate artery
The glomerulus—consisting of a tuft of capillaries surrounded by *Bowman's capsule.* It is here that blood from the afferent arteriole is subjected to high pressure filtration and most of the following constituents are removed into the capsule: water, chloride, urea, vitamin C, acetoacetate, creatinine, bicarbonate, sodium, potassium, glucose, and amino acids.
Juxtaglomerular apparatus—where pressure-sensitive receptors regulate the secretion of renin (a catalyst in the angiotensin-aldosterone-Na^+ conservation process)
Distal convoluted tubule—where Na^+ is reabsorbed in exchange for K^+ and H^+. Aldosterone is thought to mediate this process. Ammonia is also formed here and antidiuretic hormone (ADH) acts on the tubule wall to increase permeability to water.
Efferent arteriole
Peritubular capillaries
Proximal convoluted tubule—where 80% of the water, sodium, potassium, and chloride is reabsorbed from the filtrate into the peritubular capillaries. A low pressure transporting process, reabsorption of glucose, amino acids, protein, as well as Na^+ and K^+ all require active metabolic "pumping" across the tubular wall
Eventually emptying into the urinary bladder
Arcuate vein
Returning the salvaged blood constituents to the general circulation
Collecting tubule—the urine that forms is subject to further concentration by the action of ADH increasing the tubule wall permeability to water
Na^+
Cl^-
Descending loop of Henle
Highly permeable to water, the net effect is to concentrate the tubular effluent
H_2O
Ascending loop of Henle
Almost impermeable to water but highly permeable to Na^+ and Cl^-, this segment contributes to further concentration of the effluent
Vasa recta
H^+
H_2O

Figure 27-1. A juxtamedullary nephron: major characteristics of each portion indicated.

als such as protein. It does contain water and crystalloidal solutes such as electrolytes, glucose, and urea, as well as other wastes of protein metabolism. In other words, the glomerular filtrate contains water and almost all of the substances dissolved in plasma water. The rate of glomerular filtration averages about 125 ml per minute in men and 110 ml per minute in women.

Tubular Function

As the glomerular filtrate passes through the tubules, it is converted to urine by selective reabsorption and the secretion of certain substances. Of the 180 liters of glomerular filtrate all except 1 or 1.5 liters are reabsorbed. Within the limits of its renal threshold, all glucose and amino acids are reabsorbed.

The transport systems that regulate the outward movement and reabsorption of both water and solutes across the lipid bilayer plasma membrane of the renal tubular cells obey the laws governing membrane transport in all biologic systems. In addition to the passive processes of simple and facilitated diffusion, a substantial portion of exchange within the tubules is accomplished by *active processes.*

As defined thermodynamically, *transport* is *active* if it results in net movement of a solute against an electrochemical gradient. To achieve this, the transport process must be either linked directly to a source of metabolic energy (primary active transport) or linked to flux of another molecular species that in turn is coupled to an energy source (secondary active transport). [Hayes, 1978]

THE PROXIMAL TUBULES. In the proximal tubules approximately 60 to 80 per cent of the water and almost all of the glucose, amino acids, bicarbonate ions, and vitamins are normally reabsorbed. The water is absorbed isotonically so that the osmotic pressure of the fluid in the proximal tubule is about the same as in plasma. The return of water to the blood is largely by diffusion and is believed to be determined by the number of ions reabsorbed; therefore, water reabsorption is obligatory. Glucose requires an active transport mechanism. When the level of glucose in the glomerular filtrate exceeds the capacity of the transport mechanism, glucose is lost in the urine.

LOOP OF HENLE The loop of Henle connects the proximal and distal tubules and is the portion of the nephron that extends farthest down into the medulla of the kidney. It consists of two basic parts, the descending and the ascending loop. In the descending loop, sodium is pumped out of the tubular fluid and about 6 per cent of the water in the glomerular filtrate is reabsorbed. The ascending loop is almost impermeable to water.

DISTAL TUBULES AND COLLECTING TUBULES. The work of the kidney is completed in the distal and collecting tubules. As the urine leaves the collecting tubules, it contains only about 1 per cent of the original fluid that was filtered. Depending upon the level of the antidiuretic hormone, which increases the permeability of this portion of the tubule to water, water is or is not reabsorbed. As much as 10 to 15 per cent of the filtered load of sodium is reabsorbed in this area. Aldosterone is the main hormone influencing the rate of sodium reabsorption in the distal and proximal tubules.

In addition to selective reabsorption of certain substances, the tubules also secrete a variety of substances. The distal tubules and collecting ducts secrete potassium and hydrogen ions, and the proximal and distal tubules and collecting ducts can secrete hydrogen ions and ammonia. As a part of the renal excretion route of certain drugs, the tubules also secrete such substances as penicillin, phenol red, and Diodrast.

SUMMARY

The kidney is a remarkable organ. With each heartbeat approximately one fourth of the blood pumped by the heart circulates through the kidney. Each day 180 liters of glomerular filtrate are formed. In health 99 per cent of the water in the glomerular filtrate is returned to the extracellular fluid. Other substances are either absorbed or secreted as needed to maintain the constancy of the fluid environment of the cells. Depending on intake and losses from the body, the quantity of sodium excreted in the urine varies from negligible to considerable amounts. The volume of extracellular fluid is directly related to this renal control of sodium balance (Wilson, 1973, pp. 58–63).

Except for a certain amount returned by diffusion, urea is largely concentrated and excreted in the urine. In general, substances useful to the body are reabsorbed, whereas those of no use or in excess are eliminated.

The kidney closely regulates the volume and concentration of urine in relation to the quantity of water and solutes added to extracellular fluid from exogenous and endogenous sources.

With a large fluid intake, the kidney excretes a large volume of dilute urine; with a small fluid intake, it excretes a small volume of concentrated urine. When both salt and water intake are limited, the minimum volume of urine depends on the volume of nitrogenous wastes, principally urea, presented to the kidney for excretion, and the kidney's capacity to concentrate urea. About 500 ml of water are required for this purpose. The capacity of the kidney to alter the concentration and volume of urine is adaptive. Within limits, it enables the body to survive water deprivation and loss and to rapidly eliminate excesses of intake. The extent to which the kidney is able to concentrate or dilute urine or specific substances in it is a useful test of renal function. The daily requirements, sources, organs of excretion, daily average excretion, and sources of excessive loss for water and electrolytes are summarized in Table 27-2. Because all excessive losses require replacement, accurate observation and reporting of the quantity lost by any avenue are important to the welfare of the patient. Problems associated with excessive losses are discussed in Chapter 41.

TABLE 27-2 *Summary of Factors Relating to Body Water and Electrolytes*

Substance	Symbols	Normal Concentration in Serum or Plasma in mEq/L*	Estimated Daily Dietary Requirement for Adults†	Source of Intake†	Organ of Excretion	Daily Average Excretion	Sources of Excessive Loss
Water	H·HO		1,500–3,000 ml	Fluids, 1,000 ml	Skin	500–1,000 ml	Sweating
				Food, free water 1,000 ml	Kidney	600–1,000 ml	Polyuria Burn fluid High renal output failure
				Water of oxidation, 300 ml	Lung	350 ml	Mouth breathing
					Intestine	100 ml	Up to 8,000 ml of gastrointestinal secretions per day; losses via vomiting, diarrhea, fistulas, stomas
Sodium	Na^+	135–148 mEq/L	2–6g	Abundant in most foods except fruit	Kidney	110 mEq/24 hr	May be lost when excess loss of fluid from GI tract, or from kidney, or by salt-wasting diuretics or excess sweating
					Skin	5 mEq/L	Sudden profuse sweating can result in loss of 3–5 g NaCl per day when first in tropics, or febrile
Potassium	K^+	3.5–5.3 mEq/L	2–4 g	Abundant in food, especially fruit juices	Kidney	25–100 mEq/24 hr	Polyuria, excessive catabolism of cells, catharsis, diarrhea, enemas, diuretics
Calcium	Ca^{++}	4.25–5.25 mEq/L	800 mg	Milk, milk products, some seafoods, and greens	Kidney	30–150 mg/24 hr	Renal failure Inadequate intake of vitamin D Hyperparathyroidism
					Intestine	As insoluble soaps	

Magnesium	Mg^{++}	1.4–2.2 mEq/L	200–300 mg	Whole-grain cereals, nuts, meat, milk, green vegetables, legumes	Intestine Kidney		
Chloride	Cl^{-}	98–106 mEq/L		With Na as NaCl	Kidney Skin	110–250 mEq/24 hr 5 mEq/L	Losses may be excessive with vomiting, or if gastrointestinal tract suctioning continues
Standard Bicarbonate‡ (Nonrespiratory sources)	HCO_3^{-}	21–25 mEq/L		End product of metabolism	Lung Kidney		(See Acid–Base Equilibrium, p. 406)
Phosphate§	$H_2PO_4^{-}$ $HPO_4^{=}$	4 mEq/L	1,200 mg	With calcium and protein foods	Kidney Possibly intestinal tract		(See Calcium)
Sulfate§	$SO_4^{=}$	1 mEq/L		Protein foods	Kidney		
Protein+		6–8 g/100 ml	40–80 g	Meat, milk, dairy products, eggs, lentils, legumes, etc.	End products of protein metabolism excreted by kidney but not as protein		May be lost via kidney, draining wounds, ulcers, burns
Hydrogen	H^{+}			Metabolism	Kidney		

* F. K. Widmann. *Clinical Interpretation of Laboratory Tests,* 8th ed. Philadelphia: F. A. Davis Co., 1979, pp. A4–7.
† Marie V. Krause and Martha A. Hunscher: *Food, Nutrition and Diet Therapy,* 5th ed. Philadelphia: W. B. Saunders Co., 1972, pp. 111–13.
‡ J. A. Halsted. *The Laboratory in Clinical Medicine.* Philadelphia: W. B. Saunders Co., 1976, p. 116.
§ A. C. Guyton. *Textbook of Medical Physiology,* 5th ed. Philadelphia: W. B. Saunders Co., 1976, p. 40.

Fluid Compartments

The largest component of the body is water. In multicellular organisms body fluids are divided into two large compartments, the intracellular and the extracellular fluids. These two compartments are separated from each other by the cell membrane. Water diffuses more or less freely across this semipermeable membrane. The movement of solutes across the cell membrane is regulated so that the concentration of each component is maintained within a limited range. Extracellular fluid is further divided into two compartments—the intravascular and the interstitial. Intravascular fluid is the fluid component of the blood. Interstitial fluid is that found in the spaces between blood vessels and surrounding cells. Most of the interstitial fluid is a transudate formed by the filtration of blood plasma through the capillary membrane. There are collections of extracellular fluids that are not simple transudates. They are formed by the secretory activity of cells. Examples include the cerebrospinal fluid, gastrointestinal secretions, bile, and pancreatic secretions. See Table 27-3 for the distribution of body water by compartment and by percentage of total body water and body weight.

TABLE 27-3 *Distribution of body water by compartment and by percentage of total body water and body weight.**

Compartment	Per Cent of Total Body Water		Per Cent of Body Weight	
Intracellular Fluids		60		36
Extracellular Fluids		26		16
1. Interstitial-lymph	(19)		(11.5)	
2. Plasma/intravascular	(7)		(4.5)	
3. Other extracellular fluid compartments				
a. Transcellular water (secretions from epithelial cells): saliva; gastric juice; bile; pancreatic juice; ileal, cecal, and cerebrospinal fluid; and sweat		2		1.5
b. Dense connective tissues: cartilage and tendons		7		4.5
c. Bone matrix		5		3.
		100		61

* Figures derived from B. D. Rose. *Clinical Physiology of Acid–Base and Electrolyte Disorders.* New York: McGraw-Hill Book Co., 1977, Chap. 1.

In health, potential spaces such as the peritoneal and pleural cavities contain only small amounts of fluid; however, in certain diseases the quantity of peritoneal and/or pleural fluid may be large enough to interfere with body functions. Recent studies have, however, demonstrated that water and electrolytes do not move as freely from some tissues as they do from others. Bone, cartilage, and other dense connective tissues contain large quantities of water and electrolytes. Bone, for example, holds a volume of water about equal to the blood plasma. This water and its electrolytes are not freely exchangeable with other body compartments. Fluid in the interstitial spaces does not appear to be a simple solution of water and the electrolytes dissolved in it. It is held in the tissue spaces by collagen fibers and hyaluronic acid. Hyaluronic acid does not interfere with the capacity of the water to dissolve electrolytes or nonelectrolytes. It enters into the cement substance that binds cells together.

In the extracellular fluid, sodium is the most abundant cation, although it also contains calcium, magnesium, potassium, and trace elements. In the intracellular fluid the most abundant cation is potassium with other cations present in lesser amounts. Whatever the amount, however, each cation and anion has an important function. For the electrolyte components of each fluid compartment see Figure 27-2. Neither the values for concentration of individual ions nor the values for the total concentration of ions within a fluid compartment are absolute. Each can vary within a range of normal. The values included in Figure 27-2 fall within average normal concentrations of the ions in each fluid compartment. However, exact balance between positive and negative ions is obligatory to maintain electrical neutrality of body solutions (Pitts, 1963, p. 26).

FACTORS INFLUENCING THE VOLUME AND DISTRIBUTION OF WATER IN THE BODY

The volume and distribution of water in the body vary with the age, sex, and amount of adipose tissue. These differences are illustrated by the Martin family in Figure 27-3. The family is composed of five members—John Martin, aged 30; Mary Martin, aged 28; Billy, aged 9; Suzy, aged 8 weeks; and Mary Martin's mother, Mrs. Bird, aged 68. Because at all ages the intravascular fluid comprises about 5 per cent of the total body weight, the extracellular fluid, as shown in Figure 27-3 has not been divided into interstitial and intravascular compartments. The most marked difference in the distribution of water at the different age levels is in the amount of interstitial fluid. In the newborn baby, the proportion of body water

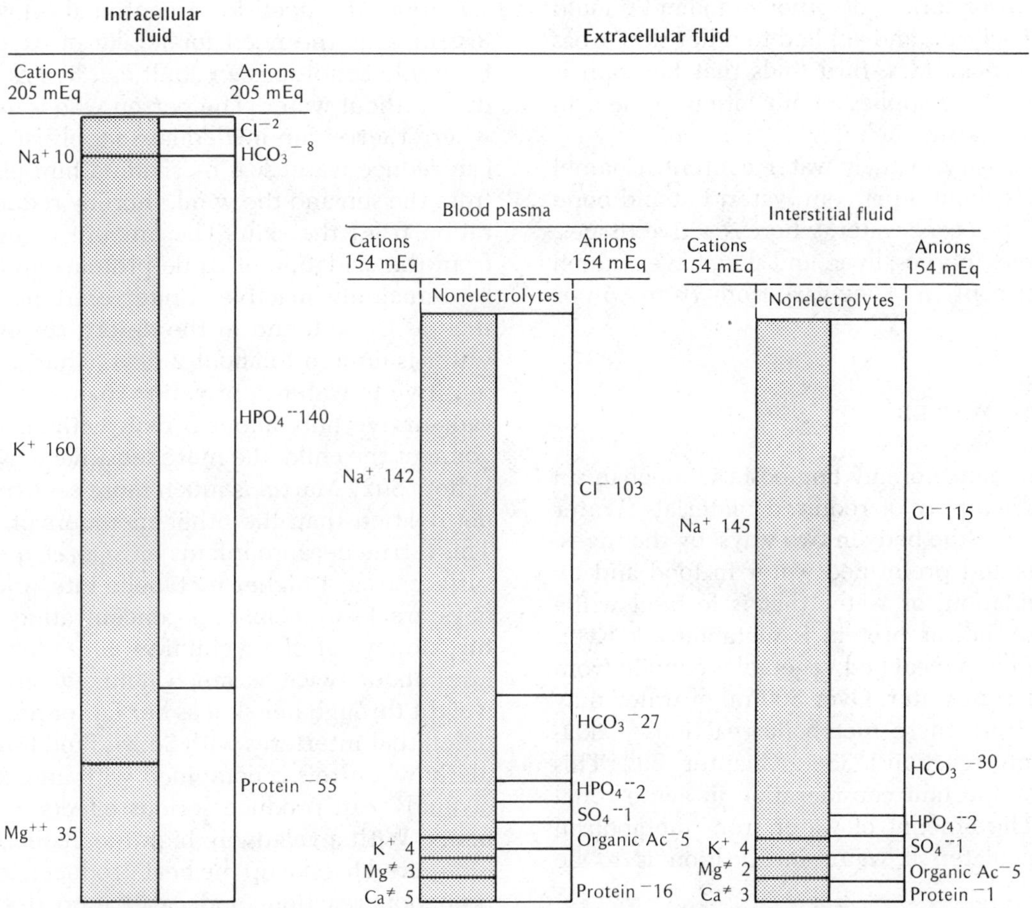

Figure 27-2. A comparison of the electrolyte composition of fluid compartments. (Adapted with permission of Abbott Laboratories from *Fluid and Electrolytes: Some Practical Guides to Clinical Use,* 1970, pp. 10–11, by Abbott Laboratories.)

in the interstitial fluid compartment is larger than at any other period in life. From Figure 27-3 the reader will note that with advancing age there is a progressive decrease in the porportion of water in the interstitial space, as well as in the total volume of water in the body. Interstitial fluid accounts for 40 per cent of 8-week-old Suzy's weight, 30 per cent of Billy's weight, and only 20 per cent of the weight of the adults. Although not shown in Figure 27-3, the water content of the body falls sharply from birth to about 4 years of age and then levels off. Maturity, in respect to water and electrolytes, is reached at about 20 years of age. Thenceforth throughout life there is a slow decline in body water. This change is also demonstrated in Figure 27-3. Although water is responsible for 75 per cent of Suzy's weight, it accounts for only 45 per cent of her grandmother's weight. Objective evidence of the loss of water in older age groups is seen in the dry skin and hair of the aged. It is also seen in their flabby muscles and wrinkled skin. The degree of dryness of the skin should be taken into consideration when planning the number and type of baths for elderly people. Men, in particular, may be troubled by dry and itching skin. For the comfort of the patient, full baths may have to be limited to one or two per week. A mild soap should be selected. Rather than alcohol,

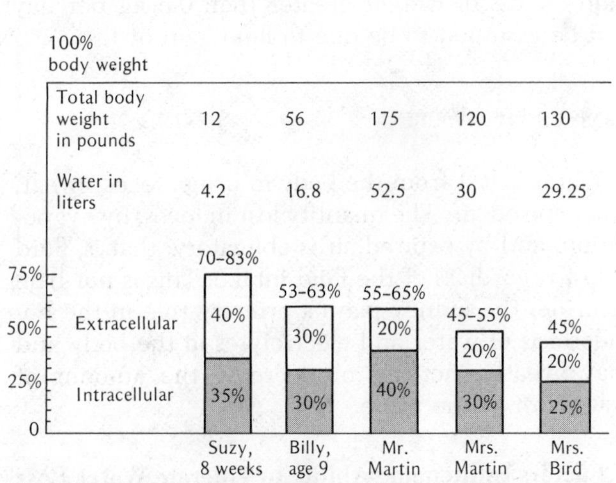

Figure 27-3. Volume and distribution of water in the body vary with age, sex, and amount of adipose tissue, as seen in the Martin family.

a hand cream or lotion, or other emollient should be used for backrubs and applied to other skin areas to reduce dryness. Mrs. Bird finds that her skin is excessively dry and applies an oily lotion to the skin of her legs and arms each day.

Tissues also vary in their water content. Enamel of the teeth is about 3 per cent water. Fat and bone are about 25 per cent water, whereas active tissues, such as muscles, nerves, liver, and skin, have a much higher water content. They vary from 70 to 85 per cent water.

Sources of Water

The maintenance of any homeostatic mechanism depends on a supply of required materials. Water is replenished in the body in two ways: by the ingestion of fluids and preformed water in food and by water of oxidation, or water that is formed while carbohydrate, fat, or protein is metabolized. Even solid foods such as meat and vegetables contain from 60 to 97 per cent water. Over 500 ml of water may be derived from these metabolic reactions (oxidation-reduction reactions). (See Chapter 29.) This water is an important consideration in acute renal shutdown. The amount of water from metabolism must be calculated if water intoxication is to be avoided.

The point at which water is normally taken from the external environment into the internal environment is the gastrointestinal tract. Any condition disturbing the function of the gastrointestinal tract may interfere with the patient's intake of fluid. Accurate measurement and recording of the patient's fluid intake, as well as losses by vomiting or diarrhea are essential. Rapid loss of weight is usually indicative of insufficient water intake. As a matter of fact, any gain or loss of weight greater than 0.5 kg per day can be assumed to be due to fluid gain or loss.

Losses of Water

Water is lost from the body in urine, feces, sweat, and expired air. The quantity lost in feces, by evaporation, and by expired air is obligatory; that is, fluid is lost regardless of the fluid intake. This is not true of urine; the kidney plays a primary role in the homeostasis of water and electrolytes in the body and may greatly increase or decrease the amount of water lost in the urine.

Factors Influencing Ability to Tolerate Water Loss

Because some water is stored and because there are effective mechanisms for its renewal and conservation, the need for a continual intake is not as urgent as is the need for intake of oxygen. Under favorable conditions an adult can live as long as ten days without water. The person who is in a situation where there is an inadequate supply of fresh water can reduce water loss by shading himself or herself from the sun and the wind, thereby reducing evaporation from the skin. The amount of urea formed from the oxidation of tissue protein can be reduced by remaining inactive. Under extreme conditions, such as those found in the desert, survival without water is limited to about 2 days. Children are more sensitive to water deprivation than are adults. They can survive only about 5 days without water. The younger the child, the more sensitive to water deprivation. Suzy Martin is much more sensitive to water deprivation than the other members of the family. This is true because infants have a relatively greater surface area, a higher metabolic rate, and their kidneys are less efficient in concentrating urine than the kidneys of older children and adults are. Suzy loses about twice as much fluid per gram of body weight through her skin as her father does. Any condition that interferes with Suzy's fluid intake, particularly when this is combined with an excessive loss of fluids, can produce serious effects within a few hours. With a relatively high metabolic rate, water is required to take up the heat produced in oxidation-reduction reactions and carry it to the surface of the body where it is eliminated. With the excessive loss of water, Suzy's temperature can be expected to rise. Because she is unable adequately to retain the volume of her blood by concentrating urine, the electrolytes become concentrated in the blood. Unless treatment is instituted quickly, the circulation may fail, and death may occur.

Water: Its Properties and Functions

Water has a number of properties that make it well suited to its role in the body. It is chemically stable. It is a so-called universal solvent. This does not mean that all substances dissolve in it, but more do than in any other liquid. It has a high ionizing power. It also has a number of properties that make it well suited to its role in temperature regulation; these include its high specific heat, its high latent heat of evaporation, and its great capacity to conduct heat. Its specific heat is the highest for all liquids.

Water functions in the body in many ways. As has been stated, it functions in temperature regulation by taking up large quantities of heat produced by cells and distributing it throughout the body. At the surface of the body, heat is lost to the atmosphere by evaporation of water and the blood is cooled. Because of the large number of substances that are soluble in water, it serves as a vehicle for the transportation of substances to and from cells. In the lung, oxygen goes into solution as it enters the blood. Carbon dioxide is in solution in the blood before it escapes into the alveoli. The volume of blood is dependent on water. Products of metabolism are diluted by water and are thus prevented from injuring cells. End products of metabolism and excesses of intake dissolved in water are excreted by the kidney. Water is necessary to the physiochemical activities of the body. Digestion of food is at least partly accomplished by hydrolysis—the breakdown of molecules through the addition of water. The chemical process within the cell takes place in water. Storage of nutrients depends on water. For each gram of protein deposited in the body, 4 g of water are needed. Growing children therefore require proportionately more water than do adults. Fat requires only 0.2 g of water to store each gram.

Water, as the principal solvent in the body, regulates the osmolality of body fluids. When water is lost from the body in excess of that ingested, body fluids become concentrated and their osmolality is increased. Because the body does not tolerate differences in osmotic pressure between the fluid compartments, water is then shifted from the compartment in which the concentration of water is greatest to the one in which the concentration of electrolyte is greatest. For example, when extracellular fluid is hypertonic in relation to intracellular fluid, water moves from the cell into the interstitial fluid, thereby dehydrating the cell. Conversely, when the interstitial fluid is hypotonic in relation to the cellular fluid, water moves into the cell, causing it to swell. Responses of the body to increased concentration of body fluids or electrolytes, as well as the role of water in the regulation of hydrogen ions, will be discussed later.

Water is essential to all body functions. It is the medium in which the physiochemical activities of the cell take place. In some bodily processes, such as hydrolysis, it is one of the reacting agents. In others, as in oxidation-reduction reactions, it may be a product. It is an essential element in the internal environment of the cell. It is the medium through which or by which all substances are transported to and from the cell and external environment. Without it, life is impossible.

The general functions of water are summarized as follows (Strand, 1978):

1. Maintenance of cellular size and form
2. Medium for chemical reactions
3. Insulation from temperature extremes
4. Electrical conduction
5. Facilitation of surface reactions
6. Fluid medium for excreted wastes
7. Lubrication

Regulation of Water

As water is removed from the cells, the cells become dehydrated. This causes drying of the mouth and pharynx and may result in the sensation of thirst. Satisfaction of the thirst by ingestion of water may correct the deficit. The kidney can also function to conserve water and protect the concentration of electrolytes in the body fluids. The chain of events leading to the correction of increase in osmotic pressure by the kidney increasing the reabsorption of water is described as follows: Osmoreceptors, especially in the supraoptic nuclei of the hypothalamus, are sensitive to increased osmotic pressure. They initiate impulses that bring about the release of the antidiuretic hormone (ADH) from the posterior pituitary gland. The antidiuretic hormone increases the permeability of the distal and collecting tubules to water and thereby facilitates and increases the reabsorption of water. A decrease in the osmolality in the extracellular fluid tends to produce the opposite effect. As the extracellular fluid becomes hypotonic in relaiton to the intracellular fluid, water moves from the extracellular space into the cells in the supraoptic nuclei; special cells in this area act like tiny osmometers, swelling when the extracellular fluid becomes hypotonic and shrinking when it becomes hypertonic. Swelling of the cells is thought to inhibit the secretion of the antidiuretic hormone and shrinking is presumed to stimulate its secretion. With a decrease in the level of ADH, the quantity of water reabsorbed in the distal and collecting tubules is reduced and the volume excreted in the urine is increased. Conversely, augmentation of the secretion of ADH increases the reabsorption of water by the distal and collecting tubules and decreases the volume of water excreted in the urine.

Whereas ADH controls the osmotic pressure of extracellular water, the volume of extracellular water is controlled by the adrenocortical hormone aldosterone, which is secreted in response to decreased renal arterial pressure and volume of blood flow. The renal afferent arteriole appears to serve as a volume receptor, responding to decreased pressure by releasing renin from the juxtaglomerular cells. (See Figure 27-1 for location of these cells.) Renin causes the formation of angiotensin II in the blood, which then stimulates the adrenal cortex to secrete aldosterone. By acting on the distal tubules, aldosterone promotes retention of sodium and water by the kidney. Potassium levels appear to have a bidirectional influence on aldosterone secretion; hypokalemia markedly retards aldosterone secretion, whereas hyperkalemia is associated with increased aldosterone secretion (Laragh, 1973).

There is evidence that a third factor, possibly a hormone, participates in regulation of extracellular water. It allows loss of sodium from the kidney when salt-retaining hormones such as aldosterone and 11-deoxycorticosterone are elevated for prolonged periods, probably by decreasing reabsorption of sodium from the proximal tubules (Goldberger, 1975).

Factors in Movement of Fluid Between Introvascular and Interstitial Compartments

As was stated earlier, body fluids are separated into compartments by the semipermeable membranes surrounding cells and capillaries. These membranes serve as the points where exchange takes place between each cell and its fluid environment (the interstitial fluid) and between the interstitial fluid and the plasma within the circulatory system. Five factors influence the movement of fluids across the capillary membrane. They are

1. Capillary permeability
2. Diffusion
3. Filtration pressure
4. Colloid osmotic pressure of the blood
5. Interstitial fluid pressure

More fluid moves from the intravascular to the interstitial compartment than returns by way of the capillary membrane. This excess fluid is restored to the blood by the lymphatic system. See Figure 27-4 for factors that influence movement of fluids across the capillary membrane.

In general, capillaries are freely permeable to low molecular weight electrolytes and nonelectrolytes, and they are much less permeable to blood proteins or other high molecular weight substances. The degree to which capillaries are permeable to proteins differs in various parts of the body. Those in the sinusoids of the liver, the heart, the lungs, and the gastrointestinal tract are quite permeable to protein. Those in the skin and skeletal muscles are much less permeable. Capillaries forming the glomeruli of the kidney are nearly impermeable to protein. The degree of capillary permeability influences the volume of water and the size of the molecules that can escape into the interstitial fluid compartment. For example, Mrs. Bird complains that on warm days her feet swell. One of the contributing factors is that, with an increase in the environmental temperature, peripheral blood vessels dilate to increase heat loss. As the capillaries dilate, permeability is increased and with it the volume of interstitial fluid is enlarged. Just as, or perhaps more, important, the filtration pressure at the arterial end of the capillary may increase, forcing more fluid out of the capillaries. A variety of physical and chemical agents increase capillary permeability. Some common examples include anoxia, some of the products of inflammation, bacterial toxins, and carbon dioxide. In any condition in which capillary membrane permeability is increased, the volume of fluid and the size of the molecules that move from the intravascular to the interstitial space can be expected to be increased.

Water and solutes move across the capillary membrane by diffusion, filtration, and osmosis. Each of these forces affects the transfer of fluid into and out of the capillary. In general, diffusion of substances to which the capillary is freely permeable occurs

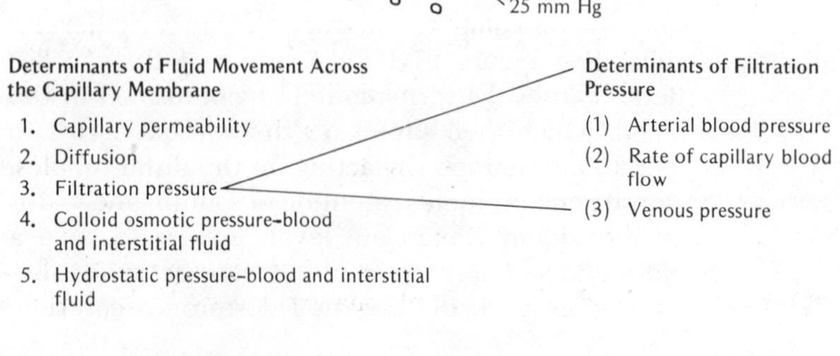

Figure 27-4. Factors that influence the movement of fluids across the capillary membrane.

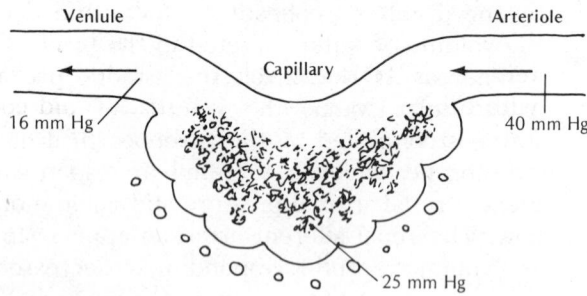

along the entire length of the capillary and takes place in both directions. An increase in the concentration of a solute in either the blood plasma or the interstitial fluids can be anticipated to be followed by an increase in the rate at which it diffuses through the capillary membrane.

Whereas substances move into and out of the capillary by diffusion, the primary effect of filtration is to transfer fluid from the capillary to the interstitial space. The filtration pressure of the blood in the capillary is determined by (1) the arterial blood pressure, (2) the rate of the flow of blood through the capillary, and (3) the venous pressure. Arterial blood pressure is affected by the volume of blood, the force of the heart beat, the resistance of the arteries and arterioles to the blood flow, and the viscosity of the blood. At the tissue level, capillary blood flow is regulated primarily by arteriolar constriction or dilatation. Constriction of arterioles decreases blood flow into the capillaries, thereby decreasing filtration pressure. Conversely dilatation of the arterioles increases blood flow into the capillary and thereby increases the filtration pressure. Because the circulatory system is a closed system, the effect of arteriolar constriction is an increase in blood pressure behind the constriction and a fall in pressure in the vessels distal to it.

Normally the hydrostatic pressure of the blood is much higher in the arteriolar end of the capillary than it is in the venous end. This results in a corresponding decrease in filtration at the venous end. The primary reason for the drop in hydrostatic pressure of the blood is that considerable energy is required to overcome the resistance offered by the capillary to the flow of blood. The effect of increasing resistance to the flow of a fluid on its movement can be demonstrated by placing water in a tuberculin syringe and in a 50-ml syringe. Water escapes from the tuberculin syringe very slowly because much of it comes in contact with the wall of the syringe and the wall offers resistance to the movement of the water. Water escapes very rapidly from the larger syringe because little of the water comes in contact with its wall. In general, the smaller the lumen of a tube, the greater the surface that comes in contact with the fluid contained in the tube and the greater the resistance to its movement.

Any condition that interferes with the flow of blood through a vein will increase the hydrostatic pressure of the blood in the capillary by increasing the volume of blood in the capillary. The effect is similar to that produced by placing a dam in a stream. The volume and pressure of fluid behind the dam are increased. This increases filtration of fluid out of the capillary. The quantity of fluid that actually leaves the capillary by filtration is determined by the relationship of the filtration or hydrostatic pressure of the blood to the interstitial fluid pressure. The greater the hydrostatic pressure of the blood in relation to that of the interstitial fluid, the greater the net filtration pressure.

The main force responsible for the transfer of fluids from the interstitial space into the capillary is created by the colloid osmotic pressure of the blood. Normally the concentration of protein is greater in the blood plasma than it is in interstitial fluid. In health, the level of protein in the blood plasma ranges from 6.5 to 8 g per 100 ml. Of this, albumin comprises the largest fraction, with an average range of from 4.0 to 5.2 g per 100 ml. Because it has the smallest molecules of the blood proteins, the effect of albumin on the colloid osmotic pressure of the blood is greater than can be accounted for by its weight. The critical factor in osmotic pressure is the number of particles per unit of water and not the size of each particle. For example, if a particle the size of a grain of sand exerts approximately the same osmotic effect as one the size of a marble, then a cupful of osmotically active particles the size of a grain of sand will have many times the effect of a cupful of particles the size of marbles.

The extent to which osmotic pressure is effective in returning fluid to the capillary depends on a number of factors. One is the difference between the colloid osmotic pressure of the blood and that of the interstitial fluid. Anything that decreases the colloid osmotic pressure of the blood or increases that of the interstitial fluid will reduce the return of fluid to the capillary. The relationship of the hydrostatic pressure of the blood to its colloid osmotic pressure will also affect the rate of exchange between the capillary and the interstitial fluid. A rise in the hydrostatic pressure in relation to the colloid osmotic pressure of the blood will increase the quantity of fluid in the interstitial compartment.

Any condition that results in a serious loss of protein from the blood can be expected to interfere with the return from the interstitial fluid compartment to the blood. Examples of conditions in which blood protein levels fall include severe and prolonged starvation and continued loss of body fluids containing protein, such as in severe burns and in kidney disorders in which protein is lost in the urine. A blood albumin level of 2 g or less is usually associated with an increase in the volume of interstitial fluid, that is, with edema. Restoration of the normal distribution of water depends on reducing the loss of protein from the body and raising the level of osmotically active substances in the blood. This is sometimes difficult to do. When the condition is severe, the patient may require intravenous infusions of blood, plasma, or plasma expanders. If able to take

Table 27-4 *Factors Influencing the Amount of Water in the Body*

Factors Increasing Water in the Body	Factors Decreasing Water in the Body
Thirst	Satiety
Retention by the kidney (ADH)	Dilution of ADH
↑ Sodium intake	Decreased secretion of aldosterone
Aldosterone	
	Decreased sodium intake
↓ Thyroid hormones	Increased loss of sodium
Heart failure	Increased metabolic rate
Edema	Lack of insulin, resulting in glycosuria
	Acidosis
	Vomiting
	Diarrhea
	Gastric suction
	Mouth breathing
	Tracheostomy
	Sweating
	Blistering of skin
	Large draining wounds
	Obesity

food by mouth, the patient should be given appropriate assistance and encouraged to eat.

The return of interstitial fluid back into the capillaries is usually not complete. The lymphatic capillaries take up excess tissue fluid and return it to the blood stream via the lymphatic and thoracic ducts. Any obstruction to the flow of fluid in the lymphatics leads to the accumulation of interstitial fluid in the tissues. Following extensive injury to the soft tissues, scar tissue formed during the healing process may obstruct the lymph channels draining the area. In tropical regions, lymph channels may be obstructed by parasites; the resulting edema can cause various parts of the body to swell so enormously that one of these diseases has been called elephantiasis. Lymphedema can also be a troublesome problem after extensive radical mastectomy. In this operation, the axillary lymph nodes are removed, thereby interfering with the flow of lymph. This can result in swelling of the hand and arm on the affected side. Whenever a patient has swelling in an extremity and there are no medical contraindications, the nurse may consider one of three measures that promote return of interstitial fluid back to the capillaries: (1) Elevation of the extremity, which decreases venous hydrostatic pressure; (2) active exercise of the part, which decreases venous hydrostatic and increases interstitial pressures by massaging action of skeletal muscles; and (3) application of full-length elasticized stocking or glove to the extremity, which increases interstitial pressure and promotes venous return.

Factors that determine the movement of water and other diffusible particles across semipermeable membranes operate consistently throughout the fluid conduits of the body. *The cell* and its homeostasis is the goal of all fluid movement, and homeostatic mechanisms at all levels operate to protect the cell. As shown in Table 27-3, about 60 per cent of total body water is contained in the intracellular compartment, but the fluid distribution with which the nurse is most directly involved is in the intravascular (7 per cent) and interstitial (20 per cent) spaces (Rose, 1977). Application of the principles of fluid movement in the extracellular compartment in assessing

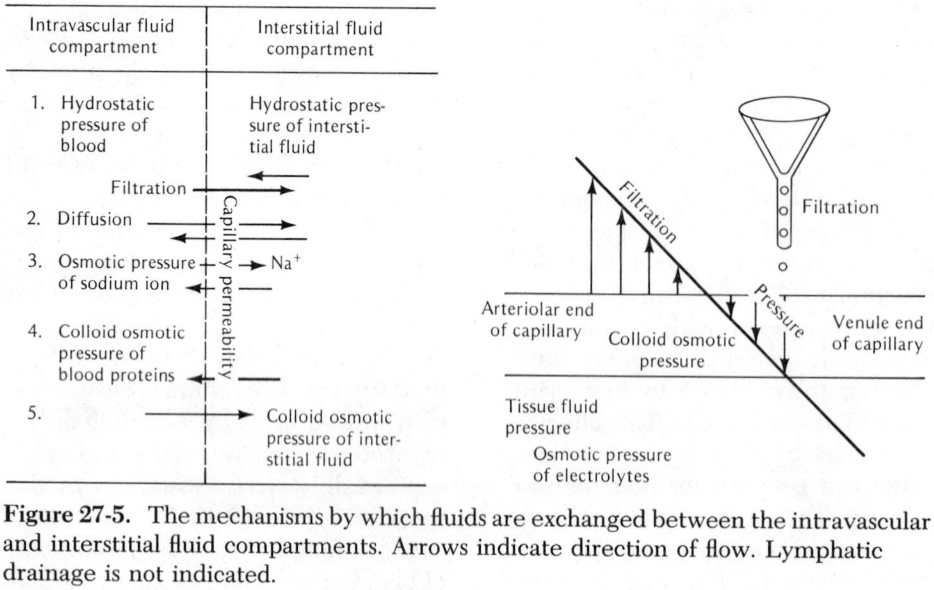

Figure 27-5. The mechanisms by which fluids are exchanged between the intravascular and interstitial fluid compartments. Arrows indicate direction of flow. Lymphatic drainage is not indicated.

and managing problems of fluid and electrolyte imbalance are discussed in Chapter 41.

Table 27-4 highlights major factors that influence the amount of water in the body.

In health a balance is maintained between the amount of fluid leaving and returning to the intravascular fluid compartment. The main mechanisms involved in exchange between intravascular and interstitial fluid compartments are summarized in Figure 27-5.

Factors in Movement of Fluid Between Intracellular and Interstitial Compartments

In most discussions of fluid and electrolyte balance, more attention is given to the mechanisms that regulate the volume and concentration of extracellular fluid than to those that control the intracellular fluid. This is partly because intracellular fluid is so difficult to obtain for study. Because all body fluids are interrelated, the state of the intracellular fluid compartment can be assumed from the studies of extracellular fluids, especially if one understands the factors that influence the movement of fluids and the behavior of the sodium and potassium ions.

As stated earlier, sodium ions have about the same concentration in plasma and in interstitial fluid. Therefore they have little effect on the movement of fluids into and out of the capillary. Sodium, however, is responsible for about one half of the osmotic pressure of extracellular fluid. Because it is present in relatively small amounts in the intracellular fluid, it is an important factor in the movement of fluid between the intracellular and extracellular compartments. Any condition that results in the retention of sodium in the body will generally be accompanied by the retention of water. Whatever the specific factor, any disorder that causes a retention of sodium in the extracellular fluids is usually accompanied by the retention of water and an expansion of the extracellular fluid volume. In persons whose mechanisms for eliminating sodium are defective or persons treated with drugs that increase the effectiveness of sodium-saving mechanisms, limitation of sodium intake can be expected to reduce water retention. For these reasons, sodium is often restricted in patients with heart and liver disorders, especially if there is edema formation. Sodium is also often restricted in patients who are treated with adrenal steroids. All salts containing sodium are interdicted, not just sodium chloride. Patients and those preparing their food should be taught to read the labels on prepared foods and medicines to see if sodium-containing salts are present. Foods, such as cured meats, to which salt has been added in preparation should ordinarily be avoided.

Electrolytes

Body fluids are composed of water, electrolytes, and nonelectrolytes. In Figure 27-2, in each set of bar graphs representing the fluid compartments of the body, cations are to the left and anions to the right. The total number of cations is equal to the total number of anions. Extracellular fluid also contains small amounts of nonelectrolytes. Unless they are greatly increased, they do not affect the behavior of extracellular fluid (Gamble, 1951). Concentrations of each electrolyte are expressed in milliequivalents per liter.

Gamble was the first to draw attention to the similarities between the composition of seawater and extracellular fluid. Although there are marked similarities, there are also significant differences. One is that seawater contains a higher concentration of most of the electrolytes. Some reasons for the changes in the electrolyte concentration of seawater were discussed previously. Other differences derive from the fact that extracellular fluid is part of a living system. As a result, it has a higher concentration of bicarbonate anion and contains protein. The latter is not found in seawater.

Function of Electrolytes Within the Body

Comparison of the composition of the fluids contained in the extracellular and intracellular compartments shows that the principal cation in extracellular fluid is sodium whereas that of the intracellular fluid is potassium. At one time scientists thought that sodium was not able to enter the cell or potassium to leave it. Evidence now indicates that sodium does enter the cell and energy is expended in preventing sodium from accumulating in the cell. The mechanism for preventing its accumulation is not clear. In conditions accompanied by starvation or semistarvation, sodium tends to replace potassium to the detriment of cellular activities. Improvement in a patient's condition may require an increase in the intake of food. The principal anions in the intracellular and extracellular fluid can also be seen to differ. The principal anion in extracellular fluid is the chloride ion, whereas that in intracellular fluid is the phosphate ion. With the exception of the red blood cell, the quantity of chloride ion found within cells is believed to be small.

All the cations and anions entering into the composition of body fluids have important functions in the body. Healthy functioning of cells depends on the maintenance of the level of each electrolyte within its so-called normal range. Deviations outside this range in either a downward or upward direction can be anticipated to have adverse effects on bodily function. Some electrolytes, such as sodium, are present in relatively large amounts. Others, such as chromium, are found only in traces. Whether the quantity is large or small, they are all essential to cell activity.

The daily average requirements, the sources of intake, the organs of excretion, and sources of excessive loss for water and the more important electrolytes are summarized in Table 27-2. Iron and the trace elements have not been included in the table. Although they are indispensable for normal function, they are not pertinent to this discussion of fluid and electrolyte balance. They will therefore be discussed in Chapters 29 and 42.

Electrolytes participate in at least four basic physiologic processes. These are (1) the distribution of water, (2) the osmolality of body fluids, (3) neuromuscular irritability, and (4) acid–base balance. The volume and distribution of water depend primarily on the presence of dissociated electrolytes and proteins. The volume of extracellular water is regulated primarily by sodium. When the concentration of sodium in the extracellular fluid rises, water moves across the semipermeable membrane of the cell in the direction of the interstitial fluid. Water thus serves to correct the increased osmolality of the extracellular fluid, thereby reducing the number of ions per unit of fluid.

Sodium Regulation

The regulation of the level of the sodium ion is complex, involving hormonal and nervous factors. Although all the hormones of the adrenal cortex increase the reabsorption of sodium, the mineralocorticoid with the most potent effect is aldosterone. Although ACTH from the anterior pituitary gland directly and profoundly affects the secretion of most adrenocortical hormones, it is not a primary factor in aldosterone production. Under appropriate circumstances, ACTH can cause aldosterone to be secreted; therefore, ACTH can be described as a sufficient but not necessary factor for its release. Aldosterone secretion is stimulated by many factors including decreased sodium, increased potassium, and increased angiotensin II in the blood flowing through the adrenal cortex.

As indicated previously, a volume receptor may lie in the juxtaglomerular apparatus. A drop in the blood pressure or blood flow through this area may stimulate the local release of renin. Renin acts on angiotensinogen, converting it to angiotensin I, which is then converted to angiotensin II. Angiotensin II then increases the release of aldosterone. With the increase in aldosterone, sodium and water are conserved and potassium is excreted. Water conservation increases blood volume and thus blood flow through the kidney. Control of sodium excretion by aldosterone is not rapid and it is not complete. Experimentally, there is a time lag between the administration of aldosterone and its effect. Further, sodium loading brings about an increase in sodium excretion that is independent of glomerular filtration rate and aldosterone secretion, a response that may be controlled by the "third factor" mentioned earlier.

Williams (1967) states that the kidney is innervated by both the sympathetic and parasympathetic parts of the autonomic nervous system. Until recently the function of the autonomic nervous system has been thought to be limited to regulating blood flow through the kidney. Williams postulates that the autonomic nervous system may well have other functions as acetylcholine (parasympathetic) increases the excretion of sodium chloride and stimulation of the sympathetic nervous system is accompanied by chloride retention.

A variety of neural stimuli and circulatory stresses cause a reduction in the perfusion of the outer cortex of the kidney. With ischemia of the outer cortex of the kidney, excretion of sodium is decreased. With increased conservation of sodium, water is also saved and the blood volume is maintained or increased. Whether or not the patient is protected by this mechanism depends on the degree of renal ischemia, how long it lasts, and what caused it.

Summary

The regulation of water and electrolytes provides an excellent example of the functioning of a homeostatic mechanism. To summarize the processes involved in the homeostasis of water and electrolytes, we will return to Mr. Martin. On a hot, sunny Saturday afternoon he mowed the lawn. Because he was exercising and the day was warm, he perspired freely. Every now and then he stopped to mop his brow. By the time he had finished, his shirt and underwear were saturated. Evaporation of sweat, because of its cooling effect, prevented a building up of heat in Mr. Martin's body. He was thereby able to keep his body temperature within physiologic limits, despite an increase in heat production that accompanied his activity and the warmth of the day. His sweat was a hypotonic solution of water and electrolytes. Let us suppose that Mr. Martin lost a liter of water in the hour he spent in mowing the lawn. As water was taken from the blood for the secretion of sweat, his blood plasma became concentrated, and developed a greater osmolality than the fluid in his interstitial space. Water was attracted across his semipermeable capillary membranes from the interstitial fluid by the increase in the osmolality of the blood. If the quantity of fluid added to the blood was not sufficient to restore its normal dilution, osmoreceptors in the internal carotid arteries and the supraoptic nuclei were stimulated. Stimulation of the osmoreceptors resulted in an increase in secretion of antidiuretic hormone (ADH). Because of the effect of ADH, Mr. Martin's kidney increased the reabsorption of water and the concentration of his urine.

If the loss of water and sodium in the sweat decreased blood volume enough to reduce the flow or pressure of the blood in the adrenal cortex, increased amounts of aldosterone would be secreted. The aldosterone in turn would cause increased absorption of sodium and water in the kidney. As fluid moved from Mr. Martin's interstitial fluid into his blood, its osmotic pressure increased. Water was then attracted from the cells to correct the situation, creating a sensation of thirst. Mr. Martin then entered the house and told his wife, "I'm thirsty. How about a pitcher of lemonade?" Later he sat on the patio and drank lemonade and ate some potato chips. The water in the lemonade helped restore his blood volume to normal and probably increased it to above normal temporarily. The salt on the potato chips helped replace the sodium chloride lost in sweating. After the volume, concentration, and distribution of his body fluids were restored to preexercise levels,

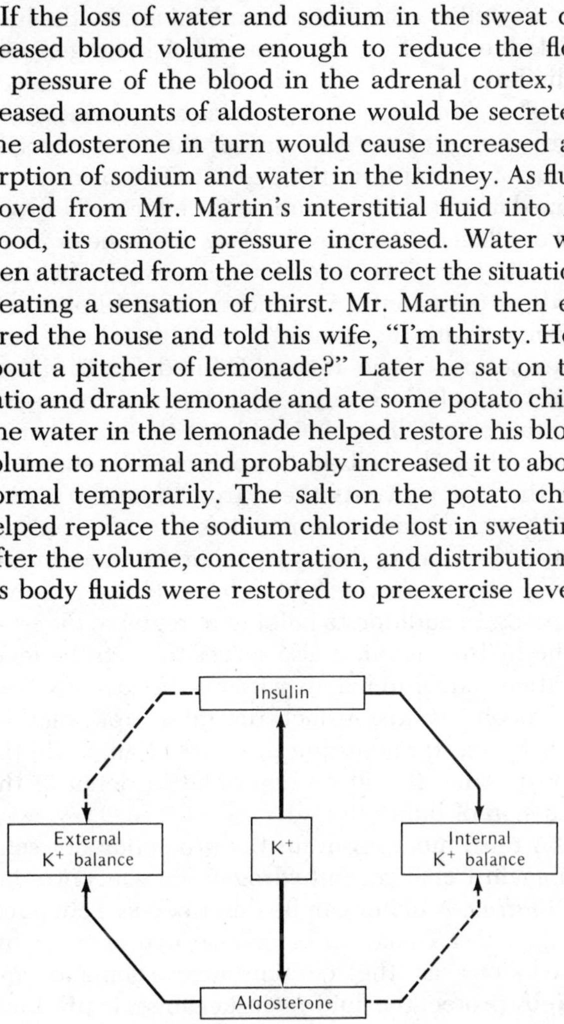

Figure 27-6. Potassium homeostasis-postulated roles for insulin and aldosterone. (Used with permission of the Massachusetts Medical Society, from The defense against hyperkalemia: The roles of insulin and aldosterone. *N. Engl. J. Med.* 299:525–32, Sept. 7, 1978, by M. Cox *et al*, Fig. 1, p. 525.)

the excess water and electrolytes were excreted by his kidneys. When blood volume was restored and the osmolality of his cells returned to normal, his thirst was quenched.

Functions of Potassium in the Body

Potassium, as the most abundant cation in the intracellular fluid, plays an important role in the maintenance of the volume of fluid within the cell. It participates in the regulation of neuromuscular irritability and in the maintenance of the hydrogen ion concentration in the blood.

Cox and his associates (1978) have proposed that the hormones insulin and aldosterone contribute to maintaining potassium homeostasis through negative feedback mechanisms. The postulated roles for insulin and aldosterone in potassium homeostasis are illustrated in Figure 27-6.

Functions of Calcium in the Body

Although calcium has little effect on the shift of fluids in the body, it has many important functions. About 99 per cent of it is found in the bone. Despite the small fraction of calcium in the blood (4.3 to 5.3 mEq/L of serum), constancy of its serum concentration is critical to nerve and muscle function. Recent research suggests that every process in which there is excitation of tissue coupled to a response depends on calcium for its action. It appears that all endocrine glands have a calcium-dependent secretion step (Raisz, 1970). Among the well-known functions of calcium are the (1) formation of bone, (2) regulation of neuromuscular irritability, (3) coagulation of the blood, (4) regulation of the irritability of the heart muscle, and (5) formation of milk.

Calcium exists in the blood in two forms. About 45 per cent is bound to the serum protein and is nondiffusible. About 55 per cent is ionized and is diffusible. Contributions to calcium homeostasis are made by the mechanisms of (1) gut absorption of dietary calcium, facilitated by adequate vitamin D, (2) tubular reabsorption of phosphate and calcium in the kidney, and (3) resorption of calcium from bone. Serum calcium concentration is regulated by a dual feedback system with parathyroid hormone (PTH) and thyrocalcitonin (TCT), a hormone produced by the thyroid. PTH acts synergistically with a metabolite of vitamin D (25-hydroxycholecalciferol, or 25-HCC) to increase movement of calcium from bone to blood; this action is stimulated by low serum calcium. PTH acts on the kidney to decrease the reabsorption of phosphate by the tubules. It also

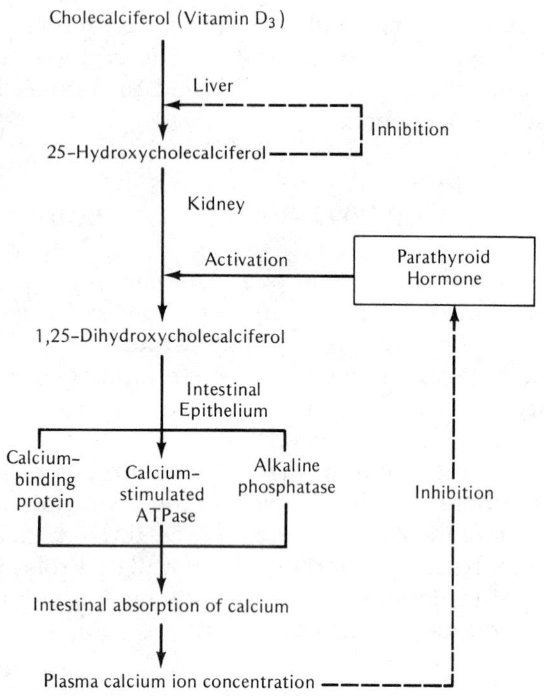

Figure 27-7. Activation of vitamin D_3 to form 1,25-dihydroxycholecalciferol; and the role of vitamin D in controlling the plasma calcium concentration. (Used with permission of W. B. Saunders Company, from *Textbook of Medical Physiology,* 5th ed., by A. C. Guyton, Fig. 79-1, p. 1053, 1976.)

increases absorption of calcium from the intestine. TCT acts synergistically with phosphate to inhibit movement of calcium from bone to blood; this action is stimulated by high levels of serum calcium (Raisz, 1970).

Intestinal absorption of calcium and phosphorus is increased by the influence of 1,25-dihydroxyvitamin D, an active metabolite of vitamin D; in conjunction with parathyroid hormone, there is increased bone resorption. See Figure 27-7 for the role of vitamin D in calcium balance. Both actions maintain serum calcium and phosphorus at levels that permit normal mineralization of newly synthesized bone matrix. Vitamin D deficiency leads to rickets in children and to osteomalacia in adults (Gallagher & Riggs, 1978).

Functions of Magnesium in the Body

Although magnesium has been known to be present in extracellular fluid for some time, its functions are still not well understood. Its concentration inside cells is second in amount to potassium. It activates many enzyme systems such as the phosphatase enzymes, and is a cofactor with thiamine in intermediate carbohydrate metabolism. It functions in calcium and phosphorus metabolism and in the regeneration of protein.

Acid–Base Equilibrium

Regulation of the Hydrogen Ion Concentration

One of the truly remarkable features of the body is that, despite continuous additions of metabolites from cells and from food, its pH is maintained at relatively constant levels. The mechanisms for regulating the concentration of hydrogen ions include (1) the dilution of the products of metabolism by a large volume of fluid; (2) the elimination of hydrogen ions, as well as other cations and anions, by the lung and kidney; and (3) the removal of hydrogen ions by buffering.

1. The *dilution* of strong acids and alkalies by a large volume of water is one of the most effective means of diminishing their effect. The principle is utilized in first aid to minimize the effects of a strong acid or alkali on tissue by flooding the tissue or structure with a large volume of running water. In other words, a teaspoonful of concentrated sulfuric acid in contact with the skin or mucous membrane produces serious tissue injury. Diluted by 10 gal of water, it has little, if any, effect. In the living organism, the extracellular fluid dilutes the strong acids produced by the cells in the process of metabolism and thereby prevents them from injuring tissues.

2. A second mechanism utilized by the body to control the level of the hydrogen ion is the *elimination of carbon dioxide* by the lung. This serves two purposes. In addition to helping to regulate the level of the hydrogen ion, it also serves to keep the level of cations equal to anions without the loss of water. This mechanism is, in fact, the most rapid method the body has for adjusting the level of anions in the blood plasma. It will be described in detail in the discussion of buffering.

3. A third mechanism for the protection of a solution against changes in hydrogen ion concentration is *buffering.* A buffer can be described as a chemical sponge. It can take up or release hydrogen or hydroxyl ions as the circumstances demand and thereby protect the fluid against changes in pH. Each buffer system for controlling hydrogen ion concentration consists of a solution of a weak acid and one of its salts, formed by neutralizing the acid with a strong base. The acid and salt are maintained in a definite relationship to each other. There are a number of so-called buffer systems in the body. They

include (1) carbonic acid and sodium bicarbonate, (2) monosodium or potassium phosphate and disodium or dipotassium phosphate, (3) oxyhemoglobin and reduced hemoglobin, and (4) acid proteinate and neutral protein (see Table 27-5). The bicarbonate fraction contributes about 50 per cent of the total buffering potential of the blood. All the buffer systems function in essentially the same manner. As in nature, the strong take from the weak. In the presence of a strong acid, the following events take place:

1. The cation from the salt of the weak acid and the strong base (sodium or potassium, for example) combines with
2. The anion (chloride, sulfate, phosphate, acetate, and so on) from the strong acid to form a salt, and
3. The hydrogen ion from the strong acid (hydrochloric, phosphoric, lactic, acetoacetic) combines with
4. The anion from salt of the weak acid to form
5. A weak acid

TABLE 27-5. *Distribution of Buffer Systems*

Buffer System	Blood	Tissues
Oxyhemoglobin–reduced hemoglobin	X	
Carbonic acid–sodium bicarbonate	X	
Acid protein–neutral protein	X	X
Monosodium or potassium phosphate–disodium or dipotassium phosphate		X

The weak acid ionizes less completely than the strong acid that it replaces, that is, it does not release hydrogen ions as readily as the stronger acid. Hydrogen ions are therefore removed from the solution. Stated simply, as the result of buffering, the strong acid is replaced by a weak acid and a neutral salt. In a weak acid, a larger proportion of the substance remains in the molecular form and fewer hydrogen ions are released than in a strong acid.

To clarify further, and to apply the manner in which buffer systems function in the body, the carbonic acid–sodium bicarbonate system is described below. This system plays an important role in the protection of the extracellular fluid from changes in the hydrogen ion concentration. Carbonic acid is a weak acid. Sodium bicarbonate ($NaHCO_3$) is a salt formed by the neutralization of carbonic acid (H_2CO_3) with sodium hydroxide (NaOH), a strong base. In health, one molecule of carbonic acid is maintained in the blood for every twenty bicarbonate ions.

When an acid stronger than carbonic acid is formed in, or ingested into, the body, it ionizes to the hydrogen ion and the appropriate anion. The anion combines with the sodium ion to form a salt. The hydrogen ion unites with the bicarbonate anion to form the weak carbonic acid. For example, if hydrochloric acid (HCl) is added, the following reaction takes place:

$$HCl + NaHCO_3 \rightleftarrows NaCl + H_2CO_3$$

Regulation of the Bicarbonate Anion

The level of the bicarbonate anion in the blood plasma is regulated by the excretion of carbon dioxide by the lung, which in turn regulates the quantity of carbon dioxide dissolved in the blood. The more carbon dioxide dissolved in the blood, the higher the level of the bicarbonate anion and carbonic acid, and vice versa.

When the level of chloride, sulfate, phosphate, or organic acid anions increases, they combine with sodium ions, thereby reducing the number of sodium cations (alkali reserve) available to combine with bicarbonate anions. The bicarbonate ion then combines with hydrogen ions to form carbonic acid, which in turn can break down into water and carbon dioxide. As the amount of carbon dioxide increases, the depth and rate of respiration also increase.[2] With an increase in the depth and rate of respiration, the carbon dioxide in the alveolar air decreases, and carbon dioxide moves from the blood to the alveoli. As the level of carbon dioxide in the blood plasma drops, more carbonic acid in the presence of carbonic anhydrase decomposes to carbon dioxide and water.[3] This results in a lowering of the level of the bicarbonate and the hydrogen ions in the blood plasma.

As the carbon dioxide and the hydrogen ion concentrations decrease, the respiratory center is depressed and the process is reversed. Respiration diminishes in rate and depth. The partial pressure of carbon dioxide in the alveoli increases. This is followed by an increase in the level of carbon dioxide in the blood. Finally, this is reflected by an increase in the bicarbonate ion in the blood.

As previously stated, the immediate source of the bicarbonate ion in the blood plasma is sodium bicarbonate ($NaHCO_3$) and hydrogen carbonate or carbonic acid (H_2CO_3). The quantity present in the mo-

[2] $CO_2 + H_2O \rightleftharpoons H_2CO_3\ (H^+ + HCO_2^-)$—reaction catalyzed by carbonic anhydrase.

[3] The pressure of a gas within a container is inversely proportional to the size of the chamber.

lecular form, that is, as hydrogen carbonate, can be increased by adding more of the bicarbonate ion in the form of sodium bicarbonate. Conversely, the amount of hydrogen carbonate that ionizes can be increased by decreasing the level of sodium bicarbonate in the blood. This results from what is known as the *common ion effect.* Additions of sodium bicarbonate to the blood decrease the number of free hydrogen ions in the blood by decreasing the ionization of hydrogen carbonate. The same effect can be produced by inhaling carbon dioxide or by holding one's breath.

Just as increases in the level of other anions result in a lowering of the level of the bicarbonate ion, a depression in the level of other anions is compensated for by an increase in the bicarbonate ion. Thus, a fall in the level of the chloride ion in the blood is compensated for by an increase in the bicarbonate ion. Although the levels of the chloride and other anions in the blood plasma are subject to change, there do not appear to be as active mechanisms for their upward or downward adjustment as there are with bicarbonate. This may result in an "anion gap" indicative of metabolic acidosis. An "anion gap" is said to exist when the sum of the chloride and bicarbonate ions is less than the serum sodium minus 12.

$$[Cl^- + HCO_3^-] < [Na^+ - 12]$$

This formula allows an estimate of the increase in unmeasured anions, such as phosphate, sulfate, proteinates, and organic acids such as ketone acids and lactic acid (Frawley, 1970).

To return to Mr. Martin for a moment, though the day was hot, he hurried as he mowed the lawn. This required a considerable expenditure of energy. In the process of obtaining the energy, he formed and released into his extracellular fluid a considerable volume of organic and inorganic acids. More specifically, hydrogen ions and the corresponding anions were added to his extracellular fluid. To adjust the level of anions to that of the cations, principally sodium, in his blood, some of the bicarbonate anion in his blood was eliminated by the lungs as carbon dioxide. In the process, hydrogen ions were converted to water and therefore had no effect on his acid–base equilibrium. The anions from the acids that were stronger than carbonic acid combined with sodium to form salts. This resulted in a reduction in Mr. Martin's alkali reserve, that is, in the quantity of sodium ion in the form of sodium bicarbonate in the blood. With a reduction in the bicarbonate in the blood, the capacity of the blood to carry

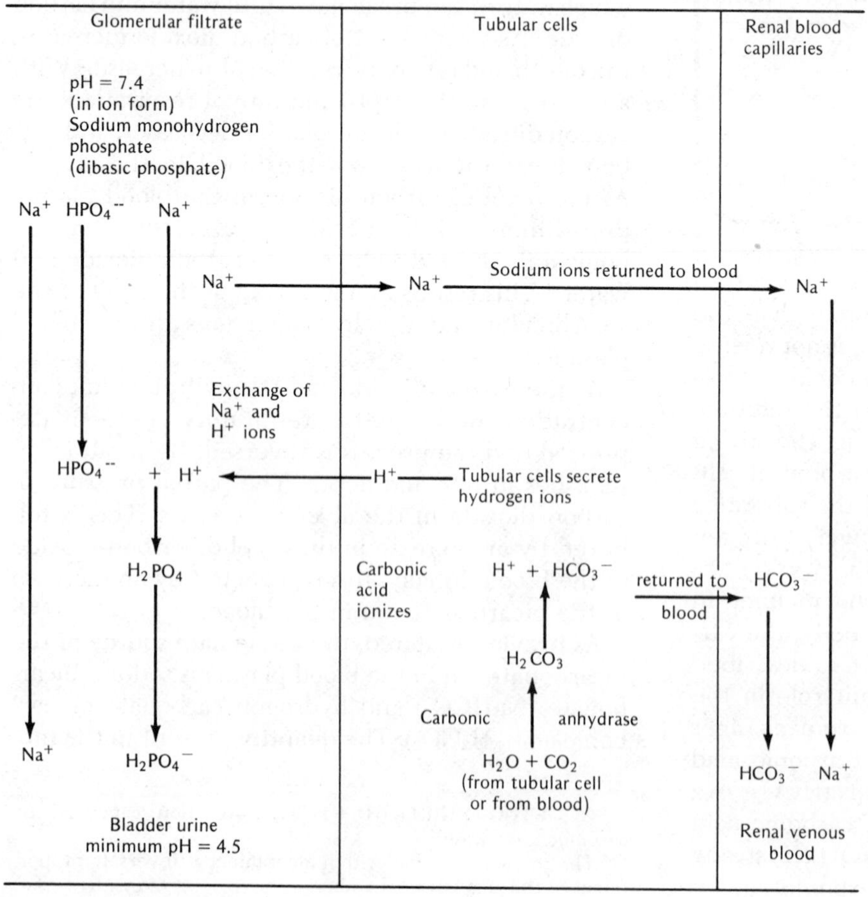

Figure 27-8. Mechanisms by which urine becomes acidified by changing the dibasic phosphate to monobasic or dihydrogen phosphate. (Modified from Davenport and adapted with permission of Macmillan Publishing Company, Inc., from *Anatomy and Physiology,* 15th ed., p. 683, by D. C. Kimber *et al.,* 1966.)

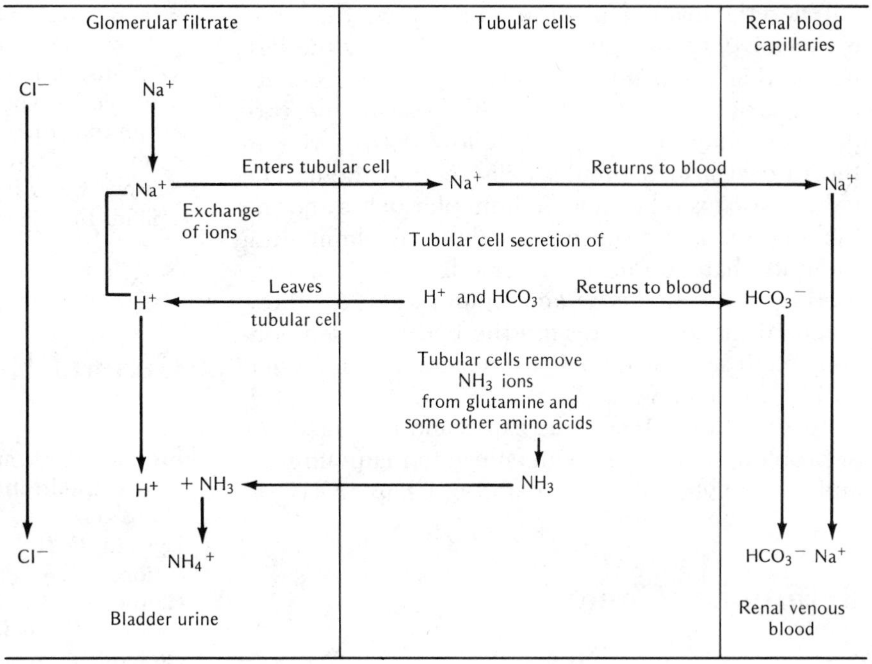

Figure 27-9. Formation of ammonia by the kidney. (Modified from Davenport and adapted with permission of Macmillan Publishing Company, Inc., from *Anatomy and Physiology,* 15th ed., p. 684, by D. C. Kimber *et al.,* 1966.)

carbon dioxide was diminished. Carbon dioxide and hydrogen ions accumulated in Mr. Martin's body, including the area of his respiratory center. His respiration increased in rate and depth, and the partial pressure of carbon dioxide in his alveolar air fell. The tension of carbon dioxide in the blood then became higher than in the alveolar air, and carbon dioxide therefore diffused from the blood to the alveoli to equalize the pressure on the two sides of the membrane. With a lowering of the tension of carbon dioxide in the blood, the depth and rate of his respirations diminished. As a result, the partial pressure of carbon dioxide in his alveolar air again rose and, as a consequence, the level of carbon dioxide and the carbonic acid in his blood plasma also rose.

Role of the Kidney in Maintaining the Acid–Base Equilibrium

By regulating the level of carbon dioxide in the blood plasma, the lung plays an important role in acid–base equilibrium. However, neither the buffer system nor the lung is able to control completely the hydrogen ion concentration. The kidney plays a significant part in this by selectively reabsorbing or rejecting both cations and anions. Its role in the maintenance of the concentration of sodium and potassium in body fluids has previously been discussed. The kidney tubules utilize three mechanisms to control the hydrogen ion. They reabsorb the bicarbonate ion from the glomerular filtrate, acidify urinary buffers, and secrete ammonia. Because ammonium ions can replace sodium or other cations in the urine, they are part of the mechanism for the excretion of "strong" anions without losing necessary cations. The kidney reduces hydrogen ions by combining them with bisodium phosphate to form monosodium phosphate. By these mechanisms, the kidney eliminates the hydrogen ion and conserves sodium and potassium as well. The functions of the various parts of the nephron and the processes utilized by the kidney in the excretion of the hydrogen ion and the conservation of the sodium ion are summarized in Figures 27-8 and 27-9.

Though the kidney is able to excrete either an alkaline or an acid urine, the urine is usually acid. The lowest pH at which urine is excreted is 4.5. Only weak acids are found to any extent in the urine. Strong acids, such as hydrochloric and sulfuric acids, are not present in the urine as free acids. They are excreted as sodium or ammonium salts. The acid buffers are responsible for much of the acidity of the urine.

Summary

The mechanisms for maintaining a normal pH include the taking up or release of hydrogen ions by the buffer systems, increase or decrease in ventilation by the lung, and elimination or conservation of hydrogen and bicarbonate ions by the kidney. A decrease in ventilation reduces the elimination of carbon dioxide and favors the formation of carbonic acid. An increase in the rate and depth of respiration has the reverse effect.

When the level of the bicarbonate ion in the blood is excessive, reabsorption of bicarbonate by the kidney is decreased and the quantity of bicarbonate in the urine is increased. An increase in the production of hydrogen ions is followed by a rise in the rate at which tubular cells secrete them. The kidney also excretes monosodium phosphate and the hydrogen ion, and conserves sodium by eliminating the phosphate ion in the monosodium form and excreting other anions as ammonium salts. All these mechanisms serve to restore the hydrogen ion concentration so that the pH of the blood is maintained within normal levels.

Further discussion of the cause and management of problems associated with failure to maintain fluid and electrolyte balance is found in Chapter 41.

References Cited

Brenner, B. M. and Beeuwkes, R., III. "The Renal Circulations." *Hosp. Prac.*, **13** (July 1978), 35–46.

Carson, R. *The Sea Around Us.* New York: Oxford University Press, 1950, pp. 13–14.

Cox, M., Sterns, R. H., and Singer, I. "The Defense against Hyperkalemia: The Roles of Insulin and Aldosterone," *N. Engl. J. Med.*, **299** (Sept. 7, 1978), 525–32.

Epstein, F. H. "Metabolic Requirements for Renal Function," *Hosp. Prac.*, **14** (June 1979), 93–102.

Frawley, T. F. "Axioms on Metabolic Considerations in Postsurgical Patients," *Hosp. Med.*, **6** (Jan. 1970), 107–21.

Gallagher, J. C., and Riggs, B. L. "Nutrition and Bone Disease," *N. Engl. J. Med.*, **298** (Jan. 26, 1978), 193–95.

Gamble, J. L. *Lane Medical Lectures: Companionship of Water and Electrolytes in the Organization of Body Fluids.* Stanford, Calif.: Stanford University Press, 1951, p. 12.

Goldberger, E. *A Primer of Water, Electrolyte and Acid–Base Syndromes,* 5th ed. Philadelphia: Lea & Febiger, 1975, pp. 30–31.

Guyton, A. C. *Textbook of Medical Physiology,* 5th ed. Philadelphia: W. B. Saunders Co., 1976.

Hays, R. M. "Principles of Ion and Water Transport in the Kidney." *Hosp. Prac.*, **13** (Sept. 1978), 79–88.

Laragh, J. H. "Potassium, Angiotensin and the Dual Control of Aldosterone Secretion," *N. Engl. J. Med.*, **289** (Oct. 4, 1973), 745–46.

Pitts, R. F. *Physiology of the Kidney and Body Fluids.* Chicago: Year Book Publishers, 1963, p. 147.

Raisz, L. G. "Calcium Homeostasis and Bone Metabolism," *Hosp. Prac.*, **5** (May 1970), 74–84.

Rose, B. D. *Clinical Physiology of Acid-Base and Electrolyte Disorders.* New York: McGraw-Hill, 1977, pp. 16–18.

Routh, J. I. *20th Century Chemistry.* Philadelphia: W. B. Saunders Co., 1953, p. 28.

Stein, J. H. "Hormones and the Kidney," *Hosp. Prac.*, **14** (July 1979), 91–95, 99–105.

Strand, F. L. *Physiology: A Regulatory Systems Approach.* New York: Macmillan Publishing Co., 1978, p. 27.

Williams, R. L. "A Re-evaluation of the Role of the Autonomic Nervous System upon Renal Function from the view of a Pharmacologist," *Perspect. Biol. Med.*, **10** (Winter 1967), 257.

Wilson, R. F. *Fluids, Electrolytes, and Metabolism.* Springfield, Ill.: Charles C Thomas, Publisher, 1973, pp. 4–5.

General References

Brenner, B. M., and Humes, H. D. "Mechanics of Glomerular Ultrafiltration." *N. Engl. J. Med.*, **297** (July 21, 1977), 148–54.

Epstein, F. H. "Metabolic Requirements for Renal Function." *Hosp. Prac.*, **14** (June 1979), 93–102.

Galton, L. "PG—A Powerful Medical Weapon." *Parade,* (Feb. 17, 1980).

Giebisch, G. "Coupled Ion and Fluid Transport in the Kidney." *N. Engl. J. Med.*, **287** (Nov. 2, 1972), 913–19.

Ganong, W. F. *Review of Medical Physiology,* 9th ed. Los Altos, Calif.: Lange Medical Publications, 1979.

Goldberger, E. *A Primer of Water, Electrolyte and Acid-Base Syndromes,* 5th ed. Philadelphia: Lea & Febiger, 1975.

Haussler, M. R., and McCain, T. A. "Basic and Clinical Concepts Related to Vitamin D Metabolism and Action." *N. Eng. J. Med.*, **297** (Nov. 10, 1977), 1041–50.

Haussler, M. R., and McCain, T. A. "Basic and Clinical Concepts Related to Vitamin D Metabolism and Action." *N. Engl. J. Med.*, **297** (Nov. 3, 1977), 974–83.

Kokko, J. P. "Renal Concentrating and Diluting Mechanisms." *Hosp. Prac.*, **14** (Feb. 1979), 110–16.

Kolanowski, J. "Influence of Glucose, Insulin, and Glucagon on Sodium Balance in Fasting Obese Subjects." *Persp. Biol. Med.*, **22** (spring 1979), 366–76.

Kuntz, I. D., and Zipp, A. "Water in Biological Systems." *N. Engl. J. Med.*, **297** (Aug. 4, 1977), 262–66.

Levinsky, N. J. "The Renal Kallikrein-Kinin System." *Circ. Res.*, **44** (1979), 441.

Monitoring Fluid and Electrolytes Precisely, Horsham, Pa.: Intermed Communications, 1978.

Peart, W. S. "Renin-Angiotensin System." *N. Engl. J. Med.*, **292** (Feb. 6, 1975), 302–6.

Penzias, A. A. "The Origin of the Elements." *Science,* **205** (Aug. 10, 1979), 549–55.

Sharer, J. E. "Reviewing Acid–Base Balance." *Am. J. Nurs.*, **75** (June 1975), 980–83.

Stein, J. H. "Hormones and the Kidney." *Hosp. Prac.*, **14** (July 1979), 91–95, 99–105.

Stroot, V. R. et al. *Fluids and Electrolytes: A Practical Approach,* 2nd ed. Philadelphia: F. A. Davis Co., 1977.

Tilkian, S. M. et al. *Clinical Implications of Laboratory Tests,* 2nd ed. St. Louis: C. V. Mosby Co., 1979.

Widmann, F. K. *Clinical Interpretation of Laboratory Tests,* 8th ed. Philadelphia: F. A. Davis Co., 1979.

Worthington, L. "What Those Blood Gases Can Tell You." *RN,* **42** (Oct. 1979), 22–27.

28

Transportation of Materials To and From Cells*

It is proved by the structure of the heart that the blood is continuously transferred through the lungs into the aorta, as by two clacks of a water bellows to raise water. It is proved by the ligature that there is a passage of blood from the arteries to the veins. It is therefore demonstrated that the continuous movement of the blood in a circle is brought about by the beat of the heart. Is this for the sake of nutrition, or the better preservation of the blood and members by the infusion of heat, the blood in turn being cooled by heating the members and heated by the heart?

WILLIAM HARVEY

Overview

Health and, indeed, life itself is dependent upon adequate metabolism of the body's cells. The processes of conception, birth, growth, restoration, and homeostasis all depend on the transport of a continuous supply of materials that are essential to the cells for catabolic and anabolic processes. Normal cellular metabolism is maintained when each cell receives and utilizes a sufficient supply of essential materials including glucose, oxygen, amino acids, vitamins, and hormones. The waste products of metabolism must be removed from the cells and eliminated to maintain favorable physical and chemical conditions of the fluid environment surrounding the cells. Excesses of materials supplied, or of substances produced, must be stored or eliminated. Substances produced by specialized groups of cells such as hormones must have a means of distribution if the substances are to influence the activity of other cells. Thus, the circulatory transport system serves as the supplier of materials to cells, remover of waste products from cells, and distributor of specialized cellular products.

In previous chapters, discussion has centered on how the organism acquires needed materials from the external environment and the mechanisms involved in maintaining the constancy of the internal environment. Reference has been made to the importance of transportation of materials to the cells. Anything that alters the transport of these essential materials to the cells deters normal metabolic processes and subsequent cellular function. Unless the required substances can be taken into the internal environment and distributed to cells, life ceases or pathology ensues.

This chapter is devoted to the factors essential to the transport of materials from one part of the body to another. It will focus on the requirements for normal transport and the factors that affect altered transport.

Transport of Materials to Cells

Essential materials, required to meet the metabolic and chemical needs of cells, are transported in the blood through the vascular system. The blood

* This chapter was revised by Elizabeth Ford Pitorak, R. N., M. S. N., Clinical Nurse Specialist, Lake County Memorial Hospital, Willoughby, Ohio, and Judith A. Wood, R. N., M. S. N., Assistant Professor of Nursing, Case Western Reserve University, Frances Payne Bolton School of Nursing, Cleveland, Ohio.

serves as the modifiable medium of exchange. Some of the materials transported in the blood are in solution and some are formed elements. Others are in chemical or physical combination with the formed elements.

The vascular system is a closed circuit consisting of the elastic and distensible arteries that convey blood from the heart to the tissues, and the veins that carry blood from the tissues back to the heart. As the arteries approach the cells, they branch into smaller structures; first, they branch into the arterioles and then into microscopic capillaries that are only one endothelial cell in thickness. It is at the capillary level that the purpose of transport of essential materials is accomplished. From the capillary, materials pass through the semipermeable capillary wall into the interstitial fluid and subsequently through the semipermeable cell membrane. Waste and other products produced are returned to the blood in the same manner.

Factors Affecting Blood Transport

The primary determinant in the maintenance of adequate blood flow through the vascular system is the *cardiac output.* Other factors that provide for a sufficient quantity and quality of blood flow to the tissues are the *blood volume* and the *blood viscosity.* Additional factors that contribute to adequate movement of blood through the system are the *velocity* of blood flow and the *resistance* to flow afforded by the blood vessels. Each of these many factors are interrelated, so that totally they contribute to a sufficient quantity and quality of blood flow to the tissues and provide for adequate movement of blood through the vascular system.

Cardiac Output

The cardiac output is the quantity of blood pumped from the left ventricular chamber into the vascular system in liters per minute. In the normal heart the volume of blood pumped from the left ventricle into the aorta is essentially the same as the volume of blood pumped from the right ventricle into the pulmonary artery. It is the left ventricle, however, to which reference is made when discussing the cardiac output. The cardiac output is the product of the stroke volume and the heart rate. The stroke volume is the milliliters of blood ejected with each left ventricular contraction. In the normal adult, the stroke volume is approximately 50 to 100 ml, and the heart rate is 60 to 100 beats per minute; thus the mean cardiac output at rest is approximately 5 to 6 liters per minute.

The normal cardiac output varies between the sexes, among individuals of different body size, among age groups, and with amount of exercise. In general, the cardiac output is slightly less for females than for males of the same body size. The cardiac output is greater the larger the size of the body. Cardiac output increases from birth through childhood until the normal adult cardiac output is reached at puberty. After puberty, the cardiac output gradually diminishes with each year of life.

During periods of exercise, the stroke volume may exceed 150 ml per ventricular contraction. Coupled with an increased heart rate, the cardiac output may approach 25 liters per minute. In the well-trained athlete, the cardiac output may reach five to six times the resting level, or up to 30 to 35 liters per minute (Guyton, 1976, p. 296). An important characteristic of the healthy heart is the ability to adjust the cardiac output to meet the metabolic needs of the tissues.

The stroke volume, and thus the cardiac output, is dependent upon the contractile power of the left ventricle to propel a sufficient quantity of blood into the systemic circulation and also upon the quantity of venous blood returned to the right atrium. Because the vascular system is a continuous circuit, the amount of blood that the left ventricle ejects depends on the amount received from the pulmonary circulation through the pulmonary veins and left atrium. The amount of blood that leaves the pulmonary circuit depends upon the amount received from the pulmonary artery, right ventricle, and right atrium. The flow of blood returning through the peripheral veins to the vena cava is supported by the contraction of skeletal muscles and the valves of the peripheral veins. A decrease in the pressure in the thoracic cavity during inspiration as well as reduction of pressure within the heart following systole also aid in the return of blood to the heart. The effects of pathology on the cardiac output as related to the stroke volume, changes in the heart rate and rhythm, and the venous return will be examined in subsequent pages.

Blood Volume

There must be a sufficient volume of blood in the vascular system for the left ventricle to eject an adequate quantity of blood into the systemic circulation with each systolic contraction. The *mean blood volume* in a normal average-sized adult is approximately 5 to 6 liters. This value varies with the sexes and with body weight. Generally, a female's blood volume is less than that of a male of the same body weight because of her lesser muscle mass and greater adipose reserve. Adipose tissue has little vascular volume; therefore the greater the obesity, the less the blood volume per unit weight regardless of the individual's sex (Guyton, 1976, p. 426).

One can note that the mean values of the blood volume and the cardiac output are comparable in the normal adult. This need not be the case, however. For example, in the initial stages of hemorrhage an individual may have a normal cardiac output for a short period of time even though blood volume is lost. Although the stroke volume of the left ventricle diminishes because of blood volume loss, compensatory mechanisms become operant to increase the heart rate as a means to preserve the cardiac output. As the blood volume continues to diminish because of loss, however, the cardiac output will decrease also. It is not unusual for the patient with heart failure to have a normal or greater than normal blood volume because of sodium and water retention, yet his or her cardiac output is less than normal because of an inability of the left ventricle to propel effectually a sufficient quantity of blood with each systolic contraction.

Blood Viscosity

The viscosity of the blood influences the quantity of blood available to the tissues as well as the actual flow of blood through the vessels. Blood is a viscous fluid composed of plasma and cells. Plasma fluid alone, minus the cellular components, is about one and one half times as viscous as water, largely because of the concentration and types of proteins present. The largest contributors to blood viscosity, however, are the erythrocytes, which comprise 99 per cent of the cells in the blood. The viscosity of whole blood is about one and one half to two times that of water, thus more pressure is required to force blood through a given structure than would be required to force water through the same structure (Guyton, 1976, p. 426). Blood viscosity affects flow most dramatically through the microcirculation. It is at the capillary level that the viscosity of blood is increased markedly because of the decreased velocity of flow through the microscopic structures.

With decreased flow, as occurs in some pathologic conditions, the quantity of blood available to carry essential materials to the tissues is diminished. It will be noted subsequently that in some individuals the percentage of erythrocytes increases markedly so that the blood viscosity can increase as much as one and one half to two times that which is normal. In this instance blood flow can become partially or totally obstructed through the smallest vascular structures. In other individuals the percentage of erythrocytes is diminished; thus the blood viscosity decreases. In this instance the transport problem is not related to quantity of blood flow to the tissues but rather to the quality of the blood in which there is a lack of oxygen carried by the erythrocytes.

Blood Flow Velocity

The movement of blood through the vascular system differs markedly from the flow of fluids through rigid tubes. The reason is that blood vessels are distensible in receipt of blood propelled through the system by the force of ventricular contraction. Further, blood is not a perfect fluid, but a liquid containing cellular elements. Despite these differences, certain physical principles utilized to describe fluid flow are an aid to understanding blood flow velocity.

Blood flow velocity is influenced by a pressure gradient in the circulatory system, the viscosity of the blood, and the resistance to flow afforded by the caliber of vessels receiving the blood. The influence of the blood viscosity on flow velocity has previously been noted.

Blood, as any fluid, flows in a system from a higher to a lower pressure. In the vascular system the pressure is highest in the left ventricle–aorta during systole and lowest in the right atrium. Considering the influence of the pressure gradient isolated from the viscosity and resistance factors, the greater the pressure gradient, the greater the velocity of flow. The converse is also true.

Normal blood flow in vessels is laminar. A thin layer of the fluid component of blood in direct contact with the vessel wall barely moves. The velocity of flow is greatest in the center of the vessel. Contrary to what one might think, the velocity of flow is less in the capillaries than in the larger vessels because of the tremendous *total* cross-sectional area of the microcirculation. The mean velocity blood flow in the aorta is 40 to 50 cm per second, which can increase up to 120 cm per second during systole. In the capillaries the mean velocity flow is approximately 0.07 cm per second (Ganong, 1977, p. 439). In the venous system the velocity flow increases to its maximum in the venae cavae, but this velocity is never as great as in the aorta.

When the pressure in a capillary is reduced, a point is reached at which flow ceases because of factors that promote collapse of the vessel. With a reduction or absence of blood flow as a consequence, essential materials are unavailable to cells for metabolic processes. Summarily, those factors that decrease blood flow velocity and thus diminish transport of oxygen and other materials to cells include decreased pressure gradient in the system, increased blood viscosity, and increased peripheral vascular resistance.

Peripheral Vascular Resistance

The final factor that contributes to an adequate movement of blood through the vascular system is the *peripheral vascular resistance* (PVR). The PVR is defined as the force that opposes blood flow through vessels. Resistance to flow is created primarily by the diameter of the blood vessels into which the blood is propelled. The arterioles are the most important structures that determine the PVR, because of the larger amount of smooth muscle and lesser amount of elastic tissue that constitute these structures. Even the slightest change in the diameter of the arterioles has a marked effect on the PVR and thus the blood flow through the vessels. As the arteriolar lumen decreases in size, the PVR increases and blood flow to an area diminishes. In addition, a larger proportion of the blood in the vessel comes in contact with the arteriolar wall, which offers further resistance to the movement of the blood. With an increase in the arteriolar lumen, the converse generally is true.

Other factors that influence the PVR and subsequent blood flow to tissues are the blood viscosity, the distensibility of the arterioles, and the activity of the autonomic nervous system. It has been noted that only extensive changes in viscosity produce effects on the PVR (Ganong, 1977, p. 433). With sufficient increase in viscosity, the PVR increases and blood flow diminishes.

The ability of blood vessels to distend in response to a quantity of blood also influences the PVR. The greater the distensibility of blood vessels, the less they contribute to the PVR. Vascular distensibilities differ greatly in various portions of the vascular system. Arteries are less distensible because of their construction and therefore contribute more to the PVR. For this reason they are called *resistance vessels.* Pathology, such as is noted with the atherosclerotic process, can effect even less distensibility with an increased PVR and decreased blood flow to tissues. On the other hand, veins are more distensible than arteries because venous walls are less muscular and more elastic; thus veins contribute less to the PVR. In fact, the veins are an important blood reservoir and as such are called *capacitance vessels.*

The activity of the autonomic nervous system is the major determinant of the PVR. The normal PVR occurs when sympathetic and parasympathetic impulses simultaneously stimulate the arterioles through the action of the neurohumoral mediator substances. The ratio of sympathetic to parasympathetic impulses stimulating the blood vessel is approximately 3:1. Thus, under normal circumstances, the sympathetic nervous system exerts the greatest influence on the PVR. If the sympathetic nervous system exerts even greater influence, as occurs during episodes of stress, vascular tone and thus the PVR increase in most parts of the body with a resultant decrease in blood flow to cells. Contrary to what one might deduce, however, greater parasympathetic activity has almost no effect on systemic blood vessels and reduction in the PVR (Guyton, 1976, p. 774).

Summarily, the primary factor that effects an increased PVR and decreased blood flow to cells is a decrease in the diameter of arterioles subsequent to (1) increased blood viscosity, (2) decreased arteriolar distensibility, and (3) increased sympathetic nervous system control of the vessels.

It can be noted that regulation of the PVR with resultant blood flow to cells is a consequence of a variety of regulatory mechanisms. The effect of greater parasympathetic control is a decrease in vascular tone in various vascular beds. Parasympathetic activity, however, is questionable as a significant factor in effecting a decreased PVR.

Regulation of the PVR and resultant blood flow is possible in individuals as a consequence of a variety of regulatory mechanisms. Under conditions of rest and moderate activity, tissues regulate blood supply in accordance with metabolic needs. Under emergency situations or with greatly increased activity, blood flow can be modified in relation to the needs of all body cells or to a particular group of specialized cells. Vital structures such as the heart, brain, and kidneys are nourished despite greatly increased oxygen demands of other parts of the body.

Factors Effecting Alterations in or Failure of the Transport System

Like other tissues in the body, the cellular components and structures that comprise the transport system are susceptible to alterations as a result of malformation, disease, or injury. The result is partial or total failure of a portion or all of the transport system. Regardless of the specific factor that causes altered transport, the result in all instances is an inadequate quantity or quality of blood to metabolizing cells. In other words, essential materials are not made available to cells and end products of catabolism are not removed; hence optimal cellular function is deterred.

The types of situations that effect altered blood transport can be categorized by phenomenon or by structure.

Types of Alterations by Phenomenon

The types of alterations by phenomenon that result in an ineffectual transportation system are (1) alterations in blood cellular components necessary for materials transport; (2) obstructions to blood flow within the transport system; (3) reduction of blood flow through the transport system; (4) insufficient power to propel blood through the transport system; (5) alterations in distensibility of the vascular structures; and (6) alterations in regulatory mechanisms affecting transport.

Types of Alterations by Structure

Alterations in the transportation system categorized by structure include those associated with the (1) components of the blood, (2) blood vessels, and (3) heart. Although the categorization of structural alterations will be utilized in the presentation of transport alterations and failures in Unit IX, reference will be made to phenomena in each instance. Implications for nursing assessment–intervention will be discussed.

Manifestations of Alterations

Manifestations resulting from malformation, disease, or injury to the transport system depend on the degree to which the metabolic needs of cells are met and specific tissues affected. As long as the activity of an individual is within the adaptive capacity of the circulatory system, there may be no symptoms or few, if any, observable signs indicating alteration of transport. The affected tissues may receive an adequate quantity and sufficient quality of blood to function at rest or during mild to moderate activity. If the activity status of the individual increases further, however, the supply of essential materials may not meet the cellular demand and clinical manifestations occur. Examples of this phenomenon include the individual with an alteration in the blood cellular components necessary for transport. If an individual has a blood hemoglobin level that is half that of normal, the individual may be comfortable during the resting state. If the individual climbs a flight of stairs, however, he or she may become severely dyspneic and prostrate. Consider the individual with diminished arterial blood flow to a lower extremity because of the arteriosclerotic process. Walking one half block may be without incident, but walking an entire block may result in severe calf pain. These and other pathologic processes will be examined in detail in subsequent pages.

The manifestations of an altered transport system result from a deficit in the supply of oxygen and nutrients to cells and from an excess accumulation of carbon dioxide and acid metabolites in the affected tissues. The effects of altered transport will also be influenced by whether the disturbance involves the entire body or is limited to a localized area of tissue. Disorders of the blood components or heart frequently affect the function of the body as a whole. Signs and symptoms are likely to be the result of disturbances in the functions of organs particularly sensitive to oxygen deprivation or carbon dioxide excess. Eventually all systems and organs will be affected. Lesions involving blood vessels may have either local or systemic effects. In some diseases of the blood vessels, as in atherosclerosis, the disorder may be more or less generalized, but its effects are more marked in some organs than in others. Survival of affected cells is possible when the transport alteration is relative; however, death of cells or of the entire organism quickly follows complete failure of the transport system.

Implications for Nursing Practice

It has been noted that the purpose of the transport system is to carry essential materials to cells for metabolic processes and to remove the end products of metabolism. It becomes obvious that every cell, organ, and physiologic system in the body is dependent on the transport system for support of metabolic activities.

From the preceding discussion, certain principles and objectives can be derived to guide nursing practice with individuals experiencing real or potential threats to the components of the transport system. The nurse must have command of certain knowledges in order to plan, implement, and evaluate comprehensive care for those with whom the nurse works. The nurse must know (1) what are the primary and secondary factors that cause alterations in the components of the transport system and thus diminish essential materials to cells, (2) what are the consequences and manifestations when alterations occur in the transport system, and (3) what means are employed appropriately to maintain or enhance transport of essential materials to cells. It was noted previously that primary causes of transport system alterations or failure are a consequence of malformation, disease, or injury. Secondary factors that impinge on the efficacy of the transport system are the effects of other illnesses or therapies. Often the manifestations exhibited are a result of multiple causes. Consider, as an illustration, the patient with generalized atherosclerosis who experiences a myocardial infarction with subsequent left ventricular failure as the primary insult on the transport system. Because neither the patient's heart nor arteries may be able to adapt to the activities of daily living, bedrest is temporarily prescribed as well as a digitalis preparation to increase the contractility of the heart.

The immobility associated with bedrest predisposes to venous stasis and formation of thrombi in the veins, thus diminishing venous return and further predisposing to pulmonary embolization. Pressure, particularly over the bony prominences, impedes arterial circulation and may lead to tissue injury due to the limited transport of essential materials to cells. The patient may develop toxicity to the digitalis preparation and develop irregularities of the cardiac rhythm which further deters the efficacious transport of essential material to cells. Thus the prescribed therapies of bedrest and medication serve as secondary factors that further compromise the transport system. Hence a situation of multiple causation is created, albeit unknowingly.

The consequences or manifestations of transport alteration or failure may be localized, affecting specific groups of cells, or generalized, affecting the overall body. Consider, as an example of localized manifestations, the patient who develops an arterial occlusion of the right femoral artery. The manifestations of transport failure will be specific to the right leg initially and may result in cellular death with need for amputation of the limb unless surgical intervention for removal of the thrombus intercedes. Consider, as an example of generalized manifestations, the patient with cardiogenic shock whereby the cardiac output drops to less than one half normal because of massive myocardial damage. All cells in the body are deprived of essential material and hence the generalized manifestations affecting multiple systems such as generalized lethargy, fatigue, liver dysfunction, and so on result. The nurse must be aware that activity exacerbates the degree of presenting symptoms. It is also important to remember that any disturbance of circulatory function, whatever the origin, will create some degree of anxiety in the individual. Anxiety also influences the magnitude of the individual's physiologic and psychologic response to the illness.

The cardinal physiologic principle that oxygen delivery to cells must equal oxygen utilization for normal cellular processes to occur guides the nurse in planning, implementing, and evaluating interventions for the patient with alterations or failure of the transport system. Nursing interventions to maintain or enhance the supply of essential materials to cells are planned to achieve one or more of the following objectives:

1. Promotion of an increased oxygen supply to support or improve the functional capacity of the affected organ(s)
2. Reduction or elimination of the primary and secondary factors that impinge on the transport system and that increase oxygen demand or decrease oxygen supply
3. Reduction of activity for a part or the entire body to decrease oxygen demand and thus minimize the disparity between oxygen delivery and utilization
4. Provision for an adequate supply of essential materials to the body for support of cellular metabolic activities
5. Provision of an environment that affords the individual maximum physiologic and psychologic comfort and rest
6. Protection of the individual from pathophysiologic and emotional disturbances that place added stress on an altered or failing transport system
7. Provision of a rehabilitation program to meet the individual's restorative, maintenance, and learning needs

The aforementioned knowledges, principles, and objectives will not only aid the nurse to understand and support the medical diagnostic and therapeutic plan but also guide the development, implementation, and evaluation of the nursing plan of care. For many years the focus in nursing has been on the physical and psychological care of patients with morbidity from pathologic disorders. Greater emphasis is now being placed on the role of the nurse in health promotion-maintenance and prevention of illness. Thus, a primary function of the nurse is education of the individual and the public for prevention and early recognition of cardiovascular morbidity.

The nurse must recognize that diseases of the cardiovascular system are the largest single cause of death in the United States. In 1979 the American Heart Association reported that approximately 40 million Americans are affected by diseases of the heart and blood vessels, which accounts for about 1 million deaths each year (American Heart Association, 1979, p. 2). Despite the strides made in prevention and early detection of disease as well as reduction in mortality, cardiovascular diseases account for 52 per cent of all deaths—more than all other causes combined. Cardiovascular diseases are a primary cause of morbidity and disability found in all age groups and in all walks of life. Although the incidence increases from birth, the greatest morbidity and mortality occur in individuals who are in their productive years of life.

References Cited

American Heart Association. *Heart Facts.* Dallas: American Heart Association, 1979.

Ganong, W. *Review of Medical Physiology,* 8th ed. Los Altos, Calif.: Lange Medical Publishers, 1977.

Guyton, A. C. *Textbook of Medical Physiology,* 5th ed. Philadelphia: W. B. Saunders Co., 1976.

Harvey, W. Quoted in *Lives in Science.* A Scientific American Book, New York: Simon & Schuster, 1953, p. 189.

General References

Adams, C. W. "Recognition and Evaluation of Cardiogenic Shock." *Heart & Lung,* **2**:6, (1973), 893–95.

Adler, J. "Patient Assessment: Pulses." *Am. J. Nurs.,* **79**:1 (1979), 115–32.

Alexy, B. J. "Monitoring Cardiovascular Status with Noninvasive Techniques." *Nurs. Clin. North Am.,* **13**:3 (1978), 423–35.

Fowkes, W. C., and Hunn, V. K. *Clinical Assessment for the Nurse Practitioner.* St. Louis: C. V. Mosby Co., 1973.

Hurst, J. W., ed. *The Heart, Arteries and Veins,* 4th ed. New York: McGraw-Hill, 1978.

Hurst, J. W., and Schlant, R. C. *Examination of the Heart: Inspection and Palpation of the Anterior Chest.* New York: American Heart Association, 1970.

Lehman, J., Sr. "Auscultation of Heart Sounds." *Am. J. Nurs.,* **72**:7, (1972), 1242–46.

Leonard, J. J., and Kroetz, F. W. *Examination of the Heart: Auscultation.* New York: American Heart Association, 1967.

Littman, D. "Stethoscopes and Auscultation." *Am. J. Nurs.,* **72**:7 (1972), 1238–41.

McInnes, B. *The Vital Signs; with Related Clinical Measurements: A Programmed Presentation,* 3rd ed. St. Louis: C. V. Mosby Co., 1979.

Prior, J., and Silberstain, J. *Physical Diagnosis—The History and Examination of the Patient,* 5th ed. St. Louis: C. V. Mosby, 1977.

Redman, B. K. "Client Education Therapy in Treatment and Prevention of Cardiovascular Diseases." *Cardiovasc. Nurs.,* **10**:1 (1974), 1–6.

Roberts, S. L. *Behavioral Concepts and the Critically Ill Patient.* Englewood Cliffs, N.J.: Prentice-Hall, 1976.

Rogove, H. J., Weil, M. H., Thompson, M., and Blair, C. "Cardiopulmonary Resuscitation (CPR) in the Hospital." *Cardiovasc. Nurs.,* **13**:2 (1977), 7–12.

Schroeder, J. S., and Dailey, E. K. *Techniques in Bedside Hemodynamic Monitoring.* St. Louis: C. V. Mosby Co., 1976.

"Standards for Cardiopulmonary Resuscitation (CPR) and Emergency Cardiac Care (ECC)." *J. Am. Med. Assoc.,* Supplement, 1974, **227**:7 (1974), 833–68.

29

Nutrition—Metabolism of Carbohydrates, Lipids and Proteins

Spurred by hunger from his remote past, man suffered, starved, struggled for food, survived, and is there to tell the tale. But only just.

SINCLAIR, 1962

Overview

For their survival and maintenance of functions, cells require a continuous supply of oxygen, water, and nutrients. Oxygen, of course, must be furnished moment by moment, whereas the need for food is less acute. Nutrients are stored to a varying degree within the body so that the cells may be constantly supplied. Cells are able, within limits, to sacrifice some of their substance for use as energy and to adapt energy output to energy intake. Despite some degree of protection against a lack of food intake, continued deprivation threatens survival. Moreover, unless the supply of food more than meets minimum requirements, growth, health, and productivity are threatened.

The earliest written record describing the effects of hunger caused by famine could be written today in many parts of the world. The following record was found on a stone in the tomb of an Egyptian Pharaoh:

> Pharaoh: From my throne I grieve over this calamity. During my reign, the Nile has failed to flood for seven years. Corn is scarce and there is no other food. My people thieve and pillage their neighbors. Those who would run cannot even walk. Children weep and the young falter and totter like old people. Their legs drag or give way under them. Their spirits are broken. My council chamber is deserted, my food stores have been pillaged and emptied. It is the end of everything (*World Health,* 1963).

Revised by Gloria J. Smokvina, R.N., Ph.D., Associate Professor of Nursing, Purdue University Calumet, Hammond, Indiana.

An exact understanding of several terms is essential in order that the nutritional needs of people can be described. All too often the words *nutrition* and *diet* are used synonymously.

Nutrition. A term that includes all the bodily processes involved in the ingestion and metabolism of foods. Good nutrition implies that the supply of food is adequate in quantity and quality to maintain the life and physiologic functions of the cells.

Nutrients. Those substances in foods that are required for cell functions; for example, amino acids, fatty acids, carbohydrates, minerals, and vitamins are nutrients.

Diet. The regimen of food required to support nutrition. A good or nutritious diet is one providing all the nutrients to sustain good nutrition. Whether such a regimen results in good nutrition depends on many other factors. The food must be eaten, digested, absorbed, transported, and finally utilized by the cells.

Nutritional status. The condition of health of the individual as influenced by the utilization of the nutrients (*Manual for Nutrition Surveys,* 1963). It can be determined only by correlating the information from a careful medical and dietary history, a thorough physical examination, appropriate biochemical tests on blood, secretions, and excretions, and x-ray or endoscopic examinations.

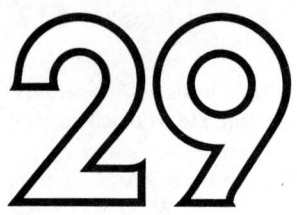

Nutrition and Health

Health, well-being, strength, and the ability to resist and recover from disease are all influenced for good or ill by the nutritional state. Not only is nutrition a significant factor in the capacity to survive, but adequate nutrition is also essential for productive and zestful living. Health is threatened by either an excess or a deficiency of food. As with other homeostatic mechanisms, within limits the individual is able to adapt to variation in supply. Although the nature of the effects differ, either a deficiency or an excess in supply of food may impair structure and function.

Nutritional therapy is a primary consideration for deficiency diseases and for errors of metabolism such as diabetes mellitus, phenylketonuria, hyperinsulinism, and others. It must be carefully adjusted to the body's ability to metabolize nutrients and to eliminate wastes, for example, protein-restricted, potassium-restricted, and sodium-restricted diets for renal failure. Nutritional therapy is supportive in the care of all patients.

In addition to problems of supply of food per se, selection of food is also a factor. The American public is constantly exposed to unjustified claims about foods and diets, as well as vitamin and mineral supplements. Communications media present information in the form of scientific or pseudoscientific articles or reports of research and in advertisements. The accuracy and validity of some of these are open to question and others are actually misleading or false. For example, a newspaper quoted two "nutrition experts." The first is purported to have said that the average person who eats a variety of foods is supplied with all the nutrients that are needed. He or she does not require extra vitamin or mineral supplements, and money spent for unnecessary food supplements is wasted. The second was cited as saying that few, if any, diets contain an adequate quantity of vitamins and minerals. To be well nourished, supplementation is necessary. What is the average lay person to believe? What, if any, function does the nurse have in interpreting present-day knowledge to the public? The first responsibility of the nurse is to be well-informed about food and factors which influence its availability, accessibility, acceptability, ingestibility, and digestibility.

Information Required by the Nurse

The maintenance of the nutrition of cells involves the same general processes and structures as do other homeostatic conditions. Food must be available in adequate quantity and quality and of the type accepted as being suitable to eat. Food requires a special service facility, the digestive system, to receive and to transfer nutrients from the external to the internal environment. Because many of the nutrients contained in food are not in an absorbable form at the time they are eaten, foods must undergo digestion, which consists of a series of physical and chemical changes by which nutrients are prepared for absorption. The residue remaining after digestion and absorption is then excreted from the alimentary canal.

Like oxygen, nutrients must be transported to the cells where they are utilized. The various nutrients provide cells with materials required for energy, for building or replacement of cell structure, and for the regulation of cellular processes. Excesses of supply are stored for future use or are excreted. Cells are, within limits, capable of adapting to differences in supply. Like other physiologic needs, the need for food must be met before higher needs can be manifested. Ill health can result from an imbalance between food intake and cell requirements. The causes for this imbalance are many and varied. There are few, if any, illnesses of any length or severity in which nutrition is not of significance.

An understanding of the nutritive processes of the body is necessary but not sufficient for effective nutritional care. Of paramount importance is knowledge of the factors affecting the food supply and of physiologic, psychological, cultural, and socioeconomic influences on food acceptance. To reach people of all socioeconomic classes with nutrition information and to motivate them to alter the quantity and quality of foods consumed requires application of principles of education and use of all media of communication and techniques of teaching. Discussion will begin with factors affecting food supply and habits and will then move to factors related to the digestion and utilization of nutrients. Major problems will be discussed in Chapter 46.

Food Supply, Nutritional Status, and Food Habits

Factors in the Supply of Food

Food Scarcity

Despite a plethora of food in a few areas of the world, such as in the United States, a lack of sufficient food to meet minimum nutritional requirements is one of the most critical public health problems in the world. In the densely populated developing countries, the vast majority of the population is adapted to a chronic state of undernutrition. In fact, the effects of nutritional deficiency may be accepted as a normal condition. For example, in the Andean Altiplano, where goiter caused by a deficiency in iodine has been present for generations, dolls are made with the characteristic neck deformity of goiter, which indicates that it is accepted as usual or normal.

Insufficient food is not a new problem, nor is it subject to easy solution. For thousands of years people in most parts of the world have led a hand-to-mouth existence. Most, if not all, of their energy is expended in obtaining just enough food to sustain life. Food supply, and with it survival, are continuously threatened by drought, floods, windstorms, and pestilence. Lack of facilities for preserving and transporting food may result in relative abundance during the warm months of the year and scarcity during the cold winter months. In other areas, hunger is always present. Food supplies are limited to plants and animals indigenous or native to the region. As is true in the United States, not all plants and animals suitable for food are utilized.

Agriculture and Food Supply

In the early history of humankind and among some present-day primitive societies, the principal methods for obtaining food were hunting and fishing or gathering berries, nuts, and roots. One of the most significant steps in the progress of humankind was the cultivation of plants and animals as sources of food. The cultivation of plants and animals is known as agriculture. Not until agriculture became a reality did the prevention of periodic or continual hunger become a real possibility. In addition to increasing the supply of food, the development of agriculture has other farreaching effects. Successful cultivation of sources of food made it necessary for people to give up being nomads and to settle in one place. Once an individual was able to produce more than enough food to feed himself or herself and the members of the immediate family, some members of the group were released for other activities. Thus specialization was born. In addition to the food producers or farmers, others became butchers, bakers, carpenters, and teachers. As the food supply became relatively secure, people had time and energy to think of ways by which the external environment might be changed or improved. Without the development of agriculture, the industrialized societies of today would be impossible.

However, shortages and high prices of agricultural commodities have given rise to concern about long-term world food prospects. An extreme view sees the world population growth as rapidly outrunning the capacity to feed people (World Hunger, 1974). A moderate view sees agricultural surpluses ending and rapidly giving rise to an increase in real food prices. As a result, the present levels of food consumption cannot be sustained (Brown & Eckholm, 1974).

Food Preservation

Despite the importance of the development of the tools and techniques essential to modern agriculture, food supply also depends on suitable means for its preservation and distribution. Without suitable means of preserving food, it is likely to deteriorate in quality or actually spoil before it reaches the consumer, who may live far from where food is produced. Food preservation also makes it possible to save perishable foods for use throughout the year. Modern methods of food preservation combined with efficient and economical methods of transportation make possible the distribution of food far from its site of production. The accomplishment of all these goals requires highly trained and skilled labor. Thus in Big City one Sunday in January, the menu consisted of fresh chicken from Alabama, lettuce from Arizona, potatoes from Idaho, peas from Minnesota, and ice cream and butter from Wisconsin.

Food Distribution

Although remarkable progress has been made in developing methods of food production, preservation, and transportation, too little available food remains a problem in much of the world. Sinclair (1962) states that, according to one estimate, one third of the population eats three quarters of the food of the world. This means that about two thirds of the people subsist on one quarter of the available food. Many factors contribute to the unequal availability of food. In some parts of the world food supplies are limited by either a lack of, or a failure to exploit, natural resources. An increase in food supplies in these areas depends on the modernization of agricultural methods, the introduction of suitable methods of food preservation, and the development of transportation facilities. The introduction of suitable methods of home preservation of foods by drying, smoking, and pickling, and in some instances by home canning, may do much to bring about immediate improvement in the supply of food.

World Nutrition Problems

Insufficient quantity and quality of calories and protein, protein-calorie malnutrition (PCM), is the world's dominant nutritional problem. PCM is often associated with other deficiencies such as vitamin A deficiency (Jelliffe & Jelliffe, 1975). In developing countries nutrition and food supply is related to cultural practices and complicated interrelationships of politics, economics, and world trade. PCM occurs more than is appreciated in disadvantaged communities in the U.S. as well as Asia, Africa, and Latin America. Studies over the past decade lend support that serious undernutrition does plague the American poor, especially the minority ethnic groups, Indians living on reservations, migrant workers, and the aged (Freeman, 1975). Preschool children and mothers are especially vulnerable to the effects of malnutrition, the mortality rate being especially high among infants and young children in the most seriously affected countries. Lack of a sanitary food supply and pure water, poor disposal of sewage, and filth among the undernourished result in a high morbidity and mortality rate, even from infections that are not ordinarily serious. Malaria, a major world health problem increases the nutritional requirements of the people it infects, rapidly debilitates the already undernourished, and keeps millions from producing the food that is desperately needed. Marasmus, a disease resulting from the body's attempt to adapt to severe calorie and protein deprivation, and kwashiorkor, a disease of protein deficiency that occurs when the body's defenses break down, are both common in underdeveloped countries.

Conversely, in the present century overnutrition (PCM "plus") is becoming a problem in the more affluent countries. This gross imbalance between food intake and physical expenditure also affects life expectancy, increases disease susceptibility, and decreases productivity.

Programs for Nutritional Improvement

The nutritional problems in the poor countries of the world almost seem to defy solution. These countries produce too little food for their populations and they do not have the money to purchase the food they need. The United States has continued to play a significant role in helping to combat malnutrition through the Food for Peace program. The Departments of Agriculture and State, including the Agency of International Development (AID), implement this program by providing shipments of food surpluses under arrangements with governments of receiving countries or with United Nations organizations. In addition the United States, through voluntary and governmental agencies, has conducted surveys of nutritional status and provided technical assistance in agriculture, food processing and marketing, and education.

Several groups in the United Nations are directly concerned with global problems of nutrition, namely, the Food and Agriculture Organization (FAO), World Health Organization (WHO), United Nations Children's Fund (UNICEF), and United Nations Educational, Scientific, and Cultural Organization (UNESCO). Through these organizations the efforts include the provision of food supplies, technical assistance, family planning for control of population growth, and general and home economics education.

Factors Influencing Food Acceptance

Food acceptance is determined by the physiologic response of the senses, biochemical changes taking place in the body, and the many meanings that food holds for the individual. In the following pages some of the physiologic, biochemical, psychological, social, economic, and educational factors affecting the acceptance of food will be discussed. References have been included at the end of this chapter for those who would like to explore one or more of these aspects in greater detail.

Desire for Food

Appetite, hunger, satiety, and *anorexia.* Terms used to indicate some aspects of desire for food. *Appetite* and *hunger* are sometimes used synonymously but they are not the same physiologic state.

HUNGER. The most basic drive for food. There is an awareness of the need to ingest food that is accompanied by increased salivation and food-searching behavior. It is associated with unpleasant or even painful contractions of an empty stomach or intestine. As hunger increases, it occupies more and more of the attention of the individual. For example, Mr. Francis arrived at his hotel late last night. He had not stopped for dinner because he expected to eat after arriving at his destination. The dining room was closed, as were all the nearby restaurants. After retiring, Mr. Francis tried to sleep, but he could not. He finally arose and drove 20 miles to find an all-night restaurant where he ate a large meal. Despite the consumption of a high-calorie meal, Mr. Francis continued to experience hunger pangs for an hour or so after eating.

The extent to which the physiologic changes characteristic of hunger are initiated by biochemical changes in the body is not completely understood. Hunger, however, is one of the frequent manifestations in certain hormonal imbalances such as hyperthyroidism, as well as both hyper- and hypoinsulinism. In the preceding example the individual did not experience a desire for any particular food; the need was for food. In certain disorders, the individual is aware of a craving for a special food. For example, in adrenal insufficiency, the patient is often aware of an increased need for consumption of sodium chloride.

APPETITE. Implies a psychic desire for food and is a pleasant sensation. Unlike hunger, it may persist after sufficient food has been ingested to appease hunger. It is conditioned by previous experiences and habit as well as by the sight, smell, and taste of food. For example. Mr. Francis arrives home in the evening. As he enters the house, he smells the aroma of his favorite stew. His mouth waters as he anticipates eating his dinner, although he has eaten a big lunch and is not particularly hungry.

Appetite and hunger also appear to be affected by the hormonal responses to a severe injury or to a major surgical procedure. During the adrenergic and glucocorticoid responses to injury, appetite and hunger are suppressed and anorexia is the rule. In fact, the sight or smell of food may induce nausea and other unpleasant sensations. During the glucocorticoid withdrawal phase, appetite begins to return. During convalescence, appetite may, unless curbed in time, be so great as to lead to an excessive gain in weight.

Satiety is defined as a state of satisfaction or lack of desire for food following its ingestion. Unless an unusually large quantity of food is ingested, it is a pleasant state. For example, after eating a big dish of stew, Mr. Francis leaned back from the table, relaxed and comfortable. *Anorexia* is descriptive of an abnormal state, because it implies an absence of hunger under circumstances in which it should be expected. At lunchtime John, aged 14, refuses to eat, saying, "I'm not hungry." Because he has not eaten since breakfast, and then only lightly, his mother asks him, "Are you ill?" John has anorexia. He is not hungry under circumstances in which he should be. When his mother investigates further, she finds that he has a fever and a rash.

The Senses and Food Acceptance

The sensations of taste and smell also affect appetite and the acceptability of food. Everyone has experienced the lack of enjoyment of food which accompanies a common cold. Inasmuch as taste and smell enable the individual to identify poisonous substances, these senses are protective. Neither sense is a completely reliable guide to the selection of foods that are safe. Familiar foods that are prepared in accustomed ways taste and smell "good." Unfamiliar foods, most particularly those with strong odors, are rejected because they taste and smell "bad." Thus Limburger cheese is a delicacy to one person and spoiled cheese to another.

Taste

As more knowledge is gained about the sensation of taste it becomes apparent that it is not a simple sensation. It is believed that the tongue is only one of several structures responsible for the sensation of taste. Cranial nerves innervate the taste buds of the tongue and tonsillar pillars. In addition the sensation of taste is complemented by the senses of smell and vision. It appears that the tongue is most sensitive to salt tastes and sweet tastes whereas the palate is most sensitive to sour and bitter tastes (Henkin, 1969). Alterations in any of these structures through disease or injury may result in an alteration in taste.

Taste is determined not only by the chemical properties of food but also by the metabolic state of the eater, and in this respect taste plays a role in the maintenance of the internal environment. Theoretically, the biochemical state of the body may influence taste acuity by influencing the penetration of the tastant through the taste pore and its membrane to the taste bud. Experiments with human subjects indicate that a 5 per cent sucrose solution is more palatable than a 30 per cent solution unless the subject has received insulin or is fasting, underweight, or obese (Lepkovsky, 1973). People with dentures, gonadal dysgenesis, and pseudohypoparathyroidism have a decreased sensitivity to sourness and bitterness, whereas patients with adrenal cortex insufficiency have a lowered threshold for the detection of all tastes (Henkin, 1969). Other alterations of taste with disease states may exist. Knowledge of these facts should alert nurses that the belief that "my body tells me just what I need" is not always true. People must use their intellect as well as senses and at times it may be essential to assist patients to realize this.

Although illness is responsible for the change in the taste of food, something can be done to improve the acceptability of food to the patient. Because a clean, moist mouth minimizes the loss of taste, the patient should be provided with the opportunity to brush his or her teeth or have them brushed before food is offered, and the mouth should also be cleansed after meals to remove food particles. The nurse can also relate the change of the taste of the food to the illness. The change of taste is usually temporary and taste will return as the patient recovers. When the consumption of food is important to recovery, the patient should be encouraged to eat. Eating is a way in which the patient can help himself or herself to recover. Recognition by the nurse that eating is difficult when food tastes different from the usual may also strengthen the efforts of the patient.

Smell

Although few people distinguish between the sensations of taste and smell, much of what is loosely called taste results from the odor of food. Odors may also be responsible for unpleasant sensations associated with food. Most persons are aware that when they have a cold, food seems "flat" or tasteless. In healthy persons, the fragrance of baking bread or broiling steak arouses pleasant sensations. To the sick person, these same odors may be highly unpleasant. Odor is often accepted as an indication of the safety of a food; for example, meat smells fresh or spoiled. Canned food should be smelled before tasting it. If it has a peculiar smell, canned food should be discarded without tasting. Appetite may be depressed by disagreeable odors and stimulated by pleasant ones. Patients with foul-smelling wounds may find eating difficult. Keeping dressings clean and minimizing the odor may do much to promote appetite.

Texture

Smooth, creamy foods are preferred to lumpy or grainy foods. Cooked vegetables that are tender yet slightly crisp are likely to be more acceptable than those that are soft, mushy, water soaked, or stringy. Generally speaking, young children like soft, smooth foods. Many older people also prefer soft foods because they may have poorly fitting dentures or find biting and chewing painful. However, diets that are varied in texture are more likely to be nutritionally adequate than those that are restricted to soft foods. Moreover, chewing of foods helps to improve dental hygiene.

Temperature

The temperature at which food is served also influences its acceptability. Despite provisions made in hospitals to ensure the correct temperature of the food served, foods do not always arrive at the bedside of the patient at either the proper temperature or the proper consistency. For example, hot foods such as coffee, soups, and entrees are all too frequently tepid by the time they reach the patient. Cold foods, such as gelatin salads and ice cream, may melt before they are served to the patient and are therefore unacceptable. When a tray must be delayed, hot food should be kept hot or heated and cold food should be refrigerated during the delay. Attention to the condition of the food at the time it is presented to the patient not only increases the likelihood of its being eaten, but affords an opportunity to reinforce the feeling of the patient that what happens to him or her is important to those responsible for care.

Maintenance of Homeostasis with Respect to Food Intake

Hormonal Regulation

Hunger, in addition to producing unpleasant gastric contractions, is accompanied by feelings of weakness, emptiness, and sometimes headache and nausea. That a low blood glucose level is related to the gastric contractions has been known for many years. Such hunger contractions were intensified when insulin was given. On the other hand, glucagon, another hormone produced by the pancreas, has the effect of inhibiting gastric contractions. Glucagon exerts its action by releasing glycogen from the liver, thereby increasing the blood glucose level. (See Carbohydrate Metabolism.)

The gastric responses to hunger are correlated with metabolic and neurologic factors in the brain. These are complex mechanisms that are not fully understood. Satiety and feeding or appetite centers have been identified in the hypothalamus. Experimental work indicates that the primary function of the ventromedial nucleus (satiety centers) of the hypothalamus is to regulate the size of the fat depots in the adipose tissue. A decrease in fat depots below a set level results in an increased absorption of calories from the small intestines (Lepkovsky, 1973). It has been shown that the food intake of the animals is closely correlated with the rate of glucose utilization. The satiety centers have a high affinity for glucose and are extremely sensitive to the availability of glucose in the blood. When the satiety centers take up glucose this is translated into an electrical impulse to other centers of the central nervous system and in turn translated into sensations of hunger or satiety. The satiety centers act as a brake to control the feeding center (lateral nuclei).

Psychological and Social Factors

Despite the significance of biochemical and physiological factors in influencing the acceptability of food, psychological factors are probably even more important. Although knowledge of the psychological and social factors in eating is incomplete, there is an increasing literature emphasizing that eating is motivated not by logic but by feelings. Mead (1953) summarizes the psychological, social, and cultural aspects of food as follows: "In most societies, food is the focus of emotional associations, a channel for interpersonal relations, for the communication of love or discrimination or disapproval; it usually has a symbolic reference."

Food has several universal functions. One function

is to attain social status and social prestige. Others are to help a person cope with stress, to reward or punish others, to initiate and maintain interpersonal relationships, and to express socioreligious ideas (Leininger, 1970).

The hypothesis that likes and dislikes are more important factors in the selection of food than health is supported by a study reported by Shapiro et al. (1962). Food selection was studied in families from different income groups. All families had sufficient income to purchase an adequate diet. Little difference was found in the food selected by families of the various economic levels. In all groups, likes and dislikes far outweighed health as a consideration in food selection.

Both physiologic and psychological factors influence the acceptance or rejection of food. For example, a healthy person who has been exercising out of doors is likely to be hungry at mealtime. This same person may develop anorexia on being frightened or angry. The person is neither likely to feel like eating nor to be hungry while in the acute phase of an illness or in pain. When at all possible, painful procedures should be performed between meals and not just before or during meals. One reason for encouraging activity in the chronically undernourished is to increase appetite and hunger.

Not only do many factors influence what people eat, but their behavior is affected by whether they are hungry or well fed. They may be irritable, withdrawn, or restless when hungry, and happy and relaxed when well fed. Shakespeare relates human behavior to food when he has Caesar say, "Let me have men about me who are fat; sleek-headed men and such as sleep o' nights. Yon Cassius has a lean and hungry look; he thinks too much; such men are dangerous."

If the nurse is to be really effective in helping people to meet their nutritional needs, she or he must know not only what people should and do eat but what food and eating mean to them, as well as what some of the possible consequences of suggested changes may be. Clear distinctions between the cultural, social, and psychological aspects of food and eating are not easy to make. Some of these will be discussed and illustrated in the following sections.

Cultural Influences

Among many potentially nutritious plants and animals available as food, only a few are used by any group of people. An explanation offered to account for this failure to use all suitable and nonpoisonous plants and animals as food is that the definition of food is of cultural origin. Some plants and animals are designated as being fit for human consumption without regard for their nutritional value. In some cultures, there are religious prohibitons against certain foods. In Moslem countries pork is forbidden. Hindus do not eat beef. Even in the absence of religious proscription, nutritious foods may be rejected. To most Americans, horse meat is not fit for human consumption. In America sweet corn is a treat; in France it is considered fit only for animals. In the southeastern United States grits are served with every meal. In the North they are seldom, if ever, eaten. Children learn very early which plants and animals are not acceptable to eat. Not quite 5-year-old Mary supported this by commenting during a conversation about the use of horse meat as food, "I like horses, but not to eat."

Something can be learned about the food habits of different groups by visiting supermarkets in various areas in a city or the country. For example, beef or pork is preferred to lamb in Iowa, with the result that lamb is seldom available in a market. In a community in which Jewish people are concentrated, kosher corned beef and bagels are easily obtained. In non-Jewish communities, these foods are frequently unknown. In Minneapolis during the Christmas season, lutefisk is found in every grocery store. In one section of Detroit, signs on store windows advertise mustard greens and possums. In northern Michigan, pasties—beef, potatoes, and onions enclosed in pastry and baked—remind one of the Welsh miners who brought their food habits with them when they migrated to America. To any one person, depending on conditioning, some of the preceding foods are delicacies, others are unknown, and still others are rejected as being unfit to be used as food, although all are nutritious and wholesome.

Family Influences

Within the framework of a culture, the family translates and modifies the cultural attitudes toward food an eating for its members. In the family, food is an important and continuining aspect of the mother–child relationship. From the beginning, the mother not only provides or makes available nutrients for the child, but, by the manner in which she feeds the child, shows her love and affection.

In the family, mealtime provides more than food. In a modern industrial society, the evening meal may be the only time when the entire family regularly meets together as a group. This coming together of the family contributes to morale and a sense of unity among the members. Experiences of the day can be shared, plans made, and events reviewed. For a little while each day, every person can feel a part of a group in which he or she is accepted and respected. In some families, eating food is looked on as a pleasure, and much time and effort are spent in its preparation. Foods may be prepared to please one or more of the family members. Mother communicates her love and affection by preparing the foods they enjoy. Significant events are celebrated with food, and individual members are made to feel important by being served a dish that they particularly enjoy.

In other families, eating may be merely a necessary activity; food is prepared and eaten and the dishes are washed promptly. Little or no sociability accompanies eating; for members of the family, eating is necessary to sustain life but has few other tangible values. In still others, mealtime is utilized to discipline the children and settle the problems of the day. Meals are accompanied by strife and tension instead of a relaxed atmosphere.

Whatever the attitude of the adults in the families, children develop values associated with food and eating. They learn what is and is not fit to eat and how it should be prepared. From their parents they learn not only what foods are good for them, but what foods are not good to eat. They learn to enjoy, tolerate, or reject food and eating.

In addition to defining the types of plants and animals suitable for use as food, the superstitions and beliefs adhered to by the family also designate those to be eaten during illness and how they are to be prepared. The old saying "Feed a fever and starve a cold" is well known. Milk may be eliminated from the diet of the sick because it is believed to be constipating, or, in the treatment of diarrhea, it may be boiled to make it constipating. Tea and toast are frequently believed to be suitable foods for sick people. Other foods such as rich desserts and cucumbers are designated as unsuitable.

Food and the Emotions

The individual eats to satisfy a psychological as well as a physiologic hunger. He or she may eat or refuse to eat to gain some measure of control over others. Mary Ellen feels comforted by eating when she feels depressed, lonely, or sad. She knows that she eats too much and is too fat, and she envies her slender classmates, but she continues to seek solace in food. She also knows that she gets more attention from her mother when she is fat than when she is thin. Despite the negative character of the remarks made by her mother and the fact that they increase her depression, Mary Ellen has her mother's attention.

Reward Value of Food

Some of the psychological implications of food stem from the value placed on certain foods as rewards. In the American culture, desserts such as cake, pie, ice cream, cookies, and candies have a reward value. They are served at the end of the meal after "wholesome" foods such as meat, bread, potatoes, and vegetables have been eaten. Whether or not desserts are included with the meal depends on specific conditions. They may be withheld if the individual fails to eat the foods that are "good for him" or as a punishment for some transgression. They are also used as a treat or as a reward for good behavior. They play a significant role in special events such as birthday parties, teas, and weddings. Atlhough using specific foods as rewards may accomplish a desired result at the time, this practice may also be responsible for engendering negative attitudes toward food.

Increasing recognition is being given to the knowledge that certain foods have a reward value in the planning of modified diets. For example, ice cream is included in the diabetic diet. The food industry has recognized the psychological value of candy and other reward foods and makes them available as diabetic candy and cookies. Education is needed to acquaint parents and teachers with the undesirable effects of using food as a threat or reward. The reward-and-punishment aspect of food should also be taken into account in planning to meet the food requirements of any patient. In the past, this aspect has often been neglected.

The basis for the use of food as a reward or punishment is to control the behavior of another. Thus a parent seeks to control a child by rewarding him or her with food or withholding it. The child or other individual, however, can gain some measure of control in the situation. By refusing to eat, the child may be able to arouse the concern and attention of the mother and gain some measure of control over her.

Symbolic Value of Food

A study of the symbolic reference of different foods in various cultures could easily take a lifetime. However, only a few examples will be cited. At the Seder feast which is celebrated at the beginning of the Passover, food is used to symbolize certain events in Jewish history. Three matzo crackers, or pieces of unleavened bread, are placed in a linen napkin on the table to represent the unity of Israel and to recall the departure from Egypt, which was so rapid that there was no time to take leaven. A roasted egg symbolizes life and its continuity, and bitter herbs symbolize the bitterness of slavery in the land of bondage.

In the Christian religions the egg is the symbol of the rebirth of the spiritual life through the death and resurrection of Christ. Eggs are colored and, in some cultures, highly intricate designs convert the egg into a thing of beauty.

Outside the realm of religion, certain foods are

symbolic of certain events, status, wealth, or hospitality. Although turkey is available in the United States throughout the year, it remains the symbol of Thanksgiving. In terms of status, hamburger may be eaten by family members, but except for a cookout, it is not served to guests, as it is often equated with a limited income.

Evidence of a high or low food intake can also be a status symbol. In some groups, plump children and a wife of ample proportions are accepted as evidence that "mama" is a good cook and "papa" is a good provider. In contrast, to be employed as a high fashion model, a young woman is required to restrict her food intake sufficiently to maintain a lean look.

Conditioning and Food Selection

Although the culture into which the individual is born defines what is fit to eat and how and under what circumstances foods are to be eaten, conditioning or habit influences what the individual will eat throughout life. Although some foods are accepted more readily than others and some infants accept new foods more easily than others babies learn to eat the foods offered to them. Food habits are established quite early in life. Most individuals prefer foods to which they became accustomed as young children, and they may be quite resistant to changing their food habits. Some people even prefer ill health or starvation to eating unaccustomed or unfamiliar foods or known foods prepared in unfamiliar ways. One of the difficult adjustments that international students in the United States frequently have to make is the adjustment to American food. Nor is the problem of adjusting to strange food limited to persons from other lands, because some Americans insist on familiar foods when they visit other countries.

Although the foods eaten by an individual are usually those to which he or she is conditioned early in life, most individuals eat more food if there is a variety of foods from which to select and a variety in methods of preparation. Variety is as important to the sick as to the healthy. The effects of the repeated serving of one food to hospitalized patients were well illustrated when a general hospital was given several hundred bushels of apples. Storage space was limited and the apples were served several times a week. Because most patients remained in the hospital only a short time, no problem was anticipated. However, a near rebellion occurred among patients undergoing rehabilitation following poliomyelitis. After several weeks, the monotony of almost daily servings of apples in some form resulted in these patients organizing a mass protest. Particular attention should be given to planning for variety for the patient who is chronically ill or who is faced with numerous adjustments and frustrations.

Changing Food Habits

Probably the most frequent reason for a change in food habits is illness. Travelers to parts of the world where food differs from that to which they are accustomed are likely to have to make some alterations in their pattern of eating. In the past, health workers acted on the premise that if properly instructed about what should be eaten, and if the person had enough money to buy food, he or she would have a nutritious diet. Although knowledge is of significance, it is not sufficient by itself.

After food habits are established they are very difficult to change, and they cannot be changed overnight. Immigrants change their language before they change their pattern of eating. During a period of famine in the rice-eating part of India, wheat was sent to relieve starvation, but the population preferred death by starvation to eating wheat. Not only was wheat a strange food, but the familiar methods of food preparation were suited to rice and not to wheat. Before the people could be expected to use wheat as food, they would have to accept it as being suitable to eat and learn new methods of food preparation. At best, changing food habits is a slow process. It took more than 200 years to establish the potato as a food in Europe. It had been introduced during the sixteenth century by Spanish explorers but was not accepted as a food. In the eighteenth century, Count Rumford gave the potato prestige by planting it in the royal gardens and feeding it to the soldiers. Guards were stationed about the garden, but they were instructed to look the other way when the potatoes were stolen. Acceptance was furthered by feeding the potatoes to the soldiers so that they developed a taste for them. In our present state of knowledge and with the variety of communications media available, it should be possible to change eating habits more rapidly. Nevertheless, food habits once developed, continue to be difficult to alter.

Principles Basic to Change

Several general principles should be observed by those who desire to assist others to change their food habits. The first is to study existing beliefs, values, and practices before attempting to make a change. The reason for food practices should also be identified if possible. For example, in the United States frequent causes of inadequate diets are lack of money, poor money management, lack of interest in food, insufficient knowledge, food fads, and misguided dieting. As in other parts of the world, food intake is sometimes limited by misconceptions about food or by values ascribed to it. Beliefs about certain foods may bear little relation to their actual characteristics. For example, Mrs. Thomas never serves milk with acid foods because she believes that acids curdle milk. The following illustration which was observed in a primitive culture, shows the relation of beliefs to practices. Despite the continued efforts of health workers and an adequate supply of eggs, the women refused to eat eggs. Eggs were not taboo because the men and children ate eggs. it was finally learned that the women believed that eggs made them aggressive and therefore were undesirable. Attention was given to changing this belief, and as the belief was changed, eggs were eaten by the women.

In the United States, values motivating people to eat or not to eat include staying slim, looking well, and keeping up with the neighbors. Studies indicate that the majority of people do not eat to be healthy per se. Motivation is through feelings, not logic. Unless the feelings of people about food are understood, information may fall on sterile soil. To date, relatively little attention has been paid by health workers to the factors motivating eating and to the utilization in practice of what is known.

Another general principle that must be observed if change is to be effected is to avoid direct or implied criticism of what is done or believed. The principal effect of criticism is to arouse stubborn resistance to change. An instance is related in which a public health nurse who was trying to encourage a group of mothers to feed their babies milk instead of beans was unsuccessful. Finally she suggested that the babies be given the water in which the beans were cooked. Later, when visiting the mothers, she found that they were feeding milk to their babies. When the nurse expressed surprise, one of the mothers said, "You accepted our way. We do your way."

One of the problems that nurses and other health workers have is that they expect the recipients of their services to accept their direction and advice without question. Moreover, they themselves may not follow the advice they give to others. Furthermore, nurses may not recognize that patients have at least two alternatives—to reject or to accept advice. The point of view of patients may be quite different from that of nurses trying to be helpful. Unless these differences in points of view are clarified by the nurse she or he may never know why the patient fails to "cooperate." After the point of view of the patient has been identified, alternatives can also be clarified.

At least a minimum amount of money must be available to purchase the food required for an optimum nutritional state. Persons whose incomes fall below the minimum are likely to have difficulty securing enough food of good quality and variety.

Any plan made to assist a person to change food habits should also include an exploration of the wants of the individual that are competing for his or her income. For example, a young woman with a baby had just enough money to buy a small can of peaches or a box of oatmeal. After much thought and indecision, she bought the peaches. Other individuals may want items other than food. When a person has an increase in salary, he or she may be faced with a number of alternatives. Should the new money be spent on nonfat dry milk, candy, carbonated beverages, cigarettes, liquor, or a television set? Objectively, the answer seems clear. To the individual who makes the choice, other answers may well take priority.

Nutrition plays a role in the etiology of or recovery from almost all diseases. It may be important throughout the course of an illness. The biochemical, physiological, and psychological changes taking place during illness frequently affect the desire for food. Often, the sick person is faced with a change—temporary or permanent—in the pattern of eating. Sometimes the problem is easily solved, as it was for Mrs. Brown who was wondering how she could ever adjust to a diabetic diet. She thought that she would be denied greens, cornbread, and ice cream. The green beens presented no problem. Within limits, neither did the cornbread nor the ice cream.

When significant changes are required, the patient may appear to accept the change, but may actually continue his or her usual food pattern. Mrs. Smith, also a diabetic, was such a person. At one time she was cared for by a physician who believed a diabetic person could and should eat the same food as a nondiabetic. When asked by a nurse about how confusing the change must have been, she said, "Not at all. I've followed about the same regimen all the time. Both physicians were so enthusiastic that I couldn't bear to disappoint them."

Some patients react with what appears to be unreasonable resistance to change. If the professional staff reacts with hostility or indifference, the resistance of the patient is likely to increase. If the cause of the reaction of the patient can be determined, then the patient may be more willing to modify behavior. Not infrequently the reasons for the rejection of the diet plan are reasonable, not only to the patient but, when the trouble is taken to identify them, to the nurse. What appears to be irrational behavior to the observer may be rational to the behaver. Often the diet plan can be altered in such a way as to make it more acceptable to the individual. Success is dependent, at least in part, on learning what the change means to the individual and working with him or her in making an acceptable plan suitable to his or her life style.

Nutrition and the Adolescent

Nutritional problems of the adolescent have received considerable attention. Numerous studies of the diet of teenaged girls indicate that their intake of nutrients is deficient in some respects. A number of characteristic features of adolescence influence how and what the adolescent eats. Adolescents want respect and understanding as individuals. They want those who work with them to believe in them and in their potential for becoming mature adults. They want to be liked and to do what their peers do. Because adolescence occurs at different ages in different individuals, individuals differ in rate of growth, size, and general appearance. The adolescent is concerned about the changes he or she is undergoing and relationships with members of the opposite sex and with peers. He or she worries about pimples and being attractive. Girls are concerned about becoming fat. They skip breakfast, try fad diets, and take other shortcuts to a slender figure. The adolescent is in a period in which concern with oneself is exaggerated. Adolescents want others to be interested in them and to make their interest known. They require respect. At the same time, adolescence is a period when the individual is developing an independent life. The adolescent may be torn between wish to remain a child and desire to be an adult. During adolescence one is developing one's own ideas and making plans for the future. Physiologically, adolescence is a period of rapid growth. Especially in boys, food is required to build muscles. Girls are preparing themselves for pregnancy and lactation. Boys and girls require the proper quantity and quality of food for growth and development into healthy adults, as well as for their current activities.

Nutritional Problems in Later Years

Another period of life when nutritional problems may be exaggerated is in late maturity. An individual brings to 60 years or more of life the food habits of a lifetime. Appetite may, however, be impaired by gradually diminishing activity, loss of the sense of taste, and loss of teeth. Ability to masticate food may be lessened by failure to replace teeth or by poorly fitting dentures. For some old people, money may be a real or perceived problem. Persons living on pensions, welfare, or social security may have barely enough to take care of their needs. Others have sufficient funds but fear their money will be exhausted before they die. The cost of illness or other emergencies may strain the budget to the point where the amount left for food is inadequate. Pride or lack of knowledge of the means available to supplement the income may be responsible. Sometimes the food money is spent for food for a dog or cat. To a lonely, aged man or woman, a pet may have more value than an adequate or nearly adequate diet. To be able to feed her dog, Mrs. Frisk eats meat only twice a week. She speaks with pride when she says that Skippy has a nice, juicy hamburger every day. A deficient food intake may result from a lack of incentive or energy to secure or prepare food. People who live alone, such as the elderly or the chronically ill, are especially prone to neglect their food intake. In some cities, Meals-on-Wheels have been developed to make meals available to the homebound at a reasonable cost.

Poverty among the elderly is not limited to lack of money. With the passage of time, the elderly man or woman often becomes increasingly isolated. As relatives and friends die or move away, the opportunity to share meals with others diminishes. With the decrease in or loss of the social aspect of eating, incentive for eating diminishes. The positive effects on the appetite of eating with others can be observed when company comes for dinner or the elderly person is invited out to eat. Mrs. Marshall illustrates this point very well. She lives alone in a small apartment. When she prepares her own meals and eats alone, she, in her own words, "eats like a bird." On Sundays, when she is invited to the home of her granddaughter, she eats about as well as the other members of the family. Her explantion is, "The food tastes better." The combination of well-prepared food, friendly conversation, and the example of others eating with pleasure has a favorable effect on Mrs. Marshall's appetite.

In some hospitals, particularly those for the chronically ill, group dining rooms are provided in order to create a social atmosphere at mealtime. For patients who are confined to their rooms, attention to the environment before food is served may help to improve the appetite. The presence of a family member or a good friend at mealtime, or a flower on the tray, may aid in creating a more homelike atmosphere, thereby encouraging eating. When failure of a patient to eat is a problem, attention to the social aspects of eating sometimes contributes to the solution.

Summary

Survival, growth, productivity, and health all depend on a continual supply of food. In some areas of the world the amount of food available is insufficient to support the population at much more than survival level. The reasons for the inadequate food supply include poor soil, crop failure and shortages, decline of carryover stocks in major exporting countries, increase in grain prices, and a decline in consumer incomes.

The supply of food is only one aspect of nutrition. Eating is a voluntary act and food must be judged suitable to eat for it to be accepted. This acceptance involves a variety of psychological, religious, and social factors which have little or nothing to do with the nutritional value of a substance. There are few events in the life of an individual when food does not play a part. Often improvement of the nutrition of an individual, family, or nation depends on a change in food habits. Though knowledge of how to effect change is limited, a few guides to action are suggested, including the following:

1 Take time to discover the what and why of the pattern of the group.
2 Do not criticize, because criticism only arouses stubborn resistance.
3 Remember that changing food habits is a slow process.
4 Motivation for eating is more psychological and social than it is intellectual.
5 Although knowledge of what constitutes good nutrition is usually insufficient to effect change, it is one factor in change.
6 Nutritional options must be available, accessible, and acceptable.

The Service Facility

Because nutrients are usually ingested in a complex state, foods must be subjected to a series of physical and chemical changes whereby they are converted to a state in which they can be absorbed. Large multicellular organisms such as humans have specialized structures that receive, temporarily store, and convert by chemical and mechanical means crude materials to utilizable forms, whereupon they are transferred from the external to the internal environment. The remaining residue is temporarily stored, water is absorbed, and eventually the residue is ejected at regular intervals.

Before discussion of individual organs, some of the common features of the digestive system and the effects of disturbances in function on the body economy as well as on the general nutritional state will be presented. The alimentary canal and the accessory organs of digestion function as a unit. Under nervous and hormonal control, the activity of each organ of the digestive system is coordinated and integrated so that food is in the right place at the right time for digestion and absorption to be accomplished.

The Alimentary Canal

The alimentary canal is a hollow muscular tube passing through the center of the body and extending from the mouth to the anus (See Figure 29-1). The primary functions of the alimentary canal are motility, secretion, digestion, and absorption of nutrients. Despite the importance of the regular evacuation of the residue remaining after digestion is completed, in health the alimentary canal plays only a secondary role in the elimination of substances from the internal environment.

Upper Alimentary Canal

Functionally, the alimentary canal can be divided into three general regions: upper, middle, and lower. The upper alimentary canal includes the esophagus, stomach, upper duodenum, liver, and pancreas. As do other regions, the upper alimentary canal conveys food from upper to lower parts. Its other principal functions are (1) the secretion of digestive juices, (2) the breaking up and mixing of food particles with these juices, (3) storage, (4) the beginning of chemical digestion, and (5) some absorption. The importance to life and health of the various structures composing the upper alimentary canal varies. Persons with strictures of the esophagus can and do live for many years. Removal of the stomach is compatible with life but is frequently associated with some loss of health.

Middle Alimentary Canal

The middle alimentary canal extends from the duodenal papilla to the mid-transverse colon. From the viewpoint of function, it is the most important region of the alimentary canal, for it is here that digestion is completed and absorption takes place. Our present state of knowledge indicates that adequate nutrition cannot be maintained without the

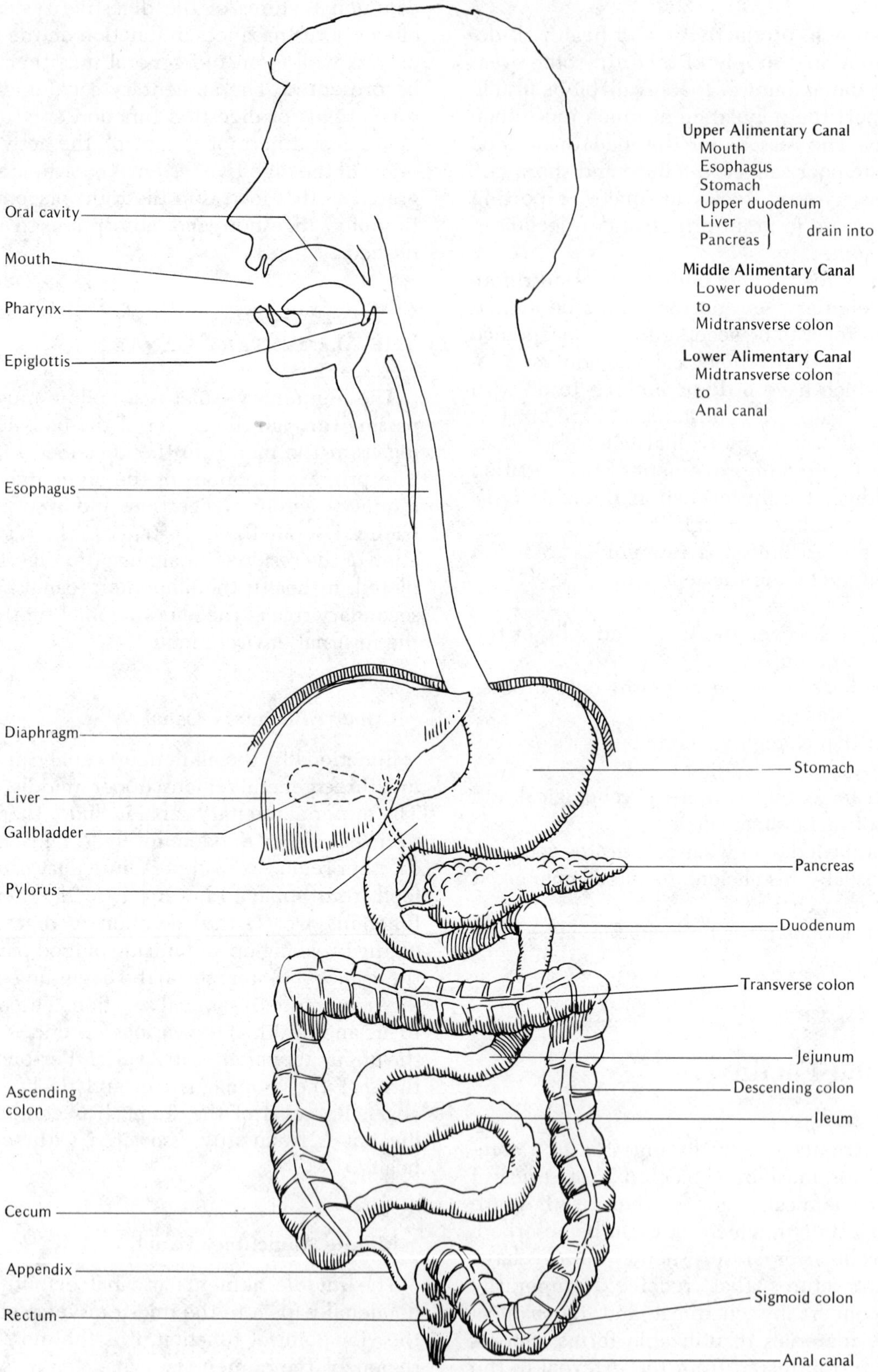

Upper Alimentary Canal
Mouth
Esophagus
Stomach
Upper duodenum
Liver
Pancreas
drain into
Middle Alimentary Canal
Lower duodenum
to
Midtransverse colon
Lower Alimentary Canal
Midtransverse colon
to
Anal canal
Oral cavity
Mouth
Pharynx
Epiglottis
Esophagus
Diaphragm
Liver
Gallbladder
Pylorus
Ascending colon
Cecum
Appendix
Rectum
Stomach
Pancreas
Duodenum
Transverse colon
Jejunum
Descending colon
Ileum
Sigmoid colon
Anal canal

Figure 29-1. The Alimentary canal.

absorbing surface of the mid-alimentary canal. The available surface for absorption in a healthy person is greater than is required, and although the small intestine cannot be removed in its entirety, some of it can be removed without threatening the nutritional status of the individual. Many nutrients can be supplied parenterally, but only by exceptional procedures can calories and amino acids be infused in sufficient quantities to meet tissue requirements. The middle portion of the alimentary canal is therefore a vital organ.

Lower Alimentary Canal

The lower portion of the alimentary canal extends from the mid-portion of the trasverse colon to the anus. Its primary function is to store refuse until it can be conveniently evacuated. The lower alimentary canal is not necessary to either life or health. An artificial opening in any portion from the lower ileum downward can be made to function satisfactorily in the elimination of wastes. Because the ascending and transverse portions of the colon absorb water from the fluid content of the alimentary canal, the lower the opening, the less physiologic adjustments have to be made. For example, the drainage from an ileostomy is watery, but the feces in the sigmoid colon are semisolid. Following an ileostomy, the lower ileum adapts by increasing water absorption, but the process of adaptation takes time and the patient needs to be protected from the loss of water and electrolytes. The skin around the ileostomy requires protection from the fluid feces. Following a sigmoidostomy, the feces may be fluid or semifluid for a few days, primarily as a result of hypermotility, but within a short time the feces assume their normal semisolid consistency.

Blood Supply

Most of the regions of the alimentary canal have a rich blood and lymphatic supply. The exceptions include a portion of the esophagus and of the colon. The parts richly supplied with blood have the advantage of healing rapidly after surgery or accidental injury. The abundant blood supply also makes hemorrhage a greater possibility when blood vessels are ruptured. Venous drainage from the alimentary canal is through the portal system which supplies the liver. In diseases of the liver in which there is obstruction of the portal venous system, varicosities of the esophageal and hemorrhoidal veins occur. Rupture of esophageal varices is attended by massive hemorrhage.

Mechanisms for Regulation of Gastrointestinal Function

The function of the alimentary canal is regulated by the nervous and hormonal systems in relation to the needs of the entire organism. The alimentary canal is exceedingly sensitive to conditions in the body as a whole. The various organs of the alimentary canal are also regulated in relation to each other. Food in one organ acts as a stimulus to alert the next organ to prepare for it or to delay the rate at which the preceding organ empties. For example, a factor in the rate at which the stomach empties into the duodenum is the degree of fullness of the small intestine. When the intestine is distended, inhibitory messages are sent to the stomach in the form of an inhibitory hormone, enterogastrone, secreted by the intestinal musosa.

Hormonal Regulation

Two groups of hormones participate in the regulation of the alimentary canal. The first consists of the hormones participating in the regulation of activities throughout the body. The second group is classified as local hormones because they are secreted by some part of the alimentary canal and alter action by stimulating or inhibiting another part. An example of a hormone of the first group is thyroxine. It increases the rate of the absorption of food and of the secretion and motility of the gastrointestinal tract. An example of a hormone of the second group is enterogastrone, cited earlier.

Nervous Regulation

The alimentary canal is richly supplied with nerves from the autonomic nervous sytem and from an intramural (within the wall) nerve plexus. This plexus extends all the way from the esophagus to the anus. It consists of two layers of neurons. The outer layer lies between the longitudinal and circular muscles of the digestive tube and is known as the myenteric (or Auerbach's) plexus. The inner layer of neurons lies in the submucosa and is known as the submucous (or Meissner's) plexus. These plexuses, often referred to collectively as the myenteric plexus, regulate many of the local actions of the digestive tube. They increase the muscle tone, the intensity and rate of rhythmical contraction, and the speed with which excitatory waves spread along the gastrointestinal wall.

The alimentary canal receives nerves from both the parasympathetic and sympathetic divisions of the autonomic nervous system. Centers in the central nervous system act through the parasympathetic and sympathetic nervous systems to increase or decrease the activity of the gastrointestinal tract. In general, these two divisions of the autonomic nervous system have opposing actions. The parasympathetic nervous system increases activity of the alimentary canal, and the sympathetic nervous system has, with three exceptions, inhibitory effects. Stimulation by the sympathetic nervous system increases the activity of the ileocecal and internal anal sphincters and the smooth muscle of the muscularis mucosac throughout the alimentary tract. The action of the entire digestive tube can be blocked by intense stimulation of the sympathetic nervous system because the wall of the gut is inhibited and two major sphincters are contracted. Inhibition of the alimentary tract is to be expected during the period immediately following severe trauma or major surgery, or during the acute phase of serious illnesses such as pneumonia. (See Chapters 18 and 22 for further discussion.) Excitement, anxiety, and fear can also stimulate the sympathetic nervous system so that it greatly diminishes the activity of the digestive tube. Attention given to minimizing the anxiety of the sick person may therefore contribute to diminishing the degree to which the alimentary canal is inactivated.

In contrast to the sympathetic nervous system, the parasympathetic nervous system increases the activity of the alimentary canal, including the secretion of digestive juices. Cannon describes the functions of the parasympathetic nervous system as being concerned with nutrition. The gut is supplied from both the cranial and sacral divisions of the parasympathetic nervous system. With the exception of some parasympathetic fibers in the mouth and pharynx, the entire cranial supply is through the vagus nerve. Whereas the loss of the sympathetic nerve supply to the gut has little or no effect on function, interruption of the parasympathetic almost always has. For example, vagotomy, a surgical procedure in which a branch of the vagus nerve is severed, is sometimes used in the treatment of intractable peptic ulcer. It is followed by reduction in muscle tone and decrease of peristaltic activity in all the following regions: the distal portion of the esophagus, the stomach, and the proximal portion of the intestine. There is also a decrease in secretions in the stomach. Severing of the sacral parasympathetic nervous system is followed by diminished tone of the descending colon, the sigmoid, and the rectum with the result that defecation is seriously impaired.

Characteristics of Movement

The rate at which the contents are moved diminishes progressively from the mouth to the anus. Motion is accomplished by smooth muscle arranged in longitudinal and circular layers. The muscle fibers lie so close together that contraction initiated at one point tends to spread to adjacent areas. The muscles of the alimentary canal exhibit the two types of contraction characteristic of smooth muscle in any part of the body—tonus contraction and rhythmical contraction. Tonus contraction determines the degree of pressure in any organ and the resistance to movement by the sphincters. Rhythmical contraction, or peristalsis, moves the contents toward the anus. Excessive tonic contractions of a segment or of a sphincter may interfere with the forward movement of the contents of the digestive tube. They may also be a source of pain.

Peristalsis

Peristalsis mixes the contents of the alimentary canal and propels them forward. Peristalsis is characterized by contraction of the muscle behind the bolus and simultaneous relaxation of the muscle ahead of it. Any increase or decrease in the activity of smooth muscle disturbs in some manner the capacity of the alimentary canal to receive, retain, digest, or absorb food.

Both the tone and the rhythmical contractions of the alimentary tract are regulated by the nervous system. As a consequence of the action of the nervous system, the rhythmical contractions of the alimentary canal can be increased or decreased in intensity or rate. In addition, peristalsis (the major propulsive movements of the gastrointestinal tract) is coordinated and the secretion of digestive juices is regulated so that each ferment is provided at the time and place it is needed.

Sphincters

Each major segment of the alimentary canal is separated from other segments by sphincter muscles. Sphincters control the rate at which the contents of the gastrointestinal tract are moved from one organ to another, and they prevent backflow. The sphincters at the inlet and at the outlet of the stomach also regulate the size of particles allowed to move forward. Food is retained in the stomach until particles are finely divided and converted into a fluid state and acidified. The resulting mixture is known as chyme.

Integrity of the Alimentary Canal

Another anatomic characteristic of the alimentary canal, of importance in understanding possible effects of disease, is that the lumen of the gut lies outside the body proper. The entire lumen from the mouth to the anus is surrounded by the body, but it is not part of it. (See Figure 29-1.) The wall surrounding the lumen of the alimentary canal either is impermeable to its contents or is permeable only to water, alcohol, small molecules, and ions. In fact, many molecules and ions require a transport or carrier system to move across semipermeable membranes in appreciable quantities.[1] Any break in the integrity of the wall therefore carries with it the possibility of the escape of the contents of the alimentary canal into the internal environment. Superficial disruption of the mucous membrane is not usually serious. If, however, the break penetrates all the layers and extends through the entire wall, the contents of the organ escape into a body cavity.

Defenses of the Alimentary Canal

Role of the Senses

As with other structural facilities serving as points of exchange between the internal and external environment, some system of defense or protection against the ingestion of harmful substances is required. The *senses* of *sight, taste,* and *smell* all function in protection. Foods are accepted or rejected on the basis of general appearance, odor, taste, and feel. Meat may be accepted when it is bright in color or rejected when it is dull red or black. If the meat smells fresh, it is more likely to be eaten than if it has a peculiar odor or is putrid. The same is true of taste. Inasmuch as these senses enable the individual to correctly evaluate the safety of a food, they are protective. Because they are subject to conditioning and are not very accurate, wholesome food may be rejected and harmful foods accepted. When there is any doubt about the safety of food, it should be rejected

The Mucous Membrane

The *mucous membrane* that extends from the mouth to the anus acts as a *barrier* to the entrance of excessively large molecules and of some microorganisms into the body proper. As in other areas of the body, the mucous membrane must be unbroken or intact. Glands in the mucous membrane secrete mucus, which tends to coat the mucous membrane lining the alimentary canal and to lessen the extent of direct contact with its contents. The mucous membrane is thereby protected from mechanical injury by fibrous foods and from the digesting action of enzymes contained in the digestive juices. As in the respiratory tract, the mucous glands in the membrane lining the alimentary canal respond to irritation by increased secretion. After a harsh laxative has been taken or hard feces are defecated, mucus can sometimes be seen in or around the stool. In a disorder known as mucus colitis, hyperactivity of the colon may be sufficient to be accompanied by the discharge of large quantities of mucus. Sometimes the sheets of mucus are in the form of a cast of the bowel. In disorders in which there is a disruption of the mucous membrane lining of the large intestine, such as in chronic ulcerative colitis, mucus secretion is also increased above the normal level. Any break in the integrity of the mucous membrane predisposes to the entrance of microorganisms and other foreign particles into the internal environment.

A *third barrier* to the entrance of microorganisms into the internal environment is the character of its *secretions.* The acid gastric juice is of particular importance. Under conditions of health, few microorganisms are found in the gastric secretions. A *fourth protection* from the invasion of microorganisms is the *phagocytosis* carried out by the Kupffer cells of the liver.

Anorexia, Nausea, Vomiting

Three closely related mechanisms serve to protect the individual against the ingestion of harmful material or remove it from the gastrointestinal tract after it has been ingested. They are *anorexia, nausea,* or *vomiting.* The person suffering from anorexia says, "I have no appetite," or "I don't feel like eating," or "Nothing tastes good." He or she may dawdle with food or force himself or herself to try to eat. Whereas anorexia is characterized by loss of appetite, nausea is an unpleasant or disagreeable sensation characterized by a revulsion for food. When food is offered, the nauseated patient says. "Take it away," or, "I can't stand the sight or smell of it," or, "It makes me feel sick even to think of it." He or she looks and feels miserable. Usually nauseated persons cannot force themselves to eat. As a rule, they have other symptoms caused by imbalance in the autonomic nervous system, such as increased salivation and secretion of mucus, sweating, and tachycardia. Evidence of increased activity of the vagus nerve may result in bradycardia and hypotension. In nausea, the tone and activity of the stomach and small intestine are probably diminished.

Although nausea and vomiting are frequently associated, they may appear independently of each other. Because of the close relationship of nausea to vomiting, factors in its cause and treatment will be discussed with vomiting. *Vomiting* is defined as the sudden forceful ejection of the contents of the stomach, duodenum, and proximal jejunum through the mouth. It is frequently, but not invariably, preceded by nausea. A projectile type of vomiting, occurring without warning nausea, accompanies rap-

[1] Fat solvent liquids such as carbon tetrachloride are readily absorbed.

idly increasing intracranial pressure, such as follows head injuries

VOMITING REFLEX. Although all vomiting results from reflex activity, the point at which the reflex is initiated varies. The basic pattern for the vomiting reflex is similar to that of any reflex. It involves a receptor connected by way of nerve fibers and cells to an effector. As in other reflexes, a group of nerve cells located within the brain, the vomiting center, regulates and coordinates the act of vomiting. Sensory receptors capable of initiating the vomiting reflex are located outside as well as within the wall of the alimentary canal. Within the alimentary canal, receptors are located in the fauces and pharynx, the stomach, and the intestine. The most acutely sensitive area is the first portion of the duodenum. Outside the alimentary canal, sensory receptors for vomiting are located in the uterus, kidneys, heart, and semicircular canals. Receptors may be stimulated by excessively irritating substances or by overdistention of an organ supplied with sensory receptors. The degree of excitability of the receptors is an element in the intensity of stimulation required to trigger the vomiting reflex. The more irritable the receptor, the easier it is to stimulate it.

Even a cursory glance at the variety of sites containing sensory receptors for vomiting and the types of conditions likely to stimulate them suggests that vomiting is a frequent event in disease. Moreover, it occurs not only in disorders involving the gastrointestinal system, but in those of the heart, kidney, uterus, and semicircular canals. Inflammatory conditions of the alimentary canal, such as acute appendicitis and gastroenteritis, frequently cause vomiting. Intestinal obstruction, mechanical or functional, also gives rise to vomiting. The vomiting associated with motion sickness results from the effects of motion on the semicircular canals in sensitive persons. Motion sickness is caused by any form of transportation in the air, on water, or on land. As in many other situations, fear and anxiety increase the tendency to motion sickness.

Because the fauces and pharynx are areas where the vomiting reflex may be triggered, care should be taken during mouth hygiene to avoid initiating the vomiting reflex by mechanical stimulation of these areas. Particular attention should be paid to this in patients who have been vomiting. Mechanical stimulation of the pharynx or fauces during the passage of a nasogastric tube or the introduction of a nasopharyngeal catheter initiates the gag reflex in many people. Procedures such as asking the patient to breathe deeply or to swallow are often beneficial as they distract the attention of the patient and help him or her to relax. Moreover, the voluntary initiation of swallowing suppresses the vomiting reflex.

Easy access to receptors initiating the vomiting reflex can be life-saving in some instances. After a toxic substance has been ingested, vomiting can sometimes be induced by stimulating the fauces with a finger or a blunt instrument. This is a commonly used technique for self-induction of vomiting. Emotionally disturbed persons sometimes induce vomiting by this method. Should a person be observed to be inducing the vomiting reflex, this fact should be recorded and brought to the attention of the physician.

Receptors in the *stomach* can be stimulated by drinking water containing an irritating substance or by the rapid distention of the stomach. A common, though not always effective, method is to drink a glass of tepid water to which a teaspoonful of dry mustard has been added. Mustard has the undesired effect of increasing any previous irritation. Distention of the stomach is accomplished by drinking ordinary tap water or starch water as rapidly as possible, and will always induce vomiting when ingested in sufficient quantities. Water has the advantage of diluting the contents of the stomach and it facilitates the removal of tonic substances.

Vomiting may also be initiated by impulses at the vomiting center by way of the *cerebral cortex*. Unpleasant sights, sounds, odors, tastes, and thoughts, as well as sensations such as severe pain, can initiate the vomiting reflex. In some persons, the sight of blood induces vomiting. It is not unusual for a person arriving at the scene of an accident where blood has been spilled to complain of nausea or actually to vomit. Fetid odors or the odor of vomitus can have a similar effect.

A third general site where vomiting may be initiated is the *chemoreceptor zone*, located in the medulla, but outside the vomiting center. At one time it was thought that circulating toxic agents caused vomiting by acting on the vomiting center. Emetic drugs such as apomorphine, toxic dosages of digitalis, and the "toxins" of acute infectious disease, as well as the retention of products normally excreted by the kidneys, are believed to induce vomiting by stimulating the chemoreceptor center. Vomiting is a problem in disorders accompanied by disturbances in metabolism such as pernicious vomiting in pregnancy, diabetic acidosis, and addisonian and hyperthyroid crises. As indicated earlier, vomiting also occurs in patients with traumatic head injuries, with infections involving the brain and meninges, and with increasing intracranial pressure.

In Figure 29-2, the location of common receptors that, when stimulated, initiate the vomiting reflex can be seen. Impulses are carried from these receptors to the vomiting center by way of peripheral, cranial, and autonomic sensory fibers. The *vomiting*

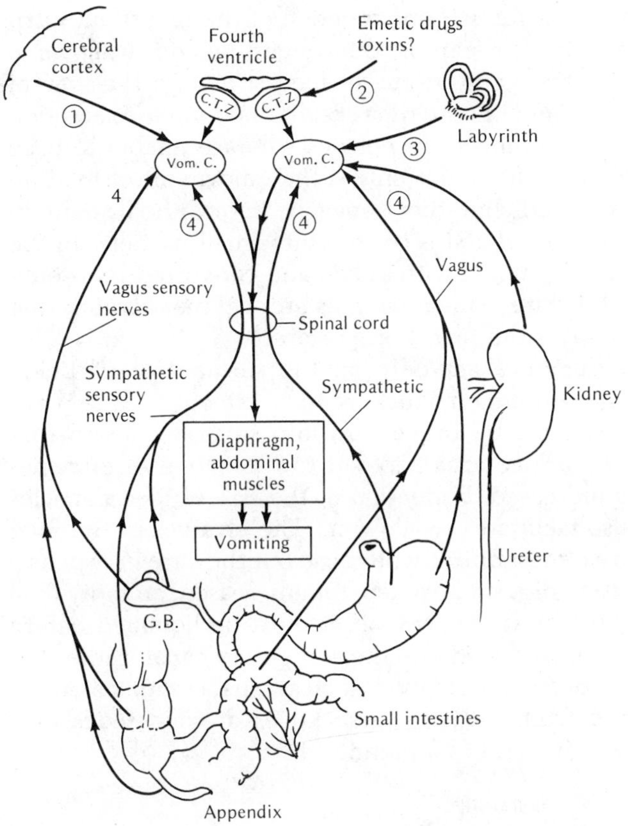

Figure 29-2. Mechanisms in the initiation of vomiting. *C.T.Z.*, chemoreceptor trigger zone; *Vom. C.*, vomiting center; *G.B.*, gallbladder; *1*, cerebral stimulation of vomiting center; *2*, drug stimulation of chemoreceptor trigger zone; *3*, labyrinthine (motion, etc.) stimulation of vomiting center; *4*, visceral afferent stimulation of vomiting center. (Adapted with permission of Macmillan Publishing Co., from *Modern Pharmacology and Therapeutics*, 4th ed., 1969, Fig. 27-1, p. 491, by Ruth D. Musser and John J. O'Neill. Copyright © by Macmillan Publishing Co., Inc., 1969).

center is located in the lateral reticular formation of the medulla oblongata. It is one of a number of visceral centers, such as the vasomotor, the defecation, the respiratory, and the salivation centers. These are all centers regulating the autonomic nervous system. During vomiting, there is additional evidence of autonomic activity, such as increased salivation, sweating, and bradycardia.

THE ACT OF VOMITING. From the vomiting center, impulses travel over efferent fibers of the vagus and phrenic nerves as well as those supplying the abdominal muscles. The act of vomiting usually begins with nausea, increased salivation, the secretion of large amounts of mucus, and what, for want of a better name, are called disagreeable sensations. During the period of nausea, the contents of the jejunum and the duodenum are emptied into the pyloric end of the stomach by strong sustained contraction of the small intestine. The pyloric sphincter and the pyloric end of the stomach contract and force the material into the body and fundus of the stomach, thus filling them. Vomiting is caused by the diaphragm and abdominal muscles contracting against the walls of the dilated stomach and forcing the contents through the open cardiac spincter into the esophagus. Vomiting cannot occur unless the cardiac sphincter relaxes. The hypopharyngeal sphincter also relaxes. The glottis is closed and is kept closed after inspiration, which takes place just as vomiting begins. Contrary to an old belief, the principal force in evacuating the stomach during vomiting is not reverse peristalsis of the stomach and esophagus, but contraction of the diaphragm and abdominal muscles. The unconscious patient, whether from general anesthesia or from some other cause, may aspirate vomitus because of failure to close the glottis during vomiting. Unconscious patients who are vomiting or are likely to vomit should be placed in a position favoring drainage from the tracheobronchial tree.

Other Defense Mechanisms

Like vomiting, *diarrhea* results in the removal of irritating substances from the alimentary canal. It is, however, almost always associated with a disease process or with an emotional disturbance. It will be discussed with disorders of motility.

Despite the effectiveness of primary defense mechanisms in preventing harmful agents from getting beyond the first lines of defense, they sometimes do. The internal environment is protected from general dissemination of injurious agents from the alimentary canal by *lymph nodes* and *phagocytes.* They function in protection just as they do in other parts of the body. The internal environment is further protected from the general dissemination of microorganisms and some potentially toxic agents by the *liver.* Bacteria in the blood circulating through the liver are destroyed by reticuloendothelial or Kupffer cells. Chemicals of extrinsic or intrinsic origin are detoxified or inactivated in the liver. To illustrate, the liver is the chief site of degradation of most barbiturates. Barbital and phenobarbital are exceptions, because they are mainly excreted by the kidney. Barbiturates excreted by the kidney have a more prolonged effect that those that are inactivated by the liver. Because persons who have severe liver damage are dependent on the kidney for the excretion of barbiturates, they are likely to experience toxicity when receiving barbiturates other than phenobarbital or barbital. Steroid hormones such as estrogen are degraded by the liver.

As in other structures in the body, tissues of the alimentary canal are capable of responding to injury by *inflammation* and by the formation of scar tissue.

Inasmuch as these responses help to limit the extent of injury and to restore the continuity of tissue, they are beneficial. Scar tissue located near or at the orifice of an organ or duct or encircling a part can cause obstruction as it contracts with maturity.

To recapitulate, in a structural facility where materials are transferred from the external into the internal environment, provisions for the protection of the internal environment from harmful agents are required. The internal environment is protected from the ingestion, absorption, and dissemination of potentially injurious substances by a variety of structures and mechanisms. The senses of sight, taste, smell, and touch can serve to warn the individual of the possible unsuitability of food or water for ingestion. Because sensory perceptions are not very accurate and are subject to conditioning, wholesome substances are sometimes rejected and harmful ones ingested. A continuous sheet of mucous membrane extending from the mouth to the anus acts as a mechanical barrier to the transfer of substances from the external to the internal environment. Mucus, secreted by the glands of the mucous membrane, provides a protective layer of material between the contents of the alimentary canal and the mucosa. Vomiting and diarrhea provide means for the removal of irritating materials. Semipermeability of the gastrointestinal mucosa as well as specific transfer mechanisms determine the size and type of materials absorbed into the internal environment. All of the above are only partly effective in preventing the absorption of injurious substances. The individual is protected from absorbed substances by phagocytic cells in the blood, lymph nodes, and liver. In addition to phagocytizing bacteria and other foreign substances, the liver decreases the activity of a variety of chemicals by altering their structures.

The mucous membrane lining the alimentary canal also requires protection from mechanical, chemical, and living agents, and from the digesting action of enzymes. It is really quite remarkable that the protective mechanisms are successful in preventing self-digestion as the protein-digesting enzymes of the alimentary canal do digest living tissue. The capacity of protein-digesting enzymes to act on living tissue can be observed when unprotected tissue is exposed to intestinal and pancreatic secretions or when the balance between the mechanisms protecting the lining of the alimentary canal from the protcolytic actions of digesting secretion is upset, as in peptic ulcer.

The Mouth

Functions

The normal entrance to the alimentary canal is the mouth, which also serves as a second entrance and exit for air. The function of the mouth in nutrition is to prepare food for digestion and swallowing. The taste and aroma of food stimulate the flow of saliva and initiate the reflexes that increase secretion in the stomach. In persons who are unable to taste or smell food, not only is the enjoyment of food diminished, but there may be some impairment in digestion. Food is broken into small particles in the mouth, mixed with saliva, and converted to a semisolid state. Saliva contains an enzyme, ptyalin, that initiates the digestion of starch.

Enzymes act only on the surfaces of particles. Therefore if enzymes are to be effective, large particles must be broken up into smaller ones so that the surface area exposed to the action of enzymes is increased. Reduction in the size of food particles also facilitates swallowing. The changes in the food are almost entirely physical, but they are indispensable to digestion. When, for any reason, an individual is unable to chew food, it must be liquefied before it is introduced into the alimentary canal. Either liquid or semiliquid foods such as milk, cream, oils, eggs, and fruit and vegetable juices or solid foods may be liquefield in a blender.

Swallowing

After food has been masticated, it passes from the mouth, by way of the pharynx and esophagus, to the stomach by the act of swallowing. Swallowing takes place in three stages. The first, or oral, phase is voluntary. The second, or pharyngeal, stage and the third, or esophageal, stage are involuntary. In the act of swallowing, food passes through the pharynx, which also serves as a passageway for air; therefore food must be transferred without entering either the nares or the glottis. Furthermore, particles too big to pass easily through the esophagus must be prevented from entering the pharynx.

Oral Stage

The first stage of swallowing is initiated after the food has been masticated and mixed with sufficient saliva to form a soft mass. It is then squeezed and rolled toward the posterior portion of the mouth by the pressure of the tongue moving upward and backward toward the palate. The tongue forces the bolus of food into the pharynx. At any time before the bolus reaches the pharynx, the act of swallowing can be stopped.

Pharyngeal Stage

As the food is pushed back, sensory receptors located in and around the pharynx are stimulated. Impulses are carried to the swallowing center located in the brainstem. Messages are sent from the brain to the pharyngeal area and a number of automatic actions are initiated. These begin with the closure of the posterior nares by the upward movement of the soft palate. This action prevents food from entering the nares. One of the characteristics of disorders wherein the soft palate is paralyzed or defective is the escape of food or fluid into the nose. In the patient who has a lesion in the nervous system, including the peripheral nerves, the escape of fluid or food through the nares should be regarded as prima facie evidence of paralysis of the soft palate. Food and fluid should be discontinued until the patient has been examined by the physician, because the patient is in danger of inhaling food or fluids.

Even more important than preventing food from entering the nares is protecting the airway below the glottis from the introduction of food. The swallowing, or deglutition, center in the brain acts to inhibit respiration as well as to facilitate the passage of food through the pharynx and into the esophagus. The glottis is closed by the approximation of the vocal cords, and the epiglottis moves backward to shield the superior opening into the larynx. The larynx is raised and moved out of the way and the esophagus is opened. All of this happens very quickly, and the bolus of food is moved rapidly through the pharynx into the esophagus. The pharyngeal stage of swallowing takes only about two seconds. Failure to closely approximate the vocal cords during swallowing always results in the introduction of food or fluid into the trachea. (See Chapter 26.) When food or fluids enter the larynx and trachea, a paroxysm of coughing or choking is initiated. Particularly in patients who have lesions in the nervous system, choking should be regarded as an indication that food and fluids should be discontinued until the patient has been examined by the physician.

Esophageal Stage

The third stage of swallowing takes place in the esophagus. After the bolus of food enters the esophagus, it is conveyed by peristalsis to the stomach. If the primary peristaltic wave, which begins when food enters the pharynx and continues over the length of the esophagus, is insufficient, secondary waves are initiated at the sites where the esophagus is distended. Peristalsis is considered to be weak in humans, and the movement of the bolus is assisted by gravity and the lubrication of saliva. Under normal conditions, the average length of time it takes food to pass through the esophagus is about 5 seconds.

Failure of Swallowing Reflex

Although the most immediate and serious danger attending failure of the swallowing reflex is aspiration of food or fluid into the airway, other problems are also created. One troublesome problem is the handling or disposal of saliva and other secretions in the mouth and upper respiratory tract. About 1200 ml of saliva are secreted per day, or about 100 ml each waking hour. When swallowing fails, saliva must be removed from the mouth by suction or by expectoration. Drooling is not only unpleasant and unesthetic, but saliva is injurious to the skin around the mouth, because a continuous state of wetness predisposes to maceration of the skin. When drooling cannot be prevented, the skin should be protected by the application of some water-repelling agent, such as petroleum jelly or zinc oxide.

The Stomach and Proximal Duodenum

Structure and Functions

The lower end of the esophagus is guarded by the cardiac sphincter, which prevents the reflux of acid chyme from the stomach into the esophagus. The esophageal mucosa is not protected against the digesting action of gastric juice, and repeated reflux of the acid gastric juice predisposes the esophagus to acid ulceration. The pyloric sphincter regulates the movement of gastric contents into the duodenum.

The functions of the stomach to be discussed are those relating to the preparation of food for absorption. The secretion of the intrinsic factor that facilitates the absorption of vitamin B_{12} is no less important in nutrition: however, because vitamin B_{12} is essential to the maturation of red blood cells, its functions are discussed in Chapter 42.

The stomach is divided into three parts: the fundus; the corpus, or body; and the antrum. The antrum is frequently, though incorrectly, called the pyloric or prepyloric region. Because the wall of the stomach has relatively little tone and the mucous and submucous coats form folds, or rugae, as the stomach empties, the size of the stomach is determined by the quantity of its contents. As food enters the stomach, it forms concentric rings with the most recently ingested food, nearest to the cardiac sphincter; food that has been in the stomach longest is nearest the pyloric sphincter.

During the time food remains in the stomach, it is mixed with the gastric secretions until a semifluid mixture called chyme is formed. When the stomach is empty and the pyloric sphincter relaxed, liquids may not remain in the stomach, but may pass immediately from the esophagus to the duodenum. When, however, a mixed diet is ingested, food remains in the stomach for varying periods of time and is slowly emptied into the duodenum. The rate of emptying depends on two factors: the fluidity of the gastric chyme, and the receptivity of the duodenum to receiving more chyme. The fluidity of the gastric chyme is determined by the type of food ingested, the completeness of mastication, the length of time food has been in the stomach, and the intensity of peristaltic waves. A meal of foods rich in fat remains in the stomach longer than a meal rich in carbohydrate but low in fat. Relatively large particles of food much be reduced in size before they can be emptied into the duodenum. The more intense peristaltic waves are, the less time chyme is likely to remain in the stomach.

Protection of Duodenum from Overloading

The duodenum is protected from overloading by regulation of its receptivity, which is determined by the quantity of chyme already present in the upper intestine, the acidity of the chyme, and the type of food in the chyme. As the duodenum fills, receptors initiate impulses that depress gastric peristalsis and at the same time increase contraction of the pyloric sphincter. A high concentration of fats in the chyme also diminishes gastric secretion. As fat or fatty acids enter the duodenum, glands in the mucosa secrete a hormone called enterogastrone, which is carried by way of the blood to the musculature of the stomach. Enterogastrone has an inhibitory effect on gastric muscle and on secretion of the gastric glands. In the presence of powerful inhibitors of the activity of the stomach, such as fat, peristalsis may be reversed and intestinal secretions regurgitated into the stomach. In general, products of protein digestion, acid, and nonspecific irritants in the duodenum act reflexively to diminish gastric activity and secretion. The effect of fats and fatty acids is mainly through the hormone enterogastrone. The coordinated functioning of the stomach and duodenum enables the stomach to be a storehouse for food and to prepare it for digestion. The duodenum is protected from overdistention and is provided with a more or less continuous stream of chyme. The importance of the regulation of the rate at which chyme enters the intestine is illustrated by the dumping syndrome, which is discussed in Chapter 46.

Gastric Secretion

Secretion into the stomach and duodenum is important in both health and disease. In the stomach and small intestine, foods undergo chemical and physical changes in preparation for absorption. Chemical reactions are catalyzed by enzymes capable of digesting not only food but also living cells. One of the factors in the activity of each enzyme is the pH of the fluid in which it works. Pepsin, an enzyme secreted into the stomach, is most active in an acid medium. In the absence of hydrochloric adic, pepsin is inactive. Chemical digestion in the stomach therefore depends on the presence of both hydrochloric acid and papsin. Direct contact with the cells lining the stomach is prevented by the secretion of mucin. Other factors, such as the blood supply to the mucosa, are also important to the defense of the gastroduodenal mucosa. Any condition upsetting the balance between digestion and protection predisposes to ulceration.

The secretion of hydrochloric acid in the stomach involves the neurogenic, chemical, and mechanical mechanisms, as well as systemically and locally acting hormones. As a result of the interaction of the various regulators, a balance between stimulation and inhibition is maintained. Digestion is accomplished, and at the same time the mucosa is protected.

Hydrochloric acid is secreted by the parietal cells in the corpus of the stomach. *Three phases, cephalic, antral,* and *intestinal* are involved. The *cephalic phase* of secretion is under nervous control. Stimulation of the vagus nerve increases the production of hydrochloric acid, whereas stimulation of the sympathetics, either by their direct effect on the acid-secreting glands in the stomach or by inhibition of the action of the vagi, lessens it. Usual stimuli initiating the cephalic phase of gastric secretion include the sight, smell, and taste of food. Even thoughts of good food, such as a thick steak or luscious lemon pie, may be sufficient to initiate the cephalic phase of gastric secretion. Impulses from distance receptors, such as the retina of the eye, travel to the cerebral cortex, where they are relayed to the hypothalamus. From the hypothalamus, secretory impulses are relayed to the glands in the stomach by way of the vagi. The cephalic phase of gastric secretion can be prevented by the sectioning of the vagus nerves. The procedure is known as vagotomy.

The *second phase* in gastric secretion is the *antral phase.* Whereas the cephalic phase prepares the stomach for food, the antral phase regulates the amount of acid secreted after food enters the stomach. The antrum does not secrete hydrochloric acid, but it secretes a hormone, gastrin, that stimulates the acid-secreting glands in the corpus of the stomach. When the acidity of the chyme is high, gastrin secretion lessens. When partial gastrectomy is performed in the therapy of peptic ulcers, the antrum is often removed, not because it secretes hydrochloric acid, but because it regulates the production of hydrochloric acid. Marginal ulcers[2] are more fre-

[2] Ulcers formed at the site of junction or anastomoses of the stomach and jejunum.

quent in patients in whom the antrum has not been removed.

The *third phase* in the secretion of hydrochloric acid is the *intestinal phase.* A hormone similar to, but not as powerful as, gastrin is believed to be secreted by the intestinal mucosa, but it has not been identified. The basis for this hypothesis is that gastric juice continues to be secreted when the stomach is empty. As indicated earlier, a high concentration of fat in the chyme entering the duodenum stimulates the production of enterogastrone, which decreases both gastric secretion and motility. Thus secretion into the stomach is regulated by nervous and hormonal factors. In health, secretion in the stomach illustrates one of the characteristics of a homeostatic mechanism; that is, a change in one direction is counteracted by increasing activity of processes acting in the opposite direction.

The mucosa lining the stomach is protected from digestion by a covering sheet of mucus. Mucous glands are located in the mucous membrane throughout the stomach. The mucosa of the duodenum is protected by alkaline mucus secreted by Brunner's glands. Secretion of mucus is constant, though the volume can be increased by the ingestion of irritating agents. Any failure to secrete mucus in adequate quantities reduces the protection of the underlying mucosa and increases its susceptibility to digestion.

In health, the mucosa of the stomach and adjacent duodenum is protected from digestion by the gastric juice, but other parts of the alimentary canal, such as the esophagus, lower duodenum, jejunum, and ileum, do not have the same degree of resistance. However, because bile and pancreatic juices are alkaline in reaction, they neutralize the acid chyme with the result that the lower duodenum, jejunum, and ileum are protected from injury.

The Middle Alimentary Canal

Structure and Function

The middle portion of the alimentary canal extends from the duodenal papilla to the midtransverse colon. It consists, therefore, of the lower duodenum, the jejunum, the ileum, the cecum, the ascending colon, and the first portion of the transverse colon. This portion of the digestive tube functions, as do other parts of the alimentary canal, to move its contents analward (toward the anus). Its specific functions are to dilute, digest, and absorb nutrients. Because the midportion of the alimentary canal is where nutrients are transported from the external to the internal environment, the most critical function of the alimentary canal as a service facility is accomplished here. With the exception of water, absorption of nutrients is largely completed before the intestinal contents reach the ileocecal valve. In terms of survival, the midalimentary tract is the most important region of the alimentary canal. Although a portion can be sacrificed, enough of the ileum must remain for the absorption of nutrients. Large quantities of fluid enter the jejunum from the duodenum and stomach, and secretions are added by the jejunum.

The ileocecal valve regulates the movement of material into the cecum and normally prevents the reflux of the contents of the colon into the small intestine. Acute obstruction of the colon distal to the ileocecal valve induces reverse peristalsis and relaxation of the valve. Reverse peristalsis may be sufficiently active to carry fecal material to the stomach, after which it is vomited. The emesis that results has a fecal odor. Needless to say, observation of the odor of vomitus is important.

The Lower Alimentary Canal

The lower portion of the alimentary canal extends from the midportion of the transverse colon to and including the anal sphincters. Because the portion distal to the ileocecal valve forms the large intestine and many of the disorders involving these structures are similar or involve the whole area, the entire large intestine will be discussed here.

The intestine, like other areas in the alimentary canal, is under control of the autonomic nervous system. Although defecation is largely a reflex action, it is subject to some voluntary control. Unless the contractions of the bowel are very powerful, defecation can be delayed for a time. The defecation reflex is similar to other reflexes in the body. Receptor cells in the rectum, which is normally empty, are stimulated by material entering the rectum. Impulses are carried to the defecation centers in the hypothalamus, where they are relayed to the intestinal muscles. Interconnections between the hypothalamus and the cerebral cortex make it possible for messages that modify the activity of the defecation center to be sent from the cerebral cortex to the hypothalamus. Feces are normally stored in the sigmoid and adjacent portions of the colon. The fecal content is moved to the storage areas and to the rectum by the same type of peristaltic action found in other parts of the alimentary canal.

A mass type of movement, known as the gastrocolic reflex, also occurs. It usually follows a meal or the ingestion of a glass or two of cold water or fruit juice on arising in the morning. The cold fluid moves rapidly through the stomach and into the deodenum and acts as a stimulus to activate the gastrocolic reflex. The entire small intestine is excited and the wave of contraction passes rapidly along the colon with the result that feces enter the rectum. Whether or not the anal sphincters are relaxed at this time will depend on the propulsive power of intestinal contractions and the cooperation of the individual with the reflex. For this treatment to be successful, the person should pay attention to the call to defecate. If he or she inhibits defecation, future efforts to defecate will be increasingly unsuccessful.

The Liver and Biliary Tract

In the preceding sections, the functions of the alimentary canal have been discussed. In addition to the secretions from glands in the mucosa of the alimentary canal, secretions from two glands external to but emptying into the duodenum have a significant role in digestion. These glands are the liver and pancreas.

Function of the Liver in Digestion

At this point, the function of the liver in digestion and absorption will be presented. Metabolic functions will be discussed later in this chapter. The liver functions in digestion by secreting bile. Because bile contains substances that are discharged into the internal environment, it is an excretion as well. Normally about 600 to 800 ml of bile are formed each day. The amount of bile synthesized varies inversely with the amount of bile acid returned to the liver through the enterohepatic circulation.

BILE. Bile formed in the liver is conveyed by a series of channels or ducts to the duodenum. Liver cells are arranged around ducts that join together to form larger ducts and finally leave the liver as the hepatic duct. The hepatic duct branches to form the cystic duct leading to the gallbladder where bile is stored and concentrated. The duct formed by the hapatic and cystic ducts is the common bile duct. It opens, usually in common with the duct of Wirsung from the pancreas, into the duodenum. The terminal portion of the common bile duct and the duct of Wirsung are known as the ampulla of Vater. The opening into the duodenum is guarded by a muscle called the sphincter of Oddi. For the structural relationships of these organs see Figure 29-3.

Storage of bile: Between meals, bile, which is secreted more of less continuously, is stored in the gallbladder, where it is concentrated. When fat enters the intestine, a hormone, cholecystokinin, is secreted by the intestinal mucosa and carried to the gallbladder by way of the blood. It stimulates the muscle in the gallbladder to contract, thus forcing the bile out into the bile ducts. At the same time the sphincter of Oddi relaxes and bile enters the duodenum along with the pancreatic juice.

Functions of bile salts: Of the constituents of bile, the only ones functioning in digestion and absorption

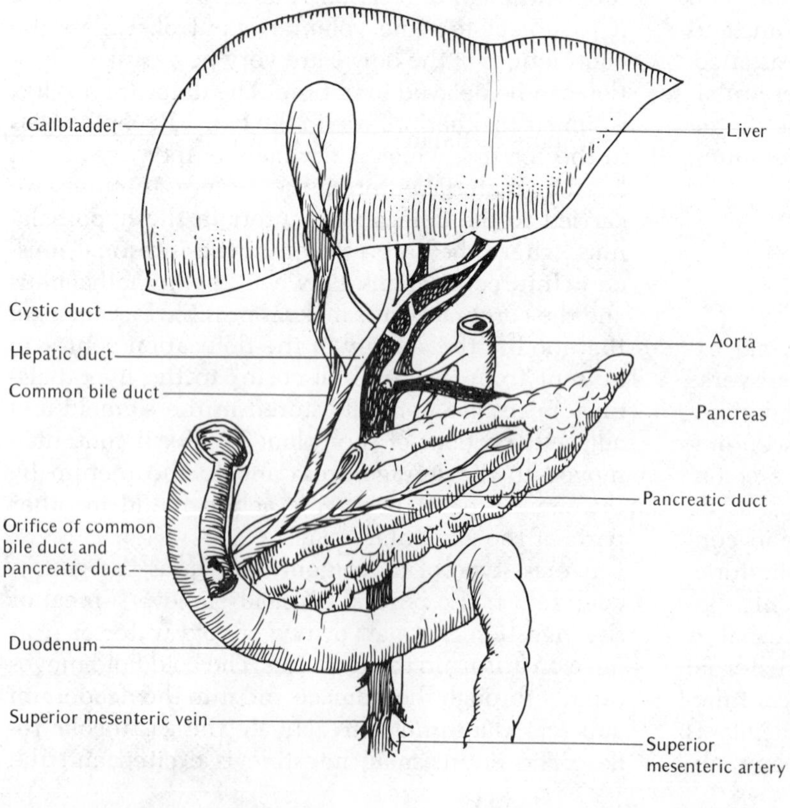

Figure 29-3. Diagram showing relationships of the pancreatic and bile ducts and their entrance into the duodenum. Where might obstructions be located to produce jaundice? (Adapted with permission of Macmillan Publishing Co., Inc., from *Textbook of Physiology,* Fig. 100, p. 278, by Caroline E. Stackpole and Lutie C. Leavell. Copyright © Macmillan Publishing Co., Inc., 1953.)

are the bile salts. Bile salts are formed by the neutralization of cholic acid in the liver and secreted as sodium and potassium salts. Bile acids are made from cholesterol and are an important means of excreting this steroid. The action of bile salts is similar to that of a detergent. They lower the surface tension of fat so that the fat globules suspended in the watery chyme can be broken up and prevented from merging again. Many small droplets offer a larger surface on which enzymes can act.

Even more important than their action in facilitating the digestion of fat, bile salts are required for the absorption of fatty acids, mono- and triglycerides, and fat-soluble vitamins. In the absorption of fats, bile salts are reabsorbed and returned to the liver to be resecreted.

Because bile is alkaline in reaction—its pH is between 8.0 and 8.6—it helps to neutralize the acid chyme entering the duodenum. Under some circumstances bile is regurgitated into the stomach, where it has a similar effect. Enzymes in pancreatic and intestinal juice require a pH of about 7 for optimum function.

Cholesterol: In addition to the secretion of bile salts, bile contains substances that are excreted from the body, such as cholesterol and bilirubin. Cholesterol is synthesized in the body and ingested in food. The liver is the chief organ in which cholesterol is synthesized but it is formed in lesser quantities in other tissues, such as the adrenal cortex, the intestines, and the skin. It appears that both in the intestines and the liver, cholesterol synthesis is primarily under the control of bile acids. Cholesterol absorption from the intestines is inefficient and slow. Although the level of cholesterol in the blood can be lowered by decreasing the quantity ingested in the diet, synthesis by the liver and other tissues prevents it from being eliminated from the blood. In fact, a lowered concentration of dietary cholesterol causes an increased synthesis of cholesterol in the liver as dietary cholesterol acts as negative feedback for hepatic cholesterol synthesis (Wilson, 1972). (See also Lipid Metabolism, page 449.)

Metabolism

Cellular Functions

The quality of nutrition depends not only on the kinds and amounts of food supplied to the body and its preparation by the digestive tract for absorption but also on the capacity of the organisms to carry out its physiologic and biochemical functions. *Intermediary metabolism* is used to describe all the changes taking place within cells of the internal environment, including the building-up, breaking-down, and functional activities. It is often thought of as those activities beginning at the point where digestion has been completed. The intestinal wall, thought of as part of the external environment, is involved in the active transport of materials and in the synthesis of many compounds, and these activities are properly included in intermediary metabolism. Thus one cannot draw a sharp line of demarcation.

Anabolism

The synthesis of larger molecules from smaller ones is known as *anabolism;* for example, the production of the various structural components of the cell itself or the synthesis of compounds secreted by the cells such as enzymes, hormones, and others. Cellular proteins are synthesized from amino acids, fats from fatty acids or glucose, and so on. The anabolic activities are energy-saving.

Catabolism

On the other hand, *catabolism* is the breaking up of large molecules to smaller ones. Thus glucose, fatty acids, glycerol, and amino acids are oxidized to yield the energy required for the synthetic and functional activities of the cell. The breakdown of energy-containing compounds yields lower energy compounds or carbon dioxide and water, and, in the case of amino acids, urea.

Metabolic Balance

Anabolic and catabolic activities take place continuously throughout life and are equal in the healthy adult who has no net change in body size. When new tissues are being added to the body, the anabolic activities exceed the catabolic activities, as during the growth of children, pregnancy, and the period of recovery from illness or injury. Catabolic processes exceed anabolic processes during weight loss whether planned or occasioned by starvation, serious illness, or trauma from injury.

Functional Activities

Among the functional activities of the cells are contraction of the muscles, the transmission of nerve impulses, the secretion of glands, the selective absorption from the intestine, and the excretion of waste products by the kidneys and other organs. Homeostasis is maintained by continuous regulation of the transport of materials across the cell membranes and of the extracellular fluid environemnt of the cells. For example, the sodium ion is continuously entering the cell, yet in health it does not accumulate there. Energy is required to prevent the sodium ion concentration in the cell from approaching the concentration of the extracellular fluid.

Energy, glucose, fatty acid, amino acid, and calcium metabolism represent just a few of the many aspects of intermediary metabolism. Space as well as the complexity of each of these aspects of metabolism permits only the briefest summary in this text. Many textbooks of biochemistry are available for the student who desires further details of a specific aspect of metabolism.

Some General Aspects of Metabolic Process

Oxidation Reduction

The chemical reactions within the cell that release energy are primarily oxidative. According to the electron theory, oxidation is a process whereby one or more electrons are given up. As a result, electrons are lost, valence raised, oxygen added, or hydrogen removed. The compound that causes oxidation is always reduced. Therefore, oxidation always involves reduction, the basic change in the latter being a gain in electrons; that is, the valence is lowered, oxygen is lost, or hydrogen is added. Thus to have oxidation reduction, a substance donating electrons and another accepting electrons must be present.

Maintenance of a Constant Supply of Materials for Metabolic Activities

The Metabolic Pool

The body maintains a supply of nutrients instantly available for the regulation of its activities and the maintenance of homeostasis. This is often referred to as the *metabolic pool,* which is an intimate combination of the nutrients available through absorption from the intestinal tract plus those that are constantly released by the catabolic and secretory activities of the cell. The metabolic pool must not be thought of as having a specific body location; it is rather that instant availability of essential nutrients at any given site to carry out any given activity. For example, the metabolic pool of amino acids would include those from the intestinal tract, those released by the breakdown of cellular proteins, and those derived from cellular synthesis. From this assortment, cells could withdraw the exact kinds and amounts of amino acids required for the synthesis of any given protein.

Nutritional Needs of Cells

Cellular function depends on an adequate supply of (1) energy-producing materials, chiefly glucose, fatty acids, glycerol, and amino acids; (2) tissue-building materials, including a complete assortment of about twenty amino acids, some fatty acids, carbohydrates, and mineral elements such as calcium, phosphorus, sodium, potassium, magnesium, and many others; and (3) materials for the synthesis of a myriad of such regulatory substances are enzymes and hormones. Many of these regulatory substances are of a protein nature and therefore require varying assortments of amino acids. Some incorporate specific carbohydrates or lipids, or both. Trace elements such as iron, manganese, fluorine, iodine, molybdenum, selenium, zinc, copper, and others are essential as are also the fat-soluble and water-soluble vitamins. In all, more than fifty nutrients are required for cellular function.

Enzymes as Catalysts

Oxidation-reduction reactions depend on innumerable enzymes, each of which acts on a specific chemical bond. Each enzyme either donates or receives electrons. The maintenance of metabolic activities depends on the capacity of the cell to synthesize enzymes and to synthesize or recover chemicals needed to keep the process going. For example, pyruvic acid ($CH_3COCOOH$) is subjected to oxidative decarboxylation and reacts with coenzyme A to form acetyl coenzyme A. The acetyl coenzyme A is combined with oxaloacetic acid to form citric acid. For the cycle to continue, oxaloacetic acid must be either recovered or synthesized. See Figure 29-4.

The activity of the enzymes is related to the concentration of materials on which they act, the pH of the environment, and the temperature. The use of hypothermia in certain surgical procedures is based on the fact that the rate of metabolism in cells is reduced by lowering of body temperature. As body temperature is lowered, enzyme activity is reduced and the rate of metabolism is diminished.

Enzyme Cofactors

Many enzymes require coenzymes or cofactors for their activity. These usually are compounds of low molecular weight that may be tightly bound as a prosthetic group to the protein part of the enzyme molecule or they may be loosely attached to the protein. Most vitamins function as coenzymes in enzyme systems that control cellular activity. For ex-

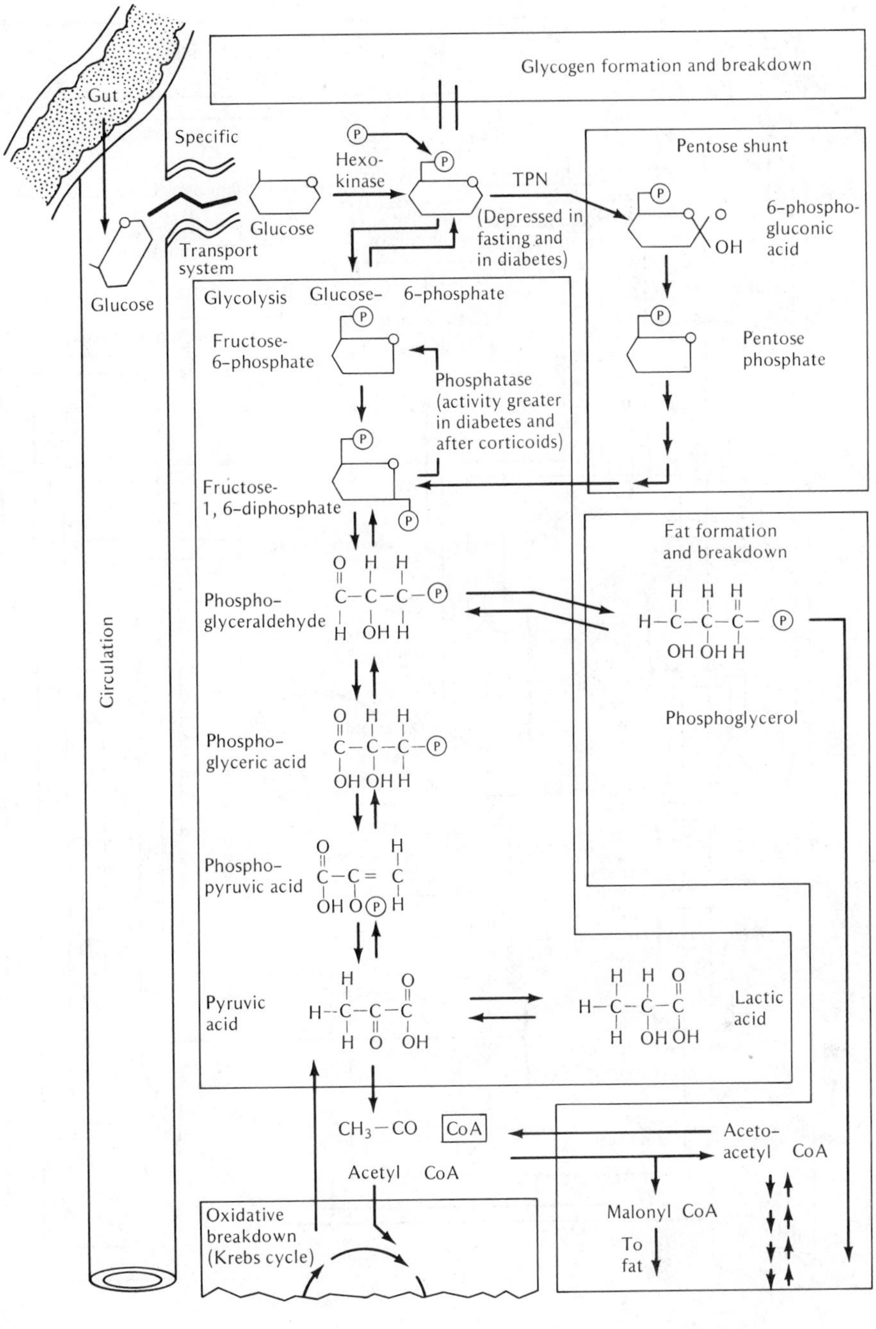

Figure 29-4. Glycolysis—the conversion of glucose to pyruvic acid and lactic acid. (Copyright 1965 CIBA Pharmaceutical Company, Division of CIBA-GEIGY Corporation. Reproduced, with permission, from *The CIBA Collection of Medical Illustrations* by Frank H. Netter, M.D. All rights reserved.)

ample, thiamine pyrophosphate, a coenzyme known as cocarboxylase, is the prosthetic group for the enzyme carboxylase. This enzyme is essential for the removal of the carboxyl group from pyruvic acid, an intermediate product in the metabolism of glucose (see Figure 29-5). When thiamine is lacking in the diet, insufficient carboxylase is available for decarboxylation to proceed, and pyruvic acid accumulates in the blood. The interference with carbohydrate metabolism at this point is serious, and, if uncorrected, leads to the classic deficiency disease, beriberi.

Riboflavin, niacin, pantothenic acid, biotin, vitamin B_{12}, folacin, and vitamin B_6 are also constituents of coenzymes and therefore are intimately associated with energy and amino acid metabolism. Ascorbic acid and vitamins E and K probably have coenzyme functions, but these are not clearly understood at the present time. The role of vitamins in enzyme activity helps to explain the correlation of dietary requirements with the caloric and protein needs of the individual. A deficiency of any of the coenzymes interferes with the metabolic machinery so that succeeding steps in anabolism or catabolism cannot take

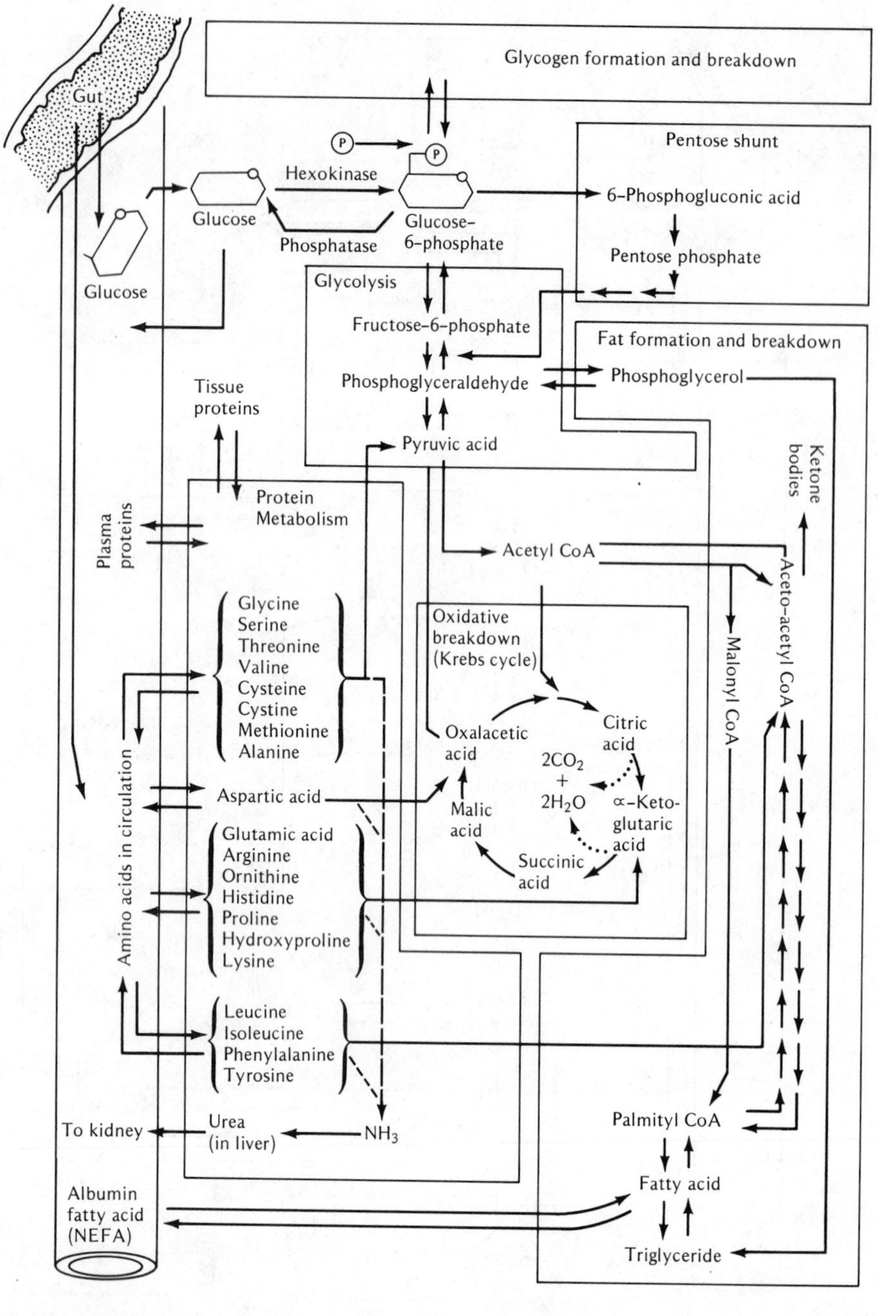

Figure 29-5. Protein metabolism. (Copyright 1965 CIBA Pharmaceutical Company, Division of CIBA-GEIGY Corporation. Reproduced, with permission, from *The CIBA Collection of Medical Illustrations* by Frank H. Netter, M.D. All rights reserved.)

place. Hence the resulting symptoms are those of multiple deficiencies rather than of specific failure of one metabolic step.

Mineral elements are also important cofactors for enzyme activity. They include magnesium, iron, copper, molybdenum, zinc, manganese, and others.

Control of the Rate of Energy Metabolism

Hormonal Controls

The rate at which enzymes catalyze chemical reactions is subject to control by hormones, or "chemical messengers." More than 20 hormones have been isolated and studied. They include those produced by the ductless glands, such as the thyroid, parathyroid, pancreas, adrenal, and pituitary. Some of their effects will be detailed in the sections that follow.

Sources of Energy

The carbohydrates, fats, and proteins of the diet are the ultimate sources of all energy for the body. In typical diets of the United States, carbohydrates furnish about 45 to 55 per cent, fats about 40 to 45 percent, and proteins about 15 per cent of the calories. In the developing countries of the world carbohydrate is responsible for as much as three fourths of the total energy value of the diet.

The body itself is provided with energy reserves that are utilized throughout each day and that can maintain the organism for a surprising length of time when no food is ingested. Glycogen constitutes a relatively small, readily available reserve, but, at best, it can supply the energy needs for only part of one day. Adipose tissue, on the other hand, furnishes a substantial and continuous reserve of energy that can, in emergency, be relied on for days or even weeks. When starvation continues, some cellular substance is also sacrificed to supply calories. Because of the loss of fat and other tissue substances, weight declines. The loss of weight decreases the quantity of tissue requiring support; and because of a loss of strength, less energy is utilized for nonsurvival purposes. The body's own substance is thereby used more slowly and life can be further prolonged.

Energy Transfer

The central mechanism in bringing about the transfer of energy is the reversible system of adenosine triphosphate (ATP) and adenosine diphosphate (ADP). When glucose, for example, is converted to glycogen, energy is required to bring about the reaction. The energy is furnished by splitting off a high-energy phosphate group from ATP. The remaining compound, having one less phosphate group, is ADP. When glucose is oxidized to carbon dioxide and water, some of the energy set free in the reaction is used to rebuild ATP from ADP. In this way the body maintains a constant source of high-energy bonds.

This system operates in a wide range of anabolic activities including the synthesis of acetylcholine for the transmission of the nerve impulse, sugar phosphates, proteins from amino acids, urea by the liver, and ammonia by the kidney. ATP also provides the energy for the absorption of sugars from the intestine and the reabsorption of glucose by the kidney.

Muscle cells also synthesize creatine phosphate, another high-energy phosphate compound. This is an available store of energy for the contraction of the muscle fiber.

Common Denominator

Three major stages characterize the degradation of carbohydrates, fats, and amino acids to furnish energy for cellular activities. In the first, glucose, fatty acids, and amino acids are converted through a series of independent steps and catalyzed by individual enzymes, to molecules serving as "common denominators" for all. These are pyruvic acid, acetyl coenzyme A, and alpha-ketoglutaric acid. Little energy is released in this stage. These common molecules then enter the last two stages to be converted to energy, carbon dioxide, and water.

The Citric Acid Cycle

The second stage in the release of energy is known as the citric acid, tricarboxylic acid or Krebs cycle. The first molecule in the ring to be metabolized is citric acid. The molecules in the cycle are three-carbon groupings, and Krebs first described the reactions. The routes by which carbohydrates, fats, and proteins reach the cycle, as well as the changes taking place within the cycle, are shown in Figures 29-4, 29-5, and 29-6. The reactions are cyclic because the series of compounds involved are utilized and regenerated so that the chain can start over again whenever another molecule of pyruvic acid or acetyl coenzyme A is available for oxidation.

Respiratory Cycle

The third stage is known as the respiratory cycle. It consists of the removal of carbon dioxide from the body via respiration and the combination of hydrogen atoms with oxygen available through respiration into water. Each of the steps in the transfer of hydrogen to oxygen requires specific enzyme activity.

Energy Requirement

Food energy is required to maintain the resting metabolism, the body temperature, the voluntary activity, and the synthesis of new tissues. The recommended allowance for the 23-year-old male engaged in light activity and weighing 70 kg (154 lb) is 2,700 kcal, and for the 23-year-old female weighing 58 kg (128 lb) it is 2,000 kcal (*Recommended Daily Dietary Allowances,* 1974). By age 65 these allowances for men and women who have maintained their same weights and levels of activity have been reduced to 2,400 and 1,800 kcal, respectively. The 11- to 14-year-old boy weighing 44 kg (97 lb) needs 2,800 kcal, and the girl of the same weight and age needs about 2,400 kcal. These allowances take into account such factors as body size, age, activity, climate, and growth needs.

Body Size

In general, the large individual has a greater energy requirement than the small one. An obese adult, however, because he or she has less lean body mass and is less active, may not have a greater energy requirement than the person of normal size. Small animals have a higher metabolic rate than larger ones, with the result that they require more food per unit of mass. A bird or mouse requires more food per gram of body weight than an elephant. An infant, who has a relatively large surface area and

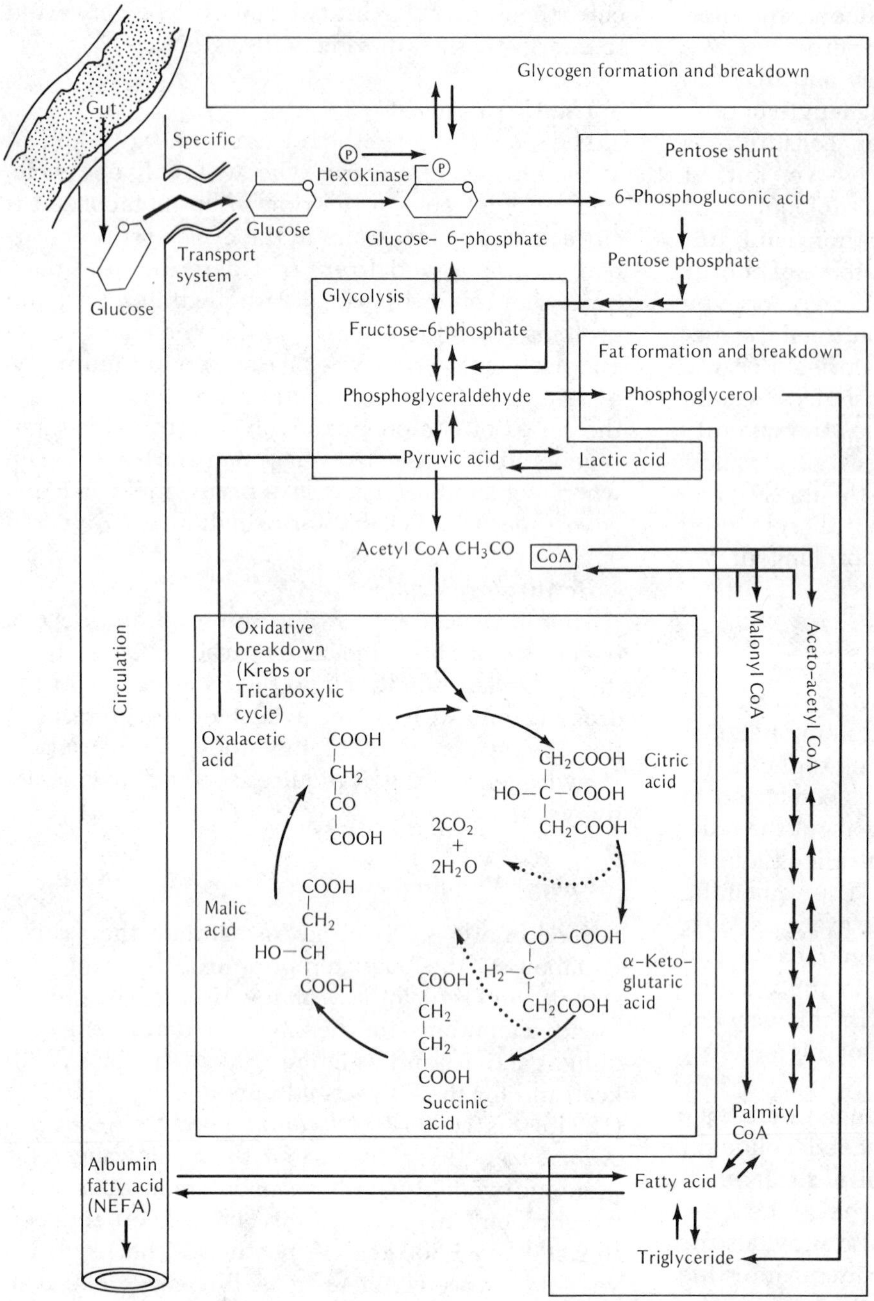

Figure 29-6. Oxidative breakdown (the Krebs cycle). (Copyright 1965 CIBA Pharmaceutical Company, Division of CIBA-GEIGY Corporation. Reproduced, with permission, from *The CIBA Collection of Medical Illustrations* by Frank H. Netter, M.D. All rights reserved.)

high rate of metabolism, requires more calories per kilogram of body weight than does the adult.

Lean Body Tissue

Males generally require more calories than do females because of greater body size and greater proportions of lean body tissue. Beginning with early adulthood (about 22 years), a steady decline in caloric need takes place. This is explained in part by the reduction in lean body mass and hence in basal metabolic rate and in part by a gradual diminution in voluntary activity. Nevertheless, there is no decrease in the number of calories required by an older person to perform any given activity. Mrs. Bird requires as many calories to walk a mile as does her 16-year-old grandson who weighs the same as she does.

Activity

Voluntary activity is an important factor in determining the energy requirement but it is somewhat difficult to make a precise estimate for the various levels of work and play. The recommended allowances have been set up for people whose activity may be described as "light." For many inactive persons in the Unites States these allowances could result in weight gain. The individual who is engaged in heavy labor might require up to 900 kcal in excess of the stated allowances.

Climate

Extremes of climate will affect the need for energy, but for most people in the United States the heating of buildings in winter and their cooling in summer together with adjustments in the clothing worn tend to equalize the calorie requirments throughout the seasons. Exposure to severe cold weather increases the calorie expenditure to maintain the body temperature, and shivering rapidly increases the energy expenditure. The wearing of heavy cold-weather clothing and footwear further adds to the energy need. Surprisingly, physically active people living in tropical areas have a higher calorie requirement than those in temperate climates at the same level of activity because of the energy needed to dissipate additional heat from the body.

Growth

Rapid growth greatly increases the calorie requirement. Infants, for example, require 100 to 120 kcal per kilogram to support their growth, their considerable activity, and their proportionately large surface area. By comparison, the calorie allowance for a 13-year-old boy is about 63 kcal per kilogram and for his 45-year-old father is only 38 kcal per kilogram.

The development of the fetus and the maternal tissues during pregnancy represents a considerable need for energy as well as for all nutrients, most especially during the last trimester. Many women decrease their activity during this period so that the addition of about 300 kcal usually suffices. Lactation would increase the need by 500 kcal.

Carbohydrate Metabolism

Dietary Sources

Wheat is the chief cereal grain in the North American diet, but corn and rice are also widely used. Potatoes and sugars are also significant sources of carbohydrate, with other fruits and vegetables contributing much smaller amounts. In worldwide use rice leads all grains. Other rich sources of carbohydrate used in some parts of the world are millet, plantain, cassava, and a variety of legumes. No specific requirements have been established for dietary carbohydrate. Moreover, no particular level of carbohydrate is most conducive to health.

Digestion and Absorption

About 98 per cent of the carbohydrate in the typical American diet is hydrolyzed to the simple sugars, chiefly glucose, and lesser amounts of fructose and galactose; the remainder is indigestible fiber. The principal mechanism for absorption is active transport, involving the phosphorylation of glucose (the addition of a molecule of phosphate available from ATP). The capillaries of the intestinal wall empty into the portal vein, which in turn carries the glucose to the liver.

Maintenance of Homeostasis in the Metabolism of Carbohydrates

Blood Glucose

The intermittent ingestion of carbohydrate and the constant requirement of the body for energy suggest the need for mechanisms to maintain homeostasis at all times. The blood glucose level, kept within a limited range, is the key to this control, just as the liver is the principal organ for the regulation of the blood sugar. A number of hormones complement or oppose one another in the maintenance of the blood sugar and in the metabolism of carbohydrate by the tissues. The nervous system is also involved in the control mechanism.

The sugar of the blood is glucose, just as the principal carbohydrate metabolized in the tissues is glucose. The relatively small amounts of fructose and galactose from digestion are converted to glucose by the liver. Normally, the blood sugar level ranges from 70 to 110 mg per 100 ml of blood. Immediately after a meal it rises to 130 mg per 100 ml or so, but drops relatively soon to the lower levels. The level of glucose at any given moment is the balance between the sources of glucose to the blood and the demands made on it by the tissues. A change in one direction is counteracted by the activation of mechanisms that correct the change. The result is change within limits. Only when there is a disturbance in these mechanisms does the blood sugar rise to abnormal levels (hyperglycemia), as in diabetes mellitus, or fall abnormally (hypoglycemia), as following an overdose with insulin.

BLOOD SOURCES OF GLUCOSE. Three general sources of supply for the blood glucose are (1) the simple sugars resulting from absorption from the small intestine; (2) glycogenolysis, or the breakdown of glycogen in the liver; and (3) gluconeogenesis, or the formation of glucose from the amino acids and other substances by the liver.

Less than 1 lb of glycogen is stored in the body, about four fifths of this in the liver. Muscle glycogen is available for glucose in the muscle cell, but it does not add to the glucose level of the blood. Glycogen reserves within the liver would be depleted within a few hours by a fasting individual in order to maintain the blood glucose. Thus the liver glycogen may be thought of as a short-term or emergency supply to meet the tissue energy needs.

When glycogen levels are depleted the blood sugar level is maintained through the breakdown of amino acids by the liver. About half of the amino acids deaminized in such a situation yield available glucose. The glycerol fraction of the fats that are broken down is also a source of glucose and accounts for about one tenth of the fat molecule.

REMOVAL OF GLUCOSE. Six ways to remove glucose from the blood are listed by West and his associates (1966): (1) by the cells for utilization as energy; (2) by the liver for storage as glycogen; (3) by conversion to fat and storage in adipose tissue; (4) for the synthesis of compounds such as lactose, mucopolysaccharides, glycolipids, and nucleic acids; (5) by glycolysis in the red blood cells; and (6) by excretion in the urine when the renal threshold has been exceeded. The renal threshold is that level of the blood glucose beyond which sugar will appear in the urine. It is somewhat variable from one individual to another, but generally it is about 160 to 180 mg per 100 ml of blood. During prolonged hyperglycemia, as in uncontrolled diabetes mellitus, the renal threshold is often above 200 mg per 100 ml. The formation of fat in the form of adipose tissue from glucose represents the body's mechanism for ensuring a long-term reserve of body fuel, as contrasted to the short-term stores available from glycogen.

HORMONAL CONTROL. The pancreas, adrenal, and pituitary glands secrete hormones that influence the blood sugar level and the metabolism of carbohydrate by the tissues. Increased blood glucose levels stimulate the secretion of insulin, the pancreatic hormone produced by the beta cells of the islands of Langerhans. Insulin increases the rate of oxidation of glucose by the tissues and the rate of glycogen and fat formation. Thus the blood sugar is lowered. Glucagon, another pancreatic hormone, probably produced by the alpha cells, increases the rate of glycogen breakdown to glucose, thereby increasing the blood sugar level.

The cortex and medulla of the adrenal gland produce a number of hormones that influence the blood sugar level. If an experimental animal is adrenalectomized, it becomes extremely sensitive to insulin, but this sensitivity is reduced when glucocorticoids are injected. Patients with Addison's disease have reduced function of the adrenal cortex and characteristically have a hypoglycemia. This is corrected when glucocorticoids are administered. The glucocorticoids secreted by the adrenal cortex increase the production of glucose and glycogen from amino acids and decrease the use of glucose by the tissues. Because the glucocorticoids are antagonistic to insulin, their administration would increase the severity of diabetes mellitus. The accelerated breakdown of amino acids brought about by the glucocorticoids results in a greater excretion of nitrogen in the urine. In fact, undesirable breakdown of tissue protein may accompany the administration of these hormones.

Epinephrine, sometimes described as an emergency hormone, is secreted by the adrenal medulla under conditions of severe emotional stress or activity. Its effect is to bring about a rapid breakdown of liver glycogen to glucose and to increase the rate of use of muscle glycogen. In extreme emotional states, the amount of hormone secreted may be sufficiently great to produce a transient hyperglycemia.

Somatostatin, a polypeptide isolated from the hypothalamus and gastrointestinal tract, is a potent inhibitor of both glucagon and insulin. Prolonged infusions of somatostatin result in hyperglycemia and hyperketonemia, but its exact role in fuel metabolism is not clear.

The hormones of the pituitary affecting carbohydrate metabolism are of two types: (1) those having a direct effect and (2) the tropic hormones having an effect on the secretion of other glands, thus indirectly affecting metabolism. Somatotropin (the growth hormone) increases the blood glucose levels by increasing gluconeogenesis, by antagonistic effects on the activity of insulin, or by the release of glucagon or other hyperglycemic factors. Adrenocorticotropic hormone (ACTH) stimulates the secretion of the adrenal cortex and thereby glucose and glycogen production by gluconeogenesis.

The thyroid hormone increases the rate of absorption of glucose from the intestine and increases peripheral utilization of glucose. Because the thyroid hormone regulates the rate of metabolism in the tissues, any excess or deficiency of the hormone would correspondingly affect the rate of glucose metabolism.

UTILIZATION OF CARBOHYDRATE. The chief source of energy to the body is carbohydrate. One gram of dietary carbohydrate, on the average, yields 4 kcal.[3] Brain tissues use glucose exclusively, and even after a short period of severe hypoglycemia the brain ceases to function, and irreparable damage may result.

Glucose is utilized as a source of energy according to the steps outlined in Figures 29-4 and 29-5. The glucose is phosphorylated by the addition of first one and then a second phosphate group and is broken down anaerobically (without the addition of oxygen) to lactic or pyruvic acid. Within the muscle cell the breakdown of glucose to lactic acid produces a small

[3] The kcalorie (kcal) refers to the kilogram calorie, which is equivalent to the heat energy required to raise the temperature of 1 kilogram of water 1°C.

release of energy that permits the muscle to operate until sufficient oxygen is brought from the blood. About four fifths of the lactic acid produced in the muscle is reconverted to glycogen, and the remainder is converted to pyruvic acid. The pyruvic acid is decarboxylated by carboxylase to acetic acid, is activated by coenzyme A, and enters the citric acid cycle, as described in a preceding section of this chapter.

Glucose is essential to prevent the excessive metabolism of fats. Whenever the breakdown of fatty acids exceeds the availability of glucose to "prime" the citric acid cycle, an accumulation of short-chain fatty acids takes place in the blood, and the condition is known as ketosis or acidosis. In the normal individual a temporary ketosis is produced by a very low-carbohydrate or low-calorie diet or by starvation. Gradually, the normal individual adjusts by increased glycogen production from amino acids. In diabetes mellitus, however, the failure to utilize glucose is accompanied by excessive breakdown of fats and their accumulation as keto acids. The effects of acidosis in diabetes mellitus are discussed in Chapter 47. Occasionally ketosis is intentionally produced in treating young children with epilepsy by using diets high in fat, somewhat restricted in protein, and reduced to less than 40 g of carbohydrates per day. A diet high in fat content (ketogenic diet) is unpleasant, and therefore difficult for patients to follow for long periods (Glaser, 1971).

Glucose is also said to be protein-sparing. In other words, when ample glucose is available through the absorption of dietary carbohydrate or from liver stores of glycogen, amino acids need not be used to form glucose.

Lipid Metabolism

Lipids include fats, oils, and many other fatlike substances. Body lipids include triglycerides or neutral fats, phospholipids, free fatty acids, cholesterol, and other substances of a fatlike nature.

Nutritional Role

The chief contribution made by dietary fats is to the energy needs of the body. Typical American diets supply about 35 to 45 per cent of calories from fats. In some parts of the world, especially in the Orient, the fat intake may account for only 10 to 15 per cent of the calories. When metabolized, 1 g of fat yields about 9 kcal. Fats improve the flavor of many foods thereby increasing food acceptability, increase the satiety value of the diet by reason of the longer time required for digestion, and serve as carriers for the fat-soluble vitamins.

Lipids are distributed in all body cells and tissues. Most of the body fat occurs as neutral fat in the adipose tissue located beneath the skin, in the abdominal area, and surrounding the organs. Adipose tissue normally represents about 15 to 20 per cent of the body weight. It is the long-term reserve of body fuel, for we have seen that the glycogen stores would suffice for less than a day in the absence of food.

Body fats serve in the cushioning of the organs and as insulation against changes in the environmental temperature. Phospholipids and cholesterol abound in active tissues and are essential for the absorption and transport of fats. Phospholipids and glycolipids are also integral components of nervous tissue. Arachidonic acid, a polyunsaturated fatty acid, is required for growth and normal skin health in infants. This fatty acid is probably required for the transport of lipids and is invovled in the permeability of the cells.

Dietary Sources

About 60 per cent of dietary fat is supplied by "invisible" sources: meats, poultry, fish, dairy products (excluding butter), egg yolks, and baked foods. The remaining 40 per cent is furnished by "visible" fats including butter, margarine, lard, hydrogenated shortenings, oils, and salad dressings.

The type of fat is an important dietary consideration inasmuch as saturated fats are believed to increase the level of the blood cholesterol whereas fats predominating in polyunsaturated fatty acids appear to have a cholesterol-lowering effect. Beef, pork, lamb, whole milk, cream, cheese made from whole milk, ice cream, butter, and egg yolk are rich in saturated fatty acids; poultry and fish contain somewhat higher proportions of the polyunsaturated fatty acid, linoleic acid. Most vegetable oils including safflower, sunflower, seasame, cottonseed, corn and soybean oils, are rich sources of linoleic acid. By contrast, peanut oil is only moderately high, and coconut and olive oils are low in linoleic acid.

By hydrogenation, oils become solid fats, the level of saturated fatty acids increases, and the level of linoleic acid is reduced. Thus even a vegetable oil high in linoleic acid is no longer a good source when it is converted to margarine or a hydrogenated shortening. Special-type margarines that have been only lightly hydrogenated are now available in most markets. It is obviously an oversimplification and error to state that animal fats are saturated and vegetable fats are unsaturated.

Phospholipids and cholesterol are readily synthesized by the liver and other organs and a dietary source is not essential. High dietary intakes of cholesterol are believed to increase the blood cholesterol levels. Rich dietary sources include egg yolk, liver, brains, kidney, shellfish, and sweetbreads. Butter, cream, whole milk, ice cream, and fatty meats are moderately high. Plant foods contain no cholesterol. The reduction of the dietary intake of cholesterol is not effective by itself in regulating blood cholesterol levels, for the enterohepatic cycle of cholesterol and bile acids serves to regulate the synthesis of cholesterol in the liver through negative feedback. Therefore, with a decreased exogenous intake of cholesterol there is an increased endogenous synthesis of cholesterol in the liver.

Digestion and Absorption

A small amount of emulsified fat may be hydrolyzed in the stomach, but the chief site of fat digestion is in the small intestine. Bile reduces the surface tension and increases the emulsification of fats so that they are more readily attacked by pancreatic lipase. The products of hydrolysis include monoglycerides, free fatty acids, and glycerol. The intestinal mucosa resynthesizes new fat so that the products absorbed include triglycerides and phospholipids, free fatty acids, and glycerol.

Normally about 95 per cent of the dietary fats are digested and absorbed. Fats high in saturated fatty acids are more slowly digested than those that are unsaturated, but there is little if any difference in the amounts that are eventually absorbed. Likewise, fried foods are more slowly digested although the completeness of digestion is not, as a rule, adversely affected.

The absorption of fats is facilitated in the presence of bile and phospholipids. Short-chain fatty acids and glycerol are water soluble and enter the capillaries of the intestinal wall and in turn the portal vein. The insoluble longer-chain fatty acids, triglycerides, phospholipids, cholesterol, and fat-soluble vitamins proceed into the lacteals, the lymph circulation to the thoracic duct, and then to the left subclavian vein.

Blood Lipids

Because they are insoluble in water, lipids are transported in the blood associated with more or less protein, phospholipid, and cholesterol. The complexes are broadly classed as alpha and beta lipoproteins. The alpha lipoproteins (high-density) remain relatively constant throughout life, but certain classes of the beta lipoproteins (low-density) increase with age.

The serum or plasma of a sample of blood taken after a meal rish in fat will be milky in appearance because of the high level of circulating lipids. After a few hours this turbidity disappears resulting from the action of clearing factors including heparin, lipoprotein lipase, and arachidonic acid.

Increased levels of certain classes of beta lipoproteins are believed to correlate with the incidence of atherosclerosis and coronary disease. The determination of total lipid, cholesterol, phospholipid, and triglyceride levels in the blood is less expensive and appears to be as useful for identifying high-risk individuals. When such determinations are ordered they should be made on blood samples drawn after an overnight fast.

Control Mechanisms for Anabolism and Catabolism of Fats

The Liver and Fat Metabolism

The key organ in fat metabolism is the liver. It shortens or lengthens fatty acid chains; synthesizes triglycerides, cholesterol, or phospholipids and attaches them to proteins for transport to the tissues; and hydrolyzes the triglycerides brought to the liver. The normal metabolism of fats in the liver proceeds only when one or more lipotropic factors are present; these are methionine, betaine, choline, vitamine B_{12} and inositol. When these factors are missing, fats accumulate in the liver.

The liver is the chief source of the ketone bodies—acetoacetic acid, beta-hydroxybutyric acid, and acetone. The acetoacetate molecule is not efficiently metabolized by the liver and passes to the peripheral tissues that normally oxidize ketones at the rate they are produced by the liver. During fasting the oxidation of endogenous fat is increased to compensate for the decreased energy available from glycogen. The production of ketones by the liver may exceed the ability of the tissues to use them so that a mild ketosis results, and 5 to 10 g of ketones may be excreted in the urine. This is corrected by giving carbohydrate to replenish liver glycogen. In uncontrolled diabetes mellitus, ketones are produced at a rapid rate but the peripheral tissues have a decreased capacity to oxidize them; in severe diabetes the excretion of ketones may exceed 100 g per day, and acidosis is severe. The ketosis is corrected by giving insulin to restore carbohydrate metabolism.

HORMONAL CONTROLS. The uptake of glucose from the blood by adipose tissue is facilitated by the action of insulin. Fatty acid and triglyceride synthesis is also stimulated by insulin. The release of free fatty acids from adipose tissue to the circulation is brought about by epinephrine, norepinephrine, glucagon, adrenocorticotropic hormone, growth hormone, thyrotropic hormone, and somatostatin.

SYNTHESIS OF FATS. Many body organs and tissues including the liver, lactating mammary glands, kidney, intestinal mucosa, arterial walls, and adipose tissue itself can synthesize fats. Adipose tissue consists chiefly of triglycerides. Contrary to widely held opinions, it is a rapidly changing tissue with free fatty acids being constantly released to the circulation and new triglycerides being resynthesized. Thus adipose tissue is effective in maintaining blood lipid levels within limits.

Fats, carbohydrates, and amino acids are donors of acetate, which, activated by coenzyme A, is the key unit in the synthesis of fatty acids. Thus an energy supply in excess of body needs, whatever the source of calories, will lead to rapid synthesis of adipose tissue. The acetate unit can be condensed with another unit to form acetoacetate; in turn, another acetate unit may be added, thereby gradually lengthening the fatty acid chain.

Various tissues also possess the ability to modify the degree of saturation of fatty acids as well as the length of fatty acid chain. Thus arachidonic acid can be synthesized from linoleic acid by adding an acetate unit and introducing two additional double bonds. On the other hand, the tissues are not able to introduce a second double bond into the oleic acid molecule to produce linoleic acid. Therefore linoleic acid is an essential fatty acid that must be present in the diet.

Phospholipids are produced by the small intestine, liver, and kidney. Cholesterol is readily synthesized from acetate units by the liver, adrenal, kidney, and lung. Just as acetate units available from excess calorie intake lead to increases in adipose tissue, so also the synthesis of cholesterol increases when calories are in excess of body needs.

OXIDATION OF FATS. Beta oxidation, first described by Knoop, is probably the main pathway for fat oxidation. According to this theory, two carbon atoms are split off from the fatty acid chain at the time. The acid (COOH) group is combined with coenzyme A and through a series of steps the acetate unit is split off. For example, stearic acid, containing eighteen carbon atoms, would eventually yield nine acetate units. The acetate units, as we have seen, may be used to resynthesize fatty acids or cholesterol, or they may be further oxidized by combining with oxaloacetate and entering the citric acid cycle to yield energy, carbon dioxide, and water. The glycerol fraction of triglycerides follows the pathway of glucose in its oxidation. (See Figures 29-4 and 29-5.)

PROTEIN METABOLISM

Nature of Proteins and Dietary Sources

Proteins are composed of 20 or so amino acids, each of which contains an acid (COOH) group and an amino (NH_2) group. Eight of the amino acids are classified as dietary essentials because they cannot be synthesized in the body. The remaining twelve or so amino acids are nonessential because the body can synthesize them, provided that some source of nitrogen is available. Proteins that contain all of the essential amino acids in sufficient amounts to synthesize new tissues as well as to maintain them are known as *complete.* Milk and milk products (except butter), eggs, meats, poultry, and fish are excellent sources of complete proteins.

When a protein lacks one or more of the essential amino acids, or has a deficient quantity of them, it is classified as *incomplete;* it is not able to meet the needs for synthesizing tissues. The proteins in cereal grains, legumes, nuts, fruits, and vegetables are incomplete. Nevertheless, cereal grains and legumes are important sources of protein because they are staple foods for much of the world's population; the amounts of these foods eaten usually meet the protein needs for the maintenance of the healthy adult. On the other hand, plant-food diets, for the most part, do not contain sufficient amounts of some amino acids to meet the growth needs of infants, children, or pregnant or lactating women or the replacement needs of people convalescing from severe undernutrition. Even a small quantity of complete protein foods eaten at the same meal with these less expensive plant-food sources will yield an amino acid combination that is satisfactory for growth needs. For example, bread is a relatively inexpensive source of protein and of calories. If bread is served with milk, the combination of amino acids will be satisfactory; nonfat dry milk is an inexpensive way to improve the protein quality of bread.

Most of the world's population has little complete protein available; the result is severe protein malnutrition among millions of infants and children. A number of approaches are being used in an effort to solve this problem: (1) Foods are developed that contain proteins from several plants. The mixtures are based on the principle that some plants are good sources of certain of the essential amino acids, whereas others supply a different assortment of amino acids. By combining the foods, the final product yields all the essential amino acids in satisfactory amounts; one food is said to *supplement* another. *Incaparina* is such a product developed in Central America for feeding infants and young children; it consists of corn and cottonseed meals, yeast, and sorghum. Many similar products have been developed in other countries of the world, using foods native to the countries. (2) Fish is an excellent source of protein and relatively inexpensive but has not been utilized as widely as it might be. Fresh fish farming has been introduced, especially in the rice-growing countries. The fish are grown in the rice paddies. Also, fish protein concentrate is now prepared in the United States and in some developing countries. This is a creamy white, practically flavor-free powder containing about 80 per cent protein. Its keeping qualities are good, an important consideration in countries of the world where refrigeration is practically nonexistent. It can be used to reinforce the protein content of breads and other foods. (3) Agricultural geneticists have developed strains of corn, rice, and wheat that are richer in some essential amino acids than the usual varieties of these grains. Lacking amino acids may be added in synthetic form to foods to improve their protein quality. (4) Leaf protein, coconuts, soya, and other oilseeds can be refined in simple village industries and flourish in many countries in which animal protein is lacking. (5) Such microorganisms as yeasts, fungi, and algae have the potential to become an important protein source. However, this is possible only where sophisticated technology exists.

Utilization of Protein

About 92 per cent of dietary proteins are hydrolyzed to amino acids in the small intestine and then absorbed into the capillaries of the intestinal wall. The amino acids are carried by the portal vein to the liver and then enter the general circulation. The amino acids are rapidly incorporated into the existing tissues or used for synthesizing new tissues; they may be used for the production of numerous regulatory compounds; they may be deaminized and used for energy or stored in the form of glycogen or fat.

Proteins are part of the structure of every tissue in the body and are components of all body fluids except sweat, bile, and urine. Tissue proteins are in a state of dynamic equilibrium; that is, cells are constantly disintegrating and new ones are replacing them. For example, the cells of the intestinal mucosa are completely replaced every few days and those of the liver almost as rapidly. The turnover rate is somewhat slower in muscle, but the large mass of muscle tissue represents a sizable daily interchange.

Proteins have innumerable regulatory functions inasmuch as they are components of enzymes and hormones. The blood proteins include hemoglobin involved in the transport of oxygen, fibrinogen as one of the factors in blood clotting, globulins that function in the defense against disease, and serum albumin for the maintenance of the osmotic pressure of the blood and fluid balance of the tissues. The amino acids have specific functions; for example, tryptophan is a precursor of niacin and of serotonin, a vasoconstrictor; methionine has lipotropic activity in the liver and is essential for the formation of phospholipids; and glycine is involved in the detoxification of benzoic acid in the liver and the formation of bile acids, purines, and fatty acids.

Proteins are also a source of energy, each gram of protein yielding about 4 kcal when oxidized in the body. Amino acids that are not used for building tissues are deaminized, that is, the amino group is split off. The remainder of the molecule is an organic acid that can enter the citric acid cycle to yield energy (see Figure 29-6), or that can be transformed into glycogen or fat. The energy needs of the body take priority over the synthesis of tissues. Therefore, if the diet does not supply sufficient calories from carbohydrates and fats, the protein of the diet as well as body glycogen, fat, and tissue protein will be used to complete the energy requirement. Under these circumstances the synthesis of tissue proteins will be curtailed. If optimum tissue building is to take place, whether in childhood or in recovery from illness, the caloric adequacy of the diet—as well as that of protein—is essential.

Most of the deamination of amino acids takes place in the liver where the amino group is used to synthesize urea, the principal nitrogen compound in the urine. The liver may also bring about the transfer of an amino group (transamination) to an organic acid, thus forming the nonessential amino acids. The kidney is able to utilize the amino group for the synthesis of ammonia that, in the form of ammonium salts, helps to conserve the sodium ion and thus aids in maintaining acid–base balance.

Nitrogen Balance

The level of protein metabolism can be determined by measuring the nitrogen balance. Because protein is approximately 16 per cent nitrogen, 1 g of nitrogen is equivalent to about 6.25 g of protein. In nitrogen balance studies the nitrogen content of the food consumed is compared with the nitrogen content of the excretions. Most of the nitrogen excreted is in the urine, chiefly as urea. The measurement of the nitrogen in a 24-hour collection of urine is a reliable indicator of the preceding metabolism of protein that has taken place. The daily excretion of nitrogen in the feces usually ranges from 0.5 to 1.5 g depending on the nature of the diet ingested. The fecal excretion includes the nitrogen from undigested protein and from bacterial cells and the disintegrated proteins of enzymes and cells of the intestinal mucosa.

If the nitrogen intake and excretions are equal, the individual is in *nitrogen balance,* which is the normal state for the healthy adult. If the nitrogen intake is greater than the nitrogen output, the individual is in *positive balance.* This means that anabolic processes are greater than catabolic processes, the expected situation in growth of infants and children, in the development of maternal and fetal tissues during pregnancy, in the production of milk during lactation, and in the recovery from illness, injury, or surgery. *Negative nitrogen balance* is an unfavorable sign for it means that nitrogen is being lost from the body more rapidly than it is supplied by the diet.

The body does not store protein in the same sense that it stores fat. Nevertheless, the tissues are able to yield some protein to maintain important functions when the intake is inadequate. These *labile* reserves permit the adult to function for comparatively long periods of time with a deficient intake of protein. For young children, the consequences of protein deprivation are much more acute.

Recommended Allowance

The recommended allowance for protein for the adult male weighing 70 kg is 0.71 g per kilogram body weight, or about 0.32 g per pound (*Recommended Daily Dietary Allowances,* 1974). Because of anabolic requirements, the needs for infants, children, and adolescents and for pregnant and lactating women are somewhat higher per unit of body weight. The calorie needs should be essentially met from carbohydrates and fats. At least one third of the dietary protein of adults should be derived from complete protein foods; one half to two thirds of the child's protein allowance is preferably furnished by complete protein foods.

Mineral Elements and Vitamins

Mineral elements and vitamins have numerous metabolic roles, many of which have been discussed in some detail in other chapters of this book. The discussion that follows is intended to summarize briefly some of the pertinent facts regarding these important body components. A number of texts in nutrition may be consulted by the student who desires more detailed discussion of one or more of these nutrients.

Scope of the Regulatory Functions

Metabolic Role

Mineral elements constitute only about 4 per cent of the body weight. Calcium alone accounts for about half of this and phosphorus for about one fourth, the bones and teeth being the chief site of the calcium-phosphate salts. Magnesium is also an important element in the bone structure, and sodium and fluorine occur in small amounts. Potassium is the chief mineral element within the cells of the soft tissues. Sulfur, a constituent of the amino acids methionine and cystine, is present in all protein tissues.

The regulatory functions of minerals are numerous, such as the maintenance of fluid and electrolyte balance, involving principally sodium, potassium, and phosphorus (see Chapters 27 and 41); the transport of materials across cell membranes—for example, phosphorus as a constituent of the phospholipids; the maintenance of nerve irritability and muscle contraction based on the precise concentrations of the sodium, potassium, magnesium, and calcium ions in the body fluids; the activity of the parathyroid and thyroid hormones, involving calcium and iodine, respectively; and the transport of blood gases by hemoglobin of which iron is an essential constituent. Trace elements, sometimes called micronutrients, are constituents of, or catalysts for, enzymes and hormones. For example, zinc is a component of insulin, iodine of thyroxine, and cobalt of vitamin B_{12}. Copper, chromium, selenium, and molybdenum were once considered to be contaminants of the diet and in the body but are now established as essential for the activation of specific enzymes.

Vitamins are organic compounds that are required in minute amounts in the diet for specific functions in the body. They differ greatly in their molecular structure, from the relatively simple ascorbic acid molecule to the exceedingly complex vitamin B_{12} molecule. Likewise, they differ in their physical and chemical properties and in their biologic functions. Generally speaking, vitamins function as coenzymes and are involved in highly specialized metabolic processes that have been described previously in this text. For example, vitamin B_{12} and folacin are required for the synthesis of red blood cells in the bone marrow (see Chapter 42); thiamine, riboflavin, and niacin are essential for the activity of many enzyme systems including those for the release of energy from carbohydrates and fats as discussed in this chapter; pantothenic acid is a component of coenzyme A that activates the acetyl group for its entrance into the citric acid cycle or for the synthesis of fatty acids and cholesterol; vitamin B_6 is essential for the metabolism of amino acids and for the conversion of linoleic acid to arachidonic acid; and so on. Ascorbic acid, or vitamin C, is essential for the formation of collagen, and thus is important in the integrity of the blood vessel walls and the connective tissues; its lack results in poor wound healing, hemorrhages, and eventually scurvy (see Table 46-3, in Chapter 46). The B-complex vitamins and ascorbic acid are stored in the body only to a limited extent. A moderate diet deficiency leads to gradual depletion of the tissues and within a period of a few months to such nonspecific signs as fatigue, weakness, neuritis, and poor resistance to infection. If the deficiency in the diet is great, the symptoms of classic deficiency disease will become manifest within months. For example, infants who are given a formula that is deficient in ascorbic acid and with no supplementary foods that are rich in this vitamin will show unmistakable signs of scurvy by the age of 6 to 8 months.

Vitamin A is essential for the integrity of the epithelial tissues, including the mucous membranes and in the regulation of vision in dim light. The liver stores vitamin A so that a person who has had a good intake will suffer few if any ill effects even after months of dietary lack. Yet it should be remembered that many people, especially adolescents, are consuming diets that fail to supply the recommended allowances. As a consequence nutritional surveys have shown lowered blood levels of vitamin A and associated night blindness. Severe vitamin A deficiency, as characterized by keratinization of the epithelium, xerophthalmia, and permanent blindness, is a major health problem particularly in the Far East.

Vitamin D is required for the utilization of calcium and phosphorus (see Chapter 41); its lack is responsible for rickets in young children. Vitamin E is important for its antioxidant properties, and vitamin K in the formation of prothrombin.

Summary

Because of the importance of food, physiologically, emotionally, and socially, it provides the nurse with a natural medium through which to convey to the patient concern for him or her as a person and as a human being. It is often through the nurse's efforts to meet patients' individual wishes and desires that the food is "transferred from the plate to the stomach." Although it may be a cliché to say "It isn't the food that is served to the patient, but what he eats that is important," it is true, nonetheless.

The theme of this chapter is summarized in the words of King (1963):

> Nutrition is the science of food, the nutrients and other substances therein, their action, interaction and balance in relation to health and disease, and the processes by which the organism ingests, absorbs, transports, utilizes, and excretes food substances. In addition, nutrition must be concerned with certain social, economic, cultural, and psychological implications of food and eating.

References Cited

Brown, L. R., and Eckholm, E. P. *By Bread Alone.* New York: Overseas Development Council by Praeger, 1974.

Freeman, H. Q. *Hunger and Malnutrition in the United States: How Much?* Washington, D.C.: Congressional Research Service, Library of Congress, May 1, 1975.

Glaser, G. H. "The Epilepsies." In *Cecil-Loeb Textbook of Medicine,* 13th. ed. Ed. by P. B. Beeson and W. McDermott. Philadelphia: W. B. Saunders Co., 1971, p. 271.

Henkin, R. I. "The Molecular Basis of Taste and Its Disorders." *Ann. Intern. Med.,* **71** (Oct. 1969), 791–821.

Jelliffe, D. B., and Jelliffee, E. F. "Human Milk, Nutrition, and World Resource Crisis." *Science,* **188** (May 1975) 557–61.

King, C. G. "A Conference on Nutrition Teaching in Medical Schools." In O. C. Johnson article. *Nutr. Rev.,* **21** (Feb. 1963), 34.

Leininger, M. "Some Cross-Cultural Universal and Nonuniversal Functions, Beliefs, and Practices of Food." In *Dimensions of Nutrition.* Ed. by J. Dupont, Boulder: Colorado Associated University Press, 1970, pp. 153–79.

Lepkovsky, S. "Newer Concepts in the Regulation of Food Intake." *Am. J. Clin. Nutr.,* **26** (March 1973), 271–84.

Manual for Nutrition Surveys, 2nd. ed. Bethesda, Md.: Interdepartmental Committee on Nutrition for National Defense, National Institutes of Health, 1963.

Mead, M. *Cultural Patterns and Technical Change. UNESCO,* (1953), p. 213.

Recommended Daily Dietary Allowances. Washington, D.C.: Food and Nutrition Board, National Academy of Sciences, National Research Council, 1974.

Shapiro, L. R., Huenemann, R. L., and Hampton, M. C. "Dietary Survey for Planning a Local Nutrition Program." *Public Health Rep.,* **77** (March 1962), 257–66.

Sinclair, M. I. "Another Man's Hunger." *World Health,* **15** (Sept.–Oct. 1962), 8.

West, E. S. et al. *Textbook of Biochemistry,* 4th ed. New York: Macmillan Publishing Co., 1966, p. 1039.

Wilson, J. D. "The Role of Bile Acids in the Overall Regulation of Steroid Metabolism." *Arch. Intern. Med.,* **130** (Oct. 1972), 493–505.

World Health, **16** (March 1963), 30.

"World Hunger: Too Little Food? Or Too Many People?" *Environmental Fund,* 1974 (Congressional Testimony).

General References

Metabolism

Bierman, E. L., and Nelson, R. "Carbohydrates, Diabetes, and Blood Lipids." *World Rev. Nutr. Dietet.*, **22** (1975), 280.
Blackburn, H. "How Nutrition Influences Mass Hyperlipidemia and Atherosclerosis." *Geriatrics*, **33** (Feb. 1978), 42.
Cummings, J. H. "Nutrition Implications of Dietary Fiber." *Am. J. Clin. Nutr.*, **31** (Oct. 1978), 521.
Schrauzer, G. W. "Trace Elements, Nutrition and Cancer: Perspectives and Prevention." *Adv. Exp. Med. Biol.*, **91** (1977), 323.
Thomas, A. D. "Alcohol and Nutrition." *Clin. Endocrinol. Metab.*, **7** (July 1978), 405.
Yek, J. K. et al. "Dietary Constituents and Somatomedin Activity." *Metabolism*, **27** (May 1978), 507.

Malnutrition

Butterworth, C. E. "The Skeleton in the Hospital Closet." *Nutr. Today*, **9** (March–April 1974), 4.
"The Fight against Malnutrition in the World." *WHO Chron.*, **31** (July 1977), 276.
Gopalan, C. "Malnutrition: The Major Health Problem of the World." *Int. J. Health Ed.*, **20** (1977), 74.
Jellifee, D. F. "Commerciogenic Malnutrition." *Nutr. Rev.*, **30** (Sept. 1972), 199.

Obesity

Bray, G. A. "The Overweight Patient." *Adv. Intern. Med.*, **21** (1976), 267.
———. "Obesity." *Dis-A-Month*, **26:**1 (Oct. 1979).
Charney, E. et. al. "Childhood Antecedents of Adult Obesity: Do Chubby Infants Become Obese Adults?" *New Engl. J. Med.*, **295** (July 1976), 6.
D'Augelli, A. R., and Smiciklas-Wright, H. "The Case for Primary Prevention of Overweight through the Family." *J. Nutr. Ed.*, **10** (April–June 1978), 76.
Felig, P. "Four Questions about Protein Diets." *N. Engl. J. Med.*, **298** (1978), 1026.
Garn, S. M., and Clark, D. C. "Trends in Fatness and the Origins of Obesity." *Pediatrics*, **57** (1976), 443.
Heydman, A. H. "Intestinal Bypass for Obesity." *Am. J. Nurs.*, **74** (June 1974), 1102.
Leon, G. R. "Current Directions in the Treatment of Obesity." *Psych. Bull.*, **83** (July 1976), 557.
Musante, G. J. "Obesity—A Behavioral Treatment Program." *Am. Fam. Physician*, **10** (Dec. 1974), 95.
Perfontaine, M., and Cormier, A. "Does Behavior Modification Work for Obese Young Adults?" *J. Nutr. Ed.*, **9** (Jan.–March 1977), 31.
Weil, W. B. "Current Controversies in Childhood Obesity." *J. Pediatrics*, **91** (Aug. 1977), 175.

Food Supply, Nutritional Problems, and Nutritional Status

Hegsted, D. M. "Priorities in Nutrition in the U.S." *J. Am. Dietet.*, **71** (July 1977), 9.
Margen, S., and Lindsey, H. A. "What to Look for in the Nutritional Examination." *Consultant*, **43** (March 1976).
Taylor, K. B. "Nutrition and Diseases of the Gastrointestinal Tract." *Prog. Food Nutr. Sci.*, **1** (1975), 225.
Walters, H. "Difficult Issues Underlying Food Problems." *Science*, **188** (May 9, 1975), 524.
"The World Food Situation and Prospects to 1985." Washington, D.C.: U.S. Department of Agriculture, Economic Research Service, Foreign Agricultural Economic Report no. 98, 1974.

Nutritional Care and Dietary Counseling

Cross, J. E., and Parsons, C. R. "Nurse Teaching and Goal Directed Nurse Teaching to Motivate Change in Food Selection Behavior of Hospitalized Patients." *Nurs. Res.*, **20** (Sept.–Oct. 1971), 454.

Recommended Reading

Donaldson, R. M., Jr. "Diets for Gastrointestinal Disorders." *JAMA*, **225** (Nov. 1973), 1243.
Dwyer, L. S., and Fralin, F. G. "Simplified Meal Planning for Hard-to-Teach Patients." *Am. J. Nurs.*, **74** (April 1974), 664.
Zerfas, A. J. et al. "Office Assessment of Nutritional Status." *Pediatr. Clin. North Am.*, **24** (Feb. 1977), 253.

SECTION THREE

Nursing Management of Common Clinical Problems

UNIT VII

The Psychosocial Aspects of Illness and Injury

An optimist is a person who sees a green light everywhere. The pessimist sees only the red light. But the truly wise person is colorblind.

ALBERT SCHWEITZER

In the preceding units the concept was developed that human beings have physiologic and psychosocial needs that must be met if the individual is to survive, grow, reproduce, and otherwise be productive. Although it is often easier to understand the complex organism called *human being* by compartmentalizing him or her according to psychological, physiological, and social functions, we must remember that humans are holistic beings—that is, beings in whom all of these parts interact to make up a unified whole. What affects one part of the person has an impact on all of him or her. Therefore, illness in any of its many forms has an effect upon humans in the psychological, physiological, and social dimensions of their being.

Each person has a physical self that not only enables him or her to react to change in the physical and social environment, but also helps to determine the limits of the individual's capacity for adaptation. Adaptation to change, within oneself or within one's environment, is dependent not only upon the individual's psychological and physiological capacities, but also upon the individual's intellectual capacity, innate and learned cognitive and coping skills, and the multitude of environmental forces that influence the way one perceives one's situation and, in turn, reacts to it. The overall capacity varies from individual to individual, and within the same individual from time to time. In short, factors that influence the process of adaptation derive from intraindividual, interpersonal, societal, cultural, and environmental forces.

Folta and Deck (1966) indicate that the health professional needs to develop a conception of life that goes beyond his or her own life in order to "become aware of and knowledgeable about the multiplicity of streams that crisscross every aspect of human endeavor" (p. 3). Rogers (1970), in her discussion of the theoretical basis for nursing, tells us that

> Professional practice is creative and imaginative. It is rooted in abstract knowledge, intellectual judgment, and

The overview of Unit VII is contributed by Jean A. Werner-Beland, Associate Professor of Nursing, Wayne State University, College of Nursing, Detroit, Michigan.

human compassion. There are no set formulas by which action is determined. Nor are there rules of thumb subject to memorization and unquestioning application. The tools of the practice are numerous, but their appropriate selection according to the needs of an individual, a family, or society is dependent upon intellectual skill (p. 122).

I would add that professional practice is also dependent upon the availability of certain tools, and upon the spiritual, psychological, social, and other factors that influence the ability of the professional to use them. In this chapter the content has been selected to provide the nurse with beginning knowledge of some of the factors to be considered if the psychosocial needs of patients with medical-surgical problems are to be met. The student of nursing should consider this a mere introduction and be reminded that much has been written elsewhere about these issues. It is not within the scope of this book to discuss the causes and effects of extreme disturbances in the interpersonal or social spheres of the individual. This unit deals with the fact that illness causes a shift in a person's equilibrium that produces a change in the way he or she functions personally, interpersonally, and so on. Although an attempt was made to speak to various issues in discrete sections of the unit, this was rarely possible. Humans cannot be compartmentalized easily.

How a person responds to illness depends upon the meaning he or she attaches to the illness as a potential life threatening event. The person is also influenced by the values that family, society, and culture place on the *sick role,* on the causal factors that thrust him or her into that role, and on relevant age-appropriate behaviors. Response is also influenced by the response of others within the health delivery system. In other words, how the person reacts to illness and how others treat him or her, depends upon an interplay of meanings that the person and significant others attach to the illness and behavior. In addition, how he or she is treated also depends upon the interplay of all these factors on the care giver.

To provide a common understanding of the points to be discussed throughout this chapter, the terms *psychology, society,* and *culture* will be defined:

Psychology is defined as, "The science which deals with the mind and mental processes—consciousness, sensation, ideation, memory, etc." (Hinsie and Campbell, 1970, p. 614). Thus psychology is primarily interested in the study of the individual as a thinking, remembering, imagining, feeling, and reacting person. In actuality, psychology is a complex field made up of many overlapping subfields, each of which looks at select factors (intrapersonal and interpersonal) that influence individual or group behavior. In nursing we are especially concerned with the wide spectrum of psychological phenomena included in ecological psychology. Ecological psychology is "concerned with both molecular and molar behavior, and with both the psychological environment (the life-space in Kurt Lewin's terms; the world as a particular person perceives and is otherwise affected by it) and with the ecological environment (the objective, perceptual context of behavior; the real-life settings in which people behave)" (Barker, 1968, p. 1).

Society refers to the association of individuals in organized relationships of mutual dependence (Biesanz and Biesanz, 1964). Biesanz and Biesanz indicate that the system of society includes the division of labor persisting within a certain time and place and the sharing of common goals. *Sociology* is "the systematic study of the development, structure, and function of human groups conceived as processes of interaction or as organized patterns of collective behavior" (Webster's Seventh New Collegiate Dictionary, 1969, p. 828). *Social* is an adjective used to describe the relationship of one person to another.

Culture, according to LeVine (1973), "is an omnibus term designating both the distinctively human forms of adaptation and the distinctive ways in which different populations organize their lives on Earth" (p. 3). Acquired behavioral characteristics or patterns of culture are the unique ways one human population as opposed to another implement their common adaptive abilities. LeVine goes on to say, "I use the term *culture* to mean an organized body of rules concerning the ways in which individuals in a population should communicate with one another, think about themselves and their environments, and behave toward one another and toward objects in their environment" (p. 4). Culture refers to understandings concerning the value of things, ideas, emotions, and actions—it even defines how one should feel and behave in various situations—during illness, when there is a reason to express joy, and so on. Culture is peculiar to humans in that it arises out of language communication (Biesanz and Biesanz, 1964). Animals such as the wolf organize into societies, but they cannot be said to posses a culture.

Sciences such as sociology and cultural anthropology deal with social action and human behavior. Together with psychology they are classified as behavioral sciences. LeVine (1973) states that this whole broad field could be assigned a complex label such as psychosocial studies, or it can be broken into its disciplinary components as we have done here for the purpose of definition.

Some application of the behavioral sciences is important in nursing in order to understand humans and their reactions in health and illness—not as isolated individuals, but as individuals who are members of a family, a society, and, in part, products of their culture. We are reminded by Folta and Deck (1966) that all cultural alternatives are not necessarily learned by everyone in a given culture. In some instances the normative requirements of the culture apply only to members of various groups as determined by geographic area, age, sex, or role.

References Cited

Barker, R. G. *Ecological Psychology.* Stanford, Calif.: Stanford University Press, 1968.

Biesanz, J., and Biesanz, M. *Modern Society,* 3rd ed. Englewood Cliffs, N.J.: Prentice-Hall, 1964.

Folta, J. R., and Deck, E. S. *A Sociological Framework for Patient Care.* New York: John Wiley & Sons, 1966.

Hinsie, L. E., and Campbell, R. J. *Psychiatric Dictionary,* 4th ed. New York: Oxford University Press, 1970.

LeVine, R. A. *Culture, Behavior, and Personality.* Chicago: Aldine Publishing Company, 1973.

Rogers, M. *An Introduction to the Theoretical Basis of Nursing.* Philadelphia: F. A. Davis Co., 1970.

Webster's Seventh New Collegiate Dictionary. Springfield, Mass.: G. & C. Merriam Company, 1969.

30

Significant Cultural and Maturational Elements in Clinical Nursing

There is a tide in the affairs of men
Which, taken at the flood, leads on to fortune;
Omitted, all the voyage of their life
Is bound in shallows and in miseries.
JULIUS CAESAR IV: 3, SHAKESPEARE

In recent years interest has increased in extending knowledge of the psychological and cultural factors that influence the acceptance, use, or rejection of health services. Many of the questions that have been and are being investigated are familiar to nurses. For example, why do some people seek medical attention at appropriate intervals whereas others do not? Even among those who appear to accept advice and follow instructions, cooperation may appear to be more complete than it actually is. The behavior among those who do not seek medical attention, or who ignore or reject advice, also varies. Some seek attention so late in the course of illness that little can be done to restore health or to reverse the disease process. Others seek attention and then openly or quietly refuse to follow recommendations or to permit themselves to be treated. The conceptual models for persuasion and attitude change can be applied in the examination of these questions. Much more work is needed if we are to understand more fully the attention, comprehension, and acceptance dimensions involved in the successful transmission of messages that relate to health care recommendations (Rosnow & Robinson, 1967). On the other side of the coin, needed treatment may be difficult to obtain. By the time the individual is admitted to a treatment facility it is possible that the point of greatest possible recovery is past. Remotivation toward participation in treatment becomes an extremely difficult task for both the patient and the health team.

This chapter was revised by Jean A. Werner-Beland, M.N., R.N., Associate Professor of Nursing, Wayne State University, College of Nursing, Detroit, Michigan.

Overview of Cultural and Maturational Elements Having Significance for the Practice of Nursing

Because illness involving hospitalization is usually regarded as an extremely disruptive situation by the patient and family, the patient can be expected to experience fear and anxiety. Frequently these feelings are related to the individual's being placed in a dependent role, and the feelings may gain expression through regressive or seemingly infantile behavior. The hospitalization may be viewed by the patient as either a stressful situation or a crisis. Rapoport (1965) distinguishes *stress* from *crisis* by stating that the concept of stress most often carries a negative connotation. In stress the person views the situation as a burden or load under which he or she will survive or break. Crisis, on the other hand, has a growth-promoting potential; it calls the person to new action, brings forth new coping mechanisms to meet the challenge, strengthens the person's adaptive capacity, and is thought to raise the individual's level of mental health. Stress, however, is thought to have great potential for reducing the individual's level of mental health (Rapoport, 1965). How a patient views an illness depends not only on inner resources but on how he or she is assisted to deal with the situation. Nurses frequently can assist patients to view hospitalization either positively or negatively depending on how they relate to the patient.

If the preceding concepts are accepted, why do those who care for Mrs. Marks consider her behavior as cooperative, courageous, and sensible and describe her as a fine woman because she takes adversity without a murmur? Why, on the other hand, is Mrs. Crane's seemingly irrational behavior equated with stubbornness, ignorance, or stupidity? Why is she looked on as childish, demanding, and lacking in self-control and self-discipline? Why does Mr. Robbin resist every suggestion or effort to help him? Why does Mr. Nelson accept the care offered without question and make no extra demands on the nursing staff? Why is Mr. Nelson described as a good patient? Why do nurses like to care for Mrs. Marks and Mr. Nelson and avoid, when possible, the care of Mrs. Crane and Mr. Robbin? Why is one person satisfied with hospital care whereas another feels that the care received was unfeeling and inadequate?

Other questions arise out of the observation that there seems to be a direct relationship between the way a person perceives an illness and the chances for recovery. Why do some patients deal with their illness realistically and engage in treatment? Why do others react with feelings of fear, loathing, or dread that seems out of proportion to the nature of their illness and that may inhibit recovery? For example, why does Mr. Hall strive to recover from a severe stroke, whereas Mr. Donald, who appears to have had a slight stroke, makes little effort to recover?

A complete answer to any one of these questions is, of course, impossible without much more information about each individual and his or her life situation. However, these illustrations suggest three general questions. Why do people behave the way they do? What purpose does their behavior serve? How can this knowledge be used in the practice of nursing?

A general answer to these questions is that people behave as they do in order to meet obvious (overt) or hidden (covert) needs. Failure to satisfy a need results in behavior that is directed toward its satisfaction. This behavior may not always seem reasonable or rational to the observer in that it does not communicate clearly and concisely what really is *the need.* Yet the goal of behavior is need satisfaction even though the behavior may fall short of obtaining the satisfaction desired. Much of the behavior that results in the satisfaction of needs is learned. What a person eats and enjoys depends, to some extent, on family and cultural background. How he or she behaves when in a situation where food is not available in the form and amount preferred is also partially dependent on past learnings. However, to add to the complexity of the individual, one cannot discount newly incorporated learnings.

Knowledge of family and cultural patterns is helpful in the identification of needs that can be met by nursing and in the selection of the manner in which care is provided. As an example, Primeaux (1977) writes that anyone caring for an American Indian patient must understand that to this patient there is little distinction between medicine and religion. "Indian medicine embodies ages of tradition and trust" (p. 91). Western-Anglo medicine, although appropriate for the disease, may have little effect upon symptoms because the treatment does not carry the element of culturally determined faith that the Indian has in tribal medicine. Primeaux states that the importance of kinship systems needs to be understood. In addition, the status position associated with age has to be understood or a non-Indian nurse may inadvertently communicate lack of respect for the patient. The health care provider must also understand the lack of future-orientation of the Indian or be continually frustrated by the Indian patient's lack of adherence to appropriate hours for taking medications and their failure to keep clinic appointments. To carry the example of the American Indian a step further, Kneip-Hardy and Burkhardt (1977), in specific reference to the Navajo Indian, point out that nurses need to be aware of the Navajo's deep concern about proper disposal of any body parts, including hair combings. Another culturally determined characteristic of the Navajo is their high regard for individual rights. The non-Indian nurse who expects to extract a health history from the relatives of a Navajo patient may experience difficulty in doing so—not because the relatives are resistive or do not understand, but because "their primary social premise might be said to be that no person has the right to speak for or direct the actions of another" (p. 96). These then are just a few examples of how the cultural variances in people influence their acceptance of and reactions to health care.

Obviously a nurse cannot be expected to know or anticipate all of the variations in patients that may arise out of differences in personal, family, or cultural patterns. However, the nurse should be aware of the dominant cultural patterns of those patients with whom she or he has contact. The nurse needs to be knowledgeable about how these patterns might interact with traditional nursing practice. Another useful guide for the nurse in recognizing and trying to understand the differences in patients is the knowledge of the influence that her or his own family and culture have had in terms of values, goals, expectations, and modes of expression. The nurse who has knowledge of the characteristic features of several cultural groups is better prepared to consider the influences that folkways and mores are having on the patient's acceptance or rejection of care. Instead of categorizing the patient's behavior as abnormal or peculiar, the nurse might find that the patient is acting in accord with cultural dictates. Considered in this light, the patient's behavior is reasonable though not in keeping with the way the nurse would behave in a similar situation.

Even in patients whose cultural background is assumed to be similar to that of the nurse, problems might arise in care delivery because the nurse fails to recognize that the illness exists apart from the disease (Kleinman, 1978). Kleinman states that the success of native healers is in the fact that "they concentrate on the social and cultural aspects of treatment dealing with sickness as a human problem that affects family functions and tears at the web of meaning that integrates day to day life, not as just an isolated event in the life of the patient" (p. 64). The failure of Western medicine, according to Kleinman, is that the symbolic and religious meaning of illness are not taken into account. He cites the case of a college professor whose disease had been treated but who failed to adhere to the medical regimen because it was the professor's personal belief that to admit he had coronary artery disease would make him an invalid. We do not know why the disease had this meaning for him, but as long as he held this belief, in spite of other explanations, he remained at risk.

According to Biesanz (1964), all cultures include an *economic system* that includes beliefs and practices governing the production, distribution, and consumption of goods and services. The economic system also encompasses the technology necessary to produce these goods and services. Every culture has a social structure that includes the family system, which, in turn, regulates sex behavior and defines rights and responsibilities regarding the procreation and education of children. Religion, systems of government, and general beliefs concerning "good" and "bad" are also included under social structure. Language, as mentioned previously, is necessary for the existence of culture and is, therefore, a universal element of cultures. Variations occur in cultures and seem to result from human adaptability, creativity, intelligence, and accidents of original choices (Biesanz & Biesanz, 1964).

Significant Elements of Culture

Although all elements of culture may be significant in patient care at one time or another, there are some elements that are generally thought to be more significant than others. These are

1. Religion
2. Patterns of family organization and child care
3. Patterns of care during birth, sickness, and death
4. Values as they relate to age and sex
5. Language
6. Orientation to time
7. Patterns of sleep and personal hygiene
8. Patterns of modesty
9. Methods of communicating satisfaction and dissatisfaction
10. Value placed on individuality and personal achievement
11. Food habits

Circumstances that influence cultural and subcultural differences in the United States include

1. Place of residence—such as city or country, North or South, and segregated or integrated
2. Socioeconomic status
3. Place of birth—United States or foreign country
4. Level of education, including professional education. As the level of education of people rises, differences among people tend to become less marked.

These elements serve as the basis for the way in which a given culture plans for and meets the problems that arise out of illness. They also affect the way in which an individual within a culture regards illness and what he or she does to prevent illness or to treat it. In other words, each person brings to every situation

1. A set of values
2. A set of expectations
3. A code of behavior—an internalized set of rules or standards that guide conduct
4. Customs and ceremonies observed
5. Manner and vocabulary by which he or she communicates nonverbally as well as verbally with other people.

An example, again from Primeaux's article on the American Indian patient (1977), points out that eye contact to the Anglo-American means that one is paying attention. To the Indian direct eye contact is considered disrespectful. Such differences easily lead to misinterpretation by the Anglo nurse who is trying to do health teaching with an American Indian patient. The nurse might interpret the patient's lack of eye contact as disinterest or lack of attention when neither is actually true.

To further illustrate and clarify the preceding statements, a folkway that is characteristic of middle- and upper-income groups in Western society will be described. The situation is one in which Mr. and Mrs. Holt invite Mr. and Mrs. Questa for supper. The language and the manner in which the invitation is extended provide information about things such as the degree of formality, purpose, and others likely to be invited. Depending on these and other factors, each person will bring a unique set of expectations about how the guests and host and hostess should behave and be treated and what constitutes hospitality. They also have a set of standards to guide their conduct, a set of customs and ceremonies they observe, and even an accepted language convention for communicating with each other.

When the expectations of both the host and the guest are the same, few problems arise. When expectations differ, the guest may arrive and find the host in his shirt sleeves and the hostess in the bathtub or find that the roast is dried out. The host and guests also have ways of expressing their satisfaction or dissatisfaction with each other. They may be sincere or they may try to cover up their true feelings. When they say good night, they may express pleasure despite the fact that the evening was dull.

Although this illustration could be expanded further, enough detail has been presented to make the point that each individual has a set of expectations, a code that guides behavior, customs observed, and a terminology for expressing meanings. Social functions are usually more mutually satisfying when the host and guests have similar expectations or when each is aware that the other has expectations different from his or her own and takes these into consideration. Moreover, when a host invites a comparative stranger into his home he attempts to learn something about this stranger. He attempts to apprise his guest of what to expect so that he can plan in terms of his or her needs. If the host values this relationship he does not show disrespect for his guest by ignoring or condemning practices that have value and meaning to the guest. For example, he does not serve pork chops to an Orthodox Jew. At the same time the host should be able to expect mutual respect from his guest. The guest, in return, does not smoke if the host disapproves of smoking and lets this fact be known.

In the care of the sick, the relationship between nurse and patient has some of the same overtones as the host–guest relationship, yet there are important differences. The nurse is a member of a service profession, and the person who comes seeking that service is called a "patient." The nurse, by virtue of her or his education, is in a position to make a decision about whether or not the service being sought can be rendered. The sick person is seeking help for some personal problem and therefore does not have the expectation of mutual give and take that is part of the social encounter. It suffices to say that knowledge of the elements of culture should be helpful to the nurse in anticipating the patient's needs and in personalizing care. In Chapter 29, attention was given to the cultural aspects of food. Because of the limitations of the scope of this book, American patterns of child care and of childbirth has not been included.

Religion

Religion is an essential consideration in the care of each patient. A simple definition of religion is that it is humankind's idea of God and our relationship to Him.[1] It includes the way in which humans show their respect and love for God. Understanding a person's religious beliefs includes knowing something about the tenets upon which that religion is founded. Almost more important to the nurse is knowledge about the way in which a person practices religion through a series of externals or rituals. These externals, in addition to being ways the individual maintains a sense of communication with a Supreme Being, also provide the person who is ill with anchor points for reality and a sense of control over his or her life. Respect for a person includes a respect for the right to practice religion to the extent that this is possible within the treatment setting. This religious practice may include certain dietary restrictions, manner of dress, or rejection of commonly accepted medical practices, to name a few. How the nurse, physician, and other care givers view the events that have religious significance for the patient, and work with the patient to incorporate these practices into plans for health care, is vitally important.

Prayer, a visit with one's clergyman, the ability to engage in a religious practice, or the opportunity

[1] See Chapter 32 for a discussion of spiritual care.

to talk with a nurse about one's concept of hope, or death and dying, may do more to allay the patient's anxiety than a prescription for a tranquilizer or a psychiatric consultation. I do not intend to demean these latter options because they are necessary for some patients, but they should not be viewed as the first option in a majority of cases. Tillich (1952) writes that ontologically rooted anxiety (i.e., anxiety that is common to all human beings and is rooted in the fact that humans are human—that they exist) makes itself known especially during times of illness because illness makes one more aware of the personal struggle of *being* versus *nonbeing.* "Much courage to be, created by religion, is nothing else than the desire to limit one's own being and to strengthen this limitation through the power of religion" (p. 73). Tillich does not deny that religion can sometimes reduce one's openness to reality, but when this occurs and has an adverse effect on health care, its dangers to the patient should be realized. Solutions are best found through the cooperative efforts of clergy, the patient and family, and health care providers.

In order to be an active participant in any aspect of the religious dimensions of a patient's life, the nurse needs to have an understanding of what is important to the patient so that the patient's religious needs can be anticipated and met. The nurse contributes to the patient's welfare by supporting the right to religious faith. This may include the fostering of hope in the patient that suffering is not in vain.

The philosopher Marcel (1965), states that "what determines the ontological position of hope—absolute hope, is inseparable from a faith which is likewise absolute" (p. 186). In speaking of the importance of religious faith—not to be confused with organized religion—Marcel writes:

> From the moment that I abase myself in some sense before the absolute Thou who in His infinite condescension has brought me forth out of nothingness, it seems as though I forbid myself ever again to despair . . . (p. 186).

Even when illness strikes one can, through faith, avoid falling into the grip of despair and hopelessness. That is what Marcel's statement means to me.

Although Tillich (1952) speaks of an individual's courage *to be* as essential for the maintenance of self in the face of adversity (and here we consider illness, disease, or disability to be an adversity), one sees that courage and hope are closely related concepts.

> Courage listens to reason and carries out the intention of the mind. It is the strength of the soul to win victory in ultimate danger, like those two martyrs of the Old Testament who are enumerated in Hebrews 11. Courage gives consolation, patience, and experience and becomes indistinguishable from faith and hope (Tillich, 1952, p. 8).

None of us would deny the patient the right to hope, nor would we deny our responsibility in assisting him or her to continue to hope even when face-to-face with grave illness or massive disability. When the nurse does recognize the closeness of the relationship between the concepts of courage, hope, and religious faith, it becomes self-evident why religion is an important consideration in nursing.

Patterns of Family Organization

Understanding patterns of family organization is important if one is also to understand certain responses that patients have to illness and to patterns of health care. Viewing the family as a system gives the nurse several guides for assessment of the roles and functions of each family member, including the patient, and the impact that illness is having on the family as a system. The patient must be considered as an integral part of the family, or, if no family exists, then perhaps as part of a surrogate family system that influences and is influenced by the illness. One of the first points to consider in making an assessment of the family is how open or closed is the family system to which a particular patient belongs. The more open the system (i.e., the more permeable its boundaries without losing the integrity or identity of the family), the more the members are likely to be change-oriented and adaptable, and the more they will be able to cope with change and to consider suggestions and alterations in plans for care. Beavers (1977) indicates that the more closed the family system boundary is, the less flexible that system will be. Any event such as illness that occurs in this relatively inflexible system will cause considerable disruption and anxiety. The occurrence of a stressful event is addressed poorly by a family that has few coping mechanisms and limited outside sources of support. A problem for the nurse might be that, although the family system is thrown into obvious disruption when one of its members becomes ill, they are so limited in the practice of accepting outside influence that they may resist any suggestions offered by the nurse or other members of the health team.

In making an assessment, the nurse should try to identify the status position and role that the patient holds in the family system. By this I mean not only the biological role of father, mother, or child, but also the psychological position that the patient holds in the family. Is this person, who is now a patient, usually the family decision maker, the favorite, the scapegoat, or what? The position which the patient holds, both biologically and psychologically, is important knowledge to have because it might help the nurse understand the family's attitude toward being involved in care plans both during and after hospitalization.

Role is important in another way. According to Parsons and Fox (1958), illness in the mother is often more disturbing to the rest of the family than illness in either the father or one of the children because in our culture, until recently, it has been the mother who provides emotional support for other members of the family. Several authors (Christopherson, 1968; Hanson, 1980; Stephens, 1963), note that culture prescribes unique sex roles for men and women. When illness forces one to give up or alter culturally prescribed sex role behavior the result can be serious—not only for the patient, but also for other members of the family whose sex role behaviors must change to accommodate those role dimensions that the patient is no longer able to fulfill. Individuals and their significant others frequently need help if they are to cope successfully with roles that result from illness or disability.

Until recently the trend toward hospitalization of the sick had been increasing. This was particularly true for those who were seriously ill or for whom illness was prolonged. Reasons given for caring for patients in hospitals include the fact that specialized services and equipment are available and that patients can be given care that would be impossible for them to receive at home. Sometimes this is true. Sociologists also suggest other reasons for caring for the sick in specialized institutions. One of these is that the institution serves to protect the family from the disrupting effects of having a sick person in their midst. In a small two- or three-bedroom house the continued presence of a seriously ill person may place great physical and emotional strain on the family. Craven and Sharp (1972) pointed out that the presence of one sick member is a more serious disrupting force in the small nuclear family, that is typical in America, than it is in the extended family systems in other cultures. In the nuclear family illness intensifies the stress load for each member. If there were preexisting problems in the family, the illness of any member compounds these problems.

The current trend is to return the sick to their homes earlier than has been the practice in the past. The success of this plan depends upon, among other things, the patient and the nature of his or her illness, the family strengths, the attitudes of family members toward each other and toward the illness, and their acceptance of the patient and the plan for home care. It also depends on provision of the kinds of services that make it possible to care for the patient at home. In addition to medical services, early referrals may be necessary for nursing care, physical therapy, housekeeping, and occupational therapy. Ambulance and other transportation services must be available to return the patient for needed outpatient services or in the event that rehospitalization is required.

Not all of the reasons for returning patients to the home environment after the shortest possible stay in the hospital are culturally determined. Rather, these reasons are more social, political, and economic in nature. Not the least of the reasons is the pressure that comes from federal and state government to review the utilization of hospital bed occupancy. There is considerable pressure from some labor unions and from industry to reduce the cost of health care, and especially the astronomical costs of hospital care. In a recent Blue Cross–funded demonstration project, whose purpose was to compare the cost effectiveness of home hospice versus hospital care for the terminally ill, the home hospice proved to be the more cost-effective (Amado, Cronk, and Mileo, 1979). The paradox in many cases, however, is that many patients experience difficulty in meeting the qualifications for needed home health care as defined by third-party reimbursers. Because of the gap between services needed and Medicare guidelines, other funding sources are often required in order for patients to be cared for at home (Lowe, 1976). This is an area where nurses need to become politically active and to be advocates for the right of patients to be cared for at home if that is their desire.

In the Anglo-American culture that makes up much of the United States, another factor that has inhibited the movement toward home health care is the fact that many in this cultural group draw away from the sick and the infirm. The terminally ill are particularly threatening because it is characteristic of this culture to deny death. There has been a slight change in attitude toward illness and death in recent years—more people are willing to look at death as a reality. Undoubtedly the proliferation of books on the subject, and especially the writings of Kübler-Ross (1969; 1975), has contributed to this greater acceptance. There also has been increased attention paid to the preparation of health care providers so that they can skillfully assess and intervene in problems arising from long-term illness, disability, and terminal illness. We have come to recognize the importance of including family members in health care planning for the patient. The education of the family to meet the needs of the patient often leads to a lower level of apprehension about accepting the patient into the home after a relatively short period of hospitalization.

Patterns of Care during Sickness and Death

Not all cultures care for their sick in the hospital. In fact they may look on the hospital as a cold and formal place that can in no way substitute for the presence of a loving family. For example, Saunders (1954) cites the instance of the young girl whose family would not permit her to be hospitalized for the treatment of tuberculosis because they believed that the sick should have the care and support of the family. The fact that the girl was capable of infecting the family was of no importance to them. Neither did they believe that she might be given better care in the hospital than at home. In other cultures support is provided by one or more of the members of the family going to the hospital with the patient and staying until he or she is well. They may cook meals and provide for personal care. Probably one of the greatest values of this practice derives from the fact that the patient shifts concern for his or her welfare to the family. They are there. They will be responsible. They will take care of the patient. Primeaux (1977) writes that to the American Indian, to be poor is to be without friends. It is very comforting to the Indian patient to have many relatives come to the hospital at one time. Therefore, if a rule of "Only two visitors at a time" is strictly enforced, the patient and family may be upset. Primeaux says that it is possible that a group of twelve to fifteen Indian family members may camp on the hospital grounds; especially if they have traveled long distances to be near their hospitalized family member. On two occasions I have observed Gypsies camping in hospital parking lots to be near their king or queen who was ill.

Practices in the care of the dying and the dead vary in different cultures all the way from placing the dying outside the village limits or deserting them to taking extraordinary measures to preserve life. Though the desertion of the sick and infirm seems cruel, in primitive societies this may be necessary to the survival of others. There are also those who question the kindness of taking extreme measures to continue life in the seriously disabled or diseased person (*Atlantic Monthly*, 1957). It seems paradoxical that we are constantly being made aware of overcrowding and overpopulation, on the one hand, and that, on the other hand, we struggle so hard to prevent some individuals from having the option of dying with dignity, without resorting to extraordinary means to preserve their lives. Mr. Zilkowski is a case in point. The Zilkowskis were in their early 60s. At one time they had money saved for retirement, had their home paid for, and had no large outstanding debts. Then Mr. Zilkowski developed emphysema and within a few years he became a respiratory invalid. His hospital bills used up all of their savings; they had to mortgage their home; and his wife was forced to go to work. In order to survive each day, Mr. Zilkowski required continuous inhalation of oxygen. Mr. Zilkowski talked quite openly about being allowed to die if he should again go into respiratory crisis. However, when he did go into crisis his wife had him rushed to the hospital where near-heroic means were used to save his life. When Mr. Zilkowski recovered sufficiently to be able to express himself he was furious that he was still alive and still being an emotional and financial burden on his wife, who consciously agreed with her husband that he and she would be better off if he did die. It must be noted that Mrs. Zilkowski had more mixed feelings than her husband about this, as evidenced by the fact that she was the one who always rushed him to the hospital. However, the message about the patient's preference to die finally got through to the hospital staff, who also had mixed feelings about who had the primary decision-making role in this case. The next time Mr. Zilkowski was brought to the hospital in crisis, he was given reasonable sustaining care and he died.

In the American culture there is a tendency to protect the young from the knowledge of death and dying. Many who die, die in hospitals, where they are separated from family members by equipment, procedures, and personnel. "Consequently the dying patient is estranged from the emotional security of the family at the point of greatest emotional trauma" (Heller, 1975).

Nurses, young and not so young, are enmeshed in the cultural taboos against recognizing and dealing with terminal illness and death. Michaels (1971) observed nurses who verbalized a desire to give emotional support to patients and their families at times of great need but who were unable to put their words into action. Personal needs of the nurse and anxiety about the circumstances with which she or he is faced often get in the way of providing the kind of nursing care the nurse knows should and wishes could be given.

By way of contrast with the Anglo taboo on death, Trelease (1975) cites his experiences as a parish priest among the Alaskan Indians. When he was called to minister to those who were dying, he found, almost without exception, that these people exhibited a willfulness about their death. "Their participation in its planning, and its time of occurrence showed a remarkable power of personal choice" (p. 33). Jewish tradition also "confronts death directly and specifically views the period of terminal illness *(Shechiv Mera)* and dying *(Goses)* as a time when loved ones should surround, comfort, and encourage the patient" (Heller, 1975, p. 39). The terminal Jewish patient is urged to face death as a real and perhaps imminent possibility. Buddhist and Hindu doctrines also encourage the acceptance of death calmly, courageously, and confidently, and to eventually come to view death as a friend. These views are quite different from the one considered typically Anglo-American, but they need to be understood if we are to work effectively with patients whose orientation to death and dying is different from ours.

One of the needs of the seriously ill or dying person is for someone to listen. Heusinkveld (1972) wrote that the terminally ill patient who is aware of his or her condition does not always wish to talk about the personal meaning that death has. That may be the first assumption that the nurse makes based on the cues given by the patient. But people use considerable denial in dealing with stress, and the dying patient is no exception. Therefore nurses need to make a concerted effort to distinguish between moments when the patient wants to talk about the seriousness of his or her condition and those times when he or she is seeking support and reassurance relative to some small improvement in body function. As long as the nurse is primarily concerned with personal fears about death and dying she or he cannot be an effective listener.

Another problem that many Anglo-Americans have in dealing with dying and death is created by the cultural values associated with the age of the dying patient. Epstein (1975), notes that nurses must look closely at the behavioral consequences of such attitudes or values. "Is it possible," she writes, "that we are less accepting of the anger and grief of a sixty-year-old woman faced with her own death than we are with similar emotions in a twenty-five-year-old woman? . . . Would we be as willing to take as much time and trouble to help an old man die as we are to help a young man die?" (p. 101). I would add that these same questions can be applied to our attitudes about patients where there is no evidence that they *are* about to die. In spite of our efforts to protect children from the knowledge of death, children see death on television and in the movies. "By the time a child is seven years old, he probably suspects that he himself will die one day. Even the child who is dying has probably guessed this fact and we only delude ourselves if we think otherwise" (Epstein, 1975, pp. 102–103). Talking with a patient who is dying and who indicates a desire to talk about his or her perceptions and concerns should be approached directly and in age-appropriate terms. See Chapter 33 for further discussion of managing the care of the terminally ill and dying person.

Values Relating to Age and Sex

The attitude of those caring for the sick aged may be adversely influenced by the fact that, in the American culture, youth is the idealized state. In some cultures youth is considered to be a handicap and age is respected because it brings with it experience and wisdom. In these cultures the aged are given status rather than being relegated to the background. In America the aged and the disabled are granted "deviant" or "minority" group status along with other minorities who are so designated because of race or sex. According to Safilios-Rothschild (1970), minority groups share the following characteristics and societal reactions: (1) they are granted a separate place in society and are encouraged to interact with their own kind; (2) the majority evaluate the characteristics of the minority group in such a way that the minority group members are designated as inferior; (3) the segregation imposed on the "minority" is rationalized as being beneficial to them because their chances for happiness are greater if they are among "their own kind"; and (4) there is a tendency to evaluate anyone with minority status on the basis of their categorical membership rather than on the basis of their individual characteristics. These four points constitute a system of stereotyping people that, in turn, serves as a distancing maneuver for the nonminority person. In this way the nonminority person is spared the effort of getting to know the minority person as an individual. Nurses and other health professionals must guard against stereotyping patients according to their minority group characteristics because such practices greatly limit the right of patients to receive care that is person-oriented and designed to take their specific needs into account. Agee (1980) writes, "Those people who view the aged as either worthless, infantalized remnants, or, as difficult, angry, embittered obligations have accepted the cultural stereotypes of aging that are essentially negative." The stereotypes about the aged influence the type of health care they receive because, "By definition, stereotyping of the aged as a group allows for no individuality and prohibits the use of critical judgment by those who hold these fixed perceptions" (Agee, 1980).

Another factor influencing the status and role of an individual in the group is sex. In some cultures the male has higher status than the female, though the reverse is true in other cultures. Certain health care practices in America discriminate on the basis of sex, although most providers of care would tend to deny this. In psychiatric care, given an instance where a husband and wife are having problems, it is most often the wife who is "treated" and resocialized to fit a mold compatible with a male-dominant view. Rehabilitation of the disabled, as another example, is primarily vocational. Because males in our culture are still considered to have employment priorities over females, it follows that the priorities for distribution of rehabilitation funds also go to males. Appropriate behavior is also defined in terms of sex. For example, in the Anglo-American culture women may cry without losing status; men may not. The Lakher of Burma will beat his wife if he has good cause and this is culturally acceptable behavior (Stephens, 1963). In the American culture this same behavior is called "spouse abuse" and is considered to be contrary to social and cultural norms. In a society such as ours what is acceptable is subject to change. Not too many years ago, "nice" women did not smoke cigarettes or wear trousers in public. Now they do both. The point is this: to satisfy patient's needs on issues relating to age and sex, the nurse needs to have some knowledge of the culturally determined values that are held by the patient. Even then one cannot generalize from one patient to another from the same or similar culture. There may be specific psychological variations that produce different behaviors and attitudes in persons with identical cultural backgrounds.

Language

Language, that intricate symbolic system through which human thought makes itself manifest (Miller, 1973), is, of course, necessary for communication. Even when two people speak the same language, difficulties in communication can arise out of the fact that it is possible to interpret words differently or that the same words may serve as the stimulus for different feeling responses in different people. Watzlawick (1978) writes that it is possible that

> the use of a specific interpersonal communication leads not merely to a change in the mood, the views, or the feelings of its recipient, as can be observed on an everyday basis, but to a *physical* change that cannot "normally" be effected deliberately (pp. 3–4).

This applies to language that comes from another outside of the self but, as Watzlawick states, "it can also be our own 'pathogenic prose' that makes us sick" (p. 4). By the same token, it must be possible to use this same language in the service of healing if we only can understand what that language might be.

All of us speak at least two languages. The first is the objective, logical, definitional language of reason. The second is the language of imagery, metaphor, synthesis, and totality (Watzlawick, 1978). Add to this complex, basic system of language a nurse who is a native Bostonian and an Italian who learned English in night school, and there is no end to the communication problems that might occur if these two people take for granted that they speak the same language. More than likely, one does not understand the idiomatic expressions of the other. Since most of us are not even conscious of the idioms we use, there is ample room for misunderstanding. Two people coming from the same geographic area, but with different cultural backgrounds can still have communication problems. For example, a recent court ruling in Michigan recognized a difference between black English and the traditional English taught in the public schools in the same town where these black children grew up. The defendants in the case charged, in effect, that American-born children who speak black English are often evaluated incorrectly by American-born teachers who speak traditional English and that the effect of this language difference has to be recognized in curriculum planning and in teaching.

Listening to what is said is an important first step toward reducing distortions in communication. Observing the nonverbal portion of communication is part of this total process. Therefore, it is not just the words, but the inflection, tone, and behavior of the individual as well that adds meaning to the verbal part of communication. People in the hospital culture, including nurses, frequently are guilty of jumping to the conclusion that they understand exactly what the patient is trying to say even before the patient has said it. This so-called mindreading ploy is both infuriating and frightening because the patient tends to think what he or she wants is discounted and begins to wonder if he or she will be heard if something *really* important does arise. When people speak different languages, some means other than verbal communication must be used. If there is someone available who speaks the patient's language, this person should be used as an interpreter. Suitable provisions must also be made to communicate with the patient who is unable to speak because of a defect in the nervous system or organs of speech. Sign language or writing may be used. Although nonverbal communication is always important, it becomes increasingly significant when caring for patients who are unable to send or receive messages through the use of speech. In such instances increased awareness of cultural factors—family and preillness patterns of the individual—is often helpful in achieving a better understanding of the person while in the hospital.

Orientation to Time

Some problems in the care of patients arise out of differences in orientation to time and the value placed on it. Orientation to time may be to the past, present, or future. This is illustrated in the literature of various peoples. For example, in our literature the ant spends the summer busily storing supplies for the coming winter months, whereas the improvident grasshopper dashes around enjoying himself. It is quite shocking to Americans to learn that there are cultures in which the ant is viewed as the foolish one and the grasshopper is wise. From the latter point of view, the present is what one has. Why expend effort for a time that may never be. A third orientation to time was held by some Chinese in bygone days. They believed that the future is behind one and therefore cannot be seen. They are said to have built pleasure gardens along the side of the streams where they sat facing downstream contemplating the past.

That not all Americans have the same view of time is borne out in a study of Koos (1954). In this study he found that respondents from class I (upper) looked toward the future; those from class II (middle) were primarily occupied with the present; and those in class III (lower) had little hope in either the present or the future. In general, middle-class Americans look at the present as better than the past, and the future is expected to be better than either. In another study, Saunders (1954) found that Spanish-speaking Americans who live in the southwestern part of the United States lived in the present or immediate past rather than in the past or the future. He states that this creates a problem in their medical care. How can they know whether they want a clinic appointment next week when they do not know how they will be feeling at that time? According to their perception of time, this is a logical conclusion. If on the day of the appointment they feel well, they see no reason to keep it.

Recently, considerable attention has been given to a type of time or timer known as biological rhythms. "Rhythms are both endogenous (internal) and exogenous (external) and occur at many different frequencies ranging from as short as a few seconds to as long as the birth-death cycle. Many endogneous rhythms, for example, blood pressure, heart rate, body temperature, and electrolyte secretion, follow daily and monthly cycles" (Tom and Lanuza, 1976, p. 569). For purposes of understanding the effect of culture on time, let us examine a few elements of time that have an endogenous beginning but are then reinforced by expectations within the Anglo-American culture. Sheehy (1976) refers to each stage of life as a *passsage,* and each passage has its own perception of time. Many young people feel that there is plenty of time, but they are restless and want to live life to the fullest. Their orientation to time is to *now,* with an ever-growing future orientation as they approach their twenties. As people grow older they begin to feel that time passes too quickly or that there is not enough time. Sheehy gives many examples involving time perceptions across the age continuum too numerous to mention here, but the reader is encouraged to explore them. Time is important nonetheless, and it is significant in understanding an individual's response to sickness and disability given his or her particular age and its accompanying cultural and social pressures. For example, Sheehy writes that the twenties and thirties are the years during which career-oriented males and females seek mastery. This corresponds roughly to Erikson's (1963) fifth and sixth stages of life—namely, identity versus role diffusion, and, intimacy versus isolation. The tasks described by Sheehy are similar to those described by Erikson. These can be summarized by saying that this is the time of life when the individual (who has mastered earlier developmental tasks) begins to feel more comfortable with the question, "Who am I?" It is a time for the individual to earn whatever credentials are needed to accomplish life goals that will gain him or her society's approval and its rewards. Imagine the effect that illness or disability would have on an individual in this age group! When the illness or disability is severe enough to pose a major threat to the accomplishment of personal or culturally dictated goals, then adjustment problems are highly probable.

There are also sex differences that affect the perception of time and the fulfillment of life goals. A woman of 40 may feel that she is emancipated from children and household chores; particularly if she has mastered the previous life stages (Erikson, 1963; Sheehy, 1976) and is moving into a phase of generativity as opposed to stagnation. She may be looking forward to using her time to take advantage of new opportunities, to resume her education, to become involved in social welfare activities, and the like. The male, on the other hand, finds 40 to be a pivotal point in his career advancement. "He often feels 'urged' to run harder in an even narrower track" (Sheehy, 1976, p. 369). At this age, time perception is still focused on external issues. Understanding the nature of these external issues and their significance to the patient adds to the nurse's perception of the total person. For the elderly, time perceptions seem to become more focused on internal issues or reminiscences. Erikson calls the period from age 60 to death the stage of ego integrity versus despair. "The quality of ego integrity arises out of the elderly person's evaluative review of his or her life, and from the acceptance of that life, with whatever joys or sorrows it held, as a necessary and worthwhile piece of work" (Grace, Layton, and Camilleri, 1977, p. 49). To the extent that the quality of ego integrity is poor, the elderly person will be unhappy and despairing. It is important that the nurse understand the developmental tasks of this age group if adequate care plans are to be developed. It seems to me that a "generation gap" is not so much a separation in years as it is a breakdown in understanding each other's perception of time and the developmental tasks that are essential to each age group.

Chapman and Chapman (1975) point to technology as being responsible for many changes, and even in the way our culture perceives time. The media rushes people with communication about *right now!* All of the prime existential questions of life are, therefore, constantly before us: "Who am I? Where am I going? What will it be like when I grow up? What is after death? How are we to survive forces that seem beyond our control?" (Chapman & Chapman, 1975, pp. 19–20). The outcome of all this is a rate of change that people have never before experienced. There is less time for leisurely reflection and problem solving. There is less of a sense of personal security for all of us even when we are well. Illness only tends to magnify this feeling.

Because many in the American culture are becoming aware of the present and what this portends for their future, there is increasing emphasis on providing for illness, old age, and death by acquiring some type of insurance or retirement package. As a result of the Depression that began in 1929, the fact that industrial workers were not always able to protect themselves against unemployment was recognized. In 1935 the Social Security Act was passed. It had three provisions based on the principle that society has an obligation to provide for the security of its people. The first provision was for unemployment compensation to be handled by the states. The second was establishment of an annuity that was to be paid at age 65 or on retirement of its members. The third provided for special categories of needy persons, including the aged, the blind, the disabled, and dependent children. The Social Security Amendments of 1965 added Medicare and Medicaid, recognizing that there are increasing numbers of elderly people in this country where there are diminishing extended family systems that will assume responsibility for the aging. In this way the government has assumed responsibility for helping people provide for the future.

The other dimension of time is the value placed on it. Time is sometimes equated with success by Americans. It is generally believed to have value in achieving success, as it can be used with profit or it can be wasted. Sayings in the American language such as "Time waits for no man" or "Time is money" indicate this. When one is employed by another, one most often sells time rather than productivity. A person may punch a time clock when he or she arrives at and leaves the place of employment. An employee is usually paid for the number of hours rather than for the units of work. There is a tendency to judge efficiency in terms of the individual's ability to appear to be busy at any given moment. Nurses are judged by this standard. Most nurses are employed for 40 hours per week. The nurse who is busy is commended. The one who is not occupied in some task and is seen talking with patients is often viewed as using time in a frivolous manner. There is probably more than one instance when a nurse has been interrupted in the course of talking with a patient about some meaningful feeling or problem. The interruption is prefaced too often by, "As long as you're not doing anything. . . . " The transmission of such values certainly encourages nurses to be utilitarian rather than humanitarian in their practice.

Because of the emphasis placed on the value of time in the American culture, it is not surprising that the sick person places great importance on having medications and treatments at the time they are scheduled. The patient frequently judges the quality of care by how closely nurses adhere to the schedule. As was seen in the previous paragraph, nurses themselves communicate that this is where the value lies. The patient not only brings some orientation to the value of time to the hospital, but he or she quickly has this orientation reinforced by the hospital value system. In our culture time carries elements of security, caring, and control, and violations of schedules may give rise to anxious feelings that gain expression through a wide range of behaviors. The hospitalized patient has the feeling that there is so little he or she can control—about the course of illness or the nature of the treatment—that the patient tends to focus on those things, such as the nurse's punctuality, over which he or she may be able to exercise some controlling influence. For example, Mrs. Pope, who was hospitalized for an extended period, was allowed to spend weekends at home provided she arrange to have a nurse administer Acthar[2] by intramuscular injection both at 8 o'clock in the morning and in the evening. When the nurse was even a few minutes late, Mrs. Pope became very agitated, thus placing

[2] Acthar (adrenocorticotropic hormone) is a trade name for an extract of anterior pituitary glands, prepared for parenteral use in doses of 25, 40, and 80 U.S.P. units. It acts by stimulating the adrenal cortex to secrete all of its glucocorticoids and its mineralocorticoids at an increased rate. The average adult dose is 40 to 50 U.S.P. units daily. See a pharmacology textbook for further information about the action and toxicity of adrenocorticosteroids.

a strain on the nurse. In this instance the nurse recognized the importance of time to Mrs. Pope and made an effort to arrive a few minutes early. Our example does not help us understand exactly what time meant to Mrs. Pope; that would require further exploration based on the nurse's observation that Mrs. Pope became agitated when the nurse was late.

The importance of time is often overlooked in discharge planning for a patient who has been hospitalized for an extended period. The patient's expectation is often that the world outside will be just as it was the day he or she entered the hospital, and the patient is surprised to find that it has changed. Especially in long-term care facilities, nurses need to help the patient maintain an intellectual awareness of the fact that time does march on. This is one of the many tasks in which the nurse can encourage continued family involvement.

Patterns of Sleep and Personal Hygiene

Some knowledge of the sleep patterns of the person may be useful when providing care. For example, the person may be accustomed to having a private room or to sharing a room with another. If the first person is in a large ward, he or she may have difficulty in sleeping, whereas the second may be lonely when alone. This does not mean that the nurse may be able to alter the situation, but she or he can be understanding of the patient's difficulties. Perhaps more attention should be given to the patient's habits of personal hygiene than is often done. Not all people come from areas where a daily bath or shower is possible. Some even live where taking a bath entails a good bit of effort and planning. Old people, especially old men, may suffer itching of the skin when they bathe more than once or twice a week. Conversely, there are those who bathe daily and are upset when they cannot. This point can be illustrated by two brothers, Allen and Bert, who were seriously ill. Allen was much upset because his nurse insisted on giving him a bath every morning. Bert was upset for an entire day because he did not have a bath. In neither instance did the patient's physical welfare depend on whether or not he had a bath. Other aspects of personal hygiene that are sometimes neglected and at other times forced on reluctant or protesting patients include the opportunity to brush their teeth, to have their hair combed, to wash their hands after using the bedpan, and to have back care.

Kira (1970) studied the importance of privacy and the bathroom. There are many points in this study that have significance for the practice of nursing. For example, Kira notes that from early childhood we are taught that excretory functions of the body are debasing. These functions are never considered in the same natural way as eating, drinking, or sleeping. The bathroom is a place where one's privacy is usually respected (unless one is in the hospital). In spite of the fact that we all go to the toilet, the activity carries with it a status hierarchy that is socially demanded and culturally accepted. For example, there is the executive washroom, or there is one toilet for six or seven passengers in the first class section of the airplane instead of one for every twenty passengers as in the coach section. The point is, that nurses should be aware of the orientation to privacy (including toileting) that the patient brings to the hospital. Many reactions of patients can be better understood if we just consider the three categories of toilet privacy that may be expected by virtue of one's socioeconomic status:

> *Low:* Expect the privacy of being heard but not seen. *Medium:* Expect the privacy of not being seen or heard. *High:* Expect the privacy of not being seen, heard, or sensed. At this level other people should not be aware of your whereabouts or your intended behavior (Kira, 1970, p. 271).

Age also has its differences in privacy needs. Because body changes create acute self-awareness, the adolescent has a strong need for privacy. Kira (1970, p. 274) states that, "in many cases embarrassment is not caused by the presence of just any person, but rather by the presence of specific culturally prohibited categories of people." This latter point is evident within the hospital culture. It is acceptable for a patient to be on the bedpan when the nurse comes in, but it is far less acceptable for the patient to be on the bedpan when the doctor comes in. I have observed nurses who reinforce this difference by "scolding" a patient, or by being overly apologetic to the doctor if he or she (and especially if the doctor is a "he") is making rounds and the patient happens to be performing one of the excretory activities of daily living.

On the other hand, the patient may have different attitudes about matters of personal hygiene than does the nurse or the doctor. He or she may naturally have a bowel movement every two days and cannot understand why he or she is suddenly expected to perform every day. The point is that health care providers need to try to learn something about the personal habits and expectations of the patient. When the nature of the illness necessitates changes in the usual patterns, then the cooperation of the patient should be enlisted. The nurse should become acquainted with those aspects of hygienic care that are essential to the welfare and peace of mind of the patient, and modify care accordingly.

Closely related to patterns of sleep and personal hygiene are the personally, socially, and culturally determined issues surrounding territoriality and privacy. Privacy was touched on previously. However, the entire matter of privacy goes far beyond one's toileting habits to how people learn to protect their privacy and territory both defensively and offensively. Sivadon (1970) indicates that the space that separates individuals is particularly significant, but it is fairly recent that the meaning of space has been studied in doctor-patient or nurse-patient relationships. Stillman (1978) identifies four types of territory that help to define behavior: (1) public territories, (2) home territories, (3) interactional territories, and (4) body territories. In nursing it is the encroachment upon an individual's body territory or intimate space that is of the greatest concern. The gynecologist who pats a patient on the face or shoulder before beginning a pelvic examination may well understand that it is less threatening to the other person if her body territory is entered gradually. The patient also may be better able to attend to advice given if she feels that her body has been respected and not just assaulted in the process of completing a procedure.

Territoriality is not unique to human beings. What is unique to the human is the learned or culturally derived differences in the way people perceive space.

> The Americans, for example, find that the Latins come too close to speak, and tend to move a comfortable distance away, but they feel then that others consider them cold. On the other hand, accustomed as they are to close neighborly relations, they are surprised, when in England, to find no particular emotional warmth in the people living near them (Sivadon, 1970, p. 415).

A current bandwagon in nursing is the rediscovery of touch. I want to caution against randomly laying hands on every person who becomes a patient. This activity might not be equally appreciated by all. As I have tried to indicate, there are innate and learned differences in the way people react to another's approach. Some of these differences are genetically determined, some are culturally determined, some come from family experiences, and others reflect psychological determinants. I, for one, do not like to be pawed over, and at the same time, I do not consider myself to be unfriendly or unresponsive. I sense that my dominant cultural influence came from my mother who was a Finn. Like many other Finns I tend to maintain my distance and move in on people slowly. I also appreciate when others behave the same way toward me. The nurse's best guideline, when it comes to touching a patient for the sake of offering comfort, is to do what seems appropriate to you at the moment. Be spontaneous with restraint. Do not go around touching and patting patients just because someone tells you "this is where it is at" in nursing. If the patient accepts your touch, and seems comforted by it, fine! If the patient recoils, or draws back, try another mode of communication to convey your caring and concern. Some of the standard nursing procedures, such as the backrub, are still the most acceptable ways of entering a patient's intimate body space in order to offer a measure of comfort. The backrub also serves as an excellent vehicle for engaging a patient in discussion about other health-related concerns.

Expression of Satisfaction and Dissatisfaction

There are innumerable ways in which people can express their satisfactions and dissatisfactions. Though either may be expressed directly, they may also be expressed indirectly. For example, a patient may smile and say that everything is fine and be sincere, or he or she may feel quite differently. Sometimes the nurse may detect something in the patient's tone of voice, expression, or position that indicates that everything is not fine. The patient may not want to hurt the nurse's feelings, may want the nurse's approval, might think that it is not safe to express dissatisfaction directly, or might think that there is no point in expressing anything because the nurse is not really interested in his or her responses. Without meaning to belabor the point, I only stress again the fact that social and cultural determinants are important. The Eskimo, for example, has a cultural norm of never being visibly irritated or upset in a face-to-face encounter (LeVine, 1973). A nurse who goes to work in an area where there is an Eskimo population needs to know this. The nurse also needs to learn how irritation is expressed, and how she or he can help the Eskimo patient communicate what is bothering him or her in terms that the nurse can understand. Many people express dissatisfaction indirectly—some by becoming demanding and hypercritical; others by withdrawing. Although knowledge of cultural norms for expression is very helpful, it is still important for a nurse to make an effort to understand individual variations and to work toward "connecting" with the individual patient in the interest of establishing the most effective communication possible.

Place of Residence

Place of residence is another factor that influences the cultural and subcultural differences in people.

In the United States there is less difference between city and country people than there once was. However, differences do continue to exist, particularly in those instances where a group is segregated or isolated, either by choice or by custom, from the remainder of the population. For example, some religious groups, such as the Mennonites and Amish, settle in communities in order to protect and maintain a way of life that is essential to the practice of their religion. One preliminary study of the behavior of hospitalized black patients being cared for by white nurses has been reported by McCabe (1960). Although she is careful to state that her conclusions are tentative, effective care of these patients appears to depend on the nurse's being aware of the patient's expectations of the nurse's behavior, as well as the nurse's own expectations. McCabe also indicates that to evaluate success in meeting the needs of black patients from southern rural areas, the nurse must know how they express satisfaction or dissatisfaction with their care. She emphasizes the importance of not stereotyping patients.

Socioeconomic Status

Despite the general conviction of Americans to the contrary, socioeconomic status does influence the expectations, aspirations, and way of life of Americans. Studies indicate that it even influences life expectancy in that the lower the income, the shorter the life expectancy. It seems safe to conclude that anything in the life of the individual that is different from that of other individuals contributes to differences in expectations, codes regulating behavior, modes of expressing and satisfying needs, and the language used. If the point that individuals differ appears to be overstressed, it is because not only patient satisfaction but also that of the nurse depends, in part, on the identification and satisfaction of individual expectations of patients.

Values

One of the important aspects of culture is its system of values. Ruesch (1951) states that many values held in America have their origin in the fact that until very recently America was a pioneer country. Moreover, the early settlers were Puritans who placed a high value on plain living, industry, self-control, willpower, cleanliness, consistency, honesty, and the assumption of responsibility. In settling the country, survival often depended on such characteristics as strength, initiative, and hard work. There was little time for pleasure. Entertainment was organized around important events in life such as a wedding, a death, or the building of a house.

According to Ruesch (1951), the American value system is based on four premises: equality, sociality, success, and change. The ideal that all people are equal has its origin in the Judeo-Christian belief that all people are equal in the sight of God. This represents a change in culture. In the ancient world the attitude toward humankind was very different. In the words of Hamilton, "In Egypt, in Crete, in Mesopotamia, wherever we can read bits of the story, we find the same conditions: a despot enthroned, whose whims and passions are the determining factor in the state: a wretched, subjugated populace; a great priestly organization to which is handed over the domain of the intellect" (1930, p. 19). The founders of our nation made their views clear in the Declaration of Independence when they said, "We hold these truths to be self-evident: that all men are created equal, that they are endowed by their Creator with certain unalienable Rights, that among these are Life, Liberty and the pursuit of Happiness." Lincoln reemphasized the belief in equality of all people in the opening sentence of the Gettysburg Address. One of the important issues in the world today stems from whose rights come first, the individual's or the state's, and from whom these rights are derived.

In application of the premise of equality to the practice of nursing, nurses are taught that they are "supposed" to give the same quality of care to all patients. What is actually taught in most health professions, including nursing, is based on white, middle-class values. This orientation makes it difficult for the nurse really to appreciate individual differences, especially when the patient subscribes to a set of values and semantic conventions that are different from those of the nurse. It is difficult to separate socioeconomic status from values. The two often go hand in hand in the formation of stereotypes. For example, several years ago the author was asked to see a young, unmarried black woman who had just given birth. The patient was described as being "emotionally upset." My initial reaction was one of surprise, and if I had verbalized my feelings the monologue probably would have been as follows: "I wonder why she is upset? From what I have heard sexual experiences out of wedlock and illegitimate kids are no big deal among the ghetto population. I wonder what she is reacting to?" When I met the patient it was not difficult to recognize that I was looking at someone who was both frightened and extremely guilt-ridden. She told me that because I was unmarried, white, and middle class, I could not possibly understand what she was going through. I told her that I did not think that what she was feeling following the birth of her baby was so unique, but that it was true that I did not understand about life in a ghetto because I had never had to live in one. But maybe, if she would fill me in on those details, I could help her with her problem. Throughout the time I worked with her she often told me that my "whiteness" was showing. Sometimes this was an indication that I had missed the point because I did not look at it through her eyes. Sometimes such a remark was her defense against my attempt to help her explore the meaning of some feeling or behavior that she had just revealed. The main point here is that I learned two things about myself: (1) that I was a wellspring of stereotypes about the values and practices of people who differed from me in some way, and (2) that I could work effectively with someone from a different background if I would just take the time to listen and learn. The third thing that we both learned was that she had as many stereotypic beliefs about me as I had about her. My favorite was when she told me that she had finally come to the conclusion that not all white women had their minds and bodies locked up in chastity belts. Because all patients are individuals, as are all nurses, perhaps the nurse can come closer to reaching the ideal of equality of care if she or he can accept the patient as a human being, recognize the patient's dignity, identify behavior that provides clues to his or her needs, consider the meaning of this behavior, and plan care to meet patient needs. To do this the nurse requires some knowledge of her or his own system of values.

The second premise on which Ruesch (1951) says the American value system is based is that of sociality. By this is meant that Americans tend to be guided in actions by the opinions of peers. They form social groups in which they work to accomplish the goals of the group. They are responsive to the pressure of the group and very much aware of their status in it. When called on to make a decision, they tend to think in terms of "What will the neighbors think?" As might be expected, health care and the way the individual behaves when sick is influenced by dependence on what he or she thinks are neighbors' approval or disapproval of his or her actions. Koos' (1954) study cites the example of a woman who called a physician to see her child with the chicken pox, not because she felt it was necessary but because she did not want her friends to think that she was neglecting the child. Children and adults are dosed with vitamins and patent medicines, not because there is objective evidence that they are required but because everyone is taking the preparation. Another message source to which high credibility is attributed is television. The commercials tell us that there is value in using preparations to help us sleep, to help us stay awake, to keep one's alimentary canal active and acid-free, and to rid one's body of any possibility of human odor. It is small wonder that most Americans are in a continuous state of anxiety about their bodily functions whether or not these are normal.

The tendency of Americans to form social groups is also evident in the health and welfare field. Organizations in the health field extend from those dedicated to research and investigation of the causes of, and education of the public about, the nature of a single disease to those in which a group of people come together in order to provide emotional support for each other as they work toward the accomplishment of a single goal such as the loss of weight.

Moreover, the value of group action is so great that Americans voluntarily tax themselves for the financial support of numerous organizations. They do this by contributing to the individual organization or to the United Way. Individuals who devote time and effort to these organizations are accorded special status in the community. They may be both approved of and envied by their peers. Certain values influence defining the goals of these groups. For instance, the strong help the weak and the weak we shall always have with us to make the strong feel stronger. Americans also place a high value on independence. Children are trained early to be independent. Dependence is accepted as concomitant to illness, but the patient is expected to work toward independence. If the individual is to receive continued assistance he or she can do so only by meeting the expectation of doing whatever is necessary to alter the situation for the better, where *better* is most often defined by others without ever asking the patients what they think is better for them.

The need to be part of a group and to have status is observable in the behavior of hospitalized patients. Persons who are hospitalized for long periods of time tend to form social groups on both formal and informal bases. Many extended-care hospitals make use of this fact when planning treatment programs. The formation of groups is encouraged as a way of providing channels through which patients can make their needs known and also get some of their needs met. For example, the need for status may be partially met by forming a group whose task is to give administration suggestions regarding patient care and general ward problems. Other groups may be used to help patients work through some feelings about illness and to prepare them for life outside the hospital. Frequently the latter groups are formed by and for individuals who share a common disability or problem. There are many examples in society of these kinds of groups—colostomy clubs, Alcoholics Anonymous, and the National Paraplegics Foundation are but a few.

Sometimes an individual achieves status by having an unusual condition or by having an unusual variation of an illness. On the other hand, the fact that a person is different or does not conform to the usual pattern may cause the patient to become anxious. After recovering the patient may boast to the neighbors that he or she had an illness that the doctors had not seen before, but during the illness he or she may have had a great deal of concern about not conforming to the norm for any diagnostic category.

The American places high value on a healthy body, on youth, and on physical attractiveness. In general, we tend to devalue those who are weak (physically or emotionally), deformed, or unsightly. At times a person may be unable to accept necessary treatment because of the effect the treatment will have, or that the person believes it will have, on appearance, capacity to function, or acceptance by the group to which he or she belongs. The need to conform to the expectations of the group is illustrated also by the concern parents have that their children meet standards that are considered to indicate that the children are developing normally. This need to adhere to "the norm" results in unnecessary anxiety on the part of parents and, in turn, places pressure on the children. Children are also sensitive to pressure from their peer group to conform, as is illustrated in the instance of 6-year-old Joey, a dark brunet, who played with light, blond children. Joey made his awareness of this difference clear when he said to his mother. "Mommy, when you were getting a boy, why didn't you get a light one?"

Recognition of the value that people place on approval from their peers, as well as their tendency to work in groups and to conform to group pressure, has significance in the practice of nursing. These are important factors to consider when the condition of the patient demands a change in pattern of living. The nurse also contributes to the care of the patient by helping members of the treatment team function more effectively as a team.

It is well to remember that in the American culture, for many people, it is more important to be liked than to like others. This is an unrealistic expectation, but the effect of this particular value system is observable. As a consequence, failure on the part of the physician or nurse to express approval may be interpreted by the patient as a lack of caring, concern, or liking or as disapproval. A hypothetical example follows: The nurse tells ten patients in the ward that they look very well this morning, but she overlooks giving the same message to the eleventh patient. The eleventh patient may interpret this in many ways, and one of the interpretations may be that the nurse is more fond of everyone else in the immediate group. Obviously, this does not mean that nurses have to treat everyone exactly the same, but they should not be too surprised if they are called on periodically to sort out patients' distortions about their intentions.

The third premise on which the American value system is based is success. Success is a yardstick by which the value of an individual is measured. This means there is generally a high value placed on achievement. There is little respect for those who rest on their oars or who are not considered to be productive. There is a tendency to believe that failure results from a lack of effort and that mastery of any problem is possible if sufficient effort and/or money is expended. Thus, the chronically ill person, or one who has lost his or her job, loses status because he or she has not expended sufficient effort to stay well or be restored to health or keep or get a new job.

There is also a tendency to measure success in terms of extremes: A baby is not just a baby who is thriving, but he or she is the biggest, the smallest, the fattest, the cutest, the cryingest, or the most voracious eater on the block. Mr. Lang was not just sick with pneumonia; he had the highest temperature, made the quickest recovery, and so on. Another measure used to indicate success is the tendency to emphasize the length of life and the status position achieved rather than the fullness or richness of it.

The fourth premise is that, for the American, life is not static but is the process of change. The result is that the American is geared for action and is ready for change. He or she values adaptability and moves from one job to another to get experience, better pay, or higher status. Our "typical American" hopes that change will improve the chances of ascending the ladder of success. Popular magazines frequently carry articles about the mobility of American society and its causes and effects. Because change constitutes moving from the known to the unknown, it is accompanied by anxiety. The degree of anxiety one experiences depends on such things as the nature and magnitude of the change, the flexibility and adaptability of the individual or the society, and the meaning associated with the change.

The attitude toward change of the person from middle-class society is reflected in expectations about what constitutes adequate and appropriate medical care. When well, the middle-class individual is often willing to spend money to finance research into the causes and prevention of illness, and when sick he or she finds it difficult to understand why answers are so slow in coming. After all, he or she is spending money on such problems and wants results. The person looks for signs that his or her condition is improving, and when they are not found or change for the better cannot be expected quickly, the person tends to become anxious and feels hopeless and helpless. The middle-class American also has great faith in the value of machines and drugs and somehow feels cheated if these are not used as part of treatment. We see on television that this drug or that machine will fix things and return them to normal in less time than it takes to run the commercial. It is no wonder, then, that the person who comes for treatment expects rapid change back to the usual state of health and functioning and has difficulty accepting changes that permanently alter the "usual."

As a basis for discussion of the role of the sick person in the American culture, some of the values that relate to Ruesch's four premises—equality, sociality, success, and change—having to do with motivation have been discussed and illustrated. There are other values that are important to many Americans. Because the values held to be important by the individual influence behavior, personalizing of patient care depends on some knowledge of what these values are. The nurse should remember that not all Americans value the same things. Understanding the place of cultural factors in reactions to illness is a principle that has application in all aspects of nursing. However, the previous examples are generalizations about middle-class culture and cannot be applied to specific individuals except as a guide for understanding one dimension of the person. Studies indicate that even in fairly homogeneous communities the values held differ from one socioeconomic group to another. For example, Hollingshead and Redlich (1958) report that the type of psychotherapy that patients expect differs with each socioeconomic group. Patients from the upper socioeconomic groups expect and profit from insight therapy. They expect to learn about why they act as they do and learn to modify their behavior. Those in the lower classes expect an authoritarian attitude on the part of the psychiatrist. They want the psychiatrist to tell them what to do. Hollingshead and Redlich qualify this by stating that there are individuals in the upper classes who cannot profit from insight therapy, whereas there are those from the lower classes who can. The authors of this study further state that psychiatrists, both because they come from the middle and upper classes and because they are trained to use insight therapy, seemed to find it difficult to work with patients from the lower classes.

Studies of the attitudes of nurses toward patients such as the one reported by MacGregor (1960) also indicate that nurses view patients in light of their own values. MacGregor concluded that the students' image of the upper-class patient tended to be that of a "spoiled, demanding, condescending person who may regard the nurse as a servant." The students' view of the lower-class patient was that of a person who is more appreciative, respectful, and less demanding." These examples are cited not in criticism of either psychiatrists or nurses but to emphasize the point that each individual tends to evaluate the behavior of others in light of his or her own values and standards. This happens even when both individuals are from a similar, though not identical, culture. Of necessity this discussion has been brief, but perhaps enough detail has been presented so that the nurse can appreciate that each person tends to perceive situations in light of his or her past learnings and experiences. It is easier to accept others who have similar values and standards of behavior than it is to accept those who differ. Individualization of the patient's care demands that the nurse try to see the situation through the eyes of the patient. The nurse should realize that she or he can never see things exactly as the patient sees them, but it is important to be aware of the necessity for trying to understand as much about the patient as is possible.

The Patient's Perception of Appropriate Illness Behaviors

In addition to having values that are important in other aspects of the life of the individual, each culture or subculture establishes rules about what it regards as sickness and the behavior and responsibilities of those who are ill as well as of those who care for them. This is illustrated in the studies of the responses of Jewish, Italian, and old Americans to pain that led Zborowski (1952) to conclude that knowledge of culture is essential to the effective care of these patients. He found that the Jewish and Italian patients were more overtly emotional in expressing pain than were the old Americans. Jewish and Italian patients differed in their response to treatment, however. When appropriate measures were instituted, the Italians were relieved of their pain and happy with the result. Jewish patients, on the other hand, were concerned about the possible implications of their pain for their future health and were reluctant to take pain-relieving medications. They were fearful that drugs might produce ill effects that would be manifested at some future time. To relieve Jewish patients' pain it was necessary to relieve their concern about what was causing the pain and to reassure them about possible delayed effects of the pain-relieving medication or about their illness. Though the observed behavior appeared to be similar for Italian and Jewish patients, the meaning was different. To be effective, the treatment had to take the meaning of the pain into account.

Zborowski (1952) also found that patients of old

American stock was similar to the Jewish patient inasmuch as they tended to be concerned about the implications of the pain for their future recovery. They differed from the Jewish and Italian patients in that they were undemonstrative in reaction to pain. They also gave the impression of trying to report on pain; that is, they appeared to be trying to be an objective observer. When they were in severe pain, the old Americans tended to withdraw from society. They might cry, but when they did they preferred to cry alone. They were observed to have a different pattern of behavior when they were with their family and friends than when they were with members of the professional staff. In the presence of family and friends they tended to minimize pain and to avoid complaining. On the ward they tried to cooperate with the staff and to behave as they thought they were expected to. They considered themselves a part of the team—doctor, nurse, and patient—in which every member had a part to play and each member was expected to do his or her share.

Not only do each individual's beliefs, customs, and value systems affect the way he or she behaves when ill, they also affect how individuals think they should be treated and how those who are responsible for their care feel about them and what they do for them. As in other areas involving human beings, multiple factors are often involved, and seemingly simple behavior may have complex meanings that are interrelated with other factors. Furthermore, the interpreter interprets in his or her own frame of reference. The patient who moans and groans when in pain may be suffering from pain that is well-nigh unbearable or may feel that this is the way to bring the pain to the attention of care givers or that the family expects him or her to behave this way. The patient may be concerned about the pain itself or its implications for the future. The nurse who cares for the patient may have been brought up to believe that pain should be borne silently, or that it is appropriate to express it, or that after it is treated one should be satisfied. The manner in which the nurse treats the patient, and the extent to which she or he is able to be helpful, will depend in some measure on the nurse's understanding of the meaning that the situation has to the patient. Respect for the rights and dignity of the individual and the right of each person to participate in plans that concern personal welfare are values that are sometimes lost in the conflict over other values.

An attempt has been made to establish the importance of knowledge of the beliefs, customs, and values of the providers of care as well as of those who receive it. It is not possible to discuss all aspects of the American culture, let alone the characteristics of its subcultures. One point that has not been introduced is that professional education creates certain barriers between those who serve and those who are served. As a result of professional education and experiences, the individual acquires a modified set of values, attitudes, vocabulary, and behaviors in regard to illness. Rather than reinforcing the distance between those who serve and those who are served, professional education should aim at assisting the learner to manipulate elements in the treatment environment so that these barriers are minimized.

The Nurse's Perception of Appropriate Illness Behaviors

Nurses like all people have needs that require satisfaction. They, like other people, learn to satisfy these needs in ways that are socially acceptable to the family, group, and culture into which they were born. When they enter a school of nursing they bring with them the values, ideals, goals, and ways of behaving they have learned. Depending on their past experiences, they bring to nursing a set of expectations for what patients ought to be like and how they ought to behave. When the students are from the Anglo-American culture, they are likely to expect that patients will respond to treatment by getting well quickly and that patients will express satisfaction with and be grateful for their care. The nursing students also bring to nursing a set of expectations based on values they have learned. This includes what they believe a good nurse is, does, and ought to be able to accomplish. Through the course of their program the goals of the students and expectations for themselves and for patients are modified or changed to conform more closely to those of mentors. Brown (1965) indicates that part of the difficulty in health care stems from the fact that health professionals do not effectively communicate with each other or with patients. Each professional group is more attuned to developing its own "uniqueness" than to understanding the needs of patients. This same author (Brown, 1965) goes on to state that "Most important, perhaps, among the causes of paucity of communication, is the fact that doctors and nurses are still trained almost exclusively to treat disease and to make patients physically comfortable. The concept of 'total patient care' is extensively promoted, but it is only in the initial stage of becoming an operational concept" (p. 15). As in other areas of nursing, all nurses need to improve their ability to identify and meet the psychosocial needs of patients through study, evaluation, and practice.

By this point the fact that illness and health have social and cultural definitions as well as biological and physiologic ones should be clear. As a result of family, group, and cultural patterns the individual learns what to regard as health or sickness. He or she learns what should be done about sickness—what kinds of measures can be expected to be effective in warding it off or in curing it. The patient learns what his or her responsibilities are when ill and what he or she should expect from others including family and the members of the patient's culture who have special knowledge and skill in matters of health and disease. Those who are given status by a society by virtue of having special knowledge and skill in treating illness also have expectations, values, and ways of behaving that they accept as being appropriate. The more nearly those of the patient and the nurse or other professional persons agree, the more satisfactory services are likely to be and the more likely both individuals are to achieve satisfaction. Conversely, the greater the disparity between the client and the giver of service, the greater the possibility that the service will not be provided in a way that is satisfactory to the recipient. Moreover, this disparity can be a source of psychological stress to the patient.

References Cited

Agee, J. M. "Grief and the Process of Aging." In *Grief Responses to Long-Term Illness and Disability.* Ed. by J. Werner-Beland. Reston, Va.: Reston Publishing Company, Inc., 1980.

Amado, A., Cronk, B. A., and Mileo, R. "Cost of Terminal Care: Home Hospice vs Hosptial." *Nurs. Outlook,* **27**:8 (1979), 522–26.

Beavers, W. R. *Psychotherapy and Growth: A Family Systems Perspective.* New York: Brunner/Mazel Publishers, 1977.

Biesanz, J., and Biesanz, M. *Modern Society,* 3rd ed. Englewood Cliffs, N.J.: Prentice-Hall, 1964.

Brown, E. L. "Meeting Patient's Psychosocial Needs in the General Hospital." In *Social Interaction and Patient Care.* Ed. by J. K. Skipper, Jr., and R. Leonard. Philadelphia: J. B. Lippincott Co., 1965.

Chapman, J. E., and Chapman, H. H. *Behavior and Health Care: A Humanistic Helping Process.* Saint Louis: C. V. Mosby Co., 1975.

Christopherson, V. A. "Role Modification of the Disabled Male." *Am. J. Nurs.,* **68**:2 (1968), 291.

Craven, R. F., and Sharp, B. H. "The Effects of Illness in Family Functions." *Nurs. Forum,* **11**:2 (1972), 188.

Epstein, C. *Nursing the Dying Patient.* Reston, Va.: Reston Publishing Company, 1975.

Erikson, E. *Childhood and Society.* New York: W. W. Norton & Company, 1963.

Grace, H. K., Layton, J., and Camilleri, D. *Mental Health Nursing: A Socio-Psychological Approach.* Dubuque, Iowa: Wm. C. Brown Company, 1977.

Hamilton, E. *The Greek Way.* New York: W. W. Norton & Company, 1930.

Hanson, E. I. "Effects of Grief, Associated with Chronic Illness and Disability, on Sexuality." In *Grief Responses to Long-Term Illness and Disability.* Ed. by J. Werner-Beland. Reston, Va.: Reston Publishing Company, in press.

Heller, Z. I. "A Jewish View of Death: Guidelines for Dying." In E. Kubler-Ross. *Death: The Final Stage of Growth.* Englewood Cliffs, N.J.: Prentice-Hall, 1975.

Heusinkveld, K. B. "Cues to Communication with the Terminal Cancer Patient." *Nurs. Forum,* **11**:1 (1972), 105–13.

Hollingshead, A. B., and Redlich, F. C. *Social Class and Mental Illness.* New York: John Wiley & Sons, 1958.

Kira, A. "Privacy and the Bathroom." In *Environmental Psychology: Man and His Physical Setting.* Ed. by H. M. Proshansky, W. H. Ittelson, and L. G. Rivlin. New York: Holt, Rinehart and Winston, 1970.

Kleinman, A. "The Failure of Western Medicine." *Hum. Nature,* **1**:11 (1978), 63–68.

Kneip-Hardy, M., and Burkhardt, M. A. "Nursing the Navajo." *Am. J. Nurs.,* **77**:1 (1977), 95–96.

Koos, E. L. *The Health of Regionville.* New York: Columbia University Press, 1954.

Kübler-Ross, E. *On Death and Dying.* New York: Macmillan Company, 1969.

Kübler-Ross, E. *Death: The Final Stage of Growth.* Englewood Cliffs, N.J.: Prentice-Hall, 1975.

LeVine, R. A. *Culture, Behavior, and Personality.* Chicago: Aldine Publishing Company, 1973.

Lowe, J. "Getting well at Home." *Modern Maturity,* **19**:4 (1976), 43–45.

MacGregor, F. C. *Social Science in Nursing.* New York: Russell Sage Foundation, 1960.

Marcel, G. "Sketch of a Phenomenology and a Metaphysic of Hope." In *Reality, Man and Existence: Essential Works of Existentialism.* New York: Bantam Books, 1965.

McCabe, G. S. "Cultural Influence on Patient Behavior." *Am. J. Nurs.* **60**:8 (1960), 1101–04.

Michaels, D. R. "Too Much in Need of Support to Give Any?" *Am. J. Nurs.,* **71**:10 (1971), 1932–35.

Miller, A., ed. *Communication, Language, and Meaning: Psychological Perspectives.* New York: Basic Books, Inc., 1973.

Parsons, T., and Fox, R. "Illness, Therapy and the Modern Urban Family." In *Patients, Physicians and Illness.* Ed. by E. G. Jaco. New York: The Free Press, 1958(b).

Primeaux, M. "Caring for the American Indian Patient." *Am. J. Nurs.,* **77**:1 (1977), 91–94.

Rapoport, L. "The State of Crisis: Some Theoretical Considerations." In *Crisis Intervention: Selected Readings.* Ed. by H. J. Parad. New York: Family Service Association of America, 1965.

Rosnow, R., and Robinson, E., eds. *Experiments in Persuasion.* New York: Academic Press, 1967.

Ruesch, J., and Bateson, G. *Communication.* New York: W. W. Norton & Company, 1951.

Safilios-Rothschild, C. *The Sociology and Social Psychology of Disability and Rehabilitation.* New York: Random House, 1970.

Saunders, L. *Cultural Differences and Medical Care.* New York: Russell Sage Foundation, 1954.

Sheehy, G. *Passages.* New York: Bantam Books, 1976.

Sivadon, P. "Space as Experienced: Therapeutic Implications." In *Environmental Psychology: Man and His Physical Setting.* Ed. by H. M. Proshansky, W. H. Ittelson and L. G. Rivlin. New York: Holt, Rinehart and Winston, 1970.

Stephens, W. N. *The Family in Cross-Cultural Perspective.* New York: Holt, Rinehart and Winston, 1963.

Stillman, M. J. "Territoriality and Personal Space." *Am. J. Nurs.,* **78**:10 (1978), 1670–72.

Tillich, P. *The Courage to Be.* New Haven, Conn.: Yale University Press, 1952.

Tom, C., and Lanuza, D., eds. "Symposium on Biological Rhythms." *Nurs. Clin. North Am.,* **11**:4 (1976).

Trelease, M. L. "Dying Among Alaskan Indians: A Matter of Choice." In E. Kübler-Ross. *Death: The Final Stage of Growth.* Englewood Cliffs, N.J.: Prentice-Hall, 1975.

Watzlawick, P. *The Language of Change: Elements of Therapeutic Communication.* New York: Basic Books, 1978.

"A Way of Dying." *Atlantic Monthly,* **199**:1 (1957), 53–55.

Zborowski, M. "Cultural Elements in Response to Pain." *J. Social Issues,* **8**:4 (1952), 10–30.

31 Maintenance and Restoration of Emotional Homeostasis

Canst thou not . . . raze out the written troubles of the brain,
And with some sweet oblivious antidote
Cleanse the stuff'd bosom of that perilous stuff
Which weighs upon the heart?

SHAKESPEARE, *Macbeth,* Act V, Scene 3

Anxiety—An Index of Psychological Stress

Because illness, particularly that which produces some degree of incapacity or requires hospitalization, is a crisis situation in the life of the patient and family, it produces psychological stress resulting in various feelings of discomfort, one of which is anxiety. Despite popular opinion to the contrary, not all anxiety is bad or undesirable, nor is it all preventable. However, much can be done in the practice of nursing to reduce the incidence of unnecessary anxiety and to provide the patient with needed support. To prevent and reduce unnecessary psychological stress the nurse needs to be aware of possible causes and must be able to recognize clues in the patient's behavior that indicate how the patient feels about himself or herself and the illness.

This chapter was revised by Jean A. Werner-Beland, M.N., R.N., Associate Professor of Nursing, Wayne State University, College of Nursing, Detroit, Michigan.

Identifying the Patient's Emotional Reaction to Illness

FOUR ASPECTS OF EMOTION

According to Sartain (1962), emotion has four aspects. The *first* is the *personal emotional experience.* These are feelings that the person is conscious of and can describe verbally. The person, in describing feelings, says, "I feel so happy that I could fly or cry" or "I feel so angry and disappointed that I want to cry." The words used to describe emotions and the ability to describe feelings verbally vary from person to person. The nurse must therefore be alert to the significance not only of what the person says but of how and why he or she says it.

The *second* aspect of emotion is that *it is also expressed through bodily changes.* These changes are those associated with altering the person to meet danger and restore the body to a state of equilibrium. They result from activation of the autonomic nervous system and that part of the hormonal system that enables the organism to respond to emergency situations. Physiological changes that may accompany anxiety include trembling or shaking, restlessness, sleep disturbances (including insomnia), loss of appetite or anorexia, inability to concentrate, irritability, and other symptoms that indicate an imbalance in the autonomic nervous system. Increases in pulse, respiratory rate, and blood pressure are common, as are increased frequency of urination and disturbances in gastrointestinal activity. Peristalsis may be increased or decreased. As a result of anxiety the patient may be nauseated, vomit, have diarrhea, suffer abdominal distention, or be constipated.

The *third* aspect of emotion is *behavior that can be observed by others.* These behaviors are expressive and should be viewed as a significant part of nonverbal communication. These behaviors involve bodily changes, too, but usually ones that can be altered consciously if the person becomes aware of them or if the emotional state changes. Skeletal muscle tension or relaxation indicates something about the emotional state of the individual. The frightened or anxious individual tenses muscles in preparation for flight or fight even when neither course is open. To illustrate, Tom was an active 18-year-old whose chest x-ray showed a well-defined lesion in the lower lobe of his right lung. Surgery was performed promptly and the diseased tissue removed. Both Tom and his parents were badly frightened. Tom did not talk about his fears but was seen lying against his pillows with his fists clenched and with obvious body tension. Deep breathing, turning, and coughing were accompanied by more than the usual amount of pain and difficulty. His cough was unproductive and the lung on the operated side was slow in reexpanding. Attempts at reassurance were of little help until one morning when the surgeon told Tom, "The reports are back from the pathologist. Your lung had a harmless little tumor in it. You are cured." The change in Tom was remarkable. He relaxed, assumed responsibility for his own care, and in other ways demonstrated that he was no longer frightened.

Behavioral expressions are especially useful when trying to identify the emotional state of the individual who is unable to talk. The nurse should keep in mind that there is no single reason people do not talk about their feelings. Some may not understand their own feelings well enough to discuss them, or they may recognize the feeling and be reluctant to discuss it because they do not know how it will be received, or they may be physically unable to talk. Facial expression is one common source of information about a person's emotional state. We frequently hear comments such as, "He talks with his eyes." "The boss is in a good mood today; he was smiling when he came in." "She looks as if she just lost her best friend," and "her face is peaceful. She must be a happy person." Though facial expression serves as a clue to the emotional state, more information is required in order to make an accurate assessment of how the individual really feels. A person may smile when he or she feels like crying or pride himself or herself on having a "poker face." Cultural and environmental factors also play a part in how a person learns to use various body or facial gestures to express emotion. In some cultures individuals learn to keep their faces immobile, and they may suffer pain and other discomfort without any change of expression. When this is the case, other means of estimating the degree of discomfort must be used. The main point here is that the facial expression is only a signal that alerts the nurse to explore its meaning. The patient is really the only person who can say what the expression means. Too often nurses are guilty of making assumptions about the meaning of the patient's behavior without actually asking the patient what it means to him or her.

Emotion may also be expressed through movements of the hands and body. In the instance of Tom, he expressed his fright by tensing his muscles and clenching his fists. Another patient may move about, twist and turn in bed, pace the floor, wring the hands, or shake his or her fists. Other emotions are also expressed through body movement. Friendliness may be shown by shaking hands, joy by clapping the hands, and so forth. Posture and step also reveal the feelings of the individual. When a person's posture is erect and the step is firm, he or she creates the impression of being healthy and feeling good about himself or herself and others. Conversely, when the person's shoulders sag, feet drag, and movements are languid, the impression is created of someone who is dejected or depressed. Clarification is necessary here as well. For example, a patient is observed picking at the edge of the covers. At this point the nurse does not actually know if the patient is anxious and needs to talk about something, is trying to get a gravy stain off the blanket binding, or is anoxic and in dire need of attention. She or he can find the answer by obtaining more information and by closer inspection of the situation.

In the American culture, where high value is placed on a healthy body and cleanliness, grooming and other evidence of cleanliness are clues to the emotional state of the individual. Uncombed and untidy hair, soiled and ragged clothing, dirty and poorly kept fingernails, or runover shoes may be interpreted as meaning that the person has a low self-opinion. Before arriving at any conclusions, one must know such things as (1) the type of work the person does, (2) the expectations of the group with whom he or she identifies, and (3) whether this appearance is a significant change associated with illness or has this been a life-long pattern. For example, a man who spends his working days greasing automobiles is likely to have a problem keeping his fingernails clean. Another may look as if he needs a shave not because he is neglecting his appearance but because he is growing a beard.

Vocal expressions of emotion may be through talking, crying, whistling, laughing, or screaming. In talking, the person's feeling is conveyed not only by what is said but by whether what is said is usual for the individual and by the tone of voice. It is also helpful to know how the person usually expresses satisfaction or dissatisfaction. Sometimes the words and tone used by a patient are offensive to the nurse. When this happens, the nurse should try to discover what the patient is trying to communicate rather than making judgments about the words themselves. When a patient is able to modify behavior, limits can be set based on the patient's needs and the situation.

In general, laughter and humor are acceptable ways of expressing feeling in the American culture. This may be related to the fact that laughter is often associated with "good" feelings such as joy. The fact is that laughter and humor may hide feelings such as sorrow, anxiety, or hostility. The patient who is always laughing and joking may be admired at first, but this "bravado" type of behavior tends to wear thin and others become suspect of the patient's motives. A little thought given to the reasons behind this behavior might reveal that the patient is frightened, or angry, or both. The last example points out the *fourth* aspect of emotion, which is *motivation.* This term refers to the fact that people are goal-directed. Our laughing, joking patient may be frightened or angry—those are his or her feelings. Because it is natural for people to want to avoid pain, we can speculate that the goal this patient seeks is to avoid the pain of personal feelings. One way the patient has learned to do this is seen in the laughing and joking behavior. Laughter is often used to relieve tension. Playwrights use humor to break the tension in a serious drama, so it is not too surprising that patients might use humor to break the tension in the serious drama of illness.

Responses to the Crying Person

Although joy and gladness may be expressed by crying, the shedding of tears is usually associated with "bad" feelings such as pain, sorrow, helplessness, and anger. Though adults have these feelings, their expression by crying is disapproved of. Moreover, when men, who are expected to be strong, cry, their behavior is regarded as being particularly inappropriate. Crying is for babies who are still dependent on their mothers and not for grown men and women who have long since reached adulthood. Nurses who find themselves with a crying adult may feel uncomfortable because they do not understand the regressive phenomenon of illness, of which crying may be one symptom. The nurse may be embarrassed because the patient is unable to control his or her behavior. The nurse may become uncomfortable because crying is viewed as a distress signal and yet she or he does not know what to do to intervene, or because a crying patient is a reflection on the quality of nursing care—or so the nurse thinks. Whatever the reason, or combination of reasons, for the discomfort, the nurse's first impulse is usually to get the patient to stop crying. Instead of concentrating on trying to stop the crying, it would be more helpful for the nurse to understand what the patient is trying to express through crying. It is also important to know the individual. Does he or she come from a subculture where crying is a fairly common means of expression? Does this patient cry easily, or is this the first time that such behavior has been noted? These are just two of the questions the nurse can ask. Usually, an effective way to find out what is going on is for the nurse to wait until the patient stops crying. She or he can indicate willingness to listen when the patient is ready to talk about his or her feelings.

It may be helpful if nurses make an attempt to understand their attitudes about crying. How do they feel when they cry? Do they ever allow themselves to cry, and if not, why not? Under what circumstances do they cry? What do they expect from others when they cry in their presence? This self-inspection does not preclude talking with the patient about why he or she cries, but it may make the situation more understandable and tolerable for the nurse. The nurse may come to understand that what the patient really wants is for someone to indicate that they care about his or her concerns. Patients may not be asking for solutions because they may know that there are no solutions available in terms of performing some technical procedure that will "cure all." On the other hand, if there is some physical comfort measure that is indicated, this should be used.

Other Expressions of Emotion

Other ways in which patients express their emotions vocally are by shouting, screaming, moaning, and sighing. These behaviors, for much the same reason as crying, may be upsetting to nurses. They are also disturbing to other patients. When this behavior is continued and is upsetting to other patients, it may be necessary to isolate the patient in a soundproof room. In one hospital the isolation of Puerto Rican women who were in labor was found to be necessary. When these women reached a certain point in labor they screamed, and their screaming was very frightening to other patients. Before placing a patient in isolation one should be certain that there is no other solution and that the isolation is for the good of the other patients or the individual patient. When isolation is necessary, the nurse has an obligation to try to identify and meet the needs of the patient. Someone should stay with the patient, or, if continuous supervision is not necessary, the patient should be told how to summon the nurse and such calls should be answered promptly. Though the welfare of others may make isolation of the patient necessary, this procedure increases the patient's need of nursing. Studies of the effects of isolation on healthy young men indicate the importance of environmental stimulation for healthy mental functioning. Downs (1974) found similar results when she replicated sensory deprivation studies using healthy subjects confined to a simulated hospital room environment.

Sometimes when the behavior is deemed unacceptable, a patient is isolated by neglect rather than by physical isolation. Mr. Jones was screaming in severe pain, but no one was paying attention to him. The reason given for the neglect was that he was "just a neurotic with a low tolerance for pain." On investigation he was found to be hemorrhaging into his urinary bladder at a spot where the bladder wall had been eroded by a bladder stone. Mr. Jones was a paraplegic and had what is called a neurogenic bladder; that is, it emptied spontaneously when it reached its capacity, which was very small. As the bladder filled, painful muscle contractions were initiated. Because blood clots blocked the urethra and prevented his bladder from emptying, the painful muscle spasms increased in frequency as the bladder wall stretched. Perhaps Mr. Jones' tolerance for pain was minimal, but he *was* suffering and needed relief. When the physician saw Mr. Jones, he scheduled him for emergency surgery. Following surgery, Mr. Jones was well controlled. This is an excellent example of the danger of categorizing patients according to their behavior without adequate investigation into its cause. That some of this man's care was inhumane should not require saying. Moreover, conclusions about the cause of a patient's behavior should not be reached without thorough knowledge of the patient and his or her situation.

There are many ways in which patients manifest their anxiety. A variety of behaviors characterized by action may be called "flight into activity." The patient makes jokes and is the life of the ward because talking relieves tension and serves much the same purpose as whistling in the dark. Pacing up and down the corridor or going from one activity to another serves a similar purpose. Careful listening may yield clues about the meaning of the patient's behavior that may make it possible to initiate action that will help allay the patient's fears.

One of the problems in planning care directed toward minimizing anxiety is that despite identification of signs and symptoms these do not in themselves identify the cause of the anxiety. Nor does the relief of anxiety always take precedence over other necessary care. The patient who is bleeding excessively will be anxious, but the problem that takes priority is the hemorrhage. At the time the most reassuring thing that can be done is to initiate prompt action to stop the bleeding. In the words of a patient who experienced this situation, "I turned on my light and the student nurse came right away. She ran and got the head nurse who ran and got the doctor. The doctor came right away and I was in the operating room before I knew what was happening—and a good thing too. I owe my life to the fact that they were on their toes."

It has been mentioned that it is not always possible to determine all the factors contributing to anxiety. Nor is it possible to relieve anxiety entirely even if such a thing were desirable. There are times in patient care when anxiety is necessary to keep the patient motivated to work toward the achievement of healthier goals. Sometimes it is necessary to stimulate anxiety in patients so they will be less willing to accept the status quo of hospitalization. This must be done with careful planning and by personnel who have considerable skill in the area of human behavior.

There are also many factors in illness and its diagnosis and treatment that are anxiety provoking but cannot be avoided. One of the greatest fears in life is the unknown. Any time the nurse can anticipate the unknown and interpret it for the patient, she or he is creating an environment that may make it easier for the patient to participate effectively in treatment. Reasonable explanations should be given to the patient, so he or she knows what is being done and why. This approach usually helps keep the patient's anxiety within reasonable bounds.

In individualizing care it is helpful if the nurse can recognize the pattern the patient uses in establishing or avoiding relationships with others. The mature adult in American culture is thought to be one who can relate to others as an equal. He or she can work interdependently or cooperatively with others and can give and take as the situation demands. In actuality this is a myth. Some people form dependent relationships, some need to dominate others, some rebel against others (especially those in authority), and some avoid forming any lasting relationships. These patterns may not be as evident when the person is well as they are when he or she is sick. The aggressive executive, for example, may deny any dependent strivings when well but may deny them even more when threatened by illness. Much has been written about the Type A coronary-prone individual and related care problems (see Chapter 43).

Patients are expected to place themselves in a dependent relationship to those who provide their care. This dependency is considered "healthy" when patients cooperate with getting the care they realistically need. The trend in health care is toward encouraging patients to participate in the decision-making process rather than expecting them to submit to decisions that others make about their care. In this view, patients are recognized as being an important element in their own recovery. That is, the recovery of the patient depends on the patient. The services of doctors, nurses, and other health workers only provide conditions under which the patient's recovery can be facilitated. Because all patients do not interact or react in the same manner, recognition of the patient's pattern should alert the nurse to some problems that may arise in his or her care. If the patient is one who characteristically rebels against others, time may be needed for talking himself or herself into doing what must be done. For this patient, pressure from another person may only increase resistance. If the pressure is too great, the patient may take a position from which no retreat can be made without considerable loss of self-esteem.

Minimizing Stress through Nursing Intervention

Florence Nightingale (1860) in *Notes on Nursing*, emphasized the need for the nurse to recognize and relieve anxiety in the patient. She wrote the following:

> Apprehension, uncertainty, waiting, expectation, fear of surprise, do a patient more harm than any exertion. Remember, he is face to face with his enemy all the time, internally wrestling with him, having long imaginary conversations with him. You are thinking of something else. "Rid him of his adversary quickly," is a first rule with the sick.

Suggesting problems to the patient can be prevented by making certain you understand what he or she is asking or wants to know. This can be done by asking for clarification or by indicating that you do not understand what is wanted. The principle here can be illustrated by the classic story about the little boy who asked his mother where his baby sister came from. The mother had been anxiously awaiting the day when her boy would raise this question, so she went into her detailed story about how his father planted the seed and so on. When she finished, she asked the boy if he understood. He said, "All I wanted to know was did she come from the hospital down the street or from the Sister's hospital?"

The question "What can we do to relieve the patient's anxiety and thus reassure him?" suggests other questions. How does one person reassure another? What does reassurance mean? Is it accomplished by telling the other person that everything will be all right? Does one person stop worrying when another says, "Leave the worrying to me"? Dictionaries define *reassurance* as a transitive verb meaning "to restore to courage or confidence, also to re-establish." Its synonyms include "to encourage," which in turn means "to inspire with courage, hope, confidence, or resolution; to help forward as well as to animate, cheer, hearten, and inspire." It is also interesting to note that synonyms of encourage include console, comfort, solace, and sympathize with. How can the nurse through the practice of nursing assist the patient to regain courage or confidence? The emphasis here is on the patient's regaining hope and confidence, not on the nurse's giving this to him or her. However, nurses contribute to this by what they do and how they do it. Wertham (1952) states that during an operation two factors contributed to decreasing his general feeling of insecurity. One was the calm, deep, authoritative voice of the surgeon. The other was the soothing effect of the touch of a woman physician as she said something to him. Though he recognized that the friends who were with him were trying to reassure him by talking and joking, he did not find this behavior at all reassuring.

Barker et al. (1953) talk of helping patients to think in terms of what they have left and what they can do rather than what they have lost and what they cannot do. This approach has great supportive value for those, for example, who suddenly become physically disabled. On the other hand, nothing is more devastating to a patient than the thoughtless statements that suddenly confront him or her with the loss and the meaning this loss has to his or her total identity. The author (then a patient) experienced the latter when a physician introduced her to another physician and added. "Before her accident, she was a nurse." This does not mean that patients should never look at the readjustments they need to make as the result of illness. They do need to assess their situation realistically but not without help that enables them to look at what is possible for them, what they need to do differently, and what they may have to defer or give up entirely.

Reassurance of the patient is frequently difficult. Sometimes it is not achieved until the patient knows the outcome of treatment. In another situation, a patient who had undergone a bronchoscopy stated that he did not think he could have withstood the procedure had the nurse not given him instructions during the procedure about what he should do and about the progress of the procedure. Here the talking related directly to what the patient could expect from himself and from the situation and was not intended to distract his attention. Though what is reassuring differs from one person to another, confidence that the situation is under control is often helpful. For some people this is all that is necessary.

Some Attributes of the Nurse Perceived by Patients as Helpful

One of the ways to learn what actions enhance the patients' confidence in their care is by listening to what they say. Some of the things that patients comment on as being reassuring and adding to their security include having nurses work with them who

1. Have the ability to assess the situation quickly and initiate prompt action when required
2. Appear to know what to do
3. Take over when the patient is overwhelmed and know how to do the "right thing"
4. Will be there when needed
5. Keep the patient informed about what they are doing and why, when they can be expected, how long they will be away, and how much time they will spend with him or her
6. Learn what the patient expects and help correct misunderstandings and misconceptions about what can be expected
7. Maintain uniformity in the performance of frequently repeated procedures and appraise the patient of changes that are planned
8. Encourage the patient in self-help in ways that are possible not because it helps the nurse per se but because in this way the patient can learn to do for himself or herself
9. Help the patient become aware of even small gains
10. Can modify their behavior in such a manner that the patient knows they are sensitive to and concerned about his or her feelings
11. Take care of the patient's personal belongings and physical environment
12. Give attention to those things that are important to the patient, such as respecting the right to some privacy
13. Keep informed about changes in the therapeutic plan even though this is not always easy—and can develop a plan for nursing care based on the therapeutic plan
14. Involve family or significant others in planning when this is indicated and acceptable to the patient

Both the person and the circumstances under which the need for reassurance arises are determining factors in the type of behavior that is to be effective. Though some suggestions can be made for the type of behavior that may be reassuring, no recipe can be given for what will always result in reassurance. Reassurance requires competence in the practice on nursing. By this is meant that the nurse knows what she or he is doing, why it is being done, and how to do it or is reassuring in the fact that she or he will seek help if something is not known. The nurse gives appropriate attention to detail not for the sake of detail but because it is important to the outcome of what is being done. The nurse thinks about what is being done, its effect on the patient, and about how it can be improved. It is important to help the patient feel valued as an individual, that needs will be met, and that he or she is in safe hands. Acceptance can be accomplished, in part, by doing for and with the patient those things that are important to his or her welfare. Because patients' welfare includes both physical and psychological aspects, care also includes both—bathing, feeding, listening, supporting, protecting, comforting, anticipating, and relieving. It also includes allowing, encouraging, and supporting the patient in assuming responsibility for personal care as soon as possible. It also involves validating the meaning of the patient's behavior and then acting appropriately.

To illustrate, a nurse answers Mr. Jason's call signal. She observes that he is irritable. She knows that irritability is common in sick people and that it indicates not what is wrong but that something is wrong. It is a warning signal. Instead of feeling personally attacked, the nurse asks herself why Mr. Jason may be irritable. Is he receiving insulin in the treatment of his diabetes? If so, is he suffering from hypoglycemia? Is he having difficulty with his oxygen intake? Does he have a low frustration tolerance as the result of brain damage? Is he cold? Is he disappointed because his wife and family have not been to visit him? Has he had too many visitors? Is he troubled about the nature of his illness, its cost, or what is going to happen in relation to his job? Is he lonely? Has he been accustomed to consuming large amounts of alcohol and is he now beginning to show signs of withdrawal? Did the patient in the next bed keep him awake all night? Is this usually the way he behaves under stress? The nurse tries to determine the cause of Mr. Jason's irritability and institutes action aimed at solving or relieving the identifiable problem. She may listen to his complaint, get him a glass of orange juice, call a social worker, or do any number of other meaningful things. What she does depends upon what the patient tells her and on her professional assessment of what the patient needs at the time.

Another illustration is the case of Mr. McGraw, who swears when he is in pain. The nurse notes the beads of perspiration on his brow and his clenched fists. She recognizes that his pain is severe and understands that swearing is his way of emphasizing its severity. The nurse lets Mr. McGraw know that she recognizes his suffering, talks with him about what he thinks will relieve it, and then does something to relieve it. Under other circumstances. Mr. McGraw's swearing may have other meanings. He may be in the habit of swearing. If his swearing really is offensive to others, the nurse may have to set limits by pointing out that his behavior disturbs others. She may ask him to try to use other, equally understandable words to convey his message.

The nurse also needs to be aware of what causes her or him to become anxious or uncomfortable. To return to Mr. McGraw, if the nurse becomes anxious, or feels that his swearing is a personal affront, she may leave him to "stew in his own juice until he can act like a gentleman." If, however, she is aware of her own discomfort and still can remain with Mr. McGraw, she may be able to take the next step, which is to find out why he is behaving this way. Her further action then can be directed toward the primary goal of meeting Mr. McGraw's needs. When she is successful in meeting the patient's needs, she also meets her own need for self-realization as a nurse.

Purposeful Conversation—A Critical Nursing Skill

Another skill needed in nursing is the use of purposeful conversation. Though all conversation has purpose, the kind we are talking about is for the specific purpose of furthering communication that is important to the improvement of patient care. Purposeful communication is an essential part of the nursing process because it makes possible the collection of information, the identification of the problem, the formulation of a plan of action, the implementation of that plan, and the evaluation of its effectiveness. What this means essentially is that the nurse becomes accustomed to thinking in a logical sequence and uses all communication skills—including conversation—to help in this.

Establishment of a Goal

The *first step* in purposeful conversation is the *establishment of a goal that is valid and sincere.* When a problem is known or suspected, the objective should be based on the desire to assist the patient rather than identifying the problem just for the sake of knowing what the problem is. Standeven (1971) writes that "the commonly described method for problem solving indicates the action to be taken but leaves out who should be involved at each step." A more effective approach to problem solving includes not only the patient but also gives consideration to out-of-view relevant others.

Dialogue

Second, purposeful conversation *implies a dialogue.* Hearing both the words and what they mean is important. Communication takes place only when the message sent is the same as the message that is received. Too often we assume that the listener understood exactly what we intended only to find that there was a major breakdown between what was intended and how it was interpreted. Listening only with the ears is perhaps too restrictive. The really skillful nurse usually has learned to listen with all the senses. One needs to hear what the speaker is saying, how he or she is saying it, and what the facial expression is. Attention should also be given to shifts in the person's conversation. What the person does not say, or skips over, may be just as important as what is said. Purposeful conversation also means that the responder may need to take time to think out a reply. To do this he or she must be able to keep the objective of the conversation in mind and to tolerate silence. Some of the world's most skillful conversationalists talk very little but listen much. This is illustrated by the taxi driver who, on discharging a passenger, said, "My, you are a good listener." During the hour's ride, the passenger had said little except "Mmm," "Not really." "You like your work," and a few other similar comments. The only purpose of the listener's responding at all was to indicate that she was following what the driver was saying and was interested in it.

In addition to listening, conversation may be facilitated by asking open-ended questions or by asking the patient to clarify what he or she has said. In using open-ended questions, the questioner tries to avoid asking the question in a way that suggests the answer. Statements such as, "I don't understand," "Could you clarify that?" or "You were saying . . . ?" or even "Oh," or "Mmm" when said with rising inflection can be used to indicate that one is interested, is following what is being said, and would like to hear more. The patient should also be given time to respond. This means that the nurse must be able to stay with the patient and wait for a response.

The nurse may suspect that something is worrying the patient and may have clues to what is troubling him or her. The nurse must put these to the test. This can be done by repeating what the patient has said or what appears to be the intent of the comment. For example, Miss Tente, a patient in her teens, appeared to be upset when the student nurse tried to instruct her in how to inject her own insulin. The student was surprised because up to this time Miss Tente had seemed eager to learn. The student suspected that Miss Tente's hesitancy might be related to something other than inserting the needle. To test her hypothesis she said, "You are troubled this morning"; then she waited. In a few moments Miss Tente started to cry. Between her sobs she told the student nurse that when she told her boy friend about her diabetes he no longer wanted to "go steady."

Use of Silence

The use of silence may give some people an opening to talk about their troubles or problems, and it has other uses as well. In the care of the seriously ill, conversation should be limited in order to conserve the patient's energy. Some seriously ill people are comforted by the closeness of having someone sit quietly by their bedside. This may give a relative or close friend an opportunity to make a substantial contribution to the patient's welfare. A relative may need some instruction in how to behave in the presence of the patient and support for his or her contribution to the welfare of the patient from nursing personnel. For example, Mr. Clark was seriously ill in a hospital located some distance from his home. His wife was notified of his illness, and the suggestion was made that she arrange to come to the hospital as soon as possible. When she arrived, she was understandably distraught. The nurse, recognizing Mrs. Clark's emotional condition and that she had been riding on the bus all night, arranged for her to wash her face and hands and apply cosmetics. Then she suggested that after Mrs. Clark greeted her husband, she might sit quietly by his bed and, if she would like to do so, hold his hand. In this instance the nurse helped Mrs. Clark compose herself and then provided some additional structure for Mrs. Clark. Action of this kind, under highly stressful conditions, served the purpose of freeing Mrs. Clark from the burden of having to make the initial evaluation of how she might be helpful to her husband.

Another frequently neglected practice of silence is what may be called friendly silence. Everyone feels good toward the other members of the group. All are comfortable and relaxed. This is the silence that says, "All is calm and serene I am glad to be with you." On the other hand, with all the emphasis on togetherness and sociability, the fact that some people need and desire an opportunity to be by themselves may be overlooked. Over the course of history the value and pain of solitude have been expressed in prose and poetry. Of modern writers few have expressed this more beautifully than Anne Morrow Lindbergh in *Gift from the Sea* (1955). In essence she says that for life to have its full meaning and purpose, time must be set aside for contemplation in peace and quiet. To quote Mrs. Lindbergh, "Here there is time; time to be quiet; time to work without pressure; time to think; time to watch the heron, watching with frozen patience for his prey. . . . Time, even, *not* to talk" (p. 116).

A purposeful conversation is one of the tools used by the nurse to establish a therapeutic relationship with a patient. The goal of a particular conversation may be to identify what is troubling a patient so that, when possible, appropriate measures can be initiated for relief. Conversation may be used to gain or to impart information, to determine the patient's expectations, to determine what the patient knows and what he or she wants to know, or to learn something about the family, work, or living conditions, as a basis for planning future care. During recovery from acute illness or during chronic illness, conversation may also provide needed diversion and recreation. Loneliness is one of the difficult problems in long-term illness. This is equally true whether the person is cared for at home or in the hospital. The patient longs for conversation with a sympathetic friend. A friendly listener may be the one bright spot in the person's day or week. Here again, attention to what the patient is saying, to what his or her interests are, and to encouraging the expansion of this interest and to bring in a bit of outside world may be a rewarding experience for patient and nurse alike. Whatever the purpose of the conversation, its goals should be known. As in the use of other techniques in the care of the patient, the goals should be defined in terms of the needs of the patient. Conversation, like other skills, is learned and can be improved. This requires practice and evaluation of each conversation. What went well? Where did I get off the track? Why? What could have been done to keep on the track? What are my real goals?

Summary of Steps Toward Establishing Significant Nurse-Patient Relationship

Throughout this chapter the goal of establishing a therapeutic or helping relationship with the patient has been emphasized. The steps in the establishment of a significant relationship, as they have been stated by Schmahl (1958), are as follows:

1. "Awareness of one's own anxiety." In addition to this, the nurse must be willing to cope with it by moving slowly, waiting, and staying with it.
2. "Sustained physical thereness." The nurse must remain with the patient when needed. This is easier to do when giving physical care. The nurse should eventually develop the ability to stay with the patient when no physical care is required.
3. "Critical listening."
4. "Open-ended questions." As emphasized earlier with regard to critical listening, attention is given not only to the obvious meanings of the words that the patient uses but to their hidden meanings. The use of open-ended questions has been discussed.
5. "Consensual validation" (p. 90). By consensual validation is meant that what one thinks something means is also what it actually does mean. This can be done by putting hunches to the test and getting feedback from the patient that validates the accuracy of the hunch.

Summary

In this chapter some of the knowledge required by the nurse to meet the psychosocial needs of patients has been presented. Because of the rapidity with which knowledge in this area is growing, no single chapter can do more than summarize the more pertinent information. The hope is that students will become interested in exploring further resources.

Throughout the chapter emphasis has been placed on the fact that human behavior is the product of multiple factors. Each individual's behavior results from reactions to and interaction with the culture. An individual's biological inheritance and structure are also a significant element in behavior, for they determine his or her possibilities for development as well as limits. A bird can fly. A human being cannot, or could not until the airplane was invented. Sophia Moore is a grown woman, but she is less than 3 feet tall. She is deeply depressed. She says, "I am a nobody. How can anyone who is small like me be anybody when to be somebody one must be big?" Sophia's size is biologically based. Her self-concept is derived from the value placed on physical bigness in the culture into which she was born. In another culture she might have been made a queen or treated as a god. In another, where smallness was the rule, she would not have been the object of any special attention. Culture is both universal and unique to humans. Though all people are of the same species and cultures have common characteristics, both humans and culture run the gamut in variety.

Illness is, however, a personal experience. How the person behaves during illness usually depends on how he or she behaves in other crisis situations in life. But the reaction also depends on the psychological meaning that illness has for the person. Other crisis situations may not have had the identical personal meaning, and therefore the reaction would be different. Studies of people who are ill reveal that not all persons react to illness in the same manner. This point is emphasized by the findings of Kaplan (1956), who studied the psychological aspects of heart disease. Some of the factors that he found to influence the reaction of the individual included (1) the personality of the patient before the illness and his or her life situation, (2) the degree or extent of the physical incapacity, (3) the abruptness of the onset, (4) the degree of severity, (5) the duration of the illness, and (6) the relationship of the patient to family and to physician. Though the subjects for this study were people having mitral commissurotomies, recent literature indicates that these factors enter into the behavior of patients with other diseases. This supports the concept that it is the patient and not the diagnosis that is of first importance in one's reaction to disease.

Failure to identify and interpret appropriately a patient's behavior may be a source of psychological stress to the patient and to the nurse. When the patient and the nurse have a common cultural heritage, their expectations and values will more likely be in agreement than when they are from dissimilar backgrounds. When the behavior of patients differs from that expected by the professional staff, the professional staff has a responsibility to accept the patient's behavior as having meaning and to adapt its own behavior accordingly. The burden should be on the professional person rather than on the patient. Application of knowledge of the psychosocial aspects of patient care should enhance the patient's feeling that he or she is accepted as an individual human being with dignity and rights. The patient should further feel safe and protected and able to depend on those who are responsible for his or her care. Skillful use of the knowledge of the psychosocial needs of patients should add to the satisfaction the nurse derives from the practice of nursing. It is one of the marks of a truly professional nurse.

References Cited

Barker, R. G., Wright, B. A., and Conick, M. R. *Adjustment to Physical Handicap and Illness: A Survey of the Social Psychology of Physique and Disability,* rev. ed. New York: Social Sciences Research Council, 1953.

Downs, F. S. "Bedrest and Sensory Disturbance." *Am. J. Nurs.,* **74**:3 (1974), 434–38.

Kaplan, S. M. "Psychological Aspects of Cardiac Disease." *Psychosom. Med.,* **118,** (May–June 1956), 221–33.

Lindbergh, A. M. *Gift from the Sea.* New York: Pantheon Books, 1955.

Nightingale, F. *Notes on Nursing: What It Is and What It Is Not,* rev. ed. London. Harrison and Sons, 1860.

Sartain, A. et al. *Psychology: Understanding Human Behavior,* 2nd ed. New York: McGraw-Hill, 1962.

Schmahl, J. "The Price of Recovery." *Am. J. Nurs.,* **58**:1 (1958), 90.

Standeven, M. "The Relevant "Who" of Problem Solving." *Nurs. Forum,* **10**:2 (1971), 167.

Wertham, F. "A Psychosomatic Study of Myself. In *When Doctors Are Patients.* Ed. by M. Pinner and B. F. Miller. New York: W. W. Norton & Company, 1952.

General References

Anxiety

Rodman, M. J. "Drugs for Treating Anxiety." *RN,* **36** (Sept. 1973), 57–68.

Pitts, F. N. "The Biochemistry of Anxiety." *Sci. Am.,* (Feb. 1969).

32 The Spiritual Dimension of Nursing

Guard the heart for it is the wellspring of life.
PROVERBS 4:23

An appreciation of the spiritual dimension of care can be seen throughout nursing history from its ancient religious origins based on the Golden Rule and Good Samaritan tradition to its modern-day practice based on the Nightingale tradition.

Nursing is an art, and if it is to be made an art, requires as exclusive a devotion, as hard a preparation, as any painter's or sculptor's work, for what is the having to do with dead canvas, or cold marble, compared with having to do with the living body—the temple of God's spirit. . . . It is one of the Fine Arts. I had almost said, the finest of the Fine Arts (Nightingale, 1872).

From the mid-1950s onward spiritual considerations in nursing curricula waned as emphasis on advancing medical technology increased. Today the critical decisions people must face in health care as a result of this very technology have brought about a refocusing on the spiritual dimensions of nursing. The spiritual dimension of nursing as presented here is based on a universal concept of spirituality rather than a particular concept of religion (Kiening, 1978). (For this latter approach see Henderson and Nite, 1978; Kelly, 1975.)

The concept of human beings presented here is as whole persons—an indivisible blending of body, mind, heart, and spirit, where distress in any one aspect affects the others (Stallwood, 1975). The nursing interventions suggested here are based on a universal concept of "inspiriting" rather than a particular concept of counseling through prayer, scripture, and religious literature. (For this latter approach see Stallwood 1975, and Fish 1978.) As used here, the term *inspiriting* is based on Sidney Jourard's concept of inspiration described in *The Transcendent Self:*

Loving care, in which someone has faith and confidence, induces hope, which in turn is a manifestation, concomitant, or cause of inspiration—a gain in spirit-titre. . . . Nursing has much to teach us here, both about the art of inspiration and about body-image correlates of spirit (Jourard, 1971).

Spiritual Dimension

Spirituality is defined as the life principle that pervades a person's entire being, including volitional, emotional, moral-ethical, intellectual, and physical dimensions, and generates a capacity for transcendent values. The spiritual dimension of a person integrates and transcends biological and psychosocial nature, giving access to the nonphysical realms of prophecy, artistic inspiration, love, and healing actions (Friedlander, 1964). Spiritual need is more encompassing than religious need. Spiritual need is that requirement which touches the core of one's being where the search for personal meaning takes place.

Written by Margaret A. Colliton, D.Sc.N., who has a private practice in New Haven, Connecticut, and administrates Wellspring, an intermediate psychiatric treatment facility whose philosophy is based on healing of the whole person.

If spiritual need is met, it becomes possible to relate to reality with hope, even in the presence of suffering (White House Conference on Aging, 1971). Spiritual help is different from emotional support. Although spiritual longing is often expressed through the emotions, spiritual help concerns itself with the relationship of a person to a higher being, a relationship through which a person may experience unconditional love, forgiveness, hope, faith, affirmation, or meaning in life (Peipgras, 1968).

Illness as Spiritual Journey

The spiritual dimension may express itself as vital through radiant health or it may express itself as gloriously indominable through devastating illness when a person transcends his or her suffering. Flannery O'Connor recounts the story of a child, Mary Ann, who lived in a hospice for persons with incurable cancer from the time she was 3 until her death at 12. Mary Ann, though disfigured with a large facial tumor, was experienced as beautiful and inspired all who knew her with a joy for life (O'Connor, 1970). Three things are necessary for a person to resolve spiritual crisis and transcend suffering with integrity instead of despair: awareness of true self, personal meaning, and relatedness to a higher being.

Awareness of True Self

Usually children, if raised in an atmosphere of love, are at one with their authentic being. In *The Brothers Karamazov,* Alyosha cautions his young friends not to lose touch with their true spirit which must be protected as the wellspring of life (Dostoyevsky, 1950). An awareness of an essential "I" who is original, existing beyond the limits of time and space and united to a larger meaning or totally integrated is expressed here by the following account of a very early childhood memory, recalled by a person exploring the roots of his later healing vocation:

> My memory reaches back into earliest childhood. I saw colors. They were bright and moved before my eyes, to and fro, sometimes darker, then again lighter. Suddenly shadows moved by. Then I winced and felt the fright move through my small body, from my head to the tip of my fingers and toes. I did not know that I lay in a baby carriage in the garden, that there were branches which moved before my eyes in the wind, and birds flying over whose voices I could hear but could not yet bring into connection with the passing shadows in the sky overhead. But apart from the fright, I felt well. I enjoyed the light, the brightness of the sky, the moving colors, and felt myself to be very fortunate and thankful. Naturally I did not know the words for this, even the little words sky, branches, and bird. They were nothing more than a kaleidoscopic picture, so beautiful, so blissful, so unique—truly the first revelation for me of the world and its beauty and the blissful feeling of fortune. I felt with my entire body the full hope of growth, a creature of nature like everything which encircled me, and I was at one with it. There was no inner and outer. I was together with everything—everything me, everything mine (Frank, 1973).

A person who has not experienced love is out of touch with his or her authentic being. In Bergman's film, *Wild Strawberries,* a very old distinguished professor, on his way to receive the ultimate academic award, inadvertently discovers that his life has been a failure because he had never been aware of his true being. In only a brief period, less than a day, but with considerable pain and turmoil, he works through this turning point, becomes aware of himself in a new way, and becomes conscious of his authentic self. With this metamorphosis, he realizes that, no matter how little life is left to him, it will be profoundly different and more satisfying. His previous comatose spiritual state has lifted and life now holds meaning. This film affirms that it is possible to evolve spiritually until death—perhaps even afterward. Though the human body becomes impoverished, the human spirit can become enriched. It is never too late to experience spiritual growth.

Awareness of Personal Meaning

The crisis brought on by illness, especially terminal illness, might be the first opportunity a person has to encounter the innermost spiritual being and, for some persons, the first opportunity to experience the meaning of their existence. Mwalimu Imara cites an example of an older woman who, in the process of dying, experienced her most creative potential in transcending the tragedy of her lifetime loneliness. Her experience of feeling unconditionally loved and accepted by the staff caring for her despite her bitter demandingness, led her to make peace with life and find meaning in her suffering (Imara, 1975). Victor Frankl based his logotherapy on the importance of discovering personal meaning. He writes

> For only to the extent that man has fulfilled the concrete meaning of his personal existence will he also have fulfilled himself. . . . The meaning which a person has to fulfill is something beyond himself, it is never just himself (Frankl, 1971).

Awareness of Relatedness to a Higher Being

The awareness of relatedness to a higher being may be experienced as a drive to self-expansion, to participation in something beyond the self. For this level of growth we are totally dependent on another—to be is to mean something to someone else. We start with nothing and cannot create this relatedness directly by ourselves. It is a blessing which must be given by another. One only has to respond to the blessing and simply accept that one is accepted: "See, I will not forget you. . . . I have carved you in the palm of my hand." (Isaias 49). With this relatedness, one's life is centered in love (a higher being); one knows what is good and can act upon it (Imara, 1975). Without this relatedness there is emptiness.

Anne Frank, in her incarceration, wrote that despite everything she knew people were basically good, and Victor Frankl writes that he survived tremendous suffering in concentration camp life because he felt connected in love. In his book *From Death Camp to Existentialism,* Frankl explains how this relatedness allowed him to hold fast to seeing himself as a person, always resisting the dehumanizing forces of the camp. The account of his struggle inspires an awareness of the innate dignity of each person and the crucial necessity for relatedness, without which morale deteriorates, immunity decreases, and illness, even death, may follow (Frankl, 1959).

Spiritual growth requires change. Since the known is familiar and the unknown risky, patients often find it difficult to acknowledge alterations in their well-being or to attempt something new. While unsuspected symptoms are developing in someone's body, the subtle changes often go unrecognized. Frequently patients, following surgery for a previously unsuspected condition, are astonished at how much better they feel than before surgery. Their customary pace had left them apparently oblivious to what must have been considerable discomfort. A person's character, life style, and spiritual state can contribute to his or her illness so that treatment may require learning a new life style, a more accurate awareness of body needs, healthier ways of coping with stress, and deeper "in touch-ness" with spiritual needs. For example, on the level of body needs, a hard-driving man, on return to work after recovery from surgery, was having trouble following his surgeon's advice not to tire himself. Through discussion of the problem with a nurse, he realized that he could only tell when he *had been* tired and that he had missed the earlier body cues for a need of rest. Such "out of touch-ness" with physical or emotional needs often means a person may be similarly oblivious to signs of spiritual needs.

An attitude which could help overcome, even prevent, such destructive self-oblivion is viewing the slowdown or constraint brought on by illness as a retreat—a chance to reorder priorities and to contemplate new directions. Meditation may help because it emphasizes resources within the individual that foster self-reliance, focus concentration, and lessen fragmentation and anxiety. Meditation is a counterpart of the "fight or flight" reflex, which has the same survival value. In the past a human being's "fight or flight" response overcame a hostile physical environment; in the present world a meditative response can overcome a hostile technical environment.

Assessment of Spiritual Resources and Needs

Each person has within his or her being powerful resources for healing; the Western attitude that the cure for any ill is to be found in sources outside the person must be overcome. Pain, and in this case spiritual pain, teaches that something needs attending to. The person yearns for wholeness, to be well, to be fulfilled. The findings in the fields of bioenergetics, psychic healing, and holistic medicine support this belief. Psychic or faith healing is essentially the body healing itself with some extra energy from a loving or inspiriting healer. To be healed one must love one's body, listen to its wisdom, be patient, and be guided by it in one's evolution.

> In some painful episodes, there is nothing the sufferer can do but give in, be as comfortable as possible, turn on good music that his own natural rhythms can flow with, and then look calmly and peacefully at this pain. This takes practice, but can happen if one remembers that the pain sensation is essentially energy that is being sent to emotional centers of the brain. In meditation, one can learn how to separate oneself somewhat from this emotional component and then to begin to go on a type of inner "trip," with the pain providing guidance for the journey. One's consciousness moves into deeper paths, and one flows with this inner direction (Schmitt, 1977).

Through pain the person is alerted to be quiet, to allow the process to ferment, and to be inspired by the quiet. In this aloneness one discovers the need for the presence and touch of another. The nurse can give this touch—her or his spirit can touch the patient's suffering spirit where healing can take place (Schmitt, 1977, pp. 621–29).

Holistic medicine, which defines wellness as a perfection in the balance of the whole person, physically, emotionally, mentally, and spiritually, also stresses the healing nature of meditation, the nurse as teacher or consultant in the healing process, and the importance of spiritual growth in healing. When health in this holistic sense is present, human potential is realized with the person experiencing the expansion and peaks of what is to be human, a harmony with nature, a fitting in and being part of one's entire surroundings near and far. The nurse's role is subtle in these matters. The nurse's guidance can be a creative work of art in helping to remove those impediments to love necessary for healing (Brallier, 1978).

Communication is impaired when the patient is unaware that his or her feeling and thinking are not united, which causes a "double message." For example, if the patient fears dependency and cannot take the risk of showing dependence by saying what he or she thinks and feels, this conflict may be converted into such physical conditions as an ulcer, high blood pressure, or a migraine headache. Productive communication, or leveling, happens in a nurturing atmosphere in which self-esteem is high: communication is direct, specific, and congruent; the rules change as need arises; there is freedom to comment on anything, and the task is appropriate and constructive.

The Importance of Trust and Hope

Helen Keller's light was uncovered because Ann Sullivan recognized it beneath the child's bewildered rage. For the nurse, it is this same kind of appreciation and faith in the patient's and one's own potential for development that leads to the trust and hope underlying spiritual communication.

Communication based on trust and hope lessens the fear of abandonment. As long as one feels connected or attached to important others and knows the isolation will be time-limited, the individual can adapt and not lose the sense of identity so necessary to well-being. When resources that help people to cope under stress break down in illness, despair may result. The need to be sick or to die is largely emotional, with the body merely carrying out or expressing great psychic pain or spiritual despair. The nurse finding the patient in such vulnerable circumstances becomes a partner with the patient in a spiritual alliance.

If the patient feels trusted to make choices that will support his or her own "becoming," he or she feels free to engage safely and openly in uninhibited discussion of diverse attitudes and beliefs without fear of rejection or disapproval. A nurse promotes freedom in stating personal views but does not manipulate, control, or inhibit the patient. If the patient should lean toward a free choice that appears to be unwise or detrimental to himself or herself or to others, the nurse intervenes to provide additional information about alternatives available and encourages further consideration. In order for this trusting communication to take place, the nurse must be sensitive to the patient's needs. (See Appendix C for signs of spiritual concerns, distress, and despair.) If his or her privacy is protected, the patient experiences a feeling of sacredness as a person which strengthens the personal integrity to face what his or her illness may bring.

Spiritual healing cannot be coercive or intrusive. It is a free-will choice on the part of the patient to say yes to life, whatever it brings. Attitudes on the part of the patient that interfere with the development of a spiritual alliance with the nurse must be respected, and too much zeal or rescue fantasy on the part of the nurse negates the patient's inherent dignity. The nurse should guard against unwarranted intrusions when the timing for spiritual intervention is not right. Such times may arise when negative feelings are too much in control, making it impossible for the patient to forgive or receive forgiveness; when defenses are strongly resisting spiritual interventions; or when spiritual problems are so buried as to be completely out of the patient's awareness. The patient's avenue to the spiritual is through free will and commitment. If faith isn't present, it shouldn't be pursued. Since faith is a gift, the patient should not feel guilty or be made to feel guilty for not having faith. Sometimes the patient has a spiritual counseling process going on with someone else and does not wish to discuss these matters with the nurse. In this case the nurse strives to affirm and cooperate with such already established assistance (Scanlon, 1974).

Patients often feel inferior when asking for help. Although society may place a negative value on not knowing something or being dependent, it is important for patient and nurse to understand, when grappling with a spiritual threat to well-being, that ignorance and dependence are as much a part of the human condition as knowledge and self-reliance. If the nurse is not experienced enough to cope with certain complexities of spiritual care, she or he serves best by seeking the help of someone who is experienced and thereby demonstrates the neutrality and potential learning involved in states of ignorance and dependence. Simply supplying solutions to problems may, at worst, be mistaken for magic, and at best, rob someone of the opportunity to learn the process of working through a problem. A common fantasy of people who are overwhelmed is that an expert will provide a "true solution." In reality no one holds the entire solution, but each person holds something of it.

In assessing what spiritual growth takes place, it is important to realize that the spiritual life is no different from other development—no step forward is maintained unless it is followed by further steps. Spiritual breakthroughs are frequently followed by backsliding toward discouragement. Thomas Merton writes of this process:

> But at the same time there is a growing conviction that joy and peace and fulfillment are only to be found in this lonely night of aridity and faith (Merton, 1950).

Physical, psychical, and spiritual health are not victories to be won once and for all, but daily struggles in which personal destiny is constantly at stake (Tournier, 1965). A guide to assessing spiritual concerns is provided in Appendix C.

The Nurse as Spiritual Partner

The spiritual dimension builds on nature and is nurtured through relationships. The person who assists another in the quest toward spiritual experience shares a creative moment wherein a transfer of spiritual energy takes place, spiritually enriching both. The nurse is in a strategic position to help persons in spiritual crises. The nurse's professional code of ethics involves a covenant to assist in meeting spiritual needs. For the nurse to respond with compassion to a patient's spiritual needs, she or he must be willing to meet the patient spirit to spirit and help in his or her experience of illness as spiritual journey.

Process

How is it that two virtual strangers, the patient and the nurse, can deal with such intimate matters as spiritual needs, with their accompanying fears, emotions, hopes, and aspirations? This deepest touch—spirit to spirit—is founded in the patient's and nurse's intimacy with body touch in physical care and verbal touch in emotional support. This touching of spirits is fostered when the patient and the nurse recognize that coming to terms with spiritual need is essential to regaining a sense of well-being. The nurse conveys this message by providing the nurturing atmosphere necessary for intimate expression through an interested, unhurried, nonjudgmental, and receptive attitude, in as quite and private a surrounding as possible. The patient cannot bare his or her soul to someone flustered, preoccupied, and scurrying about or while within eye and earshot of people not directly concerned with him or her. It takes a great deal of energy to trust and reveal oneself to another. Trust is invited by the nurse's sensitive treatment of those patients who need help to cope with overwhelming physical realities by not prying for feelings of desperation which must be avoided in order to keep going. A person's hope is crucial and should be protected as a source of energy to struggle against despair. The nurse protects hope in persons with terminal illness by discerning that individuals differ in their ability to pursue fears about such illness and by awareness that dreaded facts can be handled more easily when the individual takes the initiative to pursue them.

Many factors intertwine, enabling the nurse to behave responsively with patients. Often the emotion revealing a spiritual crisis is grief with attendant anger. An understanding of the need to grieve over a sense of loss which usually accompanies illness will help the nurse to view the patient's anger as catharsis, as health-promoting as pus being expressed from an abscess. The loss may be the death of a loved one, the knowledge of one's own impending death, a change in body image coming from illness or surgery, grave disillusionment in oneself, a significant person, or an ideal, dashed aspirations, or a change in status or property. The nurse can play a part in whether the patient uses his or her loss to reach a higher level of spirituality, maintain the existing level, or regress. By being aware that anger is a natural reaction to loss, the nurse can create a climate in which the patient feels free to express this anger rather than to internalize it to create a hopeless depression or somatic illness. Knowing that shock and disbelief may be the first response to loss, the nurse can anticipate that grieving persons may behave in a grossly disturbed manner. The fact that the person is not acting in his or her usual manner is a good sign of progression beyond denial and reaching out for help. Also, knowing that a person may fall ill in a somatic cry for help following a serious loss, the possibility of loss should be explored in eliciting the patient's history. If an unresolved loss is determined, the nurse may be able to provide the patient with an opportunity to work through the spiritual implications of the loss, thus averting psychosomatic or psychopathological solutions.

What a person values is a highly individual matter, hence to understand what is considered a loss one must listen carefully for the way the loss is expressed. Pursuing what seems discordant with the patient's general character can help the patient bring to awareness a loss that he or she may be experiencing on a preconscious level. The following examples taken from an unpublished clinical manuscript illustrate loss of self-image and loss of aspiration.

A nun relearning to walk after a bad ankle break said to the nurse, "I know this sounds wacky, but I just can't face the step exercise. If you just let me sit down and have a good cry, I think I can do it." Fortunately, the nurse understood, and the nun, after crying, managed the steps. Later the nun realized that she had learned the value of expressing her feelings about the loss of mobility from a nurse friend who had visited her in the hospital while first recovering from the fracture. During the visit the nun was very embarrassed at having "broken down in uncontrollable tears" in her friend's presence. The friend, on the other hand, was relieved because she could see what strain her friend was under in feeling that a nun had to be a perfectly composed, "good" patient.

The second example concerns a 38-year-old single patient who reacted in what seemed an inappropriate way to her doctor's recommendation that she be medicated for her high blood pressure. Although she was a bright, well-prepared teacher of nursing, she found herself asking her physician, "Is my hypertension connected with my family's high incidence of RH negative blood?" (which she herself had), "or with my mother having preeclampsia at the time of my birth?" The nurse felt humiliated by her inappropriate questions, by her unwillingness to begin the drug treatment, and by her annoyance that drug treatment had been suggested. Later she realized that her atypical behavior stemmed from her feeling a great loss that she might never be able to safely have a baby. Though 38 years old, she still aspired to marriage and motherhood and now felt devastated by the knowledge that not only age and blood type, but also hypertension made her aspiration seem hopeless.

With more overwhelming loss there is greater need for inspiriting on the part of the nurse. Also, in the spiritually overwhelmed patient, communication is more than discordant. In may be primitive and vital because the patient often feels loss of control in life and plagued with terrifying fears of destruction of all that is held dear. These fears may intensify the patient's feelings of anger, guilt, and worthlessness. If the spiritual isolation, brought on by this completely dependent, helpless, despairing position is dealt with, the patient can find meaning in suffering. Mere logical reassuring words evoked by the anxiety of the nurse hold no meaning for the despairing patient. Operating on a spiritual plane, he or she perceives the anxious feeling behind the reassurance, which reaffirms the feeling of panic.

In approaching the overwhelmed patient, rather than being falsely reassuring, the nurse acknowledges how terrible it must be for him or her to have these fears and that she or he will be available in the struggle to conquer the fears. This language of feeling—be it warmth, concern, or empathy—is the one that a spiritually overwhelmed person comprehends and responds to. These subjective responses to another person are conveyed to a large extent through nonverbal and behavioral signs. This is why it is so important for the nurse to be as conscious of her or his subjective state and reactions to patients as of the words used. The nurse needs self-knowledge when struggling to understand the patient, his or her responses, and how the two interact. The nurse needs an understanding of what effects their interactions have on the process of inspiriting, what needs they satisfy, what frustrations they engender, what anxieties they create or add to, and for what purpose they use one another in the relationship. The nurse tries to lend herself or himself to the patient as a spiritual partner to satisfy the need for relatedness in such a way that the patient will find strength to come to terms with life, gain confidence, and become more fully a person. St. Vincent de Paul acknowledged the reciprocal nature of this inspiriting by thanking anyone who allowed him to help them.

In the following poem the nurse joins the unconscious patient and by silent intention offers spiritual strength and will to live to someone who has lost it, or from whom it hangs in balance.

Each Day

Each day,
That summer,
I would pause
Before the almost too narrow door
With its neatly lettered,
almost forbidding,
sign:
INTENSIVE CARE UNIT
To hear
The unmistakable rhythmic gush of a respirator
and the steady beep of a monitor.
Then,
I would enter
And silently pray:
"Oh, God,
Help me to see past the bottles,
see past the tubes
see past the machines,
That I might see into their eyes,
see into their hearts,
And bring them some small part of my healthy self,
That they will still believe
Life is worth the living;
Life is worth the fight."

(Strumpf, 1969)

Family members, too, may have a similar wish to offer spiritual strength to a loved one who is unconscious and unable to support life alone:

My brother's wife, my only other brother, a physician, and I had to make a decision to discontinue the respirator on my brother who at forty-five had suffered a massive MI. We shared religious values and that helped, but what I agonized over was in a spiritual realm and impossible for me at the time to share with them. They had no hope for Jim because the ICU staff had given no hope. I, on the other hand, flooded with childhood memories of Jim, could not give up hope. I felt a miracle was possible and that I had to protect Jim's right to this miracle (Colliton, 1975).

Just as the giving of spiritual energy inspires the nurse, so too the nurse can become dispirited when the care of a patient completely unable to speak and supported for life merely by technology is dehumanized, unrelated, and uninspired (Johnson, 1977). No matter how isolated, unrelated, and overwhelmed with abandonment and despair the patient is, it may be possible for the nurse to become a spiritual partner with the patient in his or her struggle. The patient can thus rely on the capacities of the nurse until the sense of mastery is regained, even when the mastery is the act of saying goodbye to all that was held dear in preparation for death. For spiritual mastery is not necessarily physical recovery but rather the attainment of a sense of being at peace with oneself in facing what life brings. When a spiritual crisis is met head-on and successfully dealt with, a person achieves a state of higher inspiration, increased emotional maturity, heightened awareness of self and others, enrichment of human capacities, and a transcendence of suffering.

Commitment

Nurses must be aware of their own spiritual vulnerability before they can help a patient face his or hers. In the extreme, for example, Henri Nouwen discusses the depth of commitment necessary to a patient in spiritual despair who fears that to continue living will only prolong a miserable existence and to die might bring greater suffering through punishment. Nouwen contends that more than anything, such an alienated person needs personal response, an assurance that someone is "waiting" for him or her, whatever life holds in store for tomorrow—recovery or death:

It is indeed possible for man to be faithful in death, to express a solidarity based not just on a return to everyday life but also on a participation in the death experience which belongs in the center of the human heart. "I will be waiting for you" means much more than, "If you make it through the operation I will be there to be with you again." There will be no "ifs." "I will wait for you" goes beyond death and is the deepest expression of solidarity which breaks through the chains of death. . . . One can lead another to tomorrow even when tomorrow is the day of the other one's death, because he can wait for him on both sides (Nouwen, 1979).

In such spiritual crises there is need for the nurse to engage the patient at the spiritual level with personal concern, faith in the meaning of life, and hope that breaks through the boundaries of death. For the nurse, this commitment means that, with personal vulnerabilities, the nurse enters into a relationship with the patient in spiritual crisis to lead him or her out of confusion and fear. Such commitment beyond time creates a powerful bond in persons who touch at so deep a level. Nouwen advocates a movement from professionalism to spirituality and, by means of self-denial and contemplation, becoming a faithful witness of the Divine Healer (Nouwen, 1971). This approaches mysticism:

So the mystic, who loves all men with a universal love and who lives in all men, rejoices with those who rejoice and weeps with those who weep. This was the case with great-souled mystics like Paul himself or Pope John or Dag Hammarskjold or Gandhi. (Johnston, 1976)

Use of Self

There are several personal resources important for the nurse to be moving toward in using the self to inspirit a patient. First, the nurse must know who the patient is—his or her spiritual needs, powers, limitations, what is conducive to growth, and how to respond to the patient's needs in relation to the nurse's own powers and limitations.

The nurse needs the flexibility to modify behavior in light of assessing the results of attempts to meet the patient's needs. Patience is expressed through a participation with the patient in which the nurse gives fully of herself or himself. Honesty for the nurse is being true to oneself so that one's words, actions, and feelings are congruent, seeing the patient realistically and not as the nurse would like him or her to be. Nurses need the kind of trust that allows them to let go and risk the unknown with courage. They need the humility of being open and unpretentious enough to recognize the patient's own integrity. They need hope in the present as being alive with the sense of the possible. Since it is in the present that the nurse renders to a patient, the primacy of the process rather than of an expected product must be recognized. That the patient is moving toward transcending his or her suffering in the here and now is what is important. The nurse realizes too that it is not enough to merely desire the patient's spiritual growth; the patient has to, at some level, want such growth and the nurse must know how to foster it.

Only if the nurse understands and responds to personal needs to grow spiritually can she or he understand the patient's desire to grow spiritually. This self-understanding enables the nurse to "be with" the patient, in contrast to simply knowing him or her from outside. Admiration and spontaneous delight bring the nurse closer to the patient. Devotion, trust, patience, humility, honesty, and the primacy of the process apply not only to the nurse caring for the patient but also to the nurse's self-caring so as to prevent becoming "burnt out." The nurse's submission to self-caring is like the voluntary submission of the artist to the artistic discipline. It is basically liberating and affirming, making the nurse feel "in place" in her or his work. This feeling of deep-seated harmony with the self brings with it the basic certainty, the security, which allows the nurse to be vulnerable and give up the preoccupation with trying to be secure. It allows faith and trust to enter the nurse's life. Priorities are ordered with clarity, important connections between events are more easily seen, and what is of real importance comes into focus. An awareness of the mysteries in life is appreciated not as something to fear but as something to be realized deeply, since it unites the nurse to those in care (Mayeroff, 1971; Colliton, 1971).

References Cited

Brallier, L. W. "The Nurse as Holistic Health Practitioner." *Nurs. Clin. North Am.*, **13**:4 (Dec. 1978) 643–55.

Colliton, M. A. "Some Moral Issues in Health Care: A Personal Reflection," unpublished manuscript, 1975.

———. "The Use of Self in Clinical Practice." *Nurs. Clin. North Am.*, **6**:4 (Dec. 1971).

Dostoyevsky, F. *The Brothers Karamazov.* New York: Random House, 1950, Epilogue, Chap. 3.

Fish, S., and Shelly, J. *Spiritual Care: The Nurse's Role.* Downers Grove: InterVarsity Press, 1978, Chaps. 6 and 7.

Frank, H. "My Path to Medicine of the Whole Person." In Paul Tournier's *Medicine of the Whole Person.* Waco, Texas: Word Books, 1973, p. 62.

Frankl, V., as quoted by Milton Mayeroff in *On Caring.* New York: Harper & Row, 1971, prologue.

———. *From Death Camp to Existentialism.* Boston: Beacon Press, 1959.

Friedlander, P. *Plato: An Introduction.* Trans. by Hans Meyerhoff. New York: Harper & Row, for the Bollingen Foundation, 1964, Chaps. 2 and 3.

Henderson, V., and Nite, G. *Principle and Practice of Nursing,* 6th ed. New York: Macmillan Publishing Co., 1978, Chap. 18.

Imara, M. "Dying as the Last Stage of Growth." In *Death: The Final Stage of Growth.* Ed. by Elizabeth Kübler-Ross. Englewood Cliffs, N.J.: Prentice-Hall, 1975, pp. 147–63.

Johnson, P. "The Long Hard Dying of Joe Rodriquez." *Am J. Nurs.*, **77** (Jan. 1977), 54–58.

Johnston, W. *Silent Music.* New York: Harper & Row, 1976, p. 137.

Jourard, S. *The Transparent Self,* rev. ed. New York: Van Nostrand Reinhold Co., 1971, p. 94.

Kelly, L. *Dimensions of Professional Nursing,* 3rd ed. New York: Macmillan Publishing Co., 1975, Chaps. 14, 15, 16, and 17.

Kiening, Sr. M. "Spiritual Needs of the Psychiatric Patient." In *Mental Health Concepts and Nursing Practice.* Ed. by Lois Dunlap. New York: John Wiley & Sons, 1978.

Mayeroff, M. *On Caring.* New York: Harper & Row, 1971.

Merton, T. *What Is Contemplation?* Springfield, Ill.: Templegate, 1950, p. 17.

Nightingale, F., quoted in Jones, Miss J., *Memorials of Agnes Elizabeth Jones by Her Sister.* London: Stahan & Co., 1872, pp. vii–viii.

Nouwen, H. *Creative Ministry.* New York: Doubleday, 1971, p. 64.

———. *The Wounded Healer.* New York: Image Books, 1979, p. 69.

O'Connor, F. "A Memoir of Mary Ann." In *Mystery and Manners.* Ed. by Sally and Robert Fitzgerald. New York: The Noonday Press, 1970.

Peipgras, R. "The Other Dimension: Spiritual Help." *Am. J. Nurs.*, **68** (Dec. 1968), 2610–13.

Scanlon, M. *Inner Healing.* New York: Paulist Press, 1974, pp. 75–77.

Schmitt, M. "The Nature of Pain." *Nurs. Clin. North Am.*, **12**:4 (Dec. 1977), 629.

Stallwood, J. "Spiritual Dimension of Nursing Practice." In *Clinical Nursing,* 3rd ed. Ed. by Irene Beland and Joyce Passos. New York: Macmillan Publishing Co., 1975, p. 1088.

Strumpf, N. "Each Day." *Am. J. Nurs.*, **69** (Oct. 1969), 2176.

Tournier, P. *The Healing of Persons.* New York: Harper & Row, 1965, pp. xix–xx.

White House Conference on Aging. Spiritual Well-Being, Washington, D.C.: U.S. Government Printing Office, 1971, p. 1.

General References

Allport, Gordon. *The Individual and His Religion.* New York: Macmillan Publishing Co., 1950.

Baskerville, M. Trevor. "Another Dimension of Care: Spiritual Consolation." In *Proceedings of the National Conference on Cancer Nursing.* Chicago, Sept. 10–11, 1973, American Cancer Society, 1974, pp. 47–49.

Bermosk, Loretta, and Corsini, Raymond, eds. *Critical Incidents in Nursing.* Philadelphia: W. B. Saunders Co., 1973.

Boisen, Anton T. *The Exploration of the Inner World.* Philadelphia: University of Pennsylvania Press, 1936.

Brallier, Lynn Wilson. "The Nurse as Holistic Health Practitioner." *Nurs. Clin. of North Am.,* **4** (Dec. 1978), 643–55.

Byrne, Marjorie, and Thompson, Lida. *Key Concepts for the Study and Practice of Nursing.* St. Louis: C. V. Mosby Co., 1972.

Calestro, Kenneth M. "Psychotherapy Faith Healing and Suggestion." *Internatl. J. Psycho.,* **10**:2 (June 1972), 83–113.

Campbell, Claire. *Nursing Diagnosis and Intervention in Nursing Practice.* New York: John Wiley & Co. 1978, Chap. 30.

Cannon, Maureen. "To Sharon, with Love." *Am. J. Nurs.,* **4** (April 1979), 642–45.

Colliton, Margaret A. "The Use of Self in Clinical Practice," *Nurs. Clin. of No. Am.,* **4** (Dec. 1971), 691–806.

———. "The History of Nursing Therapy: A Reactionaire to the Work of June Mellow." *Perspectives in Psychiatric Care,* **3**:2 (1965).

Cunningham, Robert. *The Wholistic Health Centers: A New Direction in Health Care.* Battle Creek, Michigan: Kellogg Foundation, 1977.

———, and Westberg, Jill. *Report of the National Symposium on Wholistic Health Care.* Battle Creek, Michigan: Kellogg Foundation, 1977.

Curran, Charles A. *Religious Values in Counseling and Psychotherapy.* New York: Sheed and Ward, 1969.

Dickinson, Sr. Corita. "The Search for Spiritual Meaning." *Am. J. Nurs.,* **75**:10 (Oct. 1975), 1789.

Draper, Edgar, Meyer, Parzen, and Samuelson. "On the Diagnostic Value of Religious Ideation." *Arch. Gen. Psychiatry,* **13** (Sept. 1965), 202–07.

Dubos, Rene. *A God Within.* New York: Charles Scribner's Sons, 1972.

DuGas, Beverly W. *Introduction to Patient Care: A Comprehensive Approach to Nursing,* 3rd. ed. Philadelphia: W. B. Saunders & Co. 1977, Chap. 14.

Duncan, Franklin D. "Pastoral Care of Disabled Persons." In *Pastoral Care in Crucial Human Situations.* Ed. by Oates and Lester. Valley Forge, Pa.: Judson Press, 1969, pp. 147–59.

Fish, Sharon, and Shelley, Judy A. *Spiritual Care: The Nurse's Role.* Downers Grove: InterVarsity Press, 1978.

Fox, Matthew. *On Becoming a Musical Mystical Bear.* New York: Paulist, Press, 1972.

Frankl, Victor E. *Man's Search for Meaning, An Introduction to Logotherapy.* New York: Washington Square Press, 1963.

———. *The Doctor and the Soul, An Introduction to Logotherapy.* New York: Alfred A. Knopf, 1955.

———. *From Death Camp to Existentialism.* Boston: Beacon Press, 1959.

Gebbie, Kristine, M., and Lavin, Mary Ann. *Classification of Nursing Diagnoses.* St. Louis: C. V. Mosby Co., 1976.

Gould, Grace Theresa. "Compassion and Communication in Nursing." *Nurs. Clin. North Am.,* **4** (Dec. 1969), 651–99.

Gruendemann, Barbara J. "Hospital Chaplains: The "Now" Member of the Health Team," *RN,* **37**:10 (October 1973), 38.

Henderson, Virginia, and Nite, Gladys. *Principle and Practice of Nursing,* 6th ed. New York: Macmillan Publishing Co., 1978, Chap. 18, pp. 1018–60.

Hofman, Hans, ed. *The Ministry and Mental Health.* New York: Associon Press, 1960.

Hubert, Sr. Mary. "For Every Patient." *J. Nurs. Educ.,* **2** (May–June 1963), 9–11, 29–31.

Hulme, William E. *Dialogue in Despair.* Nashville: Abingdon Press, 1968.

James, William. *The Varieties of Religious Experience.* New York: Random House, 1929.

Journal of Nursing Ethics. National Center for Nursing Ethics, Vol. I (fall 1978).

Johnson, Priscilla. "The Long Hard Dying of Joe Rodriguez." *Am. J. Nurs.,* **77** (Jan. 1977), 54–57.

Journard, Sidney M. *The Transparent Self.* New York: Van Nostrand Reinhold Company, 1964.

Jung, Carl G. *Modern Man in Search of a Soul.* New York: Brace and World, 1931.

———. *Psychology and Religion.* New Haven: Yale University Press, 1964.

Karl, Thomas. *The Healing Touch of Affirmation.* Whitensville, Mass.: Affirmation Books, 1976.

Kelly, Lucie Y. *Dimensions of Professional Nursing,* 3rd ed. New York: Macmillan Publishing Co., 1975, Pt. III, Sec. 2.

Kelsey, Morton. *Healing and Christianity.* New York: Harper & Row, 1973.

Kiening, Sr. M. Martha. In *Mental Health Concepts and Nursing Practice.* Ed. by Lois Dunlap. New York: John Wiley & Sons, 1978, Chap. 7.

Kinget, G. Marian. *On Being Human: A Systematic View.* San Francisco: Harcourt, Brace, Jovanovich, 1975.

Koski, Peter. "Symposium on Cultural and Biological Diversity and Health Care," *Nurs. Clin. North Am.,* **12** (March 1977), 1–84.

Krieger, Delores. "Healing by the Laying on of Hands as a Facilitator of Bioenergetic Change: The Response of In-vivo Human Hemoglobin." *Int. J. Psychoenergetic Systems,* **1** (1976), 121–29.

———. "Alternative Medicine: Therapeutic Touch." *Nurs. Times,* **15** (April 1972), 572–74.

———. "Therapeutic Touch: The Imprimatur of Nursing." *Am. J. Nurs.,* **5** (May 1975), 784–87.

———. "Therapeutic Touch: An Ancient, But Unorthodox Nursing Intervention." *J. New York State Nurs. Assoc.,* **6** (Aug. 1975), 6–10.

———, Peper, E. and Ancoli, Sonia. "Therapeutic Touch: Searching for Evidence of Physiological Change." *Am. J. Nurs.,* **4** (1979) 660.

Kübler-Ross, Elizabeth. *Death.* Englewood, N.J.: Prentice-Hall, 1975.

Lamerton, Richard. *Care of the Dying.* London: Priory Press Limited, 1973.

Lewis, C. S. *The Problem of Pain.* New York: Macmillan Publishing Co., 1962.

Loewald, Hans W. *Psychoanalysis and the History of the Individual.* New Haven and London: Yale University Press, 1978.

Manfreda, Marguerite L. *Psychiatric Nursing,* 9th ed. Philadelphia: F. A. Davis Co., 1973, Chap. 17.

Maslow, A. H. *The Farther Reaches of Human Nature.* New York: The Viking Press, 1971.

———. *New Knowledge in Human Values.* Chicago: Henry Regnery, 1959.

———. *Religions, Values, and Peak Experiences.* New York: The Viking Press, 1971.

———. *Toward a Psychology of Being,* 2nd ed. New York: D. Van Nostrand Company, 1968.

Mayeroff, Milton. *On Caring.* New York: Harper & Row, 1971).

McGreeby, Abigail, and Van Heukelem, Judy. "Crying: The Neglected Dimension." *The Canadian Nurse.* **72** (Jan. 1976), 19.

Medicine and Religion Committee, Zumbro Valley Medical Society, Rochester, Minnesota. *Religious Aspects of Medical Care: A Handbook of Religious Practices of All Faiths.* 1976.

Meninger, Karl. *Whatever Became of Sin?* New York: Hawthorne Books, 1973.

Munley, M. Joan, and Keane, Mary C. "Symposium on Impressions of Pain: A Nursing Diagnosis." *Nurs. Clin. North Am.,* **12** (Dec. 1977), 609–68.

Murray, Ruth, and Zentner, Judith. *Nursing Concepts for Health Promotion.* Englewood Cliffs, N.J.: Prentice-Hall, 1975, Chap. 11.

Naugle, Ethel H. "The Difference Caring Makes." *Am J. Nurs.,* **73** (Nov. 1973), 1890–91.

Nelson, James B. *Rediscovering the Person in Medical Care.* Minneapolis, Minn.: Augburg Publishing House, 1976.

Nichols, Elizabeth Grace. "Jeanette: No Hope for Cure." *Nurs. Forum,* **11** (1972), 97–104.

Niklas, Gerald R., and Stafanics, Charlotte. *Ministry to the Hospitalized.* New York: Paulist Press, 1975.

Oates, Wayne E., and Lester, Andrew D., eds. *Pastoral Care in Crucial Human Situations.* Valley Forge, Pa.: Judson Press, 1969.

O'Connor, Flannery. In *Mystery and Manners.* Ed. by Fitzgerald, Sally and Robert. New York: The Noonday Press, 1970.

Paige, Roberta, L., and Looney, Jane F. "Hospice Care for the Adult." *Am. J. Nurs.,* **11** (Nov. 1977), 1812.

Parks, Colin M. *Bereavement.* New York: International University Press, 1972.

Peipgras, Ruth. "The Other Dimension: Spiritual Health." *Am. J. Nurs.,* **12** (Dec. 1968), 2610.

Perrine, George. "Needs Met and Unmet." *Am. J. Nurs.,* **11** (Nov. 1971), 2128–33.

Polcino, Anna, ed. *Intimacy.* Worcester, Mass.: Mercantile Printing Co., 1978.

Powell, John. *A Reason to Live: A Reason to Die!* Niles: Argus Communications, 1975.

Pumphrey, John B. "Recognizing Your Patients' Spiritual Needs." *Nursing 77,* **12** (Dec. 1977), 64.

Rines, Alice, and Montag, Mildred. *Nursing Concepts and Nursing Care.* New York: John Wiley & Sons, 1976.

Scanlon, Michael. *Inner Healing.* New York: Paulist Press, 1974.

Schwartz, Lawrence H., and Schwartz, Jane Parker. *The Psychodynamics of Patient Care.* Englewood Cliffs, N.J.: Prentice-Hall, 1972.

Schwing, Gertrude. *A Way to the Soul of the Mentally Ill.* New York: International University Press, 1954.

Selzer, Richard. *Mortal Lessons.* New York: Simon & Schuster, 1976.

Siantz, Mary Lou. "Bioethical Issues in Nursing,". *Nursing Clin. North Am.,* **14** (March 1979), 1–91.

Southard, Samuel. *Religion and Nursing.* Nashville: Broadman Press, 1959.

Terruwe, Anna A., and Baars, Conrad W. *Loving and Curing the Neurotic.* New Rochelle, N.Y.: Arlington House, 1972.

Tournier, Paul. *A Doctor's Casebook.* London: SCM Press, Ltd., 1954.

———. *The Healing of Persons.* New York: Harper & Row, 1965.

———. *Medicine of the Whole Person.* Waco, Texas: Word Books, 1973.

Travelbee, Joyce. *Interpersonal Aspects of Nursing.* Philadelphia: F. A. Davis Co., 1966.

Ujhely, Gertrude. *Determinants of the Nurse-Patient Relationship.* New York: Springer Publishing Co., 1968.

Vaillot, Sister Madeleine C. "Hope: The Restoration of Being." *Am. J. Nurs.,* **2** (Feb. 1970), 270.

———. "Existentialism: A Philosophy of Commitment,"*Am. J. Nurs.,* **66** (March 1966), 500–5.

Watson, Jean. *Nursing.* Boston: Little, Brown & Co., 1979.

White, John, ed. *Frontiers of Consciousness.* New York: Avon Books, 1974.

White House Conference on Aging. *Spiritual Well-Being.* Washington, D.C.: U.S. Government Printing Office, 1971.

Wygant, W. E. "Dying, But Not Alone." *Am. J. Nurs.,* **3** (March 1967), 574.

33

Terminal Illness, Dying, and Death

We hide within ourselves—except when we rend ourselves open in our frenzy—and the solitude in which we suffer has no reference either to a redeemer or a creator.

PAZ, 1965

Changing Patterns of Experience with the Terminally Ill Person

Conception, birth, growing up, maturity, aging, health, disease, and death are all aspects of life. All species have a life span. For some it is only a few days or weeks, for others it may be a century or more. There is also great variability among individuals of the same species. Some die at the very beginning of life. Others live beyond their expected time. Whatever the life span for the species or the individual, death is as certain and natural as other aspects of life.

Some things have changed, however. At the beginning of the century most persons had lived through the experience of one or more family members dying. Because the sick as well as the dying were cared for at home, children were not screened from death. They were present when family members died and were taken to funerals and wakes. Further, much of the population lived on farms and in small towns, where death of animals was a frequent event. Today babies that are born live to maturity. The proportion of the population over 65 is increasing. Some 80 per cent of those who die, die in hospitals, where young visitors are excluded. Grandparents either move to retirement areas or the young family moves to follow its work. Thus many reach maturity having little significant contact with either older people or the dying.

The word *death* has been taboo; euphemisms such as *passed on, passed away, passed,* or *disappeared behind a velvet curtain* are substituted. Recent reports indicate that the attitude toward death is changing rapidly. This can be seen in the number of books and papers published and courses and conferences presented on death and dying.

Interest in death and dying has been stimulated by a number of factors. Unlike infectious diseases from which parents either recover or die in a predictable period of time, long-term illnesses tend to have a prolonged course. Patients may be in the last stages of some of these diseases for weeks, months, or years. Modern methods of treatment may extend this period considerably. There is no denying that the burden of long-term illness, accompanied by increasing disability on the person, family, and the community, is at times considerable.

Controversial Issues

A number of controversial issues related to death and dying are being debated. Arguments are advanced to support the position taken. In some instances little consideration is given to the long-term implications of some proposals.

1. Every life is sacred. The commandment "Thou shalt not kill" is to be taken literally. Abortion,

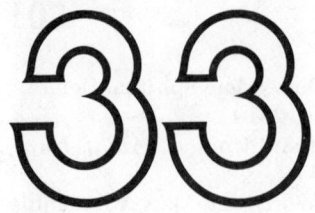

capital punishment, war, and euthanasia are morally wrong.

2. Because times change, the commandment "Thou shalt not kill" should be rewritten to read "Thou shalt not kill those who are already born and are sociologically and economically valuable."
3. The quality of life is more important than its length. Suffering serves little or no purpose and should be avoided if possible.
4. Every person has a right to be treated to the full extent of knowledge and technology. Life should be preserved at all costs and death should be delayed as long as possible or even avoided. With sufficient knowledge and technology, disease and death can be postponed or even eliminated.
5. Each person has the inherent right to determine what happens to his or her own body, be it to abort a fetus, end life, or delegate the responsibility to others. The latter is known as euthanasia. Euthanasia is of two types, negative and positive. In negative euthanasia ordinary treatment is given, but nothing is done for the purpose of hastening death. Ordinary measures include the maintenance of nutrition, comfort, relief of pain, and the like. In positive euthanasia some measure is used to hasten death in those who are hopelessly ill. Laws have been enacted in some states that allow a person to appoint a family member or a friend to make decisions about continued treatment if the person is incompetent to do so.
6. A person who is dying should be protected from this knowledge. Glaser and Strauss (1965) say "Americans are characteristically unwilling to talk openly about the process of dying itself; and they are prone to avoid telling a dying person that he is dying. This is, in part, a moral attitude: life is preferable to whatever may follow it, and one should not look forward to death unless he is in great pain." This attitude is changing.
7. Dying persons usually know that they are dying. The question is not whether they should be told, but how.

When Is a Person Dead? Who Decides?

Some answers have been suggested for the following questions: When is a person dead? Who decides? The problem of determining the moment of death was precipitated by the development of the technology for supporting respiratory and heart functions for extended periods of time. It was made acute when it was learned that organs from the newly dead could be successfully transplanted. However, the viability of these organs is dependent on continued perfusion with oxygenated blood. Therefore blood must be circulating until the organs are removed. Is the person whose heart is beating and who is breathing really dead? He or she is not if the accepted criterion of death for centuries is accepted, but is if certain newly defined criteria are met.

Brain Death

A criterion for death is that the person is dead if in irreversible coma (brain death). Among the evidences of irreversible coma cited are the following: (1) the person is deeply unconscious for a period of 24 hours, (2) there is no response to external stimuli or internal need, (3) no movements, (4) no breathing, and (5) except in some instances of spinal reflexes, no reflexes. Although some physicians support clinical evidence of irreversible coma with a flat EEG (electroencephalogram), Beecher (1970) does not think that an EEG is required. Excluded from this definition is the person who is under the influence of central nervous system depressants or whose body temperature is below 90°F. When an organ transplant is contemplated, the donor and the recipient must have different physicians. The donor's physician as an advocate is expected to defend his or her right to life, if such is possible.

The pronouncement of death in the presence of irreversible brain death is a legal as well as a medical matter. Laws have been enacted making brain death a legal criterion for death. The first court ruling establishing brain death as a legal concept was made by California's Alameda County Superior Judge William J. Hayes in the following instruction to the jury.

> A person may be pronounced dead if, based on usual and customary standards of medical practice, it is determined that the person has suffered an irreversible cessation of brain function.

Nursing the Person Whose Brain Function Has Ceased

With the growing armamentarium of biomedical equipment and procedures for life support of critically ill patients who would otherwise be dead, increasing attention has been given to the definition of brain death. The nurse working in critical care and emergency treatment settings is most likely to be involved in providing care to a person whose brain function has ceased. Nursing care of the dying patient as described in this chapter is appropriate

TABLE 33-1. ***"Harvard" Criteria for Brain Death****

1. Unreceptivity & unresponsivity. "Even the most intensely painful stimuli evoke no vocal or other response. . . ."
2. No movements or breathing. "Observation covering a period of at least one hour by physicians is adequate to satisfy the criteria of no spontaneous muscular movements or spontaneous respiration or response to stimuli . . . the total absence of spontaneous breathing may be established by turning off the respirator for three minutes and observing whether there is any effort on the part of the subject to breathe . . ." (this requires that carbon dioxide tension be normal and the patient be breathing room air for ten minutes before the test).
3. No reflexes. "The pupil will be fixed and dilated and will not respond to a direct source of bright light . . ." "Ocular movement (to head turning and to irrigation of ears with ice water) and blinking are absent." "There is no evidence of postural activity" (decerebrate or other). "Swallowing, yawning, vocalizing are in abeyance." "Corneal and pharyngeal reflexes are absent." "As a rule the stretch or tendon reflexes cannot be elicited."
4. Flat electroencephalogram. "Of great confirmatory value is the flat or isoelectric electroencephalogram . . ." (Technical guidelines including 5 μV/mm or higher gains, absence of response to pinch or noise, and 10-minute minimum recording time are added). "All of the above tests shall be repeated at least 24 hours later with no change." Hypothermia (temperature below 32.2°C [90°F]) & central-nervous-system depressants such as barbiturates must be excluded. "In situations where . . . electroencephalographic monitoring is not available, the absence of cerebral function has to be determined by purely clinical signs . . . or by the absence of circulation as judged by standstill of blood in the retinal vessels, or by absence of cardiac action. . . ."

* A definition of irreversible coma: report of the Ad Hoc Committee of the Harvard Medical School to examine the definition of brain death. *JAMA* **205** (1968), 337–40.

to the person whose brain function has ceased. The family needs continuing support, both to understand that the person is not experiencing pain and to deal with the loss of accustomed response from their loved one. The suffering experienced by families under these circumstances was well described, and appropriate help was suggested, in Chapter 32, The Spiritual Dimension of Nursing.

Although brain death is a medical determination, the nurse is usually closest to and a participant in recording the changes that signal impending cessation of brain function. Therefore, it is important to know the criteria for determining brain death. The set of criteria for brain death which appear to have the most widespread acceptance at the present time are the Harvard criteria, presented in Table 33–1.

Despite differences of opinion on criteria which must be met, it has been demonstrated that bodily death inevitably follows brain death within 3 months, despite the use of every current therapeutic life-support measure (Black, Part I, 1978).

Physical death is also defined as occurring on two levels. One is biological, the other clinical. *Biological death* is defined as the point at which organs cease to function. *Clinical death* is defined as the point at which the individual ceases to function as an organism.

Biological death may be limited to a single cell, to a part, or to an organ. Further, it takes place at different rates in different tissues and organs. In the living, certain cells die and are replaced, an area in the heart dies and is replaced with a scar, but cardiac function continues. In the dead person brain and heart cells die, but liver cells (as well as those in other organs) continue metabolic processes for varying periods of time. Even in the brain, cells in different locations die at differing rates.

SOCIAL DEATH

Social death is defined as the rejection of a dying person by society. It occurs after the physician pronounces the person terminally ill. In other words, cure is unlikely. Social death is most likely to occur after the person is institutionalized, but it may occur in any setting. Biologically and clinically, the person is alive but is treated as if he or she were dead. Friends, sometimes family members, and even nurses and physicians either avoid the person or they treat him or her as already dead (Ryder & Russ, 1977).

For Whom Do Decisions about Death Have To Be Made?

The four types of patients for whom decisions have to be made are

1. The person in acute cardiac or respiratory arrest, requiring resuscitation immediately.
2. The person whose prognosis is hopeless and who is maintained on supportive therapy.
3. The person who is dying and is a potential donor of an organ—kidney, liver, pancreas, heart—to another dying patient.

4. The person who is dying and whose life depends on the transplantation of a living organ or the use of an artificial organ.

The decision that a patient is or is not dead and the decisions about what is to be done are the responsibilities of the physician. In the absence of a physician, nurses, fire fighters, police officers, and others may be expected to institute cardiac and respiratory resuscitation. When the nurse is responsible, she or he should know which patients are to be resuscitated and should have had practice in the proper techniques and in the use of equipment. (See Chapters 40 and 44.)

Although nurses do not decide when supportive therapy is to be discontinued or which patients will serve as organ donors, they are touched by these decisions. As an example, a beautiful 4-month-old baby girl was brought into an emergency room. She appeared to have been suffocated. Heartbeat and respirations had ceased. When the mother found the baby, she was not breathing but was warm. Despite the probability that her brain was seriously injured, resuscitation was undertaken. Her heart started beating and respiration was maintained with a respirator. On checking her EEG, it was and remained flat and her pupils were fixed and dilated. There were no spinal reflexes. Should supportive therapy be continued? The physician faced with this decision paced the floor of the intensive-care unit asking himself this question. Eventually he turned off the equipment. The baby continued to breathe for 3 or 4 hours. No nurse who was present was untouched. Each felt the anguish of the physician as he made the decision to disconnect the respirator. Each felt grief at the death of the baby. Each nurse also sensed the physician's feeling of helplessness and guilt for having the machines turned off and for not being able to save the baby.

As a basis for making decisions about life and death, physicians refer to Pope Pius XII, who said that although ordinary means must be used in the treatment of the sick, extraordinary means are not required. This statement is of some help, but what is "ordinary" or "extraordinary"? That which is ordinary at one time and place may be extraordinary at another.

Stimulated by the rapid growth of the hospice movement, the International Work Group in Death, Dying and Bereavement (1979) has developed a set of assumptions and principles underlying standards for the care of terminal patients and their families. "These principles have been prepared as an aid to those who have initiated or are planning programs for the terminally ill in delineating standards of care." Many of these assumptions and principles should underly the care of all who seek care in health and illness. Certainly they should be considered whenever the terminally ill are given care.

With the introduction of machines to take over body functions and organ transplants a host of other questions are arising. As an example, most of these procedures are extremely expensive. Among the questions to be answered is how will an organ transplant be paid for? To what extent do these procedures not only extend the length of life, but enable the person to live a reasonably active life?

Who Is Involved

Despite the fact that each person dies alone, this does not mean that other people are not involved in his or her death. For there are family and friends, those upon whom he or she depends for care, as well as society. The significance of death to each differs depending upon one's age, responsibilities, and relationship to others.

The Dying Person

Who is the dying person? Strictly speaking, it is everyone, for the process of death starts at the moment of conception. Cells die and may or may not be replaced. Structures having served their purpose wither and die. The individual may die at any moment after conception. Some die quickly and for others the process of dying takes weeks or months. This person may be young or old, though in industrialized societies he or she is more likely to be old than young. The behavior of dying persons varies from the stoic who never complains to the one who is clingingly dependent, to the one who bewails or fights fate each step of the way. Individuals who are dying can be described, but because each person is an individual there is no single stereotype that fits the dying any more than there is one that fits the living.

Needs of the Dying

From research and the experience of those who work with the dying, some kinds of information have been acquired that should be useful in identifying and meeting the needs of the dying. The dying are similar in their needs to those who are healthy or sick with noncritical illnesses. They continue to have physiologic, psychological, spiritual, and social needs. In addition to the needs of all individuals, the dying have some special needs that arise from the nature of the process and attitudes toward death.

Essential Care

Rynearson (1959) summarizes the activities that are indispensable in the care of the dying patient and lists criteria for judging the adequacy of care. The indispensable care of the dying patient includes food, fluids, good nursing care, appropriate measures to relieve physical and mental suffering, and opportunity to prepare for death. The criteria to be met as suggested by Rynearson are the following:

1. He should die with dignity, respect and humanity.
2. He should die with minimal pain.
3. He should have the opportunity to recall the love and benefits of a lifetime of sharing; he and his family and friends should visit together, if the patient so wishes.
4. He should be able to clarify relationships—to express wishes—to share sentiments.
5. The patient and relatives should plan intelligently for the changes which death imposes upon the living.
6. The patient should die in familiar surroundings, if possible; if not, then quietus should take place in surroundings made as nearly homelike as possible.
7. Finally, but importantly, there should be concern for the feelings of the living.

The hygienic and physiologic needs of the dying are also of great importance and they should not be neglected. In the debilitated patient, improvement of nutrition may by itself bring about a marked change in outlook and in the ability to be active. The same is true when anemia is corrected. Exercise is usually encouraged. It prevents the loss of strength that accompanies inactivity and improves the appetite as well as the morale of the patient. Encouraging the patient to maintain as much independence as possible is also a benefit. Florence Nightingale in *Notes on Nursing* (1860, p. 85) expressed the wish that as much attention be paid to the effect of the body on the mind as the reverse. Later she stated that one of the common causes of death in chronic illness is starvation (1860, p. 92). This is no less true today than it was in Miss Nightingale's day.

Attention should be given to the maintenance of other functions, such as fluid intake, respiration, and elimination. As the patient fails, more and more of the daily activities of living, such as bathing and mouth care and protection of the skin against breakdown, will have to be assumed by others. Eventually the patient may become so weak that he or she is incontinent of urine and feces and can do little for himself or herself. For most adults this is a cause of shame and embarrassment and a threat to self-esteem. A matter-of-fact and kindly approach is usually effective in minimizing the patient's distress. Prompt attention to the soiled or wet bed is essential, as are measures to limit wetting and soiling. Attention to details that give the patient comfort benefits not only the patient but the members of the family.

Psychological Stages of Dying

In the last decade or so research has been reported on the psychological stages of dying and needs of dying patients. Kübler-Ross (1969) studied over 200 terminally ill patients. She concluded that the dying patient passes through five overlapping stages.[1] These are first stage: denial and isolation, second stage: anger, third stage: bargaining, fourth stage: depression, and fifth stage: acceptance. However, the nurse must remember that not only may the stages be overlapping, but not every patient goes through every stage. Some persons continue to deny the fact that death is approaching or to be angry with their fate until they die—or they may have a mixture of feelings. Just as the needs and approaches to the healthy person vary with the emotional state so do those of the dying. The questions to be answered are "What is important to this person at this time? Are his physiological needs being met? How can I, through nursing, help this person?" Whatever the patient's behavior, it is probably the best that he or she can do at this time.

Some investigators interpret the psychological responses of the dying somewhat differently. Death is a crisis situation in which the individual mobilizes psychological defenses that enable him or her to cope with the crisis. It is always essential to distinguish between use of a defense mechanism to help oneself and to meet other people's expectations. As an example, an individual may pretend not to know that he or she is dying because of the belief that others cannot tolerate the idea or that he or she will be better treated. Simply, individuals act as they think they are expected to act, and not as they really feel.

First Stage: Denial and Isolation

There is disagreement as to the extent to which patients who are faced with a serious illness with an unfavorable outcome use denial, that is, refusal to believe, as a defense mechanism. Certainly the extent to which it is used and the length of time varies with each individual. For the patient with whom there has been difficulty in establishing the diagnosis, even the presence of a fatal disease may actually be a relief, as it validates complaints. Probably most patients experience shock followed by a

[1] All these patients had a long-term illness, usually cancer.

period in which they cannot believe what has happened. It must be remembered that denial is a defense mechanism against anxiety. It acts as a cushion to protect the individual against unexpected bad news and allows time to come to terms with the situation and to mobilize other less radical defenses (Kübler-Ross, 1969). Although an occasional patient may use denial until he or she dies, most come to at least partial acceptance of their situation relatively soon. The statement, "It cannot be" is followed by, "Why me," and eventually, "Why not me?" Depending upon the circumstances, a patient may resort to at least partial denial at any time during illness. At the same time the patient is denying the seriousness of the illness, he or she is feeling alone. This feeling may be intensified by family members who are also frightened as well as by those who are responsible for the patient's care.

During the "It cannot be" stage, the patient looks for other solutions to problems. An error has been made or a different physician will find a more favorable diagnosis. It is during this stage that the patient or responsible family member is most likely to seek help from quacks who promise a cure. It is during this stage that *actions* as well as words promise that all possible will be done to benefit the patient.

Judgment is required in deciding the extent to which a patient's denial should be supported, particularly when it does not interfere with treatment. At times when a disease is far advanced and the patient is not believed to have much time before death, it may be necessary for the physician to make the facts known to him or her. This is likely to be a difficult time for everyone. For all patients, however, movement from denial to less drastic defenses depends on the establishment and maintenance of a caring relationship. It is in this kind of climate that the patient will be able to talk about whatever comes to mind, whether these thoughts are of better times, of the present, or of when he or she will cease to be.

Second Stage: Anger

Sooner or later most patients feel anger, rage, and envy. They ask such questions as, "Why me?" "What have I done that God should so punish me?" "Why not Jim or Mary?" This is a difficult stage as the patient displaces anger on staff and family members. He or she criticizes everyone and everything and sees rejection where kindness was meant. The food is cold, the nurse unfeeling, dull needles are selected to cause pain, sheets are rough, the physician does not know what he is doing, the hospital is inferior. His wife and children are uncaring. As in other situations, the extent and way in which patients express their anger differs from patient to patient. Those who have been tyrants when they were healthy generally continue to be tyrants when they are ill. If the staff can act on the principle that hostility breeds hostility, and that they are objects of displaced anger, they are more likely to be able to cope with the patient. If the patient feels that an effort is being made to understand his or her feelings and that those who are giving care are concerned about him or her and are not abandoning the patient in a time of extremity, a satisfactory relationship can usually be established.

Third Stage: Bargaining

Kübler-Ross (1969) says that the third stage is less well known, but may be helpful to the patient for brief periods of time. In this stage the patient promises God or someone else that certain changes will be made in his or her life in exchange for a cure or at least a delay in death. These promises vary from giving up smoking or alcohol, living a more balanced life, being a kinder spouse or better parent, to contributing to church or a worthwhile charity.

Fourth Stage: Depression

When illness and its effects can no longer be denied and the patient loses hope for a miracle, a profound feeling of loss is experienced. The fact that the patient is dying, that is, losing life, is often less important than what the loss of life means to him or her. As examples, Mr. Light was once a strong and athletic man who valued his strength, athletic prowess, and ability to support his family. He is now deeply in debt. His wife has had to seek work. Once firm muscles are flabby. Each day his weakness is greater. A once strong man, he is now almost completely dependent on others. His son and daughter will have to grow up without his loving guidance. There will be little money to pay their college expenses. He thinks of his past life and the things that he planned to do. All of his dreams have to be abandoned. As he is overwhelmed by it all, he becomes deeply depressed.

Kübler-Ross (1969) is of the opinion that depression experienced by the dying is of two types, the reactive depression and the preparatory depression. The first type results from the patient's feeling of how his or her present state differs from the past. This patient may be helped by enlisting his or her aid in making plans for dependents. In the instance of Mr. Light, his wife was encouraged to compliment him on being a good husband and father. Together they planned to sell their recently purchased house and to use the equity to reduce their debt. Because he was fully covered by Social Security, the children would have an income until they were 22 years of age, providing they did not marry and continued in school.

The preparatory depression, as the term implies, prepares the person for the next stage of dying, acceptance. This person is about to lose everything—self, hopes and dreams, and loved ones. The tendency on the part of those caring for the person is to try to cheer him or her, but this is of no help. The person should be encouraged to express grief. This is a time when procedures involving touch may be especially beneficial. Not only the nurse, but family and friends may help such patients by holding and squeezing their hands, stroking their brow, bathing them, rubbing their back, and changing their position. Family and friends may need encouragement and specific instructions to carry out even simple measures, such as hand holding. A person sitting quietly and relaxed in the room can be of benefit. In some cultures a family member is an indispensable part of the patient's care as the patient delegates all responsibility for well-being to this person. In contrast, in the American culture responsibility is vested in professionals. Therefore they have an obligation to guide the patient's family and friends so that they do what they can do. By so doing, they also help themselves by translating their grief into action.

Fifth Stage: Acceptance

Providing a patient does not die suddenly and is given some help in passing through the earlier stages (Kübler-Ross, 1969), he or she usually reaches the stage of acceptance. The person is no longer angry or depressed and has gone through a period of grieving. As implied, not all individuals reach the stage of acceptance and go on fighting until the end. Despite the tendency of families, nurses, and physicians to admire the courage of these patients, they may be unable to achieve a peaceful death. It is important to recognize behavior accordingly. In this stage, death may not be feared. It may even be welcomed. Various poets have expressed their feelings about death, such as the following:

Death stands above me, whispering low
I know not what into my ear;
Of His strange language all I know
Is, there is not a word of fear.
WALTER SAVAGE LANDOR, *On Death*

Alexander Pope in the first stanza of "The Dying Christian to His Soul" expresses a variety of feelings.

Vital Spark of heavenly flame!
Quit, O quit this mortal frame!
Trembling, hoping, lingering, flying,
O the pain, the bliss of dying.
Cease fond Nature, cease thy strife,
And let me languish into life!

John Donne, 1573–1631, in one of his sonnets says,

Death be not proud, though some have called thee
Mighty and dreadful, for, thou art not so;
For, those whom thou think'st thou dost overthrow,
Die not, poor death, nor yet canst thou kill me.
From rest and sleep, which but thy pictures be,
Much pleasure, then from thee, much more must flow,
And soonest our best men with thee doe go,
Rest of their bones, and soules delivery.
Thou art slave to Fate, Chance, kings and desperate men.
And dost with poyson, warre, and sicknesse dwell,
And poppy or charms can make us sleep as well,
And better then thy stroke; why swell'st thou then?
One short sleepe past, wee wake eternally
And death shall be no more; death thou shalt die.

In the earlier stages of dying the patient may benefit from verbal communication in which there is an opportunity to have questions answered honestly and to say what is thought and felt. In the stage of acceptance nonverbal communication plays a larger role; this includes touching, sitting quietly with the patient, attending to physical care, relieving pain, and through the manner and timing of actions the nurse and others demonstrating that they do care about the patient. During this stage the family may need more psychological care than the patient, as the dying person may ignore or turn from them with the result that they feel rejected. Small acts of kindness and attention to the needs of the relative for food, fluids, and rest help to make a difficult time more tolerable.

Irrespective of the stage of dying or who is responsible for the care of the patient, the person can be expected to experience fear and to be benefited by being treated as an individual, making his or her own decisions, and having hopes sustained.

Fear

Fear is one of the states experienced by the dying and by those associated with the dying. Although fear of death is generally considered to be common to all, it is not the only fear experienced by the dying. Despite the belief that the dying usually experience pain and suffering, this is not always true. Noyes (1971) cites a study made by Sir William Osler in which only 18 per cent of 500 patients studied suffered bodily pain. Generally this pain can be minimized by appropriate care. (See Chapter 36 for pain management.) Some fear the loss of ability to do the things that they were once able to do, as well as becoming dependent and a care or nuisance to others. Other causes of fear include altered consciousness, loss of a part of the body, disfigurement, incontinence, loss of control of oneself and of one's own affairs, and helplessness and vulnerability. Some may fear punishment in an afterlife or that when they die they will be no more. Unfortunately some, with or without reason, fear that they will be abandoned by their families and those to whom they entrust themselves for care and treatment.

Everyone participating in the care of a dying person has a responsibility to identify personal fears. One tool is open communication for the benefit of the patient and not for gaining information per se. In the words of Fielding (1962),

> When death comes slowly, fear may come fast: it can spread a conspiracy in a home: bright-eyed, stiff-smiling, and truly fearful. A silence is engendered which isolates the dying person far more surely than his malady. Two languages begin to be spoken: one in the sickroom and the other in the remainder of the house; the bedroom door may become an iron lattice filtering off the light and truth of the household from him who is in most need of them. But if the fear is described and accepted, the conspiracy shrinks to its proper dimensions; it is confined to the bed, to one man and the not-terrible whisperings of his demise. As Jacques de la Rivière said:
> "Peace lies only in the irremediable."

Need for Hope

It is important to continue to think about the person as an individual, not as a disease. It is also essential to believe that the patient who is beyond medical help can continue to be helped by nursing. Such patients should be permitted and encouraged, but not pressed, to talk about interests, accomplishments, hopes, and fears. They may want to talk about how their illness has changed them as persons. Their hope for recovery should be encouraged.

Hope is the expectation that what one wants will come to pass. It is one of the most essential supports that even realistic patients have and nothing should be done to cut off all hope. Despite overwhelming evidence to the contrary, patients with advanced disease do hope for the miracle of being restored to their life as they have known it in the past. One value of ethically managed experimental treatment programs is that they offer hope of benefit to patients and through them to others. As Mrs. Genny said, "I'm taking a new drug. Even if it does not benefit me, it may help others in the future." Her hope was supported and she believed that she was making a significant contribution to others. By making this contribution, she was giving her life purpose and meaning.

When possible and advisable, the patient should make decisions. There are many decisions in the course of the day that a patient can make. When this is done he or she continues to feel some control over the situation. It is also essential that no matter how difficult the patient, he or she not be abandoned. In fact, the angry, demanding patient may be in most need of support.

Spiritual Care

In writing about the spiritual care of every patient, Sister Mary Hubert (1963) makes some suggestions that are particularly relevant to the dying patient. Her first suggestion is kindness, thoughtfulness, gentleness, and a "personalized warm concern." Second, she suggests "frequent contacts"; staying away from the patient is easier when one is afraid or the patient is irritable and demanding, but only through contact with the patient can the nurse express real concern for him or her or be kind or thoughtful. Third, the nurse should understand her or his own attitude toward "the truths of human existence; life, suffering, old-age, and death." According to Sister Mary Hubert, suffering is one of the most frequently encountered facts of life and is the least understood. Her fourth suggestion, the encouragement of wholesome reading, may or may not be applicable. Certainly, encouragement of the patient to continue former interests and activities as long as possible is to be recommended. Finally, by prayer—the nurse may pray with the patient, help the patient to pray, offer to say a prayer for the patient—the nurse may be able to convey concern for the patient and his or her welfare. (See also Chapter 32.)

Where Do People Die

The simple answer to where people die is wherever people are. According to statistics, however, about 80 per cent die in hospitals. The remainder die in nursing homes, in hospices, in their own homes, on the highway, and at work. If the present trend continues, hospice care will be available to more people. (See Chapter 4.) In areas where home care programs are available and the family is willing and able to manage, patients may be cared for at home or alternate between hospital and home. As an example, though Mrs. Genny died in a hospital, she spent much of the 2 years after a diagnosis of metastatic cancer at home. She was hospitalized for treatments that could not be given at home and during acute episodes of illness. In some instances a patient may be hospitalized for a week or so in order for the family to get needed rest and recreation.

The advantages to the patient are not always in the hospital. Rees (1972) found that patients dying at home were more likely to remain alert until shortly before death. They were less likely to be incontinent, develop bedsores or vomiting, or have unrelieved physical distress.

A development in the hospital is the intensive-care unit where the man or woman and machine combine to prevent death or in positive terms to save lives. Here the critically ill for whom there is hope that highly skilled care and sophisticated machines can turn the tide toward life are placed. That the purposes of these units are accomplished is without doubt. Some of the more human needs are sacrificed at times in order to observe accurately the patient's status or to carry out required procedures. Patients and families are separated by machines and hourly 5-minute visits. Despite the best efforts of nurses and physicians, some patients die.

Especially when a patient is young or when great effort has been expended, failure to save a life can be a most traumatic experience for nurses and physicians alike. They experience feelings of helplessness and failure, even when they know that they did their very best. They need help in evaluating the effects of their behavior on patients and families. Nurses may need help in accepting themselves and what they are able to do. For milk to be poured from a pitcher it must continue to be refilled. Recently attention has been given to the effects that stressful situations have on the ability of care givers to function in a caring way.

The Family

Despite exceptions, the premise that the family has a commitment to the dying patient and a legitimate interest in his or her welfare is sound. Further, the nurse has a responsibility to assist the family in helping the patient utilize resources constructively. At times a family member is the first to be told of the patient's unfavorable prognosis. This person is asked to decide what should be told to the patient and how the information should be communicated. Like the patient, family members go through the stages of grief, shock, denial, anger, bargaining, depression, and acceptance. They, too, are faced with losses. These losses include not only the loss of the member of the family, but a variety of other losses. The nature of these losses varies with the sex, age, marital status, and other factors. As an example, the widow finds her status as a no longer married woman different from that of a woman with a husband. She may find herself with insufficient means to support herself and dependent children. A husband loses the emotional support of his wife. A child not only loses a parent, but may lose loving support and guidance.

Other factors complicate the life of family members. They may have to cope with real or fancied guilt and shame for past neglect or other offenses against the dying person. Long illnesses are expensive and financial resources may be exhausted. Time and energy used in the care of the sick may leave the family emotionally and physically drained. When the grieving process has been completed before the patient dies, the family may feel obligated to appear to be grieving when the death brings only relief.

Sudden death also brings with it problems to the living. The grieving process has not begun. Often the survivor(s) is still in a state of shock at the time of the funeral. Friends and relatives quickly return to their ordinary lives. The family is left to cope with their grief and the problems caused by the sudden death of the family member. Guilt for sins of omission and commission may be very strong. Surviving husbands or wives have to learn suddenly a new pattern of living. Depending upon the age and economic situation, surviving wives may have to seek work to support themselves and dependent children. The sudden death syndrome in infants causes great distress. Despite the fact that these deaths are not due to neglect, parents, relatives, and neighbors may believe they are. Thus the parents not only have to cope with the grief engendered by the loss of their child, but with guilt and shame for not having done something to prevent it. Evidence that death in the family is stressful is the fact that during the first year after a death in the family, more family members die than would otherwise be expected.

There are many ways in which the nurse can be of assistance to the family. One of the most basic is to accept them as human beings who have a legitimate interest in the dying person. Further, different people have different ways of expressing their feelings. Though some instinctively act appropriately (as defined by nurses and physicians), others need instruction. They may not know what to do or they may be fearful that they will do something that is harmful. When the patient is angry, this anger may be projected to one or more family members. Despite this behavior, he or she may need their support. In these instances the perceptive nurse supports the relative and encourages him or her to continue visits. During all stages, relatives and friends may assist with aspects of care with which they are comfortable. Assistance with moving, turning, positioning, and walking can often be given by family members. Hand holding, reading, writing letters, and sitting quietly can provide opportunities for family members and friends to feel that they are contributing to the patient's well-being. All of these situations provide an opportunity for the family to communicate their love and support to the patient.

If the family is to be supportive to the patient, it needs a source of support. Sometimes they get it from each other. More often they need some support from nurses and physicians. Family members need an opportunity to express their grief. When they are rejected or ignored by the patient they need to know that this is an expected phenomenon. It does not mean that they are unworthy. When they have spent many hours with the patient or dying has been prolonged, they may need to be encouraged to eat and to rest. A comfortable chair and foot stool could certainly be available. A cup of hot tea, or a squeeze of the hand convey an appreciation of their feelings and needs. When they are encouraged to leave, they should have a firm promise of a call should the patient's condition change. When an illness is relatively short or the grieving process has not been completed, the family may have difficulty accepting the patient's death and need much help.

A word should be said about inappropriate family behavior. First of all one should be sure that it is inappropriate. Though visiting hours are less rigid than they once were and are often relaxed for dying patients, there are instances where relatives are unnecessarily restricted. Conversely, too many people may arrive at one time, be too noisy, and make inappropriate demands on the patient. Particularly during the stage of acceptance, the patient may want nothing so much as peace and quiet with one or at the most two close family members sitting quietly in the room. Here as in other situations, the nurse has a responsibility to assess the needs of the patient and act accordingly.

Who Cares for the Dying Person

The care of the terminally ill patient is shared by the patient's family, physician, nurses, social workers, and clergyman—minister, priest, or rabbi. When available, specialists in psychology, sociology, and anthropology can be helpful to those caring for the dying. Healthy people often hesitate about having a clergyman visit a seriously ill person for the first time. They fear that the patient will be frightened and give up hope of living. Some hospitals solve this problem by employing or arranging to have a clergyman visit all newly admitted patients, unless the patient specifically asks not to be visited by a chaplain. Visits are then continued as a regular service to the patient. Catholic patients usually expect to be visited regularly. Though non-Catholics find it hard to believe, most Catholics are comforted by having the sacrament of the sick.

The Nurse

Although the nurse is not alone in the care of the dying patient and family, she or he is the one who carries the hour-to-hour responsibility. Similar to other members of the American culture, the nurse defines cure as the most important criterion of success. When a patient recovers, nurses as well as doctors take credit for the patient's success. Moreover, patients, nurses, and doctors frequently expect not only that patients should get well but that they should recover quickly and pleasantly. When they do not recover or they die, the nurse and physician feel that they must have failed in some respect.

In addition to being an agent in the cure of the sick person, nurses also expect to comfort the sick and to relieve their suffering. When they are unable to do this, they may feel that as nurses they are inadequate and feelings of anxiety are aroused. With anxiety the defenses of the person against anxiety are invoked. The psychological defenses of people sick or well are alike. Nurse and patient may both be using similar or different defenses against feelings of fear. Because the burden for adapting behavior is on the nurse, she or he must have some insight into personal feelings about death and dying. When the nurse has come to terms with these feelings, she or he should be better able to concentrate on what the patient is feeling, even when he or she projects negative feelings to the nurse. The patient can be allowed to talk about feelings, be they of anger, remorse, guilt, or regrets.

When the patient has reached that stage in illness during which the goal in care is to provide comfort, the nurse may wish to comfort him or her. At the same time the nurse may be angry with the patient. This produces feelings of guilt because nurses are taught to have kindly feelings toward patients or because the nurse is healthy and will continue to live. These problems are further compounded when the patient does not know or is not supposed to know that he or she is dying. The nurse must be continuously on guard to not reveal the true state of the patient.

The nurse is thus forced to use a variety of strategies against unacceptable feelings. The nurse's own feelings of helplessness and despair may cause denial of feelings and withdrawal from the situation and refusal to care for the patient, or the nurse may try to relieve personal feelings by being excessively solicitous. She or he may treat the patient in an impersonal or cold manner (the cool, starched look). When the nurse is excessively disturbed by the predicament of the patient and feels too strongly, the patient may be frightened and the nurse may be unable to be sufficiently objective[2] to support him or her emotionally. The nurse requires a support system to be able to come to terms with personal feelings.

As the condition of the patient deteriorates, he or she can be expected to become more and more dependent on care givers. How nurses (or others) react depends on their ability to tolerate dependency in others. Chodoff (1960) states that healthy persons often have ambivalent feelings with elements of hostility when they have contact with the helpless and disabled. In the patient who is in the terminal phase of a long-term illness such as cancer, there is no need for concern about the effects of long-term dependency on the nurse–patient relationship. The nurse must exercise judgment and sensitivity to the needs and feelings of such patients, so that they have done for them what comforts them and they are allowed and encouraged to do the things that they can and wish to do.

Other problems to the nurse in the care of patients who die or are dying include the possibility that the nurse fears that the patient would not have died if she or he had acted quickly enough or in a different manner. When a patient dies unexpectedly or dies when the nurse is giving or assisting with care, the nurse may feel responsible in some manner. When a nurse is disturbed by any of these questions, the problem should be discussed with someone who can help in exploring the various facets of the problem.

Another aspect of the care of the dying that engenders negative feelings relates to the extent to which life should be prolonged or death prevented. Though nurses are not responsible for making the decision that a given treatment should be instituted, withheld, or continued, they are affected by these decisions. For example, the nurse may be troubled when therapeutic measures are instituted that, though they have as their objective the prolongation of the life of the patient, appear to increase suffering. The physician is responsible for informing the family of the condition of the patient and suggesting to them courses of action. Much of the care of the dying patient is given by nurses. They cannot help but be affected by the decisions made relative to the patient.

[2] The term *objectivity* is herein defined as the ability of the nurse to evaluate and meet the patient's needs in such a way that he or she is helped.

In the recent past there has been and is a tendency either to neglect the care of those who are in the terminal phase of an illness or to use extraordinary measures to prolong life. There is a beginning trend toward emphasizing that much can be done to increase usefulness and comfort during the period in which the health of the individual declines. In some instances the patient is fully informed of the nature of his or her condition and what may be expected from the treatment. Attention continues to be on what can be done and on conveying to the patient that something can and will be done to help. The emphasis here is not on cure, though this possibility is recognized, but on comfort and support of the sick person. The criterion for evaluating success is not so much how many are cured, but how long an individual is maintained in a reasonable comfortable and useful state.

References Cited

Beecher, H. K. "Definitions of 'Life' and 'Death' for Medical Science and Practice." *Annual N.Y. Academy Science,* **169** (1970), 471–74.

Black, P. M. "Brain Death. Part I." *N. Engl. J. Med.,* **299** (Aug. 17, 1978), 338–44.

Chodoff, P. "A Psychiatric Approach to the Dying Patient." *CA,* **10** (1960), 30.

Fielding, G. "The Uses of Fear." *Harper's Magazine,* **224** (1962), 94.

Glaser, B. G., and Strauss, A. *Awareness of Dying.* Chicago: Aldine Publishing Co., 1965, p. 3.

Hubert, M., Sister. "Spiritual Care for Every Patient." *J. Nurs. Ed.,* **2** (1963), 9–11.

"International Work Group in Death, Dying and Bereavement. Assumptions and Principles Underlying Standard for Terminal Care." *Am. J. Nurs.,* **79** (1979), 296–97.

Kübler-Ross, E. *On Death and Dying.* New York: Macmillan Publishing Co., 1969, pp. 34–121.

Nightingale, F. *Notes on Nursing: What It Is and What It Is Not,* new ed., rev. and enlarged. London: Harrison and Sons, 1860, pp. 5, 85, and 92.

Noyes, R. "The Care and Management of the Dying." *Arch. Internat. Med.,* **128** (1971), 300.

Paz, O. "The Day of the Dead," in *Death & Identity,* R. Fulton, ed. New York: John Wiley & Sons, Inc., 1965, p. 395.

Rees, W. D. "The Distress of Dying." *Br. Med. J.,* **3** (1972), 105–7.

Rynearson, E. H. "You Are Standing at the Bedside of a Patient Dying of Untreatable Cancer." *CA,* **9** (1959), 87.

Ryder, C. F., and Ross, D. M. "Terminal Care-Issues and Alternatives." *Public Health Rep.,* **92** (1977), 20–29.

General References

Agee, J. *A Death in the Family.* New York: Avon Books, 1957.

Black, P. M. "Brain Death: Part II." *N. Engl. J. Med.*, **299** (Aug. 24, 1978), 393–401.

Breu, C., and Dracup, K. "Helping the Spouses of Critically Ill Patients." *Am., J. Nurs.*, **78** (1978), 51–53.

Cannon, M. "To Sharon with Love." *Am. J. Nurs.*, **79** (1979), 642–45.

Cawley, M. A. "Euthanasia: Should It Be A Choice?" *Am. J. Nurs.*, **77** (1977), 859–61.

Davis, A. J. "Brompton's Cocktail: Making Good-byes Possible." *Am. J. Nurs.*, **78** (1978), 611–12.

Eigsti, D. E. "Helping Parents to Deal with the Developmental Task of Death Education." *Health Values,* **2** (1978), 31–43.

Fulton, R. *Death and Identity.* New York: John Wiley & Sons, 1965.

Griffin, J. Family Decision. *Am. J. Nurs.*, **75** (1975), 795–96.

Gunther, J. *Death Be Not Proud.* New York: Modern Library, 1953.

Jackson, P. L. Chronic Grief. *Am. J. Nurs.*, **74** (1974), 1289–91.

Kobrzycki, P. "Dying with Dignity at Home." *Am. J. Nurs.*, **75** (1975), 1312–13.

Kowalsky, E. L. Grief. *Am J. Nurs.*, **78** (1978), 418–20.

Kristein, M. M., Arnold, C. B., and Wynder, E. L. "Health Economics and Preventive Care." *Science,* **195** (1977), 457–62.

Lande, S. "A Gift of Hope." *Am. J. Nurs.*, **77** (1977), 639–40.

Mills, G. C. "Books to Help Children Understand Death." *Am. J. Nurs.*, **79** (1979), 291–95.

Relman, A. S. "Michigan's Sensible Living Will." *N. Engl. J. Med.*, **300** (1979), 1270–71.

Stoller, E. P. "Effect of Experience on Nurses' Responses to Dying and Death in the Hospital Setting. *Nurs. Res.*, **29** (Jan.–Feb. 1980), 35–38.

Tolstoy, L. *The Cossacks, the Death of Ivan Illych, Happy Ever After.* Trans. Rosemary Edmonds. Baltimore: Penguin Books, 1960.

34

Rehabilitation Nursing

Life is a fatal adventure. It can only have one end. So why not make it as far ranging and free as possible?

ALEXANDER ELIOT

Overview

Rehabilitation is a process which emphasizes reeducation of the client so that he or she may participate in the activities of a normal life within the limitations imposed by physical disability. Rehabilitation should be a continuous restorative process recognizing the person's needs and goals and helping to positively integrate the person's resources physically, psychologically, socially, and vocationally within the limitations of the individual's maximum ability for participation. All too frequently rehabilitation has been thought of as a specialty. Even more unfortunate is the fact that it has been thought of as something that follows acute and convalescent care, and something that occurs only in specific settings such as a rehabilitation hospital or a specialized rehabilitation unit. One of the earliest authors on rehabilitation nursing, Alice B. Morrissey (1951, p. 26), wrote that rehabilitation extends from the bed to the job. Emphasis is placed on ability rather than disability, and we teach people to live and work with what they have left. Today the term restorative care is being used as well as rehabilitation. Both restorative care and rehabilitation have essentially the same meaning, but restorative care implies broader application to patients with all kinds of problems being cared for in a variety of settings.

Need and Setting for Rehabilitation

The need for restorative care is increasing at an amazing and frightening rate. It is increasing with the same rapidity as modern medical, surgical, and technological advances in the health care field. In every age group, the number of chronically ill or disabled persons grows yearly. Modern medical and surgical procedures, infection control, new drugs, and other advances are allowing the survival of many persons with birth defects, accidents, and disease who previously would not have survived. Older people figure more and more predominately among the chronically ill. The simple act of living longer increases the likelihood of disability in everyone.

The burden for providing restorative care rests upon the community including its acute hospitals, nursing homes, and community health agencies. Rehabilitation centers are too few in number and resources to be able to meet the needs of the population who needs restorative care. The major focus of patient care in acute care hospitals continues to be life-saving priorities and often leaves the less dramatic but urgent restorative needs of the patient unmet; yet an increasing proportion of the patient population in the acute care facility are those in need of restorative care (Schizkedanz & Mitchell, 1972).

This chapter was contributed by Rita H. O'Neill, R.N., M.S., Associate Professor of Nursing, College of Nursing, Southeastern Massachusetts University, North Dartmouth, Massachusetts.

Restorative care is a component of care in all settings where professional nurses practice: intensive and intermediate care units, as well as extended, long-term, and home care. The client with a functional disability may be compromised by failure of the system's regulatory mechanisms to adequately process existing input. The client may be unable to perform the activities which are considered essential to daily living (activities of daily living, ADL), and nursing activities may be necessary to help the client cope with and overcome these problems. The nurse is mainly concerned not with the disease the client has but rather with how it affects the client. Her or his responsibility is to know how to help the client deal with the problem. A nursing approach is influenced less by whether the client has a medical diagnosis of arthritis or hemiplegia than by whether the nurse knows how to deal with a painful extremity versus a paralyzed one.

The Rehabilitation Team

Rehabilitation is a service provided in a variety of health care institutions and community agencies. To meet the total needs of the client physically, psychologically, socially, and vocationally, many specialties or disciplines must combine their services and function as a team. The rehabilitation team is generally composed of the following health care professionals: a physiatrist, that is, a physician who specializes in physical medicine and rehabilitation; a professional nurse; a social worker; a physical therapist; an occupational therapist; a psychologist; a vocational counselor; a nutritionist; and a speech therapist. In the modern rehabilitation department, a handicapped person, when admitted, is first evaluated by each member of the team in order to determine the individual's physical, mental, social, and vocational abilities. The team takes a dynamic approach and concerns itself not as much with the negative aspects of the person's disabilities as with the positive aspects of the person's remaining abilities. When the various members of the rehabilitation team have made the evaluation, they join in a group conference to develop a comprehensive program to assist the client in making the most of his or her remaining abilities. The team may function in a general hospital or a specialized rehabilitation center.

At the time of injury or illness, the disabled person usually receives initial care in a general hospital. After the acute period of illness, the person may be admitted to an institution that specializes in rehabilitation or another unit within the acute care hospital. Almost all persons requiring extensive rehabilitation services will require a more lengthy stay in an institution than is generally allowed in the acute care hospital. Whether the person receives rehabilitation care in a specialized rehabilitation center or in a rehabilitation unit of a general hospital, what is most important is that the team approach be utilized and that the team's philosophy be directed toward rehabilitation. No agency, rehabilitation center, or hospital, even when using the team approach, can totally meet the needs of the disabled person. The disabled person and family will definitely need to be involved in the rehabilitation process. Community agencies, official and nonofficial agencies, such as the Visiting Nurse Association, Office of Vocational Rehabilitation, and others, will be involved as the person's need and goals indicate.

Rehabilitation Nursing

In order for the patient to receive the greatest benefit from a rehabilitation program, it is imperative that nurses perceive rehabilitation as a process that begins when a patient first suffers from acute disease, trauma, or the early symptoms of progressively debilitating disease. Over 50 per cent of the patients in most acute care hospitals have one or more chronic diseases and about 25 per cent of these are over 65 years of age (Stryker, 1977, p. 17). All persons who have sustained trauma or pathology that affects their interaction with the environment require rehabilitation. They need our assistance to refashion their life styles as their life processes continue in an altered direction.

The elements of rehabilitation nursing need to be viewed as part of basic nursing rather than as a specialty. Those who work at rehabilitation centers where patients are severely disabled naturally require additional knowledge in this field of nursing. However, this is a matter of degree and depth of knowledge rather than one of learning a completely new body of knowledge (Stryker, 1977). A comparison might be made with the nurse who works in the coronary care unit. The degree and depth of her or his knowledge in cardiovascular nursing is different from the nurse on the medical unit, but it is not a completely new body of knowledge concerning cardiovascular nursing. The same applies in the area of rehabilitation nursing.

The major objectives of rehabilitation nursing are prevention and restoration. Prevention is the major emphasis of Chapter 49, which is devoted to disuse syndromes. The second objective is to restore as much function as possible to the injured or diseased part. This is the area of rehabilitation in which the nurse working in a rehabilitation center will have a greater depth of knowledge than a nurse working in a nursing home, extended care facility, public health agency, or general medical-surgical area of a hospital.

One of the most important qualities of a rehabilitation nurse is the possession of an attitude of wholeness, a holistic approach to humanity. An honest holistic approach is essential if one is to reach and rehabilitate effectively patients and their families. Their overwhelming loss is the prime consideration in working with these patients. Loss with its resultant deformity, dysfunction, or absence of function implies that these patients are no longer whole if a part is gone or if what remains is malfunctional or nonfunctional. If these patients are to refashion their lives, a holistic approach is imperative (Rotkovitch, 1976, p. 141). In addition to this most important quality of a holistic approach, the rehabilitation nurse must possess certain knowledge and skills. The nurse needs a good understanding of both the physiological and psychological effects of long-term illness in order to respond appropriately to patients' needs during the various stages of adjustment to a disability. Also, she or he needs knowledge of anatomy, physiology, and pathophysiology, especially of the nervous system and musculoskeletal system. The nurse will have to communicate with patients who may have difficulty in expressing themselves and understanding others. In addition, the rehabilitation nurse needs to be an expert in certain skills. These skills involve position changes, transfer techniques, and range-of-motion exercises which are essential in planning and delivering nursing care as well as in patient and family teaching.

The rehabilitation nurse must know and use community resources. In the community, the public health nurse will both find rehabilitation candidates and follow those who have completed a program. Public health nursing follow-up is a key factor in maintaining rehabilitation gains in many instances.

A major role of the rehabilitation nurse is that of patient and family teaching. Both the patient and family usually have a great deal to learn. The patient may need to learn new ways of performing activities of daily living (ADLs) such as dressing, bathing, eating, and toileting. He or she may need to learn how to care for a catheter, how to catheterize himself or herself, or how to walk again.

Coordination is also a key role of the nurse responsible for the care of patients who receive attention from various members of the rehabilitation team. The patient needing rehabilitation services will often be receiving care from physical therapists, occupational therapists, speech therapists, and others. It is necessary to coordinate the learning from the various therapists into the patient's activities throughout the day.

In many rehabilitation centers, a broadened scope of independent nursing practice has been encouraged and developed. The Loeb Center in New York, under the leadership of Lydia Hill, pioneered in the concept of nursing as an individual therapy that can upgrade care and decrease hospital stay. At the Rehabilitation Institute in Chicago, every full-time registered nurse is a nurse therapist who is responsible for specific individuals' plans of care throughout their stay and who continues to work with the patient, family, or other care givers after discharge whenever possible. Primary nursing is another means of better utilizing the skills of the nurse. Each nurse is responsible for her or his caseload from admission to discharge, plans and gives patient care, writes nursing orders for other care givers to follow, communicates directly with the physician and other disciplines, and is both responsible and accountable for the patient load.

Psychological Reactions to Physical Disability

A successful rehabilitation program depends upon psychological adaptations. There are certainly many factors that affect a person's adjustment, and all these factors cannot be considered here; however, there are certain factors that will influence the patient's adjustment and must be considered in the nursing assessment in order to anticipate patient problems and help the person cope with his or her adaptations. The grieving process and the concept of body image can be used as a frame of reference in dealing with rehabilitation patients. Our culture places high value on beauty, good physical condition, youth, and physical ability. This emphasis pervades our entertainment and leisure activities. When someone has a physical disability, feelings of frustration and shame often dominate until new understandings develop. The impact of chronic illness is further complicated by the fact that it does not go away. Each person will attach a particular meaning to illness, consciously or unconsciously. Some people view illness as punishment, whereas others may view illness as a release from an intolerable situation or a concrete reason for dependency.

Kübler-Ross's (1975) stages of the grieving process are used as a frame of reference in working with rehabilitative patients. In order to repattern their life processes in view of actual or anticipated loss, patients must be assisted in reaching resignation or acceptance (Kübler-Ross, 1975, p. 142). This is a necessary concomitant to realistic rehabilitation—a psychological necessity, not a weakness or self-indulgence. Persons faced with a loss of major body function and/or parts will proceed through a series of phases, much like those experienced in mourning. The duration of each phase may differ, and a person may skip a phase or plateau. It is the job of the staff to understand that it is important for patients to feel comfortable in expressing their anger, anguish, depression, and other feelings at each phase in order for progress to occur (Stryker, 1977, p. 35).

Dr. Kübler-Ross's stages are milestones in a patient's rehabilitation journey. Initially, denial, sometimes associated with shock and disbelief, is evident. This may be manifested by withdrawal or anxiety. The person is fearful not only about the specific loss, but also about his or her total life's orientation. How will the person be able to care for himself or herself? What about family and job? Will he or she be sexually adequate? What about bowel and bladder control? These questions, often unanswerable at this time, are overwhelming. Dr. Kübler-Ross sees two components: a protective coping one, assisting the patient to cooperate with therapy; and an active, destructive denial, when the patient refuses medication, surgery, and therapy. The nurse must listen, try to understand the patient and attempt to be supportive throughout this period. This is a difficult time for the patient's family and they too require a great deal of encouragement from the nurse. This denial period gives the patient time to gather new strength to deal with the task of coping with the disability. Staff must be careful not to confront patients with too much reality too soon.

Anger—the "Why me? Why this diagnosis?" stage—is usually most trying for staff but is very beneficial for the patient who may begin to verbalize and express many fears. The nursing staff may need assistance from clinical nurse specialists to realize that the anger expressed by the patient is not directed toward them personally but rather toward the patient's situation. The healthy, motivating aspects of anger should be realized to help the patient move on to the next stage.

In bargaining, the third stage, various members of the rehabilitation team are joined with physicians and God in being able, in the patient's eyes, to perform miracles. Awareness of loss or impending disability is increased in this "Yes, me, but . . ." stage. This is particularly applicable for the patient facing radical surgery or amputation. Depression sets in during the latter stage and brings rehabilitation patients to an all-important period of grief. The reality of the disfigurement or loss becomes imminent; separation from the former body image of wholeness begins, and prerequisites for acceptance of loss can be met.

The stage of resignation or acceptance—"Yes, me"—is the opportune moment to involve the individual in active participation in the rehabilitation program. Here the long, hard job of helping the patient realistically to repattern his or her life begins. Acceptance may be considered the restorative plan of rehabilitation, where patient and nurse set practical goals and direct their mutual efforts toward accomplishing them.

In adapting to a disability, a patient must begin to enlarge his or her scope of values. What seemed important yesterday may become unimportant today. Most persons with a severe disability say that they eventually become far better persons as a result of the kind of soul-searching and analysis required in their adjustment to living with a disability. Dorothy Smith's recent research on survivors of serious illness confirms this change in values in those who have also survived acute illnesses (Smith, 1979). New values with deeper meaning will emerge. As a person identifies and re-examines the normal values held by society, he or she will be able to subordinate the ideal of a perfect physique as deeper and more enduring values emerge.

This stage of acceptance arrives for some after months, for others after years, and for a few never. People accept things in many ways. One might cope with a disability and yet have unrealistic goals. Another might appear to accept the diagnosis but deny the implications of the disability. Some experts feel that a goal of the patient's total acceptance is unrealistic. As the patient begins to work through this initial shock, depression, fear, and anger, he or she begins to develop an inner acceptance and to move toward social integration. The patient realizes that his or her total life style, although responsive to the reality of the problem, does not allow for personal gratification. He or she begins to experience satisfaction from what can be done rather than defeat from what cannot be done. Acceptance means giving in to the treatment, but it does not mean constricting one's interests or remaining unnecessarily dependent (Stryker, 1977, p. 38).

No matter how brilliantly conceived a rehabilitation program may be, it will be worthless unless the patient is involved. He or she must be motivated positively—and this is the essence of rehabilitation. Whereas the rehabilitation team is the body of the process, positive patient motivation is the soul. The driving force must come from within the patient even though the team makes evident the patient's potential and provides continued teaching, support, and encouragement.

A revision of self-concept is necessary for a patient to become positively motivated. The patient is no longer the same physical being of earlier times. Until such time as this all-important fact is recognized and comprehended, no changes in how the patient now views himself or herself will occur. In too many instances we expect patients to have had a secure and positive self-concept prior to their disability. The patients are what they were before their injury—only more so. If patients were cognizant of their strengths and weaknesses, such an awareness will tend to continue. If, however, they had not found their role previous to the disability, it will be extremely difficult to do so now. (This is the major reason disabled adolescents, not having finalized a concept of self, are often so frustrating to work with.) The patient's present situation and premorbid personality are essential factors in revising the self-concept. We cannot expect changes in self-concept or positive motivation to occur rapidly. This is a process that requires greatly differing lengths of time and that will depend on the individual. Determining whether or not a person is positively motivated is a very difficult undertaking and cannot and should not be done by one person.

The team must be at once flexible and consistent. The staff must be alert to the patient's manner of expressing just where he or she is in the adjustment process. They must know when to move ahead and when to leave the patient alone. They must be aware of the time when he or she becomes an active participant. Or they must accept the decision that the person is not a rehabilitation candidate. Only by being objectively observant can they appraise; only by being adaptable can they function; and only by being consistent can they establish a working relationship with the patient.

Preparing the Patient and Family for Discharge

As plans for the patient's care begin to be formulated, the nurse should keep in mind the patient's ability for self-care and begin to evaluate the kind of support that will be available in the home setting and whether it will allow the patient to function safely. A devoted family with strong bonds of affection greatly improve the patient's potential for adjusting to the disability and progressing in independent self-care. The family is included in giving care gradually. Knowing when the family is ready is not always easy. When family relationships are disturbed, the patient's illness can place even greater strain on family ties. For those patients with no family members available to care for them, discharge often means placement in another type of institution, either a nursing home or long-term care facility. Community support systems such as day care should be exhausted before institutional placement becomes a reality for the patient who truly desires discharge to his or her home. Whether the patient is in a hospital, nursing home, or a rehabilitation facility, discharge planning for continuing care should be well under way long before the patient is ready for discharge. The following elements should be included in discharge planning:

1. Establish early contact with the family to first observe therapy, and then participate in the care giving.
2. Involve family in the rehabilitation team conferences.
3. Familiarize the family with self-care techniques and assistive devices.
4. Teach the family the procedures the patient should perform regularly, such as range of motion exercises and techniques for activities of daily living.
5. Arrange day and/or weekend passes to assess the patient's ability to function at home, and determine whether his or her rehabilitation program needs to be altered.
6. Schedule follow-up visits with the rehabilitation team to assess the patient's function and adaptation to the home.

When planning the physical environment for home care, the family should be discouraged from making early and expensive alterations in their home. The exact changes required can best be determined by occupational and physical therapists. Because of the financial strain disabilities bring about, their recommendations are geared toward adapting what is presently in the home as opposed to purchasing expensive equipment. Furthermore, only toward the end of hospitalization can the need for all necessary changes and devices be determined. Often very little in the way of alteration is required.

References Cited

Kübler-Ross, E. *Death: The Final Stage of Growth*, Englewood Cliffs, N.J.: Prentice-Hall, 1975.

Morrissey, A. B. *Rehabilitation Nursing.* New York: Putnam and Sons, 1951.

Rotkovitch, R., ed. *Quality Patient Care and the Role of the Clinical Nurse Specialist.* New York: John Wiley & Sons, 1976.

Schizkedanz, H. R., and Mitchell, P. *Restorative Nursing*

in a General Hospital. Springfield, Ill.: Charles C Thomas, Publishers, 1972.

Smith, D. W. "Survivors of Serious Illness." *Am. J. Nurs.,* 79 (March 1979), 441–46.

Stryker, R. *Rehabilitation Aspects of Acute and Chronic Nursing Care,* 2nd ed. Philadelphia: W. B. Saunders Co., 1977.

Stryker, Ruth. *Rehabilitative Aspects of Acute and Chronic Nursing Care,* 2nd ed. Philadelphia: W. B. Saunders Co., 1977.

Wright, Beatrice A. *Physical Disability: A Psychological Approach.* New York: Harper & Row, 1960.

General References

Rehabilitation

Bonner, Charles, ed. *Homburger and Bonner's Medical Care and Rehabilitation of the Aged and Chronically Ill,* 3rd ed. Boston: Little, Brown & Co., 1974.

Burnside, Irene. *Nursing and the Aged.* New York: McGraw-Hill, 1976.

Christopherson, Victor A., et al. *Rehabilitation Nursing: Perspective and Applications.* New York: McGraw-Hill, 1974.

Downey, John, and Low, Niels, eds. *The Child with Disabling Illness.* Philadelphia: W. B. Saunders Co., 1974.

Hirschberg, Gerald, Lewis, Leon, and Vaughan, Patricia. *Rehabilitation. A Manual for the Care of the Disabled and Elderly,* 2nd ed. Philadelphia: J. B. Lippincott Co., 1976.

Kübler-Ross, Elizabeth. *Death: The Final Stage of Growth.* Englewood Cliffs, N.J.: Prentice-Hall, 1975.

Licht, Sidney. *Rehabilitation and Medicine.* Baltimore: Waverly Press, 1968.

Little, Dolores E., and Carneval, Doris L. *Nursing Care Planning,* 2nd ed. Philadelphia: J. B. Lippincott Co., 1976.

Long, Janet. *Care for and Caring about Elderly Persons; A Guide to the Rehabilitation Approach.* Philadelphia: J. B. Lippincott Co., 1972.

Marram, Gwen, et al. *Primary Nursing.* St. Louis; C. V. Mosby Co., 1974.

Marriner, Ann. *The Nursing Process: A Scientific Approach.* St. Louis: C. V. Mosby Co., 1975.

McCollum, Audrey T. *Coping with Prolonged Health Impairment in Your Child.* Boston: Little, Brown & Co., 1975.

Morrissey, Alice B. *Rehabilitation Nursing.* New York: G. P. Putnam & Sons, 1951.

Redman, Barbara. *The Process of Patient Teaching in Nursing.* St. Louis: C. V. Mosby Co., 1969.

Rotkovitch, Rachel, ed. *Quality Patient Care and the Role of the Clinical Nursing Specialist.* New York: John Wiley & Sons, 1976.

Rusk, Howard A. *Rehabilitation Medicine,* 4th ed. St. Louis: C. V. Mosby Co., 1977.

Schizkedanz, H. Ruth, and Mayhall, Pamela. *Restorative Nursing in a General Hospital.* Springfield, Ill.: Charles C Thomas, 1972.

Strauss, Anselm. *Chronic Illness and the Quality of Life.* St. Louis: C. V. Mosby Co., 1975.

Periodicals

Alfano, Genrose. "There Are No Routine Patients." *Am. J. Nurs.,* **75** (Oct. 1975), 1804–07.

Anderson, M. "Rehabilitation Nursing Practice." *Nurs. Clin. North Am.,* **6** (June 1971), 303.

Burnside, Irene. "Listen to the Aged." *Am. J. Nurs.,* **75** (Oct. 1975), 180–84.

Crisler, J. R. et al. "An Integrated Rehabilitation Team Effort in Providing Services for Multiple-Disability Clients." *J. Rehabil.,* **45** (Jan.–March 1979), 34–38.

Eggert, F. M. et al. "Caring for the Patient with Long Term Disability." *Geriatrics,* **32** (Oct. 1977), 102–3.

Eisenberg, M. G. "Psychological Aspects of Physical Disability: A Guide for the Health Care Educator." *NLN Publication,* **114** *League Exchange* (1977), 1–32.

Forsland, C. K. et al. "A Behavioral Approach to Physical Rehabilitation: A Case Study." *J. Psychiatric Nurs.,* **16** (May 1978), 48–51.

Fozzard, E. L. "The Psychosocial Needs of the Neurologically Disabled." *J. Neurosurg. Nurs.,* **10** (Sept. 1978), 92–94.

Hackler, E. S. "Expanding the Role of Nurses in Rehabilitation." *Geriatrics,* **31** (May 1976), 77–79.

Joyce, A. et al. "Preventive Nursing Interaction with the Elderly." *J. Gerontol. Nurs.,* **4** (Sept.–Oct. 1978), 28–34.

Madden, B. W. "Rehabilitation: Principles, Philosophy, Practice." *Nurs. Dig.,* **5** (Summer 1977), 35–40.

Murray, E. W. "Rehabilitation of the Mentally Ill." *Nurs. Mirror,* **145** (Dec. 1977), 39–40.

Owens, J. F. et al. "Cardiac Rehabilitation: A Patient Education Program." *Nurs. Res.,* **27** (May–June 1978), 148–50.

Perlman, L. G. "Rehabilitation in the 1980's in Serving Persons with Invisible Handicaps Such as Cancer, Heart Disease, Epilepsy." *J. Rehabil.,* **45** (Jan.–March 1979), 16–21.

Rusk, H. A. "Rehabilitation Medicine: Knowledge in Search of Understanding." *Arch. Phys. Med. Rehab.,* **59** (April 1971), 156–60.

Shintz, L. C. "Psychological Adjustment to Physical Disability: Trends in Theories." *Arch. Phys. Med. Rehabil.,* **59** (June 1978), 251–54.

Symposium. "The Special Needs of the Elderly." *Geriatrics,* **31** (May 1976), 51–103.

Thomas, Linda. "Sensory Deprivation: A Personal Experience." *Am. J. Nurs.,* **73** (Feb. 1973), 266–69.

Westin, M. T. et al. "The Family's Role in Rehabilitation." *J. Rehabil.,* **45** (Jan.–March 1979), 26–29.

Wojtowicz, G. "Rehabilitation Nursing in Long-Term Care." *J. Gerontol. Nurs.,* **3** (May–June 1977), 62–63.

UNIT VIII

Alterations in Regulatory and Response Mechanisms

Etiology of Disorders in Regulation

All internal and external injurious agents discussed in Unit III, as well as psychogenic disorders, can produce malfunction, injury, and disease of regulatory structures. Particularly in the brain, disturbance in the blood supply is a frequent source of injury. Traumatic injury to the brain and other parts of the nervous system is not infrequent. Neoplasms involving endocrine glands differ from those in other parts of the body inasmuch as they sometimes secrete the hormone of the parent gland, thus causing signs and and symptoms of hyperfunction. Regulatory facilities are also subject to defective development that may be of genetic origin, or they may result from a lack or excess of required materials or injury at a critical point in the process of development. Disturbances may also result from the failure of a target cell to respond to agencies controlling its function. For example, in some instances hyperactivity of the adrenal cortex appears to result from the failure of the gland to respond to the governing influence of the adrenocorticotropic hormone (ACTH). Diabetes mellitus may be caused, in some instances, by loss of sensitivity of cells to insulin.

Disturbances in regulation with alterations in physiologic or psychological behavior may arise out of the manner in which the individual perceives his or her situation. Thus harmless things or situations may be the source of malfunction. Six-year-old Bobby Tears presented an extreme example of disturbed function caused by a harmless event. When he was 2 years old, he was knocked down by a dog. Except for an abrasion on his elbow, he was not hurt physically. However, for years, if even the most sedate and harmless old dog approached him, he became terrified and developed nausea and vomiting, followed by prolonged anorexia. In contrast, disturbances in regulation can result in effects that are interpreted as being of psychological origin when they actually have a physical basis. As a result, they may be ignored or misinterpreted. For example, Mr. Heron had physiologic manifestations that were thought to be of psychological origin but that were actually caused by a neoplasm causing pressure on his spinal cord. One of the major manifestations experienced by Mr. Heron was a lack of desire to void until his urinary bladder contained approximately 3,000 ml of urine. The nurse can contribute to the identification of the nature of the patient's medical problem by careful description of observations including the circumstances under which the signs and symptoms presented by the patient occur.

Before the effects of injury or disease of specific regulatory structures and functions are discussed, the general implications of disturbances in regulation will be presented.

Results of Failure of Regulation

The general consequence of failure of regulation is an inability of the organism to adapt appropriately to its environment. Except at the time of death, failure of adaptation is not complete, but there is an inability to maintain one or more functions within the central range referred to as normal. Function may be *hypo-*, *hyper-*, or *disorganized.* Because most important physiologic processes are subject to more than one regulatory mechanism, a disturbance in one is likely to unbalance others. Sometimes this is useful to the organism; at other times it may be harmful. Depending on the nature of the offending agent and the site of its action, the condition may be temporary or permanent. When a disturbance is of limited duration, the care of the patient is directed toward protection from the effects of adaptive failure until such time as the patient is restored to health. When a disability is of a long-term or permanent nature, the patient and family require instructions and support so that the patient can learn how to live as fully as possible within the limits imposed by the disorder. Because a long-term illness involving one member of a family usually affects the lives of the others, any assistance to the patient is likely to have a beneficial effect on the family as well.

The Nurse's Responsibilities in Caring for a Patient with Regulatory Dysfunction

The nurse has an important role in the care of patients with disturbances in regulation. Attention should be given in the nursing plan of care to modifying the environment of the patient so that the effect of the regulatory disability is minimized. This may be done by modifying the environment of the patient so that needs are met with a minimum of effort on his or her part, or by supporting a defective adaptive mechanism. For example, Mr. Olena is admitted to the hospital in an unconscious state as the result of a cerebrovascular accident. His capacity to protect himself from injury is minimal. His survival depends on identifying the sources of injury and protecting him from them. One of the most immediate and serious threats to his well-being is the inability to maintain a clear airway. Measures must be instituted and carried out regularly to promote drainage of the tracheobronchial tree and to prevent aspiration of pharyngeal and gastric secretions. Because Mr. Olena is unable to protect his tissues from the effects of pressure, this must be done for him. His future recovery also depends on his extremities being maintained in good alignment and position, so that joint and muscle function is preserved. Passive exercise of extremities is essential to preserving joint and muscle function.

In contrast to Mr. Olena, whose survival depends on others modifying his environment so that his needs are met, Mr. Esbo requires care directed toward supporting a failing adaptive mechanism. Mr. Esbo, who is obese, secretes insufficient insulin to utilize normal amounts of glucose. If his requirements for insulin can be reduced, his own insulin-secreting capacity may be adequate to his needs. One of the objectives in his care is, therefore, to lessen the demands on his islet cells to secrete insulin. The methods employed are a diet limiting the quantity of carbohydrates as well as the number of calories. By reducing the carbohydrates in his diet, his insulin requirement is lessened. The reduction in his calories should lead to a loss of weight and, with it, a decrease in his insulin requirement. Should these measures be inadequate to maintain the level of glucose in his blood within physiologic limits and to prevent the excessive use of fat and protein for fuel, insulin may be prescribed to supplement his own supply.

This Unit discusses the consequences and management of overwhelming challenges to cellular, neurochemical, thermal, and immunologic regulation and response. Although the essential life processes protected and facilitated by *effective* function of the regulatory and response mechanisms inevitably are also altered by alteration in these mechanisms, discussion of alterations in essential life processes is the focus of Unit IX. It is important for the nurse to realize that this separation is possible only for purposes of analysis; interaction and interdependence of all psychobiologic processes are continuous and essential to health.

35

Problems with Chemical Regulation

Disorders of Cellular Chemistry

All disordered function and disease in the body involves some alteration in the chemistry of biologic processes. Sometimes the alteration is circumscribed in time or in extent of cells affected, and therefore is either (1) correctable by homeostatic mechanisms without significant disruption, or even awareness, of the individual, or (2) slow to develop or extend sufficiently to produce manifestations detectable either by the individual or by techniques used in comprehensive physical examination. In the latter instance, when cellular disorder exists prior to its clinical manifestations, disease is said to be in the *prepathogenic period,* that stage of development in which host, agent, and environment interact to produce a continuing stimulus to disease. The prepathogenic period precedes tissue changes and is the period during which measures should be instituted to prevent a disease or delay its onset. (See discussion of the natural history of disease, Chapter 2.)

Education is the major strategy to prevent avoidable chemical alterations in cellular metabolism which characterize the prepathogenic period. In 1979, then-Secretary of the Department of Health, Education, and Welfare, Joseph Califano predicted that prevention of disease will be the second public health revolution in the history of the United States.

The goal of education for health promotion is control of those factors that are known to place the individual at risk for the major killing and disabling diseases such as heart disease, cancer, stroke, trauma secondary to accidents, and the multifarious consequences of abuse of alcohol and other substances. Scientific research supports the importance of several simple personal habits which contribute to cellular, and subsequently tissue, alterations that lead to the major diseases: smoking, drinking, abuse of over-the-counter and prescription drugs, poor eating habits and excessive caloric intake, irregular sleep and exercise patterns, and irresponsible use of motor vehicles (Surgeon General's Report, 1979).

Another target of disease prevention in the 1980s is regulation of chemicals within the environment which expose the individual unknowingly to potential alteration of cellular function. The common chemical poisons of extrinsic origin were discussed in Chapter 12. Of particular concern to an aroused public are unsafe disposal of toxic industrial wastes and the chemicals added to food for preservative and other effects. The nurse contributes to prevention of disease due to chemical poisons by

1. Participating as a partner with other informed citizens to establish and monitor the effectiveness of regulatory agencies, through the political process
2. Obtaining a careful and comprehensive health history which specifies environmental considerations
3. Engaging in individual and group teaching to help people reduce those factors known to put people at risk for the major killing and disabling diseases by helping them to modify the high-risk personal habits elaborated previously

The search for biochemical causes of disease has been a major research emphasis in the last decade and has extended even to research in mental illness. For example, the consistent antidopamine effects of virtually all antipsychotic agents now in use support the idea that overactivity of dopamine synaptic neurotransmission in the limbic forebrain may be an important aspect of schizophrenia (Baldessarini, 1977). Research on monoamine oxidase activity in persons diagnosed as chronic paranoid schizophrenics suggests that this disorder may be separate from other forms of shizophrenia, at least in part because of biochemical characteristics (Potkin et al., 1978). Nursing implications of the link between behavior and cellular biochemistry will evolve as the research frontier describes and explains more basic mechanisms of behavior. However, today the critical application of this linkage is found in the nurse's responsibilities in drug administration and related patient and family teaching; every drug that enters the internal environment of an individual is a substance that will affect biochemical processes in some way. The nurse must know how it is intended to work, how it should be taken or administered, what the potential hazards are, and how to deal with adverse effects. It is also the nurse's responsibility, in consultation with the physician and possibly the clinical pharmacist, to ensure that the person taking the drug possesses the same working knowledge of its intended and possible adverse effects.

Disorders Caused by Abnormal Chromosomes

The chromosomes may also be responsible for congenital malformations. Despite the involvement of the material of inheritance, they are not hereditary in the usual sense of the word. Neither are these disorders environmental. They arise from a defect in the mechanism by which the hereditary material is transmitted from parent to offspring.

Chromosomal abnormalities include the following: (1) Inversion—a disorder in which genetic material crosses over in a single chromosome. As a result, the genes are arranged in an abnormal order. (2) Deletion—a piece of a chromosome is broken off and lost. (3) Translocation—parts of two dissimilar chromosomes are broken off and relocate. Translocation is similar to inversion, except that chromosomal material is relocated in a different chromosome. (4) Nondisjunction—the failure of two homologous chromosomes to segregate during meiosis. A number of disorders have been demonstrated to be caused by nondisjunction. (5) Crossing over—the exchange of genetic material between two homologous chromosomes. Crossing over occurs during meiosis.

A number of disorders have been demonstrated to be caused by one or the other of the preceding. Mongolism usually results from the fertilization of an ovum containing two number 21 chromosomes (a small somatic chromosome). The resulting zygote contains three chromosomes, instead of a normal pair. Most patients with Klinefelter's syndrome who have been studied have two X chromosomes in addition to one Y chromosome. The resulting individual is a male who is tall, has enlarged breasts, and produces few, if any, sperm. In this instance, the individual may inherit the abnormality, that is, nondisjointed chromosomes, from either his father or his mother. In another chromosomal disorder, males with an XYY karyotype are said to be abnormally aggressive and to be more frequently involved in crimes of violence than normal XY males.

There are a number of other disorders known to result from a failure in the process whereby the hereditary material is passed from the parent to child. The type of resulting abnormality depends on the nature of the defect. These disorders are not hereditary nor are they environmental in the usual sense of these terms. They may result from the effect of an illness or a drug at a critical stage in the development of a gamete. Examples include certain virus infections. A number of drugs, including LSD, have been believed to damage chromosomes. In mongolism the age of the mother appears to be a predisposing factor, for the incidence of mongolism rises steeply as the age of the mother increases. The nurse may be able to reinforce the assurance given by the physician that anomalies caused by an abnormality in the process of meiosis are not hereditary. Children born later are likely to be normal.

Genetic Disorders

The observation that some diseases occur in some families more frequently than in others is not new. Increased biochemical and physiologic knowledge of the nature of heredity has made it possible to identify the reason in some instances. At this time genetic disorders are classified as (1) common disorders of complex etiology, (2) disorders caused by a mutant gene or simply inherited disorders, and (3) disorders caused by abnormal chromosomes.

Common Disorders

Many common disorders, such as hypertension, allergy, peptic ulcer, some types of neoplastic disease, as well as others, have a genetic component in their etiology. Possibly there is a direct or indirect genetic component in most, if not all, diseases.

Disorders Caused by a Mutant Gene or Simply Inherited Disorders

A large number of disorders, some of which occur frequently and others infrequently, are caused by a mutant gene. Among them are the hemoglobin abnormalities such as sickle-cell anemia and thalassemia. Also in this group are the inborn errors of metabolism.

As carriers of the hereditary characteristics of the individual, genes have an important influence on the health potential and longevity of the individual. There is some evidence to support the belief that heredity determines the reserve capacity of the tissues and organs of individuals. It also predisposes individuals to diseases such as the ones previously mentioned. Whether certain other diseases, in which heredity appears to be a factor, develop depends on the interaction of the individual with the environment. For example, a person who inherits a limited reserve of insulin-secreting cells may protect himself or herself from diabetes mellitus by avoiding obesity. Conversely, a combination of a hereditary tendency, overeating, and underexercising favors its development. It is probably safe to say that, directly or indirectly, heredity plays a role in most disease states.

Because genes direct the synthesis of proteins and proteins act as enzymes or catalysts in chemical reactions, an abnormal gene may result in the failure to metabolize some substance. For example, phenylketonuria (PKU) results from the failure of the individual to metabolize one of the common amino acids, phenylalanine, because of a deficiency in the enzyme phenylalanine hydroxylase. In the absence of this enzyme, phenylalanine accumulates in the blood and the other body fluids. Unless the defect is discovered early in infancy, the phenylalanine injures the brain, causing mental retardation. If the condition is discovered early enough in the life of the child, the damaging effects to the child can be prevented by a diet low in phenylalanine. There is one negative aspect: any offspring of an individual with phenylketonuria will carry the trait.

Heredity and Drugs

The discovery that there is a relationship between genetic constitution and the effects of some drugs has implications for drug therapy. One drug that has been studied is isoniazid (INH). Some individuals have been identified who inactivate INH quickly; others inactivate it slowly. As might be expected, those who inactivate INH quickly have a less satisfactory response to a given dosage than do those who inactivate it slowly. Barbiturates and certain other drugs are highly toxic to persons with a relatively mild hereditary disorder known as porphyria variegata.

Genetic Counseling

One of the problems facing the individual who may be a carrier or who has a hereditary defect is whether or not to marry. Despite the inability of the nurse to give the patient a definite answer to this question, she or he can be of help by encouraging the patient to seek advice from the physician. In some instances the family physician will be able to provide the person with the desired information. In others, the person may be referred to a physician who specializes in medical genetics.

Five types of knowledge help the physician to predict whether or not a genetic disorder is likely to be inherited and what the chances are that it will be: (1) the manner in which the defective gene is inherited, (2) the ability to identify abnormalities in the absence of disease, (3) the frequency of the defective gene in the population, (4) the character of the gene and the age at which the disorder manifests itself, and (5) the hereditary background of the individual seeking advice.

As an example of the first, sons of a father with a sex-linked disease such as hemophilia will not have hemophilia unless they develop a mutant gene. His daughters will carry the gene, but are not likely to develop hemophilia. It is possible to identify carriers of the sickle-cell anemia trait by subjecting their erythrocytes to hypoxic conditions in a test tube; abnormal cells undergo sickling. Some genes such as those for galactosemia occur infrequently. Knowledge of such factors as (1) whether the disorder is caused by a single gene or several; (2) whether or not the gene is dominant, incompletely dominant, or recessive; and (3) the age at which the disorder is manifested is extremely important to making a satisfactory prediction. As an example, a dominant gene is responsible for Huntington's chorea, but the disorder does not usually develop until after the person is 50 years of age. Finally, the gene for cystic fibrosis is recessive but occurs quite commonly in the population. If two people with a history of cystic fibrosis in the family marry, the possibility of their having children with cystic fibrosis is as high as one in four. Because children with cystic fibrosis are now living to be adults, all of their children can be predicted to be carriers.

PREVENTION AND THERAPY

The prevention of genetic disorders is not easy. Theoretically, diseases in which carriers can be identified could be eliminated in one generation by preventing them from reproducing. The elimination of thalassemia is being attempted in Italy. Persons with diabetes in both families are discouraged from marrying.

Therapy of genetic disorders is often difficult. As stated previously, the damaging effects of PKU may be limited by a diet low in phenylalanine. Diabetes mellitus may possibly be prevented by the prevention of obesity and controlled so that the individual can live a more or less normal life.

SUMMARY

Genes, as the units responsible for the hereditary characteristics of the individual, may transmit abnormal as well as normal traits. Although a person carries one or more abnormal genes, he or she is not certain to develop a hereditary disorder. A variety of factors influence the expression of hereditary diseases. These include (1) the character of the gene—dominant or recessive, (2) the effects of heredity on the reserve capacity of tissues or organs, and (3) the conditions in the environment of the individual. Each of these points has been discussed and illustrated.

Enzymes in Disease

As knowledge of the nature and actions of enzymes has grown, interest in them as causative agents in disease as well as in its diagnosis and treatment has been stimulated. In the last 30 years or so, knowledge of enzymes has increased at a phenomenal rate.

As indicated earlier, the presence of a mutant gene may deprive the organism of an enzyme required by the cell to catalyze a step in a biochemical reaction. This can result in the accumulation of partly utilized materials in the tissues or in the formation of an abnormal or defective protein. It can result in failure to digest or to absorb nutrients or in failure to clot blood. It also suggests the possibility that enzymes may be involved in disorders of growth. One recurring and as yet unsubstantiated theory relating to cancer is that the enzyme pattern in malignant neoplasms differs from that of healthy tissue. What actually happens in the absence of an enzyme depends on the process that is blocked by the lack of the required enzyme. Because all biochemical processes are dependent on enzymes, the variety of disorders having their origin in some disturbance in the enzyme system appears to be great.

Because enzymes appear to be dependent on the physical and chemical conditions in their environment, many disorders may have adverse effects on the functioning of enzyme systems. Most enzymes function at a narrow range of temperature and hydrogen ion concentration. The injury to tissue in hyperpyrexia may result from the effect of elevated temperature on enzyme systems. Failure to convert the hydrogen atom to water when oxygen is deficient may be the cause of death in shock.

Certain poisons, such as salts of cyanide, are highly lethal because they inactivate respiratory enzymes. Without respiratory enzymes, oxidation-reduction reactions proceed at such a slow rate that insufficient energy is released to carry on the activities of the cell. Death occurs within a matter of minutes.

The removal of a glandular organ either by disease or by surgery may also be responsible for a deficiency of one or more enzymes. For example, when the pancreas is surgically removed in the treatment of cancer, enzymes secreted by the pancreas are not available for the digestion of fats, proteins, and carbohydrates. Because the pancreas is the principal source of lipase (fat-digesting enzyme), the individual has a problem in the digestion of fat unless lipase is replaced. The most serious problems that arise following pancreatectomy do not stem from a lack of insulin, but from the absence of the digestive enzymes secreted by the pancreas.

ENZYMES IN DIAGNOSIS

Knowledge of the action of enzymes is employed in the diagnosis and treatment of disease. Their use in diagnosis is based on the hypothesis that enzymes produced by a cell remain in the cell until the cell disintegrates, or until there is sufficient alteration in energy-producing pathways to alter the cell membrane and increase its permeability to the point where enzyme leakage occurs. As the cell breaks up, enzymes are released into the blood. Through the use of appropriate laboratory tests, the increase in the level of the particular enzyme in the blood serum can be demonstrated. Some examples include the elevation of serum amylase in acute pancreatitis, the elevation of the serum *acid* phosphatase in cancer of the prostate, and the elevation of lactic dehydrogenase in acute myocardial infarction. In all these disorders cell membrane permeability may be increased or cells may undergo necrosis and disrupt the cell membrane, releasing enzymes into the blood.

Enzymes in Therapy

Not only are enzymes useful in establishing the presence and sometimes the site of a disease process but they have a variety of uses in therapy. They may be administered to replace enzymes that are deficient or to modify the effect of a disease or treatment. For example, pancreatic enzymes may be given to the patient who has had a pancreatectomy. Hyaluronidase, an enzyme that digests hyaluronic acid, may be administered with subcutaneous fluids or local anesthetics to facilitate absorption. Agents containing protein-digesting enzymes are sometimes applied to wounds to aid in their débridement. An enzyme, fibrinolysin, has been studied to determine its effectiveness and safety in the treatment of intravascular clotting.

Besides the introduction of enzymes into the body, treatment may involve the inhibition of enzymes already present. For example, a number of modern diuretics are effective because they block an enzyme system. The organic mercurial diuretics are believed to interfere with the enzyme systems required for the reabsorption of sodium and fixed anions. Water loss is secondary to the loss of electrolytes. Acetazolamide (Diamox) inhibits carbonic anhydrase, an enzyme catalyzing the hydration of carbon dioxide. As a result, hydrogen ion is not available to substitute for sodium and potassium ions. These cations are excreted in the urine as bicarbonate salts. When the excretion of sodium increases, water is excreted.

The special problems of patients who have a deficiency or lack of essential enzymes are related to the fact that many of these disturbances have a genetic basis and continue throughout the life of the individual. In these conditions the capacity of the individual to adapt on the biochemical level is in some way deficient. In some instances, as in phenylketonuria, the nature of the disturbance is known and, if discovered early enough, can be controlled. In others, control is not yet possible.

The objective relating most specifically to the nursing of these patients is to assist the patient and family to gain the knowledge and skill required to control the progress of the disease, when this is possible. When the course of the disease cannot be altered, the nurse should direct the attention of the patient and family toward living as full a life as is compatible with the disorder and toward preventing unnecessary disability. For the nurse to be of maximum assistance to the patient and family, she or he should have some understanding of the cause and nature of disorders of enzyme systems, and be familiar with the objectives and means of therapy. Because of the nature and prognosis of these disorders, the nurse will undoubtedly require competence in the expressive role of nursing.

The field of enzymology and its applications to health and disease is rapidly expanding. The literature in the field is enormous. Because enzymes function in regulation at the biochemical level, their effects are widespread and profound. By their action or lack thereof, they influence the capacity of the organism to adapt to its environment. Lack of, or alteration in, the activity of enzymes may be the cause of disease. Likewise, disease may alter the activity of enzymes. Without enzymes, life cannot exist.

Endocrine Disorders[1]

Causes of Endocrine Disorders

Cells of the endocrine glands are subject to the same types of injury from physical, biological, and chemical agents as other structures in the body (see Unit III). As a result, the endocrine glands express the same types of pathology as other structures of the body. Structures and function are impaired when a gland is deprived of its blood supply. Infection and autoimmune disorders may have a similar effect. Unfavorable genetic or environmental conditions may result in an absence of, or insufficient, tissue to secrete an adequate supply of a hormone or hormones. Failure to control the growth potential of the secreting or supporting cells of a gland may result in a benign or malignant neoplasm. When secreting cells are involved, alterations occur in the level of secretion of the hormone(s) elaborated by the affected gland. Either hypo- or hypersecretion may result. The effects of neoplasms as space-occupying and metastasizing lesions depend on the location of the gland involved. A neoplasm of the thyroid gland may obstruct breathing or swallowing.

A disturbance in the functioning of an endocrine gland may result from malfunction in the regulating

[1] Contributions to this section of the chapter were made by Judith Landry Valone, R.N., M.S.N., Ob-Gyn Clinical Nurse Specialist, Brookline, Massachusetts.

mechanism or from failure to respond to regulation. To illustrate, Cushing's syndrome is a disorder resulting from hyperactivity of the adrenal cortex. The hyperplasia of the gland, along with its hypersecretion, could be the result of excessive stimulation caused by oversecretion of ACTH or of failure of the adrenal cortex to respond appropriately to controlling mechanisms. Thus it continues to secrete despite a decrease in the secretion of ACTH. Other endocrine disorders may be caused by failure of end organs to respond appropriately to a hormone. Inappropriate secretion of a hormone (one is ADH)[2] occurs in certain types of malignant neoplasms and a variety of other disorders not of endocrine origin (Bartter, 1973).

Because hormonal disturbances are usually characterized by the hypo- or hypersecretion of a hormone or result from the imbalance between or among hormones, the first objective in the therapy of patients with hormonal disturbances is to restore hormone balance. When a disorder is characterized by hypofunction, one or more of the following approaches may be used to maintain function. The first and most frequently employed is the replacement of the deficient hormones. In some instances the individual's requirements for the hormone may be lessened. Finally, measures may be utilized to stimulate the production of the hormone by the individual. For example, among the factors in the etiology of diabetes mellitus is a deficiency in insulin supply. Diabetes may be treated by replacing the deficient insulin, by reducing the individual's insulin requirements, or, if he or she is middle-aged or older and diabetes is not too severe, by stimulating the islet cells to release insulin (see Chapter 47).

In patients with conditions characterized by hyperfunction, therapy is directed toward returning secretion to normal levels. This may be accomplished by the surgical removal of all or a part of the secreting tissue or by blocking the production of the hormone. When all the tissue is extirpated, or destroyed, the individual is treated by the same general methods employed in the therapy of persons with hypofunction.

When patients require continued therapy with hormones, they should be observed for symptoms and signs indicating over- and underdosage. They should also be taught why they require the hormone, what effects are to be expected, and what to do should untoward symptoms develop; sensitivity to hormones differs from person to person and in the same person from time to time. Symptoms of overdosage are comparable to those found in disease states characterized by hyperfunction. In addition to the factors mentioned, patients also should be instructed about how to administer their own medication and why a regular schedule is required. Some endocrine disorders make it necessary for the person to modify one or more aspects of life style. Emphasis in the instruction should be on helping the patient to develop the knowledge and competence that he or she requires to manage the disease. Success in management of some of the more common endocrine diseases frequently depends on the willingness and ability of the patient and family to assume responsibility for the management of the disease. Physicians and nurses can and should act as teachers and consultants. Instructional plans should therefore help to prepare the patient to assume the necessary responsibility. To be successful the instruction should take into account what the patient can and will be able to do. Some patients respond better to a structured program, whereas others do better when responsibility is delegated to them. A highly elaborate teaching plan may not be effective unless it makes provision for the individual patient's home and work situations.

[2] ADH is antidiuretic hormone from the posterior pituitary.

Characteristics Common to All Endocrine Dysfunction

The following features tend to be characteristic of all endocrine dysfunction. They are features that tend to influence greatly the individual's self-perception, and even the ability to perceive himself or herself and others as previously. Consequently, they have a direct effect on the individual's ability to cope with stress and thus provide guidelines to the type of assistance which may be required from the nurse.

1. Functions which are normally regulated automatically begin to demand attention and volitional control.
2. Dysfunctions tend to develop and re-equilibrate *slowly*.
3. Dysfunctions tend to be accompanied by changes in appearance, disposition, and even personality, thus producing an altered self-concept and alterations in the response of others to the individual affected.
4. Dysfunctions always have a degree of chronicity, even when treated successfully: for example, the need for insulin for the diabetic or substitution hormones following removal of all or part of a gland. The individual has either to take substitution hormones, control extremes of demand, or both to avoid overstressing an impaired hormonal delivery system.

Methods Utilized in Diagnosis of Endocrine Disease

1. Laboratory tests
   a. Direct measurement of the concentration of the hormone in the plasma, blood, or urine
      (1) Immunoassay
      (2) Chemical assay
   b. Indirect methods
      (1) Tests to determine the blood or plasma level of a metabolite influenced by the hormone
      (2) Capacity of the gland to respond to an increased load
      (3) Intake or output of a metabolite or product of metabolism
      (4) Capacity of end organs to respond
2. Nonspecific tests—water test
3. Clinical manifestations—signs and symptoms

It would appear that the way to establish the nature of an endocrine disorder would be to measure the level of a specific hormone in the blood. Because of the exceedingly small quantity of hormones as well as for other reasons, not all hormones in the plasma can be measured. Hormonal secretion may be estimated by measuring the amount of the hormone or its degradation products in the urine.

From the measurement of plasma or urinary hormone levels, the physician may be able to determine (1) the quantity of hormone secreted, (2) the rhythmicity—normal or abnormal—of secretion, and (3) how the gland responds to various types of stimuli, inhibitory as well as excitatory. Stimuli may be physiologic. For example, glucose is a physiologic stimulus for insulin secretion, while tolbutamide[3] is a pharmacologic stimulus.

Even when it is possible to measure the level of a hormone in the blood, other tests may be required to establish the nature of a disorder. Failure may not be caused by inadequate secretion but by inactivation of the hormone or failure of the end organ to respond. As an example, in growth-onset or juvenile diabetes, insulin output is inadequate or even absent. In the maturity-onset type, the individual may have elevated plasma insulin levels. This type is sometimes referred to as high output failure. The difficulty lies not in the quantity of insulin secreted, but in one or more of the following possibilities: (1) the secretion of inactive insulin, (2) the inactivation of insulin by an antagonist, or (3) the failure of the muscle and fat cells to respond to insulin in a normal manner.

[3] Orinase (trade name for tolbutamide) is an oral hypoglycemic sulfonylurea compound used to stimulate islet cells of the pancreas to secrete insulin in treatment of maturity-onset diabetes mellitus. See Chapter 47.

One of the common methods utilized in the diagnosis of endocrine disorders is the determination of the level of one or more metabolites regulated by a particular hormone in the blood or urine. As examples, hyperglycemia and glycosuria are both present in diabetes mellitus. Low sodium combined with elevated potassium is found in adrenal insufficiency.

Abnormalities found in some disorders may not be evident under all circumstances. In some instances the reserve capacity of a gland can be determined by placing stress on its capacity to adapt to an increased load. To illustrate, in some individuals the blood glucose is within normal limits unless the glucose-regulating mechanism is taxed. The glucose tolerance, that is, the reserve capacity to secrete insulin, can be tested by comparing the quantity of glucose in the blood before and after a meal or the ingestion of 100 g of glucose. Further strain may be placed on the capacity to utilize glucose by cortisone.

In the patient with a mild adrenal insufficiency, signs and symptoms can be precipitated by withholding sodium chloride. Because the patient will continue to lose sodium chloride in the urine, acute adrenal insufficiency may be precipitated. Careful observation and immediate reporting of (1) any drop in blood pressure, (2) nausea and vomiting, (3) diarrhea, (4) weakness, (5) restlessness, or (6) irritability must be included in the plan of care.

Some abnormalities seen in endocrine disorders are nonspecific. All the preceding signs and symptoms occur in many other types of disorders. The interpretation of indirect laboratory tests is complicated by the fact that hormones are not solely responsible for any one function. The basal metabolic rate is an example. Under normal conditions the thyroid is responsible for about one third of the total rate. Other factors are responsible for the other two thirds. Moreover, basal conditions are difficult to achieve during the performance of the test. For most indirect laboratory tests a single negative result is not generally relied on, especially when there is reason to believe that the patient has an abnormality.

Uses of Hormones

Naturally occurring hormones and their synthetic analogues are used (1) to correct a deficiency, (2) to aid in diagnosis of an endocrine or metabolic disorder, and (3) as a drug. Thus insulin is administered in the therapy of diabetes mellitus. ACTH may be used to determine the secretory ability of the adrenal cortex. Finally, some hormones are administered for their pharmacologic effects. Large doses of cortisone or one of its relatives may be administered in the treatment of very different disorders, such as septic shock, acute lymphoblastic leukemia, and rheumatic fever.

Although there are many disorders involving hormones, only those hormones most directly affected by disease of the pituitary, adrenal, thyroid, parathyroid, and female endocrine glands will be included in the following section. For purposes of illustration, considerable detail is included in discussing hypo- and hypersecretion of the adrenal cortex and hypo- and hyperthyroidism, as well as common disturbances of the female sexual cycle.

The Pituitary Gland (Hypophysis)

Panhypopituitarism

In a strict sense the pituitary gland is not essential to life. Hypophysectomized animals not given any hormone substitution may live for months or years, provided they are protected from environmental stress. They must be kept in a warm, air-conditioned room, protected from infection and from too much physical exercise. In panhypopituitarism, whether induced by disease or by the complete removal of the gland, the manifestations result from the deficiency of the antidiuretic, the thyroid, the adrenocortical, and the gonadal hormones. Of these, the first three are of the most significance to survival and health, and they must therefore be replaced. Because the thyroid gland contains a supply of hormones, after hypophysectomy a patient may not require an exogenous supply of thyroid hormones for months. The other hormones, however, are necessary immediately. In most instances, the patient will require hormone replacement therapy for the remainder of his or her life.

The Adrenal Gland

Hyperfunction of the Adrenal Medulla

A neoplasm known as a pheochromocytoma is associated with hyperfunction of the adrenal medulla. A functioning pheochromocytoma is characterized by hypertension that may be either paroxysmal (periodic attacks) or continuous. The character of the hypertension depends on whether the tumor secretes constantly or intermittently. The clinical manifestations depend on whether the tumor secretes epinephrine or norepinephrine, or both. Mrs. Lanera presented a classic picture of a patient with the paroxysmal type of hypertension caused by pheochromocytoma. Between attacks she lay quietly in bed. During an attack she appeared to be acutely anxious. She said that she felt shaky and that her head ached. She thrashed about in bed and complained of her heart's pounding (palpitation). She felt nauseated, and vomited and perspired profusely. Her blood pressure rose to 200 mm Hg systolic and 135 mm Hg diastolic. She did not have paresthesia or tetany.

Because there is a possibility for cure and patients having this condition are frequently young, the diagnosis is important. The urine is examined for excessive catecholamines or their metabolites. Various pharmacologic tests are available to detect the presence of a pheochromocytoma. Unfortunately, deaths have occurred as a result of these provocative tests and as many as 25 per cent of cases are missed. For example, following the administration of histamine the healthy person's blood pressure falls, the skin flushes, and he or she is likely to have a headache. In the patient with pheochromocytoma, the blood pressure usually, though not always, rises.

In patients whose blood pressures are above 170/110, drugs that block the effect of norepinephrine on the blood vessels may be employed to establish the diagnosis. The best known is phentolamine hydrochloride (Regitine Hydrochloride). When a dose of 5 mg of phentolamine is administered intravenously to a patient with pheochromocytoma, the blood pressure falls immediately. The maximum decrease is reached in 2 to 5 minutes and lasts for 10 minutes or longer. A fall of 35 mm systolic and 25 mm diastolic or more is considered to be positive; that is, it indicates the presence of pheochromocytoma.

The treatment of pheochromocytoma is the surgical removal of the tumor. Preoperatively the patient can be protected from severe hypertension by the regular administration of phentolamine. Because the manipulation of the lesion during the operative procedure may cause the release of epinephrine and/or norepinephrine, the blood pressure of the patient may rise to critical levels. Because the patient can be protected from an excessively high blood pressure by the administration of phentolamine, the blood pressure of the patient should be monitored continuously. In the immediate postoperative period the patient may have episodes of hypotension, and occasionally a patient suffers severe shock. Norepinephrine or another pressor amine may be prescribed by the physician to elevate the blood pressure. The blood pressure of the patient should be observed frequently until it is stabilized. Because stabilization may not occur for 2 or 3 days after surgery, the patient requires monitoring for a longer period than most postoperative patients. When the patient gets out of bed, he or she should be cautioned to change from the supine to the upright position slowly so that the blood vessels have time to adapt. Dizziness and a feeling of faintness are indicative of hypotension. Depending on the severity of these symptoms, the patient may have to be returned to bed. Certainly the patient should be protected from falling. In the absence of irreversible shock, patients usually make an uneventful recovery. Unless both adrenal glands are removed, adrenal steroid therapy usually is not required. Adrenomedullary secretions do not have to be replaced, regardless of whether one or both glands are excised. As far as can be determined, the adrenal medulla is not essential to life. When both adrenal glands are removed, the adrenergic response to stressing situations is somewhat lessened, but the sympathetic nervous system still reacts.

Adrenocortical Hormones

The adrenal cortex is generally considered to be essential to life. In the absence of adrenocortical secretions the individual has difficulty in adapting to even mild degrees of stress. This includes all types—variations in temperature, exercise, changes in position, infections, burns, and emotional stresses. The degree of susceptibility varies somewhat from individual to individual. Exposure to severe stress, however, can be expected to induce a shocklike state characterized by prostration and peripheral circulatory failure. Death follows unless the deficient hormones are replaced. Life can be maintained in the absence of adrenocortical hormones if electrolytes and nutrients are carefully controlled.

Methods used to diagnose the functional status of the adrenal glands include (1) direct measurement of the adrenocortical hormones or their degradation products in the plasma or urine, (2) response to ACTH stimulation (glucocorticoids), (3) plasma or serum levels of metabolites regulated by these hormones, (4) cellular elements in the blood, and (5) response to loading or withholding substances regulated by one or more hormones and the signs and symptoms presented by the patient.

Some of the commonly used tests to evaluate the secretory functions of the adrenal cortex are summarized in Table 35-1.

Table 35-1. ***Diagnostic Tests Used to Evaluate Adrenocortical Status in Adrenal Insufficiency and Adrenocortical Hypersecretion***

Adrenal Insufficiency	Hypersecretion
1. Direct measurement of adrenocortical hormones or degradation products in the urine and plasma	
Low values for 24-hour excretion of 17-hydroxycorticosteroids and 17-ketosteroids	Elevated 17-hydroxycorticosteroid (17-OHCS) in plasma and urine
Low plasma 17-hydroxycorticosteroid	
Low plasma cortisol	
2. Response to ACTH stimulation. In panhypopituitarism, the administration of ACTH is followed by increased urinary excretion of adrenocortical hormones. In failure of the adrenal cortex, there is a minimum or no increase in the secretion of adrenocortical steroids. In a healthy person, the eosinophil count drops 70% or more.	Increased 17-OHCS when caused by adrenal hyperplasia, decreased by dexamethasone administration
3. Blood, plasma, or serum levels of metabolites regulated by hormones	
Elevated serum K	Reduced serum K
Reduced serum Na	Normal serum Na
Reduced serum Cl	Reduced serum Cl
Reduced CO_2 combining power	
Low fasting blood glucose	Hyperglycemia and intermittent glycosuria
Normocytic anemia	Normal hematocrit
4. Cellular elements in the blood (eosinophils moderately elevated). Depending on the degree of insufficiency, values may range from low normals to marked changes in values. Does not drop in response to ACTH.	Eosinopenia Lymphopenia
5. Response to loading or withholding a substance regulated by one or more hormones. Water loading or withholding sodium. Seldom used.	

Adrenocortical Insufficiency

Manifestations of disorders of the adrenal cortex result from the effects of hypo- or hypersecretion. Adrenal insufficiency may result from atrophy, destruction by a chronic disease such as tuberculosis, or by an immunologic process, hemorrhage into the gland, or surgical removal of both adrenal glands. It may be secondary to failure of the anterior pituitary gland. Although tuberculosis was formerly a more common cause of adrenal insufficiency than it is now, it still is responsible for a significant number of cases. Secretion of hormones by the adrenal cortex is depressed by the administration of exogenous hormones; withdrawal of hormone therapy may leave the patient in a state of relative deficiency. During the period immediately following withdrawal, the person is likely to be more susceptible to infection than usual. At one time adrenal insufficiency and other disorders of the adrenal cortex were believed to be extremely rare. Because of improved methods of diagnosis, disorders of the adrenal cortex are being identified with greater frequency. Whereas they were once believed to be rare, they can no longer be so considered. Most of the effects of adrenal insufficiency are caused by a deficiency of the mineralo- and glucocorticoids. Some of the signs and symptoms are caused by disordered electrolyte balance. Others stem from disordered metabolism of protein, fat, and carbohydrates.

The clinical manifestations of adrenal insufficiency were described by Thomas Addison more than 100 years ago and consequently this condition was called Addison's disease. It was not, however, until the adrenocortical steroids were isolated and synthesized that marked progress was made in understanding their role in the regulation of body activities or in controlling the manifestations of the disease. Before the introduction of adrenocortical extracts, the prognosis of a person with Addison's disease was extremely poor. Since adrenocortical hormones have become available, it is much improved.

Untreated adrenal insufficiency is characterized by weakness (asthenia), easy fatigability, and hypotension. Weakness is one of the most outstanding symptoms. In the beginning it tends to be worse on some days than on others. Eventually, it becomes so severe that the patient is confined to bed. Finally, even bedrest does not afford relief. Hypotension is also a common finding. The majority of patients have blood pressure readings of less than 110/70. In extreme cases it may be as low as 80/50 or even lower. A change in the color of the skin to brown, tan, or bronze is the most striking physical change that can be observed directly. The pigmentation may be diffuse, involving exposed and unexposed areas of the body, or it may appear in patches or freckles. Bluish-black or slate gray discoloration of the mucous membranes may also occur. Disturbances in the function of the gastrointestinal tract may give rise to anorexia, nausea, vomiting, diarrhea, constipation, and abdominal pain. Weight loss is a common finding. As might be expected, mental changes may be prominent. Depression, irritability, lethargy, apprehension, and anxiety are common.

Medical Therapy of Adrenocortical Insufficiency

Despite differences in specifics, the general approaches to the treatment of patients with chronic adrenal insufficiency are similar to the treatment of diabetes mellitus. Hormones are available that can be employed to replace those that are lacking. Whether or not the patient is maintained in a satisfactory state of health frequently depends on the patient. As in other disorders in which there is a permanent deficiency state, the patient must understand that therapy must continue for the rest of his or her life. The patient must follow a prescribed routine and remain under medical supervision. Because more hormones are required during the stress of illness, the patient must understand this and know what to do. He or she should carry a card providing information such as name, address, diagnosis, and the medications being taken. The patient should also be registered with a national medical alerting system.

In some patients, adrenal insufficiency can be controlled by the administration of cortisone (or hydrocortisone) by mouth. The dosage is administered in divided doses to mimic the higher production of cortisone in the morning hours and, the lower production in late afternoon. Because of the local effect on gastric mucosa, the patient is instructed to take the medications with meals, if possible, and with milk or antacids, if food is not available. In other patients, replacement of mineralocortical function is also necessary. A potent salt-retaining steroid such as a fluorohydrocortisone or desoxycorticosterone acetate is required in addition to cortisone to maintain electrolyte balance. The first is administered orally in small dosages of from 0.1 to 0.2 mg daily. The administration of desoxycorticosterone is more complicated. The dosage is first established by determining the effects of daily intramuscular injections on blood pressure and serum electrolyte concentration. After the requirements of the patient have been determined, desoxycorticosterone may be administered by deep intramuscular injection once every 3 to 4 weeks or by intraoral tablets or buccalets placed in the mouth two or three times per day. Because absorption is less complete from the mucosa of the mouth than when the drug is administered intramuscularly, the daily requirement is two to three times that established for intramuscular injection. The patient who receives desoxycorticosterone should be instructed to weigh himself or herself regularly because overdosage causes edema as a consequence of retention of the sodium cation. In marked overdosages of desoxycorticosterone, hypertension and congestive heart failure may be induced.

Adrenocortical failure secondary to failure in anterior pituitary function differs from primary adrenal insufficiency in that there usually are disturbances in thyroid and gonadal function as well. Disturbances in electrolyte balance, though present, are often less severe. As in primary adrenal insufficiency, the characteristic features are weakness, inability to cope with stress, poor resistance to infection, and the tendency to spontaneous hypoglycemia (Randall & Rynearson, 1961). These effects can usually be controlled by small doses of cortisone.

The most serious event in chronic adrenal insufficiency is the development of acute adrenal insufficiency or crisis. In this condition all the signs and symptoms of adrenal insufficiency are intensified. Although prevention is to be preferred to therapy, the survival of the patient in acute adrenal insufficiency depends on prompt and vigorous treatment. Because an increased supply of adrenocortical hormones is required to cope with stress, any condition that makes extra demands on the individual can be anticipated to predispose to adrenal crisis. The dosage of hormones should be increased during infection, gastrointestinal upsets, trauma, surgery, and any other condition that is likely to increase the need of the individual for adrenal hormones. The patient should also be instructed to add excess amounts of salt to his or her diet during periods of stress or excessive sweating, such as rigorous exercise, unusually hot weather, or gastrointestinal upsets. When the condition occurs, all signs and symptoms of adrenal insufficiency worsen. Unless it is corrected promptly, the patient goes into vascular shock and dies. The nurse should be alert to and report any evidence of an intensification of signs and symptoms, such as increasing weakness or a lowering of the blood pressure.

Therapy in adrenal insufficiency has three objectives: (1) to raise the level of adrenal hormones in the circulation, (2) to support the heart and vascular system, and (3) to control infection. To raise the level of hormones in the circulation, the patient is given 100 to 200 mg of hydrocortisone in 1,000 ml of 5 per cent glucose in physiologic saline. The first 250 ml are administered over the first 30 to 60 minutes. The remainder is administered slowly over a 4- to 8-hour period.

Nursing Responsibilities in Caring for a Person with Adrenocortical Insufficiency

Observation combined with a careful description of the emotional and physiologic status of the patient cannot be overemphasized. Objectives on which to base the nursing care plan include (1) to contribute to the accomplishment of the medical objectives, including the protection of the patient from infection, and (2) to maintain conditions of the physical, emotional, and social climate so that demands made on the patient to adapt are reduced to a minimum. The contribution of the nurse to the medical objectives includes the supervision of the treatments and observation of their effects on the patient. The patient should not be left alone. Observation of vital signs by the nurse or monitors and reporting of significant changes are important. Any drop in the blood pressure of the patient is likely to be significant because it may be at a critical level at the time treatment is initiated. Because hyperthermia is a problem in some patients, hourly recordings of temperature may be requested by the physician.

It is important to eliminate as much as possible all forms of stimuli, because the patient in adrenal crisis is unable to adapt to even minor stresses. As a consequence, a situation that might be of no importance to a healthy person or one who is experiencing other types of illness may have an adverse effect. Attention should be given to details such as maintaining the temperature of the room between 70° and 75°F, protecting the patient from drafts and from bright lights, and providing a comfortable bed. The room should be quiet. Loud noises and talking should be avoided. Until the crisis is past, physical care should be kept to the minimum required for the comfort of the patient. The patient should do nothing for himself or herself; whatever care is required should be administered. This includes moving and turning as well as activities such as mouth care and feeding. Conversation should be kept to the minimum required to give directions to the patient or for brief explanations of what is to be done. Persons with infections, including family members and hospital personnel, should be excluded from the environment. An environment that limits the demands made on the patient to adapt contributes to recovery.

Hypersecretion of the Adrenal Cortex

The adrenal cortex secretes a number of hormones, each of which has different physiologic effects. Consequently the clinical manifestations in disorders characterized by hypersecretion will depend on which hormones are oversecreted. In either hyperplasia or adenoma of the adrenal cortex, oversecretion of one hormone may predominate, or there may be a variable mixture of hormones. Three clinical syndromes of hyperfunction are usually described. They are Cushing's syndrome, adrenogenital syndrome, and primary aldosteronism. Cushing's syndrome results largely from the hypersecretion of cortisol. Large doses of cortisol or one of its analogues, when administered over a time, produce effects similar to Cushing's syndrome. In primary aldosteronism, as the name implies, synthesis of aldosterone is excessive. The adrenal virilizing syndrome includes all the disorders of sexual development that can be attributed to abnormal adrenocortical function.

Cushing's Syndrome

Cushing's syndrome is a state manifested by a group of signs and symptoms resulting from the inappropriate secretion of cortisol. The disorder may be caused by an adenoma, by a highly malignant neoplasm of the adrenal cortex of one gland, or by the diffuse hyperplasia of both glands. In some instances no abnormality of the adrenal gland is readily identifiable. Hyperplasia is usually caused by overstimulation of the adrenal cortex by ACTH. In some instances the adrenal cortex may fail to respond to the regulating effects of ACTH.

The characteristic features of Cushing's syndrome are a peculiar type of obesity in which fat is distributed in pads between the shoulders (buffalo hump) and around the waist (girdle or truncal obesity); moonface; hypertension; easy fatigability and weakness; purplish striae over the obese areas; thin and fragile skin that is easily subject to ecchymosis; a ruddy color of the face and neck; glycosuria as a result of disturbance of carbohydrate metabolism; acne and hirsutism in women; oligomenorrhea or amenorrhea in women; or impotence in men. The patient is frequently irritable and changeable in mood. In addition to the clinical manifestations, almost all persons with this disorder have a high level of 17-hydroxycorticosteroid in the plasma and urine.

MEDICAL THERAPY is directed toward reducing the level of adrenocortical secretion. Some patients respond favorably to irradiation of the pituitary gland. Others require surgical treatment.

After undergoing adrenalectomy, the patient's temperature, pulse, blood pressure, and central venous pressure should be monitored for 36 hours because cardiovascular collapse is a real possibility. Evidence that shock is developing, and in some instances disorders contributing to its development, includes (1) fever, (2) hypotension, (3) falling or rising central venous pressure, (4) tachycardia, and (5) nausea and vomiting. Patients undergoing total adrenalectomy must continue under competent medical supervision for the rest of their lives. A therapeutic plan identical to that of the patient with Addison's disease is indicated.

NURSING THERAPY. The objectives on which the nursing care plan is based include (1) to make observations that will be helpful to the physician in establishing accurate medical diagnosis and medical plan of treatment, (2) to provide the patient with a physical, emotional, and social climate that is safe and supporting, and (3) to assist the patient in acquiring the knowledge and skill that will be needed to maintain physiologic functioning should this be required.

One of the simplest and at the same time most difficult responsibilities in the care of the patient with Cushing's syndrome is the collection of urine specimens. Because adrenal hormones are excreted in the urine and some of the effects of the disease or its therapy are reflected in the composition and quantity of the urine, accurate and complete measurement and collection of all urine voided by the patient are important. Besides the collecting and recording of urine output, the intake of water and food should also be recorded. Despite the apparent obesity of the patient, he or she usually suffers from effects of the loss of protein and potassium, because an excess of adrenocortical hormones increases protein catabolism. Excessive potassium is lost in the urine and sodium is retained. The patient should be encouraged to eat the diet that has been prescribed. When a low-sodium, high-potassium diet is prescribed, the nurse should check the patient's tray to be sure that it contains the appropriate food.

The patient with Cushing's syndrome has a tendency toward emotional lability (fluctuation in mood). Depression and moodiness are common. The nurse should identify the types of situations that are disturbing and record them on the nursing care plan. The patient should be observed for evidence of depression, for suicide is not an uncommon occurence. Some patients continue to be depressed after surgical removal of the adrenal gland. Observations made by the nurse indicating a depressed state should be reported promptly to the physician.

The tendency toward masculinization with hirsutism in women and obesity are frequent sources of emotional stress. Patients in whom the disorder is caused by a benign adenoma or hyperplasia of the adrenal cortices can be given reasonable assurance that following treatment they can expect to be restored to their former selves. Weakness, accompanied by the frustration of not being able to carry on their usual activities, is also distressing to patients. At times weakness is the most outstanding symptom. Friends, as well as members of the family, often have little sympathy for the patient. They do not see how anyone who is fat can be as weak as the patient claims to be. The family should be helped to understand that weakness and obesity are, in fact, compatible.

Primary Aldosteronism

Another disorder caused by hypersecretion of the adrenal cortex is primary aldosteronism. It usually results from an aldosterone-secreting tumor of the adrenal cortex. The principal features of this disorder are hypertension, renal and electrolyte abnormalities, muscle weakness, and an increase in the concentration of the salt-retaining hormone in the urine. Sodium is retained and potassium is lost from the body in excessive quantities. Aldosteronism is treated by surgical removal of the neoplasm. Recovery is complete when the tumor is benign. The nursing care of the patient is essentially that of any patient undergoing adrenal surgery.

Adrenal Virilizing Syndrome

Adrenal virilizing syndrome results from the excessive production of androgens by the adrenal cortex. These androgens are then converted to testosterone, the effect of which is virilization. This syndrome results from hyperplasia, adenomona, or carcinoma of the adrenal cortex. A congenital form of adrenal hyperplasia, known as adrenogenital hyperplasia, results from a fundamental enzyme defect. An excessive amount of ACTH stimulation produces hyperplasia of the adrenal cortex with resultant elevated levels of adrenal androgens.

Signs and symptoms associated with adrenal virilizing syndrome depend upon the age of onset and the sex of the patient. At birth in the female infant, ambiguous genitalia present; in the male, the syndrome is manifested by premature virilization. In the adult female, hirsutism, acne, temporal balding, deepening of the voice, increasing muscle mass and strength, decreased breast size, atrophy of the uterus, amenorrhea, enlargement of the clitoris, increased heterosexual drive, and development of the male habitus are associated with excessive androgen production. Virilizing syndromes are difficult to detect in the adult male (Williams et al., 1977).

Treatment is dependent upon the particular cause of the overproduction of androgens. Adrenogenital hyperplasia is suppressed by the daily administration of glucocorticoids. The surgical removal of an adenoma or carcinoma of the cortex removes the source of the excess androgens. However, in cases where carcinoma exists, long-term survival is rare.

Summary Guidelines for Nursing Management

In the absence—either absolute or relative—of adrenocortical hormones, the capacity to cope with stress of all types is lost. Hypersecretion of adrenocortical hormones leads to serious defects in the adaptive capacity of the individual. Clinical manifestations of disorders involving the adrenal cortex depend on which hormone predominates or is hypersecreted. The nursing of patients with disorders in which there are abnormalities in the secretion of the adrenal steroids should be based on the knowledge that *they have difficulty in coping with stress of all types* and that they have *increased susceptibility to infection.* Many of the most serious effects are caused by disordered electrolyte balance. Other nursing responsibilities include the making of observations contributing to the medical diagnosis and the carrying out of that part of the medical regimen usually assigned to nursing. When the disorder experienced by the patient is incurable, the nurse has an important role in assisting the patient to acquire the knowledge and skills that are needed to maintain life and health.

The Thyroid Gland

Diagnostic Tests of Thyroid Function

A wide variety of tests are available to assess different aspects of thyroid function. Those tests may be divided into five major categories: (1) direct tests of thyroid function, (2) tests related to the concentration and binding of thyroid hormones in the blood, (3) metabolic indexes, (4) tests of homeostatic control of thyroid function, and (5) others (Ingbar & Woeber, 1977, p. 505). Often several of these tests may be used to obtain a reliable picture.

Direct Tests of Thyroid Function

1. *Thyroid radioactive iodine uptake* (RAIU) is the most commonly used test to measure functional activity of the gland. The patient is given a tracer dose of ^{131}I (radioactive iodine) mixed with water to drink. The iodine is absorbed into the blood from the alimentary canal. As the blood circulates through the thyroid gland, ^{131}I is trapped in it. The rate at which ^{131}I is concentrated in the thyroid gland is measured by monitoring with a counter of radioactivity. The ^{131}I not trapped by the thyroid is excreted in the urine. Testing the functional capacity of the thyroid with ^{131}I is possible because the cells of the gland are unable to distinguish between radioactive and nonradioactive isotopes. Trapping of iodine increases in hyperthyroidism and decreases in hypothyroidism. ^{131}I is valuable in identifying areas of hyper- and hypoactivity. Because the rate of uptake of iodine may be influenced by the previous ingestion of iodine by the patient, the physician will want to know whether the patient has been taking iodine-

containing drugs before the test is undertaken. Drugs that depress thyroid activity also inhibit the removal of iodine from the blood and will therefore influence the outcome of the test.

Concentration and Binding of Thyroid Hormones in the Blood

1. *Serum T_4 concentrations determinate* is perhaps the most important and most widely available test of thyroid function. The amount of T_4 is measured by radioimmune assay or by competitive binding analysis. Since a large percentage of T_4 is bound to several transport proteins, especially thyroxine-binding globulin (TBG), abnormal results of this test may reflect hyper- or hypofunction of the thyroid or an alteration in the serum concentration of the binding proteins. Normal values fall within the range of 5 to 12 μg/dl (Kaplan & Utiger, 1978).

2. *Serum protein-bound iodine (PBI) concentration.* Thyroid hormones are transported in an unstable combination with the globulin fraction of the serum proteins. The concentration of the thyroid hormones in the blood serum can be determined by precipitating the protein to which they are attached. The laboratory test by which this is done is known as the protein-bound iodine (PBI). The normal level is from 4 to 8 μg of protein-bound iodine per 100 ml of blood serum. In hypothyroidism the level may drop to less than 1 μg. In hyperthyroidism it may rise to as much as 20 μg. This test is much less specific than serum T_4 concentration. A variety of conditions of nonthyroidal origin can lead to abnormally high or low values. For this reason, this test has been largely replaced by measurements of T_4.

3. *Serum T_3 concentrations,* measured by radio immunoassay, measure the amount of stable T_3 in the patient's serum to displace T_3 from anti-T_3 antibody. The normal range is 70 to 200 ng/dl. Since the conversion of T_4 to T_3 takes place in peripheral tissue, a wide variety of acute and chronic diseases can alter T_3 concentration while T_4 concentrations are within the normal range.

4. *Alteration in TBG concentration or T_3.* A test being used with increasing frequency determines the ability of serum to bind resins of tri-iodothyronine or erythrocytes labeled with ^{131}I. Serum from the patient is incubated with the labeled material. In thyrotoxicosis, binding is high. In hypothyroidism it is low. This test has the advantage of being simple to do. All that it requires from the patient is a sample of blood.

Metabolic Indexes

1. *Basal Metabolic Rate (BMR).* The basal metabolic rate is based on the observation that a healthy person of a given age, sex, and surface area utilizes a predictable amount of oxygen when well relaxed and fasting. The results of the BMR are expressed in the percentage of deviation from the norm, which is no or zero deviation. Rates below the average are reported as minus; those above the average as plus. The normal range is from a −15 to a +15.

Ideally the patient who undergoes a BMR should have a good night's sleep and not be disturbed in the morning. To ensure sleep some physicians prescribe a sedative such as secobarbital at the hour of sleep. The patient who is in the hospital is not disturbed in the morning before the test is performed. The outpatient is provided with an opportunity to rest before the test is started. Breakfast is delayed until after the test is performed. The patient should be told the purpose of the test and that he or she will be directed to breathe through a tube placed in the mouth. In addition to instructions about how the test is performed and how to prepare for it, patients who must be absent from work or employ a babysitter should be told about how long the test will take.

Since other tests of thyroid function have been introduced, the BMR is used less frequently than formerly. True basal conditions are difficult to attain; many conditions alter the BMR and a single BMR determination has only about a 50 per cent chance of being accurate.

2. *Serum cholesterol.* Decreases in serum cholesterol are suggestive of hyperthyroidism, whereas elevations are usually present in hypothyroidism.

Tests of Homeostatic Control

1. *Thyroid-stimulating hormone.* The level of thyroid-stimulating hormone (TSH) is very sensitive to alterations in thyroid hormone. Measurement of TSH, by radioimmunoassay, is a means of determining the relationship between hypothalamic-pituitary function and thyroid function. Hypothyroidism of thyroid origin is characterized by elevated levels of TSH, whereas hypothyroidism of hypothalamic-pituitary origin is characterized by undetectable or low normal levels of TSH.

2. *Stimulation and suppression tests.* Administration of thyrotropin-stimulating hormone (TRH) tests the ability of the pituitary to respond to hypothalamic stimulation. This test distinguishes between hypothyroidism of hypothalamic and pituitary origin.

Suppression of thyroid function, as measured by lowered levels of TSH and decreased RAIU, following the administration of exogenous thyroid hormone assesses the normal homeostatic mechanism.

Other Diagnostic Tests

Many other diagnostic tests may be utilized to estimate thyroid function. The presence of circulating antibodies against various thyroid components, such as antithyroglobulin antibody and long-acting thyroid stimulation (LATS) as well as imaging by scintiscanning to localize sites of abnormal function may provide the physician with data upon which a diagnosis may be based.

Like other disorders, those involving the thyroid gland may either be easily identified or require extensive investigation. Unfortunately no single test gives a uniformly valid answer. Often only when a number of tests are combined with the patient's history and observations of behavior can the diagnosis be made.

Disorders of the Thyroid Gland

Disorders of the thyroid are manifested by changes in the size and structure of the gland and by an inappropriate increase or decrease in the production of hormones. The condition in which the size of the gland is increased is known as goiter.

Goiter

Goiter may be accompanied by normal, hypo-, or hypersecretion of thyroid hormones. Locally, as a space-occupying mass, a goiter may interfere with swallowing or breathing by causing compression and displacement of the esophagus or trachea. Compression of the recurrent laryngeal nerves may also lead to hoarseness. In our culture the enlargement of the neck is considered unsightly, and as such it may be a cause of psychological stress. In areas of the world where goiter is endemic and common, it has been accepted as evidence of health and beauty. In the Andean Mountains in South America, where goiter was the rule, dolls were made with enlarged necks like that observed in the person with a goiter.

As a result of epidemiologic studies, scientists have learned that the incidence of goiter is high in areas where the soil has been leached of its supply of iodine. Its incidence is low where the diet includes iodine-containing foods. For example, in mountainous and inland areas the incidence of goiter is high. In regions where the land is sprayed by seawater or where an appreciable part of the diet is from the sea, the incidence of goiter is low. Goiter may also have a genetic basis. A defect in any one of the enzyme systems involved in the synthesis of thyroxine may result from the presence of a mutant gene. As in other disorders, multiple factors influence whether or not goiter develops. It is much more common in females than in males. It is more likely to develop during those periods in the life of the individual when the iodine requirement is increased. Thus goiter is more likely to appear during puberty or pregnancy and in individuals whose protein intake is excessive. In some women who develop goiters during pregnancy, the condition disappears at the termination of the pregnancy. Infections in the gastrointestinal tract may contribute to the development of goiter by interfering with the absorption of iodine.

Goiters caused by a lack of iodine can be prevented by the regular intake of water or salt to which iodine has been added. When the addition of iodine to water or salt was first proposed, the furor was no less than it is today over the introduction of fluorides into public water supplies. Nurses have a responsibility to instruct homemakers to use iodized salt because it is one of the simplest forms of primary prevention available.

TYPES OF ENLARGEMENT. Enlargement of the thyroid gland may be diffuse or nodular. Although not very common, goiter may also be caused by a malignant neoplasm. In all types of goiters, hormone production may be within normal limits, deficient, or excessive. The general effects resulting from disorders of the thyroid depend on the extent to which the output of thyroid hormones is below or above the normal range. Conditions characterized by *hypofunction* include cretinism and myxedema. Cretinism characteristically occurs in infants and young children, myxedema in older children and adults. (Hypothyroidism may be present in the absence of either.) In disorders characterized by alterations in the secretion of the thyroid gland, there is a tendency to classify them as hypo- or hyperthyroidism or thyrotoxicosis rather than by name, such as cretinism or myxedema. Hypothyroidism may be caused by failure of the thyroid gland to develop as a consequence of a congenital developmental defect or from a pre- or postnatal immunologic disturbance. Infection, surgical removal of the gland, or therapy with ^{131}I may reduce the quantity of tissue below that required for normal functioning. Hypothyroidism may be secondary to failure of the anterior pituitary to produce TSH, or to failure of the hypothalamus to secrete TRH.

Conditions characterized by *hyperfunction* include exophthalmic goiter, or Graves's disease, and toxic nodular goiter. In exophthalmic goiter disease, the thyroid gland is diffusely enlarged. In nodular goiter, parts of the gland are increased in size. In exophthalmic goiter, the eyes protrude and the disorder is usually more severe than in nodular goiter. The question of why the thyroid gland hyperfunctions has not been answered. All the signs and symptoms observed in hyperthyroidism except the exophthalmos can be produced by excessive dosages of thyroid hormones.

The presence of excessive dosages of thyroid hormones reflect the disruption of the normal mechanism of homeostasis. Considered among the possible mechanisms of dysfunction are (1) the excessive stim-

Table 35-2 *Effects of Hyposecretion and Hypersecretion of the Thyroid Hormones*

	Hypothyroidism	Hyperthyroidism
Conditions with which associated	Cretinism—infants, young children Hypothyroidism without myxedema (atrophy or destruction of the thyroid gland); surgical extirpation	Exophthalmic goiter or graves's disease: a triad of hyperthyroidism with a true goiter, ophthalmopathy and dermopathy
	Myxedema—older children, adults	Toxic nodular goiter
Basic physiologic disturbance	Decrease in thyroid hormones at some stage of their production	Increased production of thyroid hormones and possibly other substances
Effects of alteration in level of thyroid hormones	1. Reduction in heat production 2. Failure of mental and physical growth in infants and children 3. Disturbances in the metabolism of proteins, lipids, carbohydrates, water, and minerals, with abnormal collections of water, salt, and protein in tissues	1. Production of heat rises 2. Deranged carbohydrate metabolism with glycosuria 3. May be increased use of fat and protein as fuel
Signs and symptoms:		
Speech	Swelling of tongue and larynx—a deep halting, slurred, hoarse speech	Rapid and excited; may be hoarse from local pressure on recurrent laryngeal nerves
	Occasional decreased auditory acuity	
Skin	Thick, puffy, dry	Warm, moist, and flushed; increased sweating; palmar erythema
Hair	Dry, brittle, sparse; may be alopecia of outer third of eyebrows; may be premature graying	Hair soft and silky, occasional loss from temporal areas
Nervous system and mental and emotional state	Often apathetic and lethargic, may be hyperirritable; cerebration slow; in older children and adults intelligence is retained; condition returned to normal when hormones are replaced; patients with myxedema may develop psychosis, infants and young children, mental retardation	Hyperactive; nervous; emotionally labile; tears are caused by trivialities; hypersensitivie, hyperirritable; tense, jittery, restless; has forebodings of disaster; occasionally depressed, but is agitated and restless at the same time; fine tremor of extended hands or tongue
Body fat and weight, appetite	Increased weight; weight may not increase because appetite usually decreases	Loss of weight depends on relationship of food intake to metabolic rate: usual picture includes increased appetite and food intake with accompanying weight loss
Susceptibility to cold	Increased	Decreased—susceptible to heat, excessive sweating
Circulatory system (includes heart and blood vessels)	Increased capillary fragility; bruises easily; heart may be enlarged and fail; cardiac output decreased; blood pressure decreased; weak heartbeat; increased circulation time	Sinus tachycardia; increased cardiac output; palpitation; increased systolic blood pressure; decreased circulation time; atrial arrhythmia; cardiac failure is not infrequent; wide pulse pressure; dyspnea
Gastrointestinal tract	Constipation; hypophagia; low glucose absorption rate	Anorexia, nausea, vomiting, and diarrhea; hyperphagia
Muscle	Weakness; hypotonia Slowing of motor activity	Weakness; muscle fibrillary twitching, tremors; muscle wasting

TABLE 35-2 *(Continued)*

	Hypothyroidism	Hyperthyroidism
Eyes		Protruding eyeballs (proptosis); infrequent blinking, lid lag; failure of convergence; failure to wrinkle brow on looking upward
Immune mechanism	Infection-susceptible; subnormal phagocytic capacity of leukocytes	Infection-susceptible
Menstruation	Menorrhagia	Oligomenorrhea; amenorrhea
Subjective symptoms	Vague aches and pains; cramps, arthralgic pain; some have constant rhinorrhea or coryza	Loss of strength, weakness exhibited during ADL
Characteristic laboratory findings		
Uptake of ^{131}I in percentage of uptake	Not discriminatory, may fall within the normal range 5–30%	Vales >30%
Concentration and binding of thyroid hormones in blood		
Serum T_4 (normal range 4–12μg/100 ml)	Decreased	Elevated
Serum T_3	Decreased	Elevated
Protein-bound iodine	Decreased	Elevated
Metabolic index BMR (normal −15 to +15)	Decreased	Elevated
Serum cholesterol concentration	Elevated	Lowered
Homeostatic control serum TSH	Elevated in hypothyroidism of thyroid origin Lowered in hypothyroidism of hypothalamic and pituitary origin	Undetectable amount in thyrotoxicosis: exception is TSH-secreting tumors
Therapy	Thyroid U.S.P. or some other form of thyroid hormone	1. Inhibit the activity of thyroid tissue (lessen the synthesis of thyroid hormones)(goitrogens) a. Propylthiouracil b. Methylmercaptoimidazole (Tapazole*) c. Iodine 2. Reduce the amount of functioning thyroid tissue a. Radioactive iodine (^{131}I) b. Surgical removal

ulation of thyroid gland by TSH, (2) the synthesis and release of thyroid hormone independent of the normal negative feedback system, and (3) an inherited, isolated defect in the immune surveillance system of the genetically predisposed individual which allows the production of thyroid autoantibodies (Volpe, 1978, pp. 3–4). These autoantibodies take the form of thyroid-stimulating immunoglobulins (IgG) and are referred to as long-acting thyroid stimulator (LATS). A cause and effect relationship between emotional stress and the precipitation of hyperthyroidism has not been established. However, authorities believe that stress may well induce hyperthyroidism in genetically predisposed individuals. The mechanism is unknown but may well involve the hypothalamic-pituitary axis or the depression of the immune surveillance system (Volpe, 1978, p. 19).

The individual who is in a hypothyroid state has

an inadequate capacity to adapt to changes in his environment. The individual with hyperthyroidism makes inappropriate adaptations to his or her environment. The hypothyroid individual complains bitterly when in a cool environment. The one who is hyperthyroid behaves as if it were hot even when the environmental temperature is cool as judged by a person who is euthyroid. Some of the differences between the effects of hypo- and hypersecretion of the thyroid hormones are summarized in Table 35-2.

To illustrate the problems of the patient who is experiencing severe hyperthyroidism, Mrs. Thinis, aged 28, sought medical attention after her husband gave her the alternative of seeing a physician or a lawyer. Patients with hyperthyroidism frequently find their way to an internist by way of a psychiatrist or a lawyer. For some time she had been increasingly irritable, tense, and jittery. She screamed at her husband and children at the slightest provocation, accused her husband of being unfaithful, and was upset for hours over insignificant things. Despite a change in her eating pattern from one of moderation to eating huge meals and frequent between-meal snacks, she was continuously hungry and did not gain weight.

During her visit to her doctor, Mrs. Thinis sat on the edge of her chair, jumped at a slight noise, and talked rapidly and in an excited manner. At one point she burst into tears. Mrs. Thinis told her physician that she was certain that her husband planned to leave her. On examination her hands were found to be wet, her pulse rapid, and there was some lid lag (the eyelid moves more slowly than the eyeball) and widening of the palpebral fissures of her eyes. She states that her mother had recently commented about her looking popeyed.

After examining Mrs. Thinis, her physician decided to hospitalize her for further study and to initiate a plan of therapy. In less acutely ill patients, many of the diagnostic tests can be made in the clinic or office of the physician. In the instance of Mrs. Thinis, the physician felt that she needed to be placed in a quiet, nonstimulating environment where she could get as much rest as possible. He arranged for her to be in a private room for a few days and prescribed the following:

1. Clinical laboratory investigation to determine the level of circulating thyroid hormones and the activity of the thyroid gland
2. Diet—high calorie, high carbohydrate, high protein
3. Thiamine chloride
4. Administration of a sedative to combat nervousness, irritability, and hyperactivity

From the description of Mrs. Thinis and knowledge of the effect of hyperthyroidism, it was clear that her capacity to adapt to her environment was impaired in a number of respects. Among those that were of immediate importance in making the nursing care plan were disturbances in her capacity (1) to adapt to increases in environmental temperature, (2) to control her emotional and muscular responses, and (3) to maintain a food intake adequate in quantity and quality to her needs. Other factors to be considered in the making of the nursing care plan include the fact that Mrs. Thinis sweated continuously and her heart rate was rapid. Both sweating and tachycardia were adaptive. The sweating protected her from an excessively high body temperature by increasing the heat loss. Her heart rate also contributed to heat loss by circulating the blood through the skin. It served further to increase the supply of oxygen and nutrients to the cells and to remove the products of metabolism. The increase in the rate of metabolism and the associated tachycardia placed a burden on the heart. When tachycardia is continued over a long period of time or the patient has a previously damaged heart, it may precipitate heart failure.

The Nursing Objectives in Caring for a Patient with Hyperthyroidism

The objectives on which the nursing care plan for Mrs. Thinis was based were

1. To modify her physical and emotional environment so that her need to adapt was minimized
2. To provide her with food adequate in quantity and quality to her needs
3. To replace fluid lost from the body
4. To provide the family with the knowledge and support they needed to be helpful to the patient.

The most important modifications of Mrs. Thinis's physical surroundings were those directed toward facilitating the loss of heat and preventing unnecessary stimulation. The radiator was shut off and the window opened. In hot, humid weather an air-conditioned room adds much to the comfort of the patient and reduces the strain on the heat-eliminating mechanisms. The severly thyrotoxic patient may be placed in an oxygen tent. He or she benefits not only from the higher-than-normal concentration of oxygen, but also from the low enviromental temperature. Sponging the patient's face and hands and arms several times a day adds to his or her comfort.

Mrs. Thinis's bed was prepared by removing the blanket and spread, leaving only the top sheet. The rubber sheet was removed. If this is contrary to hospital policy, the rubber sheet should be placed under the mattress pad. A contour sheet was placed over the mattress in order to facilitate keeping the bottom sheet free from wrinkles. The nurse suggested that Mrs. Thinis might find pajamas more comfortable than a gown, as a top sheet would be unnecessary should she be too warm. Because Mrs. Thinis was restless and perspired profusely, her bed frequently required straightening and changing. Every effort was made to convey to Mrs. Thinis that these procedures were for her comfort.

Because Mrs. Thinis overreacted to emotional and physical stimuli, her need for rest was greater than that of many patients. The nature of her illness contributed to the difficulty in providing conditions favoring rest. Every effort was made to prevent sudden and loud noises. Talking and laughing outside her room were avoided, because Mrs. Thinis tended to be suspicious. When she heard voices outside her room, she would get out of bed and go to the door to check on the talkers. The fact that the conversation had nothing to do with her did not alter her disquiet. Mrs. Thinis was found to be less restless and more relaxed in bed when she had some nonstimulating activity to do. Because she liked to knit, her husband brought her needles and yarn. She was encouraged to select a relatively simple pattern and to alternate periods of rest and activity. When rest is an important objective and the condition of the patient interferes with resting, the program should be adapted so that he or she obtains as much rest as possible.

The fact that Mrs. Thinis was hyperirritable and easily upset for extended periods of time by minor incidents contributed to the difficulty in securing rest for her. Mrs. Thinis was given her bath and assisted with all aspects of her care despite her apparent ability to do many of these things for herself. Because Mrs. Thinis's frustration level was low, her light was answered promptly and every effort was made to get her medications to her on time. Topics that were disturbing to her were avoided in conversation, and this information was relayed to all the personnel in the unit. As is not infrequent, some of her visitors were upsetting to her. As a result all visitors with the exception of her mother and husband were asked not to stay more than 10 minutes. The method of handling this problem differs with the wishes of the patient and family. The objective is to protect the patient from unnecessary stimulation. The nurse who was responsible for Mrs. Thinis was well suited to her requirements. She had a quiet, low-pitched voice. Her manner was unhurried and relaxed. Because tension tends to be communicable, a tense nurse is likely to add to the tension of the patient. The same nurse was assigned to care for Mrs. Thinis over a period of time, which enabled her to learn what was important to the patient and to utilize this information in meeting her needs. The patient also had an opportunity to develop confidence in the nurse. As the nurse identified Mrs. Thinis's needs and ways of meeting them, she recorded this information on Mrs. Thinis's nursing care plan so that it was available to others as required. Because of the severity of Mrs. Thinis's clinical manifestations and her need for rest, her physician ordered phenobarbital, 30 mg four times per day. Not all patients with hyperthyroidism need sedation. It is necessary only in those who are seriously ill.

One of the most important responsibilities of the nurse who cared for Mrs. Thinis was to make certain that all personnel—professional and nonprofessional—and the patient's family understood that Mrs. Thinis's behavior was part of her illness. Adjustments should be made by the person caring for the patient, rather than by the patient. If Mrs. Thinis's behavior was accepted as part of her illness, then attention could be given to modifying her environment in such a way that stimuli inducing the behavior were avoided. Reactions to the patient's irritability and hypersensitivity with anger or irritation only act to intensify her symptoms.

Mrs. Thinis was similar to many patients with hyperthyroidism in that her appetite was enormous. To satisfy it and to provide her with the extra calories she needed, she was given a diet high in calories, carbohydrates, protein, and vitamins. The high-carbohydrate and high-vitamin content of the diet also help to protect the liver from damage. Liver glycogen tends to be depleted in hyperthyroidism. Mrs. Thinis ate well. She disliked soft-boiled eggs and became upset when they were served to her. Therefore her nurse made a point of checking her breakfast tray before it was served. Because she was hungry between meals, she was served sandwiches and milk mid-morning and afternoon and before retiring. Fresh ice water was kept at her bedside at all times.

Occasionally a patient has a poor appetite despite hyperthyroidism. Under these circumstances, particular attention should be paid to increasing the patient's food intake. Food that he or she likes should be provided. Between-meal feedings, unless they result in a decrease in appetite, may increase the intake of food.

Medical Therapy

In the selection of the method of therapy, the physician considered the degree of hyperactivity of Mrs. Thinis's thyroid gland and the status of her cardiac function, as well as her age and her personal preference. He also considered the possibility of each possible therapeutic method's effecting a cure, and what, if any, harmful effects it might have. Among the therapeutic methods to be considered were drugs suppressing the synthesis of thyroid hormone, surgical removal of the thyroid gland, and treatment with radioactive iodine. Because Mrs. Thinis was only 28 years of age and still of childbearing age, radioactive iodine was eliminated as a possible choice. In patients who are 40 years of age or older, ^{131}I (radioactive iodine) is frequently employed in the treatment of hyperthyroidism.

The plan finally decided on for Mrs. Thinis was to prepare her for surgical removal of a part of the thyroid gland at a later date. To decrease the synthesis of thyroid hormone, 100 mg of propylthiouracil and 10 minims of Lugol's solution were prescribed to be administered three times per day. To maintain the concentration of these drugs at a constant level they were administered at 8-hour intervals—8:00 A.M., 4:00 P.M., and 12:00 midnight.

That iodine is useful in the treatment of disorders of the thyroid has been known since antiquity. During the Middle Ages, persons with enlargement of the neck were treated with burnt sponge or seaweed. Not until 1916 did the now classic experiments of Marine and Kimball prove that iodine could be used in the prevention of goiter. When it is administered to patients with hyperthyroidism associated with a diffuse enlargement of the thyroid gland (Graves's disease), the thyroid gland undergoes involution and the storage of colloid is promoted. Maximum effects are obtained 10 to 15 days after therapy is initiated. Iodine inhibits the release of thyroid hormones from the thyrotoxic gland more rapidly than agents that inhibit hormone synthesis. The effects of iodine therapy are temporary, because the patient returns to the hyperthyroid state. In fact, the degree of hyperthyroidism may be intensified by increasing the amount of hormone stored in the thyroid gland.

The introduction of thiouracil, followed by its safer analogue, propylthiouracil, and other antithyroid drugs, made it possible to induce a more or less permanent remission of hyperthyroidism.

According to Goodman and Gilman (1975), antithyroid drugs act by preventing the binding of iodine in the organic form; as a result the effects of hyperthyroidism are reversed. Therapy is initiated by administering 300 to 450 mg of propylthiouracil daily. The total dosage is divided into three so that the patient receives 100 to 150 mg three times during the 24 hours (Ingbar & Woeber, 1977, p. 514). Proper spacing is essential for effectiveness when the drug is given every 8 hours. After the patient becomes euthyroid, the dosage is reduced until the maintenance dosage is achieved. In about 50 per cent of persons treated for hyperthyroidism with propylthiouracil, a permanent remission of the disease is induced. In patients in whom remission does not occur, signs and symptoms diminish and the general state of health improves.

Patients receiving antithyroid drug therapy must be informed of possible side effects. The most common symptoms are mild skin rashes and pruritus. The use of antihistamines, along with antithyroid medication, is usually successful in controlling these symptoms. Agranulocytosis is rare but lethal if not recognized quickly. However, leukopenia is not uncommon during drug therapy. A patient experiencing any evidence of infection, including fever, sore throat, stomatitis, abdominal pain or furuncles should be taught to notify the physician immediately (Braverman, 1978).

Mrs. Thinis responded rapidly after therapy was initiated. After 3 days of treatment she was discharged from the hospital with the expectation that she would continue drug therapy and a high-calorie diet for 6 or 8 weeks. After her hyperthyroidism was controlled and her general health status was improved, she was to have a subtotal thyroidectomy.

RADIOACTIVE IODINE. Over the last 30 years the availability of ^{131}I has altered significantly the therapy of hyperthyroidism and has become the most commonly used treatment modality. Because the thyroid gland removes iodine from the blood and concentrates it in itself, radioiodine is useful in the diagnosis and treatment of disease of the thyroid. Because iodine is readily absorbed from the gastrointestinal tract, it is administered by mouth. The amount of iodine concentrated in the thyroid gland can be tested with a Geiger or similar counter. In hypothyroidism little iodine will be concentrated in the gland. In hyperthyroidism the quantity will be excessive. Iodine not absorbed by the thyroid gland is excreted in the urine. Because the quantity of radioiodine used in diagnosis is very small, no precautions are required to protect the nurse or others giving care to the patient. Because larger quantities are used in therapy, the patient should be isolated. (See Chapter 11 for precautions to use with persons being treated with radioactive substances.) Therapy with ^{131}I has several important advantages. It is easy to administer and it results in the highest rate of cure of all forms of therapy. Although there may be some increase in symptoms on the fourth or fifth day, radioiodine is less likely to cause a serious exacerbation of the hyperthyroid state than other forms of treatment. The temporary increase in the degree of hyperthyroidism is explained as follows: Radioiodine produces some degree of thyroiditis with necrosis of thyroid cells. With the disintegration of cells of the gland, there is an increase in the release of the thyroid hormone stored in the gland.

Radioiodine has three disadvantages. Because it requires special equipment for its storage and handling, it is available only in medical centers. It may have an adverse effect on the germ plasm, and it may be carcinogenic. To avoid the possibility of either of these effects some physicians prefer not to treat patients younger than 40 or 45 years of age with ^{131}I. After evaluation of patients treated with ^{131}I, smaller dosages are now being used and are found to be effective.

THYROIDECTOMY. Although surgery is employed less frequently in the treatment of hyperthyroidism than it once was, it is still the treatment of choice for some patients. Furthermore, some of the hazards accompanying surgery on the thyroid gland have been lessened since introduction of the goitrogenic drugs, as most patients will become euthyroid after therapy with them. As a result of the use of the goitrogenic agents, there has been a marked reduction in the incidence of thyroid crisis following operation and a marked improvement in the mortality rate. Because these drugs reduce the metabolic rate and improve the general status of the patient, time can be taken to improve his or her nutritional state. Furthermore, emotional calm and confidence that the patient's needs will be identified and met promptly have positive effects.

The basic principles underlying the care of the surgical patient are presented in Chapter 51. Following any operation, the site and nature of the operative procedure have an important bearing on the needs of the patient and the possible complications. On returning from the operating room Mrs. Thinis was placed in low semi-Fowler's position with her head well supported. In her preoperative preparation she had been taught that she should avoid either extending or flexing her head or her neck. She had also been taught to brace her head with her hands when she moved. This action served to prevent unnecessary pain and strain on the suture line. Until she was up and about she was turned every 2 hours. Deep breathing and coughing were encouraged at the same time. Her vital signs were checked every 15 minutes for 2 hours, then every 4 hours for 24 hours. She was helped out of bed the evening of the day of surgery. In preparation for getting up she was instructed to brace her head and assisted to the "dangling" position. After a few minutes she was assisted off the edge of the bed and helped to walk.

As soon as Mrs. Thinis was able to swallow, she was encouraged to drink high-carbohydrate fluids. She was given glucose in water intravenously. As is usual in patients following thyroidectomy, she complained of discomfort on swallowing.

Complications to which Mrs. Thinis was particularly predisposed were hemorrhage, leading to respiratory obstruction, paresis or paralysis of the vocal folds, tracheitis, parathyroid failure, and thyroid crisis or storm. The fact that the thyroid gland has a rich blood supply increases the possibility of hemorrhage. Although external hemorrhage is possible, bleeding into the tissues is more common and more dangerous. To detect external bleeding, dressings should be checked each time the patient is seen. Because water flows downhill, the back and lower portions of the dressings are likely to be stained first. To detect bleeding early, she was asked each time she was observed if her dressing felt comfortable. Had she had a feeling of fullness or tightness in her neck, the physician should have been called immediately. If hemorrhage is allowed to continue, the patient can be expected to become dyspneic and to have other symptoms indicating respiratory obstruction. When the symptoms progress rapidly, the nurse should loosen the dressing before the physician arrives. Because hemorrhage into the tissues surrounding the trachea can be expected to cause respiratory obstruction, a tracheotomy tray was placed in Mrs. Thinis's room before she returned from the operating room.

The recurrent laryngeal nerves that supply the vocal cords may be injured during the surgical procedure. When one nerve is injured, the sole effect is hoarseness, which improves with time. Should both nerves be injured or severed, a tracheotomy may be required for the relief of respiratory obstruction. Because of the possibility of traumatizing the recurrent laryngeal nerves at the time of surgery, some surgeons check the condition of the vocal cords immediately after the operation by observing them. When they are in good condition and the patient develops hoarseness within 24 to 48 hours after surgery, it is almost certainly because of swelling in the region of the glottis and can be expected to subside. Following thyroidectomy, hoarseness should be reported promptly to the surgeon.

A third complication following thyroidectomy is hypoparathyroidism. It may be caused by the removal of all or some of the parathyroid tissue or by the combined effect of edema and swelling of the remaining tissue. Evidence of this complication is not likely to be present before 24 hours or to develop after 48 hours.

A complication once common in patients who were severely thyrotoxic was *thyroid crisis* or storm. Thyroid crisis or storm can and does occur before surgical therapy, as well as in the immediate postoperative period. In either event, it is a serious condition and is accompanied by a high mortality rate. In thyroid crisis all the symptoms of hyperthyroidism are exaggerated. The pulse rate rises to 140 or 200 beats per minute. There is also a rise in the rate of respiration and in the body temperature. In severe thyrotoxicosis, the temperature-regulating center loses control of body temperature and the temperature continues to rise until the time of death. Treatment during thyroid crisis is directed toward supplying cells with oxygen and glucose and preventing hyperpyrexia.

Supportive therapy includes intravenous glucose and saline, vitamin B complex, and glucocorticoids (to avert or treat adrenocorticoid insufficiency). The patient is placed in a cooled, humidified oxygen tent and a hypothermia blanket is utilized to facilitate heat loss. When a hypothermia blanket is not available, continuous sponging with cool water or the application of ice packs can accomplish the same effect. Whatever method is used must be sufficiently vigorous and continued long enough to prevent the exposure of the cells to the effects of prolonged hyperpyrexia.

Drug therapy during thyroid crisis includes the administration of (1) antithyroid medication to induce the blockade of hormone synthesis, (2) iodine to prevent the release of thyroid hormones from the thyrotoxic gland, and (3) an adrenergic antagonist, propanolol, to alleviate the peripheral effects of excess thyroid hormone. Certain cardiac medications may be necessary to treat cardiac failure whereas intravenous pressors may be required to treat shock.

Thyrotoxic patients treated by *subtotal thyroidectomy* experience postoperative suppression of the hypothalamic-pituitary-thyroid axis. In a follow-up study of 100 thyrotoxic patients treated with propranolol (Inderal) before and immediately after surgery, Toft and his associates (1978) found that 80 per cent were euthyroid at 12 months; 14 per cent developed permanent hypothyroidism; and 6 per cent relapsed to the thyrotoxic state. Postoperative thyroid function was related to the estimated weight of the remnant of thyroid gland after surgery. In caring for the postthyroidectomy patient, the nurse must observe closely for manifestations of both hypo- and hyperthyroidism.

A source of stress for some patients is the scar resulting from the incision. Mrs. Thinis was concerned that she might be left with an unsightly scar. She was reassured that she could expect the scar would, after a time, be no more than a fine line. The incision is usually made so that it follows the lines of the neck. Some surgeons use skin clips to further decrease scarring. Although the newly formed scar can be expected to be red, it will shrink and fade with the passage of time. Women who wish to cover the scar may do so by wearing a necklace or scarf.

Exophthalmos

A complication accompanying hyperthyroidism in some patients is exophthalmos. It is associated with the disease and is not a complication resulting from surgical or other forms of treatment. In exophthalmos the eyeballs protrude or appear to do so. The mechanism that is responsible remains unsettled. Apparently the mechanism responsible for the seeming protrusion is not the same in all individuals. In some patients there is no forward displacement of the eyeball. In others there is. When there is true forward displacement, it is caused by edema and fibrosis of orbital tissues. It does not appear to be related to the severity of the hyperthyroidism, nor is its progress affected by thyroidectomy. In fact, in some instances, exophthalmos seems to get worse following thyroidectomy. Although progressive exophthalmos is a self-limiting process, the eye may be lost before a remission occurs. If the eye is to be saved, it is imperative that the cornea be protected from drying. The patient should be taught to close his or her eyes consciously at regular intervals to moisten the eyeball with tears.

In mild disease, simple measures, such as elevation of the head of the bed and tinted glasses to provide protection from the sun, wind, and foreign bodies are sufficient. The administration of diuretics to reduce edema may be necessary. A 1 per cent solution of methycellulose or plastic shields may help prevent corneal drying in patients unable to oppose their eyelids to sleep. In severe disease, large doses of prednisone may be necessary to reduce edema and infiltrative components.

Other Disorders of the Thyroid Gland

One not uncommon disorder of the thyroid gland is simple goiter. In the early stages of simple goiter, the thyroid gland is diffusely enlarged. There is usually no change in function, though occasionally hypofunction occurs. Simple goiter is most likely to develop during periods when additional thyroid function is required, such as puberty or pregnancy. Although intake of iodine is inadequate and the enlargement tends to disappear, it may persist; it then almost always becomes nodular. When the gland is greatly enlarged, it may compress the surrounding structures. Simple goiter is treated with thyroid hormone.

Mrs. Grivin, aged 50, illustrates fairly well the pattern by which simple goiter develops into a nodular goiter. She was born and reared in a large city in the Great Lakes region. Her mother had been thyrotoxic in 1918. At age 13, Mrs. Grivin had an enlarged thyroid gland that was diagnosed as a simple goiter of the iodine-deficiency type. She was treated with 15 drops of potassium iodide three times per day for 3 months. Although the gland decreased in size, she continued to have some asymmetrical enlargement of the gland.

At the time of Mrs. Grivin's admission to the hospital for a thyroidectomy, she had an extensive nodular goiter. Study with ^{131}I indicated that thyroid function was normal. There was no clinical evidence of hyperthyroidism, though for the 3 months previous to her hospitalization her thyroid gland had been progressively enlarging. During the 3 weeks immediately preceding her admission to the hospital, she had had difficulty in swallowing and had been hoarse. Total thyroidectomy was performed to relieve pressure on the esophagus and the recurrent laryngeal nerves.

With the exception of developing parathyroid tetany, Mrs. Grivin made an uneventful recovery. The manifestations and treatment of hypoparathyroidism are discussed in relation to the parathyroid gland. Because it was necessary to remove all of her thyroid gland, she will have to have thyroid hormone for the remainder of her life. Should she neglect this for a period of time, signs and symptoms of hypothyroidism could be expected to develop.

Hypothyroidism

The clinical manifestations of hypothyroidism are summarized in Table 35-2. Not all persons with hypothyroidism develop a full-fledged picture of cretinism or myxedema.[4] In mild hypothyroidism the patient may complain of mild aches and pains, easy fatigability, inability to control emotions, and, in women, menstrual disturbances. The patient may be pale in appearance. Because the symptoms experienced by the patient are common to many disorders, the fact that he or she is suffering from hypothyroidism may be missed. The most serious consequence of hypothyroidism is a type of heart failure known as myxedema heart. It can be prevented by continued and adequate dosages of thyroid hormone. Probably the most important reason for the correction of hypothyroidism and maintenance of the euthyroid state is that it is essential to the feeling of well-being and productivity of the individual. A patient who complains of symptoms of or whose appearance suggests hypothyroidism should be encouraged to seek medical attention. Patients such as Mrs. Grivin should be helped to understand why they should take their medication every day for the rest of their lives. Because the effects of thyroid hormones are initiated slowly and continued for some weeks, the patient may feel well for a time after discontinuing the medication and conclude that it is no longer required. The patient should be encouraged to continue under regular medical supervision.

[4] The generalized edema typically found in myxedema is explained primarily by extravascular accumulation of albumin and other plasma proteins. Formation of exudates in serous cavities characteristic of myxedema may be explained by inadequte lymphatic drainage (Parving, 1979).

When making a nursing care plan for the patient with hypothyroidism, the ways in which he or she fails to adapt to the environment should be identified. Plans should then be made to modify the physical and emotional environments. Unlike the patient with hyperthyroidism, the one with hypothyroidism is intolerant to cold. He or she is comfortable only when the temperature is relatively high. At night the patient sleeps in a flannel gown and bed socks and has three or four woolen blankets on the bed. If he or she has an electric blanket, the heat is turned on high. When in the hospital, despite the complaints of roommates that the room is too warm, he or she desires several blankets on the bed.

Because the patient with hypothyroidism has a dry skin, soap should be used sparingly, and cream or oily lotion may add to comfort. To prevent bruising the patient, care should be taken when handling him or her. Furniture should be placed so that the chance of bumping into it is minimized.

Although patients are often apathetic and lethargic, they may be hyperirritable, and their ability to maintain their emotional control may also be disturbed. As in the care of other patients, the nurse should adapt behavior to the needs of the patient. The apathetic and lethargic patient cannot be hurried or stimulated to move quickly. Hyperirritability too is part of the illness. Fortunately, the patient can be approached with optimism. When he or she is treated with thyroid hormones, the condition can be corrected. The form of drug prescribed alters the rate at which the patient should be expected to improve. It may take as long as ten days to 2 weeks for signs of definite progress to be evident. The dosage of hormone has to be adjusted to each patient. See Table 35-3. As stated previously, patients with a hypofunctioning gland are more sensitive to the thyroid hormones than are those with normally functioning glands. Signs and symptoms of overdosage are those of hyperthyroidism. One precaution relates to the increased sensitivity of hypothyroid individuals to drugs such as morphine or codeine. When they are prescribed by the physican, dosages should be lower than they are for persons who are euthyroid.

To recapitulate, the manifestations of disorders of the thyroid have their origin in the effects of the expanding lesion on the tissues in the vicinity of the thyroid and in alterations in the level of production of thyroid hormones. Mrs. Grivin illustrated two of the effects of a goiter on the surrounding tissue. She was hoarse (pressure on the recurrent laryngeal nerve) and she had dysphagia, or difficulty in swallowing. Had the condition been allowed to continue she might have developed respiratory obstruction.

She also exemplified one of the causes of hypofunction of the thyroid gland, because she had a total

TABLE 35-3. ***Available Preparations, Usual Maintenance Dosage and Thyroid Hormone Levels During Maintenance Therapy****

Preparation	Composition	Tablet Strengths	Maintenance Dose	Serum Hormone Levels T_4	Serum Hormone Levels T_3
Levothyroxine Sodium	T_4	0.025, 0.05, 0.1, 0.15, 0.2, 0.3, and 0.5 mg†	0.1–0.2 mg daily or 1–2 mg weekly	normal	normal
Liothyronine (Levotriiodo-thyronine) Sodium	T_3	5, 25 and 50 μg‡	25 g two or three times daily	low	elevated
Thyroid U.S.P.	20–35 μg T_4 and 8–14 μg T_3§ per 60 mg (1 grain)	15, 30, 60, 90, 120, 180, 240, 300 mg	90–180 mg daily	low normal	usually elevated
Thyroglobulin	20–35 μg T_4 and 11–21 μg T_3 per 60 mg (1 grain)	15, 30, 60, 90, 180 and 300 mg	90–180 mg daily	low normal	usually elevated
Liotrix	Euthyroid: 60 μg T_4 and 15 μg T_3	½, 1, 2, and 3 "grain equivalents"	1.5–3.0 "grain equiva-lents"	low normal	often elevated
	Thyrolar: 50 μg T_4 and 12.5 μg T_3				

* Taken from W. E. Cobb & M. D. Jackson. "Drug Therapy Reviews: Management of Hypothyroidism." *Am. J. Hosp. Pharmacy,* **35** (Jan. 1978), 52, Table 1.

† Parenteral preparation: lyophilized powder 0.5 mg, with mannitol 10 mg and 5 ml normal saline as diluent.

‡ Parenteral preparation: powder (for solution) 114 μg/ml; not commercially available, but Smith Kline & French Laboratories will supply kit upon request for use in myxedema.

§ Range of $T_{4:3}$ ratio is 2–3.1 for pig glands and 3–4.5:1 for beef or sheep glands.

thyroidectomy. She should not develop signs and symptoms of hypothyroidism if she continues to take thyroid hormone for the rest of her life. The manifestations of hypothyroidism are the result of a lack of the thyroid hormones. The manifestations of hyperthyroidism, as exemplified by Mrs. Thinis, arise from an excess of thyroid hormones. Patients with either hyper- or hypofunction of the thyroid gland are unable to adapt appropriately to certain aspects of their environment.

Parathyroid Disorders

The parathyroid glands are also subject to disease and to injury; disturbances in the structure of the parathyroids may be accompanied by disordered function. Benign neoplasms are the most frequent cause of hyperparathyroidism. Inadvertent removal of the parathyroid gland during surgery of the neck, particularly thyroidectomy, and idiopathic atrophy and the most frequent causes of hypoparathyroidism. In both hyper- and hypoparathyroidism, homeostasis of calcium and phosphate is disturbed. Specific effects depend on the direction of the change in secretion.

The clinical manifestations of hyperparathyroidism are diverse. (Patient with hypercalcemia, 1973). This disorder, though by no means rare, is often discovered accidentally. Frequently the disturbance that causes the patient to consult a physician is bilateral renal lithiasis (kidney stones or calculi).[5] With the increased secretion of the parathyroid hormone, the activity of the osteoclasts in the bone is enhanced. If the quantity of calcium phosphate stored in the bone is decreased and the concentration of calcium in blood is elevated as calcium is removed from the bone, its density is reduced (osteoporosis). Occasionally the loss of mineral from the bone is so great that there are areas of cystic degeneration resulting in a disorder known as osteitis fibrosa cystica. With the demineralization of the bones, they become fragile, thus predisposing to fractures. Hyperparathyroidism can, however, exist without changes in the bones provided the intake of calcium is sufficient to prevent excessive demineralization of bone.

By an elevation in the level of calcium in the blood, its excretion in the urine is increased. When conditions such as concentration or alkalinity of the urine favor precipitation, stones form.

Symptoms experienced by patients with hyperparathyroidism include bone pain, particularly in the back; muscular weakness; anorexia; and vomiting. The high level of calcium and phosphates in the blood results in increased excretion of these substances by the kidney. Polyuria follows because water excretion increases with the loss of calcium. With polyuria, polydipsia is to be expected. A vast number of other signs and symptoms may occur, especially in patients in advanced stages of hyperparathyroidism.

When hyperparathyroidism is caused by a benign neoplasm, the disorder is cured by surgical removal of the neoplasm. Because the glands are small and the neoplasm may also be small, the surgeon may have difficulty in finding it. Hyperplasia of the parathyroid glands is a possible, though less frequent, cause of hyperparathyroidism. It may be either primary or secondary to some other disorder. For example, in advanced kidney disease in which the kidney no longer reabsorbs normal amounts of calcium, the parathyroid gland undergoes hyperplasia.

Much of the nursing of the patient with hyperparathyroidism is similar to that of any sick person who is undergoing diagnosis and possible surgical treatment. In the care of patients in whom bone changes are evident, care should be taken to prevent placing stress or strain on bones when they are being moved either in bed or from the bed to the wheelchair. Attention should also be given to providing the patients with an adequate supply of water.

The management of patients with chronic hypoparathyroidism is directed to the goal of increasing the level of calcium in the blood and reducing the amount of phosphate ion to relieve the symptoms of increased neuromuscular irritability. Therapy involves the administration of vitamin D, usually as ergocalciferol (vitamin D_2), in doses of 50,000 to 100,000 units per day and calcium as citrate, lactate, or gluconate in doses adequate to achieve blood calcium levels of 8.5 to 9.0 mg/100 ml (Potts, 1977).

To reduce further the level of phosphates in the blood, the patient may be placed on a low-phosphorus diet. Foods high in phosphorus include milk products, cauliflower, and molasses. Aluminum hydroxide, 0.6 g three times per day, may be administered to decrease the absorption of phosphates from the intestine.

In nursing the patient with acute hypoparathyroidism, or the one who is predisposed to it, attention should be directed toward detecting signs indicating increased neuromuscular irritability. Treatment should then be given promptly. Should the patient have a convulsive seizure, care of the patient during the seizure is no different from that of convulsions from other causes. The seizure can be terminated by the administration of calcium gluconate intravenously. This should, therefore, be done promptly.

[5] Hyperparathyroidism is not, however, the sole cause of this condition.

Female Sexual Cycle Disturbances—Disorders of Menstruation

Overview

Persons with abnormal vaginal bleeding constitute a major portion of gynecologic practice (Danforth, 1977, p. 792). Bleeding from spontaneous abortions and from polyps or other pathologic processes account for only 25 per cent of abnormal vaginal bleeding (Goldfarb & Little, 1980). Thus the remaining 75 per cent have to be placed in the category of dysfunctional uterine bleeding (DUB), that is, abnormal bleeding which has no organic cause such as inflammation, neoplasia, or pregnancy. A common explanation for a number of cases of DUB is that we are dealing with anovulatory forms of bleeding.

Bleeding associated with pathologic lesions of the uterus or adnexa, and with blood or systemic diseases would be excluded from this anovulatory category. Brewer (1967) has advised against the use of expressions such as *functional uterine bleeding, metropathia hemorrhagica,* and *anovulatory bleeding* because their meaning is not always clear and they cause confusion. Although a nonorganic etiology is essential by definition, DUB can coexist with organic pathology such as benign and malignant neoplasms.

Dysfunctional Uterine Bleeding (DUB)

Dysfunctional bleeding may be characterized as too long, too profuse, and too frequent, or it may be intermenstrual spotting. It occurs most often in adolescent girls and climacteric or premenopausal women, but it may occur during the reproductive period. If a definite delimiting time element is important, it would seem reasonable to consider bleeding at menstruation, occurring over a period of 3 months, as abnormal (Brewer & DeCosta, 1967).

Etiology

The two principal causative factors of DUB are

1. An endocrine dysfunction
2. The inability of the endometrium to respond in an ordinary manner

This etiologic concept proposed in 1967 by Brewer and DeCosta still stands.

Willson et al. (1975) state that

> The underlying cause of DUB is still uncertain, but in most cases it is associated with failure of ovulation and a consequent hormonal imbalance. Ovarian dysfunction may be caused by either a primary defect or pathologic lesion within the ovary itself or it may be secondary to malfunction of other endocrine glands, notably the hypothalamus, pituitary and thyroid.

Speroff et al. (1978) contend that, in considering abnormal menstrual bleeding, it is usually impossible to reduce the issue of etiology to a single factor. The normal ovulatory function of the menstrual system relies on a dynamic coordination of complex actions. Abnormal function may represent discordance at all levels.

Kempers (1977, p. 1) introduces the subject of dysfunctional uterine bleeding as follows:

> Dysfunctional uterine bleeding is abnormal bleeding which has no organic cause, e.g., neoplasia, inflammation, or pregnancy. The bleeding results from a disturbance in the usually finely synchronized hormonal secretory activity. Although the term has frequently been used to signify anovulatory forms of bleeding, it also describes disturbances in ovulatory forms of bleeding. Although a nonorganic etiology is essential by definition, it can coexist with organic pathology such as malignant and benign neoplasms. Dysfunctional uterine bleeding occurs most frequently during puberty and in the perimenopausal years, is less common during the adult reproductive years, and is among the most frequent of all gynecologic complaints.

Kempers's modified clinical classification of dysfunctional bleeding, with the accompanying terminology, is useful for the following discussion of these disturbances. See Table 35-4 for Kempers's classification of dysfunctional bleeding. A summary of follicular and luteal defects that result in DUB appears in Table 35-5.

Terminology[6]

Menorrhagia or Hypermenorrhea: excessive uterine bleeding in both amount and duration of flow, occuring at regular intervals.

Hypomenorrhea: decreased menstrual flow occurring at regular intervals.

Metrorrhagia. Uterine bleeding, usually not excessive, occurring at irregular intervals.

Menometrorrhagia. Frequent, irregular, excessive, and prolonged episodes of uterine bleeding.

Polymenorrhea. Frequent, regular episodes of uterine bleeding, occurring at intervals of less than 18 days.

Oligomenorrhea. Infrequent, irregular bleeding episodes, occurring at intervals of more than 45 days.

[6] Definitions are derived from Kempers, 1978, p. 1.

TABLE 35-4. ***Kempers' Classification of Dysfunctional Bleeding****

Ovulatory
Midcycle spotting
Polymenorrhea (short proliferative and/or secretory phases)
Oligomenorrhea (long proliferative phase)
Corpus luteum insufficiency and luteolysis
Premenstrual spotting
Menorrhagia, hypermenorrhea
Polymenorrhea
Corpus luteum prolonged activity (irregular shedding and persistent corpus luteum)
Oligomenorrhea
Menorrhagia, hypermenorrhea
Anovulatory
Oligomenorrhea
Hypermenorrhea
Menometrorrhagia

* Taken from R. D. Kempers. "Dysfunctional Uterine Bleeding." In *Gynecology and Obstetrics,* Vol. 1. Ed. by J. J. Sciarra. Hagerstown, Md.: Harper & Row, 1977, Chap. 12, p. 12–2.

Intermenstrual bleeding. Episodes of uterine bleeding between regular menstrual periods.

Kempers's classification of dysfunctional bleeding (Table 35-4) and his explanation of it are a methodic and didactic approach to a most intricate subject. The subsequent presentation will follow its orientation rather closely.

Ovulatory DUB.

Ovulatory DUB is more typically found during adult reproductive years than is anovulatory dysfunctional bleeding. In one study of 3,000 ovulatory cycles, 13.5 per cent were found to be irregular. Midcyclic spotting in cycles of normal length is common and approximately 94 per cent of ovulating women may have microscopic uterine bleeding of this type. Of those women who have periodic intermenstrual pain, 20 per cent also have associated frank intermenstrual bleeding. This bleeding is attributed to estrogen withdrawal associated with the decrease in estrogen at midcycle following follicular rupture. In general, preovulatory circulating estrogen levels are usually reduced one third or one fourth at the time of ovulation. The midcyclic bleeding is usually self-limiting and requires no specific therapy.

Ovulatory dysfunctional bleeding may manifest as either polymenorrhea or oligomenorrhea. Polymenorrhea, or menses occurring at intervals of less than 18 days, is considered to be abnormal. However, cycles occurring as frequently as every 18 to 21 days occassionally may be considered normal; there are women who have regular cycles at these intervals and have perfectly normal secretory endometrium obtained on biopsy. The polymenorrhea of DUB in ovulatory cycles may result from either a short proliferative phase, a short secretory phase or, in some instances, both. The short proliferative phase may result from ovarian hypersensitivity, and the diagnosis can be established by finding evidence for early ovulation in the form of earlier-than-expected shift in basal body temperature, normal secretory endometrium on biopsy prior to menses, and normal midluteal progestational vaginal smears. In the later reproductive years, particularly in the premenopausal period, it is not uncommon to encounter cycles with premature degeneration of the corpus luteum, resulting in a shortened secretory phase. In these circumstances, polymenorrhea is the usual manifesta-8tion, but the bleeding pattern can progress to oligomenorrhea and amenorrhea as the result of ovarian failure. The diagnosis of the short secretory phase is made by establishing that the postovulatory elevation in basal body temperature, the serum progesterone or urinary pregnanediol secretion have decreased prematurely and that the endometrial biopsy reveals midsecretory endometrium out of phase with the days of the cycle. (See Chapter 15, Figure 15-4 and Table 15-2).

Ovulatory bleeding associated with a long proliferative phase is usually manifested as oligomenorrhea. The delay in ovulation in these cycles may result from early ovarian failure or infrequent ovulation associated with the polycystic ovary syndrome (*S*tein-*L*eventhal syndrome). The underlying mechanism seems to be a decreased follicular response to gonadotropins. Frequently this results from abnormal ratios between follicle-stimulating (FSH) and luteinizing (LH) hormones. It is the type of dysfunctional bleeding frequently seen at the extremes of the reproductive years. It has been suggested that in this situation the estrogenic activity follows one of two patterns:

1. The estrogen levels rise slowly during the follicular phase and exhibit an abrupt rise prior to ovulation.
2. The estrogen levels rise much earlier and are maintained at an elevated level for an abnormally long period of time prior to ovulation.

In the former type the follicles require an abnormally long period for maturation, whereas in the latter type the follicles are arrested in later stages of development for an unusual length of time.

The diagnosis is made by finding that (1) the basal

Table 35-5. ***Follicular and Luteal Phase Defects that Result in Dysfunctional Uterine Bleeding****

	Follicle Maturation	Ovulation	Luteal Phase	Endometrium	Menstrual Pattern	Functional Diagnosis
	Early/Late		Early/Late			
NORMAL (FUNCTIONAL) UTERINE BLEEDING						
1	Normal	Normal	Normal	Normal biphasic changes	Eumenorrhea	Normal ovulatory cycle Perfect biphasic cycle
2	Normal and short	Normal	Normal	Normal biphasic changes	Eumenorrhea	Short normal ovulatory cycle not shorter than 22 days
3	Normal and prolonged	Normal	Normal	Normal biphasic changes	Eumenorrhea	Long normal ovulatory cycle not longer than 34 days
DYSFUNCTIONAL UTERINE BLEEDING						
I Ovulatory Group						
4	Short	Normal	Normal	Accelerated Proliferation Normal secretory changes	Polymenorrhea	Premature follicle maturation cycles shorter than 22 days "Polyovulation"
5	Prolonged	Normal	Normal	Retarded proliferation Normal secretory changes	Oligomenorrhea	Delayed follicle maturation cycles longer than 34 days "Oligoovulation"
6	Normal	Normal	Normal/ Slightly delayed	Combined secretory & proliferative changes in early folicle phase	Menorrhagia after regular interval	Delayed involution of corpus luteum
7	Normal	Normal	Normal/ Delayed	Prolonged secretory changes	Menorrhagia after slightly prolonged interval	Short-term corpus luteum persistence
8	Normal	Normal	Normal/ Missing	More prolonged secretory changes with marked pseudodecidual reaction	Severe menorrhagia after more prolonged interval	Long-term corpus luteum persistence (pseudocyesis)

9	Normal	Normal	Inadequate	Inconsistent, atypical changes throughout luteal phase	Eumenorrhea with or without interval variations	Luteal phase inadequacy "imperfect biphasic cycle"
II Subovulatory Group						
10	Normal or prolonged	Normal or missing	Normal or missing	Normal biphasic changes or proliferation only	Eumenorrhea alternating with oligo- and/or hypomenorrhea	Ovulation alternating with anovulation
III Anovulatory Group						
11	Normal	Missing	Missing	Proliferation only	Menorrhea with normal or shortened interval	Anovulation "Perfect Monophasic Cycle"
12	Normal/ slightly delayed	Missing	Missing	Proliferation only with mild hyperplasia	Metrorrhagia with prolonged interval	Short-term follicle persistence
13	Normal/ Delayed	Missing	Missing	Proliferation only with variable degrees of marked hyperplasia	Severe metrorrhagia following more prolonged interval	Long-term follicle persistence
14	Deficient	Missing	Missing	Poor proliferation only	Oligohypomenorrhea	Deficiency of follicle maturation "Imperfect Monophasic Cycle"
15	Deficient/ Deficient or missing	Missing	Missing	Early proliferation gradually changing to atrophy	Secondary amenorrhea first degree	Ceasing follicle maturation
16	Missing	Missing	Missing	Nonfunctioning, atrophy	Secondary amenorrhea second degree	Ceased follicle maturation absence of cycle

* From Arronet, G. H. "Arrata WSM: Dysfunctional Uterine Bleeding." *Obstet. Gynecol.*, **29** (1967), 97–107, as adapted for Danforth (1977, p. 797).

body temperature shift occurs later than expected, coupled with a luteal phase which persists for the expected 14 days, and that (2) the endometrial biopsy on the twenty-sixth day shows secretory endometrium.

Corpus luteum insufficiency (luteal phase defect).

In this unusual disorder there is an inadequate amount of progesterone production although the estrogen production seems to be unimpaired. Clinically it is associated with infertility and repeated first-trimester abortions. It may be the etiologic factor in approximately 3.5 per cent of infertility cases. Among patients with habitual abortion, a luteal phase defect was present in approximately 35 per cent of cases. The associated bleeding is variable as either menstrual spotting, menorrhagia, hypermenorrhea, or polymenorrhea.

The diagnosis of corpus luteum insufficiency is made by a combination of basal body temperature graphs, serum progesterone levels, and endometrial biopsies. The basal body temperature is not a reliable means of establishing the diagnosis, although it can alert the clinician's suspicion. If the abnormal luteal function is severe enough, the basal body temperature may show little if any biphasic quality. Serial serum progesterone values obtained during the luteal phase are helpful in establishing the diagnosis when practical from the economic and time standpoint. However, clinical studies in patients with this condition have shown that progesterone levels are decreased whether the luteal phase is short or normal (Speroff, 1978). Perhaps the single most consistent method of diagnosing the condition is to obtain an endometrial biopsy on the twenty-sixth day of a 28-day cycle. If this biopsy is found to be out of phase by 2 days or more, similar biopsy studies should be obtained in the subsequent cycle. If the second cycle is out of phase, the diagnosis is strongly suspected.

Dating of the menstrual cycle is generally based on the most advanced elements of the endometrium such as glands, stroma, and vessels, and in corpus luteum deficiency, the discrepancy in dating reflects a retarded pathologic picture.

The pathogenesis of the corpus luteum defect may relate to multiple etiologies. Jones (1968) has classified these as follows: (1) primary ovarian defects; (2) primary central defects of the hypothalamic-pituitary axis; (3) primary metabolic defects; and (4) specific defects in luteal cell steroidogenesis.

PRIMARY OVARIAN DEFECTS: A small proportion of luteal defects are the result of primary ovarian defects. Occassionally, patients with luteal phase defects are infertile and also experience premature menopause. Since premature menopause is related to a disturbance in oocyte maturation, it was suggested that certain patients with luteal phase defects represent failure of proper follicular organization during embryogenesis as a consequence of abnormal ova. This would explain why these patients failed to achieve pregnancy despite adequate substitution therapy.

PRIMARY CENTRAL DEFECTS: Central factors probably account for the majority of corpus luteum disturbances. Inadequacy of hypothalamic LH-releasing factor, pituitary LH, or both, are etiologic and may result specifically from hereditary defects of the central nervous system or pituitary gland, neurogenic scars, psychogenic trauma, stress, or they may be secondary to nutritional or chronic disease factors. If normal follicular development is impaired, corpus luteum development and function will likewise be impaired. Thus, if the rising levels of FSH are inadequate for follicular maturation, the corpus luteum function will likewise be inadequate. Clinically this is encountered frequently in the perimenarche and when using exogenous gonadotropins for the induction of ovulation. However, not only is proper maturation of the follicle necessary but also an adequate LH surge is required for normal luteal function.

The corpus luteum requires the continuous presence of small amounts of LH for its maintenance. Secretory capacity nevertheless declines 9 to 11 days after ovulation. To prolong luteal function over the usual 14-day span, repeated injections of LH are required if LH is used for the ovulatory stimulus. On the other hand, if human chorionic gonadotropin (HCG), which has a longer half-life and luteotropic action, is used to induce ovulation, a single large administration is sufficient to maintain the corpus luteum. Thus, although it has been thought that the life span and steroidogenesis of the corpus luteum was independent of FSH and LH secretion and that it functioned automatically once it had been formed, it is now evident that residual tonic LH is an important factor in the maintenance of the 14-day luteal span. Therefore, inadequate tonic LH may be etiologic in some instances of the short luteal phase defect.

PRIMARY METABOLIC DEFECTS AND STEROIDOGENESIS: Metabolic factors may be etiologic. Inadequate blood oxygenation as seen in patients with tetralogy of Fallot is considered an etiologic factor. It is believed that poor oxygenation is responsible for inadequate steroidogenesis. The defect in oxygenation is also associated with abnormal steroidogenesis of the placenta in these patients.

Corpus Luteum Luteolysis.

Certain progestational steroids as well as estrogens and stilbesterol can inhibit corpus luteum function, an action attributed to a direct effect of the agent on corpus luteum steroidogenesis. Under the influence of estrogens, the corpus luteum can secrete prostaglandin which is also luteolytic for the luteal cells. Thus the corpus luteum may have an inherent mechanism for terminating its existence.

Corpus Luteum Prolonged Activity (irregular shedding, persistent corpus luteum).

Prolonged levels of progesterone excretion may result in a menstrual dysfunction termed *irregular shedding,* which is manifested as menorrhagia, hypermenorrhea, and, in some instances, oligomenorrhea. Irregular shedding is considered to represent ovulatory cycles in which cyclic menstrual flow is prolonged. The cause is though to be incomplete lysis of the corpus luteum with mild elevation of progesterone levels during the menstrual phase of the cycle, which prevents complete sloughing of the endometrium.

The diagnosis of irregular shedding can be made by means of endometrial biopsy on the fifth day of bleeding; the specimen reveals secretory endometrium along with regenerating endometrium. Irregular shedding is best treated by suppression of ovulation with oral contraceptives for a month or two (Goldfarb & Little, 1980).

Prolonged life of the corpus luteum can also result in ovulatory dysfunctional bleeding. Persistent corpus luteum (Halban's disease) is characterized by a variable delay in menses, usually lasting for less than 4 weeks, but occasionally for up to 6 months. The delayed bleeding is due to persistent secretion of estrogen and progesterone at levels sufficient to maintain the endometrium. The endometrium may show a pseudodecidual change histologically. When bleeding occurs, it may be prolonged and irregular because of the fluctuation of estrogen and progesterone secretion. Adnexal pain may be associated with bleeding within a corpus luteum cyst which may be mistaken for an ectopic pregnancy, but it is self-limiting and tends not to recur (Goldfarb & Little, 1980).

Anovulatory Dysfunctional Bleeding.

Ninety per cent of DUB is anovulatory bleeding and occurs most commonly at the extremes of the reproductive years. In the majority of cases, the bleeding is due to estrogen withdrawal or to estrogen breakthrough. Examples of estrogen withdrawal bleeding are those that occur following bilateral oophorectomy (with preservation of the uterus) or after the discontinuation of estrogen administration in similar patients. Two characteristic patterns of estrogen secretion associated with estrogen breakthrough bleeding have been described. In one type there is a steady urinary secretion of 30 μg of estrogen per day throughout the cycle with a failure of estrogen to peak at midcycle or to drop premenstrually. In these cases there is a gradual thickening of proliferative endometrium which outgrows its blood supply, or there may actually be "teetering" of estrogen above critical levels, ultimately causing the unpredictable menometrorrhagia. In the second type there is marked fluctuation of the estrogen levels with a urinary excretion that may exceed 100 μg of estrogen per day and that persists until there is a rapid fall in estrogen secretions. The abnormally high estrogen levels through much of the cycle have been attributed to abnormal FSH–LH ratios, with an absolute midcycle LH deficiency. Utimately, through feedback inhibition, the high estrogen level inhibits the gonadotropins, and estrogen withdrawal bleeding ensues. In these situations the menorrhagia is often preceded by amenorrhea and there is associated persistence or a delay in rupturing of follicular cysts. Nevertheless, even with the fluctuating estrogen levels, relatively regular cycles may be seen. One study reported the finding of normal-length cycles in 50 per cent of anovulatory cycles, while 28 per cent were associated with oligomenorrhea and 22 per cent with polymenorrhea.

Menstrual patterns associated with anovulatory cycles may be either oligomenorrhea, hypermenorrhea, or menometrorrhagia. Given (1961) divided anovulatory oligomenorrhea into five stages. Stage 1 consists of patients with at least eight cycles per year. Their estrogen levels rose and fell normally or remained high. The endometrium was either proliferative or hyperplastic. As the stages increased, the oligomenorrhea became more profound. Stage 4 patients had only two or three menses per year, the estrogen levels were nonfluctuating, and the endometrium was hyperplastic. Finally in stage 5 there was complete amenorrhea and the endometrium was atrophic. Although 10 per cent of the 150 patients in Given's study were in stage 1, 40 per cent were in stage 5. This latter stage is similar to the progression of events associated with impending ovarian failure or menopause. Similarly, this type of bleeding is frequently associated with the polycystic ovary syndrome (S-L syndrome).

A second characteristic bleeding pattern associated with anovulatory cycles is menorrhagia or hypermenorrhea.

A third pattern associated with anovulatory cycles is menometrorrhagia. This is frequently the bleeding characteristic of benign cystic hyperplasia. The bleeding disorder named *metropathia haemorrhagia* by Schroeder in 1915 followed histologic studies in which he showed that the abnormal persistence of unruptured follicles in the absence of corpora lutea produced hyperplasia of the endometrium due to the persistent and unopposed estrogenic stimulation. It has since been shown that prolonged unopposed estrogen stimulation may result in cystic hyperplasia which may ultimately progress to adenomatous hyperplasia with the associated risk of carcinoma of the endometrium. Bleeding from this type of endometrium may not always occur uniformly but can involve scattered portions at different times and without being synchronous. The vascular adenomatous hyperplastic tissue is fragile, partly because of its excessive growth, but largely because it lacks structural rigidity. The excessive bleeding that ensues is due not only to the large quantity of tissue available for sloughing but also to the asynchrony in the bleeding opening up multiple vascular channels. There is no rhythmic vasoconstriction of the spiral arteries to assist in stasis. Healing is the result of exogenous estrogen effect (Kempers, 1978, p. 6).

The fundamental disturbances associated with anovulatory dysfunctional uterine bleeding can be (1) central, due to hypothalamic hypophyseal factors; (2) peripheral, due to ovarian factors such as defective uteroidogenesis or functioning ovarian tumors; or (3) constitutional, due to nutritional deficiencies, chronic illness, and metabolic disease such as hypothyroidism and diabetes. One study reported that 77.5 per cent of these patients had evidence of pituitary, adrenal, ovarian, or thyroid dysfunction. In patients with anovulatory menometrorrhagia, it is particularly important that obvious organic lesions be ruled out. Organic pathology that is frequently missed in these cases includes submucous fibroids, pelvic inflammatory disease, incomplete abortion, precocious puberty, endometrial polyps, and malignancy.

Diagnosis of DUB

Obviously, Kempers's modified classification involves the concomitant discussion of the clinical orientation toward diagnostic approach and tests for each characteristic pattern of dysfunctional uterine bleeding.

Treatment of DUB

In dealing with this final topic of dysfunctional uterine bleeding, after the lengthy and extremely informative discussion of the components of Kempers's classification, these words from Goldfarb and Little (1980, p. 666) are offered:

> The essence of the science of medicine is identification of the physiology and pathophysiology of an abnormal process and determination of the intervention that will arrest the abnormal and promote the normal state. Knowledge of the endocrinology of the menstrual cycle, its aberrations, and the availability of specific hormones to imitate or replace the endogenous secretions makes abnormal bleeding much more a medical than a surgical problem. The use of dilatation and curettage can then be reserved for cases in which the administration of drugs is predicted to be ineffective or fails to resolve abnormal bleeding.

In conclusion, the clinician will be frequently made aware that the term dysfunctional bleeding is as difficult to define as the bleeding is to cure (Brewer & DeCosta, 1967).

Guidelines to Nursing Management

The nurse frequently has the opportunity to prepare a woman for participation in two common tests: (1) graphing basal body temperature; and (2) endometrial biopsy.

Basal Body Temperature Charts.

This exceedingly simple, yet tedious, activity can provide presumptive evidence of ovulation. The woman is instructed to take her temperature each morning at approximately the same time, prior to engaging in any activity, such as getting out of bed, smoking, or drinking water, since even these activities will affect the accuracy of the readings. During ovulatory cycles the thermogenic effect of progesterone causes an elevation of the basal body temperature during the luteal phase of the cycle. With the fall of progesterone production at the end of the luteal phase, the basal body temperature falls to preovulatory levels. No such predictable patterns are discernible during anovulatory cycles.

Endometrial Biopsy.

This is an office procedure most commonly performed without anesthesia. The instrumentation does cause some pain; however, this is transient. The administration of oral analgesics or a paracervical block may be necessary with certain women because of either a low pain threshold or a high anxiety level.

The particular behaviors demonstrated by a woman experiencing disturbances in the female sexual cycle depend upon her perception of the problem, her level of understanding of reproductive function, and the availability of resources to help her cope with the problem. Certain behaviors, however, can be anticipated based on the endocrinologic nature of the dysfunction and the involvement of sexually-related concerns. Behaviors consistent with mild anxiety, anticipatory grieving, and a threat to self-concept are frequently demonstrated by this female population.

Mild anxiety is the result of the woman's fear of the unknown. There is anxiety regarding the potential significance of the problem in relation to general health and the reproductive potential of the individual, if she is still of childbearing age. There is also anxiety surrounding the diagnosis and treatment of such problems. Finally, anxiety is generated by the woman's lack of comfort in describing symptoms associated with the female sexual cycle. It must not be forgotten that the female sexual cycle and related reproductive physiology have been shrouded in superstition and misinformation for centuries. Entry into the health care system for the investigation of reproductive dysfunction may be the first time a woman is faced with open discussion regarding issues of sexual and reproductive function. A problem of terminology frequently presents itself. The woman lacks the appropriate medical terminology to describe her problem adequately and is embarrassed by her own terms. As the nurse engages in history taking, the opportunity is afforded to demonstrate acceptance of the woman's terminology and to begin the process of education as the nurse relates the terms used by the woman to appropriate anatomic or physiologic terms. The nurse can, therefore, decrease the woman's anxiety, at least in part, by increasing her ability to communicate effectively with other health care professionals. These actions also demonstrate the acceptability of the woman's problem and the appropriateness of seeking professional care.

Problems of reproductive dysfunction are rarely acute or of short duration. Rather, the long-term efforts to deal with reproductive dysfunction, such as infertility, can lead to surprise, denial, isolation, guilt, and grief reactions among the female population (Manning, 1979). Efforts must be made by all members of the health team, including the nurse, to provide an environment supportive of women's emotional needs. Since contact with this population is almost entirely on an outpatient basis, the nurse must establish a relationship over time which integrates the emotional and educational needs of women. Since long intervals between visits may be required to adequately document problems or to evaluate the effectiveness of specific therapy, the woman must be encouraged to initiate contact with the nurse for further clarification of specific therapy or for continued emotional support should the need arise. Community resources as well as hospital-based services must be coordinated to meet the long-term needs of this population.

References Cited

Baldessarini, R. J. "Schizophrenia." *N. Engl. J. Med.*, **297** (Nov. 3, 1977), 988–95.

Bartter, F. C. "The Syndrome of Inappropriate Secretion of Antidiuretic Hormone (SIADH). *DM,* (Nov. 1973).

Braverman, L. E. "Therapeutic Considerations." *Clinics Endocrinol. & Metabol.*, **7** (March 1978), 221–40, 222.

Brewer, J. I., and DeCosta, E. J. *Textbook of Gynecology,* 4th ed. Baltimore: Williams & Wilkins Co., 1967, p. 137.

Danforth, D. N., ed. *Obstetrics and Gynecology,* 3rd ed. New York: Harper & Row, 1977.

Given, W. P. "Functional Menstrual Disorders: A Study of 150 Patients." *Fertil. Steril.*, **12** (1961), 282.

Goldfarb, J. M., and Little, A. B. "Current Concepts: Abnormal Vaginal Bleeding." *N. Engl. J. Med.*, **302** (March 20, 1980), 666–69.

Goodman, L. S., and Gilman, A., eds. *The Pharmacological Basis of Therapeutics,* 5th ed. New York: Macmillan Publishing Co., 1975, pp. 1410–20.

Ingbar, S. H., and Woeber, K. A. "Diseases of the Thyroid." In *Harrison's Principles of Internal Medicine,* 8th ed. Ed. by G. W. Thorn et al., New York: McGraw-Hill, 1977, pp. 501–19.

Jones, G. S. "Luteal Phase Defects," in *Progress in Infertility,* Behrman, S. J. and Kistner, R. W., Eds. Boston: Little, Brown & Co., 1968, pp. 299–325.

Kaplan, M. M., and Utiger, R. D. "Diagnosis of hyperthyroidism." *Clinics Endocrinol. & Metabol.*, **7**:1 (March 1978). 97–113, 102–6.

Kempers, R. D. "Dysfunctional Uterine Bleeding." In *Gynecology and Obstetrics,* **Vol. 1.** Ed. by J. J. Sciarra. Hagerstown, Md.: Harper & Row, 1977. Chps. 12, p. 12–2.

Parving, H-H. et al. "Mechanisms of Edema Formation in Myxedema—Increased Protein Extravasation and Relatively Slow Lymphatic Drainage." *N. Engl. J. Med.*, **301** (Aug. 30, 1979), 460–65.

Patient with Hypercalcemia." *Diagnostica,* **26** (Feb. 1973), 21–24.

Potkin, S. G. et al. "Are Paranoid Schizophrenics Biologically Different from Other Schizophrenics? *N. Engl. J. Med.*, **298** (Jan. 12, 1978), 61–66.

Potts, J. "Disorders of Parathyroid Glands." In *Harrison's Principles of Internal Medicine,* 8th ed. Ed. by G. W. Thorn et al. New York: McGraw-Hill, 1977, pp. 2014–25, 2025.

Randall, R. V., and Rynearson, E. H. "Clinical Aspects of Anterior Pituitary Failure. *Postgrad. Med.*, **29** (Jan. 1961), 25.

Speroff, L. et al. *Clinical Gynecologic Endocrinology and Infertility,* 2nd ed. Baltimore: Williams & Wilkins, 1978, pp. 158–60.

Surgeon General's Report on Health Promotion and Disease Prevention. *Healthy People.* (PHS) Publication No. 79-55071, Washington, D.C.: Department of Health, Education, and Welfare, 1979.

Toft, A. D. et al. "Thyroid Function after Surgical Treatment of Thyrotoxicosis. *N. Engl. J. Med.*, **298** (March 23, 1978), 643–47.

Volpe, R. "The Pathogenesis of Graves' Disease: An Overview." *Clinics Endocrinol. & Metabol.*, **7**:1 (March 1978), 3–29, 3–4.

Williams, G. H. et al. "Diseases of the Adrenal Cortex." In *Harrison's Principles of Internal Medicine,* 8th ed. Ed. by G. W. Thorn et al., New York: McGraw-Hill, 1977, pp. 520–57, 543.

Willson, J. R. et al. *Obstetrics and Gynecology,* 5th ed. St. Louis: C. V. Mosby Co., 1975.

General References

Frantz, A. G. "Prolactin." *N. Engl. J. Med.,* **298** (Jan. 26, 1978) 201–7, 206–7.

Kato, J. et al. "Effect of Clomiphene on the Uptake of Estradiol by the Anterior Pituitary and Hypophysis." *Endocrinol.,* 82 (1968) 10–19.

Marshall, J. "Induction of Ovulation." *Clin. Obstet. & Gynecol.,* **21** (March 1978) 147–62 158.

Novak, E. R. et al. *Novak's Textbook of Gynecology,* 9th ed. Baltimore: Williams & Wilkins, 1975.

Reid, D. E. *A Textbook of Obstetrics.* Philadelphia: W. B. Saunders Co., 1962.

Romney, S. L. et al. *Gynecology and Obstetrics: The Health Care of Women.* New York: McGraw-Hill, 1975.

Sciarra, J. J. *Gynecology and Obstetrics,* Vol. 1. New York: Harper & Row, 1977.

Taymor, M. D. "Evaluation of Anovulatory Cycles and Induction of Ovulation." *Clin. Obstet. & Gynecol.,* **22** (March 1979), 145–67.

36

Problems with Neural Regulation

Neurological Assessment of Persons with Impairment of Neural Regulation

It has been emphasized repeatedly that careful observation and reporting are critical to effective nursing care of the person with alterations in neural regulation. The axiom that we see what we look for, and we look for what we know, is nowhere more applicable than in assessing neurological function. Initial contact with the person should be used to begin a comprehensive assessment of status; information gathered at that time serves as a baseline against which subsequent changes can be interpreted. Elements in assessment of the person with known or suspected alteration of neurologic function include a thorough history as related by the patient (or a person who knows him or her well) to describe patterns of sleep, activity, eating, and elimination, with special emphasis on mental state, speech, and any episodes of loss of consciousness, with or without convulsions. The traditional neurological examination tests for six functions: cerebral, cranial nerves, cerebellar, motor, sensory, and reflex (Alexander & Brown, 1976). Understanding the preceding discussion of the organization of the nervous system is but a first step toward developing beginning skill in neurological assessment. The reader is referred to the references in Chapter 8 on physical examination, each of which includes a full description of equipment and techniques to evaluate neurological function.

Impaired neurological function can result from inherited metabolic defect, vascular disease, infection, tumor, or trauma. Current research about mental illness is focusing on the relation between genetic and environmental factors (Kety, 1979). In short, any of the injuring agents described in Unit III can alter neurological function, and are apt to exert their injuring effects on nerve cells before other types of tissue are injured. (Principle 3: The more highly specialized a tissue, the less able it is to survive severe and sudden deficits in supply.) But whatever the nature or cause of the person's neurlogic response or impairment, intervention is likely to be safer and more effective when ongoing observation and assessment proceed from an initial comprehensive appraisal of the person's status.

Continuous observation of the patient who has neurological disease or accidental or surgical trauma is a critical nursing responsibility. Bolin (1977) proposes that a total picture of the patient's neurological status can be derived from checking:

1. Reaction of the pupils to light
2. Response of all four extremities to various stimuli
3. Level of consciousness

A guide and recording format for neurological assessment has been developed and tested at Colorado General Hospital which is concise and complete, and allows quantification of observations for quick comparison of time-series observations. A scale is described for each of five states or variables. On each scale, the zero point represents absence of evidence of efferent function. See Table 36-1 for ordinal and nominal scaling of the five variables used to assess patients' neurological status.

Analysis of data over a 2-year period suggested

TABLE 36-1. ***Rating scale for assessing the status of neurological patients****

Variable	Ordinal Scale	Nominal Scale—Definition
1. Reaction of pupils to light	2	Equal, react(s) briskly
	1	Smaller, react(s) slowly
	0	Greater, no reaction
2. Level of consciousness (LOC)	5	Alert and oriented x3—awakens easily; oriented to person, place, time
	4	Alert and partially oriented—awakens easily but oriented in only 1 or 2 spheres
	3	Lethargic but oriented—slow to arouse, possibly slurred speech, but oriented x3
	2	Lethargic and disoriented—slow to arouse, oriented in only 1 or 2 spheres or completely disoriented
	2	Restless/combative (confused)—spontaneously thrashing about in bed; striking out at others; inattentive to commands
	1	Responds to stimulation only—exhibits only some type of withdrawal or posturing to stimulation
	0	Unresponsive—no response of any kind
3. Stimulus-response (SR)	5	Responds to commands—appropriate response to orientation questions, compliance with hand grasp, toe wiggling, and so on
	4	Responds to name—opens eyes to name, or gives some indication that he or she hears you (nods, moves, etc.) but does not follow all commands
	3	Responds to shaking—responds only to vigorous physical stimulation
	2	Responds to pin prick—responds to light pain applied with pin to trunk or extremities to elicit either withdrawal or posturing
	1	Responds to deep pain—responds only to mandibular pressure, periorbital rub, sternal rub, or pinch
	0	No response—nothing elicited by any stimulus
4. Type of response (TR)	3	Complex withdrawal—withdrawal and attempt to remove stimulus
	2	Simple withdrawal—only withdrawal from stimulus
	1	Posturing—decorticate: head, arms, and hand flexed decerebrate: head extended, arms extended and pronated, back arched
	0	Flaccid—no response
5. Motor All four extremities are rated:	2	Spontaneous use—moves designated extremity or extremities with or without any stimulation
Right upper(RUE)	1	Moves to stimulus only—response only to touch, pin, or deep pain
Right lower(RLE) Left upper(LUE) Left lower(LLE)	0	No movement—nothing
		Weakness of any extremity is described in the area designated on the recording format for the particular extremity.

* Adapted with permission of the American Journal of Nursing Company, from "Assessing the Status of Neurological Patients." *Am. J. Nurs.*, 77 (Sept. 1977), 1479, by K. L. Bolin.

that average scores during the first few weeks of intensive care were prognostic (Bolin, 1977, p. 1479):

Average Score	Prognosis
18–20	Patient will probably be able to function at home with some assistance
10–18	Patient will eventually go to a nursing home
Below 10	Patient is likely to die in the hospital

Nursing Actions Dependent on Assessment

1. Report and record changes in levels of consciousness in behavioral terms. (Changes indicating improvement are as significant as those indicating deterioration.)
2. Safety precautions.
   a. Maintain clear airway. In any patient whose consciousness is depressed, maintenance of a clear airway takes a high priority. (See Chapters 40 and 52.)
   b. Protect the patient who is unable to swallow from his or her own secretions and test ability to swallow before offering fluids. (See Chapters 40 and 46.)
   c. Maintain patient in (prescribed) position.
   d. Turn every 1 to 2 hours. (See Chapter 49.)
   e. Prevent patient from lying on arm when in the side-lying position. (See Chapters 49 and 52.)
   f. Breathing exercises if patient can cooperate. (See Chapter 40.)
   g. Mouth care. Give particular attention to the area around the uvula in patients who breathe through their mouths for lengthy periods of time. Crusts forming in and around the uvula may break off and be aspirated. (See Chapter 52.)
   h. Skin care. (See Chapter 49.)
   i. Side rails, padded if necessary.
   j. Removal of cigarettes, matches, or other harmful objects if patient is confused or delirious.
3. Maintain fluid and food intake. (See Chapters 41, 45, and 46.)
4. Attention to indwelling urinary catheter. (See Chapter 52.)
5. Protect conjunctiva and cornea from exposure to drying.
   a. Remove secretions as indicated.
   b. Bandage the eye.
   c. Request and instill methyl cellulose eye drops ("artificial tears").

Whenever an individual is subjected to stress from any source, be it from psychological, physical, or biologic agents, the sympathoadrenal medullary axis is activated to some extent. In Unit V we discussed implications of this repsonse as part of the nursing responsibilities to support an individual's total effort to avoid, defend against, or respond by repairing injury.

Care of Confused Persons

Given the narrow range of alteration in available oxygen and glucose within which cerebral cortical neurons can continue to function effectively, it is not surprising that *confusion* is one of the patient problems most frequently encountered by the nurse. All of the injurious agents described in Chapter 4 are capable of altering, directly or indirectly, the supply of oxygen and glucose to cells. Common causes of acute confusional states in physically ill individuals include infections and metabolic diseases; surgical and nonsurgical trauma; cardiovascular disease; intracranial vascular, neoplastic or infectious disease; drug intoxication and withdrawal; and senility, alone or in combination with other stated conditions (Adams & Victor, 1977).

Dodd (1978) has developed an assessment tool to document mental status of a hospitalized patient, using descriptions of behavior in five areas proposed to be characteristic of four categories of mental status: *orientation, confusion, disorientation,* and *delirium.* The five types of behavior described for each mental status category include awareness of time and place; awareness of and response to pain; recognition and response to visual and tactile stimuli; and intactness of recent, intermediate, and long-term memory. Although the types of behavior used by Dodd to describe mental status may not be equally applicable to assessment of persons in settings and circumstances other than hospitalization for physical illness, her approach to standardization of measurement of this important functional state is a valuable contribution.

Caring for the confused patient can be perplexing and frustrating to all concerned, including the patient. When approaches are appropriate, manifestations of confusion can be markedly reduced or even eliminated completely. Doctor Trockman, a psychiatrist interested in the alterations of mental status experienced in physical illness, recommends ten ways to help the patient until confusion clears (Trockman, 1978):

1. Ensure adequate sensory reception through the use of eyeglasses, hearing aid, radio, or television. Increase nightime stimulation for sundowners.
2. Maintain familiar surroundings. Provide individual personal contact as needed.
3. Communicate face-to-face with simple, direct, descriptive statements. Do not use complex questions or explanations.
4. Explain what you are doing when giving physical care. Do only what the patient cannot do himself.
5. Moderate the amount of anxiety to keep it tolerable. Encourage realistic optimism.
6. Focus initially on areas of competent functioning to aid internal reorientation.
7. Provide new information slowly and in small doses to help the patient to think logically.
8. Do not respond to delusional material without reinforcing reality.
9. Protect severely agitated patients with constant staff attendance or mittens and restraints. Consider medication for patients who are agitated, delusional, or very frightened.
10. Maintain a tolerant, calm, unflustered manner. Accept the confusional state as a partially adaptive one by which some people cope with devastating insults to their physical and emotional integrity.

Care of Persons with an Altered Level of Consciousness

Granted that a disturbance in the level of consciousness is more likely to be associated with some disorders than with others, it is a possibility in any seriously ill or toxic individual. The first responsibility of the nurse is to watch over the patient in order to detect any changes in the mental state of the patient, which may change with great rapidity. He or she may appear to be alert when seen at one time and 5 minutes later be stuperous.

A great number of intrinsic (internal) and extrinsic (external) factors may depress or alter cerebral function. Probably the factor responsible for CNS depression most frequently encountered by the nurse is administration of anesthetics to persons whose medical problems are treated surgically. (See Chapter 51 for nursing care of patients in the postanesthesia period.) Other factors responsible for altered level of consciousness include (1) intracranial pathology (vascular thromboses or hemorrhage, cerebral edema, neoplasm or infection); (2) cranial or skull lesions and injuries; (3) metabolic disorders in which the homeostatic conditions of cells are altered (hypoglycemia, diabetic ketoacidosis, renal failure, liver failure, or iatrogenic disorders in which the levels of electrolytes such as potassium, hydrogen, and calcium are abnormal): (4) respiratory or circulatory disorders, which result in a failure to supply needed materials or to remove products of energy metabolism; and (5) toxic chemicals, including drugs and microbial products that have a depressing effect on the brain. All of the preceding as well as others may be accompanied by some alteration in the patient's state of consciousness.

The level of consciousness is the most important single indicator of cerebral function. The nurse must be able to detect changes as early as possible. According to one estimate, approximately 3 per cent of patients admitted to city hospitals have a disturbance in level of consciousness. Many more develop an alteration after admission. A point that must be emphasized is that the terms *conscious* and *unconscious* are abstractions. They are used differently in general medicine, psychiatry, psychology, and philosophy. The nurse should also know that mental function cannot be divided into clear or distinctive stages between consciousness and unconsciousness.

The nurse observes the patient to gather data to answer two major questions: (1) What is the direction of change, that is, is the patient improving or getting worse? (2) What is (are) the possible cause(s) of loss of consciousness? Descriptions of behavior are likely to be more helpful than naming a stage in answering these questions. In general the level of consciousness is assessed by noting the patient's response to various types of stimuli—verbal, tactile, visual, and painful. As the patient loses consciousness, he or she goes from alert and purposeful behavior to purposeless behavior. As improvement occurs, the reverse is true. Bolin's (1977) guide to neurological status description and evaluation, described in the previous discussion, will help increase accuracy of descriptions and patterning of changes in neurological status.

When observing for skeletal muscle response, the nurse should note the patient's ability to move voluntarily on command in the following ways: extremities, smile, puckering of lips, hand grasp, eye movements, change of position. The patient's ability to swallow and control of elimination of urine and feces must also be assessed, as well as the condition of the skin, mouth, eyes, and ears.

The following definitions may be helpful in predicting, recognizing, and describing altered states of consciousness.

Conscious. Alert, awake, aware; responds promptly to visual, auditory, tactile, and painful stimuli. Oriented to time, place, and self. Responds spontaneously to questions. In respect to orientation, awareness of time is first to be lost and awareness of self is last to disappear. Response to simple commands such as "squeeze my hand" is lost following disorientation to self. A point to be kept in mind is that when a person is in a strange environment or sleeping patterns are disturbed, he or she may not know the hour of the day or the day of the week. Fully conscious patients may comment about "losing track" of time. On the other hand, gross misjudging of time is usually significant. A patient may appear to be fully alert and reveal some loss of awareness by making an irrelevant remark. As an example, Mrs. Alpha, aged 84, was hospitalized for the treatment of congestive heart failure. She was given digitalis and diuretics. Her serum postassium was 3 mEq/L. The only indication of a disturbance in mentation was a comment to her nurse. She believed that it was 1915 and that she was in the hospital to have a baby. Her nurse reminded her that it was 1979. The nurse also gave her orange juice to drink and reported and recorded the incident. The patient's judgment may be tested by asking him or her to interpret a well-known saying such as "The grass is greener on the other side of the fence." The nurse should try to select statements that will have meaning to the patient and remember that the higher the patient's intelligence and level of education, the more difficult it is to test judgment. Others, such as family members, report failing judgment before a physician or nurse can detect it.

Confusion. The state of an individual who is unable to recognize and respond to the environment in a normal manner. For example, Mr. Penn thinks that his nurse is his granddaughter. Conversely, some patients believed to be confused are not when all the facts are known. [See Dodd (1978).]

Lethargy. Drowsiness, somnolence, a dull sluggish state. The patient can be aroused and may be clear mentally, but is frequently somewhat confused. Answers questions with sentences, but slowly.

Obtundation. Dull, lacks mental acuteness. The patient can be awakened but little more. Uses gestures but few words.

Stupor. The patient can be aroused only by vigorous and continuous stimulation; he or she may move spontaneously and respond to painful, loud noises and bright light. Response is usually by withdrawal, but the patient may be combative. Bowel and bladder control varies. Able to locate site of painful stimulation.

Semicoma. The patient responds only to painful stimuli by mass movement.

Coma. Varies from moderate coma to deep coma. In moderate coma the patient has rudimentary reflex motor responses. In deep coma all psychological and motor responses are lost. The patient is incontinent of feces and urine.

Delirium. A self-limiting state associated with an acute brain syndrome. It is characterized by fluctuating levels of consciousness. The patient is disorientated as to time, place, and person. He or she may experience anxiety to the point of panic. When this anxiety is severe, the patient may attempt suicide. Hallucinations, especially of the visual type, may occur. The patient may fear that he or she will be poisoned or harmed in some way.

Sleep. A state of cortical inactivity reflected in an electroencephalogram characterized by slow random waves. The production of this state physiologically depends upon a complex interplay between the cerebral cortex and the central reticular formation in which the alerting influence of the central reticular formation upon the cortex temporarily falls into abeyance. Electrical stimulation of an area of the hypothalamus can induce sleep (Bannister, 1973). Sleep and wakefulness are cyclical states occurring under predictable conditoins; a sleeping person can be fully awakened by an unusual stimulus. The amount of stimulation required varies with the depth of sleep.

An all too common error is the presumption that any patient admitted in a stuporous or comatose state and who has the odor of alcohol on his or her breath is intoxicated. The patient may or may not be. As a result he or she may be allowed to die from the effects of some treatable disorder such as hypoglycemia or a subdural hematoma.

Care of Persons with Increased Intracranial Pressure (IICP)

In the adult, there is no potential for expansion of the skull when the need arises. The skull has many foramina in it provided for the entry or emergence of blood vessels and nerves, but they are well sealed off. The fontanels have long been closed, and the suture lines are too tight to be split open again. The only major opening in the skull is the foramen magnum. There can be no increase in bulk of any element within the head except at the expense of something else (Monro-Kellie doctrine) (Elliott, 1963, p. 402). Therefore increase in intracranial pressure must occur with increase in intracranial bulk from any cause, and if this is long continued, the brain is pressed downward into the foramen magnum. The resulting pressure on the medulla oblongata partly or completely cuts off its blood supply *(pressure conus)*, and death occurs almost immediately as a consequence of respiratory failure.

Increased intracranial pressure may develop slowly, as in the case of a tumor growing above the tentorium, or very rapidly after a *head injury.*[1] or rupture of an intracranial aneurysm, with intracranial bleeding that frees a high-protein fluid eager to attract and hold water in a box that is already full.[2] Intracranial pressure rises in inflammatory diseases of the nervous system such as encephalitis. In any condition where there is arteriolar spasm, the volume of blood circulating in the capillaries is reduced, and they become highly permeable. This can occur in acute nephritis and in malignant hypertension, and results in an edematous brain. Anything that blocks, partly or completely, the normal course of cerebrospinal fluid will cause pressure to rise. This could be a tumor that presses on the channels, gluey inflammatory exudate from meningitis that seals the foramina of Magendie and Luschka or absorptive areas in the meninges over the cortex. Whatever the cause, the patient is likely to demonstrate some characteristic signs. Although some signs may be caused by local pressure, they depend much more on the fact that the more crowded the nonexpansible space becomes within the cranium, the more limited will be the blood supply, and hence the oxygen, to each cell. The point of no return for the cells of the cerebral cortex in respect to lack of oxygen comes quickly, and for the cells of the brainstem a little later, but none can stand starvation for long, and the patient's symptomatology reflects their faltering.

[1] *Head injury* is trauma to the scalp, skull, meninges and/or brain, with severity defined by effect on brain function. A definition of a *severe brain injury* is one that causes amnesia of more than 24 hours (Meyd, 1978).

[2] Intracranial bleeding, or *subarachnoid hemorrhage* (SAH), is confirmed by lumbar puncture that reveals blood in the CSF. The stiff neck and severe headache associated with SAH are due to meningeal irritation. A frequent cause is rupture of congenitally weak or bulging artery(ies) *(aneurysm)* of the circle of Willis. Immediate goals of treatment are (1) to stop bleeding by reducing the pressure of cerebral blood flow and interfering with fibrinolysis and (2) to prevent or reduce IICP. If the patient survives the critical 7 to 21 days after bleeding, the long-term goal is to prevent rebleeding. This may be accomplished by (1) long-term hypotensive drugs or (2) surgery: excision of the aneurysm or ligation of the common carotid artery.

Persons with increased intracranial pressure have headache. They need to have their heads elevated somewhat and often to be given acetylsalicylic acid compounds and caffeine. Elevation assists venous return from the head and caffeine is a cerebral vasoconstrictor agent and so decreases the headache. The nurse will find no orders to give opiates that decrease respiratory rate and efficiency, already depressed by the disease process. As congestion increases, the blood pressure will rise and the rate of pulse will slow down, because of ischemia of vasomotor centers. The patient, who may have been restless and irritable earlier, becomes lethargic and slow in verbal responses. Later he or she may be stuporous. In stupor the individual is not alert to the stimuli which would ordinarily elicit responses, but can be roused with some effort. As pressure continues, respirations may become arrhythmical with periods of apnea, and the patient falls into a coma from which he or she cannot be roused; and at last, unless relieved, the hard-pressed bulb can no longer send forth stimuli to produce any respiration.

At any point in this sequence of events, the nurse may note signs referable to involvement of cranial nerves other than X and should be alert to these and report them: A dilated pupil that fails to constrict on exposure to a light, drooping of one eyelid (III), and facial weakness (VII) should not only be recorded, but also the time at which these signs were first observed. These signs, and others, are not necessarily results of the increased intracranial pressure itself but are indicative of changes going on and of further involvement that the nurse, being present, may be the first to note.

Patients with increased intracranial pressure are required to have continuous or very frequent (every 5 to 30 minutes) observations of their pulse, respiration, and blood pressure. Recording should be done on a graphic flow sheet, for economy of time of both the recorder and the reader of the information. Regardless of who is assigned the task, it is the professional nurse's duty to know the trend of the record so that the physician may be notified if this trend becomes adverse. A record of vital signs that shows a consistent slowing of pulse and respiration accompanied by a rising blood pressure should be called to the physician's attention and not just left for him or her to find.

The subarachnoid screw is a new device inserted directly in the cerebrospinal fluid (CSF) of the cranial subarachnoid space via a burr hole in the skull, thus permitting a direct reading of intracranial pressure (Johnson & Quinn, 1977). Cerebrospinal fluid pressure is converted by a transducer into electrical current, which records pressure readings on an oscilloscope, in a manner similar to electroencephalogram and electrocardiogram tracings. Nursing responsibilities include the following:

1. Careful preparation of the patient and family for the purpose and process of the procedure
2. Maintenance of sterility of the entire system to prevent infection
3. Strick adherence to specified procedure for safe and accurate readings of intracranial pressure (See Johnson & Quinn, 1977, p. 450.)
4. Prevention of any leaks in the system that could either introduce saline and increase intracranial pressure or drain CSF and lower intracranial pressure
5. Close observation of neurological signs, *not to be replaced by ICP monitoring.*

When patients have surgery for some difficulty that lies intracranially below the tentorium and within the confines of the posterior fossa, the bone that is removed is not replaced. Often the dura is not resutured at the end of the operation. Several blood vessels will have been clipped during the surgery, and the blood supply may be temporarily somewhat less than normal. Edema may build up in the area in the hours after operation and endanger the patient's respiration temporarily, for the patient may be subjected to considerable compression of the bulb thereby. It is safest always with patients who have had craniotomies of this sort to keep the head in alignment with the body at all times including those moments when he or she is being turned. The rules are simple: (1) have as many persons as are necessary to turn without twisting the patient, and (2) leave the patient supported on the side so that his or her nose is in line with the xiphoid process. If the patient is an infant, one nurse can safely accomplish the turning alone; but if he is a man, this may require four nurses, with one person whose sole duty is control of the head. The infant's large head and narrow shoulders usually permit lining up nose and xiphoid very simple, securing the position by a small folded pad under the side of the chin. A child's head, being relatively smaller in relation to the shoulders than the infant's will need one or two folded pillowcases; and the athlete with heavy broad shoulders will need to have considerable height to the support under the head to bring it in line. When the work of adjusting the patient's position has been well done, he or she should be so perfectly balanced that there is no need for a pillow at the back although there is no objection to this, if the patient wants it, after correct position has been attained.

Two primary objectives of nursing care of the person who is predisposed to or exhibiting signs of IICP are (1) close observation, reporting and recording of behavior, and (2) protection from any events that may (a) increase cerebral arterial blood flow or (b) decrease venous return. Because muscular activity tends to increase cerebral arterial blood flow, the conscious patient should be instructed to lie quietly and to avoid sudden movements. The physical environment should be kept free of disturbing stimuli, such as strong odors, bright lights, clutter, extremes of temperature, loud or annoying noises, and disturbing people. The nurse should precede all procedures with a quiet, concise description of what she or he is about to do, requiring as little response and participation from the patient as possible. Because flexion or extension of the head on the body interferes with venous return, the patient should neither raise the head nor feed himself or herself. He or she may be allowed one thin pillow to keep the head and neck in a neutral position. Because elevation of intrathoracic pressure interferes with venous return, activities that involve holding the breath after a deep inspiration, such as coughing and straining during defecation or urination, are particularly dangerous. Medication may need to be requested to suppress cough and soften stool.

Mitchell and Mauss (1976) state seven ways to protect patients at risk from sudden increases in intracranial pressure:

1. Maintain fully patent airway.
2. Maintain adequate ventilation
   a. Monitor blood gases
   b. Auscultate chest
   c. Suction if necessary for 15 seconds maximum
   d. Hyperinflate with O_2 before suctioning (with MD consultation)
3. Position carefully
   a. Avoid prone position
   b. Prevent neck flexion
   c. Avoid extreme (90° or greater) hip flexion
   d. Elevate head 15–30°.
4. Prevent Valsalva's maneuver
   a. Stool softeners to prevent constipation
   b. Avoid enemas
   c. Instruct alert patient to exhale while turning, moving in bed
5. Prevent isometric muscular contraction
   a. Assist patient to move up in bed
   b. Instruct patient not to push against foot board
6. *Do* perform passive range of motion exercises to joint.
7. Plan nursing care procedures so that those that might precipitate increased pressure are not performed together.

The importance of conscientious observation and the above regimen in the prevention of respiratory fail-

TABLE 36-2. *Antiepileptic Drugs**

Drugs of Choice	Indications	Usual Adult Maintenance Dose, mg./day and (Dose Range)	Desirable Blood Concentration µg/ml.	Side Effects and Adverse Reactions
Phenytoin—new generic name for diphenylhydantoin (Dilantin)	generalized convulsive seizures, all forms of partial seizures; often in combination with primidone and/or phenobarbital	300 (200–600)	15–25	drowsiness, gastric distress, gingival hyperplasia, rash, megaloblastic anemia, ataxia, diplopia, fever, hirsuitism
Phenobarbital (Luminal)	generalized convulsive seizures, all forms of partial seizures; often in combination with phenytoin	90 (60–400)	10–30	drowsiness, rash, ataxia
Primidone (Mysoline)	generalized convulsive seizures, all forms of partial seizures; often in combination with phenytoin and/or phenobarbital	750 (500–1500)	5–15	drowsiness, dizziness, rash, megalobastic anemia, ataxia, diplopia, nystagmus
Ethosuximide (Zarontin)	generalized nonconvulsive seizures, especially petit mal; used in mixed seizure states with phenytoin	750 (500–2000)	30–100	gastric distress, nausea, vomiting, anorexia, dermatitis, drowsiness, dizziness, blood dyscrasias
Alternative Drugs				
Carbamazepine (Tegretol)	generalized convulsive seizures, partial seizures, especially psychomotor; also used for treatment of trigeminal neuralgia	800 (600–1600)	3–6	headache, drowsiness, dizziness, feelings of inhibition, gait disturbances, blood dyscrasias
Mephenytoin (Mesantoin)	generalized convulsive seizures, all forms of partial seizures	300 (300–800)		drowsiness, rash, blood dyscrasias
Mephobarbital (Mebaral)	same as phenobarbital			drowsiness, irritability, rash
Trimethadione (Tridione)	generalized nonconvulsive seizures—petit mal, myoclonic and akinetic; often used with phenytoin and phenobarbital	900 (900–2400)	600–800	drowsiness, gastric distress, rash hemeralopia, blood dyscrasias, nephrosis
Paramethadione (Paradione)	generalized nonconvulsive seizures, especially petit mal; sometimes useful for psychomotor seizures	900 (900–2400)		gastric distress, rash, photophobia, blood dyscrasias
Methsuximide (Celontin)	generalized nonconvulsive seizures, especially petit mal; sometimes useful for psychomotor seizures	900 (600–1200)		drowsiness, headaches, anorexia, blood dyscrasias, ataxia
Phensuximide (Milontin)	generalized nonconvulsive seizures, sometimes useful for psychomotor seizures	1500 (1000–4000)		dizziness, hematuria, nausea, rash

TABLE 36-2. *(Continued)*

Drugs of Choice	Indications	Usual Adult Maintenance Dose, mg./day and (Dose Range)	Desirable Blood Concentration μg/ml.	Side Effects and Adverse Reactions
Phenacemide (Phenurone)	only used in resistant cases because of toxicity; all types of seizures, especially psychomotor	3000 (1000–6000)		liver damage, psychotic behavior, nausea, rash
Acetazolamide (Diamox)	sometimes useful for petit mal seizures; in all seizure disorders as an adjuvant to control seizures related to menstrual cycle	750 (500–1000)		anorexia, dizziness, drowsiness
Dextroamphetamine Sulfate (Dexedrine)	used with some antiepileptics to counteract sedative effects; some therapeutic effect in petit mal	(15–30)		anorexia, irritability, insomnia

* Used with permission of the American Journal of Nursing Co., from "Epilepsy: A Controllable Disease." *Am. J. Nurs.*, **76** (March 1976), 388–97, 395, by M. A. Bruya and R. H. Bolin.

ure resulting from pressure conus in susceptible patients cannot be overemphasized.

Care of Persons Subject to Seizures

Many times disease in the nervous system is accompanied by seizures, convulsions, or fits, three terms that should be equally useful, although the shortest one seems, nowadays, to be regarded as undignified. A seizure is a symptom, not a disease. *Seizure* is a transitory disturbance in consciousness or in motor, sensory, or autonomic function that is due to uncontrolled electrical discharges in the brain. The terms *seizure* and *epilepsy* are used synonymously (Bruya & Bolin, 1976, p. 388). Myth and social discrimination still surround the diagnosis of epilepsy, despite massive public education efforts, legislative advances, and good control of seizures with modern drug therapy. Compliance with prescribed antiepileptic medication results in significant control in 70 to 80 per cent of all patients (Bruya & Bolin, 1976, p. 393).

Major nursing responsiblities in the care of epileptic patients is to help both patient and family restore control (1) by understanding and avoiding precipitating factors, and (2) by developing a system to guarantee that the patient consistently takes prescribed medication. Of vital importance in the system for taking antiepileptic drugs is knowledge of their side effects, how to minimize them, and what to do if they persist. See Table 36–2 for indications, dosage, and side effects of antiepileptic drugs in common use.

ACUTE CARE

Until the nurse has had some experience with patients who are subject to seizures, she or he may fail to recognize those of a minor nature *(petit mal)* that often have no, or only a slight, motor component. The experienced person will recognize the momentary lapse of focus, the fading out of the voice, and the little meaningless movements of a part as manifestations of a seizure and will record the occurrence. No one can fail to note or recognize a major convulsion, but the inexperienced nurse may be frightened and rendered incompetent when first seeing one. Fear reduces effectiveness, and the patient who has seizures may need some assistance from the nurse. The physician, too, may need a careful description of the attack.

Although the patient may be in bed when the attack starts, it is quite likely that he may not and that he or she will fall down. In a large percentage of major *(grand mal)* attacks, the person is immediately unconscious and in a state of generalized tonicity, with teeth clenched, body stiff, and no respiratory exchange occurring at all. Although this phase lasts only a few seconds, it is long enough for the face to become very turgid in appearance and for saliva to collect in great quantity. Shortly, the fit shifts to rhythmical jerking, the clonic phase; the patient breathes adequately, and the color clears. This clonic phase lasts from moments to many minutes. Gradually, the rhythmical jerking becomes slower and slower and finally stops, and the patient shows signs of returning consciousness, often making random movements accompanied by attempts at verbalization, but the patient seems confused and still incompetent. Complete recovery from the attack is usual after a period of sleep, although headache for a few hours is not uncommon.

Because, at the onset of the attack, clenching of the jaws occurs at once, there is no possible way to prevent the patient's biting the tongue if it was between the teeth when they clamped together. Neither is there any way to prevent the patient from "turning black in the face and foaming from the mouth," for he or she is not breathing. No attempt should be made to force a wedge between the teeth. To do so results in bruising the gums and has been known to break a tooth. These few moments can be employed more usefully in loosening the collar and belt. After this, one cannot do better than to drop to the floor, kneeling at the patient's head, and taking it firmly in hand, prop it either on one's own thighs or on a jacket or sweater placed underneath it, turning the head so that saliva can run out and the tongue drop forward away from the airway. It is now possible to insert a padded wedge, but this is rarely useful. By this time the convulsion will be in the clonic phase and one can protect the patient's head from pounding up and down on the floor or pavement throughout the attack. Although a postseizure headache may be the rule, it is certainly not made less severe by preventable banging. It is neither useful nor advisable to restrain the patient during the attack other than to control the head. Urinary incontinence often occurs during the seizure, and sometimes fecal as well. No attempt should be made to move the patient until the seizure is over unless attendant circumstances make this imperative. Furniture or other encumbrances should be moved away. When the attack is over, the patient should be helped to a quiet place and permitted to sleep until he or she wakes, when activities may be resumed as before, if the patient feels able.

Certain convulsions are focal in nature. They start at a point and spread. This type of seizure may indicate a localized lesion in the brain and is often immediately preceded by paresthesias in the part that will shortly begin to twitch. Patients subject to such attacks often have time to walk to a bed and lie down and even to put a wadded face cloth or hankerchief between their teeth before the attack begins. They are usually conscious for the early part of the seizure, but, when it spreads to become generalized, are likely to become unconscious briefly.

These attacks should be carefully and completely described by the nurse, especially if one has not already been observed by the patient's physician. This is not easy to do the first time, and a nurse should not be chagrined at failing to note everything, so long as she or he is accurate in reporting what has been seen. The following will illustrate a description.

> Patient came to me looking scared and said, "Rub my left hand." I did so and walked with her to her bed where she lay down, and immediately the fingers of the left hand began rhythmical twitching. This spread to involve wrist, whole arm, and then left leg, and then the whole body. The patient seemed to watch the jerking until the attack became generalized, at which time she was apparently unconscious. I did not time the attack but estimate it to have been altogether about a minute and one half, with the period of unsonsciousness about 15 seconds. The patient was alert again shortly after the attack. Her left-hand grip was weak and remained so for an hour.
>
> [Signature]

Care of Persons Undergoing Diagnostic Procedures

Diagnostic procedures such as lumbar puncture, pneumoencephalogram, and ventriculogram are not always accorded the seriousness they deserve and are needlessly uncomfortable. One who is to have a lumbar puncture should be helped to the appropriate position on the side with thighs flexed on the abdomen, back bowed, but with the lumbar spine kept parallel to the edge of the treatment table. The patient must keep the "up" shoulder from falling forward or the spine will rotate. If the nurse slips her or his arm under the patient's neck, stoops, and opposes a shoulder to the patient's, it will make this easy for the patient and will secure the shoulder. At the same time the nurse can slip the other arm around the back of the patient's knees to help him or her remain in the hip-flexed position.

Lumbar puncture is primarily a diagnostic procedure that is absolutely indicated (1) when central nervous system infection is suspected, in order to identify the organism, and (2) before using anticoagulants to treat a transient ischemic attack (TIA) or an evolving stroke, to be sure the neurologic signs are not due to cerebral hemorrhage instead of ischemia (Posner, 1973). Lumbar puncture can also be used to introduce into the CSF medications that cross the blood–brain barrier poorly. This procedure is safe, relatively simple, and painless when the patient is placed and maintained in the proper position, and when the physician's technique is careful. However, possible complications for which the nurse must watch closely for 24 to 48 hours following the procedure include headache, backache, evidence of pressure conus, signs of epidural hematoma in patients with bleeding tendencies, reaction to anesthetic agent, and signs of meningitis that may result from a contaminated needle. Whenever high pressure is found at the time of spinal puncture, observation of the patient should be constant for at least 24 hours (Posner, 1973, p. 21).

Patients who are to have air or oxygen injections into the ventricular system either directly through a burr hole in the skull or by the lumbar subarachnoid space should have forewarning of post-procedure headache and know that they will be asked afterward to turn from side to side. The injected air, being light, tends to pocket in the uppermost ventricle. There is no mechanism for absorption in the ventricle; the gas will have to go the regular route. (See Figure 16–2). Recovery from the procedure is slow if the patient refuses to roll, and rolling over hurts for the first day.

Both these procedures have hazards. Gases such as air or oxygen are foreign bodies to these tissues and produce cellular reaction. Sudden withdrawal of considerable fluid from below reduces pressure in the spinal canal, the fluid in the cranial cavity rushes toward the area of reduced pressure, carrying the medulla with it, causing death from respiratory arrest. Therefore encephalogram is not done when there is any considerable increase in intracranial pressure. It is especially hazardous if the cause of pressure lies below the tentorium, as in cerebellar tumor. If visualization of the ventricles is important, the ventriculogram may be safer, for the tentorium provides a roof between, and the pressure changes incurred by the procedure are less likely to produce medullary compression. Uncomfortable and unfavorable responses may occur in response to these air injections whether or not the report is "negative." Every patient subjected to these examinations deserves intelligent observation and thoughtful care, which will necessarily include watching for signs of generalized increase in intracranial pressure, as a response to the irritation from the injected gas, and especially for depressed respirations.

Feeding the Physically Dependent Person

In normal healthy existence, one ordinarily swallows while in a sitting or standing position when the head is in line with the body. It is not difficult, however, to swallow when the head is slightly flexed forward, as one does in using a drinking fountain; but to twist the head sharply to the side and eat is so difficult that one always returns one's head to the midline, or nearly, before swallowing. Persons who are recumbent in bed are therefore at a disadvantage in respect to ease of swallowing. The position is unnatural. If aware of her or his own behavior in respect to this normally automatic act, the nurse will be careful to make eating as easy as it can be for the patient in bed. This will always include having the patient's head in line with his or her body and, unless specifically contraindicated, somewhat elevated. If this elevation cannot be allowed, the patient should be carefully placed in a side-lying position for safety, because it is very difficult for a small nurse to assist a large patient, who is lying perfectly flat on his or her back, quickly enough to avoid serious aspiration if choking occurs while attempting to swallow. The patient who has a neurologic problem may be trying to cope not only with a position that is mechanically unfavorable but with an organic difficulty in the act of swallowing too.

In some clinics, after craniotomy no patient is permitted anything by mouth until "tested for swallowing" by the surgeon. The observant nurse will note that the physician who is doing this has put the patient well over on the side, has made sure the patient's mouth is clear, and has the suction tip in one hand and a teaspoon of water in the other. The physician then introduces water carefully and watches intently to see how successfully this act of swallowing is completed. If swallowing is impossible for the patient at this time, it is easy for the physician to suction the fluid back. Even when a patient is permitted feedings after a successful test, the nurse should appreciate the recent difficulties and act to make eating as safe and as easy as it can be.

Neurologic patients often have trouble with vomiting, both those with lesions in the appropriate areas in the brainstem and those with generalized intracranial pressure. If the reasons for this vomiting cannot be remedied promptly, the individual's nutrition suffers. Careful observation of time and circumstances that provoke emesis is needed. The patient's self-observations in this regard may be helpful and should be sought. There are often patterns of serving food to the patient that will result in more calories being retained than just by giving the three meals a day in the routine manner at the routine hours. If, for instance, radical change of posture provokes trouble, it may be advisable to get the patient out of bed before breakfast so that the episode will be over some time before breakfast is served. If the man has had trouble after his regular full meals but manages successfully a dry ham sandwich at 3:30 every afternoon, it will be worth trying to give him only solids at meals and his fluids in between. There are no rules for guidance except those of careful observation, resourcefulness, and concern for the patient's welfare. Remember that the patient's trouble is in the brain and not the digestive tract; and if the nurse either withholds food because of vomiting or fails to meet the basic nutritional needs of the patient through supplying again the calories that were lost—and chlorides along with them—there may arise problems of electrolyte balance to add to those already present. (See Chapters 41 and 46.)

Nursing Involvement with Sensory Stimulation and Deprivation

Living things gain their knowledge of how to adapt to life through sensory experience. The body of the sea anemone is stimulated by the incoming tide and puts forth its tentacles to catch food that the fresh inflow of water will bring. The intelligent, highly trained and practiced college youth sights the football coming his way and runs to place himself in position to complete a play, the strategy of which he fully comprehends, and to which he can make a number of adaptations. Bruner, who is quoted in J. A. Vernon's monograph on experiments in sensory deprivation, says, "We deal with our environment by a set of models or expectancies that have been gradually acquired since birth. They are based on previous experience" (Vernon, 1963, p. 200). The needs and experiences of the sea anemone and of the college football player are widely different, but for both, the essential elements are present. The coelenterate will not act appropriately without the stimulus of the changing environment, nor will the man.

Sight is a dominant sense for those who can see, and the nurse should give attention in basic care to supporting ocular defense mechanisms. It has been estimated that a sighted person obtains 90 per cent of the sensory information from the external environment through the eyes. The ocular defense mechanism includes tears, the conjunctiva, and eyelid action. The conjunctiva is rich in all immunologic components (Baum, 1978). When ocular defenses are intact, nursing care should address structuring the environment in such a way that light, color, texture, and people provide visual stimulation appropriate to the sensory needs of the patient's general condition; that may require an enrichment, rearrangement, or depletion of sources of visual stimulation to the patient. When ocular defenses are impaired, the nurse must include provisions to prevent irritation, infection, and ulceration of the poorly defended eye.

The sense of touch has been referred to earlier as all-important and it is of considerable significance to nurses. The animal has means for receiving touch just about everywhere on the body surface and a variety of tracts by which it ascends to the brain. He or she has, in the reticular formation, means for alerting wide areas of the cortex and for involving the cranial nerves: in the cerebellum and basal ganglia the animal has means for completing the integration and plan for control. Tracts descending in the spinal cord inform the muscles by way of the neuron of the final common path, and activity takes place.

Stimulation of the body surface of the newborn animal by the mother's tongue as she licks it dry is followed by defecation and the getting underway of its digestive tract. If deprived of this or comparable stimulation by mechanical means, digestive activity does not occur and the baby animal dies. The child who is born deaf or blind has a devastating handicap because of the sensory deprivation and will need extraordinary incitements to learning by the stimulation of the remaining major senses, sight or hearing and touch, if he or she is to come eventually to respond adequately to life. When a previously well person suffers illness or mutilation of any considerable degree, the environment changes, body image may be considerably modified, and his or her life as a patient may markedly change the sensory inflow on which so much behavior is based. It is only this last that will be considered here in reference to some common nursing situations.

The baby girl who at a few months of age is noted to have congenitally dislocated hips has fully half of her body, about which she has been learning since birth, encased in a rigid plaster for many months. She no longer has the experience of kicking, hitting her legs together, and learning to play with her feet, thereby getting to know all about this half of her body, because it is no longer available to her. She does not gain experience in reciprocal motion, in learning the feel of textures and of varying weights and pressures upon her legs. The environment of the lower half of her body is homogeneous, receiving few stimuli, offering her little to evaluate and therefore little from which she can learn.

From these facts arise two situations of concern to the nurse. This very young child who has necessarily suffered deprivation of sensory experience will have very little knowledge to go on when she is released from her cast, mechanically sound, and undertakes the task of learning to walk. Her performance cannot be compared to that of her 3-year-old contemporary who happens to break a leg, is in a cast for a few weeks, and is running around again without difficulty shortly after being released. Although the sensory and motor deprivations are serious, they are unavoidable under the circumstances, and the child's nurses will do everything they can to stimulate her senses in other areas, giving her toys she must manipulate, food to handle, stories to listen to, people to talk to, and a change of environment by moving her from place to place.

The human being finds a homogeneous situation unendurable and will strive to change it in any way available. If a new environment cannot be built the individual will rid himself or herself of the old in order to effect some sort of change, and the change the individual can most easily make is to fall asleep. The nurse will recognize that for this child, or for patients of any age, 2-hour naps morning and afternoon and 12 hours of sleep at night are indications not for keeping curtains down but for raising them both literally and figuratively.

Early sensory deprivation prevents the formation of adequate models and strategies for dealing with the environment, as illustrated in simplest form by the foregoing example of the baby with dislocated hips who is deprived before she has had much chance to learn. Normal adults, however, who were experimentally deprived by isolation in a dark room, demonstrated marked upset of their ordinary discriminative and evaluative abilities. Bruner found that these men failed to identify common foods or to enjoy eating. They gauged time poorly, they slept to excess and dreamed beyond their usual patterns, and suffered various hallucinatory phenomena. All these men knew that the confinement was temporary and that change and normal life would return, yet when sensory input was sharply reduced, integration was inadequate and the behavior faulty or bizarre (Bruner, 1961).

The sick individual, more or less sensorily deprived, may not be confident that everything will be all right again in the future and, being sick, does not have normal forces to help in making the best adjustments. He or she needs the help of others, certainly of the nurses.

An elderly man who has recently had a stroke with resulting hemiplegia and aphasia has lost what once he had opportunity to develop fully. Recovery of useful motion and speech will be hard and will advance very little with nurses who handle him as little as they can and who give their meager care in silence. Unless there is sensory input there will be little output. "Mr. Abdou, I am washing your arm and hand. Now I am bending your wrist up. I'd like you to help me to do this and I'll tickle it a little so you will feel it better." The stroke has deprived Mr. Abdou, and his nurse knows that his hand and arm can become increasingly remote from him and thereby harder to rehabilitate without stimulation and continued awareness. The fact of deprivation creates a situation that "upsets the balance of the regulating system, namely, the ascending reticular arousal system (ARAS). When this happens perception is disrupted, attention gives way to distractibility, and interest to boredom. Behavioral performance is either held in abeyance or becomes highly stereotyped and not adaptive" (Lindsley 1961).

The man who has had the stroke will be helped to regain lost motor patterns as well as more subtle interests and abilities by appropriate sensory stimulation and other therapy. But it is not only deprivation that results in poor or undesirable responses but also what Lindsley calls sensory distortion and sensory overload. All represent disturbances within the ARAS by which the higher parts of the brain are poorly informed and do not integrate and respond normally.

There are diseases during which one aims to reduce sensory stimulation for the very reason that there is hyperesthesia. With hyperesthesia, undesired and harmful motor responses occur from any kind of sensory stimulation. Tetanus is one such disease, and acute meningitis another. Certainly, too, there are times when tactile stimulation can be damaging or make it hard for the patient. Inconsequent sensory stimulation can result promptly in dramatic emotional disturbance (Riesen, 1961). Examples of the sad truth of this crowd the mind: the sudden change of affect to one of withdrawal or seemingly unprovoked weeping by the patient who has overheard what was not meant for his or her ears (inconsequent auditory input), and the anger and increased agony of the one who, being in great pain, has been severely jarred when the bed is knocked by a passing portable x-ray machine. It is in daily routines of care that nurses often needlessly fail their patients. To darken a room simply because the patient is ill is as thoughtless as it is totally irrational, the more so if the patient is chronically or progressively ill. It is not uncommon for someone to darken a room for the patient's afternoon rest and then never reenter it to raise the shades. The patient, awakening from a postprandial nap to a dreary twilight, makes no effort to move or undertake any occupation and so slips farther down the slope toward apathy. Human beings seek light from early infancy throughout life: when they are ill, it should not be denied them.

With increasing years and attendant diminution of sensory perception, acuity of sight and hearing especially, one may expect less accuracy in interpretation than formerly. This is especially the case when there are concomitant arteriosclerotic changes in the brain. In general, people in their own homes or familiar surroundings adapt satisfactorily to these gradual losses as they have to other changes within themselves throughout life. With illness and transfer to an unfamiliar environment in a hospital where they are attended by many persons who are strangers and are subjected to procedures and a daily mode of living that is foreign, often in noisy surroundings, the elderly become the victims not only of the illness that has put them in hospital but also of the effect of the altered environment on sensory systems less acute than they used to be, and, therefore more prone to provoke inaccurate or false integration and response.

Some elderly patients struggle with the confusion, asking for repetition of what they do not hear or understand, complaining and demanding frequently, and refusing to be conquered by circumstances with which they need help. These patients are not really difficult; one has only to give the help and to respond to the demands and clarify what is irritating or confusing. One can identify the shadows of the waving branches outside that make queer patterns on the wall, and explain the meaning of the squawking loudspeaker that is so offensive and sounds like Donald Duck calling the doctors.

Patients who have no courage or energy to struggle are those whose needs are greater and who demand much more acuity on the part of those who care for them. In childhood, in old age, and at any age in time of severe illness, common sensory experiences may become distorted and terrifying. We expect this in childhood and are prepared for it; with the aged and severely ill, the possibility of confusion is not to be forgotten and can be anticipated. "Mrs. Elder, do you enjoy watching the play of the shadows of those lilac branches on your wall or does it annoy you? I can move your chair so you can see them more easily or not at all." "Mr. Olds, I think that the loudspeaker that calls the doctors has been bothering you. It distorts voices dreadfully, I know, but it will soon be turned off for the night."

The elderly patient, being often worn and tired, easily deals with the altered environment by withdrawal from it. He or she sleeps, dozes when urged out of bed, accepts everything wanly, and does not seem to seek to communicate at all. From such a patient, already withdrawn, breeziness and chatter will rarely receive a favorable response. One must work from a more basic level than that of verbal interchange. Often the nurse's best approach is through touch. Physical care of a simple kind given with dignity and gentleness conveys feeling to the patient and is a means of communication of an elemental and very fundamental nature. By acceptance of this feeling, the patient is stimulated to respond, perhaps not with speech but by some change of position made to assist the nurse in his or her care. This move is the nurse's satisfaction and success; she or he has comprehended the patient's needs, can now formulate plans for working to meet them, and by this slight response from the patient, the nurse sees that the first goal has already been achieved.

Altered Motor Function

As indicated in Chapter 17, loss of any degree of mobility has immediate and devastating consequences for one's independence and autonomy. Problems with mobility are detailed in Chapter 50.

Care of Persons in Pain

Probably no human experience is more illustrative of the highly complex, integrated, and holistic pattern of neurologically regulated behavior than pain. One of the most common manifestations of illness is pain and fear of pain. In the minds of many people some illnesses, such as cancer, as well as certain treatments, such as surgery, are practically synonymous with pain. The nurse has a significant role in both the prevention and relief of pain.

To fulfill that role with understanding, the nurse requires some knowledge of (1) the nature of pain, (2) the anatomy and physiology of pain, (3) what constitutes the pain experience, (4) the factors increasing the suffering caused by pain, (5) the physiologic and emotional responses to pain, (6) signs or other evidence of pain, and (7) the measures useful in the therapy of pain.

The fact that pain is a private and personal experience is not to be denied. No one except the person who is in pain knows how much pain he or she has, or its exact nature, or what the pain means to the person. There is a poverty of words in the English language to describe pain. The words used by the patient to describe pain are chosen on the basis of what he or she thinks is happening. Words such as crushing, boring, burning, prickling, or gnawing are used. For many centuries and until recently, pain was not classified as a sensation but as the antithesis of pleasure. Despite extensive study, pain had never been defined to the satisfaction of all scientists. Most definitions, however, include the following points: (1) pain is a sensory perception; (2) pain has a psychic component; (3) pain is unpleasant; (4) pain, even when it is localized, involves the whole person; and (5) pain is useful to the extent that it causes the individual to seek help in determining its cause and in securing relief. On the other hand, fear of pain may cause a person to delay seeking necessary treatment.

Prejudices of Providers which Interfere with Assessment and Management of a Person's Pain

Although there are many critical factors that contribute to the pain experience, which must be assessed by gathering objective date (e.g., vital signs, skin color and moisture, pattern of anagesics administered), the patient's *verbal report of pain* (a subjective datum) is *more reliable* than any physiological indicator (Jacox, 1979, p. 895). Perceptual dissonance is a major hurdle facing the nurse who wishes to give appropriate emphasis to the verbal report of pain as a basis for providing help to relieve the pain; this obstacle exists because "the ability of one person to interpret accurately what is felt by another is complicated when the attitudes of the assessor and the person being assessed differ" (Jacox, 1979). Three major prejudices of health professionals about pain and analgesia pose obstacles to accurate assessment and to effective management of pain (Jacox, 1979, pp. 898–99):

1. Expectation that patients experiencing chronic pain display the same behaviors as those experiencing acute pain
2. Belief that the cell is more reliable than the person, that is, in order to hurt, one's pain must have an organic basis
3. Unnecessary conservatism in the use of narcotic analgesics because of an unreasonable and undocumented concern for iatrogenic addiction

The third prejudice, analgesic conservatism, is evidenced by reported practices with surgical patients; physicians underprescribed narcotic analgesics, and nurses administered less than patients could have received in conformity with the inadequate pain prescriptions (McCaffery & Hart, 1976).[3]

[3] For an excellent discussion of optimal use of narcotics, alone and in combination with potentiating drugs, in the treatment of acute pain, see M. McCaffery and L. L. Hart. "Undertreatment of Acute Pain with Narcotics." *Am. J. Nurs.*, **76** (Oct. 1976), 1586–91.

Anatomy and Physiology of Pain

Knowledge of pain as a sensation has come about during the last 100 years or so. Keats and Lane (1963) state that most of the progress in the treatment of pain has been made in the therapy of specific pain. Nonspecific pain is one of the unsolved problems in clinical medicine. To illustrate the magnitude of the problem the *Physician's Desk Reference* for 1979 lists approximately 140 systemic analgesics. Until relatively recently the anatomy of pain has been described in terms of specific pain receptors, pain fibers, and pain centers in the central nervous system. Melzack (1961) states that the modern view of pain is not that it is a single sensation but that it is a complex experience that involves the total individual. The anatomy of the sensory perception of pain is fairly well known; that of the complex experience is just beginning to be identified. Knowledge of the latter is at the point where there is sufficient knowledge to test hypotheses. There are two pathways that carry pain impulses to the central nervous system, one conducting impulses rapidly and the other conducting them slowly. Like other sensory perceptions, pain impulses are transmitted from receptors to spinal tracts by way of mixed peripheral nerves. Keats and Lane (1963, p. 4) also state that pain impulses are transmitted over two sets of nerve fibers, both of which are present in all peripheral nerves. In one system, known as the A delta fibers, the fibers are large and myelinated. They conduct impulses rapidly. In the other, or the C fibers, the fibers are small and unmyelinated and they conduct pain impulses slowly. The two systems contribute somewhat differently to the pain experience. The A delta fibers alert the individual to the presence of pain and localize it. The C fibers contribute to the suffering in pain. Keats and Lane summarize the pain pathways as shown in Figure 36-1. The A delta fibers, which are myelinated, pass more or less directly to the thalamus and the sensory areas in the cerebral cortex. The collateral system connects with the reticular formation and provides for slower conduction than does the main pathway. In addition, it has many diffuse connections with many centers in the brain. These fibers are unmyelinated. The suggestion has been made that the role of the collateral system is to integrate information from many sources and to modify the reaction of the individual to pain. Melzack (1961, p. 44) states that fibers have been identified that go from the brain to message-carrying nerve pathways in the spinal cord. These fibers modify impulses coming into the spinal cord over sensory fibers. As a consequence, impulses may be suppressed and never get beyond the level of the spinal cord, or be altered so that the message that is delivered is different from the one that originated the impulse.

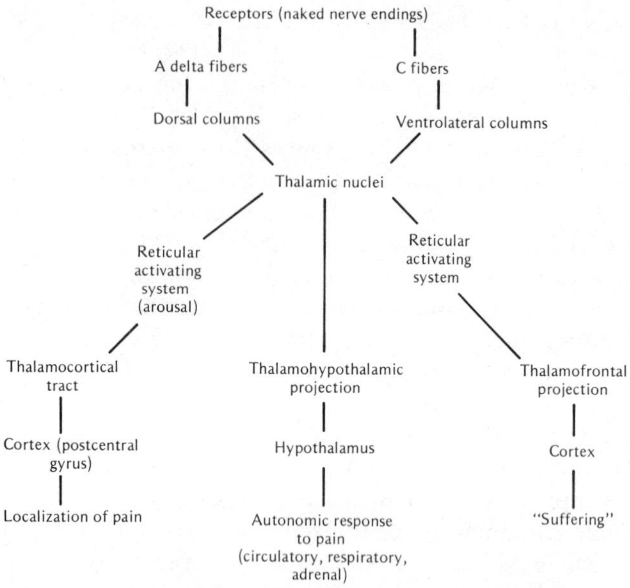

Figure 36-1. Schema of pain pathways. [Adapted with permission of Year Book Medical Publishers, Inc., from The Symptomatic Therapy of Pain. *Dis.-a-Month,* June 1963, p. 7, by Arthur S. Keats and Montague Lane.]

According to Melzack's gate-control theory of pain, a portion of the sensory nerve impulse entering the spinal cord or brainstem passes over a dense network of interconnecting internuncial neurons. Although not proved, this may be the point at which memory, thoughts, and emotion modify sensory messages after injury. There is experimental and psychological evidence to support the assumption that higher centers in the brain do modify sensory nerve impulses at various lower levels. In time, the pathways whereby higher centers influence lower centers will undoubtedly be identified.

Sensation of any type requires not only pathways for the conduction of impulses and centers for their interpretation and integration but receptors that are sensitive to painful stimuli. Formerly it was believed that there were specific pain receptors in the skin. The current view is that the skin contains widely branching bushy networks of receptors that overlap one another and are stimulated by noxious stimuli, including stretching of the tissue. When the stimulus approaches the point of tissue damage, the resulting sensation is interpreted as pain. The point at which the individual interprets sensory stimulation as pain is known as sensory pain perception. In our present state of knowledge, the thalamus appears to function in the awareness to pain. The thalamus has, however, connections with many areas of the brain. The cerebral cortex is presumed to function in the localization of pain and in the recognition of its nature, severity, and significance.

The Pain Experience

Common Types of Pain

Pain is the most common and compelling symptom for which patients seek medical help. Engel (1970) describes eight clinical characteristics of the pain experience:

1. Pain is a private, subjective experience, information about which can come only from the sufferer.
2. Pain is not a pure sensation.
3. Generally speaking, pain correlates with the intensity of stimulation.
4. Pain includes an affective quality of suffering, discomfort, distress, misery, torture, and punishment.
5. Only those parts of the body which have an afferent nerve supply belonging to the dorsal root system or their analogues in the cranial nerves can give rise to pain.
6. Both consciousness and attention are necessary for the experience of pain.
7. Psychological factors significantly influence how and when pain is experienced and reported.
8. Social and cultural influences modify how different peoples react to and report pain.

Based on the clinical characteristics of pain described above, Engel (1970) proposes the following definition:

Pain is a basically unpleasant sensation referred to the body which represents the suffering induced by the psychic perception of real, threatened, or fantasied injury.

Engel counsels wisely that the clinician never deals directly with pain, per se, but rather with the patient's statements about his or her pain.

Headache

Possibly the most common type of pain experienced by modern man is headache. Of all patients who present headache as the chief complaint to primary care practitioners, it is estimated that about 90 per cent of them are suffering from muscle contraction headaches (Pearson, 1976, p. 12). Guyton (1976, p. 674) states that emotional tension often causes many of the muscles of the head, including especially those muscles attached to the scalp, and the neck muscles attached to the occiput, to become moderately spastic; it is postulated that this tugging causes headache. The pain of the spastic head muscles supposedly is referred to the overlying areas of the head and gives one the same type of headache as do intracranial lesions. Since the brain itself is almost totally insensitive to pain, much, or most, of the pain of headache probably is not caused by damage within the brain itself (Guyton, 1976, p. 673).

Headaches fall into two major categories by origin: (1) those that arise from stimulation of intracranial structures; and (2) those that occur with stimulation of tissues that lie on the outside of and adjacent to the skull (Wolff, 1970, p. 62). As indicated previously, the second type are the most common, that is, those vascular headaches of the migraine type and the headaches from sustained muscle contraction accompanying vasoconstriction and associated with anxiety and emotional tension. Headaches associated with fever and septicemia probably rank next in frequency, and then come those due to nasal, paranasal, and eye disease. The headaches of meningitis, aneurysm, brain tumor, and brain abscess, although important and dramatic, are much less common (Wolff, 1970, p. 89).

Pearson (1976), a nurse practitioner, has developed a guide to the very important history, as well as physical findings, necessary to analyze the symptom of headache. Pearson's protocol identifies (1) the data to be collected, (2) the type of headache suggested by the findings, and (3) the appropriate action to take based upon the assessment. Pearson's protocol is highly recommended to the reader.

When headache is due to muscle contraction, the most effective remedy is to relieve the spasticity of the neck and shoulder muscles. Heat, massage, and exercise involving leg muscles will often alleviate the pain of tension headache. (See Chapter 21, discussion of measures to relieve muscular tension.)

Dysmenorrhea

Next to headache, one of the most prevalent types of pain is *dysmenorrhea* (menstrual cramps). It is estimated that 30 to 50 per cent of women of childbearing age suffer from dysmenorrhea, with a resulting loss of more than 140 million working hours each year (Marx, 1979). Growing evidence suggests that the cause may be overproduction by the uterus of prostaglandins, which activate uterine contractions, after "turning off" the synthesis of progesterone; through their stimulation of smooth muscle contractions, prostaglandins at elevated levels can also account for the nausea, vomiting, diarrhea, fatigue, and nervousness which often accompany dysmenorrhea. The following steps in the cause of dysmenorrhea provide another illustration of the intimate interrelationship of neural and endocrine function (Singh, 1975):

1. Estrogen is released from the ovary.
2. Prostaglandins are synthesized in the mature endometrial cells.
3. After ovulation, the ovaries are stimulated to produce progesterone as well as estrogen.
4. Growth of myometrium is stimulated, and uterine muscle relaxation is effected.
5. At the onset of menses, necrosis allows the escape of prostanglandins.
6. In the presence of high concentrations of prostaglandins, spastic uterine muscle contractions begin.

Clinical trials of potent prostaglandin synthesis inhibitors for relief of dysmenorrhea are very encouraging; the drugs are classified as nonsteroidal, anti-inflammatory drugs currently registered by the Food and Drug Administration for treatment of arthritis, but not for dysmenorrhea (Marx, 1979).

Low Back Pain

Low back pain is the most common chronic pain syndrome in the United States, accounting for more than 18 million physician office visits a year (Clark et al., 1977). A major contribution to the high incidence of low back pain in the United States is undoubtedly our high incidence of obesity, sedentary life style, and generally poor posture. The best prevention for low back pain is a regular program of activity to maintain muscle tone, a diet which provides only the calories required for energy expenditure, practice of good posture while walking and sitting, and use of proper body mechanics when lifting or moving objects.

Cervical Spine Syndrome

Cervical spine syndrome is an increasingly common cause of pain in an era of frequent trauma from automobile collisions, which account for 90 per cent of cervical disorders, and increased longevity accompanied by osteoarthritis.

The cervical spine is affected by the same forces as other weight-bearing joints. Clinical signs of injury result from irritation or compression of cervical nerve roots in or about the intervertebral foramina before the roots divide into anterior or posterior rami, or from soft tissue injury. The signs do not indicate the initiating cause but rather the effects of pathological changes.

Depending on the location of the lesion(s), the symptoms in order of frequency include: head, neck, shoulder, and arm pain; paresthesias, numbness, tingling, pins and needles sensations; neck and shoulder stiffness and weakness; and muscle atrophy and loss of grip.

Factors predisposing to cervical syndrome include aging, immobility, emotional stress, and mental and physical fatigue which increase nervous tension and anxiety. With aging, water content of the discs and articular cartilages decreases and they lose resilience. There is a loss of muscle as well as fibrous connective tissue from ligaments. These changes diminish the stability of the spine, although function may continue as long as undue stress is not placed on the discs. Stability is also lessened by atrophy of muscles and ligaments as the result of prolonged bedrest (Hogan & Beland, 1976).

Initially, the pain caused by cervical spine syndrome often is not accompanied by physical findings and is not usually responsive to single or short-term intensive therapy. As a result, the victim may go from one physician or clinic to another, seeking unsuccessfully for acknowledgment and relief of pain, while structural damage progresses and pain intensifies. Health professionals tend to be more persuaded by physical findings than by subjective reports, and more gratified by patient problems which respond promptly to treatment than those in which progress is made in miniscule steps over a long period of time.

The objectives of treatment are to relieve pain, restore function, and help the patient learn to protect his or her neck, thereby reducing symptoms and preventing recurrence. These objectives can be met by moist heat, traction, immobilization, and analgesics and muscle relaxants to relieve pain and muscle spasm. Treatment at home is possible, even preferable, with nursing assistance to improvise traction devices and adapt daily activities (Hogan & Beland, 1976).

Altered Perceptions of Pain

The integrity of sensory mechanisms is essential to the perception of pain. Occasionally a child is born who lacks pain and temperature receptors in the skin. Although this deficit does not interfere with the survival of the child, he or she lacks one of the mechanisms for learning to protect himself or herself from injury. More common is the individual who, because of disease, injury, or therapy, is deprived of structures or functions enabling perception or interpretation of pain sensations. The individual then must learn how to protect the tissues thus deprived from injury and to inspect them for evidence of injury. For example, Melvin Gale suffered a transection of his spinal cord at the level of the first lumbar vertebra. He was completely paralyzed below the point of injury. For the remainder of his life, measures must be instituted for the protection of the paralyzed parts of his body from the effects of pressure and other injury. As soon as his physical condition permitted, he was taught the importance of moving and turning himself regularly, of checking the temperature of bath water with his hand or a thermometer, and of inspecting his skin for evidences of pressure or injury. In contrast, Mr. Roberts, who was paralyzed as a result of acute anterior poliomyelitis, did not have this problem. Despite his flaccid paralysis, he was sensitive to painful stimuli. In fact, during the acute stage of his illness, his skin was so sensitive that his nurse was frequently reminded of the princess who could feel a pea though it was covered by seven mattresses.

A third example is that of Mr. Westwind, a 68-year-old man with trigeminal neuralgia. As a result of this disorder, Mr. Westwind had suffered paroxysms of excruciating pain for years, unsuccessfully treated by drug therapy. To relieve him of his pain, the surgeon cut all the sensory branches of the trigeminal nerve. The trigeminal nerve is sensory to the skin and mucosa of the head, to the teeth, and to the cornea of the eye. Mr. Westwind was therefore deprived of the ability to detect foreign bodies in, or injury to, the eye, or to detect stimuli indicating the possibility of injury to the skin of his head or to the buccal mucosa. In his care, provisions were made to protect the structures thus deprived of sensation and to teach Mr. Westwind what he needed to know and do to protect himself from injury. Part of his instruction was to inspect his eye at least three times a day for evidences of irritation. He was also taught to inspect the inside of his mouth and tongue after each meal for food remaining in his mouth and for evidences of injury and to protect the affected side of his face from overexposure to cold. Fortunately most patients with trigeminal neuralgia do not require that all branches of the trigeminal nerve be cut for relief of pain. The branch supplying the cornea of the eye can usually be saved, and when it is, special protection of the eye is unnecessary.

Mr. Gale and Mr. Westwind have been used to illustrate some of the problems that arise when an individual is deprived of the sensory nerve supply. Tissues are no longer warned that they are being exposed to noxious stimuli. Plans for the nursing of the patient should include provisions for the protection of the tissue from injury and for the instruction of the patient in self-protection. The basic protective measures are those that prevent injurious agents from coming in contact with the tissue or that limit the length or degree of exposure. Because there is always a possibility of injury, the affected area should also be regularly inspected for evidence of inflammation.

Intractable Pain

Perhaps the most eloquent definition of intractable pain is provided by a nurse who lived with the pain and suffering of trigeminal neuralgia (Eland, 1978):

Chronic intractable pain is a long-term, perhaps a lifetime, condition where pain serves no useful purpose and where the usual methods for dealing with it are ineffective or inappropriate. It is as vicious as any cancer, ravaging the entire body and affecting the whole person—psychologically, physiologically, and emotionally. Without wanting to sound overdramatic, I can honestly say that the world of chronic pain is truly a living hell where, little by little, people are destroyed until they hardly recognize their former selves.

The Psychic Component

In humans, the psyche can be the sole stimulus to great pain. Ideas, loss, disillusionment can cause a person great suffering, driving him or her even to violence against others and self. This type of pain is eloquently described by Sobel (1976):

Human violence is that act which occurs when a blow is struck against life. Its roots lie not in man's fighting behaviors, for these are normally applied toward constructive ends, but in the pain which affects men's hearts (and in man's) efforts to control pain.

More commonly, the psychic component is known as the reaction to pain. It includes what the person thinks and feels about pain as well as what he or she does about it. Interest in the psychic component in the pain experience has been stimulated by the observation that, despite similar bodily injuries, the degree of pain varies from individual to individual or even in the same individual at different times. Melzack (1961, p. 42) illustrates that point by quoting the studies of Beecher. During World War II, Beecher was surprised to find that among seriously injured soldiers admitted to a combat hospital, only one in three complained of pain severe enough to require morphine. Moreover, many of these men denied having any pain at all. After the war, he studied a group of civilians who had incisions similar to the wounds received by the men in battle. In this group, four out of five stated that they had severe pain and wanted something to relieve it. From these findings Beecher concluded that factors other than the extent of the wound determine the degree of pain experienced by an individual. One of the most fundamental factors is the meaning that the pain has for the person. The soldiers were grateful for having escaped from the field alive. In contrast, civilians regarded their situations as a serious misfortune or even a catastrophe. Instead of being saved from death, they were facing the possibility of serious injury, pain, and even death. On the battlefield, injury results in the relief of anxiety. The patient facing surgery or some other painful experience has an increase in anxiety. In the words of Crowley (1962, p. 61), three factors contribute to the production of anxiety in the patient in pain: "They are the threat to the self, the loneliness of pain, and the element of the unknown in pain." These sources of anxiety contribute to the quality of the first of McCaffery's (1972) three phases of the pain experience: (1) anticipation, (2) experience, and (3) aftermath of pain. The nurse can effect a significant reduction in the distress experienced by a person in all three phases of the pain experience.

Factors Influencing Behavior of a Person in Pain

Because culture influences the way in which people view the various events in life, it also influences what the individual regards as painful and how he or she reacts to pain. Mark Zborowski's studies of the cultural components in responses to pain are cited in Chapter 31. In the United States, the group of people who place a high value on health regard pain as an indication for seeking medical attention. They expect that the cause of the pain can be determined and the condition treated successfully. The behavior of the patient in pain is in part attributable to culture and training. In many American families, girls may cry when in pain, but boys are told that men do not cry and that they should bear pain like a man. In some cultures, such as certain tribes of American Indians, children are taught from infancy to bear pain without giving evidence of suffering. Procedures such as hypodermic injections that cause other children to cry out are tolerated without any display of emotion. Other patients are also seen who, as a result of culture and training, bear pain silently. The only evidence that they are in pain may be a drawn facial expression, beads of perspiration on the brow, or a quickened respiratory or pulse rate. Others express their pain openly.

Patients with deep religious faith may tolerate conditions that are ordinarily associated with severe pain with little evidence of pain. This is explained by the meaning that the religious faith of the patient gives to pain. He or she may believe that pain has a spiritual purpose and that suffering should not be wasted. (See Chapter 32, for assessment of spiritual needs.) Care should be taken to make sure that patients who have pain receive attention. Patients who do not express their pain freely may be overlooked. Those who are noisy and demanding may also be neglected, because of the tendency to regard them as overdemanding, neurotic, or childish.

Pain is increased by anything that focuses attention on it. Conversely, any condition or event that distracts the attention of a patient, tends to lessen pain. Hundreds of examples ranging from the trivial to the dramatic could be used to illustrate this point. The pain of minor burns and scratches in children is relieved by a kiss, a dab of colored antiseptic, or a tape bandage. A small child that has fallen and bumped his head may pick himself up and start to play again only to start crying when his mother, looking anxious, asks him where he hurt himself. Athletes, soldiers, and even ordinary lay people may, at the time of an emergency, carry out a necessary activity and completely ignore or be oblivious to the pain of serious injuries. Mr. All, who was burned, is a good example. Despite serious burns he returned to his apartment to rescue his son. After his son was safe, he fainted. The pain-relieving effect of distraction and activity is quite often seen in patients. When the nurse enters the room, the patient complains of pain and general discomfort. By the time the nurse has bathed the patient, placed him or her in a comfortable position, and administered whatever care is required to improve general comfort, very little pain may be experienced. A similar effect of distraction frequently is seen in elderly people who spend much of their time alone. When a visitor first arrives, Mrs. Cotton complains of the pain in her joints and other discomforts. By the time the visitor is ready to leave, her pain may be all but forgotten. The nurse frequently uses distraction to lessen a patient's pain or discomfort. She talks to him during a procedure or instructs him to do something such as to take a deep breath or to squeeze her hand.

When the pain experienced by the patient is mild or moderate, diversions such as music, reading, visiting, or crafts may serve to distract the attention of the patient from pain. This is not meant to be a universal prescription, however. In the patient who is suffering severe pain, attempts at diversions may increase the tension of the patient. Diversion should be employed when it is indicated and avoided at other times. In general, patients who are acutely ill, including those who have recently undergone major surgery, should be protected from overstimulation and fatigue. What they need is a quiet, calm, and restful atmosphere combined with a feeling that they can trust those responsible for their care to meet their needs. Less acutely ill patients, and particularly those with long-term illness, may be benefited by diversional activities that are suited to their state of health and personal interests. These patients should also be protected from overfatigue, as fatigue lowers the tolerance of the patient to pain.

The fact that the effectiveness of analgesic drugs is increased by telling the patient that the drug will relieve pain has been demonstrated by experimental study. In some patients pain can be relieved by the assurance that the injection or pill he or she is receiving will relieve pain. This is known as the placebo effect. This does not mean, as it is generally interpreted to mean, that the patient does not have pain. By reassuring the patient that something is being done for the pain, attention is distracted from the pain and apprehension is relieved. A nurse is appropriately utilizing the placebo effect when she or he says to the patient while administering a pain-relieving medication, "I have something [a hypodermic or pill] that will relieve your pain." Occasionally the physician prescribes an injection of water or saline for its placebo effect, but a nurse should never make the decision to give a patient a placebo without such an order. Psychological factors are of importance in all patients who have pain. They should be utilized to the benefit of the patient.

Another factor in the suffering caused by pain is the feeling of the patient that he or she has or does not have some degree of control over the pain. To provide the patient with a feeling of having some control over pain, some physicians allow certain of their patients to keep analgesics, such as acetylsalicylic acid, at the bedside. When the patient is in pain and the nurse is responsible for the administration of an analgesic drug, she or he can add to the sense of security of the patient by administering it promptly.

When movement aggravates pain, as it is likely to do, every effort should be made to prevent unnecessary pain. Attention should be given to minimizing both the sensation of pain and the fear of pain. The first step is to prepare the patient for what to expect and for what is expected of him or her. For example, "We have come to turn you to your other side. We will use the turning sheet. You can help by holding your spine 'stiff as a poker.' " Suggestions made by the patient should be treated with kindness and respect. Therefore when the patient says, "I always keep my neck from moving by placing my hands on each side of my face," the nurse responds by saying, "Fine, we will tell you when we are ready and then you can help." The nurse should use discretion in following the suggestions of the patient; one that is harmful should not be followed. The patient should be told why the suggestion is rejected in such a way that self-esteem is maintained. Courtesy and tact should be characteristics of the behavior of the nurse at all times.

The patient who has been, or is, in pain is frequently reluctant to move. Whether or not movement of the patient is essential at a particular time depends on the needs of the patient and of the situation. If harm is likely to result to the patient if not moved, then he or she should be encouraged to move or to permit himself or herself to be moved. Often allowing a patient to wait for a short time in order to provide an opportunity to mobilize resources will lessen reluctance. The patient should be assured that enough competent assistance is available so that he or she will be moved with a minimum of discomfort. The number of persons required to move a patient is not always the deciding factor. One or two skillful nurses who are trying to do what must be done gently may be all that is required. Finally, the patient should know why he or she should move or be moved at this particular time. Sometimes the reluctance of the patient results not so much from lack of acceptance of what has to be done but from the illness.

The patient's fear of pain can be minimized by providing care in such a manner that he or she knows that those who are providing care will do their best to protect the patient from unnecessary pain. All care should be characterized by gentleness, steadiness, and smoothness. Force, haste, or rough, jerky movements have no place in the care of the patient in pain. Noise, confusion, and ineptitude are disturbing to the patient in pain and should therefore be eliminated. In patients who have a painful illness, expressions of negative feelings are common. The nurse should try to accept these as part of the illness and continue to treat the patient with kindness and consideration. Undue levity and boisterousness should be avoided. Although the nurse does not help the patient by being as depressed by the pain as the patient is, neither is excessive cheerfulness helpful. What is generally beneficial is a combination of acceptance of the fact of the suffering of the patient and an air that implies that something can and will be done to lessen it.

ANALGESIA

Analgesia is the relief of pain. Actions taken to relieve pain are based upon (1) its location, severity, and duration; (2) the factor(s) that seem to be causing it; (3) the extent to which the patient's normal pattern of living is disrupted by it; and (4) the nature and effectiveness of any previous methods to relieve the pain. These factors are considered in the pain assessment guide in Figure 36-2.

Medical management of pain includes the use of psychological, physical, and chemical measures to remove or modify the stimulus to pain, or to block the transmission of pain impulses.

Psychological Measures

Exciting results are emerging from a multidisciplinary approach to the analysis and management of the behavior of persons with chronic pain. The basis of effective treatment is comprehensive assessment. At the Pain Clinic of University Hospital, Seattle, Washington, nurses participate in the behavioral analysis that consists of four profiles of (1) present performance patterns, (2) personality, (3) social learning patterns and reinforcers, and (4) drug intake patterns. These profiles are considered in conjunction with medical evaluation by an anesthesiologist, neurosurgeon, orthopedist, and psychiatrist, with appropriate additional consultation. In patients who exhibit major dysfunction with little or no evidence of pathology, application of principles of learning, referred to as behavior modification, has had gratifying results.

Physical Measures

In patients with chronic pain who are found to have incurable pathology, or in whom lesser measures fail to relieve pain, physical measures are used to slow or interrupt transmission along pain pathways. Transmission may be affected by application of electrical or thermal energy. (See Chapter 11 for effects of these agents on cells.) Application of electrical energy for the relief of pain is called *electroanalgesia*, and its mode of action is believed to be explained by the gate theory of pain. In electroanalgesia, electrical stimulation is applied directly to the dorsal column for the control of severe, chronic pain for which all other means have failed. In dorsal column stimulation (DCS), electrodes are implanted into the epidural space and connected to an external transmitter which is operated by the patient. Central nervous system pain syndromes and those involving peripherally injured nerves respond most often to DCS; relief of cancer pain with this technique is not impressive (Gramse, 1978). As indicated earlier, Melzack's gate theory proposes that

> there are specialized afferent fibers that inhibit pain messages from reaching the brain. These fibers, when stimulated, may shut a hypothetical gating mechanism in the spinal cord that both passes pain signals to the brain and also modifies them in accordance with rebounding messages from these higher centers. The theory itself is still in dispute—but electronic stimulators implanted in the region of the dorsal column reportedly have brought relief to many human patients suffering chronic, intractable pain (Pain, 1970).

The gate-control theory has helped to explain and legitimatize some previously suspect techniques for relief of chronic pain, such as hypnosis; acupuncture; and electrical stimulation. Figure 36-3 schematically represents how these three techniques produce pain relief.

24-Hour Pain Profile

If situation indicates, complete the following:

Sex: M F

Age: ________

Hospital day: ____________ Diagnosis: ____________

Postop. day: ____________ Surgery: ____________

Location: ________________________

Quality

(√) _____ Dull aching
_____ Throbbing
_____ Sharp/stabbing
_____ Burning
_____ Boring
_____ Pressing
_____ Stinging
_____ Cramping
_____ Gnawing
_____ Pricking
_____ Steady
_____ Shooting
_____ Other (describe)

____

Associated Manifestations

(√) _____ Crying
_____ Decreased activity
_____ Vital sign changes
_____ Sweating
_____ Muscle rigidity
_____ Tense facial expression
_____ Impaired mental processes/ concentration
_____ Other (describe)

____

Times of pain medication
(List for 24 hours)

Your inference of cause of pain
(Describe)

Quantity

(√) _____ Mild
_____ Severe
_____ Intolerable
_____ Other (describe)

____

Onset

_____ Gradual
_____ Sudden

Duration
(periodicity, interval, frequency)

____

Aggravating factors

(√) _____ Time of day
_____ Visiting hours
_____ Laughing/coughing
_____ Moving
_____ Other

Alleviating factors

(√) _____ Spontaneous
_____ With distraction or suggestion
_____ Heat or cold

Medication

(√) _____ Tranquilizer
_____ Nonnarcotic analgesic
_____ Narcotic
_____ Oral
_____ Parenteral

Quality of pain relief

(√) _____ Low
_____ Moderate
_____ High

Figure 36-2. Guide to assessing a person's pain. Variables and values in this Guide were identified by R. N. students in a course, "Evaluation and Measurement in Clinical Nursing," Wayne State University College of Nursing, 1972, taught by Prof. J. Y. Passos.

The type and location of surgical procedures to interrupt pain pathways are shown in Figure 36-4. Nursing care of patients undergoing any of the surgical procedures indicated follows the principles for care of any surgical patient; in addition, special observations and attention must be given to protecting the patient from loss of any sensory or motor function that may be a known or unintentional concomitant of the procedure.

Chemical Measures

There is some evidence from the frontiers of research that one day the body's own biochemistry may be mobilized to combat pain, through the action of *endorphins,* which are a group of substances manufactured by the body that appear to act as physiological opiates. If the body's production of these substances can be stimulated, or if the substances can be isolated, purified, and synthesized, they could become the powerful nonaddictive pain relievers of the future (Restak, 1977).

However, at present, by far the most common chemical measures used to relieve pain are analgesic medications. The means by which different drugs relieve pain differ. They act by (1) removing the cause of pain, (2) decreasing consciousness, (3) lessening the conduction of impulses over pain fibers, (4) raising the threshold for pain perception, and (5) lessening the awareness, or appreciation, of the significance of pain.

The effectiveness of analgesics is dependent entirely upon the *intensity* of pain and not at all on the site or origin or the particular mechanism inducing the pain (Wolff, 1970, p. 95). This makes it imperative that the nurse frequently reassess pain intensity, against a baseline description of intensity by the patient, if measures to relieve pain are to be effective.

Some common misconceptions held by both pa-

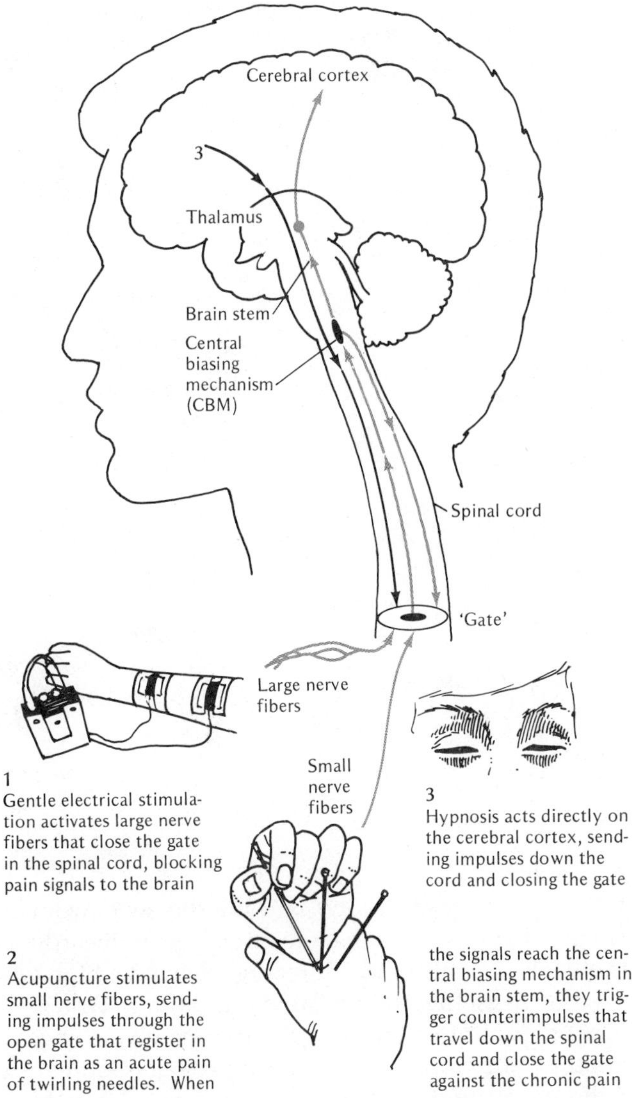

Cerebral cortex
3
Thalamus
Brain stem
Central biasing mechanism (CBM)
Spinal cord
'Gate'
Large nerve fibers
Small nerve fibers
1
Gentle electrical stimulation activates large nerve fibers that close the gate in the spinal cord, blocking pain signals to the brain
3
Hypnosis acts directly on the cerebral cortex, sending impulses down the cord and closing the gate
2
Acupuncture stimulates small nerve fibers, sending impulses through the open gate that register in the brain as an acute pain of twirling needles. When
the signals reach the central biasing mechanism in the brain stem, they trigger counterimpulses that travel down the spinal cord and close the gate against the chronic pain

Figure 36-3. Techniques for chronic pain relief based on the gate-control theory. (Used with permission of Newsweek, Inc., from The new war on pain. *Newsweek*, Apr. 25, 1977, pp. 48–58, by M. Clark *et al.* Diagram by Harry Carter, p. 50.)

tients and staff about the regular use of narcotic analgesics are fear of addiction, discussed previously, and an expectation that a drug will have an instantaneous onset and extended duration of action (Silman, 1979). Addiction occurs rarely in patients treated with narcotic analgesics during hospitalization. Knowledge about onset, peak, duration, and side effects of analgesics are the responsibility of the nurse caring for the patient in pain; this information is available in pharmacology textbooks, the *Physicians' Desk Reference*, or from the pharmacist in most hospital and long-term care facilities. DiBlasi and Washburn (1979) found that the welfare of the patient in pain was dramatically improved by (1) planning specific actions to minimize known side effects, such as increased fluids and fiber to prevent constipation, and by (2) scheduling activities that required patient participation to coincide with *peak action* of the analgesic.

The drugs most commonly used to suppress consciousness are the general anesthetics. Although they can be utilized to suppress pain of all types, their use is limited almost entirely to the operative period of surgical therapy. Local anesthetics are most frequently employed to prevent pain during a surgical procedure, but they may also be used to relieve pain that does not respond to the more usual methods of treatment. Procaine, when injected into a nerve, interrupts the transmission of nerve impulses. The procedure is known as a nerve block and is employed to prevent pain incident to making a surgical incision or in the treatment of painful diseases. In the instance of Mr. Westwind, a patient with trigeminal neuralgia, alcohol injected into his gasserian ganglion relieved the pain for about a year.

Modell (1961) classified analgesic drugs as the greater, or addictive, analgesics and the lesser, or nonaddictive, analgesics. The most important member of the first group is morphine. Its substitutes, such as meperidine hydrochloride and methadone hydrochloride, are also useful. The lesser, or nonaddictive, drugs fall into four groups. They are the salicylates, antipyrine, the coal tar derivatives, and cinchophen. Drugs that are not of themselves analgesics may contribute to the relief of pain when combined with an analgesic by decreasing the capacity of the patient to evaluate pain and the meaning of pain. Thus a patient may be given acetylsalicylic acid (aspirin) in combination with phenobarbital or one of the so-called tranquilizers, such as chlorpromazine.

Aspirin

Aspirin is probably the world's favorite medicine, as a result of both physicians' prescription and laymen's self-medication. The American public alone consumes an estimated 37 million pounds of aspirin and related compounds each year, at a cost of $500 million (Farr, 1972). Aspirin and other salicylates are used primarily to relieve pain of moderate intensity and to lower fever, through action on the CNS. Although the precise way in which aspirin affects the nervous system to relieve pain is not known, what has been learned is that aspirin works better for somatic pain (headache, sprains, toothache, arthritis, and so on) than for visceral pain (intestinal cramps, colic, and gastric distress) (Farr, 1972, p. 63). Aspirin is *not* a harmless drug. Studies have demonstrated its ability to inhibit formation of the prostaglandins by interfering with their synthesis. Prostaglandins are a family of hormonelike substances present in

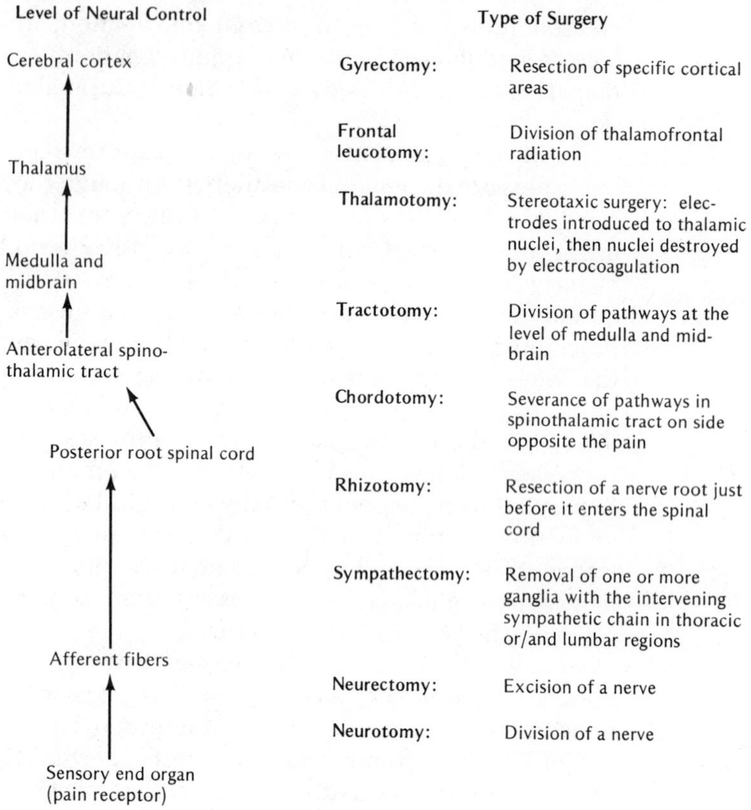

Figure 36-4. Location and type of surgical procedures to interrupt the transmission or perception of pain impulses.

all tissues of the body and have the capacity to contract or relax smooth muscles in the lung, gut, bowel, uterus, and blood vessels. They act in the CNS to cause fever and are probably involved in the process of inflammation. (See Chapter 25.) People with known hemorrhagic problems, or who are under severe or prolonged stress, should avoid aspirin and probably use instead for their minor pains and fever such drugs as sodium salicylate or acetaminophen (Tylenol) (Farr, 1972).

Any pain, if severe or persistent enough, will eventually cause character deterioration, with emergence of psychological abnormalities. Treatment for alleviation of persistent pain begins with peripheral, or local, measures such as applications of heat or cold, exercises, modification of clothing or activity patterns. Spinal cord and central nervous system procedures are limited to those persons in whom peripheral treatment has not been beneficial. Surgical treatment should be considered before narcotic addiction develops (Jannetta, et al., 1973).

Conditions Lessening a Person's Ability to Tolerate Pain

Pain that is long continued reduces the capacity of the person to tolerate pain. Miss Smart illustrates this point very well. She is a middle-aged woman with a diagnosis of subacute bacterial endocarditis; the bacteria causing the infection showed a high degree of resistance to available antibiotics. To try to control the infection, Miss Smart was given one or another antibiotic by intramuscular injection every 2 hours around the clock. Before too long, Miss Smart's body was studded with painful spots. Her ability to tolerate pain and discomfort was reduced to the point that she screamed at the slightest touch or jarring of her bed. Fatigue, sickness, debility, and repeated painful procedures reduced her tolerance to pain to an exceedingly low level. After the injections were discontinued and her condition improved, she was able to tolerate pain as well as most people.

Pain is a subjective experience. Because every person is different, each patient can be expected to behave in an individual manner when in pain or in a pain-provoking situation. There is abundant psychological and experimental evidence to indicate that psychological factors are of great importance in the pain experience. To prevent and relieve pain, the way the patient feels and thinks about the pain must be taken into account. The nurse cannot always know why one patient has more or less pain than does another, but she or he can assume that there is a reason. The nurse can modify the care of the patient so that unnecessary pain is avoided. Pain cannot always be eliminated, but it can be made more bearable by kind and thoughtful care.

The nurse has another responsibility to the patient who is in pain, and that is to observe pain and its effects. Pain may originate in superficial or visceral structures or in the central nervous system. Superficial pain is initiated by the effect of an injurious agent on the skin. The points at which tissue damage and pain occur have been demonstrated to be very close. Sensitivity of the skin to painful stimuli varies from anesthesia, to hypesthesia, to hyperesthesia. In anesthesia, the skin is insensitive to painful stimuli. In hypesthesia, a greater-than-normal stimulus is required to evoke pain. In hyperesthesia, the skin is abnormally sensitive. Anesthetic and hypesthetic skin lacks the normal protective mechanisms against heat, cold, pressure, and trauma. Depending on the extent and location of these areas, protective measures may be required in the protection of the patient. Hyperesthesia is common in acute febrile diseases and in neuritis. In the latter condition the skin may be exquisitely painful over the affected area. Stimuli that would not ordinarily cause any discomfort may result in severe pain. The area may even have to be protected from the weight of bed coverings by a cradle. Hyperesthesia of the edges of a wound is common, and when it occurs, the patient can be assured that it is expected and will disappear in time.

With severe superficial pain, certain defense mechanisms of the body are mobilized. There is an increase in the activity of the sympathetic nervous system and in the production of epinephrine, with a resultant tachycardia and peripheral vasoconstriction. With the increase in the heart rate and vasoconstriction, the blood pressure can be expected to rise. In patients who do not express their discomfort either verbally or by a change in facial expression, the nurse may have to depend on evidences of increased sympathoadrenal activity, such as sweating, tachycardia, and a rise in blood pressure, to detect pain. A generalized increase in muscular tension may also indicate pain.

Pain can be deep, such as that occurring in bones or viscera. Pain in bones is often dull, aching, and localized. Pain in the viscera is usually dull and diffuse. Pain impulses arising in deep muscles and in the viscera are often mediated by nerves that also convey sensations from various areas of the skin or other viscera. This contributes to difficulty in identifying the origin of the pain. For example, difficulty may be encountered in distinguishing between the pain of cholelithiasis, peptic ulcer, and myocardial infarction. A type of sensation often called referred pain may accompany pain in the viscera. This referred pain occurs in the superficial structures supplied by the same sensory apparatus as the organ that is diseased or injured. The explanation usually given is that the brain is unable to locate the specific origin of the pain and therefore projects it to the skin. The following are illustrations of disorders characterized by referred pain. In tuberculosis of the hip, pain is frequently referred to the knee. In myocardial infarction, pain may be referred to the neck, the shoulder blades, and the left arm. The patient may have so much pain in the shoulder that he or she hesitates or refuses to move the arm and, as a result, develops a frozen shoulder. In subphrenic abscesses, the pain is often referred to the top of the shoulder.

Severe deep pain differs from superficial pain in that it is more likely to cause failure in homeostatic defense mechanisms. Weakness, hypotension, pallor, sweating, bradycardia, and nausea and vomiting are common. These signs and symptoms can be observed in patients with a variety of thoracic and abdominal conditions. Examples include myocardial infarction, perforations of abdominal viscera, and biliary or renal colic.

Central pain is a type of pain that is perceived in the mind of the individual and for which there is no apparent peripheral cause at the time the pain is experienced. The classic example is phantom limb, a condition in which a patient has pain and other sensations in an amputated limb even when he or she can see that the limb has been removed. For example, one patient asked to have a pillow in his bed to support his amputated leg. He had the feeling that he had to hold his leg up off the bed. Such a sensation can occasionally be relieved by placing a pillow in the bed where his leg would have normally rested. Many patients have sensations that appear to originate in the amputated extremity. Although these sensations usually eventually disappear, occasionally they persist for years, and they may be so severe that the person is incapacitated. There have been encouraging results from efforts to relieve phantom limb pain with electroanalgesia (Melzack, 1970).

The manner in which pain is elicited differs with different types of tissues. The skin is sensitive to cutting, burning, pricking, and trauma. Severe pain is induced in skeletal muscles by ischemia. This is the basis for Mr. Elderly's pain during exercise. He has severe atherosclerosis that limits the ability of the arteries to increase the blood supply to his legs during exercise. When he walks for a block or so, he develops a severe cramplike pain, which is known as intermittent claudication in the calf of his leg. Pain in the skeletal muscles can also be caused by prolonged contraction and by the injection of irritating substances into them. Ischemia is also the cause of pain in the heart muscle. The ischemia may be relative or absolute. In atherosclerosis or as a result of arterial spasm, the capacity of the coronary arteries to deliver blood to the heart muscle may be inadequate. When Mr. Plump increases his activity, he develops a cramplike pain in his chest. Essentially Mr. Elderly and Mr. Plump have a similar problem. Both of them have pain because their arteries are unable to deliver sufficient blood to maintain muscular activity. In both, pain is protective inasmuch as it acts as a warning. With the onset of pain they stop whatever they are doing; they rest and allow their muscles to recover. They also learn to avoid activities that precipitate the pain. When an artery supplying a muscle is obstructed, pain continues for some time. It is not relieved by rest or by drugs that dilate arteries and increase the blood supply.

Pain in the gastrointestinal tract may be caused by trauma to the mucosa and by stretching or spasm of smooth muscle. The intestine and stomach can be cut or burned without giving rise to pain. Stretching or spasm of smooth muscle in the biliary and urinary tract usually causes severe pain. Arteries also give rise to pain when they pulsate excessively as in migraine headaches or in arteritis.

Observation of the patient is necessary in the collection of information on which the nurse bases the judgment that the patient does or does not have pain of sufficient degree to require relief. From her observations of the patient, the nurse also decides on the course of action to take to treat the pain experienced by the patient. The first step is to determine whether or not the patient is in pain. When a patient is asleep or resting quietly, there is not likely to be pain. When the patient is aroused he or she may complain of pain and then lápse back into sleep. The belief that all postoperative patients and patients with cancer have pain is erroneous. Keats (1956) cited a study of another investigator who found that 44 per cent of 237 patients did not complain of pain after operation. In his own series he found that 21 per cent of 104 patients who had either a gastrectomy or colectomy received no more than one dose of an analgesic during the entire postoperative period. Some of these patients received none. Despite the preceding, it is invalid to conclude that a patient who does not complain of pain is comfortable.

When the patient complains of pain, he should be asked to indicate its location and to describe it. The patient may be asked to point to the painful area. Leading questions should be avoided as they may result in the patient giving misleading information. The question should be phrased so that the cause of the discomfort experienced by the patient can be determined. The resulting answer may indicate that the patient is in pain or is sleepless; is suffering from discomfort from a nasal oxygen catheter; has a sore throat, headache, or backache; is in an uncomfortable position in bed; has an overdistended bladder; or has some condition other than pain from an operative incision or relating directly to the disease. The selection of the method of treatment should be based on the cause of the discomfort. Information should be elicited about any situation or condition that provokes or relieves the pain. For example, Mrs. Robin continued to complain of pain 5 or 6 days after a gastroenterostomy. Her nurse noted that the pain was always precipitated by Mr. Robin's visit. About the same time, Mrs. Robin also made the comment that she always felt so good after she had a "hypo." Both facts were reported to her physician. As Mrs. Robin was showing early signs of addiction to morphine, the drug was discontinued and other therapy prescribed.

The quality of the pain and other characteristics of the pain should be noted and recorded, preferably in the words used by the patient. The mode of onset of the pain, its duration, severity, and time of onset are all important. When the character of the pain experienced by the patient changes or pain appears in a new or unexpected area, this information should be reported to the physician. Whether this is done immediately or delayed until the next regular visit of the physician depends on the possible significance of the pain. Severe pain or pain and other symptoms and signs indicating involvement of the viscera should usually be reported before an analgesic drug is administered, as the drug may mask the patient's pain and thus eliminate an indispensable factor in helping the physician to identify the nature and location of visceral involvement.

Other Indications of Pain

In addition to the description of the pain by the patient, there is usually other evidence to indicate that a patient has pain, for example, restlessness, discomfort indicated by facial expression, hands pressed over the painful area, moaning or other sounds indicating pain, irritability, refusal to move or moving carefully, perspiration, and anorexia. When the pain is severe, the blood pressure may be elevated or depressed and the pulse and respiratory rate altered. Not all these effects are unique to pain. Restlessness is also common in hypoxia, and it is important to rule out the possibility of respiratory difficulty before any analgesic, especially a narcotic, is given. Anorexia occurs in many types of illness. When pain is long continued, it contributes to the debility of the patient by decreasing food intake. In just a few weeks, Mr. Westwind (trigeminal neuralgia) lost 25 pounds. Each time he tried to eat, a paroxysm of pain was precipitated. Therefore he refused to eat. Pain, even when it is not induced by food, is so all-encompassing that everything else becomes unimportant.

Observation of the patient should continue after measures have been taken to relieve pain. Observation should be directed toward determining the success or failure of the treatment and any undesired effects. Some of the drugs used to relieve pain depress the respiratory and other centers in the brain. Patients with borderline cardiovascular function or hypovolemia may go into shock soon after intramuscular or intravenous narcotics are given. Such patients should be given narcotics only in small amounts or not at all. A patient may have an idiosyncrasy to any one of these drugs. When the patient exhibits unusual behavior shortly after a drug is administered and his or her behavior improves after a period of time, the probability is that there is a relationship between behavior and the reaction to the drugs. Examples have been cited earlier in the chapter. Patients who have severe pain are often afraid that the pain will continue or return or that the pain indicates they have a serious illness from which they will die. They are afraid to allow themselves to relax and to go to sleep. When they are under the watchful eye of a nurse whom they trust to meet their needs, they have less need to remain alert. The external environment of the patient should also be controlled so that the therapy has an opportunity to be effective. A quiet, cool, but not cold environment is usually conducive to rest. For some patients the feeling of safety is increased by having a relative or good friend sit quietly at the bedside. The relative may require some instruction as to how he or she should behave and some recognition of the value of his or her contribution to the patient. Furthermore, the nurse should continue to assume the responsibility for the care and supervision of the patient. The relative should supplement, not replace, the nurse.

Pain and fear of pain are common to most illness. The extent to which each aspect predominates varies with the individual and with the cause of illness. Pain is useful because it serves to warn the individual that something is wrong and spurs the person into appropriate action. It is harmful when it frightens the individual so much that action is avoided or when it exhausts physical and psychological resources.

The nurse's responsibilities in the care of the patient as they relate to pain are summarized in the following objectives:

1. To care for the patient so that preventable pain is avoided.
2. To evaluate the nature and cause of the patient's pain, so that appropriate measures may be instituted.
3. To convey to the patient that the nurse (nurses) can be counted on or trusted to meet his or her needs.
4. To continue to offer comfort and support to the patient whose pain persists despite the best efforts of all concerned.

Reference has been made repeatedly to the necessity for the nurse to evaluate the degree of pain experienced by the patient; failure to do so resulted in the following tragedy. The patient, who was approximately 40 years old, had been an actress as a child but was now destitute. She was divorced and lived with her mother. She had developed a severe proctitis as a consequence of large doses of radiation in the treatment of cancer of the cervix. Because of her dependent behavior, she was seen by a psychiatrist who described her as being immature and childlike. Despite her pleas for relief of what is known to be an exquisitely painful condition, pain-relieving medications were unfortunately withheld until she became mentally disorganized. Although Mrs. Child Actress is an extreme example, the incident is uncommon only in degree. When a patient says he or she has pain, the complaint should be treated seriously. Insofar as possible, the causes should be determined and appropriate treatment undertaken.

Nursing Involvement with Substance Abuse

There is epidemic abuse in the United States of voluntarily ingested substances, most of which are used by people who are trying either (1) to screen out the frustration and suffering in their lives by depressing central nervous system function, or (2) to bolster and extend flagging energy by stimulating central nervous system function. Chapter 5 discussed the importance of assessing the adaptive consequences which may follow the persistent practice of excessive use or ingestion of substances such as food and tranquillizers (See Figure 5-4); Chapter 12 discussed injurious effects of alcohol and a number of other chemical injuring agents. Brief mention needs to be made here of a national pastime which is probably taking its toll on the neurological health of the entire adult society.

Probably the most flagrant abuse of CNS stimulation in the United States results from the love affair of Americans with the coffee break. This may well contribute to the incidence of hypertension and other cardiovascular renal disease, due to the effects of caffeine. Even the quantity of caffeine in two to three cupsful of coffee has been shown to elevate plasma renin activity by over 50 per cent within 3 hours in previously noncoffee drinking subjects (Robertson et al., 1978). Even though tolerance develops in coffee drinkers to such caffeine effects as diuresis, parotid gland secretion, bradycardia, and sleep disturbance (Robertson et al., 1978), the wear and tear on the cardiovascular system of chronic excessive use of caffeinated coffee justifies the nurse in working diligently to help patients and families to understand the long-term health cost of this beverage habit and to try other beverage alternatives.

Summary

Stimulus, receptor, arousal system, integrator, and effector—if any are absent or weak, the response is lacking or inappropriate. The nurse whose care is based on thorough initial and ongoing assessment of the person's total behavior, including neurologic function, is in a position to enhance or weaken the force of the circuit.

References Cited

Adams, R. D., and Victor, M. "Delirium and Other Acute Confusional States." In *Harrison's Principles of Internal Medicine,* 8th ed. Ed. by G. W. Thorn et al. New York: McGraw-Hill, 1977, pp. 145–50.

Alexander, M. M., and Brown, M. S. "Physical Examination. Part 17: Neurological Examination." *Nurs. 76,* **6** (June 1976), 38–43.

Bannister, R. *Brain's Clinical Neurology,* 4th ed. New York: Oxford University Press, 1973, p. 139.

Baum, J. L. "Current Concepts in Ophthalmology: Ocular Infections." *N. Engl. J. Med.,* **299** (July 6, 1978), 28.

Bolin, K. L. "Assessing the Status of Neurological Patients." *Am. J. Nurs.,* **77** (Sept. 1977), 1478–79.

Bruner, J. S. "Cognitive Consequences of Early Sensory Deprivation." Paper No. 13 in *Sensory Deprivation: A Symposium Held at Harvard Medical School.* Cambridge, Mass.: Harvard University Press, 1961, pp. 195–207.

Bruya, M. A., and Bolin, R. H. "Epilepsy: A Controllable Disease." *Am. J. Nurs.,* **76** (March 1976), 388–97.

Clark, M. et al. "The New War on Pain." *Newsweek,* (April 25, 1977), 48–58, 48.

Crowley, D. M. *Pain and Its Alleviation.* Berkeley: University of California Press, 1962, p. 61.

DiBlasi, M., and Washburn, C. J. "The Management of Pain: Using Analgesics Effectively." *Am. J. Nurs.,* **79** (Jan. 1979), 74–78.

Dodd, M. J. "The Confused Patient: Assessing Mental Status." *Am. J. Nurs.,* **78** (Sept. 1978), 1501–03.

Eland, J. M. "Living with Pain." *Nurs. Outlook,* **26** (July 1978), 430–31.

Elliott, H. C. *Textbook of Neuroanatomy.* Philadelphia: J. B. Lippincott Co., 1963.

Engel, G. L. "Pain." In *Signs and Symptoms,* 5th ed. Ed. by C. M. MacBryde and R. S. Blacklow. Philadelphia: J. B. Lippincott Co., 1970, pp. 44–45.

Farr, R. S. "Aspirin: Good News, Bad News." *Sat. Rev. Sci.;* **55** (Nov. 25, 1972) 60–63.

Gramse, C. A. "Dorsal Column Stimulation." *Am. J. Nurs.,* **78** (June 1978), 1022–25.

Guyton, A. C. *Textbook of Medical Physiology,* 5th ed. Philadelphia: W. B. Saunders Co., 1976.

Hogan, L., and Beland I. L. "Cervical Spine Syndrome." *Am. J. Nurs.,* **76** (July 1976), 1104–07.

Jacox, A. "Assessing Pain." *Am. J. Nurs,* **79** (May 1979), 895–900.

Jannetta, P. J. et al. "The Neurosurgical Approach to the Relief from Pain." *Curr. Prob. Surg.* (Feb. 1973).

Johnson, M., and Quinn, J. "The Subarachnoid Screw." *Am. J. Nurs.,* **77** (March 1977), 48–50.

Keats, A. S. "Postoperative Pain: Research and Treatment." *J. Chronic. Dis.,* **4** (July 1956), 72–73.

Keats, A. S., and Lane, M. "The Symptomatic Therapy of Pain." *DM,* (June 1963), 3.

Kety, S. S. "Disorders of the Human Brain." *Sci. Am.,* **241** (Sept. 1979), 202–18.

Lindsley, D. B. "Common Factors in Sensory Deprivation, Sensory Distortion and Sensory Overload." Paper No. 12 in *Sensory Deprivation.* Cambridge, Mass.: Harvard University Press, 1961, p. 177.

Marx, J. L. "Dysmenorrhea: Basic Research Leads to a Rational Therapy." *Science,* **205** (July 13, 1979), 175–76.

McCaffery, M. *Nursing Management of the Patient with Pain.* Philadelphia: J. B. Lippincott Co., 1972.

McCaffery, M., and Hart, L. L. "Under-Treatment of Acute Pain with Narcotics." *Am. J. Nurs.,* **76** (Oct. 1976), 1586–91.

Melzack, R. "Phantom Limbs." *Psychol. Today,* **4** (Oct. 1970), 63–68.

Melzack, R. "The Perception of Pain." *Sci. Am,* **204** (Feb. 1961), 49.

Meyd, C. J. "Acute Brain Trauma." *Am. J. Nurs.,* **78** (Jan. 1978), 40–44.

Mitchell, P. H., and Mauss, N. "Intracranial Pressure: Fact and Fancy." *Nurs. 76,* **6** (June 1976), 56.

Modell, W. *Relief of Symptoms,* 2nd ed. St. Louis: C. V. Mosby Co., 1961, pp. 86–100.

"Pain." *Med. World News,* **11** (Dec. 11, 1970), 26–32.

Pearson, L. B. "A Protocol for the Chief Complaint of Headache." *Nurse Practitioner,* **2**:1 (Sept.–Oct. 1976), 12–16, 37.

Posner, J. B. "Sure and Careful Lumbar Puncture." *Consultant,* **13** (Nov. 1973) 17–21, 17.

Restak, R. "The Brain Makes Its Own Narcotics!" *Sat. Rev.,* (March 5, 1977) 6–11.

Riesen, A. H. "Excessive Arousal Effects of Stimulation after Early Sensory Deprivation." Paper No. 3 in *Sensory Deprivation.* Cambridge, Mass.: Harvard University Press, 1961, p. 40.

Robertson, D. et al. "Effects of Caffeine on Plasma Renin Activity, Catecholamines and Blood Pressure." *N. Engl. J. Med.,* **298** (Jan. 26, 1978), 181–85.

Silman, J. "The Management of Pain: Reference Guide to Analgesics." *Am. J. Nurs.,* **79** (Jan. 1979), 74–78.

Singh, E. J. et al. "Levels of Prostaglandins in Human Endometrium during the Menstrual Cycle." *Am. J. Obst. & Gynec.,* **121** (April 1, 1975), 1003–06.

Sobel, D. E. "Human Violence." *Am. J. Nurs.,* **76** (Jan. 1976), 69–71, 70–71

Trockman, G. "Caring for the Confused or Delirious Patient." *Am. J. Nurs.,* **78** (Sept. 1978), 1495–99.

Vernon, J. A. *Inside the Black Room,* New York: Clarkson N. Potter, 1963, p. 200.

Wolff, H. G. "Headache." In *Signs and Symptoms,* 5th ed. Ed, by C. M. MacBryde and R. S. Blacklow, Philadelphia: J. B. Lippincott Co., 1970, pp. 62–98.

General References

Haynes, U. A. "Nursing approaches in Cerebral Dysfunction." *Am. J. Nurs.,* **68** (Oct. 1968), 2170–76.

Kety, S. S. "Disorders of the Human Brain." *Sci. Am.,* **241** (Sept. 1979), 202–18.

LeBow, M. D. *Behavior Modification: A Significant Method in Nursing Practice.* Englewood Cliffs, N.J.: Prentice-Hall, 1973.

Oldendorf, W. H., Braum, S. H., Oldendorf, S. Z. "Blood-Brain Barrier: Penetration of Morphine, Codeine, Heroin and Methadone." *Science,* **178** (Dec. 1, 1972), 984–86.

"Psychosurgery: Legitimate Therapy or Laundered Lobotomy." *Science,* **179** (March 16, 1973), 1109–12.

Robinson, J., ed. *Coping with Neurologic Problems Proficiently,* Horsham, Pa.: Intermed Communications, 1979.

Siesjo, B. K. "Cerebral Metabolism in Cerebral Hypoxia and Ischemia." *Curr. Concepts Cerebrovasc. Dis.,* **8** (March–April 1973), 5–8.

Soulairac, A., Cahn, J., and Charpentier, J., eds. *Pain.* London: Academic Press, 1968.

Wolff, H. G., and Wolf, S. *Pain,* 2nd ed. Springfield, Ill.: Charles C Thomas, 1958.

Zborowski, M. *People in Pain.* San Francisco: Jossey-Bass, 1969.

Sensory Impairment

Cullins, I. "Techniques for Teaching the Patient with Sensory Defects." *Nurs. Clin. North Am.,* **5** (Sept. 1970), 527–38.

Ellis, R. "Unusual Sensory and Thought Disturbances after Cardiac Surgery." *Am. J. Nurs.,* **72** (Nov. 1972), 2021–25.

Glass, D. C., Cohen, S., and Singer, J. E. "Urban Din Fogs the Brain." *Psychol. Today,* **6** (May 1973), 94–99.

Jackson, C. W., and Ellis, R. "Sensory Deprivation as a Field of Study." *Nurs. Res.,* **20** (Jan.–Feb. 1971), 46–54.

Ohno, M. I. "The Eye-Patched Patient." *Am. J. Nurs.,* **71** (Feb. 1971), 271–74.

Zuckerman, M. et al. "Sensory, Deprivation versus Sensory Variation." *J. Abnorm. Psychol.,* **76** (1970), 76–82.

Motor Function

Flacke, W. "Treatment of Myasthenia Gravis." *N. Engl. J. Med.,* **288** (Jan. 4, 1973), 27–31.

Flechsig, L. "Living with Cerebral Palsy." *Am. J. Nurs.,* **78** (July 1978), 1212–13.

Hawken, M., and Ozuna, J. "Practical Aspects of Anticonvulsant Therapy." *Am. J. Nurs.,* **79** (June 1979), 1062–68.

Plummer, E. M. "The MS Patient." *Am. J. Nurs.,* **68** (Oct. 1968), 2161–67.

Head Injuries

Kurze, T., and Pitts, F. W. "Management of Closed Head Injuries." *Surg. Clin. North Am.,* **48** (Dec. 1968), 1271–78.

Ransohoff, J. "Treatment of Ruptured Supratentorial Aneurysms." *Curr. Concepts Cerebrovasc. Dis,* **8** (Sept.–Oct. 1973), 21–26.

Tate, G. Assessment and Direction of Nursing Care for Patients with Acute Central Nervous System Insult." *Nurs. Clin. North Am.,* **6** (March 1971), 165–71.

Torres, H., and Ferguson, L. "Acute Head Injuries." *Am. Fam. Physician,* **2** (Dec. 1970), 89–98.

IICP

Bordeaux, M. P. "The Intensive Care Unit and Observation of the Patient Acutely Ill with Neurologic Disease." *Heart and Lung,* **2** (Nov.–Dec. 1973), 884–87.

Hinkhouse, A. " Craniocerebral Trauma." *Am. J. Nurs.,* **73** (Oct. 1973), 1719–22.

Jones, C. "Glasgow Coma Scale." *Am. J. Nurs.* **79** (Sept. 1979), 1551–53.

Pain

"Aspirin as an Anti-Prostaglandin." *Med. World News,* **12** (Aug. 6, 1971), 13–14.

Baer, E., Davitz, L., and Lieb, R. "Inferences of Physical Pain and Psychological Distress." *Nurs. Res.,* **19** (Sept.–Oct. 1970), 388–401.

Black, S., and Friedman, M. "Effects of Emotion and Pain on Adrenocortical Function Investigated by Hypnosis." *Br. Med. J.,* **1** (Feb. 24, 1968), 477–81.

Brena, S. "Intractable Pain: Getting to the Root of It." *Med. -Surg. Rev.,* **7**(July 1971) 24–31.

Casey, K. L. "Pain: A Current View of Neural Mechanisms." *Am. Sci.,* **61** (March–April 1973), 194–200.

"Challenge to the 'Gate' Theory of Pain." *Med. World News,* **14** (Oct. 12, 1973), 53–55.

Coyle, N. "Analgesics at the Bedside." *Am. J. Nurs.,* **79** (Sept. 1979), 1554–57.

Dalessio, D. J. "Vascular Headache Syndromes." *Curr. Concepts Cerebrovasc. Dis.,* **7** (Jan.–Feb. 1972), 1–6.

Davitz, L. J., and Pendleton, S. H. "Nurses' Inferences of Suffering." *Nurs. Res.,* **18** (March–April 1969), 100–7.

Fordyce, W. et al. "An Application of Behavior Modification Technique to a Problem of Chronic Pain." *Behav. Res. Ther.,* **6** (1968), 105.

Harvey, S. "Clinical Bulletin: New Relief for Menstrual Discomfort." *RN,* **42** (Sept. 1979), 116.

Hinton, J. "Sedatives and Hypnotics." *Practitioner,* **200** (Jan. 1968), 93–101.

Kim, S. "Pain: Theory, Research and Nursing Practice." *Advances in Nurs. Sci.,* **2** (Jan. 1980), 43–59.

Millard, L. "Low Back Pain: Guide to Evaluation." *Hosp. Med.,* **14** (Sept. 1978), 79–90.

Pain. "Part I: Basic Concepts and Assessment." *Am. J. Nurs.,* **66** (May 1966), 1085–1108.

Pain. "Part II: Rationale for Intervention." *Am. J. Nurs.,* **66** (June 1966), 1345–68.

Piercey, M. L. "Assessment of Low Back Pain." *Nurs. Practitioner,* **1** (March–April 1976), 18–21.

Richards, W. "The Fortification Illusions of Migraines." *Sci. Am.,* **224** (May 1971), 89–94.

Wilson, W. P., and Nashold, B. S., Jr. "Pain and Emotion." *Postgrad. Med.,* **47** (May 1970), 183–87.

Drugs

American College of Neuropsychopharmacology—Food and Drug Administration Task Force, "Neurologic Syndromes Associated with Anti-Psychotic-Drug Use." *N. Engl. J. Med.,* **289** (July 5, 1973), 20–23.

Clark, M. et al. "Drugs and Psychiatry: A New Era." *Newsweek,* (Nov. 12, 1979), 98–104.

Grinspoon, L., and Hedblom, P. "Amphetamines Reconsidered." *Sat. Rev. Sci.,* **55** (July 8, 1972), 33–46.

Hill, J. B. "Current Concepts: Salicylate Intoxication." *N. Engl. J. Med.,* **288** (May 24, 1973), 1110–13.

37

Problems with Thermal Regulation

The snow so chilled him that he immediately fell so extremely ill, that he could not return to his lodgings (I suppose then at Graye's Inn) but went to the Earl of Arundel's house at High-gate, where they put him into a good bed warmed with a pan, but it was a damp bed that had not been lain-in in about a year before, which gave him such a cold that in 2 or 3 days as I remember Mr. Hobbes told me, he died of suffocation."

CATHERINE DRINKER BOWEN

Catherine Drinker Bowen: *Francis Bacon, The Temper of a Man*

Boston: Little, Brown and Company. 1963.

Two Abnormalities in Body Temperature

Body temperature varies widely among individuals as well as in the same individual from one time of day to another. Environmental conditons also affect body temperature. Depending on the circumstances, a healthy person's temperature may range from 35.8°C (96.6°F) to 37.8°C (100°F). Particularly at the upper limits of normal, there is some overlapping between what in one person may be a normal temperature and in another hyperthermia or fever. In general, persons who are ill with a temperature of 37.4°C (99.2°F) or above may be suspected of having a *low-grade fever. Hyperthermia* is usually considered to be a temperature of 41.1°C (106°F) or above. Similarly, persons whose temperatures are below 35°C (95°F) may be *hypothermic* (Hayber, 1980).

Fever

The nurse should keep in mind that fever is not a disease but part of the body's response to tissue injury. Fever is associated with two quite different situations. In the more common and usually less serious one, the individual behaves as if his or her temperature-regulating center were reset at a higher level. Body temperature continues to be regulated, but it is regulated at a level above normal. In the other type of fever, as a result if injury or disease of the hypothalamus or midbrain, temperature regulation fails and the temperature continues to rise unless external measures are employed to increase heat loss. When the condition injuring the heat-regulating center is temporary and tissues are protected from excess heat, recovery is possible. For example, in thyroid crises, or heat stroke, temperature regulation may fail. If body temperature is controlled within levels tolerated by the tissues, until such time as the thyroid hormone level falls toward normal, the patient may be saved.

Pathogenesis

Although fever has been recognized as a cardinal sign of disease since the time of Hipprocrates, why it occurs or what purpose it serves is not known. A number of theories have been advanced to explain fever. The one most generally accepted is that fever results from the effects of pyrogenic (fever-producing) substances liberated by injured cells. The body responds to tissue injury with an inflammatory process. The exudate formed in inflammation has been demonstrated experimentally to contain a substance that, when injected, induces fever. If this theory is correct, then fever, whether it occurs in the patient with cancer, diphtheria, an infection in a crushing wound, or an infarction in the heart or lungs, has a common denominator.

The following chemical agents are presently believed to activate fever associated with disease: endotoxins, viruses, bacteria, antigen–antibody complexes, delayed hypersensitivity antigens, and steroids. Each of these agents is believed to stimulate the production of endogenous pyrogen (EP), probably from polymorphonuclear leukocytes (PMNs) in the blood. Other cells in the body that can also release EPs include monocytes, lymphocytes, and the Kupffer cells of the reticuloendothelial system (RES) (Petersdorf, 1977). Circulating EPs presumably serve as the "final common pathway" in producing fever, by stimulating prostaglandin production in the brain; prostaglandins turn up the body's hypothalamic thermostat, causing fever (Dinarello & Wolff, 1979). See Figure 37-1 for the course of fever production. However, the weight of evidence suggest that the common *contributory factor* in all febrile diseases, whether or not those diseases are infectious in origin, is *tissue injury* (Petersdorf, 1977, p. 60). See Unit III for detailed discussion of tissue injury and the agents that produce it.

It is not always possible to determine the cause of a fever. All febrile patients, including those in whom the etiology of fever is uncertain or unknown, must be protected from thermal injury to cells. Pending a definitive diagnosis, febrile patients may be diagnosed as having "fever of unknown origin" (FUO). Criteria for the diagnosis of FUO include (1) an illness of at least 3 weeks' duration, (2) temperatures exceeding 38.3°C on several occasions, and (3) no established diagnosis after 1 week of hospital investigation. The majority of cases of FUO are ultimately found to be due to one of three causes: (1) infections (40 per cent), (2) neoplastic disease (20 per cent), and (3) collagen–vascular disease (15 per cent) (Jacoby & Swartz, 1973).

The nurse can make a valuable contribution to diagnosis and treatment of patients with FUO by talking to the patient or parent about preceding events that might be related to the major causes of FUO. The majority of febrile illnesses in children are caused by viral infections. In assessing the nature and severity of a febrile episode in a child, it is imperative to obtain a good history and a careful examination, to perform a minimum of laboratory tests, and to avoid unnecessary antibiotics (Tomlinson, 1978). Interpreting the significance of fever of children requires an understanding of the factors that produce normal variations. Normal variations of temperature in children are presented in Figure 37-2.

The Value of Fever

Experiments with nonhuman vertebrates show that fever does reduce the lethality of disease, as long as the core body temperature does not exceed some limit characteristic of the species (Case, 1979, p. 390).

Although the value of fever in humans is in most instances not known, in certain chronic conditions, such as neurosyphilis, some gonococcal infections, and rheumatoid arthritis, fever is followed by an improvement in the patient's condition. It is uncertain whether fever helps to kill microorganisms; it is certain that very high temperatures are harmful. When rectal temperature is over 41°C (106°F) for prolonged periods, some permanent brain damage results; over 43°C, heat stroke develops and death is common (Ganong, 1973, p. 1972).

To the extent that fever has adaptive value, the traditional home remedy of taking aspirin at the first sign of elevated temperature may actually be counterproductive; aspirin is now known to inhibit production of prostaglandins, which appear to be the chemicals that raise the hypothalamic thermostat and thus produce fever (Brody, 1979). See Figure 37-1 for prostaglandins in the course of fever.

Description of Fever Patterns

The onset of fever may be abrupt with a shaking chill, or fever may develop without the patient being aware of its presence. The course may be constant or fluctuate greatly. Fever may terminate suddenly with a drenching diaphoresis or it may decline slowly. It may last a predictable period of time or

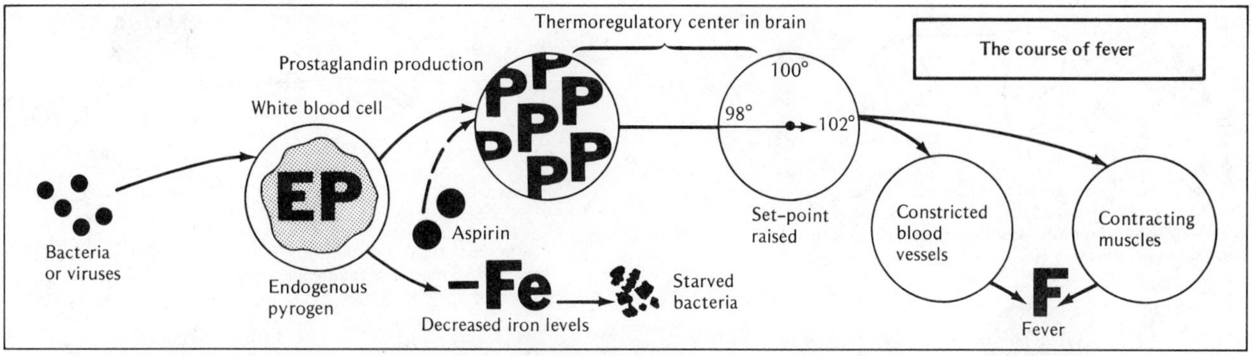

Figure 37-1. The course of fever. From "Fever," *Human Nature,* (Feb. 1979), 66–72, by C. A. Dinarello & S. M. Wolff, p. 69.)

continue indefinitely. It may disappear only to return. When this occurs it may mean that the patient is developing a complication or it may reflect the nature of the disease causing the fever. As an example, malaria is characterized by attacks of chills and fever alternating with afebrile periods. The length of time between attacks of chills and fever varies from 48 to 72 hours, depending upon the species of malarial parasite.

Three Stages of Fever

Fever progresses through three distinct phases (Davis-Sharts, 1978):

1. *The cold or chill stage*—body temperature is rising.
2. *The hot stage*—body temperature is being maintained at the new elevated level. The fever is said to be "running its course."
3. *Defervescense*—fever breaks, and the stage continues until body temperature returns to the person's normal level.

Physiologic Changes Responsible for Febrile Temperatures

Heat production is increased in much the same way as in exercise. Heat loss, however, does not increase to the same degree. In fact, the body responds much as it does when exposed to cold. The peripheral vessels constrict and limit the circulation of blood through the skin. The person may shiver and his or her muscle tone increase. The muscles attached to the hair in the skin contract and elevate the hair; accompanying this are elevations of the skin commonly called goose pimples. The person feels cold and piles blankets on or turns the electric blanket on high even when the room is hot. When the temperature of his or her tissues reaches the new level, shivering stops and the patient may feel warm. Whereas during the chill it was pale, the skin becomes pink. A new equilibrium between heat production and heat loss has been set. Return of body temperature to normal levels is preceded by the regulator being reset at a lower level. The mechanisms responsible for the lowering of the body temperature are the same as those accompanying exercises; that is, sweating and vasodilatation occur.

The mechanisms responsible for the elevation of the temperature in patients who have a chill are easy to explain. The mechanisms responsible in the patient who does not have a chill are less clear. Elevation in temperature may be brought about simply by a decrease in heat loss. It is also possible that the metabolic processes are stimulated by a specific fever-producing substance. Of all the discomforts accompanying fever, chills and sweating are probably the most unpleasant.

What Are the Nurse's Responsibilities in Caring for the Patient Who Has a Chill

When a patient has a chill or a rapidly rising temperature, temperature should be checked frequently enough during and after the chill to determine the height and trough of the fever. For example, during the chill the temperature may be measured every 10 minutes. After the chill ceases, it may be measured every half hour until the last reading is no higher or is lower than the preceding one. Readings may then be taken every 2 to 4 hours until the patient maintains a normal temperature. Whatever the hospital routine, temperature determinations may be necessary at more frequent intervals than those prescribed by the physician. When the temperature of the patient is rising very rapidly or is at a very high level, his or her safety may depend on frequent determinations and on the institution of effective

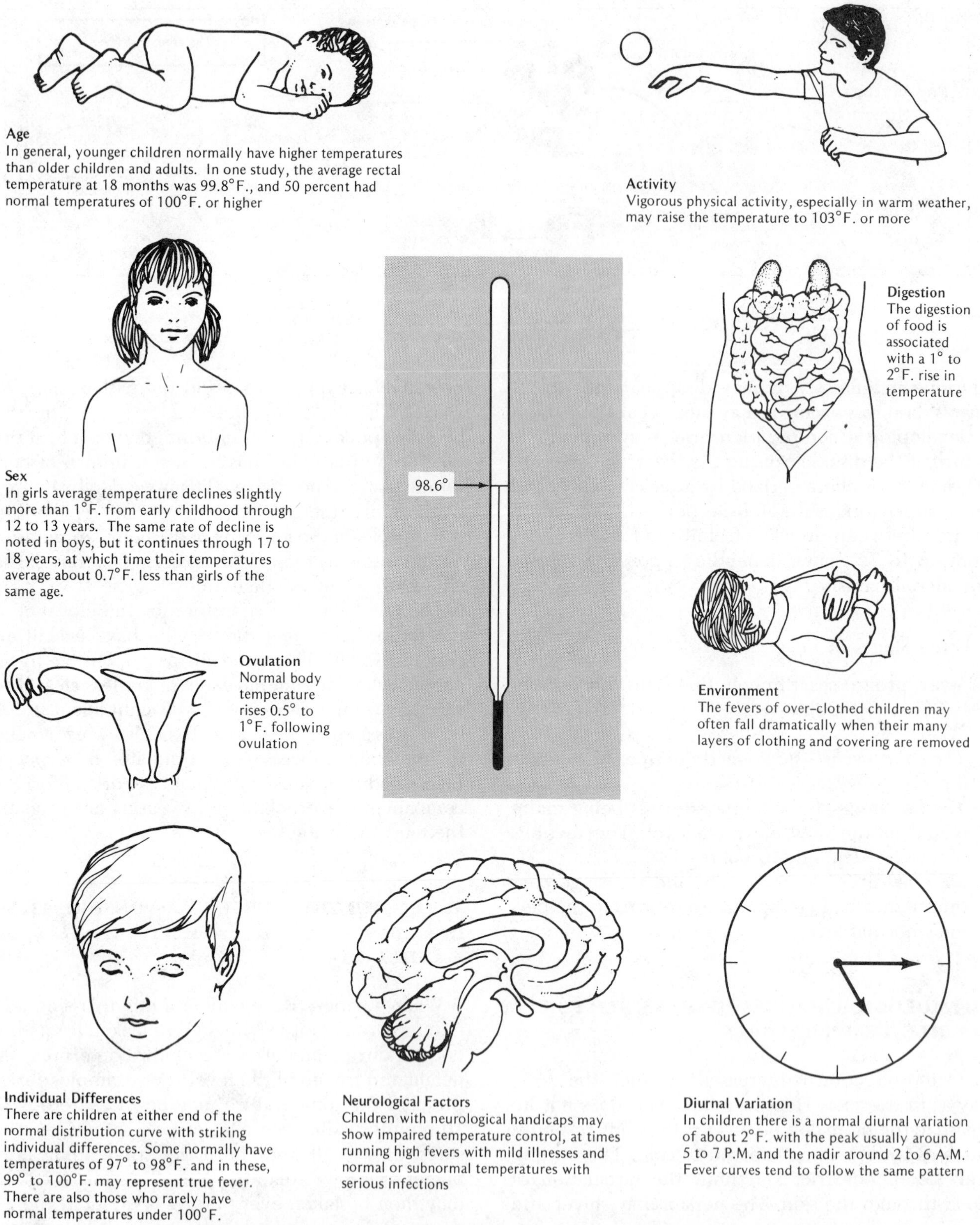
Age
In general, younger children normally have higher temperatures than older children and adults. In one study, the average rectal temperature at 18 months was 99.8°F., and 50 percent had normal temperatures of 100°F. or higher
Activity
Vigorous physical activity, especially in warm weather, may raise the temperature to 103°F. or more
Digestion
The digestion of food is associated with a 1° to 2°F. rise in temperature
98.6°
Sex
In girls average temperature declines slightly more than 1°F. from early childhood through 12 to 13 years. The same rate of decline is noted in boys, but it continues through 17 to 18 years, at which time their temperatures average about 0.7°F. less than girls of the same age.
Ovulation
Normal body temperature rises 0.5° to 1°F. following ovulation
Environment
The fevers of over-clothed children may often fall dramatically when their many layers of clothing and covering are removed
Individual Differences
There are children at either end of the normal distribution curve with striking individual differences. Some normally have temperatures of 97° to 98°F. and in these, 99° to 100°F. may represent true fever. There are also those who rarely have normal temperatures under 100°F.
Neurological Factors
Children with neurological handicaps may show impaired temperature control, at times running high fevers with mild illnesses and normal or subnormal temperatures with serious infections
Diurnal Variation
In children there is a normal diurnal variation of about 2°F. with the peak usually around 5 to 7 P.M. and the nadir around 2 to 6 A.M. Fever curves tend to follow the same pattern

Figure 37-2. Normal variations of temperature in children. (Used with permission of Hospital Publications, Inc., from "Evaluation of the febrile child." *Hosp. Med.* 14:50–63, July 1978, by W. A. Tomlinson, p. 51, Fig. 1.)

measures of control. When a battery-powered rectal probe is available, it is preferable to use this method of continuous monitoring of body temperature. Constant stimulation of the patient by repeated insertions of a thermometer is thus avoided, and a more accurate and continuous reading of body temperature is available to trace progress and guide therapy.

Although instances have been recorded in which patients have survived temperatures as high as 44.4°C (112°F) for a short period of time, a temperature as high as 42.2°C (108°F) for an extended period of time can be expected to do permanent damage. Furthermore, when temperatures exceed 41.0°C (105.8°F), regulatory mechanisms cannot be depended on to resist further rise. (See Chapter 20, Figure 20-5, for limits of negative feedback mechanisms to maintain required body temperature.) Excessively high temperatures endanger the body by irreversibly inactivating essential enzyme systems and by producing permanent alterations in the structure of body proteins. Therefore when a patient's temperature is elevated to, or approaches, 40.56°C (105°F) and continues to rise, measures are instituted to reduce it.

When the heat-regulating centers are injured, the only effective measures are those that increase heat loss by increasing the temperature gradient between the skin and the external environment. To increase the difference in temperature gradient, measures are instituted to increase the evaporation of moisture from the skin, or the patient is placed in a cold environment, so that the heat moves from tissues to the surrounding media. Thus the patient may be sponged liberally with water or alcohol. When the skin is cool, the sponging should be accompanied by rubbing in order to encourage the circulation of blood through the skin. Another point to be remembered when giving a sponge bath is that it should be continued for as long a period of time as is necessary to lower the temperature. A quick "splash" may do more harm than good as it may only stimulate heat production. In young children temperature may be effectively lowered by cooling rectal irrigations, and by immersion in a tub of water a few degrees cooler than body temperature.

For the patient whose temperature is dangerously high, placing him or her in a tub of iced water may be life-saving. When hypothermia blankets are available, a patient may be placed between them. "Space suits" that may be either cooled or warmed are also available. When electrical equipment such as the hypothermia blanket is used, the nurse maintains vigilance through tactile confirmation of readings on temperature gauges. Equipment breaks down, and a faulty reading can lead either to freezing or burning the person's skin. These procedures must be prescribed by the physician. When drastic measures are taken to reduce body temperature, regular and frequent checking of the patient's temperature and pulse are essential. Because the temperature continues to fall after the decline is established, the physician should be asked to indicate the level at which the temperature-reducing procedure should be discontinued. During the chill, the patient should be covered and protected from drafts. A hot-water bottle applied to the feet and an ice cap to the head may increase the patient's comfort.

Signs and Symptoms of Fever

The signs and symptoms accompanying fever result from (1) the increase in the metabolic rate as a result of the elevation in body temperature, (2) the response of the cardiovascular and respiratory systems, (3) the nonspecific responses of the body to injury, and (4) the nature of the causative agent.

As the metabolic rate rises in fever, utilization of calories and protein catabolism increases. Unless carbohydrate and protein intake is increased in proportion to the elevation of body temperature, weight loss occurs. Attention to the patient's food intake is of particular importance when fever lasts more than a few days. Weight loss does not need to occur, providing the patient's food intake is adequate.

Another effect of the increased metabolic rate is increased sweating. As much as 3 liters of water may be lost each day by the patient with fever. Salt is also lost. To maintain fluid balance, the patient must be given assistance to replace this fluid. The higher the temperature, the more fluid is lost and the more help is needed to ingest sufficient fluids to keep fluid intake equal to fluid loss. An inadequate fluid intake is accompanied by a low output of concentrated urine and sordes in the patient's mouth. When fluid intake is adequate, he or she does not develop sordes and excretes at least 1000 ml of urine daily. In those patients who have drenching sweating (diaphoresis), comfort is increased by sponge baths and by replacing wet with dry clothing and linen. In patients who continue to feel chilly, such as those with influenza, bathing may increase discomfort.

The cardiovascular and respiratory responses to fever are those one expects when the metabolic rate is increased. They include an increase in the heart and respiratory rates and dilatation of the peripheral blood vessels. As a result of the vascular changes, the patient appears flushed and complains of the feeling warm. In the patient with a limited cardiac reserve, the extra burden placed on the heart by the increased heart rate may precipitate heart failure.

Among the nonspecific responses to fever are nausea, vomiting, and diarrhea. The leukocyte count may be elevated above 12,000 cells or be lower than 5,000 cells per cubic millimeter of blood. There may be an increase in the sedimentation rate.

Although patients who have a fever may have few or no subjective symptoms, they may feel unpleasantly warm, have headache and malaise, muscle aching, and photophobia, and feel miserable. For the relief of headache, applying an ice cap to the head or sponging the patient's face may be helpful. Protection of the patient with photophobia from bright light is essential and may lessen the headache. The physician may prescribe aspirin for the headache. However, some patients prefer the headache to the sweating that follows the ingestion of aspirin. Adults tolerate fever quite well unless it continues for an extended period of time.

In addition to the signs and symptoms that accompany fever, the patient is likely to have others that are related to the condition causing the fever. For example, the sputum of the patient with pneumococcal pneumonia has specific characteristics. The type of fever and the length of time it lasts are related to the fact that the pneumococcus is the causative agent. In many disorders in which fever occurs, the type of fever as well as the length of time it lasts is generally predictable.

The possibility that the cause of the fever may be an infectious agent should not be overlooked in those patients in whom there is a problem of differential diagnosis. Measures appropriate to the prevention of the spread of infection to personnel and to other patients should be instituted. These measures should take into account the avenues by which organisms leave the host, vehicles whereby they can be transported to others, and portals of entry to others. (See Chapter 10.)

Types of Heat Disorders

Heat disorders fall into three overlapping categories (Summertime, 1979):

1. *Heat cramps,* which are painful muscle spasms set off by a chemical imbalance. Prevention and treatment are the intake of salt and water, particularly prior to strenuous exercise.
2. *Heat exhaustion,* which is usually manifested by fainting accompanied by profuse sweating.
3. *Heat stroke,* which almost always occurs when both temperature and humidity are high. Heat stroke may be regarded as an end stage of prolonged heat exhaustion. *Collapse* occurs *with the absence of sweating.*

Figure 37-3 illustrates the physiologic responses to heat stress, tracing those events that lead to heat cramps, heat exhaustion, and heat stroke. Heat stroke is a medical emergency, and should be treated promptly with intravenous fluids and ice water immersion (Summertime, 1979). In heat stroke resulting from either direct thermal injury of the myocardium or increased pulmonary vascular resistance, the heart may not be able to meet the elevated circulatory demand. Therapy must (1) rapidly reduce body temperature and (2) support the cardiovascular system (O'Donnell & Clowes, 1972).

Hypothermia

Just as the tissues can, within limits, tolerate temperatures higher than the normal range, they can tolerate temperatures that are lower. Healthy tissues can survive slow cooling to 20°C (68°F). However, the rate and moisture associated with cooling are critical factors in determining whether or not tissue injury results. With fast moist cooling, ice crystals form that damage capillary endothelium, thus increasing capillary permeability. Intravascular fluid leaks into interstitial spaces, erythrocytes concentrate and clump in the capillaries, blood flow is obstructed, and tissue destruction ensues.

The usual response to cold is shivering and constriction of the peripheral blood vessels. It is possible for peripheral vasoconstriction to contribute successfully to conservation of core temperature while at the same time producing such pronounced peripheral ischemia that local tissue injury, or *frostbite,* results.

Frostbite

Emergency treatment for frostbite is to rewarm the affected areas rapidly, either by immersion in water or by application of wet compresses, using water at temperatures of 100 to 110°F (37.8 to 43.3°C). Cooler water will delay rewarming dangerously, and warmer water can damage tissues further (Gedrose, 1980).

Factors Affecting Development of Hypothermia

Shivering is accompanied by an increase in the production of heat and by changes decreasing heat loss. When these mechanisms are adequate or the environmental temperature is not too low, they may

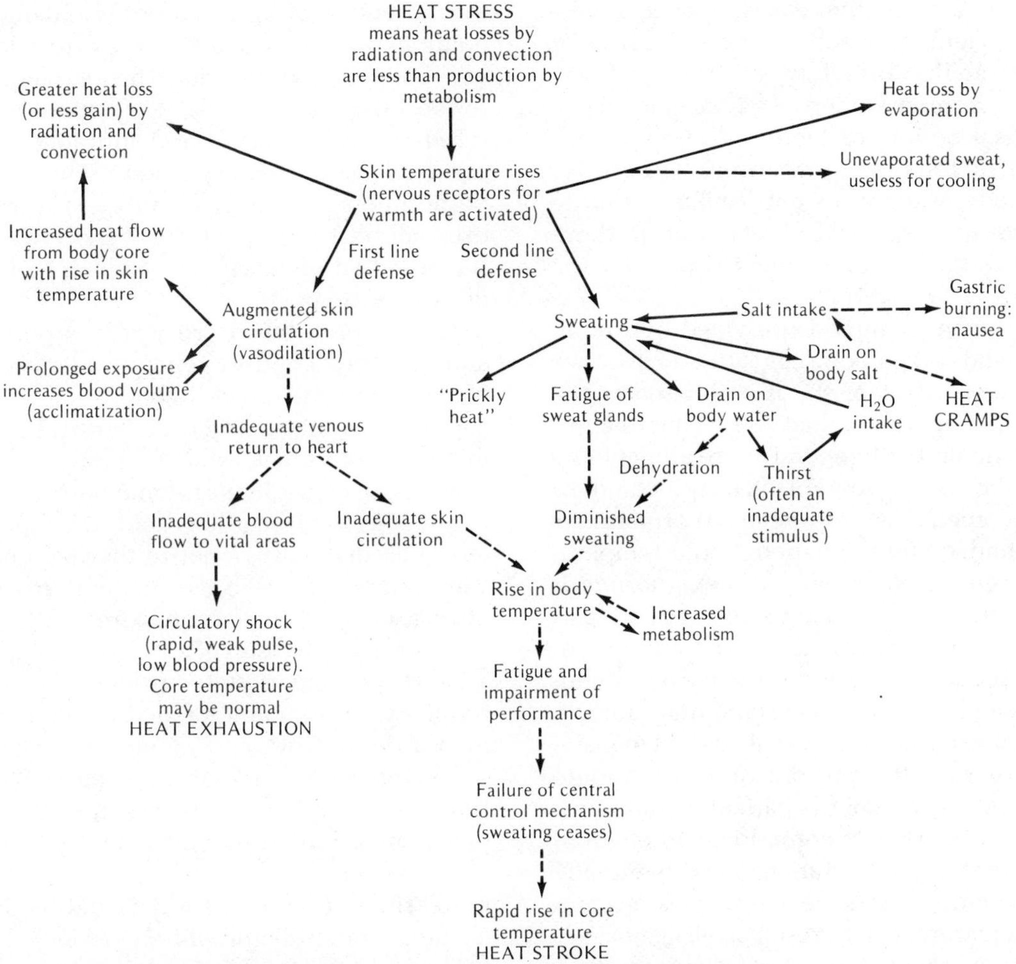

Figure 37-3. A chart indicating the physiologic responses to heat stress in man. Solid lines indicate usual responses, and the directions of the arrows show cause and effect relationships. Broken lines denote events leading to injury. (Adapted with permission of Academic Press, Inc., from "Resistance to Heat in Man and Other Homeothermic Animals," in *Thermobiology*, A. H. Rose, ed., 1967, p. 490, by H. S. Belding.)

be sufficient to maintain body temperature within normal limits. The greater the insulation, either by fat or clothing, the lower the environmental temperature at which heat production increases. Heat conservation is aided by increase in body weight. If cold persists, shivering ceases but extra heat production is maintained by enzymatic activity of muscles, liver, and other organs. The optimum diet for severe cold is not known. But regardless of a person's dietary pattern, sudden exposure to cold results in loss of adipose tissue (Barnett & Mount, 1967).

When heat loss exceeds heat production, hypothermia (abnormally low body temperature) ensues. Our extremities can withstand external temperature changes of 30° to 40°, but our core body temperature cannot tolerate fluctuations greater than 2° or 3° without significant physiological alterations occurring (Gedrose, 1980).

When Core Temperature Falls Below	Usual Consequences
98.6°F (37°C)	Decreased pulse, respiration and blood pressure Decreased metabolism
80.°F (26.7°C)	Numbness and loss of sensation
77–70°F (25–21.1°C)	Coma and death

As an example of the type of situation which places people at high risk for hypothermia, a hunting party is lost in the woods or mountains or on the prairie in freezing or near-freezing weather. The seriousness of their predicament depends not only on the temperature of the environment but on the adequacy of their clothing, whether or not it is wet or dry, and their ability to find or construct a shelter for protection from the wind. As indicated previously, water is a better conductor of heat than air. As air warms, it tends to form an insulating layer around the body; water does not. Chilling is more rapid when evaporation takes place and/or there are air currents than when clothing is dry and the air is still.

A more common example is provided by the elderly person who is exposed to cold after a fall either outside or indoors. If he or she is inebriated at the time, heat loss is increased because alcohol causes vasodilation. Should the temperature reading of any patient be 95°F, the lowest reading on a standard clinical thermometer, a low-reading thermometer should be obtained and the patient's true temperature determined. Another cause of hypothermia is depression of the nervous system by drugs such as morphine and the barbiturates. Hypothermia can occur as a consequence or complication of many clinical disorders and altered homeostatic mechanisms, as well as from exposure to unusual cold. Manifestations of hypothermia that are probably appropriate to the low metabolic rate of the patient include slow pulse, atrial arrhythmias, hypotension, and oliguria. Although each of these alterations may eventually require treatment, unless rewarming is accomplished first, treatment may result in drug toxicity or circulatory overload when normal temperature is restored.

Rewarming may be accomplished by either active or passive methods. *Passive rewarming* methods place the patient in an environment slightly warmer than his or her body temperature, thus preventing additional heat loss and allowing heat production mechanisms to raise core body temperature. *Active rewarming* is accomplished by either internal or external rewarming methods. With external methods, the patient may be immersed in hot water or placed between thermal blankets. This method may lead to "rewarming shock" as a result of peripheral vasodilatation. Internal, or core, methods apply heated fluids directly to the core organs in greatest danger of injury from cold. Methods of application include peritoneal dialysis (see Chapter 41), cardiopulmonary bypass, and thoracotomy with lavage of the mediastinum. Risks of these procedures dictate that their use be restricted to life-saving situations (Hudson & Conn, 1974).

A hypothermic patient is passively rewarmed by being placed at ordinary room temperature and being covered with light bed covering. His or her temperature should rise about 1° to 2°F per hour. As the patient warms, the patient is in danger of developing hypovolemic shock as the arterioles dilate. To prevent this complication the physician may prescribe intravenous fluids. They should be administered slowly because rapid infusion of fluids may overload the circulatory system. The skin of the hypothermic patient is susceptible to heat. Therefore external heat is applied cautiously. The skin should be inspected regularly for reddening or other signs of overheating.

The patient's blood pressure, temperature, pulse, and possibly central venous pressure should be checked regularly. The hypothermic patient is susceptible to ventricular fibrillation and cardiac arrest in addition to shock as he or she warms. Therefore, rewarming of the hypothermic person must include continuous electrocardiographic monitoring; regardless of cardiac status prior to thermal injury, the rewarming process itself can trigger dysrhythmias and, ultimately, cardiac arrest (Gedrose, 1980). This hazard is probably a result of a shift in the oxygen dissociation curve which resulted from the cooling, thereby reducing the amount of oxygen delivered to the myocardium. Defibrillation efforts are not successful unless the body temperature is at least 28°C (82.4°F) [Baughman & Bangs, 1979]. Cardiac irregularities may also be caused by metabolic acidosis, which occurs as a consequence of anaerobic metabolism. Irregularities of pulse or EKG should be promptly reported. A defibrillator and emergency drugs should be on hand to use if needed.

Prevention of Frostbite and Hypothermia

The best management of frostbite and hypothermia is prevention through education. Major points to emphasize include the following (Gedrose, 1980):

1. *Evaluate the weather.* Special attention should be paid to the wind chill factor when temperatures are near freezing.
2. *Wear the proper clothing.* Multiple layers of loose-fitting, natural-fiber clothes provide the best protection against the cold.
3. *Heat the home adequately.* With the supply and cost of home heating fuels, this is a massive risk factor, particularly for the elderly on fixed incomes. Recommended home temperatures may be very difficult to maintain without obtaining heating fuel subsidies for persons at risk of hypothermia in cold climates.

Age	Recommended Room Temperature
65–75 years	65°F (18.3°C)
Over 75 years	70°F (21.1°C)

Older persons who survive accidental hypothermia show an impairment of their thermoregulating mechanisms that persists for up to 3 years, thereby increasing their vulnerability to subsequent episodes of hypothermia (Finch & Hayflick, 1977).

Other practices against which to caution people who are, or may be, exposed to cold environments include the following (DeLapp, 1980):

1. Use of alcohol, which causes peripheral vasodilation
2. Use of nicotine, which causes peripheral vasoconstriction
3. Remaining outside in wet clothing, even when wet from perspiration, which increases heat loss by conduction
4. Excessive washing and shaving of the face prior to exposure, which increases the risk of frostbite by compromising skin integrity

Artificial Induction of Hypothermia

The method employed to induce hypothermia depends on why it is used, how long it is to be maintained, and the equipment available. Hypothermia is induced by three methods: (1) *external or surface cooling,* (2) *internal or body cavity cooling,* and (3) *extracorporeal cooling.*

The fastest method of external cooling is by immersion of the trunk and extremities in a tub of iced water. Because they are easier to use, refrigerated blankets are more commonly used for surface cooling. These blankets contain coils through which a refrigerant is circulated.

Hypothermia or even freezing of body cavities such as the stomach has been used to treat diseases such as peptic ulcer. The purpose is to decrease the activity of the acid-secreting glands. In the hands of physicians skilled in the technique, it may be beneficial to some patients.

In open heart surgery, blood is cooled by circulating it through the cooling system of the pump oxygenator. The same system is used to warm the patient after the procedure is completed.

Effects of Hypothermia

As the body temperature falls, the metabolic rate also falls. The most important effect of the decreased metabolic rate is that the oxygen requirements of the tissues are likewise decreased. Experimental evidence indicates that when tissue temperature is decreased to 30°C, oxygen consumption is reduced by about 50 per cent (Gauging a Safe 'Time Out,' 1973). One of the important uses of hypothermia is therefore in surgical procedures requiring interruption of the circulation to important structures, such as the brain. By induction of hypothermia, the length of time the circulation is stopped can be prolonged. It is used in open heart surgery and in operations on the aorta to protect the brain from the effects of hypoxia. It is also employed in the therapy of patient with serious injuries to the brain as well as in the treatment of uncontrolled hyperthyroidism.

The Nurse's Responsibilities in Caring for the Patient Who Undergoes Hypothermia

The responsibilities of the nurse vary with the method used and the length of time hypothermia is maintained. When hypothermia is induced by circulating the blood through a pump oxygenator, most of the responsibility is borne by the physician and the technician who runs the pump. When the blanket is used and the patient is maintained in a hypothermic state for several days, much of the responsibility is delegated to the nurse.

Shivering

One of the problems in hypothermia is the control of shivering. It must be controlled as the temperature will not fall unless heat loss is greater than heat gain. In the conscious patient, shivering is a source of great discomfort. The patient should be observed regularly for evidence of shivering, which starts with a quivering of the chest muscles. One of the phenothiazines, usually chlorpromazine, is prescribed, to be given before hypothermia is instituted and every 2 hours as needed. Other drugs such as Demerol may be prescribed to reduce discomfort.

In all phases of hypothermia—induction, maintenance, and warming—regular and accurate observation of the patient is essential. During induction and also during rewarming the temperature tends to overshoot the desired mark.

Observation

The nursing care of the patient who has had hypothermia artificially induced is similar to that in which hypothermia is accidentally induced. When induction is artificial, the temperature, blood pressure, central venous pressure, and rate and rhythm of the pulse should be monitored continuously. The blood pressure and pulse rate are expected to decrease. Especially during the warming period, ventricular fibrillation and cardiac arrest are possible. Irregularity of the pulse may herald this event. Urine output diminishes. The urine has a low specific gravity. Because hypothermia depresses the activity of tissues, bodily responses to infection may be diminished. Respiratory infections may develop in the absence of the usual signs and symptoms.

The size and shape of each pupil as well as their response to light should be noted. Because tearing is likely to be minimal, the condition of the conjunctiva should also be observed. Irrigations of the eyes and/or applications of eye patches may be necessary to keep the cornea moist and protect the eyes from injury.

Drugs

With the depression of metabolism and of organs such as the liver and kidneys, reactions to drugs may well be abnormal. Absorption may be delayed or the mechanisms for their destruction or elimination impaired. The nurse should know the expected as well as the toxic effects of drugs given to the patient.

To illustrate, Mrs. Molly McRobin was admitted to the emergency room for treatment of a stab wound to her chest. Although she was fully conscious at the time of her admission, she soon lapsed into unconsciousness from which she never recovered. She was rushed to the operating room, where she was found to have cardiac tamponade caused by bleeding into the pericardial sac, and she experienced cardiac arrest for a period of from 5 to 10 minutes.

Because of the injury to the temperature-regulating centers in the hypothalamus, Mrs. McRobin was unable to control her temperature and it began to rise. To prevent damage to the brain by hyperthermia and to decrease its oxygen requirements, Mrs. McRobin was placed on a hypothermia blanket. At this time Mrs. McRobin was deeply unconscious and she was dependent on the nurse to meet her physiologic needs. Observation not only of the status of the patient but of the functioning of all the different types of equipment was necessary. Although the only aspect of Mrs. McRobin's care that will be discussed is the hypothermia, she required special attention to maintenance of oxygen supply, fluid intake and output, nutrition, mouth care, protection of her skin, and attention to position and body alignment. To maintain her joints in a functional condition, her extremities were moved slowly and passively through normal range of motion daily. Because ventilation is impaired by hypothermia, the nurse made certain that tracheostomy and respiratory assistance were available, should the patient require them. Also, a regular turning schedule was established.

Because Mrs. McRobin was unconscious, the procedure could not be explained to her. Her mother, her only visitor, was informed, however. Before Mrs. McRobin was placed on the blanket, she was bathed and her skin was covered with a thin layer of lanolin to lessen the possibility of frostbite. After she was on the blanket, she was given partial baths as needed. Cool water was used. Patting rather than rubbing motions were used in drying her.

Although the patient may be placed between two hypothermia blankets, Mrs. McRobin was placed on one. The patient may be placed directly on the blanket or the blanket may be covered with a sheet. The latter practice is more aesthetic and may be more comfortable for the patient; when the sheet is tucked under the sides of the mattress, it may also help to keep the blanket in place. By such placement of the blanket or sheet, the rate of cooling is reduced by trapping air, which insulates the skin from the blanket.

As prescribed by Mrs. McRobin's physician, the thermostat on the blanket was set at 32.2°C (90°F). To observe her temperature, a rectal probe was introduced and connected to a battery-operated thermometer. Her temperature could be determined at any time by switching on the machine. The blanket operates automatically. Because the patient's temperature drops about 2°F after cooling is discontinued, the machine should turn off before the desired temperature is attained. It should also turn on when the temperature starts to rise.

Although not a problem with Mrs. McRobin, the restless patient may move off the blanket. When this happens, either the patient or the blanket must be moved so that the patient is reclining on it.

The blanket itself requires some care. Tape rather than safety pins should be used to fasten tubing to sheets. A punture, of the blanket will allow the refrigerant fluid to escape and render the blanket useless. Hot water or strong chemicals should not be applied to the blanket as they may damage the plastic covering. The blanket can be washed with soap and tepid water or a solution of benzethonium chloride. It should not be folded when stored, but it should be rolled loosely and placed on a flat surface.

Summary

The purpose of this chapter has been to discuss some of the needs of the patient who has problems in the control of body temperature or in whom hypothermia is induced. As a basis for understanding the nature of these problems, the homeostatic mechanisms utilized by the body in maintaining temperature were reviewed in Chapter 20, and were related in this chapter to the mechanisms that are involved in hyperthermia and hypothermia. Suggestions have been made as to how this content applies to the care of patients in general and to those with alterations in body temperature. Students who are interested in pursuing the study of temperature regulation in its various aspects will find references at the end of the chapter.

References Cited

Barnett, S. A., and Mount, L. E. "Resistance to Cold in Mammals. In *Thermobiology.* Ed. by A. H. Rose New York: Academic Press, 1967, pp. 411–77.

Baughman, D., and Bangs, C. "The Frozen Patient: Handle with Care." *RN,* **42**:(Nov. 1979) 38–44.

Brody, J. E. "As New Uses Arise, Aspirin Remains a 'Wonder Drug,'" *The New York Times* (Oct. 30, 1979).

Case, J. F. *Biology,* 2nd ed. New York: Macmillan Publishing Co., 1979, pp. 385–90.

Davis-Sharts, J. "Mechanisms and Manifestations of Fever." *Am. J. Nurs.,* **78**:(Nov. 1978), 1874–77.

DeLapp, T. D. "Taking the Bite Out of Frostbite and Other Cold Weather Injuries." *Am. J. Nurs.,* **80** (Jan. 1980), 56–60, 57.

Dinarello, C. A., and Wolff, S. M. "Fever." *Human Nature,* (Feb. 1979), 66–72.

———. "Pathogenesis of Fever in Man." *N. Engl. J. Med.* **298** (1978), 607–12.

Finch, C. E., and Hayflick, L., eds. *Handbook of the Biology of Aging.* New York: Van Nostrand Reinhold, 1977, pp. 645–50.

Ganong, W. F. *Review of Medical Physiology,* 6th ed. Los Altos: Lange Medical Publications, 1973.

Gedrose, J. "Prevention and Treatment of Hypothermia and Frostbite." *Nurs. 80,* **10** (Feb. 1980), 34–36.

"Gauging a Safe 'Time-Out' for Stopped Hearts." *Med. World News,* **14** (Jan. 26, 1973) 62E.

Hayter, J. "Hypothermia Hyperthermia in Older Persons." *J. Gerontol. Nurs.,* **6** (Feb. 1980), 65–68.

Hudson, L. D., and Conn, R. D. "Accidental Hypothermia." *JAMA,* **227** (Jan. 7, 1974), 37–40.

Jacoby, G. A., and Swartz, M. N. "Fever of Undetermined Origin." *N. Engl. J. Med.,* **289** (Dec. 27, 1973), 1407–10.

O'Donnell, T. F., Jr., and Clowes, G. H. A., Jr. "The Circulatory Abnormalities of Heat Stroke." *N. Engl. J. Med.,* **287** (Oct. 12, 1972), 734–37.

Petersdorf, R. G. "Chills and Fever." In *Harrison's Principles of Internal Medicine.* Ed. by G. W. Thorn et al. New York: McGraw-Hill, 1977, pp. 59–68.

Summertime—When the Thermometer Reads Hot." *Harvard Med. School Health Letter,* **4**:10(Aug. 1979), 1–2.

Tomlinson, W. A. "Evaluation of the Febril Child." *Hosp. Med.,* **14** (July 1978), 50–63.

General References

Atkins, E., and Bodel, P. "Fever." *N. Engl. J. Med.,* **286** (Jan. 6, 1972), 27–34.

Brown, N. K., and Thompson, D. J. "Nontreatment of Fever in Extended-Care Facilities." *N. Engl. J. Med.,* **300** (May 31, 1979), 1246–50.

Kluger, M. J. "The Evolution and Adaptive Value of Fever." *American Scientist* **66** (Jan.–Feb. 1978), 38–43.

———. "The Importance of Being Feverish. *Natural History,* **85**: 1 (Jan. 1976), 71–76.

Petersdorf, R. G. "Disturbances of Heat Regulation." In *Harrison's Principles of Internal Medicine.* Ed. by G. W. Thorn et al. New York: McGraw-Hill, 1977, pp. 53–59.

38

Problems with Infections

Until the present we have lacked a rational strategy applicable to overcoming infectious disease. In 1907, Paul Ehrlich pointed to the future development of a specific chemotherapy which killed the parasite without harming the host; the selectivity and efficacy of the sulfanilamides and various antibiotics in treating bacterial disease were only discovered in the late 1930's and subsequent decades.

COHEN
Cohen, S. S.: "A Strategy for the Chemotherapy of Infectious Disease," *Science* 197:431 (July 29) 1977.

The Nurse's Responsibilities in the Control of Infectious Diseases

In this chapter information has been selected to further the understanding of the nurse of some of the important problems involved in the control of diseases caused by microorganisms. No attempt will be made to describe in detail all the infectious diseases to which humans are heir. Such information is readily available for many sources. Four diseases that are problems in the United States will be used to illustrate points being made (staphylococcal disease, syphilis, tuberculosis, and viral hepatitis). Not all information will be included for each disease. Emphasis is on the prevention and control of an infectious disease rather than on the care of the patient who is sick. Nursing of the person who is ill with an infectious disease has two general aspects, the care of the person who is sick and the prevention of the spread of disease to the nurse and others. The underlying principle of the control of infectious disease in the hospital or in the community is that of direct action against the factor(s) promoting the existence of the disease, with emphasis on procedures that have the greatest promise of breaking the chain of transmission. The more knowledge we have of the natural history of each disease, the easier it is to determine where the chain of the disease process can be broken successfully. On occasion an effective control measure has been based, not on considerable knowledge of the disease, but on astute observation of what was occurring in nature. Jenner observed that cowpox gave protection against smallpox and advocated this preventive measure nearly a century before the germ theory originated.

This chapter has been revised by Jean Stallwood-Hess, R.N., M.S.N., Associate Professor, College of Nursing, Wayne State University, Detroit, Michigan.

Knowledge Base for Practice

To fulfill responsibilities in the prevention and control of infectious disease, the nurse needs a body of knowledge that will enable her or him only to

1. Keep abreast with changes in knowledge of the factors in prevention and the control of infectious disease.
2. Develop procedures and practices based on the knowledge required for the protection of patients, personnel (including self), and the community.

3. Evaluate, or participate in the evaluation of, practices employed in the control of infectious disease.
4. Accept changes in established procedures when change or changes are indicated.
5. Carry our procedures that are for the protection of all concerned by consistently practicing aseptic technique.
6. Develop and/or participate in the health care agency educational program.
7. Participate in the health care agency program to control infection
   a. By identifying problems in the control of infection.
   b. As a participating member of the infection control committee.
      (1) Report to the committee problems in the control of infections.
      (2) Report to the nursing staff the deliberations of the committee.
      (3) Make suggestions in the committee on the problems and possible solutions.
   c. By making suggestions to the nurse member(s) of the committee on the problems and proposing suggestions as to how the problems might be solved.
8. Act as a case finder.
9. Participate in community programs of prevention.
10. Participate in health consumer education supporting the rational use of antimicrobial agents.

The preceding is indeed an imposing list of responsibilities. To fulfill them, the nurse requires knowledge, experience, interest in learning, and a willingness to alter practice when new discoveries indicate the need for change. In addition, the effective prevention and control of infectious disease frequently depends not on the nurse alone or on a single measure, but on the cooperation of a large proportion of the community and a variety of procedures. The specific major responsibilities of the nurse will vary according to the work setting. Some of the special responsibilities of nurses employed in the hospital will be discussed in a later section on hospital-acquired infections. Nurses employed by schools, health departments, visiting nurse associations, and health maintenance organizations have the opportunity to play an important part in case finding, encouraging prevention through the use of vaccines and other immunizing agents, and working with people to maintain or improve their general level of health and thus their resistance to infection.

One of the essential elements in the effective prevention and control of infectious disease is application of the concept that a change in practice is difficult if not impossible to effect unless the person who desires to bring it about understands what the beliefs and values are that support existing practice and can effectively communicate the reasons why change is desirable. Understanding this concept is important in the United States because of the diverse character of the population. Further, more and more nurses are traveling to distant lands to assist people to improve their health practices. Because not all persons have the same beliefs or system of values, one element in the success of nurses working with people from different cultures is the ability to put this concept into practice.

Legal Aspects

In this age of markedly increased numbers of lawsuits against hospitals, doctors, and nurses, the nurse can help protect herself or himself from legal action by strict attention to aseptic techniques and all other professional aspects of infection control. It is the nurse's responsibility to use ordinary, reasonable care in nursing activities. The court has held a nurse negligent for using an unsterile needle, from which a patient developed an infection (Creighton, 1975). As nurses move into extended roles and assume more responsibility for independent judgments, such problems can become more serious.

A few examples of situations in which adverse legal rulings against nurses and their employers may occur are mentioned by Dubay and Grubb (1978):

1. Nurses' failure to wash hands resulting in cross-infection among patients
2. Use of improperly sterilized or unsterile operating or injecting equipment
3. Negligence in not calling a superior when a problem arises that might lead to an infection
4. Improper care of wounds
5. Reprocessing and reusing a disposable article that is unsterile

Legal cases regarding nosocomial infections have increased significantly during recent years and include almost all categories of infections. Many cases have been settled out of court, but some have come to trial.

The risk of iatrogenic infections is increasing because of newly developed techniques of diagnosis and treatment during the past 10 years. Data gathered by the National Nosocomial Infection Survey and the Center for Disease Control have shown that approximately 50 per cent of all infections are associated with instrumentation related to diagnosis and treatment—catheterization, hyperalimentation, and mechanical respirators, to name a few. The duty and challenge of combatting the risk of infection by exercising "ordinary care" in the legal sense, must be met (Morris, 1979).

Realistic and practical hospital policies and procedures regarding infection control are important. Well-documented records regarding routine surveillance activities are helpful as evidence that "ordinary care" was exercised by adhering to infection control policies and procedures (Morris, 1979).

With regard to causation of infections, the plaintiff must prove that alleged negligence of the hospital led directly to his or her infection and that he or she would not have the infection except for the hospital's negligent acts. In the future, more sophisticated "detective hunts" may be conducted by plaintiffs and defendants. Questions such as:

"Which is a 'bad bug'? Is it masked by another 'bad bug'? Is the real 'bad bug' the bug underneath? Why does it do harm? Is the harm due to the hospital's negligence, or is it due to the patient's idiosyncracy or to an unforeseeable, intervening event." (Morris, 1979, p. 193)

It is not the purpose of this chapter to discuss malpractice cases, but one will be cited as an example to highlight the lack of proper aseptic technique by personnel which exposed a hospital to liability. The plaintiff had been placed in a two-bed room with a patient who had displayed signs of a staphylococcal infection and he too developed a staphylococcal infection while hospitalized. Nurses and attendants who cared for the two patients during the period of 8 days did not wash their hands between contacts with the men *or* when leaving the room. The court evidence demonstrated that modern hospitals are alert to risks of cross-infection and that personnel are taught to employ aseptic technique in handling patients with suspected staphylococcal infections. Lab reports did not confirm identical staphylococcal infections, but indicated that cross-infection may have occurred. The jury found this was what had happend. Although infections cannot always be traced to a hospital's negligent acts, liability may be incurred if personnel do not observe accepted standards of infection control (Cohen, 1978, p. 21).

Nosocomial or Hospital-Acquired Infections

An infection acquired by a patient after hospitalization is defined by the Center for Disease Control as a nosocomial infection. The infection was neither present nor incubating at the time of admission unless related to a prior admission. Some nosocomial infections may not produce clinical symptoms until after discharge of the patient from the hospital. All other infections seen in hospital are considered community-acquired.

INCIDENCE

One reason for the present concern about nosocomial infections is the observation that the incidence of infection in hospitals is higher than it was just prior to the introduction of the "wonder" or antimicrobial drugs. Finland (1970) has reviewed changes in the major serious bacterial infections seen at Boston City Hospital, based on the criteria of blood stream invasion and fatality, for selected years between the presulfonamide year 1935 and 1965 following the introduction of wider-spectrum semisynthetic penicillins. The number of bacteremic patients increased steadily until 1947, leveled off during the next 4 years, and then increased rapidly and steadily with an increase of 80 per cent from 1957 to 1965. The case fatality rate of bacteremic patients declined dramatically after the introduction of the sulfonamides, and again to a less marked degree after penicillin and streptomycin became widely used. But between 1947 and 1965 mortality has increased slowly but steadily. Although Finland did not comment on the source of the original infections, he did comment that the organisms that have increased or newly appeared as causes of bacteremic infections in hospitals are rarely seen as causes of community-acquired infections.

Bennett and Brachman (1979) state that approximately 5 per cent of patients admitted to acute care hospitals develop a nosocomial infection, and 3 percent of the infections result directly in the death of the patient. They further state that data accumulated over recent years indicate that as much as half of all nosocomial infections may be preventable. Estimated direct annual cost of these infections exceeds $1 billion with indirect costs possibly doubling this figure.

INFECTING ORGANISMS AND SITES

Since the introduction of antibiotics, there have been dramatic changes in the species of organisms associated with nosocomial infections. The major shift has been from frank pathogens to species that have been considered part of the normal biota of the upper respiratory and alimentary tracts. Klainer and Beisel (1969, p. 431) use the term *opportunistic* in reference to indigenous biota and other usually nonpathogenic organisms that produce infections when the host's defense mechanisms are altered. They relate the increase of such infections to newer medical knowledge by which life can be prolonged for people with debilitating illnesses and by which tissues and organs can be transplanted, as well as the development of many new diagnostic and therapeutic techniques.

Selwyn (1972, pp. 642–46) has described the changing patterns in hospital infection. Hemolytic streptococcal infections, already waning, virtually were eliminated by the arrival of the sulfonamides in the late 1930s. *Staphylococcus aureus* emerged during the 1940s and rapidly developed resistance to newer antibiotics. By the early 1960s gram-negative organisms and opportunistic bacteria and fungi had become the major causes of infection. The explanation Selwyn gives for these changes are similar to those given earlier: older and more seriously ill patients, complicated surgery, immunosuppressive drugs, plus the careless use of antibiotics.

More emphasis is put on the development of drug resistance among bacteria by many authors. The gram-negative bacilli with more extensive natural resistance to the commonly used antibiotics are selectively favored, so that *Pseudomonas, Klebsiella,* and *Proteus* are all too often responsible for hospital-acquired infections. Resistance frequently develops for multiple antibiotics, through mutation or acquisition of genetic material transferred from resistant to susceptible organisms when they are closely adjacent, as in the bowel.

Diseases of viral etiology are of importance in any discussion of hospital-acquired infections. There are many reports of the transmission of hepatitis in dialysis units and by blood transfusion. Rubella has spread within hospitals. Ample opportunities exist for the transmission of virus-caused respiratory disease in pediatric units. In one hospital one fifth of the uninfected contact infants under 18 months of age acquired parainfluenza virus type 3 infection during hospitalization (Mufson et al., 1973, pp. 141–47). Even though most of these infants were admitted because of respiratory tract illness, about one third developed a new, mild respiratory illness and as a group they remained in the hospital longer than contact infants who were not infected.

Site specificity of infecting organisms is controlled to some extent by such factors as mode of transmission and the particular insults sustained by the host's defense mechanisms. *S. aureus* is ubiquitous and can infect many sites but is frequently associated with skin, wound, and burn infections. *Pseudomonas* is becoming increasingly prevalent as a cause of nosocomial infections. Finland (1970, p. 429) noted the steady increase in enterobacterial infections and the high mortality associated with them, especially *Escherichia coli, Proteus, Klebsiella,* and *Enterococcus.* The list of organisms and the sites from which they can be recovered is lengthy. It includes yeasts, fungi, and anaerobic organisms as well as the more commonly encountered bacteria.

Urinary tract infections usually follow catheterization or some type of instrumentation of the urinary bladder. *E. coli, Proteus,* and *Klebsiella* are frequent invaders. Commonly cultured organisms from respiratory infections are *P. aeruginosa* and *Klebsiella.* The dynamic nature of nosocomial infections is demonstrated by the experience at one hospital. Before 1956, 65 per cent of surgical wound infections were caused by gram-positive cocci, particularly *S. aureus.* Since then, such infections have been caused increasingly by gram-negative bacilli, such as *E. coli, Aerobacter aerogenes, Klebsiella, Proteus, Pseudomonas, Serratia,* and anaerobic gram-negative bacteroids (Altemeir, 1971, p. 85).

Predisposing Factors

Some of the specific factors predisposing to nosocomical infections have been indicated in the preceding discussion. To a great degree these are factors that alter the host's resistance and thus increase susceptibility. In a recent review of hospital infections, Eickhoff (1977) stated that serious hospital infections are most common in the very young and in the elderly, but age is probably a major risk factor only in the premature infant. He summarized the determinants, or factors, as anatomic, metabolic, immunologic or hematologic, cardiovascular, respiratory, and antibiotic.

Anatomic determinants are those procedures or conditions that disrupt the integrity of the skin or endothelial surfaces, and thus deprive the patient of one defense against infection. Burns and foreign bodies do this. Invasive procedures categorized as (1) percutaneous procedures, (2) surgical procedures, and (3) procedures that enter a body orifice provide risks of infection. Examples of percutaneous procedures are: intramuscular and subcutaneous injections; catheters inserted in arteriograms; needles used for amniocentesis, thoracentesis, paracentesis, and lumbar puncture; long-term intravenous infusion tubes and stop cocks, central venous pressure lines; peritoneal dialysis and external cardiac pacemakers. Examples of surgical procedures are discussed in later chapters. Examples of entering a body orifice are: insertion of endotracheal tubes, suction catheters, urinary catheterization, and vaginal and rectal examinations (Wineland, 1979, pp. 54–56). During any of the procedures the host may be colonized by new and/or resistant organisms.

Metabolic determinants include both inborn errors of metabolism and those that develop during life. Inborn errors may cause chronic liver disease and thus interfere with protein metabolism and the integrity of body tissues. Diabetes mellitus is a disorder of carbohydrate metabolism, but this is so intertwined with the fates of proteins, fats, water, and electrolytes that it can seriously disturb nutritional status. Diabetics probably do not develop more infections than normal people, their increased risk comes from such accompanying conditions as acidosis, vascular insufficiency, and renal failure. Both bacterial and fungal invasion of the skin are apt to be more dangerous and dramatic than in normal people, in part because of the high glycogen content of the skin, or because of ineffective phagocytosis resulting from acidosis.

Immunologic and hematologic determinants have an effect on patients with such diseases as leukemia and lymphoma and autoimmune diseases. The use of immunosuppressive drugs for organ transplants has created new problems of hospital infection. These factors predispose to endogenous as well as exogenous infections. They include x-ray therapy, the use of cytotoxic drugs and corticosteroids. Other factors include hemolytic disease, and agammaglobulinemia.

Eickhoff (1972) classified as *cardiovascular determinants* those surgical procedures accompanied by hypotension and shock, which in turn increase the patient's risk of acquiring an infection. Respiratory determinants include such diseases as influenza, emphysema, and other chronic obstructive pulmonary conditions. These may have a direct influence on the defense mechanisms of the host, and in addition they result in a greater exposure to antibiotics and inhalation therapy. Antibiotic determinants affect the microflora, not the host, and have been discussed previously.

In addition to predisposing factors that alter the resistance of the patient-host, *the opportunities for exposure to pathogenic organisms are intensified in the hospital.* The population density will be greater than in the patient's normal surroundings. A room may be shared with from one to twenty or more people. The number of hospital personnel and visitors spending time in the patient's immediate environment further increases the possibility of being exposed to infection. The areas in the hospital where infection rates are highest are those in which contact between patient and personnel is the greatest. The increasing complexity of patient care in the hospital makes a contribution to setting the stage for nosocomial infections. The patient is cared for by a large number of highly skilled people who go throughout the hospital caring for various other patients. He or she is moved about the hospital for diagnostic and therapeutic reasons, and exposed to complicated equipment shared by other members of the hospital population.

This discussion has presented some of the circumstances predisposing patients to hospital-acquired infections. As stated earlier, all people, including nurses, are susceptible to infection. By identifying the risk factors that increase the likelihood of patients developing an infection, measures can be instituted to protect patients and personnel.

Sources of Infection

Microorganisms enter the hospital in or on people, in or on inanimate objects, in air, and in or on animals or insects. Within the hospital *three general groups of people act as sources for microorganisms.* The first group includes patients who are admitted for treatment of a septic condition or who are carriers of pathogens. The second group includes patients who are negative at the time they are admitted but who acquire an infection after their admission to the hospital. The person may become a carrier or develop an infectious disease. The third group is composed of various hospital personnel. They, too, may act as carriers or develop *overt disease.*

Modes and Vehicles of Transmission

Food and Water

Food may serve as a vehicle for the transmission of microbes and their products and thus be a source of disease. An example of the first is the *Salmonella* group of bacteria and of the second is the enterotoxin of the *Staphylococcus aureus.* The only procedures of value are to prevent the contamination of food and to refrigerate it if it is not eaten as soon as it is prepared. The sanitary handling of food lessens the chances of introducing microorganisms and refrigeration minimizes bacterial growth.

Water drawn from the tap in the hospital can usually be considered safe for consumption. It can become a vehicle for the transmission of pathogens if it is not dispensed to patients in a safe manner. Ice cubes have been found to contain pathogens although this is a rare occurrence. The bedside water pitcher can become contaminated easily. These pitchers should have wide necks so that they can be thoroughly cleaned and should be made of a material that can be sterilized. They should be covered when on the bedside stand. Ice cubes should be handled with tongs.

Equipment

One way in which exogenous organisms are transmitted to the patient is on or in the equipment used in his or her care and in supplies. Serious outbreaks of *Pseudomonas* infection have been traced to such varied items as humidifiers, skin lotions and creams, sink traps, floor mops, and shaving brushes. Inhalation therapy equipment can be a vector of hospital-acquired pneumonia. When humidifiers and small-volume nebulizers are used, each patient should have fresh tubing and equipment as long as needed. Nebulizers with large reservoirs are a great hazard, and must be sterilized or decontaminated every 24 hours.

The prevention of transmission of infection by equipment involves individualizing all parts that come in contact with the patient or the patient's secretions. Equipment that is not discarded after use should be thoroughly cleaned by healthy, trained personnel who understand the importance of each detail and take pride in doing a competent job. Postoperative pneumonia caused by *Pseudomonas* has been traced to anesthetic equipment and the people who clean it. All types of equipment from thermometers to cardiac bypass machines should be checked at regular intervals for the efficiency of disinfecting techniques.

When air conditioners are used in rooms where there is more than one patient, room air should not be recirculated. Inside air should be exchanged for outside air.

Catheterization

Catheter-induced urinary tract infections are the most prevalent and preventable of serious gram-negative infections in hospitals. To emphasize this statement, Bennett (1979, p. 245) states that data from CDC's National Nosocomial Infections Study reveals the most important underlying site for nosocomial secondary bacteremias are urinary tract infections. They further indicate that there are 37 million acute care hospital admissions per year and 10 per cent of these have indwelling catheters (3,700,000). Eight to 10 per cent of the 3,700,000 have significant bacteriuria each year with risk of further problems.

Organisms can be pushed into the bladder when the catheter is inserted, apparently can be carried up the inserted catheter in air bubbles, and can work their way up the mucous lining of the urethra. One way to help prevent such infections is by scrupulous catheterization technique. Great care should be taken to avoid contamination of the catheter at the time of insertion; it should be lubricated adequately to avoid trauma to the mucous membrane of the urethra; and the smallest possible catheter should be used.

The patient who requires an indwelling catheter presents other needs. A sterile closed drainage system with an antiseptic added to the collecting container should be used. A rigid collecting container should be used for ambulatory patients. The tubing leading from the bladder should be below the level of the bladder but above the level of the urine. The meatus should be washed with a bacteriostatic agent before insertion of the catheter. The area around the meatus should be cleansed at least twice daily with antiseptic. The catheter should be generously lubricated before it is inserted. Measures to increase the relaxation of the patient such as asking him or her to take a deep breath at the time of insertion generally decreases constriction of the urethra. To prevent pushing bacteria normally present in the terminal meatus into the urinary bladder, the urethra may be irrigated by inserting a sterile bulb syringe about three fourths of an inch into the urethra and irrigating it with 1 oz of 1:1,000 aqueous benzalkonium chloride solution or using an antibacterial lubricant. To prevent the upward ascent of bacteria in the tubing, fluids should be forced when the patient can take fluids by mouth.

The protection of the patient who must be catheterized or who has an indwelling catheter is facilitated by measures (1) to prevent or limit the number of organisms introduced into the bladder, (2) to prevent trauma to the urethral meatus and bladder, (3) to prevent the reflux of urine into the bladder, and (4) to maintain drainage from the bladder to the collecting container. (See Chapter 17 for further discussion of the patient with an indwelling urinary catheter.)

Airborne Infections

The air may become directly or indirectly contaminated and serve as a vehicle of transmission of hospital-acquired infections. Pathogenic organisms from human sources found in air originate primarily in the respiratory tract, but some can come from skin or clothing. When considering the respiratory system as a portal of exit for pathogenic organisms, it was stated that there are two basic mechanisms by which they escape: in large droplets, which settle and become incorporated in dust, and in droplet nuclei. Dust particles become resuspended by air movement such as that caused by people moving or by sweeping. The organisms in them can resist drying but usually are susceptible to strong light. They include staphylococci, streptococci, and tubercle bacilli, among others. Each dust particle can contain several organisms. Because of their size and settling speed, they are usually deposited in the upper respiratory tract. Dustborne infections are associated with places more than the immediate presence of an infectious patient. The room that has housed an infectious tubercular patient can be a source of infection to others for hours or days after the patient has left, unless it is thoroughly cleaned.

In contrast, each droplet nucleus probably contains only one pathogenic organism. Because of their small size and slow settling, they can reach the alveoli and deposit their contents there. For disease to be transmitted by droplet nuclei, some proximity between the infected host and the susceptible person is usually required. This mechanism is considered to be the principal vehicle of the tubercle bacillus and probably of many of the viral upper respiratory diseases.

Blankets, sheets, pillows, and mattresses of infected patients and carriers rapidly become contaminated with pathogenic organisms. Not all investigators agree on the extent to which they act as vehicles of transmission for the pathogens. Blankets and sheets may be soiled with drainage from a wound. Patients with nasal staphylococcal infections have been shown to be prolific dispersers of staphylococci, which ride on minute particles of human skin (Noble & Davis, 1965, pp. 16–18). It has been demonstrated that during the process of bed making, large numbers of bacteria are released, up to 50 *S. aureus* particles per cubic foot in a 1,000-cubic-foot room and other aerobic flora between 10 and 100 times this level (Noble, 1962, pp. 552–58). Obviously careful attention must be paid to disinfection of hospital beds and bedding.

One of the most commonly used measures in the control of airborne infection is the wearing of masks. Masks are worn to accomplish two purposes. One is to prevent the contamination of the external environment by microorganisms from the respiratory tract of the person wearing the mask. In terms of the links in the chain of the infectious process, the mask stands between the point at which a microorganism leaves the infected host and the point at which it finds a vehicle for its transmission. This is the basis for wearing a mask in the operating room or in the newborn infants' nursery or for having the patient with a cold, tuberculosis, or other respiratory infection wear a mask. A mask may also be used to guard a portal of entry. In this instance a nurse or doctor wears a mask for protection from microorganisms discharged by the patient.

The construction of the mask and the way it is worn determine its effectiveness. The selection of a satisfactory mask is difficult. Wide variations occur in the filtration efficiency of masks not only from one manufacturer to another, but also in certain instances from mask to mask of the same manufacturer (Dineen, 1971, pp. 812–14). The mask should always cover the mouth and nose and be tied firmly in place. It has been said that a mask should be replaced when it becomes damp, but Dineen (1971) has demonstrated that even when masks were worn for as long as 8 hours and became thoroughly damp, there did not seem to be any loss of filtration capacity. The present-day use of disposable masks eliminates the need for disinfection between use. Modern fabrics in masks, such as special paper or plastic, are porous but quite effective.

Other measures are available to help control airborne infection. The concentration of microorganisms in the air can be reduced by proper ventilation. Florence Nightingale advocated ventilation as a measure in the care of the sick. It is still frequently neglected. Particularly in the operating room, air-conditioning systems may be used to remove the respired air and add clean air. Newer central ventilation systems are designed to filter air if it is to be reused.

There is a direct relationship between quantity of airborne particulates, the pore size of air filters, and the rates of air exchange. State and federal recommendations influence use of filters such as the High Efficiency Particle Air (HEPA) filters which eliminate microorganisms or particles greater than 0.5 microns regardless of the presence of a unidirectional flow of air (Fahlberg, 1979, p. 39). Hospital air is conventionally provided at a rate of two air exchanges per hour to patient rooms, and preferably exhausted through patient bathroom vents. Six air changes per hour is recommended for isolation rooms (Mallison, 1979, p. 90). For areas in the hospital in which very clean air and protection from airborne infection are essential, such as the operating room and laboratory, a unidirectional ("laminar") air flow system with controlled temperature (68 to 74°F) and humidity (50 to 70 per cent) offers much potential (Lidwell, 1971, p. 207). The whole room is, in effect, a short wind tunnel with low velocity.

Riley (1972, pp. 421–23) has suggested that upper-air irradiation with ultraviolet rays can minimize the spread of airborne infections throughout the hospital without exposing the occupants to excessive doses. However, there is some disagreement from others (Mallison, 1979, p. 90) about its effectiveness. Air movement in the enclosed atmosphere of a building results largely from convection currents related to temperature gradients, and that corridors, stairwells, and elevator shafts serve as huge ducts to convey air to different parts of a building. One point that is too often neglected in the control of airborne infection is keeping doors closed. Air currents carry droplet nuclei wherever they go. Although we do not know what proportion of hospital-acquired infection is spread this way, it is probably fairly high.

Hands: Healers and Killers

In general, each individual has a unique characteristic bacterial flora on the hands which is quite stable. Common organisms include gram-positive *Corynebacterium* acnes, diphtheroids, and nonpathogenic staphylococci (Larson, 1979, p. 59). The opportunistic gram-negative organisms normally inhabiting the intestinal tract which have emerged as pathogens, do not usually inhabit skin but can contaminate hands.

The hands, therefore, may act as vehicles in the transmission of organisms. Patients at greatest risk from contaminated hands are newborn infants, those with catheters, and surgical patients (Mallison, 1979, p. 89). The source of contamination may be discharges from the nasal mucosa of carriers or discharges from open lesions, as well as urine and feces. Contamination of the hands may therefore result from direct contact with a lesion or its discharges or from contact with dressings covering septic wounds, bed coverings, or the clothing of the patient. Measures should be carried out to prevent the hands from being contaminated or to remove any microorganisms present on them.

To protect the person who is changing dressings, covering draining wounds, sterile disposable gloves should be worn. The dressings should also be discarded in such a manner that no one handles them after they are removed. For example, they may be placed on several thicknesses of newspaper and wrapped so that the outside of the package is kept very clean. Or they may be put in a plastic bag. Whatever technique is utilized, it should be based on the certainty that discharges from infected lesions are teeming with virulent microorganisms.

Because it is impossible to prevent contamination of the hands in all instances, hand washing is essential to the removal of microorganisms. To be truly effective, it must be performed properly and after each patient contact. Each hospital will have its preferred technique but the general principles are the same. A special cleansing agent is usually advocated. (The F.D.A. has recently restricted use of hexachlorophene, which has long been the most popular cleansing agent for hand washing in hospitals.) The hands should be washed under running water, and dried on a paper towel. It is questionable whether more complicated procedures are an added protection. Data show that the routine quick hand wash usually employed by busy aides and nurses is effective in removing patient-acquired organisms. The technique usually employed in this study was described as "wetting hands with tap water, dispensing a small unstandardized amount of pHisoHex on one palm and spreading it over the hands in two or three brisk washing movements, rinsing with tap water and drying on a paper towel which was subsequently used to turn off the faucet" (Sprunt el at., 1973, pp. 264–65).

Properly performed, hand washing is an essential step in the prevention of the spread of bacteria from patient to patient. But the burden is not all on the nurse. The practice of hand washing by patients helps prevent self-infection and the infection of others, as well as reducing contamination of the environment. This is particularly important when many of the patients are ambulatory.
A study of Pollock et al., revealed over 50 per cent of hospitalized patients were found to carry gram-negative organisms on their hands (1972, pp. 668–71).

Prevention and Control of Hospital-Acquired Infections

A program for prevention and control of hospital-acquired infections requires consideration of the following (U.S. DHEW, 1970, p. 32.):

1. Standards, recommendations, and requirements of the Public Health Service, state and local health departments, and other organizations, such as the American Hospital Association and American Academy of Pediatrics.
2. Infection control committee responsibilities
3. The hospital population
   a. Patients
   b. Hospital personnel
   c. Students
   d. Visitors
   e. Volunteers
   f. Persons delivering items to patients
4. The physical environment and facilities
5. Environmental sanitation
6. Aseptic practices and procedures

Implications for nurses will be included in the discussion, especially the role and function of the infection control practitioner.

No respectable hospital, concerned with the care, treatment, and cure of its patients, is pleased to think those patients can acquire a complicating infection during their hospitalization. Concern and action for the prevention and control of nosocomial infections were stimulated by the significant increase in staphylococcal infections that occurred in hospitals during the middle and late 1950s. In 1958, the Joint Commission on Accreditation of Hospitals and the American Hospital Association recommended that each hospital appoint an infection control committee. A program for surveillance of nosocomial infections has been conducted under the aegis of the Hospital Infections Section, Epidemiology Program, of the Center for Disease Control. They suggest that the membership of the infection control committee should include the hospital epidemiologist, representatives of the major clinical departments, the pathologist or microbiologist, the infection control practitioner, the director of nursing, and a representative of the hospital administration. Other members of the hospital community should be encouraged to attend, such as representatives of the housekeeping and dietary sections. The functions of the committee include policy setting and implementation. The two key members of the committee would be the hospital epidemiologist, whether or not he or she has that specific title, and the infection control practitioner.

Surveillance refers to continuous day-by-day scrutiny of all factors related to the occurrence of infection within the hospital. It involves infection case finding through communication with hospital personnel, infection control rounds with special attention given to patients with fever, those on antibiotic therapy, those having high-risk procedures, or underlying serious pathology. Eickhoff (1977) suggests four benefits from an effective surveillance program: (1) identification of pathogens responsible for a specific hospital infection, (2) estimation of endemic levels of hospital-acquired infection in the hospital, (3) prompt recognition of all epidemics, and (4) prompt implementation of personnel and hospital hygiene practices.

Infection Control Practitioner

The concept that infection control was a separate area in nursing developed in England in 1960 (Davis et al., 1963, pp. 1321–22) and was so successful that it was adopted in the United States a few years later. Kicklighter (1973, pp. 48–56) calls this person a nurse epidemiologist, and considers her or him to have a vital role in infection control.

This nurse may also be titled infection control nurse, surveillance officer, or infection control practitioner. The latter seems most prevalent in the literature. She or he is responsible for facilitating implementation of Joint Commission on Accreditation of Hospitals' (JCAH's) Standards for Infection Control (Krause & Pappas, 1979, p. 2).

The infection control practitioner applies a broad base of theoretical knowledge to clinical expertise in nursing. Her or his functions as discussed by Krause and Pappas (1979, pp. 2–6) are representative of primary, secondary, and tertiary prevention. They include the following:

1. Observing, advising, educating, and guiding the infection control practice of all health professionals
2. Conducting surveillance on high-risk patients
3. Utilizing methods of epidemiological study to investigate the existence and extent of a problem
4. Acting as a behavior model, a facilitator, a change agent, a teacher, and a consultant to personnel and various committees
5. Being involved in the research process through participating in studies of others; utilizing research of others through scientific literature review, analyzing findings, and assimilating or applying findings in current infection control program
6. Evaluating professional and personal growth and seeking to evaluate effectiveness of the hospital's infection control program
7. Acting as hospital liaison with local health department and other health care facilities, such as alerting a nursing home of transfer of an infected patient—type of infection, mode of transfer and containment measures necessary
8. Playing an important role in the era of risk management in today's "malpractice suit–happy" society by effectively practicing the above mentioned functions

Hospital Populations

Patients should be questioned at the time of admission about recent exposure to infectious diseases, either at home or in the community. If there is any indication that any patient may be incubating such a disease, or physical examination indicates it, chemotherapy and/or isolation may be indicated. If isolation is recommended, the reasons should be explained to the patient very carefully, so that he or she will not feel rejected in addition to the other emotional problems of adjusting to the hospital situation.

The number of personnel required to provide patient care has been greatly increased. This mere increase in numbers increases the possibility that they may be a source of infection for the patient. Every hospital needs a sound health program for its personnel including pre-employment physical examinations, basic services such as immunizations and the administration of gamma globulin if indicated, and medical consultation for any with symptoms of infection. Orientation and in-service education programs should stress the importance of personal hygiene and health status, alertness to possible signs of infection in themselves and patients, and the principles and importance of asepsis. Competent supervision should be provided to be sure personnel do not serve as a source of infection.

Currently, there is increasing concern in the area of formal educational programs designed to prepare an effective infection control practitioner. The academic community is slowly addressing this need. Wayne State University, Detroit, Michigan, has a master's program to prepare a nurse epidemiologist.

Students of nursing and other related disciplines, should have the same knowledge about their potential as sources of infection, and ways to prevent this happening, as personnel. They are potential future employees of a hospital. Volunteers should be taught some principles of aseptic techniques if they have any direct contact with patients, such as the importance of good hand washing and alertness to infections in themselves.

Visitors present a more difficult problem, because there is no way they can be screened for the presence of an active infection. But if they come to see a patient in isolation, they should be instructed in the procedures that will prevent them from acquiring the infection, such as thorough hand washing and gowning techniques. Most hospitals today do not allow delivery people to have direct contact with patients.

Environmental Sanitation

Every facet of the physical environment within a hospital has some influence on the welfare of the patient. However, *it is now widely accepted that effective patient care practices consitute the most important single factor for minimizing nosocomial disease, rather than environmental control programs* (Stamm, 1976, p. 60). Programs of *routine* environmental surveillance are not only time-consuming and expensive, but they tend to generate much data that are difficult to interpret and may even be misleading. Therefore, the preferable alternative is to maintain surveillance of nosocomial infections in patients and employees (Mallison, 1979, p. 91).

One major area of environmental sanitation vital to the control of infection comes under the heading of housekeeping. Although nurses are no longer directly responsible for cleaning, they should utilize their knowledge to make certain that the environment is clean. The workers who are involved in cleaning should understand the importance of their work for infection control and why cleaning procedures must be done in a specified way. Many hospitals today use commercial laundries, and this has eliminated some of the labor but none of the responsibility for seeing that bedding and such is not a source of infection. Each hospital should have a system for handling contaminated linen so that their workers are protected, and it should be sent out in such a way that laundry workers are not endangered. Blankets have been recognized as important vehicles in the transmission of infection, so they are thoroughly washed and sterilized after the discharge of a patient. In some hospitals blankets are oiled to encourage particles to adhere to the fibers. Pillows and mattresses pose special threats, especially because staphylococci are resistant to drying. In some Danish hospitals they and the entire bed are sterilized before being used by another patient. General cleaning techniques should include wet mopping or mopping with a mop treated with a substance that causes dust to adhere to it. Double-bucket floor cleaning systems are recommended with thorough drying of mops (Mallison, 1979, p. 89). The same procedure should be observed in dusting. In the past the use of vacuum cleaners has been frowned upon because they stir up dust, but newer designs are removing this objection.

Aseptic Practices

Aseptic practices are those carried out to decrease the number of pathogens and to prevent the transmission of potential pathogens from one person to another. They are essential for infection control and must be observed by all personnel providing any services or supplies for any patient. It does no good for the professional staff to set and carry out fairly rigid procedures and precautions to control hospital cross-infection if other personnel perform their duties as though the germ theory had never been discovered.

Aseptic practices range all the way from such commonsense items as providing each patient with clean, freshly issued supplies and equipment to the most elaborate isolation techniques for very infectious patients. Every hospital will have established procedures for ensuring good asepsis. These will include how supplies are to be properly sterilized or decontaminated and distributed; the disposal of wastes; and how food is to be served. A handwashing routine should be meticulously observed before and after any body contact with a patient. Special precautions should be observed when dressing changes are made. The list is endless.

Personnel who give patient care should be free from infection and they should observe high standards of personal hygiene. Patients should be encouraged to practice personal cleanliness when they are able, such as thorough bathing and hand washing to reduce opportunities for self-infection or infection of others. They can be taught the proper use of paper

TABLE 38-1 *Summary of the Interrelationship of Factors that Produce Four Infectious Diseases in Humans*

	Staphylococcal Disease	Syphilis	Tuberculosis	Infectious Hepatitis
Causative agent	*Staphylococcus* (numerous strains)	*Treponema pallidum*	*Mycobacterium tuberculosis*	Hepatitis virus A (other strains include B and non-A and non-B)
Distribution	Worldwide (ubiquitous)	Worldwide	Worldwide	Worldwide; highest incidence in fall and winter
Nature, characteristics				
1. Ability to survive outside host	More resistant to drying than most nonspore formers; pathogenic strains resistant to antibiotics	Fragile—exists outside host only moments; susceptible to penicillin; adequate dose usually terminates infectiousness within 24 hours	Capable of long-term survival; resistant to disinfection; acid-fast; susceptible to sunlight, ultraviolet light	Resistant to moderate degrees of heat such as 56°C; to pasteurization; to many chemicals; can survive at room temperature for 6 months and −10° to −20°C for years; destroyed by heating to 100°C for 30 minutes, or by ethylene oxide (liquid or gas)
2. General description	Host susceptibility important; multiplies rapidly in tissues, causing multiple focal abscesses and necrosis; coagulase-positive agent may survive within phagocytes	Highly infectious; systemic from onset; overt manifestations in primary and secondary stages; years of asymptomatic latency may or may not result in serious manifestations; after 2 years not usually communicable by sexual contact; can be transmitted from mother to fetus	Primarily chronic respiratory infection; miliary in some areas	Varies; often subclinical especially in children; icteric phase frequently; liver involvement from minimal to destruction by extensive fibrosis
3. Hosts	Humans, carriers and obviously infected; possibly animals	Humans, universally susceptible	Humans; cattle in some areas	Humans; chimpanzee

4. Characteristic lesions	(a) Impetigo and pyoderma of infants, and umbilicus of newborn; (b) mastitis in postpartum patients; (c) surgical wound infections; (d) infections in debilitated patients such as pneumonia, bacteremia; (e) furuncles, carbuncles, infected decubiti and paronychia; (f) pyelonephritis, endocarditis, parotitis	Primary stage—chancre; secondary stage—lymphadenitis, skin rashes, moist condylomata; late syphilis—gumma; congenital—varies from marasmus to apparent health	(a) First infection—usually asymptomatic; mild inflammation in small area of lung, spread to lymph nodes, caseation necrosis, hypersensitivity, calcification-Ghon complex; (b) reinfection—frequently endogenous; bronchogenic spread of lesions with caseation necrosis and fibrosis; little lymph node involvement	See general description; infection originates in intestinal tract
5. Vehicles and conditions of transmission	Airborne droplets or droplet nuclei, skin scales; contact with heavily contaminated air, probably contaminated articles	Open lesions; vaginal secretions during primary and secondary stages; blood; direct contact with infectious lesions, genito-oral, genitorectal, mouth to mouth, fondling of children; transplacental; needle prick; break in skin	Droplets or droplet nuclei; secretions from infected organs; milk from diseased cattle; personal contact but usually requires extended intimate exposure; crowded living conditions	Fecal-oral route; infected blood and saliva through skin or mucous membranes into circulatory system; insect vectors; blood transfusions; contaminated needles and syringes from illicit drug use
6. Incubation period		2–10 weeks chancre develops; in 3–6 weeks secondary stage—about 3 months from time of infection	4–6 weeks	15–40 days—usually 30–38 days but may be as long as 50 days
Human host: 1. Age, sex, race 2. Genetic, personality 3. Habits, customs 4. Defenses—general and specific	All susceptible, especially newborn, elderly, debilitated, wounded, traumatized, burned; fair degree of immunity or resistance	Majority of cases in 15- to 24-year age group; both sexes equally susceptible; sexual promiscuity, homosexuality	Susceptibility high in children under three years; highest incidence in older nonwhite males; some evidence of genetic susceptibility; more among undernourished	Infection especially common among children of lower socioeconomic group living under overcrowded conditions; poor sanitation; institutionalized children
5. Portal of entry	Skin; wounds; respiratory tract	Mucous membranes; breaks in skin	Respiratory and gastrointestinal tracts	Mouth
		Placenta		Breaks in skin and mucous membrane

(Continued)

TABLE 38-1 *(Cont.)*

	Staphylococcal Disease	Syphilis	Tuberculosis	Infectious Hepatitis
6. Portal of exit	Open lesion; skin; anterior nares	Chancre; mucous patches; moist condylomata; blood	Respiratory tract; urine	Feces; blood
7. Immunity	Not well understood; most adults have some immunity; hypersensitivity may result from infection	Cannot be reinfected if untreated	Varies with individual; largely cellular, BCG may provide partial immunity	Probably life-long following disease; passive immunity may be induced with human gamma globulin
8. Carrier state period of communicability	Duration varies; indefinitely in some, intermittently in others	Untreated, basically primary and secondary stages; pregnancy	Duration of open lesions in lung	Blood: variable feces; days to weeks, not clearly known, but may be prior to onset of symptoms
9. Prevention	Meticulous aseptic technique; no one with any lesion should care for patients; isolation regulations vary; antibiotic therapy for carriers with susceptible strains	Postexposure treatment; condoms; education	Chemoprophylaxis for disease and those newly tuberculin test positive; BCG immunization for high-risk groups	Sanitary, uncrowded living conditions; personal hygiene; gamma globulin; for patient and exposed contacts; modified isolation to prevent spread by feces or blood
		Compulsory serological tests for marriage licenses, pregnant women, military personnel, and others		Possible home care for uncomplicated cases

wipes when they cough, sneeze, or expectorate and to discard used wipes directly into a moisture-proof bag.

The control of the spread of nosocomial infections is neither quick nor easy. The procedures that are available are not glamorous; no newspaper is likely to headline them as producing a miracle. They are based on the application of principles of hygiene and antiseptic and aseptic techniques. Everything that comes in contact with a patient, be it an oxygen tent or a mask or a bed sheet, should be treated as being contaminated. The nurse should have some knowledge of the organisms likely to be encountered such as their ability to survive outside the human host, how long and under what conditions, and how the organisms can be destroyed. Such knowledge will help in carrying out measures designed to break the chain of infection.

Isolation Procedures

The infection control committee formulates isolation policies and guideline criteria for categories such as strict isolation, respiratory isolation, protective isolation, enteric precautions, and wound and skin precautions. Currently, most hospitals use these five categories of isolation based on degree of communicability and modes of transmission.

The use of the word "isolation" may produce negative images in the minds of patients, families, and friends, so a sensitive nurse will explain the rationale for isolation (strict, especially), answer questions, and seek to allay fears (Kellerhals, 1979, p. 68). Written material provided to reinforce verbal information will assist greatly.[1]

In summary, hospital-acquired infections as well as other infections are a very old problem. But the infections that are most prevalent at this time in the United States are different from those of the past. The discovery of the sulfonamides and then of penicillin and other antibiotics encouraged the hope that humans could be victorious in their struggle with microorganisms. Instead, antibiotic-resistant strains have flourished as a result of the disturbed ecological equilibrium. The increasing number of elderly patients, many with debilitating diseases, has decreased the hosts' resistance to their own organisms. This susceptibility is often increased by lengthy, complicated surgical procedures and/or the use of immunosuppressive and cytotoxic drugs. As a result, the importance of considering all the factors influencing the infectious process when planning the control of pathogens is of great importance. The indifferent application of medical and surgical asepsis, stemming from false overconfidence in miracle drugs, must be reversed. Specific methods useful in the destruction of microorganisms have not been discussed. References giving such specific information are at the end of the chapter.

Nurses are responsible for helping to minimize nosocomial infections. They have an obligation to participate on the infection control committee, to cooperate in control measures, and to study ways to improve methods of control. They also have a responsibility to participate in educational programs in the institution so that more effective control measures can be instituted and effected. In protecting themselves and others nurses should ask the questions "Who is protected from whom? Why? From what? How?"

To conclude, Table 38-1 summarizes the interrelationship of factors that produce four infectious diseases in humans. They were chosen as representative of a variety of problems and illustrative of the basic questions just mentioned that a nurse must ask.

[1] Kellerhals's article in *Topics in Clinical Nursing,* July 1979, is an excellent reference on details related to five isolation categories.

References Cited

Altemeir, W. A. "Current Infection Problems in Surgery." In *Proceedings of the International Conference on Nosocomial Infections.* Chicago: American Hospital Association, 1971, p. 85.

Bennett, J. V., and Brachman, P. S. *Hospital Infections.* Boston: Little Brown & Co., 1979.

Cohen, M. "Why Support an Infection Control Program in Today's Monetary Crises." *Association for Practitioners in Infection Control,* **6**:1 (March 1978), 19–21.

Creighton, H. F. *Law Every Nurse Should Know.* Philadelphia: W. B. Saunders Co., 1975.

Davis, N. C. et al. "The Infections Control Sister." *Lancet,* **2** (Dec. 21, 1963), 1321–22.

Dineen, P. "Microbial Filtration by Surgical Masks." *Surgery, Gynecology, Obstetrics,* **133** (Nov. 1971), 812–14.

Dubay, E. C., and Grubb, R. D. *Infection, Prevention and Control,* 2nd ed. St. Louis: C. V. Mosby Co., 1978.

Eickhoff, T. C. "Hospital Infections." *DM* (Sept. 1972).

Eickhoff, T. C. "Nosocomial Infections." In *Infectious Diseases.* Ed. by P. D. Hoeprich. New York: Harper & Row, 1977, pp. 27–33.

Fahlberg, W. J. "Environmental Control of Transmission of Hospital-Acquired Infection." In *Infection Control, Topics in Clinical Nursing.* Ed. by E. Larson. **1**:2 (July 1979), 39.

Finland, M. "Changing Ecology of Bacterial Infections as

Related to Antibacterial Therapy." *J. Infect. Dis.*, **122** (March 1970), 419–31.

Kellerhals, S. A. "Isolation for Person-Environment Protection: Rationale and Utilization." In *Infection Control, Topics in Clinical Nursing,* Ed. by E. Larson. **1**:2 (July 1979), 67–75.

Kicklighter, L. "The Nurse Epidemiologist." *Hospitals,* **47** (Jan. 1, 1973), 48–56.

Klainer, A. S., and Beisel, W. R. "Opportunistic Infection: A Review." *Amer. J. Med. Sci.*, **258** (1969), 431.

Krause, S. L., and Pappas, S. "The Nurse Epidemiologist: Role and Responsibilities." In *Infection Control, Topics in Clinical Nursing.* Ed. by E. Larson. **1**:2 (July 1979), 1–6.

Larson, E. *Infection Control, Topics in Clinical Nursing,* **1**:2 (July 1979), xi.

Lidwell, O. M. "Hospital Uses of Unidirectional (Laminar) Air Flow." In *Proceedings of the International Conference on Nosocomial Infections.* Chicago: American Hospital Association, 1971, p. 207.

Mallison, G. F. "The Inanimate Environment." In *Hospital Infections.* Ed. by Bennett and Brachman. Boston: Little, Brown & Co., 1979, pp. 81–91.

Morris, R. C. "Legal Aspects of Nosocomial Infections." In *Hospital Infections.* Ed. by Bennett and Brachman. Boston: Little, Brown & Co., 1979, pp. 181–94.

Mufson, M. A. et al. "Acquisition of Parainfluenza 3 Virus Infection by Hospitalized Children. I. Frequencies, Rates and Temporal Data." *J. Infectious Dis.*, **128** (Aug. 1973), 141–47.

Noble, W. C. "The Dispersal of Staphylococci in Hospital Wards." *J. Clin. Pathol.*, **15** (Nov. 1962), 552–58.

Noble, W. C., and Davis, R. R. "Studies on the Dispersal of Staphylococci." *J. Clin. Pathol.*, **18** (Jan. 1965), 16–19.

Pollock, M. et al. "Factors Influencing Colonization and Antibiotic Resistance Patterns of Gram-Negative Bacteria in Hospital Patients." *Lancet,* **2** (Sept. 30, 1972), 668–71.

Riley, R. L. "The Ecology of Indoor Atmospheres: Airborne Infection in Hospital." *J. Chron. Dis.*, **25** (Aug. 1972), 421–23.

Selwyn, S. "Changing Patterns in Hospital Infection." *Nursing Times,* **68** (May 25, 1972), 642–46.

Sprunt, K., Redman, W., and Leidy, G. "Antibacterial Effectiveness of Routine Hand Washing." *Pediatrics,* **52** (Aug. 1973), 264–65.

Stamm, W. E. "Elements of an Active, Effective, Infection Control Program." *Hospitals,* **50** (1976), 60.

U.S. Department of Health, Education, and Welfare. *Environmental Aspects of the Hospital. Vol. 1. Infection Control,* Public Health Service Publication No. 930-C-15, 1970, p. 32.

U.S. Department of Health, Education, and Welfare. *Isolation Techniques for Use in Hospitals,* 2nd ed. Superintendent of Documents, Stock # 017–023–00094–2. Washington, D.C.: U.S. Government Printing Office, 1975.

Wineland, M. D. "Invasive Procedures and Infection Control." In *Infection Control, Topics in Clinical Nursing.* Ed. by E. Larson. **1**:2 (July 1979), 53–57.

General References

Abelson, P. H. "A View of Health Research and Care." *Science,* **200**:4344 (May 26, 1978), 845.

Aber, R. C., and Bennett, J. V. "Surveillance of Nosocomial Infections." In *Hospital Infections.* Ed. by Bennett and Brachman. Boston: Little, Brown & Co., 1979, pp. 53–61.

Bagshawe, K. D., Blowers, R., and Lidwell, O. M. "Isolating Patients in Hospital to Control Infection." *Bri. Med. J.*, Part I, **2** (Aug. 26, 1978), 609–12; Part II, **2** (Sept. 2, 1978), 684–86; Part III, **2** (Sept. 9, 1978), 744–48; Part IV, **2** (Sept. 16, 1978), 808–11.

Bennett, J. V. "Incidence and Nature of Endemic and Epidemic Nosocomial Infections." In *Hospital Infections.* Ed. by Bennett and Brachman. Boston: Little, Brown, & Co., 1979, pp. 233–38.

Chavigny, K. "The Scope of Hospital Epidemiology." In *Infection Control, Topics in Clinical Nursing,* Ed. by E. Larson. **1**:2 (July 1979), 77–84.

Cohen, S. S. "A Strategy for the Chemotherapy of Infectious Disease." *Science,* **29** (1977), 431–32.

Clark, E. G., and Danbolt, N. "The Oslo Study of the Natural Course of Untreated Syphilis: An Epidemiologic Investigation Based on a Re-study of the Boeck-Bruusgaard Material." *Med. Clin. North Amer.*, **48** (May 1964), 613–23.

Dowling, H. F. *Fighting Infection: Conquests of the Twentieth Century.* Cambridge, Mass.: Harvard University Press, 1977.

Eickhoff, T. C. et al. "Surveillance of Nosocomial Infections in Community Hospitals. I. Surveillance Methods, Effectiveness, and Initial Results." *J. Infectious Dis.*, **120**:3 (Sept. 1969), 305–17.

Kaslow, R. A. et al. "Staphylococcal Disease Related to Hospital Nursery Bathing Practices—A Nationwide Epidemiologic Investigation." *Pediatrics,* **51**:2 (Feb. 1973), 418–25.

Lemon, S., and Pagano, J. S. "Fulminant Pneumonia." *Hosp. Med.*, **13** (Jan. 1977), 79–112.

Maki, D. G. "Septic Thrombophlebitis, Part 2." *Hosp. Med.*, **13** (Jan. 1977), 6–29.

McArthur, B. J. "Administrative Proposals Useful in the Prevention of Infections in Intensive Care Units." *Current Topics in Critical Care Med.*, 3 (1977), 192–98.

McArthur, B. J. et al. "Stopcock contamination in an ICU." *Am. J. Nurs.*, **75**:1 (Jan. 1975), 96–97.

Peter, G., and Smith, A. "Group A Streptococcal Infections of the Skin and Pharynx. Part I." *New Engl. J. Med.*, **297** (Aug. 11, 1977), 311–17. Part 2, **297** (Aug. 18, 1977), 365–70.

Reimann, H. A. "Infectious Diseases: Annual Review of Significant Publications." *Postgrad. Med. J.*, **49** (May 1978), 325–43.

Richman, A. "Infectious Hepatitis." *Hosp. Med.*, **14** (March 1978), 72–87.

Rivkind, R. J., "Legal Responsibilities in Infection Control." *Association for Practitioners' in Infection Control,* **6**:1 (March 1978), 23–25.

Robinson, M. "Viral Hepatitis—Update." *Association for Practitioners in Infection Control,* **6**:1 (March 1978), 10–17.

Robinson, W. S., and Greenburg, H. "Hepatitis B." In *Infectious Diseases.* Ed. by P. D. Hoeprich. New York: Harper & Row, 1977, pp. 609–17.

Turner, J. G. "The Nurse Epidemiologist: Selection and Preparation." *Supervisor Nurse,* **9**:4 (April 1978), 33–41.

Whitehead, J. E. M. "Bacterial Resistance: Changing Patterns of Some Common Pathogens." *Bri. Med. J.,* **2** (April 28, 1973), 225.

Wilson, M. E., Mizer, H. E., and Morells, J. A. *Microbiology in Patient Care,* 3rd ed. New York: Macmillan Publishing Co., 1979.

Zieg, G. "Current Treatment of Gonorrhea." In *The Drug Therapy Newsletter,* **3**:2, published by Drug Information Center of Harper-Grace Hospitals, 1979.

39

Problems Resulting from Failure to Regulate the Proliferation and Maturation of Cells

The cancer story, so old to us, is always new and devastating to the patient. To this illness, so fraught with gravity, he brings his old problems and weaknesses. We can help him by recognizing rather than belittling his situation, and by remembering that all patients are individuals with varying degrees of illness and maturity, with different backgrounds and sources of emotional support. We can help the patient most by our own attitudes, so readily perceived, for these transcend words.

(BARCKLEY, 1967)

Overview

Cancer is an important chronic disease. This is true not only because it ranks second as a cause of death, and sometimes causes a lengthy and costly illness, but also because of the many fears that it engenders in people. It is probable that cancer is not a single disease but a group of diseases in which multiple factors are involved in its causation. Whatever its pathogenesis, the manifestations are the result of failure to control the proliferation (growth) and maturation of cells. Because of the nature of this disease, nursing has much to offer in all its stages; from prevention to the care of the dying patient. In fact, few diseases provide a greater test of the skill and competence of the nurse.

PURPOSE OF CHAPTER

The purpose of this chapter is to present current information about neoplasia and to make some suggestions about how it can be implemented into nursing practice. Before beginning a discussion of cancer and cancer nursing it is necessary to be reminded of a point that has been emphasized throughout this text. In health, all body structures and functions are regulated so that the needs of individual cells and tissues as well as of the total organism are met, despite changes in the environment to which the person is exposed.

HISTORICAL REVIEW

Cancer is neither a new disease nor a disease of civilization per se. Evidence indicating the presence of an osteoma (a benign neoplasm) has been found in the vertebrae of a dinosaur that lived some 50 million years ago. References to neoplasms are found in the earliest medical literature. They were described by the Egyptians in 1200 B.C. Neoplasms were known to Hippocrates.

Not only is cancer a disease of antiquity, but it is not unique to humans; it occurs in both plants and animals. Cows, chickens, parakeets, horses, monkeys, dogs, fish, amphibians, and laboratory animals such

This chapter has been revised by Carole A. LaFleur, R.N., M.S.N., Chief, Advanced Clinical Practice, Visiting Nurse Association of Metropolitan Detroit, Detroit, Michigan.

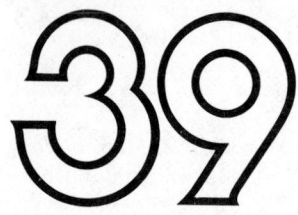

as mice, rats, and rabbits develop neoplasms. Because of the contributions of these animals to the study of disease, they might be included with the dog as best friends of man. When cancer, as well as other types of neoplasms, is viewed as a phenomenon of growth, neither the fact that it is of ancient origin nor that it occurs in species other than humans should be surprising. In all living creatures it has one essential characteristic: the organism is unable to control the growth and proliferation of cells.

Advances in the study of oncology were closely tied to the development of the achromatic microscope in the study of normal and diseased tissue and to techniques for preparing and staining tissues for microscopic examination. Microscopic study allowed for demonstration of the fact that neoplastic cells generally resemble the tissue from which they arise and are characterized by abnormal proliferation of cells, which infiltrate and destroy contiguous tissues and transplant to distant sites as metastases (del Regato, 1977).

This modern concept of cancer as a disturbance in cellular growth, is not much more than 130 years old. It probably had its origin in the work, published in 1838, of Johannes Muller, who is credited with the first description of the cellular nature of cancer. Virchow, some 20 years later, gave impetus to the idea by describing the characteristic changes in cancer cells. Continued progress in the study of cancer cells required that tumor tissue be available. From 1876 to the turn of the century Novinsky, Hanau, and Moreau paved the way in experimenting with transplantation and growth of tumors in laboratory animals. In 1903 Jensen's systematic work on transplantable tumors initiated the efforts of diligent cancer research (del Regato, 1977).

Previous to the discoveries of Muller and Virchow, the relationship of cancer to certain occupations had been observed. In 1775, Sir Percivall Pott reported his observation that chimney sweeps in London, who were consistently exposed to soot, had an exceptionally high incidence of cancer of the scrotum. In the sixteenth century, men working in mines in the mountains of Saxony were known to develop a progressive and fatal disease. Not until later, however, was the disease identified as cancer. The discovery that pitchblende was the causative agent did not come until still later. In 1895 another occupational cancer hazard was reported by Ludwig Rehn, who observed the occurrence of bladder cancer among aniline dye industry workers. Legal prohibitions and improvements in industrial hygiene regulations have controlled though not eliminated the problem of chemical bladder carcinogenesis. More than 500 chemical agents are now known to be carcinogenic.

Legislation

Probably no disease in the history of the United States has been given more attention by politicians and legislators than cancer. Evidence of the interest shown by legislators in cancer control is demonstrated by the laws that have been passed. A summary of important cancer-related legislation and some results follows (Rettig, 1977):

1922—Cancer research was initiated in the United States Public Health Service (USPHS).

1937—Congress established the National Cancer Institute within the USPHS.

1965—The Heart Disease, Cancer, and Stroke Amendments were passed.

1971—The National Cancer Act was enacted—goals of the act included *(a)* increasing understanding of cancer; *(b)* developing improved means of prevention, diagnosis, and treatment; *(c)* development of a network of cancer care centers throughout the United States; *(d)* authorization of fifteen such comprehensive cancer care centers.

1974—The National Cancer Act of 1971 was reauthorized and the limitation on the number of cancer centers was removed.

1978—National Cancer Act was extended.

1979—Twenty comprehensive cancer centers were in existence throughout the United States.

What Is Cancer?

Cancer is a disturbance of cellular growth characterized primarily by excessive proliferation of cells without apparent relation to the physiological demands on the organism involved (International Union Against Cancer Committee on Professional Education, 1973).

The cell, like other structures, responds to conditions in its environment. It alters its activities in relation to its food supply to the demands made on it, and to potentially harmful agents. Depending on the quantity and nature of the injuring agent, the cell may recover, be altered in some manner, or die. The inherent characteristics of the remaining cells determine whether dead cells are replaced by like cells or by fibrous connective tissue. Certain cells can adapt to an unfavorable environment by undergoing metaplasia.

Furthermore, cells may appear to recover following injury, but at some later time, sometimes many years later, they are transformed into less differentiated cells that no longer look or behave like normal cells. Exactly what happens in the process whereby healthy cells are transformed to neoplastic cells has been very difficult to identify.

Proliferating cells often but not always lose their ability to differentiate. They often mutate and become abnormal. The result is unrestricted growth of cells that are often poorly differentiated and without useful function. Even if they retain their original function they rarely contribute to the patient's welfare and often damage the body by flooding it with excessive amounts of their products.

Definitions

Some of the terms to be used in our discussion will first be defined.

Anaplasia. The transformation of cells to a less differentiated or more primitive embryonic type, with greater capacity for multiplication but less ability to specialize.

Neoplasm. A new growth that can be accompanied by a loss as well as a gain in cells. For example, malignant neoplasms of the stomach are sometimes in the form of ulcers.

Tumor. The word *tumor* is frequently used interchangeably with *neoplasm.* Strictly speaking, they do not have identical meanings. A tumor is a swelling that can be caused not only by an increase in the number of cells in a tissue but by inflammation or an accumulation of blood or fluid in a localized area of tissue.

Benign neoplasm. The word *benign* takes its origin from the Latin word *benignus; bene* means "well" and *gnus,* "kind." When the word *benign* is used to describe a disease, the implication is that it is relatively harmless. A benign neoplasm is therefore one that is not of itself deadly. It may, however, cause harm by virtue of its location and by the fact that it occupies space.

Malignant neoplasm. The term *malignant* has its origin from the Latin *malignans,* which means "evil." Similar to the adjective *benign malignant* may be employed to characterize any type of disease. Malignant diseases are ones in which death is probable, unless something can be done to halt or alter their course. The separation between benign and malignant neoplasms is not always clear-cut inasmuch as many benign neoplasms, because of their location or size, can be fatal. On the other hand, some malignant neoplasms can run a relatively long course. Some of the significant differences between benign and malignant neoplasms will be discussed in greater detail where the characteristics of neoplasms are presented.[1]

Cancer. Often used synonymously with *malignant neoplasm.* Garb (1968) defines *cancer* as a "condition in which abnormal cells develop, multiply, and invade normal tissue, interfering with normal functions and eventually causing death unless adequate therapy is given early."

Carcinoma—Malignant. Neoplasms arising in tissues originating in the ectoderm or entoderm of the embryo are called carcinomas.

Sarcoma. Malignant neoplasms (fleshy tumors) having their origin in tissues that are formed from the mesoderm, or mesenchyme.

Oncology. The study of tumors. The word is often used more broadly to include all aspects relating to tumors, including the prevention, diagnosis, and treatment of patients with tumors.

Incidence and Mortality of Malignant Neoplasms: Past and Present Trends

According to probabilities published by the American Cancer Society, the chances for Americans of one day developing cancer are one in four. The chances of eventually dying of cancer are better than one in seven (ACS, Cancer Statistics, 1978).

Incidence

Most authorities express the opinion that the incidence of cancer is probably the same all over the world, but the actual occurrence of the disease is difficult to verify because statistics are not reliable in many regions. Furthermore, because of lack of trained medical personnel, many persons who develop cancer may not be identified.

In some countries a smaller proportion of the people may be dying from cancer than in other countries because the average length of life is shorter. However, certain types of cancers are known to occur in some areas more commonly than others, such as liver cancer in South Africa and China, choriocarcinoma in Southeast Asia, and an unusual lymph node cancer in children, in so-called Burkitt's lymphoma, in the rain forest regions of Africa. In the United States lung cancer is the leading cause of death from cancer and cancer of the stomach is steadily declin-

[1] The words benign and malignant are adjectives used to describe the character of a variety of situations, conditions, diseases, and even people.

ing. In Japan cancer of the stomach is the leading cause of death from cancer, but lung cancer is rising in incidence.

The probability of eventually developing cancer including carcinoma in situ is increasing in all race-sex groups in the United States. The probabilities have increased in all groups compared with similar figures from 1949 to 1951. The sharpest increase in probabilities in both males and females is for the development of lung cancer (ACS, Cancer Statistics, 1978).

The most recently reported years' (1973–1976) incidence rate of cancer in the United States for all race-sex groups was 323.8 per 100,000 population or a total of 68,623 Americans (refer to Table 39-1). The incidence rate is higher in males than it is in females. Cancer of the lung and bronchus leads in incidence for all race-sex groups. Lung and bronchus leads in incidence for males and breast leads in incidence for females (Young and Pollack, 1978). It is interesting to note that the incidence of breast cancer during 1973 was 80.2 per 100,000 and in 1974 it increased to 92 per 100,000. During the next 2 years, from 1974 to 1976, it fell to 80. The rise in reported incidence rates of breast cancer from 1973 to 1974 could be attributed in part to the publicity given to the open manner in which wives of the president and vice-president of the United States, Mrs. Gerald Ford and Mrs. Nelson Rockefeller, publicly communicated their diagnoses and treatments of breast cancer. It seems that as the notoriety surrounding these women and their diagnoses of breast cancer diminished, so too did the general concern among women for early detection of breast cancer.

Mortality

The probability of eventually dying of cancer are greater for males, both white and nonwhite, than they are for white and nonwhite females. This is a reversal of the situation observed in 1950. Some possible reasons for this trend include more rapid decreases in other causes of death among women, easier accessibility to cancer sites in women, and emphasis on educational programs for women to facilitate early recognition and detection of neoplasm.

Accessibility of site does not of itself guarantee a reduction in the mortality rate from cancer. The death rate from cancer of the breast remains essentially the same, despite extensive educational programs intended to facilitate early detection of neoplasms in the breast. By way of contrast, the programs for the early detection of cancer of the cervix have been accompanied by a decrease in mortality rate from this cause.

Cancer statistics published in 1979 again show cancer to be second only to heart disease as the leading cause of death in the United States. It is now the leading cause of death among women aged 35 through 54 years and it causes more deaths than any other disease in school-aged children (Silverberg, 1979). The number of deaths reported as due to cancer in 1979 was 377,312. At this rate approximately 1,034 persons per day or 43 per hour die of cancer.

Mortality rates for males with cancer are considerably higher than those for females (refer to Table 39-1). The leading causes of cancer deaths when combining statistics for both sexes, are lung and bronchus, colon, and breast. For males the leading

TABLE 39-1. ***Incidence Rates, Mortality Rates, and Leading Sites of Cancer Occurrence***

Group	Incidence Rates (per 100,000 population)	Leading Incidence Sites	Mortality Rates (per 100,000 population)	Leading Mortality Sites
All race-sex groups	323.8	1. Lung and bronchus 2. Breast 3. Colon	175.8	1. Lung and bronchus 2. Colon 3. Breast
All males	371.4	1. Lung and bronchus 2. Colon and rectum	215	1. Lung and bronchus 2. Colon 3. Pancreas
All females	297.5	1. Breast 2. Colon 3. Lung and bronchus	137	1. Lung and bronchus 2. Colon

Table compiled from: American Cancer Society, *Cancer Statistics*, 1978; Young, Asire, and Pollack, 1978; Silverberg, 1979.

causes are lung and bronchus, colon, and pancreas; for females, lung and bronchus, and colon (Young, Asire, and Pollack, 1978). Several factors contribute to the high mortality rates for cancer of the lung and bronchus. They include a high incidence (see discussion on smoking), the inaccessibility of the site for early detection and diagnosis, and the failure of present methods of treatment.

Whites and nonwhites are both experiencing an increase in cancer mortality, but it is increasing at a greater rate in the nonwhite population (Schottenfeld, 1975). Possibly, the quantity and quality of health care available to different groups are responsible for some of the differences. Mortality is higher in cities and in industrial areas than it is in rural and less heavily populated areas. It also varies with different regions of the United States. For example, the middle Atlantic, New England, and east north central regions have demonstrated high mortality rates (Schottenfeld, 1975). On the other hand the mountain region of the United States recorded the lowest mortality rates (Schottenfeld, 1975). The increased mortality rates among persons living in the industrial and populous areas very likely are related to exposure to carcinogenic-linked agents which are by-products of industrialization and population; for example, hydrocarbons, radiation, food additives, and pesticides. Conversely, inavailability of health care facilities in rural, less populated areas may be a factor in the reporting of lower mortality rates.

Factors Related to Incidence and Mortality

The increase in the number of persons having a diagnosis of cancer is not believed to be caused by a significant rise in its actual incidence. Similar to other chronic diseases a number of factors have contributed to the increase in the number of persons diagnosed as having cancer. Some can be explained on the basis of improved diagnostic methods and facilities. The number of persons having a diagnosis of cancer is greater in areas having good medical facilities than in areas with poor facilities. The total is increased by the fact that formerly diseases such as leukemia and Hodgkin's disease were not classified as cancer, as they now are. With the lessening of the infant mortality rate and decrease in mortality from acute communicable diseases, more persons are living to be of an age when the incidence of cancer is highest. Another factor contributing to the increase in the total number of persons having cancer is the fact that the population is rising.

Although the incidence of cancer tends to rise with age, the disease occurs in all age groups from infancy to old age. As a cause of death, cancer is second only to accidents in children 1 to 14 years of age (*Cancer Statistics,* 1978). More than half the deaths from cancer occur in persons over 55 years of age (*Cancer Statistics,* 1978). The common sites in which cancer occurs differ with age. Leukemia and cancer in the brain, nervous system, and kidney are types most frequently found in children. Among persons in older age groups, cancer of the breast, skin, lung, gastrointestinal tract, and genital organs are most common.

In evaluating the rise in the number of deaths due to cancer, factors that contribute to the increasing number cannot be overlooked. These include improved methods of statistical reporting, rising population size, and advances in earlier recognition and diagnosis of disease.

Survival

Despite the emphasis on cancer as a cause of mortality, it should be remembered that a considerable number of patients are living and well many years after the diagnosis and treatment of cancer. To illustrate, acute leukemia generally is accompanied by an unfavorable prognosis, yet of 157 long-term survivors of acute leukemia, 103 are living and well and free from any evidence of the disease from 5 to 17 years after diagnosis (Burchenal, 1968).

Commonly, patients with a diagnosis of cancer who are alive and well at the end of 5 years after treatment are considered cured. The figure of 5-year cure is useful, however, only for the more rapidly growing cancers because some slower-growing cancers can recur or persist without any treatment for decades.

There have generally been improvements in the 5-year survival rates for both black and white cancer patients, with the exception of white females with cervical cancer. The greatest improvements among black patients were for cancer of the breast, prostate, bladder, and rectum; among white patients the greatest improvements were for those with cancers of the bladder and prostate (Axtell, Asire, & Myers, 1976). Relative survival rates for all cancer patients combined, indicate that the percentages are improving, though slowly. To illustrate, 5-year survival rates of patients diagnosed between 1950 and 1959 were 39 per cent for white patients and 29 per cent for black patients. Five-year survival rates for patients diagnosed between 1960 and 1966 demonstrated a slight improvement to 40 per cent for white patients but a slight drop to 28 per cent for black patients. Though the data are incomplete for patients diagnosed from 1967 to 1973, the evidence so far supports improved 5-year survival rates—41 per cent for white patients and 32 per cent for black patients (Axtell, Asire, & Myers, 1976). The improvement in overall survival rates might be attributed to an earlier diagnosis; that is, a diagnosis while the tumor is localized, which allows for more effective treatment. Improved management techniques in treating cancer patients must also be considered.

In looking more closely at the 5-year survival rates for the leading incidence sites of cancer in males and females, one notes the following (refer to Table 39-2). Cancer of the lung, which leads in incidence rates for males, shows a 28 per cent 5-year survival rate if the disease is localized, but only an 8 per cent rate for all stages of disease. Cancers of the colon and rectum, which were second and third in incidence for males, are reported as one category, and demonstrate a 71 per cent 5-year survival rate if the disease is localized and 44 per cent for all stages of disease (*Cancer Statistics,* 1978). For females, breast cancer is first in incidence, followed by colon and lung. If the breast cancer was localized, the 5-year survival rate was 85 per cent; for all stages it was 65 per cent. The 5-year survival rates for females with cancer of the colon and rectum were 72 per cent for localized disease and 46 per cent for all stages. In females with cancer of the lung, the 5-year survival rate for localized disease was 51 per cent, but only 13 per cent for all stages (*Cancer Statistics,* 1978).

Survival rates for Hodgkin's disease are rising steadily as a result of better patient evaluation and improved treatment with chemotherapy and radiation. Results of chemotherapeutic programs such as MOPP, which is an acronym for Mustargen, Oncovin, procarbazine, and prednisone, are now capable of inducing complete remission in approximately 80 per cent of patients. Approximately 75 to 95 per cent of patients with early-stage Hodgkin's disease can expect to achieve long-term survival beyond 5 years (Canellos, 1979). Patients with more advanced disease who are treated by total nodal radiotherapy will have a five-year disease-free survival rate of from 40–60 percent but the addition of chemotherapy will improve these figures (Canellos, 1979). Canellos (1979, p. 30) states that the combination of radiation and chemotherapy in patients with intermediate stages of Hodgkin's disease are all potentially curable.

Maier et al. (1977) reported a 10-year survival rate of 49.5 per cent for a group of 219 patients with medullary cancer of the breast. Improvements in the 5-year and longer survival rates supports the emphasis on early detection, diagnosis, and clinical management. Advances in clinical management reflect the growing appreciation among health care professionals of the contributions of various disciplines in evaluating and treating the cancer patient. Clinical management and care of the cancer patient is further enhanced by modern diagnostic procedures, recognition of the importance of accurate diagnosis in the staging of cancer, technical improvements in therapeutic procedures, rational use of systemic methods of therapy, especially, adjuvant to regional treatment, and recognition of the importance of rehabilitation as an aspect of cancer patient management (Lawrence and Terz, 1977).

Enhanced clinical management and care of the patient combined with improving attitudes of health care personnel and the public toward cancer should continue to have positive benefits for the cancer patient. The recognition of rehabilitation as an important aspect of the cancer patient's care should ensure that the patient will be receiving the assistance and support necessary to live as fullfilling a life as possible with the disease. With increasing cancer survival rates and an emphasis on rehabilitation as a vital component of care, cancer is coming to be recognized as a chronic disease for which much can be done to improve the patient's condition and to prolong his or her useful life.

TABLE 39-2. ***Five-Year Survival Rates for Cancers of Leading Incidence***

Sex	Cancer Site	Stage of disease (percentage) Localized	All Stages
Male	Lung	28	8
	Colon and rectum	71	44
Female	Breast	85	65
	Colon and rectum	72	46
	Lung	51	13

Compiled from: American Cancer Society, *Cancer Statistics,* 1978.

Pathophysiology of Neoplastic Disease

Homeostasis of Cell Proliferation and Differentiation

In the discussion of homeostasis thus far, emphasis has been on the maintenance of conditions in the internal environment favorable to cellular activity. Homeostasis is also dependent on the ability to maintain the structure and function of tissues. The continuity of tissues and the maintenance of function require that cells lost as a result of wear and tear and of injury be replaced. Fundamental to this replacement is the capacity of cells to proliferate (multiply) and to differentiate into mature tissue. As with other homeostatic mechanisms, the usefulness of the capacity of cells to multiply depends on (1) the ability of the organism to regulate the proliferation and maturation of cells and (2) the appropriateness and adequacy of the response. The potential for growth of the different types of tissues varies. Some, such as fibrous connective tissue and reticular cells, are not only able to proliferate but they can differentiate into a number of types of tissue cells. Other types of tissue cells are capable of proliferation, but they can mature only into cells similar to the parent cell. The example of the ability of epithelial cells to proliferate and mature into some type of epithelial cell has been previously cited. Immature epithelial cells differentiate into the various types of epithelial tissue. In the examples just cited, tissue cells have a great potential for growth. In other types of tissues, such as nervous tissue and striated muscle, the potential for growth, is exceedingly limited.

In healthy tissues, the process whereby cells multiply follows a predictable pattern known as mitosis. In mitosis the cell undergoes a complicated series of changes in which each chromosome is divided and two new, or daughter, cells are formed.

The cell cycle extends from completion of one cell division to completion of the next. There are four basic phases in the cell cycle: G_1, S, G_2, and M. The first phase is G_1 (G for growth or gap). During the first phase enzymes, structural proteins, and cell organelles are synthesized. It extends from completion of the previous cell division to the beginning of chromosome replication. DNA synthesis occurs at the end of G_1 and continues as the S (synthesis) phase. The S phase usually lasts 6 to 8 hours. It is followed by a 2 to 3-hour G_2 phase during which macromolecules of the cells are prepared and arranged for the occurrence of mitosis. The period of the actual mitosis and cell division is called the M (mitosis) phase. It usually lasts for less than an hour and the cell is again returned to the G_1 phase (see Figure 39-1).

The G_1 phase is the least well-defined and probably the most crucial in understanding regulation and rate of cell replication. During this phase the initiation of DNA synthesis is determined. Once DNA synthesis begins, the cell proceeds rather quickly to completion of division and production of two daughter cells. The G_1 phase also determines the length of the cycle, since other time phases are fairly fixed. Some rapidly proliferating cells such as bone marrow have a very short G_1 phase, whereas others such as muscle or neurons have an extensive or permanently arrested G_1 phase (Lessner, 1978). Knowledge of the cell cycle is applied practically by the nurse in understanding actions of the various chemotherapeutic agents because they attack tumor cells during different phases of the cell cycle. (Refer to discussion on chemotherapeutic agents. See Figure 39-1.)

Depending on the potentialities of the cell and environmental conditions, new cells may be a replica of the parent cell or may differ in some respect from it. The ways in which a daughter cell can differ at maturity from the parent cell are predictable. The daughter cells fit into the overall organization of the tissue. For example, the type of epithelial cells entering into the formation of a mucous membrane may be altered by exposure to an unfavorable environment. Following a tracheostomy, transitional cells in the mucous membrane lining the trachea undergo metaplasia and are replaced by a thick layer of squamous epithelium. The change is adaptive, as squamous cells are better able to survive chronic irritation than are transitional cells. The pattern for metaplasia is predictable and the resulting tissue organized and functional.

As with other homeostatic mechanisms, the multiplication of cells occurs in reponse to a need and ceases when the need is met, which indicates that the potential for growth of cells is subject to regulation. Not all the factors in the regulation of growth are understood. The growth of some tissues is influenced by both intrinsic and extrinsic factors. Among the extrinsic regulators are certain hormones; adjacent cells also appear to exert a growth-inhibiting influence on each other.

Many examples could be cited in which cell proliferation occurs in reponse to a need and ceases when the need is met. One such example is wound healing. Other examples include the continuous replacement of worn-out erythrocytes and leukocytes. The pro-

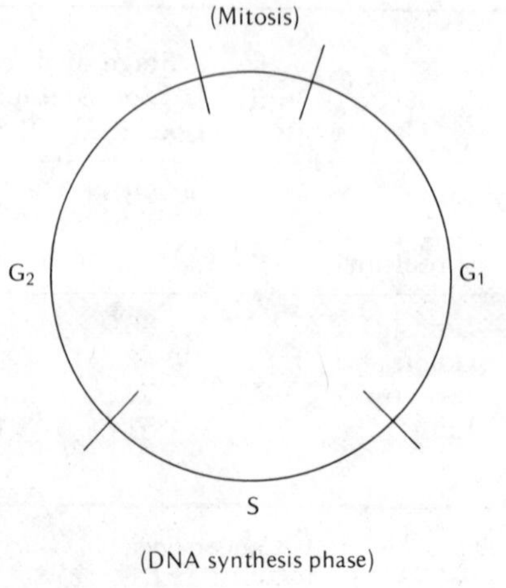

Figure 39-1. The cell cycle.

duction of either erythrocytes or leukocytes may be greatly increased in response to appropriate stimuli. The production of erythrocytes is increased following acute hemorrhage or an exposure of the organism to a lowering of the oxygen tension in the atmosphere. Infection initiated by one of the pyogenic cocci, such as the pneumococcus or meningococcus, is accompanied by an outpouring of neutrophils. When the demand for either erythrocytes or neutrophils is very great, cells may be released from the bone marrow at an earlier stage of development than is usual. Following hemorrhage, the level of not quite mature erythrocytes—the reticulocytes—rises from the usual 2 per cent or less to 10 per cent or more. This same response can be observed in the patient who is treated for certain types of anemia. Shortly after a hemorrhage occurs, the reticulocyte count rises rapidly. The rate at which the level of mature erythrocytes rises is slower. As the normal level of erythrocytes is approached, the reticulocyte count drops to normal. This is therefore evidence of a mechanism operating to control the proliferation of erythrocytes. The extent to which the reticulocyte count is elevated, under conditions such as those cited, is an indication of the capacity of the bone marrow to produce blood cells.

In conditions under which the neutrophils are markedly elevated, the proportion of nonfilamented or nonsegmented leukocytes to filamented or segmented leukocytes is increased. Nonfilamented leukocytes are the not quite mature form of white blood cells. Like reticulocytes, they represent a normal stage in the development of leukocytes. When the situation calling for the increase in leukocytes is controlled, the normal level of leukocytes is restored.

The process whereby cells multiply and produce cells that are the same type and form as those found in the tissue or organ is known as hyperplasia. It occurs in response to an extracellular stimulus. With the removal of the stimulus the multiplication of cells ceases; that is, in hyperplasia the multiplication of cells is controlled. The cells are typical of the tissue from which they arise and are organized into a normal or healthy pattern, and multiple tissue elements are often involved. For example, in the healing of a wound, neutrophils, macrophages, fibroblasts, epithelial cells, and capillaries participate in the formation of the scar.

How Abnormal Cell Growth Differs from Normal Cell Growth

The principal differences between the normal replacement of cells and abnormal growth are as follows: the proliferation of cells is homeostatic when the multiplication of cells (1) occurs in response to an appropriate stimulus, (2) is adequate to the requirements of the organism, (3) differentiates or matures into normal functioning tissue, and (4) ceases when the need of the organism is met. In contrast, the proliferation of cells is abnormal when it (1) occurs in response to an inappropriate stimulus; (2) is inadequate to or in excess of, the needs of the organism; (3) results in immature and abnormal cells; and (4) continues growth without regard for the needs of the organism—the well-being and possibly the life of the individual are threatened. Malignant neoplasms may cause widespread toxic effects even at a time when the lesion is more or less localized.

Tumor cells may exist in a sterile vegetative state where they continue to survive but are unable to proliferate. Other tumor cells are not dividing, but have the capacity to proliferate. An insufficient supply of nutrients will prohibit a tumor cell from proliferating. The noncycling cells are considered to be in G_0, which is a subphase of G_1. *Growth function* is the term used to describe the proportion of proliferating tumor cells (Lessner, 1978).

Though there are important differences between normal and neoplastic cells, difference in rate of growth is not one of them. In both normal and abnormal tissues, the rate of growth may be slow, rapid, or moderate. As examples, the bone marrow can produce erythrocytes at an extremely rapid rate. Cells in the gastrointestinal mucosa reproduce rapidly. Liver cells multiply at a fairly rapid rate. Conversely, cells of the brain, heart, and kidney do not reproduce at an appreciable rate. Neoplasms arising in the latter organs tend to grow more rapidly than the parent cells. Those occurring in epithelial cells of the skin and the gastrointestinal mucosa often grow more slowly than healthy epithelial cells.

Neoplastic cells differ from normal cells in a variety of ways. The structure and organization of cells in a neoplasm may be similar in many respects to that of healthy tissue, or they may be so different that there is little or no resemblance to normal tissue. For example, in glandular structures, goblet epithelial cells are arranged in an orderly fashion around the ducts. In some neoplasms, this pattern may be disturbed but still recognizable. In others, the pattern of organization and the character of cells are so abnormal that most, if not all, resemblance to normal tissue is lost. Some of the characteristics of neoplastic cells are the following: (1) Abnormal cells tend to be larger, with a disproportionately large nucleus, than normal cells. (2) Cells tend to vary in size and shape. (3) There is a high frequency of mitotic figures within the nucleus. (4) Although neoplastic cells have been observed to have abnormalities in the number and appearance of chromosomes, chronic myelogenous leukemia is the only disorder with a consistent chromosomal change.

Table 39-3. *A Brief Classification of Neoplasms*

Type of Tissue	Type of Neoplasm: Benign	Malignant
Connective tissue		
1. Fibrous	Fibroma	Fibrosarcoma
2. Cartilage (chondroblast)	Chondroma	Chondrosarcoma
3. Bone (osteoblast)	Osteoma	Osteogenic sarcoma
4. Fat (lipoid tissue)	Lipoma	Liposarcoma
Muscle tissue		
1. Smooth muscle	Leiomyoma	Leiomyosarcoma
2. Striated muscle	Rhabdomyoma	Rhabdomyosarcoma
Epithelial tissue		
1. Squamous cells	Papilloma or wart Epidermoid cyst Sebaceous cyst	Squamous cell carcinoma
2. Basal cell	Little adenoma or sweat gland adenoma	Basal cell carcinoma
3. Pigmented layer	Mole or nevus	Malignant melanoma
4. Gland cells (adeno-)	Adenoma	Adenocarcinoma
Nervous tissue		
1. Nerve tissue	Neuroma	Neurofibrosarcoma
2. Glia		Glioma
3. Meninges	Meningioma	Malignant meningioma
4. Nerve sheath	Neurofibroma	Neurofibrosarcoma
Endothelial tissue		
1. Blood vessels	Hemangioma	Hemangiosarcoma
Lymphatic and hematopoietic tissues		Hodgkin's disease Leukemia Lymphoma Lymphosarcoma
Mixed tumors	Dermoid cysts	
Tumors derived from embryonic cells well differentiated	Teratoma	Malignant teratomas

An important characteristic of neoplasms is that they serve no useful purpose. Some neoplasms arising in glands do produce the secretion of the gland, but this usually results in an excess of the secretion. Neoplasms arising in endocrine glands are frequently, though not always, functional. For example, neoplasms in the thyroid gland may secrete the hormones of the thyroid gland, thus causing symptoms and signs of hyperthyroidism.

Neoplasms, like other living tissues, require nutrient materials for their growth and survival. They are dependent on the host for their food supply. They grow without regard to the needs of the host and frequently at his or her expense. Slow-growing neoplasms may exist for extended periods of time without interfering with the nutrition of the host. Rapidly growing ones are likely to be accompanied by severe emaciation and debility of the host. Neoplasms in the alimentary canal may further interfere with nutrition by their mechanical effect. The maintenance of nutrition is one of the common problems in the care of patients with certain types of neoplasms.

Summary

Although the cells in some malignant neoplasms are fairly normal in appearance and in organization, they may be so abnormal and immature that there is little or no resemblance to healthy tissues. Cells differ from healthy cells in size, shape, and staining characteristics. Whereas healthy cells are similar in size and shape, neoplastic cells may demonstrate great variability. In normal mitosis, each parent cell divides into two daughter cells, but in tissues taken from a malignant neoplasm, cells can sometimes be seen to be dividing into a number of cells, for example, three, four, or six. Neoplastic cells behave as if they were mutants with an impaired sensitivity to the organizing influence of adjacent cells. They disregard the normal regulators of growth; they often continue to multiply without limit or regard for the needs of the organism as a whole, and not infrequently at the expense of healthy cells. The extent to which neoplastic cells differ from healthy cells varies.

Naming Neoplasms

For the most part, the system for naming neoplasms is relatively simple. The suffix *oma* is derived from the Greek and is used to denote a tumor or neoplasm. Benign neoplasms are usually classified as to site of origin. In a few instances, the term for the type of cell is used. In general, the word is formed by adding *oma* to the combining form, indicating the type of tissue. To illustrate, a benign neoplasm of fibrous tissue is a fibroma. There are some exceptions. Gliomas, which have their origin in the neuroglia, are almost always, if not always, malignant. Malignant neoplasms are also commonly classified as to site of origin. For the purpose of illustration, a brief classification of neoplasms is given in Table 39-3. For anyone wishing to examine a complete list, the *International Classification of Diseases* (U.S. DHEW, 1968) is suggested.

When the origin of the neoplasm is uncertain, this system of naming may not be very helpful, however. For example, malignant melanoma, a tumor of pigment cells in the skin, may originate from one of two cells; melanocyte, a skin cell that actually originates from nerve tissue, or from melanophore, a pigment containing cells of the lower skin layers. In any individual tumor the exact determination of the origin is difficult and therefore leads to confusing multiplicity of the names. Terms such as *melanosarcoma* and *melanocarcinoma* have been used; however, both of them probably should be abandoned for the better term *malignant melanoma.*

When more than one tissue enters into the formation of a neoplasm, the combining forms for each type are used. For example, the so-called fibroid tumor of the uterus is actually a *letomyofibroma,* because it contains smooth muscle and fibrous connective tissue.

Many terms are used to describe the character of the neoplasm. The term *polyp* or *polypoid* is used to indicate that a neoplasm extends from a mucous membrane into the lumen of a tube. Some polyps have a stem or stalk similar to a cherry. The stalk is called a peduncle and the polyp is said to be pedunculated. Other polyps are attached to the surface by a broad base. The term used to indicate this characteristic is *sessile.* Some neoplasms grow around the wall of tubular organs; that is, they are annular growths. Annular neoplasms tend to obstruct the tube by constricting or reducing the size of its lumen. Some neoplasms stimulate the production of large amounts of fibrous connective tissue, which causes the neoplasm to be firm or hard. A firm, hard neoplasm containing a large quantity of connective tissue is called *scirrhus.* There are many other terms used in the description of neoplasms. Satisfactory definitions can usually be found in a medical dictionary.

How Benign and Malignant Neoplasms Differ

Table 39-4 represents a number of important characteristics in which benign and malignant neoplasms differ.

The capsule enclosing a neoplasm is formed of fibrous connective tissue as a result of the local tissue

Table 39-4. *A Comparison of Selected Characteristics of Benign and Malignant Neoplasms*

Characteristic	Benign	Malignant
1. Capsule	Usually	Rarely
2. Manner of growth	Expansive	Infiltrative
3. Rate of growth	Usually slow and restricted; extent limited	Compared to healthy tissue may be slow or rapid and unrestricted; varies greatly from patient to patient and with the type of lesion
4. Tendency to recur after removal	Rarely	Frequently
5. Characteristic of cells	Fairly normal	Varying degrees of abnormality; immature and abnormal in appearance and organization
6. Mitotic activity	Little	Usually great; mitosis is abnormal
7. Metastasis	Never	Usually
8. Vascularity	Slight	Moderate to marked

reaction to the abnormal growth of cells. Occasionally the cells inside an encapsulated neoplasm are found to be malignant, but this is a rare occurrence. It is not known whether the connective tissue capsule has its origin in the connective tissue of the organ in which the tissue has arisen or whether it arises from the tumor itself. The capsule helps to explain why benign neoplasms are usually accompanied by a better prognosis than are malignant neoplasms. The capsule tends to confine the neoplastic cells, and the removal of an encapsulated neoplasm is not only easier but it causes less damage to healthy tissue. Because encapsulated neoplasms grow by expansion rather than by infiltration, their principal effect is pressure. Although some benign neoplasms such as ovarian cysts grow to enormous size their growth is usually limited. Benign neoplasms do not spread to distant parts of the body, and, with rare exceptions, they do not recur. Although some benign neoplasms eventually become malignant, this does not occur very frequently. Few, if any, persons escape having one or more benign neoplasms during their lifetime; most of them are of no significance.

Because of their manner of growth, malignant neoplasms, as the term implies, may cause death. Some malignant neoplasms, but not all, can be eradicated by present methods of treatment. Furthermore, not all malignant neoplasms behave alike. Some types may be present for many years and never cause any known ill effect. Others are so rapidly progressive that despite what appeared to be prompt diagnosis and treatment, death occurs only a few weeks after their presence becomes known. The differences in the behavior of malignant neoplasms are well illustrated by the different types of cancer occurring in the skin. Three types have been identified: basal cell carcinoma, which tends to remain localized; squamous cell carcinoma, which spreads through the lymphatics to the lymph nodes; and malignant melanoma, which has often produced systemic disease by the time it is identified.

Metastasis

As commented on previously, malignant neoplasms tend to infiltrate or invade the surrounding tissue as they grow. They tend to disseminate throughout the body, or metastasize. A single cell or a small group of cells separate from the parent cell and are transported by way of the lymph and blood streams to distant parts of the body. When the cells survive and lodge in a site favorable for their growth, they multiply. The new growth is not detectable, however, until it reaches a size of about 1 cm in diameter, at which time it contains about 500 million cells. The time taken to produce a detectable tumor will depend on the length of the reproductive cycle for the neoplastic cell. If it is 10 days, it will take 10 months for the original cell to grow into a nodule 1 cm in diameter. If the cycle is 30 days, it will take almost 3 years for a detectable nodule to develop. This explains why it may take months or even years for a metastatic neoplasm to appear after surgeon removes a primary growth.

Major Problems

The major problems seen when caring for patients with malignant tumors are caused by the propensity of the tumor growths to spread locally, regionally, and distantly. Little is understood about the biochemical, immunologic, genetic, and hormonal mechanisms involved in the process of metastasis. The metastatic process undoubtedly is a complex series of events that involves: (1) tumor cell separation, (2) survival during circulation in the blood and lymphatic systems, (3) adhesion to and penetration through endothelial walls, (4) establishment of secondary tumors in tissue surrounding vessels, and (5) the eventual establishment of metastasis to more distant sites (Clark, 1979). In order to establish a metastatic lesion, four factors or events must be present and occur (Clark, 1979):

1. Alteration in structure of the malignant cell membrane
2. Separation of a cell cluster from the primary lesion
3. Arrest in and/or infiltration through the lymphatic or vascular vessels
4. Growth of micrometastasis

Invasive Behavior

Theories based on mechanical considerations and possible enzymatic activities are offered to explain the first factor necessary for metastasis. For example, the initial spread of a tumor and invasion of normal tissue is not obviously seen by growth and extension of the tumor itself. The mechanical expansion of the tumor facilitates penetration into a cavity or fluid environment such as the blood, lymph, or spinal fluid. Other characteristics of malignant cells have been offered to explain its potential for metastasis. George Eaves of the University of Leeds School of Medicine has demonstrated that highly malignant cells will penetrate a sheet of normal cells (Nicolson, 1979). There is also evidence that malignant cells possess an increased mobility. It is believed that the increased mobility is a result of decreased linkage between tumor cell membrane and normal tissue cell membrane proteins and glycoproteins (Clark, 1979).

Evidence suggests that the invasive behavior of tumor cells may be facilitated further by their enzymatic destruction of the normal connective matrix between cells (Nicolson, 1979). It is speculated that these proteolytic enzymes enhance modification of the cell periphery, which makes it possible for the malignant cells to escape regulatory controls of growth (Clark, 1979). Treatment of cells with proteolytic enzyme inhibitors has shown cessation of growth. Though there is evidence to support increased release of proteolytic enzymes from malignant tumor cells, other studies have demonstrated little difference between normal and malignant cells (Clark, 1979; Nicolson, 1979). Clearly, no one factor can explain the invasive ability of malignant cells. Most likely it is a combination of characteristics of malignant cells including mechanical factors, cell mobility, and enzymatic factors.

Separation of Cells from Primary Tumor

The second step in establishment of metastatic lesions is separation of the cell or cluster of cells from the primary tumor; that is, before metastasis can occur malignant cells must become detached from the original tumor. Factors that facilitate and allow this detachment are not understood, but evidence suggests that malignant cells have a reduction in the normal adhesive forces that bind cells together. This reduced adhesiveness of malignant cells allows for separation from the tumor and thus tumor cells are freed to implant at another site. Theories attempting to explain these changes in the malignant cells are not conclusive but may support the presence of enzymatic activity which allows malignant cells to invade normal tissues and to migrate. For example, it is believed that the surface of malignant cells possess a proteolytic enzyme that can activate plasminogen into plasmin, which is capable of splitting fibrin (Williams, et al., 1977). Ossowski et al. (1973) demonstrated that chicken embryo fibroblasts in culture were not able to solubilize fibrin but showed marked fibrinolytic ability after infection by a Rous sarcoma virus. Clark (1979, p. 793) speculates that "the limited specific proteolysis carried out by plasmin on other proteins could be involved in the generation of pharmacologically active peptides such as those involved in vascular permeability and perhaps others yet to be discovered."

Penetration into Lymphatic or Blood Vessels

With these possible explanations in mind, let us move to the third step in establishment of metastatic lesions—arrest in and/or infiltration through the lymphatic or vascular vessels. Penetration into the lymphatic system and the blood allows for widespread and distant metastasis. It should be noted here that some tumors are able to spread without benefit of the blood and lymphatic systems. Metastasis is also accomplished by implantation. For example, tumors arising from the ovaries are able to spread by implantation on the abdominal or pelvic peritoneum. Also on occasion tumors of the oral cavity have been known to break away and implant in the tracheobronchial tree (del Regato, 1977). During surgery for removal of a malignant neoplasm, cells may also be carried from the original site and implanted to another area, including the incision.

Since the lymphatic and blood systems are connected, tumor cells can pass back and forth between the two systems. Malignant cells are probably released continuously into the blood as the tumor grows. The mechanism that allows this is unknown. Using electron microscopy Chew et al. (1970) studied rat tumors of lung, liver, pituitary, and brain tissue. Though they concede that their observations varied from organ to organ, they, nonetheless, observed some common patterns. These observations are summarized by Clark (1979, p. 794):

1. Platelet cells almost always associated with the malignant cells when they enter the vessels.
2. Small amounts of fibrin usually appeared and located on the platelet mass.
3. While the tumor cells were still in the vessel the platelet fibrin mass disintegrated leaving tumor cells exposed but closely adherent to the endothelium.
4. After variable time intervals the tumor cells are able to leave the vessel as a result of destruction of the endothelium and basement membrane at multiple points.
5. Tumor cells invade the surrounding tissue through the vessel defects.
6. Tumor cell multiplication continued throughout this process so that a group of malignant cells was formed outside of the vessel space.

Fidler (1975) suggests that there is a "cancer coagulative" factor which causes the thrombus formation around the circulating tumor cells. He further speculates that adhesion to the endothelial wall could result from hypercoagulability properties, increased levels of fibrinolysin inhibitors, and formation of fibrinogen and fibrin clotting. Local injection of fibrinolysin or heparin have been shown to reverse malignant cell clumping, attachment, and penetration, thereby reducing the incidence of metastasis (Clark, 1979). In any event it seems "that malignant cells induce dramatic changes in the adhesion of endothelial cells of blood vessels to their underlying extracellular matrix—the endothelial cells retract, leaving free spaces through which the malignant cells can escape into the vascular system" (Nicolson, 1979, p. 68).

Immune Response

The role of the immune response in the metastatic process is not clear. Many tumor cells have specific antigens on their surfaces (Avis et al., 1979). Evidence suggests that immune response genes of the host may influence effective, ineffective, or nonresponse to the tumor antigens, but this genetic analysis is in a very early phase of development (Klein, 1976). Macrophages are also a part of the host's immunologic response. According to Hibbs (1975), use of an activator such as Bacille Calmette Guerin (BCG) stimulates the lymphocytes that originate in the thymus to initiate macrophage function to defend the host against malignant cells.

In spite of the poorly understood defense of the host against malignant cells in the blood, the fact is that the majority of malignant cells released into the blood die very quickly. Injection of melanoma cells whose DNA had been labeled with radioactive iodine into peripheral veins of mice demonstrated that within a few minutes most of the injected cells were arrested in the lung and died there. This occurred in the lung because it was the site of the first capillary system the cells encountered. A few of the cells continued to circulate but within a day's time only 1 per cent of the injected cells were alive. After 2 weeks only one tenth of 1 per cent of the radioactive cells injected were still alive (Nicolson, 1979).

Implantation at Distant Site

The fourth step of the process is growth of the micrometastasis or its implantation at a distant site within the host. Survival in the new tissue environment is dependent on establishment of a blood supply for the tumor cells to deliver nutrients and remove cellular waste products. Vascularization of new tumors is thought to be stimulated by "tumor angiogenesis factors," which are released by malignant cells (Folkman, 1976). Folkman (1975) distinguishes between an avascular and a vascular phase as the micrometastasis establishes itself. During the avascular phase the cell receives nutrition and eliminates waste by diffusion to and from the extracellular fluid. Examples of avascular tumors are carcinomas in situ; for example, an in situ carcinoma of the uterine cervix. These tumors can remain dormant for years, but with the onset of the vascular phase; that is, the establishment of a vascular supply for the tumor cells, cell proliferation takes place.

Probably only a few of the malignant tumor cells are capable of all the interactions that seem to be necessary for metastasis. Only a small fraction of cells that extend from a primary tumor penetrate a body cavity or enter the lymphatic and blood systems, and of those only a few survive transport and successfully implant in distant tissue. This suggests that the few that survive to metastasize may be a highly specialized subpopulation of malignant cells. Perhaps the constant attack of the host's defense mechanisms may be responsible for the natural selection development of a subpopulation of malignant cells that have highly malignant properties (Nicolson, 1979). The International Union Against Cancer (UICC) (1973) lists 273 types of cancer. Presumably cells of each type of cancer have unique cell membrane characteristics. The task is to find what is common either for groups of tumors or for each type (Clark, 1979).

In summary, cancer metastasis is a very complex process. There are five separate and sequential events that lead to development of a distant metastatic tumor (Nicolson, 1979):

1. Extension into surrounding tissues
2. Penetration of body cavities and vessels
3. Release of tumor cells for transport to other sites
4. Reinvasion of tissue at the site of arrest
5. Manipulation of the new environment to promote tumor cell survival, vascularization, and tumor growth

Sites of Metastasis

Certain organs seem to be preferred sites for metastasis. The site of metastasis is primarily determined by the lymph and blood drainage of the original cancer site; however, it is possible that local conditions within some organs are more favorable to cancer growth than others. Injury to the tissues appears to predispose the tissue or make it more susceptible to metastasis. Besides the lymph nodes the four most common sites of metastasis are the lung, the liver, the bone, and the brain. Cancers with venous drainage directed to one of the venae cavae tend to metastasize primarily to the lungs (various sarcomas, carcinomas of the liver, lower rectum or anus, and kidney). The venous drainage carries metastasis from the cancers of the digestive tract through the portal vein into the liver. Tumors originating closely to the intercostal or paravertebral veins tend to spread to the bones (carcinomas of the breast, prostate, thyroid, and kidney). The tumors of the lung metastasize through the arteries and therefore can spread anywhere. Because of a very high blood flow rate through the brain and lung, metastasis commonly appears there. Cardiac meta-

TABLE 39-5. ***Sites of Metastasis***

Site of Metastasis	Organs from Which Metastasis Originates								
	Breast	Colon	Kidney	Liver	Lung	Pancreas	Prostate	Stomach	Thyroid
Bone	✓		✓		✓		✓		✓
Brain	✓		✓		✓				
Liver	✓	✓			✓	✓	✓	✓	
Lung	✓		✓	✓				✓	
Heart	✓	✓	✓		✓				
Skin	✓	✓	✓		✓			✓	

For reasons not understood, malignant neoplasms may spread early in one person and late in another.

stasis has been reported in various studies. In a study done by Baker, Al-Sarraf, and Vaitkevicius (1972), of 975 patients with disseminated malignancy, 138 patients, or 14.4 per cent, had cardiac metastasis, which was found at autopsy. From the preceding, the reader can note that neoplasms from some organs metastasize to a number of organs; for example, cancer of the breast can metastasize not only to the bone but also to the lung, brain, or liver. The sites of most commonly encountered metastasis are summarized in Table 39-5.

As emphasized, a characteristic feature of malignant growth is its tendency to metastasize, or to set up secondary growths at points distant from the primary site. Some tissues appear to provide conditions that are more favorable to metastasis than others. Injury to tissue favors metastasis. The routes by which neoplasms spread are those by which materials are distributed throughout the body.

Recurrence

No discussion of the characteristics of malignant neoplasms would be complete without a comment about the tendency of malignant neoplasms to recur. As with other characteristics, the likelihood of recurrence varies considerably for different types of malignant neoplasms and from one person to another.

A concept introduced to explain the behavior of malignant neoplasms is that of *biological predeterminism.* By this term is meant that the course and behavior, or natural history, of a cancer is determined at the time of its inception. A slow-growing neoplasm with little power of invasion can be expected to retain these characteristics, whereas a rapidly growing and/or highly invasive neoplasm has the potential for rapid growth and invasiveness from the start. The earlier-cited example of the different types of malignant neoplasms of the skin illustrates the concept of biological predeterminism exceptionally well.

Variability

A point that must be emphasized about malignant neoplasms is that, despite their general characteristics, there is great variability in their behavior in different individuals. For example, cancer cells are found in the prostate without any evidence of invasion to surrounding tissue or spread to distant parts. The fact of their presence may have been unknown to the patient or the attending physician until after death, when the prostate is examined at autopsy. Other neoplasms, such as malignant melanomas, are highly malignant from the start. Despite a small primary lesion, malignant cells may be distributed throughout the body before the primary lesion is known to be active. What appears to be the same type of lesion also behaves differently in different individuals. There is a growing appreciation that each person who has cancer is an individual and that the way in which the disease behaves in each person is also unique.

To illustrate differences in the course of malignant neoplasms in two different people, Mr. Bernard and Mr. Lester will be described. Mr. Bernard, who died last week, had always been a healthy and active man. Five weeks before his death, he complained of feeling ill. When, after a week or so, he continued to feel weak and tired, he consulted his physician who, after appropriate studies, made a diagnosis of acute leukemia. Mr. Bernard did not respond to any of the therapeutic measures and he failed rapidly.

Mr. Lester lives across town from Mr. Bernard. Eight years ago, he was found to have chronic leukemia. Unlike Mr. Bernard, he has responded well to therapy. Although he seldom feels entirely well, he has been able to continue his employment as an accountant and to support himself and his family. Recently he has not been feeling as well as he did in the past. How long he will be able to work is a matter for conjecture. Although many elements in the lives of Mr. Bernard and Mr. Lester are similar, the manifestations of leukemia have been quite different.

Grading and Staging

Grading and staging are two criteria for evaluating tumors and they are based on different characteristics. Grading refers to the microscopic appearance of the tumor cells—specifically to their degree of anaplasia. Most tumors are described using four grades. Grade I tumors are well differentiated and closely resemble the normal parent cell. Grade IV tumors are so anaplastic that it becomes difficult to recognize and identify their cell of origin. Grades II and III are intermediate. Many times the numerical classifications of Grades I through IV will be replaced by description of the tumor as well differentiated, moderately differentiated, poorly differentiated, or undifferentiated.

The staging of cancer is based on the extent of its spread, not on the microscopic appearance. The TNM system of staging has been established by the International Union Against Cancer (1962). "T" represents the primary tumor; "N" refers to involvement of the lymph nodes; "M" refers to distant metastasis. With each of these letters, subscript codes are utilized to further describe the extent of the cancer. Following is the TNM classification as described by the International Union Against Cancer (1973):

- TIS Carcinoma in situ
- TO No primary tumor present
- T_1 Tumor 2 cm or less in its largest dimension, strictly superficial or exophytic
- T_2 Tumor more than 2 cm but not more than 5 cm in its largest dimension or with minimal infiltration of the dermis, irrespective of size
- T_3 Tumor more than 5 cm in its largest dimension or with deep infiltration of the dermis, irrespective of size
- T_4 Tumor involving other structures such as cartilage, muscle, or bone
- NO No palpable nodes
- N_1 Movable homolateral nodes
  - N_{1a} Nodes not considered to contain growth
  - N_{1b} Nodes considered to contain growth
- N_2 Movable contralateral or bilateral nodes
  - N_{2a} Nodes are not considered to contain growth
  - N_{2b} Nodes considered to contain growth
- N_3 Fixed nodes
- M_0 No evidence of distant metastasis
- M_1 Distant metastases present including lymph nodes beyond the region in which the primary tumor is situated or satellite nodules more than 5 cm from the border of the primary tumor

Staging is not an exact science, though agreement has been reached concerning many anatomic sites; for example, the TNM system is widely used for breast, gynecologic, and laryngeal cancers and for Hodgkin's disease.

Several cancer sites or organs such as bile ducts, small intestine, urethra, liver, adrenal, eye, gallbladder, and penis, have not yet been defined by stage. Preliminary staging is underway for other sites, such as salivary glands, thyroid, and pancreas (American Joint Committee for Cancer Staging and End-Result Report, 1977).

Staging and grading tumors is the responsibility of the physician. The nurse, however, must be aware of definitions of the various grades and stages. The precise definitions for each grade or stage varies slightly from the previous general definitions and is dependent on the location of the cancer. (Refer to pathology texts or a manual for staging cancer, such as that published by the American Joint Committee for Cancer Staging, 1977.) The nurse's knowledge of the stage or extent of disease provides vital information about prognosis and treatment as the patient's nursing management is planned.

The Papanicolaou smear test has become a standard part of the physical examination. (Refer to discussion on Gynecological Examination.) Following are definitions of cytological grading and staging which are obtained from a Pap smear. These are examples of precise definitions for a cancer site based on the general definitions of the TNM system.

Cytological Grading from Papanicolaou Smear (Holland and Frei, 1973, p. 1737):

- Grade 1—Smear contains only normal cells
- Grade 2—Some atypical cellular features; for example, vacuolization, cytoplasmic granulation, double nuclei, and nuclear enlargement, but none suggestive of a malignant cell
- Grade 3—Cells having abnormal features, suggestive of but not definite for malignant cells
- Grade 4—Containing malignant cells
- Grade 5—Malignant cells, more bizzare than Grade 4

Staging from Papanicolaou smear (Holland and Frei, 1973; Rubin, 1978, American Joint Committee for Cancer Staging and End-Result Reporting, 1977):

- Stage O—Carcinoma in situ
- Stage I—Carcinoma strictly confined to cervix
  - IA—Microinvasive carcinoma, preclinical phase
  - IB—All other cases of Stage I

Stage II—Carcinoma extends beyond cervix, but not to the pelvic wall or lower vagina
IIA—No obvious parametrial involvement
IIB—Obvious parametrial involvement
Stage III—Carcinoma has extended to the pelvic wall; no free space between the tumor and the pelvic wall on rectal examination; tumor involves the lower third of the vagina
IIIA—Involves the lower third of the vagina, but has not extended to the pelvic wall
IIIB—Extension to the pelvic walls and/or ueretheral obstruction
Stage IV—Carcinoma has extended beyond the true pelvis or has involved the mucosa of the bladder or rectum
IVA—Spread to adjacent organs
IVB—Spread to distant organs

Squamous cell carcinoma of the uterine cervix can be staged by clinical examination alone, but cancers such as adenocarcinomas of the large bowel require examination of resected specimens for staging (Rosai & Ackermann, 1979).

Both grading and staging serve as a guide to prognosis of cancer. Generally prognosis deteriorates as cells become less differentiated and as the stage of the disease progresses (Rosai & Ackermann, 1979). Another advantage of staging is that it allows for comparison of treatments for various stages and their survival rates (Horton & Hill, 1977).

Factors in the Cause and Promotion of Cancer

As in most other chronic diseases, knowledge of the factors in the etiology of cancer is incomplete. Similarly, causes of cancer can be classified under the general headings of susceptible host, injuring or carcinogenic agents, and the elements in the environment bringing the host and agent together. The concept of necessary and sufficient cause probably applies to some cancers. In the etiology of cancer, no single element is known to be required for its development. Whatever the factors are in its etiology, they must be of sufficient degree to initiate malignant change and to allow the abnormal growth to continue. The differences in susceptibility of various individuals to the effect of smoking cigarettes appears to illustrate the concept of sufficient causation. Not all individuals who smoke cigarettes develop bronchogenic carcinoma; a few who do not smoke do. The length and intensity of exposure are both elements, however, as the incidence of bronchogenic carcinoma rises with the length of time the individual has smoked and as the number of cigarettes smoked increases. (U.S. DHEW, 1977). Individual susceptibility varies, but bronchogenic carcinoma develops when the injury to the cells is sufficient to overcome the protective mechanisms of the individual. In many cancers multiple factors probably interact to cause the disease.

Intrinsic Factors

Host Susceptibility

Among elements presumed to affect the susceptibility of the host are genetic constitution, age, hormone balance, immunity, nutritional status, and precancerous lesions. Data on the possibility that heredity is a factor in cancer are derived from several sources: the occurrence of certain types of cancer among close relatives, so-called cancer families, and the development of cancer strains of experimental animals.

Genetic Factor

Accurate knowledge of the genetic factors in cancer among human beings is difficult to obtain. Persons who are predisposed to cancer may die from some other cause before the disease develops. For many reasons, information gained about disease and cause of death among family members tends to be unreliable. Persons may not know what caused the death of members of preceding generations. Some persons withhold information about family members who have had cancer because they believe it is caused by venereal disease or results from an activity that is unclean or sinful. There are undoubtedly a variety of reasons for the unreliability of data reported by persons relative to a history of cancer in the family.

Genetic factors appear to influence the development of cancer either by the effect of a specific gene or as a consequence of the genetic constitution of the individual. Neoplasms for which there is known to be a familial tendency are relatively rare. They include von Recklinghausen's neurofibromatosis, osteochondroma, and pheochromocytoma. There are a few lesions that are not of themselves malignant, but they undergo malignant degeneration when they are exposed to specific conditions. As an example, xeroderma pigmentosa is hereditary, but neoplastic change is dependent on exposure of the skin to sunlight. Besides the disorders in which evidence of genetic factors is reasonably clear, there are studies indicating that a tendency to cancer of the breast is inherited. The transmission of the tendency to cancer of the breast is not consistent enough, however, to make accurate predictions possible. Although a few cancer families have been identified, the extent to which genetic factors are responsible is not known.

Heredity may predispose to cancer, not by a specific gene or genes, but by the effect of the genetic constitution of the individual. In keeping with this concept, susceptibility to or protection from cancer depends on the effects of genes on bodily processes. As one example, mutant or abnormal cells are known to be formed by persons who do not develop cancer as well as by those who do. Heredity may be a factor in the efficiency of defense mechanisms against abnormal cells. Theoretically, at least, the genetic constitution of an individual may alter the manner in which his or her cells respond to or metabolize potentially carcinogenic agents. In one individual the product of the metabolism of a carcinogen may be harmless and in another it may be harmful. Another possibility lies in the ease with which the cells of an individual throw off the restraints on growth. In the vast majority of persons heredity is only one of a number of factors interacting to protect the person from, or to predispose him or her to neoplasia. Whether or not a given individual develops cancer depends on the net result of all these factors.

Other evidence implicating heredity as a factor in the etiology of cancer is that the neoplasia is universal in nature. Strains of experimental animals, such as mice, have been developed that demonstrate a high degree of susceptibility not only to cancer but to cancer in certain sites. Even among these animals, in some instances the tendency to the disease requires additional etiological agents to ensure its development. In studies with strains of mice inbred to develop spontaneous tumors of the breast, multiple factors are required for the mice to develop mammary cancers with any degree of consistency.

Certain malignant neoplasms are associated with specific abnormal chromosomes. Chronic myelogenous leukemia occurs more commonly in individuals with one chromosome 21 having one short arm. Children with Down's syndrome (mongolism) usually have forty-seven chromosomes rather than the normal number. They have an unusually high incidence of leukemia. Apparently their chromosomal abnormalities increase their susceptibility to leukemia.

In a study involving two sets of identical twins, Wilms tumor was diagnosed in only one of the twins from each set. These findings support the hypothesis that development of Wilms's tumor requires the occurrence of more than one successive mutational event (Mauer et al., 1979).

Recent findings suggest that cancer occurs more commonly among married couples. Payan (1979) observed an increase in incidence of cancer of the same organs and histopathologic types among a group of married couples he studied. These findings suggest the importance of including the spouse of the cancer patient in the family history.

Despite a growing body of knowledge about heredity as a factor in the development of cancer, exact information about how it influences its development is far from clear. For most individuals, their genetic constitution is presumed to protect them from or to predispose them to not only cancer but other diseases. In most instances, additional factors are involved.

Hormones

Hormones have long been suspected of influencing susceptibility to cancer. In 1889, Schinzinger suggested that hormones might be important in the development of cancer of the breast in women. (Hardy, 1958).

In 1918 Loeb (Hardy, 1958) demonstrated that the incidence of cancer of the breast in cancer-susceptible strains of female mice could be prevented by removing their ovaries.

Since then, chronic estrogen administration in rodents has been shown to produce uterine, cervical, mammary, renal, adrenal cortical, pituitary, ovarian, and testicular neoplasms (Holland and Frei, 1973). That cancer of the breast is extremely rare in males and is the leading cause of death from cancer in the female is well known. The exact role of hormones in the induction of cancer is not clear. Knowledge is not available as to whether hormones act as inciting agents or whether they prepare the tissue so that it responds to carcinogenic agents. The hormones found to be carcinogenic in animals are those that have an influence on the growth of certain tissues.

Diethylstilbesterol (DES), a synthetic estrogen receiving much publicity of late, was used to prevent abortions in the 1950s. Evidence today suggests that adenocarcinoma of the vagina in young women is related to prenatal ingestion of DES by the mother (Herbst, et al., 1971). The nurse should promote regular gynecological examinations among daughters of women who took DES during pregnancy. Hormones from the ovaries, testes, and adrenal cortex are necessary to the growth of some cancers. In addition to promoting growth of specific tissues, these hormones are all steroids and their chemical structure is similar to that of the carcinogenic hydrocarbons. The significance of these relationships is not known. That a relationship exists between certain hormones and the development of cancer is supported by animal experiments. Breast cancer has been induced in male mice of susceptible strains by castrating them and implanting ovaries under their skin or by the prolonged administration of excessive dosages of female hormones (del Regato, 1977, p. 19). Some cancers have been induced in animals by upsetting hormonal balance. From available knowledge, certain hormones are necessary to the growth of some cancers. Other hormones inhibit for a time the growth of some cancers. Thus a deficient supply of hormone might be a factor in the development of certain neoplasms. After a time a neoplasm whose growth is inhibited by a hormone adapts to its presence, and it is no longer restrained by it. From this and other evidence, hormones appear to be one of the multiple factors entering into the genesis of cancer.

In a report of a large case control study, Antunes et al. (1979) demonstrated that the overall risk of endometrial cancer was six times greater for women who were taking estrogen than for women who were not. Women who were on estrogen for 5 years or more showed a fifteenfold risk. Excessive risk was present for both diethylstilbestrol and conjugated estrogen users. In addition, the risk associated with cyclic use was as great as for continuous use.

Age

Authorities disagree as to the influence of age on susceptibility to cancer. Some interpret the fact that the incidence of cancer increases with age as evidence that age influences susceptibility, whereas others do not. The age at which the peak incidence for cancer in various sites occurs differs. Although some of these are benign rather than malignant, some types of new growths, such as Wilms's tumors of the kidney, teratomas, neuroblastomas, neurofibromas, chondromas, hemangiomas, and nevi, are often congenital. Leukemia, which was once presumed to have its highest incidence in young children, actually occurs more frequently in adults than it does in children, and the rate is increasing, (*Cancer Statistics,* 1978). In children, leukemia is more likely to be more acute and the course shorter than in adults. Acute lymphatic leukemia is, however, primarily a disease of childhood. Hodgkin's disease occurs most commonly in young adults.

Sex

The incidence of some sites of cancer is influenced or determined by sex. As examples, cancer of the breast is common among women but occurs rarely among men. Cancer of the stomach and lung is more common among men than among women. Not all the reasons for sex differences are known.

Racial Factors

The distribution of certain cancers varies among different racial and ethnic groups. For example, African blacks have higher rates of cancers such as Burkitt's lymphoma, Kaposi's sarcoma, and carcinoma of the esophagus than do blacks in the United States. Japanese women show a very low incidence of breast cancer compared with American women. Blacks and others with darker skin pigmentation seem to be protected from melanomas and skin cancers which are thought to be induced by exposure to the sun's rays. Although there is some evidence that race may be a factor in cancer susceptibility, genetic factors and environmental exposure cannot be overlooked as significant factors in accounting for racial distribution of cancer (Holland & Frei, 1973).

Precancerous Lesions

Certain lesions in the body appear to increase host susceptibility to cancer. The presence of one neoplasm increases the likelihood of developing another. The person who develops cancer in one tissue is more likely to develop another one than is the person who has never had a cancerous lesion. Another type of lesion, the so-called precancerous lesion, may also predispose to cancer. These are lesions that at their inception are not cancerous but that tend to undergo malignant degeneration. Among the more common precancerous lesions are (1) large burn scars, particularly those resulting from third-degree burns; (2) nevi, especially moles near the juncture of the two sides of (midline) the body; (3) senile keratosis, a disease of the epidermis involving the horny layer; and (4) leukoplakia, a disorder characterized by the development of a white patch or patches on the buccal mucosa inside the cheek or on the female vulva.

Immunity

On the basis of several types of observations, there has been recurring interest in the role of immunity in cancer. Not all persons require the same degree of exposure to carcinogenic agents to develop cancer. Among those who do there is definitely a host response. Spontaneous regression occurs in 1 of 100,000 cases. Some persons have a desmoplastic, that is, fibrous tissue, reaction. Among others, the disease is manifested by rapid growth and spread. Mutant cells developing in healthy persons are rapidly destroyed. Whether or not each of the preceding represents immunity or an immune response is not clearly established.

As mentioned earlier, a neoplastic cell's structure is altered from a normal cell's structure. The changes in the surface of a neoplastic cell should allow for recognition of the cell's surface by the host's defense mechanisms and for the consequent mobilization of the body's defense mechanisms and elimination of the altered cell. Research with laboratory animals and results of immunosuppressive treatments in humans suggest that compromised immunologic integrity enhances the frequency of tumor development. It is not understood if this is a result of the inability of the immune system to destroy the altered neoplastic cell or if it is a failure of the immune system to restrain antigenic agents such as viruses which may be causing the neoplastic growth. Neoplastic growth may also reflect a failure of the surveillance mechanisms to recognize and destroy the neoplasm (Holland & Frei, 1973).

The occurrence of spontaneous regression of human neoplasms (Bakemeier, 1978) has led to much investigation in host defenses against tumors. The possibility that natural immunologic mechanisms play a role in protecting against malignant neoplasms has also gained acceptance because of reports of higher incidences of cancers in those having immunologic deficiencies, whether congenital, acquired as part of another disease, accidental, or latrogenic. Patients who have Hodgkin's disease have evidence of immunologic deficiency, but there is a difference of opinion relating to the prevalence of second unrelated malignant neoplasms in this disease. (Cancer and Immune Mechanisms, 1973).

Conversely, laboratory findings indicate that the use of an immunorestorative drug, Thiahendazole, in the perioperative period resulted in improved cytotoxic response and with a significant decrease in metastases. In other words, immunotherapy seems to be an effective adjunct to cancer surgery (Lundy et al., 1979). These findings lead support to the theories suggesting that tumor growth can be inhibited or permitted to develop, depending on the condition of the host's immune mechanisms.

Extrinsic Factors

Carcinogens

In addition to host susceptibility, a variety of chemical, physical, and living agents are associated with neoplasia. More than 500 substances have been identified that are carcinogenic; that is, they induce malignant change in cells when applied to tissue for a sufficient period of time. No one knows how carcinogenic agents act. They may overstimulate the cell or release it from the inhibiting influence of growth regulators. Not all persons who are exposed to carcinogenic agents develop cancer. Knowledge of carcinogenic agents is important, however, for many are subject to control. The chances of developing cancer in certain sites can be lessened by reducing or eliminating contact with carcinogenic agents.

Carcinogenic chemicals include a great variety of organic and inorganic substances. Some of them contaminate the air in industrial and urban areas. Among the organic chemicals are aromatic compounds, such as tar, soot, asphalt, crude patallin oil, lubricating and fuel oils, as well as aromatic amines such as benzol and aniline dyes. Inorganic chemicals include nickel, asbestos, and arsenicals.

Physical carcinogens include heat rays, ultraviolet light, and ionizing rays and particles.

Living agents implicated as carcinogens include viruses and *Schistosoma haematobium.*

Two recently discovered carcinogens that are possibly related to human cancer originate from "natural sources." (Cancer and Immune Mechanisms, 1973). One is aflatoxin, which is produced by the mold *Aspergillus flavus.* This grows on damp peanuts, corn, cottonseed, and other food crops that are not properly harvested or stored. Aflatoxins are related to cancer of the liver in poultry and fish. The other natural carcinogen is cycasin, which is found in the cycad nut. Cycasin, it was discovered, needed bacterial flora to afford the active metabolite in the production of cancer of the liver and kidney in rats.

Habits and Customs

Because the habits and customs of a people determine to a large extent the carcinogens to which they are likely to be exposed, they are important in carcinogenesis. Some habits and customs seem strange because they are unfamiliar. All people, including Americans, have some customs and habits that result in their exposure to carcinogens. From many examples that could be cited, only a few have been selected. In England, the incidence of cancer of the scrotum, which was common among chimney sweeps in the eighteenth century, was reduced by teaching the men to bathe frequently. This form of cancer is absent among similar workers in Japan because they practice meticulous cleanliness. In Kashmir, mountaineers carry charcoal-burning stoves under their cloaks to keep themselves warm. The stoves are supported on the upper areas of the abdomen. Burns of the abdomen and chest are frequent. There is a high incidence of cancer in the burn scars. Cancer of the cheek is frequent in those who chew betel nuts. Cancer of the lip is more frequent among pipe smokers than among nonpipe smokers. More than twenty-five scientific studies in ten countries have demonstrated a high degree of relationship between the smoking of cigarettes and the risk of developing cancer.

CIGARETTE SMOKING. Few subjects have been studied more intensively during the past two decades than the relationship of cigarette smoking and health. The risk of developing lung cancer is ten times greater for cigarette smokers than for nonsmokers, and that risk increases proportionately with the number of cigarettes smoked per day, total lifetime number of cigarettes smoked, number of years smoking, age at initiation of smoking, and depth of inhalation. The occurrence of lung cancer has been increasing for the past 30 years. It is currently the number-one cause of cancer deaths among males (Silverberg, 1979). Historically women smokers smoked fewer cigarettes per day than men, and consequently the lung cancer rate was lower. However, over the past 30 years women have been smoking more heavily and there has been a 400 per cent increase in women's lung cancer mortality rates (U.S. DHEW, 1977).

The fact that fewer women die from lung cancer than men is explained by the following: (1) fewer women smoke than men, (2) more women who smoke are under 50 years of age than men (lung cancer in men has its highest incidence in the 65 to 74 age group), and (3) women's smoking habits are different. They are not as likely to smoke cigarettes down to the end where the tars and nicotine are proportionately higher. They do not inhale as deeply. They smoke more filter-tip cigarettes and low tar and nicotine cigarettes than men (U.S. DHEW, *Health Consequences of Smoking,* 1968, p. 97).

Although tar and nicotine are two chemicals known to be present in cigarettes, studies indicate that tobacco smoke contains several thousand compounds. Of these, 700 to 800 have been identified (U.S. DHEW, *Health Consequences of Smoking,* 1968, p. 90). Despite the evidence that cancer of the lung and other organs can be prevented by the elimination of smoking, the application of this knowledge is highly complex. Some aspects of this problem include the following: (1) children, especially boys, may start smoking as early as 8 or 9 years of age; (2) children of parents who smoke are likely to follow their example; (3) people who smoke appear to do so for many reasons, and therefore a single approach to the problem is not likely to solve it, and (4) because the incidence of cancer caused by smoking is correlated with the length and degree of exposure, the development of cigarettes as well as of smoking habits that lessen exposure to tar and nicotine should be encouraged. Generally less tar and nicotine are inhaled with filter-tipped cigarettes. Tobacco is being developed with a lower tar and nicotine content than that previously grown. Avoidance of inhaling cigarette smoke and discarding the cigarette after it is half smoked also reduces exposure. Rapidly burning and porous cigarette papers reduce the degree of exposure.

Cigarette smoke interacts with other environmental and occupational contaminants which are also associated with increased incidences of cancer. The interaction of these pollutants produces a greater risk of developing lung cancer than exposure to just one of the contaminants. For example, nonsmoking workers in uranium mines and in the asbestos industry have only slightly increased lung cancer rates than nonsmokers in general, but workers in these occupations who smoke have greatly elevated lung cancer rates. It is estimated that cigarette-smoking asbestos workers have 92 times the risk of developing lung cancer than nonsmokers, and uranium miners who smoke have 10 times the risk of nonsmoking uranium workers (U.S. DHEW, 1977). Not only is cigarette smoking linked with cancer of the lungs; it is also linked with cancer of the larynx, pharynx, oral cavity, esophagus, pancreas, and bladder. Rief (1976) calculates that deaths caused by cancers in these various sites could have been reduced anywhere from 23 to 81 per cent if the patients had not been smokers. Winkelstein (1977) suggests that smoking may also be a risk factor in cancer of the uterine cervix and recommends that additional observations be made to determine the correlation and ultimately the cause-and-effect relationship. Researchers have demonstrated that the combined effect of alcohol and tobacco usage significantly increases the risk of cancer, particularly cancer of the larynx, lung, esophagus, and oral cavity (McMichael, 1978; Wynder, 1977).

Oncogenic Viruses

Of the possible causative agents in cancer, none is of greater interest than the possible role of viruses. Interest in the virus as an etiological agent in cancer is not new for at least 50 years ago Rous[2] demonstrated that a virus caused sarcoma of the breast in chickens. Until recently, however, there was no evidence that a virus acted as a carcinogenic agent in any species except birds and fowl. Since Bittner's discovery in 1936 that the milk factor was a necessary condition to the development of cancer of the breast in mice, a number of neoplastic diseases in animals have been shown to be of virus origin. (Bitt-

[2] Dr. Peyton Rous shared the Nobel Prize in medicine and physiology in 1966 for his fundamental research in this area.

ner, 1946–47). Included among these are leukemia in mice and papillomatosis in rabbits. Warts and papillomas in humans, though nonmalignant growths, are of virus origin. Until recently no virus had been found in a human malignant neoplasm; this fact had been taken as positive evidence against the virus as an initiating factor in cancer in human beings. A herpes-type virus (HTV), the Epstein-Barr (EB) virus, is believed to be the cause of Burkitt's lymphoma, cancer of the lymph glands, which occurs primarily in African children. Another kind of HTV, type 2, is suspected as a cause in cervical cancer (del Regato, 1977, p. 22). A common virus located in the nose and throat of humans, adenovirus 12, can cause cancer in hamsters (Holland & Frei, 1973, p. 18).

To date viruslike particles have been isolated from human tumor material, but no virus has been isolated that has been shown to cause cancer in humans. Establishing proof of the neoplastic-inducing properties of viruses in humans will be especially difficult because humans cannot be employed as a host to study the viruses suspected of oncogenesis. The question still remains unanswered as to why cancer-causing viruses have not been isolated in humans.

There is a growing body of scientific evidence indicating that a virus or viruses may be the principal cause of leukemia in human beings. Interest in the virus as a causative factor in leukemia has been stimulated by the occurrence of clusters of individuals ill with leukemia in a number of communities. One such instance occurred in Niles, Illinois, where thirteen individuals were discovered concentrated in one area; this number is many times the expected incidence (ACS, *Facts about Leukemia*, 1963).

Even if a virus proves to be a factor in some or all cancers, there is no evidence to suggest that cancer is contagious in the ordinary sense of the word. It is not disseminated in the same manner as measles, chickenpox, or the common cold. It is not transmitted by the blood, as healthy people have been transfused with blood from patients with leukemia without subsequently becoming ill. Mothers with leukemia have healthy babies. Neither a physican nor a nurse has ever been known to develop leukemia after caring for a patient with it.

Despite the possibility that viruses are a factor in the development of some cancers, a number of factors contribute to the difficulty in identifying their presence in tissues even when they are there. There is evidence to indicate that viruses can be present in the tissues in the absence of morphological evidence that they are there. They are apparently able to assume a latent form and to resume their virulent characteristics when conditions are favorable. Studies have demonstrated that cells transformed by certain cancer viruses, such as the Rous sarcoma virus, appeared to be able to transmit the genetic material of the virus from one generation of tumor cells to another without producing the virus in the infectious form. For the infectious form to appear, the tumor cells had to be subjected to special conditions (Link Viral Genes to Cancer, 1963). The discovery that some viruses that infect animals enter into the genetic DNA is also of more than passing interest. Some viruses, such as the Rous sarcoma virus, are RNA viruses.

Other Factors

Other Habits and Customs

Practices by certain groups may alter the incidence of cancer. As an example, cancer of the penis has a low incidence in Jewish and Moslem men. This is believed to be related to the practice of early circumcision.

Cross and his associates (1968) reported a study in which cervical smears were made on over 5,000 women who were considered to be typical of the U.S. rural population. The socioeconomic and medical standards of the group were similar. Almost half of the group were Amish, a religious group that has practiced strict endogamy and monogamy for many generations. The incidence of cancer of the cervix was lower for the Amish than for other women. The authors interpret this finding as indicating that the marital behavior of the Amish may limit the spread of an agent important in the etiology of cancer.

Cancer of the skin is more common in persons whose skin is exposed to the rays of the sun, such as farmers and sailors, than it is among indoor workers. Exposure to the rays of the sun probably accounts for the observation that cancer of the skin is more common among persons living in the southern than in the northern part of the United States.

Those who live in cities and industrial areas of the United States have a higher incidence of cancer than those who live in rural areas. Among the factors presumed to contribute to this difference is that those who live in cities are exposed to an atmosphere contaminated by smoke and automobile exhaust gases. From these examples, the conclusion that customs and habits are a factor in cancer appears valid, for they determine to some extent the carcinogens to which the individual is exposed and the degree of exposure.

Certain occupations also increase the likelihood of exposure to chemical and physical carcinogens. A large number of chemical agents of organic and inorganic origin have been implicated as carcinogens. Included among organic chemicals that have been demonstrated to be carcinogenic in animals are the carcinogenic hydrocarbons found in tar and soot. The aromatic amines and benzol as well as many other chemicals are potentially carcinogenic. Among the inorganic chemicals with carcinogenic powers are the arsenicals, chromates, nickel, and asbestos. Many of these chemicals are either used in industrial processes or are products or by-products of these processes. Knowledge of the carcinogenic potential of chemicals is essential to the protection of workers and the members of the community. Protection involves the development of effective procedures for eliminating or minimizing contact and a program to teach workers how to use them.

A number of physical agents are known to be carcinogenic. The effect of long-continued exposure to ultraviolet light or to the rays of the sun has already been mentioned. Ionizing radiation, whether produced by x-ray or from natural or artifically produced radioactive isotopes, is of increasing significance. The increased use of ionizing radiation in hospitals, in industry, and in national defense increases the amount of and the number of opportunities for exposure.

A significantly higher death rate from leukemia among radiologists has been demonstrated in comparison to a group of nonradiologist physicians. More recent studies, however, do not indicate an excessive mortality rate from leukemia among younger radiologists. This improvement is thought to be partly attributable to improved radiological practices, which are reducing the occupational hazards of exposure to radiation (Travis, 1975).

Survivors of the bombing of Hiroshima and Nagasaki demonstrate a marked increase in incidence of leukemia in persons subjected to the highest dosages of irradiation from the bomb—10 per cent of that group developed leukemia (Burch, 1976).

These findings suggest that the increasing ionizing radiation in our atmosphere is contributing to the rising incidence of leukemia in the United States.

The role of physical or mechanical injury of the tissues in carcinogenesis has been a subject for debate. The possibility of a single injury being a causative factor in cancer is believed to be remote. When a neoplasm is found following an injury, the probability is that it was there at the time the injury occurred and the injury served to call the attention of the person to it. Following tissue injury, the rate of growth of a neoplasm is sometimes accelerated. This occurs frequently enough that some lay people are aware of the possibility. Some authorities discount the importance of chronic mechanical irritation as a significant etiologic factor in cancer. Others regard the fact that cancer develops in old burn scars and in cells forming the walls of draining sinuses as evidence supporting chronic irritation as an etiologic agent (Holland & Frei, 1973).

Living agents may also act as etiological agents. Leukoplakia is sometimes, though not always, associated with syphillis. Cancer of the liver is more common in those parts of the world where a type of flat worm, the liver fluke, is ingested in the drinking water. The fluke invades the liver, where it sets up housekeeping.

Summary

Two factors are involved in the development of cancer. One is a susceptible host. The other is an agent or group of agents capable of injuring the cell. Except in those rare instances in which cancer appears to result from the action of a specific gene, the induction of cancer depends on the action of multiple factors. Knowledge of the epidemiology of cancer has been expanded significantly. Epidemiologic studies are directed toward the identification not only of carcinogenic agents and of the characteristics of individuals who develop cancer but of the characteristics of those who do not. Present evidence points to the conclusion that cancer does not have a single cause and is not really a single disease but that it is the result of the interaction of multiple factors, some of which have their origin in the host and others in the environment (See Figure 39-2).

To emphasize the natural history of cancer, its course has been compared to that of an infection. Although there are significant differences, the course of cancer has many aspects in common with infectious disease. They both involve a susceptible host, injuring agents, and conditions in the environment bringing the two together. The degree to which host susceptibility and the pathogenicity of inciting agents are significant factors in etiology differs among infectious diseases as well as neoplastic ones. In some infectious diseases, such as measles, the nature of susceptibility is largely a matter of the presence or absence of immune bodies. To date, evidence that immunity plays a significant role in cancer is not clear-cut. Because of the scientific interest in this field, answers may be found to questions about it. In infections such as tuberculosis, factors other than immunity affect susceptibility. This is probably also true in cancer. In neither tuberculosis nor malignant neoplasms are all the factors in etiology understood.

In infection, the causative agent has its origin in the external environment and is a necessary condition of disease; a microorganism is the inciting agent. In cancer, the relationship of the injuring agent to the development of the disease is not as clear and

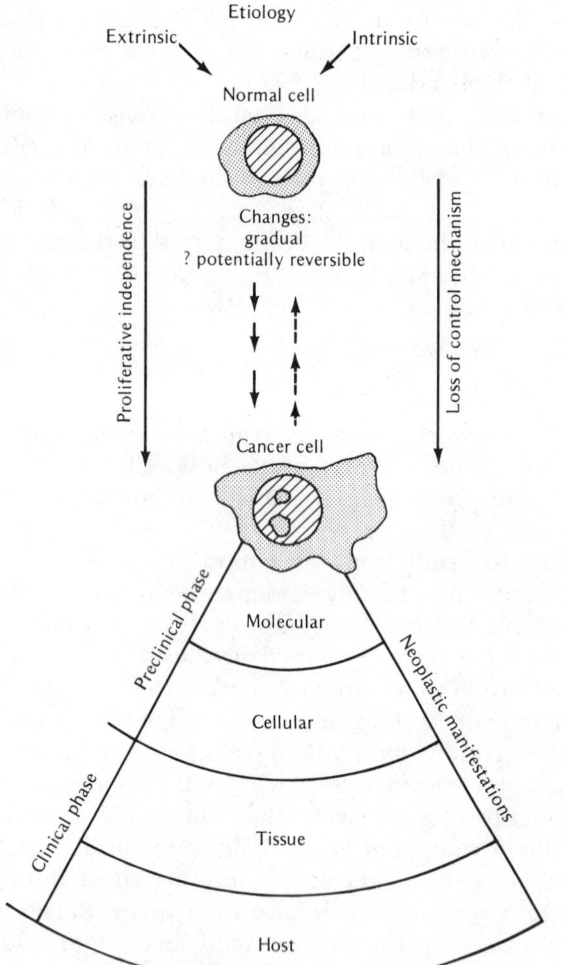

Figure 39-2. Stages of cancerogenesis: (1) neoplastic reaction of normal cell to etiologic factors, (2) neoplastic conversion of normal cell to cancer cell, and (3) manifestations of established cancer cell and malignant tumor. (From Lewin, Isaac: Neoplasia. In Talso, Peter J., and Remenchik, Alexander P., editors: *Internal Medicine*, St. Louis, 1968, The C. V. Mosby Co., Fig. 9-1, p. 150.)

possibly not as direct as in infection. The injuring agent may have its origin in the internal environment as well as in the external environment. It may serve as an inciting or a promoting agent. An inciting agent is one that induces changes in the cell that result in cancer. A promoting agent acts to support or favor cellular growth after cancerous change has taken place.

In both infectious and neoplastic disease a period of time elapses between the moment a microorganism enters the body or a cell is injured and the development of overt disease. In infectious disease, this is known as the incubation period. During the incubation period, the organism establishes itself in a favorable tissue, multiplies, and overcomes the body defenses against its growth and spread. Disease does not occur unless the microorganism is able to proliferate to the point where it can cause some type of cellular injury either directly or by means of its products. In the development of cancer, the periods between the time the cell is injured and the overt disease develops are known as the induction and lag periods. Two theories have been advanced to explain this observation. One is that this is the length of time required by the cell to establish a new metabolic pattern. The other is that time is required for the cancer cell to overcome the restraining influences on proliferation.

In both infectious disease and in cancer, clinical manifestations depend on the multiplication of cells—microorganisms or cancer cells—to the point where they or their products injure tissue cells. In infection, the body recognizes the microorganism as foreign or alien and mobilizes both specific and nonspecific defense mechanisms. Apparently, the body also recognizes abnormal or mutated cells and destroys them. When the body defenses are adequate, microorganisms or abnormal cells are destroyed and the individual returns to or maintains his or her health. In addition, in some, though not all, types of infection, the body develops a sort of recognition system that enables it to protect itself against future attacks. Cancer differs from infection in that, after the stage of overt disease is reached, the body does not appear to have an adequate system of defense against it. There have been a few authenticated instances in which cancer in a person with overt disease disappeared, but these are rare. They are, naturally, of great interest. If the reason for the regression of the cancer could be determined, this knowledge might be useful in prevention and therapy of disease in other individuals. When cancer reaches the stage of overt disease, cancer cells are more or less unresponsive to factors regulating the growth, reproduction, and differentiation of cells. Therefore unlike an infection, the body is unable to limit the extent of injury or, by itself, to restore health.

In some types of infectious processes, the infection has its origin in a localized site. Whether or not the infection remains legalized or spreads to distant points depends on the virulence and invasiveness of the microorganism and the adequacy of the defenses of the body. When the body is unable to localize the infecting microorganisms, they may infiltrate the surrounding tissue or enter the blood and lymphatic vessels. The microorganisms entering the blood and lymphatic system may be destroyed by cells in the blood or in lymph nodes or they may be deposited in distant tissues. There they may be destroyed or conditions may favor their multiplication. When this is true, a secondary or metastatic infection is established. Cancer cells behave in a similar manner. From the available evidence, cancer usually has its origin in a single cell or group of cells. For a period of time, it remains localized at the site of origin. It may never go beyond this site and may even regress.

Cancer Research

Cancer research strategy as developed under the National Cancer Program has seven objectives (Rauscher, 1974). The first four objectives center on cancer cause and prevention. They include: (1) reducing the effectiveness of external agents for producing cancer; (2) modifying individuals in order to minimize the risk of cancer development; (3) preventing transformation of normal cells to cells capable of forming cancers; (4) preventing progression of precancerous cells to cancers, the developing of cancers from precancerous conditions, and spreading of cancers from primary sites. Research directed at accomplishing these objectives ranges from identification of carcinogenic agents in the environment, to genetic and metabolic studies, to cell biology investigations, to development of models in order to more precisely study the cancer process.

The fifth objective centers on cancer detection and diagnosis and intends to develop the means to achieve accurate assessment of *(a)* the risk of developing cancer in individuals and populations and *(b)* the presence, extent, and probable course of existing cancers. Research methods here include epidemiological studies, improved techniques of population screening, identification of individuals most likely to develop cancer, and clinical testing of diagnostic procedures.

The sixth objective centers on cancer treatment. Its aim is to develop the means to cure cancer patients and to control progression. Therapeutic modalities being researched include surgery, radiation, chemotherapy, immunotherapy, combination therapies, and new drugs or chemical agents.

The seventh objective centers on the means to improve the rehabilitation of cancer patients. Studies in this area are designed to look at individual rehabilitation and how to provide cancer patients with up-to-date comprehensive rehabilitation services no matter where they live.

Ultimately the intention of the National Cancer Research Program is to put usable knowledge and tools into the hands of cancer care practitioners as quickly as possible (Rauscher, 1974).

Signs and Symptoms of Neoplastic Diseases

The signs and symptoms accompanying cancer, as well as benign neoplasms, are caused by the local mechanical effects of the primary and metastatic growths and by the total biochemical impact of the disease. Except in neoplastic diseases that are manifested as a generalized disease from the beginning (such as leukemia), the early signs and symptoms are usually caused by the local mechanical effects of the primary lesion. Because of the availability of modern surgical techniques, it is usually possible to remove the primary lesion, so that it is seldom the direct cause of death. Death is usually caused by the extensive derangements of normal biochemical functions associated with the systemic or metastatic stage of the disease (Burch, 1976). The effects observed in late cancer are similar to those seen in generalized sepsis—another point of similarity between infection and cancer.

Local Tissue Effects

The manifestations due to local tissue effects occur by virtue of the four basic characteristics of a malignant neoplasm (Talso and Remenchik, 1968): (1) expansive growth, (2) infiltrative growth, (3) destructive growth, and (4) necrosis of the tumor. Expansive growth is found most frequently in patients with cancer and usually presents itself before other manifestations are evident. Most of the discussion will relate to the signs and symptoms it causes which are swelling, obstruction, and pressure. The tumor forms and distorts anatomic structure, which is a direct result of the mechanical effects of expansive growth. When expansion produces obstruction and pressure phenomena, loss of function ensues.

How soon symptoms develop, as well as their nature, depends on the anatomic and functional characteristics of the involved organ or structures. Such factors as the size and distensibility of the space containing the neoplasm influence the period of time elapsing before the neoplasm causes signs and symptoms. The location of a lesion in a hollow or tubular organ also influences its effect. For example, a lesion near the outlet of the stomach causes symptoms earlier than one in the fundus. A neoplasm growing around a tubular organ causes a greater degree of obstruction than one projecting into it. Each of these points is illustrated later.

Because neoplasms are formed of masses of cells, they generally occupy space and cause clinical manifestations by (1) interfering with the blood supply of tissue, (2) interfering with the function of an organ, and (3) activating compensatory or defensive mechanisms.

As stated earlier, the size and distensibility of the space or organ containing a neoplasm influence the nature as well as the earliness with which manifestations of disease occur. The examples that follow are intended to clarify the mechanical effects of expansive growths.

Mike Sunny, aged 11, has a rapidly growing neoplasm in his cerebellum. As the neoplasm increases in mass, it occupies space and presses on the tissues of the cerebellum.[3] The earliness with which local pressure is exerted is influenced by the fact that the cerebellum is surrounded by a rigid bony wall, the skull; it does not distend to accommodate the increase in the contents of the cranial cavity. Furthermore, the location of this particular neoplasm is such that it obstructs drainage of cerebrospinal fluid from the ventricles, causing the fluid to accumulate within the ventricles and thus further raise the intracranial pressure. Because the size of the cavity containing the brain is fixed, increased resistance to the flow of blood through the brain is a consequence of an elevation in intracranial pressure.

The manifestations presented by Mike are caused by an inadequate supply of blood to the cerebellum and other parts of the brain and by the activation of mechanisms to maintain the blood supply of the brain. The signs and symptoms presented by Mike indicate disturbances in the function of the cerebellum as well as evidence of alterations in cardiorespiratory function, which tend to overcome the resistance to the flow of blood to the brain. (See Chapter 36, for further discussion of disturbance in the function of the cerebellum and for signs and symptoms of increased intracranial pressure.)

In contrast to Mike, who had an expanding lesion within a fixed space, Mrs. Thinly had a neoplasm in a space that is highly distensible. Mrs. Thinly had a benign ovarian cyst, which, at the time it was removed, weighed more than 40 lb. It was so large that it overfilled a basin about the size of an ordinary dishpan. The day before Mrs. Thinly was admitted to the hospital she had done the family wash and cleaned the house. For some months previous to seeking medical attention she had noticed a gradual increase in the size of her abdomen which she attributed to the fact that she had had several children and was getting old. Until the tumor reached considerable size, it had little effect on function because the abdominal wall distended to accommodate the increase in contents. As the size of the tumor increased, however, the intra-abdominal pressure rose, causing pressure against the diaphragm and decreasing the capacity of her stomach and other abdominal organs. She experienced some shortness of breath, swelling of the feet, and loss of appetite. Because of her loss of appetite she lost weight. After the tumor was removed, she weighed 85 lbs, but she made a rapid and uneventful recovery. Because the neoplasm was benign, she was cured.

[3] In the cerebellum the space is less confining than that enclosing the cerebrum. Because the neoplasm is malignant, it also invades the surrounding tissue, but at this point the effect of a space-occupying mass is under discussion.

Mike Sunny and Mrs. Thinly have been described to illustrate how the rigidity or distensibility of the space in which a neoplasm grows influences its effects. At the time Mike Sunny's skull was opened, the neoplasm was about the size of a small orange, and it was already threatening his life by its effect on the blood supply to his brain. In contrast, because of the distensibility of the abdominal wall, Mrs. Thinly had a very large neoplasm that had little effect on the blood supply to the tissues in the abdominal cavity. Signs and symptoms observed in Mrs. Thinly were mainly caused by the interference with the functions of the respiratory and digestive systems.

Obstruction

Mr. Timothy Thomas illustrates what happens when the diameter of a tubular structure is decreased by a space-occupying mass. Mr. Thomas had a carcinoma of the prostate that, as it increased in cell mass, caused pressure on the urethra, thus increasing the resistance to the flow of urine. Any tubular structure may be obstructed by the pressure created (1) by a neoplasm external to it, or (2) by a neoplasm extending from the lining membrane into the lumen of the tube, or (3) by a neoplasm arising in the wall and encircling it as it grows. Both benign and malignant neoplasms may obstruct by creating external pressure on a tubular structure or by extending into its lumen from the lining tissues. Neoplasms arising in the wall and encircling the lumen of a tube, such as the large intestine, are usually malignant.

In the instance of Mr. Thomas, obstruction of the urethra was caused by a neoplasm in tissue external to it. Whatever the cause of the obstruction, its primary effect is to interfere with the passage of the tube's contents. When the obstruction of a tubular structure develops slowly enough, the portion of the tube preceding the obstruction dilates, and the muscle layer in its wall hypertrophies. Muscular hypertrophy occurs as a result of the increase in resistance to the movement of the contents of the obstructed tube; it is therefore a compensatory mechanism. Eventually, as the degree of obstruction increases, the lumen will be blocked and the tube will cease to function as a passageway. Chronic obstruction, whatever its cause, predisposes to infection of the organ drained by the duct and, if unrelieved, to its destruction.

To return to Mr. Thomas, who has an obstruction of the urethra caused by a carcinoma of his prostate gland—as the neoplasm enlarged, it encroached on the lumen of the urethra, thus impeding the passage of urine. To overcome the effect of the increase in resistance caused by the narrowing of the urethra, the muscle in the neck of the bladder hypertrophied. As the urethra narrowed, Mr. Thomas noted that he had difficulty in starting to void and that the urinary stream was small. He also had a feeling of urgency and seldom felt that he had really emptied his bladder. As time passed and the obstruction increased, the bladder did not empty at the time of voiding. Urine accumulated and became infected. The bladder was distended by the accumulated urine. Eventually, if the obstruction is allowed to continue, the ureters and the pelvis of the kidney become distended with urine and all the structures—urethra, bladder, and kidneys—become infected. The outcome of unrelieved obstruction along the urinary tract is kidney failure.

The effects of obstruction of the alimentary canal and of the ducts emptying into it are discussed in Chapters 46 and 52, and will not be pursued here. One effect meriting some consideration is that neoplasms in the alimentary canal usually impair nutrition before those located in other parts of the body. Patients with obstructing lesions in the upper alimentary canal not infrequently experience a rapid loss in weight and are markedly dehydrated and anemic because of impaired intake of food and fluids.

Because the effects of obstruction of ducts forming the tracheobronchial tree and the biliary tract are covered in Chapters 40 and 46, they will not be discussed here.

Another mechanical effect of neoplasms results from pressure created by the neoplasm on the overlying mucous membrane. Pressure on any tissue decreases its blood supply. With impairment in its nutrition the mucosa atrophies, and if the pressure is severe and unrelieved, it ulcerates. Ulceration predisposes to bleeding in benign as well as in malignant neoplasms. For example, some patients with leiomyofibromas located in the submocosa of the wall of the uterus (fibroids) are predisposed to profuse bleeding. Tumors located in the deeper layers of the wall of the uterus do not usually result in hemorrhage. To illustrate, Mrs. Beech has a leiomyofibroma located in the submucosa of the wall of the uterus. As a consequence of pressure, the blood supply to the mucosa overlying the tumor was impaired. It atrophied and eventually ulcerated. During her menstrual periods she experienced heavy bleeding, or menorrhagia. Despite the benign nature of leiomyomas, Mrs. Beech's health and possibly her life were threatened by repeated hemorrhage. Because she has multiple fibroids (leiomyomas) and she is bleeding excessively, she has been advised by her physician to have a hysterectomy.

In the preceding discussion, the manner in which neoplasms cause signs and symptoms by their mechanical effects has been presented. As space-occupying masses, they create pressure on tissues, thus impairing their blood supply; they obstruct the lumen and interfere with the function of tubular organs; and when they are pedunculated, they are likely to twist on their pedicles. All of these are local effects and may be caused by either benign or malignant neoplasms. Specific signs and symptoms depend on the location of the lesion, the degree to which function is disrupted, and the extent to which compensatory or defense mechanisms are mobilized.

Systemic Effects

Benign and malignant neoplasms may also be accompanied by systemic effects. Malignant neoplasms cause symptoms by utilizing nutritional elements required by normal cells. They continue to grow as long as the host remains alive. This is true even in the most emaciated patient. The rate of growth is sometimes slowed by undernutrition, but growth continues. Why malignant cells have a competitive advantage over normal cells is not known. They seem to require more of some types of amino acids and vitamins than do normal cells, but little more is known.

Cachexia

One of the most striking effects of advanced cancer is severe cachexia. In lay terms, the individual literally becomes skin and bones. The patient appears to be, and is, suffering from severe starvation. One explanation offered to account for cachexia is that the food intake of the individual is insufficient to support the neoplasm and the individual. Although an inadequate intake of food may be a contributing factor, it is probably not the sole cause of cachexia, as forced feeding is often unsuccessful in correcting it. It is probable that cachexia, as well as other manifestations of terminal cancer, is caused by derangements in the biochemical functions of the body. Whatever its cause may be, every reasonable effort should be made to encourage the patient to eat, particularly protein-containing foods.

Bleeding and Anemia

As indicated earlier in this chapter, malignant neoplasms differ from benign neoplasms in a number of ways. Whereas benign neoplasms are usually localized to the area where they originate, malignant neoplasms tend to invade the surrounding tissue and to be disseminated throughout the body. Some of the effects of malignant neoplasms are caused by the invasion and replacement of healthy tissue at the site of the primary growth or of metastasis. The specific effects of metastasis depend on the site affected. For example, in cancer of the lung, either primary or metastatic, the destruction of lung tissue eventually leads to asphyxia of the patient. In leukemia, the abnormal cells invade and destroy the bone marrow as well as other vital structures. As the bone marrow is invaded and destroyed, its capacity to produce erythrocytes and thrombocytes fails; this predisposes to anemia and bleeding.

Bleeding not only accompanies ulceration, but it can also be the result of the erosion of one or more blood vessels. The amount of blood lost at a time may be micro- or macroscopic. Any evidence of abnormal bleeding such as purpura (petechias and ecchymoses), gingival bleeding, hematuria, and gastrointestinal bleeding should be investigated as it may indicate the presence of a malignant neoplasm.

Blood in the stool or urine or any unusual bleeding from the vagina should be investigated for evidence or absence of cancer. Eventually the continued loss of blood leads to anemia, with its characteristic signs and symptoms. Bleeding is not the only cause of anemia in cancer, as anemia occurs in advanced cancer in the absence of any significant loss of blood.

The most common causes of anemia in the cancer patient include: (1) blood loss; (2) toxic depression—infection, inflammation, uremia, and "tumor toxin"; (3) radiotherapy and chemotherapy; (4) myelophthisis (replacement of bone marrow by neoplasm); (5) nutritional problems—faulty intake, storage, synthesis or loss of nutrients; (6) decreased erythropoiesis; (7) increased hemolysis (Horton & Hill, 1977). Metastasis to the liver or bone marrow may reduce the capacity to replace blood cells. Treatment of cancer by radiotherapy or chemotherapy is usually accompanied by some degree of depression of the bone marrow, thus predisposing to anemia. With the exception of pallor, the signs and symptoms are those of circulatory distress. They are tachycardia, palpitation, dyspnea, dizziness, easy fatigability, and weakness.

Infection

A number of the manifestations accompanying malignant neoplasms are caused by their tendency to outgrow their blood supply. As in healthy cells, cells in malignant neoplasms die unless their nutritional needs are met. Death or necrosis of cells on the surface of a neoplasm predisposes to ulceration. Ulceration predisposes to infection and bleeding and is one of the important causes of pain. Ulceration with its concomitant effects can sometimes be observed in the patient with advanced and neglected cancer of the breast. Large, infected ulceration, often with foul-smelling drainage, occur over the affected area. Signs and symptoms accompanying tissue necrosis and/or infection include fever, leukocytosis, elevation of the sedimentation rate, anorexia, and malaise. Because these symptoms and signs are nonspecific, a patient who manifests them without an obvious cause should be investigated for cancer.

In addition to infections of ulcerated lesions, the patient with metastatic cancer is predisposed to infections of the lung and urinary tract. These infections are frequently caused by obstruction of a bronchus, a ureter, or the urethra. Curing of the infection depends on relief of the obstruction and use of appropriate antibiotics. Nursing measures that can and should be instituted to prevent obstruction of the airway by secretions in the bedfast patient are discussed in detail in Chapters 26 and 40.

Fever

Fever may result directly from the neoplastic growth or secondarily as a result of obstruction or infection caused by the tumor. Tumors that cause fever directly include lymphomas, hypernephromas, and tumors metastatic to the liver, especially those originating in the gastrointestinal tract. Pelvic tumors, for example, tumors of the prostate, uterine cervix, bladder, uterus, and ovary, have a high incidence of fever indirectly related to cancer (Horton & Hill, 1977).

Infection is a major cause of fever in patients with cancer. It is uncertain if the fever is due to an immune deficiency resulting from the tumor itself or if it is resultant from a compromised immune response caused by chemotherapy or radiotherapy.

Patients with acute leukemia are likely to develop infections because their leukocytes are unable to phagocytose microorganisms. Patients with chronic lymphatic leukemia are more susceptible because of their hypogammaglobulinemia status.

It is not clearly understood how tumors produce

fever directly; however, endogenous leukocyte pyrogens have been discovered. It is known that a variety of cells produce these pyrogens, including polymorphonuclear leukocytes, blood monocytes, peritoneal and alveolar macrophages, and phagocytic cells of the reticuloendothelial system. It is thought that the tumor cell or factors within the cell such as viruses, antigens, enzymes, and carcinogenic agents may stimulate production of the endogenous pyrogens (Horton & Hill, 1977).

Endocrine Gland Tumors

As stated earlier, neoplasms arising in glands (adenomas) may elaborate the secretion of the gland. When this occurs, symptoms of hyperfunction occur. Functioning tumors may be benign or malignant. At least in the thyroid gland, hyperfunction is more likely to be associated with a benign than with malignant neoplasms. The symptoms manifested depend on the gland which is affected by tumor growth. For example, if the adrenals are affected, signs and symptoms of Cushing's syndrome will be seen. Tumors involving Beta-type cells of the pancreatic islet cells will produce hypoglycemia whereas alpha-type cell involvement will produce hyperglycemia.

Paraneoplastic Carcinoid Syndromes

Nonendocrine malignancies are also capable of producing clinically important endocrine syndromes. The metabolically active hormones and metabolic syndromes produced "ectopically" by nonendocrine tumors make up what is called paraneoplastic syndromes and they occur in 15 per cent of all hospitalized patients with advanced malignancy (Horton & Hill, 1977). Six syndromes have been identified to exhibit well-defined and isolated hormone production, though the tumors are generally metabolically inactive: (1) hypercalcemia and parathormone excess commonly seen in renal cell carcinoma, squamous cell lung carcinoma, and ovarian carcinoma; (2) water intoxication and antidiuretic hormone (ADH) excess commonly seen in oat cell tumors; (3) hyperadrenalism and adrenocorticotropic hormone (ACTH) excess seen in oat cell lung tumors with some reports of occurrence in prostatic cancer; (4) thyrotoxicosis and thyroid-stimulating hormone (TSH) excess seen in trophoblastic tumors, such as, placental tumors; (5) hypoglycemia and insulinlike production occurs in nonpancreatic tumors which are of mesenchymal derivation involving the retroperitoneum or pleural-based tumors of the thorax; (6) erythrocytosis and erythropoietin excess seen in renal cell carcinoma with Wilms's tumor and occasionally in liver carcinoma (Anderson, 1979).

Prognosis of these tumors is generally poor, because it is unusual for the tumors to be definitively excised, for the thyrotoxic syndrome associated with choriocarcinoma, which is very sensitive to chemotherapy (Anderson, 1979). However, therapeutic management of the paraneoplastic complications can be controlled; for example, by administration of glucose for relief of signs and symptoms of hypoglycemia. It is, therefore, very important to recognize the signs and symptoms manifested by a patient with one of the various neoplastic syndromes.

Carcinoid syndrome is caused by tumor secretion of several hormones which cause flushing, leading to chronic telangiectasia, cyanosis, and pellegralike skin lesions. Additional clinical manifestations include diarrhea, abdominal cramps, borborygmi, bronchospasm and dyspnea, right-sided cardiac valvular disease, and congestive failure. Carcinoid tumors may originate from the foregut, midgut, or hindgut (Horton & Hill, 1977).

Neurological Disorders

Manifestations of neurological disorders occur in patients with neoplasms. Central nervous system symptoms occur most often in patients with tumors of the lung, female genital organs, and breast. Most patients die within a year after the appearance of central nervous system symptoms, which include ataxia, incoordination, nystagmus, dysarthia, personality changes, diplopia, and pain (Horton & Hill, 1977).

Two major types of peripheral nerve disorders are recognized. The first is a mild symmetrical sensory peripheral neuropathy that can occur in the late stages of neoplastic disease. The second is a mixed neuropathy which involves both sensory and motor nerves. This neuropathy may be present before the cancer is diagnosed and may be accompanied by orthostatic hypotension; it may progress from muscle weakness to severe paralysis. Both of these nerve disorders may have occasional brief remissions (Horton & Hill, 1977).

Pain and Cancer

Because pain has been discussed in some detail in Chapter 36, it will be considered here only as the pain experience specifically relating to cancer and the cancer patient.

In many patients, cancer is not painful at the onset of the disease. Unfortunately, the extent and degree to which pain is a problem among cancer patients is very difficult to define. There is a paucity of accurate date from epidemiologic studies on the incidence and magnitude of pain among cancer patients. Data suggest that severe pain is experienced by 60 to 80 per cent of hospitalized cancer patients (Bonica, 1978). Regardless of the lack of epidemiologic data on cancer pain, the belief that cancer and pain are synonymous contributes to the dread and fear of cancer that permeates our society.

As stated in Chapter 36, the discomfort caused by pain has two sources. One is the pain sensation and the other is the meaning that the pain has for the individual. Studies of persons who are in pain-inducing situations demonstrate that the meaning that pain has for the individual frequently determines the degree of suffering experienced. The belief that pain is inevitable and frequently so severe that it is intolerable can of itself increase the severity of the pain experienced by the patient. When nurses and physicians are convinced the pain is an unavoidable aspect of cancer, it may result in a narrow or unimaginative approach to the care of the patient. The care may be such as to reinforce the fears of the patient, and other causes of discomfort may be missed or neglected. Not only does a morbid fear of pain add to the suffering of the patient who has been diagnosed as having cancer, but it may prevent persons who suspect that they have it from seeking medical attention. Persons who do not have cancer therefore experience unnecessary discomfort and those who do may delay until such time as metastasis has occurred. There are undoubtedly other negative aspects of the all too common belief that pain and cancer are synonymous.

When pain does occur in cancer patients, it is usually the result of one or more of six mechanisms of the disease. As the mechanisms which cause pain are discussed, two categories of pain can be specified: continuous and incident. Continuous pain is constant, unremitting, and often of such extreme intensity that it dominates the person's entire existence, disturbing sleep, thought, and activities of daily living. Relief of this pain is more successful in early stages, when it is localized, by destruction of nerves, cordotomy, or chemical neurectomy. As the malignant disease becomes more widespread, analgesic medication is used as necessary (Mehta, 1973). Incident pain is periodic, equally severe at the start, but becomes gradually less intense with time and can be initiated by unpleasant or intermittent stimuli. Unlike continuous pain, it can be exacerbated by movement or improved by rest. Many times it can be relieved by treating the precipating factor; for example, draining an abscess, stopping hemorrhage, or immobilizing a pathological fracture (Mehta, 1973).

The nature of cancer and the metastatic process should make it clear that cancer patients who are having pain will likely experience more than one of these types of pain concurrently. This means that any given cancer patient with pain may be experiencing incident and continuous pain simultaneously.

Bonica (1954; 1978) identifies the following tumor mechanisms as being causitive of cancer pain: (1) compression of nerves by tumor or bony fragments from metastatic fracture of bone. This type of pain is incident in nature. It is commonly experienced in the lumbosacral plexus related to pelvic tumors; in the brachial plexus related to superior sulcus tumors; and as intercostal neuralgias related to mediastinal or retroperitoneal tumors. This mechanism and type of pain is also experienced after vertebral collapse, sudden massive hemorrhage, large pleural effusions or localized edema (Mehta, 1973). (2) Infiltration of tissues including nerve endings and blood vessels. Pain experienced from this mechanism is continuous and is referred to as sympathetic pain. It leads to irritation of nerve endings and is felt as a continuous burning or discomfort with an approximately even level of intensity. The sensation may be accompanied by numbness. The location of this kind of pain will be dependent on the location of the tumor. For example, the patient with breast cancer likely will experience continuous pain in the upper extremity because of infiltration of the plexus, nerves, and blood vessels of the axilla, whereas the patient with cancer of the uterus or uterine cervix will experience pain in the back and lower extremities because of lumbosacral plexus involvement. (3) Visceral pain is related to obstruction of structures such as the stomach, colon, rectum, gastrointestinal, urinary, and biliary tracts. Visceral pain is an example of continuous pain sensation. It is experienced as a vague, ill-defined, dull ache. The pain is caused by tumor obstruction of an abdominal or pelvic organ that has become distended, inflamed, or ischemic (Mehta, 1973). Surgical removal of the tumor most likely will bring relief (Shawver, 1977). (4) Vascular pain is considered to be incident pain. It is caused by tumor occlusion of blood vessels, which results in venous engorgement, arterial ischemia, or both. Vascular pain is typically experienced as sudden, sharp, and intermittent. Retroperitoneal and pelvic tumors could cause this type of pain in the perineal area and lower extremities (Shawver, 1977). (5) Distension of the tumor into hollow organs or other tissues surrounded by pain-sensitive structures, such as fascia or periosteum, causes a tension pain with sensations of the incident type. The pain is actually caused by the tumor's stretching a fascial or peritoneal lining (Mehta, 1973). The pain is experienced as severe and localized. Patients with cancer of the uterine cervix experience this type of pain in the uterosacral ligaments (Shawver, 1977). (6) Necrosis, infection, and inflammation cause pain which is considered to be of the continuous type. It can be excruciating and it is experienced as severe, persistent, and unrelenting. Tumor in a hollow abdominal organ such as the stomach or bowel can cause a rupture of the organ which results in contamination of the peritoneal cavity and the resultant severe pain of peritonitis. Patients experiencing this type of pain are in severe distress and require immediate treatment (Mehta, 1973).

MEDICAL MANAGEMENT. Cancer pain is a patient problem that both physicians and nurses must manage. According to Murphy (1973) medical treatment of pain requires "intelligent appraisal and a systematic plan for relief that will conserve the patient's physical, mental, and moral resources as long as possible" (Murphy, 1973, p. 187). Selection of an appropriate pain control plan requires that the physician evaluate: (1) the severity and duration of pain; (2) the nature of the disease; (3) probable life expectancy; (4) temperament and psychological state; and (5) occupational, domestic, and economic background of the patient (Rowlingson, 1978, p. 317). Implicit in assessing these areas is an evaluation of the location and mechanism of pain, type and grade of neoplasm, structures it may invade, the physical and mental condition of the patient, the patient's obligation to society and family, and availability of various methods of pain relief (Murphy, 1973, p. 187).

Medical management of pain in cancer patients involves two major approaches: (1) tumor therapy to diminish or irradicate the neoplasm and (2) symptomatic therapy which does not affect the neoplasm. Tumor therapy includes palliative surgery, irradiation, hormonal therapy, and ablation of endocrine glands, immunotherapy, and chemotherapy. Symptomatic therapy includes analgesics, psychological techniques, neurosurgery, and nerve blocks (Murphy, 1973).

PALLIATIVE SURGERY. Palliative surgery is indicated to relieve pain and eliminate odor, for example, from ulcerations. It is also indicated to remove tumor obstruction of a hollow organ or of a large blood vessel. Irradiation has been used successfully to relieve pain in cancer patients with bony metastases. It has also been useful in carcinomatous pleurisy, pulmonary metastases, and skin metastases. Sometimes irradiation will be combined with other methods; for example, surgery and endocrine therapy; castration or hypophysectomy by radiation, surgical, or chemical means have been used to control tumor growth, eliminate metastases, and relieve pain. Steroids also are useful in controlling pain in cancer patients. Chemotherapy, by controlling tumor growth and metastases, has been successful in controlling pain in cancer patients (Murphy, 1973).

Systemic analgesics are frequently used to control cancer pain. It is considered good practice to use the least potent analgesic that is able to produce adequate relief. It is not necessary to give cancer patients opiates all the time. Mild to moderate cancer pain can be controlled with aspirin and other nonnarcotic agents. Use of analgesics in combination with sedatives, hypnotics, and tranquilizers is especially advantageous with cancer patients because their complaint of pain includes manifestations of fear and anxiety. Use of an hypnotic also promotes rest, which many times is crucial for cancer patients. When nonnarcotics are unable to control the pain, the physician likely will move the patient to a mild narcotic such as Codeine or Talwin. Strong narcotics are used when the other systemic analgesics and methods of therapy are ineffective or not applicable. It must be kept in mind that patients may develop an early tolerance to narcotics and may require massive doses to control pain in the late stages of disease. Examples of such drugs would be Demerol, Dolophine, Dilaudid, and Pantopon (Murphy, 1973).

Hypnosis, techniques of self-relaxation, and other methods of cognitive control are also being used with varying degrees of success to control cancer pain. Neurosurgical control of pain includes rhizotomy, sympathectomy, spinothalamic tractotomy, stereotaxic procedures, nerve blocks, and transcutaneous nerve stimulation (see Chapter 36).

Nursing Management of the Cancer Patient with Pain

Thorough nursing assessment of cancer pain is vital for two basic reasons: (1) it provides the data base necessary to rule in or out a nursing diagnosis of alteration in comfort-pain or discomfort (Third Conference for Nursing Diagnoses, 1978) and (2) it is essential for adequate nursing management of cancer pain. The process of assessment itself will provide relief of pain for some clients. The patient should be assessed for pain as soon as he or she is admitted to nursing service so that a baseline evaluation is available for future comparisons. As mentioned earlier, many cancer patients do not experience pain. With such patients, the nurse in a nonfrightening manner should instruct the patient that she or he is to be informed if the patient does begin experiencing pain or discomfort.

If the cancer patient is experiencing pain, two major areas should be assessed: (1) the nature of the pain and (2) the impact or effect of the pain on the individual and family (Shawver, 1977). Information ascertained concerning the nature of the pain should include type of sensation, location, intensity, duration, and precipitating factors. The effect of the pain should include physiological and psychosocial observations. Physiological observations include alterations in blood pressure, pulse, pallor, drawn face, restlessness, and a dull glassy look in the eyes. In the psychosocial area, the nurse may observe changes in mobility patterns, changes in activities of daily living, changes in disposition, and narrowing focus of attention.

In order to assess knowledgeably the cancer patient's pain, the nurse must know the size, location, and extent of the tumor. She or he must also be aware of the degree and location of metastasis. This knowledge is vital because new locations of pain may indicate further spread of disease.

Listening is key in data gathering concerning pain. Asking the patient to describe his or her experience and using the family as a resource for additional information is essential, especially in psychosocial assessment of pain. Ongoing assessment of the cancer patient's pain cannot be overemphasized. It is necessary for evaluation of the success of nursing and medical interventions being used to control the pain.

Pain associated with cancer in the early stages of disease is usually not severe, frequently intermittent, and generally fairly easily managed. During this time the pain can usually be controlled with interventions such as mild analgesics, diversion, exercise, and application of heat or cold.

DRUGS IN THE TREATMENT OF PAIN. When drugs are required for the relief of pain, they must be prescribed by the physician. In selecting a drug or drugs, the physician usually considers the following points: (1) Is the pain severe? (2) Does it come in episodes or is it continuous? (3) How much anxiety does it produce and how anxious is the patient? (4) What is the patient's life expectancy? (5) What can be done about the cause of the pain? In a patient with good life expectancy, can the cause of pain be completely removed? Drug addiction can become a problem; therefore nonaddicting drugs should be used when possible and, in some instances, patients are requested to tolerate some pain. On the other hand, when the cause of a patient's pain cannot be removed and, particularly, when the patient's life expectancy is short, withholding narcotics is cruel. For a patient who is no longer employed and who no longer is required to function as the breadwinner or family mother, the control of pain is more important than the avoidance of drug addiction, which, in a terminal cancer patient, very rarely represents a serious management problem.

The nurse has the responsibility for preparing the patient so that he or she is in a comfortable position for observing the effects of the drug. Drugs are usually ordered at either specific times or at specific time intervals. The nurse should therefore observe the length of time that the patient is relieved. Because of daytime activities, patients often require less medication during the day than at night. In some instances, small doses of a pain-relieving medication given every 2 hours provide more relief than do large doses given every 4 hours. Part of the benefit from the drug comes from the faith of the patient in its effectiveness. Nothing should be done to interfere with this by either word or deed. Occasionally a well-intentioned, though misguided, nurse decides to protect the patient from the danger of addiction by prolonging the time the patient has to wait for medication or decides to withhold the narcotic portion of prescription. The result of the first may well be that the patient receives little or no benefit from medication because the pain has become intolerable. The result of the second is that the faith of the patient in the power of the medication to relieve his or her suffering is destroyed.

Unless the patient is presenting evidence of toxicity from the drug, the prescription left by the physician should be adhered to. Any problem related to the drug or drugs the patient is receiving should be discussed with the physician before a change is made. In the use of drugs for the control of pain in the patient with cancer, the objective is to regulate selection and use so that the patient is provided relief over the course of the illness.

The Brompton's cocktail has been used recently in the country for control of intractable pain of terminal cancer patients (Valentine, 1978; Miaskowski, 1978). It was developed at the Brompton Chest Hospital in England. The mixture of Brompton's cocktail used in this country typically contains morphine (10 to 90 mg), cocaine (10 mg), 98 per cent ethyl alcohol (2.5 ml), flavoring syrup (5 ml), and water. Typically the cocktail is given every 4 to 6 hours around the clock. An anti-emetic may be given with the syrup if nausea is a problem (Miaskowski, 1978).

In summary, although pain is not inevitable to cancer, it does occur. Even patients who do not experience pain are almost certain to fear they will. There are a few areas in which a kind, gentle, thoughtful, compassionate, and creative nurse can do more to prevent human suffering. The prescription of drugs and treatment by surgical and chemotherapeutic means are the prerogative of the physician. Whether or not the drugs are effective often depends on the quality of nursing care the patient receives. Furthermore, by attention to the hygienic, physiologic, and psychosocial needs of the patient, pain and suffering from pain can be minimized.

NURSING IN PAIN RELIEF. Though our society

is oriented to the use of drugs for pain relief, there are alternative methods of intervention which the nurse can use very effectively. Shawver (1977) divides them into three approaches: (1) physically based approaches, (2) cognitively and emotionally based approaches, and (3) supporting and providing coping resources.

The objectives of nursing intervention in the physically based approaches are to reduce the perception of the painful stimulus. Actions used to reduce the painful stimulus will depend on the cause of the pain. In a situation where the pain is caused by the tumor growth itself, the nurse should direct attention toward reducing the intensity of the pain since obviously she or he cannot remove the tumor. Nursing actions that can be employed to reduce the painful stimulus include repositioning of body parts, mobility as tolerated, and use of heat and cold (Shawver, 1977).

As an example, Mr. Sands had metastatic cancer involving the ribs and sternum. Even touching his chest with a sheet caused him to cry out in pain. His nurse was able to prevent unnecessary pain by placing a large cardle over his torso as a support for the bed covering. When she moved and turned him she was gentle and moved him slowly. She supported his head and arms in a relaxed position, so that they did not pull on his thorax. Mrs. Lottie had metastatic cancer involving her cervical vertebrae. Although she had a neck brace, she found it uncomfortable. Mrs. Lottie and her nurse worked out a plan for turning her so that pain was prevented and the brace was not required. Mrs. Lottie supported her head with her hands as she turned. After she was turned, pillow supports were used to keep her head in alignment. Pain was prevented by the identification of the situations causing it and by the utilization of effective nursing measures.

Distraction is used to reduce perception of painful stimulus. Nursing interventions include encouraging the patient to exercise, perform activities of daily living, and participate in social events (Shawver, 1977). Activities such as these also serve to enhance the patient's self-concept and general sense of well-being.

The major goal of the cognitively and emotionally based approaches is to reduce the degree and amount of anxiety associated with pain. Shawver (1977) suggests this goal can be met in two ways: (1) by supporting the patient in using coping behaviors that have been successful in the past and (2) by providing the person with additional coping resources. These methods will assist the patient in achieving a greater feeling of control over the situation, thereby contributing to a reduction in at least the mental pain he or she is experiencing. The point should be made that it is unrealistic to completely separate physical and mental pain in a patient, but the artificial dichotomy is made here for clarification of nursing approaches and interventions.

Supporting and providing resources uses provision of information as a means to help the patient in coping with cancer pain. Information about the treatment plan or what to expect during and after procedures can be very helpful for patients coping with pain. Teaching patients relaxation techniques or providing opportunities for them to communicate how they are feeling are also very helpful. Additional resources may occasionally become necessary, for example, referral to a mental health resource for counseling.

Psychological Effects

The psychological suffering experienced by a patient who has or suspects he or she has cancer can be overpowering. As mentioned previously, the psychological effects extend to persons who do not have cancer, inasmuch as many fear that their illness or ill health is caused by cancer. The family is also affected by a diagnosis of cancer in a family member. Their response to the diagnosis and to the individual affects the behavior of the sick person. The psychological effects are those resulting from the manner in which the individual perceives the entire cancer experience, that is, its nature and effects and outcome, as well as the measures utilized in its diagnosis and treatment. The sociological effects of cancer stem from group attitudes toward it and its nature, effects, and treatment. Each person reading this book has attitudes about cancer and its effects and curability that were learned from the groups of which he or she is a part. These attitudes influence how persons feel and behave when faced with a diagnosis of cancer in themselves or in another individual. Their behavior toward another individual is also influenced by the way in which the individuals define their role in the situation. The quality of care that a patient receives is affected by the attitude of all who have a relationship with him or her—family, neighbors, nurses and physicians, and the community.

Any person who has a diagnosis of cancer can be expected to be under severe emotional stress. For most persons in the United States, the diagnosis carries with it a threat of prolonged and painful course, ending in death. Because of the extended course of illness and the nature of the treatments, cancer is often an economic burden not only to the patient but also the family.

On the discovery of a lesion or symptom that suggests cancer, most persons experience fear. With the fear, the person may have a variety of feelings—a sense of doom, anger, helplessness, shame, and disgrace. He or she may feel trapped or abandoned.

The emotional response of the person with cancer depends on the specific nature of the cancer, its site, treatment, and course. In the cancer disease process, the symptoms or manifestations of the disease are as important as the diagnosis in determining the patient's response (Tiedt, 1975). The fear and anxiety experienced by the patient in response to a diagnosis of cancer and/or its symptomatic manifestations in the person are extended to family, friends, neighbors, and community.

Nurses also have culturally derived attitudes toward cancer and what nurses ought to be able to accomplish in the care of the sick. To be successful in identifying and meeting the needs of the patient, nurses are helped by knowing what their own feelings are. The aim of nurses is not to avoid feeling but to manage feelings in such a way that they can attend to those of their patients. Nurses should try to take a middle course so that they are able to identify the needs of the patient and to meet them in ways that are helpful. Neither feeling too strongly with the patient nor isolating themselves from him or her will enable nurses to achieve this goal with any degree of consistency.

The person who suspects or knows he or she has cancer can then be expected to experience fear and its attendant feelings. How the person reacts to this fear depends on the way in which he or she customarily behaves when under severe stress and the quality of support given by family. If the fear is reasonable, the person may be stimulated to seek medical attention and follow through with the recommendations of the physician. In contrast, unreasonable fear leads to denial, disorganization, confusion, and panic. Denial is a very common reaction. It may be strong enough to convince a cancer patient that he or she is suffering from some other ailment. This conviction exists even after all the diagnostic studies have been completed and even after cancer therapies have been administered. Sometimes this denial mechanism will prevent the patient from seeking help or accepting appropriate treatment when it is offered. When denial is complete, the patient may grasp at straws, seek new treaments, and ask for constant reassurance. Such patients ask not to know that they have cancer but to be reassured that they do not. Like many psychological reactions, the denial can also be useful, particularly to patients with cancer having a poor prognosis or terminal patients. The denial of hopelessness will frequently help the patient to remain cheerful and productive in spite of incurable cancer. A skillful physician or nurse can utilize the denial to increase the patient's comfort, whereas uncontrolled denial may force the patient to delay the diagnosis and treatment and drive him or her to consult "quacks" who promise cure.

Another possible source of stress is that treatment of cancer frequently involves the loss of important functions and organs. These may be important not only to the patient but to the members of the family, friends, and the community. The lesion, because of its location or the nature of its treatment, may be the cause of psychological stress. Either benign or malignant neoplasms may cause disfigurement. Nevi or birthmarks on the exposed surface of the body may be the cause of more or less psychological stress.

In addition to the psychological stress caused by a diagnosis of cancer, neoplasms located in certain sites may be responsible for additional stress. Neoplasms located in the head and neck not only cause obvious disfigurement, but the removal of the lesion is usually accompanied by some degree of mutilation and loss of function, including loss of the ability to swallow, to speak, or to breathe normally. After laryngectomy the patient may feel that because of the loss of speech he or she is something less than human. About 70 per cent of persons who have had a laryngectomy can learn esophageal speech. It takes about 12 months for the patient to reach the stage of maximum intelligibility. Some patients who cannot learn esophageal speech may be able to use an artificial larynx. It differs from the esophageal speech, which provides an internal source, by providing a sound source external to the human vocal folds.

The loss of the breast causes disfigurement and some loss of function of the muscles moving the shoulder and the arm. It also predisposes to edema of the arm on the affected side. The structural deformity can be corrected by a prosthesis. Because the breast is a symbol of femininity, the woman may feel that she is less of a woman after mastectomy. A variety of prostheses are available from which a woman can select one best suited to her.

The removal of reproductive organs of either the male or female is usually accompanied by some feeling of loss of identity. The man who loses his testes is likely to feel that he is less a man, just as a woman who loses her uterus, breast, or ovaries feels less a woman.

The psychological problems created by a colostomy are discussed later, in the study of Mrs. White. The discussion of the needs of the patient who is in the terminally ill phase of the disease was included in Chapter 33.

Some of the factors causing psychological stress in the patient who has a diagnosis of cancer have been presented. Further discussion of psychosocial aspects of care are included in later sections of the chapter. For a more detailed discussion of the effects of severe psychological stress and what the nurse can do to help the patient, see Unit VII.

TELLING THE PATIENT. A problem growing out of the fact that cancer can and often does create a high degree of psychological stress among members of the family, nurses, and physicians is the question of whether or not the patient should be told about a diagnosis of cancer. In few, if any, other diseases, is there any question about withholding the nature of the diagnosis.

Jablon (1976) presents reasons for and against telling the cancer patient of the malignant diagnosis. Following are the reasons identified by Jablon for concealing a diagnosis of malignant neoplasm:

1. Awareness of the diagnosis of cancer produces too great an emotional burden.
2. Most cancer patients do not want to know the truth about their illness.

Jablon's reasons arguing for informing the cancer patient of the diagnosis include:

1. It is impossible to deceive a cancer patient effectively about the diagnosis.
2. Most cancer patients suspect their diagnosis and become aware of it at some point. The attempts to conceal it breed distrust, resentment, and emotional isolation in the patient.
3. Many patients have known their diagnosis and have had the strength to continue productive living.
4. Most lay people are to a degree emotionally and knowledgeably irrational about illness. If the patient suspected cancer but has been told otherwise he or she is left alone to harbor irrational fears.

Often the cooperation of the patient in the treatment requires that the patient know what the diagnosis is. Although physicians may not inform the patient of the nature of the illness, some member of the family is informed. Practice among physicians varies. In cancer, as in other diseases, the physician carries the responsibility for informing the patient of the nature of the diagnosis and the treatment required. At one time it was common practice not to tell the patient unless there was some reason to do so. Some physicians still rarely tell a patient about a diagnosis of cancer. Oncologists usually tell their patients and feel strongly that patients should be told except in rare instances. Many physicians try to make their decision on the basis of whether the patient wants to know and how the knowledge will affect him or her.

Though it is the physician's responsibility to inform the patient of the specific diagnosis, medical treatment plan, and prognosis, the nurse is responsible for knowing what the patient's diagnosis and treatment plan are and for ascertaining what information has been given to the patient and family. The nurse can also be an effective patient advocate since she or he has a unique collection of knowledge of the patient's situation and is in a key position to provide input, including the patient's perception of the situation, to those who make decisions concerning information given to the patient (Kastenbaum, 1978).

The key problems in making this decision are (1) perceiving the unique way each patient will integrate the information and (2) judging therefrom the course of medical information to be provided for the specific patient (Jablon, 1976). What and how much to tell the patient defies generalization. Whatever is said must be individualized to the patient and circumstances and the clinical oncology care team should speak with one voice to provide consistency (Bagshawe,1975).

SOME HARMFUL EFFECTS OF WITHHOLDING INFORMATION ABOUT A DIAGNOSIS OF CANCER. In the past there has been much argument about the harmful effects resulting from the patient's learning of cancer; not too much consideration has been given to the harmful effects of his or her not knowing. Making an issue over whether or not to tell the person who has cancer fosters the urge to secrecy. It also suggests that the situation of the person is hopeless and that there is something mysterious about cancer. The fact that patients know that they may not be told may cause some persons to distrust the information given them. It is not unusual to hear persons say that they are not certain whether they have or have not been told the truth about their illness. Patients who are not told that they have cancer sometimes obtain this information through questions and statements made to a nurse or physician. When the patient is not told, this creates the necessity for treating the patient as if nothing were wrong. The patient's questions have to be answered without giving any information. This, in turn, creates a barrier between the patient and the professional staff. The patient is cut off from seeking information, help, and comfort, from those who, by preparation, should be able to help. A patient may be told by a visitor or another patient that he or she has cancer. This can be, needless to say, an exceedingly traumatic experience. Furthermore, uncertainty usually causes more discomfort than certainty. Imagination, unless disciplined by reality, can do terrible things to an individual. According to the accounts of persons writing about their personal experience with cancer, the lives of some persons have become richer and more meaningful after they know they have cancer. Not knowing may have an adverse effect on the course of the disease, inasmuch as the patient who does not know that he or she has or has had cancer may fail to keep appointments for care and for follow-up examinations.

As mentioned earlier, telling the patient he or she has cancer can, for many people, be very upsetting. In some people it may cause a disruptive panic and possibly lead to suicide. Actually, suicide is quite rare among patients who have cancer and its risk can be virtually eliminated by giving the patient the necessary information tactfully and sympathetically, as well as explaining to the patient all the aspects of the disease—not only unpleasant ones but also the hopeful ones.

At the present time, two factors determine whether or not a given patient is told he or she has cancer. One is the feelings of the physician. The other is the distress of the patient. Unless there is an important reason for telling them, patients are not told when they indicate that they do not want to know that they have cancer. If they never refer to cancer as a cause of their illness, or if they ask to be reassured that they do not have cancer, this is taken as an indication that they do not want to know. Conversely, when patients ask the direct question, "Do I have cancer?" they are answered in the affirmative.

Frequently the intelligent patient who is not using powerful denial mechanisms probably knows that he or she has cancer by the time the physician has established the diagnosis. In some of these patients, the condition is worsened by fostering denial mechanisms. They want to know whether or not they have cancer. Physicians who do inform these patients of their status try to do so in a manner that fosters their hope. Although they tell the patient the truth, they do not usually go into all the future possibilities. A friend with cancer of the breast was told by her surgeon that he had removed her entire breast because she had some abnormal cells. Over the course of the next 2 or 3 years she learned the extent of her disease. She commented later that in the beginning she did not believe that she could have tolerated knowing the full truth, but by learning it gradually, she had come to accept her situation. With time she was able to accept that she had cancer.

McIntosh (1976) interviewed patients with diagnosed but undisclosed malignancy to ascertain their awareness of their condition and their desire for more information about it. He found 88 per cent of the patients either knew or suspected they had a malignant tumor, but the majority did not wish to augment that knowledge. Only a minority who knew or suspected they had cancer actively sought any information about their prognosis. These findings suggest that many patients prefer the anxiety of uncertainty to factual information concerning their diagnosis and prognosis. The uncertainty may be used to retain hope and to construct a hopeful conception of their condition from clues that are available to them (McIntosh, 1976).

To summarize, whether or not, and how, the patient is told depends on the patient and the situation. The physician and the family of the patient weigh the factors that enter into the decision. Not only the personality of the patient but also the prognosis has to be considered. The support that may be obtained from the family and even the personality of the physician are important factors. There is not, at this time, a single answer to the needs of all patients. Decisions should be based on what will in the long run, make it possible to meet the needs of the patient. One day the problem of telling or not telling the patient will cease to exist. Under all circumstances, every effort should be made to convey to the patient that much can and will be done to promote his or her welfare and the approach to the patient with an incurable cancer should be similar to the approach used in treating patients with other chronic diseases.

Phases in the Life Cycle of the Patient with Cancer

The life cycle of the cancer patient has been depicted as occurring in seven phases (*Cancer Bulletin*, 1959). To these seven should be added another, the first or preventive phase. The phases, as listed, included (1) early diagnosis, (2) recommended treatment, (3) comprehensive treatment, (4) follow-up education for the patient, (5) regular follow-up by the physician (6) rehabilitation, and (7) adequate terminal care. Not all patients who have a diagnosis of cancer progress through all these phases.

The discussion is organized as follows: (1) the elements in primary prevention; (2) the phase of secondary prevention, detection, and diagnosis of cancer; (3) the phase of curative and palliative treatment; (4) tertiary prevention or continuity of care; (5) the phase of terminal illness. Although rehabilitation begins the moment the individual enters the clinic or physician's office, it continues throughout all phases of the patient's life. Separate consideration will be given to this phase as it relates to continuity of care out of the hospital.

In all phases of the patient's illness, the nurse tries

to convey to the patient that something can and will be done to improve his or her condition. This does not always mean that life will be prolonged, but that, whatever the probable outcome, the quality of life can be improved. The goals for each patient should take into account the phase of the patient's illness, psychological and physiologic resources, and the nature and extent of treatment. Persons who happen to have cancer are people. They have the same basic needs as do all people. Because of the manner in which cancer and its treatment are perceived, patients with cancer can be expected to be under severe stress. Each patient behaves as an individual. To meet the needs of patients, the nurse requires knowledge and competence in all nursing skills. These include skill in observing, in communicating, in providing care in such a manner that the patient feels accepted and respected, in teaching the patient and family members, in planning and organizing the patient's care, and in performing the procedures required in his or her physical care.

Observation is a continuous process directed toward the identification of the patient's physiological and psychological needs. From observation, data are collected that indicate improvement or deterioration of the patient's condition or the development of complications. Instruction of the patient is planned to achieve three goals. First, the patient continues to have regular medical supervision for the remainder of his or her life. Second, within the limits of the patient's capacity, he or she continues as an active and productive member of the family and community; the patient should not be unnecessarily invalided. The third objective is an aspect of the second—if the patient can accept in perspective whatever limitations are imposed by treatment, he or she can be helped not to allow them to become the focus of life. The other aspects of nursing will be integrated throughout.

PRIMARY PREVENTION

In the control of cancer, prevention is the keynote. As in other chronic diseases, prevention is of two types, primary and secondary. In primary prevention the objective is to eliminate conditions predisposing to its development. In the present state of knowledge evidence points to multiple factors interacting to cause cancer. A problem in prevention is to identify those factors that are controllable. Through the use of epidemiologic studies, some of the agents in the external environment have been identified as carcinogenic. As they become known, methods can be developed to eliminate them or to protect persons from their effect. Much has been accomplished in industry to protect workers from carcinogenic chemicals. A familiar example from the health field is provided by the precautions that are taken to protect workers from exposure to ionizing radiation. The basis for, and the nature of, these precautions have been discussed elsewhere. At times knowledge about the significance of a factor is less clear-cut, or the findings of epidemiologic studies are difficult to implement. For example, the incidence of cancer of the lung is higher in urban than in rural areas. Many factors may well enter into this difference. Among these is the higher concentration of smoke discharged into the air from all sources—houses, stores, industrial plants, and automobile exhaust gases. Both smoke and exhaust gases contain carcinogenic hydrocarbons. To reduce the pollution of the air by potentially harmful substances, public education is required. The public must accept, demand, and be willing to pay for whatever is required to do this. Furthermore, permanent control of air pollution depends on continued supervision and enforcement of regulations. In the primary prevention of cancer, much has been accomplished to protect workers from the carcinogenic effects of agents used in industry. A beginning has been made in the protection of the general public from known carcinogens.

Equally difficult or possibly even more difficult to accomplish is the primary prevention involving a major change in a custom or habit. As an illustration, the Surgeon General's report stated that cigarette smoking is an etiologic agent in cancer of the lung. Most of the deaths from this disease could be prevented by eliminating smoking. Yet many persons continue to smoke. Knowledge of hazards, especially when cause-effect relationships are not immediately observable, is not enough to effect changes in the habits of all people. Many other factors are involved.

A secondary type of primary prevention is based on the identification and removal of precancerous lesions. These have been discussed previously. One of the reasons cited for the decrease in the incidence of cancer of the cervix is that women receive better obstetrical care than in the past. By preventing injury of the cervix and providing early treatment of lesions that develop, the chances of development of cancer of the cervix are reduced.

Primary prevention of cancer is the ideal method of control. The most extensive and effective applications of the principles of primary prevention have been made in industry in the protection of workers from carcinogenic chemicals. Some cancer is prevented by treatment that eliminates the possibility of development of a precancerous lesion or by the removal of suspicious lesions. Applications of primary prevention, though significant, are limited by knowledge of the direct and indirect causes of cancer.

The nurse assists in primary prevention by (1) supporting research projects, not only those directly related to cancer, but those directed toward understanding the nature of cell growth; (2) supporting community efforts to improve environmental conditions; (3) practicing self-protection in situations in which there is a possibility of exposure to carcinogens; and (4) observing and reporting precancerous lesions in herself or himself and others and encouraging others to do likewise.

Secondary Prevention

The secondary prevention of cancer is based on the identification of a cancer while it is still a local rather than a systemic disease. In this stage of disease, malignant change has taken place, but cancer cells have not been distributed throughout the body. In terms of the life of the patient with cancer, this is the first phase. In the past the presumption has been that if cancer could be detected, diagnosed, and treated early enough, then its harmful effects could be prevented. Emphasis has been placed on early diagnosis and adequate treatment. In some patients, cancer can be and is detected while it is a local disease. It can be eradicated and the patient cured. In other patients, with the present methods of diagnosis, cancer is a systemic disease by the time its manifestations are evident, and possibly from the beginning. At first sight, this is shocking. It serves to emphasize the fact that cancer is not a single disease with one cause and one method of treatment. Control depends on more knowledge than is now available. Some patients can, however, now be cured by early diagnosis and adequate treatment. Many patients can have their effective lives prolonged. In the American culture the tendency to want one complete answer that works universally appears to contribute to a person's disappointment when the problem turns out to be complex. In whatever phase the patient is when cancer is discovered, much can be done to improve the condition. There is also the possibility that some discovery will be made that will reverse the disease process.

In the present state of knowledge, the patient's best hope of cure lies in early diagnosis followed by adequate treatment. Slaughter (1960) emphasizes the difficulty in establishing a diagnosis of early cancer. One characteristic of early cancer is that it has not invaded the surrounding tissue. According to the American Cancer Society publications, about one half of the persons who have cancer could be cured if treatment were initiated early enough.

The Cancer Examination

Ideally, every woman over the age of 35 and every man over the age of 45 should have a physical examination every year. According to Dr. Emerson Day (1960) of the Strang Clinic, the cancer-detection examination should include the following:

- History
  - Family
  - Environment, habits, illness
  - Review of Systems
- Physical
  - Skin and lymph nodes
  - Head and neck
  - Breasts
  - Lungs
  - Abdomen
  - Genitalia
  - Rectum—colon
  - Extremities
- Laboratory
  - Hemoglobin or hematocrit
  - White blood cell and differential counts
  - Urinalysis
  - Chest x ray
  - Vaginal and cervical smears
  - Tubeless gastric analysis
  - Stool guaiac

Although the physician is responsible for making the medical diagnosis, the nurse should know what constitutes a thorough examination and why it is desirable. This knowledge is of value to the nurse as a person and in practice as a professional person. In working with patients, the nurse requires this information in order to prepare them for what to expect and for what is expected of them. The examination is planned to elicit two types of information. One is directed toward identifying any condition that predisposes the patient to cancer and the other toward determining whether the patient has any signs, symptoms, or tissue changes pointing to the presence of cancer.

The information is utilized in two ways. The more obvious is that it is necessary to the medical diagnosis of the condition of the patient. The other is that, as data are collected about many patients, the data are subject to analysis and then conclusions are drawn as to their relevance. For example, the conclusion that a relationship exists between cancer of the lung and smoking is based on information obtained from the medical histories of many patients and the statistical analysis of the information.

Most physicians agree that specialized medical training is not required to do a thorough cancer examination. Any physician who is convinced that a thorough examination is important should be able to perform it satisfactorily. The first step is to obtain the family and personal history of the patient. Have other members of the family had cancer? If so, where? Did they recover or die from it? In the personal history, such data as where the person lives, whether or not he or she is exposed to carcinogens at work, whether the patient smokes and what, and whether he or she drinks alcoholic beverages are pertinent. For women, the menstrual history as well as obstetric data are desired.

A review of systems is made to elicit any information about previous signs or symptoms that the patient has observed. Unless this is done, the patient may not remember them or may think that observations he or she has made are insignificant. By the review of each system, one by one, the memory of the patient is refreshed and the patient is given an opportunity to relate observations. Patients do not always understand why this is necessary. This is especially true when they seek advice for a symptom or sign in one part of the body. The nurse may help the patient by treating the patient's question courteously and answering it or by referring it to the physician.

The physical examination consists of the palpation and visual inspection of organs to determine changes in color, texture, contour, and function and of listening to the heart and lungs. The physician performs the examination systematically so that no part is missed. The examination often begins with inspection of the skin for evidence of an increase or decrease in tissue and for changes in its appearance. Although the physician examines the entire skin surface, special attention is paid to areas exposed to sun, to the palms and soles, to the genitalia, and to areas subject to repeated trauma, as these are the sites where cancer of the skin most commonly occurs. The skin is observed for small, scaly lesions, small ulcers or sores, lumps, senile keratoses, nevi, pigmented moles, and burn scars. Basal cell carcinoma usually makes its appearance as a small scale that later disappears and leaves a sore that increases in size. Squamous cell carcinoma may also start with a scaly lesions or a small lump or an encrusted nodule. It is frequently preceded by senile keratosis, a condition in which there are patches of horny hypertrophy of skin in the aged. They often occur on the face. Nevi, or pigmented lesions, in areas subject to chronic irritation or that have undergone a change in size or color, are ulcerated, or bleed, should be viewed with suspicion. Any person with a lesion that is suspected of being a malignant melanoma should consult or be referred to a surgeon who is experienced in treating melanomas.

The palpation of the superficial lymph nodes is an essential part of any cancer-detection examination. Enlargement of lymph nodes may point to lymphomas or leukemia or to cancer in structures drained by the lymph channels supplying the node. An increase in size in a node or group of nodes may be the first evidence of the disease.

A cancer-detection examination of the head and neck includes the inspection of the skin and the oral and nasal cavities, the visualization of the larynx, and the palpation of the oral cavity, the areas containing lymph nodes, and the thyroid gland.

One of the most publicized cancer-detection examinations is that of the breast. There has been a widespread promotional program to teach women how to examine their own breasts. Many physicians instruct their patients in the procedure. Teaching women to examine their own breasts regularly and systematically each month is based on the expectation that women will be able to detect cancer while the disease is still localized in the breast. It is estimated that 95 per cent of cancers of the breast are discovered by the patient. Even though breast cancer before the age of 25 is rare, the American Cancer Society advocates young girls to begin breast self-examination on a regular monthly basis, as a practice begun early in life is inclined to become an established habit. Instructions for breast self-examination may be obtained from the American Cancer Society or from a local branch of the society. The woman is instructed to report immediately any findings of lumps or changes in the contour or skin of the breast or secretions from the nipple. The physician follows essentially the same pattern in examining the woman's breast that he or she teaches her to follow. Some patients require special types of examinations. They include those whose breasts, because of the size or because of the cystic changes, are difficult to examine as well as patients coming from cancer-prone families. The recent introduction of mammography and xerography has been shown to be helpful. Because of relatively high amount of radiation utilized for these diagnostic tests, until further advancements in these techniques are made, they should not be used routinely for examination of every woman.

In the early 1970s thermography was being used experimentally to detect breast cancer. Although it was recognized that the method could not be used to make a specific medical diagnosis, it was hoped that an abnormal thermogram would serve as a prescreener to identify breast cancers with a noninvasive, quick, inexpensive technique (Libshitz, 1977). However, a recent study by Moskowitz et al. (1976) severely questions the efficacy of thermography as a screening tool for a minimal and Stage I breast cancer. His findings suggest that thermography may be no more accurate than random selection (Moskowitz, 1976). It seems before thermograms become realistic diagnostic tools, more research is required in methods to improve thermography; that is, the techniques necessary to detect differences in thermal gradients between normal and abnormal breast tissue must be refined.

The most essential tool in the detection of lung cancer is the chest x ray. Because the lung is a common site of metastasis, the chest x ray is useful not only in detection of primary cancer but in estimation of its prognosis. In persons who are predisposed to lung cancer by their work or personal habits, cytological examination of bronchial secretion may be performed. The presence of abnormal cells in the sputum is an indication for further examination. Physical examination of the chest is also essential. Partial obstruction of a bronchial tube by a neoplasm may cause a wheezing sound as the air passes through accumulated secretions. Furthermore, the partial obstruction may result in the incomplete expansion of a segment of the lung.

The abdomen is palpated to determine the presence of any lumps or increase in size of abdominal organs. Because the liver is a frequent site of metastasis, it receives special attention. If there is evidence of abnormality of the liver or spleen, scintigraphy can be used to confirm the diagnosis without the use of invasive procedures (Drum, 1973).

Vaitkevicius and Moghissi (1968) reported that the number of patients who were detected and operated on each year for carcinoma in situ by the staff of the Department of Gynecology at Wayne State University rose from 0 in 1953 to119 in 1966. During the same period the percentage of patients with invasive carcinoma decreased from 100 per cent to 12 per cent. They advocate that cytologic screening be carried out on a yearly basis beginning at age 20, or younger if the patient is sexually active. They further stated that no woman need ever develop invasive carcinoma of the cervix.

The theme of the Uterine Cancer Control Program of the American Society is "Let No Woman Be Overlooked." The program is directed particularly at women in the lower socioeconomic groups, and to all menopausal and postmenopausal women who have never had a Pap test.

A 21-year cervical cancer control program yielded the following trends in mortality and morbidity. Screening was most successful in younger age groups. There was a drop in screening success after age 45, with a marked decrease after age 60. Women at highest risk for cervical cancer in the low socioeconomic quartile had a better initial screening rate than women in the two middle-income quartiles, and the women in the low socioeconomic quartile had the highest rate for subsequent rescreening. The greatest decrease in morbidity and mortality was in women below 50 years of age. Morbidity rates decreased most among women aged 30 to 39 and 50 to 59, with a decrease of 70.8 per cent and 69.0 per cent, respectively. There was no change in mortality rates for women 70 years and older (Christopherson, 1976).

GYNECOLOGICAL EXAMINATION. In preparation for a gynecologic examination, a woman should be instructed not to take a vaginal douche. Immediately preceding the examination, she should be asked to empty her urinary bladder. The bed or examining table should be screened and the patient should be draped, so that the genitalia are exposed, but the surrounding area is covered. The patient should lie on her back with her hips flat on the bed or table. When the patient is on an examining table, the hips should be brought to the edge of the table and the legs and thighs supported by stirrups. When the patient is examined in bed, the thighs should be raised so they are perpendicular with the bed. The feet should be resting with the soles flat on the bed. During the examination, the knees are moved outward.

At the beginning of the examination, the external genitalia are inspected for nevi, leukoplakia, ulcerative lesions, and other abnormalities. The vaginal mucous membrane and cervix are examined. The speculum that is used is moistened with water rather than jelly, as the jelly interferes with the cytologic examination. Cells are obtained for the vaginal Papanicolaou smear by aspirating secretions from the posterior lateral fornices with a vaginal pipette. The secretions are then spread thinly on a glass slide. The slide is immediately placed in a jar containing equal parts of 95 per cent alcohol and ether. Material for the cervical smear may be obtained by swabbing the surface of the cervix with a cotton applicator and by inserting the cotton into the cervical os and gently rotating it. Another method is to scrape the cervix with a wooden tongue depressorlike device. Material may be obtained from the cervical os by a specially designed cervical scraper. The material obtained from the cervix is spread thinly on a glass slide. The slide is immediately placed in the jar containing equal parts of 95 per cent alcohol and ether or it is fixed by spraying its surface with a commercially available spray fixative. The latter method is a much more convenient way of handling the slides.

The physician also investigates the pelvic organs by means of a bimanual examination. As the prefix *bi* implies, two hands are used. One hand is placed on the abdomen, and one or more fingers of the other hand are placed in the vagina. By exerting pressure, the physician can determine changes in the size and conformation of various structures.

When areas of the cervix present a suspicious appearance, biopsy may be done to establish the diagnosis. Some physicians do a punch biopsy of the suspicious tissue. This can be performed in the outpatient clinic or in the office of the physician as well as in the hospital.

Cancer-detection examination for men should include an investigation of the male reproductive system. This examination should include the inspection and palpation of the external structures and the palpation of the internal organs. Cytologic examination may be made on fluids obtained by aspiration from the testes or from a hydrocele. Prostatic fluid may be obtained by massaging the prostate. Every physical examination on an adult male should include the digital examination of the prostate per rectum. From this procedure the physician can identify changes in the size of a part or the entire gland as well as the presence of nodules. Although the enlargement of a lobe or the entire gland is often a benign condition, unless corrected it can cause serious harm by obstructing the flow of urine from the bladder.

RECTAL AND SIGMOID EXAMINATION. The digital examination of the rectum serves a further purpose in that some 50 per cent of lesions in the large bowel are within reach of the examiner's finger. For this reason the physical examination of every adult should include this procedure. Because some lesions are beyond the reach of the examiner's finger and cannot be felt, the examination of the rectum and colon should include a proctosigmoidoscopy. It is estimated that two thirds of the lesions in the rectum and colon can be diagnosed by this method. In the proctosigmoidoscopy, a lighted tube is introduced through the anal sphincter into the rectum and sigmoid. The walls of these structures are directly visualized and abnormalities such as polyps, ulcerations, and narrowing of the lumen are noted. This is a relatively simple and safe procedure that can be performed in the office of the physician or in an outpatient clinic. Some physicians instruct the patient to take an enema the night preceding the morning of the examination. The purpose of the enema is to cleanse the bowel. The importance of cleansing the bowel to the success of the examination should be stressed. Others prefer to do the examination without any special preparation and remove any feces in the area at the time of the examination. The reason for the omission of enemas is that the solution may injure the mucosa lining the bowel and increase the activity of the intestine. The latter makes the performance of the procedure more difficult.

For the performance of the proctosigmoidoscopy, the patient must be placed in a knee–chest position. The process of assuming this position can be strenuous, and the patient may feel embarrassed. To assist the patient into the knee–chest position, he or she should lie face down on a table that can be adjusted to the proper position or the patient may be instructed to assume the proper position on the table. When the patient assumes the knee–chest position, he or she should turn onto the abdomen with the left arm under the chest. The hips are elevated by bringing the legs up so that the patient rests on the knees, and shoulders. When in proper position, the thighs are perpendicular to the table and they form one side of a triangle. The other two sides of the triangle are formed by the back and the table. Because a proctosigmoidoscopy takes about 5 minutes, the patient should not be placed in position until the physician is ready. As with other procedures, unnecessary exposure of the patient should be avoided by draping and screening. Although the procedure is safe, relatively simple, and leaves no after effects, the introduction and movement of the tube may cause cramping. The patient should be reassured that the discomfort is to be expected and that it will cease as soon as the procedure is completed.

LABORATORY EXAMINATIONS. The laboratory examinations performed as part of a cancer-detection examination are for the purpose of uncovering clues indicating the presence of cancer in the body as well as pinpointing its location. At the present, there is no single test for the identification of early cancer.

Originally carcinoembryonic antigen (CEA) was thought to be present only in patients with colorectal carcinoma (Reynoso, 1972). The antigen was later demonstrated to be present in inflamed colonic mucosa and polyps (Isaacson & LeVann, 1976). These findings tend to support the concept of carcinoma in situ in adenomatous polyps and the transition from polyp to cancer. Recently elevated serum concentrations of CEA have been found in patients with locally advanced and/or metastatic medullary thyroid carcinoma (DeLellis et al., 1978).

Enzyme studies may be helpful both in the diagnosis and in the evaluation of the effects of therapy in patients with malignancies. These tests may indicate the appearance of a metastatic tumor lesion long before it becomes clinically apparent. Elevated phosphatase may indicate either primary or metastatic bone malignancy.

Evidence indicates that adenosine triphosphatase may be elevated in mammary carcinoma (Buell, 1976). Elevated alkaline phosphatase isoenzymes have also been observed in patients with carcinoma of the stomach (Miki et al., 1976). Researchers in cancer enzymology caution that further study must be done and that the presence of elevated enzymes must be interpreted with caution (Buell, 1976).

Some laboratory tests, though not specifically for cancer, should be part of every cancer-detection examination. Every examination should include a hemoglobin or hematocrit determination. An unexplained anemia is often the first symptom in cancer of the gastrointestinal and urinary tracts. A leukocyte count combined with a determination of the types of leukocytes (differential white count) may provide evidence of leukemia or lymphoma. A complete urinalysis may provide information indicating the presence of a neoplasm in the kidney or urinary tract. The finding of microscopic amounts of blood in the urine is especially significant. Occult (hidden) blood in the feces may indicate a malignant lesion somewhere along the gastrointestinal tract.

Exfoliative cytology is an extremely valuable method of detecting cancer and other pathologic conditions in humans through microscopic examination of body fluids and secreta. The following is but a brief number of the kinds of secreta that can be examined by this method and from which a diagnosis can be made: bone marrow aspirate, oral smears, breast secretion, bronchial aspirate and lavage, sputum, and vaginal and cervical smears. Tests of this nature do not take long to perform and are not usually uncomfortable for the patient.

IMPLICATIONS OF SUSPICIOUS LESIONS. The discovery of suspicious lesions, signs, or symptoms may make further investigation necessary. The methods used are those enabling the physician to visualize the lesion directly or indirectly and to obtain tissue for microscopic examination. X-ray, endoscopic, and tissue examinations are made. These procedures have been described in other chapters and will not be repeated. The point that many of these examinations are sources of physical and psychological stress bears repeated emphasis. The patient should be prepared for what to expect and for what is expected of him or her. When the patient is required to prepare for a diagnostic procedure, he or she should be given written, as well as verbal, instructions.

The location of lesions and their general character may be indirectly visualized by x-ray or fluoroscopic examination. The progress of lesions may be followed by either endoscopic examination or x-ray or both. For example, a patient is found to have an ulcer in the stomach. At the time of the initial examination, it appears to be a benign lesion on both the gastroscopic and x-ray examinations. Although ulcers occurring in the stomach can be benign, they are usually viewed with suspicion. Following treatment, the patient is again examined to determine any changes in the size of the ulcer. Failure of the ulcer to diminish in size and to give other evidence of healing is presumptive evidence that the lesion is not benign.

BIOPSY. The diagnosis of cancer is confirmed by the finding of cancer cells by microscopic examination. When tissue is removed for this purpose, the entire procedure is called a biopsy. When the lesion can be reached from the surface of the body either directly or through a small incision, the procedure itself is relatively minor. Cells may be obtained in body fluids by using a needle or by introducing a punch into the tissue or by cutting out a piece. Tissue is removed from the uterus by scraping. At times a body cavity, such as the abdominal or the thoracic cavity, must be opened to obtain the necessary tissue. In the emphasis on the biopsy as the critical procedure in establishing the diagnosis of cancer, the point may be missed that it is equally useful in establishing that a patient does not have cancer. For example, only four out of ten lumps in the breast are cancerous. Neither are all lumps in other organs malignant. When they are, treatment is initiated promptly. When they are not, the patient can be reassured that there is no cancer.

At the time a diagnosis of cancer is made, the characteristics of the cancer and the extent of its spread are evaluated. This information is useful in estimating the prognosis of a patient. The characteristics of cancer are determined by macroscopic and microscopic examination. The macroscopic examination yields information about the size, shape, consistency, and location of the neoplasm. From looking at and feeling the growth, information is gained about whether the neoplasm (1) extends into or grows around an organ, (2)is separate from or has invaded the surrounding tissue, (3) is hard or soft, (4) is ulcerating or intact, and (5) has spread to distant points. The microscopic examination provides information about the character of the cancer cells and the degree to which they resemble or differ from healthy cells. It is also useful in determining the extent of metastasis. With few exceptions, the more cells differ from healthy cells in character and organization, the more rapidly they grow and the faster they metastasize.

CANCER DETECTION. Because the outlook of patients with neoplasms that respond to therapy depends on early diagnosis and treatment, every individual is important in a cancer-control program. There is disagreement among physicians as to the advisability, practicality, and possibility of every person having an annual or biannual cancer-detection examination. Some physicians suggest that those in the high-risk groups, women over 30 or 35 years of age and men over 40 years of age have yearly examinations. A family history of cancer, a past history of cancer, smoking, and employment in a hazardous occupation (involving exposure to carcinogens) are suggested as indications for a regular checkup.

Every individual has a responsibility in cancer detection. Many see a physician only when they are obviously ill. To help people recognize signs and symptoms that indicate the possibility of cancer, the American Cancer Society has prepared and distributed a list known as the Seven Warning Signals. These signs and symptoms are not positive proof that cancer is present, but prompt action is required to prevent unnecessary damage. The warning signals are

C hange in bowel or bladder habits.
A sore that does not heal.
U nusual bleeding or discharge.
T hickening or lump in the breast or elsewhere.
I ndigestion or difficulty in swallowing.
O bvious change in wart or mole.
N agging cough or hoarseness.

(If you have a warning signal see your physician!) There are a number of other warning signals. These are, however, the important ones. Prompt reporting of any of these does not necessarily ensure that the cancer is in an early stage. Prompt reporting plus regular medical examination with follow-through on advice given is the best protection available.

Cancer detection depends on people and facilities. The term *people* encompasses everyone, not only the person who suspects or knows he or she has cancer but also professional personnel who understand the nature of cancer and its manifestations and have the skills that enable them to identify suspicious lesions or changes. To participate in cancer detection a lay person must know what to look for and where to go for help. He or she also needs to know that help is available if sought. Professional personnel must have the conviction that cancer detection is important and that it makes a significant contribution to the well-being of people. Following the stage of cancer detection, persons with suspicious lesions go on to diagnosis.

Therapy in Cancer

With diagnosis, therapy follows. Three types of therapy are available. They are surgery, radiation, and chemotherapy. In the treatment of any patient, any one or a combination may be used. The plan of treatment is based on the condition of the individual patient; on the nature, extent, and location of the lesion; and on what can be expected from a given therapeutic agent. That is to say, therapy is individually tailored. The initiation of a plan of therapy is contingent on its acceptance by the patient. Occasionally a patient prefers taking his or her chances with cancer over the treatment that is suggested. This the the patients right and must be respected as such. In this event the plan has to be modified so that it becomes acceptable to the patient. Some patients, given time and support that recognizes their right to make their own decisions, will eventually agree to the original plan. The outcome is not always as bad as anticipated. For example, Mrs. Friend had a malignant melanoma on the sole of her left foot. At the time of diagnosis, the recommendation was made that she have a high leg amputation, but she refused to have the operation. Instead of dying within a few months, she lived for 10 or 12 years. She lived, for the most part, an active life. Sometimes children whose parents refuse amputation for the treatment of melanoma live for a number of years after the diagnosis is made. In other instances where parents allow the amputation to be done, the activity of the disease is increased and death comes soon thereafter. Although patients and parents do not always make what appears to be, at the time, a wise decision, the result is not inevitably bad. Whatever the outcome, however, they have the right to their choice. This right should be respected.

The underlying philosophy of all cancer treatment is to improve the quality and/or length of life of the patient (Lawrence and Terz, 1977). If the stage of cancer is such that a long-term cure cannot be achieved, the goals of treatment are directed at (1) management of disabilities produced by disease and (2) achievement of the highest quality of life possible despite limitations in function and decreased life expectancy (Lawrence and Terz, 1977). The term *cure* is used cautiously. Although the physician may be reasonably certain that all cancer cells have been eradicated from an individual who has cancer, he or she cannot be positive. Terms are coined to express this caution in the use of the word *cure*. Thus patients who are alive and well at the end of 5 years are said to have a 5-year cure. Those who are alive and well at the end of 10 years have a 10-year cure. The patient who is alive and well at the end of 5 years is presumed to be cured, but this is not a certainty.

In patients with advanced and progressive disease, therapy has as its objective the amelioration of the condition of the patient. The same methods are used as in the curative treatment of cancer. The criterion for success is that the patient be objectively or subjectively improved. Although palliative therapy is sometimes neglected, there is much that can be done to improve the well-being and comfort of the patient for whom there is little chance of cure.

For example, Mrs. Jane Merriweather, who had a large abdominal mass, was short of breath on the slightest exertion, she was anorexic, and when she did force herself to eat, she usually became nauseated and vomited. She was losing weight and strength rapidly. She looked and felt sick and discouraged. Soon after x-ray treatment was initiated, improvement was noticeable. On palpation of her abdomen, the tumor could be felt to be smaller in size. Even Mrs. Merriweather had objective evidence that the tumor was regressing as she could again wear dresses with belts. She gained weight. Subjectively she felt better. She was able to carry on moderate activity without becoming short of breath. She felt encouraged and stronger. Her appetite improved and she began to enjoy her meals. The basis for the use of x-ray in the treatment of Mrs. Merriweather was palliation. The x-ray did not, and was not expected to, cure. Mrs. Merriweather did have, however, several months in which she was relatively well.

Surgery

The surgical treatment of cancer goes back some 3,500 years. The Greeks and Egyptians have recorded the surgical removal of tumors (ACS, *Essentials of Cancer Nursing,* 1963). Hippocrates and his school attempted a classification of tumors (470–375 B.C.) and Celsus (53 B.C.–7 A.D.) distinguished between benign and malignant tumors (Raven, 1977).

The first successful operation for cancer was performed in 1882, when Bilroth removed a cancer of the stomach. The history of the advances that contributed to the development of modern surgery is outlined in Chapter 51. Suffice it to say that as knowledge of ligatures, anesthesia, asepsis, and the physiologic needs of humans, as well as techniques for meeting their needs, has increased, more and more extensive surgery has been possible. As a consequence, cancer in any body cavity or any part of the body may be removed surgically. Some of the problems arising from the surgical treatment of cancer are similar to those that arise in the surgical treatment of patients for other conditions. In addition, there are problems that arise out of the fact that the diagnosis is cancer. Then, too, the surgical procedure is often, though by no means always, more extensive than it is in the treatment of noncancerous conditions.

OBJECTIVES OF SURGICAL TREATMENT. The primary objective of the surgical treatment of cancer is the extirpation of the primary growth and the tissues to which it has extended. In the performance of the operation, the surgeon tries to encircle the growth without cutting into it in order to prevent its spread. Since learning that cancer cells can be found in the venous blood draining the neoplasm and the surrounding area, some surgeons tie off these veins before attempting to remove the cancer. The extent of the operation selected depends on the natural history of the cancer, the condition of the patient, and the stage of the disease. For example, a slow-growing cancer that spreads locally by invading the surrounding tissue, such as an early basal cell carcinoma, may be succesfully removed by simple excision. In squamous cell carcinoma, however, the lymph channels and nodes are excised in addition to the primary lesion, because it spreads through the lymphatics. In treatment of malignant tumors involving an extremity, the removal of an entire limb may be necessary to permit cure of the patient.

PALLIATIVE SURGICAL THERAPY. A second objective of surgical treatment is palliation. Although palliative treatment is not expected to cure the patient, it is primarily performed to increase the patient's comfort or well-being and in many instances it can prolong the patient's life.

The lesion itself may be removed, or rerouting or short-circuiting operations may be done to relieve symptoms of obstruction. The nerve supply to an area may be interrupted to relieve pain or muscle spasm. The indication for the removal of the neoplasm is that it is necrotic, infected, or bleeding. Ulcerated and infected lesions are the common cause of pain in cancer. When the lesion is at the surface of the body, the control of odors is difficult. Removal of the growth may result in relief of pain and in a general improvement of the patient. The effects of obstruction have been discussed previously.

Another type of palliative surgery is based on the observation that the growth of some tissues is dependent on certain hormones. Cancer of the breast sometimes regresses after oophorectomy. Castration in the male may be of benefit in cancer of the prostate. Adrenalectomy and hypophysectomy are also of benefit in selected patients. In these operations, the beneficial effect is presumed to result from removing a condition favorable to the growth of the neoplasm. The possibility exists that as more is learned about the factors favoring the establishment of metastatic growths these and other organs may be removed before, or at the time, the local growth is excised. If this should come to pass, then the operation would be curative.

The same principles apply to the preparation of any patient for a surgical procedure whether or not he or she has cancer. The patient requires emotional, physiological, and physical preparation. The patient needs to know what to expect and what is expected of him or her. The patient needs to be able to trust those responsible for care and to know that they can be counted on to meet his or her needs. In patients who are admitted one day and undergo a surgical procedure the following day, there is little time to develop a trusting relationship. Each step or act in the process of the admission of the patient is therefore exceedingly important. When people are under stress, they tend to magnify and personalize behavior that under happier circumstances would pass unnoticed or be dismissed as unimportant.

Patients who require special preparation because of the location of the lesion or because of the need to repair physiologic deficits may be in the hospital some days before surgery is scheduled. Improvement in the patient's physiologic status may be essential to survival. The correction of anemia and protein and other nutritional deficiencies as well as restoration of water and electrolyte balance and/or relief of obstruction, is often a required part of preoperative preparation.

IONIZING RADIATION. Ionizing radiation is also utilized to eradicate cancer cells or in palliation. In either event it may be used alone or in combination with surgery or chemotherapy. It may be used prior to an operation to reduce the size of neoplasm or after a suitable period to destroy the cells that remain behind.

The principle upon which use of ionizing radiation as a treatment is based is the belief that the cell varies in degree of radiosensitivity with age during the mitotic cycle. Characteristics of radiosensitivity in relation to the cell cycle are as follows: *(a)* cells are most sensitive during mitosis (M phase) or close to mitosis; *(b)* G_2, the time between DNA synthesis and M, is thought to be as sensitive as the M phase; *(c)* resistance to radiation is greatest during the S phase (Lawrence & Terz, 1977). Although all cells, regardless of whether they are dividing or not, are equally damaged by radiation, the nondividing cells are frequently able to repair the radiation-induced damage, whereas cell division prevents such repair and often multiplies radiation injury. Many of the radiated cells will not die until they try to divide. This may occur sometimes as long as several months after radiation has been completed. Ionizing radiation may be applied to an area or may be administered as a radioactive isotope solution. The latter is used in a few instances in which the body removes the isotope from the blood and concentrates on a selected tissue or when the radioactive solution can be directly applied to tumor-affected areas. Radioactive iodine is useful in the treatment of cancer of the thyroid because the body removes the iodine from the blood and concentrates it in the gland or in the tumor originating from the thyroid. In addition the half-life of iodine is 8.1 days, which makes it suitable to practical use. Radioactive gold and radioactive phosphorus are sometimes injected into the pleural cavity to treat malignant effusions.

Patients may be extremely apprehensive about beginning a course of ionizing radiation. Explanation to the patient is imperative and may make the difference between its being a horrible ordeal or one that is easily tolerable. It must indeed be frightening to lie on a table, looking into the face of a massive machine, and to be all alone with the lead door closed. Some radiation therapy departments have attempted to improve the atmosphere in the treatment area by painting murals on the walls. Some have a system by which they can see and communicate with the patient. The patient knows that someone is near and he or she can be told how much longer the treatment will be.

The patient and family should know the expected side effects. Hearsay from friends can be detrimental to any positive aspects of the treatments. Patients may express considerable fear about what will happen as a result of radiation treatments. Patients fear "radiation burns,"[3] loss of hair, and nausea and vomiting. Side effects are dependent on the area to which the radiation is directed. As an example, patients who receive cobalt treatments for a lesion on the vocal cord, can expect skin reactions on the neck over the area of treatment. The skin will develop an erythema that may later turn brown, then a dry epidermis may occur, followed by a moist epidermis. The area that is denuded weeps constantly, but in a few days covers over with circular islands of new epidermis. A sore throat may occur, and this can be relieved by using a gargle. Hoarseness will probably ensue but will disappear about 3 weeks after treatments are completed.

Irradiation sickness is rare and usually occurs only when large areas of the body are irradiated or when excessive doses are directed to moderate-sized fields. The effects of this phenomenon are anorexia, nausea, vomiting, lassitude, pallor, lividity, profuse perspiration, and, in extreme cases, chills (del Regato, 1977, p. 98). The effects of ionizing radiation, the measures required for the protection of the patient and personnel, the nursing needs of the patient, and the therapy are discussed in Chapter 11.

CHEMOTHERAPY. Modern chemotherapy is the newest form of cancer therapy. Although some of our chemotherapy agents had been used by the ancient Egyptians and Greeks, their rational use became commonplace only in the second half of this century. Specifically, the modern era of cancer chemotherapy was initiated by C. P. Rhoades when he published his observations that nitrogen mustard had significant anticancer effects (Rhoades, 1946). Since that time chemotherapy has evolved as a major means of therapy. The tendency to consider che-

[3] The term *radiation burn* is a misnomer, as it actually refers to the chemical reaction that takes place in the skin.

motherapy to be a final resort of the terminally ill cancer patient has been replaced to include chemotherapy as an integral part of treatment even at the time of initial diagnosis. Chemotherapy is the primary treatment of diseases such as choriocarcinoma, acute and chronic leukemia, Burkitt's lymphoma, and multiple myeloma. It is used as an adjuvant in the treatment of many other kinds of cancer, for example, breast cancer, Wilms's tumor, and osteogenic sarcoma, to name a few. Apparent cures have been achieved with chemotherapy, for example, patients with some stages of Hodgkin's disease have benefited by extension of life (Cannellos, 1979).

Though chemotherapy has advanced rapidly in the past three decades, it is not to be considered established or conventional and should be directed by a qualified clinical oncologist (del Regato, 1977).

INVESTIGATIONAL DRUGS. Nurses frequently care for patients who are receiving investigational drugs (M.D. Anderson Hospital and Tumor Institute, 1972), which includes "any drug which has been approved for investigational use by the Food and Drug Administration" and is available only for research studies carried out by a limited number of qualified investigators. These drugs are not commercially available. They may be referred to as phase I, phase II, or phase III study drugs.

Phase I study. This indicates that the correct dose and known side effects of the drug are not determined. The goal of a phase I study is to discover all known side effects and to determine what the correct dosage should be.

Phase II study. Patients receive a dose that is known to be effective. The goal is to discover in which tumor categories the drug is effective.

Phase III study. Both the dose and types of tumor in which the drug is effective are known. The objective is to compare one drug therapy with another drug therapy in a specific disease to determine the best therapeutic regimen.

Once the investigational drugs have passed through phases I, II, and III, they may become commercially available, which indicates that they can be obtained through regular drugstores and pharmacies throughout the nation by any licensed physician. Some drugs are available commercially in one dosage form, such as oral, but another form, such as injectable, may be under investigation.

CHEMOTHERAPEUTIC AGENTS. The five major classifications of chemotherapeutic agents are alkylating agents, antimetabolites, plant alkaloids, antibiotics, hormones, and miscellaneous agents (refer to Table 39-6).

Alkylating agents are the largest and oldest group of chemotherapeutic agents (Greenspan, 1975). They are thought to act by binding the two DNA strands, and thus preventing the separation of the two strands of the coiled double helix which is necessary for cell replication. Alkylating agents can kill cells in any phase of the cycle including G_0, but rapidly replicating cells are most sensitive (del Regato, 1977). Alkylating agents rarely produce optimal effects without being combined with other agents that affect a specific phase of the cell cycle (Lawrence & Terz, 1977). Alkylating agents have been demonstrated to be useful in treating Hodgkin's disease and other malignant lymphomas, acute and chronic leukemia, cancer of the lung, breast, and ovary, malignant melanoma, various sarcomas, neuroblastomas, retinoblastomas, and malignant gliomas (del Regato, 1977).

Antimetabolites affect cells by inhibiting the biosynthesis of nucleic acids which are essential components of DNA and RNA (Lawrence & Terz, 1977). This mechanism prevents both cell multiplication and function. These agents are effective when the cell is in the synthesis (S) phase. The rate of destruction of cells by antimetabolites is determined by the life span of the cells since these agents are effective only during the S phase of the cell cycle. Antimetabolites have been shown to be useful in the treatment of acute leukemia, osteogenic sarcoma, squamous cell cancer of the upper respiratory tract, lung and uterine cervix, Burkitt's lymphoma, and cancer of the breast and testes (del Regato, 1977).

Plant alkaloids are derived from the periwinkle root (Vinca). Their mechanism of action is thought to be one of mitotic inhibition by interfering with spindle formation in metaphase (Greenspan, 1975; Lawrence & Terz, 1977). Plant alkaloid's action by mitotic inhibition makes treatment more effective if they are combined with other categories of agents (Lawrence & Terz, 1977). They have been demonstrated to be effective in treatment of childhood lymphoblastic leukemia, Hodgkin's disease, malignant lymphomas, cancer of the breast, rhabdomyosarcoma, neuroblastoma, Wilms's tumor, and Ewing's sarcoma (del Regato, 1977).

Antitumor antibiotics are nonspecific in terms of their effect on the cell cycle. They are thought to act by binding DNA to block RNA production, thereby preventing cell replication (Lawrence & Terz, 1977). Antibiotics are useful in various squamous cell carcinomas including upper respiratory passages, penis, cervix, and vulva. They have also been used in Hodgkin's disease, malignant lymphomas, testicular tumors, renal carcinoma, soft tissue sarcomas, osteogenic sarcomas, carcinomas of the breast, ovary, and thyroid, transitional cell cancer of the bladder, Ewing's sarcoma, and neuroblastomas (del Regato, 1977). Antibiotics are frequently used as adjuvant to surgery and radiation therapy (del Regato, 1977).

Specific actions of the miscellaneous drugs is unclear. Some are thought to interfere with cellular synthesis of protein, for example, L-asparaginase which hydrolyzes L-asparagine and prevents protein synthesis. It is unclear how steroid hormones inhibit cancer growth, but speculation is that they may interfere at the cell membrane level. These drugs are used in treatment of a wide range of malignancies and accompanying complications. Adrenal corticosteroids have been useful in autoimmune hemolytic anemia accompanying chronic lymphogenous leukemia, hypercalcemia, hemorrhage associated with thrombocytopenia, increased intracranial pressure in patients with brain metastases or those with cord compression. Estrogens have been used in patients with metastatic prostatic cancer to produce remission and relief of symptoms (del Regato, 1977). To determine if a patient will be responsive to endocrine therapy, the tumor tissue or cells in fluid are tested for the presence of the estrogen receptor protein estrophilin. Tumor tissue containing the estrogen receptor responds favorably to endocrine therapy in two thirds of patients, but when the estrogen receptor is absent, the response is negligible (del Regato, 1977). Generally, this classification of drugs is used most frequently in breast cancer, prostatic cancer, hypernephroma, and leukemias (Lawrence and Terz, 1977).

MODALITIES OF TREATMENT WITH CHEMOTHERAPY. Anticancer chemotherapy is prescribed using basically three approaches: (1) regional chemotherapy; (2) adjuvant chemotherapy; and (3) combination chemotherapy.

Regional chemotherapy involves intra-arterial infusion, fractionated or continuous, for regional perfusion of anatomic locations by means of extracorporeal equipment. Currently the method is being used for treating squamous cell carcinoma of the head and neck, recurrent and metastatic melanoma, and primary and metastatic carcinoma of the liver. Though regional arterial chemotherapy is being used it is believed at this time that it will not be a major factor in clinical cancer therapy (Lawrence & Terz, 1977).

The Watkins USCI chronometric infusion pump (U.S. Catheter and Instrument Corp., 1971) is an example of a regional infusion pump. It is a compact self-contained portable apparatus. It injects 5 ml of medication per 24 hours through a fine plastic catheter that passes into a blood vessel or to a body cavity. It is useful for a long-term continuous drug therapy in ambulatory patients, and for intra-arterial or intravenous infusion of antimetabolite drugs for the chemotherapy of cancer.

The pump is small and can be easily contained in a carrying harness. The pump needs to be wound every 8 hours. This is usually done by the nurse in the hospital; at home it is suggested that patients set their alarms to remind them to wind the pump. The key should be kept in the same safe place. In the hospital the key is taped to the bedside table. Initially patients are disturbed by the constant ticking; eventually the ticking becomes such a part of them that the lack of ticking is disturbing. Husbands, wives, and children may have difficulty adjusting to such constant ticking. When traveling, especially by plane, a letter from the physician is needed explaining the device, and the necessity for the patient to use it. Patients are likely to incur stares from others whenever they are in public places where the pump mechanism is audible. Patients should be encouraged to return for clinic visits as scheduled for refilling of the pump. They need to be instructed regarding precautions necessary to prevent the pump's mechanism from becoming wet. Bathing in the tub is usually allowed, but the pump should be inserted into a plastic bag and placed on a chair beside the tub; catheters are sufficiently long to permit this. If water should get into the mechanism the pump will stop, and the catheter may become plugged.

Not only is it imperative for the nurse to be knowledgeable about the side effects and the toxic effects that may be exhibited by the patient, but the patient and family must know what side effects to expect in the hospital and after discharge. Many of the side effects are not evident until several days after the patient is discharged. The patient and family should know what might happen, and what can or should be done for each side effect. Medications that may be necessary to relieve these side effects should be ordered by the physician before the patient is discharged. This information should be in writing so the patient can refer to it. An example of one format is given in Table 39-7.

Because chemotherapeutic drugs affect the hematopoietic system, blood studies are required at specific intervals. The physician will inform the patient how often and what blood studies are necessary. Patients do not necessarily need to return to their treatment center to have the blood studies done. They should be told that they may go either to a medical laboratory or to a local hospital to have these tests performed. This will spare the patient unnecessary traveling and waiting. Wherever the laboratory work is done, the patient should request that the results

TABLE 39-6. *Agents Used in Cancer Chemotherapy**

Agents	Principal Routes of Administration	Usual Dose	Side Effects	Late Toxic Manifestations
Alkylating agents				
1-(2-chloroethyl)-3-cyclohexyl-1-nitrosourea (CCNU)	Oral	100–300 mg	N and V†	Leukopenia and thrombocytopenia (3–6 weeks after administration), anorexia
Cyclophosphamide (Cytoxan, CTX)	Oral IV	50–400 mg	N and V (slight)	Alopecia, hemorrhagic cystitis, WBC depression
Phenylalanine mustard (melphalan, Pam, Alkeran)	Oral IV Intra-arterial	2–24 mg	Rare N and V	Myelosuppression
Nitrogen mustard (HN_2, mustargen)	IV Intrapleural	3–30 mg (every 2 weeks)	N and V, thrombophlebitis along vein of injection, skin slough if injection outside of vein	Myelosuppression
Triethylenethiophosphoramide (thio-TEPA, TSPA)	IV IM Bladder infusion	15–30 mg	Mild N and V, headaches, fevers	Prolonged myelosuppression
Antimetabolites				
5-Azacytidine (AzaC)	IV	150–1000 mg × 5 days 1 × a month	N and V, diarrhea, fever	Bone marrow depression
Cytosine, Arabinoside (Cytosar, ARA-C, C.A.)	IV Subcut. Intrathecal	50–1000 mg	N and V	Myelosuppression, hepatic toxicity
5-fluorouracil (5 FU)	IV	250–1500 mg × 5 days	N and V	Stomatitis, anorexia, diarrhea, alopecia, myelosuppression
6-Mercaptopurine (6-MP, Purinethol)	Oral IV	50–150 mg		Stomatitis, skin eruptions, fever, myelosuppression, liver dysfunction
4-Amino-N^{10} Methylpteroylglutamic acid [Methotrexate (MTX)]	Oral IV IM Intrathecal	10–50 mg × 5 days		Ulceration of oral mucosa, alopecia, myelosuppression, hepatic toxicity
Antitumor antibiotics				
Adriamycin (Adria)	IV	30–240 mg 1 × every 3 weeks	Necrosis and sloughing outside of vein, thrombophlebitis, fever, N and V	Oral ulcerations, alopecia, bone marrow suppression, possible cardiotoxicity

Actinomycin D, Dactinomysin (Cosmegen, ACT-D, DACT)	IV	0.5–2.0 mg 1 × every 3 weeks	N and V, severe tissue damage if given outside of vein	Alopecia, stomatitis, diarrhea, myelosuppression
Bleomycin (Bleo)	IV IM Subcut.	15–50 mg, 1 − 2 × weekly 1 − 2 mg per day	Occasional hypotension, fever 101–104°F., chest pain, rare anaphylaxis manifested by urticaria and asthma	Pulmonary fibrosis, symptoms of pneumonia, alopecia, stomatitis, swelling, reddening of skin, pressure and trauma points, pain in fingertips, weakness, anorexia, N and V, pigmentation, nail changes
Daunorubicin (Daunomycin, Rubidmycin, Dauno)	IV	60–200 mg	Severe sloughing of tissue if given outside vein, fever	Alopecia, stomatitis, myelosuppression, tachycardia, heart failure, respiratory distress
Imidazole Carboxamide Dimethyltriazeno (DIC, ICT)	IV Intra-arterial	200–1,500 mg × 5 days	N and V	Delayed myelosuppression, Rare: "Flu-like" symptoms, photosensitivity
Imidazole carboxamide mustard (BIC, Imidazole Mustard, TIC Mustard)	IV	300 mg–3g	N and V	Myelosuppression (3–5 weeks after first day of therapy)
Mithramycin (Mithracin)	IV	0.5–4 mg	N and V, facial flushing, epistaxis	Increased BUN, prothrombin and liver enzymes; confusion → delirium; punctate dermatitis; stomatitis; anorexia; malaise; minimal myelosuppression
Mitomycin C	IV	1–40 mg 1 × every 8 weeks	N and V	Profound thrombocytopenia, leukopenia
Procarbazine (Matulane)	Oral	50–350 mg a day	N and V, neurologic symptoms	Marrow depression, skin toxicity, desquamation
Miscellaneous drugs Vinblastine sulfate (VLB, Velban)	IV	4–30 mg	Persistent pain if injected outside of vein, causes necrosis if extravasates	Myelosuppression, neurotoxicity (high doses)
Vincristine sulfate (VCR, Oncovin)	IV	0.5–3.0 mg	Persistent severe pain lasting several weeks if injected outside vein	Neurotoxicity (loss of DTR, numbness of fingers and toes), alopecia, weakness of hands and feet, cranial nerve paralysis and severe constipation with abdominal pain
bis-(b-chloroethyl) nitrosourea (BCNU)	IV	100–400 mg every 6 weeks	N and V, pain along vein of injection	Delayed myelosuppression, liver and renal toxicity (at higher doses), pigmentation of skin along veins

(Continued)

TABLE 39-6 *(Cont.)*

Agents	Principal Routes of Administration	Usual Dose	Side Effects	Late Toxic Manifestations
1-(2-chloroethyl)-3-(4-methylcyclohexyl)-1-nitrosourea (Methyl-CCNU, MeCCNU)	Oral (to be given on empty stomach)	150–500 mg every 6 weeks	N and V	Anorexia, bone marrow depression
Guanazole	IV	10–70 g a day × 5 days	N and V, fever	Stomatitis, diarrhea, myelosuppression, alkalinization of blood, skin toxicity, pigmentation and desquamation
L-Asparaginase (L-ASP)	IV	2—10,000 IU a day	Urticaria after previous exposure, anorexia, nausea, hypofibrinogenemia	Coagulation defects, hepatic toxicities, hyperglycemia, pancreatitis, CNS depression
Hormones and steroids				
Estrogens:				
Diethylstilbesterol	Oral	1–3 mg a day	N and V	Fluid retention in patients with cardiac, liver, renal disease; gynecomastia; changes in libido; uterine bleeding
Progestational agents				
Medroxyprogesterone acetate (Provera)	Oral IM	100–200 mg a day, 200–600 mg 2 × weekly	None	Changes in epithelium of the female genital tract and the acinar cells of the breast
Hydroxyprogesterone (Delalutin)	IM	1 g twice a week to 5 g a week		
Androgens				
Testesterone propionate (Perandren)	IM	50–200 mg per day, total weekly dosage 200–1200 mg	None	Virilization, fluid retention, change in libido
Fluoxymesterone (Halotestin)	Oral	10–40 mg a day		Same, plus oral absorption and hepatic toxicity
Prednisone	Oral	40–120 mg a day	Gastric irritation	Diabetes mellitus, fluid and sodium retention, potassium loss, psychosis
Prednisolone	IM	40–120 mg a day		*Rare:* osteoporosis, striae, purpura, truncal obesity

† N and V = nausea and vomiting.
* Information adapted from *Investigational Drug Data Sheets* (Houston: The University of Texas at Houston, M. D. Anderson Hospital and Tumor Institute, 1973).

TABLE 39-7

Side Effect	Action
Gastrointestinal tract	
Nausea and/or vomiting	Use of antiemetic; choice of foods—bland, small amounts
Diarrhea	Selection of foods—decrease intake of juices Medication (order from doctor) Kaopectate Lomotil (use *only* as directed)
Surface ulcerations	Xylocaine viscous, Chloraseptic before meals, these decrease taste of food, but make it more comfortable to eat Cook's ointment Foods—bland, avoid citrus juices Soft touthbrush or rinse mouth only
Mouth coated, does not hurt	Liquid or soft foods (dry foods difficult to eat)
Bone marrow	
Anemia	Choice of foods—basic four, liver
Leukopenia	Prevent infections, stay away from persons who have colds or other contagious disease
Thrombocytopenia (bleeding)	Report to your doctor any bleeding
Hair follicles	
Alopecia	No brushing, gentle combing Wigs Nightcaps

be both phoned and mailed to their physician. Many of the medical laboratories will provide home calls for patients who are too ill to travel even short distances. Patients can consult the yellow pages of their phone book to locate the laboratory nearest them.

ADJUVANT CHEMOTHERAPY. Adjuvant chemotherapy involves combining treatment modalities for better results. Combination of systemic chemotherapy with localized surgical or radiation therapy allows the physician to deal with the microscopic cancer that would not be controlled by the regional treatment of surgery or radiotherapy. Success of adjuvant chemotherapy has varied with different malignancies. For example, clinical data support good control using adjuvant chemotherapy for Wilms's tumor, embryonal rhabdomyosarcoma in children, osteogenic sarcoma, Ewing's sarcoma, and some testicular cancer (Lawrence & Terz, 1977). However, no benefit has been shown for cancer of the lung, gastric cancer, or cancer of the bladder (Lawrence & Terz, 1977). Recently some success has been demonstrated with patients who have cancer of the breast (Salmon & Jones, 1977).

COMBINATION CHEMOTHERAPY. Combination chemotherapy involves the simultaneous administration of two or more anticancer agents. Generally when planning combination therapy, the oncologist will use agents that have different modes of action and differing patterns of toxicity. The rationale is that this will reduce the possibility of drug resistance and achieve an additive effect from the individual agents. Combination chemotherapy has been very useful in treating lymphatic leukemia in children, Hodgkin's disease, carcinoma of the breast, and gastrointestinal cancer (Lawrence & Terz, 1977). Cancer chemotherapeutic agents presently available have serious toxic effects. Nurses need to be aware of the expected side effects of the drugs and toxic effects that are known and to be alert to those that are unknown at the present time. Because patients may be receiving a combination of drugs, nurses need to be especially keen observers.

Normal tissues that have a high rate of cellular proliferation are most severely affected by the drug action. These tissues include the normal bone marrow elements, the gastroinstestinal epithelial cells, cells of the hair follicles and of the skin. Clinically, evidence of toxicity is seen as follows:

Bone marrow: anemia, leukopenia (infection), thrombocytopenia (bleeding).
Gastrointestinal tract: nausea, vomiting, surface ulcerations, diarrhea.
Hair follicles: alopecia (Cline, 1971).

Some drugs cause severe irritation to tissues with which they come in contact. They should be administered only by a physician or a nurse thoroughly instructed in their use, and every effort should be made to prevent the drug from escaping into surrounding tissues. However, appropriately selected patients and careful use of these drugs often produce worthwhile remissions that may last several years.

Because of the extreme toxicity, occasionally these drugs are used locally, either by administering them directly to the tumor or to the blood vessels supplying the tumor. In this manner the systemic toxic effects of these drugs can be minimized and sometimes completely eliminated. Such is the case in patients who have hepatic carcinoma. They may have either a transbrachial or a transabdominal catheter, which is threaded through to the hepatic artery. In this way a larger dose of medication can be delivered directly to the liver. Pumps are necessary to supply the drug to the liver against the arterial force.

The IVAC 200 infusion controller (Melton, 1973) is an instrument that controls the gravity flow of intravenous fluid. A flow rate of 5 to 60 drops per minute can be obtained. (See Figure 39-3 for illustrations of this and the following pumps.)

The IVAC 500 (Melton, 1973) infusion pump administers fluid by peristaltic action at rates of 1 to 99 drops per minute, either intravenously or intra-arterially. Other than its pumping action, it operates essentially as the controller.

The desired drops per minute are obtained by setting the dial on the front of the machines. These machines are equipped with a "catseye" drop sensor, which counts each drop. A blue light blinks as each drop falls. If for any reason the drop rate cannot be maintained, the instrument will change into an alarm mode. When this occurs the tubing closes and there are both audible and visible signals that alert the nurses. An alarm sounds and an orange alert light goes on. By means of a special attachment, the alarm could sound through the hospital call system. The alarm mode goes into action if

1. The pump cannot maintain the selected drop rate.
2. The drops are not detected by the "catseye" sensor.
3. The intravenous has infiltrated.
4. The bottle is empty.
5. There is crimped tubing.

The IVAC controller has proved a valuable asset not only in delivery of chemotherapy drugs at a desired rate of flow, but also in anesthesiology, labor control, and cardiac treatment. It has been used in various kinds of fluid therapy, such as hyperalimentation.

The IVAC 500 is used for arterial infusion of drugs for treatment of solid tumors, such as for primary or metastatic tumors of the liver.

The Holter pump (Extracorporeal Medical Specialties), series 900, is a small lightweight pump that has an integral rechargeable battery but that can also operate with AC current. It can control flow rates within the range of 2.5 ml per hour to 210 ml per hour. Its accuracy is ±3 per cent. The fluid is stretched over rotating rollers. The flow rate is selected by setting the dial, which locks in place to prevent accidental change in flow rate, to control the rotor speed. One primary advantage of the Holter pump is that when patients leave the unit for treatment or studies the flow rate is not interrupted.

The catheter site needs frequent observation for signs of infiltration, which can be extensive, because of the positive pressure of the pump. Positive pressure infusion carries the risk of air embolism. It is essential to prevent the bottle from running dry. There is no automatic shutoff or alarm; therefore a potential danger exists of air being pumped into the vascular system (Cort, 1970). One institution offset this possible hazard by using a second "piggy back" bottle to serve as a safeguard.

Immunotherapy

Immunotherapy of human cancer is currently under investigation. Several techniques are being studied. One technique is active immunization (see Chapter 10). In this technique tumor cells from the patient or from other patients with a similar type of tumor are used to extract soluble antigens from them after they have been rendered inactive by radiotherapy or cytotoxic drugs. These antigens are used for specific active immunization. Another method of active specific immunization involves tissue culturing the patient's tumor cells and placing the patient's lymphocytes in contact with the cultured tumor cells. This process is called "immunogenic training" and the lymphocytes are subsequently reinfused into the patient (del Regato, 1977).

Some substances are used as active nonspecific immunizations because they produce general stimulation of the immune response. A common example of this is Bacillus Calmette Guerin (BCG). The BCG vaccine is applied via a skin scarification technique or it may be injected into the tumor (del Regato, 1977). Some success in using BCG has been reported in treating acute lymphocytic and myelocytic leukemia, chronic myelocytic leukemia, and malignant melanoma (Best et al., 1974).

Controlled Environments

HOST. Patients receiving radiation therapy and/or chemotherapy frequently have their white blood cell counts drop to dangerously low levels. Nurses

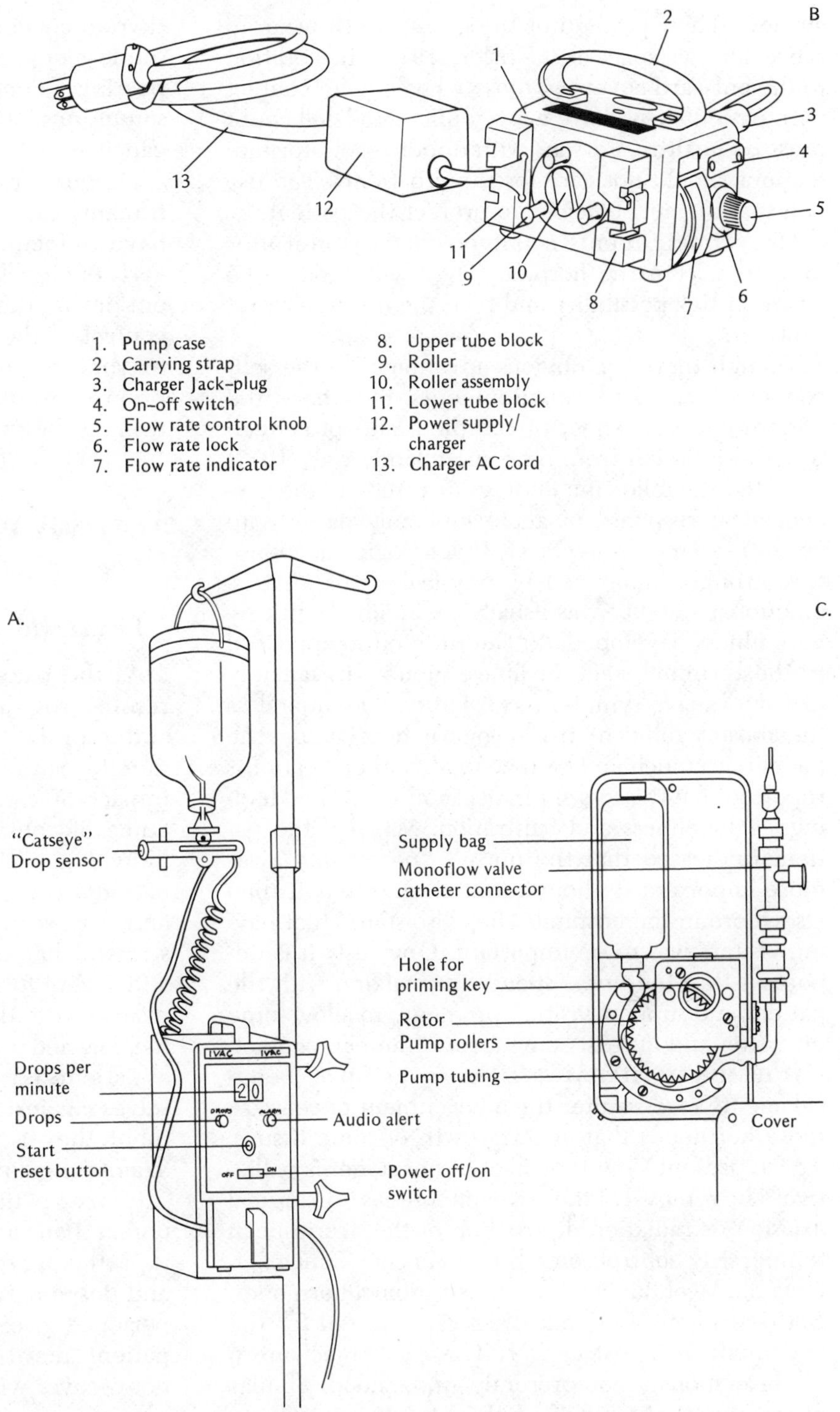

Figure 39-3. A. Diagram of IVAC controller (Adapted with permission of IVAC Corporation, San Diego, Calif.) B. Diagram of the Holter pump (Holter® 900 Series Pump). (Photograph was supplied through the courtesy of Extracorporeal Medical Specialties, Inc., Royal & Ross Roads, King of Prussia, Pa. 19406.) C. Diagram of the Chronofusor. (Adapted with permission of USCI, a division of C. R. Bard, Inc., Billerica, Mass.)

need to observe the laboratory results for this occurrence. Some institutions automatically place patients in reverse isolation when their white blood cell count drops below 2,000 cells per cubic millimeter. The reason for this isolation should be carefully explained to the patient and visitors. Self-contained germ-free units are designed and used at some cancer treatment centers. Such environments are useful in the treatment of patients who are taking chemotherapeutic agents that cause leukopenia (Yates & Holland, 1973). The purpose of such units is to minimize patients' exposure to infectious organisms.

At Roswell Park Memorial Hospital "germ-free" units are in operation. All materials within the unit are sterile, and cross-contamination from the nurse to the patient is prevented by the laminar (vertical) air flow. Those who enter these units must wear an attire like a "space suit" (Isler, 1972). In addition to the outward covering, those who come in contact with patients who have a low white blood cell count must be healthy. Persons with upper respiratory infections should not care for these patients. The use of a mask is not sufficient to protect the patient.

Many times patients' counts do not drop until after discharge from the hospital. They will need to be aware of this possibility and take the necessary precautions.

Though there are obvious advantages to the self-contained germ-free environments, they have the undesirable side effect of complete and prolonged physical isolation from others. Holland et al. (1977) reported the following findings in a study of the psychological response of acute leukemia patients to germ-free environments: (1) Psychological response was strongly influenced by physical status; that is, emotional stability was usually maintained until severe illness developed. (2) Delirium often appeared in the terminal stage of illness along with anxiety and depressive symptoms. (3) Patients identified as the most significant psychological deprivation the inability to touch and be touched by others. Patients reported that this loss of physical contact caused feelings of loneliness and frustration. Many of the patients indicated that the nurse's "personality" was more important to them in the germ-free unit than elsewhere in the hospital. They also stated that having visitors was more important. Obviously it is important that the nurse spend time talking with the patient and support visiting privileges to allow some diversion and at least some form of human contact.

HORMONAL THERAPY. The main group of chemical agents used to alter the environment of cells are those hormones that affect growth of some tissues. At the present time the effect of hormones is palliative. The removal of the estrogen sources (by surgical excision or radiation destruction of the ovaries) can temporarily control some breast cancers. Similar effects can be obtained by administration of hormones. Both estrogens and androgens can be used for the treatment of breast cancer. The exact mechanism of the action is not presently understood. Similar effects can be obtained with these hormones in treatment of cancer of the prostate. Adrenocortical hormones such as cortisone can also induce remission of these tumors as well as temporary control of some forms of leukemia and lymphoma.

Because a number of agents are capable of producing such tumor remissions, the fact that the patient no longer responds to one of the previously effective agents does not mean that he or she will not be responsive to another. Thyroid hormone has recently been shown to be effective in suppression of thyroid cancers in young individuals. For some reason it is not effective in treatment of identically appearing cancers in older patients. Progesterone sometimes helps patients with endometrial or renal cancers.

Despite progress in the control of cancer much remains to be accomplished. Not all patients who have an incurable form of the disease are diagnosed early enough to receive maximum benefit from present-day methods. New methods are required for the control of the types of cancer that do not respond to surgery, radiation, or chemotherapy. Further progress awaits greater knowledge of the factors controlling the growth of normal cells.

Tertiary Prevention: Continuity of Care

Living with Cancer

As the patient recovers, he or she is helped to resume responsibility for meeting personal needs and to prepare to return to the family and the community. Sutherland, in discussing the psychological impact of cancer surgery, emphasizes the importance of considering every patient in the light of individual problems. Each person makes an individual adjustment to the kind of cancer experienced and its treatment. Sutherland et al. (1952) also stresses that the cancer patient is under a special and severe form of stress. The psychological mechanisms of the defense ultilized are those the patient has learned to use in coping with the world. Just as patients use avoidance and denial to defend themselves against anxiety before diagnosis and treatment, they use it after surgery to protect themselves against the anxiety induced by the therapy.

Cancer patients have been observed to use more denial than cardiac patients; it is speculated the goal is protecting themselves from a reality of frustration and despair (Levine & Ziegler, 1975). They also experience grief, depression, and dependency. Some patients may be so seriously depressed that they cannot recover without help. For most patients, depression is a forerunner of recovery. Instead of becoming depressed, some patients express their anger by projecting their feelings to the members of the family and the nursing personnel.

In cancer and its treatment, many factors may cause psychological stress. The fact that the disease is cancer rather than some other disease is one. Stress is particularly likely to arise out of treatment when the effects of treatment are obvious or when a bodily function is altered in a way that is obvious to the individual and/or to others. The patient often experiences shock when he or she realizes the extent of the operation or the nature of the change in function. He or she becomes concerned about how this change in appearance or function will affect relationships with family members, friends, and co-workers. This concern extends to how this change is going to affect the ability to make a living.

The Family

In the study by Sutherland et al. (1952) of the problems in living created by colostomy and what patients did to solve these problems, the authors emphasize that one of the most significant factors is a supportive spouse or home situation. The adjustment of the patient was in general more rapid and more satisfactory when the husband and wife relationship was favorable. In families where the relationship had been poor before the colostomy was performed, the relationship deteriorated after it. These findings point to the desirability of utilizing family members whose feelings toward the patient are positive in his or her rehabilitation. Nurses are not responsible for the nature of family relationships of their patients, but they can and do observe these relationships. This information can be used in planning to meet the needs of the patient. Recognition of the importance of the family to the rehabilitation of the patient should result in including them in plans made to meet the needs of the patient. Sutherland et al., 1952, p. 868) state that the family must understand the needs of the patient and why they are important if they are to give him or her adequate support. The family may require considerable interpretation. To fulfill their supportive role, family members need to have their efforts recognized and appreciated.

Giacquinta (1977) had identified four stages families must face in coping with cancer: (1) living with cancer, (2) restructuring the living-dying interval, (3) bereavement, (4) re-establishment. At this time only Stage I will be discussed. The remainder of the stages will be discussed with terminality. For each phase Ciacquinta identifies phases through which the family must progress, hurdles they must overcome, and goals of nursing intervention for each phase-hurdle combination.

In Stage I, living with cancer, the family must deal with the impact of learning the cancer diagnosis, overcome the functional disruptions caused by the role dilemmas related to the cancer illness, attempt to gain intellectual mastery over the cancer process by searching for meaning and reassurance that it cannot happen to another family member, inform others of the diagnosis, and acknowledge emotions related to profound changes caused by the diagnosis of cancer. Goals of nursing intervention for Stage I include: fostering hope, for example, by fostering hope in the treatment approaches being used or by encouraging families to separate thoughts and feelings; fostering cohesion by promoting use of family support systems, interaction among members, and co-operation; fostering security by supporting the family system in maintaining its identity, integrity, and continuity; fostering courage by supporting within-family communication and support of each other; fostering problem solving by supporting and encouraging the family in continuing to make daily decisions and assisting them to recognize that they are making them (Giacquinta, 1977).

The Nurse and Stage I

Sutherland et al. (1952) also reported that patients regarded a warm and supporting relationship with the nurses as important in changing their attitude and aiding in their recovery. The desire of the nurse to be helpful and willingness to devise measures that improve the feeling of well-being of the patient are imperative. Attention to details that increase the physical comfort of the patient is sometimes neglected. Because lower needs must be met before higher needs can be manifested, the undernourished or dehydrated patient cannot be expected to feel encouraged; neither can the patient whose bed is wet with urine or feces. As an illustration, Mrs. Karlin had an ileostomy in the treatment of chronic ulcerative colitis. She wore an ileostomy bag that was glued to the skin with a type of adhesive. For the seal to be effective, both the skin and the rubber disk that attached to the skin had to be perfectly clean. Any soiling of either meant that the intestinal contents leaked under the rubber disk and out onto the skin of the abdomen, thus soiling her clothing and the bed linen. Because the contents of the ileum are liquid, enzymes contained in them come in intimate contact with the skin and cause irritation. Continuously wet or moist skin also loses its resistance to irritation. Mrs. Karlin was asked to speak to a group of nurses about the quality of care that she received. Her major criticism stemmed from the fact that, until her physician taught her to care for the apparatus herself, she was never dry. After she assumed responsibility for her own care, she was never again wet. This patient suffered psychological stress and physical injury not because nurses were unkind or unfriendly but because a basic physical need was neglected.

To be helpful, the nurse must be able to allow the patient to become dependent without becoming unduly anxious. She or he must also be able to tolerate projection of the negative feelings of the patient and still remain accepting and kindly. This is not always easy to do, especially when the nurse has tried very hard to meet the needs and wants of a patient who still continues to be critical and dissatisfied. The behavior of the patient is, however, his or her way of coping with an intolerable situation. The nurse who can accept it as such is in a better position to be helpful to the patient. Such nurses will have less need to punish the patient or themselves for the patient's behavior. One nurse was able to help herself when she was caring for a highly critical patient by saying to herself, "There must be a reason, there must be a reason." To her surprise, when the nurse had convinced herself that the behavior of the patient was reasonable, her relationship with the patient improved.

Another technique that sometimes helps is a group conference in which persons responsible for the care of a patient discuss the nature of the problem presented by the patient. Knowing that others are also aware of the problem is often of help. Conferences may involve only the nursing staff on the unit, or they may include members from the interdisciplinary team. The purpose is essentially the same, planning together to develop methods of meeting patients' needs.

Observation of the behavior of the patient is also the responsibility of the nurse. Continued disruption in sleeping and eating patterns after the acute phase of illness or treatment is indicative of depression. Depression may also be accompanied by disturbances in cardiovascular function, which is evidenced by tachycardia and palpitation. Patients, especially women, often cry. Although some depression is to be expected, severe or prolonged depression is not (see Chapter 19).

To summarize, a warm and friendly relationship between the nurses and patients facilitates recovery. This relationship is characterized by mutual trust. The patients know that they and their welfare are important to the nurses and that insofar as possible the nurses will try to meet their needs.

In the restoration of the patient to health, attention must be given to the physiologic needs of the patient. If the neoplasm has been in the gastrointestinal tract or has affected its function, the patient may be both dehydrated and undernourished. Loss of weight, fatigue, and weakness may be evident. Anemia present before surgery may be a continuing problem. The ingenuity of the nursing and dietary staff is often taxed in finding ways to improve the nutritional status of the patient. In addition to trying to serve the patient foods that he or she can and will eat, a number of other activities may be helpful. One is to be sure that the patient who wears dentures has them and that they are clean. Exercise improves not only muscle tone but also morale and the appetite. Ventilation of the room and getting the patient into a chair or into a position that facilitates eating may be of help. Eating in a community dining room may create a social atmosphere conducive to eating. Continued refusal of the patient to eat may be evidence of depression.

In addition to the psychological and physiologic rehabilitation of the patient, the patient is helped to resume responsibilities for the daily activities of living and for special requirements that result from having or having had, cancer and from its treatment. As the patient resumes increasing responsibility for meeting his or her own needs, the nurse should try to communicate that (1) the shift indicates progress toward recovery, (2) the nurse is standing by to give assistance if the patient really needs it, (3) the nurse has faith in the patient's ability to care for himself or herself, (4) the nurse will not interfere with the patient's efforts unnecessarily, (5) the nurse appreciates the struggle that he or she is making, and (6) recognizes successful efforts.

The nurse should try to avoid any behavior that suggests to patients that responsibility for their care is shifted to them because the nurse is too busy or does not want to care for them. The nurse should be sure that the patients know what is expected of them and what they should expect. She or he is also responsible for supervising patients' care so that their needs are met.

Transfer from Hospital to Home

To meet the needs of patients who have cancer more effectively, nurses must make ongoing assessments. It is imperative that the nurse be aware of the home situation. With whom does the patient live? Who will care for him or her at home? Does the patient even have a home? Unless nurses have visited patients in their homes they cannot begin to realize the problems the patient may encounter. There may be no family or significant others who can assist the patient in the home. Such things as bathing, preparing meals, doing housework, caring for children, or climbing stairs may be impossible for the patient. Intricate planning must be accomplished to afford maximum support for patients who are too well to be in the hospital but are too sick or weak to perform the normal activities of daily living.

Physicians and nurses need to teach patients concerning their diagnosis, procedures, equipment, medications, and activity. As an example, Mrs. Kelly, who was discharged following an almost 3-month hospitalization, exclaimed: "Oh, what is really confusing me is when to take my pills. You know here in the hospital the nurses brought them to me, and I didn't pay any attention to the times." Such confusion can be alleviated by making a chart for the patient, listing the name of the drug and possibly even the color or taping one of the pills to the chart in that place, writing in the times it is to be taken, and making a workable schedule for the patient. An X can be placed in the square or the time the drug was taken if it is a PRN medication. This chart can be taken to the physician on subsequent visits and will serve as a guide for increasing or decreasing medication. This is a simple chart that can be made several days in advance of discharge, or hospitals could have available preprinted forms for use by all patients who are discharged with medication.

Another example is Mrs. Black, who had colon carcinoma with liver metastasis. She was receiving chemotherapy through a transabdominal hepatic artery catheter, by means of a Watkins pump. She became very depressed and expressed some of her fears to a nurse in the outpatient department. She didn't know how she was progressing, or if the medication was doing any good. She was worried because she had no appetite and was continually nauseated. She did not know the side effects of her chemotherapy and she found it difficult to communicate with her doctor. She was fearful of pulling out the hepatic artery catheter, therefore she did not attempt even small chores at home. She had not been out shopping in several weeks. The nurse was able to be an advocate for the patient, discussed her concerns with the doctor, who was able to alleviate her fear of pulling out the hepatic artery catheter. Mrs. Black experienced unnecessary mental anguish. If there had been open communication between the doctor, nurse, and patient about the pump, the security of the catheter, her medications, and activity, she might have been less fearful. Mrs. Black also would have benefited by having a visiting nurse after she was discharged.

Before being dismissed, the patient should learn to carry out required procedures. The groundwork for the instruction of the patient begins when he or she first contacts members of the health team with a suspicion of illness and continues throughout all phases of care. By the time the patient is ready to be taught to care for personal needs he or she should have developed confidence in nurses and physicians. The nurses and physicians should also know what the patients want to know, what they already know, and something about their home and work situation, as well as their goals. The instructor should know that people learn more slowly when they are excessively anxious (see Chapter 19 and Unit VII). The instructor should be prepared to repeat over and over, patiently and simply, the instructions to be followed. The nurse who instructs the patient should also be skilled in the performance of the procedure being taught to the patient; otherwise, the patient will distrust the nurse and may even hold her or him in contempt. The patient should practice the procedure with the equipment and materials that are available at home, and he or she should learn how to care for the equipment. Enough time should be allotted for practice so that the patient has an opportunity to develop some degree of confidence in his or her ability to cope with the required procedures.

All cancer patients require some discharge planning, though, some require less than others. The needs for discharge planning arise from the cancer disease process itself, the medical regimen, procedures which have been performed or will be performed, surgical interventions either curative or palliative, nursing diagnoses and nursing regimens, and various factors of the patient's home environment including psychosociocultural and economic factors.

Nursing Management

Nursing management of a nursing diagnosis of impairment and/or lack of knowledge is again very important in discharge planning. Specific areas of knowledge deficits which the nurse must address include: (1) Medications for pain and chemotherapeutic agents. It is important that the patient be aware of safe use of the drugs and side effects and measures to minimize side effects. (2) Treatments to be done in the home or on an outpatient basis. For example, the patient and family must be taught to care for skin lesions whether from metastasis, decubitus ulcer, or radiation therapy. If the patient is receiving radiation therapy, he or she should be informed about how to minimize skin damage (see Chapter 49) and of side effects and measures to relieve them. (3) Diet and nutrition. Nutrition for the cancer patient will be handled in more detail later, but it should be pointed out here that the nurse is responsible for teaching the cancer patient about nutritional need and requirements. (4) Community resources. The nurse is responsible for informing the patient and family of resources in the community from which they can get help. Food supplements, supplies, and equipment are available through the American Cancer Society and local cancer foundations, for example, in Michigan, the Michigan Cancer Foundation.

VISITING NURSE SERVICE. In communities where a visiting nurse service is available, referral of the patient to this agency should help the patient to bridge the gap between the hospital and the home. Problems that did not occur to the patient earlier may arise; minor adjustments may assume major proportions. Even patients (and their families) who seem to be well prepared for discharge frequently require some help and emotional support after discharge. In cities where home care programs are available, co-operation between the hospital and visiting nursing service often makes possible the early discharge of patients. In some instances a home care program reduces the cost of illness and facilitates the rate at which the patient recovers. When a patient is discharged from the hospital early, supervision of his or her care and provisions for required assistance become imperative.

In some communities, persons who have had surgical procedures such as colostomy or laryngectomy are organized into a society for the purpose of mutual support. Members of these organizations are eager to assist persons facing surgery and to aid in their adjustment afterward. In some areas, classes are available for laryngectomized patients to learn esophageal speech. Physicians may arrange for a person who has made a successful adjustment to laryngectomy or colostomy to visit each patient who is facing a similar procedure and to continue visits thereafter. The Reach to Recovery Program of the American Cancer Society is a rehabiliatation program for women who have had breast surgery. Upon authorization of her physician a volunteer, who is a mastectomee, will visit patients, either in the hospital or at home, who have had breast surgery. Nurses may also make these arrangements. When they do, they should be acquainted with the wishes of the physician as well as with the nature of the adjustment made by the person called upon to help. Information about local organizations can be obtained from the local division of the American Cancer Society.

In the care of the patient with cancer, the objectives are to eradicate the disease and to assist the patient in returning to as normal a life as the condition permits. To meet the patient's needs during detection, diagnosis, and treatment, attention should be given to (1) needs as an individual, (2) needs resulting from cancer and its effects, (3) needs resulting from the method of treatment, and (4) needs resulting from the effects of the treatment on the emotional and physiologic condition of the patient.

Employing the Person with Cancer. Patients may express concern to nurses or physicians about remaining in their same positions at work or being rehired elsewhere. Employers also may have concerns about patients with cancer being a liability. Based on a 14-year study by the Metropolitan Life Insurance Company, indications are that persons who are treated for cancer can be selectively hired for positions for which they are physically qualified. Their work performance is comparable to that of others who are hired at the same age for like assignments. It further revealed that company expense was not increased noticeably by excessive absences, reduced productivity, or increased mortality (Metropolitan Life Insurance Company, *Statistical Bulletin*, 1973).

The Nurse's Responsibility in Caring for Patients with Widespread and Progressive Disease. At the time of diagnosis or at any point thereafter, cancer may be found to be widespread and progressive. Hope for cure or even for prolonging the life of the patient is not expected; that is, death is the probable outcome. For this reason this phase in the life of the cancer patient is called terminal. The use of the word *terminal* is unfortunate as it suggests that the patient's situation is hopeless, whereas this phase may extend over weeks, months, or years. The result has been that patients in this phase of illness have been and still are neglected. The tendency has been to give preference to those in whom cure is a possibility. Despite the improbability of cure, nurses can do a great deal to improve the condition and the well-being of the patient.

The basic ingredient in the care of the patient with widespread and progressive disease is the firm conviction that much can and must be done to help the patient. Emphasis is placed not on cure but on what can be done. Hope is encouraged, not hopelessness and despair. Objectives for the patient's care are (1) to encourage and support the patient's efforts to remain independent and useful, (2) to maintain physiologic function, and (3) to prevent and relieve suffering. As is often the case, some of the same procedures contribute to the accomplishment of more than one objective and are appropriate in all stages of the disease.

Common problem areas seen in cancer patients at any stage of the cancer process, but especially in patients where the disease is widespread and progressive include information, coping, comfort, nutrition, mobility, elimination, protective mechanisms, ventilation, and terminality (ANA, 1979). In providing nursing service to these patients, several nursing diagnoses related to these problem areas present themselves and must be managed. Following is a discussion of common nursing diagnoses made when caring for cancer patients with widespread and progressive disease, the goals of care, and nursing orders (Campbell et al., 1979).

Information

For the patient problem area of information, the obvious nursing diagnosis to be made is impairment and/or lack of knowledge. Nursing goals of care include (1) provision of information, interpretation and clarification of the cancer disease process so that the patient and family can attain maximal self-management and participate in decisions of care and (2) reduction of anxiety resulting from lack of factual information. Nursing orders in managing a cancer patient with this diagnosis include (1) assessing the information and misinformation the patient and family have about the disease process and therapy; (2) assessing the patient's and family's previous experience with cancer; (3) teaching related to the disease and its impact on the body, effects of therapy and possible side effects, and community and personal resources that can provide information and/or services; (4) repeating information as often as necessary for comprehension and when appropriate giving written instructions related to the care.

Coping

Coping is a major patient problem area (see Chapter 19 and Unit VII). As discussed earlier, the emotional stressors can be overwhelming. Common nursing diagnoses manifested in this area include alteration/impairment in individual coping, alteration/impairment in family coping, grieving, and disruption of spiritual integrity.

Altered or impaired individual coping in the cancer patient is frequently related to emotional depression, hostility, shame, despair, denial, fear, or anxiety. These responses are common and are in reaction to the diagnosis of cancer (Mundinger, 1978). Nursing goals in assisting such patients include (1) promotion of functional coping mechanisms to achieve individual homeodynamics and (2) promotion of individual development and maintenance of a positive concept of self, significant others, and environment. To accomplish these goals, the nurse must (1) assess for failing coping processes; (2) establish a rapport and trusting relationship with the patient; and (3) encourage the patient to verbalize thoughts and feelings concerning his or her condition.

Families too face a crisis when cancer becomes widespread and assaults the integrity of the family system (Giacquinta, 1977). Nursing goals in managing a nursing diagnosis of altered or impaired family coping include (1) promotion of open communication among family members; (2) promotion of identification of and performance of care needs; (3) promotion of family support of patient and each other. Nursing orders include (1) family assessment of response to the patient with the cancer diagnosis; (2) exploration with the patient and family of their need-response patterns of communication by assisting them to recognize expectations of each other, encouraging them to express resentments concerning the patient's diagnosis and illness, and assisting them in planning for redistribution of roles and tasks; (3) assistance of family members to problem solve and make decisions; (4) as necessary, referral to community counseling services.

Grieving can be a very normal, healthful response unless it is unresolved (see Unit VII). The cancer patient and each family member are at risk for a nursing diagnosis of grieving because each faces real and/or threatened losses related to the disease process, such as, loss of life, loss of body part(s), loss of a loved one, and loss of functional abilities. Nursing goals for managing patient and family grieving include (1) promotion of the patient's and family's passage through the grief process to resolution while maintaining personal integrity and (2) provision of assistance to the family in identification of the need for and implementation of family reorganization necessitated by the patient's illness. Nursing orders include (1) assessing the patient's and family's degree of incapacitation or destructiveness; (2) having the patient and family define the loss (actual or threatened); (3) encouraging expression of feelings and thoughts concerning fears and sadness associated with loss or change; (4) altering the environment to make it as pleasant and secure as possible through use of lighting, music, and personal belongings.

Cancer patients, especially those with widespread disease, are likely to struggle with basic spiritual factors such as the meaning of life and death, questioning why this illness happened to them or doubting the compassion of a Superior Being. If a nursing diagnosis of disruption of spiritual integity is made, the nurse's primary goal is to assist the patient and family to explore the meaning of the patient's illness within the context of their spiritual belief in an attempt to achieve a sense of peace and comfort. Nursing orders include (1) identification of spiritual beliefs before illness and changes since illness; (2) provision of a safe nonjudgmental atmosphere; (3) encouraging expression of feelings related to the relationship between illness and spiritual beliefs and practices; (4) referral as appropriate, for example, to a clergyman (see Chapters 7, 19, and Unit VII).

Comfort

Comfort is a significant problem area for cancer patients. Nursing diagnoses made in this area are dependent on the severity of symptoms and will be either alteration in comfort-discomfort or alteration in comfort-pain. Refer to the previous discussion in this chapter for the nursing management of the cancer patient with a nursing diagnosis of pain.

Nutrition

Because of increased caloric demand by tumors and the nausea, vomiting, and anorexia which frequently accompanies the disease process and many of the antitumor therapies, nutrition becomes a significant cancer patient problem. Common nutrition-related nursing diagnoses which present themselves are altered nutritional requirements–less than required and body fluids depletion—dehydration.

Nursing goals for a diagnosis of altered nutritional requirements–less than required include (1) reversal of the malnourished/catabolic state and (2) restoration of adequate nutrition to all cells. Nursing orders include (1) ongoing assessment of the patient's nutritional state using parameters such as height, weight, measurement of arm muscle circumference, and measurement of triceps skin fold; (2) implementation of techniques of nutritional support such as (a) Implementing measures which enhance food intake and retention for patients with intact intestinal function; for example, mouth care before meals, small feedings of favorite foods, use of oral antiemetics one-half hour before meals or injections 10 to 20 minutes before meals, high protein, high caloric foods, and varied flavors and consistency of foods. (b) Administering parenteral nutrition to restore the anabolic state may become necessary if the patient is unable to consume sufficient nutrients orally or by tube. Total parenteral nutrition (TPN) generally refers to intravenous hyperalimentation of a hypertonic dextrose, crystalline amino acid solution through the subclavian vein. The TNP must be ordered by the physician, but the nurse is responsible for caring for the patient when he or she is receiving it (see Chapter 46).

If the patient's mouth is sore because of stomatitis, an order for an anesthetic mouth rinse should be obtained from the physician. The patient who has stomatitis should avoid highly seasoned foods and citrus foods and juices. Bland foods, puddings, ice creams, eggs, and soft foods may cause less distress. Commercially available instant breakfasts may also be used. These contain many of the minimum daily requirements. It is important to remember to plan the diet regimen to be consistent with the patient's and family's cultural, social, and ethnic practices and in line with any other prescribed special diets. Food supplements may be used to ensure adequate food intake; for example, commercial liquid or powdered food supplements including instant breakfast. Supplemental elemental diets may also be used.

It may become necessary to provide nutrition for the patient via gastric tube feeding. Commercially prepared feedings can be used or tube feedings can be prepared by blenderizing an appropriate diet.

Dietitians and nurses collaborating with the patient can most effectively arrive at decisions about foods the patient can and will eat. If the patient needs to be fed, nursing personnel should be available to feed him or her while the food is hot. Cold food loses its appeal.

Hyperalimentation

Some consideration is being given to the feasibility and potential advantages of sending cancer patients home on hyperalimentation. Suggested advantages include maintenance of nutrition despite the gastrointestinal toxic side effects of antitumor chemotherapies and radiation. There is a positive correlation between nutritional status and potential for response to chemotherapy (Englert & Dudrick, 1978). As yet, however, TPN for cancer patients at home is not a common practice primarily because of cost (Englert & Dudrick, 1978) and because it entails more risks such as infection than other techniques.

Fluid Intake

In the cancer patient, a nursing diagnosis of body fluids depletion-dehydration is usually secondary to the patient's inability to ingest and/or retain adequate fluids and nutrients. Nursing goals for such patients include (1) maintenance of a fluid balance which facilitates optimal hydration and (2) prevention of fluid and electrolyte imbalance. Primary nursing orders include (1) ongoing assessment of the patient's hydration status and (2) implementing of measures that will increase fluid intake, for example, modifying flavors, frequently offering the patient small sips of fluid, using ice chips, foods high in water content such as citrus fruits and melons, fluids of varied consistency such as popsicles, soups, jello, and ice cream.

Mobility

Mobility can become a serious problem area for cancer patients. Limited mobility in patients with widespread disease frequently results from weakness related to poor nutrition or from cord compression caused by metastatic tumors to the spine, usually in the epidural space. The symptoms experienced by the patient are neck, back, and root pain, and slowly or rapidly progressive quadriplegia or paraplegia. Motor weakness usually precedes the development of numbness. Sphincter control is impaired or may be lost by the time there is moderate or severe weakness in the extremities. In cord compression there is most often a sensory loss that is caudal at the beginning and that slowly rises to the level of the lesion. X-rays of the spine and myelograms are used to locate the area of metastatic disease in the spine and spinal canal. These tumors occur most often in the thoracic region. If the pressure on the cord is relieved in less than 24 hours after the occurrence of paraplegia, the paraplegia is usually reversible. It is essential that signs and symptoms be recognized early and that treatment begin promptly. (*Rehabilitation of the Cancer Patient,* 1972). Mobility and function are affected in patients who have bone metastasis and are predisposed to developing pathologic features. Most of these fractures involve the femur of the hip. Internal fixation and radiation therapy are generally the choice of treatment.

Nurses can teach patients who have bone metastasis certain measures to decrease the incidence of fractures. They should be cautioned against falling, climbing on chairs, lifting heavy objects, reaching, and twisting. Women who have small children should be encouraged to let the child crawl up on their laps, rather than lifting them. Many patients have found vacuuming and carrying groceries difficult to accomplish (McCorkle, 1973). Nurses need to be aware of possible dangers in the patient's environment and develop measures to prevent, or decrease the incidence of pathologic fractures.

Nursing Diagnoses and Orders

Frequent nursing diagnoses made in the problem area of mobility are impairment in mobility and variation in functional performance. The primary goal of nursing management for a diagnosis of impairment in mobility is promotion of safety and optimal mobility and independence consistent with limitations imposed by illness. Nursing orders include (1) implementation of an activity/exercise schedule (collaboration with physical therapy and occupational therapy is very helpful in planning an activity exercise schedule); (2) implementing a skin care program as necessary (see following discussion on nursing diagnosis of impaired skin/mucous membranes); (3) implementing a pain control program (refer to previous discussion on management of pain in the cancer patient); (4) modifying the environment as necessary to be as safe as possible; for example use of an electric bed, trapeze bar, transfer board, and placing necessary objects within reach; (5) teaching the patient and family good body mechanics, bathroom safety (shower chair, rubber mats, safety bars, elevated toilet seat) and energy saving techniques.

Often the cancer patient has an altered ability to participate in self-care activity, for example, a patient with cancer of the right breast who has excessive lymphedema will be restricted. For such patients a nursing diagnosis of variation in functional performance is appropriate. The primary nursing goal is promotion of the patient's participation in personal and therapeutic self-care activities consistent with limitations imposed by illness. Nursing orders include (1) ongoing assessment of the patient's functional status; (2) encouragement of the patient to perform those activities which he or she can; (3) provision of necessary assistive equipment, for example, overhead trapeze, wheelchair, walker, elevated toilet seat, bathroom bars, and tub mat; (4) collaboration with occupational and physical therapy as necessary; (5) use diversional activities; (6) patient and family teaching concerning use of equipment and resources for obtaining equipment in the home, causes of patient's limitations and measures to correct and/or manage, such as positioning, transfer, and energy saving techniques.

Elimination

Alterations in elimination, both urinary and bowel, are seen in cancer patients. These alterations are a result of direct tumor growth, metastasis, or cord compression, or they may result from therapeutic measures such as surgery (colostomy and ileal conduit) or side effects of radiation and chemotherapy (anorexia, nausea, vomiting which all cause fluid loss).

A nursing diagnosis of alteration in urinary elimination should state specifically what the alteration is, for example, retention, incontinence, or diversional method. Nursing goals should be directed at the specific problem, but generally should prevent and/or control the alteration in urinary elimination in a manner that promotes optimal renal function and comfort. Nursing orders should include (1) ongoing observation of the quality and quantity of urine; (2) implementing of measures to promote urinary output and/or correct urinary alteration and its effects, such as prescribed medications, dietary and fluid regimens, and use of assistive devices such as urethral catheters.

Some cancer patients, especially those with cancer of the bladder or tumors obstructing the urinary system, will have a diversional method of urinary elimination such as an ileal conduit, ureteral catheters, nephrostomy tubes, or suprapubic catheters. If a nursing diagnosis of altered urinary elimination-diversional method is made, the primary nursing goals are (1) maintenance of urinary output necessary to facilitate optimal renal function and prevent urinary tract infection (see Chapter 38) and (2) facilitation of safe management of the diversional method of urinary elimination. Nursing orders include (1) ongoing assessment of the status and function of the diversional method; (2) evaluation of the effectiveness of the catheter or stoma appliance; (3) observation of the quality and quantity of urine; (4) careful attention to skin care around the stoma; (5) patient and family teaching regarding *(a)* adequate urinary elimination and the need to report changes; *(b)* measures to promote maintenance of urinary output such as adequate fluid intake; *(c)* catheter irrigations and medications, techniques for managing the diversional method such as skin care, irrigations, hygienic measures; *(d)* resources for obtaining equipment and supplies; *(e)* adaptation techniques for sexual activity as appropriate.

Alterations in bowel elimination as constipation, diarrhea, or diversional methods are seen in cancer patients. A nursing diagnosis of alteration in bowel elimination-diversional method (usually colostomy or ileostomy) is commonly associated with tumors, primary or metastatic, of the bowel which necessitate surgical resection and a colostomy or ileostomy procedure. The primary nursing goal for a nursing diagnosis of alteration in elimination-diversional method is promotion of safe management of the diversional method in a manner consistent with the patient's life style. Nursing orders include (1) ongoing assessment of the status and function of the diversional method including observation of the quantity and nature of the ostomy drainage; (2) inspection of the stoma and skin care around the stoma including cleansing, thorough drying, use of skin shields such as stomahesive or Karaya rings and absorbant powders such as Karaya powder; (3) referral to community resources such as the American Cancer Society or local cancer foundations for informational materials, dressings, supplies and to local groups such as ostomy clubs for support; (4) patient and family teaching concerning adequate bowel elimination and need to report changes, techniques for managing the diversional method such as skin care, irrigation procedures, hygienic measures, stoma dilation, adaptation techniques for sexual activity if necessary and appropriate, measures to promote elimination such as adequate fluid intake, physical activity, and preventing flatus or odor by avoiding foods such as cabbage, corn, nuts, carbonated beverages, chewing gum, onions, beans, fish, and asparagus.

A nursing diagnosis of alteration in bowel elimination-diarrhea in cancer patients is frequently related to chemotherapy, radiation therapy, bowel obstruction, infectious process in the bowel, stress, or diet. Nursing goals are directed at (1) prevention and/or control of diarrhea in a manner that promotes optimal bowel function and comfort and (2) maintenance of fluid and electrolyte balance. Nursing orders include (1) regular assessment of the quantity, quality, and frequency of bowel elimination; (2) implementation of measures to control the diarrhea such as *(a)* providing a diet to increase calories and decrease peristalsis (high protein, high carbohydrate, bland, low residue), *(b)* decreasing the patient's stress if possible, *(c)* administering prescribed medications, such as anticholinergic drugs and tranquilizers; (3) monitoring intake and output; (4) providing skin care as needed (thorough cleansing and drying, use of powder and emollients); (5) offering patient and family teaching regarding *(a)* causes of patient's diarrhea, *(b)* factors that contribute to the diarrhea, and *(c)* measures to control the diarrhea.

A nursing diagnosis of alteration in bowel elimination-constipation in cancer patients is usually related to such factors as bowel obstruction, lack of bulk or poor fluid intake in the diet, or decreased mobility. The primary nursing goal is the prevention and/or control of constipation in a manner that promotes optimal bowel function and comfort. Nursing orders include (1) regular assessment of bowel function; (2) implementation of measures to control and/or prevent constipation such as *(a)* diet regimen of increased fluids and foods higher in residue, *(b)* physical activity and exercise program, *(c)* stool softeners, laxatives, exercise program, *(d)* encouragement of a regular time for evacuation; and (3) patient and family teaching regarding causes of the constipation, factors that contribute to constipation, and measures to promote bowel elimination.

Protective Mechanisms

Protective mechanisms such as the immune, hematopoietic, integumentary, and sensory-motor systems are affected by the cancer disease process and/or therapy. Common nursing diagnoses concerning protective mechanisms made in cancer patients include alteration in protective mechanism-infection, alteration in composition of body fluids, and impairment in skin/mucosal integrity.

A nursing diagnosis of alteration in protective mechanism-infection can be seen in patients receiving radiation therapy or chemotherapy as a complication of the bone marrow depression caused by therapy, in cachexic patients, or in patients who have open wounds secondary to surgery or cancerous lesions. The nursing goals are twofold: (1) prevention or early detection of the infectious process and (2) promotion of healing to minimize systemic effects. Nursing orders include (1) ongoing monitoring to detect infectious process; (2) ongoing assessment of existing infectious process; (3) patient and family teaching regarding *(a)* causes of potential or existing infection; *(b)* signs and symptoms of infection, *(c)* monitoring techniques, such as taking temperatures, or specific observations as appropriate, such as changes in sputum or drainage, *(d)* factors to promote prevention of infection such as adequate fluid intake, position change, and measures to reduce environmental contamination.

A frequent actual or potential nursing diagnosis seen in cancer patients is alteration in body fluid composition. Many times the alteration is related to bone marrow depression caused by chemotherapy or radiation therapy, obstruction, ascites, or changes in third space fluids. Altered composition may be changes in electrolytes, RBCs and hemoglobin, platelets and clotting factors, pH, or serum proteins (see Chapter 41).

Hypercalcemia

Hypercalcemia is a fairly common alteration in body fluids in cancer patients. Patients who have bone metastasis are more likely to develop hypercalcemia than other patients. The process of metastatic bone destruction causes an extremely large calcium load in the blood, which may eventually exceed the kidneys' capacity to excrete it. It is important that careful observation be made for any elevation of the calcium level in the blood. Symptoms of hypercalcemia are nausea, vomiting, polyuria, dehydration, personality changes, lethargy, and finally coma. Muscle weakness and easy fatigability are also seen. Hypercalcemia is treated by hydration of up to 4 liters in 24 hours with fluid containing a high proportion of sodium, if the cardiovascular system will permit this, and if the patient is urinating. The patient should be mobilized. Electrolyte imbalance should be stabilized. Drug treatment may include diuretics, phosphates, mithramycen, cortisone, and calcitonin (Hill & Hickey, 1973).

Nurses must be ever watchful for indications of this complication so that early preventive measures may be taken. Because hypercalcemia usually develops when the patient is at home, both the patient and family need to know of the early signs and symptoms and need to be instructed to call the physician should these occur.

Nursing Goals

General nursing goals are (1) restoration of the body fluid composition to a homeostatic state (see Chapter 27 and 41) and (2) prevention of secondary complications resulting from the alteration in body fluid composition. Nursing orders must be specific to the altered component of body fluids, but generally they should include (1) ongoing assessment of signs and symptoms of the alteration in composition of body fluids; (2) implementation of measures appropriate to preventing and/or controlling the alteration in body fluids and their sequelae; (3) patient and family teaching regarding *(a)* factors that influence alteration in composition of fluids such as vomiting, diarrhea, wound drainage, inadequate food intake, chemotherapy, radiation therapy, and drugs, *(b)* signs and symptoms of impaired clotting mechanisms, *(c)* relationship between altered composition in body fluids and optimal body function, and *(d)* interventions to prevent and/or control bleeding tendencies.

Impairment of skin and mucosal integrity is a frequent nursing diagnosis made in cancer patients. Generally the diagnosis is related to other nursing diagnoses, such as immobility or altered nutrition–less than required, tumor growth, radiation, or chemotherapy. General nursing goals are (1) promotion of optimal skin/mucosal integrity and (2) prevention of complications secondary to the interrupted skin/mucosal integrity. Nursing orders include (1) ongoing assessment of the patient's skin/mucosal status; (2) patient and family teaching of measures to promote and maintain the skin/mucosal integrity, (3) development and implementation of a plan to maintain and promote skin/mucosal integrity. The following discussion suggests some specific nursing measures to use and teach.

Nursing Measures

Mouth Care

When patients are experiencing stomatitis it may be too painful for them to do more than rinse their mouths with an anesthetic solution. Any brushing of the teeth can be accomplished by using a soft toothbrush or cotton-tipped applicators.

Patients who have crusting in their mouths, and are mouth breathers, perhaps because of coma, may benefit by the use of Cook's ointment (de Gutierrez-Mahoney & Carini, 1970). This is an absorbable antiseptic, and its use will assist in keeping the mouth moist, free of crusting, and sweet smelling.

Decubitus Ulcers

Care of decubitus ulcers consumes an astronomical amount of nurses' time, as well as causes the patient increased debilitation and the family tremendous frustration (see Chapter 49). It has long been known that preventing decubiti is much easier than healing one once it begins. Patients have already received insults to their body. To develop an additional opening that allows entry for microorganisms and subsequent infections, thereby causing increased discomfort, seems entirely unnecessary. Ongoing inspection of the patient's skin condition is therefore essential. This should be done each shift by the professional nurse. The nurse should teach the patient and family various exercises that may be implemented to decrease further the likelihood of skin breakdown. Both the patient and the family are involved in a meaningful part of health care. Family members may sit by the bedside for hours each day, feeling helpless and useless. The nurse can help to reduce these feelings by suggesting some things they can do to assist in the patient's care. Some suggestions are

1. To remind the patient to do isometric exercises at least every 2 hours. Contracting and relaxing muscles in all body parts is an excellent method to enhance muscle tone and increase circulation.
2. To encourage the patient to use the overhead bar to exercise the arms.
3. To suggest the patient turn from side to side every hour.
4. To reposition the bed, unless contraindicated, from a sitting to a lying position every 2 hours. This assists in redistributing the body weight, thereby decreasing pressure.
5. To encourage the patient to reach with one hand under the mattress or to the side rail and to pull, thereby effecting a lifting, rolling motion of the body every 2 hours.
6. To massage the bony surfaces every 3 hours or more.

Early utilization of such preventive measures as alternating pressure mattresses, lamb's wool, silicone pads, water beds, and/or Circ-o-Letric beds may also reduce the incidence of decubitus ulcers.

Patients' activity orders may read "Up ad lib.," but the patient is too weak or tired or may otherwise simply lack motivation to get out of bed. Patients with an "up" order may spend as much as 23 out of 24 hours in bed. Nurses should observe how often the patients are out of bed; if they need assistance to get up, and when in bed if they assume the same position most of the time. It is easy for nurses to be sympathetic when the patient says, "I'm too tired to get up now," to allow the patient to stay in bed and to write in the nurse's note, "Patient refuses to get out of bed." This is not being kind to the patient, for patients who are immobilized in this way rapidly develop complications of bedrest.

Patients may suffer extreme weakness so that any active motion will be exhausting. Nurses, together with patients, should decide on a schedule of activity that is spaced to conserve the patient's energy as much as possible.

Preventing decubiti is a 24-hour occupation; therefore nursing care plans should be such that each shift is sharing in the prevention. This becomes extremely difficult for the afternoon and night shifts because there are fewer personnel. Use of turning teams during these times may be one method of utilizing staff more effectively. Two people can accomplish turning in a manner that is faster and more comfortable for the patient. Visiting hours in most institutions extend well into the afternoon shift. What better way for nurses to teach family members care of the patient than to utilize them in assisting to turn the patient, to get him or her up, and to walk the patient? Families are not "in the way" but are a real asset to patients and to nursing personnel. This does not mean that families should assume total care of the patient when they visit, but this time does provide an opportune time to teach them the care they will be doing when the patient is discharged.

Should a decubitus develop, intensive measures for treatment are immediately necessary. Early treatment may consist of exposure to the air and light and of keeping the area dry and clean. Chlorpacten soaks have been used effectively in some institutions. Debridement may be essential before treatment can begin in the more extensive decubiti. Packing the ulcer with commercially available white granulated sugar and covering the area with gauze pads has been effective in healing about 80 per cent of the cases reported by Barnes (1973). The rationale for its use is that the granules cause "local injury" and initiate wound repair processes; granulation tissue formation is stimulated, the acid pH of the sugar solution increases vasodilatation; and the sucrose solution that is hyperconcentrated is also bactericidal. Whatever method is used, the patient benefits because something is being done to keep him or her off the broken-down area. Cleanliness, hydration, and nutrition are very much a part of prevention and healing of decubiti.

Control of Odors

When the lesion remains open, the most important general measure is cleanliness. The agent used to cleanse the lesion should be prescribed by the physician. There is usually no reason for not cleansing the area around the lesion with soap or detergent and water. Moreover, when the patient has a draining and foul-smelling wound, the nurse should take whatever initiative is required to see that it is cleansed. An inexpensive deodorant is buttermilk. This may be applied as compresses to wounds, or it can be used as an irrigation. Yogurt dressings have also been useful. The rationale for their use is to fight bacteria with bacteria. Odors originate from dead tissues and the effects of infection. These odor-producing organisms require an alkaline medium. Buttermilk and yogurt organisms produce an acid medium and this acid prevents the odor-forming bacteria from growing and multiplying (Barkley, 1964).

Dressings should be changed when soiled and replaced by clean ones. If bed linens or patient attire is soiled, it also should be changed. Because odor often permeates the plastic mattress cover, it should be throughly washed and dried with every linen change. Soiled dressings should be removed immediately from the room. When wounds are treated by exposure to the air, the patient should be draped and screened so that he or she is protected from view. Ventilation of the room, with precautions to prevent chilling the patient, reduce the intensity of odors. When deodorizing agents and devices are used, they should supplement and not substitute for keeping the wound clean.

Ventilation

Ventilation is a patient problem area for cancer patients, especailly those with cancer of the lung. The nursing diagnosis typically made is alteration in respiratory function. It is frequently related to other nursing diagnoses such as impaired mobility or variation in functional performance. It may also be related to other factors such as drugs used for pain control, obstructions, effusions (pleural or peritoneal), chemotherapy, or radiation-induced pulmonary fibrosis, anemia, anxiety, or fear. The primary nursing goal is to maintain and/or promote ventilation that facilitates optimal respiratory function. Nursing orders include (1) ongoing assessment of the patient's respiratory status; (2) planning and implementing measures that facilitate optimal respiratory function, for example, *(a)* coughing and deep breathing exercises, *(b)* using oxygen therapy as ordered, *(c)* correct body alignment, *(d)* suctioning techniques as necessary, *(e)* pain control, *(f)* chest physiotherapy, *(g)* energy-conserving measures, *(h)* control of anxiety and pain; (3) patient and family teaching concerning *(a)* factors that influence respiratory function, *(b)* signs and symptoms of altered respirations, *(c)* measures to facilitate optimal respiratory function, *(d)* emergency action plan if patient develops respiratory distress, especially if the patient is being cared for in the home.

Body Fluid Retention

Another problem area for many cancer patients is excessive retention of body fluids. The problem can be related to multiple possible causes for example, renal failure, cardiac failure, elevated or decreased serum proteins, blocked lymphatics as a result of tumor growth, or surgery and steroid therapy. If a nursing diagnosis of body fluids excess is made, the general nursing goal is to maintain and/or promote a fluid balance that facilitates optimal hydration and comfort. Nursing orders include (1) ongoing assessment of the patient's fluid status; (2) development of a nursing plan and implementation of measures appropriate to the etiology which decrease fluid excess such as *(a)* elevation of body part, *(b)* use of ace bandages or elastic hose as appropriate, *(c)* administration of medications, such as diuretics as ordered, *(d)* a restriction of sodium intake, *(e)* an increase in protein intake; (3) implementation of measures that protect the body or the affected part(s) from injury.

Dealing with Terminality

To achieve the objective of caring for the terminally ill person the nurse requires some understanding of her or his own feelings toward death. Most healthy people feel uncomfortable in the presence of the dying and the dead. The words *dead* and *death* are avoided whenever possible. Instead words and phrases such as *passed away, passed on* and *expired* are used. Nurses, because of their own fears, may spend as little time as necessary with the dying patient. Many patients fear dying alone. It is then that the presence of the nurse is so important. The meaning of touch becomes very significant, holding the patient's hand, wiping the brow, turning him or her ever so gently from one side to another, assuring the patient that he or she will be cared for and will not be abandoned. Families, too, need considerable support. They need to talk out their fears and sometimes their guilt feelings. (See Unit VII, especially Chapter 33.)

When the patient becomes comatose more of the nurse's attention is directed to the family. Families often exhaust their own reserve by spending most of their time at the hospital. Nurses should be aware of this. A nurse who has developed a close working relationship with a patient and family can suggest that the family member not come in as often. She or he can advise them to stay home and get more rest. Arrangements can be made for them to call the hospital and discuss the patient's condition with the nurse. Family members will probably welcome such advice. On the other hand, some patients desire that their husband or wife not leave them. If this is the case, arrangements should be made to provide sleeping accommodations. Hospitals may furnish cots that can be placed out of the way in the patient's room, or a recliner lawn chair could serve as a bed for a short time.

Family members might be reluctant to leave their loved one even for the time necessary to eat. A member of the nursing staff could volunteer to stay with the patient for that length of time, thereby relieving the family member. Nursing staff could supply coffee or offer to get the family something to eat. All of these considerations let the family know that nurses do care and they do want to help. Clergy need to be involved as members of the interdisciplinary team from the time the patient is admitted. The patient, when realizing he or she is going to die, may desire to talk with a religious advisor who can assist in making peace with God. Because patients may be too ill to read or pray, nurses can give comfort by praying with or for the patients, and by reading Bible passages or other religious material to them.

Patients may have other unfinished business that needs attention. When at all possible wills should be made; this will alleviate family hassles and guilt feelings thereafter. Arrangements need to be made for children, and sometimes older persons for whom the patient is responsible. Severed relationships need to be reconciled. Financial matters need to be settled. All of this planning causes tremendous emotion for both the patient and family. However, once these decisions are made, and unfinished business resolved, a feeling of relief and calm can be sensed. Until recently little has been available in the medical literature about the care of the dying. See Chapter 33 for a more detailed discussion of the care of the dying patient. At this time a nursing diagnosis of disruption of spiritual integrity might appropriately be made and a plan implemented.

As mentioned earlier, Giacquinta (1977) has identified four stages families must face when dealing with the crisis of cancer. Stage II, restructuring the living-dying interval is very important as the family begins to deal with the patient's terminality.

The first phase of Stage II is reorganization. During this phase role responsibilities must be redistributed among family members because of the changes caused by the cancer illness. The nursing goal here is to foster co-operation among family members by supporting them as they define family goals and redistribute the role responsibilities (Giacquinta, 1977).

Framing memories is the second phase of Stage II. This is a time for remembering the person's life history. The nursing goal is to foster the family's efforts to crystalize the patient's identity and relationships through time. Activities which may be useful to the family include looking at pictures and scrapbooks and family story telling (Giacquinta, 1977).

As the patient's vital signs decompensate and it becomes increasingly clear that death is imminent, a nursing diagnosis of impending death can be made. At this point in the patient's life the primary emphasis is on maintaining comfort. The goals are (1) to assist the patient and family for whatever time is left to identify changing needs and (2) to achieve optimal physical and psychological comfort. Nursing orders include (1) participation in determining the patient and family's preference as to the setting of care—hospital, home, hospice, extended care facility; (2) assessing the potential caregiver's ability to manage the care, especially if home is the setting of choice; (3) patient and family teaching concerning *(a)* the meaning of changes in the patient's physical and functional status, *(b)* reprioritizing of patient's needs to promote comfort versus maintaining or improving status, *(c)* methods of managing supportive care, and *(d)* expected changes in patient status.

The third family crisis stage is bereavement. Separation and mourning are the two phases of this stage (Giacquinta, 1977). During separation the patient's consciousness diminishes and awareness of the environment disappears. The family truly experiences the loneliness of separation. The nursing goal at this time is to fostor intimacy among family members so that they can support each other through the grieving process (Giacquinta, 1977).

Mourning of the loved one following death is the second phase of Stage III. The grief of mourning is experienced differently by each family member. The nursing goal of this phase is to foster relief among the members. Very likely the family members have reached their limit of endurance and may at least initially need to admit their relief that the patient has died (Giacquinta, 1977).

A nursing diagnosis of bereavement can very appropriately be made during this stage. The major nursing goals are (1) to facilitate the family's passage through the mourning process and (2) to prevent or minimize incapacitating or destructive behavior. Nursing orders include (1) ongoing assessment of the family member's response to their loss and their potential to proceed through the bereavement process; (2) encouragement of family members recalling the patient by describing the bereaved person's physical and personal traits and by encouraging family members to relive good experiences; (3) utilization of the bereaved person's personal objects to elicit feelings; (4) provision of a safe, accepting environment for ventilation of feelings; (5) referrals as necessary, to clergy or mental health resources.

Stage IV, the final stage families face in the crisis of cancer is re-establishment. The only phase of this stage is expansion of the social network. It occurs after completion of mourning and successful resolution of grief and bereavement. Only then can the family re-enter the social environment and extend beyond themselves. The nursing goal is to foster relatedness so that self and family estrangement and meaninglessness can be overcome. The nurse can assist the family members to look back on their family life with acceptance and self-respect and to be open to experiencing their changing identities.

To this point information useful in understanding the needs of patients with cancer and their families has been stressed. In the following section we will discuss the needs of Mrs. Reed, who had cancer of the breast treated by radical mastectomy; Mrs. White, who had cancer of the sigmoid colon treated by combined abdominal perineal resection, and Mr. Paul, who had cancer of the larynx treated by laryngectomy.

Patient Situations

As you read through the situations, identify the nursing diagnoses and care plans you would make.

The Patient with Breast Cancer

During her regular monthly examination of her breasts, Mrs. Reed found a small lump in the upper outer quadrant of her right breast. For a moment she thought that she must be mistaken, but it was there. After a sleepless night, she made an appointment with Dr. Smith, her family physician. He confirmed the fact that there was a lump and suggested that she see Dr. Surgeon for diagnosis. He reminded her that tumors in the breast are frequently harmless. Mrs. Reed asked if there was any hurry about seeing the surgeon. Dr. Smith suggested that Mrs. Reed not delay but make an appointment to see the surgeon within the next week.

Mrs. Reed was admitted to the hospital the day before the biopsy was to be performed. Because the extent of the operation was to be determined by the biopsy, she was prepared for a radical mastectomy. Dr. Surgeon had explained to Mr. and Mrs. Reed that this was a possibility and so she was not surprised. A biopsy was performed, and a frozen section of the neoplasm was made. It proved to be malignant. Dr. Surgeon then proceeded to perform a radical mastectomy (a less radical procedure varying from a lumpectomy to a simple mastectomy might have been selected).

In planning Mrs. Reed's nursing care, four major elements were considered. First, Mrs. Reed is an individual human being who reacts or behaves in an individual manner; second, at the time Mrs. Reed was admitted, the nature of her illness was uncertain, but following biopsy the diagnosis was established as cancer; third, Mrs. Reed had an extensive surgical procedure; fourth, the operation was a radical mastectomy. The information required to meet the first three is presented elsewhere. The discussion that follows relates principally to meeting Mrs. Reed's requirements arising from having radical breast amputation. All elements had to be taken into account in meeting her needs for nursing.

In the postoperative period the nursing care required by Mrs. Reed was accomplished by planning to meet the following objectives: (1) to facilitate her emotional adjustment to the removal of her breast, (2) to heal her wound, and (3) to maintain the function in her right arm.

When Mrs. Reed recovered from the anesthetic she was overwhelmed by the extent of the procedure. Her entire breast had been removed along with lymph channels, axillary lymph nodes, and the pectoral muscles. Her chest and the upper part of her right arm were swathed in dressings.

In a radical mastectomy a large area of tissue is removed and many blood vessels are disrupted. This results in the formation of a large amount of fluid exudate in the wound area. Although some fluid in the wound is to be expected, large amounts delay healing, and the fluid must be removed before healing takes place. Surgeons meet this problem in different ways. One is, as was done for Mrs. Reed, to apply a large pressure dressing over the area to lessen the exudation of fluid and to prevent it from accumulating in the wound. This fluid drains from the wound into the dressings. When the dressings become saturated, they may be reinforced by the nurse. Because hemorrhage is always a possibility, the nurse must decide when the quantity of drainage is excessive. In general, the wound exudate is a strawberry colored fluid that is blood-tinged. Obvious bleeding is bright red in color and should be immediately reported to the physician. Changes in vital signs, such as a fall in blood pressure and an increase in pulse rate, are also indicative of hemorrhage. When there is external evidence of bleeding, the nurse should not wait for the pulse and blood pressure to change before reporting the bleeding to the physician. A point to remember when checking dressings for blood or other fluids is that water runs downhill. Therefore the part of the dressing next to the bed should always be checked. This same principle is also used to facilitate drainage from a wound.

A second method employed by some surgeons to remove the wound exudate is to insert catheters into the wound to which gentle suction is applied by a suction machine or a commercial device known as a hemovac (see Figure 39-4). As wound exudate is suctioned into the hemovac, pressures are gradually equalized. To maintain suction the drum must be emptied of drainage and the negative pressure reestablished. The inside of the hemovac is sterile; care must be taken to maintain this sterility when the drum is emptied, as the serosanguinous exudate being suctioned from the wound provides an ideal medium for the proliferation of microorganisms.

Characteristics of drainage are easily observed through transparent walls of the drum; all pertinent

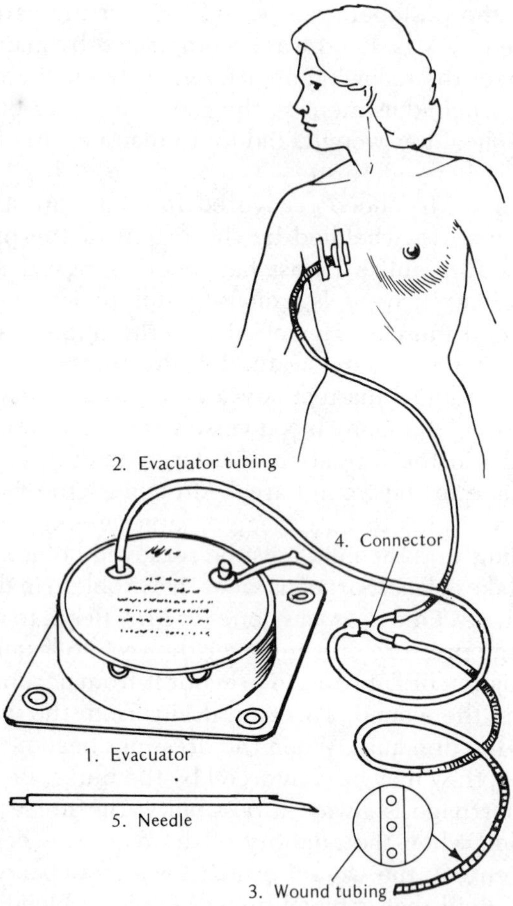

Figure 39-4. The Snyder hemovac, a light, simple, commercial device with gentle suction used for the removal of fluid exudate of extensive wounds. *1,* Evacuator; *2,* evacuator tubing; *3,* wound tubing; *4,* connector; *5,* needle. All wounds, clean or septic, are completely closed. Wound suction is continuously applied from the insertion of the tubes, through the wound closure, and until the tubes are removed. Drip and suction for closed circulation are started as soon as the tubes are placed and before wound closure is started. Drip and suction never cease during wound closure, during transportation of the patient from surgery, or until the permanent attachment to the mechanical pump is made for continued use. If tubes are to be left in for some time, as for patients with circulatory problems, the check-rein suture is used. Otherwise no suture is used. In either instance it is a great convenience to have the wound dressing completely separated from any attachment to the tubes. Manipulation, inspection, and removal of tubes can then be done without disturbing the wound dressing. Keep tubes in line with their skin exits. Do not curl them to put pressure on the skin holes or the skin will become irritated or will slough. Pad lightly between skin and tube but put adhesive directly against and over the tube to anchor it firmly to the skin. (Adapted courtesy of Snyder Laboratories, Division of Snyder Manufacturing Co., Inc., New Philadelphia, Ohio.)

facts about drainage are reported and recorded when the drum is emptied.

Because of materials used in its construction, the hemovac cannot be resterilized. It is discarded after use for a single patient. No dressing, or only a small dressing, is applied. The catheters may be left in place for 3 or 4 days. The patient may be taught how to disconnect the suction so that he or she is free to walk about.

When Mrs. Reed was returned from the operating room, she was placed in bed with the head of the bed elevated to about a 15° angle. Her right arm was abducted at the shoulder, rotated internally with the forearm flexed at the elbow, and elevated. Some surgeons ask that the arm be abducted at the shoulder and that the forearm be flexed at the elbow with the hand above the head. Others place the arm across the chest of the patient and bandage it in that position. The latter position reduces the tension on the wound and therefore is favorable to wound healing, particularly when a skin graft has been done. The first two positions are for the purpose of maintaining the function of the arm. In all three positions the arm should be supported so that unnecessary strain and discomfort are prevented. In the first two positions, elevation also supports venous return and prevents stasis of fluid or edema of the arm. The removal of the lymph nodes and channels as well as the inflammatory response in the operated area interferes with the drainage of fluid from the arm.

Whatever the position of the arm, it should be supported so that there is no unnecessary pull on the muscles. A pillow should be placed along the side of the chest and under the arm that is strapped over the chest, as well as under those parts requiring elevation. The pillows or supports should be placed so that they support the arm of the patient.

Because the patient can and should move about, the supports tend to become disarranged and require readjustment. The first criterion to be used in checking their placement is, because water runs downhill, that the most distal portion—in this instance the hand—should be higher than the portion proximal to it. In checking the position of Mrs. Reed's arm, her hand should be higher than her elbow and her elbow higher than her shoulder. One of the common errors in elevating the arm is to allow the elbow to be lower than the shoulder, with the result that fluid tends to accumulate at the elbow and cause swelling. The second criterion is the following: Do the muscles of the arm appear to be relaxed? Does the patient appear to be comfortable? When the patient looks uncomfortable, the arm is probably in poor position. The degree of the elevation, as well as the alignment of the arm, should be checked. No matter how comfortable the position of the patient is at the time the pillows are arranged, she does not stay comfortable. Even if she does, one position soon becomes fatiguing. Therefore the plan for the nursing of the patient should include provision for regular checking and changing of the patient's position.

At the same time, the hand and arm should be checked and any evidence of swelling of the hand or interference with the circulation noted. You will remember that the dressing extended over the upper part of Mrs. Reed's arm. As emphasized in Chapter 9, when swelling is allowed to continue in a part surrounded by a fixed or nondistensible wall, first the venous return and then the arterial circulation are interrupted. With a loss of the arterial blood supply, death of tissue follows.

In addition to hemorrhage and swelling of the hand and arm, pneumonia is a possible complication in the early postoperative period. This can usually be prevented by encouraging the patient to move about in bed and to deep breathe and to cough. Mrs. Reed was encouraged and assisted to move and to cough, and she recovered without developing respiratory complications.

Mrs. Reed had some pain in her incision which was controlled by meperidine hydrochloride (Demerol) 75 mg on request, but not more often than every 4 hours. Dr. Surgeon had informed Mrs. Reed that she could have a pain-relieving medication when she needed it. She required meperidine hydrochloride only twice.

One of the objectives following radical breast amputation is to restore the arm on the affected side to full usefulness. Two problems require control to achieve this objective. One is the prevention of limitation of motion of the arm by the scar tissue formed in healing of the wound. The other is to prevent or limit edema of the hand and arm. The restoration of the arm to full usefulness, by preventing disability caused by contractures, is accomplished by arm exercise. When exercises are to be started and what type are to be used at a given point are decisions made by the surgeon. Some surgeons start exercises early, whereas others prefer to wait until wound healing is well under way. When the quantity of tissue that has been excised is extensive, the amount of skin left to close the wound may be marginal, and additional tension on the incision may interfere with healing.

In the early postoperative period Dr. Surgeon asked that Mrs. Reed's arm be put through the normal range of motion without forcing abduction. Mrs. Reed was fearful, and arm movement was painful. Dr. Surgeon reassured her that the movement of her arm would not produce harmful effects and was necessary to recovery. The nurse reinforced Dr. Surgeon's statements. The first few times that Mrs. Reed exercised her arm, the nurse supported it and abducted and adducted it slowly and gently. She also encouraged Mrs. Reed to alternately flex and extend her elbow as well as her wrist and fingers. Because movement of the arm is painful, arm movements should be started slowly.

Dr. Surgeon requested that a Reach to Recovery volunteer visit Mrs. Reed to explain and demonstrate the prescribed arm exercises. The volunteer, Mrs. Wilson, came on the third postoperative day. She was about the same age as Mrs. Reed, was also married, and had a teenage daughter. Because Mrs. Wilson had a mastectomy she could understand the fears Mrs. Reed was experiencing and could help to allay these. The volunteer gave Mrs. Reed the Reach to Recovery kit which included a ball, a rope, a temporary prosthesis, and the booklet Reach to Recovery (Lasser, 1969).

Mrs. Wilson explained and demonstrated the various exercises outlined in the booklet. Mrs. Reed was taught to do wall-climbing, pendulum, pulley, broom-raising, and rope-turning exercises.

Mrs. Wilson told her about the various breast forms available, and where these could be purchased. She gave her suggestions for brassiere and clothing adjustments. Mrs. Wilson left her phone number in the event Mrs. Reed wanted or needed some additional help. Mrs. Reed was very encouraged by the visit. It was good to see someone who had had the same kind of surgery look and act so normal. Mrs. Reed was especially grateful for the temporary prosthesis, which was light and soft and could be pinned inside her gown without fear of causing injury to her incision. She did not look as lopsided now.

As soon as the physician's prescription permits, the patient should be encouraged to carry on her usual activities with her arm. These include feeding herself, washing her face and hands, brushing her teeth, and combing her hair. These activities serve a double purpose. They not only exercise the arm, but they improve the morale of the patient. They are more effective than countless words in convincing the patient that the arm will in fact be restored to usefulness. The fact that the use of the arm is painful at the beginning should be recognized. The patient can be assured, however, that within a relatively short period of time pain on use will disappear and by exercising she is helping with her own recovery. As the nurse cared for Mrs. Reed, she tried to communicate to Mrs. Reed the fact that she did appreciate her discomfort but that movement of the arm was necessary if she were to recover its full use. Each day the nurse assisted or supervised Mrs. Reed in doing her arm and shoulder exercises.

To do the wall-climbing exercises, Mrs. Reed stood facing the wall, and as close to it as possible, with her feet about 8 inches apart. Both hands were placed against the wall at shoulder level. Then using the fingers, the hands parallel to each other, she climbed the wall until her arms were completely extended. When this exercise was started, Mrs. Reed was unable to extend her right arm fully. This was to be expected. The nurse made a small mark on the paper placed on the wall, so that Mrs. Reed could check her progress. In the beginning the nurse encouraged Mrs. Reed to take her time as she performed the exercise and to repeat it ten times. In performance of the pendulum exercise, Mrs. Reed stood with her feet 8 inches apart, and bent forward, allowing her arms to hang to the floor. At first she let her arms dangle, and then she swung them back and forth. Eventually she was able to swing them in circles.

To perform the pulley exercises, an 8-ft length of rope is placed over a door, a shower curtain rod, or a suspended pulley. The patient then alternately raises and lowers each arm. The arms are in adduction and extended.

To perform the broom-raising exercise, any horizontal bar similar in weight to a broomstick may be used. The stick or broom handle is grasped by both hands with the hands about 2 ft apart. The broom is then raised until the arms are fully extended. Then it is brought down behind the head of the patient. This exercise is somewhat harder to do than some of the others. The patient should therefore be encouraged to try it only once or twice the first few times and to gradually increase the number of times that it is performed.

The rope-turning exercise is performed by turning a rope, ribbon, or string that has been tied to a doorknob or other suitable object. The patient holds the rope in the hand on the affected side with the arm straight in front of her and places the other hand on her hip for balance. Then she moves the rope in a circle without turning her elbow or wrist. As the function of her arm improves, she will be able to form larger and larger circles.

Some surgeons refer patients to physical therapy for instruction and supervision of arm and shoulder exercises. In teaching the patient, emphasis should be placed on the objective: to return the arm to its normal function. Although some patients require support and urging to return to full activity, others need to be cautioned against overuse of the arm. This is true especially in the beginning. As the patient returns to normal activity, the need for special exercises is lessened.

One of the expressed or unexpressed problems of the patient who has a radical mastectomy is the loss of the breast and the resulting disfigurement. The patient should be encouraged to discuss with her surgeon the earliest time that she can start wearing a brassiere and then to shop for the type that is suitable and comfortable for her. Mrs. Reed was very much concerned about the extent of her operation and its effect on her appearance. The surgeon and nurse both tried to reassure her that the operation was similar to what is usually done. The nurse reminded Mrs. Reed about the types of brassieres now available. They are sold in department stores and at specialty shops. They are made with a variety of fillers and in different sizes. Fillers contain fluid or are made of sponge rubber and other similar materials. For the patient who feels lopsided, the filler containing fluid may be preferred; the shape of the breast also changes with position. The patient should be encouraged to select a brassiere that is comfortable and fits her individual requirements.

Patients should be encouraged to resume normal activities after they return home. There is some evidence that patients tend to regress immediately after they go home and to be more dependent than they were in the hospital. If the family accepts the behavior of the patient, the increase in dependency is usually short-lived and the patient soon begins to assume more responsibility. Actually, there is some evidence that the patient who is permitted to be dependent recovers more rapidly than the one whose family is not as accepting.

Before Mrs. Reed was discharged from the hospital, the nurse taught her how to examine her remaining breast for any abnormalities. Patients who have cancer in one breast have a high incidence of developing cancer in the other breast (del Regato, 1977). In preparation for discharge, plans should be made with her and a family member about when she will visit the physician. If x-ray therapy is planned and the patient knows this, she may have questions, some of which the nurse may answer. Others may need to be referred to the physician. Some increase in anxiety at this time can be expected.

The patient who faces or has a radical mastectomy has a special problem. The operation itself involves removal of a large amount of tissue and disruption of many blood vessels. The nursing care has among its goals to preserve and strengthen the self-esteem of the patient as well as to contribute to the accomplishment of the medical goals to heal the wound and restore the function of the arm. The accomplishment of these goals depends on the application of knowledge of the patient, the effects of cancer, and the nature of the operation to the care of the patient.

Dr. Surgeon told Mr. and Mrs. Reed that, as her strength returned, she should resume full activity. Household activities that involve reaching and stretching and full movements of the arm are especially helpful.

The family may require some instruction for support. They should know what is to be expected of the patient, how they can be helpful, and that the patient may not be very active for a week or so after she returns home. The Reach to Recovery Program includes the sending of letters to husbands, teenage daughters and sons. It assures them that their wife and mother is the same person she was before surgery. The letter also suggests some specific ways in which each family member can be helpful. One way the family can be helpful to the patient is by making a conscious effort to note and to comment on progress and efforts made by the patient.

In most women the breast has significance as a symbol of femininity. Some of the patients will equate the loss of the breast with the loss of their attractiveness to their husbands. This often creates major psychological problems. Many of these problems can be solved by the reassurance of a thoughtful husband.

The Patient with a Colostomy

Mrs. Alan White, an active, vivacious, charming, fastidious, intelligent, and well-educated woman of 65, and Mr. White had been married for 39 years. Mr. White's income allowed them to enjoy many comforts in life. Mrs. White was active in community affairs. The day following her sixty-fifth birthday, Mrs. White had an appointment with her family physician for her annual physical examination. She had always been a healthy woman, neither overly concerned about her health nor neglectful of it. At the time of the examination, she told Dr. Olds that she had had some discomfort in her abdomen but that she found it difficult to describe. She had had some flatulence that she considered to be embarrassing. She had also recently been constipated. On physical examination Dr. Olds found that Mrs. White's general state of health was good. Her weight, 125 lb, was the same as for the previous year. Her hemoglobin level was 13.8 g, which was also unchanged. Her leukocyte count at 7,500 cells per cubic millimeter was within normal limits.

The proctoscopic examination revealed a narrowing of the bowel at the junction of the rectum and sigmoid. At one point there was an ulcerated area. On x-ray of the large bowel, Mrs. White was found to have an encircling, or annular, lesion. Because of these findings, Dr. Olds referred Mrs. White to Dr. Surgeon. He suggested that he make an appointment for her to see Dr. Surgeon as soon as possible. Mrs. White's immediate reaction was a common one: to seek to delay the diagnosis. Mrs. White desired to defer an appointment with Dr. Surgeon until after she returned from a planned vacation to Florida. She thought nothing bad could happen in three months. Dr. Olds was firm, but kindly, as he urged her to delay the trip. She was quiet for a moment, and then said, "You think I have cancer, do you not?" Dr. Olds did not evade the question. He answered by saying, "Yes, I think so, but I think that it is an early cancer. If it is removed now, there is a good possibility that it can be entirely removed. Dr. Surgeon is a competent surgeon. You will be in good hands." Mrs. White decided she would like to discuss the situation with her husband before making any decisions. Dr. Olds agreed that she should talk it over with her husband. He recognized Mrs. White's need to maintain some control over her situation and her reliance on her husband. Furthermore, in the difficult days ahead she would need the help, support, and understanding of her husband as well as the knowledge that she had made her own decision.

Sutherland et al. (1952) emphasize the importance of a supportive spouse in the eventual adjustment of the patient to the colostomy. In his studies of families where rapport was poor before the operation, the relationship deteriorated afterward; in a series of patients, four out of fifty-seven patients who had colostomies had to live away from home because they were unacceptable to their families. Both patients and family members studied tended to hide the fact of the colostomy from others. Of the fifty-seven patients referred to above, twenty-five had not allowed even other family members to see the colostomy. Even when the patient was willing to allow family members to see the colostomy, they sometimes refused to view it.

That evening she discussed with Mr. White the outcome of her visit to Dr. Olds. They decided to visit Dr. Olds together the next day. At this time Dr. Olds urged her not to delay treatment. An appointment was made with Dr. Surgeon for the following day. Mr. White accompanied Mrs. White for her appointment with Dr. Surgeon to provide support to her. Dr. Surgeon confirmed Dr. Old's suspicions and explained to both Mr. and Mrs. White the need for prompt surgery as well as the type of procedure that would probably be necessary. He explained that the left half of the bowel would have to be removed and that a colostomy would have to be performed. Despite her expectation that an operation would be imperative, she felt overwhelmed and confused when Dr. Surgeon stated that she should prepare to enter the hospital without delay. She later told members of the family that she felt that she was in a fog. She went through the necessary motions, but they were automatic. Mr. White was also upset but tried to hide his feelings and to comfort Mrs. White. He made all the essential arrangements for her admission to the hospital.

Mrs. White was fortunate because Mr. White was a kindly and dependable man who gave her understanding and support through the months that followed the diagnosis and treatment of her disorder.

The large intestine is among the five common sites for cancer, and the rectosigmoid is the most common site for the large intestine. According to the *1973 Cancer Facts and Figures,* 47,000 persons were expected to die from the effects of cancer in the colon and rectum in 1973. It was also estimated that cancer of the colon and rectum would be the site of the greatest number of new cases of cancer in 1973, as 79,000 persons were expected to be diagnosed with this malignancy for the first time. Almost three out of four patients could be saved by early diagnosis and proper treatment. The incidence of cancer of the rectum is higher in men than in women, whereas the reverse is true in cancer of the colon. One half of the cancers of the colon and rectum can be diagnosed by the examiners finger. Two thirds of the cancers of the colon and rectum can be diagnosed by the sigmoidoscope (del Regato, 1977). Therefore the majority of these lesions can be diagnosed early, when they can still be cured. When discovered early, the cure rate by surgery is greater than the cure rate of most other tumors.

Symptoms accompanying cancer of the colon and rectum vary with the location of the lesion. Symptoms of obstruction are more commonly associated with lesions on the left than on the right side. Water is absorbed from the feces as they pass through the large intestine, and the narrowing of the lumen of the intestine offers more resistance to the semisolid feces than to liquid feces higher in the intestine. Symptoms include, as in the instance of Mrs. White, vague abdominal distress and a change in the bowel habit including constipation, obstipation, and diarrhea. Especially in low left-sided lesions, the shape of the stool changes and becomes smaller in diameter, ribbon-shaped stools are not uncommon. Hemorrhoids frequently accompany left-sided lesions. They may, in fact, be an early warning sign. Bright-red blood can be observed in the stool in left-sided, but not in right-sided lesions. Anemia accompanies lesions located on either side. Anemia of unexplained origin may be the first indication of cancer of the rectum. Weakness and general debility occur as the cancer progresses. Mrs. White had not experienced any of these effects.

The treatment of cancer of the large intestine, like treatment of cancer in other parts of the body, is directed toward the eradication of all cancer cells. The same methods—surgery, ionizing radiation, and chemotherapy—are used. Treatment of cancer on the left side often, though not always, includes a colostomy. Cancer of the right bowel can usually be treated without a permanent colostomy; the diseased portion of the bowel is removed and the ends are anastomosed (joined).

The purpose of the colostomy in all instances is to provide an avenue for the discharge of intestinal contents. It may have a single opening, as in the instance of Mrs. White; it is then called a single-barreled colostomy. When the proximal and distal loops are brought to the surface, it is known as a double-barreled colostomy. Occasionally there is difficulty in identifying the proximal loop for irrigation; the surgeon should be asked to identify it when this is the case. When the distal loop is irrigated, the patient discharges the fluid via the rectum.

Prior to her surgery, Mrs. White was visited by the enterostomal therapist who would be responsible for teaching her the proper care of the stoma. The stomal site was marked by the therapist preoperatively, which served as a positive suggestion that Mrs. White would survive the surgery. In selecting the stomal placement, the most important consideration is proper fitting of a permanent collection appliance. Other important factors are physical freedom, aesthetic considerations, and visibility to the patient (*Rehabilitation of the Cancer Patient,* 1972).

Mrs. White was treated by a combined abdominal perineal resection. In this operation a left hemicolectomy is performed. All of the bowel distal to the splenic end of the transverse colon is removed. In Mrs. White's case, the distal end of the remaining bowel was brought through the abdominal wall to form the colostomy.

During the performance of this operation, Mrs. White had three incisions: a stab wound for the formation of the colostomy; an anterior incision for the exposure, exploration, and preparation of the area for the removal of the lesion; and, finally, a perineal incision for the completion of the removal of the tumor and the surrounding tissue. (Readers who are interested in the details of the operation are referred to the References.)

The surgeon had two objectives relating to the nature of the cancer and its site. His first objective was to remove all of the tumor bearing tissue, including the lymph channels and nodes draining the area. The second was to prevent the dissemination of cancer cells in the lumen of the bowel or through the veins draining the area. Dr. Surgeon also had in mind a third objective, which he was unable to achieve, that is, to preserve, if possible, the anal sphincters.

Throughout all phases of Mrs. White's experience as a patient with cancer, the objectives on which her nursing care was based took into account (1) her needs as an individual human being, (2) the fact that she was diagnosed as having cancer, (3) the fact that she had had an extensive surgical procedure, and (4) her resultant colostomy.

Factors considered in meeting Mrs. White's needs for nursing as they relate to the first three points have been discussed previously. The discussion will be limited to the steps in the eventual adjustment of Mrs. White to her colostomy.

Time is required to adapt to major changes in one's way of life. Although the social, psychological, financial, and health factors were favorable, she required time to adjust to the fact of the colostomy and to develop confidence that she would be able to control its behavior.

For the first two or three days following the operation, Mrs. White's needs were similar to those of other patients who had had extensive abdominal surgery. Dr. Surgeon had reassured both Mr. and Mrs. White that, as far as he could tell, all of the tumor had been removed. Mrs. White's postoperative progress was most satisfactory. On the morning of the third postoperative day, Mrs. White passed flatus through the colostomy. Although this indicated that normal physiological functioning of the gastrointestinal tract was returning, it also reminded Mrs. White that she was no longer able to control defecation. This aroused the fear that she might not be able to travel again because of the danger of involuntary defecation. As Mrs. White recovered physically, she became more and more aware of the physiologic alterations in her alimentary canal. As the function of the bowel returned, flatus and liquid feces were discharged through the colostomy stoma. This was very distressing to her and she became discouraged and depressed and had difficulty sleeping at night. She had little appetite. The enterostomal therapist visited her each day and as Mrs. White expressed some of her fears the therapist attempted to allay these by answering her questions frankly and clarifying any misconceptions that she had. Mrs. White was still apprehensive about caring for and irrigating her colostomy. Plans were made, through a local Q.T. club, for a person who had had a colostomy to visit her, someone who would be able to understand the fears she was experiencing and help her deal more effectively with these frustrations.

Mrs. White's behavior was by no means unusual. Some degree of depression usually accompanies serious illness and treatment by a major surgical procedure. Furthermore, the patient who has a colostomy may suffer additional shock from seeing the colostomy for the first time, from the involuntary discharges, and from the irrigations. A more or less severe emotional reaction is to be expected, because of what a colostomy means to many individuals. Some of these meanings stem from the fact that one of the important achievements in the life of a child is the attainment of control of his or her sphincters. Removal of the rectum with the ensuing loss of the ability to control defecation has consequences that go beyond the physiologic aspects. These consequences are largely emotional. In a few instances they may be so serious that, despite thoughtful and careful management, the life of the patient is permanently disrupted. In most instances, however, patients can be helped so that unnecessary restriction is prevented.

From the fourth day to the seventh day the colostomy moved erratically. A soft disposable postoperative pouch was applied as needed. Instructions on management of her colostomy began about the seventh postoperative day. During this time the therapist taught her care of the skin around the stoma, proper placement of the bag over the stoma, and irrigation of her colostomy. Although Mrs. White could have used the natural method of colostomy control, she decided in favor of the irrigation method. Her surgeon and the enterostomal therapist had planned that she learn how to irrigate regardless of the method she decided to use. They explained to Mrs. White that there might be occasions when it would be necessary to irrigate her colostomy, which is actually no more than an enema given through the stoma.

Two weeks after the operation Mrs. White was discharged from the hospital. She had made a good physiologic recovery. She had learned how to care for her colostomy and how to irrigate it, and had been assuming total care of herself since the tenth postoperative day. A visiting nurse referral had been made to assist Mrs. White in making the transition from hospital to home.

Most authorities emphasize that no special diet is required. A well-balanced diet in amounts necessary to maintain the desired weight and strength should be the objective. Patients may find that certain foods, especially those that are high in roughage, such as raw cabbage and fresh fruits, or very rich foods do stimulate peristalsis. The patient should be encouraged to eat a variety of foods. Mrs. White gradually added different foods to her diet. Eventually she found that by limiting the amount, she could eat almost anything but highly seasoned foods. She rarely had diarrhea, but when she did, she selected foods low in residue. She used as a reference *A Guide for Colostomee Rehabilitation* (Michigan Cancer Foundation, 1971).

Although Mrs. White was able to care for herself she was not without some fears. Because she was afraid of spillage, Mrs. White felt that she should wear a colostomy bag. This was a disposable plastic pouch that had a self-adherent backing and that was further secured by micropore tape.

Despite the reassurance of her surgeon that in time the colostomy would become regulated and that she would not require a bag, she found this difficult to believe. As is usual, in the early postoperative period Mrs. White had many liquid stools from her colostomy. As time passed, the number of defecations diminished and the contents became less fluid and more formed. In the early postoperative period, the bowel responds by increasing its activity and allowing less time for the absorption of water, resulting in liquid feces. As the activity of the bowel diminishes, water is absorbed and the stool becomes formed. The period in which her bowel was adapting to the artificial opening was a very trying time for Mrs. White, as it is for most patients. When a colostomy bag is applied soon after the colostomy starts to function, the patient is protected from spillage of intestinal contents on the wall of the abdomen, provided, of course, that it is properly applied. When absorbent dressings are used, they should be changed as soon as they are soiled. The skin around the colostomy should be washed and dried and a water-repellent powder applied. Low-lying areas such as the groin should be checked and washed as necessary. In the reapplication of dressings, the fact that water runs downhill should serve as a guide to their placement. Dressings should be fluffed to increase the surface for absorption and placed around the colostomy forming an encircling mound. They have little value when they are piled on top of the colostomy. When the bed linens are soiled, they should be changed. After the patient is clean and dry, the room should be aired.

At the time the dressing is changed, the skin around the colostomy should be observed for signs of redness or excoriation. This may be a result of too large an opening in the appliance; the stoma shrinks after surgery, causing the intestinal contents to irritate the skin. When the patient has an anterior abdominal incision, the dressing should be protected from, and checked for evidence of, soiling. Any abnormalities discovered should be reported to the surgeon.

Mrs. White needed to determine the best time for her to irrigate her colostomy. After some trial and error she decided to irrigate at night as this allowed time for any solution left in the intestine to be discharged. The irrigation took about 1 hour each evening. During her first 2 weeks at home Mrs. White had the assistance of a visiting nurse who came in twice a week. By that time Mrs. White had developed sufficient confidence in her ability to care for herself without the services of a visiting nurse. Total rehabilitation usually takes several weeks after discharge from the hospital, but it is usually complete in about 3 months following the operation.

After about a year Mrs. White and her husband took a trip around the world. She took a bottle of paregoric and the names of physicians that she could consult with should she need their services. Although she took a colostomy bag, she had graduated to wearing a piece of soft tissue lubricated with a small quantity of petroleum jelly over the colostomy. She wore an elastic girdle to hold it in place. During the entire trip, she spent only 1 day in her hotel room because of diarrhea. This was the only time that she needed her colostomy bag. When she returned home, she resumed her social and community activities.

Not all patients make as complete an adjustment to a colostomy as did Mrs. White. She was fortunate in that, as a person, she had the inner resources that made it possible for her to recover from the emotional shock created by having a colostomy. She was most fortunate in having an understanding and supporting husband as well as the financial resources to provide for her needs. Her medical and nursing care also contributed to her recovery. As a result of these and other factors, Mrs. White made a complete recovery.

Not all patients make as complete a recovery as Mrs. White. This is reflected in some degree of curtailment of their activities. Reasons given include fear of spillage, feelings of being unacceptable to others, the fear of being offensive because of odor, the fear of gas escaping, and the time required for irrigation. An occasional patient spends the entire day irrigating his or her colostomy. The problems confronting the patient are those illustrated by Mrs. White. They include (1) acceptance of the colostomy as necessary and manageable, (2) irrigations, (3) what is worn over the colostomy, and (4) diet—to the end that the food intake is adequate in quantity and quality. The overall objective should be to help the individual with a colostomy to learn to manage it so that, although it is necessary to remaining alive, it does not become the focus of his or her life.

Some of the factors in the patient's acceptance of the colostomy have been presented in the discussion of Mrs. White. To these might be added that patients regard a warm and supporting relationship with nurses as important in changing their outlook and aiding in their recovery. Moreover, an operation such as a colostomy lowers the self-esteem of the patient. Attention should be paid in the care of the patient to preventing further decrease in self-esteem by the way in which care is given.

All patients should be taught to irrigate their colostomy. Whether they use the method routinely or use the natural method, it may be necessary on occasion to irrigate. If patients are initially taught this procedure, it will not cause as much stress if and when it is required.

Patients who have a natural bowel movement at a regular time each day do not need colostomy irrigations. The patient who does not, or who, like Mrs. White, feels, more secure by irrigating the colostomy, uses the irrigation method. When irrigation is required, the patient and, if possible, a member of the family should be taught the procedure to be followed before the patient leaves the hospital. The equipment that the patient expects to use should be procured and the patient should use it when learning to irrigate the colostomy. Such factors as whether the patient has a bathroom that he or she can use and the time of day it is available should be considered in selecting the time to irrigate the colostomy.

The enterostomal therapist or nurse who instructs the patient should be competent and skillful. The patient can be expected to be highly anxious, and the anxiety decreases ability to learn. As a result, instruction may need to be repeated over and over. Learning is also easier when the person providing the instruction is understanding and supporting. A person under stress is likely to interpret the behavior of the nurse in personal terms. If the nurse is incompetent or appears to find the performance of the procedure distasteful, this behavior is likely to increase the anxiety of the patient and impair his or her ability to learn. Many hospitals have developed a procedure that they have found to be satisfactory. For hospitals lacking such a procedure, both the American Cancer Society (*Care of Your Colostomy*, 1976) and the Michigan Cancer Foundation (1971) have booklets that may prove helpful. Each booklet outlines a procedure for colostomy irrigation adapted for use at home. This same procedure can also be followed in the hospital. The instruction of the patient should be based on the fact that the purpose of the colostomy irrigation is the same as that of an enema. The same general principles apply in both instances. There is one important difference. The anal sphincters normally prevent the fluid from returning immediately. Because there is no sphincter at the opening of the colostomy, fluid may return as rapidly as it is introduced. A guard is required to prevent the backflow of fluid while it is introduced. A guard can be made by cutting off the tip of a rubber bulb syringe (ear syringe) and making an opening in the opposite end. The catheter is then introduced through the upper part of the bulb and down through the tip of the syringe. The position assumed by the patient during colostomy irrigation usually differs from that suggested for an enema. The patient sits on the toilet or a low stool and uses the toilet or a pail to catch the return. A plastic sleeve or conduit placed over the colostomy is helpful to direct the flow of the contents of the colon into the appropriate receptacle. Before the catheter is introduced, the air should be removed and the catheter lubricated as for an enema. When there is resistance to the passage of the catheter, force should not be used as the bowel can be perforated by its forcible introduction.

Because the colon does not contain any nerve endings, perforation does not always exhibit immediate pain. If resistance is felt, the clamp on the tubing should be opened and water allowed to flow into the intestine as the tube is introduced; the water opens the lumen of the bowel. Deep breathing and relaxation also allow for easier insertion of the catheter.

Because the opening into the colostomy may narrow with the passage of time, some surgeons teach patients to dilate the colostomy by inserting a finger into its opening and gentle rotating it.

The amount of solution required to effectively cleanse the bowel varies. Some patients use as little as a pint, whereas others use a quart or more. Some physicians advise patients to use warm water, whereas others suggest 2 tsp of salt or 1 tsp of baking soda be added to a quart of water. The frequency with which different individuals require irrigation also varies. Occasionally an individual has a regular evacuation and remains clean and dry in between. Some patients irrigate daily. Others irrigate only every second or third day. Timing is something that the patient has to learn by experience. After the patient becomes adept in the performance of the procedure, the total length of time required should not be more than one half to three quarters of an hour. If the patient consistently takes more than an hour, he or she should be encouraged to discuss this problem with the physician or with the enterostomal therapist. The patient should aim toward the development of a regular routine and schedule that is followed. The patient should be assured that after adjustment, the schedule does not have to be followed slavishly. Moreover, the time selected for the irrigation should take into account the needs of other members of the family as well as those of the patient. The time selected should be one that enables the patient to be comfortable and relaxed. The colon is sensitive to the feelings of the person. Feelings of pressure or tension have an adverse effect on the activity of the bowel.

The patient should be prepared for the difficulties

that are encountered in the performance of the procedure. Painful cramping is caused by the too rapid introduction of fluid into the intestine or by too large a volume; the flow of water should be stopped and the height of the fluid container lowered.

Just as with an enema, the results obtained from a colostomy irrigation may be inadequate. This may be caused by constipation or by fatigue or nervous strain. When the fluid does not return after a suitable interval, there is no need to be concerned about it, most of the fluid will return later. Some of the water will be absorbed by the colon, and the patient will notice a temporary increase in the frequency of urination. If the flow is just slow to return, massage of the abdomen may hasten its return.

Because the mucous membrane lining the colostomy is fragile, irritation may cause a small amount of bleeding, which is not unusual. Physicians vary in their recommendations to patients about what type of covering to wear over the colostomy. Some recommend that a colostomy bag be worn. Others suggest that a small, flat dressing (cloth, paper tissue, or a square cut from a disposable diaper) be worn. Gauze may be too rough and irritating. A small amount of petroleum jelly placed over the colostomy stoma lessens irritation. A girdle, supporter, or micropore tape may be used to hold the dressing in place.

With the exception of odors caused by escaping flatus, odors can be controlled by avoiding foods that the patient finds causes odor, and by scrupulous attention to cleanliness. The skin around the colostomy should be thoroughly washed with soap and water, and any equipment used must be kept clean. Equipment includes not only the colostomy bag, if one is worn, but girdles and irrigating equipment. There are deodorizing agents that can be taken by mouth or inserted into the colostomy pouch that will assist in combating odor.

Despite careful instruction of the patient and a member of the family before discharge from the hospital, the patient frequently requires, or benefits from, some assistance in adjusting to the home situation. In communities where a visiting nurse service is available, referral of the patient for this service should be considered. Patients are seldom fully recovered at the time of discharge. The home situation and family relationships may differ from those perceived by nurses and physicians who care for the patient in the hospital. For example, Mrs. White, who was well prepared, felt more secure by having this service available to her, for a short while. During the period of adjustment, the members of the family frequently require help in understanding the needs of the patient and their role in helping. The visiting nurse is accustomed to working with patients and their families in the home situation. She or he can guide them in working out practical and acceptable solutions to problems as they arise.

In communities where there are colostomy clubs, some persons gain comfort and help from other members of the club. They learn that they are not alone, as many others have a similar problem. They have an opportunity to learn from each other and to give each other mutual support.

The successful management of a colostomy by an individual requires knowledge, skill, and confidence that it can be managed without its being an undue burden. Whether or not the patient eventually achieves success depends on the patient, family, and the quality of professional services that are received during the entire period of illness and recovery. There are a few patients who are, despite excellent management, unable to adjust successfully with appropriate assistance. The adjustment of the patient is facilitated by all the members of the health team working with the patient and the members of the family to meet the needs of the patient at each stage of the recovery.[4]

The Patient with a Laryngectomy

Mr. Paul, a 60-year-old man, had suffered increasing hoarseness for a number of months. After seeking medical attention it was discovered, following a biopsy, that he had a large malignant laryngeal tumor. Mr. Paul refused a laryngectomy; therefore radiation therapy was given. This provided only temporary relief and soon he developed dyspnea and his voice was barely audible. The nurse asked Mr. Paul why he did not want to have the surgery. He replied that he "did not want to be a guinea pig so doctors could learn to do the operation" on him. After talking for a while longer Mr. Paul finally said, "When I have no more voice, I am no more a man." Thus the deeper meaning of loss of voice was revealed. To be voiceless meant a loss of manhood, not merely a surgical procedure and loss of his voice.

Because the voice is such a personal and powerful part of an individual's life, the loss of voice is a very real threat to the person's self-image. When deprived of the ability to speak, a person often feels less like an individual and may begin to suffer emotional difficulties. A man may equate the loss of his voice with the loss of his masculinity, as in the case of Mr. Paul. When a laryngectomy is performed, the man not only loses his masculine-sounding voice, but no longer possesses the fixator of the thorax, which

[4] Mrs. White died recently at age 90 from causes unrelated to cancer.

enables him to lift heavy objects. During the period of adjustment following surgery, and until other methods of communicating are developed, the man's resentment may increase, and he may experience ego deflation and depression.

As previously stated, Mr. Paul had developed progressive hoarseness, which is the main symptom of cancer of the larynx. Other symptoms are a feeling of having a lump in the throat, which is especially noticeable when swallowing, and dyspnea. Shortness of breath develops late, and obstruction of the airway indicates far advanced disease. Because Mr. Paul refused surgery the tumor's size had increased to the point that he experienced a partial airway obstruction.

The larynx is unique in that it contains a combination of functions, such as respiration, deglutination, phonation, communication by intelligible speech, and expression of emotions.

Through a local cancer society, plans were made for a laryngectomee (a person who has had the larynx removed) to visit Mr. Paul. Mr. Allen, using esophageal speech, talked with him about his fears and frustrations. He explained that there were some 25,000 laryngectomees in the United States, including about 3,000 women, and that most of them had returned to society as useful citizens. He told him that although cancer of the larynx was increasing by 4 to 5 per cent each year, it was one of the most curable cancers. He also tried to assure Mr. Paul that he could speak again by learning esophageal speech. Sixty-five per cent of laryngectomees speak effectively using this method. Sometimes an electrolarynx, a mechanical device, is used by persons before esophageal speech is learned, or by the 35 per cent who for various reasons cannot learn this method of speaking.

Although the nurses and physicians supported Mr. Paul in his decision not to have surgery, it became obvious that his respiratory obstruction was increasing with each passing day, and that a tracheostomy would be necessary to maintain life. Finally Mr. Paul decided in favor of the surgery. The surgeon again explained a total laryngectomy to him. The entire larynx (voice box) would be removed, including the epiglottis and the cricoid cartilage. (When possible, partial laryngectomies are performed.) The surgeon further explained that following surgery Mr. Paul would breathe through an opening in his neck called a stoma. He also told him that he would be able to learn esophageal speech a few weeks after surgery. The nurse who was present when the surgeon talked to Mr. Paul remained to answer any questions and to clarify what the surgeon had said.

The person who is diagnosed as having cancer of the larynx experiences three main fears. The first fear is of the diagnosis and surgery that will be necessary. Second is a fear of the actual operation, and the physical alteration caused in the body. The third, and most distressing fear is that of the loss of the voice (Stanley, 1967).

The nurse explained the postoperative exercises: coughing, deep breathing, turning, and moving his legs. She briefly discussed with him the use of the suction machine, the humidifier, intravenous therapy, and nasogastric tube feeding. She told him that he would have medication to reduce the pain. The nurse anticipated that Mr. Paul would indeed be frightened if he awakened following surgery to this strange new world of machines, sounds, and functions. She knew it was important to prepare him for these changes, but not in such detail that new fears might emerge. She allowed Mr. Paul time to ask questions and gave direct answers when she could. He expressed concern about being unable to speak and to make his wants known after surgery. He also expressed his worries about losing his job as a carpenter, about the loss of friends, and about how his family would accept him. The surgeon and nursing staff allowed him to discuss his concerns. After the surgeon had talked with his employer he was able to assure Mr. Paul that his job was secure.

It is difficult for the patient to communicate via writing for the first 24 to 48 hours following surgery because he is too weak and too uncomfortable. Therefore the nurse had a discussion time with Mr. Paul and his family, and a few of his close friends, to develop means of keeping communication open particularly during the first period after surgery.

A standard "request list" was individualized for Mr. Paul by adding specific notations. It was placed between plastic material that would make it easier to handle and that would prevent smudging from handling or from spills of liquids. The size of the lettering was sufficiently large to permit ease in reading. By means of the "request list" Mr. Paul would need only point to those things he wanted. Mr. Paul also decided he would prefer a "magic slate" to paper and pencil. A card index system is another form of the "request list." In this arrangement, requests are written on 3 x 5 in. index cards and assembled in alphabetical order. The cards are attached with metal rings, and alphabetized tabs are placed on the index cards; this allows the patient to turn quickly and easily to requests. For the patient who is unable to read, pictures may be drawn or cut from magazines and pasted on a sheet of paper or on separate cards. The patient can then locate the picture that symbolizes his wants.

The intracommunication system was explained to Mr. Paul and his family. The key on the intracommunication system box was marked to indicate that Mr.

Paul was unable to speak. Thus when the call is answered from the desk Mr. Paul can be told that someone will be there. Because he is unable to call out to gain notice, he may feel insecure. He was also given a hand bell to assist him in gaining someone's attention.

The nasogastric tube was inserted the morning prior to surgery. Mr. Paul knew that he would be fed by this means temporarily after his laryngectomy. Mr. Paul was premedicated and left for the operating room at 8 A.M. His wife and daughter accompanied him to the elevator. They then went to the surgical lounge to wait till the surgery was completed. Meanwhile, the nurse who was preparing the unit for his return obtained a suction machine, the suction catheters, and the necessary solutions for rinsing the catheters between suctioning. A humidifier was placed by the bed to increase the moisture of the inspired air, to prevent crusting and drying of secretions in the tracheostomy tube and in the trachea. A tracheostomy tube clean-up tray was placed in readiness, as the inner cannula may need cleaning every 4 hours for the first 24 to 48 hours following surgery. Secretions are much more copious in the immediate hours following the operation, both because of the edema and increased secretions resulting from the surgery and because of the trachea, which is attempting to rid itself of the foreign laryngectomy tube. The "request list" along with a "magic slate" were tied to the side rail. Mr. Paul returned to his room at 2:30 P.M. He was positioned in a 45° angle. He was coughing and needed immediate suctioning. The obturator for the laryngectomy tube was labeled and taped to the head of the bed. The dressing was observed for signs of bleeding. The intravenous site was observed for infiltration and for the amount remaining in the bottle. The bell cord was attached to his gown. Mr. Paul was restless, turned his head from side to side, and winced. Mr. Paul pointed to the word *pain* on the "request list" and pointed to his neck. After checking the chart the nurse noted that Mr. Paul could have meperidine hydrochloride, 100 mg every 3 to 4 hours for pain, and he had not received any since surgery. It took about one half hour for the medication to take effect and reduce the pain for Mr. Paul. His wife and family stayed until late that evening. Mr. Paul was sleeping when they left.

Mr. Paul began nasogastric feedings on the first postoperative day and tolerated them well. He continued to need suctioning every hour, which was performed very gently to decrease injury to the fragile mucous membrane. The inner cannula of the laryngectomy tube was removed for cleansing every 4 hours. Strict asepsis was maintained to reduce the development of infection around the stoma or within the trachea. The skin around the stoma was cleansed four times a day. A 4 x 4 in. telfa pad was placed around the outer laryngectomy cannula. This decreased irritation to the suture line as pads of this composition do not interfere with wound healing. By the second postoperative day, Mr. Paul was ambulating four times a day and was doing part of his bath. The nurse was now having him assist with the nasogastric feedings; within a couple of days he could acomplish this for himself. Mr. Paul continued to be more independent. He was communicating by using both the "request list" and the "magic slate." He also had devised a method by which he could communicate via the telephone with his wife by tapping with a coin a certain number of times, according to their code.

Oral hygiene was carried out diligently. Brushing his teeth three times a day and using a mouth wash as many times made Mr. Paul much more comfortable. Mr. and Mrs. Paul were learning how to suction the laryngectomy tube and how to clean the inner cannula. The home care coordinator had been notified well in advance of the discharge and discussed care in the home with Mr. and Mrs. Paul. The nasogastric tube had been removed and Mr. Paul was tolerating oral foods and fluid well. The speech therapist talked with Mr. Paul and made arrangements for him to attend classes to learn esophageal speech.

In preparation for his discharge Mr. Paul was given an identification card for a "neck breather," which was obtained from the American Cancer Society. He was instructed to carry it with him at all times. Medic-Alert was explained, and the name and address were provided should Mr. Paul desire to secure an identification bracelet from this source. Information was given to Mr. Paul regarding the International Association of Laryngectomees. This association has 150 Lost Chord or New Voice clubs in the United States.

Mr. Paul was given bibs to cover his neck stoma which would prevent dust and dirt from entering the trachea. His wife was given instructions and a pattern for making these bibs. Samples were obtained from a local cancer foundation. A suction machine was borrowed from the local Cancer Society 2 days prior to discharge so that Mr. and Mrs. Paul could become familiar with it, as often one machine varies slightly from another. A humidifier was borrowed from a daughter.

At the time of discharge Mr. Paul was able to cleanse his own laryngectomy tube and to suction himself. Arrangements were made for a visiting nurse to be in the home the day following discharge, to answer any questions, to observe the ease with which transfer was made from hospital to home, and to assist and guide in his care. Mrs. Paul stated that she felt more secure knowing that a nurse would come to the home to "check on things."

Six weeks following his laryngectomy Mr. Paul attended speech classes to learn esophageal speech. After 4 weeks of class Mr. Paul was unable to use the esophageal voice effectively. He became very frustrated and feared he would never be able to speak again. The speech therapist and Mr. Paul's physician agreed to let Mr. Paul purchase a mechanical device so that he might be able to speak. They are simple to use and supply the individual with an instant voice. Both physician and speech therapist thought this would encourage Mr. Paul, cause him to relax, and allow him to learn esophageal speech more easily. Three weeks later Mr. Paul was speaking using esophageal voice and was able to communicate to a degree with others.

Cancer Quacks

No discussion of the problems created by neoplasms is complete without some consideration of why people consult cancer quacks and of the kinds of information useful in distinguishing between a quack and a bona fide physician. First, quacks are not unique to cancer. They seek out people who have a health problem that is not easily solved by available methods of treatment. Any long-term and disabling illness provides the quack with an opportunity to offer sick people hope and to exploit their feelings to his or her own ends. Sometimes a quack treats many types of disease including arthritis, cancer, diabetes mellitus, and gout.

Possibly cancer offers a more fertile field for the quack than many other diseases because people all too often regard cancer as a mysterious and hopeless disease having a poor prognosis. Knowledge or even a suspicion that cancer is a possibility may cause the person and the family to go into a state of panic. This may result in the person grasping at straws and seeking help from someone who promises cure—the cancer quack.

When a person consults a cancer quack for diagnosis and treatment, he or she may be "cured" because cancer is not present. Persons who do have cancer may lose valuable time or undergo treatments that spread rather than eradicate the growth. Persons who are in the terminal phase of cancer may experience an extended period of declining health. As the patient and members of the family observe this failure to respond to treatment, their anxiety increases as they wonder whether all that can and should be is being done. When they are told or read about a "doctor" who not only promises but is able to cure persons who are seriously ill with cancer by injections of a magic solution or rays of a mysterious light, they may be sorely tempted to consult him or her.

Approaches that cancer quacks implement include drugs, mechanical devices, nutritional approaches, and occult techniques.

Two drugs that are commonly used by quacks for prevention and cure of cancer are krebiozen or carcalon and amygkalin or Laetrile. Food and Drug Administration analyses of krebiozen has shown it to be composed of mineral oil, amyl, alcohol, and a creatine derivative. It has no proven anticancer activity (ACS, *Cancer Quackery*, 1977).

Laetrile has been receiving much publicity lately but it has been known for better than 50 years. It was first described in 1920 by Ernst Krebs, Sr., who reported "substantial results" in treating cancer patients with advanced disease. (Horton & Hill, 1977). He used betacyanogenic glucoside (amygdalin), which was derived from apricot kernels. The substance was too toxic for general use, but Ernst Krebs, Jr., a biochemist, made the chemical safe for human parenteral administration in 1952. In 1962 it was called 1-mandelo-nitrile-betaglucuroniside. Ernst Krebs, Jr., named the drug Laetrile because it was a laevorotary nitrile (Horton & Hill, 1977).

Use of Laetrile as a treatment is based on the trophoblastic theory of cancer; that is, there is only one kind of cancer, therefore, a single miracle drug can be used for all types. Because the drug has received such widespread publicity it is currently under investigation by several reputable research institutes. To date there has been no proven anticancer activity in humans and use of Laetrile is illegal in the United States. Because of its cyanide content, large doses of Laetrile may be toxic.

Hoxsey is another chemical agent used by quacks for cancer treatment. It contains ingredients such as cascara, prickly ash, potassium iodide, red clover, buck thorn, alfalfa, sugar syrup, and water.

All of these chemicals are available and legal in certain foreign countries. Many cancer patients spend great sums of money traveling to these countries to purchase the treatments.

Mechanical devices include ozone generators which produce a gas for inhalation that supposedly cures the cancer and Down instruments which cure via remote control. Use of these machines has decreased in recent years, but many cancer patients still turn to them (Burkhalter, 1977).

Nutritional approaches run the gamut from ingestion of particular kinds of food to fasting. The regimens are offered for prevention and/or cure of cancer. The diets may recommend only raw vegetables or periods of fasting from 3 to 45 days while ingesting only water. Other regimens include combinations of various nutritional supplements, fasting, and colonic enemas (Burkhalter, 1977). Although these approaches may not be harmful per se, they can delay seeking legitimate interventions and treatment that may be helpful.

Some cancer quacks create a faith cult around themselves and their methods. Occult techniques used include seances, trances, and incantations. "Psycho-surgeons" who claim to be able to perform surgery without incisions represent a form of occult cancer quackery (Burkhalter, 1977). None of these methods is proven.

One form of protection of the patient and family is the kind of supportive care that convinces them that all that can be done will be done. Among the values to patients who participate in studies of drugs and other treatments for cancer is that they are offered hope that they will be benefited in time. Perhaps at least as important is the interest that medical and nursing personnel express in their behavior and progress. Many patients take pride in knowing that they may die making a contribution to knowledge of the prevention and treatment of cancer.

Use of unproven methods is deletereous to patients because it can give them a false sense of security and prevent them from seeking methods of early detection and treatment; they may stop conventional proven methods of radical treatment; and the cost can ruin families financially.

The Pure Food, Drug and Cosmetic Act became more forceful in 1962 by the addition of the Kefauver–Harris amendments, which place the burden of proof upon the proponent of a remedy. Under this law those wishing to distribute an unproved remedy for investigational purposes in interstate commerce must file an acceptable plan with the federal Food and Drug Administration.

Legislation has been passed in only eight states to control worthless cancer remedies within state boundaries. California was the first state to pass such legislation, in 1959 (ACS, *Cancer Quackery*, 1977, p. 15).

To help people avoid cancer quacks, the American Cancer Society has prepared the following list of common characteristics of quacks that the public should be aware of when selecting or rejecting a physician to diagnose and treat cancer (*Cancer News*, 1973, pp. 20–22):

1. They guarantee a cure in all or at least a vast majority of cases.
2. Their "cures" are secret.
3. Their "cures" are "natural" or based on some principle supposedly overlooked by all other researchers.
4. They present testimonials.
5. They claim that they are being persecuted by the "medical monopoly" or are generally being conspired against.
6. They are avid for publicity and advertise their nostrums and services.

The American Cancer Society and the local county medical society are sources of information about many quacks.

In addition to using public education, the nurse also helps to prevent patients from seeking attention from quacks by the practice of her or his supportive role. Patients and their families desperately want to have something done that offers hope. They want evidence that something is being done. They want to feel that those who care for them care about what happens to them. The quack offers this hope and exploits the feelings of the patient and family to his or her own ends.

There are at least six things the nurse can do to help patients who may be tempted to seek treatment from a cancer quack (Burkhalter, 1977): (1) Give the patient your time. That is probably the primary commodity that the quack offers that the patient truly needs. Treat the patient with dignity and support his or her integrity. (2) Know what quackery is and the various forms of it which may be offered to the patient. Be prepared to provide correct information to the patient when the opportunity arises. (3) Maintain an open attitude so that the patient will not feel embarrassment in asking your opinion concerning unproven methods. This will provide a channel of communication through which the patient can get correct, current information. (4) Maintain a nonjudgmental attitude, especially if the patient is coming to you after having had an experience with quackery. (5) If there are unproven methods being used in the community, report them to the health department and support legislation to control use of unproven methods. (6) Offer hope. If cure or control is not a possible outcome, at least support hope for a quality of life which includes maintenance of dignity and self-worth.

In all phases in the life of the patient with cancer, the nurse contributes to the care of the patient through supportive and therapeutic roles. She or he has a part to play in prevention and in detection of cancer as well as in the phases in which the patient has overt disease. In whatever stage of illness, the nurse has much to offer the patient. This is true even, and particularly, in the care of patients who have widespread and progressive disease.

References Cited

American Cancer Society. *Cancer Quackery—Laetrile.* New York: American Cancer Society, 1977.

American Cancer Society. *Cancer Statistics.* New York: American Cancer Society, 1978.

American Cancer Society. *Facts about Leukemia.* New York: American Cancer Society, April 1963.

American Cancer Society. *Essentials of Cancer Nursing.* New York: American Cancer Society, 1963.

American Cancer Society. *Care of Your Colostomy.* New York: American Cancer Society, 1976.

American Cancer Society. "Combating Cancer Quackery." *Cancer News,* **27** (Spring 1973), 20–22.

American Joint Committee for Cancer Staging and End-Results Reporting. *Manual for Staging of Cancer.* Chicago: American Joint Committee, 1977.

American Nurses Association. *Outcome Standards for Cancer Nursing Practice.* Kansas City, Mo.: American Nurses Association, 1979.

Anderson, N. "Paraneoplastic Syndromes: A Clinical Approach." In *Program of the Course in Management of Advanced and Metastatic Cancer.* Boston: Harvard Medical School, June 7–9, 1979.

Antunes, C., Stolley, P., Rosenshein, N., Davies, J., Tonascia, J., Brown, C., Burnett, L., Rutledge, A., Pokempner, M., and Garcia, R. "Endometrial Cancer and Estrogenase." *New Eng. J. Med.,* **300:**1 (1979), 9–13.

Avis, F., Avis, I., Hindsley, J. P., and Houghton, G. "Interactions of Cancer Cells with Antibodies and Other Tumor Factors." In *Fundamental Aspects of Metastasis.* Ed. by L. Weiss, Amsterdam-Oxford: North Holland Publishing Co., 1979, pp. 191–204.

Axtell, L., Asire, A., Myers, M. *Cancer Patient Survival Report Number 5.* Bethesda, Md.: U.S. Department of Health, Education, and Welfare, Publication No. (NIH) 77–992, 1976.

Bagshawe, K. D., ed. *Medical Oncology: Medical Aspects of Malignant Disease.* London: Blackwell Scientific Publications, 1975.

Bakemeier, R. "Basic Principles of Tumor Immunotherapy." In *Clinical Oncology for Medical Students and Physicians a Multidisciplinary Approach.* Ed. by P. Rubin, New York: American Cancer Society, 1978.

Baker, L. et al. Electrocardiographic Changes in Cancer Patients with Cardiac Metastasis." A paper presented at the Grace Hospital Clinic Day at Raleigh House, Southfield, Mich., May 1972.

Barkley, V. "Nursing the Patient with Cancer, an Exercise in Timing." *Cancer,* **17** (May–June 1967), 127.

Barnes, J. W. "Sugar Sweetens the Lot of Patients with Bedsores." *JAMA,* **223** (Jan. 8, 1973), 122.

Best, R., Zbar, B., Borsos, T., Rapp, H. "BCG and Cancer, Part 1," *New Engl. J. Med.,* **290:**25 (1974), 1413–20.

______. "BCG and Cancer, Part 2." *New Engl. J. Medicine,* **290:**25 (1974), 1458–69.

Bittner, J. "The Causes and Control of Mammary Cancer in Mice." *Harvey Lect.,* **42** (1946–47), 224.

Bonica, J. J. "Cancer Pain: A Major National Health Problem." *Cancer Nurs.,* **1:**4 (1978), 313–16.

Bonica, J. J. "The Management of Pain of Malignant Disease with Nerve Block." *Anesthesiology,* **15:**1 (1954), 134+.

Buell, R., Tremblay, G., Rowden, G. "Distribution of Adenosine Triphosphatase in Infiltrating Ductal Carcinoma and Non-Neoplastic Breast." *Cancer,* **38:**2 (1976), 875–87.

Burch, P. *The Biology of Cancer a New Approach.* Lancaster, Eng.: MTP Press Ltd., 1976.

Burchenal, J. H. "Long-Term Survivors in Acute Leukemia and Burkitt's Tumor," *Cancer,* **21:**596, Apr. 1968.

Burkhalter, P. "Cancer Quackery." *Am. J. Nurs.,* **77:**3 (1977), 451–53.

Campbell, J., Doublsky, J., McNally, J., and LaFleur, C. *"Nursing Protocols for Hospice Home Care."* Detroit: unpublished manuscript. Copyright, June 1979.

"The Cancer Program Workshop." *Cancer Bull.,* **11** (May–June 1959), 47.

"Cancer and Immune Mechanisms." *JAMA,* **224** (May 28, 1973), 1286.

Canellos, G. "Diagnosis and Treatment of Hodgkin's Disease." *Resident and Staff Physician,* a desk reference issue. (1979), 26–31.

Canellos, G. "Treatment of Leukemias." *Resident and Staff Physician* (Jan. 1979), 47–55.

Chew, E. C., Josephson, R. L., and Wallace, A. C. "Morphologic Aspects of the Arrest of Circulating Cancer Cells." In *Fundamental Aspects of Metastasis.* Ed. by N. Weiss, Amsterdam: North Holland Publishing Co., 1970, 120-150.

Christopherson, W., Lundin, F., Mendez, W., and Parker, J. "Cervical Cancer Control." *Cancer,* **38:**3 (1976), 1357–66.

Clark, R. L. "Systemic Cancer and the Metastatic Process." *Cancer,* **43:**3 (1979), 790–97.

Cline, M. *Cancer Chemotherapy Vol. I: Major Problems in Internal Medicine.* Philadelphia: W. B. Saunders Co., 1971.

Cort, D. F. "Positive Infusion Control in the Treatment of Burns in Children." *Br. J. Plastic Surgery,* **23** (Oct. 1970), 395–97.

Cross, H., Kennel, E., and Lilienfeld, A. "Cancer of the Cervix in Amish Population." *Cancer,* **21** (Jan. 1968), 102.

Day, E. "What Is an Adequate Cancer Check-up?" *Postgrad. Med.,* **27** (March 1960), 275.

de Gutierrez-Mahoney, C., and Carini, E. *Neurological and Neurosurgical Nursing,* 5th ed. St. Louis: C. V. Mosby Co., 1970.

DeLellis, R., Rule, A., Spiler, I., Nathanson, L., Tashjian, A., and Wolf, H. "Calcitonin and Carcinoembryonic Antigen as Tumor Markers in Medullary Thyroid Carcinoma." *Amer. J. Clin. Pathology,* **70:**4 (1978), 587–94.

del Regato, J. A., and Spjut, H. J. *Cancer Diagnosis, Treatment and Prognosis,* 5th ed. St. Louis: C. V. Mosby Co., 1977.

Drum, D. "Scintigraphy of the Liver and Spleen." *Postgrad. Med.,* **54:**7 (1973), 118–23.

Englert, D., and Dudrick, S. "Principles of Ambulatory Home Hyperalimentation." *Amer. J. Intravenous Therapy*, (Aug.–Sept. 1978), 12–28.

Extracorporeal Medical Specialties. *New Holter Precision Roller Pumps Series 700.* King of Prussia, Pa.: Extracorporeal Medical Specialties, Inc.

Fidler, I. J. "Mechanisms of Cancer Invasion and Metastasis." In *Cancer: A Comprehensive Treatise, Vol. IV.* Ed. by F. Becker. London: Plenum Press, 1975, pp. 101–31.

Folkman, J. "Tumor Angiogenesis." In *Cancer: A Comprehensive Treatise, Vol. III.* Ed. by F. Becker. London: Plenum Press, 1975, pp. 355–88.

Folkman, J. "The Vascularization of Tumors." *Sci. Am.* **234:**5 (1976), 59–73.

Garb, S. "Neglected Approaches to Cancer." *Sat. Rev.* (June 1, 1968), 54.

Giacquinta, B. "Helping Families Face the Crisis of Cancer." *Am. J. Nurs.*, **77:**10 (1977), 1585–88.

Greenspan, E., ed. *Clinical Cancer Chemotherapy.* New York: Raven Press, 1975.

Hardy, J. D. "Pathophysiology in Surgery." Baltimore: Williams & Wilkins Co., 1958.

Herbst, A. L., Ulfelder, H., and Poskanzer, D. C. "Adenocarcinoma of the Vagina: Association of Maternal Stilbesterol Therapy with Tumor Appearance in Young Women." *New Engl. J. Med.*, **284:**16 (1971), 878–81.

Hibbs, J. B., Jr. "Role of Macrophages in Resistance to Cancer." In *Immunological Aspects of Neoplasia.* Baltimore: Williams & Wilkins Co., 1975, pp. 305–27.

Hill, C. S., and Hickey, R. "Drug Therapy of Hypercalcemia in Cancer Patients." *Drug Therapy Bull.* (Jan. 1973), 19–21+.

Holland, J., and Frei, E. *Cancer Medicine.* Philadelphia: Lea and Febiger, 1973.

Holland, J., Plumb, M., Yates, J., Harris, S., Tuttolomendo, A., Holmes, J., and Holland, J. "Psychological response of Patients with Acute Leukemia to Germ Free Environments." *Cancer,* **40:**2 (1977), 871–79.

Horton, J., and Hill, G., eds. *Clinical Oncology.* Philadelphia: W. B. Saunders Co., 1977.

International Union Against Cancer (UICC). *TNM Classification of Malignant Tumors.* Geneva: UICC, 1962.

International Union Against Cancer (UICC) Committee on Professional Education, eds. *Clinical Oncology a Manual for Students and Doctors.* Berlin: Springer-Verlag, 1973.

Isaacson, P., and LeVann, P. "The Demonstration of Carcinoembryonic Antigen in Colorectal Carcinoma and Colonic Polyps Using an Immunoperoxidase Technique." *Cancer,* **38:**3 (1976), 1348–56.

Isler, C. "The Cancer Nurse: How the Specialists Are Doing It." *RN,* **35:**2 (1972), 4.

Jablon, R., and Volk, H. "Revealing Diagnosis and Prognosis to Cancer Patients." In Turner, E., ed. *Differential Diagnosis and Treatment in Social Work,* 2nd ed. New York: The Free Press, 1976, pp. 394–402.

Kastenbaum, B., and Spector, R. "What Should a Nurse Tell a Cancer Patient?" *Amer. J. Nurs.*, **78:**4 (1978), 640–41.

Klein, C. "Tumor Immunology: A General Appraisal." In *Scientific Foundation of Oncology.* Ed. by T. Symington and R. L. Carter, London: William Heinemann Medical Books Ltd., 1976, pp. 497–504.

Lasser, T. *Reach to Recovery,* rev. ed. New York: American Cancer Society, 1969.

Lawrence, W., and Terz, J., eds. *Cancer Management.* New York: Grune and Stratton, 1977.

Lessner, H., ed. *Medical Oncology.* New York: Elsevier North Holland, 1978.

Levine, J., and Ziegler, E. "Denial and Self Image in Stroke, Lung Cancer, and Heart Disease Patients." *Consult. Clinical Psychol.*, **43:**6 (1975), 751–57.

Libshitz, H. "Thermography of the Breast." *JAMA,* **238:**18 (1977), 1953–54.

"Link Viral Genes to Cancer." *Pub. Health Rep.*, **78** (July 1963), 568.

Lundy, J., Lovett, E., Wolinsky, S., Couran, P. "Immune Impairment and Metastatic Tumor Growth." *Cancer,* **43:**3 (1979), 945–51.

Maier, W., Goldman, L., Kaplan, C., Tyson, R. "A Ten Year Study of Medullary Carcinoma of the Breast." *Surgery Gynecol. Obstet.*, **144:**5 (1977), 695–98.

Mauer, T., Pendergrass, T., Borges, W., and Honig, G. "The Role of Genetic Factors in Etiology of Wilms's Tumor." *Cancer,* **43:**1 (1979), 205–8.

McCorkle, M. "Coping with Physical Symptoms in Metastatic Breast Cancer." *Am. J. Nurs.*, **73:**6 (1973), 1034–38.

McIntosh, J. "Patients' Awareness and Desire for Information about Diagnosed but Undisclosed Malignant Disease." *Lancet* (Aug. 7, 1976), 300–3.

McMichael, A. J. "Increases in Laryngeal Cancer in Britain and Australia in Relation to Alcohol and Tobacco Consumption Trends." *Lancet,* (June 10, 1978), 1244–46.

M. D. Anderson Hospital and Tumor Institute. *Investigational Drugs Data Sheets.* Houston: The University of Texas, 1972.

Mehta, M. *Intractable Pain.* Philadelphia: W. B. Saunders Co., 1973.

Melton, P. *IVAC 500 Infusion Pump.* San Diego: IVAC Corporation, 1973.

Melton, P. *The IVAC 200 Infusion Controller.* San Diego: IVAC Corporation, 1973.

Metropolitan Life Insurance Company. "Employing the Cancer Patient." *Statistical Bull.*, **54** (June, 1973).

Miaskowski, C. "The Brompton Cocktail." *Cancer Nurs.*, **1:**6 (1978), 451–55.

Michigan Cancer Foundation. *A Guide for Colostomee Rehabilitation.* Detroit: Michigan Cancer Foundation, 1971.

Miki, K., Oda, T., Suzuki, H., Niwa, H. "Alkaline Phosphatase Isoenzymes in Intestinal Metaplasia and Carcinoma of the Stomach." *Cancer Res.*, **36:**11 (1976), 4266–68.

Moskowitz, M., Milbrath, J., Cartside, P., Zermens, A., and Mandel, D. "Lack of Efficacy of Thermography as a Screening Tool for Minimal and State I Breast Cancer." *New Engl. Med.*, **295:**5 (1976), 249–52.

Mundinger, M. "Nursing Diagnoses for Cancer Patients." *Cancer Nurs.*, **1:**3 (1978), 221–26.

Murphy, T. "Cancer Pain." *Postgrad. Med.*, **53:**6 (1973), 187–94.

Nicolson, G. "Cancer Metastasis." *Sci. Am.*, **240**:3 (1979), 66–76.

Ossowski, L., Unkeless, J. C., Tobia, A., Quigley, J. P., Rifkin, D. B., and Reich, E. "An Enzymatic Function Associated with Transformation of Fibroblasts by Oncogenic Virus: II Mammallian Fibroblasts Cultures Transformed by DNA and RNA Tumor Virus. *J. Exper. Med.*, **137** (1973), 112–26.

Payan, H. "Cancer in Married Couples." *S. Med. J.*, **72**:1 (1979), 17–19.

Rauscher, F. J., Jr. *National Cancer Program: Report of the Director.* Bethesda, Md.: U.S. Department of Health, Education, and Welfare, Publication No. (NIH) 74–472, 1974.

Raven, R., ed. *Principles of Surgical Oncology.* New York: Plenum Medical Book Co., 1977.

Rehabilitation of the Cancer Patient. Chicago: Yearbook Medical Publishers, 1972, pp. 143–45.

Reif, A. E. "Public Information on Smoking: An Urgent Responsibility for Cancer Research Workers." *J. Nat. Cancer Institute,* **57**:6 (1976), 1207–10.

Rettig, R. A. *Cancer Crusade.* Princeton, N.J.: Princeton University Press, 1977.

Reynoso, G., Tsann, M., Holyoke, D., Cohen, E., Nemoto, T., Wang, J., Chanung, J., Guinan, P., Murphy, G. "Carcinoembryonic Antigen in Patients with Different Cancers." *JAMA* **220**:3 (1972), 361–65.

Rhodes, C. P. "Nitrogen Mustards in the Treatment of Neoplastic Disease. Official Statement." *JAMA,* **131** (1940), 656–58.

Rosai, J., and Ackermann, L. "The Pathology of Tumors, Part III: Grading, Staging, and Classification." *CA-A J. Clin.,* **29**:2 (1979), 66–77.

Rowlingson, J. "Management of Cancer Pain." *Cancer Nurs.,* **1**:4 (1978), 317–18.

Rubin, P., ed. *Clinical Oncology for Medical Students and Physicians, a Multidisciplinary Approach,* 5th ed. New York: American Cancer Society, 1978.

Salmon, S., and Jones, S., eds. *Adjuvant Therapy of Cancer.* New York: North-Holland Publishing Co., 1977.

Schottenfeld, D. *Cancer Epidemiology and Prevention Current Concepts.* Springfield, Ill.: Charles C Thomas, 1975.

Shawver, M. "Pain Associated with Cancer." In *Pain a Sourcebook for Nurses and Other Health Professionals.* Ed. by A. Jacox. Boston: Little, Brown, 1977, pp. 373–89.

Silverberg, E. "Cancer Statistics." *CA—A Journal for Clinicians,* **29**:1 (1979), 6–21.

Slaughter, D. P. "What Is Early Cancer?" *Postgrad. Med.,* **27** (March 1960), 271–73.

Stanley, L. "Meeting the Psychological Needs of the Laryngectomy Patient." *Nurs. Clin. North Am.,* **3**(Dec. 1967), 520.

Sutherland, A. et al. "The Psychological Impact of Cancer and Cancer Surgery." *Cancer,* **5**:9 (1952), 857–72.

Talso, P., and Remenchik, A. *Internal Medicine: Research on Mechanisms of Disease.* St. Louis: C. V. Mosby Co., 1968.

Third National Conference for Nursing Diagnosis Classification. April 5–9, 1978, St. Louis, Missouri.

Tiedt, E. "The Psychodynamic Process of the Oncologic Experience." *Nurs. Forum.* **14**:3 (1975), 264–77.

Travis, E. *Primer of Medical Radiobiology.* Chicago: Yearbook Medical Publishers, 1975.

U.S. Catheter and Instrument Corp. *Watkins USCI Chronofusor.* New York: C. R. Bard, 1971.

U.S. Department of Health, Education, and Welfare. *Health Consequences of Smoking.* Bethesda, Md.: U.S. Department of Health, Education, and Welfare, 1968.

U.S. Department of Health, Education, and Welfare, Public Health Service. *International Classification of Diseases Vol. II.,* 8th rev. Washington, D.C.: U.S. Department of Health, Education, and Welfare, Public Health Service, 1968.

U.S. Department of Health, Education, and Welfare. *National Cancer Program: the Strategic Plan.* Bethesda, Md.: U.S. Department of Health, Education, and Welfare, Publication No. (NIH) 74-569, 1974.

U.S. Department of Health, Education, and Welfare. *The Smoking Digest: Progress Report of a Nation Kicking the Habit.* Bethesda, Md.: U.S. Department of Health, Education, and Welfare, 1977.

Vaitkevicius, V., and Moghissi, K. "The Pap Test Can Save More Lives: Comments about Research in Detroit, Nation." *Michigan Med.,* **67**:3 (1968), 315–18.

Valentine, A. "Caring for the Young Adult with Cancer." *Cancer Nurs.,* **1**:5 (1978), 285–389.

Valentine, A., Steckel, S., and Weintraub, M. "Pain Relief for Cancer Patients." *Amer. J. Nurs.,* **78**:12 (1978), 2054–56.

Williams, D. ed. "Biological Mechanisms in Metastasis." In *New Aspects of Breast Cancer, Vol. III.* Ed. by B. A. Stoll. London: William Heinemann Medical Books, 1977, pp. 95–110.

Winkelstein, W. "Smoking and Cancer of the Uterine Cervix: Hypothesis." *Amer. J. Epidemiol.,* **106**:4 (1977), 257–58.

Wynder, E. L., Mushinski, M. H., and Spivak, J. C. "Tobacco and Alcohol Consumption in Relation to the Development of Multiple Primary Cancers." *Cancer,* **40**:4 (1977), 1872–78.

Yates, J., and Holland, J. "A Controlled Study of Isolation and Endogenous Microbial Suppression in Acute Myelocytic Leukemia Patients." *Cancer,* **32**:6 (1973), 1490–98.

Young, J., Asino, A., and Pollack, E., eds. *SEER Program: Cancer Incidence and Mortality in the United States.* Bethesda, Md.: U.S. Department of Health, Education, and Welfare, Publication No. (NIH) 78-1837, 1978.

General References

Ambrose, E., and Roe, F. eds. *Biology of Cancer,* 2nd ed. Chichester, Eng.: Ellis Harwood Limited, 1975.

American Cancer Society. *Reach for Recovery.* New York: American Cancer Society, 1977.

American Cancer Society. *Unproven Methods of Cancer Management.* New York: American Cancer Society, 1971.

Ariel, I., ed. *Progress in Clinical Cancer, Vol. VII.* New York: Grune and Stratton, 1978.

Beck, S. "Impact of a Systemic Oral Care Protocol on Stomatitis after Chemotherapy." *Cancer Nurs.*, **2**:3 (1979), 185–99.

Benoliel, J., and McCorkle, R. "A Holistic Approach to Terminal Illness." *Cancer Nurs.*, **1**:2 (1978), 143–49.

Bloomquist, L., and Lewis-Hungstiger, M. "To Care for the Child at Home: Discharge Planning for the Child with Leukemia." *Cancer Nurs.*, **1**:4 (1978), 303–8.

Blues, K. "A Framework for Nurses Providing Care for Laryngectomy Patients." *Cancer Nurs.*, **1**:6 (1978), 441–46.

Bodansky, O. *Biochemistry of Human Cancer.* New York: Academic Press, 1975.

Bradbury, S. *The Microscope Past and Present.* London: Pergamon Press, 1968.

The Cancer Letter. Reston, Va.: Cancer Letter, Inc. **4**:42 (1978), 1.

Carroll, R. "BCG Immunotherapy by the Tine Technique: The Nurse's Role." *Cancer Nurs.*, **1**:3 (1978), 241–46.

Chew, E. C., Josephson, R. L., and Wallace, A. C. "Morphologic Aspects of the Arrest of Circulating Cancer Cells. In *Fundamental Aspects of Metastasis.* Ed. by L. Weiss. Amsterdam: North Holland Publishing Co., 1970, pp. 120–50.

Clark, R. L., and Howe, C. D., eds. *Cancer Patient Care at M.D. Anderson Hospital and Tumor Institute.* Chicago: Year Book Medical Publishers, 1976.

Cucuzzo, R. "Method Discharge Planning." *Supervisor Nurse,* **7**:1 (1976), 43–45.

Fisher, S. "Psychosexual Adjustment Following Total Pelvic Exenteration." *Cancer Nurs.*, **2**:3 (1979), 219–25.

Gargaro, W. "Cancer Nursing and the Law." *Cancer Nurs.*, **1**:3 (1978), 249–50.

Gottlieb, A., Plescia, O., and Bishop, D. *Fundamental Aspects of Neoplasia.* New York: Springer-Verlag, 1975.

Hushhower, G., Gamberg, D., and Smith, N. "The Nursing Process in Discharge Planning." *Supervisor Nurse,* **9**:9 (1978), 55–58.

Jacox, A., ed. *Pain, a Sourcebook for Nurses and Other Health Professionals.* Boston: Little, Brown, 1977.

Kennedy, B., Tellegen, A., Kennedy, S., and Havernick, N. "Psychological Response to Patients Cured of Advanced Cancer." *Cancer,* **38**:5 (1976), 2184–91.

Kennedy, P., and Luedke, D. "Adenocarcinoma of Unknown Origin." *Postgrad. Med.*, **65**:1 (1979), 151+.

Lee, R., Cumley, R., and Hickey, R. *The Yearbook of Cancer 1978.* Chicago: Yearbook Medical Publishers, 1978.

Lovejoy, N. "Preventing Hair Loss during Adriamycin Therapy." *Cancer Nurs.*, **2**:2 (1979), 117–21.

McCaffery, M., and Hart, L. "Undertreatment of Acute Pain with Narcotics." *Am. J. Nurs.*, **76**:10 (1976), 1586–91.

Miller, M., and Nygren, C. "Living with Cancer-Coping Behaviors." *Cancer Nurs.*, **1**:4 (1978), 297–302.

Newlin, N., and Wellisch, D. "The Oncology Nurse: Life on an Emotional Roller Coaster." *Cancer Nurs.*, **1**:6 (1978), 447–49.

Rhodes, J., Biship, M., Benfield, J. "Tumor Surveillance: How Tumors May Resist Macrophage-Mediated Host Defense." *Science,* **203**:4376 (Jan. 12, 1979), 179–81.

Rundles, R. W. "Principles of Palliation." *Resident and Staff Physician* (Jan. 1979), 75–77+.

Sheehan, M. "Reflections of a Cancer Nurse." *Cancer Nurs.*, **1**:4 (1978), 309–11.

Smith, D., and Chamorro, T. "Nursing Care of Patients Undergoing Chemotherapy and Radiotherapy." *Cancer Nurs.*, **1**:2 (1978), 129–34.

Steckel, R., and Kagan, R. *Diagnosis and Staging of Cancer: A Radiologic Approach.* Philadelphia: W. B. Saunders Co., 1976.

Sutherland, A. "Psychological Impact of Cancer Surgery." *Pub. Health Rep.*, **67**:11 (1952), 1143.

Sutnick, A. J., and Engstrom, P. P., eds. *Oncologic Medicine: Clinical Topics and Practical Management.* Baltimore: University Park Press, 1976.

Symington, T., and Carter, R. L., eds. *Scientific Foundations of Oncology.* Chicago: William Heinemann Medical Books Publication, 1976.

Warren, B. "Adjuvant Chemotherapy for Breast Disease: The Nurse's Role." *Cancer Nurs.*, **2**:1 (1979), 32–37.

Watson, P. "Psychological Aspects of the Cancer Experience." *Canadian Nurse,* **74**:7 (1978), 45–48.

UNIT IX

Alterations in Essential Life Processes

When regulatory and response mechanisms are inadequate to deal effectively with the existing quantity, quality, and duration of stressors impinging upon the individual from internal and/or external environments, the ability of the individual to sustain essential life processes is altered in some way. Alteration in any one of the essential processes of gas exchange, fluid and electrolyte balance, transportation of materials to and from cells, nutrition, and excretion of waste products will affect other processes in some way.

The interrelationship of essential life processes is alluded to, to a greater or lesser extent, in each of the following chapters. Common clinical problems in which there is alteration in all processes are illustrated with detailed discussion of shock, diabetes mellitus, severe burns, and postoperative complications. Special attention is given to the effect of disuse syndromes and immobility on altered essential life processes.

40

Problems with Removal of CO_2 and/or in Maintaining the Supply of O_2

People don't think about their lungs very often. The lungs are supposed to go on silently doing their job. And yet, things can happen. A person who is well can get into serious trouble with pneumonia. A person with emphysema can land in the hospital with a seemingly mild respiratory infection. A fireman can die from noxious fumes.

American Lung Association Bulletin

"Lung Failure—How and Why It Happens." American Lung Association Bulletin **66**:2 (January–February), 1980.

Overview—Special Techniques of Respiratory Care

In Chapter 26, many of the techniques used in respiratory care were discussed. Included were breathing exercises, postural drainage, aerosol therapy, airway suctioning, and oxygen therapy. This chapter will deal with some additional therapeutic techniques and some techniques whose purpose is diagnostic.

Tracheal Intubation

Patients who require tracheal intubation present special nursing care problems. The most common reason for inserting a tracheal tube is to provide a route for continuous mechanical ventilation. Some patients who do not require mechanical ventilation may also require tracheal intubation. These are patients with severe upper airway obstruction or patients in whom ready access to the lower airway is necessary to maintain airway patency. Tracheal tubes are inserted into the trachea through the upper airway (commonly called endotracheal tubes) or a direct incision into the trachea (tracheostomy tube). With a few exceptions such as chronic, permanent tracheostomies following laryngectomy, tracheal tubes in adults are cuffed. The cuff or balloon is located above the distal end of the tube. This balloon, when inflated, prevents aspiration from the upper airway and provides a closed system in those patients who require continuous mechanical ventilation.

It is usual practice initially to insert an endotracheal tube. Should an artificial airway be required for an extended period, a tracheostomy is done. The endotracheal tube can produce some laryngeal damage because of friction produced by its rubbing against the cords. This type of damage is alleviated by the tracheostomy. Some authors believe that an endotracheal tube should not be left in place more than 72 hours; others have delayed doing a tracheostomy for 14 days or more with no adverse effects. The use of the endotracheal tube prevents the need for a surgical procedure and allows for more optimal functioning of the patient's own airway defense

This chapter has been revised by Gayle A. Traver, R.N., M.S.N., Associate Professor of Nursing, College of Nursing; Assistant Professor of Medicine, College of Medicine, University of Arizona.

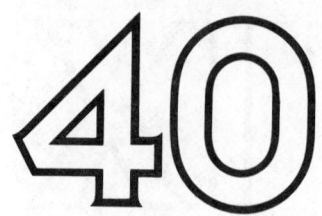

mechanisms immediately upon removal of the tube.

Because both types of tubes bypass the upper airway and require an inflatable cuff, they represent some special nursing care needs and also present the possibility of some special problems for the patient. It is, of course, evident that whenever a patient has such a tube in place and the cuff is inflated, speech would not be possible as air is not allowed through the vocal cords. The nurse must be aware of the patient's inability to speak and perform care in an appropriate manner. As previously discussed, the tube also inhibits the patient's defense mechanisms—cough, mucociliary clearance, and filtering. In addition, the inflated cuff can produce pressure necrosis of the airway. This pressure irritation and necrosis of the trachea can result in the development of a tracheal stricture because of fibrotic tissue laid down during the healing process.

Today most cuffs are designed so that only minimal pressure (less than 20 cm H_2O) is exerted against the tracheal wall. These are called low-pressure or high-compliance cuffs. Even with the new cuffs however, care must be taken during inflation to prevent excessive pressure build-up in the cuff and the resulting damage to the trachea. The cuffs are inflated according to two basic techniques. One is the minimal occlusive pressure technique whereby the cuff is inflated just until there is no air leak around the tube. The other technique is the partial seal technique whereby a slight air leak is allowed around the tube and the ventilator is adjusted to compensate for this volume loss. In both techniques it is advantageous to inflate the cuff carefully during the inspiratory phase of ventilation to ensure that the cuff is not overinflated. Injection of air into the cuff should stop as soon as it is evident that there is no air leak present. The intracuff pressure is then measured to ensure that the pressure is not too high. In some settings it is routine practice periodically to deflate the cuffs on such tubes. When the cuff is deflated, the nurse must be careful that aspiration of upper airway secretions does not take place. Therefore the upper airway is suctioned to clear it of obtainable secretions before the cuff is deflated. That catheter is then discarded and a new sterile catheter is placed on the suction line. Air is withdrawn from the cuff during the inspiratory phase on the ventilator or while bagging if the patient is not on a ventilator. This technique tends to "blow" secretions into the upper airway. If material does gain access to the lower airway, it should be immediately aspirated. If the patient does not have a low pressure cuff in place, but rather one of the high pressure cuffs, cuff deflation should be carried out every hour.

For patients who require intubation but are not being ventilated, the nurse should deep breathe the patient at least every hour with a self-inflating or anesthesia bag. Such a procedure prevents the development of atelectasis.

Positive Pressure Breathing

Positive pressure breathing has become an important part of respiratory care. Positive pressure breathing is, by definition, the application of positive pressure to the airways during some phase of the ventilatory cycle. There are a variety of modifications of positive pressure breathing and a variety of clinical indications for the use of such apparatus. The pressure changes during spontaneous breathing and the various modifications are shown in Figure 40-1.

IPPB

The most common approach to positive pressure breathing is intermittent positive pressure breathing (IPPB). In other words, positive pressure is applied during the inspiratory phase of ventilation (Figure 40-1). This application of pressure increases the pressure gradient between the atmosphere and the alveoli and should thereby theoretically increase the volume delivered to the alveoli. Intermittent positive pressure breathing has also been purported as a means of improving gas distribution within the lung and as a means of improving bronchial hygiene.

Intermittent IPPB treatments have been used to promote airway clearance, facilitate deep breathing, and to administer bronchodilators. Today many of these uses are being questioned. IPPB treatments have been used frequently in the prevention and treatment of postoperative complications. Present research, however, has demonstrated that this treatment modality is no more effective than deep breathing and coughing in preventing or treating such pulmonary complications (Bartlett, Gazzaniga, and Geraghty, 1973). In fact, some persons recommend that the correct breathing techniques would be much more effective in clearing an atelectatic area because the negative pressure produced around all areas of the lung would encourage flow to the atelectatic area. With positive pressure breathing, the air flow is more likely to follow the path of least resistance, and therefore flow goes to the normal area, leaving the affected area unventilated.

Intermittent positive pressure breathing has also been used as a mechanism of bronchial hygiene in the treatment of patients with pneumonia and various chronic obstructive pulmonary diseases. This use

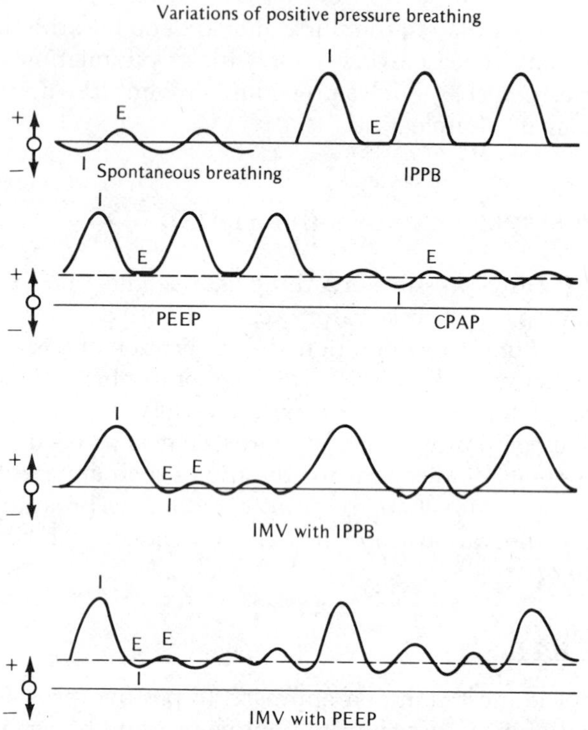

Figure 40-1. Variations of positive pressure breathing. In spontaneous breathing, airway pressures drop below atmospheric with inspiration (I); with expiration (E), airway pressure rises. With IPPB, positive pressure is added during inspiration, expiration is at atmospheric pressure. The addition of PEEP means that a positive pressure is maintained throughout the respiratory cycle; positive pressure during inhalation assures volume delivery; during expiration pressures fall but are still kept above atmospheric. CPAP maintains a positive pressure on the airway but the patient generates his own volume change; therefore pressures fall during inspiration and rise during expiration—the same pattern as seen during spontaneous breathing only at a higher baseline. The two IMV nodes show the combination of machine assisted breaths and spontaneous breaths with and without PEEP.

has also been questioned. First of all, an IPPB machine used for treatments does not actually deliver a water or saline aerosol to the patient and therefore is not effective in adding water content to the airway. The large flow generated through the machine causes evaporation of the nebulizer output and therefore especially dry air is administered to the patient. The nurse should realize that, even though an aerosol is visible at the mouthpiece when the main flow is off and nebulizer on, the aerosol will not be visible when the machine is "tripped" on (inspiratory flow is generated through main tubing). In addition, much of the humidifying effect of the nasopharynx is bypassed because the patient is mouth breathing. Perhaps the best indicator of this common misconception about IPPB treatments is the frequent comments of patients that their IPPB treatments "give them dry, scratchy throats." Second, if the desired effect is simply one of deep breathing, the patient can usually be taught to take a deep breath without the assistance of the machine. If cough is the desired outcome, the patient must still be taught how to deep breathe and cough in addition to being taught how to use the apparatus. It is then questionable why it is necessary to use the machine, if the therapeutic objectives can be reached by simply teaching the patient to deep breathe and cough.

IPPB has also been advocated as a means of delivering bronchodilators and other medications to the lower airways. The theoretical basis was that the pressure would provide better distribution of the medications. However studies have demonstrated that bronchodilators administered via compressor units (hand or electrically powered) are just as efficient as are those bronchodilators administered via an IPPB apparatus (Goldberg and Cherniack, 1965; Dolovich, et al., 1977). Therefore the use of IPPB equipment for such treatments, in that it involves greater patient costs and greater problems of sterilization and maintenance without documented benefit is questioned.

Another use of intermittent positive pressure breathing treatments (administered on an intermittent basis) has been in the care of patients with carbon dioxide retention. It has been shown, however, that an IPPB treatment has less effect on lowering carbon dioxide retention in patients with severe disease than it does in those persons with minimal or no disease (Birnbaum, et al., 1966). In addition, if a lowering of the carbon dioxide level does occur during the treatment, these values have returned to baseline level within anywhere from 20 minutes to 2 hours after the treatment. Therefore if such treatments are to be effective in patients, they must be given at 1-hour intervals or even more frequently. This treatment regimen again becomes very uneconomical for the patient and very difficult for those caring for the patient, be it at home or in the hospital. Again, it must be realized that deep breathing and teaching of the correct breathing pattern to such patients will often decrease their carbon dioxide level (Petty & Guthrie, 1971).

If in any of the preceding examples the patient cannot be taught to deep breathe, IPPB may be considered as a means of increasing the depth of respiration periodically. In some instances several deep breaths by a self-inflating bag (which is a means of providing IPPB) are sufficient and, in some, more sophisticated IPPB apparatus is necessary. What method is used is frequently dependent on the nursing assessment of the situation and/or the nurse's skill in teaching the patient. The important thing to remember is that alternatives are available and that the nurse should not assume that the IPPB will "make" the patient deep breathe.

Continuous Ventilation

Intermittent positive pressure breathing as a means of continuous ventilation has become a mainstay in the care of those patients who are unable to maintain their own ventilation at acceptable levels. Mechanical ventilation with intermittent positive pressure breathing is therefore instituted in those patients with acute respiratory acidosis who are unable to maintain ventilation. (See section on carbon dioxide retention and ventilatory failure). When intermittent positive pressure breathing is used for mechanical ventilation, there are two basic types of ventilators available. These are the volume-set machine and the pressure-set machine. In the pressure-set ventilator, such as the Bennett PR-II or the Bird Mark VIII, pressure can be manipulated and set by the operator. Volume is variable and follows the preset pressure. Such a mechanism means that these machines do not deliver a constant volume to the patient. Volume will vary with the compliance or resistance of the system (including both machine and patient), requiring that the patient be carefully monitored in order to ensure adequate ventilation. For example, if airway resistance increases as in bronchospasm, the volume delivered to the patient will decrease even though pressure remains constant. In the volume-set machine the volume is determined by the operator, and pressure, as a variable, follows the constant volume delivered. These machines therefore ensure the delivery of a constant and reliable tidal volume to the patient. Most of the volume-set machines also have a pressure limit and blow-off valve. Such a setting allows the operator to set an upper limit of pressure that would be acceptable during the delivery of the preset volume. Whenever that limit is reached, the additional volume is then vented to the outside and not delivered to the patient. This setting, if coupled with an alarm system, is frequently used by the nurse to indicate a change in the patient's status, rather than the peak acceptable pressure. For example, if the peak pressure is 30 cm water during delivery of the tidal volume, the nurse should set the pressure limit at 35 to 40 cm of water. Then, whenever the patient coughed, accumulated secretions, and so on, the pressure would rise and the alarm would sound as the pressure limit was met.

In addition, all ventilators (pressure-set or volume-set) must have a means of providing 100 per cent humidity at body temperature. They should also be capable of assisting ventilation (the patient's spontaneous inspiratory efforts trigger the machine on) or controlling ventilation (automatic cycling). For further discussion of the pros and cons of specific ventilators, the reader is referred to specific respiratory care and inhalation therapy texts listed in the bibliography.

PEEP

Ventilators can also be set to deliver positive end expiratory pressure (PEEP). By convention, the term PEEP is usually used to indicate that there is positive pressure applied during inspiration (IPPB) in order to attain the tidal volume desired and also positive pressure at end expiration (See Figure 40-1). Now, instead of expiration being at atmosphere pressure as with IPPB, alone, a positive pressure is also exerted during the expiratory phase of ventilation. The major use of PEEP has been in the treatment of the patient who has a stiff lung (low compliance) and is at the same time extremely difficult to oxygenate. In other words the patient requires inspired oxygen levels of greater than 50 per cent in order to maintain even minimal oxygenation levels. The use of PEEP often enables much more adequate oxygenation at much lower inspired oxygen levels. This situation is one where mechanical ventilation is instituted for severe hypoxemia even if carbon dioxide retention is not present.

It has been proposed that one of the reasons that such types of patients are difficult to oxygenate is that they are breathing at very low lung volumes and that small airways tend to collapse. Therefore, because blood flow is continuous, the blood that flows through those areas of lung is not oxygenated. When this blood is then mixed together with the oxygenated blood, the overall result is that the patient is hypoxemic. This is referred to as a shunt mechanism. PEEP is usually not required unless the shunt is greater than 30 per cent. In such cases, the introduction of the positive end expiratory pressure maintains a larger lung volume at end expiration (FRC), because pressures at end expiration never reach atmospheric pressure. This volume then serves as a splinting mechanism for the small airways so that collapse does not occur. The overall result is therefore that oxygenation improves. It must be noted that this technique is not usually that effective in patients with chronic obstructive pulmonary disease and floppy compliant lungs, such as is the case in emphysema. In such patients the rate of complications, such as mediastinal and subcutaneous emphysema, pneumothorax and decreased cardiac output is much higher.

CPAP

Continuous positive airway pressure (CPAP) is a means of providing an end expiratory pressure plateau during spontaneous breathing (See Figure 40-1). Instead of breathing from an inhaled gas source at atmospheric pressure, the inhaled gas is kept at a constant, predetermined pressure above atmospheric. Extra positive pressure is not exerted during inspiration and the patient's tidal volumes will depend on his or her own respiratory efforts. This technique has been used extensively in the neonate with idiopathic respiratory distress syndrome and is now being used in the adult. In the neonate the technique can often be used without tracheal intubation, but in the adult, a cuffed endotracheal tube is required.

IMV

Intermittent Mandatory Ventilation (IMV) is another adaptation of mechanical ventilation. This technique allows the patient to breathe spontaneously, without ventilator assistance, with periodic breaths delivered at a preset rate from the ventilator (See Figure 40-1).

The machine-delivered breaths may constitute almost all of the minute volume, or the IMV rate may be set very low (1 to 4 breaths per minute) so that the majority of the minute volume is determined by the patient's spontaneous, unassisted breaths. Synchronized IMV (SIMV) simply means that the machine-delivered breaths are synchronized with the patient's spontaneous inspiratory efforts rather than being delivered at random times during the patient's respiratory cycle.

Although originally conceived to facilitate the weaning of a patient from mechanical ventilation, IMV is now used much more extensively. This technique is thought to prevent the loss of respiratory muscle strength due to lack of use. Therefore, even if the patient's spontaneous tidal volume is much too low to maintain alveolar ventilation, the ventilator may be set in the IMV mode with a relatively high machine rate but still allowing the patient to take periodic spontaneous breaths without machine assistance. In addition IMV has helped to prevent some of the mechanical-ventilation-induced hyperventilation. Large tidal volume ventilation (10 to 15 ml/kg) is preferred so as to prevent atelectatic changes. For example, for a 70-kg man, a tidal volume of 700 to 900 cc is often used. In order to maintain an adequate alveolar ventilation, a rate of only 10 may be required. Yet many patients are tachypneic because of their disease. (Remember that the rate and volume are adjusted to attain the desired P_{CO_2}.) In such situations, with the ventilator in the assist mode, the patient would soon be overventilated, often to the point of a severe alkalemia, because the large tidal volume would be delivered with every breath. In the past the options available in such situations were (1) to sedate the patient to the point of abolishing the respiratory drive or paralyzing him or her and then using a control mode or (2) to add dead space to the ventilator tubing so that the patient would rebreathe his or her own expired air. Both options have serious drawbacks, and therefore IMV is now frequently used in such situations. The ventilator-delivered breaths provide the beneficial high tidal volume and the rate can be adjusted so that respiratory alkalemia does not develop.

The ventilator mode of IMV can be used for patients on simple intermittent, positive-pressure ventilation or for those requiring PEEP. For those patients requiring PEEP, the spontaneous breaths still have the positive pressure plateau on expiration with the inspiratory phase dependent on patient effort. To reduce the patient's work of breathing, continuous positive airway pressure (CPAP) is maintained.

Monitoring

Patients who have severe respiratory dysfunction require careful monitoring of their respiratory status. For chronically ill patients, monitoring of respiratory function is done by periodically assessing spirometry and blood gases. For patients who are acutely ill and hospitalized, more techniques are used.

Periodic blood gas analysis is used to assess the gas exchange function of the lung. The frequency of blood gas analysis depends on the severity and lability of the dysfunction. In some acute care settings oxygenation is continuously monitored either by an intraarterial sensor or ear oximeter. In all situations blood gases must be carefully noted and kept in the chart in sequential order. One blood gas alone and its interpretation can often be erroneous. What is important for both the nurse and the physician is to know the direction of serial blood gas changes. Just as the physician can use blood gases to help in diagnosing and in a therapeutic approach to the patient's problems, so can the blood gases help the nurse in determining and assessing nursing care intervention. For example, accumulation of secretions can cause a decrease in the P_{O_2}; hyperventilation with severe alkalosis can result in tetany; a decreased P_{O_2} can cause restlessness. With the data from the blood gas analysis, there must also be a description of the conditions under which the blood was drawn: for example, What was the inspired oxygen concentration? Had a bronchodilator just been administered? Was the analysis done to determine the effect of a specific intervention—postural drainage, turning, and so on? For patients on ventilators, the respiratory rate and tidal volume delivered should be noted as well as the level of PEEP. For patients on IMV the rate and volume of both the machine-delivered and spontaneous breaths should be noted. Decisions regarding patient care must be made considering the result of the blood gas analysis and all the factors which could be influencing those results. Only then can knowledgeable decisions be made.

More sophisticated measures of gas exchange may also be done. These include the measurement of the difference between the ideal alveolar oxygen and the arterial oxygen tension. This measurement, called the $A\text{-}aD_{O_2}$, is used to assess the amount of ventilation—perfusion mismatching. Calculation of the actual shunt may also be done. Another measure of the gas exchange function is the V_D/V_T. This measurement, ratio of dead space to tidal volume, allows one to see how much of each breath is wasted ventilation or dead space and how much participates in alveolar ventilation.

Monitoring of lung mechanics is also done. The most basic, but important, measurement is respiratory rate. Other measurements which are easily obtained are the vital capacity, tidal volume, and minute volume. There are a variety of devices which can be attached to a mouthpiece, mask, or an endotracheal tube for this purpose. As with blood gases, notation of the circumstances under which the measurement was made should be noted, that is, on or off ventilator, position, after bronchodilator, and so forth. Another measure of mechanical function is the maximal inspiratory force (MIF). This measurement allows some assessment of respiratory muscle strength. As the patient inhales deeply from functional residual capacity, the inspiratory air flow is cut off. The patient therefore develops a negative airway pressure which can be measured. Normal maximal inspiratory pressures should be -75 to -100 cm H_2O. Patients who fall markedly below this level may not have adequate muscle strength to maintain ventilation; the MIF should be more than -25 cm H_2O to maintain adequate spontaneous ventilation. In terms of ability to physically move the thorax, the nurse should also carefully monitor the patient's respiratory pattern. In cases of severe muscle fatigue or extreme diaphragmatic dysfunction, patients will often develop a dysynchronous respiratory pattern; the diaphragm and intercostals contract in series, one after the other, rather than together. A final measure of lung mechanics that is made when patients are on ventilators is compliance. Since compliance is the change in volume divided by the change in pressure, this measurement is easily obtained. The change in pressure is the pressure required to generate the volume change; this measurement is available from the ventilator. The volume is the tidal volume delivered. Thus, if it takes more pressure to produce the same tidal volume, the nurse knows that the lung is becoming stiffer; if less pressure is required, the lung is becoming more compliant.

In addition to monitoring the gas exchange and mechanical function of the lung, in acute care settings it is also necessary to monitor oxygen delivery. This aspect becomes especially important in patients with primary or secondary cardiovascular dysfunction. When high pressures are required for mechanical ventilation, cardiac output can be affected. Since intrathoracic pressures are higher than with spontaneous ventilation, venous return to the right heart can be compromised. In addition, under certain conditions, the pulmonary vasculature is compressed. These factors may, in some patients, result in decreased cardiac output. In addition to measuring cardiac output, mixed venous oxygen levels provide an assessment of actual oxygen delivery to the tissues. Mixed venous blood, drawn from the pulmonary artery via a Swan Ganz catheter, has a normal oxygen tension of 40 mm Hg. If the mixed venous oxygen is abnormally low or there is an abnormally high content difference between the arterial and mixed venous bloods, it indicates a low cardiac output and poor oxygen delivery.

These monitoring techniques, especially of gas exchange and lung mechanics, are especially helpful in the decision of whether or not the patient requires mechanical ventilation. Similarily they are extremely helpful to the nurse when a patient is being weaned from mechanical ventilation. The nurse should know what the measurements mean and how they can be accurately obtained. For example, fatigue can lead to decreased alveolar ventilation in some patients. If early changes in lung mechanics can be detected and treated, the gas exchange abnormalities may be prevented. It is much more meaningful to report a decrease in vital capacity and decreased MIF than to simply say you think the patient looks tired. Your original observation is only the beginning of the assessment.

Diagnostic Techniques

In this section of special techniques used in respiratory care, it is important to mention some of the special diagnostic procedures frequently used with pulmonary patients. The routine chest radiographs (a PA and lateral view) are the most common. In addition, there are other views and radiographic techniques, such as obliques, decubitus, and tomograms, that can add helpful data. Skin testing is another type of diagnostic tool. Skin testing is another type of diagnostic tool. Skin testing may be for an immediate reaction, such as is seen in allergy testing. In such a test a small drop of the antigen is placed on the patient's skin. A small gauge needle is then used gently to prick and lift the skin. No bleeding should be produced. The appearance of a wheal within several minutes demonstrates a reaction to that specific allergen. For diseases such as tuberculosis, coccidioidomycosis, and histoplasmosis skin testing is done to test for delayed hypersensitivity with an intradermal injection of the antigen. At 48 hours the presence of induration (10 mm or more) signifies a positive skin test and prior experience with the antigen. The induration is reported in millimeters. (Erythema is *not* reported.)

One of the most common of the diagnostic techniques is the examination of sputum. Sputum is examined for several purposes. First, the sputum may be examined for several purposes. First, the sputum may be examined for the presence of certain of the white blood cells. For example, an infection will demonstrate the presence of more polymorphonuclear or pus cells in the sputum. Various allergic responses that have pulmonary manifestations are also evident by the presence of eosinophils in the sputum. The most common of the sputum examinations are the examination of sputum for the presence of bacteria and for the culture of the sputum in order to identify these various bacteria. For any of these examinations, the nurse must be able to ensure that the material being examined is actually sputum from the lower airways and not just saliva or oral secretions. In addition, an adequate amount must be available so that the appropriate examinations can be made. If a sputum sample cannot be obtained by having the patient deep breathe and cough, additional techniques are available to the nurse. First is the administration of aerosol prior to deep breathing and coughing. If routine aerosol therapy is unsuccessful, an ultrasonic aerosol of hypertonic saline (10 per cent) may be administered. This aerosol is very irritating and causes a bronchorrhea. It should be remembered, however, that hypertonic saline aerosols cause a great increase in airway resistance, especially in patients with hyperactive airways, as is the case with asthmatic patients. Therefore hypertonic aerosols should not be used in such situations nor should they be used for sputum cytologies as they can distort cell morphology. Another technique that can be used to obtain sputum for examination is postural drainage. If all other means are unsuccessful, tracheal suctioning and bronchoscopy can be used. Most laboratories like several milliliters of sputum for examination. The sputum is smeared on a slide and examined microscopically for the presence of organisms. It must be remembered that it is not unusual for organisms to be present because the sputum expectorated has passed through the upper airway. Because the upper airway has many natural bacterial inhabitants, they will also be seen in the sputum. There are some distinctive organisms that can often be diagnosed simply from the morphology seen on smear. In the majority of cases, however, exact identification of the organism requires culturing techniques whereby the organism is actually grown and identified via various morphologic and biochemical tests. At the same time that the culture is done, the organism can be tested for its sensitivity to a variety of antibiotics. In addition to smear and culture techniques for bacteria, special culturing techniques can be used for the various fungi. Although results from most bacterial cultures are available within several days, cultures of acid-fast organisms *(M. tuberculosis)* may require 10 days to several months, because of the slow growth rate of the organism.

In addition to the use of sputum collections for the detection of infection due to bacteria or fungi, sputum can also be examined for the presence of abnormal cells. This latter examination is known as sputum cytology examination. Many times a tumor in the airway sloughs cells that are then carried by the sputum. The sputum can be examined for the detection of these malignant cells and is therefore used in the diagnosis of cancer. Another method of diagnosing cancer that involves the airways is the use of diagnostic bronchoscopy. The bronchoscope is used to visualize the tumor, which is often growing into the airway. Forceps may then be passed through the bronchoscope and a small biopsy of the abnormal area taken. With a biopsy, an actual cell block can be made and this method, because it gives a piece of tissue rather than just sloughed cells, can be used to diagnose cell type of the tumor much more specifically than can a sputum examination. It is important for the nurse to realize that during a bronchoscopy, washings are also done and that the patient will often expectorate a great deal of sputum postbronchoscopy. It is therefore important to collect this sputum in the postbronchoscopy period, for it is frequently the material that is diagnostic.

For pathologic conditions that do not specifically involve the airways, other diagnostic procedures are used. For those diseases that produce a pleural effusion (fluid in the pleural space) a thoracentesis can be done to remove that fluid. This fluid can then be examined to detect the presence of actual bacteria and also to determine the amount of protein and other substances in the fluid. In addition at the time of the thoracentesis, a biopsy of the pleural surface can be made. This biopsy can be examined in terms of detection of malignant cells present and it can also be cultured to determine the presence of an infecting agent. In other disease processes, a lung biopsy may be required. This technique can be used in some of the interstitial diseases, in lung infiltrates of unknown cause, and in isolated coin lesions that are suspected to be malignant. Several techniques are used to do a lung biopsy. One is the percutaneous lung biopsy whereby a variety of types of equipment can be used to obtain a piece of lung by inserting a needle through an intercostal space into the lung parenchyma in order to remove a piece of lung tissue. The other method is to do a small thoracotomy and be able to visually remove a piece of tissue. The latter technique, of course, results in a larger piece of lung tissue available for examination and also allows visualization of the area of lung removed so that there is greater potential of obtaining a piece of tissue that is pathologically involved. Another technique that can be used involves various biopsy procedures that allow the physician to obtain tissue from the lymph nodes. Such techniques are especially common in assessing the operability of a patient with cancer. (If the tumor has metastasized to the lymph nodes, the patient is usually considered inoperable.) Mediastinoscopy can be done whereby a mediastinoscope can be inserted into the mediastinum through a small incision at the suprasternal notch and the mediastinum can be visualized as well as a biopsy taken. Biopsies may also be done of the supraclavicular lymph nodes if there is evidence of extrapulmonary metastasis of the tumor.

Nursing Assessment Guide

Just as the physician does a history and physical in obtaining information from a patient for diagnostic purposes, so should the nurse use these skills, history taking and physical assessment, to plan for and evaluate nursing care. The performing of a history and physical requires both knowledge and skill. The actual techniques cannot be skillfully used without a knowledge base. First, you have to know what questions to ask; then once you have received information from a patient, that information must have meaning so that you are guided in a specific direction in order to obtain additional information. Although it is common now in the discussions of the expanded role of the nurse to hear much more about the nurse's use of the history and physical, it must be remembered that these are skills that the nurse should be able to use regardless of the situation or role practiced. It is important, however, to recognize that there is a difference between the way the physician and the nurse use these skills. Both roles require many of the same skills, but they are used toward a different purpose. The physician uses the skills of history taking and physical examination to determine a diagnosis for the patient. The nurse uses the skills of history taking and physical assessment to deal with the therapeutic problems that the patient presents. For example, the nurse will want to determine the patient's knowledge of the disease, the patient and family's coping mechanisms, specific nursing interventions that would be appropriate, and the effects of these nursing interventions. In other words, the nurse's assessment may be of limited breadth but increased depth in that she or he is concentrating on the specific therapeutic problems of the patient. The physician is concerned with arriving at a diagnosis and instituting a therapeutic regimen. The carrying out of the general plan of care, including both preventative and therapeutic care in such a way that it is adapted to the individual, is the role of the nurse.

A general guide for the assessment of the patient with pulmonary dysfunction is presented in this section. The reader is cautioned that not all questions are appropriate for every patient, nor is the use of each of the assessment skills appropriate in any given situation. Interviewing techniques mean that as certain pertinent data become available, the nurse would ask further questions in that area. If no answer is received that indicates something is a problem, then there is not that much sense in asking further questions. For example, if the patient denies sputum production, it is not useful to ask what the color of the sputum is or how much is produced per day. On the other hand, if the patient does indicate that there is sputum production, then it is important to determine how much, what color, and so forth. In addition to these interviewing techniques, the assessment guide also includes data about various physical assessment findings of the patient. These would include the use of inspection, palpation, percussion, and auscultation. Too many times nurses have strictly relegated these skills to the physician, and yet they are extremely important in the determination of the effectiveness of nursing intervention. For example, are there sounds indicating the presence of secretions before postural drainage and do they disappear after postural drainage? Chest auscultation may then be one way of assessing the effectiveness of a nursing treatment. If a patient complains of pain, the nurse should be able to use palpation to determine the area of pain and describe it more carefully in order that further action may be taken. To clarify the data that can be gained from the specific skills used in physical assessment, a brief discussion of inspection, palpation, percussion, and auscultation of the chest will be presented at this point.

Inspection simply means that you look at the patient and determine if there are any abnormalities present. For example, Does the patient have a kyphosis or scoliosis that may affect posture and respiratory pattern? What is the patient's respiratory pattern at rest? Is there cyanosis present that might indicate poor oxygenation? Meaningful inspection of the patient can supply the nurse with a wealth of pertinent data that should be incorporated into the patient's plan of care. Too often the nurse "looks" at the patient but does not truly see him or her. Frequently what one sees can be some of the most important data gathered.

Palpation indicates the use of touch and vibratory sense to determine the presence or absence of abnormalities. For example, areas of tenderness or pain can be localized by palpation. In examining the chest, palpation is used to assess vocal fremitus—how well the vibrations produced during speech are transmitted to the chest wall. In the abnormal situation it is not uncommon to be able to "feel" the vibrations produced as air flows through large airways that contain secretions. Such a technique is often used during percussion and vibration. As the secretions are moved to larger airways, they can often be felt under the nurse's hand and indicate the need for further work on that area of the lung.

Percussion is a tapping of the chest to determine areas of increased or decreased sound transmission. For example, is the sound obtained during percussion dull or hollow? Percussion can be used to delineate organs of different densities, such as outlining the lung, heart, and so on. It can also be used to detect changes in density that vary from normal. For example, percussion will often demonstrate areas of dullness over a pleural effusion or consolidated pneumonia, because the tissue under the area of percussion does not contain air.

Auscultation of the chest is used to identify the presence or absence of normal breath sounds and the presence of abnormal adventitial sounds. Breath sounds consist of three types: (1) vesicular, (2) bronchovesicular, and (3) bronchial sounds. Vesicular sounds are heard over the majority of the chest and are heard as a soft swishing sound, which is louder during inspiration; expiratory sounds are short and nearly silent. Bronchial breath sounds are normal only over very large airways such as over the trachea; if they are heard in other parts of the chest they are considered abnormal and indicate areas of compression of lung tissue. In bronchial breathing, inspiration sounds short and relatively quiet whereas expiration is long and loud. Bronchovesicular sounds are heard near the scapulae and supraclavicular areas where larger airways are near the chest wall. In bronchovesicular sounds, inspiration and expiration are of nearly equal duration, although expiration usually sounds louder. If heard over other areas of the lung, these are abnormal sounds and indicate compression of lung tissue. An absence of all breath sounds indicates that no air is being moved in that area. For example, if an endotracheal tube is inserted into the right mainstem bronchus, there would be an absence or decreased volume of breath sounds heard on the left.

Adventitial sounds are abnormal sounds that are superimposed upon the normal breath sounds. They are usually subdivided into crackles (rales), rhonchi, and pleural sounds. Crackles are discontinuous sounds that are more evident on inspiration. Their presence may indicate retained secretions or pulmonary edema. Rhonchi are harsher, more sonorous sounds that are more evident on expiration. They are continuous sounds. Rhonchi indicate retained secretions or obstruction in the larger airways. Wheezing, which is also classified as a rhonchus, is a musical sound heard on expiration and is caused by narrowing of airways. Pleural sounds are high-pitched, squeaking sounds caused by irritation and rubbing together of the pleural surfaces.

Table 40-1 is a general guide to the assessment of the patient with pulmonary disease. What specific questions are asked or which skills are used will depend on the actual patient care situation and the goals of the nurse. Remember that the problem often determines what data base is required. For this reason, each area of data collection includes comment as to some of the reasons for obtaining the data and its possible significance. It must also be remembered that the nurse can obtain the data base from a variety of sources. If the nurse is the first person to see the patient, the responsibility of obtaining certain parts may be considered a nursing function. In other situations, much of the data base will be gathered by other persons (physicians, admitting personnel) and the nurse will have it readily available in the chart; in others many of the historical aspects of the data base can be obtained via a self-completion questionnaire that the patient fills out. It should also be noted that the majority of the historical data is considered subjective data, whereas physical assessment, laboratory findings, x-rays, and other special tests are objective data. The original data base often uses the headings of history and physical findings. From this data base the patient's problems are defined. Follow-up notes are then written in terms of each problem with notations of the subjective and objective data that are pertinent to that problem. From that data an assessment is made and plans for future intervention delineated. Examples of the use of data will be presented in the case studies.

TABLE 40-1. ***Guide to Assessment of the Patient with Pulmonary Disease—the Data Base***

Data to Be Obtained	Selected Examples of Rationale and Significance
I. Patient identification	I. Baseline information
II. Informant	II. For later comparison and evaluation of reliability, personnel need to know from whom the information was received.
III. Chief complaint	III. Too often the nurse's perception of the patient's problem is the one that receives emphasis, not the patient's. For example, instituting the use of the bicycle for exercise therapy is not reasonable if the patient's concern is the ability to climb stairs.
IV. Present illness	IV. This is the patient's statement of his or her symptoms and how they affect the patient and his or her life. Here the nurse will receive input that serves as a basis for further data collection.
V. Past physical history (related to pulmonary)	V.
A. Does the patient have a cough? If yes, how frequently? only with a cold occasionally but not on most days What kind of cough? dry wet Are there precipitating factors the patient can identify?	A. Because cough is a common symptom of many respiratory diseases, it must be quantified and qualified. Often a history of cough is difficult to elicit. The patient may ignore the so-called smoker's cough as not applicable, or say he "clears his throat" but doesn't cough. Therefore care must be used to ensure an accurate history. A history of frequent cough or chest colds indicates the possible need for improved bronchial hygiene; further data may or may not support that impression.
B. Does the patient produce sputum? If yes, how frequently? only with colds occasionally but not on most days on most days in small amounts on most days in large amounts What color? yellow green clear Is the sputum always the same color or does it change? Under what circumstances does it change? Is there blood in the sputum? never for years only recently Is the blood in red streaks or in larger volumes of blood?	B. Sputum production, like cough, must be quantified and qualified. The nurse must describe the frequency, amount, consistency, and color of sputum produced. It should be remembered that many of these qualities are difficult for the patient to determine. If the patient is unsure of volume, the number of tissues used per day is of help. As to color, smell, and consistency, many patients do not look at their sputum. It is therefore helpful to have the patient expectorate some sputum into a cup or tissue so that it can be observed. This technique not only allows the observation of the sputum, but demonstrates the fact that "coughing and spitting" are acceptable and that sputum should be observed.
C. Is the patient short of breath at rest? with activities of daily living with mild exercise only with strenuous exercise Has shortness of breath made him or her do less slow down Does the patient feel well except for intermittent, short periods of acute shortness of breath?	C. Many patients do not appear short of breath at rest, but will be short of breath with exertion. Additionally, many patients may not recognize their shortness of breath because they have gradually limited their activity to prevent inducing shortness of breath. It is often helpful to find out "what the patient does" as compared to "what he or she used to do."

(Continued)

Table 40-1. *(Continued)*

Data to Be Obtained	Selected Examples of Rationale and Significance
D. Does the patient smoke? If no, did he or she smoke in the past? When did he or she start? stop? What did the patient smoke? If yes, what does the patient smoke? How much?	D. Because smoking appears to be related to the development of many pulmonary diseases, smoking history is extremely important. Because incidence of diseases is related to the amount of cigarette smoking, findings are usually summarized in terms of "pack years." One pack year equals one pack per day for 1 year. If the patient smoked two packs a day for 1 year he or she would have a history of 2 pack years. Similarly, if the patient has stopped, it is important to know when and why. (Many patients stop because of shortness of breath, hemoptysis, and so on, not just because it seems like a good idea.) Smoking history may also indicate a need for patient education.
E. Does the patient have any known or suspected allergies? If yes, to what? What symptoms does the patient have when exposed to the allergens?	E. Allergies play a role in many of the immunologic diseases of the chest, asthma being the most common. Data here may disclose areas where further teaching is necessary to avoid allergens, for example.
F. Has the patient ever had TB? If yes, when was it last active? How was it treated? How long were medications taken?	F. Many patients who had TB prior to the 1940s received no chemotherapy and may require chemotherapy at this time. Also, because of the lack of any specific treatment, many patients who had TB prior to the 1940s have a great deal of scarring associated with the healing of their disease and this "scarring" could be limiting their present activity.
G. Does the patient have swelling of the ankles or legs? If yes, only occasionally or most of the time? If yes, does he or she ever take any "water pills" for this problem?	G. Right-sided heart failure may occur secondary to pulmonary dysfunction and cor pulmonale. Edema of the feet, ankles, or legs may be due to right-sided heart failure. It may, however, also be due to other causes such as varices, liver disease. Therefore other causes must be considered. In the situation where the patient has cor pulmonale and right-sided heart failure, he or she is usually hypoxemic and at least occasionally acidemic. Therefore a history of "swelling" makes the nurse suspicious that the patient may be hypoxemic.
H. Has the patient ever had chest surgery? If yes, When? Where? Why?	H. There may be a variety of reasons for doing a thoracotomy, including diagnostic and therapeutic. The nurse should know why it was done, as it may influence present care of the patient. Knowing geographically where it was done allows the gathering of further information, such as slides of tissue, pathology reports, and pre- and postop course.
I. What medicines does the patient take? (Include drugs found most helpful and drugs that cannot be tolerated.)	I. Be sure that the patient is free to include nonprescription drugs and "home remedies." Oxygen and respiratory therapy equipment should also be included. Many times patients take over-the-counter drugs that could be potentially detrimental (for example, cold tablets with antihistamines in the chronic bronchitic). If the patient has certain "home remedies" that work and are not detrimental, do not degrade them.

TABLE 40-1. *(Continued)*

Data to Be Obtained	Selected Examples of Rationale and Significance
J. When was the patient's last chest x-ray and where?	J. It is often necessary to obtain old films for comparison with present x-rays for diagnostic and therapeutic reasons.
K. Any other comments that the patient might have regarding past medical history.	K. Never assume your questions have gained all pertinent information the patient has for you. Always be sure to leave an "open-ended" question that the patient can use for free response.
VI. Family history A. Parents age state of health if not living, age at death and cause of death B. Siblings age state of health if not living, age at death and cause of death	A. Some respiratory diseases have a hereditary basis in which case familial information may be helpful. It may also provide guidelines for teaching. For example, in the patients who have a family with a history of alpha$_1$-antitrypsin deficiency (see case study on emphysema) a special effort would be made to have them stop smoking and avoid other pollutants.
VII. Social History A. Birthplace and geographic history	A. Some pulmonary diseases are endemic to certain geographic areas, making a geographic history of possible diagnostic value. (Examples are coccidioidomycosis and histoplasmosis.)
B. Occupational history	B. Certain occupations involve exposure to allergens and pollutants that may cause disease (silicosis, asbestosis, farmer's lung, and so on). It is not always sufficient to know the patient's last or present occupation because previous exposure may now be causing symptoms. In addition, the specific job of the patient must be identified in order to make any assumptions about the exposure. For example, knowing that the patient worked in a mine is not sufficient; you must know what type of mine, and what the specific job in that mine was (whether the patient worked at the face, for example).
C. Marital history Duration of marriage Spouse age state of health present residence Children age state of health present residence If married, present husband/wife relationship	C. This information can be of special help to the nurse in plans for patient teaching, family involvement, and long-term follow-up. In addition to the basic history, the nurse needs to gather data regarding the patient-spouse relationship. Is the patient overly dependent upon the spouse? Does the spouse force the patient to be dependent? Much of these data are very personal to the patient and it is often inappropriate to question the patient specifically on the first visit. Much can be learned by observation and as the patient gains confidence in the nurse, he or she may pose questions that imply problems regarding these personal aspects of life, if they exist. The important thing to remember is that pulmonary diseases, especially the chronic diseases, have a great impact on the patient-spouse relationship (or significant other relationships). This impact can range from the social role to the economic role to the interpersonal role to the sexual role. On the other hand, the nurse should not make a problem when one does not exist!

(Continued)

Table 40-1. *(Continued)*

Data to Be Obtained	Selected Examples of Rationale and Significance
D. Social and economic status Standard of living Extent of education Special financial problems Present housing with descriptions (how many rooms, what size, arrangement, stairs, heating, and cooling systems, and so on) General life style, avocations Number of persons in household and their relationship to patient	D. These data are of help to the nurse in planning patient and family education and long-term follow-up. For example, if the patient has special financial problems, every effort is made to use effective yet inexpensive modes of therapy; referral to other agencies that can offer some financial assistance may be needed. The description of the patient's present housing may indicate that modifications are required to enhance the patient's level of function at home. For example, the patient's room may be on the second floor and he or she may be unable to climb stairs; a dry heating system may contribute to tenacious sputum in the winter months. The plan of care must be feasible in the patient's home environment and life style. You don't recommend the use of the shower for aerosol therapy if the patient's home does not have a shower.
E. Reaction to illness What is the patient's understanding of the illness? What is the patient's understanding of the treatment? What are the patient's and family's coping mechanisms?	E. This aspect of the history is especially important in the care of the patient with chronic disease in order to plan patient education. There are times, however, when the gathering of this data should be delayed. For example, if the patient is admitted to the hospital with a superimposed infection with acute shortness of breath, he or she does not want to talk about his or her understanding of the illness, but wants someone to help in breathing. The nurse may make the observation that the patient delayed seeking medical help for too long a period that implies some lack of understanding of the illness and its treatment. Direct questioning and teaching should, however, be delayed until someone has dealt with the acute symptoms.
VIII. Physical assessment (pertinent to pulmonary problems)	
A. Vital signs temperature pulse respiration blood pressure	A. Changes in vital signs may, for example, indicate infection, cardiac arrhythmias, respiratory distress.
B. Inspection of the chest What is the degree of respiration excursion? Is there any abnormal anatomic configuration? Are accessory muscles used on inspiration; on expiration? Are retractions present? What is the predominant respiratory pattern (thoracic or diaphragmatic)? Does the respiratory pattern change with activity?	B. These observations provide the nurse with information regarding the need for exercises and how to teach breathing exercises, areas needing emphasis. In the more acute situation, it provides data as to the extent of respiratory distress and may provide indications for positioning of the patient in order to alleviate some of the distress.

TABLE 40-1. *(Continued)*

Data to Be Obtained	Selected Examples of Rationale and Significance
C. Palpation of the chest	C. Areas of pain or tenderness, as previously described, can be detected and delineated. For the nurse, this information may indicate the need to splint the chest when the patient coughs, need to alter percussion technique with postural drainage, and so on.
D. Percussion of the chest	D. Areas of differing density, as previously described, can be assessed. In addition to delineating areas of dullness such as seen in a consolidated pneumonia, abnormal findings may indicate fluid accumulation as in pleural effusion or air in the pneumothorax. These latter data may be helpful to the nurse in evaluating the function of chest tubes—is air and/or fluid being removed?
E. Auscultation of the chest Are normal breath sounds present absent distant Is there expiratory slowing? Are adventitial sounds present? If so, what type? Where? Is there wheezing with forced expiration?	E. These findings may help the nurse to plan for care (that is, need for improved bronchial hygiene) and to evaluate the care given (determine if adventitial sounds change after postural drainage).
F. Inspection of the skin and extremities Is cyanosis present? Is clubbing present?	F. Cyanosis may indicate oxygen lack and need for oxygen therapy. Clubbing is often associated with pulmonary diseases such as fibrosis and cancer of the lung.
G. Is peripheral edema present? H. Is liver tenderness present?	G&H. Because patients with pulmonary disease may develop cor pulmonale and right-sided heart failure, observations must be made for significant clinical findings.
I. Mental status	I. Is the patient alert and oriented? A change may indicate hypoxemia or acidemia and the need for further nursing intervention.
IX. Laboratory data	
A. Spirometry, especially FEV_1 and VC	A. These data are of assistance in evaluating care and planning for teaching of breathing exercises and cough.
B. Chest radiographs	B. X-rays are used to evaluate present status or changes in pulmonary and other radiographic infiltrate findings. The nurse can use reports to help in planning for care as in postural drainage and to evaluate care.
C. Blood gases at rest and with exercise	C. The results provide data as to the patient's status and limitations of gas exchange that are present at rest and/or exercise; the nurse can use this data to help in patient education and rehabilitation, for example, can you expect the patient to increase exercise without supplemental oxygen? If the patient tends to be hypercapneic, the nurse should observe him or her more closely for heart failure. In general, these studies document the need for oxygen therapy and response to that therapy.

(Continued)

Table 40-1. *(Continued)*

Data to Be Obtained	Selected Examples of Rationale and Significance
D. Blood count	D. Patients who are chronically hypoxemic may have secondary polycythemia. An increased hematocrit and hemoglobin may indicate the need for blood gases and other observations related to hypoxemia. An elevated white blood count with a shift to the left (increase in polymorphonuclear neutrophils) indicates a response to infection. The presence of eosinophils is seen in certain allergic responses.
E. Electrolytes	E. Abnormalities of serum K+ and Cl^- levels may be observed in response to pH changes and diuretic therapy, both common in chronic pulmonary patients. In patients who have low serum K+ levels, in addition to the need for medication, the nurse can encourage the patient to include such foods as orange juice and bananas in order to increase K+ levels.
F. EKG	F. The EKG may indicate cardiac abnormalities of right ventricular hypertrophy and P pulmonale. An EKG is often needed to evaluate an irregular pulse which may be seen in lung diseases.
G. Skin tests	G. Skin tests for TB (PPD), coccidioidomycosis (coccidioidin), histoplasmosis (histoplasmin), and specific allergy skin tests are done to evaluate present and/or past exposure to the sensitizing allergen and the resulting immunologic response.

Selected Case Studies

The following case studies have been selected as representative of the major problems of pulmonary dysfunction affecting the adult patient and as examples of the range of nursing interventions required in the care of the pulmonary patient. A complete data base is not included for each case, nor is there a complete discussion of the progress of all problems. Rather, the data have been limited to those pertinent for the specific problem and stage of acuity being presented. Interspersed throughout all the case studies are discussions of the data and plans, to help the reader understand why those specific data were obtained and why any specific intervention was planned.

Chronic Obstructive Lung Disease (COLD)

Two case studies of patients with chronic obstructive lung disease (COLD) will be discussed. One patient is in an ambulatory care setting; the other is hospitalized during an acute exacerbation. In addition, the patients demonstrate slightly different pathologies, one having less bronchitis and more emphysema than the other. It is important for the nurse to recognize the range of COLD in terms of pathology and the wellness-illness continuum. The patient must not be categorized.

Patient A: Data Base

History and Physical

Mrs. Burns is a 55-year-old female with COLD who was referred to the chest clinic for evaluation by her private physician. She has a history of increasing shortness of breath over the last 10 years. She had been a schoolteacher, but 2 years ago had to retire because of her inability to "keep up" at work. She now has shortness of breath with mild exercise, for example, she can only walk one city block on the level before having to rest. Except for a slight morning cough and colds (about four per year), she denied cough and sputum production. Mrs. Burns used to smoke one to one and one-half packs of cigarettes a day but quit 2 years ago because of her increasing shortness of breath. She has a total of 30 pack years.

Mrs. Burns's mother and one brother have a history of lung disease which was described as being "like asthma." The mother died at age 50. The brother, age 57, is still working but is under medical care for his lung disease and has frequent colds for which he must miss work. Mrs. Burns has three children, ages 30, 33, and 35, who are all living and well. They live in another area of the country. Mrs. Burns lives in the city with her husband in a small one-story home which they own. Her husband, age 65, has just retired.

On physical examination, Mrs. Burns had a respiratory rate of 24 per minute and a pulse of 110. She was short of breath after walking down the hall to the examining room. Her respiratory pattern was upper thoracic and demonstrated use of accessory muscles on both inspiration and expiration. The shoulder girdle was elevated and she sat in a slightly forward flexed position. On chest auscultation, breath sounds were distant with expiratory slowing. There were no crackles or rhonchi. The rest of the physical examination was within normal limits.

Laboratory Data

RADIOGRAPHS. PA and lateral views of the chest show a hyperinflated chest with areas of hyperlucency. There are no infiltrates. The heart size is within normal limits.

BLOOD COUNT AND ELECTROLYTES. Within normal limits.

ALPHA$_1$-ANTITRYPSIN LEVEL. Decreased in the heterozygotic range.

EKG. Shows a sinus tachycardia at a rate of 100.

Pulmonary Function Studies

	Baseline	After Isuprel	Predicted
VC	2,500 cc	2,740	3,240
FEV_1	710 cc	770	2,127
FEV_1/VC	28%	28%	>70
MVV	34 L/min	40	104

Blood Gases

	P_{O_2} (mm Hg)	Sa_{O_2}	P_{CO_2} (mm Hg)	pH
Normal	85–95	95–97%	38–42	7.4
Rest	66	90	38	7.43
Exercise	58	86	42	7.40

PROBLEM. COLD with alpha$_1$-antitrypsin deficiency.

PLAN. Oral bronchodilators (aminophylline). Inhaled bronchodilators (β_2 sympathomimetics). Tetracycline prn for infections. Refer to nurse for patient teaching and long-term surveillance.

DISCUSSION. This patient has an obstructive ventilatory defect as demonstrated by her pulmonary function studies (FEV_1/VC less than 70 per cent), which cannot be corrected by bronchodilators. In addition, no specific cause for the obstructive defect was found. This criterion, of a persistive obstructive ventilatory defect for which no specific cause is known, is the basis of the diagnosis of COLD.

The chronic obstructive lung diseases include emphysema and chronic bronchitis. (Yet it must be remembered that a patient may have emphysema or chronic bronchitis without have COLD.) Emphysema is defined pathologically as destruction of the lung parenchyma distal to the terminal bronchiole. Chronic bronchitis, on the other hand, is described symptomatically and refers to the patient who coughs and raises sputum on most days for a minimum of 3 consecutive months each year for at least 2 years. Other diseases such as bronchiectasis or tuberculosis which may produce the same symptoms must be excluded. Clinically, this patient has both diseases, but the symptoms indicate more emphysema than bronchitis: there is minor sputum production; the prime complaint is shortness of breath; there is mild hypoxemia but no hypercapnia; the x rays show areas of hyperlucency which may indicate areas of lung destruction; and there is the etiologic factor of alpha$_1$-antitrypsin deficiency. Alpha$_1$-antitrypsin deficiency is sometimes present in those patients where the emphysema is diagnosed at an earlier than usual age (in the third or fourth decade rather than the fifth or sixth decade) and is typified by areas of lower-lobe destruction rather than the more common finding of upper-lobe destruction. In patients heterozygous for this trait, as exemplified by this patient, there are still no definitive data available to predict which patients will have severe emphysema.

Medications

Medications for the patient being discussed include bronchodilators. Even though airway obstruction is not completely reversible, bronchodilators will often have some beneficial effect. The dosages of the bronchodilators must be tailored to each patient. Especially in the ambulatory care setting, it is important that maximum therapeutic effect be attained without intolerable side effects that might cause the patient to discontinue the medication. The oral aminophylline preparations and their derivatives may also cause side effects at dosages necessary for effective therapeutic bronchodilation. In addition, the absorption of these drugs from the gastrointestinal tract and breakdown in the body is highly variable. To ascertain whether or not therapeutic levels have been attained an aminophylline blood level is often necessary. If blood levels are too high, in the toxic range, the drug should be stopped for a day and then restarted at a lower dose rather than the dosage simply be cut.

The sympathomimetics are also given to produce bronchodilation. These drugs are most commonly given orally and/or by inhalation. The newer drugs act on β receptors, which means they are good bronchodilators without as much cardiac stimulation as the older drugs. These drugs also produce side effects of nervousness, shakiness, and insomnia. Therefore, especially with the oral drugs, dosage is gradually increased, which usually decreases side effects. For patients who use an inhaler, the nurse must carefully instruct the patient in its use. The patient exhales normally. Then, *as* he or she breathes in deeply and slowly, the inhaler should be depressed, aerosolizing the medication. This movement is often difficult to coordinate. If the patient aerosolizes the drug after inhaling or during expiration it will not be carried into the lung and therapeutic effect will be lost.

Patients with obstructive lung disease are given antibiotics for acute infections. The broad-spectrum antibiotics such as the tetracyclines are usually used. The patient is instructed to start the antibiotic whenever sputum becomes yellow or green, as the change in color is usually the first sign of infection. If the sputum does not begin to clear after two days of antibiotic therapy, the patient is instructed to call the physician for additional therapy.

Other Therapy

Other general areas of therapy include exercise programs and patient education. Patients with obstructive lung disease often become "pulmonary cripples" before their time. Once they are labeled with the diagnosis of chronic obstructive lung disease or "emphysema" they believe nothing can be done for them. They often tend to reduce their activity so as not to stress themselves or induce shortness of breath. The end result is that they lose muscle bulk and, therefore, decrease their ability to perform any exercise including activities of daily living. These patients are encouraged to increase their exercise tolerance. This may be done through a formal program or simply by increasing those activities the patient enjoys, such as walking. Knowing the level of arterial oxygen tension and saturation on exercise aids the nurse in determining how much exercise can be encouraged in a patient. If the patient without oxygen supplementation desaturates his or her blood on exercise, such a program would not be encouraged, or would be encouraged only if oxygen supplementation was given.

Patient education takes a variety of directions. Basically, however, the goal is to teach the patient how to control his or her own disease. For example, when the patient loses control and has increased anxiety with increased shortness of breath, the result is often an increased respiratory rate, aggravating the shortness of breath. The patient who is more secure in the ability to control the disease does not experience as much anxiety during shortness of breath and, therefore, can prevent the symptoms from worsening. In order to teach the patient how to control shortness of breath, the nurse must be sure that the patient has some understanding of the disease and some understanding of how breathing exercises relate to the control of symptoms produced by that disease. The specific therapeutic goal is improving the patient's pattern of respiration. In addition, the patient must know how to cough effectively so that when there is no sputum he or she can raise it, and thus avoid greater difficulty. The patient is also taught how to recognize exacerbations of acute bronchitis or heart failure early so that treatment can be started immediately rather than waiting until the symptoms become so severe that hospitalization is required. Other patient education factors include suggestions on how the patient can manage better at home, both in handling daily activities and in increasing general physical tolerance. All of these factors will, as an end result, teach the patient how to gain some control of the disease. He or she may then feel in charge of having the disease rather than disease being in charge of him or her. Concurrently, the plan of care developed must be adjusted to the individual patient so that it is effective, as simple as possible, economical, and acceptable to the patient and family.

Patient Visit to Nurse

SUBJECTIVE. The patient appears to be depressed; states that she cannot do the things she enjoys doing.

OBJECTIVE. Respiratory pattern is inefficient at rest with increased use of the accessory muscles. Respiratory rate is increased and depth of respiration appears to be decreased with walking. On auscultation, breath sounds are decreased with expiratory slowing; there are no rales or rhonchi. With deep breathing and coughing a small amount of clear mucoid sputum is produced.

ASSESSMENT. Blood gases showed some drop in P_{O_2} during exercise, but not enough to prevent an exercise program. There is no present problem of heart failure. This patient may be able to increase her exercise tolerance with breathing exercises that would allow her to reduce her respiratory rate and therefore maintain depth of respiration during activity. In the same respect, this program may help with activities of daily living. As exercise tolerance and ability to maintain normal activities increase, it is hoped that the depression will decrease. Sputum production is scant and does not pose a problem to the patient at this time.

PLAN. (1) Obtain more data on specific activities which cause patient's increased shortness of breath. (2) Teach breathing exercises; stress slow rate and diaphragmatic pattern. (3) Teach patient to observe sputum so that episodes of increased sputum production or change in sputum color can be immediately treated. (4) Plan frequent visits for the next several weeks. To return in 2 days.

DISCUSSION. In caring for this patient, the nurse has planned frequent visits for her period of initial contact with the patient. These frequent visits will not only offer more teaching sessions where the patient can be taught about her disease and treatment, but will also allow her to understand that there are personnel available to give her help. Many times patients with obstructive pulmonary disease are extremely fearful, have been shuttled from one health facility to another, and believe that no one really cares for or wants to help them. By frequent contact with the patient and teaching the "little things" that will help at home, the nurse demonstrates to the patient that there are things that can be done for her and that someone cares enough about her to spend time going over these aspects of her care. Some examples of the "little things" are how to take a deep breath; how to raise secretions by doing a prolonged exhalation; and how to increase tolerance for taking a shower by first using bronchodilator inhalation.

As the patient gains greater understanding of her illness and its treatment, the frequency of visits can be slowly decreased. At this stage the nurse is encouraging the patient to take over the responsibility for her own care. Visits can become more infrequent as the patient becomes more independent in providing surveillance of her disease and her response to it. The patient is assured that help is available while gaining the added hope that she can now exert some control over her own symptoms and can function at a much higher level. The subjective improvement of the patient may not necessarily be demonstrated in pulmonary function tests or arterial blood gases. It is not uncommon for the patient to remark after such a patient education program that now she or he is no longer frightened. The patient understands the disease and knows what to do to help himself or herself. Therefore the patient often feels much better, is able to do more, and does not get into serious problems from exacerbations. With good patient education and a patient who is at a relatively stable stage of the disease, the number of visits can be decreased to intervals of several months. These visits may be periodically interspersed with telephone calls from the patient just to inform you that he or she is "still feeling well." These phone calls provide the patient with confidence that he or she is doing the right things and the knowledge that the nurse is still concerned about the patient's wellbeing.

The ultimate goal is to improve the quality of life. Emphysema is a slowly progressive disease for which no cure is known. Quality care, however, will maintain the best physiologic function possible for the individual and improve and maintain capability to function at the highest possible level. The patient must feel that he or she is a contributing member of society. It is not infrequent that the patient's sources of gratification must be changed as capabilities change, but the patient must feel like a worthwhile person.

Chronic Ventilatory Failure Complicated by Superimposed Acute Ventilatory Failure

Patient B: Data Base

History and Physical

Mr. Jones called the Chest Clinic this morning and reported that he has been having increased shortness of breath over the last several weeks. He is producing more sputum, which is now yellow, and has developed swelling of his ankles. The clinic secretary made an appointment for the patient to see a physician that morning.

Mr. Jones is a 60-year-old retired construction worker who lives alone in a mobile home. He has a 15-year history of cough and sputum production and for the last 8 years has been having increasing shortness of breath. Chronic obstructive lung disease was diagnosed 8 years ago after spirometry demonstrated an FEV_1/VC ratio of 55 per cent with an FEV_1 of 700 cc. The studies did not show significant improvement after the administration of bronchodilators. Mr. Jones has been smoking since age 20, one and one-half to two packs per day. He has been unable to stop smoking but has reduced his cigarette smoking to one pack per day this past year. He raises approximately 1 ounce of sputum per day. Although when he is well the sputum is clear, he has chest infections with yellow to green sputum at a frequency of six to eight times a year that respond well to broad-spectrum antibiotics. The patient also has corpulmonale with intermittent right-sided heart failure that has required diuretic therapy.

Mr. Jones's present illness started 2 weeks ago with a cold. About 10 days ago his sputum production increased and became yellow and it is now yellow-green; his shortness of breath also increased. The patient has not been taking antibiotics. Five days ago he noted that his shoes were tight and that his ankles were swelling. A neighbor who accompanied the patient to clinic noted yesterday that the patient appeared very fatigued and lethargic, and would frequently doze off. In clinic the patient is tachypneic and has mild cyanosis of the oral mucous membranes.

On physical examination the vital signs are temperature 37.8°C, pulse 110 and irregularly irregular, respiratory rate 26, and blood pressure 140/90. On chest auscultation there is expiratory slowing and scattered crackles and rhonchi throughout both lung fields. Cardiovascular findings are an S-3 and an S-4. Peripherally, the JVPs are filled above the clavicle with the patient in the upright position. The liver is tender and enlarged. There is bilateral 3+ ankle and pretibial pitting edema.

Laboratory Data

RADIOGRAPHS. Show a hyperinflated chest. The heart is enlarged in comparison with old films and there is a left-lower-lobe infiltrate.

BLOOD COUNT AND ELECTROLYTES. Show a white blood count of 15,000 with a shift to the left (increase in per cent of polymorphonuclear neutrophils); the hematocrit is 50.

CHEMISTRIES. Show a sodium of 145, potassium of 3.4, and chloride of 90.

EKG. Shows P pulmonale, right ventricular hypertrophy, and frequent premature atrial contractions.

Blood Gases

P_{O_2}	Sa_{O_2}	P_{CO_2}	pH
40	73%	65	7.28

The patient was admitted to the medical unit with the following problem list:

1. COLD—chronic bronchitis.
2. Left-lower-lobe pneumonia.
3. Ventilatory failure.
4. Cor pulmonale and heart failure.

The plan of care included the following:

1. Oxygen at 2 liters per minute by nasal cannula; draw arterial blood gases 30 minutes after oxygen started.
2. Bronchodilators. IV aminophylline; aerosolized bronchodilator qid.
3. Antibiotics.
4. Sputum culture.
5. Intravenous fluids.
6. Diuretics.
7. Measures of airway care, including aerosol, postural drainage, deep breathing, and coughing.

DISCUSSION. This patient has a history of sputum production that is not related to a specific cause and is therefore consistent with the diagnosis of chronic bronchitis. In addition, he has COLD as evidenced by the persistent obstructive defect on his pulmonary function tests. The frequent bronchitic infections, hypoxemia, CO_2 retention, and heart failure are also frequently seen with the diagnosis of chronic bronchitis.

The patient's present admission was precipitated by acute bronchitis, pneumonia, and heart failure. The diagnosis of infection has been made by the elevated white count with a shift to the left, the elevated temperature, increased sputum production with change in color, and the x-ray, which shows the pneumonic infiltrate in the left lower lobe. The heart failure was diagnosed by the increase in heart size, increased venous pressure, and peripheral venous congestion exemplified by the enlarged liver and the peripheral edema. The history, EKG, and presence of hypoxemia and acidemia are consistent with the diagnoses of cor pulmonale and chronic bronchitis. Hypoxemia and acidemia result in an increased pulmonary vascular resistance, which then leads to an increased pulmonary artery pressure. This increased resistance places an additional load on the right ventricle, which will then hypertrophy and dilate in order to maintain cardiac output. This condition of right ventricular hypertrophy secondary to a primary pulmonary disorder is defined as cor pulmonale. When the right ventricle is no longer able to maintain cardiac output, the condition is termed right-sided heart failure, which this patient has.

The blood gases, in addition to demonstrating severe hypoxemia and acidemia, also indicate that the patient has probably had carbon dioxide retention for some time because there is partial compensation of the pH. A patient with acute carbon dioxide retention with a P_{CO_2} of 65 would have a pH in the approximate range of 7.2 to 7.25. Because the patient's pH is 7.28 it can be assumed that he may have had chronic hypercapnia that is now being complicated by an acute ventilatory failure. The elevated hematocrit indicates that this patient may also be chronically hypoxemic. Both of these findings, chronic hypoxemia and chronic carbon dioxide retention, are relatively common in chronic bronchitis and cor pulmonale.

This patient is being treated with low-flow oxygen. The objective of this therapy is to increase the oxygen content of the blood and thereby oxygen supply to the tissues without depression of the hypoxemic drive, which could lead to further carbon dioxide retention. The oxygen therapy will also help to treat the right ventricular failure and cardiac arrhythmias precipitated by the hypoxemia. The patient should, therefore, he observed carefully for both his ventilatory and cardiac responses to the therapy. The findings of acidemia and hypoxemia and their related cardiac abnormalities demand that the patient's ventilation be improved concurrently with his oxygenation. Aminophylline is being given as a bronchodilator in order to increase ventilation and stimulate respiration. The measures of bronchial hygiene, if effective, will help to improve oxygenation and make ventilation more effective. The specific nursing interventions may have to be modified so that the patient can tolerate them. If the sputum is too tenacious to be expectorated with deep breathing and coughing, aerosol therapy may be needed. If a bland aerosol is indicated, this patient will probably require an aerosolized bronchodilator prior to the treatment. Because this patient already has some cardiac arrhythmias, he must be closely observed for his cardiac response to the bronchodilators. If the preceding measures are still not effective in promoting airway clearance, postural drainage with percussion and vibration may be instituted. Because the patient is in respiratory distress and heart failure, he may not be able to tolerate the head-down or prone positions. Therefore the positions are modified to patient tolerance.

Throughout this initial phase of therapy the patient is observed carefully for any changes in the level of consciousness that could be secondary to decreased ventilation and/or oxygenation. No narcotics or sedatives should be given at this time, nor should the patient be allowed to sleep for extended periods of time, which would depress ventilation. One of the major prerequisites for successful therapy is nursing personnel who can keep this patient awake and breathing until the underlying cause of his acute ventilatory failure is treated.

It is evident from his symptomatology that this patient has an increased volume in the extravascular fluid compartment. For this reason diuretic therapy is given. At the same time, however, it is not uncommon for the patient to require fluid therapy. This patient is receiving intravenous fluids and aerosol therapy, which also adds to the total fluid intake. There are several reasons why these patients often need regulated fluid therapy. Because the patient has been ill for some time, it is not unusual that he has decreased his oral fluid intake because of shortness of breath, (He cannot hold his breath long enough to swallow.) In addition, he is febrile, has an increased respiratory rate, and is probably mouth breathing. All of these factors lead to increased insensible water loss and drying of the respiratory mucosa. Therefore IV fluids are given carefully so as not to overload the system further but to keep water inake adequate to maintain the function of normal defense mechanisms of the airway. It must be remembered that the patient's heart failure is not due to an intrinsic cardiac disorder but is in response to primary pulmonary disease. Therefore treatment must be aimed at the pulmonary dysfunction. It should also be noted that this patient is not receiving a digitalis preparation. The basic reason is that his heart is responding normally to the increased load; it is the pulmonary problem that is producing the load and that must therefore be treated. In addition, these patients are usually hypoxemic and hypokalemic, increasing their incidence of digitalis toxicity.

Nurse's Admission Note

SUBJECTIVE. Patient is short of breath; restless; skin color dusky. According to friend accompanying patient, patient is confused.

OBJECTIVE. Respiratory rate 36; pulse 110 and irregular; temperature 38°C, blood pressure 130/90; sputum thick and yellow; increased use of accessory muscles of respiration.

PLAN. Give oxygen as ordered. Position patient in high Fowler's; try resting arms on overbed table in order to fix shoulder girdle and improve respiratory pattern; deep-breathe and couth q 30 to 60 minutes. Verbal and physical stimuli to keep patient awake.

DISCUSSION. At this stage of the patient's illness, the nurse's objectives for the patient are to improve oxygenation, improve ventilation, and conserve energy. Her observations and judgment will be crucial to determining the amount of activity needed to improve the patient's pulmonary status without placing unwarranted stress on his cardiovascular system.

M.D.'s Note

Thirty minutes after admission:

OBJECTIVE. Blood gases P_{O_2} 58 (on 2 liters per minute) P_{CO_2} 63; per cent sat. 87 per cent; pH 7.3.

ASSESSMENT. Oxygen therapy has raised P_{O_2} and Sa_{O_2} to acceptable levels.

PLAN. Continue as before.

Nurse's Notes Four Hours Later (only selected nurse's notes are presented)

SUBJECTIVE. Patient fatigued, lethargic, difficult to arouse; color remains good.

OBJECTIVE. Respiratory rate 30, patient not coughing. Numerous crackles and coarse rhonchi throughout both lung fields. Percussion and vibration done in right and left lateral positions with bed flat followed by nasotracheal suctioning productive of large amounts of thick, yellow sputum.

ASSESSMENT. Patient will need increased stimuli to maintain ventilation; suctioning used as a stimulus as well as a means of maintaining airway patency; patient more alert after suctioning.

PLAN. Observe closely, if respirations decrease in rate or depth or if it becomes difficult to arouse the patient, call the physician for a blood gas order.

DISCUSSION. As patients become fatigued their respiratory rate and depth decrease. It is important not to confuse these findings with improved status. Although the patients' respiratory rate is returning to a more normal rate, they appear less air hungry and appear to be "resting," they are actually worsening. Often stimulation of the patient to produce deep breathing and coughing is sufficient to reverse this decreased ventilation. This stimulation requires a vocal, aggressive nurse in order to be effective. Should this patient not have responded to the nursing intervention, blood gases would have been done *stat* to provide a more precise evaluation of gas exchange status and to plan further therapy.

Within the next 12 hours the patient improved and the following note was written:

Note

SUBJECTIVE. Patient alert.

OBJECTIVE. Temperature 37.6°C; pulse 90 and regular; respiratory rate 24; blood pressure 126/94. Sputum being raised more easily; remains yellow. Suctioning no longer required.

Blood Gases

P_{O_2} (on 2 liters per minute)	P_{CO_2}	pH
60	58	7.36

PLAN. Decrease frequency of deep breathing and coughing to every 1 to 2 hours. Allow for periods of sleep.

DISCUSSION. The patient is now improving; for example, his arrhythmias have disappeared (by EKG) as his oxygenation has improved. Although the selected nurse's notes demonstrated the course of problem 3, the status of the patient's other problems have also showed improvement. Diuresis occurred with oxygen therapy and diuretics and the patient has lost 3 kg. The patient must still be observed closely for, if he retains secretions, his oxygen tension will again fall as may ventilation and he will return to his previous state. Continued aggressive nursing intervention based on knowledgeable observation and judgment will help to ensure the patient's continued improvement.

ASTHMA

Data Base

History and Physical

Sally Brown, a graduate student, was seen in the emergency room for an asthmatic attack. She stated that she has had a history of asthma since childhood and had positive skin tests to a variety of allergens including grasses and house dust. She knew of no specific or unusual exposure that may have precipitated this attack. The patient stated that she takes aminophylline and bronchodilator inhalations intermittently at home. Over the last 24 hours she had increased her bronchodilator inhalations to every 3 hours with no relief. She is not on steroids now but has been in the past.

On physical examination she was seen to be a young woman in acute respiratory distress. The vital signs showed: temperature 37°C, pulse 120 and regular, respiratory rate 30, blood pressure 135/84. The patient was audibly wheezing and diaphoretic. She was sitting upright and using accessory muscles for ventilation with forced expiration. Auscultation of the chest demonstrates expiratory and inspiratory wheezing throughout both lung fields.

PROBLEM. Acute ashmatic attack.

TREATMENT. Epinephrine, subcutaneously; aminophylline, IV; corticosteroids, IV.

DISCUSSION. Asthma is a disease characterized by hyperreactive airways. There is intermittent airway narrowing which is relieved spontaneously or with treatment. During an asthmatic attack there is airway obstruction caused by the bronchoconstriction, increased production of viscous mucus, and mucosal edema. Cough is also a common symptom and is precipitated as a response to the airway irritation.

Asthma is often classified as being atopic (allergic), nonatopic (nonallergic), or mixed. The individual with atopic asthma demonstrates a type I allergic response. A type I response is an immediate allergic reaction. The IgE-sensitized mast cells liberate mediators when exposed to the specific allergen. The onset of this reaction is immediate and the duration lasts from 1 to 1½ hours. This reaction is the basis for the immediate response to prick tests. The asthmatic demonstrating this type of allergy to inhaled allergens will have an immediate asthmatic response to the allergen, but if exposure is terminated the response should spontaneously remit.

In the nonatopic (nonallergic) individual there is no specific demonstrable allergic cause of the asthma. Various irritants (infection, cold, exercise) may initiate an attack or there may be no specific causal relationship identified. The onset of nonatopic asthma is usually during the adult years and it is common to find an elevated eosinophil count in these patients. In many patients with asthma there appears to be both atopic and nonatopic factors involved.

Treatment of asthma includes a variety of interventions. Most specific is the treatment of the patient for whom a specific allergen that causes all the patient's asthmatic attacks has been identified. In such an instance, of course, treatment is to avoid that specific allergen. In other cases drug therapy is used. The sympathomimetic drugs are used to decrease the mucosal edema and to relax the bronchial musculature. Some of these drugs affect both aspects, edema and musculature, whereas others act mainly on the bronchial musculature. In patients where the asthma has caused a decrease in the oxygen tension and the pH, these drugs must be given more cautiously. Another class of drugs are the theophylline drugs and their derivatives including the aminophylline preparations. These drugs, when given in combination with the adrenergic drugs, tend to have a potentiating effect. They will also effect relaxation of the bronchial musculature but act at different points than do the adrenergic drugs.

Steroids may also be given in situations where response to the bronchodilators is inadequate. The steroids may help to block the late immune response and therefore prohibit prolonged bronchoconstriction. Some patients respond to inhaled steroids such as Vanceril. This steroid is not absorbed systemically and therefore does not result in the adverse systemic effects of steroid therapy.

Another important measure in these patients is hydration so that secretions can be kept as thin as possible in order to aid expectoration. Postural drainage with percussion and vibration is also very helpful in some of these patients although in the acute phase it may precipitate more wheezing. Tranquilizers are ordered in some patients but must be given cautiously, for if the patient has a very severe asthmatic attack, which could result in an elevated carbon dioxide tension, the tranquilizer is a potentially dangerous drug. A drug released for use in the United States in 1973 is disodium cromoglycate. This drug has been effective in some patients and blocks the release of the mediators that produce the attack. It is given as a prophylactic drug rather than as a specific measure for treatment of an acute asthmatic attack. The cromolyn is administered by a special inhaler called a spinhaler.

The nurse who is with the patient makes the following note minutes after the medications are started:

Note

SUBJECTIVE. Anxious and restless; very dyspneic.

OBJECTIVE. Respiratory rate 36; audibly wheezing; using forced expiration.

ASSESSMENT. No apparent response to treatment yet.

PLAN. Stay with patient; do breathing exercises with pursed-lip exhalation in order to help patient gain more effective and efficient pattern and to slow respiratory rate.

DISCUSSION. The anxiety precipitated by an asthmatic attack often serves to increase the patient's respiratory rate. In turn, this increase in rate requires a shorter expiratory time. The result is an attempt to increase the force of expiration, which can significantly increase airway obstruction in airways that are already narrowed by mucus and bronchospasm. Breathing exercises can help to slow the expiratory rate and therefore not aggravate the obstruction. Using pursed-lip exhalation also helps to keep airways open and improve ventilation. In addition, pursed-lip breathing often makes the wheezing less audible to the patient and therefore also serves to decrease anxiety. Perhaps the most important aspect is that someone remains with the patient to help her. She is not left alone nor is she faced by a nurse or other personnel whose response to the asthmatic attack is anxiety and purposeless hyperactivity.

M.D.'s Note

One-half hour later:

SUBJECTIVE. Breathing easier, appears less anxious.

OBJECTIVE. Pulse 90; respiratory rate 20; wheezing no longer audible; some expiratory wheezing on auscultation; cough producing clear mucoid sputum.

ASSESSMENT. Responding to therapy.

PLAN. Discontinue IV after all of the fluid in; discharge from emergency room after therapy completed; schedule appointment in clinic for this week in order to continue follow-up, which would include patient education program, and better control of medications.

DISCUSSION. This patient will require continued follow-up if she is to be able to function well with her asthma. The teaching of breathing exercises in a quieter situation, not one involving an acute asthmatic attack, can be helpful in aiding the patient to exert some control over her disease. If when she first begins to wheeze she can do breathing exercises and therefore not worsen the airway obstruction by the forced expiratory pattern, she may be able to maintain a lower level of anxiety and not further aggravate the asthmatic attack. In addition, more follow-up will need to be done concerning the incidence of asthmatic attacks and the necessity for such long-term therapy as bronchodilators or cromolyn in order to keep the patient as symptom-free as possible and able to maintain her activities.

TUBERCULOSIS

Data Base

History and Physical

Mr. Calkins, a 35-year-old county engineer, has been informed that his recent yearly chest x ray was abnormal and that he should see a physician. Mr. Calkins is married, with two children, ages 12 and 15. He and his wife own their own home in the suburbs. As a county engineer most of his work hours are spent out-of-doors. The patient feels well and has no symptoms except for a slight morning cough which has not bothered him. He is concerned about the recent abnormal x-ray. He has had yearly x-rays for the last 5 years, all of which have been normal until now. He does not remember ever having been skin-tested for tuberculosis. The rest of the past medical history is noncontributory and the physical examination is within normal limits.

PROBLEM. Abnormal chest x-ray by history.

PLAN. Chest x-ray, full size PA and lateral today; get old films; PPD intermediate; return in 48 hours to have skin test read.

On the patient's return 2 days later the physician makes the following note:

M.D.'s Note

SUBJECTIVE. No change; no known exposure to tuberculosis; minimal sputum production.

OBJECTIVE. X-ray demonstrates a right-upper-lobe infiltrate involving the posterior segment; old films are normal; PPD intermediate read at 48 hours showed 30 mm of induration.

ASSESSMENT. Infiltrate and positive PPD without other specific findings make tuberculosis the prime diagnostic probability. Other possibilities that must be ruled out include bacterial infection and fungal infection.

PLAN. Induced sputum for smear and culture; smear and culture for AFB × 3; fungal culture × 3; return appointment in 3 days.

DISCUSSION. Tuberculosis is an infectious disease that may have multisystem involvement, but whose classical manifestation is pulmonary. The cause of the infection is a microbacterium, usually *Mycobacterium tuberculosis.* The incidence of new cases of tuberculosis is declining in this country, but still remains a problem in many areas.

Mycobacterium tuberculosis is usually transmitted by a droplet nuclei produced by an individual with active tuberculosis. Because active tuberculosis may not produce any symptoms, persons can be unknowingly exposed to the disease. Simple exposure to an individual with active tuberculosis, however, does not mean that the disease can be transmitted. The exposed individual must be in a susceptible state and be exposed to a high enough concentration of organisms in the environment that, as he or she breathes, droplet nuclei will reach the alveolar level. These droplet nuclei consist of a microbacterium in a minute quantity of water. The droplets, as first produced from the respiratory tract of the patient with active tuberculosis, are usually large (greater than 50 microns). The droplet nuclei are produced by evaporation of these particles to much smaller dimensions. The larger particles (greater than 50 microns) are filtered by the normal airway defense mechanisms and therefore do not reach the alveolar level where they can cause disease. The small droplet nuclei are capable of reaching the alveoli. Even if the organism does reach alveolar level, it may not cause active tuberculosis. In many persons, body defense mechanisms are mobilized in response to the invading organism, and the organism is walled off and never allowed to become active. The past occurrence of such a phenomenon is characterized by a positive PPD skin test. PPD is a purified protein derivative of the microbacteria. When the antigen is injected intradermally, it is "recognized" because of the body's previous contact with the organism. An immune reaction takes place locally and produces a wheal or induration; crythema is not considered a positive reaction. Induration of greater than 8 to 10 mm is considered a positive reaction. A positive skin test alone does not necessarily indicate the presence of active pulmonary tuberculosis, but shows evidence of previous contact with the antigen. The diagnosis of active disease is made by sputum smears and cultures that specifically identify the microbacteria, and by a progressive worsening of the lesion by x-ray. It should be remembered that in culture *Mycobacterium tuberculosis* is a slow-growing organism and 2 to 12 weeks may be required before cultures can be reported as positive or negative.

During this phase of therapy, it is important for the nurse to understand the patient's anxiety about the report of the abnormal chest film and the tests being performed by the physician in order to make a diagnosis. Many persons are still extremely frightened by the word tuberculosis and it conjures up many misconceptions. The nurse must therefore be supportive in explaining what the skin test means and why it is being done in this patient's specific situation. Adequate information given to the patient will be of great help in maintaining contact with the patient so that a specific diagnosis can be made and therapy prescribed as indicated.

Physician's Appointment

SUBJECTIVE. No change.

OBJECTIVE. Sputum smear for AFB (acid-fast bacilli or *Mycobacterium tuberculosis*) is positive showing few organisms.

ASSESSMENT. From recent x-ray changes, skin tests, and sputum, this patient is diagnosed as having minimally active tuberculosis.

PLAN. Start isoniazid (INH) and ethambutol (EMB). Do skin tests and chest x-rays of family. Recommend prophylactic INH therapy.

DISCUSSION. Treatment in most cases of tuberculosis requires only chemotherapy. Within a week after starting the drug, in patients with the susceptible organism, the disease is usually no longer contagious. For this reason, persons no longer require hospitalization in a sanatorium for extended periods of time as in the past. For many patients with minimal tuberculosis and a home setting that does not involve exposure to chronically ill persons or very young children, the patient never needs to be hospitalized and after a short period of time can return to work. Patients with moderately advanced disease often do require hospitalization, but in a general hospital not a sanatorium. In the general hospital the nursing care need not be as technically involved as was once thought necessary. During the first week or two the patient is usually placed in isolation. Isolation for a patient with tuberculosis only requires that the patient be in a room with nonrecirculating air and that the door be closed. This system prevents the droplet nuclei from being carried to others on the air currents. In the majority of cases the nurse need not wear a mask, as the droplet nuclei that cause infection are small enough to pass through the mask. In addition, the patient is reminded or taught to cover the mouth and nose when he or she coughs or sneezes. Particles thus impact and are not allowed to become airborne. If the patient cannot or will not cooperate with this technique, a mask should be placed on the patient. When the droplets are first expelled, before evaporation, the majority are large enough to be deposited on the mask worn by the patient.

In addition to specific treatment of the patient, good care requires follow-up of the patient's contacts. In the patient with active pulmonary tuberculosis who is smear- and culture-positive, the contacts who should be examined include household contacts and other close contacts. (Close contact is defined as 10 to 20 hours of exposure or more every week for the last 3 months.) It is questionable as to whether other more casual contacts need to be investigated. These contacts are then followed by skin testing or x-ray. If the original skin test is positive, then x-rays should be used for follow-ups; if the skin test is negative the follow-up can be done by simple skin testing. Close contacts are in most instances offered prophylactic INH therapy for 1 year.

In addition to being involved in the investigation of contacts of the patient, the nurse should also be closely involved in the patient's care regimen. It is extremely important that he understand his disease and the need for the therapy he is taking. Because the patient does not have any symptoms, he often finds it very difficult to take medication every day for such extended periods of time (a minimum of 1 year). Therefore the professional staff must make an in-depth assessment of the patient's motivation to follow such a plan of care. In the case of this patient, it was decided that he could be depended upon to follow his treatment regimen and that he could be allowed to undergo all his therapy in the home situation. His children are old enough that he can be treated at home without endangering them. If the children were infants, the original treatment would be done in the hospital setting. Also, because the patient works out-of-doors, the danger of transmission to persons in the work situation is negligible.

THORACIC TRAUMA

Data Base

History and Physical

John Roger, age 22 years, was brought to the emergency room by ambulance following an automobile accident.

VITAL SIGNS. Temperature 36.8°C, pulse 110, respiratory rate 30, blood pressure 110/74.

Examination demonstrated multiple contusions and lacerations on the right side of the body involving the chest, abdomen, and right leg. The patient complained of chest pain which was accentuated by attempting to take a deep breath. There was decreased excursion of the right hemithorax. The patient was short of breath and his color was dusky. Nasal oxygen was started and the patient's color improved. There was tenderness to palpation over the right anterior hemithorax. Auscultation revealed decreased breath sounds with crackles on the right side. The rest of the physical examination, including the neurologic, was within normal limits. Intravenous infusions were begun for fluid replacement, blood gases were obtained, and the patient was sent to x-ray. Blood gases demonstrated a P_{O_2} of 50 and 3 liters of oxygen by nasal cannula, a P_{CO_2} of 45, and a pH of 7.37. The chest x-ray demonstrated fractures of the second through the sixth anterior ribs on the right. There was a small pleural effusion on the right, but no pncumothorax noted. There was an infiltrate on the right side, which was interpreted as a lung contusion by the radiologist. During the x-ray procedure, the patient progressively became more short of breath and complained of further chest pain; the respiratory rate increased to 36, depth of respiration decreased, and his color became more cyanotic. At this point, the patient was intubated, placed on a volume respirator, and transferred to the surgical intensive-care unit with a diagnosis of chest trauma and a flail chest.

DISCUSSION. Rib fractures can produce a wide spectrum of pulmonary dysfunctions. In simple rib fractures such as may be precipitated by coughing, no specific treatment is needed. In other cases, such as thoracic trauma, there may be several rib fractures but if they do not interfere with the mechanical functioning of the lung to a significant degree, they also can be treated conservatively with periodic deep breathing and coughing, and allowed to heal naturally. In more severe cases where there are more extensive rib fractures, and especially in those also associated with contusions of the lung or pleural effusions, more aggressive therapy is needed. In the flail chest, where there is a "floating" segment of rib the rib fractures deter optimal mechanical functioning of the lung. Because of the rib fractures, the thoracic wall on the affected side can no longer be expanded with contraction of the inspiratory muscles. Therefore the lung parenchyma on that side is compressed and ventilation is decreased. Flail chest can often be observed by looking at the patient. As the patient inhales, the affected side does not expand as much as the nonaffected side and, in severe cases, the affected side can be seen to "cave in" on inspiration. Lung contusion and pleural effusion add significantly to the problem of lung compression. In the effusion the fluid in the pleural space limits lung expansion, and with the contusion there is escape of blood and fluid into the alveolar spaces. The lung contusion therefore causes obstruction, decreased area for gas exchange, and loss of fluid, which can lead to circulatory collapse. The net result is decreased ventilation with hypoxemia and hypercarbia.

In the severe case of thoracic trauma with flail chest the preferred treatment is positive-pressure ventilation. The patient is intubated and placed on a volume ventilator. Because positive pressure is added for lung inflation, the ventilator serves to splint the chest so that the affected side can be expanded on inhalation. In severe cases where positive-pressure ventilation alone is not sufficient to maintain ventilation and oxygenation, positive end expiratory pressure can be added so that positive pressure and lung volume are maintained in the chest on both inspiration and expiration. (See the section on positive-pressure breathing.)

Treatment of the lung contusion is aimed at supportive measures (maintenance of ventilation and circulation) until the contusion clears. The pleural effusion is usually drained. In many cases, a simple thoracentesis is all that is needed; the fluid is drained and does not reaccumulate. If there is a bronchopleural fistula (caused by tearing of pleura and lung by a fractured rib), with pneumothorax or rapidly reaccumulating fluid, chest tube drainage may be necessary.

Nurse's Note

On admission to the surgical intensive-care unit the nurse made the following note regarding the problem of flail chest:

SUBJECTIVE. Patient restless; will respond to verbal direction.

OBJECTIVE. Temperature 37°C, pulse 120 and thready, blood pressure 108/74, IV running, patient has a nasoendotracheal tube in place and is being bagged on 100 per cent O_2. On transfer to unit, patient was placed on a volume ventilator with a respiratory rate of 10, a tidal volume of 800 cc, and FI_{O_2} of 50 per cent.

PLAN. Restrain patient, obtain arterial blood gases in 15 minutes per physician's order, give medication for pain, institute airway care measures, including suctioning as needed. Monitor respiratory rate and tidal volume.

DISCUSSION. At this point, the major nursing efforts are directed toward maintaining the patient's ventilatory support and correcting the circulatory collapse. The patient has been placed on a volume ventilator at large tidal volumes with a rate of 10. Should he continue to be extremely restless and agitated because of pain, his spontaneous respiratory rate may be greater than 10, which may lead to respiratory alkalosis. By giving the patient medications to reduce the pain induced by the deep breathing required by the mechanical ventilation and as a result of trauma, the patient may well slow his rate and tolerate ventilation at much lower peak pressures. Therefore the response would be more adequate ventilation and also less of an effect on his circulatory status by the high airway pressures generated by the respirator. The blood gases are obtained within 15 minutes in order to allow for equilibration of P_{O_2} and P_{CO_2} changes and to ensure that the level of ventilation begun is adequate for the patient. When the patient is first placed on mechanical ventilation, it is often necessary to draw blood gases at frequent intervals in order to establish the correct ventilation therapy.

It is also the nurse's role to maintain airway patency. The nurse has restrained the patient to prevent him from removing or dislodging any intravenous lines or the endotracheal tube necessary to maintain airway patency and ventilation. In addition, the patient will require suctioning. On x-ray it appears that this patient has a lung contusion, seen as an alveolar infiltrate on the right side of the chest. Suctioning will not remove the blood from the alveolar level but, as secretions accumulate and more fluid in the airway occurs, it is important that this material be removed when accessible so that gas exchange can take place as effectively as possible. Previous blood gases have shown that the patient is hypoxemic. Therefore the nurse realizes that every time she removes the patient from the ventilator in order to suction him, his P_{O_2} will drop and, in addition, the suctioning procedure itself will further lower the O_2 level. She should therefore pre- and postoxygenate the patient any time that suctioning is done in order to maintain the level of oxygenation. In addition, the patient is turned and postural drainage is done. Turning must be done carefully with support of the chest wall on the right where the rib fractures are located. The patient is turned from his unaffected side to his back, because the fractures eliminate the possibility of a full right-side turn. The turning from side to back will help to drain secretions and accumulated fluid just as does postural drainage. When percussion and vibration are performed, only the unaffected side is done. It must be remembered that secretions must be at a relatively high position in the tracheal bronchial tree to be accessible to the suction catheter. Therefore these techniques are used to move the secretions upward.

Physician's Progress Notes

PROBLEM. Flail chest.

SUBJECTIVE. Patient remains restless after pain medication.

OBJECTIVE. Blood gases Pa_{O_2} of 90 on 50 per cent O_2, Pa_{CO_2} of 25, and pH of 7.55. Patient spontaneously tripping ventilator at a rate of 14 to 16.

ASSESSMENT. Blood gases demonstrate acute hyperventilation with respiratory alkalosis. Patient's medication has not significantly reduced respiratory rate, even with adequate oxygenation. There is a need to maintain large-volume ventilation (large tidal volumes) to stabilize the chest, so mechanical dead space will be added to the ventilator.

PLAN. Add 75 cc of dead space; check arterial blood gases in 15 minutes.

DISCUSSION. The addition of dead space means that the patient rebreathes some of his or her own expired CO_2. The purpose is to continue high lung volume ventilation without lowering the P_{CO_2} and producing alkalosis. The nurse must be alert to any decrease in ventilation as a result of a decreased respiratory rate. If the ventilation does decrease because of a decrease in respiratory rate, it may be necessary to remove the dead space or control the respiratory rate so that CO_2 retention does not occur. Another approach to this problem would be to institute IMV. In some cases of severe flail, however, the spontaneous breaths are considered too detrimental in terms of chest wall stability. A third approach is to increase sedation to the point of depressing ventilatory drive.

The P_{O_2} is within an acceptable range although it is not desirable to maintain a patient on 50 per cent O_2 for long periods. Ensuring the removal of accumulated secretions and fluid from airways will help to raise the Pa_{O_2}. It must also be remembered that an increase in the P_{CO_2} will cause a decrease in the Pa_{O_2}. Some persons might consider adding PEEP at this time.

The repeat blood gases demonstrated partial correction of the respiratory alkalosis and are in an acceptable range: P_{O_2} 85, P_{CO_2} 32, and pH 7.46.

Nurse's Note

The next day the following note is made by the nurse:

SUBJECTIVE. Patient responding; no longer restless, color good.

OBJECTIVE. Vital signs: temperature 37°C, pulse 90, blood pressure 120/80, respiratory rate 10. Sputum has increased in amount and is more tenacious. Sputum color remains clear with minimal blood streaking. Crackles throughout right chest and at left anterior base.

PLAN. Ensure adequate humidification of airway by checking temperature of main line humidifier on respirator; add periodic tracheal irrigation.

DISCUSSION. It is not unusual for the patient who has endured thoracic trauma and has had bleeding into the lung to exhibit a temperature in the posttrauma period. At present, the patient does not appear to have an infection because the sputum is remaining clear, even though it has become more tenacious and difficult to remove. Because it is known that the patient has bled into the lung, which provides an optimal medium for the growth of bacteria, infection is a constant threat. (The patient is on prophylactic antibiotics.) Therefore optimal airway care is extremely necessary in order to remove secretions from the airway, for if retained they could lead to a complicating pneumonia. By keeping the temperature of the inspired air near body temperature, humidification will more nearly approximate 100 per cent. Because the secretions are becoming more tenacious, tracheal irrigation is done to make their aspiration easier.

After 5 days the patient demonstrates less asynchronous movement, MIF, and VC are in acceptable range. The patient is then placed on IMV to facilitate weaning from the ventilator. Over the next 3 days the IMV rate is gradually decreased and the patient carefully monitored. By the nineth day postaccident the patient is extubated and able to maintain ventilation spontaneously. It will take much longer for the ribs to heal completely. Because of continued discomfort and infringement on mechanical function the patient is encouraged to periodically deep breathe and cough. Frequently, wrapping a towel around the patient's chest and letting him use it to increase stability on deep breathing and coughing helps. The patient crosses his wrists holding the left side of the towel with the right hand and the right side with the left hand. With coughing the hands are pulled so that there is pressure around the entire chest circumference. The tension is relaxed, but contact of the towel and chest wall is maintained with inspiration.

Bronchogenic Carcinoma

Data Base

History and Physical

Mr. Robert Snow is a 49-year-old architect who recently saw his physician for his yearly physical exam. On the physical exam no abnormalities were found; however, the report on the chest films showed a nodular lesion in the right upper lobe, anterior segment. On receiving this abnormal x-ray report the data from the recent physical exam were reviewed and the following data noted:

Physician's Note

The patient has had a morning cough for several years; there has been no change in cough or sputum over the last few months. The patient gives a smoking history of 40 pack years and is presently smoking one pack per day and, in addition, is smoking a pipe. There is no history of tuberculosis or other chest diseases. Review of the radiology reports of past chest x-rays demonstrates that they were all read as normal; in retrospect, however, there is the possibility that there was a small lesion in the area where the nodule is now seen.

PROBLEM. Right-upper-lobe lesion, anterior segment, on x-ray.

PLAN. Tuberculosis and fungal skin tests; sputum for AFB smear and culture; sputum for fungal culture; sputum × 3 for cytology; tomograms of the right upper lobe.

DISCUSSION. Because this lesion on x-ray is nodular and because there is a possibility that it may have been present 1 year ago, the prime diagnostic possibility is a neoplastic lesion.

Bronchogenic carcinoma is the most common fatal malignancy in males in the Western Hemisphere. Although bronchogenic carcinoma is more common in the male, its frequency in the female is increasing as the incidence of smoking among women increases. Bronchogenic carcinoma is most common in those persons in their fifth and sixth decades who have a history of cigarette smoking. The lesion is more commonly seen in the right lung than in the left lung and is more commonly seen in the upper lobe than the lower lobe. A bronchogenic carcinoma usually arises in a segmental bonchus and then extends from that point to adjacent areas.

It must be remembered that there are other types of malignancies found in the lung, including alveolar cell carcinomas, Hodgkin's disease, the lymphosarcomas, and the metastatic neoplasms. In addition, the bronchogenic carcinomas can be classified into different cell types. These include squamous, adenocarcinoma, large-cell undifferentiated, and small-cell undifferentiated.

At the present time the preferred treatment of carcinoma of the lung is surgical excision. In instances where the lesion is inoperable (where there is hilar involvement and/or metastases to other areas, or where the patient is not physiologically able to tolerate the surgical procedure) radiation therapy or chemotherapy may be used as prophylactic treatment to reduce the symptomatology.

The presenting symptoms of the patient with carcinoma will vary greatly. Some patients, such as the one presented in this case study, have no specific symptoms but the lesion is detectable by x-ray. It may be that this lesion is producing some cough, but because of his or her usual productive morning cough, the patient may not be able to recognize any change. Other patients will present with more symptomatology, such as increased sputum production, hemoptysis, general malaise, and weight loss. In the patient being discussed, the diagnosis of carcinoma is highly probable because of the radiographic appearance of the lesion. In addition, the patient has a long history of cigarette smoking, which is very common in the patient with bronchogenic carcinoma of the squamous type. Occupational exposure to various carcinogens may also be pertinent. Included are exposure to asbestos, radioactive material, arsenic, and certain of the ores such as nickel. In the present case, the patient's occupational history did not indicate any such exposure.

A specific diagnosis of carcinoma can be made in a variety of ways. The first diagnostic methods used involve noninvasive techniques such as x-ray studies and sputum for cytology. The x-ray cannot be specifically diagnostic but can give further clues as to the origin of the lesion, be it infectious or neoplastic. The cytologies can yield a specific diagnosis of a malignancy. During this period of diagnostic studies to confirm or reject the diagnosis of carcinoma, it is important that the patient be allowed the time to verbalize concerns. Even though cancer may not be the prime diagnostic possibility in some patients who demonstrate a lesion on x-ray, the patient usually suspects the possibility of a neoplasm and is frightened and anxious about it. Those caring for the patient must be able to assess his or her psychological response to the abnormal finding, the need for further studies, and the ability to cope with the available information. The patient's questions must be answered but the manner in which the responses are given must be adapted to the individual patient. Of prime importance is the personnel's communication to the patient that it is acceptable to ask questions and that the questions will be answered.

OBJECTIVE. On the patient's next visit the following data were available: Fungal cultures were negative; fungal skin tests were negative; tuberculosis skin test demonstrated 6 mm of induration; and the tuberculosis smear was negative. The sputum cytology was negative; the tomograms of the right upper lobe demonstrated a multilobular mass containing a small cavity; there was no calcium present.

ASSESSMENT. A tissue diagnosis is still needed. Because of the location of the lesion on x-ray it may be accessible with the fiberoptic bronchoscope.

PLAN. Fiberoptic bronchoscopy to attempt visualization and possible biopsy of the lesion. Bronchial washings and postbronchoscopy sputum will also be collected for culture and cytology.

OBJECTIVE. The results of the bronchoscopy demonstrated a reddened area in the right-upper-lobe bronchus. There was a slight narrowing of the orifice leading to the posterior segment. A biopsy of the reddened area was taken and bronchial washings of the right upper lobe were obtained. The pathology results of the biopsy were negative. The bronchial washings taken during bronchoscopy were positive for squamous cell carcinoma.

PLAN. Discuss findings with patient and family and encourage admission for surgery. Do spirometry.

DISCUSSION. The nurse can play an important role during a bronchoscopy by giving the patient a great deal of support during the procedure. Topical anesthesia is very effective in alleviating discomfort; however, because the bronchoscopist must be constantly visualizing the tracheobronchial tree through the bronchoscope, the nurse can play an important role by closely observing the patient's response. If the patient's position seems uncomfortable, if he or she is becoming extremely anxious, or if the patient's vital signs change, the nurse can make these observations known to the bronchoscopist and allow the patient to know that someone is watching and is concerned about him or her. The nurse had instructed the patient to refrain from eating before the procedure, and afterward he is cautioned not to eat or drink until he has recovered his gag reflex, which usually takes several hours. Findings such as were demonstrated in this case are often difficult for the patient to accept. The patient will usually realize from what is being done (a biopsy being taken) that something unusual was seen. Yet the bronchoscopist cannot say that a lesion that is a carcinoma has specifically been observed; he or she can only say that there is a reddened area. Therefore the patient is left with a great deal of doubt. He or she has gone through an unusual procedure and still does not have an answer. The patient must be given a great deal of support and must realize that anxiety is normal and acceptable and that he or she will be informed of the test results (biopsy, for example) as they are available.

When the data from the bronchoscopy became available, the patient returned to the physician and was given the information that was available. This included the fact that on x-ray there was a single nodule and that the sputum obtained during the bronchoscopy demonstrated some malignant cells. Because of the location of the lesion and the lack of involvement of other areas, surgery was recommended for the removal of the lesion. The patient and family were accepting of the need for surgery, and plans for admission within several days were made.

Prior to admission, spirometry was done. The patient has never complained of shortness of breath and is not short of breath with mild exercise (walking). However, because he has a long smoking history and a history consistent with chronic bronchitis, spirometry is done to rule out obstructive airway disease that would increase operative risk. The results of the spirometry in this patient were within normal limits.

Nurse's Note

On admission to the surgical unit the following nurse's note was made:

SUBJECTIVE. Patient and wife state that the patient is admitted to have surgery for a lung tumor. They are able to discuss the diagnosis calmly and describe the diagnostic procedures that have been done very intellectually.

ASSESSMENT. The patient and wife appear to accept the diagnosis on an intellectual basis but their lack of expression of emotion is very noticeable. At this time, it is difficult to tell their true understanding or acceptance of diagnosis.

PLAN. Allow opportunity for patient and wife to discuss the upcoming surgical procedure and what this means to them. Start preoperative teaching, including the need for and how to deep breathe and cough, the need for chest tubes postoperatively, and information regarding the surgical intensive-care unit. Check with physicians regarding any anticipated special problems during the pre- or postoperative period.

DISCUSSION. It is not uncommon to have a patient admitted to the hospital shortly before the surgical procedure is to be performed. The result is that there is very little time to do adequate preoperative teaching. In some cases the patient is admitted a week or so preoperatively in order that certain preoperative measures can be handled more effectively and efficiently in the hospital setting. An example is the patient who has borderline pulmonary function and a secretion problem. Admission a week prior to surgery would allow for more aggressive measures of bronchial hygiene to be initiated to bring the patient to an optimal physiologic state before surgery. In this case, as with most cases, however, this extended period of time is not available and preoperative teaching must be done within 1 or 2 days. The procedures carried out after surgery are often very familiar to the staff nurses and are therefore not adequately explained to the patient. One so-called routine measure, but one that is often omitted, is to teach the patient preoperatively about the need to deep breathe and cough postoperatively. Preoperative teaching both gives the patient instruction in technique and conveys concern about the problem. There is no reason for a patient to take deep breaths postoperatively if no one really thinks it is important. The maneuver causes discomfort and the patient probably does not see what the benefit is. On the other hand, if during both the pre- and postoperative period, the staff has explained why deep breathing with coughing is important and has demonstrated how it should be done (including splinting), the patient is much more likely to try to deep-breathe and cough for them. Physiologically, deep breathing with coughing is the optimal method of improving lung expansion, and other equipment (IPPB, blow bottles) is usually not necessary. The patient should also be informed about the equipment that he or she will find in the room, such as IVs and chest tubes. Depending on the type of chest tube drainage used, the noise produced by the apparatus should be explained to the patient so that he or she is not frightened. The nurse should also check with the physician on whether there are any anticipated pre- or postoperative problems. This would include, as previously mentioned, the need for preoperative bronchial hygiene. If the physician anticipates that the patient will be intubated and ventilated in the immediate postoperative period or if other problems are anticipated, then the patient should be warned, for example, that there is a possibility of having a tube in the throat and a machine to help in taking deep breaths.

Patient was scheduled for a right upper lobectomy the following day with a preoperative diagnosis of carcinoma of the lung. The postoperative diagnosis confirmed the carcinoma of the lung and the right upper lobe was removed. No other involvement was found. Postoperatively the patient did not require mechanical ventilation. Chest tubes were in place, IVs were running, the patient was monitored for cardiac rate and rhythm, and transferred to the surgical ICU.

Nurse's Note

Several hours after admission to the surgical intensive-care unit this nurse's note was written (as in other case studies not all notes are reported here):

SUBJECTIVE. Patient prefers to lie on unoperative side; complaining of chest pain, color good.

OBJECTIVE. Breathing shallow, vital capacity measured to be 1.8 liters (preoperative VC 4.0 liters); cough is weak; chest tubes draining serosanguineous fluid and small amount of air.

ASSESSMENT. Patient may be able to increase depth of respiration and cough more effectively if pain is reduced; although patient prefers lying on unoperative side, must encourage movement from side to side.

PLAN. Turn side to side every 2 hours; give pain medications followed by deep breathing with coughing.

DISCUSSION. Chest tubes are inserted after a surgical procedure involving an incision through the pleura in order to maintain the mechanical functioning of the lung. When air and/or fluid accumulates in the pleural space (between the parietal and visceral pleura), the normal mechanical relationships that allow for optimal expansion of the lung (as discussed in the section on mechanics) will be inhibited. The accumulation of the air or fluid will produce a more positive pressure in the pleural space. This pressure then acts on the lung, forcing it to lose volume. Therefore a chest tube(s) is inserted to allow for removal of both air and fluid from the pleural space in order to maintain optimal lung function. It must be remembered that the postoperative thoracotomy patient is not the only patient requiring chest tubes. Patients may have a spontaneous pneumothorax that allows entrance of air into the pleural space because of a fistula connecting the bronchus and the pleural space. In other situations there may be trauma to the chest allowing outside air to rush into the pleural space. In cases where the accumulation of air and/or fluid in the pleural space is of great enough quantity that mechanical functioning of the lung is inhibited, chest tubes are inserted. (It must be remembered that in some cases of pleural effusion the fluid can be aspirated with a needle and syringe on a one-time basis; providing there is not rapid reaccumulation, chest tubes are not necessary. In other instances where there is a very small spontaneous pneumothorax and mechanical functioning of the lung is not severely limited, chest tubes are not necessary and normal reabsorption of the air is allowed to take place.)

After thoracotomy one or two chest tubes may be inserted. The tubes must be located so that both air and fluid are removed. Because the air will rise, it is often necessary to place one chest tube higher in the thorax for the removal of air and one lower in the thorax for the removal of fluids. Whether one or two chest tubes are used depends on the preference of the surgeon and any possible anticipated complications. In the case of a pneumonectomy, no chest tubes are usually inserted so that fluid can accumulate and fibrosis may occur. This process allows for the filling of the space left by the removal of the entire lung. In the case of a segmental resection or lobectomy, as long as the fluid and air are removed, the remaining lung will usually expand to fill the space left by the excised area of lung. The nurse must be aware of the location of the chest tubes and the surgeon's rationale for this location in order to make pertinent observations in the postoperative period as to the effectiveness of the tubes.

The chest tubes can be connected to a variety of types of drainage systems. In all instances the intention is to maintain a pressure gradient preventing atmospheric air from entering the pleural cavity and maintaining drainage from the pleural space to the outside. The simplest drainage system, and one that is used on many patients who have a spontaneous pneumothorax requiring a chest tube, is one-bottle water seal drainage. Here the chest tube is connected to a container located below the level of the chest and the end of the tube is placed below the water level in the bottle. The reservoir is always kept below the level of the chest so that by gravity drainage fluid will flow downward and, in the same way, fluid is not allowed to enter the chest from the water seal. The water seal maintains a vacuum whereby atmospheric air is not allowed to enter the chest. In most postoperative cases suction is applied to the system to allow for more rapid removal of the air of fluids. A variety of systems, one-, two-, and three-bottle, may be used to provide this type of drainage. The nurse must be familiar with the system in use so that the correct observations can be made. *Observations basic to care of any patient with chest tubes* in place requires that

1. The chest tubes are always below the level of the bed to prevent backflow.
2. A closed system of drainage is maintained so that atmospheric air is not allowed to enter through the tubes. This closed system requires that all connections be taped and that Kelly clamps be available to clamp off the chest tubes should the system be intentionally or unintentionally exposed to atmospheric pressure. It should be realized however that in patients with a large bronchopleural fistula, clamping chest tubes is dangerous. The air can escape from the lung to the pleural space and build up excessive amounts of pressure.
3. Observations be made to ensure that the chest tubes are patent. Such observations would include seeing a rise and fall in the fluid level of the column, which is submerged under the water. This fluctuation of fluid level should be synchronous with the patient's respiration. If such fluctuation is not seen, the chest tube may be plugged and require milking or stripping in order to remove any clots or other material that may be occluding the tube. When there is a large amount of serosanguinous drainage, the tubes are often stripped and milked on a routine basis.
4. Observations be made on the amount of drainage and the amount of air removed. The removal of air from the pleural space is determined by the amount of bubbling seen in the drainage system. (Continuous bubbling with no fluctuations may mean there is a leak in the system.)
5. Observation for any signs or symptoms of a mediastinal shift, which would occur if air and fluid accumulated in the pleural space to such a degree that the mediastinum shifted to the opposite side.

This shift can produce a kinking of the great vessels and result in tachycardia, blood pressure changes, and shock.

Other postoperative measures include deep breathing with coughing as previously cited, early ambulation, and shoulder exercises to regain muscle strength in those large muscles that required incision during the surgical procedure. Deep breathing is done to promote full lung expansion in order to prevent atelectasis and to promote clearance of secretions. The patient can usually deep breathe more effectively if the nurse's hands are used to splint the incision. Some pressure is placed on the chest during both inspiration and expiration. The hand on the unoperative side exerts a varying pressure (greater during expiration) in order to promote lung expansion. At the same time the forearm can be used to control the use of the abdominal muscles by applying pressure over the upper abdomen during expiration. It is not uncommon that patients who have had a thoracotomy do not want to lie on the operative side because of the fear of lying on the chest tubes. With careful positioning, however, the patient can be positioned on the operative side and will often generate a higher vital capacity when lying on the operative side (Caruso, 1973). Even though a larger vital capacity is generated on the operative side, it is important to turn the patient from side to side for good expansion of all areas of the lung.

Follow-up Summary

After several days the drainage from the pleural space ceased and the chest tubes were removed. Chest x-rays showed that the patient had good expansion of the lung on the operative side. The patient was alert and deep breathing and coughing well. He was transferred to a surgical unit and within a week was discharged home. Any patient who has had a diagnosis of cancer will require very close follow-up to ensure that there is no unseen tumor not removed and that there are no metastases. The patient is therefore encouraged to maintain close medical supervision and continuing care.

Summary

The goals of this chapter have been to explain the scientific basis for many of the problems produced by pulmonary dysfunction and to discuss and demonstrate the nursing care measures that are indicated. Not all nursing care measures or techniques or types of pulmonary dysfunction have been included. By understanding basic reasons for nursing care measures, however, it is hoped that the reader will be able to apply this knowledge to a variety of conditions or situations in which the nurse is involved. Only when nursing care practices are based upon scientific theory can we have better standards for the development of criteria for the quality of care in addition to simply the quantity of care, and therefore develop direction for the improvement of nursing care measures. Through the ages, nurses have hastened to protect the rights and the uniqueness of the individual. However, if we cannot generalize nursing care from a scientific base, we are, in actuality, hurting rather than protecting the individual. We must delineate the quality of the care based on scientific facts so that nursing can move forward and not just continue to provide care because that is the way it has always been done. The uniqueness of the individual is still maintained in terms of his or her unique physiologic and psychological response to the variables in the situation. However, based on a knowledge of the variables and the patient's ability to respond to them, the nurse must scientifically determine what care will be provided. In this manner, this chapter has attempted to provide not simply techniques of nursing care, but an approach and a method of determining what that nursing care should be. All of the sciences involved in the delivery of health care are constantly changing. Therefore any attempt to describe a specific technique in a specific situation is self-limiting. Only by obtaining a base of scientific fact and an understanding of how to apply this knowledge in the care of the individual patient will the nurse be able to meet the future needs presented by the patient and the nursing profession.

References Cited

Bartlett, R. H., Gazzaniga, A. B., and Geraghty, T. R. "Respiratory Maneuvers to Prevent Postoperative Pulmonary Complications." *JAMA*, **224** (May 14, 1973), 1017–21.

Birnbaum, M. L., Cree, E. M., Rasmussen, H., Lewis, P., and Curtis, J. K. "Effects of Intermittent Positive Pressure Breathing on Emphysematous Patients." *Am. J. Med.*, **41** (Oct. 1966), 552–61.

Caruso, M. E. "The Effect of Lateral Positioning on Vital Capacity in Postoperative Thoracotomy Patients." Unpublished M.S. thesis, University of Arizona, College of Nursing, Tuscon, Ariz., 1973.

Dolovich, M. B., Killian, D., Wolff, R. K., Obminsky, G., and Newhouse, M. T. "Pulmonary Aerosol Deposition in Chronic Bronchitis: Intermittent Positive Pressure Breathing Versus Quiet Breathing." *Am. Rev. Resp. Dis.*, **115** (March 1977), 397–402.

Goldberg, I., and Cherniack, R. M. "The Effect of Nebulized Bronchodilator Delivered with and without IPPB on Ventilatory Function in Chronic Obstructive Emphysema." *Am. Rev. Resp. Dis.*, **91** (1965), 13–20.

Petty, T. L., and Guthrie, A. "The Effects of Augmented Breathing Maneuvers on Ventilation in Severe Chronic Airway Obstruction." *Resp. Care,* **16** (May–June 1971), 104–11.

General References

Ashbaugh, D. G. et al. "Continuous Positive Pressure Breathing (CPPB) in the Adult Respiratory Distress Syndrome." *J. Thorac. Cardiovasc. Surg.*, **57** (Jan. 1969), 31.

Ayres, S. M. "Cigarette Smoking and Lung Diseases." *Basics of RD,* **3**:5 (May 1975).

Barlow, P. B. "Treatment of Tuberculosis." *Basics of RD,* **5**:1 (Sept. 1976).

Beaumont, E. "Up-to-Date Survey of Tracheal Tubes." *Nurs. 76,* **6** (Nov. 1976), 66–72.

Behnke, R., et al. "Resources for the Optimal Care of Acute Respiratory Failure." *Circulation,* **43** (June 1971), A185–A189.

Blair, E., Topuzler, C., and Deane, R. S. "Major Blunt Chest Trauma." *Curr. Probl. Surg.*, (May 1969).

Bryant, L., Trinkle, J. K., and Dubilier, L. "Reappraisal of Tracheal Injury from Cuffed Tracheostomy Tubes." *JAMA,* **215:4** (Jan. 1971), 625–28.

Burrows, B. et al. "Patterns of Cardiovascular Dysfunction in Chronic Obstructive Lung Disease." *N. Engl. J. Med.*, **286** (April 27, 1972), 912–18.

Bushnell, L. S. "An Adverse Effect of Respiratory Therapy." *Anesthesiology,* **29** (1968), 1085–86.

Butler, E. K. "Dyspnea in the Patient with Cardiopulmonary Disease." *Heart and Lung,* **4**:4 (July–Aug. 1975), 599–606.

Campbell, E. J. M. "Oxygen Therapy in Diseases of the Chest." *Br. J. Dis. Chest,* **53** (1964), 149.

Carr, D. T., and Rosenow, E. C. "Bronchogenic Carcinoma." *Basics of RD,* **5**:5 (May 1977).

Colgan, F. J., Mahoney, P. D., and Fanning, G. L. "Resistance Breathing and Sustained Hyperinflations in the Treatment of Atelectasis." *Anesthesiology,* **32** (June 1970), 543–50.

Crosby, L. J., and Parsons, L. C. "Measurements of Lateral Wall Pressures Exerted by Tracheostomy and Endotracheal Tube Cuffs." *Heart and Lung,* **3**:5 (Sept.–Oct. 1974), 797–803.

Curtis, J. K. et al. "IPPB Therapy in Chronic Obstructive Pulmonary Disease." *JAMA,* **206**:5 (Oct. 28, 1969), 1037–40.

del Bueno, D. J. "Recognizing Fat Embolism in Patients with Multiple Injuries." *RN,* **36**:1 (Jan. 1973), 48–55.

Diener, C. F. "Evaluation of Disability and Assessment of Operative Risk." *Med. Clin. North Am.*, **57** (May 1973), 763–70.

Ditthrenner, Sister M., and Herbert, W. M. "Regimen for a Thoracotomy Patient." *Am. J. Nurs.*, **67**:10 (Oct. 1967), 2070–75.

Dudley, D. et al. "Psychosocial Aspects of Care in the Chronic Obstructive Pulmonary Disease Patient." *Heart and Lung,* **2**:3 (May–June 1973), 389–93.

Ellison, L. T. "Evaluation for Pulmonary Resection." *Chest,* **62**:5 (1972), 525.

Ferris, B., Jr. "Chronic Bronchitis and Emphysema: Classification and Epidemiology." *Med. Clin. North Am.*, **57**:3 (May 1973), 637–50.

Fink, J. N., and Sosman, A. J. "Therapy of Bronchial Asthma." *Med. Clin. North Am.*, **57** (May 1973), 801–8.

Fitzgerald, L. M. "Mechanical Ventilation." *Heart and Lung,* **5**:6 (Nov.–Dec. 1976), 939–49.

Fitzgerald, L. M., and Huber, G. L. "Weaning the Patient from Mechanical Ventilation." *Heart and Lung,* **5**:2 (March–April 1976), 228–34.

Fitzgerald, M. X., Carrington, C. B., and Gaensler, E. A. "Environmental Lung Disease." *Med. Clin. North Am.*, **57**:3 (May 1973), 593–622.

Fleischner, F. G. "Recurrent Pulmonary Embolism and Cor Pulmonale." *N. Engl. J. Med.*, **276** (June 1967), 1213–20.

Fuks, M. F., and Stein, A. M. "Better Ways to Cope with COPD." *Nurs. 76,* **6** (Feb. 1976), 29–38.

Gernert, C. F., and Schwartz, S. "Pulmonary Artery Catheterization." *Am. J. Nurs.*, **73** (July 1973), 1182–85.

Guenter, C. A., and Welch, M. H. *Pulmonary Medicine,* Philadelphia: J. B. Lippincott Co., 1977.

Hopewell, P. C. "Adult Respiratory Distress Syndrome." *Basics of RD,* **7**:4 (March 1979).

Hudson, L., and Sbarbaro, J. "Twice Weekly Tuberculosis Chemotherapy." *JAMA,* **223**:2 (Jan. 8, 1973), 139.

Hudson, L. D. "The Acute Management of the Chronic Airway Obstruction Patient." *Heart and Lung,* **3**:1 (Jan.–Feb. 1974), 93–96.

Hugh-Jones, P., and Whimster, W. "The Etiology and Management of Disabling Emphysema." *ARRD,* **117**:2 (Feb. 1978), 343–78.

Jones, R. N., and Weill, H. "Occupational Lung Disease." *Basics of RD,* **6**:3, (Jan. 1978).

Kersten, L. "Chest-Tube Drainage System." *Heart and Lung,* **3**:1 (Jan.–Feb. 1974), 97–101.

Kettel, L. et al. "Treatment of Acute Respiratory Acidosis in Chronic Obstructive Lung Disease," *JAMA,* **217:11** (Sept. 1971), 1503–08.

Kettel, L. J. "The Management of Acute Ventilatory Failure in Chronic Obstructive Lung Disease." *Med. Clin. North Am.*, **57**:3 (May 1973), 781–92.

Kinley, C. E. "Tracheostomy in the Adult." *Int. Anesthesiol. Clin.*, **8** (Winter 1970), 859–73.

Klastersky, J., Geuning, C., Mouawad, E., and Daneau, D. "Infections in Patients with Tracheostomy." *Chest,* **61**:2 (Feb. 1972), 117–20.

Kory, R. C. et al. "Comparative Evaluation of Oxygen Therapy Techniques. *JAMA,* **179** (March 10, 1972), 767–72.

Law, J. "The Fat Embolism Syndrome." *Nurs. Clin. North Am.*, **8**:1 (March 1973), 191–98.

Lefcoe, N., and Carter, P. "Intermittent Positive Pressure Breathing in Chronic Obstructive Pulmonary Disease." *Can. Med. Assoc. J.*, **103** (Aug. 1970), 279–81.

Lertzman, M. M., Cherniach, R. M. "Rehabilitation of Patients with Chronic Obstructive Pulmonary Disease." *ARRD*, **114**:6 (Dec. 1976), 1145–65.

Levy, M. M., and Stubbs, J. A. "Nursing Implications in the Care of Patients Treated with Assisted Mechanical Ventilation Modified with Positive End Expiratory Pressure." *Heart and Lung*, **7**:2 (March–April 1978), 299–305.

Meador, B. "Pneumothorax: Providing Emergency and Long-Term Care." *Nurs. '78.* **8** (Nov. 1978), 43–45.

McCombs, R. P. "Diseases Due to Immunologic Reactions in the Lungs." *N. Engl. J. Med.*, **286** (June 1972), 1186–1245.

Nealon, T. F., and Ching, N. "Pressure of Tracheostomy Cuffs in Ventilated Patients." *N.Y. State J. Med.*, **71**:16 (Aug. 1971), 1923–26.

Peterson, L. D., and Green, J. H. "Nurse-Managed Tuberculosis Clinic." *Am. J. Nurs.*, **77**:3 (March 1977), 433–38.

Petty, T. L. *Intensive and Rehabilitative Respiratory Care.* Philadelphia: Lea & Febiger, 1971.

Petty, T. L. "Pulmonary Rehabilitation." *Basics of RD*, **4**:1 (Sept. 1975).

———. "Respiratory Failure and the Heart." *Heart and Lung*, **1**:1 (Jan.–Feb. 1972), 84–89.

Petty, T. L., and Guthrie, A. "The Effects of Augmented Breathing Maneuvers on Ventilation in Severe Chronic Airway Obstruction." *Respir. Care*, **16** (May–June 1971), 104–12.

Pflug, A. E., Cheney, F. W., Jr., and Butler, J. "The Effects of Ultrasonic Aerosol in Pulmonary Mechanics and Arterial Blood Gases in Patients with Chronic Bronchitis." *Am. Rev. Respir. Dis.*, **101** (May 1970), 710.

Powaser, M. M., et al. "The Effectiveness of Hourly Cuff Deflation in Minimizing Tracheal Damage." *Heart and Lung*, **5**:5 (Sept.–Oct. 1976), 734–41.

Rasmussen, D. L. "Black Lung in Southern Appalachia." *Am. J. Nurs.*, **70** (March 1970), 509–11.

Riby, R. "The Hazard Is Relative." *Am. Rev. Respir. Dis.*, **96** (Oct. 1967), 4.

Robertson, K. J., and Guzzetta, C. E. "Arterial Blood Gas Interpretation in the Respiratory Intensive-Care Unit." *Heart and Lung*, **5**:2 (March–April 1976), 256–60.

Robin, E. "Abnormalities of Acid-Base Regulation in Chronic Pulmonary Disease with Special Reference to Hypercapnia and Extracellular Alkalosis." *N. Engl. J. Med.*, **268**:16 (April 1963), 917–22.

Rogers, R. A., and Juers, J. A. "Physiologic Considerations in the Treatment of Acute Respiratory Failure." *Basics of RD*, **3**:24 (March 1975).

Selecky, P. A. "Tracheal Damage and Prolonged Intubation with a Cuffed Endotracheal or Tracheostomy Tube." *Heart and Lung*, **5**:5 (Sept.–Oct. 1976), 733.

Shapiro, B. A., Harrison, R. A., and Trout, C. A. *Clinical Application of Respiratory Care.* Chicago: Year Book Medical Publishers, 1975.

Stevens, P. "Positive End Expiratory Pressure Breathing." *Basics of RD*, **5**:3 (Jan. 1977).

Thurlbeck, W. M. "Chronic Bronchitis and Emphysema." *Med. Clin. North Am.*, **57**:3 (May 1973), 651–68.

Wade, J. F. *Respiratory Nursing Care.* St. Louis: C. V. Mosby Co., 1973.

Weg, J. G. "Tuberculosis and the Generation Gap." *Am. J. Nurs.*, **71**:3 (March 1971), 495–500.

Weiss, W., Cooper, D. A., and Boucot, K. R. "Operative Mortality and Five-Year Survival Rates in Men with Bronchogenic Carcinoma." *Ann. Int. Med.*, **71**:1 (1969), 59.

Winter, P. M., and Lowenstein, E. "Acute Respiratory Failure." *Sci. Am.*, **221**:5 (Nov. 1969), 23–29.

Youmans, C. R. et al. "Recognizing and Managing Flail Chest." *Postgrad. Med.*, **48** (Oct. 1970), 87–93.

41

Problems with Maintaining Fluid and Electrolyte Balance

Let your boat of life be light, packed with only what you need - - - - - - and a little more than enough to drink; for thirst is a dangerous thing.

JEROME KLAPKA JEROME

From *Three Men in a Boat* (1889) Chapter 3, from Bartletts p. 788

Overview

A recurring theme of the units in Sections 1 and 2 has been the phenomenal capability of the body's regulatory and response mechanisms to protect, maintain, and restore dynamic equilibrium of the body's fluid internal environment, thus facilitating regulation and maintenance of essential life processes. Therefore, when symptoms of fluid and electrolyte imbalance appear, they are usually treated as presumptive evidence of disease, and the person manifesting the symptoms needs to be under the care of a physician.

The physician shares with the nurse the responsibility for making observations on which to base decisions about the fluid needs of the person who is under medical care. When the patient is hospitalized or exhibits signs or symptoms of fluid imbalance, the physician is usually responsible for the prescription of the amount, character, and route of administration of the patient's fluid intake. The nurse is usually responsible for the administration of the fluids and for determining and meeting the related needs of patients.

This chapter will be limited to knowledge essential for nurses to (1) observe and report with clarity the signs and symptoms and the deviations from normal behavior that the patient presents, (2) interpret the signs and symptoms indicating a deviation from health that constitute nursing problems, (3) administer fluids in a safe and effective manner, and (4) select the course of action that will help the patient attain the goal that is realistic for him or her, as total care is planned.

Disturbances in Body Fluid and Electrolyte Balance

The capacity to maintain the stability of body fluids is greatest during youth and early middle life and is least at the extremes of life. Many illnesses are accompanied by some disturbance in water and electrolyte balance. In some illnesses the disturbances are minor. In others, the recovery of the patient may depend on the ability to correct disturbances and to restore and maintain the normal regulatory mechanisms. In these patients the regulation of fluid and electrolyte balance may be a major objective of the therapy. The constancy of the fluid environment of cells, as well as of the intracellular fluid, depends on (1) the supply of required materials; (2) the regulation of intake, transportation, and storage; and (3) the excretion of excessive wastes and/or excess of required materials.

Disturbances in fluid and electrolyte balance may result from hypo-, hyper-, or disorganized function. A disturbance in the capacity of one organ to regulate one mechanism may set into action a chain of events leading to widespread and complicated disturbances.

Disturbances in body fluids are usually characterized by some change in volume, concentration, osmotic pressure, or hydrogen ion concentration. The specific effects on the patient will depend on such factors as whether the disturbance is local or general, how severe it is, and its effects on other components of the body fluid. Disturbances seldom occur in a single component. They are usually multiple and often complicated. Each substance entering into the composition of one of the fluid compartments has a significant function. Alterations in the level of any one component of body fluids outside the so-called normal range is likely to be attended by adverse effects and changes in other compartments.

The most frequent disturbances in fluid and electrolyte balance are those resulting from an excess or deficit of water or of sodium, potassium, calcium, or hydrogen ions. The effects of a disturbance on a particular person or patient will depend on (1) the direction and degree of change, (2) the effects the disturbance has on the other components of the system, and (3) the effectiveness of the body's mechanisms for correcting or adapting to the disturbance. For example, as Mr. Martin (see Chapter 27 for reference to the Martin family) mowed his lawn, he lost increased amounts of water and electrolytes in sweat, which is a hypotonic solution of sodium chloride. His mechanisms for adapting to these losses were efficient and he was able to maintain the stability of his extracellular fluids.

Effects of Illness on Fluid and Electrolyte Equilibrium

In illness there are many causes of disturbances in fluid and electrolyte equilibrium. They fall into the following categories: (1) a simple deficit or excess in the supply of water and/or electrolytes; (2) inability to ingest or to absorb water or electrolytes; (3) failure of the kidney to eliminate excesses of exogenous or endogenous origin; (4) excessive losses through the skin, gastrointestinal tract, lung, or kidney; (5) loss of fluids through abnormal avenues or as the result of injury to tissues, as in surgery and other trauma, fistulae, burned tissues, blood loss, or inflamed serous membranes; (6) disturbances in the transportation system; and (7) shifts of fluid from one compartment to another, as in ascites, edema, burns, or acute gastric dilatation. The ultimate effect on the individual patient will be determined by how these changes affect the volume, distribution, osmolality, and concentration of fluid and electrolytes in each compartment.

Water Deficit

Probably the most frequent disturbance in water and electrolyte balance is a simple deficit of water, with output of water exceeding its intake.[1] This may simply be the result of an inadequate intake or an excessive output. This leads to an increase in the concentration and osmolality of the extracellular fluid. Water may be lost alone or in combination with electrolytes. Sweating causes proportionately greater loss of water than of sodium chloride. Diarrhea in the early stages has the same effect. In breathing, water with little or no electrolyte content is lost. Patients who breathe rapidly and deeply lose more water from the lungs than those who breathe normally. Water losses can be expected to be further increased in patients who breathe through their mouths. Often patients who have increased loss of water through respiration are those who have difficulty in replacing water by their own efforts. Lethargic, comatose, or confused patients are especially likely to develop water deficits unless attention is paid to keeping up their fluid intake. Patients with fever also lose increased amounts of water. Loss of water from the skin is of two types: insensible water loss and sweat (sensible water loss). Insensible water loss refers to loss of water directly from the skin or other body surfaces without our being aware of its presence. This water loss results in little or no electrolyte loss. In contrast, sweat can be seen and felt and has a sodium and chloride content which is about one third or one fourth of that which is found in the plasma. Thus, increased insensible water loss caused by excessive respiration or fever without sweat, is pure water loss. Increased loss of sweat, on the other hand, can result in significant deficits of both water and salt. Maintenance of adequate fluid intake under these circumstances is essential and may require careful planning, patience, and effort for persons whose homeostatic mechanisms and/or independence are impaired.

Physiologic Effects of Loss of Water

In any condition in which the loss of water from the body exceeds that of intake, water is lost from

[1] One classification of disorders of sodium and water balance defines *water deficit* or *depletion* as an increase in serum sodium above 145 mEq/L. [R. C. Atkins, C. D. Leonard, and B. H. Scribner: "Management of Chronic Renal Failure," *DM*, (March 1971), 9.]

the extracellular fluid. As a result, the remaining extracellular fluid becomes hypertonic in relation to the intracellular fluid. Water can then be expected to move from within the cell to the more concentrated extracellular fluid. This results in *cellular dehydration.* In the person who is conscious and competent, the most prominent and reliable symptom is thirst. When water is available and the patient is able to ingest and absorb it, the condition is easily corrected by drinking water.

When the loss of water continues without a comparable loss of electrolytes, the amount of available intracellular fluid may be insufficient to correct the water deficit in the extracellular fluid. This results in an increase in the level of hemoglobin, nonprotein nitrogen, sodium, and other electrolytes in the blood. The hematocrit, that is, the proportion of red blood cells to the blood plasma, also rises. The kidney adapts by excreting a small volume of concentrated urine. In patients with normal kidneys, a urine output of less than 500 to 800 ml per 24 hours is usually indicative of an insufficient intake of water. As dehydration increases, skin and mucous membranes become dry and parched. The tongue becomes wrinkled and furry. Sordes, collections of dried secretions and other debris, are formed in the mouth and on the lips. When fluid losses are great, water may even be taken from extracellular spaces, such as the eyes, with the result that the eyeballs become soft. In infants and young children, fever may result from dehydration alone. Irritability, muscle twitching, and eventually drowsiness and coma result as the brain becomes progressively dehydrated.

Boylan and Marbach (1979) suggest the checklist questions at top right of page to help detect *early signs of dehydration.* The more "yes" answers the nurse obtains, the greater the probability of dehydration, and the greater the need for careful attention to measures to increase the person's fluid intake.

- Does the patient complain of thirst?
- Are his lips and/or conjunctiva dry? Are his mucosa sticky?
- Is his tongue swollen?
- Are his eyeballs sunken? Does he have dark circles underneath his eyes?
- Is his temperature above normal?
- Is his blood pressure below normal?
- Is his urine output lower and more concentrated than usual?
- Is he constipated?
- Is he losing weight?
- Does he seem unusually agitated or disoriented?
- Is he nauseated or vomiting?
- Has he recently experienced diarrhea? Excessive urination (such as that associated with uncontrolled diabetes mellitus)? Diaphoresis?
- Is he hyperventilating?
- Is he producing large amounts of sputum?
- Has his food and fluid intake decreased?
- Do lab studies, if available, show: Elevated hematocrit? Elevated hemoglobin? Urine specific gravity above 1.030? Elevated BUN, serum sodium, or serum protein? Decreased urine chloride (below 50 mEq/l)?

When any condition disturbs the balance between the intake and output of water so that more water is lost from the body than is replaced, the extracellular fluid is decreased in volume and becomes hypertonic in relation to the intracellular fluid. Because the body does not tolerate differences in osmotic pressure, intracellular fluid moves from the cell to the extracellular fluid. The increase in osmotic pressure in certain cells stimulates the sensation of thirst. As a result of decreased blood flow through the kidney and increased secretion of the antidiuretic hormone, the kidney secretes a small volume of concentrated urine. Scanty production of urine is *oliguria* and, although it is always associated with dehydration, the presence of oliguria does not always signify dehydration but may be due to other abnormalities. See Figure 41-1 for some practical considerations for evaluating the significance of oliguria. When dehydration is allowed to persist for a long period, the body's mechanisms for adaptation fail. Circulatory collapse followed by death is the result.

Prevention of Water Deficit

For many patients, the prevention of a deficit of water involves little more than providing adequate amounts of water in a clean and palatable form. Water offered to patients in carafes has not always met the latter criteria. In 1958, Walter et al. reported a study in which the water provided to patients was often grossly contaminated with microorganisms, unpalatable, and possibly unsafe for drinking. Two practices contributed to the contamination of the water. The carafes in which the water was served had narrow necks. This made thorough cleaning difficult. Ice used to chill the water was handled by hand rather than with the tongs provided for this purpose. The net result was that patients were served foul-smelling, potentially unsafe water.

Among the criteria that should be used in establishing, or evaluating the safety of, a procedure for providing patients with drinking water are (1) shape of the carafe—wide opening to facilitate cleaning, and a cover to prevent airborne and other contamination of water; (2) source and transfer technique of ice—readily available source of ice chips or cubes, to prevent having to chip by hand, and use of a scoop, tongs, or similar tool to prevent transfer of ice to carafe by hands; and (3) frequency of cleaning and sterilizing carafe—personnel and equipment ad-

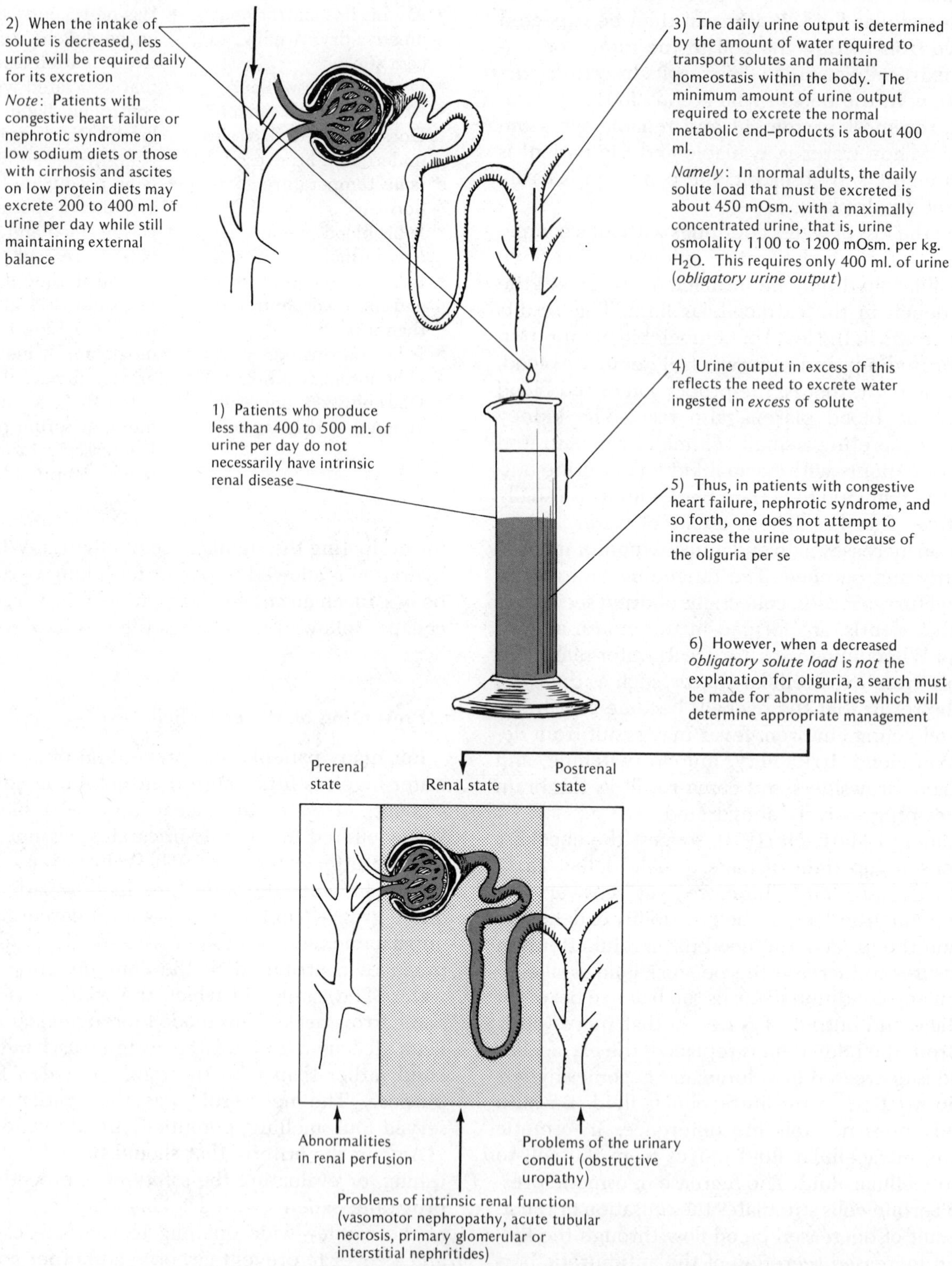
2) When the intake of solute is decreased, less urine will be required daily for its excretion
Note: Patients with congestive heart failure or nephrotic syndrome on low sodium diets or those with cirrhosis and ascites on low protein diets may excrete 200 to 400 ml. of urine per day while still maintaining external balance
3) The daily urine output is determined by the amount of water required to transport solutes and maintain homeostasis within the body. The minimum amount of urine output required to excrete the normal metabolic end-products is about 400 ml.
Namely: In normal adults, the daily solute load that must be excreted is about 450 mOsm. with a maximally concentrated urine, that is, urine osmolality 1100 to 1200 mOsm. per kg. H2O. This requires only 400 ml. of urine (*obligatory urine output*)
4) Urine output in excess of this reflects the need to excrete water ingested in *excess* of solute
1) Patients who produce less than 400 to 500 ml. of urine per day do not necessarily have intrinsic renal disease
5) Thus, in patients with congestive heart failure, nephrotic syndrome, and so forth, one does not attempt to increase the urine output because of the oliguria per se
6) However, when a decreased *obligatory solute load* is *not* the explanation for oliguria, a search must be made for abnormalities which will determine appropriate management
Prerenal state
Renal state
Postrenal state
Abnormalities in renal perfusion
Problems of the urinary conduit (obstructive uropathy)
Problems of intrinsic renal function (vasomotor nephropathy, acute tubular necrosis, primary glomerular or interstitial nephritides)

Figure 41-1. Oliguria and the obligatory urine output: Some practical considerations. (Used with permission of Hospital Publications, Inc., from Acute oliguria: A logical approach to diagnosis. *Hosp. Prac.* 15:22–43, Sept. 1979, by A. R. Nissenson, Fig. 1, p. 27.)

equate to collect, wash, sterilize, refill, and replace carafes at least once every 24 hours.[2]

Some patients require assistance with meeting their need for water. The nurse may have to help patients who, because of their age or the nature or degree of their illness, are unable to meet their own need for water. The amount and type of assistance needed by patients vary greatly. The apathetic, the confused, or the very ill patient will require more attention than the patient who is alert and thirsty. The patient may be completely dependent on the nurse. When the patient is unable to drink unless water is placed in his or her mouth, a cup with a spout, a teaspoon, or a drinking tube filled with water may be used. When water is placed in the mouth, care should be taken to adjust the patient's position so swallowing is favored and the danger of aspiration of fluid is minimized. The sitting position is most satisfactory. When a patient is in the supine position, the head should, if possible, be turned to the side. Those on mechanical respirators should be instructed to swallow during expiration. Another patient may only require that fluids be placed within easy reaching distance and an explanation of why a given fluid intake is desirable. Some patients will more willingly drink water that is iced. Others refuse to drink water, but will take other types of fluids such as ginger ale, broth, or tea. Whatever the problem, the nurse has a responsibility not only to identify it, but also, within the limits of the situation, to try to find a solution.

Attention should be given to the distribution of the patient's fluid intake over the ordinary waking hours. The patient should be observed for signs and symptoms indicating that the need for water is being met. In addition to the absence of thirst, a urine output of at least 500 to 800 ml in 24 hours, lack of irritability, moist, clean mucous membranes and good skin turgor are all indications that the patient's fluid intake is adequate. Conversely, a urine output of less than 500 ml, irritability, dry, cracked mucous membranes, with sordes on the lips and in the mouth, and dry skin that remains peaked when pinched (poor turgor) are indicative of an inadequate fluid intake. Day-to-day loss of more than a pound of weight indicates an insufficient intake of water or an excessive loss of fluid.

As stated earlier, a deficit of water in the body is reflected in a decrease in the volume of extracellular fluid and a corresponding increase in its concentration. Unless the loss of fluid, including whole blood, is great or continued, the condition is corrected by an increased fluid intake and/or by dehydration of cells. The body's mechanisms for adapting to changes in the volume of extracellular fluid are such that the blood volume is kept relatively constant. When, however, the loss of water from the body is excessive, blood volume cannot be adequately maintained. The seriousness of the situation depends on whether or not the individual can ingest and digest sufficient fluid to restore blood volume, on the nature and cause of the loss of body water, and on the extent to which the decrease in the volume of blood interferes with the nutrition of vital structures.

Except for the small amount of endogenous (internal) water of oxidation that results from metabolism of carbohydrate, protein, and fat[3] humans rely solely on the ingestion of fluids and food (exogenous source) to satisfy their water requirements. For persons who cannot or should not take fluids by mouth, the prevention or replacement of water deficit must be accomplished by some form of *infusion* (the act or process of pouring in water or other fluid) that bypasses the appropriate structures or system(s). In correcting water deficits, it must be remembered that hypertonicity of extracellular fluid always implies cellular dehydration. Water deficits should be corrected cautiously, to avoid the danger of brain swelling, because brain cells are protected by producing their own intracellular solute to "hold" water, in the presence of loss of extracellular fluid (Feig & McCurdy, 1977).

Medical science has shown infinite inventiveness in finding ways to introduce tubes into natural and manmade orifices of the body, through which fluids are introduced to meet the water and electrolyte requirements of the sick individual. The critical requirement is that the fluid enter an organ or space from which it can be absorbed and transported to body cells. A few of the most common methods, routes, and indications are mentioned here. For the person who is unconscious or who has some oral or pharyngeal defect that interferes with mastication or swallowing, a tube can be passed through the nose into the stomach for feeding. (See Chapter 51 for insertion of, and care of the patient with, a *nasogastric tube*.) When the esophagus, cardiac sphincter, or the stomach itself is involved in pathology, a tube can be introduced into the stomach through a surgical opening in the abdominal wall *(gastrostomy tube)*. Occasionally, small amounts of fluid are instilled slowly via a rectal tube into the rectum, to

[2] Many institutions have adopted the use of disposable carafes that meet the first criterion. However, even when the carafe can be discarded after a specified number of days or at the end of a patient's stay, the procedure should still satisfy the second and third criteria.

[3] Metabolism of 100 calories yields 14 ml of endogenous water.

be absorbed through the lining of the large bowel *(rectal instillation)*. Fluid may be introduced via a large bore needle directly into the interstitial space, usually in the area of the thighs *(clysis)*. But by far the most common route of administration for fluids in persons unable to take them by mouth is by *intravenous infusion*.

Intravenous Fluid Administration

Parenteral is a nonspecific term indicating some route other than the gastrointestinal canal (*para,* "contrary to," + *enteron,* "intestine") for administering fluids, nutrients, or medications. Because intravenous infusion is the most prevalent parenteral route used in preventing and correcting water and electrolyte deficit, the nurse must understand the purposes, principles of flow, and problems associated with administration of intravenous fluids.

PURPOSES. An intravenous infusion may provide the sole supply, may supplement oral intake, and/or may replace excessive losses of water, calories, electrolytes, and colloids. It may also serve as a medium for rapid-acting drugs.

PRINCIPLES OF FLOW. The principles that govern the flow of intravenous fluids (IVs) include those that control the flow of fluids in any open-ended system.

1. *Flow is directly proportional to the pressure exerted by the head of the fluid.* The head of an IV is the reservoir (bottle or bag) from which the fluid flows. The fuller the reservoir, and the higher it hangs above the level of the patient's heart, the faster the flow.
2. *Flow is inversely proportional to the viscosity of the fluid.* Viscosity of a fluid is a function of the attraction of its molecules for each other. The more viscous the fluid, the slower the flow. To illustrate, if all aspects other than viscosity are comparable in two systems used to administer fluid, an IV of 5 per cent dextrose in water will flow faster than either packed cells or whole blood.
3. *Flow is directly proportional to the size of the lumen of the tubing and of the needle. Lumen* is the passageway of a tubular structure. The larger the lumen of IV tubing and needle,[4] the faster the flow.
4. *Flow is inversely proportional to the pressure of the medium surrounding the exit from the system.* Point of exit from the IV system is the tip of the needle or intracatheter within the vein. Pressure of the medium surrounding the exit exerts a back pressure against the flow of IV fluid. The higher the venous pressure, the slower the flow.
5. *Flow is faster when the conduit (tubing) is straight than when it is coiled.* Straight tubing allows linear flow, whereas coiled or twisted tubing creates turbulent flow. (See Chapters 26 and 28 for applications to the movement of gases and the transportation of fluids.)

[4] There may be a plastic tube or *intracatheter* instead of a needle within the vein.

ASSOCIATED PROBLEMS. In the process of receiving an intravenous infusion, the patient is subject to injury by various mechanical, chemical, and biological agents. Whether the nurse actually starts the IV or only assists by preparing the patient and the equipment, nursing responsibility for preventing or minimizing the hazards of injury to the patient begins the moment a particular IV is ordered and extends beyond removal of the IV to include observation of the response to the patient.

It is imperative to remember that although parenteral injections are everyday procedures to hospital personnel, that is not necessarily true for patients. Patients receiving them are often very ill and present special problems not only because they are seriously ill, but also because intravenous injections carry special risks.

Nursing responsibility for the safe and effective administration of IV fluids is directed toward (1) preventing infections, (2) minimizing mechanical trauma to blood vessels and surrounding tissue, (3) observing for evidence that the therapeutic objectives of IV fluids are being achieved, and (4) preventing circulatory overload.

Prevention of infection is first addressed by maintaining the sterility of all parts of the fluid system, from needle to fluid reservoir. Thorough surgical skin preparation over and around the venipuncture site reduces the introduction of microorganisms with venipuncture. Once the infusion is running, every effort should be made to keep the system closed. When fluid or medication must be added, by interrupting the continuity of the system, procedures should adhere to strict surgical asepsis. Should infection develop, there may be redness, swelling, heat, or pain (signs of inflammation) at the venipuncture site and/or elevation of body temperature, pulse, and respiration. (See Chapters 25 and 38.) For patients on continuous IV therapy, the Center for Disease Control recommends that IV administration sets be changed at least every 24 hours, preferably at the time of bottle change (Change IV Sets, 1972).

Minimizing mechanical trauma to blood vessels and surrounding tissue is possible both during and after venipuncture. Whenever venipuncture is to be performed on veins of the upper extremities (which are the most frequently used sites for IVs), the arm least used by the patient should be selected, to reduce irritation of the vein by inadvertent movement of the arm, and to reduce patient discomfort and frustration. The following technical aspects of venipuncture minimize trauma to the vein. (1) Application of the tourniquet should be tight enough and long enough to produce adequate palpability of the vein, without interrupting arterial blood flow. To promote venous distention, the patient may be directed to make a fist and the surface of the arm may be stroked from the periphery toward the intended puncture site. (2) The angle of the needle should be parallel with the vein, or at a 10° to 20° angle, to prevent penetrating through the blood vessel. (3) The needle should be sharp, without burrs, and have a gauge[5] adequate to the viscosity and desired flow rate of fluid to be administered. (4) Penetration of the vein by the needle should be accomplished by decisive, firm, and steady pressure. (5) In the event that the vein is punctured but not entered on the first try, go to another vein. After the vein is entered, tubing is patent and fluid flowing, the needle is secured to the skin by tape at or near the hilt of the needle, and a loop of tubing proximal to the needle is taped to the skin to prevent drag on the needle and thus trauma to the vein. When venipuncture site lies near a joint, a firm surface such as an armboard should be used to stabilize and prevent flexion of the extremity, thus preventing perforation of the vein. Measures taken to stabilize the needle in the vein should be carried out in such a way that there is no interference with venous return.

During IV therapy the most common cause of tissue injury is infiltration of fluid into interstitial spaces. By frequent gentle palpation around the puncture site, the nurse can detect early signs of increasing fluid in the tissues. In addition, the patient will usually complain of discomfort or pain as fluid infiltrates the interstitial space. At the first sign of infiltration, the infusion should be discontinued and restarted in another vein to minimize tissue injury. Application of heat to the infiltrated tissue may facilitate reabsorption of fluid and relief of pain.

A frequent cause of unnecessary trauma to the vein is repeated venipuncture when an IV slows or stops, and the nurse assumes the needle is not in the vein. Before removing and restarting an IV, the nurse should first create a negative pressure in the tubing to get a backflow of blood, either by squeezing the gum rubber tubing near the hilt of the needle or, when this is not possible or successful, by lowering the fluid reservoir (bottle or bag) below the level of the heart.

[5] Lumen size of needles is scaled inversely, i.e., #25 is very narrow gauge, appropriate for subcutaneous injections, and #15 is very large gauge, appropriate for blood transfusions.

Another cause of chemical trauma to the vein is drug therapy. The nurse should ensure that IV drugs are properly diluted and infused at the recommended flow rate.

Achieving therapeutic objectives of IV fluid administration is enhanced when the nurse knows the hydration and electrolyte status of the patient, the volume and composition of fluid to be administered, the medical indication(s) for IV therapy, and when she or he calculates and maintains a flow rate sufficient to achieve the therapeutic objectives without overloading the patient's circulation.

White (1979), a registered pharmacist, has prepared for nurses a quick-reference pocket guide to twelve common IV formulations, which answers four critical questions:

1. What will the fluid do for your patient?
2. How does it achieve its effects?
3. How would you know if something went wrong?
4. What would you do about it?

Preventing circulatory overload requires close observation of the patient and the flow rate of the IV. Although all patients should be observed regularly throughout the period when fluids are being administered, observation is of special importance in those whose homeostatic mechanisms are inadequate or defective. Precautions should be taken to make certain the patient gets the correct solution, in the proper amounts, and at the rate consistent with fluid and electrolyte needs of the patient and with the ability to absorb fluid. The rate may be prescribed by the physician, or it may be left partially or totally to the discretion of the nurse. When the rate at which fluids are to be administered is prescribed, some method should be used to simplify checking. For example, a marker may be placed on the bottle of solution, indicating the number of drops per minute or milliliters per hour. Devices are available that can be set to regulate the rate of flow automatically.

In the regulation of the flow of the solution, both the number of drops per minute and the size of each drop are significant in the determination of the number of milliliters delivered per hour. Most intravenous sets have tubing in the drip chambers that deliver 10 to 20 drops per milliliter. Microdrip tubing sets usually deliver 45 to 60 per milliliter. Individual manufacturers usually provide this data on the package. No matter how carefully the rate is set, it can be expected to change, especially if the patient changes the position of his or her hand or arm. The following formula is helpful in calculating the flow rate required to ensure the patient a given fluid volume within a prescribed time period.

$$\text{Flow rate in gtts per min} = \left[\frac{\text{Total volume in ml}}{\text{Total time in hr}}\right] \div \left[\begin{matrix}\text{60 min}\\ \text{per hr}\end{matrix}\right] \times \left[\begin{matrix}\text{gtts per ml}\\ \text{delivered by}\\ \text{IV drip}\\ \text{chamber}\end{matrix}\right]$$

To illustrate, Mr. Ray, a 48-year-old postoperative patient, returns to his room from the recovery room, following abdominal surgery for removal of a calculus ("kidney stone") in his right ureter. He has an IV of 5 per cent dextrose in water running, with 900 ml remaining in the bottle. Postoperative orders indicate that the IV should run for 3 more hours. You find on the IV set package that this drip chamber delivers 15 drops per milliliter. What should the flow rate be to enable Mr. Ray to receive the total volume within the next 3 hours?

$$\begin{aligned}\text{Flow rate} &= \left(\frac{900}{3}\right) \div 60 \times 15\\ &= \left(\frac{300}{60}\right) \times 15\\ &= 5 \times 15 = 75 \text{ gtts per min}\end{aligned}$$

The rate of flow of parenteral solutions affects both the comfort of the patient and the stability of the fluid and electrolyte balance. Rate of flow is a factor not only in the comfort and fluid balance of the patient, but also in the patient's safety. The rate at which fluids can and should be administered varies with the condition of the patient and the concentration of the solution. As much as 600 ml of an isotonic solution can be safely administered in an hour. Under emergency situations the rate may be increased so that the patient receives as much as 2,000 ml per hour. The patient must, however, be under constant supervision. The concentration and the composition of the fluid also affect the rate at which it can be safely administered. Hypotonic solutions should not be given. Solutions with less than 5 per cent glucose or with a concentration of cations or anions less than 150 mEq per liter can be considered hypotonic. Hypertonic solutions should not be administered at a rate faster than 200 ml per hour. The maximum rate of flow for glucose solutions is 0.5 g per kilogram of body weight per hour. A more rapid rate results in glycosuria and the loss of potassium. If the fluid load is too great for the heart, kidneys, and lungs, the patient may develop *pulmonary edema,* and the rate of infusion will have to be decreased. Sensitive indicators of fluid overload include a sharp increase in central venous pressure and/or a marked decrease or increase in hourly urine volume. Elderly persons tolerate a rapid infusion rate poorly, primarily because of reduced compliance of their circulatory system and progressive impairment of cardiac and renal function. Pulmonary edema is one of the most serious risks to the patient related to rate of flow of parenteral fluids or blood transfusions. This danger is greatest in those receiving repeated blood transfusions, in elderly patients, and in persons who have a limited cardiac or renal reserve.

Pulmonary Edema

The basic mechanism of *acute pulmonary edema* is an impairment of contractile strength of the left ventricle which may occur acutely as a result of a sudden increase in the workload of the heart caused by fluid overload, hypertension, or valvular disease. The pump failure of the left ventricle and its inability to empty itself adequately (reduced ejection fraction and stroke output) result in lowered cardiac output, increased left ventricular end-diastolic volume and pressure, increased pulmonary blood volume, increased left atrial and pulmonary venous pressures, and, finally, a high pulmonary capillary pressure.

The hallmark of pulmonary edema is the severe rise in the pulmonary capillary pressure (measured at the patient's bedside by a Swan-Ganz catheter inserted in the pulmonary wedge position) to a critical level exceeding 30 to 40 mm Hg. This high pressure exceeds the osmotic pressure of the blood and results in transudation of fluid through the alveolar capillary walls into the alveolar spaces and interstitial tissues. The presence of fluid in the alveolar spaces and interstitial tissues interferes with alveolar gas exchange, mechanically impairs the expansion of the lungs, and increases bronchial and bronchiolar secretions. All of these factors, in turn, result in impaired ventilation, reduced vital capacity, and anoxemia (Dack, 1978). See Chapter 44 for further discussion of this cause of ventilatory impairment and its treatment.

The hazard of pulmonary edema as a consequence of fluid overload can be reduced by maintaining a slow rate of flow of blood or solution. Patients receiving parenteral fluids or blood transfusions require regular and frequent observation for prevention and early detection of pulmonary edema. Should the patient develop shortness of breath, or wheezing, or a persistent cough with or without frothy sputum, or a sense of pressure in the chest, or a marked increase in pulse or respiratory rate, the flow of the infusion should be slowed to a rate sufficient only to keep open the vein, and the physician called immediately. Throughout the time when a patient is receiving an infusion, the urine output should be measured at least hourly so that the status of the patient's output in relation to intake will be known.

Intravenous infusions and blood transfusions should be slow enough to prevent blood volume from suddenly increasing. When there is a question about the rate at which a solution should be administered, the nurse who is responsible for the care of the patient should consult with the patient's physician.

Blood Transfusion

The patient who receives a blood transfusion is exposed to all the risks of patients receiving intravenous fluids, plus the hazards of incompatible or contaminated blood (discussed in Chapter 52). An additional hazard common to all infusions for which the risk is greater with blood transfusion is air embolism. The possibility of air embolism is greatest when using a Y-type set, which is ideal for giving blood and IV solution alternately. To prevent air embolism, the nurse should never permit either container to empty completely. When either container is running, its upper clamp must be wide open and the clamp to the other container securely closed. This prevents air from entering the system via the blood bottle. Flow is regulated only *below* the Y, by a clamp which should be placed as close to the patient as possible. Before the first container is completely empty, its upper clamp is closed tightly. Only then may the clamp to the second container be opened.

Except in serious emergencies, blood is usually transfused at a rate of about 500 ml, each 2 to 4 hours. In dire emergencies, however, it may have to be given under pressure at rates up to 100 ml per minute. Care must be taken not to introduce air or fibrin clots. If at all avoidable, drugs should never be administered with blood or injected into blood transfusions or the intravenous tubing used for the transfusion. If this must be done, one should be certain that the drug is compatible with the blood and its constituents. Calcium should never be given in blood or in the same tubing with the blood because it neutralizes sodium citrate used as an anticoagulant, and causes clotting.

IV Fat

When the substance to be administered intravenously is a fat emulsion, there are at least eight points to guide the safe and effective administration of the IV fat (Wilson & Cooley, 1979, pp. 63–64):

1. Check the history and physical examination for signs and symptoms of disturbances in fat metabolism. If present, DO NOT ADMINISTER THE IV FAT.
2. Evaluate the patient to rule out: anemia, coagulation disorders, abnormal liver function, pulmonary dysfunction. If present, *monitor closely* during IV administration. Lipemia should clear between IVs; if this fails to occur, no more IV fat should be administered.
3. Store preparations appropriately:
   Intralipid 10%—refrigerate at 39.2–46.4°F (4–8°C) until used
   Liposyn 10%—store at room temperature
4. If the emulsion bottle shows any of the following DISCARD THE BOTTLE:
   "Oiling out"—separation into layers
   "Creaming"—separation into fat globules
   Frothiness
5. Prime the IV tubing slowly to prevent air bubbles and loss of large amount of emulsion.
6. Never filter IV fat, as it will clog the filter.
7. Begin the IV at a slow rate to provide time for possible evidence of allergic manifestations to develop, which necessitates the immediate termination of the infusion.
   Initial rates:
   For adults = 1.0 ml/minute
   For children = 0.1 ml/minute
   Observe closely for the following symptoms:
   dyspnea, cyanosis, hyperlipemia, hypercoagulability, transient increase in liver enzymes, nausea and vomiting, flushing, increased temperature, sweating, sleepiness, headache, chest and/or back pain, pressure over the eyes, dizziness, irritation of IV site, thrombocytopenia (especially in infants)
8. Discard partially used bottles to prevent contamination.

IV Precautions

General precautions cited by White (1979) for all IV products include:

1. Follow aseptic technique.
2. Use a local anti-infective agent in caring for the venipuncture site.
3. Check the flow rate several times a shift.
4. Change the set and tubing every 24 hours or other specified frequency.
5. Watch for signs of:
   a. Circulatory overload—edema, labored breathing, congestive heart failure
   b. Air embolism
   c. Nosocomial infection
   d. Thrombophlebitis

IV products included in a twelve-product basic file:

Dextrose in water	NaCl in water: 0.9%, 0.45%, 3%
KCl in ampules	$NaHCO_3$
Balanced electrolyte solutions	Lactated Ringer's solution
1/6 molar Na lactate	Mannitol
Ethyl alcohol in 5% D/W	Dextran 70, 40 in NS, or 5% D/W
Protein hydrolysate	Fat emulsion

IV INCOMPATIBILITIES The proliferation of intravenous solutions and additives increases the probability of intravenous incompatibilities. Predicting the possibilities of intravenous incompatibilities involves many factors. To anticipate certain common situations, the nurse may find the following guidelines helpful (Morris, 1979):

1. Is the diluent for the drug of special formulation?
2. Are there cautions in bold print in the package insert on how to reconstitute or further dilute the drug? If so, it probably indicates a problem and the directions should specify what solutions should be used.
3. Is the drug a penicillin, for example, carbenicillin, ampicillin, methicillin? If so, it is sensitive to hydrolysis by acids or bases.
4. Does the medication contain calcium or its salts? If so, it probably should not be combined since calcium will precipitate many drugs.
5. Nothing should be mixed with blood or blood products.
6. Does the additive or solution have an excessively high or low pH? If so, it will probably cause compatibility problems.
7. Avoid adding any *additional* drugs to total parenteral nutrition (hyperalimentation) solutions.
8. Whenever possible, avoid mixing more than one antibiotic in the same IV solution. The chances of incompatibility are greater as the number of drugs involved increases.
9. If you do not know the compatibility of the drugs to be mixed and cannot obtain any information concerning their compatibility, DO NOT MIX THEM.

In some hospitals, patients are instructed to call the nurse when the intravenous solution stops running or when the bottle becomes nearly empty. Before a patient is asked to do this, however, the nurse should be sure the patient is emotionally and physically well enough to assume this responsibility. Moreover, the nurse should not rely on the patient and should continue to observe him or her closely. Calls for help should be answered promptly. If there is any evidence of increased anxiety, the nurse should resume full responsibility for observing the fluid level. The importance of this to the sick patient is illustrated by an excerpt from a letter written by Mrs. Blonde, who wrote to a friend concerning her experience in a hospital after a cholecystectomy: "to have to supervise every step of your own care when you feel rotten is, to say the very least, very disturbing. I had to be sure that I stayed awake to watch the IVs and blood, because, sure as anything, if I dropped off to sleep they would run dry. This happened even after I had discussed it with the head nurse and she had assured me that I could relax because they would watch it very closely." Whether Mrs. Blonde's physical safety was threatened is not known; certainly, she felt unsafe and neglected. Energy she should have been using for recovery and rest was expended in protecting herself against possible injury.

Attention should be given to the patient's general comfort. When necessary, the patient should be assisted in moving and turning. When a patient receiving intravenous fluids is ambulated, enough assistance should be available to give the patient the help required. The patient should be told what to expect and what is expected of him or her. This may be an everyday procedure to the nurse, but this is not true for the patient.

When properly monitored, intravenous fluids constitute a highly effective means of preventing or correcting water deficit. However, in high-risk patients whose IV therapy is unwisely selected or inadequately monitored, water excess may result.

WATER EXCESS

Water may be found in the body in excess as well as in deficit. With an excess of water there is an increase in the volume of water in one or more of the fluid compartments. This then alters the osmotic pressure relationship between the intracellular and the extracellular fluid compartments. Since materials from the external environment enter and leave the body by way of the extracellular fluid, an excess of water is usually first reflected in a change in the extracellular fluid volume.[6] Neither the healthy nor the sick will ordinarily drink themselves into water intoxication, but they may occasionally be persuaded to do so. In the sick, the usual source is water administered by intravenous infusion. Water of oxidation may contribute to the total quantity of water in the body. Water intoxication need not develop if attention is given to the fact that the patient's fluid intake is in excess of the total fluid output. Chances for errors of measurement are great within existing practices for measuring and recording 24-hour fluid intake and output. Therefore an ongoing record of the patient's weight is probably the best single measure of the patient's fluid status, particularly as evidence for or against the storage of water. A gain in weight by a patient who is ingesting a limited amount of food should create more than a suspicion that water intake is exceeding its loss. For each

[6] A recent classification of disorders of sodium and water balance defines *water excess* as a lowering of serum sodium levels below 130 mEq/L. (Atkins et al., 1971, p. 9.)

pound of weight gained, about a pint of fluid is retained. Tarail (1959) states that, in the absence of food intake, a patient should be expected to lose about 14 oz per day.

To obtain an accurate weight, a balance scale should be used, with the patient being weighed at the same time each day and with the same amount of clothing. When at all possible, the patient should be weighed in the morning before breakfast, after having emptied the bladder. If he or she is able to stand on a scale, the simplest way is to remove all clothing except a hospital gown, and have the patient step onto a paper towel that has been placed on the scale. If the patient is weighed on a bed scale, the same amount of covering can be used each day, or it can be weighed each time and subtracted from the total. The scale should be balanced before the weight is taken. Accurate weighing of the patient contributes data that, when added to other facts, can be used to judge the patient's response to therapy. Improperly done, the weight obtained is worthless. It may even be the basis for making harmful changes in therapy. To state this another way, the value of the information obtained by weighing a patient depends, as do the data in any scientific investigation, on the care with which the variables are controlled.

Reduced Serum Osmolality

An excess of water dilutes the sodium (hyponatremia) and other osmotically active substances in the extracellular fluid. This dilution results in hypotonicity and a decrease in the osmolality of the extracellular fluid. As a consequence of the loss of osmotic activity, water moves from the extracellular fluid into the cell, causing it to swell. The symptoms presented by the patient have their origin in disturbed cerebral function. Initially, these symptoms are probably caused by the swelling of neurons. They include disturbed thought and behavior. If the condition is allowed to progress, coma and death may follow. In general, the severity of the symptoms is related to the rapidity of change and not to the extent of the hyponatremia or the dilution. For example, slow development of hyponatremia from the use of diuretics is generally fairly well tolerated. Rapid development of hyponatremia with excess water infusions may cause convulsions and death.

As has been previously emphasized, thirst is a reliable indicator of the need for water. For a variety of reasons, the quantity of water ingested may be insufficient or in excess of the needs of the individual. In health, the kidney does a remarkably efficient job of removing or conserving water. Under most circumstances, water intoxication is not likely unless the renal mechanisms for the elimination of water fail. The fault may be in the kidney itself, in the overproduction of the antidiuretic hormone, or the result of an impairment in the circulation of blood through the kidney. The first few days after surgical procedure, or following a serious injury, patients are susceptible to overloading with water. As stated earlier, overloading is dangerous because it predisposes to circulatory failure with pulmonary edema and disturbed cerebral function. This is the reason accurate recording of intake, output, and weight is important during this period.

Prevention and treatment of water intoxication include the limitation of the patient's water intake, so that water is not allowed to accumulate in the body. In patients with acute renal failure, this may mean the patient receives as little as 300 to 500 ml of fluid in 24 hours. Careful observation and recording of the patient's intake, output, and weight provide information about the patient on which his or her needs for fluid can be based. Urine may be collected and measured hourly as well as every 24 hours. Because specific gravity of urine is determined by the capacity of the kidney to concentrate urine, each specimen of urine may be tested for specific gravity.

Hyponatremia, or Sodium Deficit

Hyponatremia (less than 135 mEq/L) may be associated with a contracted or expanded extracellular fluid volume and with an adequate or inadequate circulation. One classification of these conditions is as follows:

1. Inadequate circulation and reduced extracellular fluid volume, including
   - a. Excessive losses from the gastrointestinal tract—severe diarrhea, vomiting, gastrointestinal fistula, or ileostomy.
   - b. Excessive sweating.
   - c. Adrenal insufficiency.
   - d. Diabetic acidosis.
   - e. Salt-losing kidney disease.
   - f. Excessive use of diuretics usually combined with overconscientious restriction of sodium intake.
   - g. Burns.
2. Inadequate circulation and excessive extracellular fluid volume, including
   - a. Congestive heart failure.
   - b. Liver disease.
   - c. Nephrotic syndrome.

3. Adequate circulation and excessive extracellular fluid volume, including
   a. Inappropriate secretion of antidiuretic hormone associated with decreased aldosterone secretion, increased urine osmolality, and excessive loss of sodium in the urine.
   b. Excessive administration of water with inadequate salt.

The major causes of sodium depletion are of two types: extrarenal (urinary sodium low); and renal (urinary sodium high) [Levy, 1978]. Specific causes of each type are summarized in Table 41-1. The most important homeostatic response to sodium depletion is conservation by the kidney of salt and water in an attempt to replenish vascular volume.

Signs and Symptoms

Hyponatremia is usually associated with an increased blood volume and is generally the result of excessive intake of water and inadequate intake of salt. The syndrome of hyponatremia with hypovolemia is quite uncommon, but very serious. When this syndrome develops acutely, the symptoms are those of circulatory collapse. There is a low plasma volume, a high hematocrit, hypotension, oliguria, thready pulse, tachycardia, and collapsed neck veins. In advanced cases, the eyeballs become soft and the eyes appear to be set deep in their sockets.

Table 41-1. *Major Causes of Sodium Depletion**

EXTRARENAL (urinary Na low)
1. Gastrointestinal causes
a. Vomiting
b. Diarrhea
c. External drainage or suction (iatrogenic)
d. Small bowel obstruction
2. Skin Na loss
a. Excessive sweating
b. Extensive burns
RENAL (urinary Na high)
1. Diuresis
a. Drugs
b. Endogenous substances with osmotic activity (e.g., glucose)
2. Mineralocorticoid deficiency
3. Chronic renal failure (with salt wasting)
4. Relief from obstructive uropathy (bilateral)
5. Recovery phase of acute renal failure
6. Various types of interstitial nephropathy (e.g., medullary cystic disease)
7. Syndromes of inappropriate ADH secretion

* From M. Levy. "The Pathophysiology of Sodium Balance." *Hosp. Prac.*, 13 (Nov. 1978), 95–106, 101.

When sodium deficits develop slowly, as might be the case in the patient on a restricted diet, particularly during hot weather, manifestations are less dramatic. They may include cramps, fainting on assuming the upright position as the result of postural hypotension, or simple general lethargy. The onset of hot weather, with the attendant increase in perspiration, may precipitate a sodium deficit in patients who have been on a prolonged regimen of diuretics and salt restriction. The nurse supervising the care of these patients, in either the hospital or the home, should be alert to this possibility and should not too quickly dismiss the patient's complaints of fatigue or loss of energy, or of feeling faint on arising in the morning, as being due to spring fever. What the patient needs is not sulfur and molasses, but an increase in salt intake. Symptoms should be reported to the physician.

These combined deficits require replacement of both sodium and water. It should be remembered always that most patients with hyponatremia actually have increased amounts of body and plasma water. Treatment in these instances requires hypertonic solutions. Fluids may be administered by mouth or by intravenous injection. The salt content of oral fluids may be increased by giving them in the form of bouillon or soup. If fruit juices are administered, they should have salt added to them. When the loss of sodium is proportionately greater than the loss of chloride, sodium bicarbonate or lactate may be administered. Intravenous fluids containing sodium bicarbonate and sometimes sodium lactate may also be used. Control of the rate of administration is important. Too rapid administration leads to an increased loss of electrolytes, and thus defeats the purpose of the treatment. In patients who undergo prolonged gastric or intestinal suction, physiologic saline solution should be used to irrigate the tube to prevent the loss of sodium and chloride ions that can occur if water alone is used as an irrigating fluid.

Hypernatremia, or Sodium Excess

As is to be expected, an increase in the retention of sodium in the body results in the retention of water and an increase in the extracellular fluid volume. Sodium concentration in such patients is often low in spite of an increased total body content of sodium because body water is generally increased. This produces a generalized edema. The most immediate and serious results are edema of the lung and an overloading of the circulatory system. Generalized edema occurs when the body's homeostatic mechanisms for eliminating excess sodium break down. As stated previously the kidney regulates the level of the sodium ion in extracellular fluid. Kidney function depends on an adequate blood flow and the presence of aldosterone. The level of aldosterone depends on the relationship of the quantity secreted by the adrenal cortex to the rate at which it is destroyed by the liver, and other regulatory mechanisms may be involved as well. Therefore sodium excess becomes a problem in (1) renal failure accompanied by salt retention, (2) disorders in which circulation of blood through the kidney is inadequate, such as congestive heart failure, (3) cirrhosis of the liver, (4) disorders characterized by overproduction of aldosterone by the adrenal cortex, and (5) patients who are treated with large doses of adrenal corticoids. In all these conditions there is sodium retention and with it an increase in the volume of extracellular fluid. It should be stressed that the increase in body water often exceeds the increase in sodium, thereby producing hyponatremia.

Prevention and treatment of sodium excess are directed toward correction of the condition causing sodium retention, combined with the restriction of sodium intake. The degree to which salt intake is reduced varies. In some patients, all that is required is to eliminate the use of salt in cooking. In others, all salts of sodium are prohibited. This includes sodium as bicarbonate, lactate, or benzoate. These patients should be taught to read the labels on foods and medicines and to reject those to which any sodium salt has been added. In the patient with congestive heart failure, restoration of the normal force of the heartbeat by digitalis, together with a restricted salt intake and diuretics to increase water and salt elimination, may be accompanied by remarkable changes in the patient. For example, Mrs. Martin, who suffered from a severe degree of cardiac insufficiency, lost 50 lb or 25 liters of fluid during her first week in the hospital. She entered the hospital short of breath to the point of orthopnea. She was also cyanotic and nauseated. Within a week she was no longer orthopneic at rest. Her color and appetite were also improved.

Although an excess of sodium ion in the extracellular fluid predisposes to edema by holding water, it is not the only factor in edema (edema is the abnormal retention of fluid in the interstitial spaces or in serous cavities). It results when the balance between the quantity of fluid entering the interstitial space is greater than that leaving it. The physiologic factors having a role in the movement of fluids across the capillary membrane and conditions associated with edema are listed in Table 41-2. It should be remembered that more than one mechanism is frequently involved.

Table 41-2. *Summary of Physiologic Factors and Conditions Associated with Edema*

Physiologic Factors		Conditions Associated with Increase in Interstitial Fluid Volume (Edema)
1. Capillary permeability	↑	a. Inflammation—increases capillary permeability b. Acute nephritis c. Burns
2. Hydrostatic pressure in the capillary	↑	a. Local venous obstruction, as in the use of constricting bandages or casts pressing on vein, swelling, varicose veins, and so on b. Generalized increase in venous pressure, as in congestive heart failure
3. Colloid osmotic pressure (decrease in blood proteins)	↓	a. Nephrosis b. Starvation c. Burns d. Chronic diarrhea e. Acute nephritis, but not a usual cause
4. Sodium retention	↑	a. Congestive heart failure b. Salt-saving nephritis c. Increase in level of adrenocortical hormones (endogenous) (exogenous) (1) Aldosterone (2) Desoxycorticosterone (3) Cortisone, hydrocortisone, and so on d. Following trauma (1) Surgical procedures (2) Burns (3) Fractures
5. Lymphatic drainage	↓	Lymphatic obstruction Cancerous lymph nodes, removal of lymph nodes, elephantiasis such as follows parasitic invasion of lymph channels

Location of Edema

The location of edema depends on the nature of the cause and whether it is localized or generalized.

In the presence of an intact cardiovascular system, fluid leaves and enters the intravascular space via the capillary membrane. To predict the pressure, and therefore the fluid shift, changes in the intravascular and interstitial compartments, the nurse may be assisted by thinking of the intravascular space as an open system, in service of the cell, in which changes in one site are inevitably transmitted in a predictable direction and with predictable fluid distribution consequences. See Figure 41-2 for a schematic diagram of the intravascular space as an open system. Generally, edema appears first in tissues that are poorly protected against the effects of hydrostatic pressure, such as the skin and subcutaneous tissues, and in dependent parts of the body. As a consequence, edema is found in the feet and ankles of those who are up and about and in the buttocks and sacrum of the bedridden. The influence of gravity on the distribution of edema fluid can sometimes be observed in the patient who has marked generalized edema. In the morning, after the patient spends the night on a lowered headrest, the eyelids may be so swollen that the patient has difficulty in opening his or her eyes, but there may be little or no pedal edema. Later in the day, and after sitting upright, the swelling around the eyes is much less marked but the feet may be greatly swollen again.

Edema of the lungs *(pulmonary edema)* is a possibility in patients with limited cardiac or renal reserve or in conditions accompanied by capillary injury such as infections involving the lung. When the hydrostatic pressure of the blood in the pulmonary capillaries rises so it is equal to, or exceeds, the colloid osmotic pressure of the blood, transudation of fluid into the lung tissue takes place. Pulmonary edema is always a serious condition. Manifestations depend on the extent to which the hydrostatic pressure is increased and the rapidity with which the condition develops. In milder cases, the patient can be expected to have moist rales and shortness of breath. In severe cases, the alveoli may fill with so much fluid that adequate ventilation is difficult or impossible. Essentially, the patient drowns in his or her own fluid. In patients who are predisposed to pulmonary edema, the possibility of this catastrophe can be reduced by modifying the fluid intake in relation to output.

As indicated earlier, the risk of pulmonary edema is greater when a person is receiving fluid intake parenterally than when eating and drinking. Additional risk factors and special considerations related

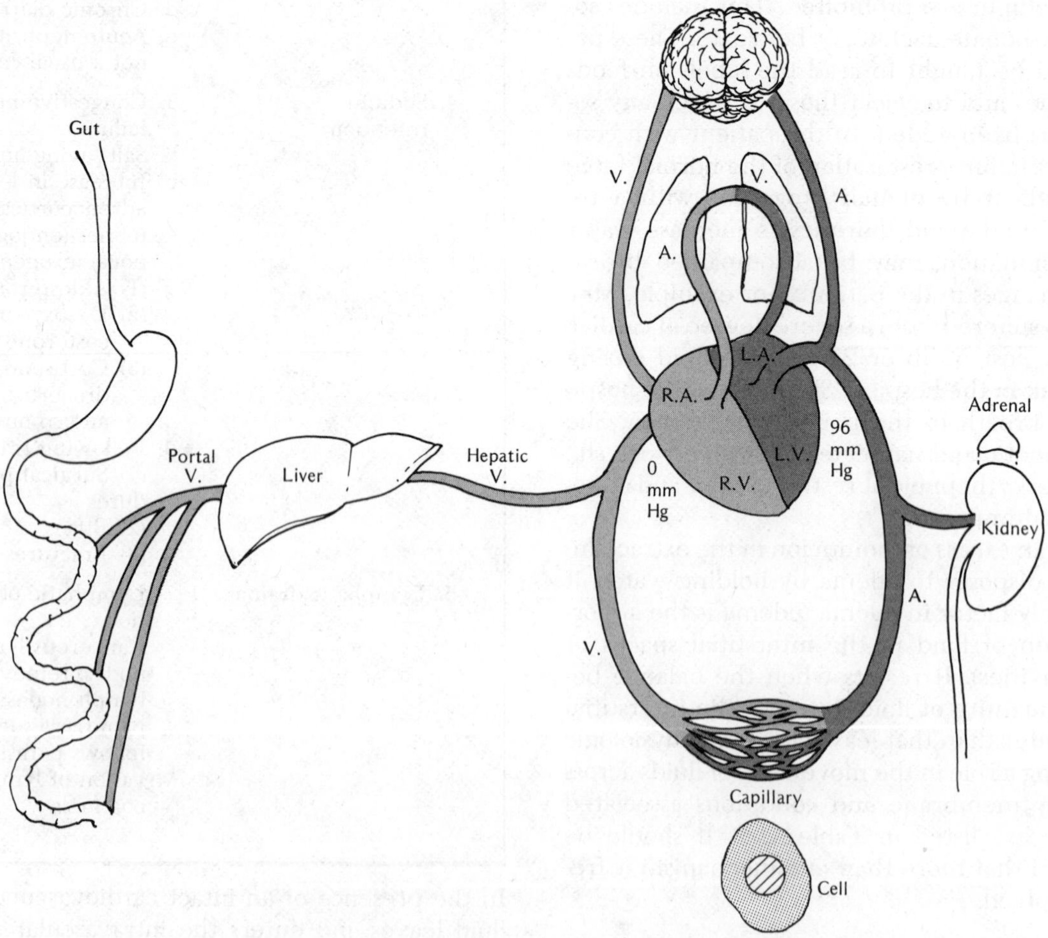

Figure 41-2. Schematic diagram of the intravascular space as an open system in the service of the cell.

to pulmonary edema are presented in the preceding discussion of parenteral fluid administration.

Edema in tissues other than the lung interferes with their nutrition by limiting the flow of blood to them. This renders the tissue more vulnerable to injury. In the bedfast patient with edema of the sacrum and buttocks, special attention to these areas is required to prevent the development of decubiti. Prevention of decubiti is especially difficult when the patient is orthopneic as a result of pulmonary edema. In orthopnea, the patient's breathing is so difficult that the patient is comfortable only when he or she sits leaning forward. Because the patient is short of breath and miserable, he or she resists changes in position; this continued pressure on edematous tissue leads to tissue breakdown. Prevention taxes the best efforts of the nurse. Small shifts in position, the use of an alternating pressure mattress, a flotation pad, or a water or air bed may be helpful in the prevention of decubiti. (See Chapter 49.)

Patients with generalized edema are often undernourished. When measures are initiated that are successful in eliminating edema fluid, the patient generally becomes thin or even emaciated. Improvement of the patient therefore depends not only on the elimination of edematous fluid, but also on improvement of nutritional state. In some patients, edema lessens as the patient's nutrition is rectified. This is especially true if the serum albumin is less than 3 per cent. The feeding of the patient is therefore an important aspect of nursing care, and the patient frequently has little interest in food. The person who has hypoproteinemia often feels lethargic, and sodium restriction prescribed to help control edema formation makes the food served less palatable than a normal diet might be. If the patient has difficulty finishing meals, the nurse should consider such modifications as small frequent feedings.

The edema or swelling following injury is discussed elsewhere. This is also true for the effects of edema in specialized organs such as the brain. The effect of edema fluid in any structure that is enclosed in a limited space is that it reduces the blood flow to the part, thereby interfering with its nutrition.

A variety of terms are used to describe the location of edema fluid. A severe and generalized edema is called *anasarca*. Accumulation of fluid in the peritoneal cavity is called *ascites*. In the pleural cavity, it is called *hydrothorax*, and an accumulation in the pericardial sac is known as *hydropericardium*. In all these conditions, the fluid takes up space normally occupied by an organ or system, thereby interfering with its function. The clinical effects depend on the site and quantity of the edema fluid.

Diuretics

Among the most commonly used diuretics for relief of severe and persistent edema are ethacrynic acid and furosemide. Although ethacrynic acid (Edecrin) and furosemide (Lasix) are not chemically related, because of the distinctive characteristics of their mode of action they are used with similar indications and in similar observations must be made to detect early signs of fluid and electrolyte imbalance for both. These two drugs are sometimes classified as *high-ceiling* or *loop diuretics*. Their three distinctive features are (White & Williamson, 1979):

1. They concentrate their action on the ascending loop of Henle in the renal tubules.
2. They achieve a rapid onset of action, as quickly as 5 minutes following IV injection.
3. They continue to act regardless of changes in acid-base balance.

Because of their rigorous effectiveness, they are valuable for treating persons with persistent fluid retention who have become resistant to other diuretics, particularly those in whom edema is due to congestive heart failure, hepatic cirrhosis, and renal disease. In acute pulmonary edema, their IV preparations rapidly counteract the pulmonary congestion.

Loop diuretics not only interfere with reabsorption of sodium and chloride but also tend to prevent reabsorption of potassium, HCO_3, and other ions. Consequently, there is a constant threat of fluid and electrolyte imbalance for which the nurse must be observant. Subjective and objective symptoms characteristic of *hypokalemic alkalosis*, the most likely imbalance, include the following:

Objective	Subjective
Dry mouth	Thirst
Weakness	Muscle pain
Muscle fatigue or cramps	
Lethargy	
Drowsiness	
Restlessness	
Hypotension	
Oliguria	
Tachycardia and other arrhythmias	
Vomiting	Nausea

To minimize the danger of hypokalemia, potassium intake is often increased during treatment with loop diuretics (White & Williamson, 1979).

Summary Case

The factors that enter into the development of edema and its effects will be reviewed in relation to Mrs. Bird, who was admitted to the hospital in congestive heart failure. Mrs. Bird has been selected because multiple factors appeared to play a role in the development of edema in her case. For many years Mrs. Bird had essential hypertension. For the last few months she noticed that her ankles were swelling and that she became short of breath when she walked up a flight of stairs or simply walked rapidly. On medical examination, she was found to have cardiac insufficiency on the basis of long-standing essential hypertension.

All the factors responsible for the development of edema in the patient with cardiac insufficiency are not understood. Authorities appear to agree that, as a result of a decrease in the force of the heartbeat, blood flow to the kidney is diminished. Mrs. Bird's heart was unable to pump all the blood brought to it. This increased venous hydrostatic pressure, and fluid tended to accumulate, especially in her feet, when she was standing. When the heart failure is severe, fluid with a low protein content (transudate) tends to accumulate in the peritoneal and pleural cavities. Mrs. Bird's condition may have been aggravated by an increase in the production of aldosterone by the adrenal cortex. Aldosterone secretion tends to increase in any condition associated with decreased blood flow through the kidney. As a consequence, the volume of her extracellular fluid rose. As the blood volume enlarged, the hydrostatic pressure of the blood rose further. With the elevation in hydrostatic pressure, filtration of fluid from the capillary to the interstitial space exceeded that removed from it. This, combined with the inability of the kidney to remove the necessary amount of water and salt, resulted in edema.

In the treatment of Mrs. Bird, the physician had two principal objectives. One was to improve the function of the heart. The other was to support the body's physiologic mechanisms for the elimination of salt and water. The first objective was achieved by treating Mrs. Bird with digitalis. To support her physiologic mechanisms for the regulation of sodium and water, she was placed on a low-sodium diet, and a diuretic to increase her renal excretion of salt and water was also given.

Objectives of Nursing Care

The objectives on which the nursing care of Mrs. Bird was based included (1) making pertinent observations as the basis for modifications in the medical regimen and the nursing care of Mrs. Bird, (2) reducing the work of the heart by meeting her physical and emotional needs, (3) preventing the breakdown of edematous tissue, (4) carrying out those aspects of the medical regimen that are the responsibility of the nurse so that the therapy is effective, and (5) as Mrs. Bird recovers, participating in a program to prepare her to return home and to activity.

The observation of Mrs. Bird was directed toward gathering information about how she was responding to her illness and to the therapy, and how she regarded her illness. Her nurse was interested in what Mrs. Bird expected in relation to her illness, hospitalization, nursing, and medical care. Because Mrs. Bird was obviously ill and apprehensive when she was admitted, she was given complete physical care. Every effort was made to reassure Mrs. Bird that her needs would be met promptly and to prepare her for what to expect. Her environment was controlled so that all unnecessary stimuli were eliminated. Planned periods of rest were provided. Visitors were restricted to the members of her immediate family. Arrangements were made for the hospital chaplain to visit her every day. As her general condition improved, a number of effects were noted: (1) she felt better, (2) she had a marked diuresis and lost 50 lb during the first week of hospitalization, (3) she could breathe comfortably in a recumbent position, and (4) her appetite improved and her activity was increased. After each increase in activity, the nurse checked her pulse and noted her respirations. Had her pulse rate risen more than ten beats per minute, or continued to rise, the nurse would have reduced her activity during that time. She also explained to Mrs. Bird that the reason for her increased activity was that she was improving. As Mrs. Bird improved, her daughter was also included in discussions of planning for Mrs. Bird's convalescence after her discharge from the hospital. Further and more detailed discussion of the care of the patient in congestive heart failure may be found in Chapter 44.

OTHER ELECTROLYTE IMBALANCES

In addition to affecting the distribution of body fluids, certain ions regulate neuromuscular irritability. Elevated levels of sodium and potassium increase neuromuscular irritability and responsiveness, whereas decreased concentrations of them decrease it (Brazier, 1972). Potassium affects the functioning of cardiac and skeletal muscle, and possibly smooth muscle. The irritability of the myoneural junction is decreased by increased concentrations of calcium, magnesium, and hydrogen ions. It is increased by decreased levels of calcium and magnesium (*Fluid and Electrolytes,* 1972).

Potassium Imbalance

Because of the difficulties involved in measuring the level of potassium in the cell, the state of potassium balance is inferred from its level in the blood plasma. The blood plasma level may or may not give an accurate picture. It may be normal or even elevated in the presence of a deficiency of potassium in the body. This is most likely to be true in conditions in which the cells are deprived of an adequate supply of oxygen or when fluids and electrolytes are lost in excessive quantities. Common examples include diabetic ketoacidosis and gastrointestinal disorders associated with the continued loss of secretions. Prolonged or severe gastrointestinal distention after surgery is occasionally due to poor motility caused by hypokalemia. Alterations in the level of potassium in the blood in either direction have an adverse effect on the function of the heart with the result that the patient may die suddenly from heart failure. It should also be remembered that electrolyte concentrations affect the activity of certain drugs. For example, digitalis is more likely to be toxic in patients low potassium and/or high calcium levels in the blood.

Mary Kay illustrates some of the causes and effects of low potassium levels in the body. She was admitted to the emergency room with a tentative diagnosis of acute appendicitis. On examination, her urine was found to contain glucose, acetone, and diacetic acid. Further investigation revealed that she was in diabetic acidosis. For some time she had been drinking large amounts of water (polydipsia) and voiding large quantities of urine (polyuria). Her blood sugar was 700 mg per 100 ml of blood plasma, and her carbon dioxide content was 10 mEq per liter. The level of potassium in her blood was 4.0 mEq per liter. To correct severe dehydration she was given 10,000 ml of fluid intravenously in a period of about 10 hours. Despite the fact that metabolism of glucose was reestablished by insulin therapy and her hypovolemia corrected, she was not given adequate potassium. As acidosis is corrected, blood potassium levels tend to fall. Also, as glucose enters the cells with the help of insulin, potassium also enters the cells, causing further hypokalemia. Her respirations became shallow, her pulse weak and rapid, and her color ashen. When adequate amounts of potassium were added to her intravenous fluids, her condition rapidly improved.

Renal mechanisms that regulate potassium homeostasis tend to favor excretion, which helps to explain why clinical states involving potassium deficits (hypokalemia) are more common than those involving potassium excess (hyperkalemia). Causes of hypo- and hyperkalemia are summarized in Table 41-3 (Cohen, 1979).

The body's mechanisms for conserving potassium are not as effective as they are for sodium. Some potassium continues to be lost in the urine, even with a low intake and low blood and tissue levels. Further, potassium loss is accentuated in metabolic alkalosis, which may be induced by excessive loss of hydrochloric acid caused by vomiting or nasogastric suction. Certain types of treatment aggravate potassium loss. These include enemas, mercurial diuretics, sodium bicarbonate, and the adrenocortical steroids. Patients who have been in the habit of taking drastic cathartics or enemas may also suffer from a deficiency of potassium.

Low levels of potassium may cause failure of cardiac, skeletal, and possibly smooth muscle. The sensitivity of the heart muscle to digitalis (Goodman & Gilman, 1975, p. 670) is increased when there is hypokalemia, and symptoms of toxicity may occur at dosages of digitalis that are ordinarily therapeutic. For this reason, a major part of the treatment for digitalis toxicity is a salt of potassium such as potassium chloride. Symptoms and signs of potassium deficiency include tachycardia, cardiac arrhythmias, altered EKG patterns, hypotension, muscle weakness, tetany, and paralytic ileus. In severe potassium deficiency the contractility of the heart muscle may be so impaired that the heart stops in diastole.

Treatment of Potassium Deficiency

The treatment is to replace the potassium that has been lost. Fruit juices, especially unstrained orange juice, bouillon, and meat broths, are rich in potassium. As soon as the patient eats a varied diet, potassium is promptly restored. When the patient is unable to take fluids by mouth, potassium may be given by intravenous infusion. Care should be taken to limit the rate of infusion of potassium in patients who have a limited renal reserve, so that blood levels do not become excessive. Intravenous infusions containing potassium require extremely careful supervision. The patient should also be observed for any signs or symptoms indicating hyperkalemia. The symptoms include paresthesias, which may be of the scalp rather than of the extremities, muscle weakness, and cardiac arrhythmias. Death may result from cardiac failure, with the heart stopping in systole.

Disorders in which hyperkalemia most commonly occurs are acute or chronic renal failure, too rapid administration of potassium, and adrenal insufficiency. Careful attention to the rate at which potassium salts are administered by intravenous injection cannot be overstressed. In adrenal insufficiency, hyperkalemia can usually be controlled by the administration of the adrenocortical hormones.

In patients with renal failure, the blood level of potassium may be more difficult to control. When

TABLE 41-3. *Causes of Hypo- and Hyperkalemia**

Causes of Hypokalemia (Potassium Depletion)	Causes of Hyperkalemia
Decreased intake	**Increased excretory burden**
Increased renal execretion	Dietary
Diuretics	Iatrogenic
Potent saluretic agents	Cell breakdown
Osmotic diuretics	**Decreased excretory capacity**
Carbonic anhydrase inhibitors	Acute renal failure
Acid-base disturbances	Chronic renal failure
Alkali loading	Hyporeninemic-hypoaldosteronism
Diabetic ketoacidosis	Adrenal insufficiency
Renal tubular acidosis	Potassium-sparing diuretics
Hyperadrenocorticism	Renal transplant
Cushing's syndrome	**Transcellular redistribution**
Primary aldosteronism	Acid-base disturbances
Edema-forming states	Exercise
Malignant hypertension	Diabetes mellitus
Bartter's syndrome	Drug-induced
Magnesium deficiency	Familial hyperkalemic periodic paralysis
Extrarenal losses	
Gastric losses	
Large intestinal losses	
Enterocutaneous fistula	
Biliary drainage	
Profuse sweating	

* Information from J. J. Cohen. "Disorders of Potassium Balance." *Hosp. Prac.*, **14** (Jan. 1979), 119–28, 122, and 124.

the failure is of short duration, control may be accomplished by eliminating all potassium intake and maintaining the patient at complete bedrest. Since most foods contain some potassium, the diet may be limited to glucose and vegetable oil, neither of which contains potassium. Elimination of potassium by the gastrointestinal tract may be increased by the ingestion of cation exchange resins, which have no potassium. Unfortunately, many patients do not tolerate these very well.

Abnormalities in the EKG, which usually appear when the serum potassium level reaches 7 to 8 mEq per liter, constitute an emergency that must be treated to prevent cardiac standstill. Treatment is aimed at promoting rapid transfer of potassium into the cells. Administration of 1 liter of a 10 per cent glucose solution with 30 to 40 units of insulin and, in acidotic patients, administration of 150 to 300 mEq of sodium bicarbonate will usually produce a marked reduction in plasma potassium level and prompt improvement in the EKG (Schwartz, 1979). To antagonize the effect of potassium on the heart, 2 g of calcium lactate may be useful. When calcium is used, it cannot be given in the same solution with sodium bicarbonate because precipitation of the calcium ion will result.

Calcium and Magnesium Imbalance

As with other elements of body fluids, calcium may be present in deficit or in excess. Deficits of calcium may be in the total quantity or in the proportion that is in ionized form. In alkalosis, the proportion of calcium in the ionized form diminishes; in acidosis, it rises. Tetany results when the amount of ionized calcium in the blood is low. This in turn may be caused by alkalosis, excessive loss of calcium, or inadequate calcium intake. For example, tetany develops in susceptible persons who induce respiratory alkalosis by overbreathing. It is seen in infants and very young children with rickets, as a result of a lack of calcium and/or vitamin D. In adults, tetany may follow injury or removal of the parathyroid glands during thyroid surgery or following the removal of an adenoma of the parathyroid gland. In the absence of the parathyroid hormone, the level of calcium in the serum falls. In advanced renal disease, the kidney loses its ability to conserve calcium. As a consequence, it is lost from the blood. Whatever the cause, a decrease in the level of calcium in the blood is followed by a heightening in neuromuscular irritability.

Often the first symptoms of impending tetany are

paresthesias about the mouth or in the fingers or toes. With an increase in muscular irritability, the hands and feet assume a characteristic position which is referred to as carpopedal spasm. In infants, spasms of the glottis may interfere with breathing. In patients whose blood level of calcium remains just above the critical point, tapping over the facial nerve in front of the ear causes a twitching of the muscles of the face. If the face muscles twitch, this is called a positive Chvostek sign. Muscle spasm is accompanied by considerable pain and discomfort which can be relieved by the intravenous administration of calcium gluconate or calcium chloride. Calcium solutions should be given very slowly and are very dangerous in patients who are getting digitalis-like drugs.

TABLE 41-4. ***Major Causes of Four Types of Osteopenia and the Usual Serum Chemistry in Three Types (all except malignancies)****

Etiology of Ostopenia by Type	Usual Serum Chemistry in Three Types: Serum Calcium	Serum Phosphate	Serum Alkaline Phosphatase	Urine Calcium
OSTEOPOROSIS				
Primary				
Senile or postmenopausal (involutional)				
Idiopathic				
Juvenile				
Secondary				
Cushing's syndrome	Normal	Normal	Normal	Normal or ↑
Chronic renal failure				
Chronic liver disease				
Turner's syndrome				
Immobilization				
Heparin therapy				
Alcoholism				
Diabetes mellitus				
OSTEOMALACIA				
Dietary lack of vitamin D				
Gastrointestinal malabsorption				
Anticonvulsant therapy				
Chronic liver disease	Normal or ↓	↓↓	↑	↓
Chronic renal disease				
Renal tubular acidosis				
Hypophosphatemic osteomalacia (phosphate diabetes; vitamin D-resistant osteomalacia)				
Vitamin D-dependent osteomalacia				
Tumor osteomalacia				
OSTEITIS FIBROSA				
Primary and secondary hyperparathyroidism	↑	↓	↑	↑
Thyrotoxicosis				
MALIGNANCIES				
Myeloma				
Metastatic bone disease				

* Adapted from "Differential Diagnosis of Osteopenia." *Hosp. Prac,* 13 (Nov. 1978), 65–72, by G. R. Mundy, tables on pp. 69 and 72.

Though the function of the calcium ion in muscle irritability and excitability has been stressed, irritability is the function of the relationship of several ions. This relationship is expressed by:

$$\frac{Na^+ \quad OH^- \; K^+}{Ca^{++} \; Mg^{++} \; H^+}$$

Thus muscle irritability is increased as the levels of sodium, hydroxyl, and potassium ions are increased in relationship to calcium, magnesium, and hydrogen ions. Relationships as well as particular levels are significant. Occasionally, patients with normal calcium levels will develop a tremor that comes and goes, and marked, sudden, irregularly occurring jerks or twitches. Hypomagnesemia may be the cause of the symptoms. If so, the tremor in the outstretched arms may resemble the so-called hepatic flap, mental aberrations may be pronounced, and reflexes may be hyperactive. However, true tetany will not result from magnesium deficiency unless there is concurrent hypocalcemia (Frawley, 1970). Symptoms of hypomagnesemia usually respond readily to administration of magnesium sulfate or chloride (Sleisenger, 1979). Magnesium deficiencies may be important in the development of delirium tremens and should be watched for in patients with severe burns or excessive gastrointestinal fluid loss.

Osteopenia

It is important in medical diagnosis to differentiate the demineralizing bone diseases, especially osteoporosis from osteomalacia, since osteomalacia is highly treatable. Osteomalacia in adults is the same fundamental disorder as rickets in children; there is a failure of normal mineralization of the bone matrix, and the nonmineralized bone matrix (osteoid tissue) is present in excess amounts (Mundy, 1978). Osteopenia ("lack of bone") is a generic term for radiologic decrease of the mass of mineralized bone, implying no particular pathology. The four major types of osteopenia are osteoporosis, osteomalacia, osteitis fibrosa, and malignancies (Mundy, 1978). Major causes of the each type of osteopenia are summarized in Table 41-4, with the usual serum chemistry patterns for all except malignancies.

Osteoporosis, the most common cause of osteopenia, affects several million postmenopausal women and elderly people in the United States. Medical treatment of osteoporosis is by use of therapeutic agents that inhibit resorption of bone. Four drugs or drug types used are sodium fluoride, estrogens, anabolic steroids, and calcitonin. Despite the availability of drugs of all four types, none is presently approved by the Food and Drug Administration for treatment of osteoporosis (Wallach, 1978).

For osteomalacia, vitamin D, with or without adjuncts, is the therapy of choice (Avioli, 1979).

Osteosclerosis (Abnormal hardening of bone)

Excessive fluoride ingestion, which usually occurs when its concentration in drinking water exceeds 20 parts per million, leads to osteosclerosis and, occasionally, to calcification of ligaments and neurologic signs due to bony overgrowth (Gallagher & Riggs, 1978).

Clinical Manifestations of Acid-Base Imbalance

Depending on their origin, deviations in the concentration of the hydrogen ion are classified as metabolic or respiratory.

Failure to control the hydrogen ion concentration so that the pH is maintained between 7.35 and 7.45 results in acidemia or alkalemia. The condition is said to be compensated as long as the ratio of bicarbonate to carbonic acid is maintained at about 20:1. As can be seen in Figure 41-3, in acidosis the ratio of bicarbonate to carbonic acid is less than 20:1; in alkalosis the ratio is greater than 20:1. In the presence of an increase or decrease in hydrogen ion concentration, mechanisms for its control act to produce changes that restore the ratio of carbonic acid to bicarbonate.

Guides to Assessment of Acid-Base Imbalance

To obtain the information needed to determine the person's acid-base balance, the nurse will find the following table on page 752 helpful (Shrake, 1979):

Restoration of acidosis and alkalosis to normal acid-base balance are accomplished through either respiratory or metabolic compensatory mechanisms, depending upon whether the imbalance is metabolic or respiratory in origin and upon the status of all buffer systems at the onset of the acidotic or alkalotic state. It is suggested that the learner reproduce Figure 41-4 to use as a pocket-card to guide in interpretation of laboratory and clinical data indicative of acidosis and alkalosis. There are three centrally useful laboratory values on which to base the judgment about the patient's acid-base status: the pH, P_{CO_2}, and bicarbonate. The grid in Figure 41-4 allows available laboratory values to be plotted in such a way that the patient's acid-base status can be estimated.

Figure 41-3. Possible changes in $H-HCO_3$ to HCO_3 in acidosis and alkalosis.

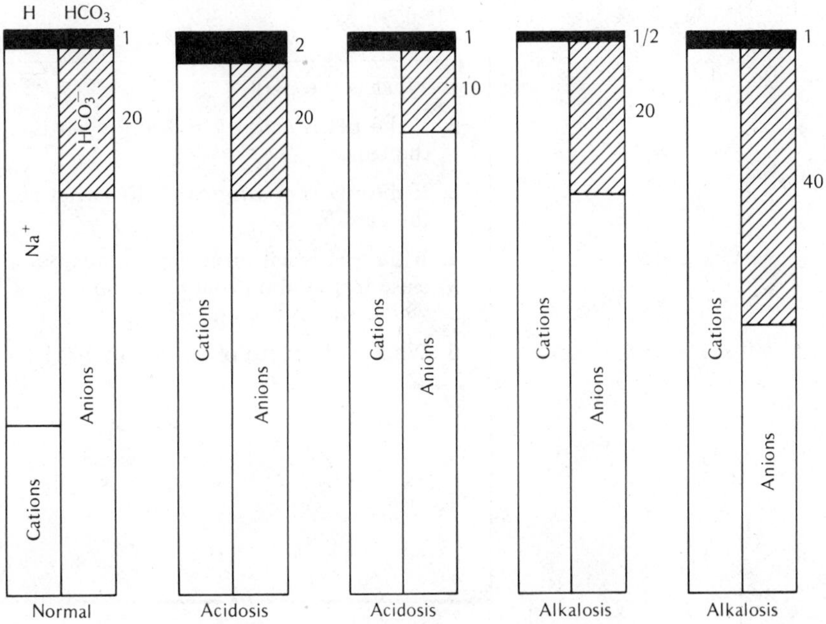

Designation of metabolic or respiratory acidosis or alkalosis can assist the nurse in seeking and interpreting concomitant clinical data.

Metabolic Acidosis

In metabolic acidosis, the ratio of bicarbonate to carbonic acid is decreased by a reduction in the quantity of sodium available to combine with bicarbonate; the quantity of sodium in combination with anions other than bicarbonate is increased. A characteristic feature of metabolic acidosis is therefore a decrease in the alkali reserve.

Regulation of the bicarbonate anion, a critical element in the body's major buffer system, was presented in Chapter 27. As stated previously, the level of the bicarbonate ion varies inversely with the level of other anions; for example, a fall in the level of the chloride ion is compensated for by an increase in the bicarbonate ion, and increases in other anions result in a lowering of the level of the bicarbonate ion. Although the levels of the chloride and other anions in the blood plasma are subject to change, there do not appear to be as active mechanisms for their upward or downward adjustment as there are with bicarbonate. This may result in an "anion gap" indicative of metabolic acidosis. The anion gap is

Figure 41-4. Grid for estimating acid-base status from any 2 of 3 blood chemistry values: pH, HCO_3, and PCO_2.

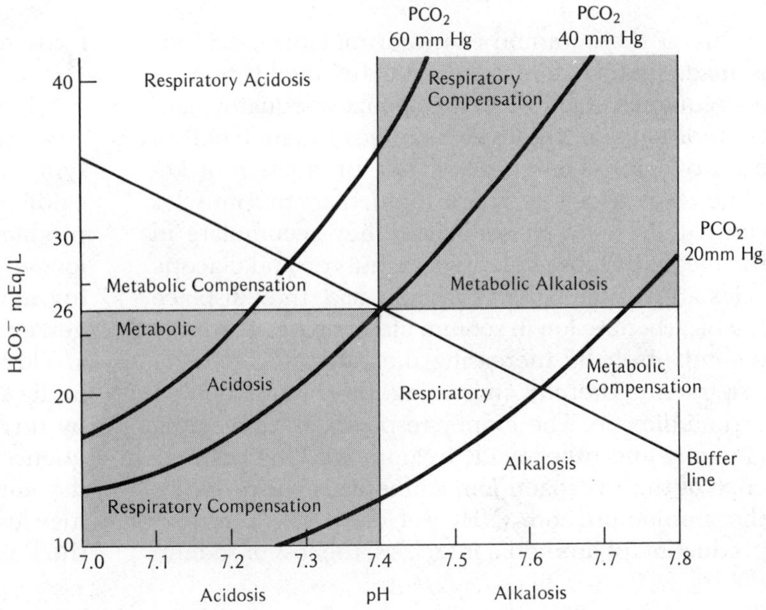

Questions	Significance of Possible Answers
1. What is the pH?	Normal = 7.35 − 7.45
2. If the pH is *acidotic* (<7.45), what is the cause	Respiratory: $P_{CO_2} > 45$ mm Hg Metabolic: $HCO_3 < 22$ mEq/L
3. If the pH is *alkalotic* (>7.45), what is the cause?	Respiratory: $P_{CO_2} < 35$ mm Hg Metabolic: $HCO_3 > 26$ mEq/L
4. If the pH is within normal limits but close to the abnormal borderline, which way is it leaning?	Direction suggests *compensated* acidosis or alkalosis
5. What is the state of oxygenation?	Know the fractional inspired O_2 (FI_{O_2}) Room air = 21% Hypoxemia = $P_{O_2} < 80$ mm Hg, *except* for newborns and old people. For people over 60 years of age, subtract 1 mm of Hg from the normal values for every year over 60.

determined by the concentrations of unmeasured anions and unmeasured cations. It is conventionally estimated as the difference between

$$[Na^+] \text{ or } [Na^+ + K^+]$$
and
$$[Cl^- + HCO_3^-]$$

Normally, about two thirds of the unmeasured anionic equivalency originates from the plasma proteins; the remaining one third is accounted for by plasma organic acids, phosphate, and sulfate (Madias et al., 1979). The "anion gap" is said to exist when the sum of the chloride and bicarbonate ions is less than the serum sodium minus 12 (Frawley, 1970).

$$[Cl^- + HCO_3^-] < [Na^+ - 12]$$

One of the common causes of metabolic acidosis is inadequately controlled diabetes mellitus. As a consequence of failure to metabolize adequate quantities of glucose, the liver increases the metabolism of fatty acids. This results in the production of ketonic acids at a rate more rapid than the muscles can handle. As a consequence, they accumulate in the blood. Because beta-hydroxybutyric and diacetic acids are stronger than carbonic acid, they displace the bicarbonate ion in sodium bicarbonate. The body defends itself by increasing the rate and depth of respiration, thereby increasing the elimination of carbon dioxide. The kidney responds by converting glutamic and other acids to ammonia. In the presence of the hydrogen ion, ammonia is converted to the ammonium ion. ($NH_3 + H^+ \rightleftharpoons NH_4^+$). As the production of ammonia increases, the loss of sodium and potassium decreases. Although the secretion of ammonia is a relatively slow adaptive response, it is an effective one.

Although the rate of formation of ketone acids is slower, some degree of metabolic acidosis develops when the patient has not eaten and adequate amounts of glucose are not present. Other conditions with which metabolic acidosis occurs include

1. Renal failure—phosphate and sulfate anions are retained.
2. The administration of large doses of acidifying salts, such as ammonium chloride.
3. Excessive exercise.
4. Anoxia or hypoxia.
5. Severe diarrhea in which the loss of sodium ions exceeds that of chloride ions.

Whatever the underlying cause, hyperpnea of the type known as Kussmaul breathing is the outstanding symptom; this hyperventilation eliminates carbon dioxide and counteracts the metabolic acidosis by producing a respiratory alkalosis. In severe or prolonged acidosis, the kidney mechanisms for conserving sodium and water and for excreting the hydrogen ion fail. As a result, water, sodium, and potassium are lost in excess of intake with a resultant increase in the acidosis. The situation is frequently aggravated by further dehydration from vomiting. As a consequence, the skin and mucous membrane become dry and tissue turgor diminishes. Even the eyeballs may lose fluid with a reduction in their tension. With the loss of fluid and the decrease in pH, restlessness, abdominal pain, and eventually coma develop. Unless the condition is corrected, death can occur.

Treatment of Metabolic Acidosis

Treatment of metabolic acidosis is directed toward two objectives. The first is to correct the underlying cause. The second is to restore the water, electrolytes, and nutrients that have been lost from the body. In the instance of Mary Kay, she was given insulin and glucose to enable her to metabolize glucose and to decrease the formation of ketone acids. In this way the underlying cause of her acidosis was attacked. At the same time, she received fluids containing sodium chloride and sodium lactate. Because the lactate ion is metabolized, the sodium ion becomes available to combine with the bicarbonate ion. The sodium ion thus enlarges the alkali reserve. In the beginning, the fluids are likely to be administered parenterally. It was also important to give Mary Kay some form of potassium. After the patient is able to tolerate fluids by mouth, bouillon, orange juice, or other fluids containing the necessary electrolytes may be given.

The functions of the nurse include making pertinent observations, protecting the patient from injury, performing therapeutic procedures, and providing for the comfort and well-being of the patient. Significant observations include the patient's general behavior. Is he or she conscious, drowsy, or stuporous? quiet or restless? What is the character of breathing? color? Is the patient's skin dry or moist? Examination of the urine in metabolic acidosis is extremely important. Because the urine should be analyzed frequently, an indwelling catheter is sometimes inserted so that urine can be obtained for regular half-hourly or hourly analyses. In addition to recording the rate of urine formation, it is also important to have it examined for glucose, acetone, diacetic acid, specific gravity, and pH. Samples of blood should also be checked at regular intervals for glucose, sodium, potassium, chlorides, carbon dioxide content or carbon dioxide–combining power, and acetone. Hemoconcentration of the blood is reflected by an elevated hematocrit or hemoglobin in the blood. Because these diagnostic tests require repeated venipuncture, the patient should be told why repeated venipuncture is necessary.

The common therapeutic measures have been indicated. The nurse's responsibilities in each of these have been discussed previously. After fluids are started by mouth, attention should be given to make certain the patient gets and ingests the required amounts. The patient in acidosis has a tendency to have gastric dilatation. When this occurs, the fluid ingested remains in the stomach. Later, the patient may vomit a large quantity of fluid. A feeling of fullness in the epigastric region is the common warning symptom accompanying gastric retention.

When the patient is restless and not fully conscious, more than usual attention to safety is required. Side rails may be placed on the bed to lessen the danger of falling out of bed. If the patient is very restless, the side rails should be padded. Other precautions in the patient's care do not differ materially from those for any patient who is not fully aware of his or her actions.

As in the care of any other patient, the nurse should be alert to the need of the patient for comfort and support. During the period when the patient is not fully conscious, the nurse should assume responsibility for reminding everyone involved in the care of the patient that he or she may be able to hear and comprehend what is said.

Respiratory Acidosis

In addition to acidosis of metabolic origin, acidosis may result from a failure of the body to ventilate adequately and remove carbon dioxide from the body. This type is known as respiratory acidosis. In respiratory acidosis, the level of carbon dioxide and carbonic acid in the blood plasma is increased, and the ratio of carbonic acid to bicarbonate is increased. This result in an increase in the hydrogen ion concentration in the blood. Respiratory acidosis occurs in a wide range of conditions in which there is an inadequate exchange of gases in the lungs resulting in retention of carbon dioxide in the blood. Inadequate exchange of gases in the lung may be caused by anything that depresses the respiratory center in the medulla or decreases the aerating surface in the lung. Narcotics such as morphine and meperidine hydrochloride, general anesthetics, and barbiturates all predispose to respiratory acidosis because they depress the respiratory center. Diseases such as poliomyelitis and injuries that involve the respiratory center can also be expected to do so. Emphysema, bronchiectasis, and pneumonia predispose to respiratory acidosis by decreasing the aerating surface in the lung.

As in metabolic acidosis, the kidney's mechanisms for maintaining the level of the hydrogen ions are utilized. The buffers also help. As the blood level of carbonic acid rises, some chloride moves into the red cell, leaving more sodium available to form sodium bicarbonate. The increased bicarbonate helps to restore the bicarbonate-to-carbonic acid ratio of 20 to 1. Thus the body attempts to compensate for respiratory acidosis by producing a metabolic alkalosis, and vice versa.

Prevention of Respiratory Acidosis

In the prevention and treatment of respiratory acidosis, therapy is directed toward correcting the cause. Narcotics should be given infrequently and then only in the smallest amounts required to relieve pain. When a patient is receiving narcotic drugs, he or she should be encouraged to perform deep breathing at regular intervals. In the patient with emphysema, a tracheostomy is sometimes performed to reduce the dead-air space, to facilitate the removal of secretions, or to allow the patient to be put on a respirator. Ordinarily, however, a tracheostomy allows more expiratory bronchiolar collapse, thereby causing more air trapping; this may be very detrimental to a patient with emphysema. The patient who is suffering from respiratory paralysis is placed on respirator. Because hypoxia increases the degree of acidosis, the administration of increased oxygen would appear to be indicated, especially if the hemoglobin saturation is less than 90 per cent or the P_{O_2} is less than 60 mm Hg. However, it may have disastrous effects in the patient with severe emphysema. The emphysema patient may have severe depression of the respiratory center because of a chronic hypercarbia. When this occurs, the only stimulus to respiration is the effect of hypoxia on the chemoreceptors, such as the carotid and aortic bodies. If such a patient is given oxygen, the oxygen content of the blood rises and the stimulus to respiration is lost. The reduced ventilation causes further hypercarbia, which may be enough to kill the patient by respiratory acidosis.

ALKALOSIS

In certain disorders the level of the hydrogen ion may be decreased to below normal. This results in alkalosis. Like acidosis, alkalosis may be of metabolic or respiratory origin.

Metabolic Alkalosis

In *metabolic alkalosis*, the bicarbonate anion is increased in relation to carbonic acid. This results in an increase in the ratio of bicarbonate to carbonic acid, so that there are more than 20 parts of bicarbonate ions to 1 part of carbonic acid. Another way to state this is that there is a relative increase of fixed cations in relation to fixed anions. *Metabolic alkalosis* is most commonly associated with disorders in which there is an undue loss of the chloride ion or excessive intake of sodium bicarbonate. Continued vomiting from pyloric stenosis and gastric suction are the most frequent causes of chloride depletion. Loss of chlorides from the patient on gastric suction is intensified by vigorous irrigation of the nasogastric tube. For this reason some physicians limit irrigation or ask that isotonic saline solution be used as the irrigating fluid. Fluid intake is generally limited for the same reason in the patient having gastric suction. Chloride depletion also occurs in patients who are given mercurial diuretics frequently. Loss of potassium from the body can also cause metabolic alkalosis. Almost all moderate to severe metabolic alkalosis is associated clinically with a substantial amount of extracellular-volume *contraction*, which may be the cause of an elevated anion gap (Madias et al., 1979).

The ingestion of excessive quantities of sodium bicarbonate is most likely to be observed in persons who treat themselves for indigestion and who have a limited renal reserve. Everyone, especially persons in older age groups, should be cautioned against this practice.

A characteristic sign of alkalosis is shallow breathing. This results from the body's attempt to raise the level of carbonic acid in the blood. In shallow breating, the concentration of carbon dioxide in the alveolar air is raised. This serves to raise the level of carbonic acid in the blood. The kidney also responds by excreting sodium bicarbonate in the urine and by depressing the mechanisms for the excretion of the hydrogen ion. Less hydrogen ion is secreted by the tubules. The formation of ammonia is suppressed. Phosphates are excreted as disodium rather than monosodium salts. Lactic acid and ketone acid anions are reabsorbed. They help to displace the bicarbonate ion in the plasma. The urine excreted as alkaline in reaction. Thus, the body, through the initiation of compensatory mechanisms, attempts to maintain the pH of the blood within normal limits.

Occasionally, a patient with alkalosis tends to excrete an acid urine. This is referred to as a *paradoxical aciduria* and is usually caused by hypokalemia.

Treatment in alkalosis is based on the same general principles as in acidosis. It is directed toward the correction of the cause and the support of the body's compensatory mechanisms. Several authorities emphasize that in alkalosis, potassium is lost and the condition cannot be treated successfully without repairing the deficit of potassium, especially if there is paradoxical aciduria. In addition to replacement of chlorides, attention should be given to improving the patient's nutrition.

Respiratory Alkalosis

Respiratory alkalosis occurs less frequently than other disturbances in hydrogen ion concentration. It results when the concentration of carbonic acid in the blood is decreased in the proportion to the bicarbonate anion. The most common cause is an increase in the rate and depth of respirations in the absence of an increase in the hydrogen ion or carbon dioxide. Respiratory alkalosis is an example of a disorder arising from the inappropriate use of a physiologic mechanism. This condition is most commonly seen in the nervous patient who overbreathes but may also be an early sign of sepsis or a pulmonary embolism. Because the hydrogen ion concentration of the blood plasma is diminished, the level of ionized calcium in the blood is also decreased. As a consequence, these persons frequently have symptoms and signs of tetany. Treatment is directed toward correcting the underlying cause of the condition. Respiratory alkalosis can be corrected by any measure that elevates the level of carbon dioxide in the alveoli and blood. This can be done by holding the breath or by inhaling carbon dioxide. Sedatives may be used to slow down the patient's respirations. A simple method of treatment for this is to have the patient breathe into a paper bag. As the patient breathes into the paper bag, the partial pressure of carbon dioxide rises in the bag and then the P_{CO_2} in the alveoli and blood also rises.

METABOLIC IMBALANCES

The probability of encountering metabolic alkalosis and acidosis is high when the nurse cares for persons with altered function of the gastrointestinal tract and accessory organs, particularly when those

TABLE 41-5 *Normal pH and mEq/L Content of Selected Gastrointestinal Fluids and the Imbalances Most Likely to Result from Significant Losses of each Type of Fluid**

Fluid	pH	Content (mEq./L.)	Likely Imbalances with Significant Losses
Gastric juice (fasting	1–3	Na^+ 60 K^+ 9 Cl^- 84	*Matabolic alkalosis* Potassium deficit Sodium deficit Fluid volume deficit
Small intestine (suction)	7.8–8.0	Na^+ 111 K^+ 5 Cl^- 104 HCO_3^- 31	*Metabolic acidosis* Potassium deficit Sodium deficit Fluid volume deficit
(Ileostomy-recent)		Na^+ 129 K^+ 11 Cl^- 116	Potassium deficit *Metabolic acidosis* Sodium deficit Fluid volume deficit
(Ileostomy-old)		Na^+ 46 K^+ 3 Cl^- 21.4	Above imbalances less likely—volume and electrolyte content of drainage markedly diminishes when ileostomy adapts
Bile (fistula)	7.8	Na^+ 149 K^+ 5 Cl^- 101 HCO_3^- 40	*Metabolic acidosis* Sodium deficit Fluid volume deficit
Pancreas (fistula)	8.0–8.3	Na^+ 141 K^+ 5 Cl^- 77 HCO_3^- 121	*Metabolic acidosis* Sodium deficit Fluid volume deficit

* Used with permission of W. B. Saunders Company from "Water and Electrolyte Balance in the Postoperative Patient." *Nurs. Clin. North Am.*, **10** (March 1975), 50, by N. A. Metheny.

alterations are treated surgically (Metheny & Snively, 1978). Table 41-5 summarizes the normal pH and mEq/L content of selected gastrointestinal fluids and indicates the most likely imbalances to result from significant losses of each type of fluid.

Summary

The volume, distribution, and concentration of water and electrolytes in the various fluid compartments result from a carefully regulated balance between intake and output. An increase in intake or output results in the initiation of mechanisms that very quickly correct any change from normal. Continued deficits in supply or failure in any of the regulatory mechanisms results in a loss of hemeostasis and disturbed cellular function. Disturbances in fluid and electrolyte balance result in disturbances in volume, osmolality, and the hydrogen ion concentration of body fluids. Fluid and electrolyte balance may become a serious problem in any sick person. It becomes a more serious problem when the illness persists or when the patient's mechanisms for adjusting to the situation are inadequate.

Disturbances in the acid–base balance or in the hydrogen ion concentration of extracellular fluids produce alterations in the ratio of carbonic acid to the bicarbonate ion in the blood plasma. In disorders of metabolic origin, the change is primarily in the level of the bicarbonate anion. In metabolic acidosis the bicarbonate anion is decreased. In metabolic alkalosis it is increased. In disorders of respiratory origin, the site of the disorder is in the carbonic acid fraction. In respiratory acidosis it is increased. In respiratory alkalosis it is decreased in relation to the bicarbonate ion.

The manifestations observed in these conditions result from (1) the compensatory responses to the condition, (2) the loss of water and electrolytes, and (3) the nature of the cause. The characteristic compensatory response is a change in the rate and depth of respiration. In metabolic acidosis, ventilation is increased by an increase in the rate and depth of respiration. In metabolic alkalosis, breathing becomes shallow. Alterations in breathing bring about rapid adjustments to changes in hydrogen ion concentration. When the disturbance continues for more than a few minutes, the kidney also participates in correcting the condition.

Problems Associated with Urination

It has been emphasized throughout this chapter that adequate renal function is critical to maintenance of fluid and electrolyte balance. An easily accessible parameter of renal function is the quality of urine secreted. One of the most frequent set of symptoms that leads people to seek medical help involves alterations in urination. Among the specific alterations of greatest concern to the nurse are changes in color of urine, inability to control micturition (urinary incontinence), and inability to urinate (urinary retention).

Changes in Color of Urine

The kidney is the primary route of excretion for most drugs. In veiw of the widespread use of both over-the-counter and prescription drugs, the nurse should always obtain a drug history from any person who describes or demonstrates a change in color of the urine. In addition, the nurse should prepare the person taking drugs which are excreted in the urine for the expected therapeutic and side effects. For example, many patients become alarmed if drugs they are taking turn their urine to unexpected colors, and they frequently will discontinue the drug in the mistaken belief that it is doing them harm. Table 41-6 summarizes changes in urine color produced by a number of drugs excreted in the urine. This information is used not only to put the person's mind at ease, but also to detect the person who may have discontinued the drug by noting that the urine has *not* changed color (DiPalma, 1977).

Urinary Incontinence

The muscles of the urinary bladder and the urethral sphincters operate in concert under the influence of both voluntary and involuntary control. Consequently, incontinence can result from any factor that interferes with effectiveness of the central or autonomic nervous systems at the level of innervation of the bladder, as well as from any factor that alters the structure or patency of the bladder and urethra. Depending upon the cause of urinary incontinence, the individual may be helped by one of the following methods: bladder training; surgery; or external catheterization. Baum (1978) describes external catheters for male children—and male adults—unable to control urination. A bowel training program is also provided by Baum for fecal incontinence. (See also the more detailed discussion of these problems in Chapters 49 and 50.)

Nurses are often admonished to refrain from using diapers to manage the problem of urinary and fecal incontinence in the adult, on the basis that the individual feels infantilized. Beber (1980) conducted a study of four methods of managing the consequences

TABLE 41-6 *Changes in Urine Color Produced by Some Drugs Excreted in the Urine**

Drug	Change in Urine Color to	Drug	Change in Urine Color to
Amitriptyline (Elavil, Etrafon, Triavil)	Blue-green (rarely)	Metronidazoie (Flagyl)	Darkens on standing (rarely)
Anthraquinone laxatives (cascara, rhubarb, senna)	Red-brown in acid urine, red in alkaline urine	Nitrofurantoin (Cyantin, Furadantin, Macrodantin)	Brown (occasionally)
Azuresin (Diagnex Blue)	Blue for 2–3 days	Phenazopyridine (Pyridium)	Orange-brown, orange-red, red
Chloroquine (Aralen)	Rusty yellow	Phenindione	Orange, which may disappear with acidification
Chlorzoxazone (Paraflex)	Orange or purple-red	Phenolphthalein (Agoral and others)	Pink-red (in alkaline urine only)
Deferoxamine masylate (Desferal)	Red	Phenolsulfonphthalein	Pink-red (in alkaline urine only)
Ethoxazene (Serenium)	Orange (occasionally)	Phenothiazine (Compazine and others)	Red (occasionally)
Furazolidone (Furoxone)	Brown (occasionally)	Phensuximide (Milontin)	Pink or red-brown
Iron sorbitex (Jectofer), iron salts	Darkens on standing	Phenytoin (Dilantin)	Pink-red or red-brown (occasionally)
Levodopa (Bendopa, Dopar, Larodopa)	Darkens on standing (occasionally)	Primaquine	Rusty yellow
Levodopa plus carbidopa (Sinemet)	Darkens on standing (occasionally)	Quinacrine (Atabrine)	Deep yellow, especially with acidification
Methocarbamol (Robaxin, Robaxisal)	Darkens on standing to brown, black, or green	Riboflavin	Deep yellow following large doses
Methyldopa (Aldoclor, Aldomet, Aldoril)	Darkens on standing (rarely) Red or brown if contaminated by hypochlorite toilet bleach	Rifampin (Rifadin, Rimactane, Rifamate, Rimactazid)	Bright red-orange
Methylene blue (M-B Tabs, Trac Tabs, Urised, Uristat, Urolene Blue)	Blue dye with yellow urine looks green	Sulfasalazine (Azulfidine)	Orange (in alkaline urine only)
		Triamterene (Dyrenium)	Pale blue fluorescence

* Information from "Drugs that Induce Changes in Urine Color." *RN*, **40** (Jan. 1977), 34–35, by J. R. DiPalma, p. 35.

of total incontinence, using 276 patients in seven Florida nursing homes. All persons in the study were classified as being *persistently incontinent*, defined as having three or more uncontrolled urinations or bowel movements per day. The four methods included use of disposable bedpads, frequent clothing and bedding changes, makeshift cloth "diapers," and a fitted disposable brief made of layered cellulose padding. Of the fifty-three persons who wore the fitted brief during the test period, only seven were judged to have had their quality of life impaired based on their objection to the idea of wearing a "diaper." Forty of the fifty-three who wore the fitted brief increased their social activities or expressed renewed confidence because the brief kept them dry. As one might predict, both nurses and aides rated the disposable brief significantly higher than conventional incontinence care on all the following qualities: protection of clothing and bedding; dryness of skin; patient comfort; convenience; ease of application; ease of removal; and odor containment (Beber, 1980). The nurse is obliged to determine whether or not the person being considered for treatment with a brief, or "diaper," will prefer the benefit of greater physical comfort to the possible disadvantage of a sense of outrage or humiliation.

URINARY RETENTION

Acute urinary retention poses a serious threat to kidney function. Despite documentation of the potential harm from abuse of urinary catheters, namely the almost certain development of urinary tract infection (UTI), urethral catheterization is mandatory in acute urinary retention. Some of the common causes of acute urinary retention include (Flanagan, 1976):

1. Mechanical obstruction of the urethra, due to such conditions as prostatic hypertrophy or swelling due to infection
2. Anorectal disease, such as hemorrhoids or abscess
3. Drugs which affect micturition, such as antihistamines and antispasmodics
4. The postoperative period, particularly following general anesthesia and/or a major or prolonged operative procedure

Signs and Symptoms of Alterations in Volume, Osmolality, and Hydrogen Ion Concentration

The characteristic signs and symptoms of alterations in volume, osmolality, and hydrogen ion concentration have been previously discussed. They are summarized here, not in relation to a specific condition, but in general terms. They include changes in (1) the patient's mental state and behavior, particularly increasing apathy, lethargy, and weakness, or restlessness and occasionally convulsions; (2) the skin—either increasing or decreasing turgor or dryness; (3) the mucous membranes—dryness in the mouth and sordes; (4) the urine output—polyuria or oliguria; (5) the concentration of urine, specific gravity—lowered, elevated, or fixed in the region of 1.010; (6) respiration—increased or decreased in rate or depth; (7) thirst—increased or absent; and (8) the blood—increased or decreased level of electrolytes and the nonprotein nitrogenous wastes as expressed by the blood urea, urea nitrogen, nonprotein nitrogen, or hematocrit. Any or all elements in the blood may be increased when additions to the blood exceed losses or when the intake or addition of water is below its output (Humes et al., 1979). The level of any substance in the blood will be decreased when the loss of that substance exceeds supply or when the addition of water is greater than its loss. For example, in renal failure, the nitrogenous wastes as well as electrolytes such as potassium and sodium tend to rise in the blood. In salt-wasting nephritis, the level of sodium cations may fall because the kidney's mechanisms for conserving sodium are defective. When water intake is insufficient, the hematocrit, hemoglobin, blood proteins, and electrolytes, as well as nitrogenous wastes, tend to rise.

In condition in which the body mechanisms are likely to need assistance in maintaining or restoring the normal character of the extracellular fluids, the blood and urine may be examined to determine the level of the various constituents. In disorders of the kidney, renal function tests are performed. In complicated cases where the results may give misleading information, other body fluids such as gastric juice may also be analyzed.

Useful Tests in Determining Fluid and Electrolyte Balance and Renal Function[7]

Blood Tests

1. The most useful tests of renal function include the *creatinine* and the *blood urea nitrogen* (BUN). Normal serum creatinine ranges from 0.8 to 1.4 mg per 100 ml. Serum level of creatinine reflects total body supply of creatine phosphate, an energy source for the contraction of muscle. Because creatinine is excreted through the healthy kidneys in quantities proportional to the serum content, elevation of serum levels above normal usually implies impaired renal function. Normal BUN ranges from 5 to 25 mg per 100 ml. Low values usually reflect expanded blood volume rather than diminished production of urea, whereas elevations usually indicate impaired renal function. Absorption of blood from the intestinal tract may raise the BUN, but seldom affects the creatinine levels in the blood.
2. *Hematocrit.* The blood is treated with an anticoagulant and centrifuged until the cells are packed in the bottom of the tube. The average range for packed cells is from 41 to 48 per cent. Increases in the hematocrit are associated with a loss of extracellular fluid. In severe burns, the hematocrit may be as high as 75 per cent. Hematocrits above 55 per cent increase the viscosity of blood enough to interfere with blood flow.
3. *Hemoglobin.* With a loss of extracellular fluid, the hemoglobin is increased in concentration. In patients whose hemoglobin is usually within the average range of 14 to 16 g per 100 ml of blood, the level may rise to 18 or 20 g. All patients on maintenance hemodialysis have a normochromic, normocytic anemia resulting from lack of erythropoietin-stimulating factor, decreased bone marrow production, and shorter survival of red cells.
4. *Levels of electrolytes in the blood plasma.* Electrolytes routinely measured include sodium, potassium, calcium, magnesium, and chloride. Significance of high and low values is best determined by serial measurements, with results

[7] This section draws heavily on F. K. Widmann. *Clinical Interpretation of Laboratory Tests,* 8th ed. Philadelphia: F. A. Davis Co., 1979.

interpreted in conjunction with clinical observations.

5. *Carbon dioxide content.* The measurement of carbon dioxide, carbonic acid, and bicarbonate of the plasma collected under oil is called carbon dioxide content. It is reported in volumes per cent, or in milligrams or milliequivalents per liter. When expressed as milliequivalents per liter, the normal range for CO_2 content is 25 to 32 mEq/L. To estimate the level of bicarbonate when CO_2 content is reported, subtract 1 from the total CO_2 content; the difference roughly approximates the bicarbonate level (Goldberger, 1975, p. 178).
6. *Carbon dioxide-combining power.* Plasma is equilibrated with air and then the carbon dioxide content is determined.
7. *The pH of arterial blood* may be determined to differentiate between respiratory acidosis and metabolic alkalosis.

Urine Tests

The urine should also be examined routinely in all patients.

1. The presence of increased quantities of red blood cells, white blood cells, protein, or sugar also may indicate renal impairment or disease. Casts of any type usually indicate some renal disease.
2. *Volume.* To retain their functional integrity, the kidneys must produce an obligatory urine volume of about 500 ml every 24 hours. This requires hourly secretion volumes of at least 20 to 25 ml per hour.
3. *The urine specific gravity* may be very useful to know, especially in the patient with oliguria. A decreased volume of urine with a high specific gravity usually implies dehydration or inadequate perfusion of the kidney. With a healthy kidney, the specific gravity decreases as the fluid intake increases. A fixed specific gravity of about 1.010 even when there is oliguria or hypovolemia indicates severe renal failure. So-called concentration tests may be performed to determine the capacity of the kidney to alter the specific gravity of the urine.
4. *pH of the urine.* Normally acid, but its pH may vary from 4.5 to 8.5, depending on the nature of the food and chemicals ingested by or administered to the patient.
5. *Presence of electrolytes in abnormal amounts or types.* For example, an absence of the sodium ion in the urine usually indicates a deficit of sodium in the body. The presence of the ketonic acids in appreciable amounts is indicative of acidosis in which the metabolism of fat is excessive.

Tests for Specific Renal Functions

1. *Measurement of filtration rate.* Glomerular filtration rate (GFR) is usually expressed in terms of clearance, a figure representing the amount of plasma from which some substance is totally cleared in 1 minute. Such clearing does not actually occur, nor could it be precisely measured if it did. Clearance is calculated from the ratio of substance excreted to the concentration of that substance in the plasma, that is, the amount available to the kidney for excretion. The amount excreted is readily measured; it is the concentration of the substance in the urine *(U)* multiplied by the volume of urine excreted in the selected time *(V)*. Dividing the amount excreted by the concentration in plasma *(P)* tells how many milliliters of plasma yielded that amount of material, assuming that each mililiter of plasma flowing through the glomerulus released all its substance into the urine. The clearance formula is $(U \times V)/P$ (Widmann, 1979, p. 556). Glomerular filtration rate can be measured by injecting a solute which is filtered by the glomeruli and which is not metabolized in the body or secreted or reabsorbed by the renal tubules. One such substance is inulin, a polysaccharide obtained from dahlia roots. Because inulin is neither reabsorbed nor secreted by the renal tubule, the quantity found in the urine is equal to the amount filtered by the glomeruli. If one knows both the quantity of urine excreted or collected per minute and the concentration of inulin in the urine and the plasma, then one can calculate the volume of plasma filtered. Because no single milliliter of plasma loses its entire complement of inulin (urea, creatinine) as it passes through the glomeruli, the results represent the volume of plasma required to provide the amount of a particular substance excreted by the kidney per minute. Metabolites such as urea and creatinine are also employed in clearance tests to estimate glomerular filtration rate. Because they are products of protein metabolism, the patient should be kept quiet during the performance of the test. In calculating the results of the test, the fact that some urea diffuses back into the blood has to be taken into account. The creatinine clearance test is not as accurate a measure of glomerular filtration as the inulin clearance test, but is more easily performed.
2. *Tests to determine the concentration and dilution powers of the kidney.* When water intake is restricted, the specific gravity of the urine should rise. When combined with a high intake of sodium and protein, it should rise above 1.025 or 1.030 and may rise as high as 1.048.

3. *Tests of the tubular transport capacity of the kidneys.* Certain materials enter the urine by both glomerular filtration and tubular secretion. Comparing this excretion against purely glomerular excretion permits estimation of tubular transport capacity. A single transport path is known to secrete phenolsulfonphthalein (PSP) and para-aminohippuric acid (PAH) into the urine, and also to transport penicillin, glucuronides, and such x-ray contrast media as Diodrast. Substances bound to plasma proteins do not pass the glomerular filter, but reach the tubules from the postglomerular interstitial circulation. The excretory rate of these substances varies with the renal blood flow and the degree of tubular function.

Some of the data required to evaluate the status of the patient's fluid and electrolyte balance have been presented. In short-term illnesses in patients whose health is essentially good, attention to the patient's desire for water may provide a satisfactory guide to fluid intake. In patients who are suffering from serious or long-term illness or whose capacity to adapt is limited, the problem of evaluating fluid and electrolyte status may be difficult and require many tests or procedures.

Objectives of Medical and Nursing Therapy

The physician has the responsibility for making the medical diagnosis and for establishing the plan of therapy. Treatment is directed toward removing the cause and supporting the body's mechanisms for correcting the disturbance. This includes not only restoring any water and electrolytes that have been lost, but also maintaining an adequate nutritional state.

The *objectives of medical therapy* will depend on the nature of the patient's disturbance. In general they will be

1. To maintain the volume of blood.
   a. Too little endangers the nutrition of the brain, kidney, and heart (all tissues).
   b. Too much overburdens the heart and circulation and predisposes to pulmonary edema.
2. To replace past and current losses of water and electrolytes.
3. To provide an intake of water of sufficient volume for the kidney to excrete the nitrogenous wastes brought to it.
4. To supply water and electrolytes in such amounts that dehydration or waterlogging of tissues and acidosis or alkalosis are prevented or corrected.

The nurse assists in the collection of the data on which the diagnosis and evaluation of effectiveness of medical therapy are based, participates in and supervises therapeutic measures, and provides comfort and support for the patient. For all patients, and most particularly those who have a chronic condition, the nurse assists in their instruction.

The *nursing objectives* include

1. To observe each patient for signs and symptoms indicating physiologic status.
2. To carry out in a safe and effective manner the procedures that have been ordered.
3. To care for the patient in such a manner that he or she is protected from unnecessary discomfort and feels safe, protected, and cared for.

The nurse is responsible for estimating the impact of the consequences of the illness and treatment on the pattern of living of the patient and family. When modifications are necessary for the comfort and safety of patient and/or family, the nurse is responsible for providing or assisting with instruction to help them in their adjustment after the patient leaves the hospital.

Risk Factors for Renal Failure

Drug-Related Risks

In assessing renal function, the nurse needs to know the patient's drug history. For example, aspirin and other nonsteroidal agents taken in anti-inflammatory doses can have a major reversible depressing effect on renal function (Kimberly & Plotz, 1977).

Extremely ill patients are at high risk for serious infection from such sources as arterial and venous catheters, indwelling urethral catheters, hypostatic pneumonia, and cross-infection. Treatment of infections when renal function is impaired is complicated by the fact that all antimicrobial agents are normally excreted in the urine. An important aspect of ongoing assessment of the person whose renal function is jeopardized is estimation of glomerular filtration rate (GFR) (Ziment & Koppel, 1976). Table 41-7 summarizes the purpose and significance of various levels of three tests commonly performed to estimate renal function: blood urea nitrogen (BUN), serum creatinine, and creatinine clearance.

Particularly in seriously ill patients with marginal renal function and potentially lethal infections, the selection of an antibiotic to treat an infection is based on benefit-toxicity ratios. Knowledge of which drugs are capable of inducing renal damage is vital to pre-

TABLE 41-7. ***Tests for Clinical Estimation of Renal Function****

A clinical estimate of renal function—specifically, of glomerular filtration—can be obtained by measuring a patient's blood urea nitrogen (BUN), serum creatinine, or creatinine clearance. Serum creatinine and BUN levels are determined primarily by endogenous production and renal excretion rates.

Parameter	Value for Assessing Renal Function	Severity of Renal Failure: Normal Renal Function	Moderate Renal Insufficiency	Severe Renal Insufficiency
BUN	Protein intake, caloric balance, hepatic function, and catabolic state may all affect endogenous production of BUN independently of renal function. Therefore, BUN provides a poor estimate of renal function.	5–25 mg%		
Serum creatinine	The rate of endogenous production depends on muscle mass, which varies with a patient's age, sex, and weight. But because endogenous creatinine production is usually constant for any individual patient, changes in serum creatinine provide a more accurate estimate of renal function than does BUN.	<1.5 mg%	1.5 to 5 mg%	>5 mg%
Creatinine clearance	The volume of blood cleared of creatinine by the kidney per unit of time is directly proportional to the glomerular filtration rate (GFR) and thus more accurately indicates renal function than do serum creatinine levels alone. In severe renal failure, total creatinine clearance is actually somewhat higher than that due to glomerular filtration, because at high serum levels creatinine is also eliminated by tubular secretion to a significant degree.	>80 ml/min	15 to 80 ml/min	<15 ml/min
Urine creatinine		14 to 26 mg/kg/day	14 to 26 mg/kg/day	When the patient is in a steady state, the rate of creatinine excretion equals the rate of production and remains constant even in renal failure. Under such circumstances serum creatinine remains stable. In the acute phase of renal failure or the end stage of chronic renal failure, however, creatinine excretion falls well below production, and serum creatinine rises.

* This table is adapted from "Antimicrobials when Kidneys Can't Cope," by I. Ziment & M. H. J. Koppel. *Current Prescribing,* (Aug. 1976), 32–43, table on p. 33.

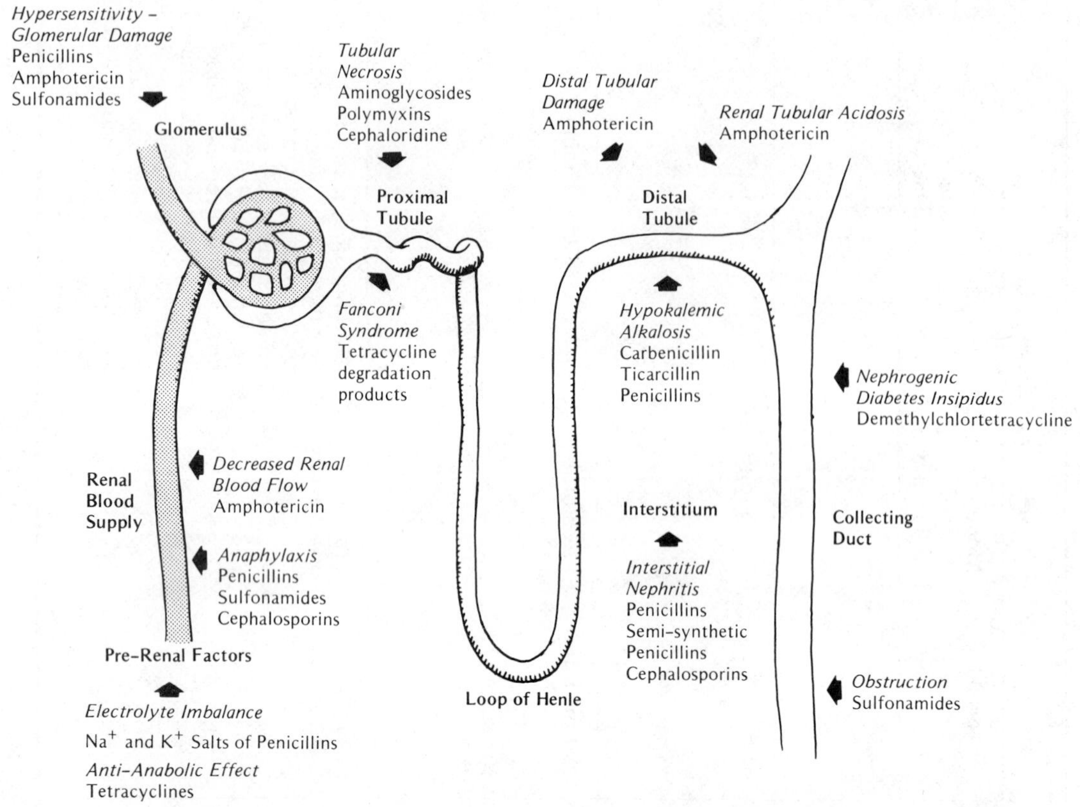

Figure 41-5. Nephrotoxic sites of antimicrobial agents. (Used with permission of the Massachusetts Medical Society, from The nephrotoxicity of antimicrobial agents. *N. Engl. J. Med.* 296:663–70, Mar. 24, 1977, by G. B. Appel & H. C. Neu, Fig. 1, p. 665.)

venting and detecting such damage. The nephrotoxic sites of some commonly used antimicrobial agents are shown in Figure 41-5.

Renovascular Hypertension

Surgical treatment of renovascular hypertension may be directed toward removing or by-passing an obstruction, thus revascularizing the kidney, or toward removing the kidney if the cause of hypertension is extensive irreversible intrarenal pathology (Novick & Stewart, 1979).

Renovascular, or "renin-dependent," hypertension has commonly been treated by renal vascular surgery and pharmacotherapy, singly or in combination. Although both have been used successfully, both have drawbacks and a substantial failure rate. Drug therapy has the disadvantages of a high rate of poor compliance and drug side effects. In addition, antihypertensive medications do not improve renal perfusion, and consequently may contribute to progressive loss of renal function (Millan et al., 1979). For renovascular hypertension associated with renal artery stenosis, excellent results have recently been obtained by dilating the stenosed renal artery by percutaneous transluminal angioplasty. Relief of renal artery obstruction is followed by improved perfusion of the kidney, suppression of renin secretion, and reduction of blood pressure to normal (Grüntzig et al., 1978).

Williams and Hollenberg (1977) demonstrated that renal perfusion can be markedly improved in persons with essential hypertension by administration of an angiotensin-converting enzyme inhibitor. Actions by which renal perfusion is believed to be effected with this class of agent include

1. Antagonism of the conversion of angiotensin I to angiotensin II
2. Generation of an increase in the plasma and tissue concentrations of the vasodilator, bradykinin (Hollenberg et al., 1979)

Renal Failure

Disturbances in water and electrolyte balance can result from disorders in gastrointestinal, respiratory, circulatory, or renal function. The first three are discussed in detail in other chapters and will not be further considered here. As are other organs, the kidney is subject to a variety of diseases that, depending on their extent and nature, reduce renal reserve or result in renal failure. Because one half of one kidney contains enough tissue to perform the ordinary functions of the kidney, there may be considerable kidney damage before evidence of renal failure develops. When one kidney is healthy, the other one can be safely removed. The manifestations accompanying renal disease depend on the nature of the cause and the extent to which renal function is impaired. For example, bacterial infections of the kidney are accompanied by signs and symptoms of infection. Whether or not renal failure occurs depends on the extent to which nephrons are destroyed by the infectious process or by the healing process. Disorders of the glomeruli usually render them more permeable to constituents of the blood. In nephroses, profuse amounts of protein are lost into the urine because the glomerular capillaries become permeable to protein. Because large quantities of protein are lost in the urine, blood protein level may fall. Many of the other manifestations observed in the nephrotic patient are due to the effects of the low blood protein. In acute glomerular nephritis, the kidney is hyperemic; some glomeruli rupture, and blood escapes into the urine.

Just before or after the renal artery enters the hilus of the kidney, it divides into a series of branches. Abnormalities in the branching of a renal artery may obstruct a ureter and impede the drainage of urine from the renal pelvis. In general, the veins draining the kidney follow a pattern similar to that of the arteries. Any condition that interferes with adequate blood flow to the kidney predisposes to renal failure. Among the conditions that may impair renal blood flow are blood loss and/or hypotension, and occlusions of the aorta at or above the origin of the renal arteries because of such factors as thrombi, emboli, and atheromatous plaques.

Acute Renal Failure

Prolonged ischemia of the kidneys or agents toxic to the kidneys may cause tubular necrosis. Whether the cause is tubular or vascular factors, tubular necrosis usually results in acute renal failure and is manifested by oliguria or anuria and rapidly developing azotemia (Levinsky, 1977).

Although many of the consequences of renal failure have been included in the discussion of water and electrolyte balance, they merit discussion and emphasis here. Renal failure may develop suddenly from prolonged ischemia of the kidney or from the effect of nephrotoxic agents. Nursing care of persons in acute renal failure is presented in relation to Mrs. Murray, a patient who responded to conservative therapy. She suffered an acute renal shutdown as the result of transfusion with about 400 ml of incompatible blood. At the time she was admitted to Hospital X for possible hemodialysis, she had been severely oliguric for 2 days. It is well to remember that even in severe renal failure, a few milliliters of urine are excreted. If there is absolutely no urine, one wonders if the renal vessels, ureters, or urethra is blocked. Blood studies and electrocardiogram indicated that Mrs. Murray had some elevation of potassium, but was not in any immediate danger. She was placed on strict bedrest; ice chips not to exceed 200 ml in 24 hours; a diet composed of glucose and Crisco; and daily weight, electrocardiogram, and blood specimens for potasium, sodium, and urea. A polyethylene catheter was introduced into the saphenous vein. It was to be kept patent with a 10 per cent solution of glucose. A micro set was used in order to minimize the quantity of solution required. An indwelling catheter was introduced, so that all urine excreted could be collected. Her total fluid intake was kept at about 500 ml plus additional volume equal to her urine output. Fortunately for Mrs. Murray, on the fifth day following the onset of oliguria, she started to excrete increasing amounts of urine. Because the ability to concentrate urine does not return as rapidly as the ability to excrete water, the urine had a low specific gravity. Despite a marked increase in the volume of urine, Mrs. Murray's blood potassium and urea did not begin to fall for a few days. During the initial period of diuresis, Mrs. Murray was carefully observed for any indication of electrolyte imbalance. Either hypo- or hypernatremia could have occurred. Neither developed. Sometimes diuresis is so extreme that the patient requires a large fluid intake. Fortunately for Mrs. Murray, her kidney function was restored rapidly enough so that hemodialysis was not required.

Mrs. Murray's nursing care was directed toward trying to make it possible for her to achieve a maximum amount of rest. Because activity increases the rate of metabolism, she was given complete care. She was turned and rubbed every 2 hours and encouraged to lie quietly. Because of the nature of her diet and limitations on her fluid intake, she was given special mouth care every 4 hours. The ice chips were divided over the 24-hour period. Because the rate of flow of the intravenous solution was important, this was noted at hourly or more frequent intervals. Strict control of fluid intake so that it does not exceed output by more than 500 ml is one of the most important aspects of the patient's care. Unless this is done, the patient may die from the effects of overhydration. Because Mrs. Murray was from out of town, she had no visitors except her husband and the hospital chaplain. Both Mr. and Mrs. Murray were concerned about the possible outcome of her illness. Nurses and physicians were aware of their concern. They encouraged Mrs. Murray's hopes and were sympathetic to her feelings of uncertainty. Through attention to meeting her immediate needs, they were able to minimize her discomfort and to convey to her that everyone was concerned about her welfare.

Not all patients in acute renal failure are as fortunate as Mrs. Murray. Recovery of the kidney may be slow and the levels of potassium in the blood may be elevated to the point of toxicity. In this event, the level of potassium and the nonprotein nitrogenous wastes in the blood may be lowered by the methods previously indicated or by hemo- or peritoneal dialysis. These procedures have other uses as well. One or the other may be utilized to remove ingested poisons such as barbiturates, salicylates, bromides, and other drugs. Dialysis procedures will be described in this chapter.

Renal failure more commonly develops slowly over the course of months and years from the effects of ischemia secondary to disease of the arterioles or arteries supplying them, from infection of kidney tissue, or from other causes. Whatever the cause or causative factors of renal failure in a given patient, the presenting signs and symptoms are due to the effect on all the organ systems of the body of the *inability of the kidney to maintain the composition and volume of body fluids.* The eventual prognosis of the patient depends on the cause of the renal failure as well as his or her ability to prevent hyperkalemia, hypertensive encephalopathy, and congestive heart failure, all of which may complicate renal failure. When the degree of injury to the kidney is such that too little renal tissue remains to perform the functions of the kidney, many patients can still be helped to lead a reasonably comfortable existence for a time by proper medical management.

The syndrome resulting from functional failure of the kidney is known as uremia or azotemia. The term *uremia* is the older and means, literally, urine in the blood. The term *azotemia* has a more limited meaning inasmuch as it refers to the presence of excessive quantities of nitrogenous compounds in the blood. The manifestations of uremia are due to the effects of the failure of the kidney to regulate the volume and composition of body fluids in total bodily functioning. As in other chronic diseases, much can now be done by appropriate medical management to extend the length of the patient's useful life.

Chronic Renal Failure (The Uremic Syndrome)

In contrast to the rapidly developing threat to life that characterizes nonspecific acute renal failure, the manifestations accompanying chronic renal failure are that the patient may be aware only of tiring more easily than formerly and having some degree of muscular weakness. The patient seeks medical attention because he or she does not feel well and may not have felt healthy or energetic for some time. Other systemic effects of chronic renal failure include increased susceptibility to infection and delayed wound healing. In children, growth and development may be retarded.

Among the most disagreeable effects of the uremic syndrome are those on the alimentary tract, as the patient experiences anorexia, nausea, and vomiting. These symptoms may be so severe that they are precipitated by the smell, sight, or even thought of food. When they are marked, they lead to marked emaciation as a consequence of failure to ingest sufficient food to meet the caloric needs of the tissues.

Nausea and vomiting can be controlled by antiemetic drugs such as chlorpromazine or one of the other phenothiazines. Every effort should be made to encourage the patient to try to eat. Some patients desire special foods and will try to eat if they are provided with them.

Particularly in advanced stages of the uremic syndrome, the breath has an ammoniacal or uriniferous odor that limits the ability of the patient to taste food. Some patients find foods with a definite taste more acceptable than bland ones. For example, Mr. Thomas, who was in the terminal phase of the uremic syndrome, requested canned clams. He could taste them because they have a strong and pungent taste. The classic fishy odor of the breath of a person in uremia has been demonstrated to reflect the systemic accumulation of potentially toxic volatile metabolities, two of which have been positively identified–dimethylamine and trimethylamine, amines which appear to be generated by the action of intestinal bacteria on choline. Treatment with nonabsorbable antibiotics has reduced breath amine levels (Simenhoff et al., 1977). The resulting improvement in breath odor has little significance for the person's uremic state, but it improves comfort and one's sense of acceptability to others.

In the later stages of uremia, ulcerations along the gastrointestinal tract are common. In the mouth they are associated with stomatitis (inflammation of the soft tissues of the mouth). Ulcerations in the stomach or more distal portions of the alimentary canal may lead to gastrointestinal bleeding. Although mouth care should be given regularly, the tissues should be treated with gentleness. Vomitus as well as feces should be observed for blood.

As the uremic syndrome develops, functioning of the nervous system is altered. In the early stages, the patient may be irritable. Later as the disorder progresses, he or she becomes apathetic, drowsy, and eventually comatose. Long-acting barbiturates and other drugs excreted by the kidney should be avoided. Muscular weakness and twitching, neuralgic or neuritic pains, headache and dizziness may be observed. In patients in whom there is some degree of hypertensive encephalopathy, failing vision or even blindness occurs.

Effects on the respiratory system are due to congestive heart failure as well as to metabolic acidosis. Dyspnea occurs as a result of the congestive heart failure, and Kussmaul breathing as a result of the acidosis.

Many of the manifestations referable to the circulatory system are caused by the hypertension accompanying renal disease. Some are, however, due to the effects of the failure of the kidney to regulate the composition and volume of the blood. The effects of hyperkalemia on the contractility of the myocardium have been previously discussed. In addition, purpura develops as a result of increased capillary fragility and alteration in the clotting mechanism. A marked and progressive anemia develops as a consequence of hemolysis and failure of hematopoiesis. Uremic pericarditis may cause precordial pain and a friction rub, or tamponade.

Changes in the skeleton include osteomalacia in the adult and rickets in the child.

The skin is also affected. One of the earliest symptoms is pruritus. The pruritus may be intense, leading to extensive self-inflicted excoriation of the skin. The severe, persistent pruritus associated with end-stage renal disease (ESRD) has been relieved within 2 to 3 weeks by safe, convenient, inexpensive, and effective treatment with ultraviolet phototherapy, using the conventional sunburn-spectrum (Gilchrest et al., 1977). Later after the level of nonprotein nitrogenous substances in the blood becomes very high, uremic frost can be seen on the skin. The white crystals are more easily seen in areas where perspiration is most abundant, such as around the mouth. They can and should be removed by bathing.

Because the composition and volume of body fluids depend on adequate renal function, the uremic patient often presents many problems, including (1) malnutrition, (2) anemia, (3) water and electrolyte imbalance, (4) hypertensive vascular disease, and (5) circulatory failure.

In nursing the patient who is in some phase of renal failure, attention should be given to the maintenance of physiologic status as well as to the patient's general comfort. Inasmuch as physiologic status can be supported, the patient's feelings of well-being will be improved. Eventually the patient becomes dependent on others to meet most if not all of his or her needs. He or she should be observed for evidence of changes in condition, and care should be modified accordingly.

In addition to measures specifically directed toward the alleviation of specific symptoms of renal failure, two other types of procedures may be of benefit to the patient. The first is a low-protein diet. The second is either hemodialysis or peritoneal dialysis.

Low-Protein Diet

Dietary intake of protein for a person with serious renal disease presents special problems. For maintenance of lean body mass, the daily intake of protein should be 1 to 1.5 gm/kg of ideal body weight, based on height and age. An adequate protein intake is reflected by a BUN serum creatinine ratio of 10:1 (Luke, 1979).

Excessive protein intake results in nausea and vomiting, apathy, weakness, increased BUN, and increased gastrointestinal and neurologic symptoms. Insufficient protein results in lowered serum albumin, muscle wasting, edema, and weight loss. Food choices should be of high biological protein value, that is, they should contain all essential amino acids for growth and repair of tissue, as are found in fish, foul, meat, eggs, and milk. Ample calories from carbohydrates and fats that do not require renal excretion of their metabolic by-products spare protein for growth and repair. The breakdown of calories should be about 15 per cent protein, 35 per cent fat, and 50 per cent carbohydrates. Since hyperlipoproteinemia is associated with some renal diseases, unsaturated fats are advised (Luke, 1979).

In the early stage of renal disease, most patients will instinctively limit protein intake. Moderate restriction to 40 to 60 g of protein a day is all that is required. As renal failure progresses, medical management aims at restricting dietary protein enough to prevent elevation of serum creatinine above 4 to 5 mg per 100 ml, and high enough to ensure the minimum 0.5 g of protein per kilogram per day needed to maintain positive nitrogen balance (Atkins et al., 1971). Protein restriction alone cannot lengthen the life of a person with end-stage renal disease. As soon as the patient shows the first sign of clinical deterioration, such as inability to perform his or her usual work or the development of neuropathy, some form of dialysis must be started (Atkins et al., 1971).

Dialysis

The last two decades have brought dramatic change in the outlook for some patients in renal failure. Significant progress has been made in regulating the composition and volume of extracellular fluids by hemo- and peritoneal dialysis. The general principles and facts on which hemo- and peritoneal dialysis are based and the main problems associated with each will be presented. No attempt will be made to describe either in detail.

Both hemo- and peritoneal dialysis are based on the principle that a substance present in different concentrations on two sides of a semipermeable membrane moves from the side of the greater to that of the lesser concentration. If the process is continued, the concentration of the substance will eventually be equalized on the two sides of the membrane. Either procedure can perform most of the kidney's functions. They can remove the wastes of protein metabolism and restore acid–base and electrolyte balance (Rosenberg, 1972, p. 7).

Dialysis fluid usually contains sodium chloride, sodium acetate (or bicarbonate),[8] calcium chloride, potassium chloride, and dextrose. Dextrose is used to maintain the osmolality between 280 and 310 m0sm/L, with higher concentrations being used when excess water has to be removed from the patient. All of the salts are added in concentrations equal to or less than their physiologic blood levels. Potassium salts are eliminated completely from the dialysis fluid with hyperkalemic patients (Rosenberg, 1972). Dialysis is usually continued for 4 to 8 hours or until the constituents in the blood are restored to normal or near-normal levels.

When dialysis was first introduced the procedure was performed by, and under continuous supervision of, a physician. With experience and improved equipment, more and more responsibility has been delegated to nurses and technicians and finally to patients and/or the members of their families. In 1972, one study estimated that about 60 per cent of patients hospitalized for treatment of end-stage renal disease were placed on home dialysis, at an annual cost of approximately $8,500 for three 6-hour treatments a week. When these treatments were performed in the hospital, the bill exceeded $20,000 annually. The average span of survival for persons on maintenance dialysis was 5 years (Brunto et al., 1972).

[8] If sodium bicarbonate is used, lactic acid may be added to adjust the pH to 7.4.

A major factor in reducing the cost of dialysis done in the home is that the number of personnel can be reduced by one third when the patient is treated at home. Home treatment has a further advantage because a patient can be treated three times instead of twice in a week. The success of home treatment depends on thorough training of the patient and appropriate supervision by the physician. Successful care of the patient also includes the nurse who prepares the patient to go home and the one who follows his or her progress at home.

One method of increasing the independence of the person requiring dialysis is a new technique of continuous ambulatory peritoneal dialysis (CAPD). The major problem with this procedure, which is highly acceptable to patients, is a high incidence of peritonitis, probably due to breaks in aseptic technique when the individual changes the reservoir and handles the peritoneal tube (Sorrels, 1979).

Hemodialysis

Currently hemodialysis is being used to (1) tide the patient over a period of acute renal failure, (2) remove toxic substances normally excreted by the kidney, (3) prepare the patient for a renal transplant, (4) maintain the composition of the blood following renal transplant until the new kidney functions well, and (5) prolong the life of the patient in chronic renal failure.

In hemodialysis, blood is circulated through cellophane tubing similar to that used for sausage casing. It is permeable to ions and molecules of small size, usually molecules with a molecular weight less than 15,000, and impermeable to large molecules such as protein, some viruses, and bacteria. These characteristics of the tubing simplify the procedure, because they allow ordinary nonsterile tap water to be used to bathe the tubing through which the blood is circulated. The tubing is placed on a device suspended in a tank of water to which is added sufficient glucose and electrolytes to make it isotonic with normal blood plasma. Most machines no longer need to be primed with bank blood, which can be the source of many complications, including hepatitis.

It is projected that by 1982 there will be 51,000 chronic hemodialysis patients (Bauer, 1980). Outbreaks of hepatitis B have become more common among both hemodialysis patients and staff, with nurses being at the highest risk among staff for acquiring hepatitis B. Strict infection-control measures, including aseptic and isolation techniques, are required to reduce this hazard. See Bauer (1980) for a description of some procedures that have been shown to reduce the risk to patients and staff of infection with hepatitis B.

THE SHUNT. One advance that has made repeated

hemodialysis practical is the tube or shunt connecting an artery and vein in an extremity; this is often referred to as a Scribner shunt. It is U-shaped; one arm of the shunt is implanted in an artery and the other in a vein, in an arm or leg. The center portion can be removed. The arterial tube is attached to a tube leading into the dialysis machine. The venous tube is attached to a tube carrying blood back from the machine to the patient. At the completion of the procedure the central portion of the tube is replaced and the blood again flows through the shunt from the artery directly to the vein.

The principal problems associated with the shunt are infection and blood clotting. Either may make repeated cannulation necessary. To lessen the possibility of infection, implantation of the shunt should be performed as a surgical procedure in the operating room. Following its implantation the area around it should be kept clean and dry. As a preliminary step in the prevention of clotting, heparin may be placed in the tubing near its insertion in the artery. Attention should be given to prevention of kinking of the tubing.

NURSING RESPONSIBILITIES. In the performance of her or his role, the nurse should be guided by the fact that all material and equipment with which the blood comes in contact must be kept sterile. Provisions should be made for the taking of blood samples. The patient should be prepared for what to expect and what is expected of him or her. Exactly what is taught to the patient depends on whether hemodialysis is used to relieve an acute or a chronic condition and whether or not the patient has previously experienced dialysis. Under all circumstances the patient should be included in any conversation carried on in his or her presence. Both the patient and family should be kept informed of progress. This is particularly important when the procedure is being performed for the first time. Because the procedure usually takes from 4 to 8 hours, attention should be given to the patient's comfort. If the patient is required to lie on his or her back throughout the procedure, the backrest may be elevated slightly. Passive exercises should be instituted and performed regularly. With the use of the shunt, the patient is usually free to move about as long as the arm or leg with the shunt does not move excessively.

Hemodialysis is not a cure, and a number of complications attend its long-term use, among them the well-known hazards of hypotension, hepatitis, circulatory overload, hypertension, anemia, cerebral edema and intracranial hemorrhage, peripheral neuropathy, and renal osteodystrophy. In addition, as experience accumulates with more patients receiving maintenance hemodialysis over longer periods of time, more subtle hazards are being identified. For example, recent reports of low SGOT (serum glutamic oxalacetic transaminase) levels in long-term dialysis patients may be due either to GOT adhering to dialyzer coils or to washout of vitamin B_6, a coenzyme of GOT (Outlook, 1973).

Peritoneal Dialysis

The general principles, objectives, and uses of peritoneal dialysis are similar to those of hemodialysis. Isotonic solutions of electrolytes are introduced into and removed from the peritoneal cavity. As the fluid bathes the peritoneal membrane, substances to which the membrane is permeable diffuse into the fluid. Although they diffuse in both directions, the net transfer is in the direction of lower concentration. Peritoneal dialysis has the advantage of not requiring any blood. Peritoneal dialysis can be carried on intermittently or continuously to maintain the concentration of substances normally removed by the kidney at physiologic levels. Because the peritoneal cavity is entered, there is danger of peritonitis and adhesions.

Several of the advantages of peritoneal dialysis over hemodialysis are that the treatment (1) can go on while the patient sits in a chair or walks around; (2) allows most patients to learn the procedure well enough within the first six sessions (about 2 weeks of hospitalization) to continue dialysis at home; (3) provides a gentler return to the normal state for initial treatment of renal failure in the very ill patient; (4) allows time for a decision on initiation of hemodialysis, and provides a means for holding patients awaiting a vacancy in available hemodialysis services; (5) provides a simpler and safer procedure for people either overwhelmed by the mechanical aspects of hemodialysis and or who dialyze at home alone; and, (6) because of its simplicity, can be learned by any nurse in an emergency (Rae & Pendray, 1973). A significant disadvantage of peritoneal dialysis is that it is more expensive than hemodialysis because of the high cost of large volumes of commercially prepared sterile dialysate. Diet following initiation of peritoneal dialysis should be permissive enough to encourage the patient to eat, because malnutrition is frequently a problem. Water intake is restricted only if serum osmolality falls markedly; sodium intake is restricted only when hypertension is difficult to control or if edema is marked; and protein intake is encouraged to aid wound healing, reduce the risk of infection, and improve the patient's morale (Rae & Pendray, 1973).

Choice of Kidney Transplantation

The nature and special problems of transplantation, as the most recent and hopeful treatment for end-stage renal disease, are discussed with other organ transplants in Chapter 24. Its availability requires renewed emphasis among health professionals on the *informed consent* of patients.

Nowhere is the concept of *informed consent* more critical than in the treatment of end-stage renal failure. One physician who had undergone chronic renal failure, dialysis, and multiple transplants urged that dialysis and transplantation be considered complementary forms of therapy, and that the patient be helped to give *truly informed consent* to one or the other, or both. He suggested that the patient be helped to decide which form of treatment he or she could best adapt to by examining the long-term requirements, constraints, and complications of each. Only then can the patient decide which form of treatment best fits the quality of life valued most by the patient, rather than by the physician. Eloquent testimony to the need for greater attention to the values of the patient is evident in the case of an 18-year-old guitarist who, after a successful transplant, stopped taking steroids because "they puff up my face" and made him unattractive on the bandstand. As a result, he lost the kidney, refused hemodialysis, and died (Calland, 1972).

The patient who is trying to decide between chronic dialysis and renal transplantation needs to know about the risks involved in each. The person considering kidney transplant has usually been maintained on dialysis, and knows well its benefits and disadvantages. Transplantation problems may be considered as renal-related and extrarenal complications (Kobrzycki, 1977):

Renal-related	Extrarenal (primarily due to immunosuppressive and/or steroid drug therapy)
Rejection of the donor kidney	Infection
Technical failures	Gastrointestinal bleeding
Acute tubular necrosis (ATN)	Hepatitis
Recurrent nephritis	Pancreatitis
	Psychological problems

Costs of Treatment for End-Stage Renal Disease

Since 1973, under the provisions of Public Law 92-603, Medicare coverage has provided for financing of treatment for people suffering from end-stage renal disease (ESRD). But the economic and social costs of ESRD can far exceed the provisions of Medicare coverage. A young couple reporting on their 4½ years of experience with dialysis and transplantation treatment for the husband found that Medicare paid only 53 per cent of the total costs; 29 per cent of over $48,000—the total cost of 4½ years of treatment—was not covered by either Medicare or private insurance (Campbell & Campbell, 1978).

By 1984, more than 55,000 patients in the United States will be on dialysis treatment for ESRD, with over 5,200 likely to receive transplants. Medical services alone for these patients will cost over $3 billion in 1984 (Guttmann, 1979, p. 975).

In 1979, the Health Care Financing Administration of the Department of Health, Education, and Welfare issued new regulations to encourage patients to seek home dialysis services instead of more costly hospital dialysis. The new regulations also encourage patients to seek a transplantation when medically feasible (*HEW Encourages Home Dialysis*, 1979). One small case-control study has documented that the first year of home dialysis for ESRD is actually more expensive than the first year of renal transplant treatment. Of even greater significance were the data on rehabilitation: all patients on home dialysis had been fully rehabilitated at the conclusion of the 5-year study, whereas only two thirds of the transplant patients had been rehabilitated (Guttmann, 1979, p. 1044). The conflicts and ambivalence experienced by persons having to make choices about treatment for ESRD require skillful assistance from the nurse and other members of the health team to formulate and face the profound ethical dilemmas involved.

What are the Causes of Renal Failure

Nearly 8 million persons in the United States are afflicted with kidney diseases and diseases related to the kidney each year. Deaths resulting from renal disease have dropped due in large part to advances in, and availability of, dialysis and renal transplant. However, renal disease deaths are substantially underreported; many deaths attributed to hypertension or septicemia are traceable to underlying renal lesions. But perhaps more important for nursing than the contribution of kidney disease to our mortality statistics is the fact that kidney disease ranked fifth in its contribution to the total estimated expenditure on health in the United States in 1965. Individuals with kidney-related diseases suffered almost 140 million days of bed disability, and roughly 16 million lost work days in 1965, totalling a cost of $1.21 billion, or 5.4 per cent of the total national health expenditure for 1965.[9]

Among the many conditions or events that may result in renal insufficiency requiring dialysis to sustain life are polycystic kidneys, lupus nephritis, hereditary nephritis, diabetic nephropathy, and traumatic injury to one or both kidneys. But the three disease processes that account for the major portion of patients who require dialysis for renal failure are glomerulonephritis, chronic pyelonephritis, and malignant nephrosclerosis (Rosenberg, 1972, p. 23). Further details about disorders of the kidney that are likely to lead to renal failure are summarized in Table 41-8.

If the nurse is to make intelligent observations and take appropriate actions related to the fluid and electrolyte status of patients in end-stage renal disease, she or he must have knowledge about disorders that may lead to renal failure. Many of the details about the disorders listed in Table 41-8 have not been included in the summary. Among them are the particular hazards to which each exposes the patient. In the section on acute glomerular nephritis that follows, the role of the nurse in anticipating and identifying evidence of developing cardiac failure or of hypertensive encephalopathy in the child or young adult with acute glomerular nephritis is outlined. Although acute glomerular nephritis is more common among children, it can and does occur in young adults. Although the following section deals with the nursing implications of a condition found predominantly in children, the author has exquisitely characterized the concurrent knowledge, sensitivity, and skill called forth from the nurse in caring for patients with end-stage renal disease, whatever the cause and whatever their age.

Acute Glomerular Nephritis[10]

Every year, especially in the springtime, nurses who are serving in medical units of children's hospitals or in the pediatric departments of general hospitals care for patients suffering from acute glomerular nephritis. Some years there are more children than in other years, but always there are several. Usually, they are from 4 to 7 years old. Although sometimes a child is very sick, often the patients are not much bothered by their symptoms. More than 95 times out of 100 they recover completely, often after little in the way of specific treatment. But of the four or five for whom this is not the happy outcome, two or three may die quite promptly. These children usually die of heart failure or hypertensive encephalopathy, which develops rapidly indeed, but not as a rule without a few signs to herald its coming. Lack of treatment that was available but not instituted because the approaching demand for it was not recognized in time by those present may be the cause for much sadness, as well as for resentment, anger, and guilt—and the child's life is lost to society.

The significant point may be found in the inference that the progression of symptoms in the child usually gives some clues to the prepared observer. The observer who is prepared both to recognize and comprehend their meaning may use these clues to the patient's advantage. A hospital unit that admits acutely sick children may be expected to have one or more professional nurses there at all hours, even though physicians may not always be at hand. These nurses should be prepared observers, able to evaluate what they see in the sick child on the basis, not just of their general knowledge of children, but of an understanding of what changes are induced in the body by acute glomerular nephritis and in what manner these changes may quickly embarrass the essential welfare of the patient. Nurses who can go this far will not often fail to take the next steps to benefit the child—acting on the orders already available and procuring the physician promptly to meet the critical medical needs of the child.

Although most children recover from acute glomerular nephritis without evident permanent injury to the kidneys, the changes that occur incident to the damaging inflammation are considerable, and the effects at the time may be severe. The sequence often starts a week or two after sore throat caused by infection with group A beta-hemolytic streptococcus type 12.[11] Toxin from the streptococcus provokes pathologic changes that have been revealed by the electron microscope in recent years. Briefly, the changes are as follows: The host produces antibody capable of reacting with this toxin (antigen), and immune complexes that are globulins result. These are laid down as nodular deposits on the epithelial side of the basement membrane of the glomerular capillary. Complement attracts leukocytes that curl up the endothelium and increase its permeability. In the inflamed capillaries there is a proliferation of*

[9] Based on analysis and interpretation of available morbidity and mortality statistics by J. C. Rosenberg, Professor of Surgery, Wayne State University, Detroit, Mich., in an unpublished proposal for a Renal Transplantation Program, 1972, p. 10.

[10] This portion of the chapter was contributed by Esther H. Read, A.B., M.Ed., R.N. Emeritus Professor of Nursing, College of Nursing, Wayne State University, Detroit, Michigan.

* (Text continues on page 775.)

[11] Although the most common causative agent of acute glomerulonephritis (AGN) is group A beta-hemolytic streptococcus, a milder form can follow infections such as (Juliani, 1979) *S. pneumoniae*, *Staphylococcus*, syphilis, toxoplasmosis, varicella, mumps, infectious mononucleosis, hepatitis B, or malaria.

TABLE 41-8. *Disorders of the Kidney that Are Common Causes of Renal Failure*

Classification	Etiology	Nature of Onset	Severity and Course of Illness	Structures Involved, Primary Disease	Major Manifestations	Major Medical or Surgical Therapy
I. Bilateral inflammatory diseases of the kidney						
A. Glomerulonephritis 1. Acute	Most frequently associated with preceding infections caused by group A beta-hemolytic streptococcus. Not a bacterial infection but an antigen–antibody reaction damaging the glomeruli. Most common in childhood and young adults but may occcur at any age	Classically, an abrupt onset occurring 1 to 4 weeks after an attack of pharyngitis or scarlatina (scarlet fever)	Evidence of healing occurs within 3 weeks. Most patients go on to complete recovery. A few die during the acute phase of the disease or progress into the subacute or chronic phase	Diffuse exudation and proliferative inflammation of the kidney glomeruli	1. Puffy eyes, swelling of feet and ankles, shortness of breath 2. Signs of congestive heart failure often prominent 3. Albuminuria 4. Hematuria. Urine may be smoky 5. Oliguria which may progress to anuria 6. Hypertension. Some degree is a common occurrence. When severe, may precipitate cardiac failure or cerebral manifestations 7. Headache 8. Malaise—abdominal pain may be colicky or steady 9. Anorexia, nausea, and vomiting 10. May be moderate to severe aching in lumbar regions 11. About one half of hospitalized patients have normal renal function. Others have some degree of retention of nitrogenous wastes	1. Treatment of infection with group A streptococci by penicillin. Penicillin is of no value unless streptococci are present 2. Bedrest until gross hematuria, edema, and hypertension have disappeared 3. Nutrition. With evidence of impaired renal function and oliguria, edema, or heart failure, intake of protein, sodium, and potassium is restricted 4. Fluid intake. In presence of oliguria, intake may be restricted. If nausea and vomiting, intake may be more liberal 5. Antihypertensive therapy. When hypertension and headaches are severe, drugs such as hydralazine hydrochloride, reserpine, or a combination of the two may be administered parenterally 6. Antiuremia therapy

2. Chronic	Failure of kidneys to heal following an attack of acute glomerulonephritis. An occasional strong familial predisposition is found	Following a latent phase that may persist for as long as 20 to 30 years or even longer. Patient develops evidence of renal failure		Few signs and symptoms of renal insufficiency until renal function falls below 20 per cent or less of normal. Inflammatory changes and scarring of the glomerular tufts	12. In renal failure, hyperkalemia (elevated blood potassium) 13. Mild anemia frequently occurs *Onset of renal failure* 1. Oliguria 2. Elevated blood urea nitrogen 3. Anemia 4. Weakness, nausea, and somnolence if oliguria persists 5. Hypertension and cardiovascular complications 6. Electrolyte abnormalities *Nephrotic syndrome or phase*—occurs sometime before death in one half of patients 1. Heavy loss of protein in urine—exceeding 5 g daily 2. Hypoalbuminemia 3. Hypercholesterolemia 4. Edema *Advanced and terminal glomerulonephritis* See discussion of renal failure	*Latent phase*—none See discussion of chronic renal failure
B. Pyelonephritis: Disease resulting from the immediate or late effects of bacterial infections of the kidney.						

(Continued)

TABLE 41-8. *(Continued)*

Classification	Etiology	Nature of Onset	Severity and Course of Illness	Structures Involved, Primary Disease	Major Manifestations	Major Medical or Surgical Therapy
1. Acute	Usually caused by the coliform group of gram-negative enteric bacilli. Frequently follows urinary tract infections. A small number caused by gram-positive streptococcus, *Proteus, Pseudomonas,* enterococcus, and staphylococcus. Infection may reach the kidney via the blood or by way of the urinary tract. Predisposing factors: 1. About one half of cases not known 2. Obstruction—prostatic hypertrophy, cicatricial tissue anomalies 3. Age and sex a. A comparatively high incidence before 18 months of age. More common in female than in male infants	Sudden		Lesion(s)—diffuse 1. Inflammation of the renal pelvis and calyces 2. Infection of renal substance, medulla, and cortex with the formation of minute abscesses 3. Healing with the formation of scar tissue	1. Sudden rise of body temperature 37.3° to 40.5°C (102° to 105°F) 2. Shaking chills 3. Aching pains in one of costovertebral areas or flanks 4. Symptoms of inflammation of the bladder: *(a)* frequency of urination, *(b)* burning pain on urination (dysuria), *(c)* passage of cloudy and occasionally blood-tinged urine 5. Tenderness in region of the kidney 6. Nausea, vomiting, diarrhea, and occasionally constipation 7. Laboratory tests: *(a)* polymorphonuclear leukocytosis, *(b)* many leukocytes in the urine, *(c)* bacteria in the urine	1. Attempt to sterilize the urine (difficult to do). Drugs employed a. Methenamine mandelate (Mandelamine) b. Nitrofurantoin (suppresses infection) c. Urotropin (suppresses infection) d. Methionine (an acidifying agent that inhibits the growth of bacteria) e. Mandelic acid f. Antibiotics such as tetracycline, chloramphenicol g. Sulfanilamides (bacteriostatic effect) h. Streptomycin (not used alone because streptomycin-resistant bacteria emerge rapidly) 2. Maintain water intake to keep urine dilute 3. Relieve or remove obstructing lesions

	b. Much more common at 18 to 40 years in women than in men 4. Instrumentation of the urinary tract including catheterization 5. Autonomic disturbances of bladder function 6. Diabetes mellitus 7. Pregnancy 8. Indwelling (Foley) catheter					
2. Chronic (one of the most common forms of chronic renal disease)	Results from the effects of scar tissue formed in the healing of an earlier bacterial infection of the kidney or from some other agent	Over half of the persons with chronic pyelonephritis have a history of attacks of acute urinary tract infection Usually onset is insidious and the progress of the disease is often slow	Fatigue, lassitude associated with anemia Signs of hypertension and congestive heart failure		1. Usually no symptoms of infection 2. Symptoms common to chronic illness Fatigue Headache (may be related to hypertension) Poor appetite Weight loss 3. Symptoms associated with failing renal function Polyuria Thirst 4. Signs of renal failure Impaired capacity to concentrate urine Elevated blood urea nitrogen	1. Eliminate urinary tract infections by drug therapy and by the removal of obstructing lesions

(Continued)

TABLE 41-8. *(Continued)*

Classification	Etiology	Nature of Onset	Severity and Course of Illness	Structures Involved, Primary Disease	Major Manifestations	Major Medical or Surgical Therapy
II. The nephrotic syndrome	1. Idiopathic 2. A phase of glomerulonephritis			In some textbooks of pathology this disease is referred to as a disease of the tubules. It is a disease in which the glomeruli are affected in such a manner that massive quantities of protein are lost in the urine	1. Profuse proteinuria secondary to loss of proteins 2. Hyperlipemia 3. Hypoalbuminemia 4. Generalized edema Other signs and symptoms depend on the cause	Idiopathic 1. ACTH and adrenal steroids. Treatment continued for 6 months or longer 2. A nutritious diet containing adequate amounts of protein. Should be sufficient to cover amounts lost in urine
III. Diseases of the arterioles (nephroscleroses) A. Benign B. Malignant	Hypertensive vascular disease	Hypertension antedates proteinuria by many years. Hematuria may occur		Intimal thickening of the small arteries and arterioles of the kidney. Eosinophilic hyaline thickening of entire walls of arterioles and prearterioles which may progress to generalized atrophy of the cortex with focal scars	Increased proteinuria and hematuria mark onset of malignant phase. Very high blood pressure, retinal hemorrhages, papilledema, heart failure, and hypertensive encephalopathy	

endothelial cells, the main pathology of acute glomerular nephritis. Disturbances of filtration result. Increased permeability means that medium-sized and large molecules will not be held back as heretofore, so that hemoglobin, and eventually even albumin, will get through the inflamed capillary endothelium; hematuria and proteinuria will appear and set the stage for the familiar symptomatology of the children (Juliani, 1979; Wrong, 1979).

Generalized vasospasm is a characteristic of this type of nephritis, and awareness of this fact contributes to understanding of some of the symptoms. When the vessels are all in spasm, the blood delivered to the kidney may be reduced in amount. Vasospasm increases peripheral resistance. Even the amount of blood that enters comes at the expense of increased effort by the heart. The arterial pressure rises, and unless the child already has a weakened heart, the pulse rate may be expected to slow somewhat because of pressure on the receptors in the carotid sinus, with resultant discharge of impulses to vasomotor centers. If the vasospasm is extremely severe, the heart muscle itself may suffer hypoxia and fail under the strain of the effort in a weakened state of pumping a large volume of blood, increased as a result of sodium and water retention, out into vessels narrowed by spasm. Cerebral anemia may result from inadequate supply to the brain as a result of the vascular spasm alone or assisted by heart failure. The child may be drowsy, or have headache, dimness of vision, or convulsions.

Children with acute glomerular nephritis do not usually look very edematous, but, if weighed, show an increase which suggests that there is a good deal of water retention consequent to the sodium reabsorption that occurs. If the child is in heart failure, not only will the edema be more marked than otherwise, but the failure further jeopardizes the child's welfare, because no organ, the heart included, is receiving the nutrition it needs.

Much of the pathophysiology is revealed by physical examination and laboratory tests, but the reports of these come late to the child's record. Concern here is for comprehension of what the sick child can demonstrate to the nurse of his or her needs for attention and understanding care.

Usually the child is of an age to talk readily. Children of 4, 5, and 6 years suffer severely in hospital from homesickness, and especially from conscious, expressed need for their mothers. Nurses cannot by any means satisfy this, but they can mitigate suffering a little by expressing sympathy for the child's unhappiness and by showing their readiness to let the child talk about his or her mother. With a little skill they can help the child to build verbal bridges to home. It is not, as a rule, helpful to try to divert a sick child when he or she is mournful, even though one can do it. This puts the child in the position of having to mourn alone, which is sad and lessens, rather than strengthens, the nurse's relationship with him or her.

In pediatric nursing one has often to do without verbal communication because the patients are too young to talk. When, however, nurses have acutely sick children who are old enough to be articulate, they are unwise indeed not to use every opportunity to demonstrate to them both by word and action interest, liking, and desire to know all about them. The children should learn that the nurse wants to know about them and to take care of them however they feel—sick, lonely, or, as they invariably reply to the casual inquirer, "fine." The relentless amuser, who cannot see a child sitting forlornly in bed without feeling constrained to try to cheer him or her up and play with the child, may not be the most helpful nurse. The child may not confide the things such nurses would like to know, for they have not shown that they like the child when he or she is unhappy; they seem always to want to change the child.

The prepared nurse, faced with the responsibility for care and professional nursing observation of a child newly sick with acute glomerular nephritis, will value understanding of children for many reasons, one of which is that it contributes to the excellence of nursing care. This is, however, but a part of all the nurse needs to know, and she or he may do well to review whatever relevant knowledge has been gained from all fields and consider the application of it to the patient.

With inflammation present in the glomeruli, the nurse expects to see evidence of blood in the urine. Because of sodium retention she or he expects the amount passed daily to be diminished. To become aware of whether or not the oliguria is becoming more severe, signaling less efficient glomerular filtration and increased water retention, the nurse realizes the need for accuracy and completeness in the recording of fluid intake and output, and not only sees that this is accomplished, but keeps informed of the relationships. If the blood pressure is elevated or the child is gaining weight or looks paler or more puffy than before, the nurse stops and observes his or her breathing. Two checks may be necessary before the nurse can be assured that this ever-useful indicator of cardiac embarrassment (increase in respiratory rate without increase in patient activity) is not a source of concern about the patient at this time. This observation has been reached by knowing that vasospasm has increased the peripheral load of the heart and may be severe enough to result in some hypoxia to the myocardium, which, emptying the chambers of the heart incompletely with each stroke, initiates the whole sequence of adjustments made by the body to compensate for the lessening efficiency of the heart muscle. Increasing respiratory rate is one such adjustment.

When, however, the nurse does observe that the child is breathing faster, she or he has something to do. First, it is to help the patient to the position of comfort and provide the pillow support needed so that no exertion is required to maintain it. Then the nurse will count the pulse, note the quality, measure the blood pressure, and procure the means of administering oxygen to assist the failing efforts of the heart. It may be that the blood pressure is rising and that the nurse already has orders provided for medication. In this event, she or he is prepared to treat the child further at once. But when there is no medical order to act upon, the nurse will do well to gain a little more information from the patient in the next 2 or 3 minutes before calling the physician. The prepared nurse will recall this sequence: vasospasm → hypertension → cerebral anemia → cerebral hypoxia → cerebral symptoms. Then, she or he will ask: Does the child have any of these? Here is the place where one *does* try to capture the attention of the child, whatever the mood, but with an objective more serious than that of simple diversion. By showing the child a small picture of a familiar object, or reviewing the illustrations of a picture book he or she knows well, a fair guess can be made as to whether the child's vision is still clear. A far better judgment can be made at the same time concerning mental alertness, for if the child and the nurse are already good friends, the child will try to respond, however ill he or she feels. By this response the child will reveal the absence or extent of drowsiness. It may be that after a sudden light tap or from a moment's close observation the nurse will see muscle twitching that may presage a convulsion soon to follow. So, within a minute or two, the nurse will have additional useful information to give the physician when he or she is immediately notified of the changes in the condition of the patient and requested to attend.

If, in the absence of a physician to note rapidly advancing symptoms, there is no nurse prepared to recognize and act upon significant changes, the child who goes quickly into heart failure may die. When needs are promptly recognized and successfully treated, the child's recovery from this emergency is quick and complete. The same is essentially true of hypertensive encephalopathy, although there is no one who would like to say that convulsions and cerebral hypoxia are conditions that one wants to see occurring often in any child.

Sometimes, when everyone has been alert, and all have given their best knowledge and skill to care and treatment, a child with acute glomerular nephritis will die. At the present time this cannot be avoided. An effort has been made here to indicate some, though not by any means all, of the pathologic changes that take place in this disease. These are changes producing symptoms with accompanying physical signs that nurses can recognize. Recognizing the signs and relating them to a disease process of which they have an understanding permits them to make judgments that are useful. It is at this point that they become free to do professional nursing.

The sick child whose parents have loaned him or her to the hospital for care has been entrusted by them to the physicians and nurses only because they believe that specialized care may, for a brief time, be better than their own. If their confidence is not to have been falsely placed, not only the physician but also the nurses, with whom the child surely will find less comfort than with his or her mother when sick, must be able to offer something that is even more important at the moment than the mother's presence. This is, for nurses, intelligent vigilance based on a knowledge of emergencies that can arise because of the stress of the child's disease on the body. Confidence that they are fulfilling their entire responsibility can be felt by nurses only when they (as well as physicians, for whom this is to be assumed) accept the thesis that all aspects of the care of the sick child are subjects for their attention and concern: "No Trespassing" signs have no proper place in pediatrics. All that each nurse knows about children, including normal growth and development, normal or pathophysiologic, techniques and skills of bedside nursing, and psychology, will be of value only when integrated and used to further the objective of all who are devoted to the hospital care of sick children. This objective is fairly met when a child is returned home well on the road to health with, as far as can be managed, few lasting scars sustained from the hazardous journey.

References Cited

Appel, G. B., and Neu, H. C. "The Nephrotoxicity of Anti-Microbial Agents." (first of three parts). *N. Engl. J. Med.*, **296** (March 24, 1977), 663–70.

Atkins, R. C. et al. "Management of Chronic Renal Failure." *DM* (March 1971), 13–19.

Avioli, L. V. "Management of Osteomalacia." *Hosp. Prac.*, **14** (Jan. 1979), 109–14.

Bauer, D. "Preventing the Spread of Hepatitis B in Dialysis Units." *Am. J. Nurs.*, **80** (Feb. 1980), 260–61.

Baum, M. E. " 'I Want to Be Dry!' The (Almost) Carefree Way to Conquer Urinary Incontinence." *Nurs. 78*, **8** (Feb. 1978), 75–78.

Beber, C. R. "Freedom for the Incontinent." *Am. J. Nurs.*, **80** (March 1980), 482–84.

Boylan, A., and Marbach, B. "Dehydration: Subtle, Sinister . . . Preventable." *RN*, **42** (Aug. 1979), 36–41.

Brazier, M. A. B. *The Neurophysiological Background for Anesthesia.* Springfield, Ill.: Charles C Thomas, 1972, pp. 35–37.

Brunto, W. et al. "The Michigan Blue Cross Hemodialysis Pilot Project: Results of a 30 Month Pilot Study." *Mich. Med.*, **71** (May 1972), 423–28.

Calland, C. H. "Iatrogenic Problems in End-Stage Renal Failure." *N. Engl. J. Med.*, **287** (Aug. 17, 1972), 334–36.

Campbell, J. D., and Campbell, A. R. "The Social and Economic Costs of End-Stage Renal Disease. A Patient's Perspective." *N. Engl. J. Med.*, **299** (Aug. 24, 1978), 386–92.

"Change IV Sets Every 24 Hours." *I.V. Tips*, No. 9. Chicago: Abbott Laboratories Hospital Products Division, Oct. 1972, p. 1.

Cohen, J. J. "Disorders of Potassium Balance." *Hosp. Prac.*, **14** (Jan. 1979), 119–28.

Dack, S. "Acute Pulmonary Edema." *Hosp. Med.*, **14** (March 1978), 112–38, p. 112.

DiPalma, J. R. "Drugs that Induce Changes in Urine Color." *RN*, **40** (Jan. 1977), 34–35.

Feig, P. U., and McCurdy, D. K. "The Hypertonic State." *N. Engl. J. Med.*, **297** (Dec. 29, 1977), 1444–54.

Flanagan, M. J. "Acute Urinary Retention." *Hosp. Med.*, **12** (Sept. 1976), 60–78.

Fluid and Electrolytes: Some Practical Guides to Clinical Use. Chicago: Abbott Laboratories, 1972, p. 20.

Frawley, T. F. "Axioms on Metabolic Considerations in Postsurgical Patients." *Hosp. Med.*, **6** (Jan. 1970), 107–21, 107–10.

Gallagher, J. C., and Riggs, B. L. "Nutrition and Bone Disease." *N. Engl. J. Med.*, **298** (Jan. 26, 1978), 193–95.

Gilchrest, B. A. et al. "Relief of Uremic Pruritus with Ultraviolet Phototherapy. *N. Engl. J. Med.*, **297** (July 21, 1977), 136.

Goldberger, E. *A Primer of Water, Electrolyte and Acid–Base Syndromes*, 5th ed. Philadelphia: Lea & Febiger, 1975, p. 178.

Goodman, L. S., and Gilman, A., eds. *The Pharmacological Basis of Therapeutics*, 5th ed. New York: Macmillan Publishing Co., 1975.

Grüntzig, A. et al. "Treatment of Renovascular Hypertension with Percutaneous Transluminal Dilatation of a Renal-Artery Stenosis." *Lancet*, **1** (1978), 801–2.

Guttmann, R. D. "Renal Transplantation." *N. Engl. J. Med.*, Part 1. **301** (Nov. 1, 1979), 975–82. Part 2. **301** (Nov. 8, 1979), 1038–48.

"HEW Encourages Home Dialysis Services, Kidney Transplants." *Physicians' Washington Report*, **1**:8 (Feb. 1979), 2.

Hollenberg, N. K. et al. "Increased Glomerular Filtration Rate after Converting-Enzyme Inhibition in Essential Hypertension." *N. Engl. J. Med.*, **301** (July 5, 1979), 9–12.

Humes, H. D. et al. "Disorders of Water Balance." *Hosp. Prac.*, **14** (March 1979), 133–45.

Juliani, L. M. "When Infection Leads to Acute Glomerulonephritis Here's What to Do." *Nurs. 79*, **9** (Sept. 1979), 40–45, 43.

Kimberly, R. P., and Plotz, P. H. "Aspirin-Induced Depression of Renal Function." *N. Engl. J. Med.*, **296** (Feb. 24, 1977), 418–24.

Kobrzycki, P. "Renal Transplant Complications." *Am. J. Nurs.*, **77** (April 1977), 641–43.

Levinsky, N. G. "Pathophysiology of Acute Renal Failure." *N. Engl. J. Med.*, **296** (June 23, 1977), 1453–58.

Levy, M. "The Pathophysiology of Sodium Balance." *Hosp. Prac.*, **13** (Nov. 1978), 95–106, 101.

Luke, B. "Nutrition in Renal Disease: The Adult on Dialysis." *Am. J. Nurs.*, **79** (Dec. 1979), 2155–57.

Madias, N. E. et al. "Increased Anion Gap in Metabolic Alkalosis: The Role of Plasma-Protein Equivalency." *N. Engl. J. Med.*, **300** (June 21, 1979), 1421–23.

Metheny, N. A., and Snively, W. D., Jr. "Perioperative Fluids and Electrolytes." *Am. J. Nurs.*, **78** (May 1978), 840–45.

Millan, V. G. et al. "Nonsurgical Treatment of Severe Hypertension Due to Renal-Artery Intimal Fibroplasia by Percutaneous Transluminal Angioplasty." *N. Engl. J. Med.*, **300** (June 14, 1979), 1371–73.

Morris, M. E. "Intravenous Drug Incompatibilities." *Am. J. Nurs.*, **79** (July 1979), 1288–91, 1291.

Mundy, G. R. "Differential Diagnosis of Osteopenia." *Hosp. Prac.*, **13** (Nov. 1978), 65–72.

Novick, A. C., and Stewart, B. H. "Surgical Treatment of Renovascular Hypertension." *Curr. Prob. Surg.*, **16**:8 (Aug. 1979).

"Outlook." *Med. World News*, **14** (Sept. 7, 1973), 15.

Rae, A., and Pendray, M. "Advantages of Peritoneal Dialysis in Chronic Renal Failure." *JAMA*, **225** (Aug. 20, 1973), 937–41.

Rosenberg, J. C. "Dialysis as a Substitute for Renal Function in Surgical Patients." *Curr. Probl. Surg.* (Feb. 1972), 43–44.

Schwartz, W. B. "Disorders of Fluid, Electrolyte, and Acid–Base Balance." In *Cecil Textbook of Medicine*, 15th ed. Ed. by P. B. Beeson et al. Philadelphia: W. B. Saunders Co., 1979, p. 1960.

Shrake, K. "The ABCs of ABGs—Or How to Interpret a Blood Gas Value." *Nurs. 79*, **9** (Sept. 1979), 26–33, 27–30.

Simenhoff, M. L. et al. "Biochemical Profile of Uremic Breath." *N. Engl. J. Med.*, **297** (July 21, 1977), 132–35.

Sleisenger, M. H. "Malabsorption." In *Cecil Textbook of Medicine*, 15th ed. Ed. by P. B. Beeson et al. Philadelphia: W. B. Saunders Co., 1979, pp. 1528–29.

Sorrels, A. J. "Continuous Ambulatory Peritoneal Dialysis." *Am. J. Nurs.*, **79** (Aug. 1979), 1400–01.

Tarail, R. "Practice of Fluid Therapy." *JAMA*, **171** (Sept. 5, 1959), 48.

Wallach, S. "Management of Osteoporosis." *Hosp. Prac.*, **13** (Dec. 1978), 91–98, 94–95.

Walter, C. W. et al. "Bacteriology of the Bedside Carafe." *N. Engl. J. Med.*, **259** (Dec. 18, 1958), 1198–1202.

White, S. J. "IV Fluids and Electrolytes: How to Head Off the Risks." *RN*, **42** (Nov. 1979), 60–63.

White, S. J., and Williamson, K. "What to Watch for When You Give Loop Diuretics." *RN*, **42** (Dec. 1979), 25–27.
Widmann, F. K. *Clinical Interpretation of Laboratory Tests*, 8th ed. Philadelphia: F. A. Davis Co., 1979.
Williams, G. H., and Hollenberg, N. K. "Accentuated Vascular and Endocrine Response to SQ20881 in Hypertension." *N. Engl. J. Med.*, **297** (1977), 184–88.
Wilson, J., and Colley, R. "Meeting Patients' Nutritional Needs with Hyperalimentation." *Nurs. 79*, **9** (Sept. 1979), 62–69.
Wrong, O. M. "Glomerulonephritis." In *Cecil Textbook of Medicine*, 15th ed. Ed. by P. B. Beeson et al. Philadelphia: W. B. Saunders Co., 1979, pp. 1390–1400.
Ziment, I., and Koppel, M. H. J. "Anti-Microbials When Kidneys Can't Cope." *Current Prescribing* (Aug. 1976), 32–43.

General References

Beeson, P. B. et al. *Cecil Textbook of Medicine*, 15th ed. Philadelphia: W. B. Saunders Co., 1979.
Broadus, A. E., and Thier, S. O. "Metabolic Basis of Renal-Stone Disease." *N. Engl. J. Med.*, **300** (April 12, 1979), 839–45.
Collins, R. D. *Illustrated Manual of Fluid and Electrolyte Disorders*. Philadelphia: J. B. Lippincott Co., 1976.
Cornfield, D. "Nephrosis in Childhood." *Hosp. Med.*, **14** (March 1978), 98–111.
Cox, M., Sterns, R. H., and Singer, I. "The Defense against Hyperkalemia: The Roles of Insulin and Aldosterone." *N. Engl. J. Med.*, **299** (Sept. 7, 1978), 525–32.
Ganong, W. F. *Review of Medical Physiology*, 9th ed. Los Altos, Calif.: Lange Medical Publications, 1979.
Goldberger, E. *A Primer of Water, Electrolyte and Acid-Base Syndromes*, 5th ed. Philadelphia: Lea & Febiger, 1975.
Gutch, C. F., and Stoner, M. H. *Review of Hemodialysis for Nurses and Dialysis Personnel*, 2nd ed. St. Louis: C. V. Mosby Co., 1975.
Guyton, A. C. *Textbook of Medical Physiology*, 5th ed. Philadelphia: W. B. Saunders Co., 1976.
Fisch, C. "Relation of Electrolyte Disturbances to Cardiac Arrhythmias." *Circulation*, **47** (1973), 408.
Friedman, E. A. et al. "Pragmatic Realities in Uremia Therapy." *N. Engl. J. Med.*, **298** (Feb. 16, 1978), 368–71.
"Helpful Hints on Blood Administration." *I.V. Tips*, No. 8. Chicago: Abbott Laboratories Hospital Products Division, Oct. 1972, p. 3.
Javadpour, N. et al. "Adrenal Neoplasms." *Curr. Probs. Surg.*, **17**:1 (Jan. 1980).
Kaplan, B. S., and Drummond, K. N. "The Hemolytic-Uremic Syndrome Is a Syndrome." *N. Engl. J. Med.*, **298** (April 27, 1978), 964–66.
Kubo, W. M. et al. "Fluid and Electrolyte Problems of Tube-Fed Patients." *Am. J. Nurs.*, **76** (June 1976), 912–16.
Law, D. H. "Total Parenteral Nutrition." *N. Engl. J. Med.*, **297** (Nov. 17, 1977), 1104–07.
Lawson, M. et al. "Long-Term I.V. Therapy: A New Approach." *Am. J. Nurs.*, **79** (June 1979), 1100–03.
Kurtzman, N. A. "Does Acute Post-Streptococcal Glomerulonephritis Lead to Chronic Renal Disease?" *N. Engl. J. Med.*, **298** (April 6, 1978), 795–96.
Manis, T., and Friedman, E. A. "Dialytic Therapy for Irreversible Uremia." *N. Engl. J. Med.*, Part. 1. **301** (Dec. 6, 1979), 1260–65. Part 2. **301** (Dec. 13, 1979), 1321–28.
Meller, S. "Hemodialysis at Camp." *Am. J. Nurs.*, **76** (June 1976), 938–40.
Michael, S. L. "Home I.V. Therapy." *Am. J. Nurs.*, **78** (July 1978), 1223–26.
Monitoring Fluid and Electrolytes Precisely. Horsham, Pa.: Intermed Communications, 1978.
Moore, V. B. "Analyzing the ABG Analysis." *Nurs. 79*, **9** (Sept. 1979), 28–33.
Nissenson, A. R. "Acute Oliguria: A Logical Approach to Diagnosis." *Hosp. Med.*, **15** (Sept. 1979), 22–43.
Raisz, L. G. "Calcium Homeostasis and Bone Metabolism." *Hosp. Prac.*, **5** (May 1970), 74–84, 74.
Relman, A. S. "Lactic Acidosis and a Possible New Treatment." *N. Engl. J. Med.*, **298** (March 9, 1978), 564–66.
Rose, B. D. *Clinical Physiology of Acid-Base and Electrolyte Disorders*. New York: McGraw-Hill, 1977.
Schwartz, S. I. et al. *Principles of Surgery*, 3rd ed. New York: McGraw-Hill, 1979.
Talbot, N. B. et al. "Application of Homeostatic Principles to the Management of Nephritic Patients." *N. Engl. J. Med.*, **255** (Oct. 4, 1956), 655–62.
Thorn, G. W. et al. *Harrison's Principles of Internal Medicine*, 8th ed. New York: McGraw-Hill, 1977.
Tilkian, S. M. et al. *Clinical Implications of Laboratory Tests*, 2nd ed. St. Louis: C. V. Mosby Co., 1979.
Wheeler, D. "Teaching Home Dialysis for an Eight-Year-Old Boy." *Am. J. Nurs.*, **77** (Feb. 1977), 273–74.

Acidosis–Alkalosis

Copeland, L. "Chronic Diarrhea in Infancy." *Am. J. Nurs.*, **77** (March 1977), 461–63.
Gennari, F. J., and Cohen, J. J. "Renal Tubular Acidosis." *Ann. Rev. Med.*, **25** (1978), 521.
"Metabolic Acid-Base Disorders: Physiologic Abnormalities and Nursing Actions." *Am. J. Nurs.*, **78** (Jan. 1978), 87–108.
Rahilly, G. T., and Berl, T. "Severe Metabolic Alkalosis Caused by Administration of Plasma Protein Fraction in End-Stage Renal Disease." *N. Engl. J. Med.*, **301** (Oct. 11, 1979), 824–28.

Calcium

Cheung, W. Y. "Calmodulin Plays a Pivotal Role in Cellular Regulation." *Science*, **207** (Jan. 4, 1980), 19–27.
Edis, A. J., and Beart, R. W., Jr. "Parathyroid Auto-

transplantation: An Innovative Approach." *Hosp. Prac.*, **14** (Jan. 1979), 78–84.

Marx, J. L. "Osteoporosis: New Help for Thinning Bones." *Science*, **207** (Feb. 8, 1980), 628–30.

Perry, W. et al. "Vitamin D Resistance in Osteomalacia after Ureterosigmoidostomy." *N. Eng. J. Med.*, **297** (Nov. 17, 1977), 1110–12.

Recker, R. R., and Saville, P. D. "Hypercalcemia and Hypocalcemia in Clinical Practice." *Hosp. Prac.*, **15** (Sept. 1979), 74–90.

Tripp, A. "Hyper and Hypocalcemia." *Am. J. Nurs.*, **76** (July 1976), 1142–45.

Intravenous Therapy

Blust, J. "Preventing Hematomas after Venipuncture." *Am. J. Nurs.*, **78** (Oct. 1978), 1675–76.

Huxley, V. D. "Heparin Lock: How, What, Why." *RN*, **42** (Oct. 1979), 36–41.

"Intravenous Therapy: A Special Feature." *Am. J. Nurs.*, **79** (July 1979), 1268–96.

Kidney Transplantation

Wolf, Z. R. "What Patients Awaiting Kidney Transplant Want to Know." *Am. J. Nurs.*, **76** (Jan. 1976), 92–94.

Renal–General

Baer, C. L. "The Growth and Development of Nephrology Nursing Practice." *Heart and Lung*, **8** (Sept.–Oct. 1979), 896–902.

Gillenwater, J. Y. et al. "Natural History of Bacteriuria in Schoolgirls." *N. Engl. J. Med.*, **301** (Aug. 23, 1979), 396–99.

Glassock, R. J. "The Nephrotic Syndrome." *Hosp. Prac.*, **14** (Nov. 1979), 105–9, 115–18, 123–29.

Wilson, C. B., and Dixon, F. J. "Immunologic Mechanisms in Nephritogenesis." *Hosp. Prac.*, **14** (April, 1979), 57–69.

Renal Failure

Appel, G. B., and Neu, H. C. "The Use of Drugs in Renal Failure." *DM*, **25**:11 (Aug. 1979).

Benson, E., and Metz, R. "Acute Renal Failure." *Hosp. Prac.*, **15** (Aug. 1979), 64–72.

Danovitch, G. M. et al. "Reversibility of the 'Salt-Losing' Tendency of Chronic Renal Failure." *N. Engl. J. Med.*, **296** (Jan. 6, 1977), 14–19.

Hetrick, A. et al. "Nutrition in Renal Failure: When the Patient Is a Child." *Am. J. Nurs.*, **79** (Dec. 1979), 2152–54.

Mitchell, J. C. "Axioms on Uremia." *Hosp. Med.*, **14** (July 1978), 6–23.

Dialysis

Anger, D., and Anger, D. W. "Dialysis Ambivalence: A Matter of Life and Death." *Am. J. Nurs.*, **76** (Feb. 1976), 276–77.

Aurigemma, N. M. et al. "Arterial Oxygenation during Hemodialysis." *N. Eng. J. Med.*, **297** (Oct. 20, 1977), 871–73.

Flegle, J. M. "Teaching Self-Dialysis to Adults in a Hospital." *Am. J. Nurs.*, **77** (Feb. 1977), 270–72.

Laborde, J. M., and Powers, M. J. "Satisfaction with Life for Patients Undergoing Hemodialysis and Patients Suffering from Osteoarthritis." *Res. Nurs. & Health*, **3** (March 1980), 19–14.

Water, Sodium, and Potassium

Fraley, D. S., and Adler, S. "Correction of Hyperkalemia by Bicarbonate Despite Constant Blood pH." *Kidney Int.*, **12** (1977), 354.

Kleeman, C. N. R. "CNS Manifestations of Disordered Salt and Water Balance." *Hosp. Prac.*, **14** (May 1979), 59–68, 73.

42

Problems with Transporting Materials to and from Cells Due to Altered Components of the Blood

Why grasse is greene, or why our blood is red,
Are mysteries which none have reach'd unto.
In this low forme, poore soule, what wilt thou doe?

—JOHN DONNE,
"Of the Progresse of the Soule"

Overview

The first component of the transportation system is the blood. The blood is the vehicle by which essential materials are distributed, whereas the heart and blood vessels provide the power and channels through which blood circulates, as well as the site of exchange between the blood and the interstitial fluid. Composed of various cellular components, the blood aids in the transportation of substances between the microcirculation and the cells.

In addition to its significance in the transport of materials, the blood serves a number of other functions. Blood flow is regulated so that homeostasis of the body fluids is maintained. The blood participates in the maintenance of its volume and composition by regulating the function of tissues and organs that contribute to blood formation. The blood also plays a significant role in regulation of body temperature and in the defense system of the body. A self-sealing mechanism protects against the loss of blood after disruption of a blood vessel wall.

Alterations in the blood cellular components or the self-sealing mechanism lead to alterations in the blood transport system. The result is insufficient quantity or quality of blood to cells for metabolic processes.

Not all alterations in blood cellular components indicate a failure of the body's homeostatic mechanisms, although the end result may still be insufficient quantity and quality of blood to tissues. In fact, in some situations if the level of blood cells were not altered, this would indicate a failure of homeostatic mechanisms. For example, the number of leukocytes should rise above normal levels in response to certain threats to the organism. This is as true with acute appendicitis as with a streptococcal throat infection. The polymorphonuclear leukocytes, particularly the neutrophils, are responsible for the rise in leukocytes with infectious processes. Inasmuch as an increase in leukocytes is the appropriate response to a threat of injury to cells, this response is homeostatic. Another example of an expected alteration in blood cellular components is when the number of erythrocytes increases above normal levels in response to a chronic deficiency of oxygen, such as in congenital heart disease or at high altitudes. A failure of the organism to increase the number of blood cells in response to an appropriate stimulus would indicate a failure in an essential homeostatic mechanism.

The disorders in function resulting from alterations in the blood cellular components include

This chapter was revised by Elizabeth Ford Pitorak, R.N., M.S.N., Clinical Nurse Specialist, Lake County Memorial Hospital, Willoughby, Ohio, and Judith A. Wood, R.N., M.S.N., Assistant Professor of Nursing, Case Western Reserve University, Frances Payne Bolton School of Nursing, Cleveland, Ohio.

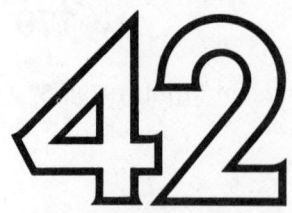

1. Failure to transport substances required by cells for metabolic processes or to remove the end products of metabolism
2. Failure of the self-sealing mechanism
3. Failure to combat the agents of infection
4. Failure to maintain the constancy of the fluid environment of cells

The effects associated with each disturbance are related to the function of the particular component involved and the rapidity with which the condition develops. Etiologic factors in disorders of the blood (blood dyscrasias) include genetic abnormalities, neoplasia or failure of the bone marrow, deficiency of materials required to form the various constituents of the blood, infection, acute or chronic blood loss, and allergic responses. As with other pathologic states, the causes of some abnormalities have not been explained.

The Components of Blood

The blood is a highly complex fluid in which the blood cells are suspended. The fluid portion or plasma comprises about 54 per cent of the total blood volume, and the cells about 46 per cent, although these figures are subject to some variation.

Plasma

The plasma and its constituents are examined in detail in Chapter 27; therefore the present discussion will be limited. Plasma, which comprises approximately 60 per cent of the blood volume, is the noncellular portion of the blood and is the vehicle that carries the other components. The high water content (over 90 per cent) enables the plasma to dissolve and carry in solution a large variety of organic and inorganic substances between the cells and the vascular system. Because of the colloidal osmotic pressure exerted by the plasma proteins, the plasma is not lost through the capillary pores even though it communicates directly with the interstitial fluid through these pores. Plasma also contains the blood proteins, albumin, globulin, and fibrinogen, as well as internal secretions, antibodies, and a variety of enzymes. Water in the plasma and other body fluids participates in the regulation of body temperature.

Cells

The cells in the blood are of three types: the erythrocytes, or red corpuscles; the leukocytes, or white blood corpuscles; and the thrombocytes, or blood platelets. The leukocytes are part of the system of defense of the body. They are discussed in Chapter 24.

The number of each of the various types of cells in the blood is determined by a balance between the production and destruction of cells. Because the number of cells per unit of blood is regulated automatically, and the cells are maintained within well-defined limits, this is another example of a homeostatic mechanism. As with other homeostatic mechanisms, the equilibrium between blood cell production and destruction may be unbalanced, resulting in a loss of homeostasis. The effects, of course, will depend on the type of cell involved and in some instances on the cause of the failure. Because of the liquid nature of the blood, cells and plasma may be lost more rapidly than they can be replaced. When the loss of blood is rapid, circulation is threatened by the loss of the blood volume as well as by the loss of cells.

The proportion of cells to the total volume of blood is determined by centrifuging whole blood. The cells settle to the bottom of the tube, and the length of the column of cells or fluid portion can be measured. The result is reported as a whole number, such as 42 or 48. The number indicates the percentage of the blood that is cells and is called the hematocrit. If the hematocrit is 42, this means that the blood cells comprise 42 per cent of the total blood volume. The remaining 58 per cent is plasma. Usually there is a direct relationship between the number of red blood cells and the hemotocrit value. In women the percentage of cells is somewhat lower than in men. The average hematocrit for women is 42 per cent, and the average for men is 45 per cent.

If the erythrocytes happen to be larger than normal or the hemoglobin concentration is above normal, the hematocrit will be higher than the corresponding red blood cell count. The hematocrit will be lower than the corresponding red blood cell count if the erythrocytes are smaller than normal or the hemoglobin content is less than normal. For example, following blood loss, the blood volume may be maintained by an increase in the blood plasma, and the hematocrit may fall below the lower limits of normal. The hematocrit should not be checked immediately following or during intravenous administration, as the hemotocrit may be decreased, depending upon the volume of fluid administered, the rate, and the volume of fluid leaving the circulatory system and entering the interstitial tissue.

Erythrocytes

The erythrocyte has several important functions. First, it transports hemoglobin and, by means of the hemoglobin, conveys oxygen from the lung to the tissues. The oxygen is loosely bound to the hemoglobin, the iron-containing pigment that accounts for a large per cent of the mass of the erythrocyte. Second, the erythrocyte contains large quantities of carbonic acid. It is largely in this form that the transport of carbon dioxide from the tissues to the lungs occurs. A third function of the erythrocyte is the buffering effect of the hemoglobin and the electrolytes contained in the cell. The erythrocyte is responsible for a large per cent of the buffering action of whole blood.

The erythrocyte is described as a biconcave disc with an average diameter of 7.2 μ. It has a thickness of about 2.2 μ at its thickest part and is 1 μ or less in its center. This shape increases its effective surface area. Erythrocytes are extremely pliable and capable of great changes in shape as they pass through capillaries. Although the erythrocyte lacks a nucleus, it carries out metabolic functions. With the advent of the electron microscope, it has been learned that the erythrocyte is composed of two separate structures, the stroma and the outer membrane (Dougherty, 1971, p. 132). The stroma, or the inner layer, is composed of lipids and proteins. It is a spongy material that is thicker than the outer membrane and is the portion to which the hemoglobin attaches in an interlacing fashion. The outer membrane, or the cell envelope, is composed of lipoproteins and in comparison with the stroma is extremely thin and pliable.

The average number of erythrocytes in a healthy man is approximately 5 million cells per cubic millimeter of blood with a range of ±600,000. In women the figure is slightly lower, with an average of 4.5 million per cubic millimeter. The range in women is narrower than in men about ±500,000. The hemoglobin fraction also varies with sex and from individual to individual. The average hemoglobin content for men is about 16 g per 100 ml of blood. For women, it is about 14 g.

The sites in which erythrocytes are formed change from embryonic to adult life. In the first weeks of fetal life erythrocytes are formed in the primitive yolk sac. Later the liver serves as the principal site for their formation, though they are also formed in the spleen and lymph nodes. As the fetus matures, the site of formation of erythrocytes shifts to the bone marrow, and by the time of birth, this is the main site of erythrocyte production. The bone marrow continues to be the site of formation throughout the remainder of the life span. Until the time of adolescence, the bone marrow in the shaft of long bones functions in erythrocyte production. After about the age of 20, it becomes quite fatty and produces no more erythrocytes, and red cell production takes place primarily in the flat bones such as the vertebrae, skull, sternum, and ribs. Because the productive bone marrow gradually lessens in amount throughout the life span, a mild anemia is not infrequent in the aged. In emergency situations in which large numbers of red cells are required, bone marrow that has stopped producing cells may become productive.

In the production of erythrocytes, or erythropoiesis, two factors are of significance: the cell itself and the hemoglobin in the cell. Many complex processes are involved in the formation of both. Many substances must be available and a number of enzymes are required to catalyze the reactions involved in the formation and maturation of the cell and its hemoglobin. In the process of development the cell goes through a number of stages. The reticulum cell in the bone marrow forms a primordial cell known as a hemocytoblast. This cell is nucleated and it does not contain hemoglobin. In the next stage the synthesis of hemoglobin is begun. As the cell develops, the nucleus shrinks in size, and the quantity of hemoglobin increases. The cell, at the stage in which the nucleus disappears and a full complement of hemoglobin is present, is known as a normoblast. Most cells contain no nuclear material at the time they enter the circulating blood. They are fully mature erythrocytes. A few cells containing fine strands of basophilic material that do find their way into the blood are known as reticulocytes. Normally, they comprise about 2 per cent of the total circulating erythrocytes. Following hemorrhage or the treatment of anemia they may account for 10 per cent or more of the total number of erythrocytes. Because they are less mature forms of erythrocytes, the presence of an increased proportion of reticulocytes to mature erythrocytes following treatment of anemia is taken as an indication of a rise in red cell production.

Red blood cell production is increased any time a condition arises where oxygen transport to the tissues is decreased. Thus any condition that causes an increase in the need for oxygen to the tissues serves as a stimulus for erythropoiesis. It is not known how hypoxia acts to stimulate erythropoiesis. Erythropoietin, or the erythropoietic stimulating factor, is formed almost as soon as the person is exposed to an atmosphere low in oxygen. Conversely when the person is exposed to an atmosphere high in oxygen, erythropoietin production ceases or falls to a very low level for a period of 24 to 36 hours. The main action of erythropoietin is to increase the rate at which stem cells are converted to hematocytoblasts. To a lesser extent erythropoietin increases the rate of all phases of red cell production, including the maturation and release of red cells. In contrast, with an excess of red cells, the formation of the erythropoietin and the production of erythrocytes are depressed.

Activity increases the oxygen need and thus serves as a stimulus to erythrocyte production. Bedridden persons are thus frequently anemic, because of lack of exercise. Erythropoiesis also is stimulated by circulatory conditions that create a decrease in the flow of blood through the peripheral vessels. Thus in prolonged cardiac failure where there is anoxia to tissues secondary to the sluggish blood flow, erythrocyte production is increased.

No specific mechanism is known for the destruction of erythrocytes. Healthy erythrocytes live an average of about 120 days. As the cell ages, its outer membrane thins and becomes more and more easily ruptured. Cell destruction therefore may be the result merely of the inability of the fragile membrane of the aged cell to withstand the pressure exerted against it as the erythrocyte passes through a capillary. Erythrocytes undergo a certain amount of deformity as they pass through capillaries, and this distortion in shape could place a strain on areas of the cell membrane. The walls of erythrocytes undergoing this process need to be strong to survive. The assumption that the aging of the membrane of the red cell predisposes it to mechanical injury is supported by the observation that poorly constructed cells with fragile membranes have shorter life span than do normal erythrocytes.

Once the wall of the erythrocyte is disrupted, hemoglobin is released. The shell of the former erythrocyte is called a ghost cell, and it is quickly removed from the blood by reticuloendothelial cells. The hemoglobin is also phagocytized by reticuloendothelial cells into globin and heme. The heme is the iron-containing fraction that further splits into iron and a pigment, biliverdin. The iron enters the iron pool of the body from whence it may be drawn to form myoglobin in the muscle or hemoglobin in new erythrocytes, or it may be stored in the liver until it is needed. The biliverdin is reduced to bilirubin, which is gradually released into the blood. Bilirubin is insoluble in water, but it combines with the blood proteins and is transported in this form to the liver. The liver separates bilirubin from the blood protein and combines about 80 per cent of it with glucuronide. Bilirubin glucuronide is highly soluble in water. The liver cells secrete it along with the other forms of bilirubin into the bile. Bilirubin is responsible for the greenish-yellow color of bile. After the bile reaches the small intestine, some of the bilirubin is converted by bacterial action to urobilinogen, some of which is excreted in the stool.

Most of the urobilinogen is reabsorbed into the portal circulation and excreted in the bile. A small amount escapes into the circulation and is excreted in the urine. An increase in the level of bilirubin in the blood may be caused by obstruction in the bile ducts or by increased red blood cell destruction. Usually the elevation is greater in the presence of obstructive lesions than in increased red cell destruction, though there are occasional exceptions. There are also other differences (see Chapter 46).

As long as blood production keeps up to the demand for red cells and the rate of red cell destruction or loss does not exceed cell production, the number of red cells found in the blood remains stable. In blood dyscrasias, the number and/or character of one or more of the blood cells is abnormal. Moreover, the alteration in the number cannot be explained as a normal response to a threat to the organism.

Deficit of Erythrocytes

Anemia is a condition that occurs when the oxygen transport capacity of the blood is below normal because of a reduction in the quantity or quality of erythrocytes and hemoglobin.

CAUSES. The anemic state may be the result of (1) inadequate production of erythrocytes because of abnormal function of the bone marrow, (2) insufficient quantity of erythrocytes because of acute or chronic blood loss, (3) inadequate maturation of erythrocytes because of absence of an essential factor, or (4) increased destruction of erythrocytes resulting from acquired or hereditary factors. Discussion of the anemias will proceed from this etiologic base.

Aplasia and hypoplasia of the bone marrow. Failure of the bone marrow to produce erythrocytes in adequate numbers may be caused by a congenital defect in which hematopoietic (blood-forming) tissues fail to develop, or as a result of injury to the marrow some time following birth. In either instance, hematopoietic tissues may be absent or insufficient in quantity, thus red bone marrow is either entirely or partly replaced by fatty or yellow marrow. In the absence of any evidence of hematopoietic activity, the bone marrow is said to be aplastic, whereas bone marrow showing less than normal activity is hypoplastic. In the absence of red-cell-producing tissue, all types of blood corpuscles, erythrocytes, granulocytes, and thrombocytes, will be decreased in number. The patient will have not only anemia, but granulocytopenia and thrombocytopenia as well. The consequences will depend on the cause of the condition. In a patient in whom there is an acute depression of the bone marrow, survival may depend on whether or not he or she can be protected from infection and hemorrhage until the bone marrow recovers from injury.

There are many possible causes of aplasia or hypoplasia of the bone marrow. Bone marrow may fail as a terminal event in leukemia or as a result of metastasis of malignant neoplasms from other parts of the body. The bone marrow is highly sensitive to a variety of chemical and physical agents. Rappeport and Bunn divide these agents into two groups: (1) predictable dose-related aplasia resulting from such drugs as antineoplastic agents and (2) idiosyncratic reactions unrelated to dose (1977, p. 1665). Among the agents in the predictable dose-related category are those utilized in the therapy of malignant neoplasms (antimetabolites such as 5-fluorouracil, cytosine, and methotrexate; alkylating agents such as cyclophosphamide, busulfan, chlorambucil, and nitrogen mustard; and natural products such as the vinca alkaloids, bleomycin, actinomycin D, and adriamycin). Additional agents that produce bone marrow damage are ionizing radiation from x-rays and radioactive elements and aromatic fat solvents, such as benzene (benzol), that are used in many industries, which also are toxic to bone marrow. Unless adequate precautions are taken to protect individuals who are using these agents, sufficient quantities may be inhaled to cause hypoplasia or aplasia of the bone marrow.

Among agents in the idiosyncratic category is a large group of chemicals, including a number of drugs. Aplasia or hypoplasia of the bone marrow occurs occasionally in individuals after exposure to one of a number of drugs or other chemical agents such as insecticides. Among the drugs most frequently associated with aplastic or hypoplastic bone marrow are the arsenicals used in the treatment of syphilis, the antithyroid drugs, antihistamines, trinitrotoluene, and preparations of gold. Insecticides have also been implicated. Before prescribing a drug reported to be associated with the development of hypoplasia or aplasia of bone marrow, it is imperative that the physician weigh the possibility of adverse effects to the patient as compared to the therapeutic effects. Moreover, the greater the possibility of injury, the greater the need for accurate observation and follow-up of the patient. The nurse has a further obligation to participate in public education to prevent needless use of or overexposure to drugs or insecticides. Children, as well as other members of the family, should be protected from the careless handling and use of drugs.

The general supportive measures of therapy required are going to be determined by the severity of the pancytopenia and the ability of the patient to tolerate this state. Red blood cell transfusions should be given as packed cells which have been stored for less than a week. The possibility of sensitizing the patient with tissue antigen not normally present on red cells arises with repeated red cell transfusions. The donor's tissue antigens accompany red cell transfusions because of their presence in platelets, white blood cells, and probably plasma. Sensitization to these antigens complicates future platelet and granulocyte transfusions or bone marrow transplants (Clift & Buchner, 1978).

If there is bone marrow failure, platelet transfusions can be started when the platelet count is 10,000 platelets/mm. The maximum effect from platelets is 6 hours after they are obtained from the donor, and they will survive 8 to 10 days in the recipient's blood. There is danger of developing antibodies to the platelets, especially if they are collected from a pooled source of platelets containing antigen from many donors. The degree to which prophylactic platelet transfusions are used varies greatly from patient to patient with marrow failure; however, this treatment modality is available.

The treatment of aplastic anemia has changed radically in the past few years due to the success of bone marrow transplants. The reader will recall that the term "transplant" means transfer from one person or part to another, and indeed the marrow is in liquid cellular form. The survival of transplant tissue is greater when there is an histocompatibility locus antigen (HLA) compatible sibling donor of the same sex. A recipient for a bone marrow transplant should be under 40 years of age. The marrow aspiration is performed under spinal anesthesia at which time approximately 500 to 700 ml of bone marrow are aspirated from various iliac crest sites. The aspirate of the bone marrow is infused into a peripheral vein of the recipient. From the blood stream the marrow migrates into the marrow spaces of the recipient's bone. How this migration takes place is unknown. Volume overload and pulmonary emboli are possible, but rare, complications of bone marrow infusions (Zimmerman et al., 1977, p. 1312).

When severe granulocytopenia is accompanied by bloodborne bacterial infections, transfusions of granulocytes can be effected to help bring the infection under control. At present the technical capacity for prolonged periods of granulocyte transfusions does not exist. Thus, granulocytes are transfused only to combat serious infective complications.

Iron-deficiency anemia. The individual who is experiencing acute blood loss through hemorrhage is an obvious example of one who has an insufficient quantity of erythrocytes and hemoglobin to support oxygen transport. Today, however, iron deficiency anemias are more likely to be associated with chronic blood loss such as with ulcerative lesions of the gastrointestinal tract. To appreciate the relationship of iron deficiency anemias to chronic blood loss, one must understand the role iron and iron metabolism play in hemoglobin formation.

Hemoglobin is formed only to the extent that iron is available to the biochemical process. If one were to look at the chemical structure of the hemoglobin molecule, it would be noted that iron is the central, most important component. Thus in the absence of sufficient iron in the body, hemoglobin formation is reduced markedly.

In the normal adult relatively small amounts of iron are absorbed in the gastrointestinal tract in comparison to the amount ingested. That which is not absorbed is excreted in the feces. The largest per cent of iron taken into the gut is in the ferric form (Fe^{+++}). The secretions of the stomach reduce the iron to the ferrous state (Fe^{++}), which is essential for absorption to take place in the small intestine. Once absorbed the iron may travel in either of two directions: (1) the iron may immediately combine with a beta globulin to form transferrin, in which form it is transported in the blood plasma, or (2) the iron may combine with the protein, apoferritin, to form ferritin, in which form the iron is stored primarily in the liver. When the quantity of iron in the plasma is low, the iron is absorbed from the stored ferritin and transported to the cells of the body where it is needed. It is at this point that iron is readily available to the hematopoietic cells for hemoglobin formation.

In the presence of iron deficiency, each erythrocyte has less than a full quantity of hemoglobin and thus the cells are smaller than normal, or *microcytic.* Because the hemoglobin is usually decreased out of proportion to the number of erythrocytes, the cells are pale in color, or *hypochromic.* Iron-deficiency anemia is therefore referred to as a *microcytic hypochromic anemia.*

Iron deficiency may result from inadequate intake or absorption, or from loss of blood, particularly chronic blood loss. One common factor predisposing to loss of blood is ulcerative lesions, either benign or malignant, of the gastrointestinal tract. Even when the quantity of blood lost at one time is small, blood loss continued over time leads to the development of anemia. In disorders involving the gastrointestinal tract, food intake is likely to be limited by a poor appetite or nausea. Vomiting and/or diarrhea may further aggravate the problem by removing ingested food from the alimentary canal before absorption can take place. Another source of anemia caused by blood loss is the female reproductive tract. Lesions involving the lining of the uterus and cervix and excessive menstruation are common factors. At the beginning of the century, iron-deficiency anemias caused by an inadequate intake of iron were common in the United States. Today, with the enrichment of cereals and flours with iron, this is less common.

Iron-deficiency anemia secondary to an inadequate intake of iron affects all age groups from infancy through adulthood. Attention to infant nutrition and early addition of iron-containing foods have lessened the incidence of iron-deficiency anemias in young children. In the 12- to 18-month age group, anemias are frequently found in children reared in families with limited income. The adolescent girl can be anemic, as she has body growth and menstruation as possible contributing factors. The adolescent's diet frequently is inadequate to meet the daily iron requirement because of erratic and nonnutritional food intake. During pregnancy it is not uncommon for anemia to occur, as twice the normal intake of iron is required.

The elderly frequently have iron-deficiency anemia secondary to multiple underlying causes. Among the various causes, blood loss represents the most common one. Chronic problems such as diverticulitis, gastric ulcers, hemorrhoids, and hiatal hernia may be responsible for chronic occult blood loss as well as acute episodes of bleeding. Drug-induced gastrointestinal bleeding caused by anti-inflammatory drugs, such as cortisone and aspirin, may result from treatment for arthritis. Also anticoagulant therapy for cardiovascular diseases carries the potential for initiating bleeding. Moreover, a faulty absorption mechanism can be associated with a total or partial gastrectomy and atrophic gastritis. Further, sufficient iron sources may be excluded from the dietary intake due to a low income, loneliness, or poorly fitting dentures. Lack of color is a clue to food sources poor in iron. Examples are chicken, rice, potatoes, cereal, milk, crackers, tea, toast, and egg. Frequently egg yolks are listed as a good source of iron; however, iron from eggs is poorly absorbed. From analyzing the above list, it is apparent that these foods are less expensive to purchase and, due to the texture, easier to chew (Flynn, 1978).

In iron-deficiency anemias, therapy is directed toward two objectives, to determine the cause and to correct the deficiency of iron. In the accomplishment of the latter objective, the simplest and least expensive salts of iron, such as ferrous sulfate, are said to be as effective as more complicated and expensive preparations. Iron is absorbed best in an acid environment, thus it should be taken between meals when the absorptive surface of the duodenum is acid. Ascorbic acid creates an acid medium which enhances iron absorption, thus oral iron should be administered with orange juice. Liquid oral iron is more palatable if it is chilled before drinking and a cold glass of orange juice is drunk after taking the iron. Some patients develop diarrhea when iron therapy is initiated. Should diarrhea occur, the drug should be temporarily discontinued and then restarted in small dosage. As the patient develops tolerance for iron, the dosage can be increased. Because iron is incompletely absorbed from the gastrointestinal tract, much of it is excreted in the stool and the stool is black. The patient should be told to expect this so that he or she will not be frightened.

Parenteral iron therapy can usually be avoided; however, in those situations where the patient is unable to take iron orally, iron dextran (Imferon) and iron sorbitex (Jectofer) can be administered. The Z-tract intramuscular technique is used to minimize pain and to prevent extravasation into the subcutaneous tissue and staining of the skin. The appropriate deep intramuscular injection sites are the gluteus maximus and ventral gluteal muscles.

Persons whose food intake has been poor in iron should also be encouraged to increase the intake of iron-containing foods in their diets. Sources of iron include organ and lean meats and shellfish. Certain fruits and vegetables are good sources, provided they are eaten frequently. The fruits include apricots, peaches, prunes, grapes, and raisins. Among the vegetable sources are green leafy vegetables. To encourage persons to change eating patterns is not always easy. Habit, limited income, misconceptions about the effects of certain foods, and lack of energy associated with ill-health often interfere with any appreciable change in the diet.

Pernicious anemia. Immature erythrocytes have a cell membrane that is poorly formed and very fragile; thus they are destroyed prematurely as compared to normal erythrocytes. As a result, the bone marrow is unable to produce adequate numbers of erythrocytes to meet the rapid destruction. The overall effect is a decrease in the quantity and quality of erythrocytes necessary to transport oxygen.

Vitamin B_{12}, or the *extrinsic factor,* is required for the growth of all cells in the body. Because erythrocyte-forming tissues grow and proliferate rapidly, the production of erythrocytes is especially affected by vitamin B_{12}. Vitamin B_{12} is stored in the liver and released as needed for the maturation of erythrocytes produced in the bone marrow. In order for vitamin B_{12} to be absorbed from the diet, the *intrinsic factor* must be present in the stomach.

The intrinsic factor is a mucopolysaccharide or mucopolypeptide that is produced in the mucosal cells of the gastric fundus. It combines with vitamin B_{12} and makes vitamin B_{12} more soluble, thus facilitating its absorption in the small intestine.

In the absence of the intrinsic factor, vitamin B_{12} deficiency results. A lack of vitamin B_{12} has two effects on erythrocyte production. The rate of production is slowed and the cells formed are abnormal.

In conditions where vitamin B_{12} is deficient, erythrocytes vary in size (anisocytic), some are larger than normal (macrocytic), and a large portion are deformed in contour (poikilocytic).

Despite defects in the maturation of erythrocytes in vitamin B_{12} deficiency, the formation of hemoglobin is normal. The macrocytic erythrocyte contains a greater-than-normal complement of hemoglobin; thus the color index for that erythrocyte is greater than normal (hyperchromic). Although macrocytic erythrocytes are present, the *total* erythrocyte count is below normal because of an increased number of reticulocytes. The overall blood hemoglobin level may therefore be below normal value. It should be noted that anemias caused by vitamin B_{12} deficiency are often classified as *macrocytic hyperchromic anemias.*

Pernicious anemia, an example of macrocytic anemia, results from the failure of the mucosal cells of the gastric fundus to secrete the intrinsic factor. In the absence of the intrinsic factor, the absorption of vitamin B_{12} is poor. Both the intrinsic and extrinsic factors must be present to prevent pernicious anemia. The most common cause for the lack of the intrinsic factor is atrophy of the gastric mucosa. Other causes would be a total gastrectomy in which the source of the intrinsic factor is removed, and gastritis or extensive neoplasia in which the gastric secretory function is damaged.

People under the age of 35 are rarely affected with pernicious anemia. As age increases both sexes are equally affected.

The physical manifestations of pernicious anemia involve primarily the nervous and gastrointestinal systems. The neurologic symptoms include symmetrical paresthesias of the toes and fingers, which can progress to a feeling of tingling, pins and needles in the hands and feet. These symptoms indicate that degeneration of the sensory fibers of the peripheral nerves has taken place. As the degenerative changes progress to include the posterior and lateral tracts of the spinal cord, lower limb weakness and difficulty in walking occur. Eventually flaccid and spastic paralysis can result. Unfortunately these neurologic changes are not reversible. Cerebral changes are common. Among these changes are dullness, loss of memory, irritability, and sometimes psychosis.

Symptoms of gastrointestinal involvement result from mucosal atrophy of both the tongue and stomach. The tongue takes on a smooth, shiny appearance and becomes beefy red. A glossitis can be present, the basis for a sore, burning tongue. Also indigestion, loss of appetite, and constipation or diarrhea are common complaints. Secondary to the gastric mucosal atrophy, achlorhydria is present.

In addition to the physical manifestations of the patient, laboratory data are important. The Schilling test is used to test for failure of absorption of vitamin

B_{12} in the intestine. With the Schilling test, 1 microcurie of radioactive vitamin B_{12} (^{60}Co—labeled cyanocobalamin) is administered orally and the 24-hour collection of urine is begun. One hour later, 1,000 micrograms (1 μg) of nonradioactive vitamin B_{12} is injected intramuscularly to "load" or saturate the liver, which serves as a storage depot for vitamin B_{12}. Thus any radioactive vitamin B_{12} that is absorbed from the intestine cannot be stored and will be excreted in the urine. Analysis of the radioactive vitamin B_{12} in a 24-hour urine sample is done. The normal individual will excrete more than 10 to 20 per cent of the oral radioactive vitamin B_{12} dose. If urinary excretion is less than 10 per cent of the oral dose, a malabsorption defect of some type is present. If the urinary excretion is less than 3 per cent of the oral dose, there is presumptive evidence of pernicious anemia.

The next step is to identify whether the absorption defect is due to lack of intrinsic factor or to gastrointestinal disease. Definitive diagnosis is secured by administering an oral preparation containing both radioactive vitamin B_{12} and the intrinsic factor. If the patient has pernicious anemia, the radioactive vitamin B_{12} and the intrinsic factor will be absorbed and normal quantities will be excreted in the urine. If the absorption defect is due to gastrointestinal disease, the urinary excretion of the radioactive vitamin B_{12} will be minimal or absent. It becomes readily apparent that the validity of the test is dependent upon the collection of all urine excreted in the 24-hour test period.

The hematologic findings associated with pernicious anemia are erythrocyte counts below 1.5 million cells per cubic millimeter of blood, anisocytosis, poikilocytosis, and a decreased hemoglobin count. Other changes that can be present are granulocytopenia with relative lymphocytosis and thrombocytopenia. The thrombocyte count usually is down to 60,000 to 70,000 cells. Also the reticulocyte index is usually well below normal. These changes would predispose to the typical signs of anemia—fatigability, weakness, pallor, shortness of breath, and faintness.

Once the diagnosis of pernicious anemia is established, some of the manifestations of the disease can be corrected and others controlled for the rest of the patient's life by regular intramuscular injections of vitamin B_{12} (cyanocobalamin). With the exception of changes in the nervous system, most of the manifestations associated with pernicious anemia respond quickly to therapy with vitamin B_{12}. Although therapy can be expected to prevent further progress of the disease and may even result in some improvement in neurologic symptoms, it will not reverse the changes that already have taken place. Initially, vitamin B_{12} can be administered at daily or weekly intervals. Later the interval is lengthened to monthly or even bimonthly administrations. The need for the patient to continue these injections for the rest of his or her life cannot be emphasized too strongly.

Today with earlier diagnosing of pernicious anemia, fewer patients require hospitalization. Those who are hospitalized usually will have symptoms of degenerative changes of the nervous system or will be too ill to be treated on an outpatient basis.

According to Chanarin (1976), with pernicious anemia significant mortality occurs among the elderly who have a hemoglobin less than 5 g/100 ml. In addition, these individuals frequently are in incipient heart failure. Whether to transfuse these individuals presents a dilemma because a sudden increase in blood volume with a transfusion may precipitate acute heart failure and pulmonary edema. If the patient is transfused, one unit of packed cells is administered over a 12-hour or longer period, and the patient is diuresed to prevent the complication of heart failure. Pertinent nursing observations include any physical signs of a cough or moist breath sounds that could be indicative of pulmonary edema. A precaution to be taken throughout the period of transfusion would be to have the patient in a Fowler's position. Accurate intake and output recordings and body weights would be parameters to monitor in documenting fluid retention or diuresis. The nursing assessment and interventions for pernicious anemia patients include the general assessment of any patient with anemia that is located at the end of this section. The following points relate specifically to the patient with pernicious anemia.

Patients who are weak or who have degenerative changes of the nervous system need to have a care plan developed that includes specific information on position change, body alignment, and range of motion exercises. Patients with pernicious anemia are prone to developing decubiti. The decubiti are thought to result from the effect of prolonged deficiency of vitamin B_{12} on somatic cells. Another contributing factor is the sensory deficits associated with pernicious anemia.

In the present state of knowledge no methods for the primary prevention of pernicious anemia are available. By giving intramuscular injections of vitamin B_{12}, the harmful effects of pernicious anemia can be prevented. It is one of the best examples of a chronic disorder that cannot be cured but that can be controlled.

Previously it was stated that the patient with pernicious anemia lacked the intrinsic factor from the gastric mucosal cells and, therefore, was unable to absorb vitamin B_{12} in the small intestine. With some individuals the intrinsic factor is not lacking, but pathology of the small intestine inhibits the absorption of vitamin B_{12} or creates a deficiency of folic acid. Examples of these situations include (1) *sprue* in which the absorbing membrane in the small intestine is defective, (2) *surgical procedures* that divert the stomach contents around the absorbing membrane or remove the small intestine, and (3) *tapeworms,* which compete with the host for vitamin B_{12}. The anemias in these conditions are similar to pernicious anemia; however, neurological changes are not characteristic features. Macrocytic anemias can also result from the toxic effects of certain drugs that cause a deficiency in folic acid. These drugs include diphenylhydantoin (Dilantin), ethanol, barbiturates, and methotrexate. An adequate dietary intake of all the B vitamins and folic acid is undoubtedly essential to hematopoiesis. These chemicals participate in a wide variety of cellular metabolic reactions essential to normal erythrocyte formation.

Hemolytic anemias. Anemia may also be the result of any disorder in which there is an excessive rate of erythrocyte hemolysis or destruction because of acquired or hereditary factors. These anemias are classified as the hemolytic anemias. The common feature of the hemolytic anemias is destruction of erythrocytes in excess of production rate by the hematopoietic tissues. The result is insufficient quantity and quality of erythrocytes and hemoglobin to meet oxygen transport requirements.

A very large number of etiologic agents have been implicated in the hemolytic anemias. Bunn classifies them as causes arising outside the erythrocyte, or extracorpuscular causes, and those associated with defects in the structure or construction of erythrocytes, or intracorpuscular defects (Bunn, 1977, p. 1651).

Among the extracorpuscular (outside-the-cell) causes are the acute hemolytic anemias caused by immune body reactions. Common examples include the transfusion of incompatible blood, and the hemolytic disease of the newborn caused by the Rh factor. Excessive hemolysis of red cells is secondary to a number of diseases, particularly those involving structures forming part of the reticuloendothelial system. Some examples include Hodgkin's disease, chronic lymphocytic leukemia, metastatic carcinomatosis, and liver disease. A variety of infectious agents are also responsible for increased hemolysis of erythrocytes as in infectious hepatitis and mononucleosis. Although not common in the United States, malaria on a worldwide basis is probably the most frequent reason for anemia caused by increased hemolysis of red cells.

A wide variety of chemicals may also be associated with increased blood destruction. The effect of some such as acetophenetidin (phenacetin), methyl chloride, acetanilid, benzene, and lead depends on the size of the dose to which the individual is exposed. Others such as the sulfonamides, quinine and quinidine, amphetamine sulfate (Benzedrine), phenantoin (Mesantoin), and vitamin K substitutes depend on hypersensitivity to the chemical agent. It may be noted that some of these chemicals may also cause hypoplasia or aplasia of the bone marrow.

Physical agents such as severe thermal burns are also associated with increased hemolysis of erythrocytes. This is one of the factors predisposing to anemia in the severely burned patient.

Besides exposure to a variety of physical and chemical agents, defects in the construction of red cells or in the type of hemoglobin also predispose to an increased rate of blood destruction. A number of these disorders are hereditary. Among them are familial hemolytic anemia (hereditary or congenital spherocytosis), thalassemia (Cooley's anemia or Mediterranean anemia), and sickle-cell anemia.

Depending on the nature of the cause, hemolysis may take place in the circulating blood or in the reticuloendothelial system. These disorders also differ widely in symptomatology, severity, and course. In some, the rate of onset may be rapid and the manifestations severe. In others, the onset is slow, and the manifestations are mild or absent. A determining factor is whether hemolysis occurs in the circulating blood or in the reticuloendothelial system. In all instances in which erythrocytes are hemolyzed at an abnormal rate, some degree of jaundice occurs. It may be barely perceptible or it may be of marked degree. It may develop slowly or rapidly, but jaundice is present to some degree. In chronic hemolytic anemias the liver and spleen are frequently enlarged, and complications such as cholelithiasis and leg ulcers may develop.

When the onset of hemolysis is rapid and a large number of erythrocytes are hemolyzed, as occurs following the transfusion of incompatible blood, the patient may have a severe shaking chill followed by a high fever, headache, and pain in the back, abdomen, and extremities. The abdominal pain may be so severe that abdominal rigidity results. When the hemolysis is significant, shock may develop. As in shock from other causes, oliguria and anuria may follow. The urine output is dark in color.

It is imperative to stop the transfusion immediately if the above symptoms occur. If symptoms of shock are present, treatment must be initiated. The remainder of the blood to be infused, a fresh sample of the patient's blood, and a urine specimen are sent to the blood bank to recheck the blood for donor-recipient ABO and Rh compatibility.

Intervention with the acquired hemolytic anemias is directed toward removal or treatment of the underlying cause. Initially, steroid therapy (prednisone) is administered for a period of months until the hemoglobin has risen to normal. Approximately half the patients with hemolytic anemia will relapse with the tapering or cessation of steroids. For those patients who cannot tolerate steroids or in whom the disease is not controlled, a spleenectomy is the second mode of therapy. In recent years patients who have become refractory to steroid therapy and spleenectomy have been treated with immunosuppressive drugs. The greatest experience has been with azathioprine (Imuran) and cyclophosphamide (Cytoxan).

Sickle-cell anemia is an inherited form of hemolytic anemia. The primary defect is in the formation of the protein portion of the hemoglobin molecule. When the sickle-cell erythrocyte is in the presence of a low blood P_{O_2}, the hemoglobin cannot combine optimally with oxygen to meet transport requirements.

The basic abnormality of the sickle-cell erythrocyte is in the globin portion of the hemoglobin molecule. During the biochemical formation of the normal hemoglobin molecule (hemoglobin A), the amino acid glutamine assumes the sixth position in both the beta chains of globin. The sickle-cell hemoglobin (hemoglobin S) differs from hemoglobin A by the substitution of the amino acid *valine* for glutamine in the beta chains. This single amino acid substitution is the only chemical difference among the 574 amino acids in the hemoglobin A and S molecules (Harper, 1973, pp. 199–200). Distortion of the erythrocyte occurs. Rather than the normal biconcave shape of normal erythrocytes, the sickle-cell erythrocytes assume a crescent shape, like a sickle, hence the name.

Sickle-cell anemia is a homozygous state where the mendelian recessive gene is received from both parents. This form of anemia affects persons from infancy to adulthood primarily in the black population. With more interracial marriages, however, Caucasians are also affected. Other groups affected, but to a lesser degree, are Puerto Ricans and persons of Greek, Italian, Spanish, Middle Eastern, and Indian ancestry. Many of these individuals possess the sickle-cell trait. When two people with the sickle-cell trait marry, each child has a 25 per cent chance of having sickle-cell anemia. Through counseling, however, persons with sickle-cell trait need to be educated to understand that the sickle-cell trait does not develop into sickle-cell anemia.

Sickle-cell trait is a heterozygous state in which the mutant gene is received from one parent. In sickle-cell trait each erythrocyte contains both hemoglobin A and S. Although the patient may experience some symptoms when the erythrocytes are in a deoxygenated environment, sickle-cell crisis usually does not occur. Diagnosis of sickle-cell trait and anemia is achieved by the clinical history, family background, sickle-cell preparation, and hemoglobin electrophoresis studies.

The symptoms of sickle-cell anemia are swelling of the hands and feet, swelling of the joints, unexplained skeletal and abdominal pain, listlessness, and fatigue. Pallor (seen as a grayish cast over brown skin) or jaundice of the skin, conjunctiva, and mucous membranes frequently are present in the chronic state. In adulthood, the "Spider body" stature characteristically is assumed, which is narrow shoulders and hips, kyphosis of the upper back, tower-shaped skull, and an increased anterior-posterior diameter of the chest.

The most feared situation with sickle-cell anemia is the pain episode. Frequently the terminology "sickle-cell crisis" is used; however, the term "pain episode" is preferred because of the lesser negative connotation. When the sickle-cell erythrocytes are subjected to a low blood oxygen tension, the hemoglobin S tends to polymerize into long chains, precipitate inside the cell, and thus become "sickled." The precipitated hemoglobin causes the cell membrane to be more fragile, which leads to a shortened life span for the cell. The normal life span of an erythrocyte is 120 days, whereas the life span of a sickled cell is 15 to 20 days. Sickled cells are rigid and inflexible cells that tend to rupture as they pass through the microcirculation. They become entangled and thus the "sickling" process occurs. The slow-moving ruptured cells promote intravascular occlusion which causes oxygen deprivation and an accumulation of acid waste products. As the tissues extract oxygen from the slow-moving blood, still more cells become sickled and a vicious cycle is created.

The factors that precipitate the pain episode are not readily apparent. They appear to occur during periods when low blood oxygen tension, acidosis, and stasis of erythrocytes are enhanced, such as (1) during periods of infection, (2) on exposure to cold, and (3) during the hours of sleep. The first sign of an infection, which can precipitate a pain episode, is fever. The physician should be notified if the temperature goes above 100 to 101°F and fluids should be forced to prevent dehydration, which precipitates the sickling process. Infections, particularly of the upper respiratory tract, should be prevented, because pneumonia with hypoxemia and respiratory acidosis could ensue. Persons with sickle-cell anemia are prone to pneumococcal infections, and the mortality from these infections can be high. Exposure to cold should be avoided as stasis of erythrocytes would more likely occur during that time. Warm nonbinding clothing is recommended. Also any type of clothing that would diminish venous return and thus deter pulmonary oxygenation should be avoided.

The *clinical manifestations of a pain episode* are the result of intravascular sickling and occlusions, particularly in the peripheral microcirculation. The patient experiences excruciating abdominal, muscular, and joint pain. Complications associated with sickle-cell anemia are cholelithiasis secondary to the build-up of bilirubin from hemolyzed sickle cells, infarction of any body organ, vascular occlusion, and cardiac failure. The sickle-cell anemia patient is prone to chronic leg ulcers at the level of the malleolus because of peripheral stasis and vascular occlusions. There is a peculiar predisposition to osteomyelitis and susceptibility to chronic infections of the urinary tract as well as pneumonia.

At present there is no known cure for sickle-cell anemia. In the event of a pain episode, the patient is (1) put on bedrest to decrease metabolic needs, (2) given liberal doses of analgesics to diminish the pain, (3) given oxygen therapy to increase blood oxygen tension, and (4) administered fluids to increase the blood volume and mobilize the sickled cells. Blood transfusions are utilized only in severe cases of anemia that have other complications, such as infection, or in the case of impending surgery. Transfusions are monitored carefully because of potential iron overload and excessive hematocrit with further increased blood viscosity. Partial blood exchange transfusions have proved helpful in some cases. In that the process of sickling is promoted by acidosis, an alkaline milieu of the blood is promoted by administration of alkaline fluids by oral and/or parenteral routes. Long-term management of the patient with sickle-cell anemia includes means to diminish intravascular stasis and promote physiologic blood oxygen tension. The patient should prevent infection, avoid exposure to cold, and avoid altitudes over 7,000 feet.

Priapism (persistent, abnormal erection of the penis without sexual desire) caused by sickling, stasis, and occlusion of venous blood flow can last for hours, days, or weeks. Prolonged episodes can result in impotence. Women are counseled against pregnancy because of the risk to both mother and fetus. Since birth control pills are contraindicated, women need to be referred to a family planning agency for alternative methods of contraception.

There has been a high mortality associated with sickle-cell anemia in early childhood. Fortunately, the morbidity-mortality rates are diminishing because of better nutritional states and prevention and early treatment of infections. Many community programs have been launched to provide public education, genetic counseling, and early screening for those with sickle-cell disease.

ASSESSMENT OF THE PATIENT WITH ANEMIA. Assessment of the patient with anemia includes analysis of the laboratory data and physical manifestations presented by the patient. Analysis not only may provide a definitive diagnosis but may serve to determine the degree of severity of the disease and indicate the response to therapy.

Laboratory data. In addition to counting the total number of each type of cell, the blood can be examined in one or more of the following ways:

- *Erythrocytes.* The erythrocytes may be studied for the total count per cubic millimeter of blood, percentage of mature cells (reticulocyte), percentage of immature cells (erythroblast) and stage of immaturity, variations in size and shape of cells (microcyte, macrocyte, anisocyte, spherocyte, and poikilocyte), and red cell fragility.
- *Hemoglobin.* The concentration of hemoglobin in grams per 100 ml of blood can be determined. The normal value for males is greater than for females, because of their higher erythrocyte count. The normal value for males is approximately 16 g per 100 ml of blood, whereas that for females is 14 g per 100 ml of blood. Each gram of hemoglobin has the potential for combination with 1.34 ml of oxygen. A hemoglobin count is the easiest and most efficient way to diagnose any anemia and to determine its severity. It also acts as a guide to the effectiveness of treatment.
- *Hematocrit.* The hematocrit measures the percentage of red cells in the total blood volume. If the red blood cells are of normal size, the hematocrit parallels the red cell count. But if the cells are microcytic or macrocytic, the red cell relationship does not hold true. In microcytic anemia (iron deficiency), the hematocrit decreases even though the red cell count may be normal because the cells pack to a smaller volume. To the contrary, in macrocytic anemia (pernicious anemia) the hematocrit is higher than the red cell count would indicate.

  The hematocrit equals three times the hemoglobin within $\pm$ 3.0 per cent. Thus, if the hemoglobin is 12.4 g/100 ml, the hematocrit should be between 34 and 40 per cent ($12.4 \times 3.0 = 37 \pm 3 = 34$ to 40 per cent). If the red cells are abnormal in size or the hemoglobin content is abnormal, the stated relationship between hemoglobin and the hematocrit will not hold true (Byrne, 1976, p. 110).
- *Erythrocyte indices.* The relationship between the hemoglobin content and the number and size of erythrocytes is important in the diagnosis of various anemic states. The erythrocyte indices that incorporate these relationships are the mean corpuscular hemoglobin concentration (MCHC), the

mean corpuscular volume (MCV), and the mean corpuscular hemoglobin (MCH).

The *mean corpuscular hemoglobin concentration* (MCHC) is the average hemoglobin content per 100 ml of *packed* erythrocytes. The MCHC value that is obtained indicates what is the per cent of hemoglobin in a 100-ml sample that is purely erythrocytes minus the plasma and other cellular components. The normal value is reported as 33 to 38 per cent or grams per 100 ml.

An erythrocyte with a normal MCHC indicates that the proper amount of hemoglobin is present for its size. These cells are called normochromic. Both microcytic and macrocytic cells can be normochromic if the hemoglobin content changes in proportion to the cell volume. If the erythrocyte volume increases more than the amount of hemoglobin, a decreased MCHC will result. These cells, classified as hypochromic, are present in iron-deficiency anemia.

Most anemias are classified as normocytic, normochromic. Among the anemias in this classification are aplastic anemia, sickle-cell anemia, and anemia present with leukemia.

The *mean corpuscular volume* (MCV) is the average size of an individual erythrocyte. The normal range is 80 to 94 cu μ (cubic microns). From this index erythrocytes can be classified as normocytic, microcytic, or macrocytic. Microcytic cells are found with iron-deficiency anemia. Macrocytic cells are present in cases of pernicious anemia and folic acid deficiency.

The *mean corpuscular hemoglobin* (MCH) is the average amount of hemoglobin per erythrocyte. The normal range is 27 to 33 $\mu\mu$g (micromicrograms). This index can reflect a change in either the MCHC or MCV. Normally there is a direct relationship between the MCV and MCH. As the size of an erythrocyte increases, so does its weight. There will be an increase in the MCH with macrocytic anemia, whereas there is a decrease in the MCH with microcytic anemia.

- *Hemoglobin electrophoresis.* The type of hemoglobin that an individual possesses can be determined by studies of structure and electrophoretic patterns. At least twelve types of human hemoglobin have been identified, examples of which are hemoglobin A (normal adult hemoglobin), hemoglobin S (sickle-cell), and hemoglobin F (fetal hemoglobin).
- *Sickle-cell preparation.* Sickle-cell erythrocytes can be identified by this test. A blood sample is deoxygenated by addition of a sodium bisulfite solution. The sickled erythrocytes, if present, can be seen under a microscope.
- *Bone marrow examination.* A sample of bone marrow is aspirated from the sternum under sterile conditions. A smear is studied for the state of hematopoietic activity, presence of abnormal cells, and the percentage and morphology of dominant cells.
- *Reticulocyte count.* The reticulocyte count indicates how well the bone marrow is producing red blood cells. The normal range is 0.5 to 1.5 per cent of the total erythrocytes. This test is especially useful in determining a patient's response to therapy for iron-deficiency and pernicious anemia. A count of 32 per cent or higher following therapy is indicative of a positive response.

  A low reticulocyte count occurs when the bone marrow is not producing red blood cells or the production is decreased, as happens with anemia, especially aplastic or pernicious. A high reticulocyte count is indicative of active red cell production. In hemolytic anemia, the reticulocyte count will be elevated because the bone marrow is rapidly replacing lost or destroyed red blood cells.
- *Icterus index.* A blood sample is analyzed for amount of bilirubin present in milligrams per 100 ml. Although this analysis does not differentiate if excess amounts are due to altered liver function or erythrocyte destruction, an increased value in the presence of other normal liver function studies may indicate a hemolytic anemia. For the direct method, the normal value is 0.05 to 1.4 mg per 100 ml. The normal range for the indirect method is 0.4 to 0.8 mg per 100 ml of blood.
- *Iron.* Analysis of the serum iron present and its ability to bind with transferrin are done in the diagnosis of iron deficiency anemia. The normal range for serum iron is 65 to 170 μg per 100 ml. The range for the total iron-binding capacity analysis is 250 to 400 μg per 100 ml of blood.

Obviously not every patient is subjected to all the preceding examinations. Moreover, in individual instances other tests may be utilized in the process of making the diagnosis. Most of these tests do not require special or elaborate preparation of the patient. The patient may need some help in understanding why blood must be removed for the purposes of examination. Even when the patient accepts on an intellectual level that blood is required, he or she may not accept it on an emotional level. This lack of acceptance is expressed in a number of ways. The patient repeatedly asks such questions as, "Is it really necessary to take all that blood?" "Doesn't the physician know that I am already short of blood?" "How can I get well when they take my blood each morning?" He or she calls the laboratory technicians, nurses, or physicians who take the blood "blood suckers." Among healthy people the loss of a few milliliters of blood can be frightening or can be perceived as dangerous. Understanding how the patient feels about the removal of blood for examination should help the nurse to be supportive. Because the anemic patient is frequently hyperirritable, taking blood may be associated with expressions of this irritability. As the patient responds to treatment, he or she will be better able to tolerate frustration and discomfort.

PHYSICAL ASSESSMENT AND NURSING INTERVENTION. Before baseline assessments of the patient are made, it is imperative to understand the pathology and underlying physiologic changes that result with the anemic state. Regardless of the etiology, tissue hypoxia is the underlying cause of the symptoms. When the blood is unable to deliver adequate amounts of oxygen to the various tissues for maintenance of metabolic processes, tissue hypoxia and cellular dysfunction occur. Obviously those systems of the body with high oxygen requirements display the most symptoms. These include the skeletal muscular, cardiovascular, respiratory, and central nervous systems.

Usually some type of exertion, which increases the oxygen demand in the body, is required before the patient experiences symptoms. The extent of symptoms is not necessarily correlated with the severity of the anemia. The patient who has a sudden severe blood loss may have more objective symptoms, because of insufficient time for other mechanisms to compensate, than the individual who has a severe anemic state that has developed over a longer period of time. Other factors that affect the severity of the patient's physical manifestations are the patient's age and general status of the cardiovascular system. The very young and the very old individuals may exhibit greater symptomatology.

Fatigue and physical weakness are the most common objective and subjective symptoms present with the various types of anemia. When the skeletal muscle cells do not receive a sufficient quantity of oxygen for catabolic processes, there is a decrease in the amount of biochemical energy (ATP) available for maintenance of optimal cellular function. Objective manifestations of fatigue include a drooping posture and slow walk. All too frequently, an increase in the pulse rate is overlooked as an important parameter when objectively assessing if the patient is becoming fatigued. Subjectively, the patient reports feeling weak and not being able to physically do as much as previously. He or she may report dizziness, shortness of breath, and perspiring associated with the fatigue as related to increased activity.

When interviewing the patient it is important to elicit information regarding the types of activity that precipitate symptoms of fatigue. One should determine the specific activities of daily living that the patient is capable of performing without causing fatigue. First, have the patient describe a normal day's activity. Also, determine such things as the following: What is the patient's normal sleep pattern? How far can the patient walk before becoming fatigued? Is the patient capable of climbing stairs? Is the patient capable of doing his or her own washing, ironing, cooking, and cleaning? Is he or she capable of working in the yard? In addition to obtaining this verbal information, it is wise to observe some of these activities. Because the patient appears well, it should not be assumed that he or she is capable of doing the activities of daily living, such as bathing and feeding; instead, observe what the patient is capable of doing without becoming fatigued. Nonprofessional personnel need assistance in making judgments regarding nursing care, as they tend to permit the patient to be too independent with activities and thus become fatigued.

The nurse must help the patient set priorities and determine what activities he or she is capable of performing independently and those that will necessitate assistance. Many patients with anemia will feel just as fatigued when they awaken in the morning as when they retire. Because of this, activities should be paced over the waking hours rather than scheduling all activities immediately upon arising. Frequent rest periods will make it possible for the skeletal muscle cells to receive a sufficient quantity of oxygen for catabolic processes. As a result, there will be an increase in the amount of biochemical energy available for cellular function, which gives the patient added strength. Patients should be taught to curtail their activity before fatigue occurs, because once fatigue is present it will take the body longer to recuperate. In addition, the slower one works, the less of a demand the body has for oxygen, thus the longer one can work. Once fatigue is present, the patient needs to be cognizant of what can be done to relieve this symptom.

Symptoms related to the cardiovascular and respiratory systems are usually present with anemia. These include tachycardia, pallor, and dyspnea. The compensatory mechanisms associated with anemia are tachycardia and an increased stroke volume, which effect an increased cardiac output. Despite many studies of the mechanism of increased cardiac output in anemia, the exact pathologic physiology is not well understood. Studies reveal that decreased blood viscosity is one, but not the sole factor that causes an increase in cardiac output. It seems likely that a decreased peripheral vascular resistance is an important factor, but the manner in which this is mediated is obscure (Fowler, 1970, p. 1381).

If the cardiac output does not compensate for the

decreased oxygen-carrying capacity of the blood, myocardial ischemia may develop, causing some patients to experience angina. This would happen more frequently in the elderly or any individual who has decreased myocardial circulation secondary to coronary vascular changes. Also cardiac failure may result from the increased workload and diminished oxygen supply to contractile cells. If this condition is not treated, varying degrees of heart failure will develop.

Pallor of certain parts of the body, such as the fingers and toenails or the mucous membranes, does indicate anemia. Despite the widespread belief that pallor of the skin indicates anemia, it is not a very reliable sign. Many factors affect the color of the skin, such as the thickness of the epidermis, the quantity and color of the skin pigment, and the number of blood vessels in the skin as well as the nature and quantity of hemoglobin carried in the blood. Some persons have naturally sallow complexions and are not anemic. Also, certain diseases are accompanied by a pallor, though anemia is absent.

As the cardiac abnormalities develop, the rate and depth of respirations increase, and the patient becomes aware of dyspnea. This symptom is correlated with a decrease in the vital capacity and respiratory reserve volume.

A patient's activity should be planned so that the activity is curtailed before dyspnea occurs. If dyspnea does occur, it may be necessary for the patient to rest upright in bed to relieve the symptom. The bedrest will decrease the oxygen requirements of cells. The upright position pulls the diaphragm down and keeps the abdominal viscera away from the lungs, thus providing for better lung expansion. Supportive oxygen therapy may be required for a brief period of time.

Varying degrees of neurologic symptoms can occur, depending on the severity and type of the anemia. Some neurologic symptoms occur in the anemic patient because the blood is diverted from the brain when standing in an upright position. These symptoms would include tinnitus, headache (pounding), spots before the eyes, fainting, drowsiness, irritability, and inability to concentrate. If dizziness or drowsiness is present, such activities as driving a motor vehicle, smoking in bed, or walking down stairs may have to be curtailed. The patient should be taught to avoid activities that would aggravate the dizziness by suddenly decreasing the blood supply to the brain. This would include sudden movements, such as bending, getting out of bed quickly, or turning quickly.

Other neurologic symptoms occur as a result of degenerative changes in the nervous system. Vitamin B_{12} is essential to maintain normal nerve cell metabolism. With deficiency, as in pernicious anemia, there is demyelination of the dorsal and lateral columns of the spinal cord, as well as the peripheral nerves. These degenerative changes are thought to be due to defective RNA synthesis. The spinal cord involvement is manifested by disturbances in sphincter control and locomotor dysfunction. Either bowel and bladder incontinence or retention may be present.

Clinical manifestations associated with the gastrointestinal tract occur secondary to the decreased nutrient and oxygen supply to cells. The symptoms include abdominal distention, flatulence, diarrhea, anorexia, nausea, vomiting, and sore mouth and tongue. When selecting a diet for the patient with the previously mentioned symptoms, consideration should be given to the amount of carbohydrates, roughage, and foods with a cathartic effect that could aggravate the gastrointestinal symptoms.

For the patient who has a painful tongue or sores in the mouth, the diet should be low in roughage and bland. In addition, hot, spicy, or highly acid foods should be avoided. For these patients special attention should be given to their mouth. When brushing the teeth, a soft brush should be used, and the teeth should be brushed gently. At times it may be necessary to apply the toothpaste with large cotton balls or with well-moistened pieces of cotton to prevent traumatizing fragile tissues that could bleed. In still other patients it may be necessary to limit the cleansing of the mouth to mouthwash. In addition, solutions such as 1 per cent hydrogen peroxide or Dobells solution can be tried. The mucous membranes of the mouth can be kept moist by rinsing with milk of magnesia, which coats the mucous membrane. The coat that forms can be removed by rinsing the mouth with water. Frequently crusts will form that can be broken up by using carbonated beverages.

Another clinical manifestation experienced by most patients with anemia is sensitivity to cold. Whether this is due to peripheral arteriolar constriction with resultant decreased peripheral cellular catabolism, reduced heat formation, or acid metabolite accumulation is still speculative. Regardless of the mechanism, the patient feels warmer and more comfortable in a warm environment or wearing extra clothing, such as sweaters and socks. External sources of heat, such as heating pads, should be avoided. With oxygen deprivation to dermal tissues, thermoreceptors may be less responsive to thermal stimuli, and the patient could become burned easily.

In long-standing anemic states, changes take place in the skin and appendages subsequent to the oxygen deprivation. The skin loses its elasticity and tone, and the hair thins. Ecchymoses and purpura may be observed in the skin. Precautions to prevent the patient from bruising should be exercised. In iron-deficiency anemia, the nails lose their luster, become brittle, and break easily.

In severe anemia, menstrual disturbances in the female and loss of libido in the male are not infrequent. The most frequent menstrual disturbance is amenorrhea, although menorrhagia can also occur. Assessment of the times and degree of bleeding should be made in order to note its contribution to the total anemic state.

An overall goal should be to protect the anemic patient from infection and trauma. Because hypoxic tissues are more prone to the invasion of microorganisms than normally perfused tissues, the patient with anemia should be protected from sources of infection. The patient should be taught to avoid crowds when illness is prevalent, to avoid contact with individuals with a known infection, and to practice good hygiene, such as hand washing. Protection from trauma is of the utmost importance, as hypoxia would only contribute to poor healing of traumatized tissue.

Therapy in anemia must be directed to the cause and pathogenesis of the disorder in each patient. In anemias caused by blood loss the condition causing the loss of blood must, if possible, be corrected. In acute blood loss the first consideration is the maintenance and restoration of the blood volume. When there is a great loss of blood with a marked decrease in its oxygen-carrying power, the cellular elements must also be replaced. In serious hemorrhage, replacement of blood cells, although not life-saving, may facilitate the recovery of the patient.

The loss of iron in chronic blood loss is the problem, not the decrease in blood volume. Therapy is directed therefore toward identifying and eliminating the cause and restoring the level of iron to normal. In iron-deficiency anemia, the patient responds to an increased intake of iron, but does not benefit from an increased intake of vitamin B_{12} unless it also is lacking. The same is true of patients who have a vitamin B_{12} deficiency. In some instances, such as in the patient with sickle-cell anemia or thalassemia, an increase in the intake of iron, particularly in the form of red cells, may actually be harmful, because the body has no mechanism by which it can eliminate iron once it is absorbed into the body. Probably the greatest harm to the largest number of people comes from the waste of money spent on "shotgun" preparations prepared to cure all blood deficiencies. In the absence of a disease of the blood or a condition causing the loss of blood, money spent for a nutritious diet is a good anemia preventative.

From this review of the effects of anemia on the various systems of the body, it is apparent that anemia has widespread effects. Some symptoms, such as those of the respiratory and circulatory systems, are compensatory mechanisms that represent adjustments to lessen the effects of the lowered oxygen-carrying capacity of the blood. Others, such as those arising in the gastrointestinal and nervous systems, are signs that pathology is present, but they are not compensatory mechanisms, and they do not add to the patient's capacity to adapt. Still others, such as loss of appetite, may aggravate the preexisting disorder.

To summarize, anemia results when blood production fails to keep up with erythrocyte destruction. The balance between the factors may be upset by a failure in blood production, by the demands for erythrocytes exceeding the capacity of the bone marrow to produce them, or by an increase in the rate of destruction of erythrocytes over the functional capacity of the bone marrow. Anemia is also caused by the loss of blood. When the loss of blood is rapid, the most acute problems are created by a loss of blood volume.

Anemias have a great number of causes. They may be primary (that is, arise from some disturbance in the functioning of the hematopoietic tissues) or they may be secondary to disturbances in other parts of the body. There are few chronically ill patients who, because of the effects of their disease on blood production or destruction or both, as well as on food intake, escape some degree of anemia. It is not unusual for the chronically ill patient with a marked degree of anemia to feel much improved after the anemia is corrected.

Excess of Erythrocytes: Polycythemia

In contrast to the anemic states in which there is a deficit of erythrocytes and/or hemoglobin, polycythemia is best defined as an abnormal increase in erythrocyte mass with a normal or increased hemoglobin level. Because of the erythrocytosis, the blood viscosity is markedly increased, which promotes a diminished velocity of blood flow through the microcirculation; thus the oxygen transport to cells is diminished.

The primary classification of the polycythemias is (1) secondary polycythemia, a consequence of recognized causes and (2) primary polycythemia (polycythemia vera), a chronic idiopathic condition. It should be noted, however, that polycythemia may also result if the plasma volume is diminished, as in dehydration, so that hemoconcentration becomes apparent. This state is known as a relative polycythemia.

Secondary polycythemia may develop as a result of a variety of conditions most of which are associated with tissue hypoxia. An accelerated erythropoiesis occurs when there is a prolonged lowering of the blood oxygen tension despite a normal or elevated hemoglobin level. The diminished oxygen tension does not stimulate the hematopoietic cells of the bone marrow directly but stimulates the kidneys to release erythropoietin, which in turn serves as the stimulus for increased hematopoietic activity of the bone marrow.

The situations that most commonly cause secondary polycythemia are of cardiac and pulmonary origins. Examples include some of the congenital heart defects in which venous blood enters the arterial circulation, thus lowering the oxygen tension, and chronic pulmonary conditions where there is a blockage of the alveolar membrane, thus inhibiting oxygen diffusion. Polycythemia has also been noted in persons with tremendous obesity (Pickwickian syndrome) and in association with primary aldosteronism and various types of cancer. There is evidence that some tumors and cysts of the kidneys liberate a substance having erythropoietinlike activity on the bone marrow. Healthy individuals, living or working at high altitudes, such as the Peace Corps workers in the Andes, may have a polycythemia proportional to the diminished oxygen tension of inspired air.

Polycythemias secondary to cardiac or pulmonary disease are accompanied by clinical manifestations of the primary disease. In this instance polycythemia is itself a symptom, and not the primary disease. Although the erythrocyte count may rise to 8 to 10 million per cubic millimeter, not all cells are normocytic. The hemoglobin level may rise, but not as high as would be expected because of the substantial number of immature erythrocytes. Reticulocytosis is present but leukocytosis is generally absent. The essential diagnostic criterion is the oxygen saturation of the arterial blood, which at rest is below 90 per cent and following exercise usually falls below 80 per cent.

Intervention with secondary polycythemia is chiefly correction or removal of the underlying cause. Elimination of the offending disorder generally results in a remission or cessation of the polycythemia. If the hematocrit rises to 65 to 70 per cent, phlebotomy may be considered as palliative therapy.

Primary polycythemia (vera) is a chronic disease of unknown etiology characterized by hyperplasia of *all* the cellular elements of the bone marrow. There is a resultant sustained erythrocytosis, leukocytosis, thrombocytosis, and elevated hemoglobin level. This state has been regarded by some clinicians as a neoplastic disease of the hematopoietic tissues analogous to leukemia. There is no evidence that diminished blood oxygen tension or erythropoietin serves as the stimulus for the excessive cell production, as occurs in secondary polycythemia. There is some thought that a "polycythemic virus" may be the cause. The incidence of this disorder is high among Jews, with males more commonly affected than females.

The blood volume can increase as much as twice that which is normal, thus causing engorgement of the vascular system. Increased blood viscosity, decreased blood velocity, and thrombocytosis promote intravascular thrombosis. Even though the increased viscosity of the blood tends to decrease the venous return, the cardiac output is usually normal. The increased blood volume tends to increase the venous return, thus counteracting the sluggish effect of the viscous blood. Another indication of decreased velocity of blood flow is a prolonged circulation time. The thrombocytosis is probably of greater importance than the increased blood viscosity in explaining the intravascular thrombosis, as the incidence of thrombosis is low in secondary polycythemia where there is also increased blood viscosity but normal levels of thrombocytes. Paradoxically, the patient with primary polycythemia tends to bleed excessively from minor cuts and bruises, which may be due to distention of the capillary and venous walls by the increased blood volume.

Assessment of the patient with primary polycythemia focuses on the clinical manifestations and differentiation of the laboratory data from those that are characteristic of secondary polycythemia. The increased blood volume is the major factor in the pathogenesis of the headache, fatigability, elevated systolic blood pressure, pedal edema, and general plethoric appearance. Splenomegaly gives rise to a feeling of fullness on the left side of the abdomen. Hepatomegaly is a common finding. Symptoms attributed to diminished blood flow and oxygen transport include dizziness, dyspnea, angina, paresthesias, visual disturbances, intermittent claudication, and itching, which is aggravated by a hot bath. The patient will usually have a ruddy cyanotic complexion because of increased amounts of deoxygenated hemoglobin in the microcirculation.

The laboratory data of primary polycythemia reveal an erythrocyte count comparable to that found in secondary polycythemia. Reticulocytosis and an increased hematocrit up to 70 to 80 per cent are noted. At this point similarities to secondary polycythemia end. In primary polycythemia the erythrocytes are normocytic. The hemoglobin level is increased but less in proportion to the increased erythrocyte count because of a low MCV and MCHC. The leukocyte count is greater than 10,000 per cubic millimeter and frequently achieves levels of 25,000 or greater. Thrombocyte levels as high as 3 million per cubic millimeter are noted. The increased production of blood cells results in an increased destruction of blood cells. This in turn gives rise to hyperbilirubinemia and hyperuricemia. The arterial saturation of the blood is normal in most instances. The oxygen saturation therefore is of little value in differentiating primary and secondary polycythemia.

At present, there is no known cure for primary polycythemia, but as with certain forms of anemia, it can be controlled. Therapeutic intervention is directed toward maintenance of a reasonable blood volume, viscosity, and thrombocyte level. When the hematocrit level rises above 55 to 60 per cent, phlebotomy with withdrawal of 500 ml of blood may be done one to two times a week. If the hematocrit remains high after phlebotomy, it may be necessary to spin down the blood obtained and replace the plasma fraction. Alkylating agents such as busulfan and chlorambucil may be used as adjuncts to phlebotomy to control the elevated thrombocyte level. In selected cases the administration of radioactive phosphorus (^{32}P) may be utilized. Radioactive phosphorus concentrates in tissues with a high phosphorus turnover such as bone marrow and suppresses hematopoietic activity. Extreme caution is exercised with this form of therapy, however, to minimize the danger of the individual developing a radiation-induced leukemia.

The patient with primary polycythemia is a prime candidate for the development of thromboembolic phenomena. Every effort should be made to keep the patient ambulatory and diminish situations that would promote decreased venous return. Planned activity patterns should take into account not only the need for ambulation but the visual impairments and paresthesia as well. Warm or cool baths would decrease the incidence of itching associated with hot water contact. In addition, the patient may need the opportunity to share the problems and concerns present with a chronic, perhaps catastrophic, illness.

The Self-Sealing Mechanism

The second function of the blood in which a disorder may occur is the self-sealing mechanism. Through the efficient operation of this hemostatic mechanism, breaks in the integrity of blood vessels are repaired before appreciable amounts of blood are lost to the extravascular tissues or external environment. Failure of the self-sealing mechanism will result in a diminished amount of blood to serve as the vehicle of transport. The blood-clotting process, a component of the self-sealing mechanism, must also be maintained within normal limits to prevent the loss of blood through bleeding tendencies and to prevent clotting tendencies that could obstruct the flow of blood to and from tissues. In either instance, if the self-sealing mechanism or clotting process fails, the result would be an insufficient quantity of blood and essential materials to metabolizing cells.

Three Participating Elements

Three elements enter into the self-sealing mechanism. They are (1) the surrounding tissues (extravascular), (2) the blood vessels (vascular), and (3) the coagulation of the blood (intravascular). Firm or nondistensible tissues tend to limit bleeding as the tissue hydrostatic pressure rises secondary to the blood entering, thus impeding blood loss. Conversely, when bleeding occurs in distensible tissues or from an area where the blood escapes from the body, tissue hydrostatic pressure may be slow to rise or may not rise at all. Consequently, bleeding involving a break in the skin, mucosa, or serous membranes is likely to be more profuse because the flow of blood is unopposed.

The second element involved in the self-sealing mechanism is the blood vessels. If a blood vessel is severed, the cut ends will constrict. With a greater degree of trauma, more vasoconstriction takes place and less bleeding occurs. Instances have been known where an extremity was amputated by accidental crushing and little bleeding occurred.

The third element in the self-sealing mechanism is the coagulation of the blood. Blood is capable of clotting when there is a break in the wall of a blood vessel, although under normal circumstances blood does not clot intravascularly.

Three Factors Preventing Intravascular Clotting

Three factors protect the blood from clotting within the normal vascular system. They are (1) the structure of the blood vessel, (2) the nature of the blood flow, and (3) the presence of anticoagulant chemicals in the blood. Normal blood vessels have a smooth endothelial lining that lessens trauma to blood cells as they are carried through the vessel. In addition there is a layer of negatively charged proteins on the intimal lining, which repels the negatively charged platelets, thereby preventing platelet adherence.

The second factor that inhibits intravascular clotting is laminar blood flow. The blood fluid has direct contact with the endothelial lining, and the cellular elements tend to pass through the inner core of the vessel. When the velocity of blood flow is slow, however, as with immobility or partial obstruction of a vessel, blood cellular elements may adhere to the vessel wall. The possibility of intravascular clotting is thereby increased.

The third factor that protects against intravascular clotting in the normal vascular system is the presence of chemicals in the blood that favor anticoagulation. Among the many substances normally found in the blood are anticoagulants and procoagulants. A balance exists between the two groups of substances, with the anticoagulants assuming greater influence, so that under normal circumstances the blood does not tend to clot. The primary anticoagulant is heparin, which is secreted by basophilic mast cells located in the pericapillary connective tissue throughout the body. Mast cells are particularly abundant in the tissues surrounding the pulmonary and hepatic capillaries. Prothrombin, which is synthesized in the liver, serves as the primary procoagulant.

Sequential Events

The self-sealing mechanism occurs in sequential steps in response to a torn or severed vessel. One author cites the sequence of events as (1) vascular spasm, (2) formation of a platelet plug, (3) blood coagulation, and (4) fibrous organization of the clot (Guyton, 1976, p. 99).

The vascular spasm associated with a ruptured or cut vessel is attributed to nervous system reflexes that initiate smooth muscle vasoconstriction. With interruption of the smooth endothelial vessel lining and disruption of the negatively charged protein layer, platelets adhere to the underlying connective tissue. The platelets liberate serotonin, which further increases the vasoconstriction, and adenosine diphosphate, which increases the stickiness of the platelets, thus additional platelets are attracted. A loose plug of aggregated platelets thus fills the tear in the vessel. The trauma to the vessel wall and the adherence of platelets serve to incite factors that initiate the clotting process. Within minutes the end of the vessel is filled with a clot. The clot that forms is usually invaded by fibroblasts, with subsequent organization of fibrotic tissue within 7 to 10 days. If, however, the blood has leaked into the extravascular tissues, substances within the tissue activate a mechanism for dissolution of the clot.

The Blood-Clotting Mechanism

Although considerable research has been conducted through the years, the precise means by which the clotting mechanism occurs is still unknown. Generally it is agreed that blood coagulation occurs in three main stages. During the first stage, a substance called *prothrombin activator* is formed in the blood. It is this first part of the clotting mechanism about which little is known. It appears that there are both intrinsic and extrinsic factors that initiate the formation of the activator substance. Platelets and other plasma cofactors serve as intrinsic factors. Thromboplastin, a lipoprotein, serves as an extrinsic factor. Physical factors that serve as extrinsic factors include trauma to the tissues, the endothelial lining of the vessels, or the clotting factors of the blood per se.

In the second stage of the process, prothrombin activator catalyzes the conversion of prothrombin to *thrombin* in the presence of calcium ions. Prothrombin is an unstable plasma protein that is continually formed by the liver in the presence of vitamin K. Thrombin is a proteolytic enzyme.

In the third stage, thrombin serves as a catalytic enzyme to convert fibrinogen to *fibrin threads* in the presence of calcium ions. The fibrin threads enmesh cellular components and plasma to form the clot. Fibrinogen is a plasma protein that is also formed in the liver.

Once a clot starts to form, it serves as the initiator of further clot formation. In other words, a positive feedback system is created. Because of thrombin's proteolytic activity, physiologists feel that it acts on some of the blood-clotting factors responsible for the formation of prothrombin activator. As a result more and more thrombin is formed, and the blood cot extends until the vicious cycle is interrupted.

The Patient with Bleeding Tendencies

Disorders of the blood that are characterized by bleeding tendencies may be due to failure of the extravascular, vascular, or intravascular elements of the self-sealing mechanism as a result of hereditary or acquired factors. Failure of any one of the three elements may result in loss of blood to the tissue spaces or external environment. The result is a diminished quantity of blood to serve as the vehicle of transport. Cells, dependent upon the materials transported by the blood, are thus deprived.

Trauma

Trauma is the most common acquired factor resulting in failure of the vascular element of the self-sealing mechanism. It has been noted that trauma to a vessel is the primary initiator of the self-sealing mechanism. When, however, trauma is coupled with a decrease in the strength of the vascular structure, the result is a loss of the transport medium into the tissue spaces. This loss of blood is characterized by dermal purpura in the form of petechiae, ecchymosis, or hematoma.

Mechanical obstructions to venous return can cause purpura such as is noted with tight garters, coughing paroxysms, and diseases of the veins. Infectious diseases associated with a high fever may induce purpura by an increase in capillary fragility. In some neoplastic and metabolic diseases, such as diabetes, capillaries are more fragile and lead to extravascular bleeding. This phenomenon is also noted with hypertension, scurvy, and food allergies and as an adverse effect of many drugs too numerous to mention.

Although fragility tests may indicate the presence of the vascular defect, laboratory tests are generally inadequate for diagnostic purposes. Similarly, therapies other than vitamin C for scurvy and avoidance of trauma are of little value.

Thrombocytopenia

The intravascular elements of the self-sealing mechanism may fail because of an acquired deficit in the quantity of platelets. Thrombocytopenia may be due to a decreased production of platelets, as with bone marrow aplasia or an increased destruction of platelets as seen in patients with splenomegaly. Other situations in which platelets are destroyed are (1) severe heart failure or hypothermia in which blood flow is stagnated, (2) uremia or bacteremia with adverse reactions to drug therapy, and (3) idiopathic or autoimmune phenomena.

The normal platelet count is 150,000 to 400,000 per cubic millimeter with the average count being 250,000 per cubic millimeter. By definition, a platelet count of less than 150,000 per cubic millimeter is classified as thrombocytopenia. When the platelet count decreases below 40,000 per cubic millimeter there is danger of hemorrhage and with a count of less than 20,000 per cubic millimeter bleeding usually will occur.

Thrombocytopenia frequently is referred to as thrombocytopenia purpura because of the characteristic petechiae and ecchymosis that occur. Petechiae are most prominent on the distal part of the lower extremities, at first, and gradually the proximal parts of the extremities become involved. Conversely, ecchymotic areas usually are present on the back, chest, abdomen, or inner thighs rather than the extremities. Generally, purpura are present; however, menorrhagia or gastrointestinal bleeding may be the only presenting clinical manifestation.

Laboratory studies utilized in the assessment process include a thrombocyte count, bone marrow studies, capillary fragility test, and bleeding and prothrombin times. The only abnormal laboratory test with idiopathic thrombocytopenia purpura (ITP) will be the platelet count. The bone marrow may show a large number of megakaryocytes which produce platelets.

In ITP there is a gamma globulin antibody produced by the B lymphocyte that coats the platelets. As the normal platelet, whose surface is altered by the gamma globulin antibody, goes through the spleen, it is sequestered and destroyed. During this process the platelet's antigen is exposed to additional B lymphocytes and more antibodies are produced. Thus, not only does the spleen destroy platelets in ITP, but it produces more antibodies which causes further destruction of normal platelets (Zeluff, Natelson, & Jackson, 1978, p. 328).

The therapy for ITP is to remove the underlying causes such as drugs and to protect the patient from further trauma. Regardless of the etiology, corticosteroids such as prednisone are used to decrease the severity of the bleeding. The mechanism of action of the corticosteroids is to decrease the phagocytosis of platelets in the spleen and to create an immunosuppressive effect. It may take weeks or months for the immunosuppressive effect in which the titer of antibodies to platelets is decreased.

If the platelet count does not dramatically increase after approximately 5 days of therapy with prednisone, a splenectomy is performed because of the danger of intracranial hemorrhage. A large percentage of patients will respond favorably to a splenectomy when they have failed to respond to steroids. After a splenectomy, the liver and lymph glands assume the platelet-destruction role of the spleen. Should ITP return after the splenectomy, chemotherapy with vincristine may be administered. A prompt and dramatic rise in the platelet count occurs with a nontoxic dose of vincristine weekly. It is believed that the drug stimulates the megakaryocytes to increase the production of platelets.

For those patients with ITP who are refractory to other modes of therapy, prolonged immunosuppressant drug therapy is being used. The drugs that have been used most widely are cyclophosphamide, azathioprine, and 6-mercaptopurine (Zeluff, Natelson, & Jackson, 1978, p. 329).

Hemophilia

Hemophilia is the best-known hereditary defect responsible for failure of blood coagulation and thus of the self-sealing mechanism. Hereditary defects in the clotting mechanism are characterized by a deficiency in a single blood-clotting factor. Of the twelve factors responsible for blood coagulation, factor VIII (antihemophiliac factor) is deficient in hemophilia. This genetic abnormality is attributed to an X-linked recessive gene so that the female serves as the carrier and the defect occurs almost exclusively in males.

Among other factors responsible for genetic defects in blood coagulation are factors XII (Hageman), X (Stuart), and IX (Christmas). The reader is referred to pediatric resources for further details on hemophilia.

Vitamin K Deficiency

Acquired intravascular defects of the self-sealing mechanism originate from a deficiency in more than a single blood-clotting factor. As an example, vitamin K is required for the synthesis of several procoagulant blood factors, particularly prothrombin. Consequently, a deficiency in vitamin K results in bleeding tendencies.

Vitamin K deficiency rarely results from inadequate dietary intake alone. Normal intestinal flora synthesize large amounts of vitamin K; thus prolonged administration of oral antibacterial agents is associated with deficiency. As a fat-soluble substance, vitamin K requires bile for its absorption. Any disorder that prevents bile from reaching the gastrointestinal tract, such as with biliary tract obstruction, results in vitamin K malabsorption and prothrombin deficiency. The intestinal malabsorption diseases also have the same effects. A common iatrogenic origin of vitamin K deficiency results from anticoagulation therapy for thromboembolic disease. Derivatives of coumarin are antagonists to vitamin K; thus they impair synthesis of prothrombin. Salicylates are similar in chemical structure to coumarin preparations and thus produce the same effect.

The bleeding manifestation of deficiency is usually a form of dermal purpura although fatal postoperative hemorrhage has been documented. Diagnosis of vitamin K deficiency is established by a significantly prolonged prothrombin time. In addition to instituting therapies for the underlying cause, intervention consists of oral or parenteral administration of vitamin K in 5- to 20-mg doses. Vitamin K should always be given preoperatively in cases on biliary tract obstruction because the first evidence of the hemorrhagic disorder often occurs when the surgical procedure is performed.

Liver Disease

Another acquired intravascular defect of the self-sealing mechanism can originate from liver disease. The liver synthesizes the primary procoagulants, prothrombin and fibrinogen; thus diffuse liver disease may produce bleeding tendencies.

The clinical manifestations are typically purpural, although bleeding from surgical wounds is common. Although the prothrombin time may be prolonged in patients with hepatic disease, administration of vitamin K appears to have little if any corrective effect. Transfusions with fresh whole blood or frozen plasma may provide transitory correction of the defect.

Disseminated Intravascular Coagulation

In order to understand disseminated intravascular coagulation (DIC), it is necessary to review selected aspects of the blood-clotting mechanism. The major steps of the mechanism that cause the formation of blood clots are (1) fibrinogen, an inactive factor, is converted to fibrin in the presence of thrombin; (2) fibrin forms a blood clot that traps erythrocytes and platelets; and (3) thrombin has to be produced constantly.

Blood coagulation, the "Cascade" of blood clotting, occurs via two pathways (intrinsic and extrinsic). The clotting process can be activated intrinsically by injury to the endothelial cell or extrinsically by damage to tissues. For activation of the *intrinsic pathway*, all the requisite factors are present in the circulating blood. An inactive compound is converted to an active compound followed by that same active compound acting on another inactive compound to convert it to an active one. The seven-step process, which is initiated by the activation of Hageman factor, continues in the above fashion until thrombin converts fibrinogen to fibrin (see Figure 42–1). Activation of the *extrinsic pathway* occurs when thromboplastin becomes available in the circulation following tissue injury. The mechanism that follows produces thrombin. Thrombin then acts on fibrinogen to convert it to fibrin and hence a clot (see Figure 42–1).

THE PLASMINOGEN SYSTEM. Not only does the body have a system for blood clotting, but it has the plasminogen system that destroys clots after the initial bleeding stops. The major steps of the plasminogen system are (1) thrombin converts plasminogen to plasmin, the enzyme of the fibrinolytic system; (2) plasmin lyses the fibrinogen clot and dissolves it; and (3) fibrin-split products (fibrin-degradation products) are the end results of the destruction of fibrin.

Disseminated intravascular coagulation (DIC) is an abnormal overstimulation of the coagulation process. Widespread small thrombi, resulting from massive fibrin formation, occur in the microcirculation. It has not been established why the abnormal process is initiated, but it is known what primary pathologies are likely to cause DIC and the mechanisms through which the clotting takes place. Researchers believe that either the intrinsic pathway is initiated by the activation of Hageman factor as seen where there is injury to endothelial cells, such as gram-negative endotoxemia and gram-positive septicemia, or the extrinsic pathway is activated by the release of thromboplastin as seen where there is tissue damage,

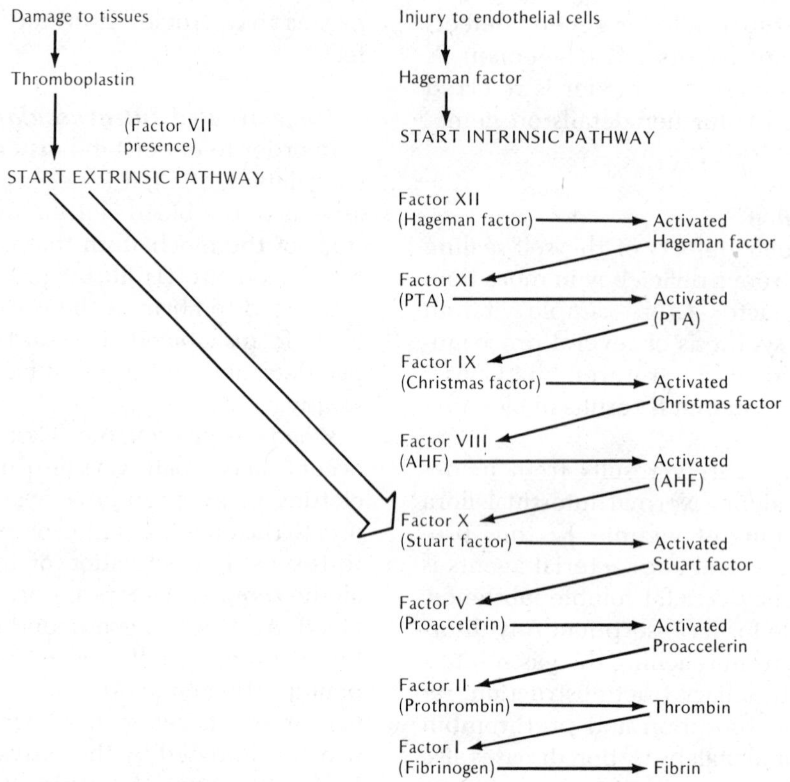

Figure 42–1. Cascade of blood clotting.

for example in neoplasms (Coleman, Minna, & Robboy, 1974, pp. 789–90). The result is that blood coagulates when it should not. In DIC, the following sequence of events takes place: (1) massive amounts of clots are occurring rapidly, thus fibrinogen is depleted by virtue of conversion to fibrin. The end result is a decreased fibrinogen level; (2) the platelets are entrapped in the clots, thus the platelet count is decreased; and (3) in the normal destruction of fibrin clots, the end products will be fibrin-split products which have an anticoagulant effect. Thus the level of fibrin-split products is elevated in DIC. The resultant effect is a tendency for generalized bleeding because the fibrinogen and platelet levels are decreased and the fibrinolytic process is stimulated by the fibrin-split products. A second problem is ischemia of organs from vascular occlusions due to fibrin thrombi. These thrombi are found more frequently in the kidneys than in any other organ.

Like fever or anemia, DIC is a symptom complex secondary to an underlying disease. It is diagnosed in patients who are usually critically ill with obstetrical or surgical problems or neoplastic diseases. One third of the patients with DIC will probably leave the hospital. The other two thirds will die because bleeding complicates an already catastrophic situation (Coleman, Minna, & Robboy, 1974).

ASSOCIATED CLINICAL SITUATION. Specific clinical situations associated with DIC are septic, hemorrhagic, or anaphylatic shock. Carcinoma of the prostate commonly is associated with DIC as are widespread terminal carcinomas of the lung or pancreas. DIC most commonly is seen in patients with gram-negative and gram-positive infections where the patient has septicemia associated with a high fever and shock. Other less common situations are tuberculosis, pulmonary embolism, fat embolism associated with bone injury, uncontrolled leukemia, renal pathology, and following surgery with cardiopulmonary bypass. There are a variety of obstetrical situations that can cause DIC. Among these are septic abortions, abruptio placentae, and retained fragments of a dead fetus.

Bleeding in any of the above high-risk patients who do not have a history of bleeding should always cause the health professional to consider DIC as a possible diagnosis. The amount of bleeding can vary to include occult internal bleeding, oozing from a wound or needle puncture, or hemorrhaging from any and all orifices. Multisite bleeding is of diagnostic importance because persons with DIC usually bleed from multiple rather than one site. Other signs of bleeding may be petechiae or ecchymosis. The patient also should be observed closely for a decrease in blood pressure, tachycardia, decreasing hematocrit, and restlessness.

DIAGNOSIS. Diagnosis is made from a composite of coagulation studies and the patient's clinical signs of bleeding. The prothrombin time (PT), used to evaluate the extrinsic pathway of coagulation, is prolonged in DIC. The partial thromboplastin time (PTT) evaluates the intrinsic pathway of clotting and usually is prolonged in DIC. The platelet count will be decreased. The fibrinogen level may be in the normal range (a relative proportion decrease) or decreased. The normal fibrinogen level is 200 to 500 mg/100 ml. Therefore, a patient's fibrinogen level may be 200 mg, a normal value, but prior to DIC the fibrinogen level had been 500 mg. For this patient, the fibrinogen level is, in reality, decreased. Another coagulation test for DIC is fibrin-split products (FSP) and the titer will be elevated with DIC.

TREATMENT. The initial step in treatment of DIC is to treat the underlying disease process, since DIC will continue as long as the underlying problem persists. Whereas the clinical and laboratory data of DIC reflect abnormalities in thrombin activity, it is logical that a part of the therapy for DIC should be to block the activity of that enzyme. The most effective antagonist of thrombin is heparin. The use of heparin therapy, however, is controversial.

Proponents of the use of heparin therapy believe that the antithrombin activity of heparin neutralizes the free-circulating thrombin. If the basic pathophysiological mechanism is the formation of fibrin clots and their destruction, it seems logical to prevent the conversion of fibrinogen to fibrin. For that interaction to take place, thrombin has to be present. Thus, if the formation of thrombin and the thrombin-fibrinogen interaction are inhibited by heparin, clot formation will be blocked. The recommended dose of heparin is 500 to 1000 units per hour via a constant infusion drip. Heparin therapy is continued as long as the underlying disease is active, usually 3 to 7 days. Inasmuch as the PTT is prolonged during the course of DIC, it cannot be used as a control for heparin therapy. The criteria used to determine the effectiveness of the heparin therapy is the cessation of bleeding. If the patient is febrile, larger doses of heparin may be required, because when cellular metabolism is increased, heparin is metabolized more rapidly. Further, digitalis, tetracyline, nicotine, and antihistamine preparations partially counteract the anticoagulation action of heparin, thus larger doses of heparin will be required. On the other hand, patients with liver and renal disease need decreased doses of heparin (O'Brien & Woods, 1978).

Once heparin therapy has been initiated, blood products may be given. Usually fibrinogen does not have to be replaced because the body has the tremendous ability to produce fibrinogen under stress. If the fibrinogen level continues to decrease, plasma and blood can be given to increase its level. Also, cryoprecipitate may be given as a fibrinogen replacement. Platelets may be given to those patients who are bleeding severely. Platelet transfusions should be stored at room temperature inasmuch as cell deterioration takes place if they are refrigerated. Prolonged administration of platelets is not advised since the development of isoantibodies can result.

NURSING CARE. The nursing care of the DIC patient can become extremely complicated. Not only is the nurse administering care to a critically ill patient, but she or he is monitoring the patient constantly for signs of bleeding. The nursing interventions are as follows: (1) monitor for signs of bleeding, (2) prevent further bleeding, (3) monitor blood loss, and (4) administer blood products and medications (Jennings, 1979). The reader is referred to the section discussing nursing interventions with bleeding problems.

Assessment of the Patient with Bleeding Tendencies

DIAGNOSTIC TESTS. Laboratory data are obtained from one or several of the following tests.

- *Platelet count.* Platelets are necessary to keep capillary walls strong. The normal range is 150,000 to 400,000 platelets per cubic millimeter. Any substantial decrease below normal will be evidenced by easy bruising. Spontaneous bleeding may occur if the platelet count is less than 50,000 platelets per cubic millimeter.

  A decrease in the platelet count is caused by either decreased production or increased destruction. Examples of conditions in which the platelet count may be decreased are idiopathic thrombocytopenia, leukemia, severe anemias, and conditions resulting from chemotherapy or radiation therapy.
- *Bleeding time.* The bleeding time can provide information as to the functional capacity of platelets and the capillaries' ability to constrict. A blood pressure cuff, maintained at 40 mm Hg, is placed on the arm and a puncture wound made on the forearm. Blotting of the wound with a gauze pad is done at half-minute intervals until bleeding stops. The normal time is within 3 to 6 minutes. A prolonged bleeding time is present with thrombocytopenia, leukemia, and aplastic anemia. An abnormal bleeding time can result if 10 grains of aspirin are ingested within 2 hours prior to the test.
- *Clot retraction.* The time and degree of an undisturbed clot's retraction in a nontreated test tube is observed as an indication of thrombocyte function. Normally retraction begins in 2 hours and is complete within 24 hours. Slow and incomplete contraction is indicative of thrombocytopenia (less

than 50,000 platelets per cubic millimeter) due to aplastic anemia, leukemia, and thrombocytopenia purpura.

- *Fibrinogen level.* The blood fibrinogen level is determined as a function of blood coagulation. The normal range is approximately 200 to 330 mg per 100 ml of plasma.
- *Clotting time.* The clotting time is utilized more as a method for control of anticoagulation therapy than as a diagnostic tool. The length of time is noted for a venous sample to clot in an untreated test tube. The usual length of time is approximately 8 to 15 minutes. The Lee—White method is utilized popularly in many hospitals to determine the therapeutic level of heparin administration. Heparin prevents clotting by inhibiting prothrombin, thrombin, and factor IX, XI, and XII, which generate thromboplastin. Heparin therapy should keep the clotting time at twice the normal value.
- *Prothrombin time.* The prothrombin time is utilized as both a diagnostic tool and as a measure of anticoagulant therapy. It measures the activity of five clotting factors; factors I (prothrombin), II (fibrinogen), V (labile), VII (prothrombin conversion accelerator), and X (Stuart). The normal prothrombin time is 12 to 15 seconds. The test also is used to monitor anticoagulant therapy with coumadin administration.

  Coumadin produces a prolonged clotting time by interfering with the function of vitamin K in the liver and by blocking the function of existing vitamin K–dependent factors II, VII, IX, and X.

  The prothrombin time should be 20 per cent of normal or 20 to 29 seconds with coumadin therapy. Coumadin acts slowly and does not affect clotting for approximately 10 hours. It will peak in 2 to 5 days and have an effect for up to 2 weeks after discontinuing the last dose.
- *Activated partial thromboplastin time (APTT).* APTT is a popularly used screening and therapeutic level test. It is used to discover clotting deficiencies other than with factor VII and platelets. The normal range is 35 to 45 seconds.

  APTT is used more frequently than Lee-White clotting time to monitor heparin therapy as it offers the same results but takes less time and is more sensitive. If a patient is receiving heparin injections q 6 h, the APTT should be maintained at 55 to 70 seconds. If heparin is given as a continuous intravenous drip, the APTT is maintained at 60 to 100 seconds (Byrne, 1976).
- *Capillary fragility test.* A clinical test to determine the fragility of capillaries is done by application of a blood pressure cuff to the arm or thigh with the pressure maintained between the systolic and diastolic pressure for a 5-minute period. Less than 10 petechiae within a circular area 5 cm in diameter is considered normal. More than 20 petechiae indicates weakness of the capillary walls or platelet defect.
- *Serum calcium level.* Although calcium is an important factor in the blood coagulation mechanism, deficiency of calcium does not result in failure of blood clotting as was once believed. The quantity of calcium required is small. Disturbances in neuromuscular functioning are noted before a calcium deficit would affect blood coagulation.

PHYSICAL ASSESSMENT. In addition to patients with known hemorrhagic tendencies, the nurse should be alert to bleeding tendencies in all individuals with pathologic disorders. Comprehensive nursing assessments could reveal a previously undiscovered tendency. The physical assessment of the patient with bleeding tendencies includes examination of the skin for purpura. Petechiae, which may occur after a blood pressure determination is taken or after application of a tourniquet for venipuncture, may be the first indication of a bleeding tendency. Bleeding from injection sites may also be noted. The patient may present ecchymoses on the extremities, of which he or she is unaware.

Bleeding or serous drainage from the nose, gums, or skin should be noted. The quantity of blood found in vomitus or with expectoration should be estimated. A first evidence of bleeding tendencies may be excessive menstrual flow, bright red or tarry stools, or hematuria. In the severest form, the patient may develop intracranial bleeding and present symptoms associated with cerebrovascular disease of varying degree. The history should elucidate any episodes of spontaneous bleeding and any unusual bleeding following dental extraction, minor surgery, or accidents.

Intervention with the Patient with Bleeding Tendencies

In addition to the specific therapies for patients with specific bleeding tendencies, precautions must be exercised for patients undergoing specific surgical procedures. Sometimes in procedures that involve the surface of a mucous membrane, a large loose clot forms while the vessels beneath the clot continue to bleed. The sheltering clot must be removed for the exposed ends of the bleeding vessels to clot and for bleeding to be controlled. Hemostatic agents, such as gel foams that contain procoagulant substances, are sometimes applied to bleeding surfaces to hasten coagulation. Common sites for this type of hemorrhage are the "dry socket" following dental extraction, the pharynx following tonsillectomy, and the bladder after prostate surgery. Following the latter type of surgery, frequent bladder irrigations are prescribed to prevent the formation of clots. If one or more clots form, they can be removed and aspirated by more aggressive irrigation techniques. Unless the continuous bladder irrigations are performed concertedly, however, the patient may lose an unnecessary quantity of blood.

Nursing the patient with a bleeding tendency can challenge the most competent nurse. The loss of even small quantities of blood evokes fear in almost everyone. A sudden large hemorrhage may frighten the nurse as well. Some of the disorders characterized by a tendency to spontaneous hemorrhage, such as leukemia, have a poor prognosis. Patient, family, and nurse live day by day in the presence of death. Family members may display a variety of emotional reactions, including panic, guilt, depression, and grief. Their demands on the nurse and physician for emotional help may be greater than those of the patient.

Perhaps the greatest challenge in administering care to patients with bleeding tendencies is making astute observations for signs of occult bleeding. The cardiopulmonary function needs to be observed closely for any signs indicating decreased tissue oxygenation or a decrease in the circulating blood volume. Significant signs would include tachypnea, orthopnea, tachycardia, palpitations, murmurs, orthostatic hypotension, and angina. The skin and mucosa must be examined carefully for color changes (pale or jaundice) and petechiae. Other covert signs of occult bleeding would include fatigue, weakness, malaise, or myalgia. Intrabdominal bleeding is manifested in the following ways: (1) the patient complains of abdominal tenderness, (2) the abdominal girth increases, (3) the patient complains of numbness and pain in the legs because retroperitoneal bleeding compresses the lateral cutaneous nerve at the second and third lumbar vertebrae (Jennings, 1979, p. 66), and (4) urine and stool have occult blood in them. Cerebral bleeding is always a possible complication when the platelet count is markedly decreased. The patient needs to be observed closely for changes in mental status, complaints of headaches or vertigo, and for signs of mental confusion.

Another goal in the nursing of the patient with a tendency toward bleeding is to prevent incidents predisposing to tissue trauma. Epistaxis is a common problem. Crusting of the mucosa of the nose predisposes to and follows episodes of bleeding. The crusting may be lessened by inserting a wick of cotton soaked with mineral oil. Only one nostril should be treated, and all excess of oil should be removed from the wick before it is inserted to prevent the possibility of aspiration.

Medications should be given orally, rectally, and through existing intravenous lines when possible. If an intramuscular injection must be given, a sharp needle of as small a diameter as is compatible with the injectable solution should be selected to minimize the danger of bleeding. The selection of the sites to be used for injection should be discussed with the physician. When repeated injections are required, the sites should be rotated according to a plan and recorded each time. Steady pressure over the injection site for a period of 3 to 5 minutes lessens the likelihood of bleeding into the tissue and the formation of a hematoma.

Mouth care is given with cotton swabs or a soft-bristled toothbrush and a mild, cool mouthwash. There is controversy over the use of a water pick. Some professionals feel that a water pick reduces the chance of gingival bleeding and others say that a water pick may cause gingival bleeding.

Straining at stool should be avoided, as a significant increase in pressure can result in a rupture of blood vessels. Stool softeners are given as well as instructions to the patient not to strain at stool.

Patients who are ambulatory should be instructed to avoid bumping themselves against furniture or other hard objects. Care should be taken to perform nursing procedures with extra gentleness. The patient should be protected from sources of infection, not only to protect him or her from unnecessary discomfort, but to minimize infection, which increases the tendency to bleed.

Another important aspect of nursing intervention is the administration of blood or elements of blood. Today whole blood is seldom administered unless large volumes of blood have been lost and both red cells and plasma need to be replaced. Instead, packed red blood cells or plasma fractions, that is, platelets, cryoprecipitate rich in factor VIII, immunoglobins, and albumin are administered. Today freshly drawn or frozen plasma which once commonly was used as a volume expander is rarely used because it can carry the hepatitis virus. Also other volume expanders are less expensive and more easily obtained. Most institutions stock albumin concentrate or plasma-protein fraction. These expanders carry less risk of hepatitis than whole blood.

During processing, all donor blood is tested for the following: (1) blood grouping—ABO and Rh blood types; (2) antibody screening, to determine whether the donor has been sensitized to red blood cells from incompatible transfusion; (3) serological test, to test for syphilis; and (4) hepatitis B surface antigen (HB_sAg) screen, to diagnose hepatitis. Because the transmission of hepatitis B is such a serious risk with transfusions, the Red Cross Blood Centers are attempting to decrease this risk by keeping a national computer file of the names of all potential donors who have had hepatitis, had a positive HB_sAg test, or donated blood for a person who developed posttransfusion hepatitis. All blood is checked against this file before it is released.

In addition to the antigen-antibody reactions with ABO and Rh incompatibility, antibodies can be produced in reaction to certain antigens found on leukocytes and platelets. Platelets and leukocytes also possess antigenic facets involving the HLA system (histocompatibility locus A). Blood typing to provide HLA compatibility is still a new field. To date, it has been shown that platelets and granulocytes appear to produce less sensitization and posttransfusion reactions if they have been matched to the HLA configuration of the recipient. The main problem is that the HLA system involves more than 50 antigens; thus it is difficult to achieve HLA compatibility.

At the completion of testing, the blood is labeled with its ABO and Rh type. In addition, negative results of syphilis, hepatitis B, and antibody screening tests are recorded on the label. At the time of the transfusion, the donor blood will be cross-matched with the recipient blood.

It is apparent that blood transfusion therapy is becoming much more sophisticated as the components and derivatives of blood obtained by fractionalization are administered. A principle that applies for one component of blood will not apply to the next. To illustrate, packed cells must be refrigerated whereas platelets are stored at room temperature to prevent cell deterioration.

The nursing interventions during the transfusion vary depending on what components of blood are administered. Before any transfusion is administered, it is imperative to verify the ABO and Rh types of both the donors and the recipient's blood. At the same time baseline vital signs are obtained, as they should be checked frequently throughout the transfusion process.

All blood products except platelets, thawed cryoprecipitate, and fresh frozen plasma should be stored in a blood bank refrigerator where the temperature is stable until immediately prior to the transfusion. If the blood cannot be transfused as soon as it arrives on the division, it should be immediately returned to the blood bank rather than stored in a refrigerator, as this could cause freezing and thawing that would result in red cell hemolysis.

The vein chosen to start the transfusion must be large enough to accommodate the needle and in a location that is comfortable for the patient. To illustrate, the veins in the antecubital fossa are easily accessible; however, elbow flexion is limited if that vein is used, whereas veins in the forearm and hand are just as suitable.

The needle size is determined by what component is going to be administered. If packed cells and blood are going to be given, at least a 19 gauge needle is necessary so that the bore will be large enough to accommodate red blood cells. On the other hand, if blood products such as platelets, cryoprecipitate, fresh frozen plasma, or albumin are going to be infused, a small-bore needle can be used. Only normal saline can be used as a vehicle to transfuse blood products containing red blood cells, platelets, or leukocytes because dextrose causes hemolysis of red blood cells.

The standard blood filter of 170 microns screens out fibrin clots and other particulate matter. If blood is more than 5 to 6 days old, microaggregate filters which screen out particles as small as 40 microns should be used. Another fact to remember when giving stored blood is that its platelet and red cell count decreases and the potassium level increases over time. Thus, any patient with a high potassium level could develop cardiac standstill.

According to Cullins (1979, p. 935), the major complications from blood transfusions are (1) hemolytic, allergic, febrile, and bacterial reactions; (2) circulatory overload; (3) embolism; and (4) transmission of infectious agents—especially hepatitis, and rarely malaria and syphilis. The reader is referred to an excellent transfusion reaction chart found in the Cullins article and to a series of articles in the May 1979 issue of the *American Journal of Nursing* on blood therapy.

Today most patients will receive packed cells rather than whole blood. This does not eliminate all risks, as there is still the risk of infection and incompatible reaction. According to Scarlato, giving packed red cells has several advantages over giving the same amount of whole blood: (1) the chance of circulatory overload is decreased; (2) the risk of reactions to plasma antigens is decreased; (3) less sodium, potassium, and ammonium are introduced into the circulation; (4) the hematocrit is raised higher; and (5) the risk of serum hepatitis is decreased (1978, p. 70).

The Patient with Clotting Tendencies

Disorders of the blood that are characterized by clotting tendencies may be due to alterations in the extravascular, vascular, or intravascular elements of the self-sealing mechanism as a result of acquired or hereditary factors. The disorders are primarily acquired vascular disturbances and as such are best discussed under alterations of the transport system associated with the blood vessels. Regardless of which element of the self-sealing mechanism fails, the result may be partial or total obstruction of blood to or from cells.

Anticoagulant Agents

The anticoagulant agents primarily utilized for disorders characterized by clotting tendencies are coumarin and heparin preparations. Coumarin derivatives (Dicumarol, Coumadin) act to diminish blood clotting by competitively inhibiting the role of vitamin K in the synthesis of the procoagulants, prothrombin, and factors VII, IX, and X. Vitamin K thus serves as the antidote when bleeding results from excessive coumarin effect.

Heparin is the more rapid-acting of the two anticoagulants. It acts in the second major phase of blood clotting by blocking the conversion of prothrombin to thrombin. Heparin has a large electronegative charge and thus is inactivated by electropositive substances such as protamine sulfate, which serves as an antidote. The specific methods of anticoagulation are discussed under the section on thrombophlebitis in Chapter 43.

References Cited

Bunn, H. F. "Approach to the Patient with Anemia." In *Harrison's Principles of Internal Medicine,* 8th ed. Ed. by G. W. Thorn, R. D. Adams, E. Braunwald, H. J. Isselbacher, and R. G. Petersdorf. New York: McGraw-Hill, 1977.

Byrne, J. "A Review of the CBC: The Quantitative Tests." *Nursing,* 6:10 (1976), 11–12.

Byrne, J: "Hematology, Part IX." *Nursing,* 7:6 (1977), 24–25.

Chanarin, I. "Investigation and Management of Megaloblastic Anaemia." *Clin. Haematol.,* 5:3 (1976), 747–63.

Clift, R. A., and Buchner, C. D. "Supportive Measures for Patients with Aplastic Anaemia." *Clin. Haematol.,* 7:3 (1978), 623–37.

Coleman, R. W., Minna, J. D., and Robboy, S. J. "Disseminated Intravascular Coagulation: A Problem in Critical-Care Medicine." *Heart and Lung,* 3:5 (1974), 789–96.

Cullins, L. C. "Preventing and Treating Transfusion Reaction." *Am. J. Nurs.,* 79:5 (1979), 935–41.

Dougherty, W. M. *Introduction to Hematology.* St. Louis: C. V. Mosby Co., 1971.

Flynn, K. T. "Iron Deficiency Anemia Among the Elderly." *Nurse Pract.,* 3:6 (1978), 20–24.

Fowler, N. "High Cardiac Output States." In *The Heart, Arteries, and Veins,* 2nd ed. Ed. by J. W. Hurst and R. B. Logue. New York: McGraw-Hill, 1970.

Guyton, A. C. *Textbook of Medical Physiology,* 5th ed. Philadelphia: W. B. Saunders Co., 1976.

Harper, H. A. *Review of Physiological Chemistry,* 14th ed. Los Altos, Calif.: Lange Medical Publishers, 1973.

Jennings, B. M. "Improving Your Management of DIC." *Nursing,* 9:5 (1979), 60–67.

O'Brien, B. S., and Woods, S. "The Paradox of DIC." *Am. J. Nurs.,* 78:11 (1978), 1878–80.

Rappeport, J. M., and Bunn, H. F. "Bone Marrow Failure." In *Harrison's Principles of Internal Medicine,* 8th ed. Ed. by G. W. Thorn, R. D. Adams, E. Braunwald, K. J. Isselbacher, and R. G. Petersdorf. New York: McGraw-Hill, 1977.

Scarlato, M. "Blood Transfusions Today, What You Should Know and Should Do." *Nursing,* 8:2 (1978), 68–72.

Zeluff, G. W., Natelson, E. A., and Jackson, D. "Thrombocytopenia Purpura—Idiopathic and Thrombotic." *Heart and Lung,* 7:2 (1978), 327–33.

Zimmerman, S., Cohen, T., Diekman, R., Calvo, C. K., and Hongsterfer, M. "Bone Marrow Transplantation." *Am. J. Nurs.* 77:8 (1977), 1311–14.

General References

Altshuler, J. H. "Disseminated Intravascular Coagulation Syndrome." In *Critical Care Nursing.* Ed. by C. M. Hudak, B. M. Gallo, and T. Lohr. Philadelphia: J. B. Lippincott Co., 1973.

Bassan, M. M., and Rogel, S. "Current Practice in the Use of Anticoagulants for Ischemic Heart Disease: A Survey of 200 Hospitals." *Heart and Lung,* 5:5 (1976), 742–46.

Doswell, W. M. "Sickle Cell Anemia: You Can Do Something to Help." *Nursing,* 8:4 (1978), 65–70.

Dougherty, W. *Introduction to Hematology,* 2nd ed. St. Louis: C. V. Mosby Co., 1976.

Foster, S. B. "Sickle Cell Anemia: Pathophysiologic Aspects." *Heart and Lung,* 3:6 (1974), 955–61.

McFarlane, J. "Sickle Cell Disorders." *Am. J. Nurs.,* 77:12 (1977), 1948–54.

Patterson, P. C., and Schumann, D., eds. "Symposium on Patients with Blood Disorders." *Nurs. Clin. North Am.,* 7:4 (1972), 711–816.

Vigran, I. M. "History of Anticoagulants." *Heart and Lung,* 3:5 (1974), 812–16.

Walker, P. "Bone Marrow Transplant: A Second Chance for Life." *Nursing,* 7:1 (1977), 24–25.

43

Problems with Transporting Materials to and from Cells Due to Altered Blood Vessels

Carrel was the first to sew blood vessels together, to keep body tissues alive in jars, to transplant animal organs, preparing the way for cardiovascular surgery and human-organ transplants.

POOLE
Gray Poole, *Doctors Who Saved Lives,* New York: Dodd, Mead & Company, 1966, p. 110.

Blood Vessels as the Conduct System for Transportation of Materials to and from Cells

Whereas the blood serves as the vehicle of transport, the blood vessels are the channels through which the blood conveys essential materials to cells and removes the end products of metabolism. For this activity to be maintained, the blood vessels must have a patent lumen, normal distensibility, and normal responses to regulatory mechanisms. Phenomena that alter the diameter of the vessels will effect alterations in the transport of materials to and from cells.

The arteries serve as the pathway through which the blood transports oxygen and needed substances to the cells. Disorders of the arteries result in a decreased or absent perfusion of groups of cells. Arterial disorders are primarily of an obstructive, nonobstructive, or vasoconstrictive nature. Alterations or failure of the transport system are related to diminished or obstructed flow through the arterial system, altered distensibility of the vascular structures, and altered regulatory mechanisms, particularly the peripheral vascular resistance.

The veins serve as the channels through which the blood removes carbon dioxide and acid metabolites from the cells. Disorders of the veins result in a decreased or very nearly absent venous return with potential accumulation of metabolic waste products and diminished cardiac output. Venous disorders are primarily due to alterations in the structure of the veins with an altered blood coagulation process. Alterations or failure of the transport system are related to diminished or obstructed flow through the venous system and altered regulatory mechanisms, particularly the cardiac output.

The effects of transport alterations from disorders of the arteries or the veins can be viewed on a continuum. For example, disorders of the arteries, such as those related to the arteriosclerotic process, produce varying degrees of oxygen deprivation to cells. With partial obstruction of arterial lumens, the dependent cells may still receive some oxygen and thus continue metabolic activities, although cellular function will not be optimal. With total obstruction, however, the oxygen deprivation will be complete, thus metabolic activities and cellular functions will cease.

Similarly, diseases of the veins produce varying

This chapter was revised by Elizabeth Ford Pitorak, R.N., M.S.N., Clinical Nurse Specialist, Lake County Memorial Hospital, Willoughby, Ohio, and Judith A. Wood, R.N., M.S.N., Assistant Professor of Nursing, Case Western Reserve University, Frances Payne Bolton School of Nursing, Cleveland, Ohio.

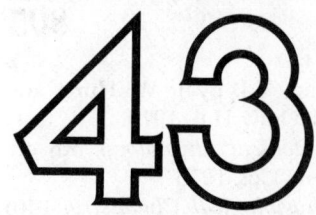

degrees of venous stasis, because of inadequate venous return. A diminished venous return with minimal to moderate venous stasis may occur with such conditions as varicose veins and venous thrombosis. In chronic venous insufficiency, the venous return diminishes further with severe venous stasis. Absence of venous return, however, with complete venous stasis may occur if a pulmonary embolus occludes the main pulmonary artery.

Structure and Function of Blood Vessels

The structure of the blood vessels varies with their location in the circuit and with their function. With the exception of the capillaries, blood vessels are composed of three layers or coats. The outer layer, or tunica adventitia, is largely areolar connective tissue. The middle layer, or tunica media, contains varying proportions of elastic and muscular tissue. The inner, or tunica intima, is also composed of three layers: a layer of elastic tissue lying next to the media, a thin layer of connective tissue, and finally a layer of endothelial cells. The walls of the large arteries, such as the aorta and the pulmonary artery, are thick and contain a large amount of elastic tissue, but relatively little muscle. In medium-sized and small arteries conditions are reversed. As arteries decrease in size, the amount of elastic tissue also decreases and their walls contain relatively more muscle.

Through regulation of the diameter of blood vessels and thus flow, the overall oxygen requirements of the body are met. Priority of flow is given to areas with high metabolic requirements; thus the special needs of local areas of tissue are met. The autonomic nervous system regulates the diameter of arteries, veins, and arterioles, but there is little evidence that it directly regulates the capillaries. The microcirculation is believed to be regulated primarily by local conditions in the tissues. Furthermore, blood is delivered to and removed from the capillaries through the regulation of the diameter of the arteries and veins and by the stroke volume and rate of the heart.

Not all the elements in the local regulation of blood flow are known. Some of the possibilities include a lack of oxygen or essential materials or the liberation of one or more substances by the ischemic tissue that are responsible for arteriolar and capillary dilatation. For example, blood vessels dilate in skeletal muscles in response to increased exercise. As a consequence of the increased blood flow, ischemia is corrected, and products that may directly dilate the blood vessels are removed. With the elimination of conditions initiating dilatation, the blood vessels automatically return to the nondilatating state.

The Veins

Structure and Function

The veins, like the arteries, are composed of three layers. The wall of a vein has a thinner medial layer that contains less muscle and elastic tissue than that of a corresponding artery. This arrangement is necessary because the pressure in an artery is greater than that in a vein. Because of the thinness of the walls, veins have a tendency to collapse when severed or when external pressure is applied. Even if a vein is obstructed by pressure, blood will continue to be propelled into it because of the higher arterial pressure. When this happens, the hydrostatic pressure in capillaries rises and transudation of fluid into the interstitial spaces takes place. The resultant effect is tissue edema. If the edema state continues, the flow of blood into the veins will be decreased.

The pressure of blood in the peripheral veins is determined by the pressure in the right atrium, and the pressure in the right atrium is dependent upon the efficiency of the heart as a pump and the resistance of the pulmonary vasculature. If the pressure in the right atrium increases, venous return is impeded with resultant higher pressures in the venous system. Similarly, a decreased right atrial pressure is reflected by a lower pressure in the venous system.

Normal valves cause the flow of blood to be unidirectional and prevent any retrograde flow. Valves have an important function in such areas as the lower extremities. When the valves are congenitally defective or are destroyed by disease, stasis of blood results in the affected limb.

The return of blood from the lower extremities is facilitated by the musculovenous pump system. With exercise the skeletal muscles of the legs compress the veins, particularly of the deep venous bed, to propel the blood back toward the heart. This system is less effective in the superficial veins; however, the valves of the communicating veins are arranged so that there is a unidirectional flow of blood from the superficial veins into the deep venous bed as it empties.

When there is a lack of skeletal muscle contraction against veins of the lower extremities for extended periods of time, the venous pressure rises in the legs and feet. This explains why continued sitting, such as long bus or automobile trips, predisposes to edema of the lower extremities. Preventive measures include getting out of the car or bus at hourly or 2 hour intervals to exercise the lower limbs. Exercises, such as flexing and extending the feet at the ankle and setting the quadriceps muscles while sitting, are also beneficial.

Assessment of the Patient with Venous Problems

Assessment of the patient with disease of the venous system includes analysis of the diagnostic tests and physical manifestations presented by the patient. The focus of physical assessment is on the lower extremities.

Diagnostic Tools

Fibrinogen Labeled with ^{131}I or ^{125}I

This is an ingenious method of detecting venous thrombosis through the administration of fibrinogen labeled with radioactive iodine. ^{131}I is administered intravenously and basal counts of radioactivity are taken over the extremity. Counts are repeated on the second and third days. If a thrombus is present, the radioactivity will increase as the fibrinogen becomes incorporated in the thrombus. Iodine is administered the day prior to the test to block the uptake of ^{131}I by the thyroid gland. Dangers associated with the test are allergic reactions to the iodine or the transmission of infectious hepatitis. Hepatitis can be prevented by labeling the patient's own fibrinogen.

Radioisotope Lung Scanning

Albumin tagged with ^{131}I or technetium 99m is administered intravenously to determine if any perfusion deficits are present within the lungs. The size of radioactive albumin particles prohibits perfusion through the pulmonary capillaries and thus the particles are present for scanning. Many institutions are using technetium 99m rather than ^{131}I as it has a shorter half-life, which permits the injection of more material. This increases the concentration of radioactive particles present to be detected with the scan counter. Limited or absent ^{131}I uptake in areas of the scan represents hypovascular areas.

Ultrasound Mapping

A newer method used to detect thrombus obstruction in veins is ultrasound. This method depends upon the physical fact that reflection of a beam of sound from a stream of blood flow will be of different frequencies as the blood flow velocity changes.

Phlebography

This diagnostic method is used to investigate venous incompetency and varicose veins in the lower extremities. Tight tourniquets are applied at the ankle and knee to obstruct flow in the superficial veins and force the injected contrast media into the deep veins. The patient performs the Valsalva maneuver to decrease venous return at the time the films are taken. The results indicate if the deep veins are patent and competent or if there is incompetency of the communicating veins.

Plethysmograph

The plethysmograph is an instrument used to study the peripheral circulation. A finger, toe, or limb is enclosed within the plethysmograph, which is connected with pressure tubing to an amplifying and recording device. The analyzed data indicate changes in the volume or velocity of blood flow in the enclosed part. Changes occur with acute venous obstruction or with alterations in the general hemodynamics of the extremity.

Physical Assessment

Size and Symmetry

Edema is probably the most common clinical manifestation present with diseases of the venous system. Swelling is best detected by observing the ankles from behind, with the patient in a standing position. Normally a concavity is present on either side of the Achilles tendon. If edema is present, the space will be obliterated in the affected extremity. With sufficient edema, pitting will occur if the tissues are indented by compression with the thumb.

By measuring the circumference of the calf of the leg, differences in the size of the extremities can be detected. Unilateral edema results from thrombophlebitis, varicose veins, or chronic venous insufficiency. Bilateral edema is more likely to result from cardiac decompensation or kidney disease; however, it could occur with varicose veins if both legs are involved.

Pain is sometimes present if the edema is severe. With edema there is a decreased venous return and an accumulation of waste products from catabolism. The acid metabolities, plus mechanical compression by the edema fluid, serve as stimuli to pain receptors.

Blood Vessels

The veins of the legs should be observed with the patient in a standing position. Tortuous, dilated, and elongated superficial veins indicate varicose veins. Dilatation of the superficial veins is present any time there is obstruction to the venous flow or loss of valves in the proximal segment of the veins. Also marked dilatation of the veins is present in an area with an arteriovenous fistula because of the increased pressure of the blood flow when an artery communicates directly with a vein. If the collateral veins take over when varicosities are present, there will be an increased number of cutaneous veins just beneath the skin. A characteristic distortion of these cutaneous veins is referred to as "venous stars." With superficial thrombophlebitis, the vein feels like a firm cord, and redness localized in the area or traversing the course of the vein is present.

Appearance of the Skin

In the presence of edema, the skin may appear shiny and taut because of expansion of the extravascular tissue spaces. The skin may also feel cool and moist to the touch because of the transudation of fluid to the external environment. With superficial thrombophlebitis, however, the skin may appear reddened and feel warmer over the inflamed vein as is noted with local inflammatory responses.

Stasis ulcers at the level of the ankle, eczematoid lesions, and/or stasis dermatitis are frequently presenting manifestations with chronic venous insufficiency. A brownish-black pigmentation of the subcutaneous tissues accompanies stasis dermatitis. In persons whose skin is normally highly pigmented, the affected tissues appear darker than the surrounding unaffected tissues.

Varicose Veins

Varicose veins are dilated veins that usually involve the greater and lesser saphenous veins of the lower extremities. As the veins dilate, pressure of the blood against the walls increases, causing further dilatation. Associated with the increase in diameter are elongation and tortuosity.

Primary varicose veins affect the superficial venous system. The exact cause is uncertain, but it is presumed that there is congenital incompetence of the venous valves, which permits retrograde flow of blood in the superficial veins. A striking feature is the familial tendency, particularly in women, although an inherited defect has not been proved. Another predisposing factor is the orthostatic increase in saphenous vein pressure with standing, thus persons who have occupations requiring extended periods of standing are prone to varicose vein formation. With increasing age there is degeneration and a decrease in the number of valves. Also there is weakness of the venous walls and valves secondary to loss of skin and tissue tone. This explains why varicose veins develop more frequently in older age groups than in the young.

Secondary varicose veins result from damaged valves usually caused by thrombophlebitis in the deep veins, with resultant venous insufficiency. With deep thrombophlebitis, damage to the valves takes place during the recanalization process following thrombosis. As the leg muscles contract, there is great resistance to venous return in a deep vein when the valves are damaged; thus the venous pressure remains high. This leads to an increased pressure in the communicating veins with resultant incompetence of the valves. This high venous pressure is reflected to the poorly supported superficial veins causing valve incompetence and secondary varicose veins.

A second cause of secondary varicose veins is any mechanism that causes an increased local venous pressure in the lower extremities. Examples would be a gravid uterus, abdominal neoplasms, and obesity. During pregnancy a humoral factor is liberated, causing relaxation of smooth muscles in the venous walls; thus dilatation of veins and incompetence of valves results. An additional factor would be that the increased blood flow from the uterus causes congestion of the iliac veins; thus the venous return from the extremities is impeded.

The clinical manifestations will vary markedly with individual patients as there is no direct relationship between the degree of severity of varices and the symptoms the patient experiences. One manifestation that may be noted is tissue edema. Normally, with exercise the musculovenous pump system propels blood through the deep veins, the popliteal and femoral, toward the heart. The pressure within the veins increases during contraction and decreases during relaxation; thus the fall in pressure permits blood to drain from the superficial venous bed through the communicating veins into the deep venous system. With incompetent valves there is a reflux of blood into the empty segments of the veins during muscle relaxation. This causes a rise in the hydrostatic pressure in the capillary beds with transudation of fluid into interstitial spaces, or edema.

Probably the most common complaint with varicose veins is aching of the muscles of the legs, particularly after standing or walking for extended periods of time. The aching results from a build-up of waste products from catabolism. Patients report that this symptom is relieved by elevating the extremities, thereby decreasing venous stasis. Less common complaints are paresthesias, such as burning, pain, and itching over the involved veins and skin around them. Unfortunately some patients scratch the skin, causing eczematoid dermatitis and pigmentation from damaging the skin.

An important part of the assessment is a thorough history taking. One should ascertain when symptoms were first noticed and how fast they progressed. Did the symptoms follow pregnancy, surgery, or a fracture of the lower extremities? Has the patient ever had thrombophlebitis? Is there a familial history of varices? What is the occupation? Are both extremities involved or just one? Does the leg swell or have sores at any time around the ankle? The previous questions help differentiate between primary and secondary varicosities. Primary varicosities usually involve both legs, whereas secondary varicosities resulting from venous insufficiency are unilateral. Persons with primary varicosities usually give a familial history or have an occupation that requires standing. Secondary varicosities resulting from venous insufficiency follow thrombophlebitis or some incident that could have caused a silent thrombophlebitis. Patients with secondary varicose veins tend to have other symptoms of venous insufficiency, such as edema or ulcers of the ankle area, as will be discussed with chronic venous insufficiency.

Different methods of examination are used to determine if the veins are competent. First the course of the great saphenous vein is traced by compressing the vein with one hand and feeling for the impulse in the vein with the fingertips of the other hand. If the impulse in the vein is felt for a distance of 20 cm above or below the level of compression, incompetence is usually considered to be present. This test alone is not considered definitive.

The other test used to determine if there is incompetence of the greater and lesser saphenous is the retrograde filling test. First the superficial veins are drained by having the patient lie on his or her back and elevate the legs above the level of the thorax. Tourniquets are applied at various levels. The patient stands erect, and the direction and rapidity of filling of the superficial veins are observed. If the vein is incompetent, there will be retrograde filling to the level of the tourniquet. Normally the vein should fill from below. Should retrograde filling occur below the level of the tourniquet, incompetence of the small saphenous, communicating, or deep veins must be considered.

The Puthes's test is used to determine the competence of the superficial, communicating, and deep veins. A tourniquet is applied to the thigh to obstruct the venous return in the long saphenous vein. The patient is instructed to walk rapidly, during which time the veins are observed. If the valves of just the saphenous vein are incompetent, the vein will empty. If the valves of both the saphenous and communicating veins are incompetent, the saphenous vein will not empty. Should the veins become more prominent as the patient walks, this would be interpreted as incompetence of the deep vein valves with reflux into the superficial venous bed.

In situations where the exact pathologic changes are uncertain, phlebograms are sometimes performed. Even though phlebograms yield information in regard to the physiologic disturbances in venous circulation, they do not necessarily influence the course of therapy.

Intervention can be either of a medical or surgical nature. As is true with any disease entity, varicose veins are treated medically for as long as possible. Elastic support stockings should be worn to decrease the capacity of the superficial venous bed, promote venous return, and reduce venous stasis. By compressing the superficial veins, the blood is forced into the deep veins, thus the rate of venous return is increased and venous stasis is decreased. Stockings that have the greatest pressure in the foot area with the pressure decreasing as it progresses up the leg are considered most effective. There are a variety of support hose on the market today, the brand name of which is not nearly as important as the method of applying them. Support hose should be put on in the morning before getting out of bed, with the leg in an elevated rather than a dependent position. If the hose have to be applied after one has gotten out of bed, it is important to get into a recumbent position, elevate the extremities, and flex the ankles to drain the venous system before applying the support hose. The same applies to putting elastic support hose or bandages on a patient. They should always be applied before the patient gets out of bed and never while the patient is sitting in a chair with the legs in a dependent position. The patient should be instructed that the use of round garters and panty girdles should be avoided, as both cause compression of the superficial veins with venous engorgement.

The patient should be counseled regarding occupation, as it could relate to the disease process. Modifications may be necessary if the occupation requires prolonged standing or sitting in one position as the musculovenous pump system would not be used during those times. Approximately every hour these persons should do dorsiplantar flexion to cause the muscle to contract against the deep veins, thus increasing venous return. Any time they sit down to relax, the legs should be elevated to promote venous return by gravity and thereby decrease the hydrostatic pressure in the veins.

Surgical intervention may be done for varicose veins when related to chronic venous insufficiency secondary to thrombophlebitis, when related to recurrent thrombophlebitis, or when desired for cosmetic reasons. The surgery of choice is stripping of the greater and/or lesser saphenous veins with ligation of the communicating veins. The ligation of the communicating veins at the site where the communicating veins join the deep veins prevents the transmission of the elevated venous pressures from the deep veins into the superficial veins with resultant secondary varicosities. Occasionally following surgery there will be small tributary veins left that are cosmetically unsightly. Injections of sclerosing agents such as Ethamoline or Sotradecol may be used to obliterate these veins. Large and extensive varicosities, however, cannot be treated in this manner.

Postoperative management includes elevation of the extremities in a high Trendelenburg position for a period of a few hours and then lowering the position until the foot of the bed is elevated about 30°. This position prevents venous stasis and thus thrombus formation. Elastic bandages will be used for the same reason.

One would assume there would be a problem with postoperative bleeding from the branches of the stripped veins; however, bleeding does not occur for the following reasons. When blood vessels are torn rather than cut, the smooth muscles in the walls of the vessels respond to the stretch stimulus by going into spasm. Second, the surgery is done with the extremities in Trendelenburg position, which decreases the amount of blood in the area and promotes hemostasis.

On the first postoperative day, the patient is ambulated. At no time should the patient be permitted to sit with the legs in a dependent position. Walking is the preferred activity, as the muscles contract against the veins and facilitate venous return. As the activity is increased each day, walking rather than sitting is encouraged.

THROMBOPHLEBITIS

The term thrombophlebitis is preferred as a generic term to refer to all lesions of the veins when the clinical manifestations of venous thrombus formation are present. Venous thrombosis (phlebothrombosis) denotes thrombus formation in a vein. The thrombus may serve as an inciting factor for a potential inflammatory response; however, inflammation usually does not occur. If the inflammatory process is present, many times it is so minimal that it cannot be detected clinically. Phlebothrombosis usually occurs in the deep veins.

In contrast, the opposite is true with thrombophlebitis. Inflammation of the veins, usually resulting from some type of trauma, serves as the inciting factor for thrombus formation. Thrombophlebitis usually occurs in the superficial veins. From a clinical viewpoint, however, it should be noted that it may be impossible to determine whether a thrombus or inflammation was the inciting factor.

A thrombus is a layered structure containing erythrocytes, granular leukocytes, and thrombocytes bound by fibrin. Thrombi appear to form secondary to a change in the vessel wall, the blood flow, or the blood. Normally platelets do not adhere to the vascular endothelium. With mechanical or chemical injury to the vessel wall, as with prolonged intravenous therapy cannulization, platelet aggregation takes place. Fibrinogen is coverted into a meshlike network of fibrin in which other blood elements are caught, and thus the thrombus forms.

Changes in the blood flow, namely stasis, occur mostly in the veins of the lower extremities because of the peculiarities of the venous anatomy. Veins have valve pockets, bifurcations, and junctions that retard the blood flow and promote local stasis. The soleal veins of the calf that lie deep in the gastrocnemius muscles have a complex venous structure that promotes venous stasis. A decrease in the use of the musculovenous pump system also causes stasis in the venous system. A typical example would be atrophy of the muscles secondary to the aging process or with arthritis. Other causes of stasis formation would be inactivity associated with congestive heart failure, bedrest, and postsurgery and postpartum convalescence.

Changes in the blood, or hypercoagulability, constitute the third factor considered in the mechanism of thrombus formation. Thrombi occur more frequently in persons who have a blood dyscrasia, such as polycythemia, malignancies, and following major operations, especially in cases of major trauma to the lower limbs, where the incidence of venous thrombosis may be as high as 40 to 60 per cent.

Several factors have been identified that predispose to thrombus formation. These include obesity, immobility, advancing age, cardiac disease, and a history of phlebitis. The exact reason why obesity increases the risk of thrombus formation is unknown. Obesity tends to limit mobility and free movements, particularly for persons confined to bed, thus contributing to venous stasis. Also certain changes in the blood could be significant as the serum lipid content tends to be higher in obese women.

Immobility includes both bedrest and prolonged sitting, such as is found with persons confined to wheelchairs. Thrombus formation also has been noted from prolonged sitting in cars and airplanes. Once again venous stasis is the underlying factor with immobility. This is why early ambulation following surgery is encouraged and why anyone immobile for periods of time should initiate means to increase venous return.

The greater incidence of thrombus formation with increasing age is probably due to a multitude of factors. The older individual tends to be more immobile and requires a longer period of time to return to full activity following bedrest or surgery. Factors that promote venous stasis in the aged individual are carcinoma, cardiac disease, changes in the venous walls, and such arterial changes as arteriosclerosis obliterans.

The following factors in cardiac cases have been identified as contributing to deep vein thrombosis. With a decreased cardiac output, there is a reduction in the arterial perfusion pressure and an increase in the venous volume, with a resultant reduction of blood flow velocity in the deep veins. Also with heart failure, there can be decreased mobility and interference with the synthesis of anticoagulants because of changes in the liver.

A previous history of thrombus formation is accepted as a predisposing factor. These persons should be anticoagulated prophylactically if surgery or a period of bedrest is required.

The clinical manifestations of superficial thrombophlebitis are a reddened, warm vein that is tender upon palpation and a minimal fever with no systemic reaction. Superficial thrombophlebitis frequently occurs in a vein of the upper arm where there has been an intravenous infusion or in the lower extremities with incompetent saphenous veins and tributaries.

Deep thrombophlebitis in the lower extremities most frequently involves the soleal veins following surgery or bedrest. Mild calf pain elicited by pressing the calf from side to side may be the only symptom. If the deep thrombophlebitis involves the major venous trunk, such as the iliofemoral, the entire extremity will be edematous with prominence of the superficial veins. Calf pain is greatly aggravated by walking. Upon palpation, the calf will be warm, and the patient will complain of tenderness. Homan's sign (pain in the popliteal space with forced dorsiflexion) may be present in about 50 per cent of the patients. Frequently students are led to believe that Homan's sign is always present with thrombophlebitis. This is not true.

At times phlebothrombosis can be present without any of the above clinical signs. In order to diagnose this condition, diagnostic tests such as ultrasound mapping, fibrinogen labeled ^{131}I, plethysmography, and phlebograms must be utilized.

Pulmonary embolism can be a complication of either thrombophlebitis or phlebothrombosis. It was previously thought that pulmonary embolus occurred only with phlebothrombosis where the thrombus was not adherent to the vein, but not with thrombophlebitis, because the thrombus was anchored to the wall of the vein by the inflammatory response. Recent studies have shown that embolism can occur with either condition.

Intervention with thrombophlebitis includes bedrest, application of heat, relief of pain, and anticoagulant therapy. Bedrest with elevation of the affected extremity is usually maintained until the tenderness and edema subside. The application of moist heat packs helps resolve the inflammatory process, relieve the pain, and afford the patient symptomatic relief.

Pain may be relieved with the use of salicylates and phenylbutazone (Butazolidin); in some cases a stronger analgesic, such as propoxyphene hydrochloride (Darvon) or codeine sulfate, is required for the first few days. Butazolidin is used for about 4 or 5 days to hasten the resolution of the inflammatory process and relieve pain. If phenylbutazone and salicylates are given in combination with anticoagulants, a synergistic effect can result; thus the patient needs to be observed closely for any signs of bleeding. Moreover, both irritate the stomach, and an antacid should be used especially when a history of ulcers is present.

Fibrinolytic therapy is a newer mode of therapy for acute thromboembolism. Streptokinase, a fibrinolytic agent, causes lysis of the clot as its primary action. In addition streptokinase reduces plasma viscosity and decreases the tendency for erythrocyte aggregation. There are variations in the way streptokinase is administered. The most common method is to administer a loading dose followed by a sustaining infusion for approximately 24 to 72 hours. Laboratory monitoring tests include streptokinase resistance test (performed prior to initiation of the therapy), thrombin, or prothrombin times. In the majority of cases, a fixed dosage schedule can be established without further monitoring. Following streptokinase therapy, heparin therapy is initiated and later converted to an oral anticoagulant (Cudkowicz & Sherry, 1978).

Streptokinase can partially or completely lyse acute thrombotic occlusions in peripheral veins that are less than 72 hours in duration. According to Cudkowicz and Sherry (1978), the restoration of the circulation is dependent upon a variety of factors; the location of the occlusion, its age and nature, the presence or absence of collateral circulation, and the presence of irreversible damage. There is suggestive evidence that early dissolving of the clot prevents valvular damage and postphlebitic insufficiency syndrome.

The major complication of fibrinolytic therapy is bleeding. Life-threatening cerebral hemorrhages and other hemorrhages severe enough to require transfusions have occurred; however, bleeding from surgical wounds, needle puncture sites, invasive procedures, and trauma is considerably more common. The bleeding is due to the fibrinolytic state, which results in a decreased fibrinogen level and the presence of fibrinogen-split products that have an anticoagulant effect.

Anticoagulant therapy is used in the treatment of deep venous thrombosis or thrombophlebitis because of the danger of pulmonary embolism. The dosage of heparin, which is administered intravenously every 4 hours, is regulated so the PTT is approximately two times the normal value. Warfarin sodium started on or about the fifth day of heparin therapy, is administered to overlap for about 4 to 5 days before the heparin is discontinued; thus the warfarin sodium has sufficient time to reach an effective level of anticoagulation. During the time warfarin sodium is administered, the prothrombin time is maintained at between two and two and a half times normal.

Dextran may be used in conjunction with anticoagulants as a prophylactic agent against extension of the venous thrombus. Much remains to be learned about the use of this plasma expander with venous thrombi. If appears that dextran coats the vascular endothelium and formed elements of the blood, thereby reducing cellular aggregation.

When edema is present, elastic support hose are worn when the patient is ambulatory. Once the edema dissipates, the elastic support hose can be discontinued.

Much discussion has been given the disease entity thrombophlebitis, but more important is how to prevent it. Leg exercises and early postoperative ambulation are desired activities in helping prevent venous thrombosis. Unfortunately the manner in which these activities are executed in most institutions is totally ineffective. For exercises to be effective, they must be done at least every hour. It has been demonstrated that the increased arterial flow in the calf that increased venous return and resulted from the muscle movements during leg exercises was short-lived; the flow fell to the basal level within 1 hour of resuming immobility.

Effective leg exercises include dorsiplantar flexion of the feet with extension and flexion of the knees. Movement of the toes is not an effective exercise, as the soleus muscle is not exercised, and inactivity of this muscle promotes venous stasis. Exercises are more beneficial if done with the extremities elevated 15°, or 4 inches, because with this degree of elevation, the venous return is doubled.

Early ambulation means to walk the patient. All too frequently the patient struggles to get out of bed, takes one or two steps, and sits in a chair with the legs in a dependent position. This is just as harmful as not getting out of bed at all. Activity should be planned so that the patient is rested and the pain controlled before attempting ambulation. The patient in severe pain is totally incapable of ambulating effectively.

A second prophylactic measure would be elastic compression. The reader is referred to the section on varicose veins for details on the application of elastic compression. Elastic compression should be applied from the toe to knee. By so doing there is an increased flow velocity through the deep veins and a decreased superficial venous bed. The venous return is increased 150 per cent if the elastic compression is applied from the toe to knee. With elastic compression applied to the groin, there is no significant increase in the venous return beyond when toe to knee hose are utilized. Also elastic compression above the knees might slip down, causing popliteal compression.

Currently the most promising approach to preventing venous thrombosis is low-dose heparin prophylaxis. The Council on Thrombosis of the American Heart Association recommends the use of low-dose heparin prophylaxis for all adults who are subjected to major abdominal, pelvic, or thoracic surgery. Low-dose heparin, 5,000 IU every 8 hours, is administered subcutaneously. The dosage is low enough so that no special monitoring is required and bleeding does not occur should the patient be exposed to trauma. The groups of patients in whom low-dose heparin appears to fail to prevent deep venous thrombosis are those patients who have major orthopedic surgery or open prostatectomy.

A routine procedure with the postoperative patient is deep breathing and coughing to improve aeration of the lungs. An equally important effect is an increased venous return, and thus prevention of stasis. When an individual breathes deeply, the intrathoracic pressure becomes more negative and venous return of blood is increased.

Pulmonary Embolism

Pulmonary embolism is an impaction of some part of the pulmonary vascular system with detached thrombi or foreign material. Most cases of pulmonary embolism occur secondary to venous thrombosis; occasionally nonthrombotic material, such as fat, air, amniotic fluid, bone marrow, and tumor particles, embolize to the lung.

Most massive emboli, which can be fatal, come from the iliofemoral channel, with a minority from the lower veins of the legs. In some situations there are no clinical signs of deep venous thrombosis, even though the embolus does come from this site; thus we have the term *silent thrombosis*.

Factors that could potentially dislodge venous thrombi would be any activity causing a *sudden* increase in venous return, such as mobility and mechanical stress following a period of immobility. This would include such activities as ambulating patients, transferring patients from the bed to chair, sudden muscular movements of previously immobile extremities, and straining at stool. During the Valsalva maneuver, which occurs with straining, there is an increase in the intrathoracic pressure, with a sudden increase in the pressure in the leg veins causing sudden distention of the large pelvic veins. Thus a thrombus may be torn away from the wall and flow up into the lungs during the negative phase.

Once a thrombus is dislodged, it travels through the great veins and right heart to the pulmonary artery. Then, depending on the size of the embolus, it becomes impacted in the main pulmonary artery, one of the main branches, or the arteries of the lower lobes. The immediate outcome depends on the length, diameter, and number of emboli. Long, wide emboli are more dangerous, as the pulmonary artery or one of the main branches could be occluded, whereas smaller and narrower emboli are more likely to occlude smaller arteries of the lung and therefore are less likely to be fatal.

Pulmonary embolism and infarction are not synonymous, for pulmonary infarction can be a resultant complication of pulmonary embolism. With pulmonary infarction there is necrosis of the lung parenchyma and resultant interference of the blood supply. Fortunately the lung has two blood supplies, the pulmonary and the bronchial arteries; thus pulmonary infarction occurs in a small percentage of the cases because of the compensatory increase in blood flow through the bronchial arteries.

The clinical manifestations of pulmonary embolism include dyspnea, tachypnea, chest pain, cyanosis, fever, hypotension, hemoptysis, tachycardia, and anxiety. The size of the embolus, however, determines the presenting symptoms.

With massive embolism there is obstruction of a segment of the pulmonary circulation with rapid onset of pulmonary hypertension and subsequent failure of the right ventricle. The patient presents a picture of acute cor pulmonale with dyspnea, cyanosis, and distended neck veins. Associated with the right ventricular failure is decreased filling of the left ventricle and a decrease in the cardiac output with diminished perfusion of the cerebral coronary arteries. Thus the symptoms of chest pain, syncope, and shock occur. The patient may die within minutes to hours following a massive embolus.

When the embolization involves smaller and medium-sized arteries, the symptoms can be transient or can be full-blown as described above. Usually there is an acute onset of a pneumonialike illness followed by increasing dyspnea with effort. In most cases the condition is resolved, and the patient completely recovers.

The clinical manifestations of pulmonary infarction vary from silent lesions to a combination of symptoms, including elevated temperature, tachycardia, tachypnea, pleuritic pain, cough, and hemoptysis. Characteristic changes in the laboratory data are an elevated leukocyte count and the triad of an elevated serum lactic dehydrogenase and elevated serum bilirubin with normal serum transaminases (SGOT and SGPT). Arterial hypoxemia, a P_{O_2} of less than 80 mm Hg in a person not receiving oxygen, is the most frequently observed laboratory abnormality. A roentgenographic examination will show elevation of the diaphram on the involved side. In addition, there may be a small pleural effusion and atelectasis.

A lung scan is done to confirm the diagnosis of a pulmonary embolus. If the diagnosis is questionable, it may be necessary to perform an angiogram. There are two methods used to perform a pulmonary angiogram. With the first method, a radiopaque medium is injected into the arm vein and serial films are taken of the lungs. The advantage of this method is that a cardiac catheterization is not necessary to perform the test. With the second method, a catheter is inserted into a peripheral vein in the upper extremity and passed through the right atrium, the right ventricle, the pulmonary artery and its branches under fluoroscopy. The advantage to this method is that pressure readings can be taken in the heart chambers and pulmonary artery in addition to cinephotography following the injection of contrast media. Both methods should demonstrate vascular filling defects; however, the results with the second method are more certain.

The initial treatment with pulmonary embolism is of a supportive nature. The patient is maintained on bedrest and oxygen is administered. Heparin therapy should be initiated immediately in all patients with pulmonary embolism to decrease the recurrence of emboli. Intravenous heparin is usually administered for 10 days because by that time clots have firmly attached to the vessel wall and organization of the clot has begun. Traditionally heparin has been administered intravenously via a heparin loc every 4 hours and the dosage is adjusted to maintain the PTT at one and one half to two times the control values. A more current approach, described by Tsou (1978), is to administer a constant infusion of heparin instead of doses every 4 hours. The advantage is the avoidance of a subtherapeutic plasma heparin level. Oral warfarin sodium is usually started on approximately the fifth day of heparin therapy and continued for varying lengths of time from 6 weeks to indefinitely.

An important adjunct to the management of pulmonary emboli is fibrinolytic therapy. Clinical studies have demonstrated that streptokinase and urokinase lyse pulmonary emboli and thereby improve pulmonary capillary perfusion and gas exchange. The reader is referred to the section on thromboembolism for details on fibrinolytic therapy. In most cases where the patient is hypotensive because of impediment to blood flow shock, vasopressor drugs are required to ensure adequate tissue perfusion and are titrated utilizing the urinary output as a measure of organ perfusion. Analgesics are used to control the pain and apprehension characteristic of persons who have a pulmonary embolus.

Surgical intervention is indicated for those patients in whom anticoagulant therapy is contraindicated or whose disease cannot be controlled with this mode of therapy. The surgery of choice is plication of the inferior vena cava by application of a serrated Teflon clip below the level of the renal veins. The external clip by its construction divides the large vena caval lumen into four or five channels; thus large, fatal emboli are blocked from traveling to the lungs. Smaller emboli, however, may still pass through the channels. With this procedure there is no significant obstruction to venous return, therefore, it is not necessary for venous collateral circulation to develop around the clipped cava.

Ligation of the inferior vena cava is the other surgical procedure performed for recurring pulmonary emboli. With ligation of the vena cava, the resultant complete obstruction causes the development of large collateral channels to carry the venous blood around the occlusion. These collateral channels can be sufficiently large to permit the passage of large fatal emboli. Because of the embarrassment to the venous system, signs of chronic venous insufficiency develop.

The nurse as a member of the health team has a major responsibility in preventing venous thrombosis which could cause a pulmonary embolus. Prophylaxis should be instituted as soon as a patient is immobilized regardless of the underlying disease process. Patients should be turned at least every hour if they are unable to be mobile. Second, leg exercises, as discussed under thrombophlebitis, should be done under supervision every hour. Also elastic stockings should be worn.

As was discussed earlier, there is danger of dislodging a thrombus when a patient has been immobilized for prolonged periods of time. During the initial ambulation of a patient, the patient should be assessed for signs of pulmonary embolism. Any patient who has been immobile and complains of sudden stabbing chest pain should be brought to the attention of the physician. Stool softeners and a diet to facilitate easy bowel elimination should be administered. The patient must be instructed not to strain at stool, and cathartics may be required. It becomes apparent that it is of utmost importance to prevent venous stasis that would create an environment conducive to thrombus formation.

Chronic Venous Insufficiency

Chronic venous insufficiency is a disorder of the lower extremities manifested by chronic edema formation and tissue changes secondary to severe venous stasis. Synonymous terms for chronic venous insufficiency are *postphlebitic syndrome, stasis edema,* and *stasis ulcer.* The situations that predispose to chronic venous insufficiency are long-standing primary or secondary varicose veins and thrombophlebitis, particularly of the iliofemoral veins.

In an extremity with a normal venous system, the venous pressure decreases and the venous return increases with walking. When valvular damage occurs, however, as in primary or secondary varicosities and deep venous thrombophlebitis, the ambulatory venous pressure increases markedly, particularly at the ankle level. Venous return is severely retarded, and the venous hydrostatic pressure rises, resulting in significant edema formation of the tissues.

A characteristic clinical picture of chronic venous insufficiency is unilateral edema that appears during the latter part of the day and disappears with recumbency throughout the hours of sleep. If the process is unilateral, the involved extremity is that which is affected by the varicosity or phlebitic process. The chronically edematous tissues may become fibrotic, thus producing a brawny induration above the level of the malleolus. This is sometimes referred to as brawny or nonpitting edema.

Resultant of the persistently elevated venous hydrostatic pressure is extravasation of blood into the interstitial spaces, which produces a brown pigmentation of the tissues from the iron component (hemosiderin) during hemoglobin disintegration. Stasis dermatitis, an itchy eczematoid rash, may appear in the area. Finally, the skin may ulcerate, producing the classic nonpainful stasis ulcer, usually at the level of the malleolus.

Once chronic venous insufficiency has developed, progressive disability usually can be expected despite treatment. The most important intervention in the management of chronic venous insufficiency is elastic support of the venous bed to promote venous return and diminish venous stasis. Elastic support stockings should be worn the rest of the individual's life to diminish potential eczematoid dermatitis and ulceration. The hose are worn while the individual is ambulatory and can be removed during the hours of sleep. The foot of the bed is best elevated 30° or 8 inches, during sleep to increase venous return.

If stasis ulcers develop, the treatment is bedrest with elevation of the extremity. Sterile moist saline compresses are utilized to promote the formation of granulation tissue. Care must be exercised to prevent iatrogenic sepsis of the ulcers. Topical or oral antibiotics may be administered if specific pathogenic organisms are cultured. Currently, a modification of the hyperbaric oxygen therapy technique is being utilized as a means of treating stasis ulcers. A plastic bag is secured around the affected limb. One hundred per cent oxygen from the standard hospital oxygen unit is introduced via catheter at 8 to 10 liters per minute for a total of 4 to 8 hours per day. The theory underlying the technique is that oxygen made available under pressure may support the metabolic processes of ischemic cells and promote healing. Definitive studies of the technique's therapeutic effectiveness are withstanding.

When ulcers do not heal with conservative medical management, surgical intervention is indicated. Debridement of necrotic tissue may be done to promote formulation of granulation tissue. Skin grafting procedures may be performed also. Either a split or full-thickness graft may be used after the ulcer and surrounding fibrotic tissue are excised. If secondary varicose veins are the cause of the chronic venous insufficiency and aggravate the response to therapy, stripping and ligation procedures may be done.

Prevention of disability is the primary goal in the rehabilitative process with chronic venous insufficiency. Specific teaching should be directed toward promoting patient understanding of the pathologic process and the adverse effects of gravity and orthostasis on the venous circulation. The rationale and method of elastic compression should be emphasized. Provisions must be made for elevation of the individual's extremities above the level of the pelvis several times throughout the 24-hour period both at home and at work. Hygienic care of the skin and prevention of extremity trauma are of utmost importance in preventing ulcer formation.

The Arteries

Structure and Function

The function of the arteries is to transport blood under high pressure to the tissues. In contrast to the veins, the walls of the aorta and other arteries contain a large amount of elastic tissue. The highly elastic structure of the aorta enables it to distend in receipt of blood as it is ejected from the left ventricle during systole. During diastole the elastic tissue shortens and aids in the propulsion of blood into the arterial circuit. With a decrease in the aortic blood volume, the biochemical energy stored in the aortic elastic tissue during distention is released in the form of kinetic energy. This energy further aids in the forward propulsion of the blood. The familiar example of the rubber band can be used to illustrate the preceding changes. An elastic band is stretched, and as it is stretched, potential energy accumulates. When the band is released, it returns to its prestretched form and, at the same time, releases kinetic energy. This energy may be used to move the propellor of a model airplane or for some other purpose. Thus the elasticity of the aorta is a factor in the continuous flow of blood through the arteries, and it also helps to protect the smaller vessels from the full force of left ventricular systolic contraction.

Upon leaving the small arteries, blood courses through the arterioles. The blood flow to the tissues is controlled almost entirely by the degree of constriction or dilatation of the arterioles. The walls of the arterioles, in contrast to large arteries, are primarily composed of smooth muscle. The muscle is innervated by sympathetic nerve fibers that are constrictor in function and to a lesser degree by parasympathetic nerve fibers that are dilatator in function. This innervation by the autonomic nervous system acts to regulate the diameter of the arteriolar lumen in response to blood volume and the metabolic needs of localized tissues.

The arterioles are only a few millimeters in length with diameters from 8 to 50 μ (microns). Each arteriole branches into smaller muscle-walled vessels called metarterioles and perfuse anywhere from 10 to 100 capillaries. The arterioles are the major site of resistance to blood flow. Changes in the arteriole walls that cause a diminished lumen result in diminished blood volume and velocity of flow to the capillaries and a significant increase in the peripheral vascular resistance.

As indicated previously, the entire function of the cardiovascular system is accomplished at the capillary level. It is here that the exchange of essential materials takes place between the blood and the interstitial fluid. The capillary wall is a single layer of endothelial cells about 1 μ thick, with an average capillary diameter of approximately 6 μ. According to Zweifach (1959), the distance from a capillary to a cell is never greater than 0.005 inch. The total length of capillaries is 60,000 miles or an average of 400 miles per pound of body weight. Thus the potential capacity of the capillaries is large enough to hold all the blood in the body.

There are many anastomosing channels between individual capillaries and between metarterioles and venules. This enables a shift of blood around a part to meet tissue needs. The flow of blood through the capillaries is regulated by the arteriolar lumen and by structures at the beginning of the capillaries, the precapillary sphincters. It has been noted microscopically that capillary channels open and close at different times. When tissues are active, the number of open channels is greater than at rest. This is another way in which the body can adapt circulatory function to meet the local needs of metabolizing cells.

Another way in which the circulation can adapt to meet local tissue needs is by collateral circulation. Tissues are protected from the effects of a diminished or obstructed arterial flow by the development and enlargement of capillaries and arterioles surrounding the deprived tissue. New capillaries develop and arterioles recanalize because of pressure gradient differences between the surrounding and affected tissues. The body part, however, may require from 1 to 6 months to increase the tissue vascularity. If the blood supply deprivation to the affected part is such that the basal metabolic needs of the tissues can still be met and if the tissues are protected from increased demands, adequate cellular function may be maintained while the collateral circulation is becoming established. If metabolic needs cannot be met during this time, however, the cellular function may cease.

Assessment of the Patient with Arterial Problems

The majority of the symptoms associated with disorders of the peripheral arteries are secondary to ischemia. The degree of clinical manifestations will vary proportionally to the degree of tissue oxygen deprivation.

Diagnostic Tests

Diagnostic test used to study the status of arteries are of two general types. In one type, the effects of various stimuli on arterial function are determined. These involve exposing the individual or a part of the body to a physiologic stimulus and observing the vascular response directly or indirectly with an instrument. In the other, tests are used to identify the location and extent of the structural change.

Reactive Hyperemia

When the blood flow through an artery is either partially or completely obstructed by external compression for a brief period of time, metabolites accumulate in the tissues and induce relaxation of the arterial tone. As the circulation is restored, because of the vasodilatation, there is an increase in the flow of blood with resultant hyperemia of the skin. Usually the artery is occluded with a blood pressure cuff for 5 minutes. Upon release of the cuff, hyperemia of the extremity should occur within 10 seconds or less. A delayed or weakened hyperemic reaction indicates organic arterial insufficiency.

Oscillometry

The oscillometer is a manometer attached to a blood pressure cuff that is used to measure arterial pulsations in the extremities. In peripheral occlusive vascular disease, it is employed to determine the point at which circulation through the deep thigh and calf vessels ceases or to compare the pulsations in the two extremities. The same data could be obtained by palpation of the pulses with the fingertips. The problem is that arteries are not readily palpable in many areas of the body.

Plethysmography

The plethysmograph is an instrument that measures the actual volume of blood entering tissues. The plethysmograph can be used to measure the actual volume of arterial blood perfusing a given area per unit time. Decrease in the rate of arterial blood flow affords data on the extent of occlusive disease.

Skin Temperature

The skin temperature is determined by a thermocouple held in contact with the skin. Conditions such as exposure to cold or heat, exercise, the ingestion of food, and the emotional state of the individual all influence skin temperatures. In an attempt to minimize these factors, the test is performed in a warm environment with the patient resting. Except when the temperature of the skin of one extremity differs markedly from that of another, the results may not be very valuable.

Arteriography

Radiopaque media are injected into an artery so that the medium can fill the arterial tree, including the collateral vessels and the runoff distal to the obstruction. Serial films are taken of the involved artery.

Physical Assessment

Pain

With peripheral arterial disease, pain is the most outstanding feature. Depending on the underlying pathology, the pain will vary in site, in duration, and with such triggering mechanisms as exercise and cold. *Persistent pain* is associated with gangrene, ulceration, sudden arterial occlusion, ischemic neuropathy, and rest pain. The pain associated with gangrene and ulceration from thromboangiitis obliterans is excruciating, whereas, if the underlying pathology is arteriosclerosis obliterans, the pain is less severe. Severe pain, present in the absence of ulceration and gangrene, can be caused by ischemia and is termed *rest pain*.

With sudden arterial obstruction as occurs from an embolus, the pain occurs abruptly and is severe. The arterial spasm associated with an embolus is responsible for the pain either directly or secondary to the ischemia.

Intermittent pain results either from changes in temperature, as occurs with Raynaud's disease, or from a decrease in the arterial blood supply to contracting muscles, as occurs with arteriosclerosis obliterans. Intermittent claudication is described by patients as tiredness, aching, or constricting pain of the affected muscle that is brought on by a specific amount of exercise or walking. The pain is relieved by ceasing the activity and resting for a few minutes. Identification of the site of the pain and the duration of the activity that initiates the pain helps in diagnosing the underlying pathology and its severity.

Obstruction of the arteries to the calves and feet, as occurs in early thromboangiitis obliterans, produces intermittent claudication of the intrinsic muscles of the feet. If the claudication involves calf muscles, it is probably secondary to atheromatous blockage of the superficial femoral arteries, whereas claudication of the thighs and buttocks is associated with obstruction in the terminal aorta and iliac arteries.

Temperature Change

The patient should be examined in a warm environment, as cold causes vasoconstriction. A change in skin temperature is more significant if it involves only one digit, foot, or localized area than if it occurs as a bilateral sign. A sudden increase in coldness of the part occurs with a peripheral embolus.

Color

The color of the skin is determined by the number and perfusion of the capillaries as well as the composition of the blood in the capillaries. Pallor occurs when capillary flow ceases because of arteriolar constriction. When the limb is elevated above the level of the heart, the pallor intensifies in an ischemic limb, whereas the color is unchanged in the normal one. With cyanosis the skin and mucous membranes take on a bluish color, which is indicative of decreased quantity or quality of blood flow. Rubor is a dull red or reddish blue discoloration of a cold extremity resulting from hyperemia. The reader is reminded that in patients with heavily pigmented skin, pallor and cyanosis may appear as leaden gray or mottling, and rubor may be seen as an intensification of skin tone.

Changes in color can be precipitated by changes in position or temperature. With Raynaud's disease the color of the digits varies from pallor to rubor with exposure to cold. With occlusive arterial disease, abnormal color changes occur in the skin with position change.

Trophic changes are manifested with chronic ischemia. The skin becomes dry, shiny, and tightly drawn over the underlying tissue with an absence of hair. The nails become thick and hardened with an accumulation of epithelial debris under the nail edges. It can also be noted that skin lesions fail to heal, and ulceration is common.

Peripheral Pulses

The pulses are used as a basis to determine the adequacy of arterial blood flow. A scale of 0 to 4 is used to grade the pulse volume, with 0 indicating an absence of pulsations; 1, marked impairment; 2, moderate impairment; 3, slight impairment; and 4, normal pulsations. Pulses are palpated to determine not only the heart rate and rhythm, but the amplitude of the pulse which reflects the elasticity of the vessel wall as well.

Peripheral pulses can be very difficult to locate and palpate, thus the examiner must assume a comfortable position. First it is most important to ascertain that the pulse being felt is the patient's and not the examiner's. As the patient's pulse is palpated with one hand the examiner simultaneously palpates his or her pulse with the other hand. A pulse can best be felt if the pressure of the examining fingers is varied. Also if the examiner's finger tips are moistened with soap, the surface friction is reduced between the fingers and the patient's skin, and the pulses can be felt more easily. Once the location of the various pulses are identified, they should be marked with a felt-tipped pen.

The peripheral pulses to be examined are the femoral, popliteal, posterior tibial, and the dorsalis pedis. The femoral pulse is palpated about 1 inch below the inguinal ligament in the femoral triangle which is midgroin. The examiner's hand on the same side of the body as the patient's leg where the pulse is being palpated is used. Also the patient must be lying flat. The popliteal pulse is located on the posterior medial aspect of the patella. To palpate it, the examiner stands on the same side as the pulse. With the patient's knee slightly bent, both of the examiner's hands are cupped behind the knee so that the finger tips of both hands can be used to palpate the pulse. The posterior tibial is located posterior to the medial malleolus of the ankle. To palpate the left posterior tibial, the examiner stands on the left side of the patient and uses the finger tips of the right hand. If the foot is dorsiflexed, the pulse will be felt more easily. The location of the dorsalis pedis artery is not constant in anatomic position and is absent in approximately 10 per cent of the population. Its usual location is on the lateral side of the first metatarsal. This pulse is palpated by standing at the foot of the bed and using the hand on the same side as the patient's foot to be palpated (Atchison & Murray, 1978, p. 38).

Arteriosclerosis Obliterans

Arteriosclerosis obliterans is an occlusive disease of the abdominal aorta and large and medium-sized arteries. It affects predominantly middle-aged or older men and postmenopausal women. It rarely affects the upper extremities. The disorder is caused by atherosclerosis of the intima with medial arteriosclerosis.

The clinical manifestations associated with arteriosclerosis obliterans are secondary to ischemia of the organ involved. The factors that influence the degree of ischemia are the degree of vessel obstruction as related to the size of the artery, the rapidity with which the obstruction occurs, and the development of collateral circulation. A slowly progressing obliteration of an artery may produce fewer symptoms and promote collateral circulation development as compared to a sudden occlusion because of thrombosis. Also the size of the artery involved will determine the degree of symptoms; thus if a small artery is involved, there can be no symptoms or only a few.

In the arterial system there are also preexisting collateral channels that can convey blood around an obstruction. Normally very little blood flows through these channels, but with obstruction there is an increase in the arterial pressure at the site of obstruction. This creates a pressure gradient that causes the collateral vessels to dilate and carry increased arterial flow.

Intermittent claudication is the outstanding clinical manifestation in arteriosclerosis obliterans of the limbs. It is described by the patient as a constricting pain, ache, or sense of fatigue occurring in certain muscles while walking. Walking causes the muscles to contract, which puts pressure on the blood vessels and further decreases the arterial flow. The pain results from the build-up of lactic acid from anaerobic metabolism which accumulates in periods of ischemia. Pain receptors also may be stimulated by bradykinin and histamine, which form in tissues during muscle cell damage (Guyton, 1976, pp. 664–65). Cessation of walking promotes removal of the acid metabolites and the decrease of pain. The pain occurs in the muscles distal to the arterial obstruction. If the atheromatous plaque is in the superficial femoral artery, the pain will be in the calf muscles. If there is blockage of the popliteal artery, the pain is in the foot. In aortoiliac disease (Leriche syndrome) the symptom of intermittent claudication is present in the thighs and buttocks and can be misinterpreted as pain involving the sciatic nerve. The severity of the claudication is determined by the distance a person can walk on level ground before the pain causes him or her to stop and rest.

Ekroth, et al. (1978) demonstrated that patients with intermittent claudication who participated in a controlled physical training program increased their walking ability. In 88 per cent of 148 patients, the walking ability was more than double the pretraining values after the training period. Development of collateral circulation has been the most common explanation given for the training effect in claudication patients; however, this study did not support that thesis. There was an increase in the patient's walking ability which could not be correlated with the degree of increased blood flow, thus the investigators cite a metabolic explanation for the change in walking tolerance. These researchers suggest that there is an increase in the metabolic capacity of muscle tissue in patients with intermittent claudication who are subjected to controlled physical training.

According to Ream (1977), the following method used to develop collateral circulation has been learned successfully by patients. The patients walk for 30 minutes two to three times daily. Should pain occur while they are walking, it is permissible to rest if the pain forces them to stop; however, they are encouraged not to stop the instant the pain starts. After resting the walk is resumed until the 30 minutes is over.

As the disease progresses, there is a gradual decrease in the individual's exercise tolerance to the point of rest pain (pretrophic pain). Rest pain, which usually involves the digits, lower parts of the leg, and foot, is worse at night. Frequently during the night these patients will hang their legs over the edge of the bed and rub them by the hour. Edema formation, secondary to the dependent position, further limits arterial flow, and the pain thus increases in severity.

Neuropathy is also present with severe ischemia. Usually the neuropathic pain will follow the distribution of the peripheral nerves and thus extend over a large portion of the lower extremity. This pain can be constant or paroxysmal and is described as a constant tingling or sharp shooting pain. A feeling of numbness, coldness, or burning may also occur. Ulceration and gangrene are sometimes present with ischemic neuropathy.

Sexual impotence, resulting from aortoiliac obstruction (Leriche syndrome), frequently is the symptom that causes the patient to seek medical advice. Therefore, when arterial disease is suspected it is important to inquire about this symptom as the patient's history is elicited.

Patients frequently complain that the involved extremity or extremities feel cold to them. A difference in the temperature of the two extremities or feet is especially significant. Whereas unilateral coldness of the involved extremity is associated with arteriosclerosis obliterans, bilateral coldness could be caused by vasoconstriction from a cold environment. Associated with changes in temperature are color changes. Pallor, cyanosis, and rubor may be present, depending on the severity of the process.

Trophic changes occur with a chronic decrease in circulation to the tissues of the limbs. There will be a decreased bulk in the gluteal muscle with Leriche syndrome. Upon physical examination loss of hair particularly on the toes and feet; atrophy of the skin which takes on a dry, shiny appearance; and a hard brittle appearance of the nails can be observed.

Skin breakdown and ulceration often result secondary to minor infections and trauma due to the reduction of arterial blood supply. Necrosis of tissue and gangrene occur as the arterial blood supply becomes occluded. Gangrenous tissue has the typical black, shriveled, dry appearance.

The quality of the peripheral pulses is significant in determining the location of the obstruction, for the pulse distal to a stenosed artery will have a low amplitude. Also auscultation of the artery is helpful as a bruit is produced by the turbulent flow of blood through a stenosed artery. Frequently it is assumed that pulses will be absent distal to an obstruction; if the obstruction is high, such as in the aortoiliac artery, collateral circulation forms around the block and peripheral pulses of good quality may persist. The reader is referred to the section on general assessment for details regarding peripheral pulses.

Diagnosis of arterial occlusive disease is based primarily upon evaluation of the presenting signs and symptoms in that the symptoms of ischemia are classical. Other diagnostic methods used include oscillometric and plethysmographic readings and arteriography. Arteriography is performed if surgery is being contemplated because it provides for precise delineation of the lesion's location, the nature of the defect, and the effect of the involvement on the dependent tissues.

The problem of preventing injury to ischemic tissue until a patient is able to develop collateral circulation is urgent. Even the slightest trauma or the mildest irritating chemical may be sufficient to upset the balance between the supply of essential nutrients and the needs of the tissues. The viability of ischemic tissue is protected by decreasing the local metabolic needs of the tissues as well as by increasing the blood flow to the ischemic part.

If a patient with an ischemic extremity is admitted to the hospital, bedrest in a constant-temperature room is usually prescribed. Measures must be instituted to prevent pressure sores or ulcers. Even relatively minimal pressure on extravascular tissues, such as the heel on the bed, exceeds the arterial pressure of an ischemic extremity. Thus this mechanical compression of the arterial flow causes further tissue ischemia.

If a patient can move about freely, there is little danger of pressure from a part remaining in one position; however, with less active patients, a regular turning and positioning schedule must be established. Devices such as alternating water mattresses must also be used to distribute the pressure evenly.

Foot Care

The prevention of ulceration and gangrene is easier than the cure. Almost all ulcerations and gangrene of ischemic extremities can be attributed to chemical, mechanical, or thermal injury or to local bacterial infection of the tissues. It stands to reason that heat in the form of hot water bottles or heating pads should not be used, nor should chemical agents be applied to the skin unless specifically prescribed by the physician. In some institutions a physician's prescription is required before toenails can be cut, and in others toenails are cut only by podiatrists. Prior to cutting the nails, the feet should be soaked in warm water to soften the nails.

Not only is the nurse responsible for trying to identify and remove possible sources of injury to the patient's feet, but the cooperation and assistance of the patient are essential. Furthermore, even when the treatment of the hospitalized patient is successful, a regimen similar to that followed in the hospital is essential if the tissues in the extremities are to be maintained in a reasonably healthy condition. The patient must know how to care for his or her extremities, especially the feet, and understand why this care is important. He or she must also be helped to understand that although physicians and nurses will do their best to assist, the main responsibility in the control of the disorder is the patient's. The patient should therefore be given written as well as verbal instructions and demonstrations of the care of the feet. He or she should have an opportunity to practice the essential procedures under supervision.

The instructions on care of the feet are appropriate for all patients who have peripheral occlusive vascular disease, including those who also have diabetes mellitus.

1. Cleanliness.
   a. Wash no less frequently than every other day in warm, soapy water.
   b. Dry thoroughly between the toes with a soft cloth. Use a patting or swabbing action.
   c. Take care not to bruise the feet or break the skin.
   d. Powder the feet if they have a tendency to perspire.
   e. Lubricate the feet with an ointment consisting of 50 parts lanolin and 50 parts petroleum jelly if they are dry.
2. Shoes.
   a. Never go barefoot. Always wear shoes when out of bed.
   b. Wear well-built shoes of soft leather.
   c. Wear shoes with a broad toe and a sensible heel. They should give the feet adequate support.
   d. Never wear new shoes more than one-half day at a time.
   e. Never wear shoes with exposed nails, defects in the lining, or any other roughened surfaces that will come in contact with the feet.
3. Hose.
   a. Wear seamless hose without holes, darns, or patches.
   b. Wear clean stockings daily.
   c. Be sure to buy hose sufficiently long. Too short stockings are as harmful as too short shoes.
   d. Lamb's wool should be worn between the toes, provided that it does not create pressure between the toes, predisposing to tissue breakdown.
4. Toenails.
   a. If you go to a podiatrist, tell him or her that you have a reduction in blood flow to your feet.
   b. Before cutting toenails, soak feet in warm, soapy water.
   c. Cut the toenails straight across and not too short, that is, not too close to the flesh.
   d. Place cotton wicks under the corners of the great toenails if there is a tendency to ingrown toenails.
5. Corns and calluses.
   a. Do not cut corns and calluses.
   b. Do not use medicated corn plasters.
   c. Have corns and calluses taken care of by a physician or a podiatrist who understands your condition.
6. Cold and heat.
   a. In cold weather, wear warm clothes and adequate foot covering to protect the feet from excessive cold. Wear loose, thick, warm socks. Do not stay out in the cold for long periods of time. Cold contracts your blood vessels and lessens the supply of blood to your feet.
   b. Do not place hot water bottles, heating pads, or other heating devices near to or on the feet or legs. Do not use any form of heat without the advice of your physician.
   c. Do not place the feet in an oven, or an electric heater, or on a radiator.
   d. If your feet are cold, warm them by wearing woolen bed socks or wrapping them in a warm blanket.
   e. Remember that your feet are sensitive to both heat and cold and that extremes should be avoided.
7. Rest and elevation of the feet.
   a. Sit down and elevate your feet on a footstool at least once every 2 hours. (Many industrial concerns allow rest periods, usually 15 minutes, for their employees. This time could be used for elevating your feet on a footstool or a chair. This is most important for the older diabetic patient who has arteriosclerosis.)
   b. Do not cross your knees or ankles when you sit.
8. Injury—any injury, however slight, may become ulcerous or gangrenous if treatment is delayed.
   a. Take care not to injure your feet. Avoid crowded places.
   b. A pillow may be used to prevent pressure on the feet by bed covering.
   c. Do not delay in consulting your physician should any redness, blistering, swelling, or pain develop.
   d. When tissue is cut or bruised, cover the part with a clean bandage.
   e. Do not use strong antiseptics, such as iodine, Lysol, carbolic acid, and bichloride of mercury. No medicine should be placed on your feet unless prescribed by your physician.
   f. Avoid sunburn and swimming in cold water or at beaches where there is a possibility of injurying the feet.
9. Athlete's foot.
   A deficient supply of blood to the feet predisposes to athlete's foot. It starts out with burning and

itching between the toes. You should report these symptoms to your physician so that treatment can be started immediately.

Too much emphasis cannot be placed on the importance of the care of the feet of the patient who has occlusive vascular disease. Attention should be centered not only on the preceding measures, but on identification of conditions in the environment that predispose to injury. Any condition that increases metabolism in tissues with an inadequate blood supply may thereby upset the balance between supply and demand and result in ulceration and gangrene.

The second objective in therapy of occlusive peripheral vascular disease is to improve the blood flow to the extremities. Interventions to achieve this goal include utilization of indirect heat, dependent position, alcohol, and abstinence from tobacco. The use of heat to promote reflex vasodilatation can be a complicated problem. The objective is to induce maximum vasodilatation without stimulating metabolism. Direct sources of heat, such as a hot water bottle and heating pad, should not be used, for they increase tissue metabolism and, because of the pathology, the arterial perfusion rate is unable to increase. By placing the patient in a warm environment of at least 80°F, however, general vasodilatation occurs, and the stimulus for vasoconstriction is eliminated. The use of a heat cradle at 90°F over an affected extremity will also increase vasodilatation. If, however, warm environmental temperature increases the pateint's pain, the heat should be discontinued.

For many years cigarette smoking has been known to cause vasoconstriction. An interesting observation has been made that when persons who are accustomed to smoking perform only the motions of smoking, their peripheral blood vessels constrict. Any influence causing even temporary vasoconstriction may have an adverse effect on already ischemic tissues. The possibility also exists that in some individuals, the blood vessels are allergic to tobacco. Occasionally it has been noted that if an individual resumes smoking, once having had a peripheral vascular ischemia, an exacerbation of the previously quiescent disease may occur. Whether or not tobacco directly enters into the etiology of occlusive peripheral vascular disease is unknown; however, it appears to intensify the effects caused by vasoconstriction.

Position can also be used to improve arterial blood flow. With severe ischemia arterial flow to the lower extremities can be improved by putting the head of the bed on 12- to 16-inch blocks. The Sander's oscillating bed has proved to be beneficial in improving the arterial circulation for some patients. Its use is more or less limited to patients who have rest pain, ischemic neuropathy, and minor noninfected ulcers or gangrenous lesions. The rationale for using the oscillating bed is that it alternately promotes arterial filling and venous return of the lower extremities without effort on the part of the patient. This bed is designed on the same principle as a seesaw with the springs attached at the center to a fulcrum so that when one end of the bed is elevated the other is depressed. The rate at which the bed oscillates can be adjusted to meet the needs of the individual patient.

One of the most effective means of producing vasodilatation is the administration of whisky. Pain relief is secured with alcohol as the vasodilating effect lasts for about 4 hours. Because of the inherent possiblility of the patients becoming alcoholic with prolonged use, some physicians rarely prescribe alcohol.

Management of ischemic pain can be a major challenge to the health care team. All too frequently the severity of the pain is underestimated and treated inadequately. Mild pain can be controlled with the judicious use of whisky in combination with salicylates. The control of rest pain is vitally important as it tends to be worse at night, causing the patient to lose hours of sleep. Barbiturates may be required in addition to salicylates and alcohol, or a more potent analgesic, including a narcotic, might be indicated. The ingenuity of the nurse is taxed to create an environment conducive to sleep.

Surgical intervention is indicated when the intermittent claudication interferes with the patient's gainful employment or when amputation seems inevitable. The operative procedures designed for vascular reconstruction include an end-to-end anastomosis, bypass graft, excision with graft replacement and thromboendarterectomy. The specific procedure is determined by the nature, extent, and site of involvement.

For patients who have pregangrenous changes of the toes and the tissue immediately adjacent the toes, a lumbar sympathectomy may be performed on rare occasions. After a sympathectomy, there is a transient increase in the blood flow to the whole limb with the blood flow returning to normal levels in the proximal parts and remaining increased in the feet. Because a lumbar sympathectomy does not increase blood flow to muscles, it becomes apparent that the symptoms of intermittent claudication will not be completely relieved with this surgery.

Following a lumbar sympathectomy, the patient may experience postsympathectomy neuralgic pain of the buttocks and thighs. The pain, which usually occurs about 10 days after surgery, can be severe. Fortunately it responds well to analgesics and always abates within 3 or 4 months, or sooner.

Aneurysmal Disease

An aneurysm is an abnormal dilatation of an artery caused by a localized weakness and stretching of the arterial media. Multiple pathologic processes can be the cause of aneurysm formation. The major one is arteriosclerosis of the medial layer; thus persons of the middle and older age groups are affected. When syphilis is the cause, the spirochete invades the media and weakens the medial wall. Syphilis has been the leading cause until recent years, but with better control of syphilis, atherosclerosis is now the leading cause. With the recent increase again in venereal disease in our society, one questions if there will be an increase in the number of aneurysms resulting from syphilis. Additional predisposing factors can be a congenital defect, trauma, and necrotizing arteritis, such as periarteritis.

Aneurysms are classified according to their anatomic pathologic features. A saccular aneurysm is a segmented dilatation of only a portion of the circumference of the aorta; thus the dilatation is saclike. The fusiform aneurysm is a diffuse dilatation of a segment of the aorta resulting from destruction of the medial layer throughout the circumference of the aorta. With a dissecting aneurysm, an intramural hematoma resulting from rupture of the vasa vasorum initiates the dissection and is followed by intimal tears. The dissection may extend proximal and/or distal to the intimal tear because of blood seeping between the layers of the media.

The various types of aneurysms by location are too numerous to discuss in detail, thus only abdominal and dissecting will be presented. The clinical manifestations depend on the site and size of the aneurysm, its effect on neighboring structures and/or upon such complications as seepage of blood or rupture. Initially, with an abdominal aneurysm, it is not uncommon for patients to be aware that they have a pulsating mass in their abdomen, but not to have any associated symptoms. As the aneurysm increases in size, vital organs in the area will be compressed, thus causing abdominal or lumbar pain. If the aneurysm ruptures into the retroperitoneal cavity, it can be fatal, or a hematoma may form thus creating symptoms that cause the patient to see a physician.

A dissecting aneurysm, regardless of its location, can either be a complication of a saccular or fusiform aneurysm or can occur in a patient with no previous history of an abnormality of the aorta. The clinical manifestations are variable. The onset is usually sudden, with a severe persistent pain frequently described as tearing or ripping. The pain usually originates in the thorax and may move progressively downward to include the thighs. Often a picture of shock with a rapidly falling blood pressure is associated.

With a dissecting aneurysm, death has been known to occur in minutes or hours, or occasionally a more chronic course is pursued. Today with the newer surgical techniques of arterial reconstruction available, it is possible to save some of these patients provided a prompt diagnosis is made.

Diagnosing any aneurysm can be difficult, for frequently the physical findings are of limited value. For example, the symptoms of an abdominal aneurysm can mimic those of an abdominal emergency such as renal colic or an intestinal obstruction. The symptoms of a thoracic aneurysm can mimic a myocardial infarction.

The most common symptom of an abdominal aneurysm is abdominal pain which is either persistent or intermittent and localized in the middle or lower abdomen. The next most common complaint is lumbar pain radiating to the flank or groin. Lumber pain is due to either pressure on the lumbar nerves or a retroperitoneal hematoma as a result of aneurysmal rupture.

A very high per cent of abdominal aneurysms are palpable. Frequently the patient will complain of a throbbing mass in the area of the aneurysm. In those situations where the aneurysm cannot be palpated, an x-ray will confirm the diagnosis. X-ray's frequently will show a curvilinear shadow of calcification on one or both sides of the lumbar spinal column. Less frequently, only a soft tissue mass can be noted.

Ultrasound examination is playing an important role in determining the size of the aneurysm as well as following an increase in size over time at regular intervals. With the advent of ultrasound, arteriograms usually play a secondary role in diagnosis for two important reasons: (1) arteriography is not without risk, because of potential rupture of the aneurysm during injection of contrast media under high pressure and (2) the results can be misleading with regard to aneurysm size if clots half fill the lumen and make the aneurysm appear small on the film because the contrast media is unable to penetrate the mural thickening. In the event that surgery is contemplated, an arteriogram is beneficial in determining the exact location of the aneurysm as well as the condition of the proximal and distal vessels. Also, it is necessary to determine if the inferior mesenteric artery should happen to be a major supplier of blood to the bowel as is true with a small number of patients, because it is normal procedure to ligate the inferior mesenteric artery during surgery.

Medical treatment is limited, with the exception of treating any underlying disease entities and limiting activity in the hope of delaying rupture of the weakened aneurysm wall. To prevent rupture the patient should be instructed to avoid all activities that result in an increase in blood pressure, such as straining during defecation, lifting heavy objects, or performing strenuous activity. In those situations where the aneurysm is believed to be very thin-walled, strict bedrest may be prescribed in a supine position.

Surgical intervention would include various forms of reconstructive surgery. For an abdominal aneurysm or a dissecting aneurysm of the thoracic or abdominal aorta, excision of the aneurysm and replacement with a prosthetic graft gives the best results. The reader is referred to the section on surgical and nursing interventions with arterial problems.

Thromboangiitis Obliterans

There is controversy as to the exact description of Buerger's disease (thromboangiitis obliterans). The disease as originally described by Dr. Buerger is now believed to have been ergot poisoning. Rye contains ergot, and until recent years rye was not refined; thus there was no control on the amount of ergot present in the rye bread. Because the disease occurred predominately in Jewish males who ate large amounts of rye bread, it is apparent how they could have had ergot poisoning.

Today the most widely accepted theory is that Buerger's disease is a premature form of arteriosclerosis obliterans with an inflammatory component of the arteries. A migratory thrombophlebitis can also be present. Thromboangiitis obliterans affects the 20- to 40-year age group, whereas arteriosclerosis obliterans occurs after the age of 45 to 50 years.

The clinical manifestations of thromboangiitis obliterans are essentially the same as arteriosclerosis obliterans. The exception is that thrombophlebitis is sometimes present with thromboangiitis obliterans.

Ergot and smoking have been identified as having a positive relationship to thromboangiitis obliterans; thus smoking and the ingestion of ergot must be discontinued if the disease is to be controlled. In some cases corticosteroids in the form of prednisone may be prescribed to control the inflammation of the arteries. The remainder of the therapy would be the same as for arteriosclerosis obliterans.

From a historical point of view, Buerger or Buerger–Allen exercises will be presented. These exercises are not used routinely today; however, some physicians may still prescribe them. In these exercises gravity is used alternately to fill the arteries and drain the veins. To accomplish this the legs are alternately elevated and lowered, with a period of rest between cycles. The cycles can be timed or the color of the extremities can be used as the criterion for determining the length of time in each position. Under these circumstances the legs are kept in the down position until rubor appears and in the up position until pallor or blanching is present. The patient should rest in the horizontal position before repeating the exercise.

Acute Arterial Occlusion

Sudden occlusion of a peripheral artery usually results from either embolization or thrombosis. Emboli can consist of air, fat, bile, amniotic fluid, tumor particles, or more commonly, thrombi that have formed elsewhere in the arterial system. The largest per cent of emboli originate within the left-sided cardiac chambers. Rheumatic heart disease with mitral stenosis predisposes to the formation of mural thrombi in the hypertrophied left atrium. These thrombi can become detached and lodge as emboli elsewhere in the peripheral arteries. The same phenomenon could occur with atrial fibrillation, regardless of the cause. Most thrombi can also form in an enlarged left ventricle secondary to cardiac decompensation and with myocardial infarction.

Thrombi that form on the walls of the arteries may detach and travel as emboli to a more distal portion of the arterial circulation. These thrombi occur in association with aneurysms and atheromatous plaques or secondary to trauma and an inflammatory process of an artery.

Arterial occlusion from an embolus is a very acute situation. The embolus travels downstream to a point where it becomes lodged due to a decrease in the diameter of the artery. Typically the point of occlusion will be at a bifurcation of the artery where the branches are smaller than the parent vessel. There are bifurcations of the aorta, the common iliac, the popliteal and the femoral arteries with the femoral artery being the most common site for an embolus to lodge.

Sudden arterial thrombosis occurs most commonly at the site of an atheromatous plaque. Trauma, such as occurs from an intraarterial needle or catheter, may also be the precipitating cause.

With sudden arterial occlusion, the blood supply to distal tissues is completely obstructed unless there is good collateral circulation. At the time of occlusion, arterial spasm proximal and distal to the occlusion occurs.

The presenting symptoms of acute occlusion are pain, numbness, coldness, tingling, and paresthesia. The pain may occur abruptly at rest and may be of an excruciating nature or develop gradually over several hours. The cause of the pain has not been completely explained. It may be caused in part, or intensified, by spasm of the associated collateral vessels. Surprisingly, in some instances pain is slight or even absent in patients with major arterial embolism. A possible explanation is that the peripheral nerves are rendered functionless by the acute ischemia.

The peripheral pulses distal to the occlusion will be absent; however, if the occlusion occurs at a bifurcation, the pulse at that point will be palpable and sometimes the amplitude is greater than normal. The increased amplitude is created by the energy of the pulse wave being transmitted to the wall of the vessel at the point of occlusion. It is only when the blood coagulates above the level of the obstruction, which usually takes hours, that the pulse is lost. In addition to loss of peripheral pulses, the affected extremity will be pale and cold, which indicates severe ischemia. Usually there is a sharp line of demarcation between the ischemic and normal tissue. Within a short period of time after onset, there may be a loss of sensory as well as motor function; thus the patient may be unable to move his or her fingers or toes, depending on the location of the occlusion. The skin may become insensitive to pain and touch.

The treatment of choice is an embolectomy, thrombembolectomy, or bypass graft if the patient's condition permits surgery. Surgery should be performed while the tissues are still viable. It is not impossible for an embolectomy to be done in the patient's room under local anesthetic if time is a critical factor. Other aspects of management include anticoagulation, relief of pain and arterial spasm, and protection of the extremity.

As soon as the diagnosis of sudden occlusion has been made, the patient should be anticoagulated with heparin to prevent the extension of the thrombus even if surgery is contemplated. If surgery is not going to be performed, the patient should be switched to an oral anticoagulant.

Because of the excruciating nature of the pain in some patients, narcotics are indicated. Also, the intravenous injection of papaverine hydrochloride into the artery proximal to the occlusion will relieve the arterial spasm. Other methods of relieving the arterial spasm are to give whisky and place the patient in a warm environment.

The ischemic extremity must be protected from injury and the flow of blood augmented. The extremity should be placed in a dependent position. When the lower extremity is involved, this can be accomplished by elevating the head of the bed on blocks. The same precautions utilized to protect the ischemic extremity of a patient with arteriosclerosis obliterans would apply.

Raynaud's Disease

Raynaud's phenomenon is a primary vascular disorder characterized by episodic constriction of the small arteries and arterioles of the extremities. Raynaud's phenomenon can occur solely as Raynaud's disease or it may be in association with a variety of other diseases. When it occurs as Raynaud's disease, the population affected is almost entirely women between the ages of 20 and 40.

The exact cause of Raynaud's disease is unknown; however, it is noted that with either emotional or thermal (cold) stimuli color changes take place in the digits. The peripheral sympathetic system overreacts to cold stimuli to the digits, causing constriction of the arterioles, with slowing of arteriolar blood flow. Depending on the degree of intermittent arteriolar spasm, the blood flow can be completely or partially obstructed to the digits.

The characteristic sequential color changes of the digits associated with Raynaud's disease are pallor, cyanosis, and rubor. Pallor occurs when there is spasm of the arterioles and perhaps the venules. During this time blood is not entering the capillaries; thus the affected part has a dead white appearance. Cyanosis, on the other hand, indicates that the capillaries and perhaps the venules are unusually dilated; thus the blood flow becomes slower and more oxygen is extracted. During the cyanotic phase, the skin will have a bluish color. Rubor is a bluish-red color associated with excessive hyperemia because of reactive vasodilatation.

The clinical manifestations of Raynaud's disease are characteristic. The onset is usually very gradual, with intermittent color changes of the skin occurring in one or two digits of the hands or feet. The color changes last only for a few minutes before returning to normal. As the disease progresses, the digits of both hands and feet can become involved. The symptoms are worse in the colder months of the year.

Pain is not associated with Raynaud's disease unless it is far advanced and ulceration of the tip of a digit is present. Paresthesias such as numbness, tingling, throbbing, and dull ache, however, can be present. During an actual attack, coldness of the digits will be present, sensory acuity is decreased, and swelling of the involved digits can occur.

Before the diagnosis of Raynaud's disease can be established, all the diseases that could have secondary Raynaud's phenomenon must be ruled out. This would include, to name a few, occlusive arterial disease; collagen diseases, such as arthritis and lupus erythematosus; and neurogenic lesions, such as multiple sclerosis and ergot intoxication. Other criteria necessary for diagnosis are (1) bilateral involvement, (2) symptoms that are precipitated by cold or emotion, (3) absence of any other disease which may be causal, (4) absence of gangrene, unless limited to minimal grades of cutaneous gangrene, and (5) at least a 2-year history of symptoms (Allen, Barker, & Hines, Jr., 1962, p. 8).

Medical intervention is not terribly successful. If the episodes of symptoms are related to emotional stimuli, perhaps professional psychological counseling can be beneficial in helping the patient cope with stressful situations. Vasodilators, such as the rauwolfia derivatives, or alpha adrenergic blocking agents, such as Priscoline hydrochloride and Dibenzyline, are beneficial in relieving the symptoms caused by vasoconstriction; however, most have unpleasant side effects that limit their use.

A regional sympathectomy is helpful in relieving the symptoms of advancing Raynaud's disease. By interrupting the vasoconstricting impulses, the arterial blood flow will be improved to the digits. The results are very good for relieving symptoms of the lower extremities; however, the results are less predictable for the upper extremities.

The nurse plays a major roll in treating the patient with Raynaud's phenomena or disease, as most of the treatment is teaching the patient the necessary prophylactic measures. The two main objectives for the patient are to avoid exposure to cold and to avoid stressful environments. Clothing must be adapted to meet the body's demands for heat in relation to the environment. Warm mittens, not gloves, should be worn in cold weather. Greater warmth can be provided if silk liners are worn inside of heavy, close-woven mittens. It is important to put the mittens on before going into a cold environment because once the digits become cold, they will not become warm again without immersing them in warm water at about 90°F. Not only is it important to keep the hands and feet warm, but the total body must be kept warm, because if the body becomes cold, vasospasm can occur in the digits. An alcoholic beverage prior to going out in extremely cold weather for extended periods of time will give some vasodilatory effect. Also handwarmers are helpful.

The hands should be protected whenever they are going to come in contact with cold objects such as frozen food or a glass with an iced beverage. To go shopping in an air-conditioned supermarket can be an ordeal for the patient even in the middle of summer. Not only is it necessary to wear warm clothing, but mittens would be necessary to handle the frozen foods. Preparation of a meal can also create additional problems. Such activities as washing lettuce or fruit in cold water can precipitate vasospasm.

The episodes of vasospasm can be relieved by putting the hands in warm water, about 90°F, because the conductivity of heat is greater through water than through air. The warming brings about a reflex reduction in vasoconstriction tone with resultant vasodilatation in the hands and feet. Smoking is forbidden, as it causes vasospasm.

For some persons with Raynaud's disease, there is an emotional element present that triggers the episodes of vasospasm. If this is known to be true, the patient should be helped to identify the emotional stimuli that trigger the episodes as well as to learn how to cope.

Surgical Intervention with Arterial Problems

A variety of surgical procedures have been designed to restore blood flow through arteries. Even though the underlying pathology can vary greatly, the operative procedures, especially for occlusive disorders, are essentially the same. Such factors as the nature of the involvement and the extent and site of the pathology are used to determine the surgery of choice.

THROMBOENDARTERECTOMY. An incision is made into the obstructed artery, and the thrombus, intima, any atheromatous plaques, the internal elastic lamina, and the inner part of the tunica media are removed.

EMBOLECTOMY. Surgical removal of an embolus lodged in an artery is called an embolectomy. An incision is made into the artery, and the embolus is surgically removed.

END-TO-END ANASTOMOSIS. The diseased portion of an artery or a severed artery is repaired, with direct anastomosis of the two remaining segments of the artery.

AUTOGENOUS VEIN GRAFT. The diseased portion of an artery is excised, and a vein graft is used to reconstruct the artery. A section of the long saphenous vein is dissected usually from the groin and used as the graft. At the time of insertion, the vein must be reversed so the valves do not obstruct arterial flow.

PROSTHETIC GRAFT REPLACEMENT. The diseased portion of the artery is resected and replaced with a dacron prosthetic graft.

BYPASS GRAFT. The diseased segment of the artery is not resected, but instead a prosthetic graft is inserted to bypass this section. The prosthetic graft is anastomosed to the side of the artery proximal and distal to the obstruction. The advantage of this surgery is the preservation of the existing collateral circulation. Thus if the graft should become thrombosed at a later date, there would be some arterial circulation to the limb.

Nursing Intervention Following Arterial Surgery

At this point the general postoperative management of the patient will not be discussed. Only those aspects of nursing care that are pertinent to vascular surgery will be presented. The following points will apply to patients who have any type of reconstruction surgery.

Adequate perfusion of a revascularized part is of utmost importance. The peripheral pulses are used as a parameter to detect any change in perfusion; thus pulses distal to the surgical site should be checked at prescribed intervals. Immediately following surgery, the location of the pulses should be marked on the patient's skin, for sometimes they are found in an aberrant location. It should be noted that for a period of a few hours after the procedure, the peripheral pulses may be distant or absent in some patients because of vasospasm or trapped air bubbles that leaked through the suture line before closure. If, however, the pulses have been present and suddenly they cannot be palpated, the surgeon should be notified immediately, for this could be the first sign of thrombosis. Today sophisticated electronic devices are used to increase the accuracy in monitoring the arterial pulsations. A popular detection method is ultrasonography with a Doppler-effect flow meter. A Doppler probe is applied to the skin over a superficial artery. This will record the presence of the pulse but tells nothing about the quality of the pulse.

Other clinical signs that could be indicative of a thrombus formation would be changes in the color and temperature of the extremity. When making observations regarding the status of arterial perfusion, the unaffected extremity should always be compared with the extremity that has had the reconstruction surgery. Sometimes the extremity that had the surgery will be warmer than the unaffected one because of hyperemia, or both extremities may feel cold if a vasopressor has been utilized. If, however, the combined signs of pallor, increased coldness distal to the site of surgery, and decreased pulses occur, a thrombus may be present and the surgeon should be notified immediately.

Some surgeons may use vasopressors following reconstructive surgery with a prosthetic graft to maintain the blood pressure approximately 20 mm Hg above the individual's normal level. The rationale is to keep the suture line taut as a means to prevent blood leakage and the accumulation of an irregular lining of fibrin that predisposes to thrombus formation.

Positioning of the patient following reconstructive surgery will vary, depending on the degree of revascularization and the location of the prosthetic graft. At times the patient will be placed in reverse Trendelenburg position for 24 hours to increase arterial flow. Conversely, sometimes it is necessary to elevate the revascularized part to decrease edema formation. Marked engorgement of the previously ischemic vascular bed can result when the influx of arterial blood exceeds the venous system's capacity to drain it. The resultant edema and stasis of the capillary bed would further impede arterial flow.

If the prosthetic graft is in the abdominal or thoracic cavity, there are no specific limitations regarding position in bed or sitting. If, however, the graft crosses a flexion point such as the groin or popliteal space, the patient is not permitted to flex that specific part for a period of approximately 10 days. Flexion would cause kinking, turbulence, and a subsequent decrease in blood flow velocity.

Revascularized parts need to be protected from injury as the poorly vascularized tissue of the distal extremity is prone to breakdown and ulceration. Also, these extremities may have blister formation resulting from pregangrenous changes of the tissue that could become infected.

Patients undergoing major vascular surgery need to have the urinary output monitored closely as there will be a rapid readjustment in the size of the vascular bed. The hourly urine output is used as a parameter to determine the rate of fluid replacement. Also, if the aorta has been clamped or resected above the level of the renal arteries, the resultant ischemia could potentially cause a decrease in the output because of renal failure.

The urinary output should not be less than 30 cc per hour for any two consecutive hours. Also specific gravity should be monitored because if the patient becomes hypovolemic, the kidney in an attempt to conserve sodium and water will put out small volumes of urine that are concentrated.

The hemodynamic status of the patient needs to be monitored closely by observing the vital signs, central venous pressure (CVP), pulmonary artery pressure (PAP) and the pulmonary artery wedge pressure (PAWP). In addition daily weights with either a portable or bed scale are important to determine any overload of fluids.

Atherosclerosis is always going to be present with the diagnosis of an abdominal aneurysm, thus complications such as myocardial infarction and cerebral vascular accident will more readily occur in these patients. The electrocardiogram needs to be monitored carefully for any signs of myocardial ischemia which could result from prolonged hypotension. Electocardiographic changes consistent with myocardial ischemia are premature ventricular contractions, inverted T waves, or ST segment depression or elevation. A neurological assessment is done frequently since the potential for a cerebral vascular accident is present. This includes pupil size and response to light; ability to move all extremities; quality of hand grasps; and orientation to time, place, and person (see Chapter 36).

As with any major abdominal surgery, respiratory complications can readily occur if preventive measures are not undertaken. These measures would include daily chest x-rays, chest physiotherapy, cough and deep breathing, and nasotracheal suctioning. Chest auscultation is done to identify adventitious sounds such as rales. According to Long (1978), many patients with abdominal aneurysms develop "wet lung" syndrome 24 to 48 hours postoperatively. It apparently results from an inflammatory response to the massive resection and a large amount of fluid accumulates in the retroperitoneal space. Consequently, the fluid leaks into the interstitial spaces of the lung. Usually this complication can be prevented by the use of a diuretic such as furosemide (Lasix).

HYPERTENSION

Despite differences in the pressure of the blood in various parts of the vascular system, there is a normal range of pressure for each part. Of particular importance to maintenance of the transportation system is regulation of the arterial and pulmonary blood pressures within physiologic limits. Persistent elevation of the pressures predisposes the vascular channels to pathologic changes that alter the quantity of blood flow to dependent tissues, and predisposes the heart to failure as the ultimate power source of transport.

Arterial Blood Pressure

The arterial blood pressure is the product of cardiac output and the peripheral vascular resistance. The blood pressure is measured in two general phases. The measure of the force with which the left ventricle ejects blood into the aorta is the *systolic pressure* and represents pressure at its highest in the arterial system. The measure of the force of the blood in the arterial system when the left ventricle and the vascular channels are relaxing is the *diastolic pressure* and represents pressure at its lowest level.

The reader will recall that the cardiac output is the product of the stroke volume and the heart rate and that the stroke volume is the amount of blood ejected into the aorta per left ventricular contraction. Thus, any factor that influences the stroke volume and hence the cardiac output affects the systolic blood pressure. Whereas the systolic pressure is a valuable source of information about the force of left ventricular contraction, it must be remembered that the pressure also is affected by the distensibility of the aorta and major vessels into which the stroke volume is ejected, the blood viscosity, and the total blood volume. The diastolic blood pressure is influenced by the peripheral vascular resistance, which represents the status of the peripheral vessels.

The *mean arterial pressure* is the average pressure required to propel the blood through the arterial system. The mean pressure, however, is not just the simple average of the systolic and the diastolic pressures. The mean arterial pressure is determined by application of the formula:

$$\text{Mean arterial pressure} = \underset{\text{pressure (D)}}{\text{Diastolic}} + \frac{\underset{\text{(S)}}{\text{Systolic pressure}} - \underset{\text{(D)}}{\text{Diastolic pressure}}}{3}$$

or, expressed in other terms;

$$\text{MAP} = \text{D} + \tfrac{1}{3} \text{ of the Pulse pressure } (\Delta\text{P})$$

Thus, if an individual has a systolic pressure of 120 mm Hg and a diastolic pressure of 80 mm Hg, the mean arterial pressure is

$$80 + \frac{120 - 80}{3} \approx 93 \text{ mm Hg}$$

The mean arterial pressure generally has replaced the diastolic pressure as the indicator of the status of the vascular system and subsequent morbidity.

As with other homeostatic mechanisms, the blood pressure is not regulated at an exact level but fluctuates within limits. Blood pressure varies among individuals as well as in the same person under different internal and external conditions. The limits of normality are determined by many factors, including the age of the individual, the condition of the peripheral vessels, the activity of the autonomic nervous system, the activity of the kidneys, the influence of various hormones, and various other factors. Each of these will be examined in relation to the factor's contribution to regulation of the blood pressure and to pathogenesis.

Age

Age is a significant factor in the level of the arterial blood pressure. It rises gradually from birth to maturity, and in many persons it continues to rise throughout the life span. In the healthy newborn infant the arterial blood pressure is approximately 56 mm Hg systolic and 40 mm Hg diastolic. Blood pressure rises rapidly during the first few days of life, and by the tenth day the systolic pressure is around 78 mm Hg. Blood pressure then rises gradually until puberty, with an average pressure of 120/80 mm Hg attained. The normal range of arterial pressure for persons up to the age of 50 years is generally accepted as 90 to 140 mm Hg for the systolic pressure, and 60 to 90 mm Hg for the diastolic.

Despite more or less general agreement as to the physiologic range for arterial blood pressure for persons under 50 years of age, there is little agreement as to the exact levels above which the arterial pressure is considered clinically abnormal. People vary greatly in the capacity of their blood vessels to tolerate pressures above established "normal" limits. Further, the age of the individual at which an elevation occurs is also of significance. For example, a blood pressure of 160/100 mm Hg is more significant in a girl 15 years old than in a woman of 60 years.

Another factor which makes the upper limit of "normal" difficult to determine is that the arterial blood pressure tends to continue to rise over the entire life span in many persons. With progressive age the systolic pressure is commonly 160 to 170 mm Hg. This increase is thought to represent decreased distensibility of the aorta and major arteries associated with the effects of aging. Some clinicians feel that because this is an expected aging phenomenon, systolic pressures of 160 to 170 mm Hg should be considered normal for this age group. Other clinicians, however, purport that the increased aortic rigidity is due to elements of the atherosclerotic process, and because this represents pathology, the systolic pressure increase should be considered systolic hypertension. Friedberg (1966) espouses the philosophy that a progressive rise in either the systolic or diastolic pressure with increasing age is not a "normal" circumstance inasmuch as a substantial number of aged persons maintain a relatively unchanged, normal pressure from earlier years.

There is agreement, however, that the higher the systolic or diastolic pressure, the higher the morbidity and mortality. There is a distinct quantitative relationship between these factors in many population studies. These statistics have predictive value when applied to a population for morbidity–mortality purposes but are of less value in anticipating the effect of blood pressure elevation on a specific individual. Some persons live to an advanced age despite a considerable elevation in arterial pressure. One of the medical endeavors deserving of considerable attention is the development of assessment tools that can predict which patients with hypertension are most likely to develop progressive vascular disease.

The lower limit of normal for the systolic pressure is as difficult to define as the upper. Unlike the individual whose systolic pressure is above the "normal" limit, the healthy person whose systolic pressure is below the accepted normal limits has a better than average life expectancy. A systolic pressure of 90 to 100 mm Hg in the absence of disease is usually not regarded as pathologic. In a sick patient, however, a lowered systolic blood pressure should be questioned and the responsible factors sought. The level at which blood pressure becomes abnormally low depends on the individual's normal pressure. Generally, hypotension is considered present in an adult if (1) the systolic pressure falls below 80 mm Hg or (2) the systolic pressure falls more than 40 mm Hg below the individual's normal resting systolic pressure. Thus if an individual's resting blood pressure is 180/110, a sudden fall to 130/70 is probably indicative of some degree of hypotension, although this blood pressure value falls within the normal range for a healthy individual.

Peripheral Vascular Resistance

Previously, it was noted that maintenance of a normal peripheral vascular resistance (PVR) involves the autonomic nervous system's ability to regulate the tone of the vascular musculature and the physiologic capacity of the vessels to respond to the autonomic stimulation. As long as the degree of stimulation and the responsiveness of the blood vessels are within physiologic limits, the PVR and the diastolic blood pressure should be within the normal range. It was also noted that even a small decrease in the diameter of arterioles results in a marked elevation of the PVR. As arteriolar resistance increases, the diastolic pressure rises, reflecting the inability of the arteriolar smooth muscle to relax. Usually, but not invariably, the systolic pressure also rises. Conversely, a loss of tone in any part of the peripheral vascular bed predisposes to a drop in the blood pressure.

The maintenance of blood pressure within physiologic limits requires that a number of mechanisms are regulated not only individually but also in relation to each other. Blood pressure remains stable as long as alterations in one or more mechanisms are effectively opposed by changes in other regulatory mechanisms. This blood pressure regulatory relationship is best exemplified by the interaction of the PVR and the cardiac output.

A reduction in the cardiac output will not result in a fall in the mean arterial blood pressure if, at the same time, the PVR increases. This phenomenon is exemplified in the intermediate states of hemorrhagic shock in which cardiac output falls because of blood volume loss and hence a decrease in the systolic pressure. As a compensatory mechanism, the sympathetic nervous system exerts regulatory control and increases the PVR; thus, an essentially unchanged mean arterial pressure is maintained. If, on the other hand, the cardiac output falls but the PVR remains unchanged, as in the initial stages of hemorrhagic shock, the mean arterial pressure falls.

Conversely, if the cardiac output increases and the PVR decreases, the mean arterial pressure can remain stable. This phenomenon may be exemplified during treatment of shock with use of volume expanders and vasodilators. If the cardiac output increases but the PVR remains the same, as in volume overload, the mean arterial pressure increases.

If both the cardiac output and the PVR diminish, as occurs in the later stages of shock, the mean arterial pressure falls. If both the cardiac output and the PVR increases, as occurs in some hypertensive states, the mean arterial pressure rises. As can be noted, multiple combinations of mechanisms are possible.

Among the factors affecting arterial blood pressure, changes in the PVR have the most profound effect. Relatively large changes are required in the blood volume, blood viscosity, or arterial elasticity before the mean blood pressure level is altered appreciably.

Autonomic Nervous System

The autonomic nervous system, principally the sympathetic nervous system, regulates the smooth muscle of arterioles, causing either vasoconstriction or vasodilatation. When impulses are transmitted along sympathetic nerves, norepinephrine is released from specialized structures in the nerve endings. Norepinephrine acts on specialized groups of cells (receptors) which are located in the blood vessel walls. Receptor stimulation effects a change in the diameter of the arteriole and thus the PVR.

Two types of receptors have been identified that are sensitive to norepinephrine stimulation. They are the alpha and beta receptors. It is felt that virtually all organs and structures innervated by the sympathetic nervous system possess alpha and beta receptors, although one or the other receptor type tends to predominate. If alpha receptors are stimulated, the response is different in various organs. The same is true if beta receptors are stimulated. For example, beta receptors predominate in cardiac tissue. When the sympathetic nervous system exerts greater control over the organism, norepinephrine stimulates the beta receptors in the heart, with a resultant increase in the heart rate.

The response of blood vessels to norepinephrine stimulation differs in the various parts of the body, depending on the predominant receptor. For example, the blood vessels of the skin and mucous membranes have a predominance of alpha receptors that effect vasoconstriction when stimulated and thus contribute to an increase in the PVR. In contrast, the blood vessels of the skeletal muscles have a predominance of beta receptors that effect vasodilatation when stimulated by norepinephrine and thus contribute to a decrease in the PVR. This variation in the response of blood vessels to sympathetic nervous system stimulation enables the body to shift blood from one region to another. Depending on the degree of sympathetic nervous system stimulation and norepinephrine release as well as the responsiveness of the vessels, the *sum* effect may be an increased, decreased, or normal PVR. Overactivity of the sympathetic nervous system and excessive systemic norepinephrine are implicated in some forms of hypertension.

Regulation of the caliber of blood vessels also is accomplished by higher nervous centers that initiate various circulatory reflexes. Centers for the regulation of circulatory reflexes are located in the medulla. The circulatory reflexes include the (1) pressoreceptor (baroreceptor, mechanoreceptor) reflex; (2) chemoreceptor reflex; and (3) medullary ischemic (CNS ischemic) reflex. Each of these reflexes is initiated by different levels of the mean arterial pressure which stimulates receptors located in the arch of the aorta and carotid arteries. Once stimulated, the aortic and carotid recceptors relay impulses to the medulla, which in turn conveys impulses to the blood vessels via the autonomic nervous system to effect constriction or dilatation and thus influence the PVR.

Other centers for the regulation of blood vessel diameter are located in the cerebral cortex and hypothalamus. Stimulation of visual, auditory, thermal, tactile, and pain receptors also effect changes in the PVR. Alterations in the PVR and blood pressure are also effected by biochemical changes, such as an altered pH of body fluids, and emotional reactions, which serve as stimuli to the sympathetic nervous system. An increase in the activity of the sympathetic nervous system has been implicated as a factor in the pathogenesis of hypertension.

Activity of the Kidney

Years of concentrated research have demonstrated that the kidney has one or more roles in the regulation of the blood pressure. Whereas much has been learned about the relationship between renal activity and blood pressure, some aspects of the specific mechanisms required further documentation. Questions such as whether the kidney autoregulates blood flow through the renal vasculature are subjects of great interest and controversy. The fact that there is some relationship between decreased blood flow through the kidney and an increased arterial pressure has been established clinically and experimentally.

The classic experiment of Goldblatt in 1934 demonstrated that degrees of renal artery obstruction through the dog kidney are followed by an elevation in the arterial blood pressure. Clinically, the same elevation in blood pressure is noted in diseases where there is a diminished flow of blood through the kidney, such as in atherosclerosis of the renal artery, acute glomerulonephritis, and chronic pyelonephritis.

It has been demonstrated that the kidney affects blood pressure in three major ways: (1) when the arterial pressure increases, the urinary output of both water and sodium increases markedly, thus regulating body fluid volume, cardiac output, and effecting maintenance of a normal blood pressure; (2) under ischemic conditions the renal juxtaglomerular apparatus releases a proteolytic enzyme (renin) that acts on a plasma protein (alpha-2-globulin) ultimately to form a highly active vasoconstrictor substance (angiotensin II); and (3) the healthy kidney secretes an unsaturated fatty acid vasodilator substance (prostaglandin E) that supports normotension.

Additional aspects of the role of the kidney in blood pressure regulation and the involved mechanisms are under continuous investigation. Examples include (1) the role of a vasodilator peptide (bradykinin) that is produced in the kidney on blood pressure regulation; and (2) the role of a renal tissue enzyme (kallikrein) on blood pressure regulation.

Hormonal Influence

The adrenal medullary hormones, epinephrine and norepinephrine, enhance the activity of the sympathetic nervous system. In addition to the norepinephrine secreted by sympathetic nerves, additional stores are liberated by the adrenal medulla during stress. Epinephrine is also secreted, which exerts a vasoconstrictor effect locally and increases the strength of cardiac contraction (inotropic effect). Both hormones lead to an elevation in blood pressure through actions on the PVR and cardiac output. These hormones probably have little effect on the blood pressure during ordinary activity but augment the effect of the sympathetic nervous system during stress.

The major hormone influencing the blood pressure is aldosterone, a mineral-corticoid produced and secreted by the adrenal cortex. The stimuli that effect release of aldosterone are (1) an increased plasma level of angiotensin II, (2) an increased fluid volume in the extracellular compartment, (3) a decreased sodium concentration in the extracellular compartment, and (4) an increased potassium concentration or ACTH secretion. Once liberated, aldosterone acts on the distal tubules of the kidney to effect sodium reabsorption in the extracellular fluid compartment and potassium excretion. In turn, there is release of the antidiuretic hormone from the posterior pituitary, which increases water reabsorption from the tubules to the extracellular compartment. With an increase in the hydrostatic pressure of the interstitial fluid compartment, fluid moves into the blood. The result is an increased blood volume causing the blood pressure to rise. Excessive aldosterone secretion has been documented as a precursor to at least one type of hypertension. (See Chapter 27 for regulatory effects of the kidney.)

Other Factors

Other factors that affect the level of the arterial blood pressure are the position of the individual, emotional state, exercise, pain, distended bladder, and the capillary fluid shift mechanism, to name but a few. The effects of position on the blood pressure will be discussed under the general assessment process. Because of sympathetic nervous system activity, the blood pressure is usually elevated when the person experiences anxiety, exercise, a distended bladder, and initially, pain. Parasympathetic activity promotes a lower blood pressure in the later stages of pain and with sleep.

Within limits, the capillary fluid shift mechanism protects the blood volume and blood pressure by rapidly removing or adding fluid to the blood. When the arterial blood volume rapidly rises, capillary hydrostatic pressure is elevated and fluid rapidly moves into the interstitial spaces, thus preventing the blood pressure from rising excessively. The reverse process may also take place. Although this mechanism is important in the protection of the individual against the effects of rapid changes in the arterial blood volume, it also can be a source of danger. In the seriously burned patient, loss of fluid into the interstitial spaces may be sufficient to cause hypotension. In some individuals a marked increase in blood volume associated with renal insufficiency leads to pulmonary edema and death. A rapid increase in blood volume also places an added strain on the pathologic heart and predisposes to cardiac failure.

Arterial Hypertension

When the level of the arterial blood pressure exceeds physiologic limits, the condition is referred to as *hypertension* or *arterial hypertension.* Whereas the World Health Organization has defined hypertension as a blood pressure of 160/95 mm Hg or greater, generally clinicians consider a pressure that exceeds 140/90 mm Hg as elevated in adults under the age of 50 years.

Depending on which component is elevated, the terms *systolic* or *diastolic hypertension* are employed, and if both components are elevated, it is called *systolic–diastolic hypertension.* Precision has succumbed to expediency in many instances, and medical personnel utilize the generic term *hypertension* more frequently.

Hypertension is not a disease per se, but rather a symptom associated with an abnormality of function and/or structure. Some clinicians employ the terms *hypertension* to denote the elevation of blood pressure in the absence of demonstrable vascular changes and *hypertensive disease* to indicate the presence of vascular disease. When the heart is involved in pathology as a consequence of the hypertensive process, the term *hypertensive cardiovascular disease* (HCVD) is utilized.

In approximately 90 per cent of individuals with hypertension, the cause is not known and the disorder is classified as primary, idiopathic, or essential hypertension. In the other 10 per cent of persons with hypertension, the elevation of the blood pressure is secondary to some known disorder. These disorders are classified as secondary hypertension.

A schema for the classification of the types of hypertension, which includes some of the disorders known to cause hypertension, is as follows:

1. Primary (essential) hypertension
   - Diastolic hypertension
2. Secondary hypertension
   a. Systolic hypertension
      (1) Increased cardiac output
      (2) Decreased aortic distensibility
   b. Diastolic–systolic hypertension
      (1) Disorders of the kidney
         (a) glomerulonephritis
         (b) pyelonephritis
         (c) renal artery atherosclerosis
         (d) polycystic kidney
         (e) renal tumors
      (2) Disorders of the adrenal gland
         (a) adrenal cortex overactivity
            - Cushing's syndrome (hydrocortisone-corticosterone overproduction)
            - Conn's syndrome (aldesterone overproduction)
         (b) adrenal medulla overactivity
            - pheochromocytoma (epinephrine-norepinephrine overproduction)
      (3) Disorders of the central nervous system
         - Increased intracranial pressure from cardiovascular accident or tumor
      (4) Disorders of the great vessels
         - Coarctation of the aorta
      (5) Toxemia of pregnancy
      (6) Drug-induced
         (a) birth control pills
         (b) amphetamines
         (c) chronic licorice ingestion
         (d) chronic use of steroid preparations
         (e) monoamine oxidase inhibitors and specific types of cheeses

Theories and Epidemiology

Investigations of the etiology of primary hypertension have been extensive, complex, and multivariable. In the vast majority of studies, the common pathophysiologic feature is an increased PVR although the definitive components of the mechanism by which this occurs is still elusive. The following is an attempt at summarization of the various theories pertinent to the etiology of essential hypertension:

1. *Hypertension results from an altered balance in the renin-angiotension-aldosterone enzymatic hormonal system.* This theory focuses on the secretion of the enzyme renin by the kidney, which catalyzes and effects an elevated plasma level of angiotensin II. Elevation of the blood pressure occurs because of angiotensin's direct vasoconstrictor effect on arterioles and by stimulation of aldosterone release with ultimately results in an expanded blood volume and increased cardiac output from sodium and water overload. It must be noted, however, that about one fourth of the hypertensive populace have diminished renin-angiotensin plasma levels. It is suggested that the hypertension may be related to an excess of mineralocorticoids other than aldosterone. Perhaps what is most clear is that the problem is increasingly complex and appears to involve several variables, and that only continued research will resolve the apparent disparities in theory.
2. *Hypertension results from genetic factors in combination with learned behaviors.* Animal studies suggest that there are certain strains of rats that are more "sensitive" to high-salt diets than others. This finding suggests the possibility of an operant genetic factor in hypertension. Anthropologic and nutritional studies have demonstrated that in several cultures where salt intake is consistently high, hypertension develops at ages earlier than in those cultures where there are low intakes of salt. This theory would then appear to be related to the next.
3. *Hypertension results from chronic sodium and water retention.* This theory focuses on the inability of the kidney to excrete sodium and water normally. The reasons for this condition are multivariable and include primary renal disease, potential genetic factors, and excessive salt intake. The end result is an expanded blood volume, increased

cardiac output and peripheral vascular resistance, and an elevated blood pressure.

4. *Hypertension results from excessive sympathetic nervous system activity.* This theory focuses on the psychologic-environmental contributions of stress to the physiologic release of excessive amounts of epinephrine and norepinephrine. In addition to the direct vasoconstrictor effects of these circulating catecholamines, norepinephrine effects the release of renin and activates the renin-angiotensin-aldosterone system.
5. *Hypertension results from insufficient renal production of vasodilatory substances.* This theory purports that the normal renal production of prostaglandin E (previously called "a vasodepressor substance") is suppressed and hence the development of hypertension.
6. *Hypertension results from some or all of the above factors.* The complexity of the etiologic picture of essential hypertension is evident. Although a single definitive otiologic factor has not been isolated, the common element among all theories is that a biochemical factor plays an important role in the development of hypertension.

Although the specific etiology(ies) are elusive, epidemiologic studies have identified certain factors that appear to predispose an individual to hypertension. The incidence of hypertension increases with age. Although uncommon before the age of 20, as much as 25 to 40 per cent of the population beyond age 50 are affected. Hypertension is slightly more common in females than in males and increases considerably after menopause. Hypertensive cardiovascular disease is more common in the male, although this may also be related to the increased incidence of atherosclerotic disease. The incidence of hypertension is greater in the black population than in the white population and frequently is more severe, although this may be due in part to the inaccessibility of health care for a variety of reasons. There is suggestive evidence of a familial tendency toward hypertension, and the incidence is greater among those who are obese.

Despite a readiness to link hypertension to urbanization and the stressors of society, definitive causal relationships have not been made. Although there is little scientific evidence to substantiate psychological disturbances as the etiologic factor in hypertension, there is documentation that elevated blood pressures occur following repeated powerful emotional experiences in many people, and existing hypertension may become more severe with environmental and emotional stress. Some characteristics that have been noted with hypertensive patients are suppressed hostility, increased dependency needs, overanxiousness, excessive rigidity, and sensitiveness. It should be noted, however, that these personality characteristics are found also in normotensive people and not all hypertensive patients manifest these traits.

General Assessment of the Patient with Hypertension

Regardless of the type of arterial hypertension, certain pathophysiologic changes are common to all forms. For this reason the general assessment of the hypertensive patient will be considered prior to discussion of the specific types. Manifestations specific to particular types of hypertension will be discussed at that time.

The clinical manifestations of hypertension are usually secondary to the effects of the elevated pressure on blood vessels in the various organs and tissues, and to the increased workload to which the heart is subjected. The consequences to the tissues are determined by the level at which the blood pressure is sustained. It has been demonstrated that with high sustained systemic pressures, the medial layer of arterioles undergoes hypertrophy and sclerosis, and thus perfusion diminishes. This initiates responses that call for an even greater increase in blood pressure in the attempt to maintain perfusion. In the heart the vascular sclerosis of the coronary arteries impairs the blood supply to the myocardial muscle, which makes the increased workload imposed by the hypertension less tolerable, and heart failure ensues. The progressive deterioration of the cerebral vessels predisposes to rupture and death from cerebral hemorrhage.

Common cerebral symptoms of hypertension are headache and a giddiness that is short of true vertigo. The headache typically occurs in the early morning affecting the occipital region with neck stiffness. It may be present only on the mornings when the individual sleeps late and may be relieved by vomiting. The mechanism of this typical headache is unexplained. With severe hypertension, personality changes may occur secondary to the vascular changes. Hypertensive encephalopathy and cerebrovascular accidents also may occur.

The hypertensive patient may experience shortness of breath, particularly on exertion, and chest pain. Presumably these are due to changes in the physical properties of the lungs and coronary arteries. Myocardial infarction or heart failure may occur without warning.

The peripheral arteries may become partially occluded or conspicuously tortuous. Common sites for tortuosity are the carotid, brachial, and radial arteries. Bleeding occurs from unexpected sites when the arterial pressure becomes excessively high. Spontaneous epistaxis and hemospermia are not uncommon. In addition to the vascular changes already mentioned, involvement of the blood vessels in the legs is noted by intermittent claudication. Nocturnal frequency is noted because of the hypertension and is not related to any underlying renal disorder. Longstanding hypertension with renovascular changes leads ultimately to renal failure and uremia.

Vascular changes of the retina are common and early occurrences. Frequently the individual has blurring of vision or scotoma initially and seeks an eyeglass prescription change. The eye examiner notes tortuosity of vessels, retinal exudates, hemorrhages, or venous thrombosis and refers the individual to an internist for further diagnosis and treatment.

Blood Pressure Measurement

The accurate determination of the arterial blood pressure is critical in the evaluation of hypertension inasmuch as with the onset of uncomplicated cases of essential hypertension, the individual is asymptomatic, hence, the term "the silent killer." Individuals can have hypertension for years before it is suspected as a result of a casual blood pressure reading. Whereas a blood pressure measurement may appear to be a technically simplistic procedure, it may be beset with error. Common errors in measurement can be avoided by overt attention to technique and knowledge of measurement error factors. A summary of the common sources of measurement error and the direction of error includes the following:

1. Blood pressures taken in the arm are lower when the individual is in a standing position. If, however, the individual sits, but is not seated for at least 5 minutes, the reading may be higher. Unless one is checking for postural hypotension, a 5-minute period is desirable between readings with position changes.
2. When a standard-size cuff is used for thigh measurements or for individuals with obese arms, the reading is falsely high.
3. When a standard-size cuff is used for individuals with thin arms, the reading is falsely low.
4. A cuff that is loosely applied produces false high readings.
5. If measurements are taken with the individual in a lateral position, a lower pressure reading may be obtained in both arms. This phenomenon is most apparent in the right arm when the patient is in a left lateral recumbent position (Foley, 1971).
6. If the arm is above the level of the heart, the reading is falsely low. The converse is also true.
7. If the sphygmomanometer is not at eye level the reading will be falsely high or low, respectively.
8. Some health professionals record the diastolic pressure as phase IV of the Korotkoff sounds, and others use phase V without indication of which phase is being reported. Until complete standardization is effected, both should be recorded, for example, 120/82/74.
9. If a pressure cuff remains inflated for a period of time before deflation, a higher reading is obtained.
10. Blood pressure readings may not be the same in two like extremities. The higher of the two readings and the extremity used should be recorded.
11. Pressures obtained by palpation are lower, by approximately 5 mm Hg, than those obtained by the auscultatory method.
12. Very fast, very slow, and irregular heart rates cause a lower reading. A series of readings should be taken.
13. During sleep the blood pressure may be as much as 20 mm Hg lower than during a resting, waking measurement.
14. A noisy, cold, or stressful environment, or painful stimuli may lead to rise in pressure of from 10 to 30 mm Hg.
15. Blood pressure may be increased following ingestion of a large meal.

Casual blood pressure measurements are to be avoided. These are single recordings that are taken without regard to the time of day and environmental factors and without special preparation of the patient. Provision should be made for serial and follow-up measurements through repeated visits or referrals. *Basal blood pressure measurements* are usually the lowest readings obtained in a 24-hour period; they are taken as soon as the individual awakens and may have diagnostic and prognostic significance.

A marked or continuing rise or fall in blood pressure generally should be regarded as abnormal, and the causative factors should be investigated. Measures then should be initiated to lower, stabilize, or elevate the pressure. It must be noted that any one causal blood pressure reading may not be significant in the total picture. Among the factors to be considered in evaluating the significance of one blood pressure reading are knowledge of the pressure level compatible with sufficient tissue perfusion, the extent of the pressure that arteries are likely to tolerate, and the usual blood pressure of the patient.

What is significant is a trend or pattern that is established with successive hourly or daily measurements. Evaluation for a trend or pattern, however, is difficult in many agencies today. This occurs because blood pressure readings are scattered throughout a patient's thick chart, and the conditions under which the measurements were taken are not recorded. The time, position of the patient, activity of the patient prior to measurement, arm used, and other pertinent factors should be recorded. A "flow chart" or summary sheet, as used in many intensive-care unit settings, is particularly helpful to facilitate evaluation of serial blood pressures.

Diagnostic Tests

In addition to the clinical history, physical assessment, and serial blood pressure measurements under various conditions, many other studies can be done to investigate the etiology of hypertension secondary to renal or adrenal dysfunction. Tests for hypertension secondary to renal dysfunction include routine urinalysis, creatinine clearance studies, 24-hour urine studies for protein and electrolytes, intravenous urogram, radioactive isotope renal scan, blood urea nitrogen and electrolytes, differential renal vein renin determinations, and renal angiography. Tests for adrenocortical dysfunction include 24-hour urine studies for 17-hydroxysteroids, 17-ketosteroids, aldosterone, and/or electrolytes; blood studies for electrolytes, and plasma cortisol, renin, and angiotensin; and an adrenal scan. Tests specific for hypertension related to adrenal medullary dysfunction are 24-hour and single specimen urine studies for catecholamines, normetanephrine, metanephrine, and vanillylmandelic acid. Rarely used now are the histamine and regitine tests because of their dangerous side effects.

Essential Hypertension

By far the most frequent type of arterial hypertension in the United States is essential hypertension for which there is no definitive cause. The American Heart Association reported that an estimated 34 million Americans have hypertension (1979, p. 10). Of that number, 90 per cent have essential hypertension. Whereas 21 to 22 per cent of white females and white males have hypertension, the percentages for black males and black females are 31 and 32 per cent, respectively. Each year the number of Americans reported with hypertension increases. This is probably due to increased screening and case-finding methods rather than a marked increase in hypertensive pathology.

Despite an elevation of the diastolic pressure and usually, though not always, the systolic pressure, the specific cause of essential hypertension is not known. The predominant feature is arteriolar constriction with an increased PVR. In the past, some authorities believed that the elevation of the blood pressure followed rather than preceded the vascular damage. It has been noted, however, that an elevated arterial pressure causes vascular injury; thus it is more generally believed that vascular sclerosis follows the hypertensive state. Whatever the sequence of events, arteriosclerosis and atherosclerosis develop at an earlier age in hypertensive than in nonhypertensive persons.

In the past, hypertension had been described categorically in terms of phases or stages, such as prehypertension, labile, benign, and malignant. This phasing was not to imply that all persons went through all phases or progressed from one to another. The categories have changed somewhat—labile, sustained, and malignant—and usage of the terms has diminished. For educational purposes, however, the phases are useful because they indicate that the development of hypertensive pathology is on a continuum.

For example, in the *prehypertensive phase,* the arterial blood pressure is within the normal range most of the time, although it may be in the "upper normal" range. The prehypertensive individual differs from the normotensive person by hyperreaction to stimuli with a greater or more sustained rise in the arterial pressure. The type of test previously used to check for this phenomenon was the *cold pressor test* whereby after a resting blood pressure, the subject's arm was plunged into a container of ice and blood pressure taken again. The degree of blood pressure elevation was used as a quasi-predictor of those who would become hypertensive. In current practice, rather than ice water, the clinical history is used with particular focus on those cardiovascular risk factors that bear a positive relationship to hypertension, such as age, sex, race, family history, obesity, alcohol consumption, physical exercise, reactions to and coping mechanism with stress, cigarette consumption, and dietary patterns. A case could be built for potential "prehypertension" if all the aforementioned risk factors were positive.

In *labile hypertension* the blood pressure is subject to fluctuation. During periods of stress the blood pressure may be elevated, but when the individual is relaxed or at rest, it may be near or at normal levels. It is not at all unusual for the patient to be admitted to the hospital with a blood pressure of 180/110 or greater and after a period of rest to find that normotension occurs. Lability is important because permanent hypertension develops more frequently than in an individual whose blood vessels do not overrespond. Persons who are in this phase of hypertension may delay the development of hypertensive complications by changes in their habits of living and reduction of risk factors. Drug therapy is, however, more often than not a requisite adjunct, particularly with quasi- or noncompliant patients.

Labile hypertension eventually becomes permanent or sustained. The term, *benign hypertension* has generally given way to *sustained hypertension* which is more accurate and descriptive. "Benign" is indeed a misnomer when one notes that cardiovascular complications are progressive in this stage although major problems are not imminent. When individuals are admitted to the hospital for aggressive treatment of hypertension, they are usually in the *malignant phase* of the hypertensive process. Currently, malignant (accelerated, necrotizing) hypertension is usually regarded as an accelerated form, or one that is unresponsive to therapy. It endangers the life of the individual often within a matter of a few years; however, with the current availability of drugs that are effective in controlling the blood pressure, prognosis in malignant hypertension has improved.

In many communities, efforts are being directed by voluntary health agencies, community health centers, industries, health planning agencies, and civic organizations toward multiphasic screening programs for the early detection of major chronic diseases including heart disease, diabetes, and hypertension. The nurse is playing an increasingly important role in these programs not only in the screening component, but in the long-term management and counseling of the individual with hypertension.

Hypertension Secondary to Renal Disease

Diastolic-systolic hypertension is common in any renal disorder in which the blood supply is impaired such as renal arterial stenosis. Hypertension is found also in disorders wherein the renal parenchyma is diseased, thus hypertension is seen even in young children with glomerulonephritis, pyelonephritis, or polycystic kidneys. In some instances whereby only one kidney is diseased and is removed surgically, the blood pressure returns to normal. When both kidneys are diseased, hypertension continues.

Hypertension Secondary to Adrenal Cortex Overactivity

Both Cushing's syndrome and Conn's syndrome (primary aldosteronism) effect diastolic-systolic hypertension. Cushing's syndrome is caused by a neoplasm or hyperplasia of the adrenal cortex, which results in hypersecretion of corticosterone and hydrocortisone. Conn's syndrome is caused by a neoplasm with hypersecretion of aldosterone. In both instances sodium and water retention result, with potentially enhanced arteriolar responsiveness and hypertension. Correction of the excessive adrenocortical hormone secretion is often followed by restoration of normotension.

Not only does hypertension occur in diseases associated with adrenocortical hypersecretion, but it may be precipitated by steroid administration in the treatment of disease. When deoxycorticosterone was first introduced in the treatment of chronic adrenal insufficiency (Addison's disease), several patients died from complications induced by the effects of rapidly developing hypertension. Persons who have adrenal insufficiency characteristically have low blood pressures.

Pheochromocytoma

Diastolic-systolic hypertension associated with hypersecretion of the adrenal medullary catecholamines is caused by a tumor of the medulla or of chromaffin tissue located less frequently in the abdomen, bladder, or chest. The tumor, known as pheochromocytoma, is usually benign and secretes both epinephrine and norepinephrine. Epinephrine affects the blood pressure primarily by increasing the strength of cardiac contraction, thus increasing the cardiac output. At the same time norepinephrine increases the PVR by effecting arteriolar vasoconstriction. The result is a marked increase in both systolic and diastolic blood pressure.

Pheochromocytoma may be present for a few weeks or several years before clinical manifestations are overt. Frequently the symptoms are present in paroxysmal attacks, varying in frequency, duration, and severity. They may occur without warning or in response to such stimuli as emotional upsets, postural changes, or physical exertion. The most frequent manifestations are pounding headache, diaphoresis, tachycardia, pallor, extreme anxiety, tremor, dyspnea, paraesthesia, vomiting, blurred vision, chest pain, and vertigo. The symptoms frequently are associated with hyperglycemia and glycosuria. One patient's blood pressure during an attack observed by the writer rose to 300/180 mm Hg. It should be noted that the highest point on the sphygmomanometer is 300 mm Hg; thus the systolic pressure could have been higher than what was recorded. Cessation of the attack results in a feeling of prostration.

Two types of chemical tests utilizing provocative and blocking agents, previously were used to diagnose pheochromocytoma. The provocative test (histamine test) utilized parenteral administration of histamine which stimulated the release of catecholamines and thus precipitated an attack. The dangers of the test are obvious. Although no longer used, the test is worthy of mention because pheochromocytoma like symptoms are seen sometimes in patients during the histalog test for gastric achlorhydria with pernicious anema. The blocking agent test (Regitine test) utilized parenteral administration of phentolamine (Regitine), which is an alpha-adrenergic receptor blocking agent, to block the action of norepinephrine on alpha receptors by competitive inhibition. Phentolamine is now used as a therapeutic, rather than diagnostic, agent. What made it possible to relinquish use of the invasive chemical tests was the development of sophisticated chemical assay methods for urinary catecholamines and their metabolites and for plasma norepinephrine.

The urinary studies obviously are perferable to the invasive chemical tests because of patient comfort and ease of collection. Twenty-four-hour urine studies are done for the amount of vanillylmandelic acid (VMA), a metabolite of catecholamine metabolism. If a pheochromocytoma exists, the amount of VMA in the sample may be as high as five to ten times normal. When the assay method was first used, it was necessary for patients to be on specific diets for compatability with the test, excluding foods containing phenolic acid such as raw fruits, vanilla, and coffee. Such is no longer the case with conversion from a colorimetric to a spectrophotometric technique; thus the only restriction is the lipid-lowering drug clofibrate (Atromid-S) which gives false negative test results.

A single voided specimen can be analyzed for the other catecholamine metabolites, metanephrine and normetanephrine. Specimens from patients with pheochromocytoma frequently exceed five to ten times normal values. Whereas in the past several drugs were documented to cause false positive tests, the only restriction with refined assay methods is chlorpromazine (Thorazine) (Sokolow & McIlroy, 1979, p. 256). The reason that the urine assays are done on the metabolites rather than the free catecholamines is that they are easier to measure and are not influenced to give false positive results by epinephrine-base drugs such as bronchodilators, cold preparations, tetracycline, and methyldopa. Methods are also now available to measure plasma norepinephrine, which is useful as a diagnostic aid per se but also assists in localizing the site of the tumor.

If the site of the tumor can be localized by radiologic studies, tomography, vena caval and adrenal venography, norepinephrine plasma studies, and urine studies, the hypertension can be cured by surgical excision of the tumor. Care must be taken during anesthesia induction and during the surgical procedure to prevent excessive catecholamine release from the tumor. Adjunct drug therapy is used pre- and postoperatively or as primary therapy in cases not amenable to surgical intervention. Combinations are used of the alpha adrenergic blocking agents, phentolamine (Regitine) or phenoxybenzamine (Dibenzyline) with the beta-adrenergic blocking agent, propranolol (Inderal).

Hypertension Secondary to Disorders of the Nervous System

Disorders of the nervous system that impinge on the cerebral blood flow usually are accompanied by diastolic-systolic hypertension. This is particularly true when the underlying pathology develops rapidly. The rise in blood pressure usually is accompanied by a decrease in heart rate, which is a cardinal sign of increased intracranial pressure. Examples of underlying pathology include head injury, neoplasm, cerebral accident, or acute inflammatory processes, all of which promote cerebral ischemia.

Hypertension Secondary to Coarctation of the Aorta

A known and curable cause of diastolic-systolic hypertension is coarctation of the aorta where at some point along the vessel the size of the lumen is reduced by a constricting muscle band. The individual is hypertensive in the blood vessels above the site of constriction and has lower-than-normal pressures below the constriction. If the constriction is below the level of the renal arteries, renal hypertension may be superimposed. Early surgical alleviation of the coarctation is necessary to return the blood pressure to physiologic limits.

Drug-Induced Hypertension

It has become apparent that there is an association between the use of birth control pills and the development of hypertension. The mechanism, although not definitive, appears to be that the estrogen-progesterone cause a rise in renin which alters the balance of renin-angiotensin-aldosterone system. The rise in pressure is slight initially but progressive over time. Cessation of pill use early in the pathologic process appears to promote normotension even in the hypertensive-susceptible individual. The effect of long-term use with subsequent cessation is less clear, although reports of a higher incidence of coronary artery disease and heart attacks at an earlier age for women who have used birth control pills suggest less than promising outcomes. It would appear that alternative forms of contraception should be considered seriously by females with predisposition to and a family history positive for hypertension.

The simultaneous ingestion of drugs that are

monoamine oxidase (MAO) inhibitors (certain antidepressive and antihypertensive agents) and cheeses has been implicated in the development of a hypertensive crisis syndrome similar to that seen in pheochromocytoma. It has been suggested that certain cheeses such as cheddar, Camembert, and Stilton contain a substance capable of liberating stored catecholamines in the presence of MAO inhibitors. Other foods and beverages implicated in this syndrome are pickled herring, chicken liver, yeast, coffee, canned figs, and beer. Wine, a favorite cheese companion, is also implicated (Goodman & Gilman, 1975). Headache is a common symptom, but death from intracranial hemorrhage has been reported. This situation is an excellent example of the multiple chemical interactions impinging upon patients about which medical personnel must develop an awareness in order to inform patients effectively.

Intervention with the Hypertensive Patient

The when and what of intervention with the individual with hypertension is determined by the level of the arterial pressure, the clinical manifestations present, the motivation of the individual, and the presence or absence of an underlying disorder causing the hypertension. Obviously, causes of hypertension secondary to another disorder are sought and remedied as possible. Cure of essential hypertension, however, is not possible owing to a lack of knowledge about etiology and pathogenesis. Thus, care measures must be employed to control or delay the progress of essential hypertension and subsequent sequelae. At best these measures appear palliative, although in some instances, such as the U.S. Veterans Administration Cooperative Study (1970), a significant decrease in morbidity and mortality has been demonstrated. The individual with hypertension *can* buy time.

Whereas philosophical differences relative to when to begin antihypertensive therapy and what modalities to use have existed among members of the medical community in the past, resolution of those differences generally has occurred with greater standardization in approach. There is little disagreement that the person with malignant hypertension having rapid acceleration of the pathogenesis should be treated aggressively with any measure to which the blood pressure responds. Consensus also exists with regard to risk factor screening for hypertension and cardiovascular disease even into the school-aged population in order to identify those at risk and to begin the educational process for modification of hazardous habits. In other words, there are certain general measures that can be initiated to delay the onset of hypertension in the prehypertensive population as well as to lower blood pressure in the labile and sustained hypertension population.

Whereas nothing can be done about the risk factors of age, sex, race, and family history, modification is possible with the factors related to dietary patterns, alcohol and cigarette consumption, physical activity, and management of stress, *provided* positive attitudinal and motivational factors are operant. The objectives to be achieved with these general measures include (1) reduction or control of body weight; (2) reduction of daily sodium intake; (3) reduction or elimination of alcohol and cigarette consumption; (4) implementation of periods of rest, relaxation, and exercise; (5) effective management of stress; and (6) development of motivation and desire to attain and maintain good health practices.

Diet and Hypertension

The dietary management of individuals with hypertension is directed to caloric reduction and sodium restriction. Weight that is on the lean side of the standard weight for a given height is desired. Reduction of the body weight in some obese hypertensive patients has resulted in a significant lowering of the blood pressure. Further, weight reduction may increase cardiac reserve in hypertensive patients with early stage heart failure.

Obviously, in any program of weight reduction an important goal is for the individual to develop eating habits compatible with maintenance of the desired weight. This frequently is easier said than done, as witnessed by the many individuals who lose large amounts of weight on various fad diets only to regain the weight plus some with resumption of former food patterns. Moreover, there are some potentially hazardous side effects of fad diets for persons with cardiovascular problems which are indicated by Food and Drug Administration (Liquid proteins, 1978) reports of sudden cardiac death among obese white women on a predigested liquid protein diet, presumably due to potassium imbalance. The nurse must be aware of counseling of obese cardiovascular patients. The reader is referred to an excellent summary of treatments for obesity by Mahan (1979).

The group-centered approach to weight reduction and maintenance has proved successful in the general population as evidenced by such groups as Weight Watchers and TOPS. Shumway and Powers (1973) report promising results with group sessions conducted by professional nurses for obese hypertensive patients as did Jones and Jenkins (1973). This would appear to be a major primary health care role of professional nurses.

A part of calorie restriction is the need to evaluate alcohol intake as a component of daily dietary intake and of perceived management of stress. Also there is a positive relationship between excessive alcohol consumption and hypertension. Counseling for alcoholism may be part of the total treatment program for hypertension. What a paradox it is that a popular fad diet for weight reduction is called the "drinking man's diet." The possibilities of abuse appear great.

In addition to the restriction of calories, sodium intake should be restricted. The rationale for this measure is that reduction of extracellular sodium and water may result in a lowering of the blood pressure by decreasing the cardiac output and thus perhaps the PVR. In the early phase of hypertension, sodium intake is not greatly restricted but is limited to elimination of all grossly salty foods with no salt used in the preparation of foods or added at mealtime. These actions would reduce the daily sodium intake to 4 to 6 g per day as compared to 5 to 10 g or greater consumed in the average American diet. The initial low-sodium diet historically used in the dietary treatment of hypertension was the Kempner rice-fruit diet, in which the sodium content was as low as 150 mg per day. The diet's components were as the name suggests and the diet was to be followed for 4 to 6 weeks. Its monotonous character plus its protein and vitamin inadequacy proved more stressful than beneficial.

As with any dietary modification whereby individuals may perceive the instructions as punitive, emphasis should be placed on what *to* eat rather than on what *not* to eat. Emphasis also should be placed on the use of herbs, spices, lemon juice, and vinegar as flavoring agents that can be used at will. The hypertensive patient requires the same instruction and assistance in meal planning as the individual with heart failure who is on a sodium-limited diet including the need for potassium-rich foods if the patient is on diuretic therapy.

Physical Activity

For most persons with essential hypertension, control is a lifetime endeavor. Hypertension control involves developing a way of life that lessens the tendency to constrict blood vessels. Moderation is the watchword with avoidance of excesses in eating, smoking, and working. For the patient who is free of complications, exercises such as walking, swimming, golf, bicycle riding, and fishing are generally recommended as a source of relaxation and as exercise to increase cardiac reserve. The form of exercise selected should be based on the interests of the patient and should be a source of pleasure, not a punishment. Moreover, the exercise program should be undertaken in the spirit of attaining relaxation and not for the purpose of competition and excellence.

Management of Stress

Periods of rest throughout the day are to be promoted as a means to diminish stressors impinging on the nervous and cardiovascular systems. The individual with essential hypertension should achieve 7 to 8 hours of sleep per night, and, if possible, relax after each meal. The patient must become aware of his or her own nervous tension and practice relaxation techniques consciously. Just telling a patient to relax frequently is of little value. Patients need specific instruction and encouragement to learn how to relax. One suggestion that can be made to a patient who is learning to relax is consciously to tense the muscles of a part of the body, such as the arm, and then consciously to let it hang limp. Isometric exercises, certain Yogic exercises, biofeedback and transcendental meditation have also been suggested to help the individual achieve more profound relaxation.

The hypertensive patient must carefully consider his or her life style and its potential contribution to physical state. The way in which this is achieved for various patients ranges from intensive psychotherapy to constructive professional relationships. Few patients will need or can afford intensive psychotherpy, nor could many psychiatrists' schedules tolerate the additional patient load. Supportive therapy may be administered by the patient's private physician. The professional nurse, however, can play a major role in this primary care area.

The attitudes of the patient toward life, work, home, family members, coworkers, and other persons all affect the level of his or her blood pressure and should be explored. Each patient may be expected to react to various aspects of life differently; a factor that is a stressor to one individual may not be so to another. Consider these potential stressors, patient reactions, and coping techniques in the following situations. An individual encounters multiple red traffic lights or a bottleneck on the freeway on the way to work. The person becomes tense and angry, and considers the situation as a personal affront. If the individual left 10 minutes earlier in the morning and made a conscious effort at muscle relaxation when approaching a red light, this might relieve one stimulus to vasoconstriction. In a second situation, an individual cares for an invalid parent and never has the opportunity to take a vacation. Despite protestations to the contrary, the individual resents the situation. By securing someone to stay with the parent for a weekend and providing relief on periodic weekends, the individual's resentment may diminish and thus the stressor.

The nurse can thus help the hypertensive patient identify circumstances that contribute to the hypertension, gain insight into behavior, and develop possible alternative actions and behavior modifications. The nurse cannot alter the environmental circumstances but can supply the emotional support to help the patient make the necessary alterations.

Learning Needs

The nurse has a major role in educating the individual and family or significant others about the many facets of the disease and therapeutic processes as one means to foster compliance with prescribed therapy to control progression of the pathologic process. Knowledge about the many facets of the disease and control measures may also help to diminish anxiety about catastrophic complications such as stroke that can result in permanent paralysis. Griffith and Madero's (1973) experience with approximately 500 hypertensive patients in a clinic setting points to the many and varied learning needs of hypertensive patients; the many misconceptions and misunderstandings about hypertension; and the problems encountered with compliance with the therapeutic regimen. Typically content areas in which individuals have learning needs include (1) what is hypertension; (2) risk factors predisposing to hypertension; (3) complications of untreated hypertension; (4) modifications of risk factors; (5) specifics of the individual's therapeutic regimen; and (6) the individual's role in follow-up and self-care. The reader is referred to Kochar and Daniels (1978) for greater specifics regarding teaching the hypertensive patient. The overall goal of the patient education program is to foster self-control and management over the chronic illness, but also recognition that medical follow-up and therapeutics are a life-long process.

Despite preparation by the physician and nurse in the hospital, office, or community health agency, assumption of responsibility for self-care is not without difficulty particularly for the elderly. Consider the many and varied problems the patient may encounter at home. Potential problematic areas include a limited income upon which additional strains are placed by multiple medications and perpetual medical care costs; apprehension engendered by the implications of hypertension; adherence to a complicated medical regimen, including meal planning and medication administration; and conflict between the medical regimen and "sure-cures" imposed by well-meaning but uninformed friends and relatives. Some patients who are responsible for daily monitoring of their blood pressure level have had insufficient practice to master the skill. Many patients are overwhelmed by the number of medications they must take and confused about how to establish a routine once they secure their filled prescriptions. Supervised self-administration of drugs and meal planning should be accomplished in the hospital setting. It also is not uncommon for a friend to propose a home remedy for high blood pressure control, such as a daily dose of dried spinach powder dissolved in seawater and the elimination of tomatoes from the diet. Within this context it is not difficult to understand why many patients discontinue all forms of therapy once the symptoms are abated and they are feeling better. Assumption of responsibility at home can be facilitated greatly by one or more visits from a community health nurse. The nurse can reinforce or initiate patient and family teaching, help the patient and family to resolve difficulties encountered, and increase the patient's and family's self-confidence.

There are no ready recipes or formulas to help health professionals deal with the problem of patient compliance with therapeutic regimens. The problem is complex and multifaceted. Why else would many individuals *not* adhere to those things which would promote a longer life? Nursing studies and literature are now being directed toward the problem of patient compliance (Foster & Kousch, 1978; Kochar & Daniels, 1978). Kochar and Daniels report a high percentage of noncompliant patients with hypertension in a metropolitan blood pressure program. The areas where counseling and education had a significant impact on compliance were reduction in alcohol and cigarette consumption. Weight control, however, was far less successful, and failure to adhere to the medication regimen was $\geq$ 50 per cent (pp. 112–113). A comprehensive review of reasons for noncompliance are presented by Kochar and Daniels.

Drug Therapy

Drugs that have hypotensive effects have been available for some time. There are a variety of potent antihypertensive drugs that can be used alone or in combination to lower the blood pressure to a desired level. In addition to lowering the resting blood pressure, an effective drug should lower the blood pressure during exercise and, ideally, during stress situations. The drug should not have undesirable side effects, nor should it interfere with the intellectual or physical working capacity of the patient when it is administered in therapeutic doses. In some patients, however, it is not possible to lower the blood pressure to a sufficient degree and at the same time avoid all adverse effects. The patient therefore may have to tolerate the side effects of the drug, if he or she is to be adequately treated.

The various antihypertensive agents are presented by physiologic category in Table 43-1. The selection of the appropriate agent, or combination of agents, for a given patient is determined by the degree of hypertension present. The object is to decrease the blood pressure to 140/90 or lower for as much of the day as possible without disabling side effects. Some trial and error is to be expected in finding the individualized combination of drugs that works for a given person when more than mild hypertension exists.

A step-wise approach is used in the initiation of drug therapy, as noted in Table 43–2. If the individual's diastolic blood pressure is 90 to 110 mm Hg at the initiation of therapy, the first agent utilized is a thiazide diuretic in combination with a low-calorie, low-salt, potassium-rich diet. If the patient has a known sulfa allergy, a milder long-acting thiazide diuretic may be used such as metolazone (Zaroxolyn). If significant potassium depletion occurs with these diuretics, a potassium-sparing diuretic such as triamterene (Dyrenium) may be employed. If the response to the thiazide preparation is inadequate, furosemide (Lasix) may be employed.

The patient taking thiazide preparations should avoid excessive water intake or a dilutional hyponatremia may occur. Similarly, if thiazides are ingested with alcohol, narcotics, or barbiturates, a postural hypotension may ensue. Further, lithium toxicity may occur in persons with manic-depressive illness on lithium carbonate due to an interactive effect (Kemp & Kemp, 1978). Patients on spironolactone should avoid excessive salicylate ingestion because aspirin inhibits the action of the diuretic (Kemp & Kemp, 1978). Patients taking furosemide should be taught to observe their skin after sunlight exposure

TABLE 43-1 *Antihypertensive Drugs*

Physiologic Category	Name	Physiologic Action	Desired Effect	Significant Adverse Affects
Diuretic agents	Chlorothiazide (Diuril)	Inhibition of carbonic anhydrase and sulfhydryl enzymes necessary to tubular reabsorption of electrolytes resulting in increased electrolyte and water excretion	Decreased extracellular fluid volume and cardiac output; relaxes peripheral vascular smooth muscle, thus decreasing peripheral vascular resistance	Hyponatremia Hypokalemia Hyperuricemia Hyperglycemia Hypercalcemia Skin rashes Sulfa allergy
	Furosemide (Lasix)	Inhibition of tubular sodium reabsorption; mechanism unclear	Decreased cardiac output and peripheral vascular resistance	Ototoxicity Hypovolemia Hypokalemia Hypochloremic alkalosis Hyperuricemia Sulfa allergy Photosensitivity
	Spironolactone (Aldactone)	Steroidal compound which competitively inhibits aldosterone at the tubular level, resulting in increased sodium and chloride excretion	Decreased cardiac output	Menstrual irregularities Hyperkalemia Hyponatremia Gynecomastia Impotence
	Triamterene (Dyrenium)	Inhibition of sodium excretion and potassium excretion although not a steroidal compound that inhibits aldosterone; mechanism unclear	Decreased cardiac output	Hyperkalemia Anemia
Adrenergic inhibitors	Propranolol (Inderal)	Blocks beta-adrenergic receptors by competitive inhibition at the myoneural junction; inhibits renin secretion	Diminished cardiac output	Bronchospasm Bradycardia Heart failure Raynaud's phenomenon Hyperglycemia

TABLE 43-1 *(Continued)*

Physiologic Category	Name	Physiologic Action	Desired Effect	Significant Adverse Affects
	Reserpine (Serpasil)	Inhibits and binds norepinephrine and epinephrine at sympathetic ganglia, thus inhibiting impulse transmission and catecholamine release at the myoneural junction	Diminished vasoconstriction and thus peripheral vascular resistance. Decreased cardiac output because of decreased heart rate	Depression Postural hypotension Bradycardia Venous pooling Edema Decreased libido Insomnia
	Methyldopa (Aldomet)	Mechanism unclear; is catabolized into alpha-methyl-norepinephrine, a less potent vasopressor than norepinephrine; appears to act by substitution of this "false transmitter" at the myoneural junction	Decreased peripheral vascular resistance	Drowsiness Depression Weakness Skin rashes Impotence Postural hypotension Liver dysfunction
	Guanethedine (Ismelin)	Blocks release of norepinephrine at the sympathetic myoneural junction; mechanism unclear	Decreased vascular tone and peripheral vascular resistance	Postural hypotension Bradycardia Diarrhea Weakness Ejaculatory inability
	Clonidine hydrochloride (Catapres)	Blocks adrenergic output at the cerebral medullary level; mechanism unclear. Inhibiton of sodium excretion	Decreased cardiac output and peripheral vascular resistance	Drowsiness Hypernatremia Rebound hypertension
Vasodilator	Hydralazine (Apresoline)	Acts directly on vascular smooth muscle to effect vasodilatation; mechanism unsure—may be related to beta-adrenergic activity	Decreased vasomotor tone and peripheral vascular resistance; greater diastolic than systolic decrease; increased cardiac output and renal flow	Headache Tachycardia Dyspnea on exertion Lupuslike syndrome
	Sodium nitroprusside (Nipride)	Acts directly on vascular smooth muscle to effect vasodilatation; mechanism presumed to be like nitroglycerine's	Decreased peripheral vascular resistance; variable effect on cardiac output	Hypotension Tubular necrosis Thiocyanate toxicity

for signs of irritation as a sign of photosensitive reaction. The skin should be protected from sunlight, and sensitized persons should avoid the sun and ultraviolet lamps.

If the patient is insufficiently responsive to step 1 therapy within about 1 month, steps 2 to 3 vasopressor therapy are added to the diuretic and dietary regimen. Propranolol and hydralazine in combination or methyldopa alone are commonly employed. Dosages are gradually increased until the desired response is achieved. If step 4 need be initiated, guanethidine is added to or substituted for the stage 2 and 3 vasopressors.

The "discovery" of propranolol (Inderal) has been a milestone in the treatment of hypertension and other cardiovascular diseases. Propranolol's primary action is as a beta-receptor adrenergic blocking agent but it also decreases renin release from the kidneys, hence the overall effect of a decreased cardiac output by decreasing the heart rate, fluid volume, and thus blood pressure. Propranolol also decreases oxygen consumption of cardiac cells and has a quinidinelike action on cardiac cells, which makes it useful as an antiarrhythmic agent for individuals with cardiac disease. Because propranolol counteracts the reflex tachycardia and increased cardiac out-

TABLE 43-2 *Step-wise Approach for Antihypertensive Drug Therapy*

Presenting Degree of Hypertension (Diastolic Pressure mmHg.)		Step	Therapy
Mild (90–110)		1	Diuretic and Diet Modification of ↓ calories ↑ salt, ↓ potassium
Moderate (110–120)	May be combined	2	Add: Propranolol or Methyldopa
		3	Add: Hydralazine
Severe (>120)		4	Add or substitute: Guanethidine

put associated with vasodilatation, it is effective particularly in combination with vasodilator drugs for control of hypertension. The usual range of propranolol dosage is 40 to 480 mg/24 hours in divided doses.

Inasmuch as propranolol is an overall beta blocking agent, not just cardioselective by action only on beta-1 receptors, its action on beta-2 receptors of smooth muscles, particularly in the bronchi, can precipitate bronchospasm, a significant side effect. Until 1978, propranolol was the only beta-blocking agent available in the United States, although several other preparations are utilized in foreign countries. The United States Food and Drug Administration (Status report on beta blockers, 1978) has reported on (1) studies of selected beta-blocking agents other than propranolol, used in foreign countries indicate tumorigenic and carcinogenic properties, and (2) approval for use of metoprolol (Lopressor), a beta-blocking agent that is primarily cardioselective.

The antihypertensive agents that act by adrenergic inhibition tend to cause postural (orthostatic) hypotension. Patients who complain of dizziness or feel faint when they assume the upright position should be taught to rise slowly to prevent syncope. When the patient is hospitalized and begins the drug therapy, particularly guanethedine, the nurse should monitor the patient's response to postural changes and assist the patient out of bed. A commonly experienced side effect of methyldopa and clonidine is drowsiness. Should this occur, patients should be aware that during the time drowsiness is present, driving or operating machinery is ill-advised. Fortunately, this effect usually dissipates with continued therapy. Patients may also exhibit mild depression. It is during this time that patients frequently become discouraged with their complicated medication routine and stop taking the drugs. Initial instruction of the patient should take this into account by discussing this likelihood and by establishing a routine that is most convenient for the patient.

Reserpine (Serpasil) is an antihypertensive agent of the adrenergic inhibitor category that has been used extensively for many years. Recent reports from the Food and Drug Administration report carcinogenic properties derived from animal studies. Although used extensively in the past, ganglionic blocking agents, such as pentolinium (Ansolysen) and mecamylamine (Inversine), are employed less frequently in current practice except in emergency cases that are unresponsive to other forms of drug therapy. In some cases, tranquilizing agents may be prescribed for the relaxing effect and to diminish the degree to which some individuals with hypertension respond to stress.

When the patient receives a large number of pills, he or she is responsible for selecting, counting, and evaluating their effect. At times the patient may feel like a walking pharmacy without a pharmacist. One error commonly made by nurses is telling the patient to take the medicines on the same schedule as when in the hospital. When a drug is to be taken at equal time intervals, such as every 6 hours in the hospital, it is usually given at 12 midnight, 6 A.M., 12 noon, and 6 P.M. The hypertensive patient, as with other patients, however, could benefit equally well from uninterrupted rest; thus the schedule for the evening medications should be modified to be administered at bedtime and immediately upon rising, with the other two doses interspersed at equal intervals.

In the classic study of elderly patients taking medications at home, Schwartz (1962) enumerates some of the problems they encountered. Among the types of errors made by patients were (1) taking medications not ordered by the physician, (2) not taking medications ordered by the physician, (3) taking medications ordered by the physician but in incorrect dosages or at the wrong time when time was a significant factor, and (4) not understanding the purpose of the medication. Schwartz questions the effectiveness of medication instruction to the newly discharged or ambulatory patient and states that better approaches must be developed. One suggestion is the use of medication calendars or clocks, or other visual aids. Certainly a period of supervised self-administration of the medication by the patient while in the hospital would prove helpful.

Hypertensive Crises

One type of hospitalization emergency with which both the nurse and patient must cope is admission for hypertension that is accelerated and predisposes to a life-threatening situation. This type of emergency is called a *hypertensive crisis.* Dhar and Freedman suggest that because accelerated and malignant hypertension share common clinical manifestations, they should be considered as on a continuum (1976, p. 571). Accelerated hypertension is manifested by a diastolic blood pressure > 120 mm Hg accompanied by retinal hemorrhages. Left untreated, malignant hypertension ensues with papilledema and convulsions leading to coma. Prompt treatment to lower the blood pressure is mandatory to abate a crisis. The most prominent types of crises are cerebral hemorrhage, renal failure, left ventricular failure, or dissecting aortic aneurysm.

The treatment of a hypertensive emergency consists of parenteral administration of antihypertensive drugs such as sodium nitroprusside (Nipride) or diazoxide (Hyperstat) for rapid lowering of the blood pressure. The doses must be carefully titrated and administered by intravenous microdrip using a constant infusion apparatus. Blood pressure readings are taken every 5 to 15 minutes. As soon as the blood pressure is lowered, oral antihypertensive agents are begun concommitantly.

Sodium nitroprusside is a peripheral vasodilating agent which, like nitroglycerin, acts directly on the blood vessel independent of the autonomic nervous system and thus effects reduction in the PVR. The duration of action is exceedingly short due to the drug's rapid conversion to thiocyanate. In those patients with severe renal dysfunction, blood cyanide levels must be monitored closely (*Physicians' Desk Reference,* 1980, p. 1474). Sodium nitroprusside is a drug with unstable properties once prepared for parenteral administration. Thus, in addition to the vigilant monitoring of the patient's blood pressure, the nurse must assume responsibility for monitoring the following: (1) only 5 per cent dextrose in water can be used as the drug's diluent; (2) the drug's properties deteriorate in the presence of light, thus the IV bottle must be covered with foil or a paper bag; (3) a freshly prepared solution has a faint brownish tint, and solutions of any other color should be discarded; and (4) fresh solutions should be prepared and initiated every 4 to 8 hours.

Treatment of hypertensive emergencies is not without potential complications. When the blood pressure is lowered, reflex mechanisms become operant. Because a reflex tachycardia will occur as the body attempts to increase the cardiac output, propranolol will be administered. Similarly, the lowered blood pressure will effect sodium and water retention, thus potent diuretics such as furosemide and ethacrynic acid (Edecrin) will be given. Care must be taken that the lowering of the blood pressure is not precipitous or additional compromising problems can ensue such as myocardial or cerebral ischemia, or renal failure.

In summary, although specific causation for primary hypertension is unknown, much can be done to slow the progress of the process and to retard the development of complications. Despite its generally deleterious effects, some individuals are able to tolerate hypertension for many years. Hypertension is similar to other chronic diseases because continued control is necessary. The burden of the therapeutic regimen is eventually borne by the patient and family. The professional nurse, however, has a major role in the detection and management of patients with primary or secondary hypertension.

Pulmonary Hypertension

Although hypertension is most frequently associated with the systemic arterial circulation, hypertension solely of the pulmonary arteries can occur. Because the characteristics of the pulmonary and arterial beds are different, however, the causes and effects of pulmonary hypertension differ from those of systemic hypertension.

Whereas blood is circulated normally through the systemic arteries under a relatively high pressure, the pulmonary circulation is a relatively low-pressure system. The normal upper limit of the pulmonary artery pressure in humans under resting conditions is approximately 30 to 25/12 to 10 mm Hg, with a mean pressure of around 15 mm Hg. The pressure in the pulmonary capillary bed (wedge pressure) is approximately 8 to 12 mm Hg. Three factors are primarily responsible for the low pressure in the pulmonary system: (1) the walls of the pulmonary artery contain relatively little muscle, (2) the pulmonary vessels are highly distensible, and (3) there is a large reserve of vessels that appear to be weakly reactive to various stimuli that normally effect vasoconstriction.

The precise level of the pulmonary artery pressure is determined by the amount of blood flow through the vessel, the resistance to flow through the vessels, and the opposing left atrial pressure. Normally the pulmonary circulation contains 500 to 600 ml of blood. An increased blood volume in the circuit will increase the pulmonary vascular pressures. Lukas (1979) points out that during exercise the mean pulmonary artery pressure increases 25 to 50 per cent when there is a two- to threefold increase in cardiac output. If, however, the cardiac output rises to four or five times the resting value, the mean pulmonary artery pressure will double (p. 1136). If the blood flow through the pulmonary vasculature is impeded at the level of the pulmonary capillaries, pulmonary veins, or left atrium, the pulmonary vascular resistance increases, causing an elevation in the pulmonary pressures.

Pulmonary hypertension may be a primary disease or secondary to another pathologic condition. Secondary pulmonary hypertension is the more common of the two forms. When the right ventricle becomes involved in the pathological process as a result of the pulmonary hypertension, the terms *pulmonary heart disease, pulmonary hypertensive heart disease,* or *cor pulmonale* are employed.

Secondary Pulmonary Hypertension

Pulmonary hypertension may result from any condition in which there is an increased resistance to the flow of blood through the pulmonary vascular bed, and/or when the right ventricle ejects more blood into the pulmonary vascular bed and left atrium than can be removed by the left ventricle. Thus secondary pulmonary hypertension is a symptom and not a primary disease. Presently recognized mechanisms and examples of pathologic conditions that cause pulmonary hypertension include the following:

1. Obstruction of the pulmonary vessels as by blood clot (pulmonary embolism), distortion (emphysema), or external pressure (intrathoracic tumors, chest deformities).
2. Loss of part of the vascular bed in the course of destructive lung disease (carcinoma, emphysema) or surgery (pneumonectomy).
3. Vasoconstriction in response to alveolar hypoxia (high altitudes, chest deformity, pulmonary disease, obesity, congenital heart disorders) and to increased blood hydrogen ion concentraion (acidosis).
4. Diminished emptying of the pulmonary vascular bed resulting from increased left atrial pressure (mitral valve disease).
5. Increased blood viscosity (polycythemia).

Pulmonary hypertension resulting from disease of the lungs is the most frequent cause of cor pulmonale in the United States. Its frequency appears to be related to the incidence of emphysema associated with chronic bronchitis. With an increase in the occurrence of emphysema and bronchitis, the incidence of cor pulmonale is also expected to rise.

The clinical manifestations of secondary pulmonary hypertension result primarily from decreased blood oxygen and increased blood carbon dioxide levels caused by ventilation-perfusion abnormalities. The degree of manifestations depends on the cause of the pulmonary hypertension as well as the degree of loss of cardiac reserve. The existence of pulmonary hypertension may be very easy to suspect in the presence of obvious pulmonary or cardiac disease; however, it may be overlooked in the absence of such obvious factors.

Undue exertional dyspnea is the most characteristic clinical manifestation of pulmonary hypertension. In severe pulmonary hypertension, chest pain, syncope, and extreme fatigability are common, reflecting oxygen deprivation of cells. A lowered cardiac output resulting from a diminished left ventricular stroke volume predisposes to cold cyanotic extremities and a weak radial–brachial pulse. The cardiac rhythm is normal initially but atrial arrhythmias may appear with distension and ischemia of the atria. Characteristic changes in the heart sounds are also noted.

Chest x-rays, although helpful, are not diagnostic. The x-ray may show contour changes of the pulmonary artery, and vascular changes in the lung fields with severe pulmonary hypertension, whereas no changes may be evident in the early stages. The electrocardiogram documents right ventricular hypertrophy when the later complication of cor pulmonale appears. Pulmonary function studies may provide useful information about the nature and severity of the underlying disorder. By far the most definitive diagnositc tool is cardiac catheterization with or without pulmonary angiography. The pulmonary artery and pulmonary capillary pressures can be measured directly, and with special techniques, the left atrial and pulmonary venous pressures can be estimated. Pulmonary blood flow and resistance can be estimated, and with injection of contrast media, the pulmonary vasculature can be visualized. The intervention with secondary pulmonary hypertension is directed to the underlying disorder. Whether the treatment is medical or surgical, the objective is to diminish the pulmonary hypertension before cor pulmonale develops.

Primary Pulmonary Hypertension

Primary pulmonary hypertension is a disease for which there is no known cause. In other words, there is a progression of hypertension in the pulmonary artery in the absence of other cardiopulmonary disorders. A genetic factor is suspected because of the tendency for the disease to occur in families. It predominantly affects young parous women between the ages of 20 and 40 years.

In some patients the pulmonary artery pressure can exceed the systemic arterial pressure at rest. In most situations the pulmonary arterial pressure is 65 to 90 mm Hg systolic. The pulmonary vascular resistance is very high, as much as twelve to eighteen times normal (Lukas, 1979, p. 1139). It has been noted that the hypertension is uniquely located in the pulmonary artery whereas the pulmonary capillary pressures usually are found to be normal. The cardiac output is diminished. The arterial blood oxygen saturation is normal or slightly low and may diminish further with exercise. The arterial blood carbon dioxide tension is usually reduced by hyperventilation. Most of the symptoms are brought on by exertion and are the same as with secondary pulmonary hypertension. In addition there may be some hemoptysis ascribed to pulmonary infarction.

The diagnosis of primary pulmonary hypertension usually can be made with certainty from the clinical picture; however, confirmation is accomplished by cardiac catheterization studies. This procedure is helpful in differentiating among other various causative possibilities when clinical data are insufficient. Other etiologic factors must be excluded, the most important of which is recurrent pulmonary embolism. Thus the patient may require extensive investigation to exclude the many and varied pulmonary and cardiac disorders. It has been noted that these patients have a propensity to die suddenly during the course of procedures that are usually well tolerated by others. Such procedures include cardiac catheterization and pulmonary angiography.

Therapeutic intervention with patients having primary pulmonary hypertension is an enigma and generally unsatisfactory. The prognosis is extremely poor, with a 2 to 8 year life expectancy from the onset of symptoms. Death is a consequence of heart failure.

Anticoagulant therapy may be used against the possibility of undetected pulmonary embolization. A few efforts have been made to reduce the pulmonary artery resistance by constant infusions of acetylcholine, bradykinin, isoproterenol, and aminophylline through an indwelling cardiac catheter. The reduction in pulmonary artery pressure is transient, however, and the adverse effects of the procedure and substance's action on other sites appear to outweigh the benefits.

Cor Pulmonale

Cor pulmonale, or pulmonary heart disease, is the term applied to hypertrophy of the right ventricle, with or without congestive heart failure, resulting from disease of the lungs or the pulmonary vasculature. Cor pulmonale was often called "emphysema heart" because it is the most common cause of pulmonary heart disease.

The clinical manifestations, diagnostic measures, and therapeutic intervention with cor pulmonale are those of right ventricular failure. The medical and nursing interventions are directed to the patient who has congestive heart failure, increased bronchial secretions, hypoxia, and hypercapnea. The reader is referred to the section on heart failure in Chapter 44, and to Chapter 40.

References Cited

Allen, E. V., Barker, N. W., and Hines, E. A., Jr. *Peripheral Vascular Disease,* 3rd ed. Philadelphia: W. B. Saunders Co., 1962.

American Heart Association. *Heart Facts.* Dallas: American Heart Association, 1979.

Atchison, J. S., and Murray, J. "Post-Vascular Surgery When Happiness Can Be a Warm Foot." *Nursing,* **8**:12 (1978), 36–39.

Cudkowicz, L., and Sherry, S. "Current Status of Thrombolytic Therapy." *Heart and Lung,* **7**:1 (1978), 97–100.

Dhar, S. K., and Freedman, P. "Clinical Management of Hypertensive Emergencies." *Heart and Lung,* **5**:4 (1976), 571–75.

Ekroth, R., Dahllöf, A., Jan Holm, B. G., and Scherstén, T. "Physical Training with Intermittent Claudication: Indications, Methods and Results." *Surgery,* **84**:5 (1978), 640–43.

Foley, M. F. "Variations in Blood Pressure in the Lateral Recumbent Position." *Nurs. Res.,* **20**:1 (1971), 64–69.

Foster, S., and Kousch, D. C. "Promoting Patient Adherence." *Am. J. Nurs.,* **78**:5 (1978), 829–32.

Friedberg, C. *Diseases of the Heart,* 3rd ed. Philadelphia: W. B. Saunders Co., 1966.

Goodman, L. S., and Gilman, A. *The Pharmacological Basis of Therapeutics,* 5th ed. New York: Macmillan Pub. Co., 1975.

Griffith, E., and Madero, B. "Primary Hypertension—Patient Learning Needs." *Am. J. Nurs.,* **73**:4 (1973), 624–27.

Guyton, A. C. *Textbook of Medical Physiology,* 5th ed. Philadelphia: W. B. Saunders Co., 1976.

Jones, Y., and Jenkins, L. "A Nurse-Directed Outpatient Obesity Clinic." *Hospitals,* **47**:22 (1973), 74–78.

Kemp, G., and Kemp, D. "Diuretics." *Am. J. Nurs.,* **78**:6 (1978), 1007–10.

Kochar, M. S., and Daniels, L. M. *Hypertension Control for Nurses and Other Health Professionals.* St. Louis: C. V. Mosby Co., 1978.

"Liquid Protein and Sudden Cardiac Deaths—An Update." *FDA Drug Bull.,* **8**:3 (1978), 18–19.

Long, G. D. "Managing the Patient with Abdominal Aortic Aneurysm." *Nursing,* **8**:8 (1978), 21–27, 26.

Lukas, D. C. "Pulmonary Hypertension." In *Cecil Textbook of Medicine,* Ed. by P. B. Beeson, W. McDermott and J. B. Wyngaarden. 15th ed. Philadelphia: W. B. Saunders Co., 1979.

Mahan, L. K. "A Sensible Approach to the Obese Patient." *Nurs. Clin. North Am.,* **14**:2 (1979), 229–45.

Physicians' Desk Reference. Oradell, N.J.: Medical Economics Co., 1980, p. 1474.

Ream, I. "Counseling Patients with Leg Pain—A Review of Peripheral Vascular Disease." *Nursing,* **7**:10 (1977), 54–57.

Schwartz, D. "Medication Errors Made by Aged Patients." *Am. J. Nurs.,* **62**:8 (1962), 50–52.

Shumway, S., and Powers, M. "The Group Way to Weight Loss." *Am. J. Nurs.,* **73**:2 (1973), 269–72.

Sokolow, M., and McIlroy, M. B. *Clinical Cardiology,* 2nd ed. Los Altos, Calif.: Lange Medical Publishers, 1979.

"Status Report on Beta-Blockers." *FDA Drug Bull.,* **8**:2 (1978), 13.

Tsou, E. "Pulmonary Embolism—A Dilemma in Diagnosis and Therapy." *Primary Care,* **5**:3 (1978), 397–409.

U.S. Veterans Administration Cooperative Study Group on Antihypertensive Agents. "Effects of Treatment on Morbidity in Hypertension; Part 2. Results in Patients with Diastolic Blood Pressure Averaging 90 through 114 mm Hg." *JAMA,* **213** (1970), 1143–52.

Zweifach, B. W. "The Microcirculation of the Blood." *Sci. Am.,* **200**:1 (1959), 54–60.

General References

DeBakey, M. E. "The Development of Vascular Surgery." *Am. J. Surg.,* **137**:6 (1979), 697–737.

Deykin, D. "Antithrombotic Therapy: Rationale and Application." *Postgrad. Med.,* **65**:1 (1979), 135–46.

Eddy, M. E. "Teaching Patients with Peripheral Vascular Disease." *Nurs. Clin. North Am.,* **12**:1 (1977), 151–60.

Fenn, J. E. "Reconstructive Arterial Surgery for Ischemic Lower Extremities." *Nurs. Clin. North Am.,* **12**:1 (1977), 129–42.

Geelhoed, G. W. "Prevention of Thromboembolism." *Am. Fam. Physician,* **19**:3 (1979), 147–53.

Gernert, C. F., and Schwartz, S. "Pulmonary Artery Catheterization." *Am. J. Nurs.,* **73**:7 (1973), 1182–85.

Inter-Society Commission for Heart Disease Resources. "Guidelines for the Detection, Diagnosis, and Management of Hypertensive Populations." *Circ.,* **44** (1961), A–270.

McConnell, E. A. "Fitting Antiembolism Stockings." *Nursing,* **8**:9 (1978), 67–71.

Pierce, P. F. "Gains and Losses of Vascular Surgery Patients." *Nurs. Clin. North Am.,* **12**:1 (1977), 119–28.

Ram, C. V. S. "Clinical Applications of Beta Adrenergic Blocking Drugs: A Growing Spectrum." *Heart and Lung,* **8**:1 (1979), 116–23.

———. "New Antihypertensive Drugs." *Heart and Lung,* **6**:4 (1977), 679–83.

Roberts, B. "The Acutely Ischemic Limb." *Heart and Lung,* **5**:2 (1976), 273–76.

Ross, S. A. "Infusion Phlebitis." *Nurs. Res.,* **21**:4 (1972), 313–18.

Ryan, R. "Thrombophlebitis: Assessment and Prevention." *Am. J. Nurs.,* **76**:10 (1976), 634–36.

Ryzewski, J. "Factors in the Rehabilitation of Patients with Peripheral Vascular Disease." *Nurs. Clin. North Am.,* **12**:1 (1977), 161–68.

Sexton, D. L. "The Patient with Peripheral Arterial Occlusive Disease." *Nurs. Clin. North Am.,* **12**:1 (1977), 89–100.

Smyth, K. "Elevated Blood Pressure and Type A in Women: A Method of Case Finding." *Image,* **10**:3 (1978), 60–69.

Taggart, E. "The Physical Assessment of the Patient with Arterial Disease." *Nurs. Clin. North Am.,* **12**:1 (1977), 109–18.

Ward, G. W., Bandy, P., and Fink, J. W. "Treating and Counseling the Hypertensive Patient." *Am. J. Nurs.,* **78**:5 (1978), 824–28.

Ziesche, S., and Franciosa, J. A. "Clinical Application of Sodium Nitroprusside." *Heart and Lung,* **6**:1 (1977), 99–103.

44

Problems with Transporting Materials to and from Cells Due to Altered Structure and Function of the Heart

"As he thinketh in his heart, so is he."
PROVERBS 23:21

Overview of Alterations in Transportation Associated with Heart Disease

The heart serves as the power source for movement of the transport medium through the vascular channels. In other words, the heart pumps the blood and essential materials through the circulatory system to the cells and provides the power for the return of metabolic waste products from the cells. The structures that comprise the heart are subject to malformation, injury, and disease, all of which may predispose the heart to failure as the ultimate power source. Alterations in or failure of the transport system resulting from cardiac disease are due to (1) diminished or obstructed blood flow through the heart as seen with valvular disorders; (2) insufficient power to propel blood through the heart and blood vessels, as in heart failure; and (3) alterations in regulatory mechanisms, particularly those that affect the heart rate and therefore cardiac output, as demonstrated by cardiac arrhythmias. The result of these phenomena is an insufficient quantity of blood to groups of cells to sustain optimal metabolic processes and cellular function.

This chapter was revised by Elizabeth Ford Pitorak, R.N., M.S.N., Clinical Nurse Specialist, Lake County Memorial Hospital, Willoughby, Ohio, and Judith A. Wood, R.N., M.S.N., Assistant Professor of Nursing, Case Western Reserve University, Frances Payne Bolton School of Nursing, Cleveland, Ohio.

Structure and Function of the Heart

The heart has been conceptualized as two pumps working side by side in unison and separated by a muscular septum. Structurally, each side consists of two chambers, an atrium and a ventricle. The left atrium and left ventricle are separated by the mitral valve, and the right atrium and right ventricle are separated by the tricuspid valve, thus, the four-chambered heart. Functionally, the heart consists of the right and left heart systems.

The right atrium receives blood from the systemic venous circulation via the superior and inferior venae cavae, and the right ventricle pumps the blood through the pulmonic valve into the pulmonary circulation where the exchange of oxygen and carbon dioxide takes place. The left atrium receives the oxygenated blood from the pulmonary veins, and the left ventricle ejects the blood through the aortic valve into the systemic arterial circulation for transport to all metabolizing cells.

The quantity of blood circulated through the right and left heart systems is essentially equal. In addition to receiving the systemic venous blood, the right heart receives some of the coronary circulation venous blood from the coronary sinus and delivers blood to the bronchial arteries. The bronchial veins empty into the pulmonary veins and thus drain into the left rather than the right atrium. It should be remembered that although the circulation is depicted in terms of the right and left heart systems and the pulmonary circulation, all portions of the circulatory system comprise one complete circuit. Each portion of the circuit is dependent on the other to maintain the cardiac output. For example, the stroke volume of the left ventricle is dependent on the amount of blood received from the pulmonary circulation, which in turn is dependent on the blood received from the right ventricle. Thus anything that interferes with the venous return or pulmonary blood flow will result in an insufficient stroke volume and cardiac output.

The wall of the heart is composed of three layers, the innermost of which is the endocardium; the outer covering is the pericardium. The middle muscular layer, or myocardium, is considerably thicker in the left ventricle than in the right because the left ventricle pumps blood into a high-pressure system. Normally the ventricles provide the main force in the movement of blood, and the atria primarily serve as reservoirs.

The heart is a rhythmically contracting organ that regularly ejects blood into the pulmonary and systemic arterial circulations. The general route of circulation, layers of the heart, and essential structures are depicted in Figures 44-1 and 44-2. Alteration in one part of the heart may directly or indirectly affect the function of other parts, including the pumping mechanism. For example, openings in the septum may be caused by failure of the interatrial or interventricular septum to close in the developing embryo. Septal defects, especially those of the ventricular septum, allow for mixing of arterial and venous blood and further subject the right ventricle to increased pressure. When combined with another anomaly, such as pulmonic stenosis or right ventricular hypertrophy, a ventricular septal defect is a cause of cyanotic heart disease or the so-called "blue baby." Septal defects predispose to failure of the pumping mechanism or heart failure, with the result of an insufficient cardiac output to meet the metabolic needs of the body.

The Cardiac Valves

The cardiac valves are flaplike structures that derive from the endocardial lining of the heart. The normal valves serve as mechanical structures that permit the blood to flow in only the forward direction through the heart and great vessels. The valves are shaped and arranged so that the pressure of blood flow in the forward direction causes the valves to open, and pressure in the backward direction on the valves from the presence of blood in a chamber or a vessel causes the valves to close.

Four valves are of importance to the normal functioning of the heart. Figures 44-1, 44-2, 44-3, and 44-4 depict the valvular structures and locations. The cuspid, or atrioventricular (AV), valves are located

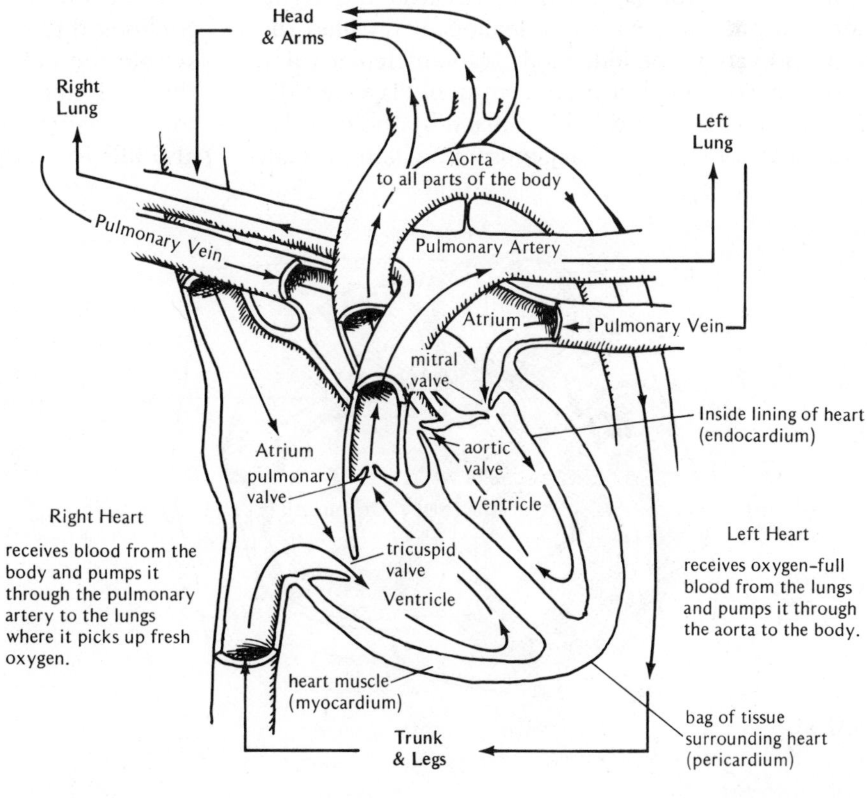

Figure 44-1. Diagram of the human heart, the veins and arteries entering and leaving it, and the route of circulation through and to parts of the body as indicated by arrows. (Information adapted with permission of the American Heart Association from *Your Heart and How It Works.*)

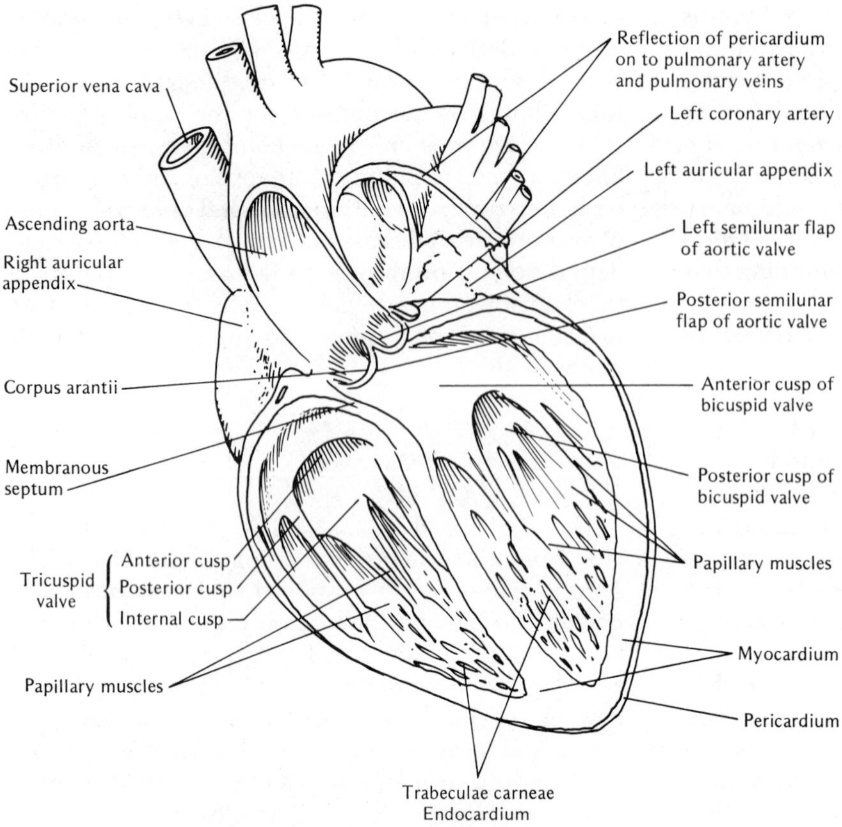

Figure 44-2. The heart seen from the front with the ventricles exposed. (Modified from Toldt. Information adapted with permission of Macmillan Publishing Co., Inc., from *Anatomy and Physiology.* 15th ed., Fig. 13-6, p. 389, by Diana Clifford Kimber, Carolyn E. Gray, Caroline E. Stackpole, and Lutie C. Leavell. Copyright © The Macmillan Company, 1966.)

between the atria and ventricles. The cuspid valve on the right side of the heart has three leaflets held in place by fibrous cords called the chordae tendineae, which in turn are anchored to the ventricular wall by the papillary muscles. Because the right-sided cuspid valve has three leaflets, it is called the tricuspid valve. The left-sided atrioventricular valve is a bicuspid valve but more commonly is called the mitral valve. It, too, is held in place by the chordae tendineae and the papillary muscles, which prevent valvular inversion into the atrium during systole. During closure of the cuspid valves there is a degree of leaflet overlapping that helps prevent the backward flow of blood.

The semilunar valves, which lie between the ventricles and the great vessels, are cup shaped. During systole the pressure of the inflowing blood collapses the cusps and thereby opens the valves. During diastole, however, the retrograde filling of the vessels also fills the cusps, bringing the edges into contact.

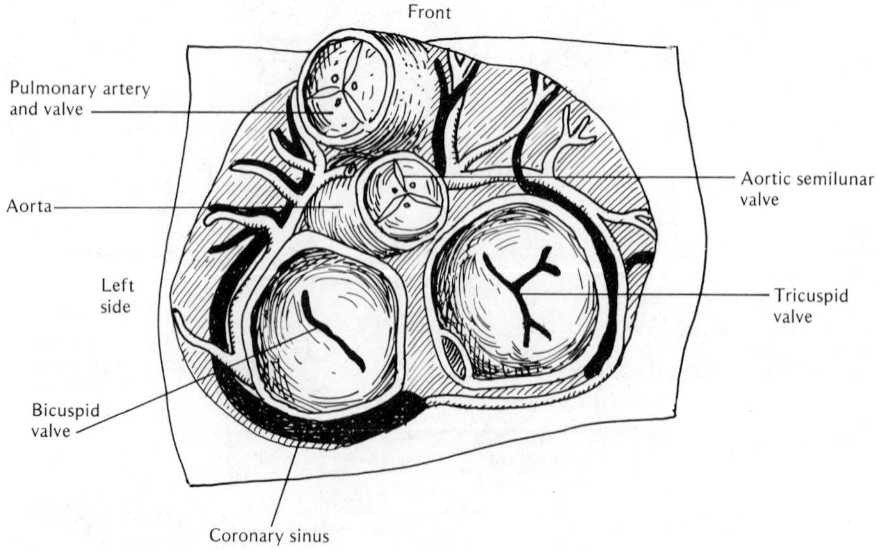

Figure 44-3. Valves of the heart as seen from a transverse view, atria removed. (Information adapted with permission of Macmillan Publishing Co., Inc., from *Anatomy and Physiology,* 15th ed., Fig. 13-8, p. 391, by Diana Clifford Kimber, Carolyn E. Gray, Caroline E. Stackpole, and Lutie C. Leavell. Copyright © The Macmillan Company, 1966.)

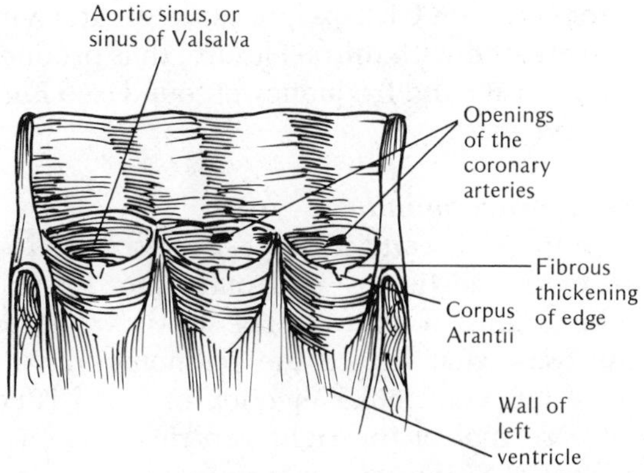

Figure 44-4. The aortic valve: sagittal dissection to show the aortic semilunar valve. The sinuses of Valsalva are three pouches or slight dilatations that are located between the semilunar valves and the wall of the aorta. These sinuses are also found on the pulmonary artery between the semilunar valves and the wall of the artery. Note the coronary ostium and the cup shape of the aortic valve leaflets. (Information adapted with permission of Macmillan Publishing Co., Inc., from *Anatomy and Physiology,* 14th ed. Fig. 225, p. 314, by Diana Clifford Kimber, Carolyn E. Gray, Caroline E. Stackpole, and Lutie C. Leavell. Copyright © The Macmillan Company, 1961.)

Thus the pulmonic and aortic semilunar valves close. Unlike the atrioventricular valves, there is no overlapping of the semilunar valve cusp edges; however, they do act to prevent retrograde flow from the aorta and pulmonary artery into the ventricles during diastole.

Valvular Defects

As a result of malformation, injury, or disease, the valvular leaflets of the atrioventricular or semilunar valves may no longer close tightly or open fully. When a valve does not close properly, it is said to be insufficient or incompetent. In lay terms, the valve "leaks." When a valve does not open fully because its orifice is narrowed or constricted, the valve is said to be "stenosed." Because valves have two or more leaflets (commissures), a valve can be both insufficient and stenosed at the same time. Deformities of the cardiac valves, which result in dysfunction, can be of a congenital or acquired origin.

Congenital Defects

Congenital valvular defects in association with other congenital cardiac defects, such as ventricular septal defect, are relatively common. Valvular deformities, however, may occur as isolated malformations. The most common are pulmonic and aortic stenosis. Congenital stenosis or insufficiency of the mitral or tricuspid valve and pulmonic insufficiency are relatively rare.

Stenosis of the pulmonic valve is recognized as one of the more common congenital cardiac abnormalities representing 10 to 12 per cent of congenital heart disease (Friedberg, 1966, p. 1230). Pulmonic stenosis denotes an impediment to blood flow from the right ventricle to the pulmonary artery. The narrowing may be at the level of the valve leaflets, subvalvular at the infundibulum, or supravalvular in the pulmonary artery. The essential hemodynamic disturbance is an increased right ventricular pressure resulting from diminished flow through the pulmonic orifice. The right ventricular hypertension leads to chamber hypertrophy and eventually right ventricular failure with a diminished cardiac output. The age for surgical intervention depends on several factors but is primarily determined by the degree of stenosis and consequent systolic pressure gradient across the valve. Although surgical intervention may take place in infancy, some procedures may take place later in life. Surgical intervention is generally effective and consists of direct enlargement of the stenotic orifice through open heart procedures.

The location of congenital aortic stenosis may also be valvular, subvalvular, or supravalvular. The flow of blood is impeded from the left ventricle through a constricted passage to the ascending aorta and systemic arterial circulation. Depending on the degree of narrowing, the hemodynamic effects may vary from no significant disturbance in circulatory dynamics to a significantly reduced cardiac output. Normally there is no systolic pressure gradient across the aortic valve. This writer can recall a 100 mm Hg systolic pressure gradient across the aortic valve in a 5-year-old boy with subvalvular aortic stenosis. The systolic pressure in the aorta was 90 mm Hg, whereas in the left ventricle it was 190 mm Hg. Clinical manifestations from a decreased cardiac output were absent at rest but present during activity. There was evidence of left ventricular hypertrophy and heart failure was feared; therefore surgical excision by open heart technique was done of the hypertrophied tissue in the left ventricular outflow tract that created the obstruction.

Acquired Defects

The most common acquired valvular defects affect the mitral and aortic valves where both stenosis and insufficiency are noted. Acquired tricuspid and pulmonic valvular defects are extremely rare. The most common of the valvular defects are sequelae of the rheumatic fever process to be discussed subsequently. These defects fall into the category of rheumatic heart disease and include both mitral stenosis and insufficiency, and aortic stenosis and insufficiency. Despite the etiology of the valvular defect, the seriousness depends on the degree of "leakiness" or obstruction of the valve, and on its location.

Auscultation of Heart Sounds

One of the major cues to valvular dysfunction is an alteration in the normal heart sounds as detected by auscultation of the heart. Traditionally, the nurse has utilized the stethoscope for determinations of the blood pressure and apical pulse. With evolution of the professional nursing role, however, utilization of the stethoscope has come to include auscultation of the heart and lungs as one means to obtain a complete data base that aids in a comprehensive health assessment of the patient. Auscultation of the heart is performed by nurses not only on the cardiac patient but also on normal individuals as part of any initial health examination. It must be kept in mind that auscultation of the heart is only one component of the entire cardiac physical examination, which also includes inspection, palpation, and percussion of the precordium.

In recent years the nurse has rather dogmatically utilized a stethoscope with a flat diaphragm, which facilitates blood pressure measurement. When auscultation of the heart is performed, however, a stethoscope with both a bell and diaphragm is required. The bell accentuates low-pitched sounds when placed very lightly on the skin. The diaphragm, on the other hand, accentuates high-pitched sounds and should be pressed very firmly against the skin. For optimal auscultation the ear pieces should fit comfortably but snugly, to minimize extraneous sounds. The rubber tubing should be as short as feasible (preferably about 12 inches in length) to enhance sound conduction. A stethoscope with binary tubing from the ear pieces to the diaphragm-bell promotes better sound conduction.

Definition

Normal heart sounds heard with a stethoscope have been described in terms of "lub-dup, lub-dup. . . ." Heart sounds are audible vibrations in the ventricles and great vessels created by the *closure* of valves and the associated blood flow. It should be noted that it is *not* the closure of the valve leaflets per se that are the audible sounds. The opening of normal valves create no audible sounds.

First Heart Sound

The "lub," or first heart sound (S_1), is associated with closure of the mitral (M_1) and tricuspid (T_1) valves at the beginning of systole. As the pressures rise in the left and right ventricles because of atrial blood influx during diastole and during systolic contraction, the mitral and tricuspid valves are forced closed. The valves close *essentially simultaneously,* with the mitral valve closing slightly before the tricuspid. The mitral component of the first heart sound is greater than the tricuspid, because greater vibrations are created with mitral closure, thus producing greater intensity and frequency of sound (see Figure 44-5, A and B).

Second Heart Sound

The "dup," or second sound (S_2), is associated with closure of the aortic (A_2) and pulmonic (P_2) valves at the beginning of diastole. The aortic valve tends to close somewhat before the pulmonic valve because the left ventricular ejection of blood is complete before that of the right ventricle. The aortic component of S_2 is thus earlier and of greater intensity than the pulmonic component (see Figure 44-5, A and B).

Timing-Intensity

S_1 marks the beginning of systole and S_2 occurs at the beginning of diastole. A critical concept to be mastered when learning about heart sounds is the timing of the heart sounds in relation to the cardiac cycle. The period of time between S_1 and S_2 represents *ventricular systole.* The period of time between S_2 and S_1 represents *ventricular diastole.* Under conditions of a normal or a slow heart rate, the time interval between S_1 and S_2 will be *shorter* than between S_2 and S_1 (see Figure 44-5A).

The intensity of a heart sound depends on two factors: (1) the *position* of the valve leaflets at the onset of systole, and (2) the *rate and amount of pressure rise* in the ventricles during diastole. For example, louder sounds are heard when (1) a valve is wide open at the beginning of systole, (2) a ventricle fills rapidly and the valve closes suddenly, and (3) the pressure is greater than in a corresponding chamber/vessel. Softer than normal sounds are produced when the converse is true. When heart sounds are depicted graphically, the height of the bar in relation to the other bars represents the intensity of the sound.

Split Heart Sounds

Valve closure normally is slightly asynchronous. When, however, the asynchronism is such that one valve of a pair closes definitively before the other, two distinct components of a single heart sound can be heard. This phenomenon is known as a *split heart sound.*

A split heart sound may be a normal or pathologic phenomenon depending on (1) which sound is split, (2) the amount of time between the split components, and (3) the relation of the split sound to the respiratory cycle. Splitting of S_2 may be normal, whereas a split S_1 is rarely normal. The time intervals between the components of the S_1 normally are too small to be audible or are shorter than the time inter-

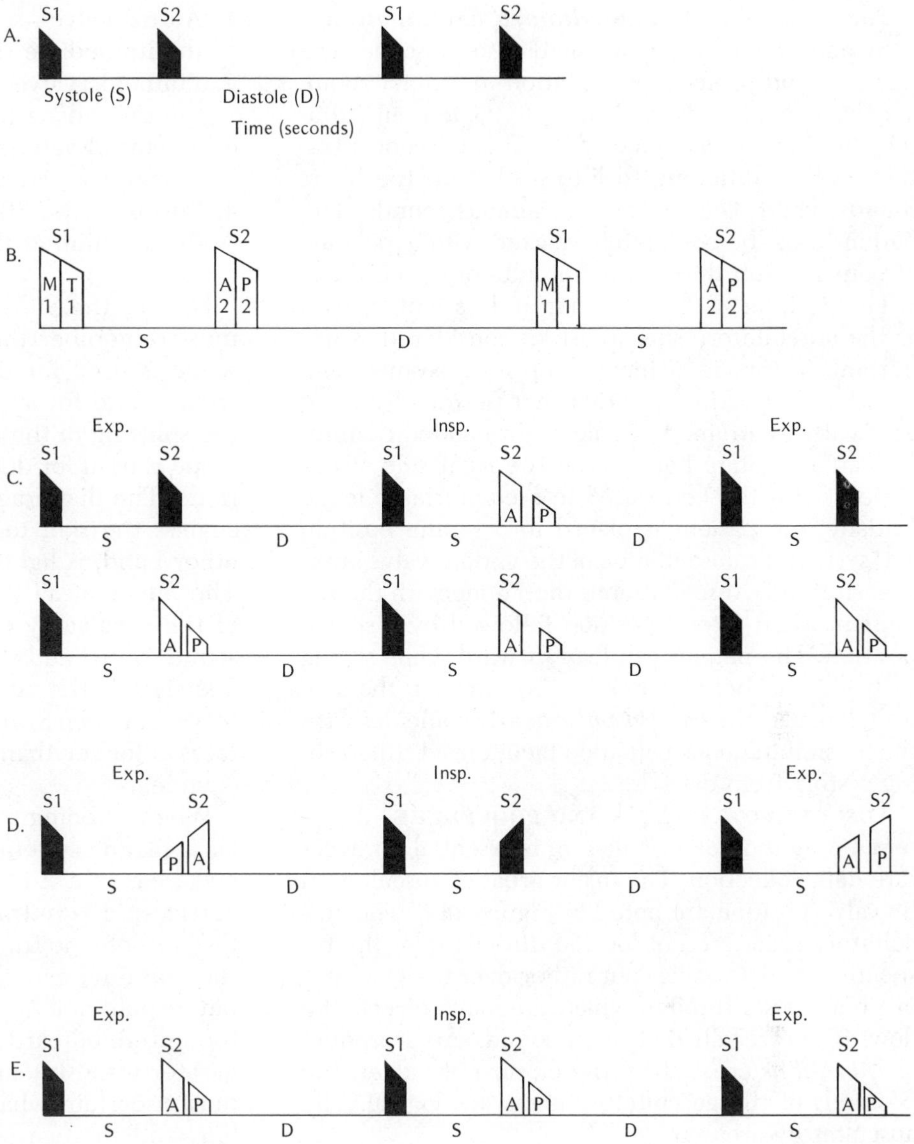

Figure 44-5. Schematic representation of the normal, and selected alterations in the normal, heart sounds. A. *Normal heart sounds:* Note that the time between the first (S1) and second (S2) heart sounds is when ventricular systole (S) occurs and is of shorter duration than between S2 and S1 when ventricular diastole (D) occurs. B. *Components of the normal heart sounds:* Vibrations created by closure of the mitral (M1) and the tricuspid (T1) valves comprise S1, while closure of the aortic (A2) and pulmonic (P2) valves comprise S2. The height of the vertical bar represents the relative intensity of the components. C. *Physiologic splitting of S2:* Asynchronous closure of A2 and P2 noted only during inspiration, or asynchronous closure of A2 and P2 which is of longer duration during inspiration than during expiration. D. *Paradoxical splitting of S2:* Asynchronous closure of A2 and P2 noted only during expiration. Note the reversed order of valve closure where P2 precedes A2. A. *Fixed splitting of S2:* Asynchronous closure of S2 during the entire respiratory cycle. Note that the difference between the second type of physiologic splitting and fixed splitting is difficult to discern and in large part is guided by other clinical manifestations.

val between the components of the S_2. Thus, judgment that a time interval between split components is longer than normal is relative to the *other* heart sound and to the heart rate. The slower the heart rate, the greater the splitting interval.

The S_2 normally is influenced by respiration. Inasmuch as closure of the pulmonic valve is influenced by the timing and amount of blood received from the right ventricle, which in turn is dependent on the venous return during the respiratory cycle, it is reasonable that respiration can likewise influence splitting of the S_2. During inspiration there is a larger amount of blood returned to the right atrium-ventricle, and thus ejected into the pulmonary artery, than during expiration. An increased volume of blood to be ejected into the pulmonary artery takes a longer period of time and thus delays closure of the pulmonic valve in diastole. Hence, P_2 follows A_2 with a time interval in between the two components; a *physiologic splitting* which is a normal phenomenon (see Figure 44-5C).

Two other types of a split S_2 are associated with various kinds of cardiac pathology. When closure of the aortic valve is delayed, as in aortic stenosis, P_2 will precede A_2 and the split will be heard best during expiration. This type of split S_2 is known as *paradoxical splitting* (see Figure 44-5D). In certain types of congenital heart disorders, such as atrial septal defect, the split S_2 is unaffected by the respiratory cycle and is always present. This type of split S_2 is known as *fixed splitting.*

Except in the circumstance of a very slow heart rate, a split S_1 usually is associated with some alteration in cardiac function. It should be remembered that both S_1 and S_2, and variations thereof, are heard best with the *diaphragm* portion of a stethoscope.

Facilitation of the Auscultatory Examination

In addition to using a reliable stethoscope, the nurse should preform auscultation in a quiet room, as extraneous sounds can obliterate the true auscultatory findings. It also takes great mental concentration and conditioning to listen solely to the heart sounds while blocking out extraneous sounds. The patient must be completely relaxed with avoidance of conversation during the auscultatory procedure.

The position of the examiner and patient, as well as the auscultatory sites, must be considered as important factors in achieving optimal results. The nurse should be in a position that permits listening ease without strain. As a rule, right-handed examiners can auscultate better if on the right side of the patient with the bed raised to a comfortable level. Initially, the patient is placed in a supine position and systematic auscultation of the various valve areas is performed. Auscultation is then done with the patient in a left lateral position followed by a sitting position. The patient can lean forward while sitting to bring the heart closer to the anterior thoracic wall. Because the *carotid pulse* nearly coincides with the S_1, simultaneous palpation facilitates distinguishing systole from diastole.

AUSCULTATORY AREAS AND PROCEDURE. A systematic method of auscultation is essential for accurate data collection. The major areas of auscultation by valve position are noted in Figure 44-6. The auscultatory areas are not located directly over the respective cardiac valves but rather over the chamber or great vessel through which the valve directs the flow. If one recalls that heart sounds are a product of *vibrations* created by the closure of valves, the positions of the auscultatory areas are logical. The auscultatory areas are

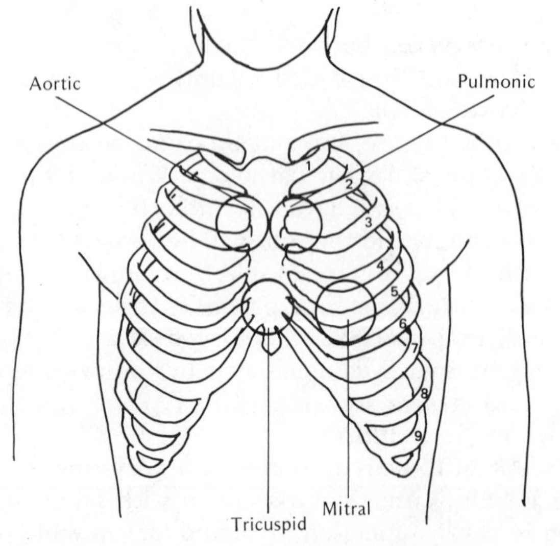

Figure 44-6. Major areas of cardiac auscultation by anatomic position of the valves.

1. Aortic valve—second right intercostal space to the immediate right of the sternum
2. Pulmonic valve—second left intercostal space to the immediate left of the sternum
3. Tricuspid valve—fifth intercostal space over the sternum superior to the xiphoid process
4. Mitral valve—fifth intercostal space to the left of the sternum at the midclavicular line

During the auscultatory examination, the nurse must remember that the diaphragm of the stethoscope is used for determination of heart rate and rhythm and for auscultation of S_1 and S_2 as well as the splitting of those sounds. The bell of the stethoscope is used for detection of extra sounds and murmurs. The diaphragm, when used, is firmly applied against the skin to obtain a seal. The bell, on the other hand, is lightly applied, to obtain an air seal. The nurse, at all times, must have a mental image of the cardiac cycle to determine when the heart sounds occur and the intervals between the sounds. Specifically, the nurse should remember that the interval between S_2 and S_1 (diastole), with normal heart rates is longer than the interval between S_1 and S_2 (systole).

When listening to the heart sounds in each valvular area, one systematically moves between contiguous areas in a Z-fashion, that is, aortic → pulmonic → tricuspid → mitral or vice versa, while "inching" the stethoscope from one area to the next. Whereas the examiner can progress from the mitral → tricuspid → pulmonic → mitral areas, it may be best for the untrained ear to progress from the lesser to the greater intensity and then back again. The listener must ascertain what is the best pattern for him or her, and this varies from individual to individual.

The general procedure for auscultation is (1) with patient in the supine position, place the diaphragm of the stethoscope over the aortic or mitral valvular area and count the heart *rate;* (2) ascertain whether the rhythm is regular or irregular; (3) auscultate for the normal S_1-S_2 sounds in a Z-fashion from area to area; (4) auscultate for the splitting of sounds in the same areas; and (5) change to the bell of the stethoscope and listen in each of the same valvular areas for abnormal sounds. The procedure is repeated for both normal and abnormal sounds with the patient in the left lateral and sitting-leaning forward positions. The latter two positions promote gravity pull of the heart close to the thoracic wall for amplification of sounds.

When learning and mastering the skills of auscultation, the nurse may listen for longer periods of time and in many areas of the precordium two to three times. Patients' perception of this act, unless otherwise informed, vary from, "There must be something terribly wrong with me because the nurse listened in sixteen *different* places." to "What a *thorough* examination I had with the many places and length of time the nurse listened." Prior to engaging in the auscultation process, the inexperienced listeners should inform the patient they are learning and less experienced in the process and will therefore take a longer period of time and listen in "more areas" but this does not mean that something is "wrong" with the patient. As time progresses and the nurse becomes more proficient with the process, "short-cuts" can be employed, such as listening in the same valvular area for normal and abnormal sounds as well as rate and rhythm all at one time.

It should be remembered that the S_1 usually is louder than S_2 at the mitral area, or apex of the heart. Similarly S_2 is usually louder than S_1 at the aortic area, or base of the heart. The nurse must record all observations of the auscultation process, however detailed they may be. Optimal auscultation entails listening to each component of the heart sounds and cardiac cycle independently with deep concentration and based on substanial knowledge.

Abnormal Sounds

The possibilities for variations in heart sounds are numerous including alterations in the normal components as well as the formation of additional sounds. A summarization of abnormal sounds includes the following:

1. *Split S_1*. Asynchronous closure of the atrioventricular valves whereby the mitral and tricuspid components can be identified individually. A split S_1 can best be heard at the lower left sternal border in the tricuspid area. (See Figure 44-7A.)
2. *Split S_2*. Asynchronous closure of the semilunar valves whereby the aortic and pulmonic components can be identified individually. *Physiologic splitting* occurs normally during inspiration. *Paradoxical splitting* occurs when aortic valve closure is delayed and is heard during expiration. *Fixed splitting occurs* when the sound is unaffected by respiration.

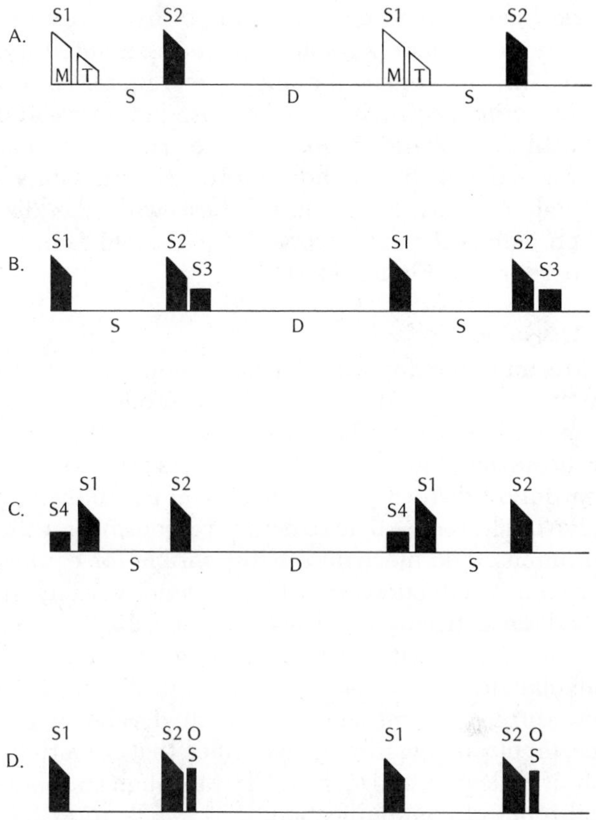

Figure 44-7. Schematic representation of selected abnormal heart sounds. A. *Split S1:* Asynchronous closure of the mitral (M1) and tricuspid (T1) valves. B. *Third heart sound (S3):* An extra sound heard in early diastole following S2. Note that an S3 can be differentiated from a split S2 by its intensity and auscultatory area. C. *Fourth heart sound (S4):* An extra sound heard in late diastole preceding S1. Note that an S4 can be differentiated from a split S1 by its intensity and auscultatory area. D. *Opening snap (OS):* An extra sound heard in early diastole following S2. Note that an OS can be differentiated from an S3 or split S2 by its intensity, pitch, and auscultatory area.

3. *S_3*. A third heart sound that may be auscultated in early diastole following S_2. It is also known as a "ventricular diastolic gallop," and results from vibrations created by filling of the left ventricular chamber when blood is still present from incomplete ventricular emptying. An S_3 may be heard normally in children and young adults. In older adults, however, it is more frequently associated with left ventricular failure. The S_3 is a dull, low-frequency sound heard best with the bell of the stethoscope in the apical area and the patient in the left lateral recumbent position. The S_3 has been characterized as sounding like "Ken-tuc'-ky" or "lubb-tup'-puh." An S_3 can be distinquished from the second component of a split S_2 by its lesser intensity. It is heard best at the apex. (See Figure 44-7B.)
4. *A fourth heart sound* that may be auscultated in late diastole immediately preceding S_1. It is also known as an "atrial diastolic gallop" and is a result of increased resistance to ventricular filling caused either by a change in chamber compliance or by an increase in the filling volume. The S_4 is a soft, low-frequency sound heard best with the bell of the stethoscope while the patient is in the supine position. Whereas an individual may have both an S_3 and S_4, one need not have an S_3 prior to or in combination with an S_4. The S_4 has been characterized as sounding like "Ten-

nes'-see." An S_4 can be distinguished from the first component of a split S_1 by its lesser intensity. It is heard best at the apex (see Figure 44-7C).

5. *Opening snap.* An abnormal sound associated with the *opening* of an inflexible atrioventricular valve that is heard shortly after S_2. It is a brief, high-intensity sound heard best with the diaphragm of the stethoscope at the lower left sternal border (see Figure 44-7D).

Murmurs

Murmurs are abnormal cardiac sounds generated by the flow of blood. The blood flow produces vibrations within the cardiac chambers or in the walls of the adjacent great vessels. Murmurs are generally heard most distinctly over the area of the individual valve or altered cardiac structure responsible for the vibrations. The mechanisms responsible for cardiac murmur production are (1) increased velocity of blood flow through normal or abnormal cardiac valves; (2) forward blood flow through a constricted valvular orifice; (3) backward or regurgitant blood flow through an insufficient or dilated valvular orifice; (4) blood flow through an orifice that has a rigid, vibrating leaflet; and (5) blood flow through an abnormal route of communication.

Among the various characteristics of cardiac murmurs are those relating to the *timing, intensity, pitch, quality,* and *location* of the murmur. Timing relates to when the murmur occurs during the cardiac cycle. Murmurs occur in either the systolic or diastolic phase of the cardiac cycle and hence the terms systolic or diastolic murmurs. Systolic murmurs are heard between S_1 and S_2, whereas diastolic murmurs occur between S_2 and S_1. It should be remembered that normally the intervals between the heart sounds are entirely silent. Further murmurs occur during the *early, mid,* or *late* phases of systole or diastole or throughout all phases. One that persists throughout all phases bears the prefix *holo-* or *pan-*, for example holosystolic. A murmur that begins in late diastole and extends through the beginning of systole is called a *presystolic* murmur. An *ejection murmur* is one which begins after S_1, peaks in midsystole, and terminates before S_2.

The intensity of murmur relates to its loudness and characteristic pattern. The intensity of murmurs has been graded to aid in standardization of a murmur's significance. The most widely accepted schema grades murmurs from I through VI. Grade I and II murmurs are heard faintly and usually have little hemodynamic significance. Grade III and IV murmurs are considered intermediate but hemodynamically significant. Grade V and VI murmurs are heard loudly with or even without a stethoscope, and are considered very significant hemodynamically. With this system of intensity of grading, the progress of a given murmur can be followed over a period of time and correlations made with the severity of clinical manifestations. Some murmurs assume a characteristic pattern or shape as related to its loudness. Some characteristic patterns are depicted in Figure 44-8. A murmur which increases in intensity after onset is a *crescendo* murmur. Conversely, one that decreases in intensity after onset is a *decrescendo* murmur. A murmur whose first portion is crescendo and whose latter portion is decrescendo is a *diamond-shaped* murmur. A murmur whose intensity is constant is called a *plateau-like* murmur.

The pitch of a murmur is described as *high* (sharp) or *low* (dull) whereas the quality of a murmur is described as *rumbling, harsh, musical* or *blowing.* The location of a murmur refers to from what auscultatory area the murmur is heard best and where, if anywhere, the murmur radiates. Certain valvular defects have characteristic "radiation" patterns. Radiation means the murmur is heard concomitantly in another area although it may be of lesser intensity. It does not imply a wavelike form. In aortic stenosis, the murmur tends to radiate to the apex of the heart and the neck, whereas in mitral insufficiency radiation occurs to the left axilla.

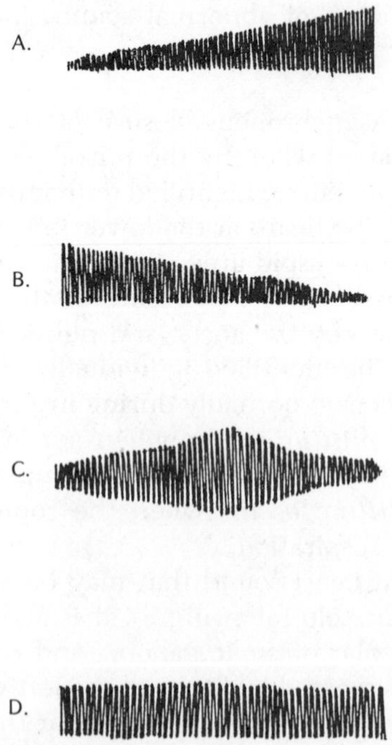

Figure 44-8. Schematic representation of selected patterns of murmurs. A. *Crescendo:* A murmur that increases in intensity from onset. B. *Decrescendo:* A murmur that decreases in intensity from onset. C. *Diamond-shaped:* A murmur that increases in intensity from onset, reaches a peak, and then decreases in intensity. D. *Plateau-like:* A murmur whereby the intensity remains constant.

In the final analysis, the detection and description of murmurs provide yet another form of data from which a comprehensive assessment of the cardiac patient is made. Unfortunately, some patients' perception of the meaning of a murmur is that the individual is now an invalid; a parent, for example, may tend to overprotect a child. Unfortunately, this even occurs with *functional (physiologic, innocent) murmurs* which are nonpathologic, due to high velocity blood flow, and usually diminish by puberty. This points out the need for education of the patient and/or the parent about "What is a heart murmur?" and "What are the implications of a heart murmur?" To refine and reinforce the reader's knowledge and understanding of murmurs, the reader is referred to two excellent programmed instruction units in the *American Journal of Nursing* (Mechner, 1977; Adler, 1977).

Cardiac Inspection and Palpation

The cardiac examination is not complete without inspection and palpation of the thorax as related to cardiac activity. In fact, inspection and palpation commonly precede the auscultatory process because some of the findings provide data about what to anticipate and look for during auscultation. A single cardiac cycle produces not only a measurable blood pressure, a palpable arterial pulse, a visible venous pulse, and audible heart sounds but palpable heart sounds as well as visible and palpable precordial movements. Because all these phenomena are the result of a single cardiac event, they should be included in the data base.

Inspection and palpation of the precordium is accomplished with the patient in a supine position at a 45° angle. Inspection is followed by palpation using the palmar surface of the hand. The primary aim of palpation is to confirm the findings of inspection; if one is unable to see a movement, sometimes it can be felt. Palpation also gives an impression of the force of cardiac contraction.

The areas of the thorax which are inspected for *pulsations* and then palpated are the (1) aortic—second left intercostal space immediate to the sternum, (2) pulmonic—second right intercostal space immediate to the sternum, (3) right ventricular—fourth left intercostal space immediate to the sternum, (4) left ventricular (Point of Maximal Impulse, apical impulse, apex beat)—fifth left intercostal space, midclavicular line, and (5) epigastrium. Terms used to describe the cardiac movements as seen and felt are *heaves, lifts, snaps,* and *thrills.*

When blood flows through a constricted area, such as a valve orifice or blood vessel, turbulence and eddies are created in the blood stream beyond the point of constriction that cause vibrations. These vibrations are felt as *thrills* and heard as murmurs. Thrills are best palpated when the patient blows out his or her breath and holds it.

Accentuated cardiac activity in the aortic and pulmonic areas are most commonly associated with valvular dysfunction. Increased activity in the right ventricular area may be associated with hypertrophy or a ventricular septal defect as examples. Examples of reasons for increased left ventricular activity are valvular dysfunction and hypertrophy.

The point of maximal impulse (PMI) is the point where the heart sound are heard the loudest and where the apical beat is frequently visible, especially in thin-chested individuals. Visibility occurs because during systole the movements of the heart push the cardiac apex against the anterior chest wall. It should be noted that the PMI may not be visible in obese patients or those with chest cage abnormalities as seen in kyphoscoliosis or emphysema. In the male this point is generally below the left nipple (Figure 44-6). Displacement of the PMI to the left and to the sixth left intercostal space toward the anterior axillary line is noted with marked enlargement of the left ventricle. This is exemplified in hypertensive cardiovascular disease and left ventricular failure. For continued study and refinement of cardiac inspection-palpation findings, the reader is referred to the *American Journal of Nursing* programmed instruction unit (Mechner, 1976).

Rheumatic Fever

Rheumatic fever is an acute or chronic inflammatory process which occurs as a sequelae of group A beta-hemolytic streptococcal infections. Although authorities are not certain of the specific etiology, it is generally agreed that rheumatic fever follows infections caused by the group A hemolytic streptococci. It has been demonstrated, however, that the streptococci are not in lesions of rheumatic fever, and the organism may or may not be recovered from the nose and throat at the time of the onset of the disease. Even when streptococci are found and eradicated by antimicrobial therapy, the course of rheumatic fever is not altered.

There is considerable evidence to suggest that the relationship between streptococcal infections and rheumatic fever is in part an antigen-antibody response. Factors to substantiate this theory are that the incubation period between the initial streptococcal infection and the development of rheumatic fever is of a sufficient duration for antibodies to be formed. Also there is an increased susceptibility to subsequent recurrent attacks of rheumatic fever with a shortened time period between the exposure to the streptococcal infection and the symptoms of rheumatic fever. According to Sellers, rheumatic fever may represent an immunologic accident in that the streptococcus acts as the original source of antigen, but an immunologically similar tissue antigen becomes the target of the antibodies (Sellers, 1970, p. 741).

The term *rheumatic fever* is derived from the manifestations resulting from inflammation of the joints. Pathology, however, is not limited to the joints nor is inflammation of the joints the most serious effect. The areas of focal inflammation are widely scattered throughout the body and have a special predilection for connective tissues. The inflammatory process predominantly affects the heart, and the small blood vessels are extensively involved. Although there are multiple manifestations of the disease, the most serious clinical implications are those of the heart.

One or all three tissue layers of the heart can be involved with rheumatic fever. With endocardial involvement, there is edema of the valve leaflets followed by secondary erosion and deposits of beadlike vegetation along the line of closure of the cusps. This involvement can extend into the chordae tendineae. All valves can be involved, and in decreasing frequency, they are the mitral, aortic, tricuspid, and pulmonic valves.

When the myocardium is affected, the characteristic lesions known as Aschoff bodies are seen. Aschoff bodies are nodules that form secondary to degeneration of collagen in the connective tissue. As the nodules age, they become fibrous and cause damage to the media of the arteries in the myocardium. Lesions similar to Aschoff bodies occur wherever the connective tissue components are found.

Rheumatic pericarditis is characterized by a serous and fibrinous exudate in the pericardial sac. Depending on the volume of exudate, a pericardial effusion can be present of sufficient magnitude to prevent venous inflow to the heart.

The exact incidence of rheumatic fever is not known, and estimates vary. Approximately 3 per cent of individuals having streptococcal infections develop rheumatic fever, with the greatest incidence between the ages of 5 and 15 years. Rarely is the process noted in persons below 2 years or over 30 years of age. Thirty to 50 per cent of the individuals who experience one attack of rheumatic fever will have one or more recurrences. Although the incidence of rheumatic fever is believed to be declining because of better detection and therapy of streptococcal infections, rheumatic fever remains an important disease among children and adults.

Among the predisposing factors of rheumatic fever are age, overcrowding, heredity, diet, and climate. Socioeconomic conditions appear to influence the likelihood of developing rheumatic fever as the incidence is highest among the lower socioeconomic groups. A lower incidence is noted in the higher income brackets. Associated with a low income are overcrowded living conditions. Overcrowding increases the opportunity for the transmission of infectious agents as several persons might sleep in the same room; thus the intensity and duration of exposure to the streptococcus for noninfected persons would be greater. In addition, with several people living in crowded quarters, there is little possibility of isolating the sick.

When the income is limited, the nutritional status of children may be inferior to that of children of a more affluent background. It is speculated that susceptibility to rheumatic fever may be increased by inadequate nutrition during early life.

A history of rheumatic fever in the family of an affected child is not uncommon. There may be a genetic basis for this. According to Sellers, studies have shown that the occurrence of rheumatic fever in children with rheumatic parents was consistent with a genetic mechanism of recessive inheritance (1970, p. 471). Another factor that appears to predispose an individual to rheumatic fever is climate. The incidence is believed to be higher in colder than in warmer climates.

The following points about the nature of rheumatic fever are useful in anticipating its clinical manifestations: (1) it is a febrile disease, (2) it is not limited to a single organ, and (3) the focal inflammatory lesions are distributed throughout the body in the mesenchymal connective tissues. The clinical manifestations can vary greatly both in variety and degree of intensity. The major manifestations are fever, polyarthritis, carditis, chorea, subcutaneous nodules, abdominal pain, and skin lesions. As with most febrile disorders, anorexia, weight loss, fatigability, and weakness can be present.

Polyarthritis is more common in the older child and adult; however, mild forms of joint pain can be present in the young child, whose complaints are frequently dismissed as "growing pains." It can be manifested in degrees of pain, varying from vague to severe, associated with acutely inflamed and swollen joints. Although the degree of pain can be slight, in some patients it is so severe that actions resulting in jarring or movement of the bed are unbearable. Among the characteristic features of the arthritis associated with rheumatic fever is that it tends to involve one joint or area at a time and to be migratory. It involves predominantly large joints such as the knees, elbows, wrists, and shoulders; however, small ones can also be involved. Fortunately the lesions of the joints are completely reversible.

As should be expected in view of the widespread involvement of connective and vascular tissues, lesions of the skin and subcutaneous tissues develop in about 25 per cent of the patients with rheumatic fever. The lesions are known as *erythema marginatum* or *circinatum, erythema nodosum,* and *subcutaneous nodules.* The lesions of erythema marginatum are red and circular. Because adjacent lesions tend to coalesce, they form larger lesions with an irregular outline. They are usually flat (macular), although some may be slightly raised (papular). The skin lesions rarely cause discomfort, although occasionally itching may be present.

Erythema nodosum is believed to be a manifestation of acute rheumatic fever. The relationship is questionable because the nodules are sometimes present when other manifestations of rheumatic fever are minimal or lacking. These lesions, which are dull red nodules, occur most frequently on the extensor surfaces of the extremities. Unlike the lesions of erythema marginatum, those of erythema nodosum are tender to touch, and the discomfort is increased with movement.

Subcutaneous nodules are firm insensitive lesions occurring over bony prominences of the various joints and tendons of the extremities. They are more frequently observed in patients with a serious form of rheumatic fever and those who have severe heart damage.

During the acute phase of rheumatic fever, the patient will usually have few symptoms indicating cardiac involvement, particularly if this is the first attack. Even though all three layers of the heart can be involved, most of the abnormal findings indicate myocardial and pericardial involvement. Endocardial involvement is not readily demonstrated during the acute phase even though scarring and distortion of the valve leaflets may be beginning. This could lead to permanent valvular heart disease.

Chorea (Sydenham's chorea, St. Vitus dance) is characterized by marked involuntary contractions of the skeletal muscles caused by central nervous system involvement. Although it is not easily described, one of the outstanding features of movement in chorea is its purposelessness. At the onset of chorea, the child may appear to be awkward and careless. He or she spills food when trying to eat and drops his or her school books and other objects. As the manifestations become more severe, the purposeless movements may be ascribed to nervousness. Eventually the movements may become so severe as to be incapacitating. Chorea may be the sole manifestation of rheumatic fever, and generally it occurs late in the course of the disease.

There is no specific laboratory test that is diagnostic of rheumatic fever. The tests that provide the most assistance are ones used to measure antibodies to streptococcal antigens. The antistreptolysin O titer will indicate if a person has had a recent streptococcal infection, but it will not differentiate between a streptococcal infection and rheumatic fever. The results of this test will be elevated in a very large per cent of rheumatic fever cases. Other laboratory data that would be elevated are the erythrocyte sedimentation rate, C-reactive protein, and lactic dehydrogenase, if carditis is present.

Just as the degree and range of possible manifestations in rheumatic fever are highly variable so is the course of the disease. Some individuals recover in 3 or 4 weeks, whereas others have some degree of rheumatic activity that persists for weeks, months, or a lifetime. People rarely die during the first attack unless they have a fulminating form of the disease in which death can ensue within a few days or weeks. Although some individuals recover completely from the first attack and never have another, one attack usually predisposes to subsequent recurrences. The extent of cardiac damage during the first attack is frequently minimal, but with each subsequent attack, the degree and permanence of cardiac damage increases.

The intervention for rheumatic fever is directed toward the alleviation of symptoms and the prevention of cardiac damage. An important aspect of preventing cardiac damage is the prevention of recurrent streptococcal infections. Today mail-in throat cultures can be done to diagnose streptococcus. The disadvantage is that if a streptococcal infection is present, treatment should be initiated before the results would be back.

Traditionally bedrest is prescribed for the duration of the acute disease process. Currently some physicians are modifying this practice and permitting greater degrees of activity because controlled studies have not proved the value of prolonged bedrest. Bedrest decreases the metabolism while the infection and fever are present as well as decreasing the cardiac workload. It may be difficult for the patient to accept prolonged bedrest, as therapeutic measures will eliminate the subjective symptoms of rheumatic fever even though the covert signs of carditis may be present. For the first 2 weeks of the acute phase, the patient is encouraged to be quiet and to have the activities of daily living performed for him or her. Gradually such activities as feeding, brushing the teeth, and combing the hair can be assumed by the patient. Depending on the degree of joint involvement and the physician's philosophy of care, bathroom privileges may be permitted once or twice a day.

Fatigue should be prevented regardless of whether the nurse performs an activity for the patient or the patient does the activity. When judging fatigue in the patient with acute rheumatic fever, the pulse is not a good parameter to use, as it could be elevated because of the febrile state or decreased because of salicylate therapy.

When the joints are painful, measures should be instituted to protect the patient from unnecessary discomfort. Bed linen should be supported with cradles so that the joints are protected from the linen's weight. Because the joints are not likely to be deformed by the disease process, the extremities can be supported in the position of most comfort. When handling the affected extremity, care should be taken to minimize movement of the joint by supporting both above and below the joint. Any therapeutic measures, such as the local applications of heat, should be carried out conscientiously, as they may afford the patient a measure of relief.

As with any febrile state, fluids will be lost through perspiration and the high rate of protein metabolism; thus the maintenance of an adequate fluid intake is important. Because of weakness and discomfort caused by the fever and pain, the appetite may be decreased. Ways of improving the appetite would be to include food the patient likes, to serve it attractively, and to provide socialization during meals. In addition to providing increased amounts of fluids, foods high in carbohydrate content should be included, for they have a protein-sparing effect.

In addition to bedrest (or modified activity), drugs are prescribed to eradicate the streptococcus organism and to relieve the symptoms and effects of the disease. The drug of choice to eliminate the streptococcal infection is penicillin; however, for those persons who have an allergic response to penicillin, erythromycin may be used. In addition to therapy to eliminate the streptococci, the patient should be protected against exposure to persons with respiratory infections who could be harboring the streptococcus organism.

Salicylates and corticosteroids are prescribed singularly or in combination to retard the inflammatory process and to decrease the tissue response. Exactly how the salicylates or the corticosteroids act is not known, but they alter the toxic effect of rheumatic fever and provide comfort for the patient. They do not, however, accelerate the rate at which the patient recovers from rheumatic fever. When the preceding drugs are administered in adequate dosages, not only do the signs and symptoms associated with the disease disappear, but the erythrocyte sedimentation rate and leukocyte count also drop. If, however, treatment is prematurely discontinued, signs, symptoms, and blood changes characteristic of rheumatic fever reappear. Because the course of the disease is unpredictable, it is difficult to ascertain if the improvement of the patient is caused by the suppressive therapy or by elimination of the cause of the inflammatory reaction. Therefore at the time drug therapy is being discontinued, the patient should be under observation so that therapy can be re-established if indications of rheumatic activity reappear.

As the patient begins to feel better, diversion appropriate for the patient's age and interest should be provided. These activities should be of the type that do not require much physical energy. In addition, social relationships should be maintained with friends and family.

Because the patient, who is usually of school age, will have restricted physical activity for extended periods of weeks to months, careful planning needs to be done in regard to educational needs. Today the trend is to permit earlier physical activity, even if a little premature, rather than have the student miss months of school. Experience has shown that even though a tutor is provided by the school board, the student tends to lose interest in school. As a result, many of these patients are school dropouts, which further complicates their adjustment to life because persons who have had rheumatic fever should have an occupation that uses intellectual skills rather than physical labor. For those who do continue in school, adjustments regarding future occupations and extracurricular activities may need to be made.

As in other long-term illnesses, the education of the patient and/or family members in the nature and effects of rheumatic fever is imperative if they are to assume responsibility for treatment of the current attack and prevent recurrences. When the home situation permits, patients may be discharged from the hospital after the acute manifestations are relieved. Even when the patient is "cured," antimicrobial therapy is prescribed. According to Sokolow and McIlroy (1979, p. 575) most patients will be on prophylactic doses of penicillin or the sulfonamides until age 30 and some advise continuing prophylaxis until age 40 to 45. The preferred method of prophylaxis is with penicillin G, 1.2 million units intramuscularly every 4 weeks. Oral penicillin 200,000 to 250,000 units daily may be used instead; however, there can be a problem of compliance with oral drugs. For those patients who are allergic to penicillin, sulfadiazine 1 g orally can be given daily.

It is possible to determine compliance with the prescribed medication regimen by doing a urine compliance test. A fresh sheep-blood agar plate is inoculated with group A beta-hemolytic streptococcus. A piece of paper dipped into the patient's urine is planted on the agar plate as well as a bacitracin disk. After incubation for 24 hours there should be a zone of inhibition around both the paper strip and the bacitracin if the patient is taking the prescribed medication. If there is a zone of inhibition around the bacitracin, but not around the piece of paper, this indicates noncompliance with the regimen to prevent rheumatic fever (Chobin, Kangos, & Miller, 1975).

Patients need to be aware of the need for good oral hygiene to prevent tooth decay and gum disease. In patients with established valvular disease, there is danger of bacterial endocarditis resulting from dental extractions unless the physician prescribes extra antibiotics during that time.

As with any type of prolonged illness, the financial drain can be tremendous. Information regarding financial aid can be obtained through the state and local health departments. Also some funds usually are available through the crippled children's services for the hospitalization of rheumatic children. Additional sources of information would be the local and state Heart Associations.

Rheumatic Heart Disease

The most common cause of acquired valvular disease is acute rheumatic involvement. It is interesting to note that some individuals who have valvular disease characteristic of rheumatic involvement will deny having had a known attack of rheumatic fever, whereas others experience a classic case. Rheumatic heart disease can be manifested as mitral or aortic stenosis and/or insufficiency. The greatest valvular involvement results with the gradual stenosis of a valvular orifice over a 20- to 30-year period.

In general, with a stenotic valve the workload of the chamber proximal to the obstruction is increased, and with an insufficient valve the work of both the chambers both proximal and distal to the insufficient valve is increased. With either stenosis or insufficiency there will eventually be clinical manifestations of cardiac failure.

The tools utilized to diagnose rheumatic valvular disease are heart sounds, clinical manifestations, electrocardiograms, x-ray changes, and cardiac catheterization results. Cardiac catheterization is the only diagnostic tool that will be elaborated on at this point. The rest will be covered under the specific disease entities.

CARDIAC CATHETERIZATION. To perform a cardiac catheterization, a catheter is inserted via cutdown into either a peripheral vein or artery. With a right heart catheterization, a catheter is inserted into a large antecubital vein and passed under fluoroscopy into the vena cava, the right atrium, the right ventricle, the pulmonary artery, and the pulmonary capillaries. The final position is the pulmonary artery "wedge" position. The "wedge" position is significant inasmuch as the left atrial pressure cannot be measured directly, but is reflected in the value of the pulmonary capillary pressure. Elevated left atrial pressure can be diagnostic of mitral stenosis or insufficiency and left ventricular failure. Other reasons to perform a right heart catheterization are to assess pulmonic and tricuspid valve and right ventricular function, to obtain pulmonary vascular pressure studies, and to identify a left to right shunt at the atrial or ventricular levels.

Left heart catheterization can be performed by retrograde passage of a catheter through either the brachial or femoral artery into the ascending aorta, across the aortic valve, and into the left ventricle. A direct left atrial measurement can be obtained by transseptal puncture and passage of a catheter from the right atrium to the left atrium, but is rarely employed. Left heart catheterization is required to diagnose mitral and aortic valvular disease as well as disease of the coronary arteries and muscle function of the left ventricle.

The more common studies performed with catheterization are pressure readings, indicator dilutional curves, oxygen concentration, and angiographic evaluations. Pressure readings are done to determine the pressure in the various cardiac chambers and the great vessels and to note pressure changes across valves. Both systolic and diastolic pressures are recorded. Also, end diastolic pressures can be recorded in the ventricles. With a stenotic valve, the pressure in the chamber proximal to the stenosis will be significantly higher than the pressure in the chamber distal to the stenosis. Pressure gradients are measured by taking continuous pressure recordings while a catheter is pulled back through a valve. Normally there is no pressure gradient across the aortic and pulmonic valve; thus if a gradient is present, it is diagnostic. A pressure gradient normally is present across the mitral and tricuspid valve, and a decrease in the gradient is indicative of stenosis. When measuring the pulmonary artery pressure, the systolic pressure is reflective of the pressure in the right ventricle and the diastolic pressure indicates the resistance in the pulmonary artery. The pulmonary artery pressure can be increased as the result of an atrial or ventricular septal defect with increased blood flow, or because of increased pulmonary resistance secondary to a pulmonary embolus or chronic lung disease. When measuring the pressure in the left ventricle, an increase in the end diastolic pressure would indicate decreased compliance as seen in constrictive pericarditis or ventricular hypertrophy, or an increase in the end diastolic volume as seen with aortic and mitral insufficiency and left ventricular failure.

Indicator dilutional curves are obtained by injection of an indicator substance at one point in the cardiac circulation with detection by a sensing apparatus at another point. With this method the obtained curves are used to calculate cardiac output and coronary blood flow and to detect shunts.

Blood samples can be drawn from any vessel or chamber during the catheterization, and the oxygen content and saturation can be measured. Septal defects with a left-to-right shunt will show blood with an abnormally high oxygen concentration in the right side of the heart, for normally the left side has the highly oxygenated blood, not the right. Also the Fick method can be used to calculate cardiac output. Samples of arterial and venous blood are obtained, and the total body oxygen consumption is measured. From this data the cardiac output is determined.

With angiographic evaluation the catheter tip is positioned in a specific area of the cardiovascular system and contrast media is injected while concomitant x-rays are taken. Cineangiography and rapid sequence filming are taken. The data will indicate chamber size and configuration, wall excursion during contraction, wall and valve thickening, direction of flow, valve motion, and ejection fraction. The ejection fraction is a comparison of the blood ejected during systole and the volume of blood remaining in the left ventricle at the end of diastole. Normally the left ventricle contains approximately 100 cc at the end of diastole and ejects 70 cc during systole. The ejection fraction is 70/100 or 70 per cent. The smaller the ejection fraction, the more incompetent the myocardium (Strong, 1977, p. 63). Abnormalities of wall excursion or motion (where part of the wall does not contract properly) develop as a consequence of a myocardial infarction or reduced blood supply to a portion of the ventricle. The abnormality of function is described in degrees of impairment as hypokinesis, dyskinesis, and akinesis.

Also during the angiographic evaluation, selective coronary arteriography may be performed. A surgical cutdown in performed in the right anticubital fossa and a cardiac catheter is introduced into the arterial circulation via brachial arteriotomy. The catheter is advanced manually to the root of the aorta under direct visualization with fluoroscopy. The catheter tip is manipulated into the right and left coronary ostia. Two to 5 ml of contrast medium are injected into each coronary artery and 35 mm cineangiographic films are taken concomitantly. Thus the entire coronary arterial system is visualized and can be evaluated. Coronary atherosclerosis is recognized by narrowing or occlusion of the arteries. Collateral vessels that bridge obstructed areas or provide retrograde filling of an obstructed artery may be visualized. During the study the catheter is introduced through the aortic valve into the left ventricle. Pressure recordings and contrast medium injection with cinematography are done to evaluate left ventricular function. The data are helpful in establishing the prognosis for the individual patient and are essential when evaluation is done for possible surgical intervention of coronary lesions. Indications for coronary arteriography are (1) acute angina attacks or an acute myocardial infarction, (2) chronic angina with pain that is increasing in frequency and severity, and (3) angina refractory to medical management.

The patient needs to have a thorough explanation of the cardiac catheterization procedure, since it will be performed under a local anesthetic. Premedication of the patient varies greatly depending upon the physician's philosophy and the needs of the patient; however, the patient will be given just enough sedation to cause only relaxation inasmuch as the patient must be cooperative throughout the procedure to follow the physician's instructions. There are some medications which can be given throughout the procedure. Frequently nitroglycerine gr 1/150 is given sublingually to promote maximum arterial dilation or to relieve anginal discomfort. Prophylactically atropine 0.5 to 1 mgm is given intravenously to counteract bradyarrhythmia caused by suppression of the sinoatrial node from the injection of contrast media into the right coronary artery. Throughout the procedure there are certain discomforts that the patient may feel. Even though a local anesthetic is used, the patient may still feel some discomfort when the catheter is moved through the vessel. If the brachial artery is used for a left heart catheterization, the catheter will be moved in a retrograde fashion through the arterial circulation. Thus the patient may experience sensations of "pins and needles" or "going to sleep" in the arm below the site of the catheter insertion, as the blood flow will be diminished. With right heart catheterization, the patient may experience some arm pain from the venospasm around the catheter. The patient also should be warned that there is a feeling of warmth following the injection of the contrast medium.

With any catheterization, premature beats may occur from the manipulation of the catheter inside the ventricles, giving the sensation of the heart doing "flip-flops." These symptoms are transitory and will subside once the catheter position is changed. During coronary angiography, the patient may be temporarily positioned on his or her side and asked to cough following the contrast media injection to facilitate dye removal and avoid asystole. Coughing also counteracts the nausea and light-headedness that sometimes follows the infection of the contrast medium. Following left heart catheterization, pulses distal to the catheter insertion site should be checked to determine patency of the interrupted artery. Sometimes the pulse will be diminished for 24 hours because of arterial spasm or site edema. In other situations there may be total loss of the radial pulse because of surgical closure of the vessel or thrombus formation. When a thrombus forms, collateral circulation usually is established; however, the extremity distal to the site of the catheter insertion should always be checked for signs of decreased circulation. The site should be observed for signs of bleeding into the extravascular tissue spaces, and thrombophlebitis. Analgesics may be ordered for site discomfort. If blood pressures are ordered postcatheterization, more accurate readings are obtained in the contralateral arm.

Possible complications, although rare, that may occur during the procedure include arrhythmias such as ventricular tachycardia or fibrillation; asystole, bradycardia, and superventricular arrhythmias; perforation of the heart, resulting in cardiac tamponade; syncopal episodes; cerebrovascular accident from air in the catheter, mural thrombi, or fragments of valvular deposits; myocardial infarction; and allergic reactions to the contrast media. The largest component of contrast media is iodine. With injections there can be immediate or delayed reactions. Immediate reactions range from nausea, vomiting, and diaphoresis to anaphylaxis. Any patient who has contrast media studies should be observed for appearance of a skin rash and diminishing urine output. Increased fluid intake should be achieved in those patients who are not on fluid restrictions to promote dilution of the contrast media in the circulatory system and excretion as well as to prevent renal crystalization.

MITRAL STENOSIS. With valvular disease secondary to rheumatic fever, there is edema of the involved valve(s) cusps. This is followed by erosion of the cusp(s) along the line of closure as a result of trauma from the closure of the edematous cusps. Along these denuded areas, fibrin and platelets are deposited in the form of beadlike vegetations.

With repeated attacks of rheumatic fever, the valve leaflets and chordae tendineae become highly deformed because of fibrous tissue formation. The leaflet commissures fuse, the chordae tendineae develop contractures and thicken, and the valve orifice narrows from a normal 4 to 6 sq cm to 2.5 sq cm or less. The resultant effect is a stenotic valve with the leaflets held downward.

The blood flow through a stenotic valve is decreased for two reasons. In the normal heart, blood flows through the opening which lies between the papillary muscles as well as the spaces between the chordae. In the rheumatic heart, however, both these channels of blood flow are reduced.

Because of the decreased diastolic blood flow from the left atrium into the left ventricle, there is a decreased stroke volume with a resultant decreased cardiac output. In addition, there will be an increased left atrial pressure with hypertrophy of the left atrium. As the stenosis becomes more severe, the pressure is transmitted backward through the pulmonary veins to the pulmonary capillaries and transudation of fluid into or around the alveoli takes place. Thus varying degrees of left heart failure will be manifested.

With long-standing stenosis there will be greater resistance to pulmonary blood flow and secondary pulmonary hypertension develops. This leads to an increased workload of the right ventricle, with resultant hypertrophy and failure.

The clinical manifestations of mitral stenosis will be varying degrees of right and left failure, depending on the severity of the stenosis. The reader is referred to the section on heart failure. Physical signs would include a diastolic murmur with a characteristic opening snap of the mitral valve, arrhythmias, arterial emboli and radiologic changes of the heart.

Atrial fibrillation is the cardiac arrhythmia that is most common in mitral stenosis. Initially it may occur in paroxysms or be preceded by other atrial arrhythmias, such as premature atrial beats, atrial tachycardia, or atrial flutter, before becoming permanent. The cardiac output in mitral stenosis is fixed at a low level. With atrial fibrillation, the cardiac output will be decreased further, as the tachycardia associated with fibrillation decreases the diastolic filling time and thus impedes atrial emptying. This is another factor that predisposes to pulmonary edema.

Systemic emboli can be a complication of mitral stenosis. Because of the left atrial hypertrophy and decreased left atrial outflow, there is stasis of blood in the left atrium, which predisposes to thrombus formation. Atrial fibrillation can further increase the tendency for thrombi formation. The emboli can lodge at any point in the arterial system, but most commonly migrate to the brain, abdomen, or lower extremities.

The radiologic changes of pure mitral stenosis would include an enlarged left atrium and pulmonary congestion. If the heart has decompensated, right ventricular hypertrophy and dilatation with pulmonary artery enlargement are noted in the hilar region.

Cardiac catheterization reveals an increased pulmonary artery and left atrial pressure with a normal left ventricular pressure. When a contrast medium is injected, it remains in the left atrium for an extended time because of the valvular obstruction. Cineangiography will demonstrate a stiff, funnel-shaped valve on diastole. Other data would include a smaller mitral valve area and a decreased cardiac output.

ECHOCARDIOGRAPHY a noninvasive diagnostic tool for cardiac problems, is based on the principle of ultrasound. Echoes from ultrasound waves are used to study and locate the movements and dimensions of cardiac structures (valve leaflets and chamber walls). Since all structures in the heart move, the reflection of the ultrasound beam will vary as it traverses the various structures causing wave forms. The ultrasound beam plots the motion of cardiac structures over a period of time. A specific echocardiographic picture represents a one-dimensional view of heart structures from a given angle. Multiple views from different angles can be taken. The end result is a composite picture of valvular function. Through echocardiography it was discovered that normally the anterior leaflet of the mitral valve moves downward toward the posterior leaflet during diastole, whereas with mitral stenosis the two mitral leaflets move anteriorly in diastole. Thus with mitral stenosis the leaflets move en bloc throughout the cardiac cycle whereas normally these leaflets move in opposite directions.

Surgical intervention can be either a mitral valvotomy (commissurotomy) or total replacement of the mitral valve done with cardiopulmonary bypass (pump oxygenator, extracorporeal circulation). Until the advent of cardiopulmonary bypass, valvotomies were done blindly as a closed procedure. With a valvotomy the fused commissures are mobilized with digital manipulation or a dilator. Also papillary muscles and chordae tendineae can be mobilized if they are fused, as frequently happens with rheumatic heart disease.

The decision of whether to proceed with a mitral valvotomy or to replace the mitral valve with a prosthetic valve ultimately is made at the time of surgery. The three basic types of prosthetic valves are the caged ball, low-profile floating disk and tilting disk. In addition porcine heterograft prostheses are being used for valvular replacement.

To date prosthetic valves have not progressed to the point where early valvular replacement is justified without first trying the conservative approach of a mitral valvotomy. Prosthetic valves add the risk of thromboembolism, malfunction of the prosthetic valve, and infection. The introduction of porcine heterograft prostheses has improved the outlook for patients requiring valvular replacement, even though thromboembolism is still a problem. Thus, the preservation of the mitral valve with an adequate palliative surgery, mitral valvotomy, is still the procedure of choice for mitral stenosis (Montoya et al., 1979).

MITRAL INSUFFICIENCY. Mitral insufficiency causes a shunting or regurgitation of blood back into the left atrium during left ventricular systole. Insufficiency can be a direct result of rheumatic valvular disease, or it can occur secondary to bacterial endocarditis, hypertrophy of the left ventricle, or rupture of a papillary muscle and chordae tendineae secondary to myocardial infarction.

With rheumatic inflammation, there are scarring and contraction of the leaflets and fusion of the chordae tendineae. The posterior leaflet becomes defective and fails to meet the large anterior leaflet; thus there is insufficient cusp tissue to occlude the valve orifice. If mitral stenosis is present, the mitral valve annulus can stretch until it becomes insufficient because of the left atrial dilatation.

If the mitral regurgitation is secondary to rheumatic involvement, all the hemodynamic changes of mitral stenosis will be present in addition to varying degrees of left ventricular hypertrophy. The left ventricle hypertrophies because of the increased left ventricular contractibility, which is an attempt to increase the stroke volume and cardiac output. Eventually the left ventricle dilates, causing greater stretching of the annulus. The cardiac output will remain decreased because of the regurgitation of blood back into the left atrium during systole.

As with mitral stenosis, the patient will demonstrate symptoms of left heart failure, and in severe cases right heart failure will also be present. (The reader is referred to the section on heart failure.)

Physical examination will reveal a pansystolic murmur and a wide expiratory splitting of S_2. The splitting of S_2 is the effect of a short left ventricular systole and closure of the aortic valve as compared to a longer right ventricular systole and closure of the pulmonic valve. On x-ray the left atrium will be greatly hypertrophied, more than occurs with mitral stenosis, and with severe regurgitation both the left atrium and ventricle will be enlarged. Also with severe regurgitation, enlargement of the pulmonary artery and right ventricle can be noted.

The echocardiogram is nondiagnostic in mitral insufficiency. In mitral insufficiency there may be an increase in the internal dimensions of the left atrium and ventricle. There is a ski-slope appearance of the anterior leaflet's diastolic closure which demonstrates combined mitral stenosis and regurgitation. This sign is helpful but not diagnostic of the disease.

Cardiac catheterization reveals increased end-diastolic pressure in both the left atrium and ventricle. With severe regurgitation the right ventricular end-diastolic pressure can be elevated in varying degrees because of right heart failure. When a contrast medium is injected into the left ventricle, there is a simultaneous appearance of medium in the left atrium and aorta as shown with cineangiography.

Surgical intervention using the open technique with cardiopulmonary bypass can be performed through either the right or left chest. In a few cases, in which the mitral leaflets and chordae tendineae are not damaged, a reduction in the size of the annulus with mattress sutures will suffice. If just the leaflet is perforated, it can be repaired with a patch.

In the majority of cases, however, the valve is also calcified and severely damaged, and repair demands a total valve replacement with a prosthetic disc valve or a porcine heterograft. A disc valve is used rather than a valve with a cage because cage valves tend to protrude too far into the left ventricle and thus interfere with ventricular contraction.

AORTIC STENOSIS. Aortic stenosis indicates narrowing of the aortic valve orifice with obstruction to ventricular outflow in systole. The most common cause is rheumatic valvulitis. Other causes include atherosclerotic changes of the aortic wall and valve leaflets and bacterial endocarditis. With rheumatic valvulitis, essentially the same pathology occurs in the aortic valve as occurs with mitral stenosis. Frequently mitral and aortic stenosis occur concomitantly.

The cusp substance itself is attacked by the disease process as well as the margin of the valve cusps. The valves become scarred with calcium deposits similar to mitral stenosis; thus they are stiff and obstruct blood flow even when there is no fusion of commissures. Calcium also accumulates in the region of the left branch of the bundle of His and may cause left bundle branch block. All three of the commissures can become fused, or just two can be fused. In either case the valve orifice is stenosed.

With aortic stenosis, left ventricular emptying will be reduced because of the obstruction of outflow. The effect is an increased velocity of blood flow as it passes through the valve orifice. During systole, the systemic arterial blood pressure can be decreased because of obstruction.

Coronary insufficiency usually results with aortic stenosis. The coronary ostia originate at the root of the aorta just above the aortic valve, thus with the lowered pressure at the root of the aorta, there is poor coronary perfusion (see Figure 44-4). Also the hypertrophied left ventricle has a greater demand for oxygen and thus for coronary flow than normal.

The patient may be symptom-free for a considerable period of time. Usually by the time symptoms are manifested, the disease is fairly far advanced. The earliest complaints are fatigability and dyspnea on exertion. As the pathology becomes more advanced, syncope, angina, and symptoms of left ventricular failure become apparent.

Symptoms of deficient cerebral blood flow are on a continuum from dizziness to syncope. The symptoms usually occur with exertion except in severe cases of stenosis where they are present without exertion. Angina pectoris frequently is present in severe cases of aortic stenosis. The angina pectoris of aortic stenosis is completely indistinguishable from that of coronary atherosclerotic heart disease. Frequently, anginal attacks are associated with syncope caused by exertion.

Dyspnea on exertion does not necessarily mean heart failure with aortic stenosis; however, x-rays may show that there is pulmonary interstitial edema when the patient has progressive dyspnea. Paroxysmal nocturnal dyspnea can be a serious sign, and if the right ventricle has decompensated, death usually occurs within 1 year. With advanced failure, patients can experience crises of restlessness, flushing, cyanosis, heavy sweating, and shock. The exact explanation for these crises is unknown, and frequently death can occur (Cobbs, 1970, p. 839).

Physical examination will reveal a diamond-shaped ejection murmur, a reduced intensity of S_2, and a loud S_4, if left ventricular hypertrophy is present. A narrow pulse pressure is typical. X-ray findings include calcification of the aortic valve as well as enlargement of the left side of the heart if stenosis is far advanced. Cardiac catheterization will reveal an elevated systolic pressure in the left ventricle. Also a pressure gradient of 50 mm Hg or more is usually present across the aortic valve.

The echocardiogram shows decreased excursion of the aortic cusps. Also dense echoes from the region of the aortic valve may be present, indicating calcification and/or fibrosis of the valve. The internal diameter of the left ventricle is increased due to stasis of blood in that chamber.

The medical treatment for aortic stenosis is limited to palliative measures for controlling heart failure and angina. There are varying opinions regarding the restriction of physical activity. The patient is usually cognizant that the symptoms are initiated by exertion; thus it is better to have the patient learn to restrict his or her own activity rather than make him or her overly anxious with imposed rigid restrictions.

Surgical treatment includes performing a valvulotomy for congenital aortic stenosis and replacing the valve with a prosthetic valve in acquired aortic stenosis. In both cases a sternotomy is done and the patient is put on cardiopulmonary bypass.

AORTIC INSUFFICIENCY. With aortic insufficiency there is regurgitation of blood during diastole back into the left ventricle through the aortic valve. Rheumatic valvulitis may attack the annulus and/or leaflets. As a result, the leaflets can become deformed, making it impossible for them to cover the valve orifice, or the annulus may become dilated, and even normal leaflets cannot close effectively. If syphilis is the cause, dilatation of both the aorta and the annulus result.

With a regurgitant aortic valve, there is both a forward and retrograde flow of blood through the valve with the resultant effect of a decreased diastolic pressure in the peripheral arteries. Because of the decrease in diastolic pressure, the coronary blood flow is decreased as the coronaries are perfused normally during diastole and now most of the coronary flow has to be during systole. Thus it is not uncommon for the patient to experience angina.

A second effect from regurgitation of blood into the left ventricle would be dilatation and hypertrophy of that chamber. Three factors account for the left ventricular hypertrophy: (1) in diastole, blood regurgitates into the left ventricle from the aorta thus increasing the volume of blood in the ventricle, (2) in systole, the distended ventricle overworks to pump the excessive volume into the systemic circulation to maintain an adequate cardiac output, and (3) diminished coronary perfusion and subsequent inadequate oxygen supply stimulates hypertrophy of cells by a mechanism yet to be explained. In contrast to aortic stenosis, the cardiac output can be increased in response to exercise.

The systolic pressure is either normal or slightly elevated; thus the pulse pressure is widened with aortic insufficiency, whereas it was narrowed with aortic stenosis. Symptoms accompanying this are "water hammer" (Corrigan) pulse and "pistol-shot" sounds over the femoral artery.

The echocardiogram demonstrates an increased internal dimension of the left ventricle. Characteristic high frequency fluttering of the anterior mitral valve leaflet during filling of the ventricle occurs. In addition there can be exaggerated movement of the interventricular septum.

Physical examination reveals a diastolic murmur that is described as decrescendo and soft. The x-ray findings show an extremely enlarged left ventricle with decompensated aortic insufficiency. Also the left atrium and right ventricle can be enlarged with signs of pulmonary vascular congestion. Cardiac catheterization reveals normal pressures in the heart unless there is decompensation of the left ventricle. Then the end diastolic pressure in the left ventricle will be elevated. The surgical intervention for aortic insufficiency is replacement with a prosthetic valve. Usually a ball valve in a cage is used.

Coronary Artery Surgery

Surgical techniques directed toward the improvement of myocardial perfusion have increased in popularity throughout the country. With the advent of coronary angiography in the late 1950s, an anatomic basis was achieved for the selection of patients in whom specific surgical procedures might be helpful. It should be noted that although these procedures have been demonstrated to improve the quality of life by providing a pain-free existence, it has not yet been demonstrated that surgical intervention improves the quantity of life significantly by extending longevity. Only longitudinal studies will provide these data over the forthcoming years.

Many surgical procedures have been developed over the years to promote direct or indirect myocardial revascularization by providing additional coronary blood flow or by relieving obstructed vessels. The first procedures were devised by Beck in the 1930s whereby the pericardium was opened, the ventricular myocardium roughened with a carpenter's file, sterile asbestos or talcum powdered on the irritated area, and the pericardium closed. The rationale for the Beck procedure was to create a chronic irritation whereby collateral circulation would develop in the ischemic myocardium. Despite some 30 years of performing the procedure, studies to document improved myocardial blood flow and significant longevity were lacking, and the procedure generally has been abandoned.

The implantation of one or both internal mammary arteries into the myocardium (Vineberg procedure) with various modifications became popular in the 1960s and is still utilized in selected cases. The purpose of the Vineberg procedure is to implant an arterial supply into a viable but ischemic area of myocardium. It has been demonstrated by coronary angiographic studies that with time a network of fine anastomotic vessels develops between the implanted mammary artery and the coronary vessels, thus improving myocardial perfusion. Today most surgeons feel that the use of an autogenous saphenous vein to do aortocoronary bypass surgery is the method of choice. Some surgeons are using the internal mammary artery and synthetic material for bypass grafts.

In order to determine who is eligible for aortocoronary bypass surgery, several factors are considered. If the patient is failing to respond to medical management and coronary perfusion deficits are demonstrated by both treadmill exercise tests and cardiac catheterization, coronary surgery is recommended (Diethrich, 1975, p. 381). In addition to identifying that a coronary perfusion deficit is present, the distribution of the coronary artery disease must be determined. Patients with diffuse disease, that is, small and sclerotic peripheral arteries with poor runoff from the major arteries, are poor candidates. Research has shown that flow through the graft and runoff to the peripheral coronary arterioles are the most important factors in determining long-term patency of the graft (Ehrlick, 1975, p. 376). Also left ventricular function is evaluated carefully by history and physical examination as well as by echocardiogram and cardiac catheterization. If the test results indicate that the left ventricle is dilated with poor contractility, the patient is considered a poor surgical risk.

One or more bypass grafts can be performed at the time of surgery depending upon the distribution of the atherosclerosis and occlusion within the coronary arteries. A piece of saphenous vein in the reversed position from venous flow is used as an autogenous graft. The saphenous vein will be slightly larger in diameter than the coronary artery. Despite the disparity in size, the vein undergoes a size accommodation as a normal physiological response of attachment to the coronary artery. The proximal anastomosis is made into the ascending aorta. If more than one graft is performed, each graft should have its own origin into the aorta. The distal anastomosis is made to the coronary artery beyond the point of obstruction. The basic principle is to bypass all obstructions and to place the graft into a portion of the artery that is relatively free of atherosclerosis. During double and triple bypass procedures, extracorporeal circulation is used. Uncomplicated single or double bypass procedures can be done on the beating heart. In addition, during the time when the anastomoses are made, the heart is put into cardioplegia. In order to obtain cardioplegia an acid solution with a high potassium concentration is instilled into the heart. The temperature of the heart is lowered to approximately 18°C at which point the metabolic needs are reduced in the heart. Thus the coronary arteries do not have to be perfused. The anastomoses can be done in a bloodless field and on a nonbeating heart.

Cardiopulmonary Bypass

The purposes of cardiopulmonary bypass (extracorporeal circulation) are to deviate blood from the cardiac chambers and great vessels to permit surgical repair in a surgical field devoid of blood and, simultaneously, to maintain normal metabolic function of the whole body. Prior to the development of pump oxygenators, intracardiac surgery in a bloodless field was limited to minutes. With the advent of the oxygenator, intracardiac operations have been extended to several hours.

The superior and inferior venae cavâe are cannulated to collect all the venous blood and divert it to the extracorporeal circuit. The blood is passed through the oxygenator, where the carbon dioxide is removed and oxygen is added. After the blood passes through the pump oxygenator, it is returned to the patient through a cannulated peripheral artery, usually the femoral or external iliac or aorta. The oxygenated blood returns in a retrograde fashion through the peripheral artery or aorta to supply the body. If the aortic valve is competent, the blood will not enter the cardiac chambers, yet the coronary arteries will be perfused. If the aorta is clamped to perform surgery on the aortic valve, the coronary arteries are cannulated and perfused. When coronary artery bypass surgery is performed, the temperature of the heart is decreased to approximately 18°C. During this time no metabolism is taking place in the myocardium; thus, the coronary arteries do not have to be perfused.

Venous blood drains from the body by gravity into the pump oxygenator; however, some blood will still enter the cardiac chambers. The venous return from the bronchial arteries and coronary sinus via the pulmonary circuit enters the left side of the heart via the pulmonary veins. This blood is collected by an intracardiac aspirator inserted into the left ventricle.

Serum hepatitis is a well-recognized clinical problem that can occur in association with blood transfusions. In the past with open heart surgery, patients were exposed to multiple sources of blood transfusions used to prime the pump oxygenator, to replace red blood cells destroyed by the pump, and to replace blood during the postoperative period. Among this earlier patient population, the incidence of posttransfusion hepatitis has been recorded in as high as 51 per cent of the cases (Prebil & Diethrich, 1974, p. 804). In light of this fact, most institutions now use a balanced electrolyte solution rather than whole blood to prime the pump oxygenator. Also in some institutions one or two units of blood are removed from the patient prior to starting the extracorporeal circulation. At the completion of the surgery the patient is retransfused with the autologous blood (Winslow & MacVaugh, 1976, p. 372). Because the blood has not been exposed to the heart-lung machine, it has good cell viability and coagulation properties. Prebil and Diethrich (1974) conducted a study of 100 patients who had cardiopulmonary bypass without the use of whole blood before, during, or after surgery. Instead, patients received electrolyte solutions, plasma expanders, and "washed" cells, as indicated. At a 4-month period following surgery all patients were checked for hepatitis and there were no cases positive for hepatitis.

During the period of cardiopulmonary bypass, the patient is heparinized intravenously via the pump to prevent blood clots from forming. At the completion of the intracardiac procedure, protamine sulfate is given intravenously to neutralize the effect of heparin. Throughout the surgery blood is sampled periodically to detect any changes in electrolytes, pH, and carbon dioxide and oxygen tensions. The degree of metabolic acidosis is constantly evaluated and treated.

Preoperative Preparation of the Cardiac Patient

Before preoperative preparation can be done, consideration must be given to the psychological response of the patient and family to the impending surgery. The emotional response of the open heart surgery patient and family tends to be more intense than other surgical patients because the heart is associated with life and death and a gamut of emotions in our society. The common use of idiomatic expressions with the word *heart* in them illustrates the significance the heart has to everyone. The fears that the patient may have preoperatively are justified, although they might not be expressed. The reason is that the risk associated with cardiac surgery is considerably greater than that associated with other types of surgery.

Another factor contributing to preoperative anxiety is that most patients requiring cardiac surgery will have had an impairment of cardiac function for a period of years, which has necessitated an alteration in their life style. Suddenly they are faced with making a decision to have an elective surgery that could enable them to live relatively normal lives. For some this could be an extremely difficult decision, as the cardiac condition has been used as a crutch. For others the alternative of having surgery could be welcome. The decision-making process may be a lonely one for most patients, as family members usually do not participate, because they are aware of the possible hazards and outcomes. Few people want to be responsible for helping to make the decision to have open heart surgery, which could result in death.

In recent years much emphasis has been placed on the preoperative preparation of the patient. For the cardiac patient more than any other patient, this emphasis has resulted in a very structured approach much of the time. There are varying opinions as to the type of preparation that should be given. On one end of the continuum are those who feel that a lack of information regarding the immediate postoperative period contributes to confusion, panic, and depression during that time. On the other end are those who feel that too much specific information about the unpleasant aspects of surgery only increases the patient's apprehension. Of utmost importance is that consideration is given to the individual needs of each patient, however varied those needs may be.

Today the majority of patients are fairly well informed regarding the nature of their surgery; they have either read about the subject or their physician has informed them. Moreover, with all the medical programs on television they have undoubtedly seen programs about heart surgery. This does not preclude, however, the possibility that the patient may have nonfactual material or misinterpretations. For example, this writer knew of a patient who thought his heart was removed from his body to perform surgery. Another patient knew that his heart was stopped during surgery but was concerned how it was restarted. This speaks to the need for clarification and reinforcement of prior patient teaching before the surgical procedure.

There are some instructions common for all patients. Each patient must assume the responsibility for coughing and deep breathing as well as using an intermittent positive pressure breathing machine (IPPB) in the recovery phase; thus the patient must understand the importance of this procedure and practice it preoperatively. Miller and Shada (1978) conducted a study where postoperatively, nineteen adult open-heart surgery patients were interviewed about their perception of important information included or not included in preoperative instructions. From the data obtained from this group of patients, it was concluded that they need (1) a clear method of preoperatively teaching patients how to breathe and relax with the mechanical respirator postoperatively, (2) knowledge preoperatively of the degree of mucus to expect postoperatively, and (3) an explicit explanation of the suctioning technique. No patients indicated a lack of knowledge with coughing and deep breathing instructions; however, even subjects who had had previous experience with deep breathing and coughing suggested that more practice was need preoperatively.

According to Meserko, preoperative group classes have proved to be most effective. The technique for deep breathing and coughing is taught, and the patients practice the exercises and breathe on the IPPB machine. As with any group teaching, however, it must be followed by assessment of the individual's learning with reinforcement (1973, p. 665). At the Texas Heart Institute, preoperative teaching is done with a cardiovascular teaching model that employs Barbie dolls in a miniature reconstruction of the recovery room. In addition to the model, plastic replicas of hearts, prosthetic valves, and pacemakers are displayed (DeVillier, 1973, p. 525). The reader is referred to the November–December 1978 issue of *Cardiovascular Nursing* for an excellent preoperative teaching guide (Romero, 1978).

It is ideal for a nurse from the intensive-care unit or recovery room to visit the patient preoperatively for several reasons: (1) to enhance the preoperative teaching done by the physician and nursing staff, (2) to evaluate the patient emotionally and physically, and (3) to provide a familiar face with which the patient can identify postoperatively. At the time of the visit the interviewer needs to ask himself or herself several questions. Although it may be the most opportune time in the interviewer's schedule to talk with the patient regarding the surgery, is it the most opportune time for the patient? Is the patient able to absorb and comprehend what is to be taught, or is he or she too preoccupied with other concerns to grasp any of the information? All too frequently nurses make the error of setting aside time to "teach the patient" without first assessing the psychological and physical climate to ascertain when the patient is ready for learning. In addition, it has been found that the choice of information to be given patients concerning their surgery is based on the nurse's concept of the patient's needs, without the patient having active involvement in determining his or her learning needs. Needless to say, many patients' needs are unknown and unmet.

The nurse should do a thorough preoperative physical assessment to obtain baseline data from which comparisons are made postoperatively. To illustrate, the radial pulse could be absent following a left cardiac catheterization. Postoperatively this could be mistaken for signs of an embolus. Preoperatively the patient could have slurred speech or a weakness in an extremity. Postoperatively these signs could be misinterpreted as manifestations of a cerebral embolus. In addition to the physical assessment, the psychological status of the patient should be noted. From the information obtained either through interviewing the patient or from the patient's chart, an operative–postoperative nursing care plan should be developed. During the operative and immediate postoperative periods this profile information can be used for subsequent assessments and care.

Nursing Care Following Cardiac Surgery

Cardiopulmonary bypass causes various physiological changes to take place. Today the hemodilution technique used to prime the pump has greatly reduced the complications following bypass; however, this technique causes a total body overload in intracellular, interstitial, and intravascular compartments. Even though the total body water has increased, there is a decrease in the effective circulatory blood volume. There are ionic shifts with a noticeable loss of extracellular potassium. In addition to losing potassium during the bypass, many patients will have a low potassium preoperatively secondary to diuretic therapy. Pulmonary function is decreased because of the loss of surfactant from the lungs during the bypass perfusion as well as localized edema secondary to the trauma of a thoracotomy. Subtle cerebral changes take place secondary to cerebral edema and cerebral ischemia from microembolism. Renal function will be affected with a temporary oliguria.

In the first 48 hours following surgery utilizing cardiopulmonary bypass, there are common problems encountered. These complications may occur in any system of the body.

When administering nursing care following cardiac surgery, it is imperative for each nurse to have a systematic way of assessing the patient. There is no one way to assess the patient. For some nurses it is easiest to use a head-to-toe approach and to assess the systems in that order. For others a review of physiologic systems comparable to the medical approach is easiest. The key to an assessment process is the systematic manner in which it is performed.

Neurologic Assessment

The level of consciousness is assessed by orientation to time, place, and person. Because the neural cells are extremely sensitive to hypoxic states, restlessness and confusion may be the first indications of hypoxia. A word of caution is in order about questioning the patient regarding orientation to time and place; the patient very frequently will lose track of time and the day. The patient will be able to recognize that he or she is hospitalized but may not know that he or she is in the intensive care unit.

Motor function should be checked, as a thrombus from a cardiac chamber or a piece of calcium from a valve could occlude a cerebral artery. Also, air trapped in the left ventricle during cardiopulmonary bypass could act as a cerebral embolus. Today the filter systems on the cardiopulmonary bypass pump have been greatly improved and fewer emboli occur. Severe cerebral edema occurs with prolonged time on the pump. These patients remain obtunded without localizing neurologic signs. Patients with larger emboli from air, clots, or atheromas may have unilateralized neurologic deficits. Thus motor function needs to be checked carefully in postcardiac surgery patients.

Respiratory Assessment

It is not uncommon for the patient to return from surgery with either an endotracheal or tracheostomy tube in place. The purpose of the tube is to provide a patent airway, permit suctioning in those patients who cannot cough effectively, prevent aspiration, and provide a means for positive pressure ventilation. In some institutions patients are routinely put on a respirator for the first 24 hours.

During the first few hours postoperatively, oxygen is administered via the endotracheal tube, mask, or nasally. The patient is oxygenated well in an effort to prevent arrhythmias, as hypoxia can stimulate premature ventricular contractions. When judging the integrity of the respiratory system, the color of the patient's lips, nail beds, and skin is noted. Color changes range from pink to cyanotic in lightly pigmented patients, and in darkly pigmented patients from normal shades of brown to gray; dusky is approximately midway on the continuum.

The patient's breathing can be assessed for depth and rate by direct observation of the movement of the chest wall. Shallow respirations can result from pain; thus a narcotic may be indicated. On the other hand, a narcotic such as morphine can be the cause of shallow respirations. The term *splinting* is used to describe shallow restricted respirations resulting from pain. Causes of increased respiratory rates are pain, acute gastric dilatation, metabolic and respiratory acidosis, bladder distention, and/or hypoxia.

Signs of respiratory distress would include flaring of the nares, sternal retraction, dyspnea, abdominal breathing, and grunting. Dyspnea or air hunger is characterized by shortness of breath; mouth breathing, including gulping of air; rapid respirations; and marked excursions on exhalation. A grunting noise upon expiration is caused by either obstruction of the airway or restrained expirations by the patient because of pain.

Among the respiratory complications are hypoxia, atelectasis, pneumothorax, respiratory acidosis, and failure. Hypoxia resulting from inadequate oxygenation has a subtle initial sign, unexplained restlessness. Hypoxia should be suspected any time a patient is restless for no obvious reason. The major causes of altered arterial saturation are ventilation perfusion defects secondary to focal atelectasis. Focal atelectasis occurs with the loss of surfactant during surgery. Atelectasis will be manifested by a temperature elevation, increased pulse rate, and altered chest excursion. With a pneumothorax there is an accumulation of air or fluid in the intrapleural space with resultant displacement of the heart and inadequate expansion of the lung. The more common symptoms of pneumothorax are decreased breath sounds on the affected side, pain, dyspnea, and cyanosis.

The lobes of the lungs should be auscultated to determine if breath sounds are present in all lobes and if there are any abnormal sounds present. Wheezing could be indicative of pulmonary edema, bronchospasm, or obstruction. Moist sounds are present when there is either excess mucus or pulmonary edema. When there is an obstruction, the breath sounds will be diminished. In addition to listening to the breath sounds, the patient's tidal volume can be checked with a respirometer.

Arterial blood gases are drawn frequently and analyzed to determine if either metabolic or respiratory acidosis or respiratory alkalosis is present. The P_{O_2} and P_{CO_2} indicate the partial pressures of oxygen and carbon dioxide in the arterial blood. The normal levels are P_{O_2}, 95 to 100 mm Hg, P_{CO_2}, 35 to 40 mm Hg, and pH, 7.35 to 7.45. Respiratory acidosis (pH below 7.35) results from inadequate ventilation and an increase in the carbon dioxide tension. On the other hand, if a patient is on a respirator and the ventilation is too vigorous, respiratory alkalosis (pH above 7.45) can occur from the decreased carbon dioxide tension.

The nurse is instrumental in preventing respiratory complications. Patients must be turned and coughed religiously at least every hour, depending on the condition of the patient. For a patient to cough effectively, he or she must be relatively free of pain. Analgesics are rarely given *too* frequently but rather *not* frequently enough. Also proper splinting of the incision is imperative for the patient to cough effectively. Either the patient or the nurse can splint the incision with his or her hands or a towel during the coughing. The splinting or application of pressure around the incision is applied during the coughing phase and not the deep-breathing phase. Sternal splitting incisions are the least painful as fewer muscle groups are cut. If the patient is unable to cough productively and clear the airway, nasotracheal suctioning is indicated.

All patients have one or two chest tubes in place to remove fluid and air that collect in the intrapleural cavity. At the close of surgery, a wide pericardial window is made to provide for drainage of the pericardial sac into the pleural space and thereby decrease the danger of cardiac tamponade. The chest tube should be milked hourly to dislodge any clots. This is done by sliding the thumb and index finger down the chest tube away from the patient. The volume of drainage from the chest tube is one means used to determine blood replacement (see Chapter 40).

Cardiovascular Assessment

All pulses (apical, radial, femoral, popliteal, posterior tibial, and dorsalis pedis) need to be checked at frequent intervals. The apical pulse is checked for rate, rhythm, and heart sounds. A rapid pulse can be associated with hypoxia, heart failure, temperature elevation, and shock, whereas a slow pulse can be indicative of complete heart block. Even though the patient is attached to a cardiac monitor, the apical pulse should be checked with auscultation to listen to the heart sounds. If a clot is present on the prosthetic valve or with dislodgment of a clot, the sounds change. With cardiac tamponade the sounds become muffled. Pedal pulses are checked for volume, not specific rate. There is danger of thrombus formation in the artery where the catheter is inserted for cardiopulmonary bypass. Also thrombi may originate in the cardiac chambers and become dislodged into the peripheral circulation.

Most cardiac arrhythmias in the immediate postoperative period are the result of a rapid shift in pH and hypoxia. The myocardial electrophysiology will be altered with changes in pH due to the shifts of intracellular and extracellular potassium, sodium, and calcium. Alkalosis (respiratory or metabolic) causes myocardial irritability, and hypokalemia can cause cardiac arrhythmias. The more common cardiac arrhythmias that are present with cardiac surgery are premature ventricular contractions (PVC's), ventricular bigeminy, premature atrial contractions (PAC), atrial fibrillation, and complete heart block. The occurrence of PVCs is the most common arrhythmia seen in patients who have cardiac surgery. They may result from myocardial hypoxia, hypokalemia, or digitalis toxicity.

When premature ventricular contractions do occur, they are treated according to their frequency, configuration (multifocal versus unifocal), and whether they occur during the vulnerable period of the T wave. Premature ventricular contractions can be seen in association with nasal suctioning. By administering 100 per cent oxygen prior to suctioning, this arrhythmia usually can be prevented. Dangerous ventricular arrhythmias are treated with a bolus of lidocaine followed by continuous lidocaine infusion. If diuresis has occurred or hypokalemia is suspected, potassium is given. If ventricular fibrillation should occur, direct-current (DC) countershock is administered.

Premature atrial contractions which commonly occur with coronary bypass surgery frequently are related to pericarditis. Premature atrial contractions can also be seen with congestive heart failure, sinus nodal injury, and pulmonary emboli. Increased frequency of premature atrial contractions may indicate impending atrial fibrillation or flutter, thus digitalization is sometimes started early.

Atrial fibrillation is most commonly associated with mitral stenosis because of left atrial dilatation. If atrial fibrillation is present prior to surgery, it may return postoperatively although temporarily converted.

Complete heart block can occur with an aortic valve replacement if a suture is inadvertently placed through the intraventricular conduction system. If this should happen or if there is question of edema interfering with conduction, a temporary internal pacemaker may be inserted at the time of surgery.

The mean blood pressure should be maintained between 70 and 100 mm Hg systolic pressure and the left atrial pressure (LAP) between 15 and 25. While elaborate electronic monitoring devices are available, most places still find a single mercury manometer for arterial pressure or a water manometer for LAP to be most useful.

According to Harken, central direct arterial pressure measurement via radial artery intracatheter, correlated with LAP monitoring, has a unique value. He cites the following examples: (1) If both the arterial pressure and LAP are elevated the patient is relatively or absolutely hypervolemic. Hypervolemia is treated with vasodilators or diuretics. (2) If both arterial and LAP are low, the patient is hypovolemic and needs volume replacement, probably blood. (3) If the arterial pressure is low and the LAP is elevated, there is left ventricular failure and the patient needs myocardial support, such as digitalis preparations, calcium, glucagon, or even isoproterenol (1974, p. 895).

When assessing the cardiovascular system, as well as any system of the body, the nurse must anticipate what the possible outcome(s) of a single change in a finding could indicate. To illustrate, occasional premature ventricular contractions may be insignificant; however, other signs need to be evaluated before that decision can be made. Do the PVCs clear when the patient is oxygenated? Frequently PVCs are a sign of hypoxia. Is the blood pressure normal or is it dropping? Is the urinary output normal or is it decreasing? A decrease in the blood pressure and urinary output would indicate that the PVCs are interfering with an effective cardiac output and thus need to be treated with antiarrhythmic drugs.

Body Temperature

An elevated body temperature could be indicative of retained pulmonary secretions, infection, hemolysis of blood from incompatible blood transfusion or postcardiotomy syndrome. An elevated temperature decreases the peripheral resistance by dilating the blood vessels. If the patient is hypovolemic and becomes febrile, there is real danger of a hypotensive state developing.

Normally fluids are forced with febrile states, but with postoperative cardiac patients, fluids cannot be forced because of the danger of overloading the circulatory system. Methods used to control febrile conditions are antipyretic medications, alcohol sponges, and hypothermic mattresses (see Chapter 37).

Total Fluid Balance

Careful control of fluid and electrolyte balance is essential. Fluids are ordered daily according to the patient's daily weight, body surface area, and metabolic demands. Initially intravenous fluids are replaced at carefully controlled flow rates on an hourly basis to prevent overloading the circulatory system. Volume overloading would increase the workload of the heart, whereas underregulating the volume would decrease the tissue perfusion.

Frequent venous pressure readings are done to determine the circulatory status. Venous pressure readings will indicate hypovolemia, hypervolemia, or such signs of complications as cardiac tamponade and heart failure. The normal venous pressure reading is approximately 8 to 15 cm of H_2O.

Low cardiac output is the most common immediate problem following cardiac surgery. Among the various causes, hypovolemia, myocardial infarction (acute), heart failure, arrhythmias, cardiac tamponade, and pulmonary embolus with hypovolemia are the most common. Hypovolemia may result from postoperative bleeding or redistribution of fluids in the vascular system. Low central venous pressure (CVP) readings are one sign of hypovolemic states.

The patient with a normal CVP who suddenly shows signs of a decreased cardiac output should be evaluated for an acute myocardial infarction which could have occurred either during or immediately following surgery. To make a definitive diagnosis, the preoperative and postoperative vectorcardiogram is compared rather than relying on enzyme levels which are poor parameters following procedures using cardiopulmonary bypass machine.

Heart failure can be difficult to diagnose postoperatively because a mild degree of the symptoms is common in the immediate postoperative period. Clues to impending heart failure are unusual dyspnea, increasing CVP, decreasing P_{O_2} and development of an S_3. As with any heart failure, taking a chest x-ray, which will reveal interstitial or alveolar pulmonary edema, is the best way to make the definitive diagnosis.

Cardiac tamponade must be suspected when signs of low cardiac output occur in association with either decreased or excessive thoracotomy drainage and an increased CVP. Again, the most reliable diagnostic tool is a chest x-ray, which would reveal an enlarging cardiac silhouette without evidence of left-sided failure sufficient to cause the clinical picture.

Urinary output is checked every hour for color, specific gravity, and volume. Occasionally hematuria may be present because of trauma from the catheter or hemolysis of erythrocytes from the cardiopulmonary bypass. The normal specific gravity is 1.010 to 1.030. High readings occur secondary to the presence of erythrocytes, oliguria, or large molecular substances such as glucose or Osmitrol. On the other hand, readings may be low because of overhydration, intentional diuresis, or the inability of the kidneys to filter waste products. Color is not an accurate indication of specific gravity.

Initially following surgery the urinary output may be increased because of the perfusion flow rates during cardiopulmonary bypass. Within a few hours the urinary output levels off to 20 to 30 ml per hour in the post-cardiac-surgery patient. An output of less than 20 ml for two consecutive hours is considered abnormally low; possible causes are hypovolemia, hypotension, and hemolysis (see Chapter 41).

Comfort Measures

For the first 24 to 48 hours postoperatively analgesics are required frequently to control the pain. Most analgesics have undesirable side effects, including depression of the cough reflex or hypotension; however, these effects do not outweigh the positive analgesic effect. At times a change of position with proper support to the back may relieve mild chest discomfort.

The patient's position in bed should be changed frequently to promote drainage of the thoracotomy tube, provide better lung expansion, and prevent pooling of pulmonary secretions and atelectasis. Position changes would include turning from side to side and into a semi-Fowler's position, depending on the patient's condition. In many institutions if the patient is hemodynamically stable, he or she will be dangled the evening of surgery and be up in the chair the first postoperative day.

Psychological Considerations

For years medical and nursing professionals have recognized the syndrome of postcardiotomy psychosis. It is not unusual for cardiac surgical patients to experience unusual sensory and cognitive disturbances during the first few days following surgery. The sensory hallucinations and illusions may occur with or without disorientation to time, place, and person. Medical means are available to correct physiologic alterations in the postcardiotomy patient such as fluid and electrolyte imbalances and hemodynamic disequilibrium that may occur in association with cardiopulmonary bypass. Nursing interventions are important in dealing with the psychosocial-environmental factors that could affect the postcardiotomy patient.

According to Harken, a new breed of diseases has been created for patients who are in intensive-care units. He coined the name, periontogenic diseases which means diseases whose genesis lie in "those things about" the patient (1974, p. 900). These may be psychological, mechanical, electrical, infectious, chemical, or human. They may be any or all combinations of these factors.

Of the periontogenic diseases, perhaps one of the most dramatic is that derived from sensory deprivation and the disruption of the normal diurnal and circadian rhythms. It is apparent that not enough attention is paid to the life patterns and cycles to which patients are normally accustomed. Frequently intensive-care units do not have windows. In addition there is no day or night; instead there is interference with sleep and all other stimuli (pain, visual, and sensory) are maximized for the patient. In addition the patient is frequently kept awake by all the treatments for 24 to 48 hours without any extended period of sleep.

Repetitious and monotonous sounds or "white noise" compound the psychological disturbances created by timelessness and loss of diurnal and circadian rhythms. There are the monitoring "beeps," alarm sounds, compounded by the patient's fear of death, loss of privacy, and loss of time (day and night).

Ellis (1972, p. 2023) also studied the area of unusual sensory experiences in postcardiotomy patients. It was concluded that the unusual sensory, emotional, and thought experiences are probably caused by multiple factors. She indicated that there could be impairment of the patient's reality-orienting capacity caused by such psychological factors as the patient's personality, family problems, or the meaning of surgery to the patient. Reality orientation could be impaired by physiologic states, such as electrolyte distrubances, pain, or drugs. It also could be impaired by unfamiliar stressful environments with either monotonous or ambiguous sounds.

From the research done by Ellis, it was recognized that unusual sensory experiences were associated with uncontrolled pain, discharge fears, the patient's clinical condition, and misperceptions of other communication problems. Ellis also found that the patients were keenly aware of reality while they were having these sensory experiences and could talk rationally about the experiences even while they were taking place.

Obviously there is no one intervention that can be used to control unusual sensory experiences that result from various causes. Of utmost importance is the need for the nurse to establish a good interpersonal relationship with the patient, control the physical environment, and help the patient become reality oriented.

Nursing care should be planned so that maximum periods of rest are provided between necessary treatment times. Some patients may not have any uninterrupted periods of sleep for several days.

Families as well as patients need psychological support during the postoperative period. For the average lay person, it is most frightening to walk into an intensive-care unit because of the vast amount of equipment and the critical conditions of the patients. To see their loved one in this environment can be most distressing. The nurse can be supportive of the family by such simple things as common courtesy, explaining what is happening, and going to the bedside with them.

In a study by Chatham, it was found that involvement of the significant family member, who had been instructed systematically to use eye contact, frequent touch, and verbal orientation to time, person, and place with the postcardiotomy patient, favorably affected the following behaviors: orientation, appropriateness, confusion, delusions, and sleep. The patients in the experimental group were more oriented to time, person, and place. They also were more appropriate and less confused as shown by speech and behaviors, had fewer delusions and had longer periods of sleep as compared to subjects in the control group (1978, p. 998).

After the patient is transferred from the intensive-care unit, the nursing care is generally the same as for any postoperative patient. Special attention is given to the diet, which is restricted in sodium content. The nurse must be cognizant of the signs and symptoms of possible complications that usually occur in the immediate postoperative period but also can occur later in the recovery phase.

Usually there are no specific restrictions regarding the patient's activity when discharged. For some patients who have lived a protected life prior to surgery because of their cardiac condition, the adjustment of the surgery can be most difficult. Other patients may need counseling regarding a change in occupation.

The Endocardium

Structure and Function

The endocardium is composed of a single layer of simple squamous epithelial cells that lie directly over a thin layer of connective tissue fibers and smooth muscle cells. The endocardium lines the chambers of the heart, is reflected over the cardiac valves, and is continuous with the endothelial lining of the blood vessels entering and leaving the heart. It serves the same function as the intima of the blood vessels by providing a smooth surface for contact with the blood. Thus the friction between the blood and the walls of the heart is lessened and the danger of blood clotting is decreased.

If the endocardium is damaged and no longer presents a nearly frictionless surface, it may serve as a site for intracardiac thrombus formation. Damage to the endocardium can result from infection, stasis, trauma, aging, infarction, or the collagen diseases. To illustrate, with a myocardial infarction that involves the endocardium, the layer becomes roughened because of necrosis of the endothelial cells and predisposes to the thrombus formation. Whenever a thrombus is present in any part of the vascular system, there is always the potential of embolization whereby the embolus will travel in the circulation until it obstructs a blood vessel. The site of obstruction depends on whether the embolus originates in the left or right side of the heart and the size of clot. An embolus originating in the left side of the heart will either partially or totally obstruct an artery in the systemic circulation, whereas an embolus originating in the right side obstructs the pulmonary circulation.

Bacterial Endocarditis

Endocarditis is an inflammation of the endocardium. The mitral and/or aortic valves are involved primarily; however, the mural endocardium of the cardiac chambers and the intima of the great vessels may be affected also. Endocarditis can be of either a nonbacterial or bacterial origin, although bacterial endocarditis is the most common. All persons with rheumatic heart disease, deformity of cardiac valves, or artificial valves are susceptible to bacterial endocarditis.

Bacterial endocarditis is classified as either acute or subacute. Acute bacterial endocarditis indicates an infection with a fulminating onset and fast progression, which frequently involves normal cardiac valves. Acute bacterial endocarditis is caused by virulent, pyogenic bacteria, such as the gonococcus, pneumococcus, nonhemolytic streptococcus, and *Staphylococcus aureus.* In contrast, subacute bacterial endocarditis is associated with organisms of low virulence, such as *Streptococcus viridans.*

Because bacterial endocarditis is not a reportable disease, there is no way accurately to estimate the overall incidence. In general there has been an overall decrease in the incidence of bacterial endocarditis since the antibiotic era. The more adequate coverage with antibiotics following genitourinary, gynecologic, and obstetric surgery and during dental manipulations has also undoubtedly reduced the incidence. Also infections, such as skin and pulmonary, must have antibiotic coverage. It should be noted, however, that there is some concern for a renewed increase in subacute bacterial endocarditis (SBE) with the advent of indwelling venous cannulas, central venous pressure catheters, and transvenous pacemaking catheters as seen in coronary and intensive-care unit patients.

The most common organism to cause bacterial endocarditis is *Streptococcus viridans,* which usually causes a subacute form of bacterial endocarditis, particularly in those individuals with a previous injury to the endocardium, such as in rheumatic valvular disease and congenital or syphilitic lesions. *Streptococcus viridans* is harbored in infectious lesions of the gums and teeth. Bacteremia can be secondary to tonsillectomies and dental extractions as well.

The second most common organism to cause bacterial endocarditis is the *Staphylococcus* organism, either *aureus* or *albus,* which most frequently causes the acute form. Endocarditis secondary to the staphylococcus organism can be a serious complication in the postoperative cardiac patient because of infection from the prosthesis or sutures. Other sources of staphylococcal endocarditis include abscesses or septic thrombophlebitis.

Streptococcus faecalis (enterococcus), an organism of low virulence, is the third most common causative organism and usually causes the subacute form. Usually it follows some type of manipulative procedure within the urethra, such as a prostatectomy, catheterization, or genitourinary infection in men 45 to 60 years of age.

The lesions of bacterial endocarditis are vegetations composed of fibrin, bacteria, and necrotic valve substance. In the majority of cases there is a predisposing lesion that permits or causes trauma to the valvular chamber or vascular lining, but in some cases bacterial endocarditis can occur on apparently normal valves. Because the lesions of bacterial endocarditis tend to form in areas of rapid, forceful circulation, the left side of the heart is more frequently involved.

The mitral and/or aortic valves are the most common sites for bacterial endocarditis, and rheumatic heart disease is almost always the predisposing factor. Even though the rheumatic involvement may not be significant enough to cause any hemodynamic changes, there will be denuded areas that will be susceptible to the bacterial infection.

The severity of damage to the endocardium will vary, depending on the virulence of the organism and the location and duration of the infectious process. The manifestations of bacterial endocarditis can range from localized valvular lesions to lesions in areas remote from the heart. Valvular lesions would include deposits of vegetation on the valves or chamber walls and in more advanced cases perforation of the cusp, as well as rupture of chordae tendineae with resultant valvular insufficiency.

A distinctive characteristic of bacterial endocarditis is the tendency for embolization; thus there can be many varied effects of the disease. If the right side of the heart is involved, the emboli will travel to the lungs, whereas left-sided involvement could result in emboli lodging in the brain, kidney, spleen, coronary arteries, or other parts of the systemic circulation.

The clinical picture of *subacute bacterial endocarditis* is varied and can mimic other diseases, both severe and insignificant. Because there are no definitive signs and symptoms early in the disease, a positive diagnosis is difficult to make. Typically the early symptoms are vague and occur gradually. The patient usually experiences a persistent low-grade fever associated with easy fatigability, malaise, or anorexia. Because the disease is caused by a variety of microorganisms, the virulence of the organism and the degree of bacteremia determine the severity of the early symptoms. Thus some patients may experience shaking chills and profuse sweats associated with the fever, whereas others may have afebrile periods.

Because the early symptoms can be so nondescript in the eyes of the patient, the disease process continues until more severe symptoms cause the patient to seek medical advice. For this reason patients with a known or suspected cardiac murmur should be counseled not to overlook signs of fever, malaise, fatigability, and anorexia, as they could be the early signs of bacterial endocarditis.

The late manifestations are development of a cardiac murmur; anemia; petechiae; arthralgia; embolization to the kidney, spleen, brain or extremities; heart failure; and renal failure. A significant soft systolic murmur is usually present and may be the only indication of cardiac involvement. A normochromic, normocytic anemia is present in a large per cent of the cases. Petechial lesions may form in any organ supplied by the systemic circulation. These lesions are believed to occur either secondary to infection of the small arterial vessels with rupture or from microinfarction with hemorrhage. They are frequently seen in the mucous membranes of the mouth and larynx, in the conjunctiva and retina, and on the skin, particularly of the hands, ankles, and neck.

The symptoms caused by emboli will vary, depending on the organ affected, the size of the obstructed artery, and the virulence of the organism. Thus there could be gross infarcts, microinfarcts, or hemorrhage secondary to the emboli. The most common site of embolic infarction is the spleen. Associated symptoms would be splenomegaly, left upper abdominal pain that radiates to the left shoulder. In rare cases the spleen may suppurate and rupture, with a resultant subdiaphragmatic abscess. The kidney is the second most common organ to have embolic involvement. The typical symptom is hematuria, and in some cases pyuria may be present. Neurologic symptoms secondary to cerebral emboli range from hemiplegia to headache, loss of memory, and confusion. The latter symptoms are caused by microinfarcts rather than by a gross infarct. Emboli also can cause peripheral vascular occlusions and thus be confused with atherosclerotic occlusive disease.

Acute bacterial endocarditis will be the same as subacute with symptoms related to infection, cardiac damage, and embolization. The major difference is that normal valves can be affected, and the course of the disease is stormier and progresses rapidly to death if therapy is not instituted.

Diagnosis is made tentatively because of a high degree of suspicion of bacterial endocarditis and is confirmed through positive blood cultures. In some cases the blood cultures will remain negative even though the patient has bacterial endocarditis. In such situations, an unexplained fever for 7 to 10 days plus a heart murmur are used as a basis for a positive diagnosis.

The aim of treatment is to eradicate the infecting organism totally within the vegetation, or exacerbation can occur. Bactericidal agents are used rather than bacteriostatic antibiotics. Only temporary remissions occur when bacteriostatic agents are used because the organisms remain deep within the vegetation, and after the treatment is discontinued, they begin to multiply. A cure can be provided if bactericidal agents, such as penicillin and streptomycin, are given in high doses over a long enough period of time. Opinion varies on what is the concentration of antibiotic necessary to kill the organism. The serum concentration should be four to ten times greater than the concentration known to kill the organism in vitro. Penicillin G or one of the newer penicillinase resistant varieties is used singly or in combination with other bactericidal agents for treatment. The usual route of penicillin administration is through a continuous intravenous drip. Oral administration has not proved to be as effective because of the variation in absorption of penicillin from the gastrointestinal tract.

Physical activity during therapy is determined according to the individual patient's situation. If there is evidence of heart failure or myocarditis, bedrest is indicated; however, if it is an uncomplicated case, bedrest is not indicated. Also bedrest is advisable when the patient is febrile.

The aim of nursing care would be the same as for any patient who has febrile periods. Because the secret to successful therapy is to eradicate the infecting organism with high doses of antibiotics, it is imperative for the nurse to administer the medication at the prescribed intervals. If the medication is given through a continuous intravenous drip, the site for the needle insertion should be one that permits maximum mobility of the extremity without dislodgment of the needle. If intramuscular injections are prescribed, a schedule for site rotation should be developed for the medication will most likely be given for a minimum of 2 weeks.

The course of the fever should be observed and

recorded because frequently the fever will spike at the same time daily. If the fever can be anticipated, therapeutic measures, such as giving a tepid sponge bath, administering aspirin, and providing fluids, can be prepared in advance.

During the acute phase when the patient is febrile, bedrest is indicated. As the patient's condition improves, ambulation is permitted even while the patient is receiving intravenous medication. Patients tire of the extended therapeutic period (2 to 6 weeks) and hospitalization. It is most difficult for many patients to appreciate the need for all the intravenous and intramuscular medication when they "feel fine."

The nurse must teach the patient regarding the disease and treatment. Any patient with a valvular disease should be cognizant of the fact that bacterial endocarditis could recur when a bacteremia is present. Thus the patient should be taught to inform any physician who might be doing a manipulative procedure, such as a tooth extraction, genitourinary instrumentation, or tonsillectomy, that they have a valvular problem, so that adequate antibiotic coverage can be provided.

After discharge, repeat blood cultures usually are done at 2-week intervals for 6 weeks. The patient must understand the necessity of keeping the physician's appointments. Also, for a period of several weeks following discharge, strenuous exercise is restricted.

The Pericardium

Structure and Function

The pericardium, or outer covering of the heart, is an inelastic sac (the pericardial sac) in which the heart lies. The pericardium is made up of two parts, the fibrous and serous layers. The pericardial sac consists of tough white fibrous tissue that is lined with the parietal layer of the serous pericardium and the visceral layer (epicardium), which is adherent to the myocardium. The fibrous layer attaches to the large vessels emerging from the heart, but not to the heart itself. Normally the visceral and parietal layer of the serous pericardium are in contact with a small amount of serous fluid lubricating the surfaces of the two layers.

The pericardium has a number of important functions. It helps to anchor the heart in position and to decrease the friction between the heart and its environment. Also the pericardium prevents overdilatation of the heart during diastole.

The pericardium can be injured by trauma, infection, inflammation, or neoplasms, with the result that fluid, blood, or purulent material may collect in the pericardial sac. As the fluid accumulates, it occupies space in the pericardial sac and reduces the capacity of the heart to relax during diastole.

Because the blood is circulated in a closed system, the decreased capacity of the heart to receive blood has at least two detrimental effects on the entire vascular system. The cardiac output falls because the left ventricle can deliver into the arterial system only the volume of blood that it receives during diastole. As a result there is decreased perfusion of tissues throughout the body. When the cardiac output is markedly decreased, the coronary circulation cannot be maintained and ventricular fibrillation ensues. A second major effect of the decreased capacity of the heart to receive blood is interference with the venous return causing passive congestion of systemic organs such as the liver. The effects of venous congestion are discussed under heart failure.

Because of the location of the pericardium, disease of other organs in the thoracic cavity may spread to it. For example, the pericardium may be infected by tubercle bacilli as well as by pneumococci. Also, disease of the pericardium may extend to and injure the myocardium, coronary vessels, and portions of the conduction system. In the process of healing, bands or sheets of fibrous tissue, with or without calcification, may encompass the heart and lead to slow cardiac failure. These bands act as splints and limit the degree to which the heart can dilate.

Pericarditis

Pericarditis is an inflammatory process of the pericardium more often than not as a consequence of another pathologic or iatrogenic process. The most prevalent type, however, is an idiopathic or nonspecific form. The most familiar causes of pericarditis in acute care settings are anterior wall transmural myocardial infarction and open-heart surgery (postcardiotomy syndrome). Robinson (1979) enumerates the following other etiologies: (1) chest trauma, (2) upper respiratory infection, (3) neoplastic disease and following radiation therapy, (4) uremia, (5) autoimmune diseases such as the collagen disorders, (6) pulmonary or mediastinal infection, (7) tuberculosis, and (8) drugs such as immunosuppressive agents, hydralazine, ergot, and anticonvulsant (Dilantin) preparation (1979, p. 73). Pericarditis has been seen recently as a sequelae of several influenzal strains effecting particularly the young and elderly. It may also occur post-cardiac resuscitation.

Whereas the cardinal components of pericarditis are chest pain, pericardial friction rub, fever, and

S-T segment evaluations in the electrocardiogram, all these "classical" features may be absent, which creates a difficult diagnostic situation. The pain of pericarditis when present has particular characteristics that help to distinguish it from other types of chest pain. This is particularly true when pericarditis is associated with myocardial infarction where pain manifestations are an important consideration in prognosis.

The visceral layer and the upper portion of the parietal pericardium are not innervated with pain fibers. On the other hand, the lower portion of the parietal pericardium is supplied with nerve fibers. The pain is presumed to be caused by inflammation of the innervated part of the parietal pericardium. In addition there can be an inflammatory process involving the diaphragmatic pleura of the lung. The pain can take on the characteristic pattern of that associated with myocardial ischemia; that is, pain radiating to the left arm, neck, or shoulder. At times the chest pain can be so severe that it resembles that of a myocardial infarction. The chest pain of pericarditis, however, usually is aggravated by deep breathing and coughing, and may be eased by sitting upright and leaning forward which is unlike the pain of myocardial infarction. The pain frequently precedes development of the friction rub.

The friction rub is heard best with the diaphragm of the stethoscope pressed firmly against the thorax at the lower sternal border. The friction rub is a consequence of the irritated visceral and parietal layers of the pericardium coming in proximity during systole and/or diastole. The sound is characteristically scratchy, crunchy, or squeaky, likened to two pieces of sandpaper or leather being rubbed together. The rub occurs only in systole or in both systole-diastole which gives it a "to-and-fro" characteristic.

Other manifestations are a consequence of the inflammatory process [fever, malaise; involvement of contiguous organs (dysphagia); guarding to diminish the pain phenomenon (shallow breathing with tachypnea, dyspnea); and the acute insult (anxiety, irritability, restlessness)]. In addition to the altered physical findings in pericarditis, there will be changes in the laboratory data and x-rays. Signs of systemic reactions to inflammation or underlying disease may be evidenced by an increased leukocyte count, elevated erythrocyte sedimentation rate (ESR), or increased serum enzymes. X-rays usually demonstrate a normal cardiac silhouette unless pericardial effusion is present, in which case there could be a symmetrical increase in the heart size. The electrocardiogram will demonstrate characteristic changes of S-T segment elevation in all standard leads with subsequent T wave inversion. Echocardiography, ultrasound recordings, are done in many centers to detect the degree of fluid accumulation in the pericardial sac and thus determine the need for intervention, such as a pericardial tap.

Complications of pericarditis include congestive heart failure, arrhythmias, and cardiac tamponade. Associated with pericarditis can be pericardial effusion with serous, purulent, or hemorrhagic fluid depending on the primary pathology. If the accumulation of fluid is slow, the pericardium stretches sufficiently with no subsequent impairment of cardiac output. On the other hand, if the fluid accumulation is rapid, cardiac chamber compression can occur with a subsequent decrease in cardiac output. Impairment of circulation because of a rapid accumulation of fluid or blood in the pericardial sac is called *cardiac tamponade.*

The manifestations of cardiac tamponade are all interrelated. Because of the increased intrapericardial pressure, the venous return to the right ventricle is decreased during diastole, and therefore there will be a decreased cardiac output. This will be manifested by a decreased systemic blood pressure and signs of shock, including a tachycardia and cold, clammy extremities. The increased pressure in the right ventricle is reflected back to the right atrium, causing an increased central venous pressure that is manifested by an engorged liver and distended neck veins. The patient appears anxious, cyanotic, and pale. A *pulsus paradoxus,* described as a waxing and waning of the arterial pressure with at least a 10 mm Hg diminution during inspiration, may be present.

Cardiac tamponade may be a life-threatening situation with need for immediate removal of the pericardial fluid. Needle aspiration of the pericardial sac is performed to establish the underlying cause of the tamponade as well as to treat the tamponade. As with any aspiration of a cavity, the nurse has a responsibility to assist with the procedure as well as to support and observe the patient during the procedure. The patient is positioned in a slightly sitting position. The preferred approach is the subxiphoid where the needle is inserted in the angle between the left costal margin and xiphoid and directed to the right shoulder. The precordial lead of the electrocardiogram is attached to the aspirating needle with an alligator clamp. This is done to monitor traversal of the various tissue layers and to determine if the myocardium is entered as evidenced by increased S-T segment elevation. Throughout the procedure, the electrocardiogram, venous pressure, and arterial blood pressure are monitored. In addition, a defibrillator should be present as ventricular fibrillation is a possible complication. Other complications would include a vagovagal arrest or laceration of the coronary artery or myocardium which could result in death.

Treatment of acute pericarditis is determined by the underlying cause and has a symptomatic orientation with general supportive measures. The choice of analgesic for pain relief is determined by the severity of pain. Large doses of morphine may be required and may not be effective. Anti-inflammatory agents such as aspirin and indomethacin (Indocin) are employed to reduce the inflammatory process. Some physicians prefer routinely to use corticosteroid preparations for the patient in severe pain who is unable to breathe deeply and assume the recumbent position (Robinson, 1979, p. 76). There is some disagreement about the use of steroids with postmyocardial infarction pericarditis because of fluid retention and retardation of scar tissue formation with aneurysm formation.

Nursing actions are directed to provision of comfort measures, alleviation of anxiety, and monitoring for the aforementioned complications. The position of the individual markedly diminishes or exacerbates the pain phenomenon. A recumbent position usually is intolerable, whereas elevating the head of the bed and leaning forward on an overhead table provides relief. A quiet environment tends to enhance comfort and allay anxiety and irritability. Sedation may be required.

Two specific types of pericarditis bear mention. Pericarditis that occurs several weeks post–myocardial infarction is *post–myocardial infarction syndrome* (PMIS), or Dressler's syndrome. A chronic fibrotic disease of the pericardium is *constrictive pericarditis*. Surgical intervention may be required with chronic pericardial effusion associated with constrictive pericarditis or other long-term forms. A shunt procedure, "pleuro-pericardial window," or a pericardiectomy may be performed.

The Myocardium

From the standpoint of function, the myocardium is the most essential part of the heart because it serves as the pump for the continuous propulsion of blood through the transport system. A number of factors contribute to the effectiveness of the myocardium as a pump. One major factor is the structure of the myocardial tissue. At one time the myocardium was thought of as a single multinucleated cell. With the advent of the electron microscope and specialized laboratory techniques for isolation of single living mammalian cells, however, it has been noted that the myocardium is composed of many cells, each with a single nucleus. The myocardial cells are arranged in a latticework fashion with branching interconnecting fibers. This arrangement helps to explain the transmission of cardiac impulses from cell to cell and the resultant wave of contraction.

A specialized property of myocardial cells is the ability to contract in response to a given stimulus. The normal stimulus is usually a cardiac impulse. Each myocardial cell contains an indefinable number of sarcomere units that are composed of interdigitating filaments of the intracellular proteins, actin and myosin. The actin and myosin filament bands slide across each other (the excitation–contraction coupling mechanism) to cause cellular contraction given the necessary conditions of (1) stimulation by a cardiac impulse, (2) mediation by intracellular calcium ions, and (3) availability of sufficient adenosine triphosphate. A reversal of the excitation–contraction coupling mechanism produces relaxation.

The all-or-none law applies to the process of myocardial contraction. When myocardial cells contract, contraction occurs to the fullest extent possible or not at all. This should not be interpreted to mean, however, that the force of contraction is always the same. The force of myocardial contraction is a function of the myocardial fiber length at the end of diastole (beginning of systole) and is explained by Starling's Law of the Heart. Stated simply, Starling's Law of the Heart means that within physiologic limits the longer the muscle fiber, the greater the strength of contraction.

Like all other tissues, myocardial cells are dependent on a continuous supply of oxygen and other essential materials to maintain metabolic processes and thus cellular function. The myocardium is more susceptible to hypoxia, however, than some other tissues. Whereas skeletal muscle cells can tolerate an appreciable oxygen debt, myocardial cells cannot. Myocardial oxygen deprivation leads more readily to permanent cellular dysfunction. Thus any disorder that deprives the myocardium of its blood supply, either in part or in whole, predisposes the myocardium to decreased efficiency as a pump.

The Coronary Circulation

Blood is supplied to the myocardial muscle mass by the right and left coronary arteries. The coronary ostia originate at the root of the aorta within the right and left anterior sinuses of Valsalva. (See Figures 44-4 and 44-9.) The right coronary artery originates from the right anterior sinus of Valsalva and principally perfuses the right ventricle and atrium. It has been demonstrated by coronary angiographic studies that the sinoatrial (SA) nodal artery originates

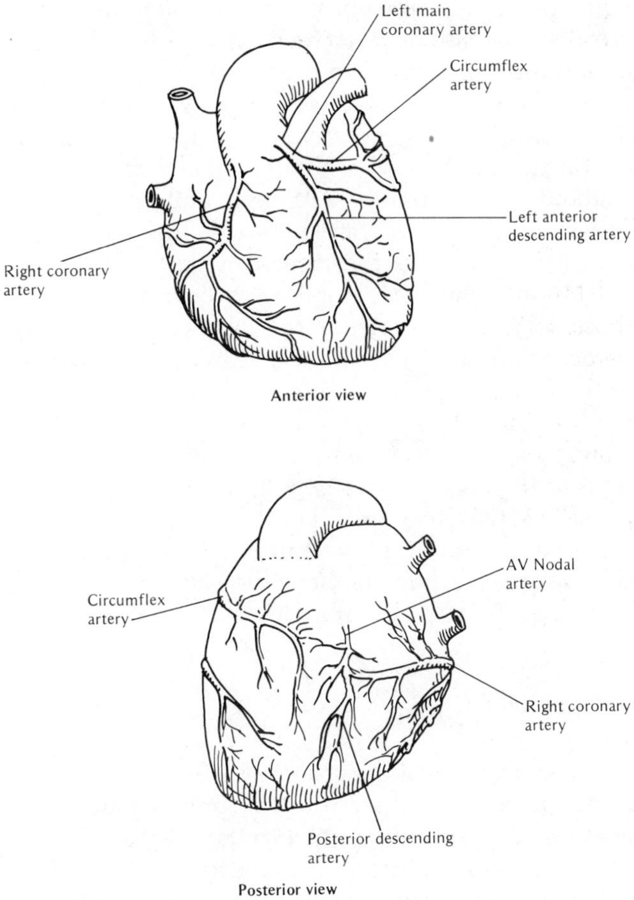

Figure 44-9. The coronary circulation: anterior and posterior cardiac views.

as a branch of the right coronary artery in the greatest percentage of human hearts. The SA nodal artery originates from the left circumflex artery in the remainder. As the right coronary artery courses posteriorly, the atrioventricular (AV) node is perfused by the posterior descending artery, a branch of the right coronary artery. In a high percentage of human hearts, the right coronary artery perfuses the inferior surface of the left ventricle.

The left main coronary artery originates from the left anterior sinus of Valsalva and principally perfuses the left ventricle and atrium via two main branches, the anterior descending and circumflex arteries. The left anterior descending coronary artery perfuses the anterior surface of the left ventricle and is the major contributor to the intraventricular septum. The circumflex coronary artery courses laterally and posteriorly, perfusing the lateral and part of the posterior surface of the left ventricle.

The right coronary artery and major branches of the left coronary artery are located in the epicardial layer of the heart and thus escape occlusion during ventricular systole. The smaller arteries penetrate into the myocardial muscle and ramify to provide arterioles and capillaries more numerous than in skeletal muscle. It has been approximated that there is a capillary for each myocardial muscle fiber.

The coronary venous system consists of smaller cardiac veins that join to become the great cardiac vein and drain into the right atrium via the coronary sinus. Although most of the venous blood leaves the myocardium via the coronary sinus, there are also vascular communications directly between the myocardial vessels and the cardiac chambers. These intraluminal channels consist of myocardial sinusoids and the thebesian veins, which open directly into the atria and ventricles.

The primary factor responsible for perfusion of the coronary arteries is the pressure within the root of the aorta during early diastole. During ventricular systole, coronary perfusion is virtually absent because of (1) occlusion of the coronary ostia by the aortic valve cusps and (2) compression of the intramyocardial coronary arterioles by the contracting myocardial fibers. During diastole, however, coronary flow and myocardial perfusion is maximal because of patency of the coronary ostia and myocardial arterioles. Thus coronary blood flow is *phasic*, occurring in *diastole* (see Figure 44-10).

Other factors that contribute to the regulation of coronary blood flow include the arterial blood oxygen tension and hydrogen ion concentration; the

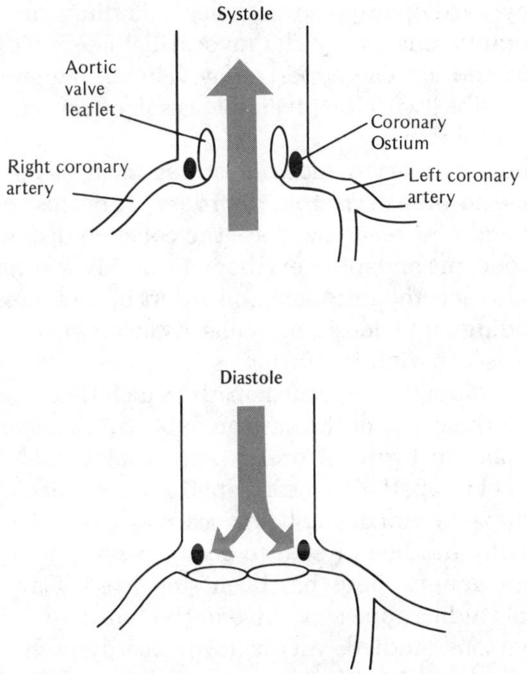

Figure 44-10. Schematic representation of coronary artery perfusion throughout the cardiac cycle: During systole, the aortic leaflets open over the coronary ostium. During diastole, the aortic valves close and retrograde aortic flow perfuses the coronary arteries.

action of certain biochemical substances; and the influence of the autonomic nervous system. Vasodilatation of the normal coronary vessel results in increased blood flow. This appears to occur with a decreased blood oxygen tension and increased hydrogen ion concentration. In general, sympathetic nervous system stimulation results in vasodilatation of the normal coronary arteries. The vasodilatation associated with sympathetic nervous system activity is thought to be due to the increased myocardial need for oxygen consequent to increased contractility and cellular metabolism. In the future, however, clarification of the contribution of alpha and beta-2 (constrictor) and beta-1 (dilator) receptor stimulation may further illuminate the complex subject of coronary blood flow regulation. To date, it merely can be noted that *many* factors appear to serve as homeostatic mechanisms for the maintenance of coronary blood flow and myocardial perfusion.

Myocardiopathy

The term *myocardiopathy* denotes a pathologic process that is localized solely in the myocardium. The myocardiopathies are most frequently classified as (1) primary (idiopathic), in which the etiology is obscure, and (2) secondary, in which the etiologic factor is more readily identifiable. Despite the presence or absence of an etiologic factor in all cases of myocardiopathy the pathologic findings are degenerative changes of the myocardial fibers with fibrosis and cardiac hypertrophy. These changes are irreversible, with the invariable result of cardiac failure and death.

The secondary myocardiopathies occur as late sequelae to other systemic disorders. The most common and best recognized are the collagen disorders, scleroderma and lupus erythematosus. Myocardiopathy also accompanies some disorders of metabolism, including amyloidosis, muscular dystrophy, and mucopolysaccharidosis (Hurler's syndrome).

The idiopathic myocardiopathies include those for which the cause of the cardiac hypertrophy is unexplainable in terms of present-day knowledge. Two forms of idiopathic myocardiopathy are familial myocardiopathy and alcoholic myocardiopathy. Myocardiopathy has been noted to occur in some families; thus a genetic basis has been suggested. Chromosomal studies appear positive in the limited number of persons studied. Alcoholic myocardiopathy has been related to the excessive ingestion of alcohol, which implies a direct injury to the myocardium by ethanol. Although it has been documented that ethanol alters cell membrane permeability and impairs metabolism during the Krebs cycle, it has also been noted that only a small proportion of individuals who are alcoholic also develop myocardiopathy. Thus the relationship of alcohol to the heart disease and the means by which such disease is produced, remain obscure. It has been noted in the primary myocardiopathies that there is a greater incidence of males affected than females. Although children are affected, most patients are between the ages of 20 and 40 years when the disease is discovered. The outstanding clinical features of myocardiopathy are those related to heart failure. Diagnosis of primary myocardiopathy is accomplished by documentation of the heart failure but also by the inability to document evidence of other forms of heart disease that would explain the heart failure. The treatment of myocardiopathy is extremely limited and only temporarily satisfactory. Intervention is directed to the heart failure until it is no longer effective. Until such time as more is known about the causes of myocardiopathy, intervention remains palliative.

Atherosclerosis

Atherosclerosis of the coronary arteries is the most frequent cause of disease of the myocardium. The general clinical term applied to the myocardial dysfunction that results from the atherosclerotic process is *coronary artery* (heart) *disease.* Atherosclerosis contributes to more deaths annually from cardiovascular disease than any other process. As noted in Figure 44-11, coronary artery disease was the principal cause of cardiovascular mortality in 1969 and 1976. More than one third of these deaths occurred in persons under the age of 65 years. The greatest mortality was recorded among males. Thus coronary artery disease resulting from atherosclerosis not only is the leading cause of death, but also strikes individuals in the prime of their productivity.

Despite the prevalence of coronary artery disease, the definitive etiology of atherosclerosis is unknown. Clinicians are currently of the persuasion that several interrelated factors are responsible. The factor that holds considerable prominence is that of a defect in lipid metabolism with resultant excessive lipids in the blood (hyperlipoproteinemia) and lipid deposition in the subintimal layer of arterial vessels. One theory holds that the lipid triglyceride and the lipidlike substance cholesterol enter the intima from the blood. There is also some evidence to suggest that other implicated lipids, the phospholipids, are synthesized within the vessel walls. Regardless of the mechanism by which deposition occurs, the lipids accumulate locally and form atheromas (atheromatous plaques), which are the hallmark of the atherosclerotic process.

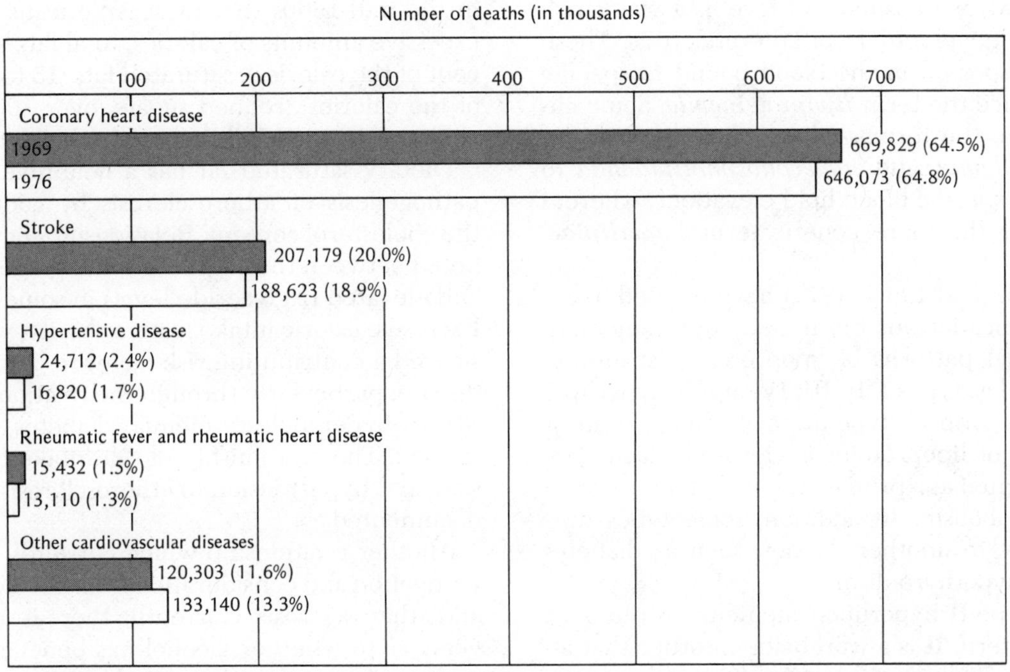

Figure 44-11. Estimated number of deaths in United States caused by specific cardiovascular diseases 1969 and 1976. (Information adapted from the National Center for Health Statistics, USPHS, DHEW, 1976)

As the process continues, calcium ions and fibroblasts precipitate from the blood and combine with the lipids; hence the characteristic "hardening of the arteries," or arteriosclerosis. As an atheroma enlarges, the diameter of the vessel lumen is diminished and partial or total obstruction occurs. The atheroma can also rupture through the intimal layer and protrude into the vessel lumen. The ragged edge of the protruding plaque can then serve as a site for fibrin and platelet accumulation, with resultant thrombus formation. It should be noted, however, that coronary vessel occlusion occurs predominantly as a result of atheromatous plaque formation per se, rather than as a result of thrombus formation.

Although authorities do not agree on the pathogenesis of atherosclerosis, there is agreement on the major sites involved. Atherosclerosis is found most frequently in vessels where there is a large amount of elastic tissue in the media. These include the coronary and cerebral arteries and the aorta.

As a consequence of the atherosclerotic process, the blood supply is diminished to the dependent tissues. The resultant phenomena will depend on the rapidity and degree of diminished tissue perfusion. When tissue perfusion slowly diminishes, as with gradual or partial obstruction of a vessel, the result is ischemia of the tissues. A sudden or complete obstruction of a vessel decreases tissue perfusion rapidly, with resultant necrosis of the dependent tissue. This process is best exemplified in the process of coronary atherosclerosis. Another consequence of atherosclerosis is a weakening of the vessel wall with subsequent aneurysm formation. The aorta is the most common site for this to occur. In those vessels where weakening is marked, the vessel may rupture and hemorrhage results. The cerebral arteries have thinner walls than those in other parts of the body and therefore are more susceptible to rupture when atherosclerotic.

Despite the lack of a definitive etiologic base for atherosclerosis, experimental, clinical, and epidemiologic studies have helped to identify multiple factors associated with atherosclerosis that appear to predispose an individual to coronary artery disease. These *risk factors* have been identified through the study of individuals and entire populations. The best known of these studies is the Framingham Heart Study (1966). It is felt that control of as many of these risk factors as possible can result in a delayed onset of coronary disease. As a result, considerable emphasis has been placed on early detection of risk factors in individuals and families through community screening and public education programs. The nurse has a primary role in case finding of the coronary-prone individual.

Hyperlipoproteinemia

Abundant evidence has accumulated over the past 20 years indicating that an elevated cholesterol, triglyceride, and/or phospholipid level is a major risk factor in the development of atherosclerosis. These fats are transported in the blood bound to specific proteins, hence the term *lipoproteinemia.* Some clinicians utilize the terms *hypercholesterolemia, hypertriglyceridemia,* and *hyperphospholipidemia* to describe the specific blood lipid elevations, whereas others prefer the more generic term *hyperlipidemia.*

Fredrickson and Levy (1972) have devised a system of classification for the hyperlipoproteinemias. The abnormal patterns of lipoprotein distribution are described as types I, II, III, IV, and V hyperlipoproteinemias. In each type a specific lipoprotein or combination of lipoproteins is elevated. Each type may be inherited as a primary familial genetic defect in lipid metabolism. In addition, some types may be secondary to another disease, such as diabetes mellitus or hypothyroidism.

Familial type II hyperlipoproteinemia is the most common pattern. It is a worldwide disorder that affects all ages. The most common finding is an elevated plasma cholesterol. If the serum triglycerides are normal, it is known as a type IIa. If the serum triglycerides are elevated, it is a type IIb. Associated with the hyperlipidemia are xanthomas and premature coronary disease. Less frequently, the type II pattern is secondary to obstructive liver disease and the nephrotic syndrome.

Type IV hyperlipoproteinemia is the second most common pattern. The most common finding is an elevated serum triglyceride level, which usually becomes evident in adulthood.There may or may not be an associated hypercholesterolemia. This pattern is associated with an abnormal glucose tolerance, premature coronary atherosclerosis, hyperuricemia, and obesity.

Laboratory testing for hyperlipoproteinemia is becoming a part of routine assessment of the cardiac patient in many institutions. In the absence of these more sophisticated procedures, blood serum cholesterol and triglyceride may be analyzed. There is concern, however, that noncardiac patients as well as known or suspected adult cardiac patients should be tested if screening is to be effective. Further, children over the age of 5 years should be tested if they are from families with histories of early coronary artery disease and hyperlipoproteinemia. With early recognition of hyperlipidemia in adults and children there can be early intervention.

Dietary Patterns

The contemporary American diet, in contrast to those of other cultures, is recognized as a significant risk factor. Stamler et al. (1966, p. 1790) reported in the mid-1960s that most Americans daily ingest excessive amounts of calories, total fats (40 to 45 per cent of the calories), saturated fats (15 to 20 per cent of the calories), refined sugars (over 100 g), dietary cholesterol (over 700 mg), and salt (10 to 20 g).

Dietary saturated fat has a definitive role in the pathogenesis of atherosclerosis by contributing to the cholesterol content. Relationships have also been noted between the excessive intake of refined sugars and elevated triglyceride levels in some individuals. Excessive caloric intake fosters obesity, which is considered a contributing risk factor to coronary artery disease, particularly through the relationship of obesity to hypercholesterolemia, diabetes, and hypertension. The relationship of salt intake to hypertension, and hypertension to atherosclerosis, also is well documented.

Another relationship which currently is under investigation and consideration is that of alcohol intake and atherosclerosis. Currently, there is some controversy as to whether alcohol has beneficial or detrimental effects on the heart and blood vessels directly and in relation to the atherosclerotic process. The answer to the controversy appears to lie in the amount, or dosage, consumed at any one time or over a period of time. There is an inverse relationship between "moderate" alcohol consumption and the development of coronary artery disease perhaps, in part, as related to the vasodilating property of alcohol on blood vessels. Conversely, with excessive alcohol consumption, the incidence of coronary artery disease increases. This may be explained by a combination of factors including an influence on the development of lipoproteinemia, myocardiopathy, and hypertension (Barboriak & Menahan, 1979, p. 738). The evidence that dietary pattern may contribute significantly to coronary artery disease, either directly or through its relationship to other risk factors, favors a preventive approach at this time.

Physical Activity

The relationship of sedentary behavior and a substantially higher mortality from coronary artery disease has been firmly established. Exercise does not retard the atherogenic process per se. Exercise promotes an improved coronary circulation by development of collateral circulation. Further, there is evidence to suggest that physical training may actually increase the diameter of the coronary vessels, thus compensating for the atherosclerotic process and decreasing the relative degree of obstruction. It is also suggested that exercising *before* the heaviest meal of the day actually curbs appetite thus decreasing food intake and contributing to weight reduction and maintenance (Alexander et al., 1978).

Age and Sex

Clinical evidence of coronary atherosclerosis may occur in the second and third decade of life, although this is not common. Studies done during the Korean War on soldiers killed during combat revealed significant coronary atherosclerosis in 77 per cent of the victims, with a mean age of 22 years (Enos, 1953). It has also been observed in the arteries of newborn infants. Generally, the incidence of atherosclerosis rises with age. The greatest incidence of overt coronary artery disease is seen in males after the age of 40 years. Coronary artery disease is unusual in females before menopause because of a normal balance of hormones. The exception would be those women who are diabetic or hypertensive. Following menopause, the incidence of coronary atherosclerosis in females approaches that of males.

Family History

A family history of early coronary artery disease has been demonstrated as a significant predictor in the detection of increased risks for blood relatives, particularly siblings. The familial predisposition to atherosclerosis is thought to be due to both genetic and environmental influences. The genetic component is noted by the familial tendency toward other key risk factors, such as hyperlipoproteinemia, obesity, diabetes, and hypertension. Environmental factors, which are both socially and culturally derived, include nutritional and smoking habits.

Blatant examples of family members sharing similar patterns of predisposition toward coronary disease has been demonstrated by epidemiological studies. For example, in one community hospital screening program of 174 family members who had blood relatives with documented coronary artery disease, the findings were (1) lipid abnormalities—23 per cent, (2) undetected hypertension—15.5 per cent, (3) overweight—44 per cent, (4) cigarette smokers—21 per cent, and (5) sedentary activity patterns—62 per cent (Manley & Graber, 1977, pp. 1048–49).

Cigarette Smoking

It has been noted that there is a greater incidence of heart attacks among those individuals who smoke cigarettes than among those individuals who do not smoke. The risk tends to increase with the number of cigarettes smoked per day. Essentially no correlation has been noted between cigar or pipe smoking and heart attacks. With cessation of cigarette smoking, the risk appears to diminish to that of a nonsmoker despite the duration of the habit.

The relationship of cigarette smoking to heart attack appears not to be one of relationship to atherogenesis per se. Rather, the relationship may be related to the influence of the carbon monoxide (CO) in the smoke to a diminished oxygen tension in the presence of atherosclerotic disease. It is significant that filters on cigarettes, although diminishing tar and nicotine, have no effect on elimination of CO. Documentation has been made of individuals with coronary artery disease experiencing anginal pain following exposure to CO in laboratory situations, in industry, and on freeways. It also has been documented that nonsmokers have CO in their blood when exposed to smoke in the air (McIntosh, Entman, Evans, Martin, & Jackson, 1978, pp. 146–47).

Another area of considerable concern is the combined relationship of cigarette smoking and birth control pill ingestion to cardiovascular disease. The risk of coronary artery disease and subsequent heart attack increased with the age of the female on oral contraceptive agents, particularly over 35 years of age, and with consumption of greater than 15 cigarettes a day (Clinical Implications, FDA, 1979, p. 6). Depending on the age of the female and the number of cigarettes consumed daily, the use of the birth control pill may be more hazardous than pregnancy per se, other considerations notwithstanding.

Despite massive public education-information programs to promote abstinence from cigarette smoking, the statistics are less than encouraging. Forty per cent of American males and 30 per cent of females smoke. The percentage of males is decreasing but the percentage of females is increasing. The number of teenagers commencing smoking (around the age of 12 years) is alarming. The old adage "one step forward, two steps back" seems apropos.

Other Risk Factors

Hypertension, as the major risk factor for coronary artery disease, was discussed in a previous section. It has been suggested that the greater the elevation in the blood pressure, the greater the number of coronary vessels involved in the atherosclerotic process (McIntosh, Eknoyan, & Jackson, 1978, p. 140). In persons who have other diseases such as diabetes mellitus, gout, and hypothyroidism, there is an increased incidence of atherosclerosis at an early age.

Although controversial, personality factors (or at least the ability to cope with stressors) appear to influence the development of coronary artery disease either directly or as related to other risk factors. Friedman and Rosenman (1974) report a definitive personality pattern (type A) in individuals who are coronary-prone. These individuals are overly ambitious and competitive, deadline oriented, time-stressed, and hard-driving. They work longer hours, smoke more, and have higher blood cholesterol levels and blood pressure. Their speech pattern is rapid, explosive, and interruptive. In contrast, the personality pattern of individuals who are less coronary-prone (type B) reflects individuals who are more relaxed and easy going and who are more moderate in their drive for achievement. It is suggested that the type A personality is twice as likely to develop coronary artery disease and recurrent myocardial infarction. It must be noted, however, that this stereotypic psychological approach is not accepted throughout the health care community.

What is most important is that studies demonstrate categorically that the more risk factors an individual possesses, the greater the risk of coronary atherosclerosis. Thus a situation of high vulnerability is created by multiple risk factors.

Because the etiology of atherosclerosis is uncertain, intervention consists of controlling those factors associated with the process. Intervention is directed toward prevention, alleviation, and/or control of risk factors; dietary modifications; and the potential utilization of serum cholesterol-lowering drugs in high-risk individuals. Although an individual cannot change his or her age, sex, and family history, control can be exerted over other risk factors. Abstinence from cigarette smoking and stressful situations is advocated as well as planned daily physical activity. Control of blood pressure, diabetes, gout, and thyroid imbalance states can be achieved by diligent medical follow-up care and individual compliance with the prescribed regime.

Dietary Management

The major thrust in prevention of atherosclerosis and coronary artery disease is directed toward dietary modification to control body weight and lipid ingestion. For the individual with an identified hyperlipoproteinemia pattern, specific dietary regimens have been developed. The dietary approach differs somewhat for individuals who primarily have elevated serum triglyceride levels and for those who primarily have elevated cholesterol levels. For individuals with hypertriglyceridemia and obesity, the primary aim of dietary management is reduction to and maintenance of the ideal body weight. There may also be dietary supplementation with a "medium chain triglyceride" substance for its lipid-lowering effect. Caloric restriction has much less effect on the plasma cholesterol. The dietary management of hypercholesterolemia is directed toward a modification in the types of dietary lipids ingested, as noted in the type II diet for hyperlipoproteinemia.

For individuals with type II hyperlipoproteinemia in which the primary problem is hypercholesterolemia, the objectives of dietary management are to obtain as high as possible a ratio of polyunsaturated to saturated fats and to decrease the cholesterol intake to less than 300 mg per day (NIH, 1970). The ratio of polyunsaturated fats to saturated fats is recommended at 2:1. The primary sources for this ratio are an increase in the foods derived from vegetable oils with a concomitant decrease in the foods containing animal fats. In order to decrease the dietary cholesterol, it is necessary to eliminate nondairy substitutes for milk, substitute skimmed for whole milk, use margarine instead of butter, eliminate or severely reduce the use of egg yolks, and restrict the intake of cheese.

One area of concern, although limited, is the effect of frequent rapid weight reduction by fad diets. There is evidence to suggest that with the employment of low carbohydrate diets, the serum lipids increase (Gotto et al., 1978, p. 133). For an individual who regains the lost weight and diets again, there is a situation of increased-decreased-increased-decreased lipid levels, or a "yo-yo" effect. What of the influence on lipid deposition and the development of atheromas during these cycles?

The American Heart Association has recommended that the national diet be altered on a voluntary basis in the interest of potential retardation of atherosclerosis. Many clinicians feel these recommendations seem prudent on the basis of current knowledge. The specific recommendations include (1) ingestion of a 2:1 polyunsaturated-saturated fat ratio up to about 10 per cent of the total calories, (2) caloric reduction for ideal weight attainment and maintenance, (3) reduction in total fat ingestion to 30 to 35 per cent of total calories and reduction of refined sugars intake to about 10 per cent of total calories, (4) reduction of cholesterol intake to less than 300 mg per day, (5) limitation of sodium intake to no more than 5 g per day, and (6) consumption of alcohol in moderation (Arlin, 1979).

In local communities, large-scale community education programs have been developed on diet and coronary artery disease. The local chapter of the American Heart Association is an excellent resource for dietary literature and consultation for professionals in the health care field as well as for the public.

Pharmacologic Management

There is lack of general agreement on the indications for pharmacologic intervention and the serum lipid level at which drug therapy should begin. It should also be noted that definite scientific data are lacking on the efficacy of drug therapy in the retardation of coronary artery disease. It would appear that the current philosophy of many clinicians is to utilize the pharmacologic agents with individuals who are in the high-risk category. Individuals in this category include those with (1) overt manifestations of advanced atherosclerosis and (2) severe primary hyperlipoproteinemia who may or may not as yet have exhibited overt manifestations of coronary occlusive disease.

One antihypercholesterolemic drug in current use is cholestyramine (Questran, Cuemid). Cholestyramine is a cation-exchange resin that, when ingested, is not absorbed from the gut. It binds bile acids in the intestine, thereby promoting bile acid excretion. Bile acids are a product of cholesterol that are totally reabsorbed in the gut. Once reabsorbed, bile acids are cycled to the liver and inhibit the further degradation of cholesterol to bile acids. If, however, the reabsorption of bile acids is inhibited in the gut, then greater cholesterol stores are broken down in the liver and thereby excreted as bile acids. The discomforts experienced by some patients related to this drug are related to the gastrointestinal tract and include distention, nausea, and constipation. Although these side effects diminish with continued therapy, stool softeners and mild cathartics may need to be considered as adjunctive therapy. One other potential side effect of cholestyramine is an interference with the absorption of other drugs such as thyroxine, phenylbutazone, warfarin, and digitoxin. It is recommended that other drugs be ingested at least 1 hour before cholestyramine administration. Cholestyramine will effect a 20 to 25 per cent reduction in the serum cholesterol level over and above that achieved by diet alone.

An antihypercholesterolemic–antitriglyceridemic agent in current use is clofibrate (Atromid-S). It may be given alone, as in type III hyperlipoproteinemia, or in combination with cholestyramine, as in type IIb. Clofibrate is thought to decrease the plasma cholesterol level by 10 per cent with therapy. Its mode of action is suggested as increasing the excretion of cholesterol by blocking gastrointestinal reabsorption, and decreasing the synthesis of cholesterol in the liver. It appears to lower serum triglyceride levels by inhibiting the transfer of triglyceride from the liver to the plasma. The Food and Drug Administration has reported recently, however, a high mortality rate among users, in a controlled study, from hepatic malignancies, postcholecystectomy complications, and pancreatitis ("New Label Restrictions," *FDA*, 1979, pp. 14–15).

Nicotinic acid (niacin) is the oldest antihypercholesterolemic, antihypertriglyceridemic agent available. Its greatest action appears to be on triglyceride levels by interfering with lipolysis at the adipose tissue site. Initially all patients flush markedly when receiving nicotinic acid and thus should be aware of this effect. The flushing usually dissipates with continued therapy. The drug should be given in divided doses with meals to diminish gastrointestinal irritation. Abnormalities in hepatic function leading to jaundice may occur with large doses and prolonged therapy.

Thyroxine has also been used in the treatment of type II hyperlipoproteinemia for its cholesterol-lowering effect. As early as the 1940s it was noted that patients with hypothyroidism had elevated serum cholesterol levels, which diminished with thyroxin therapy. Similarly, patients with hyperthyroidism were noted to have low concentrations of plasma cholesterol. This led to the use of thyroxine therapy in hyperlipidemic conditions. Although thyroxine causes an increased synthesis of cholesterol by the liver, it also produces increased excretion in the feces and increased conversion of cholesterol to bile acids. An increased cholesterol excretion and conversion greater than synthesis results in thyroxine's antihyperlipidemic effect. Thyroxine must be used with caution, however, in individuals with overt manifestations of coronary artery disease, because of its tendency to increase cellular metabolism and oxygen need. These effects promote myocardial ischemia and irritability of cells.

The use of estrogen compounds as an antihypercholesterolemic agent was suggested by the observations that young females had an appreciably lower incidence of coronary artery disease and serum cholesterol levels than young males. For a period of time estrogen compounds were administered to males with advanced coronary atherosclerosis. On these large doses of estrogens, however, the male patients experienced gynecomastia, loss of libido, impotence, and often mental depression. Lower doses were less effective for the serum cholesterol-lowering effect, and now this form of therapy is generally not regarded as worthy.

What is a "normal" cholesterol level is debatable. Some feel that although the normal range is cited as 150 to 250 mg per cent, that range is too high as it is based on what *is* rather than on what *should be.* The development of coronary artery disease is noted when the serum cholesterol level is above 220 mg per cent (McIntosh, Stamler, & Jackson, 1978). Mallison (1978) reports, however, that a physiologically normal level probably is 180 to 200 mg per cent.

Myocardial Ischemia

Myocardial ischemia (coronary insufficiency, ischemic heart disease, atherosclerotic heart disease) is a state of myocardial anoxia secondary to insufficient coronary perfusion of cells. Although the most frequent cause of diminished coronary perfusion is atherosclerosis, it may also be caused by other conditions, such as stenosis of the coronary ostium resulting from syphilis, and aortic stenosis. Anemia contributes to myocardial ischemia resulting from a disease in the oxygen available to myocardial cells. Any disorder that results in a pathologically low blood pressure, such as in circulatory collapse, will be accompanied by myocardial ischemia and can progress to death of cells. Other situations in which coronary perfusion is diminished because of low blood pressure in the root of the aorta are aortic valvular insufficiency and aneurysm of the ascending aorta.

The result of diminished oxygen to groups of myocardial cells is an increase in cellular lactic acid and a decrease in high-energy adenosine triphosphate. The consequences of the altered catabolism are a potential diminishment in cellular function and the occurrence of the primary clinical manifestation, angina pectoris.

Angina Pectoris

Angina pectoris is the characteristic pain associated with myocardial ischemia. Thus angina is a clinical symptom and not a disease. Its occurrence, however, strongly suggests the presence of underlying cardiac pathology. The presence of angina always indicates the same basic physiologic disturbance, myocardial hypoxia, whatever the underlying disease. The basic pathophysiologic mechanism suggested to explain the anginal phenomenon is related to the metabolic changes associated with cellular oxygen deprivation. The lactic acid that accumulates within the cell diffuses to the extracellular fluid environment, where it stimulates sympathetic nerves. Impulses are transmitted via the autonomic nerves to the spinal cord and to the cerebral cortex, where they are perceived as pain by the individual.

Although certain elements of the anginal phenomenon may be atypical for some individuals, angina generally has certain typical characteristics. Angina is characteristically episodic, and is precipitated by physical exertion, a heavy meal, an emotionally laden situation, and/or exposure to cold weather. The individual reaction to angina is highly variable. Those who perceive it as mild discomfort may ignore the sensation and carry on with their normal activities. Other individuals may perceive it as a sign of impending death and cease all actitivy. Many individuals attribute the discomfort to indigestion and initiate measures to relieve the gastric discomfort. Often a strong element of denial enters into the picture, which distorts the individual's perception of the situation. Some individuals may markedly limit their activity to abate future attacks.

Anginal pain is characteristically a dull, aching, or heavy sensation that begins behind the middle or upper third of the sternum (retrosternal). It is not felt on the surface of the chest wall. Among the words that patients sometimes use to describe the sensation of pain are *choking, strangling, pressing, burning,* and *tightness.* Many times patients have difficulty verbalizing the sensation and will clench their fist descriptively over the mid-upper sternum. Clinicians describe this as the "clenched fist syndrome," which is characteristic of the anginal phenomenon. Anginal pain is not typically sharp, stabbing, or throbbing, nor an intense precordial crushing sensation as is the pain associated with acute myocardial infarction.

Anginal pain seldom localizes in the sternal area, nor is it felt in the region of the cardiac apex. Instead the pain radiates to the left shoulder and left arm as the intensity increases. Usually it radiates down the medial aspect of the left arm to the wrist and fingers. It may radiate to the neck, back, jaw, or ear. Occasionally it may radiate down the right arm or both arms. Radiation does not mean that the pain progresses in a wavelike fashion from the chest to the arm, but that the pain occurs in these areas concomitantly. Although the usual anginal pattern is that the pain begins retrosternally and radiates to the left arm, some patients report situations where the pain was felt in one place only, such as the wrist or shoulder, without radiation. This writer is aware of situations where individuals sought the assistance of a dentist or otologist because the pain localized in the jaw and ear. Despite the wide radiation pattern of angina pectoris, rarely does it radiate to the face, head, scalp, abdomen, groin, or knees. These distributions more commonly are observed with the pain of acute myocardial infarction.

Although the duration of anginal pain is somewhat variable, depending on the precipitating factor, the pain usually persists no more than 3 to 5 minutes. It usually subsides with cessation of the precipitating factor or with the use of nitroglycerin. Pain that is persistent and unrelieved by rest and/or nitroglycerin may be related to another process, such as myocardial infarction, and should be investigated immediately. Usually the characteristics of angina are reasonably constant for a given patient. In other words the precipitating factor, intensity, radiation, duration, and mode of relief for the angina are fairly regular from one attack to another. Any change in the anginal pattern should be regarded with suspicion.

There are variant forms of angina in addition to

the typical, stable *exertional angina* just described. *Nocturnal angina* awakens the individual from sleep and occurs without apparent cause, although it has been demonstrated frequently that it was preceded by a dream in which the individual was stimulated emotionally or was exercising (Julian, 1979, p. 1225). *Crescendo angina* (intermediate syndrome, unstable angina, preinfarction syndrome, status angiosus) refers to angina that (1) increases in frequency or severity without apparent provocation, (2) is almost continuous at rest, and/or (3) is only transiently relieved by nitroglycerin. As with exertional angina the symptoms may be accompanied by electrocardiographic changes of S-T segment depression and T-wave inversion accompanied by an increased heart rate. It must be noted, however, that there may be *no* electrocardiographic changes. Some clinicians feel this syndrome is due to a pathologic change in a coronary artery that will develop shortly into an obstruction with subsequent myocardial infarction. Although the mechanism cannot be explained, a high percentage of these cases do develop a myocardial infarction. A variant form of unstable angina is called *Prinzmetal's angina* because of the unique electrocardiographic change of S-T segment elevation (Gronin, 1978, p. 1679).

Clinical manifestations associated with the anginal syndrome include apprehension, increased perspiration, increased heart rate, and elevated blood pressure, all reflective of increased sympathetic nervous system activity. The individual may press or rub the sternum. The individual may complain of inability to breathe or may actually hold his or her breath, although frank dyspnea is not present. In some individuals there is a paradoxical splitting of the second heart sound and a mid-late systolic murmur during the anginal attack. Belching is common and may bring some element of relief. If there has been previous experience with angina, there may be eagerness on the individual's part to take a nitroglycerin as rapidly as possible.

Assessment of Myocardial Ischemia

Many physicians feel a clinical history that is descriptive of the anginal phenomenon is virtually pathognomonic of myocardial ischemia. Other diagnostic tools that may be used to provide objective evidence of the pathologic process include the electrocardiogram and coronary angiography.

It must be emphasized, however, that the electrocardiogram may not provide definitive evidence of the myocardial ischemic process. For example, the resting electrocardiogram may be entirely within normal limits in the patient who has indisputable angina pectoris, particularly when the myocardial ischemic process begins. Only during an anginal attack or during exercise may electrocardiographic abnormalities occur in some patients. If electrocardiographic abnormalities become present, they are reflected in the ventricular repolarization phase of the cardiac complex as a depressed S-T segment and flattened or inverted T waves. These changes, if present, are self-limited and reversible. If myocardial infarction were to occur, the electrocardiographic abnormalities would gradually evolve in a typical pattern rather than rapidly return to the original pattern.

One electrocardiographic technique that has been utilized to detect myocardial ischemia is the *exercise tolerance (stress) test.* In the past the Master's two-step stair test was used. The treadmill test is used in current practice. Merrill and Froelicher (1977) cite four uses for this noninvasive test: (1) to identify the 10 per cent of the population falsely labeled as having coronary disease, (2) to evaluate the patient's functional capacity, (3) to assess the effect of medical or surgical therapy, and (4) to determine the patient's prognosis (p. 23). While the individual walks at different speeds on various graded levels, the measurements are taken of (1) oxygen consumption, (2) heart rate by electrocardiogram, (3) blood pressure, and (4) respiratory rate. These parameters are all assessed for cardiopulmonary status.

The treadmill test may be done on an inpatient or ambulatory basis. Some physicians do the test in their offices. All personnel who may be involved in the testing process, such as physicians, nurses, and technicians, must be skilled in cardiopulmonary resuscitation (CPR) techniques for the rare occasion when an emergency may occur.

Instructions prior to the testing session include (1) avoidance of smoking, drinking, and eating for 4 hours prior to the test; and (2) wearing comfortable clothes and tennis shoes during the test. After the test, the patient should rest and avoid eating, stimulants, and showers with extreme temperatures (Merrill & Froelicher, 1977, p. 27).

Another electrocardiographic technique may be used in difficult-to-document cases. *Twenty-four hour cardiac monitoring* may be done with the ambulatory patient. The person wears electrocardiographic monitoring electrodes and a battery-operated cassette tape recorder while keeping a dairy of his or her activity. The tape recording and diary are analyzed. The results often are unusual and very revealing.

With the advent of *coronary angiography,* there has been an increased disenchantment with the electrocardiogram as a diagnostic tool for myocardial ischemia. There are no specific indications for coronary angiography on which all physicians agree. Physicians range in their philosophy from a last resort approach to the almost routine use of the procedure in any patient suspected of having coronary artery disease. Some of the indications cited are (1) suspected but ill-defined coronary artery disease, (2) angina pectoris associated with valvular heart disease, and (3) evaluation for surgical revascularization procedures. The reader is referred to the section on cardiac catheterization.

In establishing a diagnosis of myocardial ischemia, especially in patients with a history of atypical chest pain, the physician may feel the necessity to order some other diagnostic studies to rule out conditions that may somewhat mimic the pain of angina. Diseases of the gallbladder and gastrointestinal tract, such as cholecystitis, esophagitis, peptic ulcer, and hiatus hernia, are most commonly evaluated. Chest wall disorders, such as costochondral junction tenderness or pectoral muscle spasm, are common mimics of anginal pain as perceived by the individual.

Intervention with Myocardial Ischemia

Intervention with myocardial ischemia will depend on the severity and intensity of the process as determined by the degree of angina pectoris experienced by the patient. In some individuals the intervention may be some adjustment in the daily living pattern that will control the anginal attacks. In others with more advanced coronary atherosclerosis and a greater degree of myocardial ischemia, there may be a need for long and/or short-acting vasodilator therapy in addition to modifications in the individual's life style. With some individuals, surgical intervention may be desirable.

The professional nurse can play a major role in the intervention process with patients who have myocardial ischemia through the processes of interviewing and patient teaching. The circumstances under which angina pectoris typically occurs need to be identified with each patient. Once identified, modification of the patient's activity pattern and/or avoidance of particular precipitating factors can be learned with adequate counseling and guidance in the attempt to reduce the frequency and severity of the anginal attacks.

In addition to known circumstances that tend to precipitate pain episodes, the nurse should talk with the patient about activities or circumstances that are *like* the known episodes as well as other kinds of activities that have potential for added stress on the heart. For example, Glasser, Clark, and Spoto (1978) report the cardiac response to "fright stress" initiated by riding a roller coaster. The authors report a case of a 39-year-old male who died of ventricular fibrillation after a ride on a popular new ride. This precipitated their research with normal subjects. Heart rates increased significantly on the ride. The investigators conclude that this kind of recreational stress should be avoided by individuals at risk for occult coronary artery disease.

Other modifiable aspects of daily life are related to the risk factors that are controllable in the attempt to retard the atherosclerotic process. These would include such aspects as cessation of smoking, reduction in body weight, reduction in saturated fat intake, participation in daily physical exercise, and control of other pathologic processes, such as diabetes and hypertension.

The nurse must keep in mind throughout the intervention process with the myocardial ischemic patient that it is not uncommon for the patient to experience some degree of depression. The experience of angina serves as a reminder that the patient is growing older and that activity is becoming restricted. Both the nurse and the patient need to assume an optimistic yet realistic attitude. With appropriate therapy and some adjustments in the daily living pattern, activity can be essentially normal. Angina may persist for many years, yet during this time, the patient can continue to work as well as enjoy his or her usual recreational activities and family relationships. There may be considerable apprehension about sexual activity, particularly on the part of the spouse. The patient and the spouse can be reasonably reassured that sexual activity can be continued as long as it does not precipitate disturbing symptoms. Some physicians prescribe a nitroglycerin tablet before and after participation in the sexual act to prevent an anginal episode.

The *pharmacologic intervention* with myocardial ischemia is primarily the utilization of drugs that act to dilate the coronary arteries. The short-acting nitrite, nitroglycerin, is utilized to abort an anginal attack. Long-acting nitrite preparations, such as isorbide dinitrate (Isordil, Sorbitrate), are used to prevent or reduce the frequency of anginal episodes as well as to aid in the development of the collateral circulation. Both the short- and long-acting nitrite preparations act directly on smooth muscle cells to effect relaxation and subsequent vasodilatation. The consequent vasodilatation increases local blood flow to the hypoxic myocardial tissue. Although the nitrites are capable of smooth muscle relaxation in the biliary, urinary, bronchial, and gastrointestinal tracts, they are usually not used for such purposes, as other antispasmodic agents are available that act more effectively at those visceral sites.

Sublingual nitroglycerin is the nitrite most widely utilized for terminating acute angina pectoris. There are many implications for patient education when nitroglycerin therapy is initiated. One of the most difficult aspects to teach is when the individual should take the medication. At the *first* sign of an anginal attack, the patient should place a nitroglycerin tablet sublingually, or buccally at the level of the third or fourth molar, and sit or lie down. Human nature, however, imposes an element of uncertainty about or denial of the chest discomfort so that the individual feels that it will go away and delays taking the nitroglycerin. This situation is comparable to the difficulty encountered initially in teaching the asthmatic patient when to utilize medicated nebulization. Once the nitroglycerin is taken, the angina should subside in 1 to 5 minutes. Many physicians advise that the patient take no more than three to four tablets at 5-minute intervals, at which point, if the pain does not subside, the patient should obtain medical assistance as the pathologic process may not be ischemia but impending infarction.

The individual should always carry some nitroglycerin wherever he or she goes, in case of an anginal episode. Many patients carry them in a saccharin or pill box. Pharmacies provide the tablets in small brown bottles which also can be used and may be preferable because there is less airspace in contact with the tablets. Air and light cause rapid deterioration of the drug's chemical properties. For this reason the patient should purchase small supplies of the medication and replace them every 3 months to avoid taking an inactive therapeutic agent. Many patients are aware when their nitroglycerin is no longer effective. One patient told this writer that the tablets no longer "stung slightly" when they began to dissolve sublingually. Nitroglycerin at the patient's bedside in the hospital for self-administration when needed should be in a similarly protective dispenser, such as a brown plastic container.

Although nurses frequently have misgivings about leaving a medication at the patient's bedside for self-administration, there is no good reason why this should not be done. Time is of the essence in the administration of nitroglycerin to abort an anginal attack. Further, the patient will assume full responsibility for this activity upon discharge from the hospital. Therefore why should he or she not do it while in the hospital? The patient should be instructed to notify the nurse when a nitroglycerin is taken so that observations can be made as to the patient's response to the drug as well as a physical and psychological assessment of the patient state.

The patient taking nitroglycerin should know what effects from the nitroglycerin may be experienced and how to minimize them. Because nitroglycerin is a generalized vasodilator, some patients may experience faintness or drowsiness resulting from a lowering of the blood pressure, and headache or visual disturbances resulting from dilatation of cerebral vessels. These effects tend to diminish with continued therapy. Nitrite syncope can develop if the patient concomitantly ingests alcoholic beverages. This can precipitate a potentially hazardous shocklike state if the individual has been drinking excessively and should be avoided. As the atherosclerotic process progresses, the patient may require larger doses of nitroglycerin to achieve relief. Although medical personnel are aware that this is related to the pathologic process, the patient may perceive it as a tolerance to the drug. The nurse should be aware of the rationale the physician has communicated to the patient for the change in dosage so that the patient is not unnecessarily alarmed. Some patients do develop a transient tolerance to nitrite compounds at which point they will be discontinued and another chemical class of vasodilator agents will be utilized for a period of time.

A number of nitrite preparations with action that is slower in onset and longer in duration than nitroglycerin are preferred for long-term use. The rationale for utilization is to abate anginal attacks by more sustained vasodilatation and development of collateral circulation.

Nitroglycerin in ointment form has regained popularity in recent years. Two per cent nitroglycerin suspended in a petroleum base when applied to the skin has a vasodilating effect that lasts for 4 to 5 hours. One inch of the ointment is squeezed onto a ruled piece of wax paper and applied to the patient's skin and secured. The site to which the ointment is applied is variable although the upper arm or chest frequently are recommended. When applying the ointment to the patient, the nurse should be careful not to get it on her or his hands because absorption with vasodilation will occur.

Another drug frequently utilized in conjunction with a long-acting nitrite preparation in the treatment of myocardial ischemia is propranolol (Inderal). It acts by occupying the cardiac beta receptors, thereby reducing the excitatory responses of the myocardium to sympathetic nervous system stimulation. The effect is a cardioinhibitory and decreased contractile response, which thereby decreases myocardial oxygen requirements. Thus it is felt that propranolol protects the ischemic heart from physical and psychic overstimulation, thereby reducing episodes of angina pectoris. Other nonnitrite smooth muscle antispasmodic drugs utilized with myocardial ischemia in lesser frequency include papaverine, theophylline, aminophylline, and persantin. The physician may also order sedatives and tranquilizers to protect the myocardial ischemic patient from the adverse effects of stress.

The prognosis for patients with myocardial ischemia is generally good. With modification of certain daily life activities and nitrite therapy when necessary, anginal episodes may gradually improve and even disappear in many patients. Most individuals with myocardial ischemia will develop an acute myocardial infarction eventually, although a period of 10 or more years may lapse from the initial anginal attack to the heart attack. Unfortunately, sudden death may occur in a significant percentage of patients with myocardial ischemia.

Sudden Death

Epidemiological studies suggest that a significant number of sudden deaths occur in the community related to coronary artery disease. Whereas the majority of these individuals have known coronary artery disease or factors known to predispose to coronary artery disease, in a significant number of individuals, sudden death is the initial and only manifestation. Most physicians and nurses are personally aware of a situation where an individual received a clean bill of health from the physician or had a normal electrocardiogram the day of or week preceding sudden death.

The mechanism of sudden death presumably is ventricular fibrillation precipitated by premature ventricular ectopic beats arising from an ischemic area of the ventricular myocardium. In 1973 De Pasquale and Bruno summarized the approaches to reduce sudden death in the community: (1) identify risk factors in the population and retard the development of coronary artery disease, (2) detect persons with coronary disease and treat prophylactically, (3) diminish the delay in individuals seeking medical assistance, (4) establish mobile coronary care units, (5) establish support units in the community and where there are crowds, and (6) eliminate arrhythmias once they have occurred. Whereas all of the approaches have been implemented in sites throughout the United States, and longitudinal studies on each demonstrate mortality reduction, it is difficult to ascertain what their collective impact has been on sudden death reduction.

The delay time of individuals seeking medical assistance is still a troublesome phenomenon. Schroeder (1978) reported that in a group of individuals, the *median* delay time was 3½ hours. The time was spent as follows: (1) deciding to seek medical care—90 minutes; (2) delay initiated by the physician telling the patient to come to the office, to try another treatment, or to wait at home for house call; (3) transport time–average time 17 minutes (standard deviation ± 49 minutes); and (4) in the emergency room awaiting disposition to the coronary care unit—76 minutes. Surely, health professionals can reduce these figures.

Regardless of the mechanism of sudden death, there is no more tragic event than the sudden termination of life in an apparently healthy person. Health professionals have a major task before them to identify those individuals who are at high risk to the phenomenon of sudden death and to develop community means to resolve the problem effectively. As De Pasquale and Bruno (1973) have stated, "although this tragedy is repeated many times a day throughout this country, and in spite of the dramatic medical advances that have occurred during the past 20 years, there are no signs that the health sciences have had a significant impact on sudden death in the community" (p. 851).

The extent of responsibility that the professional nurse can undertake in the initiation, planning, and implementation of a community-based program for preventive and emergency coronary care services is almost limitless. Communities are often slow to act when the potential for health care delivery services and human resources are not readily visible or coordinated. Professional nurses can provide a valuable community service by organizing health care providers and consumers to discuss community need for these types of medical services. The planning and implementation of such a system must be a collaborative decision of responsible nurses, physicians, consumers, and appropriate administrative and emergency service personnel. In some communities, professional nurses have assumed major responsibility for the instruction of emergency medical service personnel in the recognition and emergency treatment of the patient with myocardial infarction and associated cardiac arrhythmias. The professional nurse can also be the key factor in the operation of strategic life support units in factories, stadiums, mobile coronary care units, and most certainly hospital emergency rooms. Professional nurses also have a major responsibility to offer their services as speakers to community groups to provide public education about the various aspects of coronary artery disease.

Myocardial Infarction

Acute myocardial infarction is a clinical state resulting from deficient coronary artery perfusion of an area of myocardium with resultant cellular death and cessation of cellular function. The mechanism of cellular death is metabolic in origin. The consequence of insufficient oxygen to an area of myocardium is cessation of cellular metabolism with excessive accumulation of cellular lactic acid and absent formation of adenosine triphosphate. Consequently, there is failure of the cellular active transport system, disintegration of the cellular membrane, and release of the cellular components to the extracellular fluid environment. The excessive amount of lactic acid stimulates autonomic nerves and produces the excruciating, prolonged chest pain characteristic of myocardial infarction. The absence of cellular function causes the many complications associated with myocardial infarction, such as cardiac arrhythmias, congestive heart failure, cardiogenic shock, and other less frequent complications.

Myocardial infarction constitutes the primary cause of death from coronary atherosclerosis. It is estimated that approximately 1.5 million Americans sustain myocardial infarctions annually. Approximately half of these individuals will die, with as many as 60 to 70 per cent of the deaths occurring before the individual reaches the medical care system. The incidence of sudden death and deaths that occur before the individual obtains medical supervision constitutes the major challenge to the present system of cardiovascular care.

The Coronary Care Unit

The development of the coronary care unit has been the major contribution of the past and current decades to the management of acute myocardial infarction. The first coronary care units (CCU) were pioneered essentially simultaneously in the spring of 1962 by three physicians working independently in Kansas City, Philadelphia, and Toronto. The concept underlying the establishment of the earliest units was centralization of potential sudden death victims in areas with specially trained personnel for close observation and available equipment for emergency intervention. Thus the CCU was first established to increase the efficiency of resuscitative attempts, and there is little doubt that effectively functioning CCUs achieve this goal with remarkable success.

The earliest CCUs also provided some valuable data upon which the current concept of intensive coronary care is based. The data included (1) disturbances in cardiac rhythm are a major cause of death in patients with myocardial infarction; (2) most cardiac arrhythmias associated with acute myocardial infarction occur within the first 24 to 72 hours; (3) 50 per cent of the cardiac arrhythmias are preventable; (4) the death-producing cardiac arrhythmias are preceded by premonitory signs; (5) the death-producing cardiac arrhythmias are preventable if the premonitory signs are aggressively treated; and (6) registered nurses who are adequately educated are the key personnel in the coronary care unit.

On the basis of this data the present concept of coronary care has expanded beyond that of detection and resuscitation of patients with death-producing arrhythmias to include the detection and aggressive treatment of the premonitory signs of lethal arrhythmias. Increased emphasis has been placed on the early recognition and treatment of other complications post–myocardial infarction, particularly left ventricular failure. With this change in emphasis, the role of the nurse in the care of the patient with acute myocardial infarction has markedly expanded. Since the advent of effectively functioning CCUs with highly skilled nursing personnel, the mortality rate from acute myocardial infarction has gradually diminished in many hospitals to between 10 and 20 per cent, half that reported prior to the establishment of CCUs.

Pathology

Although it is logical to assume that acute myocardial infarction is always the direct result of the sudden obstruction of a major coronary artery, pathologic studies indicate this is not always the case. Infarction without occlusion and occlusion without infarction have been observed pathologically. In the presence of a significant collateral circulation, an acute coronary occlusion may not produce infarction. On the other hand, if an area of myocardium is dependent on collateral circulation for perfusion, a remote occlusion may produce an infarction considerably removed from the occluded site. Infarction may also result from calcific embolization as in aortic stenosis or secondary to shock and hypotension from a variety of causes.

Although a coronary occlusion may result from thrombus formation associated with rupture of an atheromatous plaque through the subintimal layer of the vessel, the largest number of occlusions are due to narrowing of the vessel lumen as a result of the atherosclerotic process. Significant coronary artery disease is usually demonstrated in the vessel directly supplying the area of infarction.

Investigative studies have demonstrated that when myocardial infarction occurs, there are three relatively distinct areas of tissue change that occur as a result of varying degrees of oxygen deprivation to the cells. The three areas are known as the zones of infarction, injury, and ischemia (see Figure 44-12). Each can be identified by characteristic changes in the electrocardiogram. The *zone of infarction* is the area of cellular death and necrotic tissue resulting from insufficient oxygen for support of metabolic processes. This area is noted electrocardiographically by the development of pathologic Q waves in the

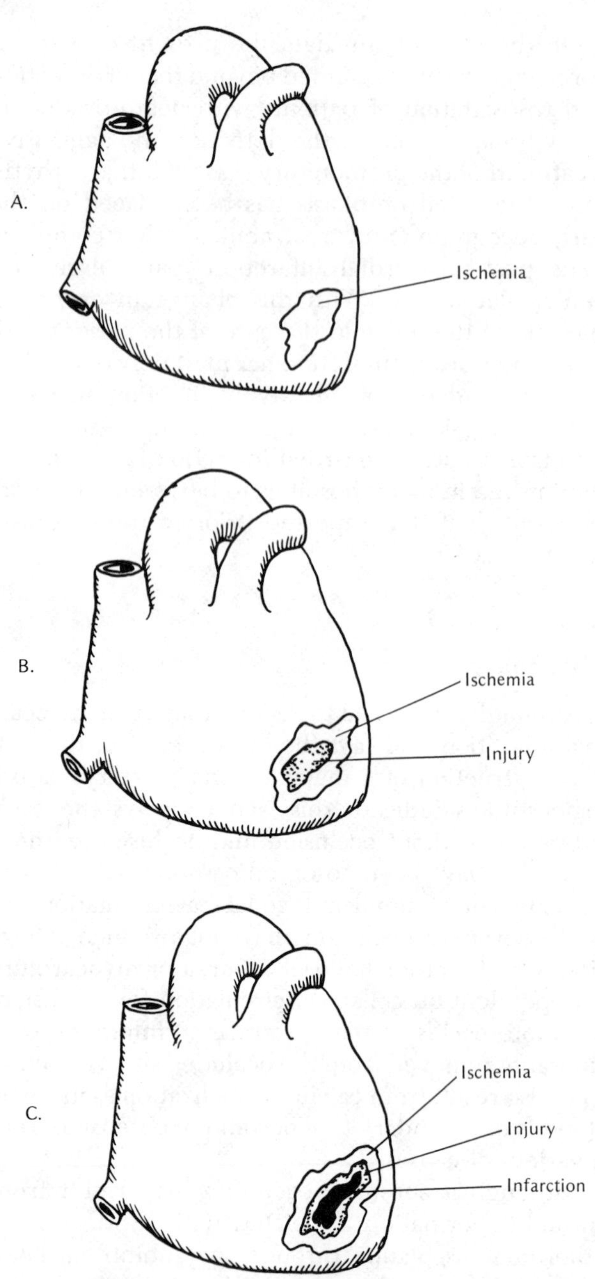

Figure 44-12. Zones of tissue change associated with: A. Myocardial Ischemia, B. Myocardial Injury, and C. Myocardial Infarction.

cardiac complex.[1] The zone of infarction is surrounded by the *zone of injury,* which is moderately deprived of oxygen but the cells are still somewhat viable and functional. The cells in the zone of injury receive more oxygen than those in the zone of infarction, but less than the zone of ischemia. The zone of injury is that which usually succumbs to infarction when it is noted that there is an "extension" of an original myocardial infarction. The zone of injury is noted on the electrocardiogram by elevation or depression of the ST segment of the cardiac complex. The zone of injury is surrounded by the *zone of ischemia,* which is minimally oxygen-deprived and represents viable cells, although potentially dysfunctional. Many of the disturbances of cardiac rhythm associated with myocardial infarction appear to originate from the zone of ischemia. This zone is noted on the electrocardiogram by inversion or flattening of the T wave of the cardiac complex.

Following infarction, the myocardial tissue undergoes various stages of recovery. Necrosis becomes evident in the zone of infarction 5 to 6 hours after the initial onset of occlusion. Within 24 hours the necrotic tissue is infiltrated with polymorphonuclear leukocytes for the phagocytotic process. By the fourth to fifth day, collateral vessels begin to enlarge and fibroblasts infiltrate the infarcted area. The zone of injury may succumb to infarction around this time or become ischemic because of enlarging collateral vessels. Within 2 to 3 weeks the fibroblasts produce connective tissue formation in the zone of infarction. The collateral circulation continues to enlarge. By this time the zones of ischemia and/or injury have regained function. Fibrous tissue formation is maximal in 2 to 3 months, and then begins to resolve, as do other forms of scar tissue. The clinical application of this data relates to the gradual and progressive activity prescribed for the patient through the various phases of convalescense.

Classification of Myocardial Infarction

Acute myocardial infarction is predominantly a disease of the left ventricle. It may also involve the interventricular septum or the papillary muscles. Rarely does infarction involve the right ventricle or the atria. The extent and location of the myocardial infarction depend on the coronary artery(ies) involved, the extent of the atherosclerotic process, the presence of collateral circulation, and the presence of previous myocardial infarction.

Myocardial infarction is classified by *extent* and by *location.* The extent of a myocardial infarction is related to the tissue layers involved. A myocardial infarction is termed *transmural* when the cellular death and necrosis extend from the endocardium to the epicardium (visceral layer of the pericardium). A myocardial infarction is termed *nontransmural* when the necrosis does not involve all three layers but is limited to the myocardium and the endocardial or epicardial layers. Nontransmural myocardial infarctions are further classified as (1) subendocardial, which involves the myocardial and endocardial layers, and (2) subepicardial, which involves the myo-

[1] The reader may wish to refer to the section on the cardiac complex (pp. 904–5) for further clarification.

cardial and epicardial layers. In general, transmural myocardial infarctions tend to be larger than nontransmural infarctions and result in more severe ventricular dysfunction. Determination of the extent of a myocardial infarction is accomplished by analysis of the component parts of the cardiac complex in the 12-lead electrocardiogram for the development of pathologic Q waves and alterations in the ST segment and T wave.

Classification of myocardial infarction by location is related to the area of left ventricle involved in the infarction process. Location is determined largely by the coronary artery involved in the occlusive process, and assessment of the location of a myocardial infarction is accomplished by analysis of various sets of leads in the electrocardiogram. A myocardial infarction is reported in terms of both location and extent. Occlusion of the left anterior descending coronary artery usually results in infarction of the anterior surface of the left ventricle near the apex and is termed an *anterior* (transmural or nontransmural) myocardial infarction. If there is electrocardiographic evidence that the interventricular septum may be involved in the process, the term *anteroseptal* myocardial infarction is employed. Occlusion of the circumflex artery generally results in infarction of some portion of the lateral or posterior surface of the left ventricle. In this case the terms *lateral* or *posterior* may be utilized. If the right coronary artery is involved, the inferior surface of the left ventricle becomes infarcted in the largest per cent of human hearts, and the term *inferior* (diaphragmatic) myocardial infarction is employed. The general locations of myocardial infarction are depicted in Figure 44-13. Variations in location are noted by terms such as *anterolateral, inferolateral,* and *inferoposterior,* which connote larger areas of involvement.

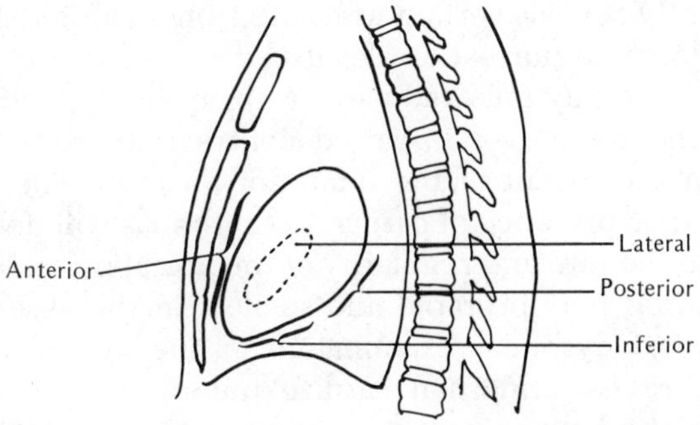

Figure 44-13. Left lateral view of the heart depicting the locations of myocardial infarction by surfaces of the left ventricle.

Assessment of the Patient with Myocardial Infarction

Diagnosis of acute myocardial infarction is accomplished by a thorough assessment of the clinical history in addition to specific laboratory and electrocardiographic data. The nurse is frequently the first professional person to have contact with the myocardial infarction patient and, as such, has increased responsibility for initiation of the assessment process. In addition to obtaining specific laboratory data and the initial electrocardiogram, the nurse must have a thorough knowledge of the typical and atypical clinical manifestations. This knowledge serves as a base for the rapid planning and implementation of interventions that are necessary with the myocardial infarction patient.

The typical clinical history reveals that the outstanding characteristic of acute myocardial infarction is severe, prolonged chest pain most often described as "crushing" or "a weight on the chest." The pain usually persists for at least one-half hour. Frequently it may persist for several hours and is relieved only by narcotics, rarely by nitroglycerin. Infarction pain may radiate more widely than that of angina pectoris. Crescendo angina may precede the acute episode by days or weeks, although the actual pain of infarction is usually of an abrupt onset. Unlike angina, which is most often precipitated by physical or emotional exertion, the pain of myocardial infarction may occur while the individual is sedentary and may even awaken the person from a sound sleep. Contrary to popular opinion, it appears that many myocardial infarctions occur when the person is at peace or beginning to relax after a sustained period of high-pitched activity rather than during a period of stress. A sense of impending doom most often accompanies the excrutiating pain.

Other symptoms associated with the pain are reflective of either increased sympathetic nervous system activity or the early development of other associated complications, such as congestive heart failure. These include apprehension, ashen color, cold sweat, and tachycardia in the absence of other cardiac arrhythmias. The patient may experience vertigo or syncope if the cardiac output is compromised. Although some patients may be restless, frequently the individual lies motionless, so as not to aggravate the discomfort. The person may rub or clench his or her fist over the sternum. Gastrointestinal symptoms such as belching, nausea, and vomiting may also be experienced, presumably because of the overlapping autonomic nerve supply to both the heart and the gut. These symptoms often serve to reinforce the patient's perception that the episode is related to "indigestion" or "ingestion of some bad food."

Examination of the cardiovascular system frequently reveals certain associated physical findings. After initial normal or elevated readings, the blood pressure may fall gradually or abruptly, depending on the degree of impaired contractility resulting from the extent of the infarction process. The absence or presence of cardiac arrhythmias will determine the rate and regularity of the apical pulse. Respirations may be rapid and shallow in the absence of overt dyspnea. Examination of the precordium may reveal abnormal cardiac pulsations resulting from the ballooning out of necrotic tissue, which is unable to contract normally with the rest of the ventricle. These movements are more likely to be noted medial and superior to the cardiac apex and tend to disappear within a few weeks unless an aneurysm of the ventricular wall develops. Auscultation of the heart sounds reveals a soft S_1 and presence of S_4 in many patients, although they may be normal in many patients. Although the body temperature is usually normal initially, a modest elevation of 100 to 101 ° F is noted, as with any infectious process, 3 to 4 days postinfarction.

Although the patient with acute myocardial infarction usually experiences severe, prolonged chest pain, it must be noted that in the atypical situation the symptoms of the acute episode may be erroneously interpreted by the patient and medical personnel. Reasons for this misinterpretation include variation in the location of the pain, low intensity of the pain, or possible absence of pain. For example, the pain may be referred to the abdomen or cranium and thus may be thought to be due to some other pathologic process. The pain may be brief and of minimal intensity, so that the individual does not seek medical care. It may not be until a much later time, when on routine medical examination an electrocardiogram reveals changes that were not previously present, that the infarction is recognized. In this instance the infarction is referred to as old or "remote." This situation typifies the story of the man who "walked through a heart attack and never knew it." When the symptoms of the acute process are minimal or absent, the term *silent myocardial infarction* is employed. The process of myocardial infarction can also be obscured by another process, which occurs simultaneously, so that the patient may be unable to communicate the symptoms. Examples of this type of situation are during a surgical procedure with general anesthesia, diabetic coma, cerebrovascular accident, psychotic state, and senescence.

Although the history and clinical manifestations provide worthy data upon which to infer that the individual has sustained a myocardial infarction, it has been noted that these parameters can be misleading or inconclusive. Other more objective data are required to reach a definitive conclusion. The electrocardiogram and certain chemical analyses of the blood may provide this data. Electrocardiographic changes are usually helpful in the diagnostic process but may be difficult to interpret in the presence of subtle changes or previously abnormal electrocardiograms. Although useful in most instances, the electrocardiogram has certain limitations.

For years the common laboratory test of the white blood cell count (WBC) and erythrocyte sedimentation rate (ESR) were utilized in the assessment process. The WBC and ESR are usually elevated in myocardial infarction, but they are usually elevated in *any* infectious or inflammatory process. These parameters therefore are influenced by other pathologic processes and are not specific to myocardial infarction. Further, in some instances the WBC and ESR may not be elevated with the acute process. Other more specific laboratory tests have become available in recent years that greatly facilitate the diagnostic process. These tests involve chemical analyses of the serum to determine the quantity of certain enzymes present.

Enzymes are proteins present in all living cells that catalyze the biochemical reactions of cellular metabolism. An enzyme temporarily combines with the substance on which it acts (substrate) to form the reaction products and then is liberated for subsequent catalytic activity. The structural configuration of an enzyme permits its combination with only one substance; thus each enzyme can catalyze only one particular biochemical reaction. It has been suggested that as many as 700 to 1,000 enzymes may exist in conjunction with a single cell. In addition, many individual enzymes exist in different forms with dissimilar physical and chemical properties yet with similar substrate specificity. These different forms are called *isoenzymes.*

Should a group of cells become injured or diseased as in myocardial infarction, the cellular enzymes are released to the extracellular fluid compartment and the serum enzyme levels rise. Normally the various enzymes are present in the serum in small, measurable amounts. Different enzymes and isoenzymes are liberated when different tissues are damaged. This is because tissues vary in enzyme concentration and composition. Serum enzyme determinations can be used to detect cellular damage as well as to suggest the site of damage if appropriate enzymes and isoenzymes are selected for study. Such enzyme studies assist in the diagnosis, prognosis, and therapy of many disease processes.

When the clinical history, manifestations, and electrocardiogram are vague or atypical, the serum enzyme—isoenzyme determinations can frequently make the diagnosis more definitive. The serum enzymes studied most frequently in patients with suspected myocardial infarction are creatinine phosphokinase (CPK); glutamic oxaloacetic transaminase (GOT), currently observed as aspartate aminotransferase (APT); lactic dehydrogenase (LDH); and to a lesser extent in some agencies, alpha-hydroxybutryic dehydrogenase (HBDH). Two other enzymes that could be analyzed if blood samples were obtained from the patient within 6 hours from the onset of symptoms are malic dehydrogenase (MDH) and aldolase.

Although isoenzymes have been identified for SGOT and MDH, the isoenzymes most frequently analyzed for presence of myocardial infarction are those of CPK and LDH. All the previously mentioned enzymes show a high incidence of elevation following a major myocardial infarction. The times at which the peak values of the serum enzymes are achieved and the duration of the elevation, however, are different. The serum enzyme determinations therefore should be analyzed daily for a period of 3 to 4 days from the onset of symptoms.

The first enzyme to reach peak values is CPK. This enzyme catalyzes the conversion of creatine phosphate to adenosine diphosphate, which is the precursor of adenosine triphosphate, the biochemical energy necessary for cellular function. Maximal serum values are achieved 12 to 24 hours from the onset of symptoms but return to normal by the third day if no extension of the infarction process has occurred. The upper limits of the normal values for CPK vary, depending upon the specific chemical test performed as do the normal values for other enzyme studies. The results must be interpreted cautiously in view of influencing variables. For example, if a patient has received multiple intramuscular injections, there may be a significant rise in the serum CPK as skeletal muscle cells also have a high concentration of this enzyme. If a patient delays seeking medical care after the myocardial infarction symptoms, the peak CPK value may not be recorded, and thus the situation can be misinterpreted. On the other hand, the early elevation of serum CPK following a myocardial infarction may assist in the prompt selection of that patient who requires the services of an intensive coronary care unit.

To clarify a clinical picture which is not definitive, a determination of the CPK isoenzymes may be done to identify the specific organ damaged. Indeed, in many hospitals, the CPK isoenzymes are analyzed from the outset, thus eliminating any generic CPK determinations. There are three CPK isoenzymes found in human cells. The isoenzyme found almost exclusively in myocardium is CPK_2.

The second serum enzyme to rise when an acute myocardial infarction has occurred is serum aspartate aminotransferase (APT), formerly SGOT. This enzyme participates in the synthesis of oxaloacetic acid, which is a critical point of entry into the Krebs cycle of catabolism. Maximal serum values are achieved in 1 to 2 days, with return to normal within 4 to 6 days. Whereas an elevation of SGOT levels is not limited to myocardial infarction due to the enzyme's prevalence also in skeletal muscle, brain, liver, and kidneys, APT is more tissue specific, hence its use currently. SGOT elevations can occur when certain drugs are used, such as anabolic steroids, Keflin, warfarin, morphine sulfate, and methyldopa.

The third enzyme to rise is LDH, which reaches maximal values within 2 to 4 days and returns to normal in 8 to 14 days. This enzyme catalyzes the conversion of lactic acid to pyruvic acid during glycolysis. Pyruvic acid is either converted to glucose or enters the Krebs cycle to produce adenosine triphosphate. Because LDH becomes elevated in a variety of other disorders, particularly in liver and renal disease, as well as certain hematologic disorders, further differentiation is needed. Electrophoretic techniques have been developed that enable the separation of LDH into five isoenzymes. The proportion of the different isoenzyme fractions varies from tissue to tissue. The LDH isoenzyme, LDH_1, predominates in cardiac tissue whereas liver and skeletal muscle have a predominance of LDH_5. Normally, the level of LDH_2 is greater in the serum than LDH_1. Within the first 48 hours of the chest pain, the presence of an elevated CPK_2 and an LDH_1 level which exceeds the LDH_2 level is virtually diagnostic of acute myocardial infarction (Scheer, 1978, p. 8).

Serum HBDH is elevated only in those same situations in which LDH_1 is elevated, thus, similar information is provided. The slow return to normal serum levels is sometimes helpful in determining the relative age of a "silent" myocardial infarction.

Numerous efforts have been made over past years to develop a prognostic indicator for patients with myocardial infarction. Correlations were attempted with electrocardiographic data, clinical history, and the usual laboratory studies to predict potential complications and mortality postinfarction but with little apparent success. Coodley (1973) now reports that a direct relationship can be found between the amplitude of enzyme rise and early mortality, as well as a relationship of elevated serum enzymes and increased incidence of arrhythmias and heart failure. Using an entirely different approach, Norris (1975) reported the development of a coronary prognostic index where outcome is predicted by summation of multiple adverse clinical factors exclusive of enzyme levels and cardiac arrhythmias. The factors used are blood pressure, age, presence of left ventricular failure, location and extent of myocardial infarction, and history of a previous myocardial infarction. The value of these tools is anticipatory intervention.

Intervention with the Myocardial Infarction Patient

Regardless of the setting in which medical care becomes available to the myocardial infarction patient, the intervention generally seeks to accomplish certain goals. Therapy is directed toward (1) alleviation of pain, (2) provision for increased oxygen available to myocardial cells, (3) provision for physiologic and psychological rest, and (4) prevention or control of complications. Ideally the patient will be admitted to an intensive coronary care setting, where mutliple assessments and interventions can be initiated immediately upon admission.

A primary objective in the intervention with myocardial infarction is alleviation and control of the cardiac pain. Such narcotics as morphine sulfate and meperidine (Demerol) are used primarily for this purpose. The resulting sedation is helpful not only in the relief of pain and apprehension, but also in the diminishment of sympathetic nervous system stimulation of cardiac cells that may predispose to potentially lethal cardiac arrhythmias. Some patients may experience pain episodically for prolonged periods of time. The pain phenomenon is dependent, in part, on the extent of myocardial damage and the degree of collateral circulation available to the zones of injury and ischemia. Repeated smaller doses of the narcotics may be necessary. It should be noted, however, that morphine has a vagotonic—vasodilator effect. Thus cardiac rate and blood pressure must be watched for diminishment with each administration. On occasion atropine sulfate may be administered concomitantly with morphine to prevent serious bradycardias, which could compromise cardiac output. Although most of the pain may be anginal in origin, the use of nitroglycerin with an actual or potential acute myocardial infarction is currently regarded with disfavor. The rationale for not employing short-acting nitrites is that vasodilatation of atherosclerotic coronary vessels in this situation may promote dislodgement of an atheromatous plaque and have potentially lethal effects.

A second general objective in the intervention with the acute myocardial infarction patient is to make sufficient oxygen available to injured and ischemic myocardial cells thus diminishing the area of potential infarction. Clinical studies have demonstrated that some degree of hypoxemia following myocardial infarction is the rule even in the absence of overt left ventricular failure or cardiogenic shock. In some instances, the hypoxemia has been attributed to alveolar collapse at the lung bases because of the use of narcotics, which depress ventilation and the sigh phenomenon; the recumbent position, which decreases the total lung volume; and/or hypoventilation from chest pain. Higgs (1968) attributes the hypoxemia to a pulmonary-shunt effect, that is, the shunting of unsaturated pulmonary blood around ventilating alveoli without the usual oxygen exchange. Regardless of the etiology of the hypoxemia, it would appear advisable to provide some form of oxygen therapy to the acute myocardial infarction patient for 24 to 48 hours following the initial symptoms. It has been suggested that oxygen concentrations of 35 to 40 per cent administered by loose-fitting nasal cannula or Venturi masks at 6 to 8 liters per minute provide sufficient oxygenation and are generally acceptable to most patients.

A third general objective in the treatment of acute myocardial infarction is to provide the patient with physiologic and psychologic rest. During the period that follows the onset of the initial clinical manifestations of myocardial infarction, the patient is in danger of sudden death from ventricular fibrillation. This death-producing arrhythmia originates presumably from the zone of ischemia. Of necessity, cardiac workload and thus oxygen utilization of ischemic cells must be decreased. This is first accomplished by placing the patient on bedrest and should be the first consideration whether on admission to the hospital or in transport of the patient to the nearest medical facility.

In transport, the patient should be protected insofar as possible from physical and emotional stimuli. Although time is of the essence in moving the patient to the hospital for treatment, the transfer should be made without the patient feeling a great sense of urgency. There should be no fast driving over rough roads with the siren screaming. Whether in transport or during admission to the hospital, the atmosphere surrounding the patient should be one of calm, gentleness, and competence. Attention should be directed to the patient and his or her responses at all times.

Considerable variation exists in activity allowances for patients admitted to the hospital with acute myocardial infarction. Generally, it is felt that minimization of the patient's energy expenditure will result in a decreased metabolic rate and therefore decrease oxygen requirements, oxygen consumption, and workload of the heart. The concept, however, was exploited in the early days of coronary care units to the point that every patient was fed, turned, bathed, and toileted by nursing personnel. In addition, the patient was placed in an environment devoid of personal objects and those that provide time orientation. He or she was, instead, surrounded by forbidding, unfamiliar monitoring equipment and strange people. Visiting by immediate family members was frequently restricted to 5 minutes three times a day. The situational stress created by such circumstances has been generally recognized by nurses and physicians who have expressed concern for the resultant physiologic effects on the patient. For example, Bogdonoff (1970) noted significant amounts of urinary catecholamines were excreted by patients during periods of situational stress, such as on transfer from the coronary care unit and on discharge from the hospital. The greatest amounts of norepinephrine and epinephrine were excreted on the day of admission to the hospital. Gentry et al. (1973) suggest that the mechanism by which psychological stress leads to an increased incidence of complications and mortality in myocardial infarction patients is via increased adrenocortical and adrenergic nervous system activity. It would therefore appear that reduction in situational stress is essential. If restriction of a particular activity creates situational stress and performance of that activity is not physiologically harmful, then consideration should be given to modification of the activity restriction.

The professional nurse has a vital role in assessment of the patient's response to activity and activity restrictions. Unfortunately, in many hospitals some rigidity still reigns with regard to patient activities. Comprehensive data on the responses of patients to activity regimens are solely needed. As an example, Merkel and Brown (1970) noted in a small sample of patients that being fed or feeding oneself did not appear to affect either the blood pressure or pulse rates of patients significantly in a coronary care unit where self-feeding restrictions were imposed frequently. It would appear that more patients could feed themselves if the nurse noted no adverse effects from the activity. A guideline for use in determination of whether an activity is too strenuous is (1) if the pulse increases 20 beats or more per minute over the preactivity pulse, (2) if the pulse exceeds 120 beats per minute during the activity, or (3) if upon completion of the activity the pulse does not return to the preactivity rate within 3 minutes. This type of assessment should be done throughout the hospitalization as a gauge of patient progress. In the acute coronary care setting another parameter that can be utilized is that provided by the electrocardiographic rhythm strips obtained from the cardiac monitor. The development of abnormal beats or rhythms during an activity may be indicative of a need for greater restriction.

The prescribed course of bedrest for a given patient will depend in large part upon the extent of the infarction, associated complications, and the patient's response to activity. Generally for the uncomplicated case, strict bedrest is maintained for the first 3 to 4 days. This regimen is followed by a gradual increase in some activities, such as partial bathing and reading. In some coronary care units these activities and others, such as shaving, chair sitting, TV watching, teeth brushing, and/or commode use, are allowed earlier but depend upon a comprehensive nursing assessment of the patient's response to the activity. Some patients, especially those with congestive heart failure, may receive the armchair treatment rather than bed confinement. The chair is reported to place less work on the heart physiologically and to negate many of the psychological adverse effects associated with prolonged bedrest (Goldstrom, 1972).

The use of the bedside commode is highly desirable for the largest majority of myocardial infarction patients. Many patients are uncomfortable in the unnatural position assumed on a bedpan. Further, studies done have demonstrated that more energy is expended in using a bedpan (4.7 Calories per minute) than the bedside commode (3.6 Calories per minute) (Gordon, 1957). Straining at stool is to be avoided because the act constitutes the Valsalva maneuver, which (1) lowers cardiac output, (2) can precipitate syncope, and (3) results in a sudden increase in venous return on completion of the maneuver. In addition, this may predispose to alterations in cardiac rate and rhythm and can promote ventricular rupture in the patient with a significant transmural myocardial infarction. To facilitate bowel elimination and prevent straining at stool, it is general practice to prescribe stool-softening agents for patients in coronary care units.

Another documented source of stress for patients is the visiting hour schedules in many coronary care units. There are about as many combinations of visiting hour schedules as there are coronary care units in the country including (1) 5 minutes three times a day; (2) 5 minutes once an hour; (3) 15 minutes three times a day; (4) one-half hour twice a day; and (5) open visiting hours. Brown (1976) documented that family visits of 10 minutes every hour were stressful to patients as evidenced by increased blood pressures and heart rates. Two interpretations of this phenomenon are possible: (1) the visits are too frequent and do not provide the patient with sufficient rest, and (2) the visits are too short for family and patient to complete family "business" and provide each other with the necessary support systems. The latter interpretation seems the more plausible. Brown concluded that the visiting time arrangments in this unit needed modification.

Hoffman, Donckers, and Hauser (1978) reported on stressors as perceived by patients in coronary care units and ways that nurses can intervene to reduce the stress. The interventions include, but are not limited to the following: (1) increased flexibility in visiting regulations, (2) effort by staff to appear unhurried, (3) placing of clocks and calendars in each room, (4) knocking on patients' doors before entering the room, and (5) decreased noise within the unit (p. 809).

In many units, staff view the patient's family or significant others as a necessary evil with which they must deal. They are often ignored or dealt with superficially at the nurses station. It cannot be overemphasized that meeting the family's psychological needs is as important in the total care of the patient as meeting the patient's needs. The family's anxieties will be transmitted to the patient unless they are diminished. Breu and Dracup (1978) cite the family's needs as (1) relief of anxiety, (2) for information, (3) to be with the patient, (4) to be helpful to the patient and participate in the care, and (5) for support and to be able to ventilate concerns.

In many hospitals the myocardial infarction patient is transferred to a convalescent unit (intermediate care, step-up unit) following the acute period. During the time spent in the coronary care unit, patients generally feel secure because of the constant surveillance of their condition by electronic equipment and highly skilled personnel. Leaving the safe environment may produce a high degree of situational stress. This writer is aware of a woman who went into ventricular fibrillation on three separate occasions when the transfer process was to take place. The patient should be prepared for the transfer from the very first day of admission. By the day of transfer the "weaning" process should already have begun. The patient should be disconnected from the cardiac monitor in advance of the transfer. Separation is also facilitated if the nurses from the convalescent unit come to meet the patient in advance and assist with the transfer process.

The purpose of the convalescent area is to provide an opportunity for close observation of the patient as activity increases. Many intermediate-care areas have means to monitor the patients' cardiac rate and rhythm by radiotelemetry monitoring systems. It is in the convalescent unit that the bulk of patient and family education regarding the disease process, risk factors, diet, medications, and activity should take place. Some aspects of teaching may begin in the acute care area with the patient who is ready to learn. Lawson (1972) outlines a comprehensive progressive activity program for the myocardial infarction patient from the day of hospital admission to a recovery point 6 months later.

The entire area of physical activity as related to the individual with a heart attack has undergone a revolutionary change since the inception of coronary care units. In the late 1950s to early 1960s it was not uncommon for a patient to be on bedrest for 2 to 3 weeks. Even in the earlier coronary care units, most activities of daily living were performed for the patient. Such is no longer the case. Williams et al. (1976) state:

> Early ambulation has resulted in a shortened hospital stay after acute MI, fewer complications, related to bed rest, psychological gains, enhanced cardiac function, and higher frequency of return to work. However, to obtain the benefits and maintain the safety of a program of early ambulation after acute MI, emphasis must be placed on proper patient selection, individualization of prescribed activity and awareness of and careful attention to potential hazards. (1976, p. 317)

Inasmuch as early mobilization after myocardial infarction does not increase morbidity-mortality, graded activity programs have become an accepted practice. In many institutions low-level treadmill testing is done prior to discharge, and the results are used for patient education of activity schedules.

One question related to activity that is frequently unasked directly but that is foremost in many patient's minds concerns sexual intercourse. Many patients, young or old, single or married, feel that they will never be able to participate in the sexual act again after a heart attack. The patient may be embarrassed or unable to ask the questions, "Will I . . . ?" "When . . . ?" The patient, however, gives many cues or double messages, such as saying, "I wonder if I'll ever be able to be a wife again to my husband?" or exhibiting sexually aggressive behavior to the nursing personnel. Some patients will not approach the physician with the question for fear the physician will feel the patient's thoughts are inappropriate. Myron Brenton (1968), a layman, has written a book, *Sex and Your Heart,* for patients, with the purpose of helping to bridge the communication gap between patients and medical personnel. The early work of Hellerstein and Friedman (1969) provided valuable data about the physiologic effects of sexual intercourse among postcoronary and coronary-prone individuals and provided the impetus for increased research in this area of activity. The finding on a limited sample of middle-aged, middle-class, Jewish males was that conjugal sexual activity between long-married spouses did not present danger for postcoronary patients. It was noted that the energy cost of sexual activity is similar to that of climbing a flight of stairs, walking briskly, or performing ordinary tasks in many occupations and is less than that utilized in performing an exercise electrocardiogram (Masters) test.

In recent years, much greater attention has been given to the area of sexual counseling. The reader is referred to the excellent articles on the topic cited in the bibliography by Puksta (1977); Scalzi and Dracup (1978); Johnston, Cantwell, Watt, and Fletcher (1978); and Cole, Lewin, Whitley, and Young (1979). Sexual activity following heart attack is no longer taboo and most of the fears can be erased.

After discharge from the hospital, progressive activity continues, with return to usual activities, including, perhaps, work on a part-time basis, generally 8 to 10 weeks from the initial onset of symptoms. It is the minority of patients who are unable to return to ordinary activities because of limited cardiac reserve and/or overt congestive heart failure. The physician and patient must decide together whether the patient is capable of returning to his or her former job. The services of a Cardiac Work Evaluation Unit may be utilized to discern the individual's work capabilities. These units have been valuable in demonstrating that 85 per cent of people with heart disease can return to gainful employment in a variety of occupations. Information about the availability of such a unit in the community can usually be obtained through the local chapter of the American Heart Association. It should be noted, however, that some individuals may lose their prior jobs as a result of inflexible workers' compensation laws and industrial insurance policies.

"Coronary clubs" are one formal pattern that has been developed to deal with the societal consequences of coronary disease. Usually organized by individuals who have had a heart attack, these coronary clubs provide an opportunity for members to exchange common experiences and problems as well as derive courage from others who have been similarly affected. Some concern has been expressed, however, that such a club may somewhat retard individuals' return to prior societal pattern by unintentionally promoting the concept of "we are different." Nevertheless, a major accomplishment of these clubs through the comraderie established has been the recognition and promotion of the need for risk-factor reduction and participation in a planned program of active physical exercise as means to prevent subsequent heart attacks. Nurses have been very instrumental in the organization and conduct of formalized group sessions for coronary patients both on an inpatient and community basis (Baker & McCoy, 1979).

Over the past 10 years, much has been written on the physiologic and psychological benefits of progressive physical activity programs for individuals with coronary artery disease and those who are coronary-prone. It has been reported that sustained physical conditioning is associated with (1) greater longevity in the general population, (2) lower morbidity and mortality rates in individuals with coronary artery disease who are physically active than in those who are sedentary, (3) slower pulse rates during emotional situations and in the performance of certain physical activities, and (4) enhanced development of coronary collateral circulation. Although individuals with coronary artery disease and those who are coronary-prone can generally enter the programs at any time, the person who has sustained a myocardial infarction may enter approximately 3 to 6 months after the initial attack. Each individual is evaluated, and an exercise program is designed that is specific for his or her cardiac status. The kinds of exercise activities prescribed vary and include such things as level or treadmill walking, jogging, calisthenics, cycling, swimming, and certain sports. Violent exercise and competitive sports are discouraged, however, because some individuals may try to prove their "wholeness" again, and the sympathetic nervous system stimulation could provoke cardiac arrhythmias and/or failure. Again, the availability of progressive exercise programs in a given community is usually known by the local Heart Association chapter.

Associated with the provision of physiologic rest as a major aim of therapy for the patient with acute myocardial infarction is the goal to provide psychological rest concomitantly. The high incidence of death from heart attacks in the United States is sufficient in itself to provoke fear in the individual who experiences chest pain. The symbolic importance of the heart to human beings has been recorded throughout history, and it is no less precious or vulnerable today despite the widespread publicity of the effectiveness of coronary care units and cardiopulmonary resuscitation in preserving life. The individual who suffers a myocardial infarction is faced with the threat of death.

The phases or patterns of behavioral adaptation that individuals and their families commonly experience to some extent following an acute myocardial infarction are anxiety, denial, and depression. The patient may also exhibit aggressive sexual behavior and/or dependency. How an individual reacts to a myocardial infarction depends upon many factors. One significant factor appears to be the age of the individual at the onset of the illness. The diagnosis of heart attack in the younger individual may be so unexpected at that stage of life that the person may take a longer time than others to accept and integrate the illness into his or her life. The young male also may exhibit a greater degree of adamant denial. This reaction is largely a result of society's value that the young male should be active, autonomous, virile, and striving to achieve. In contrast, men past 60 years of age generally appear to adapt more readily to the diagnosis and may even have anticipated such illness as a part of the aging process. This reaction may be due to at least partial resolution of the young male image. The most problematic group appears to be the 50- to 59-year-old males. In this group males appear to encounter a period of crisis in which there is open conflict over the shift from the active youth orientation to the more passive position of later years. The heart attack then accentuates these very issues with which the individual is struggling. In this group of patients there appears to be more overt anxiety, denial, depression, and noncompliance with the medical regimen.

Regardless of the age of the patient, the initial reaction is one of anxiety in response to (1) the shock and disbelief associated with the pain experience; (2) the fear of death or chronic disability; and (3) the threat to the self-image. When the patient reaches the medical facility, the anxiety may be heightened by the uncertainty of the diagnosis and prognosis; introduction into a strange, overwhelming environment; development of complications; and perhaps misinterpretation of unfamiliar words and activities (Scalzi, 1973). The nurse must be aware of the causes of anxiety in the patient and the family, assess the level of anxiety upon admission to the hospital, and intervene accordingly.

Among the general interventions directed toward anxiety reduction in this situation is maintenance of a continuous and consistent nurse–patient relationship, with the nurse demonstrating calm, concerned, competent behavior. This is not the time for the new nurse to question how the monitoring equipment works in front of the patient or a family member. The nurse will need to give the patient and family members an initial orientation to the routines, equipment, and procedures of the intensive coronary care area. This orientation may need to be repeated on several occasions, as severe anxiety and panic serve to block the patient's hearing and retention of information. The nurse should elicit questions and concerns from the patient and family as a means for allowing them open expression of anxiety. All these actions will help to establish the much-needed trust relationship between the nurse and the patient. It should also be noted that in some patients even the therapeutic relationship will not suffice to lower the patient's anxiety to the point that it is not physiologically harmful. Particularly in this instance, chemical means of control are required. In some coronary care areas each patient is routinely given a tranquilizing agent, such as Valium or Librium, three to four times a day. In other units the use of tranquilizers is determined individually by nursing–medical assessments.

One means of coping with a situation that is anxiety-producing is to deny its existence. The myocardial infarction patient may adapt to the present circumstances by denial. There was a time when denial was viewed as a destructive mechanism for coping with a perceived threat, and it was felt that the patient's denial should be eliminated. The current consensus is that denial may serve a useful purpose as long as it does not interfere with the treatment regimen or rehabilitation. Initially, denial may serve to lower the physiologic responses associated with anxiety. When, however, denial is no longer verbal but becomes translated into physiologically destructive activity, it will need to be dealt with more directly. Examples of this situation are when the patient does not comply with activity limitations or even proceeds to sign out of the hospital against medical advice.

The nurse must assess whether the denial is verbal or interferes with physiologic rest. If verbal, the nurse listens but neither reinforces the denial or attempts to enforce acceptance of the heart attack. If the denial results in increased physical activity, the nurse must assess whether it is having harmful physical effects. One approach to diminish the activity is to convey concern and allow the patient control over certain elements of care and the environment that will not cause disruptions in the medical regimen. One thing that is not helpful or useful is to threaten the patient with such statements as, "Now you'd better just own up to the fact that you've had a heart attack or you're going to do yourself physical harm," as a means to secure compliance with imposed therapeutics.

Concomitant with the phases of anxiety or denial may be expressions of direct or projected anger and hostility. It is here that major disturbances occur in the patient's relationships with family members and staff. The patient is now less able to deny what has happened and is concerned about the future, for example, loss of job and possible independence, fears of sexual impotence, premature aging, and so on. The patient is angry with himself or herself and/or "others" who may have "caused" this situation. These feelings are compounded by enforced passivity whereby the patient is placed in a dependent role and must renounce ownership of his or her body to others. Characteristically, many patients summarize this experience as "being treated like a baby."

Anger and hostility from the patient are among the responses least understood by the staff, and are perhaps the most difficult with which to deal. Many nurses feel that this patient response is a direct attack on their competence and dedication. The staff's reaction is one of avoidance or minimal contact with the patient, which then reinforces the patient's feelings of guilt and lack of self-worth. Trying to reason with the patient fails. The nursing staff must understand and accept the patient's hostility and actively promote the expression of the angry feelings, because anger turned inward becomes depression.

Few, if any, patients escape some feeling of depression. Even the patient who makes a great show of taking the situation lightly experiences some degree of depression, because of feelings of diminished self-worth and hopelessness. The patient may outwardly appear cheerful, yet still be depressed. The writer recalls one patient who typifies this point. The patient was boisterous and appeared to be carefree. About 10 days after admission, he became unusually quiet as the nurse assisted with the bath and said: "I beat it (death) this time. It was a close call, wasn't it?" His usual behavior was a façade to cover his feelings.

The intervention with the depressed myocardial infarction patient is directed toward externalization of the patient's feelings rather than internalization. The nurse must first match the patient's mood. A cheerful, jocular approach can readily reinforce the patient's guilt feelings and internal anger. The nurse can reflect observations of the patient and solicit his or her feelings about the situation. Tearfulness and crying are to be allowed and encouraged by verbal communication and the use of touch. It should be communicated to the patient that these feelings are normal and experienced by most patients. The nurse's concern and intervention can do much to prevent the onset of pathologic depression.

Although the emotional responses to a myocardial infarction are relatively consistent from patient to patient, the duration and intensity of the responses vary considerably (Scalzi, 1973). For example, the phase of anxiety may be fleeting in some patients, and they enter the hospital exhibiting frank denial. On the other hand, some patients may leave the hospital with denial, and the depressive phase does not occur until the patient has been home for a period of time. What this then says is that all psychological intervention is not done within the confines of the hospital walls. All medical and nursing personnel with whom the patient has contact after the period of hospitalization have a role to play in facilitating the psychological as well as the physiologic rehabilitation of the myocardial infarction patient.

A fourth major objective in the general intervention with the patient is prevention and control of complications associated with myocardial infarction. Although all the previously mentioned interventions contribute to this goal in varying degrees, another therapy specific to complication prevention and control is the dietary management of the patient. The dietary management of the patient with myocardial infarction is primarily aimed at prevention or control of heart failure, provision of a fuel source for cellular metabolism, and promotion of myocardial perfusion during the process of digestion. These aims are accomplished during the first 24 to 48 hours of hospitalization by a low-sodium, liquid to semisolid diet. In some hospitals although the patient is advanced to solid foods, he or she is still maintained on a low-sodium, low–saturated fat, low-risidue diet throughout hospitalization.

After the early period of diet restriction, the low-sodium component may be removed if the patient does not demonstrate evidence of congestive heart failure. Depending on the philosophy of the physician, the patient may be maintained on a cholesterol-lowering diet. Dietary instruction should be given to the patient and a responsible family member during the course of hospitalization in sufficient time to allow reinforcement of content and assistance with menu planning. Unfortunately, many physicians and nurses do not remember about dietary instruction until the day before the patient's discharge, and its effectiveness is often minimal at best.

Generally, extremes in temperatures of liquids are avoided in the acute-care setting as are the use of coffee, tea, or other cardiac stimulants. Controlled clinical studies are still needed to document the necessity of these practices. Smoking is prohibited not only because of the oxygen-fire hazard, but also because of the need to decrease cardiac stimulation. It is felt that after the patient has not smoked for 4 to 5 days, the time may be optimal to begin a teaching program on the permanent cessation of smoking.

Complications of Myocardial Infarction

The emphasis today in the treatment of acute myocardial infarction is prevention of complications through early detection and prompt, aggressive intervention utilizing highly educated professional nurses in an intensive coronary care setting. Of the many complications that can occur after myocardial infarction, those that have particular significance for the professional nurse because of expansion of the nursing role in the assessment–intervention process are cardiac arrhythmias, thromboembolic phenomenon, ventricular aneurysm, ventricular failure, and cardiogenic shock.

Cardiac Arrhythmias

Cardiac arrhythmias are the most prevalent type of complication associated with an acute myocardial infarction. Killip and Kimball (1969) report that constant electrocardiographic monitoring of patients in coronary care units has revealed that the incidence of arrhythmias in acute myocardial infarction is about 90 per cent. Seventy per cent of the patients with an acute myocardial infarction experience premature ventricular contractions, and 30 per cent of patients develop ventricular tachycardia. These arrhythmias are premonitory to the death-producing arrhythmia, ventricular fibrillation, which 10 per cent of patients develop. It was recognized that if the premonitory arrhythmias were recognized and treated aggressively, ventricular fibrillation could be abated in most instances. Further, the key to recognition and treatment was the professional nurse.

Meltzer (1965) pointed out that the need for nurses to have a working knowledge of electrocardiography was no longer a remote and farfetched idea. Rather, it was very important for nurses who care for patients with acute myocardial infarctions to interpret electrocardiographic tracings and to act on the basis of the interpretation. Today it is recognized that it is advantageous not only for nurses in acute-care settings to have a working knowledge of electrocardiography but nurses in a variety of other occupational settings as well.

Prior to any discussion of cardiac arrhythmias, a fundamental review of the cardiac conduction system and basic principles of cardiac electrophysiology is necessary. The cardiac conduction system is depicted in Figure 44-14. The cardiac impulse is initiated normally in the sinoatrial (SA) node. The SA node is a small, crescent-shaped structure composed of an indeterminate number of P (pacemaker) cells and is located subepicardially inferior to the superior vena cava. From the SA node, the cardiac impulse is transmitted via the internodal tracts to the atrioventricular (AV) node, where the structure of the node causes a delay in further transmission. As the impulse traverses the atrial walls, the atria contract essentially simultaneously with the right atrium beginning to contract slightly before the left atrium. The AV node is located subendocardially in the lowermost portion of the interatrial septum, superior to the tricuspid valve. The inferior portion of the AV node and bundle of His penetrate the interventricular septum.[2]

The impulse is conducted from the AV node to the bundle of His and then to the right, left anterior, and left posterior bundle branches. From the bundle branches the impulse reaches the Purkinje fibers. As the impulse traverses the ventricles, contraction occurs essentially simultaneously with the left ventricle beginning contraction slightly before the right ventricle. There are cells capable of pacemaking functions located in the His-Purkinje system.

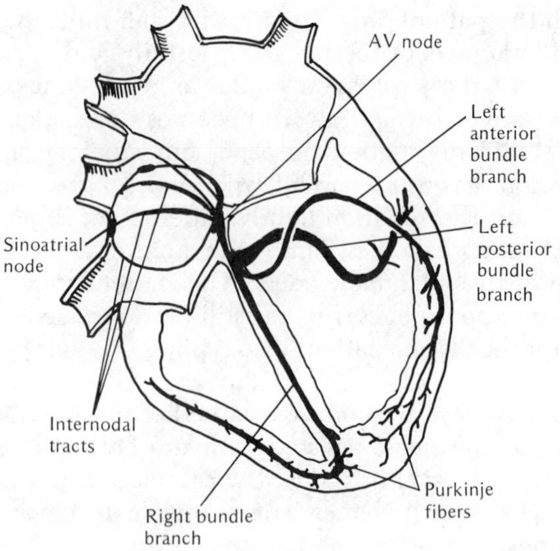

Figure 44-14. Schematic representation of the cardiac conduction system.

Under normal circumstances there are certain factors that influence the rate of cardiac impulse initiation and its transmission through the conduction system. The primary influencing factor is the autonomic nervous system. The SA and AV nodes are innervated by parasympathetic and sympathetic nerves that constantly release acetylcholine and norepinephrine, respectively. As a result, the rate of cardiac impulse initiation and transmission is within the normal range of 60 to 100 times per minute. If, however, the parasympathetic nervous system exerts greater influence on the SA node, the result is a decrease in the rate of cardiac impulse initiation and transmission. In contrast, if the sympathetic nervous system exerts greater influence, the effect is an increase in the rate of cardiac impulse initiation and transmission. Because the sympathetic nervous system also innervates areas of the atrial and ventricular myocardium, stimulation of sympathetic nerves also results in increased myocardial contractility and potentially the initiation of abnormal cardiac impulses.

Two other factors that influence the rate of cardiac impulse initiation under usual circumstances are the activity of the carotid sinus receptors and the Bainbridge reflex. When the carotid sinus receptors are stimulated by (1) a decreased pressure in the arterial system, (2) a decreased arterial blood oxygen tension, or (3) an increased arterial blood carbon dioxide tension, impulses are transmitted to the cardioaccelerator center of the medulla, which in turn sends impulses via the sympathetic nerves to increase the rate of cardiac impulse initiation. Similarly, acceleration of the heart is accomplished when the Bain-

[2] The AV node has some cells that are capable of pacemaking function primarily located at the junction of the AV node and the bundle of His. Consequently, the terminology, AV junction, is employed when referring to this potential pacemaking site.

bridge reflex is elicited. When the right atrium is distended, as with an increased venous return, the sinus node region is stretched mechanically, and the rate of cardiac impulse initiation is increased. To balance the accelerator effects of the carotid sinus and the Bainbridge reflex, the rate of impulse initiation is decreased when the carotid sinus receptors are stimulated by (1) an increased pressure in the arterial system, (2) an increased arterial blood oxygen tension, and (3) a decreased arterial blood carbon dioxide tension. It should also be noted that pathologic conditions may accentuate the effects of these normal reflex mechanisms.

The terms *cardiac impulse initiation* and *transmission* assume greater meaning when the properties of cardiac cells are examined. The heart is a complex organ that is composed of different kinds of cells. There are four basic properties possessed by the different cardiac cells. Although a cardiac cell possesses each property to some degree, each cell tends to specialize in *one* of the properties and, as such, has assumed the *name* of that property.

There are groups of cells that specialize in the property of *automaticity* (rhythmicity) and thus are called the automatic cells. Automaticity means that these cardiac cells initiate cardiac impulses spontaneously at regular intervals. The cells that specialize in the property of automaticity are (1) the SA node, which initiates impulses at a rate of 60 to 100 times per minute, (2) the AV junctional region, which can initiate impulses at a rate of 40 to 70 times per minute, and (3) cells in the bundle of His and Purkinje fibers, which can initiate impulses at a rate of 20 to 40 times per minute. The question then arises, "Why is the SA node the normal pacemaker of the heart if other automatic cells can perform the same function?" The answer is that the group of cells that initiates impulses at the fastest rate suppress the automaticity of the other automatic cells and thus assume the primary pacemaker function. If the SA node is the pacemaker of the heart, the cardiac rhythm is said to be *sinus*. If, for some reason, the rate of impulse initiation by the SA node diminishes or the rate of impulse initiation by the AV junctional tissue increases, the junctional region may become the pacemaker of the heart. The cardiac rhythm is then said to be *junctional*. Similarly, if the automatic cells in the bundle of His or the Purkinje system assume the pacemaker function because of diminished SA node or junctional region rate of impulse initiation, or acceleration of the His–Purkinje rate of initiation, the cardiac rhythm is said to be *ventricular*. Thus a "back-up" system exists in the heart whereby if one pacemaker fails, a subsidiary pacemaker is available. When all pacemakers fail, the situation created is *ventricular standstill*.

Excitatory cells specialize in the property of *excitability*. This means that given an appropriate stimulus, a cell will respond by initiating a cardiac impulse. Although there are groups of cells that appear to specialize in the property of excitability, such as in the walls of the atria and ventricles, virtually every cardiac cell possesses this property under given conditions. The primary difference between excitatory and automatic cells must be noted; excitatory cells require a stimulus to initiate a cardiac impulse, whereas automatic cells initiate impulses spontaneously at regular intervals. It will also be noted that most cardiac arrhythmias occur as a result of alterations in the properties of automaticity and excitability.

There are groups of cells that specialize in the property of *conductivity* and thus are named conducting cells. Conductivity means that these cells respond to a cardiac impulse by transmitting the impulse along the cell membrane. The obvious example of conducting cells is the conduction system. The final property is *contractility* in which the contractile cells specialize. This means that the response to a cardiac impulse is contraction. The largest muscle mass of the heart is composed of contractile cells. It should be noted that although a cardiac cell specializes in one property, the cell can assume another property under given circumstances. For example, a cell in the ventricle may specialize in contractility. At times that cell will be a conducting cell. Given an appropriate stimulus, that same cell may become an excitatory cell, and if located in the Purkinje fibers, it may need to assume pacemaking function as an automatic cell.

The ability of cardiac cells to initiate cardiac impulses is derived from the unequal distribution of electrolytes between the intracellular (ICF) and extracellular (ECF) fluid compartments. Because of these ionic concentration differences between the ICF and ECF (principally, potassium and sodium), an electrical energy difference exists between the two compartments. The electrical energy difference between the ICF and ECF, that is, *across* the cell membrane, is called the *membrane (electrical) potential*.

The membrane potential, as measured in the majority of cardiac cells, is slightly less than 100 millivolts (mV) when the cell is in a "resting" or polarized state. The existence of the potassium concentration gradient between the ICF and ECF is the primary cause of the voltage difference across the cell membrane.

Initiation of a cardiac impulse begins with the process of *depolarization* at one point of a cell membrane. The sequence of events in depolarization is as follows: (1) the permeability of the cell membrane increases at one point of the membrane either spontaneously (automatic cells) or in response to an appropriate stimulus (excitatory cells), (2) sodium moves into the cell along concentration and electrical potential gradients, and (3) potassium moves out of the cell along the same two gradients. When the amount of sodium inside the cell reaches a critical (threshold) level, a cardiac impulse is generated. The movement of the charged ions creates an electrical current. The electrical current associated with depolarization at one point of the cell membrane serves to depolarize adjacent points of the cell membrane. The wave of depolarization that is created as adjacent points of the cell membrane depolarize, represents impulse transmission. Further, depolarization of various points of a cell membrane serves as a stimulus for depolarization of adjacent cells. It is the syncytial arrangement of cardiac cells that promotes the spread of depolarization through all the cells in the heart.

The process of *repolarization* returns the cell to the "resting" state. The sequence of events in repolarization is as follows: (1) the permeability of the cell membrane decreases at a point of the cell membrane that had previously depolarized, and (2) sodium leaves and potassium re-enters the cell by the active transport system. It should be noted that a cell does not completely depolarize and then repolarize. One point of a cell membrane may be depolarizing while another point is repolarizing.

The electrical currents generated during the depolarization and repolarization of cells can be graphically recorded and are noted as changes in the membrane potential. The recording of the membrane potential changes is the *action potential,* as depicted in Figure 44-15. The cell membrane goes through various degrees of excitability as repolarization takes place. This means that stimulation of the cell membrane by an appropriate stimulus can result in the initiation of another cardiac impulse prior to the return of the cell membrane to the "resting" state. The three phases of repolarization are the *absolute refractory, relative refractory,* and *supernormal periods.* In the absolute refractory period, the cell membrane is in a phase of negligible excitability, which means that a second impulse cannot be elicited no matter what the strength of a stimulus. During the relative refractory period, the cell membrane is in a phase of limited excitability whereby a stimulus of strong intensity can elicit another impulse. The supernormal period is a phase of hyperexcitability. The cell membrane is extremely sensitive to stimuli as it has almost returned to the "resting" state, and a very mild stimulus can elicit an additional cardiac impulse.

The action potential is a graphic recording of the

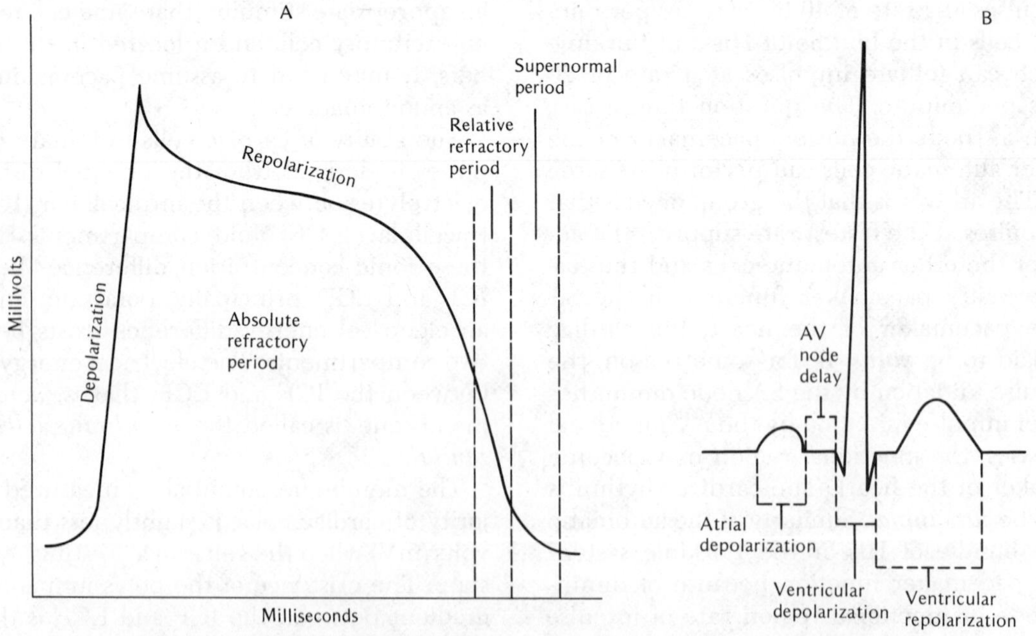

Figure 44-15. The action potential of a ventricular myocardial cell as the cell goes through the phase of depolarization and the component periods of repolarization. *B.* The "action potential" (cardiac complex) of all cardiac cells as they go through the phases of depolarization and repolarization. It should be noted that the phase of atrial repolarization takes place during AV node and early ventricular depolarization and thus is masked by the large QRS complex.

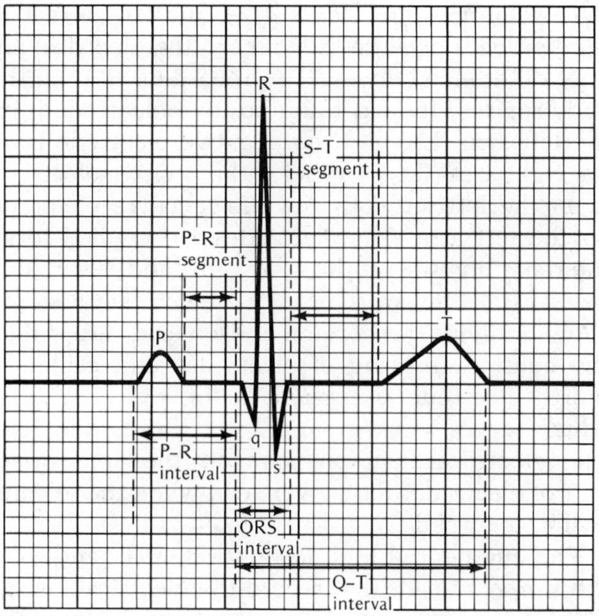

Figure 44-16. The cardiac complex and its component parts. The normal P–R interval is 0.12 to 0.20 second. The normal QRS interval is 0.06 to 0.10 second. Each little box on the horizontal axis of EKG paper is equal to 0.04 second. Each large box (five small squares) on the horizontal axis of EKG paper is equal to 0.20 second. Other waves and segments are usually not assessed in terms of time, rather the configuration is noted as well as the relationship of the wave or segment to the isoelectric baseline.

electrical activity generated by one cell as it depolarizes and repolarizes. In other words, the action potential is the electrocardiogram of one cell. Figure 44-16 shows the cardiac complex, which is a graphic recording of the electrical activity created by *all* the cells in the heart as they undergo one depolarization–repolarization. One complete depolarization–repolarization cycle of the heart is represented electrocardiographically by a P–QRS–T sequence.[3]

The straight line after the T wave and before the P wave is known as the baseline (isoelectric line) and represents a period of negligible electrical activity, or the "resting" state. The initiation of the cardiac impulse by the SA node generates negligible electrical activity and is thus not detected on the electrocardiogram. It immediately precedes the P wave, which represents atrial depolarization. The P–R segment represents the period of impulse delay as the AV node depolarizes. Once again this is a period of negligible electrical activity as noted by the isoelectric line. The QRS complex represents ventricular depolarization. Atrial repolarization occurs essentially during the time of AV node and ventricular depolarization and thus is not seen on the electrocardiogram. The ST segment and T wave represent ventricular repolarization. The ST segment and a portion of the T wave coincide with the absolute refractory period. The peak of the T wave is also known as the vulnerable period, and the peak and downstroke of the T wave essentially coincide with the relative refractory period. The terminal portion of the T wave coincides with the supernormal period.

There is a normal period of time in which the depolarization and repolarization events should take place. Measurement of the time required for atrial and AV node depolarization (P–R interval), and for ventricular depolarization (QRS interval) provide data about abnormalities in cardiac impulse transmission through the conduction system.[4] The normal P–R interval is 0.12 to 0.20 second. The normal QRS interval is 0.06 to 0.10 second. Prolongation of the P–R interval usually connotes delayed depolarization of the AV node and/or beginning of the interventricular conduction system. Prolongation of the QRS interval usually connotes altered depolarization of the interventricular conduction system. Although a small q wave normally may be present or absent in the QRS complex, the presence of a pathologic Q wave is usually indicative of myocardial infarction. The ventricular repolarization phase is not assessed in terms of length of time. Rather, the configuration of the component parts, ST segment and T wave, are examined for evidence of altered ventricular

[3] The letters P–QRS–T were arbitrarily selected from the alphabet and have no significance as abbreviations. Further, it should be noted that a cardiac complex does *not* need to have a Q or S wave to be normal.

[4] Some basic terminology and electrocardiographic concepts are requisite to measurement of time intervals. An electrocardiographic "wave" is composed of two distinct sides; one side leaves baseline and the other returns to baseline. A wave that projects *above* baseline is a *positive deflection*. Conversely, a wave that projects *below* baseline is a *negative deflection*. A deflection that does not have two rather distinct sides is not a wave. Ventricular depolarization is depicted on the electrocardiogram by both positive and negative deflections. Collectively, these waves are called the QRS complex; however, not all waves must be present for normal ventricular depolarization to have taken place. A labeling system was developed to describe the configuration of the QRS complex: (1) if the first deflection is *negative*, it is a Q wave; (2) a *positive* deflection is *always* an R wave; (3) a *negative* deflection *after* an R wave is an S wave; (4) a *second* R or S wave is a *prime* wave, e.g., R′ or S′; (5) a complex that is *solely* a negative deflection is called a QS complex; and (6) the relative size of waves is indicated by upper- and lower-case letters, e.g., R or r. This labeling system then assists in determining where to measure the time intervals. Atrial and AV node depolarization are measured from where the P wave leaves baseline to where the Q *or* R wave leaves baseline, depending on whether the QRS starts with a negative or positive deflection. In other words, measurement is from the *beginning* of atrial depolarization to the *beginning* of ventricular depolarization, which constitutes a P–R (or P–Q) interval. Similarly, ventricular depolarization is measured from where the first wave leaves baseline to where the last wave returns to baseline and constitutes a QRS interval.

repolarization.[5] The ST segment is assessed for elevation or depression above or below the baseline. The T wave is assessed for contour and projection above or below the baseline.

The electrical currents generated by the heart during the processes of depolarization and repolarization are transmitted through the body tissues and fluids to the surface of the body where the electrical activity can be recorded. The electrocardiograph is the device used to accomplish the recording. The electrocardiograph is essentially a galvanometer, which amplifies the currents detected at the skin surface and then graphically records this electrical energy as the electrocardiogram (EKG).

The recording sites on the patient's skin surface are cleansed with alcohol to remove skin oils and thus decrease the skin resistance to transmission of the impulses to the recording device. A conducting jelly is applied to the skin at the recording sites and electrodes are fastened securely. Conducting cables are attached to the electrodes and to positive and negative terminals of the electrocardiograph, thus completing a contiguous recording circuit. This same principle applies for the continuous cardiac monitoring done in intensive-care settings. With cardiac monitoring, however, the cardiac complexes are displayed directly on an oscilloscope rather than on electrocardiographic paper.

A number of different recording sites are utilized for a standard 12-lead EKG. An EKG *lead* consists of a pair of recording sites. One recording site is connected by cable to the positive terminal of the electrocardiograph, and the second site to the negative terminal. Both recording sites can thus be on the body surface as in the standard limb leads, I, II, and III. In the other nine leads, one recording site is on the body's surface (attached to the positive electrocardiograph terminal by cable), and the other is a *combination* of recording sites (attached to the negative electrocardiograph terminal by cable). It should be noted that different parts of the skin surface receive and transmit to the EKG machine different levels of electrical energy from the heart. This is because the electrical currents generated by the heart encounter resistance from the various body tissues as they traverse them. What this means then is that when one EKG lead is recorded, the electrical activity displayed on the paper is the electrical energy *difference* (electrical potential) between two recording sites.[6] Application of this principle is illustrated with the various EKG leads.

[5] See previous section on electrocardiographic evidence of myocardial infarction.

[6] This is a crucial electrocardiographic principle often misunderstood by nurses.

The standard limb leads (I, II, and III) are called *bipolar* leads because they record the electrical energy difference between two recording sites on the body surface. In lead I, the positive electrode is on the left arm (LA) and the negative electrode is on the right arm (RA).[7] In lead II the positive electrode is on the left leg (LL) and the negative electrode on the left arm. The electrodes are applied to all the recording sites at the same time, and a switching device (selector switch) on the electrocardiograph allows individual recording of each lead rather than the constant moving of electrodes and cables. A fourth electrode is applied to the right leg (RL), which serves as a "ground," not a recording site. The electrocardiograph connects the appropriate pair of electrodes for a given lead when the selector switch is turned.

The augmented limb leads (aVR, aVL, and aVF) are *unipolar* leads that record the electrical energy from one recording site on the body surface (the positive electrode) and a second site, which is "in the machine." In other words, several other recording sites are combined that algebraically sum to *zero* at the negative terminal of the electrocardiograph machine (the negative electrode). In aVR the positive electrode is on the RA; in aVL the positive electrode is on the LA; and in aVF the positive electrode is on the LL. The negative electrode is the remaining two limb electrodes paired together.

The precordial leads, V_1 through V_6 are unipolar leads that record the electrical activity from one site on the precordium. The positive electrode is a movable suction cup placed in various positions on the chest surface whereas the negative electrode is derived from a combination of the recording sites on the limbs.[8]

For constant cardiac monitoring purposes, modifications of leads II and V_1 have been devised. In these leads the electrodes are placed in various positions on the chest wall rather than on the limbs to enhance freedom of patient movement and reduce artifact from extremity movement. The reader is referred to a coronary care nursing text for the specific placement of electrodes for the modified lead II and Marriott's modified chest lead (MCL_1).

[7] Rather than speak of "an electrode attached by cable to the positive (or negative) terminal of the electrocardiograph machine," convention has lead to abbreviation of the verbiage by stating the "positive electrode" or the "negative electrode."

[8] The positive electrode for the precordial leads is positioned as follows:

V_1: fourth intercostal space at the right sternal border
V_2: fourth intercostal space at the left sternal border
V_3: equidistant between V_2 and V_4
V_4: fifth intercostal space at the left midclavicular line
V_5: fifth intercostal space at the left anterior axillary line
V_6: fifth intercostal space at the left midaxillary line

Whether performing the 12-lead electrocardiogram or placing the patient on constant cardiac monitoring, the nurse must explain the procedure to the patient, especially if this is a new experience for him or her. The unknown is a common source of anxiety, and in this case, the prospect of heart disease can evoke additional anxiety. Persons unfamiliar with electrocardiograms and monitoring sometimes interpret the procedure as involving the passage of electrical currents from the machine to themselves, that is, potential electrocution, rather than the reverse. When the patient is alert and able to communicate, the nurse must find out what the patient knows and correct any frightening misconceptions.

With the preceding as a base, some specific arrhythmias associated with acute myocardial infarction will be discussed. There are hundreds of specific electrocardiographic disorders, and the arrhythmias presented here are but an introductory sample. The normal cardiac mechanism, *sinus rhythm,* is presented in Figure 44-17A as a basis for comparison with the cardiac arrhythmias.

SINUS RHYTHM. The SA node is the pacemaker of the heart in sinus rhythm as noted by the presence of a normal P wave occurring regularly before each QRS complex in each cardiac complex. The SA node automatic cells initiate cardiac impulses regularly at a rate of 60 to 100 times per minute, and each impulse is transmitted to the ventricles. This is noted by a QRS complex following each P wave, which indicates that ventricular depolarization follows atrial depolarization. Thus the atrial and ventricular rates are the same.[9] With a normal heart rate and a normal ventricular stroke volume, there is a normal cardiac output with the resultant hemodynamic effect of adequate perfusion of all tissues and organs.

SINUS BRADYCARDIA. A commonly occurring arrhythmia associated with myocardial infarction is sinus bradycardia (Figure 44-17B). The SA node is the pacemaker of the heart as noted by the presence of a normal P wave occurring regularly before each QRS complex; however, impulses are spontaneously initiated at a rate less than 60 times per minute. Each impulse is transmitted to the ventricles as noted by atrial depolarization preceding each ventricular depolarization; thus the atrial and ventricular rates are the same, and the rhythm is regular. The electrophysiologic mechanism responsible for sinus bradycardia is decreased automaticity of the SA node. Some factors that predispose to decreased automaticity of the SA node are increased parasympathetic nervous system activity (sleep, carotid sinus pressure, increased intracranial pressure, and the oculocardiac reflex of glaucoma), hyperkalemia, and hypothermia.

Although sinus bradycardia may be a normal finding in healthy athletes, its presence in the acute myocardial infarction patient evokes some concern. This is because of the potential decrease in cardiac output associated with a slow heart rate and decreased perfusion of the coronary arteries. Sinus bradycardia is most frequently associated with an inferior wall myocardial infarction. This is because the right coronary artery perfuses the inferior surface of the left ventricle in the largest majority of hearts and provides a branch to the SA node. Occlusion of the right coronary artery may result in ischemia of the SA node and sinus bradycardia. Certain cardiac depressant drugs such as morphine, lidocaine, quinidine, pronestyl, digitalis, and propranolol (Inderal) may also contribute to diminishing the automaticity of the SA node by a variety of electrophysiologic mechanisms.

Sinus bradycardia may cause symptoms such as dizziness or syncope if the ventricular rate is very slow and cardiac output is impaired seriously. In the acute myocardial infarction patient, sinus bradycardia may precipitate or worsen pre-existing heart failure or angina. Unless coronary perfusion is maintained by an adequate cardiac output, extension of the myocardial infarction can occur. For these reasons, in the majority of acute coronary care units, there are standing orders for the intravenous administration of atropine sulfate 0.4 to 0.5 mg if a patient's ventricular rate falls below 50 beats per minute. Atropine is an anticholinergic agent that effects an increase in the heart rate. Its use is contraindicated in the patient with glaucoma and overt prostatic hypertrophy. An alternative pharmacologic agent, such as isoproterenol (Isuprel), may be considered in this instance. Atropine is useful when intervening with brief episodes of sinus bradycardia, but with prolonged periods of sinus node slowing, insertion of a transvenous pacemaker catheter may be necessary.

SINUS TACHYCARDIA. Another arrhythmia of the sinus node associated with the acute myocardial infarction process is sinus tachycardia (Figure 44-17C). The SA node retains the pacemaker function of the heart as noted by the regular presence of a normal P wave before each QRS complex; however, the rate of impulse formation is generally 100 to 150 times

[9] There are several methods to calculate atrial and ventricular rates. Two major methods utilized are the following:

1. Count the number of P waves (atrial rate) or QRS complexes (ventricular rate) in a 6-second (6-inch) strip and multiply by 10 to obtain the number of beats per minute. This method is useful primarily for irregular rhythms.
2. Count the number of small squares (0.04 second) between two successive P waves (atrial rate) or between two successive R waves (ventricular rate) and divide into 1,500 to obtain the number of beats per minute. This method is generally used for regular rhythms.

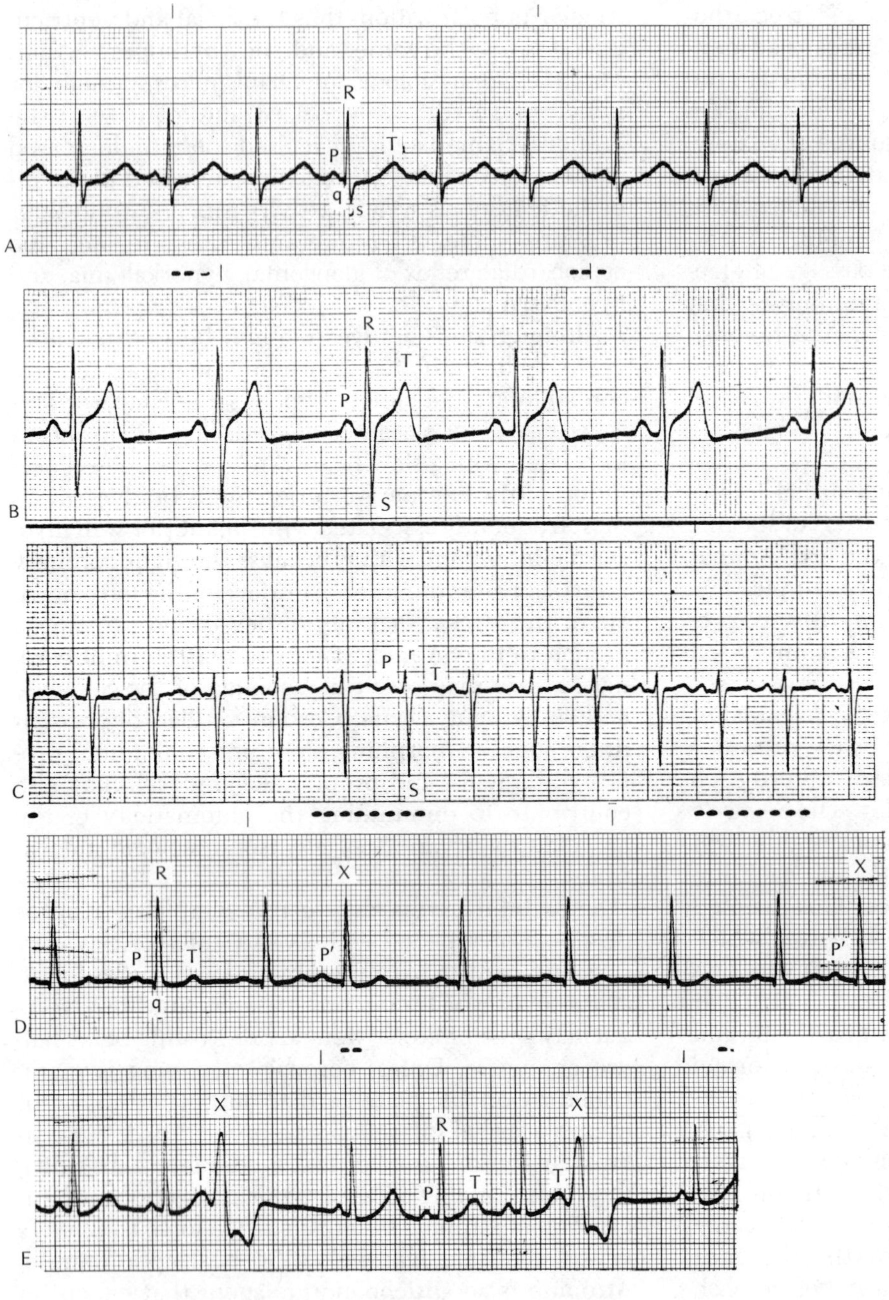

Figure 44-17. Electrocardiographic strips of selected cardiac arrhythmias. *A. Sinus rhythm:* atrial and ventricular rates of 83 per minute. *B. Sinus bradycardia:* atrial and ventricular rates of 50 per minute. The large T waves are potentially suggestive of hyperkalemia. *C. Sinus tachycardia:* atrial and ventricular rates of 115 per minute. *D.* Sinus rhythm with two PAC's: the premature beats *(X)* are preceded by P waves that are of a different configuration *(P′)* and QRS complexes that are the same as the beats from the SA node. *E. Sinus rhythm* with two PVC's: the premature beats *(X)* are not preceded by P waves, and are characterized by the wide bizarre QRS complexes and T waves which go in the opposite direction of the QRS complex of the PVC. The PVC's are also noted to occur on the downstroke of the T wave of the preceding beat originating in the SA node.

per minute. Each impulse is transmitted to the ventricles; thus the atrial and ventricular rates are the same, and the rhythm is regular. This arrhythmia is a result of increased automaticity of the SA node generally resulting from an increase in sympathetic or a decrease in parasympathetic nervous system activity.

Factors that predispose to enhanced automaticity of the SA node because of increased amounts of epinephrine–norepinephrine acting on the cells are anxiety, pain, or physical exertion. Other factors that contribute are nicotine, caffeine, hypokalemia, and increased body temperature. It has been estimated that the heart rate will increase 10 beats per minute for every 1°F increase in body temperature. Enhanced automaticity also occurs when oxygen consumption of cells exceeds oxygen delivery, as is noted with hypoxia, hemorrhage, anemia, infections, fever, shock, and hyperthyroidism. Mechanical stretching of cells, such as that which occurs with cardiac dilatation in right heart failure, also enhances automaticity.

The presence of a sustained sinus tachycardia in the acute myocardial infarction patient elicits concern. As the heart rate increases, ventricular diastolic filling time decreases, with a resultant diminished

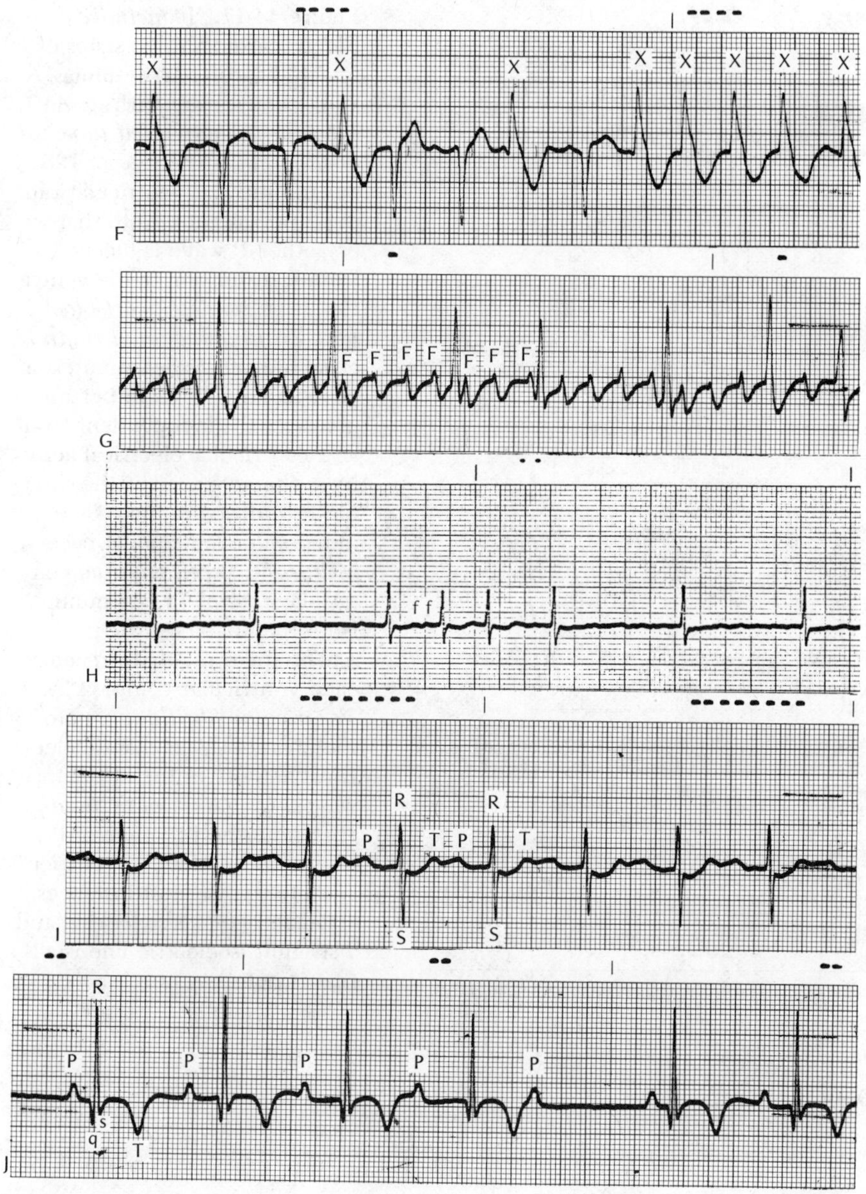

Figure 44-17. [*continued*]. Electrocardiographic strips of selected cardiac arrhythmias. *F.* Sinus rhythm with PVC's in the form of *trigeminy* leading to *ventricular tachycardia G. Atrial flutter:* atrial rate of 250 per minute and ventricular rate of approximately 70 per minute. Note the characteristic "picket-fenced" flutter *(F)* waves. *H. Atrial fibrillation:* atrial rate is not measurable and ventricular rate is approximately 80 per minute. Note the fibrillatory *(f)* waves and grossly irregular ventricular rhythm which is characteristic of atrial fibrillation. *I.* Sinus rhythm with *1° AV block:* atrial and ventricular rates of 79 per minute. The P-R interval is 0.36 second. *J.* Sinus rhythm with *2° AV block of the Wenckebach type, 5:4 conduction:* note the successive prolongation of the P-R interval (0.20, 0.30, 0.38, 0.46 second) until transmission of one P wave to the ventricles is blocked. There are five P waves for four QRS complexes. The inverted T waves are potentially suggestive of the ischemic process.

ventricular stroke volume and cardiac output. Sinus tachycardia (or any other cardiac arrhythmia with a fast ventricular rate) can therefore precipitate heart failure, angina, or extension of a myocardial infarction. Similarly, sinus tachycardia may be an early sign of heart failure, pulmonary embolism, or even cardiogenic shock.

Intervention with sinus tachycardia depends on the underlying cause. For example, initial interventions may be directed toward reduction of anxiety, fever, pain, hypoxia, hypokalemia, and so on, with promotion of physical rest. Sedation may be required and often proves effective. Digitalis preparations should not be used to treat sinus tachycardia in the absence of ventricular failure. Edwards (1972) suggests that the use of digitalis in the instance of acute myocardial infarction without congestive heart failure may cause extension of the zone of injury. The use of propranolol (Inderal) may also be considered for its beta-blocking activity. Propranolol use in this instance, however, must be approached with caution, and the patient's physiologic state must be monitored closely. This is because propranolol has a negative inotropic effect and could precipitate incipient left ventricular failure.

PREMATURE CONTRACTIONS. Another common phenomenon associated with acute myocardial infarction is the occurrence of premature contractions (beats). Under certain conditions an abnormal (ectopic) focus in the atria, ventricles, or junctional region can initiate a cardiac impulse prior to or in "substitution" of the normal SA node impulse, thus

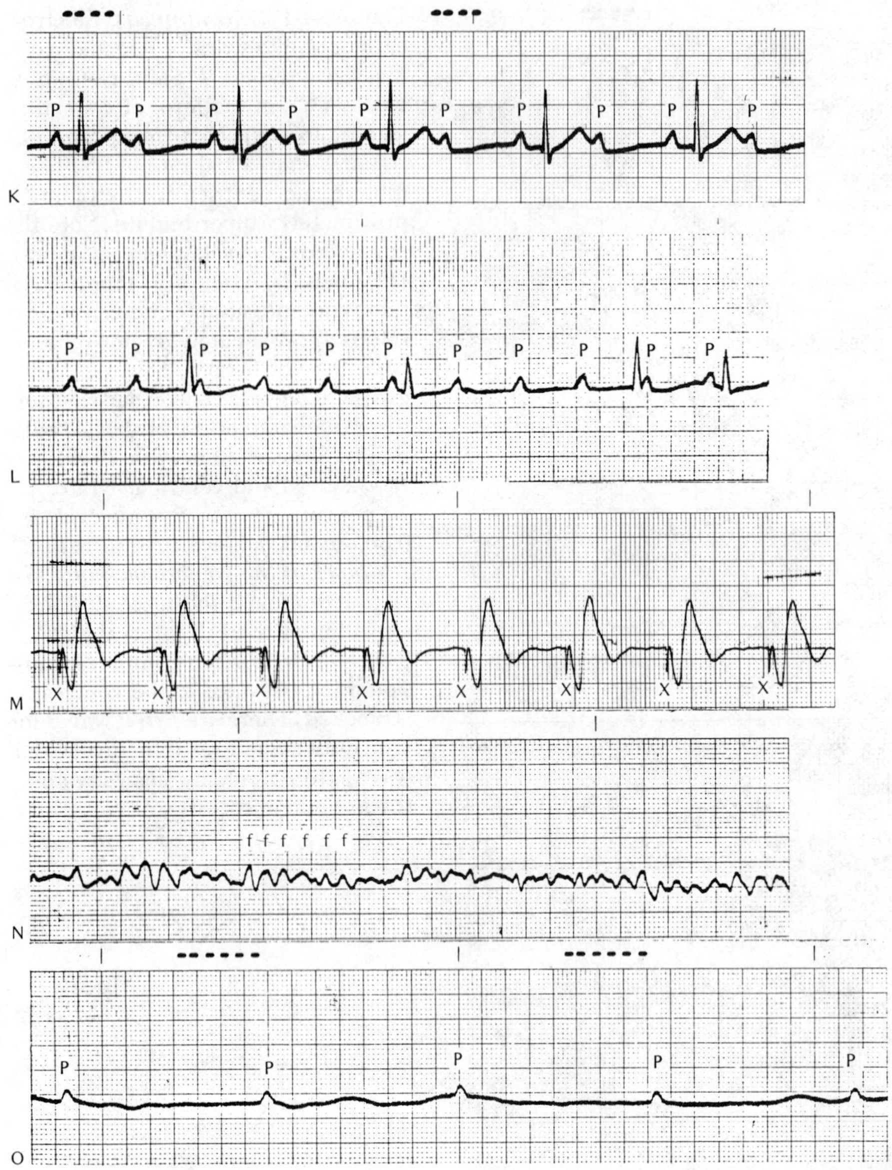

Figure 44-17. [*concluded*]. Electrocardiographic strips of selected cardiac arrhythmias. *K. Sinus tachycardia with 2° AV block of the advanced type, 2:1 conduction:* atrial rate of 125 per minute and ventricular rate of 63 per minute. Note that every other P wave is blocked from transmission to the ventricles. *L. Complete heart block with an idiojunctional rhythm:* atrial rate of 125 per minute and ventricular rate of 40 per minute. Note the independent atrial and ventricular electrical activity as characterized by the variable P-R intervals and independent junctional pacemaker. *M. Paced rhythm:* ventricular rate of 71 per minute. Note the characteristic pacemaker spike *(X)* that precedes each ventricular complex. *N. Ventricular fibrillation:* note the characteristic chaotic electrical activity of the fibrillatory waves. *O. Ventricular standstill:* note the presence of P waves but absence of ventricular activity. In most instances, atrial activity is also lacking and a straight isoelectric line is all that is noted.

creating an ectopic beat. These beats are called *premature atrial contractions* (PAC), *premature ventricular contractions* (PVC), and *premature junctional contractions* (PJC).[10] Only PACs and PVCs will be discussed in this section.

With a *premature atrial contraction* (Figure 44-17D) an ectopic focus in the right or left atrium depolarizes prior to the initiation of a normal SA node impulse and thus usurps the pacemaker function of the heart for at least one beat. This phenomenon is noted on the EKG by a beat that occurs earlier in time sequence than a normal beat from the SA node and thus creates an irregular rhythm. Initiation of the impulse from a site in the atrium other than the SA node is indicated by a P wave that is of different configuration from a P wave initiated by the SA node. The ectopic impulse is usually transmitted normally to the ventricle through the usual conduction pathways; thus the QRS complex of the PAC is the same as a normal beat arising in the SA node, and the atrial and ventricular rates of the entire cardiac rhythm are the same. The ectopic impulse temporarily depresses the SA node, which accounts for the pause that follows a PAC and that precedes the next beat from the SA node.

The electrophysiologic mechanism that accounts

[10] There is a great deal of inaccuracy in the use of the terms *contraction* or *beat,* which connote a mechanical event, when the phenomenon is actually one of premature ectopic *electrical* activity. The most accurate terminology to describe the phenomenon would be *premature atrial, ventricular,* or *junctional depolarization.* Use of these new terms, however, would create considerable confusion; thus the time-honored use of *premature contraction* will be perpetuated.

for PACs is enhanced excitability of cells. The stimuli that promote impulse initiation by atrial excitatory cells are varied. For example, PACs are not infrequent even in healthy individuals where certain substances serve as excitatory stimuli, such as epinephrine–norepinephrine in times of emotional stress and as a result of the excessive use of coffee, tea, or tabacco. Mechanical stretching of the left atrial cells accounts for PACs in patients with mitral stenosis, whereas the stretch phenomenon of the right atrial cells precipitates PACs in the patient with corpulmonale. In patients who have had a myocardial infarction, however, the occurrence of PACs is usually related to the congestive heart failure process and not to the myocardial infarction per se. For this reason it is crucial that PACs are watched for increased frequency, as they may herald the appearance of a more serious sustained, rapid atrial arrhythmia (atrial flutter or fibrillation) associated with marked ventricular failure.

The treatment of PACs depends on the underlying cause. Predisposing factors should be eliminated. When PACs occur infrequently, no intervention is usually necessary. With increased frequency of PACs, treatment for congestive heart failure may be initiated. If the PACs persist despite therapy directed toward the probable cause, antiarrhythmic drug therapy with quinidine may be considered.

Premature ventricular contractions (Figure 44-17E) may originate from one or more ectopic foci in either ventricle occurring (1) prematurely as a substitute for a beat from the SA node or (2) in addition to the normal beats from the SA node (interpolated PVC). In both instances the regularity of the cardiac rhythm is interrupted. On EKG, a PVC is noted as a beat that occurs earlier in sequence than a normal beat from the SA node. Initiation of the impulse from a site in the ventricles is noted by the absence of a P wave preceding the cardiac complex and a premature, wide, bizarre QRS complex that is indicative of an altered ventricular depolarization pathway. The T wave of the PVC deflects in the opposite direction of the QRS, which is indicative of altered ventricular repolarization.

Generally, it is assumed that the SA node depolarizes the atrium at the same time the ventricular ectopic focus impulse depolarizes the ventricles. The P wave is commonly not seen because it is masked by the large QRS deflection. The atrial and ventricular rates are then assumed to be the same. Because the AV node is rendered refractory by the PVC, the impulse initiated by the SA node cannot reach the ventricles, and a pause in the rhythm is noted following the PVC prior to the next normal beat. Occasionally the ventricular ectopic impulse may be transmitted in a retrograde manner to the atrium, and in this case an inverted P wave may be seen following the QRS of the PVC.

Premature ventricular contractions may occur as isolated beats or in an identifiable pattern. The term *ventricular bigeminy* is employed when every other beat is a PVC and *trigeminy* when every third beat is a PVC. (See beginning portion of the strip in Figure 44-17F.) The same terminology can be employed when a pattern of PACs is identified (*atrial* bigeminy, for example). There are several different types of PVCs,[11] and the reader is referred to a coronary care nursing text for more detailed information.

The electrophysiologic mechanism that accounts for PVCs is enhanced excitability of cells. Healthy individuals may experience PVCs in response to stress, various cardiac stimulants, and situations where cellular oxygen requirements are increased, such as during fever associated with minor infections. PVCs are seen with hypokalemia and cardiac trauma, and may be an early sign of ventricular failure. Ventricular bigeminy is classically associated with digitalis toxicity. In patients who have had a myocardial infarction, however, hypoxia serves as the excitatory stimulus, and the PVCs originate from the zone of ischemia.

The hemodynamic effects of PVCs depend on the frequency of occurrence. Most PVCs occur early in diastole before the ventricles have had sufficient time to fill with blood, and thus the stroke volume of the PVC is less than adequate. This may have two effects. With isolated PVCs, sufficient blood may not be ejected in systole to perfuse the extremities, and thus a pulse deficit may be noted. With successive PVCs (three or more successive PVCs are termed *ventricular tachycardia*), an appreciable drop in the cardiac output may be noted with inadequate coronary perfusion and the precipitation or potentiation of ventricular failure.

PVCs generally are regarded as a warning arrhythmia. The danger of ventricular fibrillation is imminent should a PVC occur during the vulnerable period of the preceding beat (on the T wave) or should there be a succession of PVCs. For this reason, PVCs in the patient with acute myocardial infarction are treated with the intravenous administration of a local anesthetic, lidocaine (Xylocaine), concomitant with interventions directed toward removal of predisposing factors. An intravenous bolus of lidocaine may be followed by a constant intravenous infusion of lidocaine for suppression of ventricular ectopic activity. The nurse must observe the patient for the early side effects of lidocaine toxicity and discontinue or reduce the intravenous drip should they occur. The

[11] Some of the various types of PVCs are interpolated, end-diastolic, R on T phenomenon, fusion beat, and multifocal.

early side effects include slurred speech, blurred or double vision, tinnitus, vertigo, and hypotension. As toxicity increases the patient may experience grand mal seizures and respiratory arrest. The second drug of choice for PVCs is procainamide (Pronestyl) administered intravenously. Procainamide or propranolol may be administered orally for individuals who experience PVCs because of chronic myocardial ischemia or in relation to stress.

Procainamide is used more often in the parenteral treatment of acute ventricular arrhythmias when refractory to lidocaine than for chronic suppression of PVCs due to a high frequency of adverse effects. When the drug is administered intravenously, the nurse must monitor the patient closely for profound hypotension leading to circulatory collapse, or for cardiac arrest. Immunologic reactions are not uncommon when oral administration of the drug is employed. Graboys (1979) reports that antinuclear antibody titers are elevated in 90 per cent of patients receiving the drug. Ultimately, lupus-like symptoms leading to the lupus syndrome occur in a substantial number of individuals unless use is discontinued. Other troublesome side effects are fever, insomnia, diarrhea, impotence, hair color changes, and personality changes leading to psychosis (Graboys, 1979, p. 707). Despite the prevalence of side effects, procainamide use has persisted for lack of other available chemical agents. Disopyramide (Norpace) has been released recently for clinical use and appears to hold promise because it possesses both quinidine and procainamide-like properties. As with any chronic condition, the physician must engage in the following processes: (1) evaluation of the basis of chronic ectopic ventricular activity; (2) evaluation of the need for treatment; (3) identification of the patient at risk for sudden death; (4) evaluation of the available drugs, their benefits, and potential side effects in view of the individual patient's history; and (5) selection of a pharmacologic versus a surgical intervention. In the rare instance, an overriding pacemaking device or invasive surgical intervention may be warranted to prevent a catastrophic arrhythmic death.

ATRIAL FIBRILLATION–ATRIAL FLUTTER. Two arrhythmias commonly associated with congestive heart failure are *atrial flutter* (Figure 44-17G) and *atrial fibrillation* (Figure 44-17H). These arrhythmias arise from one or more ectopic foci in the atria that usurp the pacemaker function of the SA node. The primary difference between atrial flutter and atrial fibrillation is the rate of ectopic discharge. In atrial flutter the ectopic focus depolarizes at a rate of 250 to 350 times per minute. On EKG this is characterized by sawtoothed or picket-fence P waves, which are called flutter (F) waves. It is sometimes difficult to see the flutter waves in atrial flutter when the ventricular rate is excessively fast. Carotid sinus pressure may be applied by the physician to slow AV node conduction temporarily and thereby discern the flutter waves. Thus carotid sinus pressure is not therapeutic in this instance. In atrial fibrillation the ectopic focus depolarizes at a rate greater than 350 times per minute. On EKG this is characterized by a wavy baseline or undulating P waves of varying contour and amplitude, which are called fibrillatory (f) waves. Because the atrial ectopic foci can speed up or slow down, it is not uncommon for a patient to experience both atrial flutter and atrial fibrillation concomitantly.

The rate at which the atrial impulses are transmitted to the ventricles in atrial flutter–fibrillation is dependent upon the response of the AV node to the barrage of impulses. What usually occurs is an erratic transmission of impulses to the ventricles, less erratic in atrial flutter than in atrial fibrillation. The result, however, is the half or fewer of the atrial impulses commonly reach the ventricular conduction system. The atrial rates thus exceed the ventricular rate. The cardiac rhythm in atrial flutter is either regular or irregular. The cardiac rhythm is characteristically grossly irregular in atrial fibrillation. Because the impulses transmitted to the ventricles in both arrhythmias generally follow normal ventricular conduction pathways, the QRS complex is normal in configuration and duration.

The electrophysiologic mechanism associated with atrial flutter–fibrillation is increased excitability resulting primarily from hypoxia of cells and stretch of atrial cells, as in congestive heart failure and mitral valve disease. Atrial flutter can occur in the absence of heart disease, whereas atrial fibrillation is almost always associated with cardiac pathology. The hemodynamic effects of atrial flutter–fibrillation are dependent on the ventricular rate. With ventricular rates exceeding 140 to 150 beats per minute, cardiac output and coronary perfusion are diminished, which can aggravate or precipitate heart failure. As with PVCs, a pulse deficit may be present.[12] During atrial fibrillation, the mechanical activity of the atria in response to the impulse formation, which exceeds 350 times per minute, is "quivering." This has been described as a "bag of worms." As a result, thrombus formation can occur. Not only does this quivering diminish the atrial contribution to ventricular dia-

[12] One measure of the extent to which ventricular contractions are ineffective in any arrhythmia or pathologic state is the pulse deficit. The pulse deficit is most accurately determined by the simultaneous counting of the apical and radial pulse rates by two individuals. Because of the irregular pulse in atrial flutter–fibrillation, the pulse rates should be counted for at least a full minute.

stolic filling, but more important, it predisposes to systemic and pulmonary embolization.

One intervention employed with atrial flutter–fibrillation is cardioversion (direct current precordial countershock), the aim of which is to restore sinus rhythm. Cardioversion is indicated in atrial and ventricular tachyarrhythmias, which compromise cardiac output and coronary perfusion. In cardioversion, direct current is discharged through the chest wall over the heart to terminate the arrhythmia. The machine is synchronized so that the electrical current is discharged during the R wave (ventricular depolarization) and not during the T wave (vulnerable period), as this could cause ventricular fibrillation. The electrophysiologic mechanism by which cardioversion achieves the desired effect is as follows: (1) when passed through a group of cells, an electrical stimulus of sufficient intensity and duration will increase the permeability of the cell membranes so the cells will depolarize at the same time; (2) the "premature" depolarization of an ectopic focus by electrical stimuli will decrease the excitability of the focus; and (3) during the period of time in which the ectopic focus is depressed, the SA node may regain control as pacemaker of the heart.

Cardioversion is the most predictably effective therapeutic intervention for atrial flutter. In the majority of cases, atrial flutter will convert to sinus rhythm. It is less predictably therapeutic with atrial fibrillation. Failure of atrial fibrillation to convert to sinus rhythm is noted particularly when the atria are markedly distended because of chronic congestive failure or mitral stenosis prior to surgical intervention, and with hypokalemia. These patients are the "chronic fibrillators."

The nurse's role with cardioversion is before, during, and after the procedure. Prior to cardioversion, the nurse–physician team should see that the procedure has been explained to the patient and legal authorization obtained. The nurse should check and notify the physician if the patient's serum potassium is not within the normal range. The nurse should also note the time of the patient's last dose of digitalis. Digitalis preparations should be discontinued 24 to 48 hours prior to the procedure. It has been noted that patients receiving digitalis preparations have a greater tendency to develop ventricular arrhythmias during the procedure. Prior to the induction with intravenous Valium for sedation, the patient's dentures should be removed, vital signs taken, and a 12-lead EKG performed.

During the procedure the nurse has primary responsibility for monitoring electrical safety procedures. Particularly at the point of electrical discharge, there should be no contact of medical personnel with the patient or the bed. This writer is aware of a situation in which a hospital orderly was touching the bed at the time of electrical discharge and developed ventricular fibrillation. The medical team then had to defibrillate the orderly right then and there as he lay on the floor. In some hospitals the nurse may perform the cardioversion under the supervision of the physician in accordance with agency policies. Following the procedure, another electrocardiogram is obtained, as well as the vital signs. The nurse must observe the patient during recovery from the sedation.

Despite the seeming appropriateness of terminating atrial fibrillation, this is not always possible or even desirable, particularly with chronic fibrillation. If effective contraction of the atria were restored, thrombi could be dislodged. Although uncommon, the occurrence of cerebrovascular accidents during the cardioversion procedure has been noted, presumably because of dislodged left atrial thrombi. When cardioversion is contraindicated, pharmacologic therapy may be employed to lessen the effect of the arrhythmia. Digitalis is a common drug employed in the treatment of atrial fibrillation. It does not usually abolish the fibrillation, but it slows the heart rate and lessens the pulse deficit. Quinidine sulfate is also utilized in this instance and for maintenance therapy following successful cardioversion.

Quinidine is prescribed for its electrophysiologic action of decreasing the excitability of ectopic foci by prolonging the refractory phases of cellular repolarization, and also thereby slowing impulse transmission. Quinidine also decreases automaticity and diminishes contractility, which speaks to its cautious use in patients with heart block and ventricular failure. A number of individuals experience gastrointestinal disturbances of nausea, vomiting, and diarrhea. These discomforting symptoms usually can be controlled with food or antacid ingestion at the time of medication administration, and with antidiarrheal agents. Over a period of time, many patients develop a tolerance to the gastrointestinal symptoms. Because quinidine is an alkaloid of cinchona, it may also cause symptoms of cinchonism, or quinine poisoning, which include vertigo, tinnitus, headaches, and weakness. Dosage reduction often abates the symptoms of cinchonism. A considerable number of patients are hypersensitive to quinidine and develop "serum sickness" type manifestations after beginning a course of quinidine therapy. The first symptom noted is most often drug fever. Frequently medical personnel do not relate the fever to the quinidine but rather seek to relate it to less frequent complications following myocardial infarction, such as pericarditis or postinfarction syndrome, until a skin rash develops. Other adverse effects associated with hypersensitivity are thrombocytopenia purpura, acceleration of cardiotoxicity, asthma-type reactions, and cardiovascular collapse. Discontinuance of the drug as soon as possible is imperative. If antiarrhythmic therapy is to be continued, substitute agents, such as Pronestyl and/or Dilantin, may be employed. It becomes obvious that any patient beginning a course of quinidine therapy should be under careful and regular observation. This observation can be facilitated and accomplished by the professional nurse in a variety of occupational settings.

HEART (AV) BLOCKS. As a result of myocardial infarction, and a variety of other acquired and congenital cardiac conditions, the passage of impulses through the AV node and interventricular conduction system can be impeded or partially or completely obstructed. The heart (AV) blocks are one type of conduction defect. The level of impedence or obstruction to impulse transmission can be at the AV node, bundle of His, or bundle branches. Block or impedance of impulse transmission to the ventricles at the level of the AV node and/or bundle branches is frequently associated with myocardial infarction. The severity of impulse obstruction is indicated by degree, such as 1° AV block, 2° AV block, and 3° AV (complete) block.

In *1° AV block* all atrial impulses are transmitted to the ventricles but with impeded conduction through the AV node. On EKG this phenomenon of delayed AV node conduction is characterized by a P-R interval greater than 0.20 second (Figure 44-17I). The underlying *rhythm* of the heart is undisturbed by delayed conduction through the AV node. The SA node is still the pacemaker of the heart, as noted by the presence of regularly occurring normal P waves, and each impulse is transmitted to the ventricles as noted by the presence of a QRS complex following each P wave. Thus the atrial and ventricular rates are the same, and the underlying basic rhythm of the heart is still either sinus rhythm, bradycardia, or tachycardia.

The electrophysiologic mechanism associated with 1° AV block is delayed AV node depolarization resulting from (1) ischemia, as with right coronary artery atherosclerosis and myocardial infarction of the inferior left ventricular wall; (2) vagal stimulation, as with carotid sinus pressure and digitalis; (3) drug toxicity, as with quinidine and Pronestyl; (4) fibrosis or degeneration of the AV nodal cells, as in Lev's and Lenegre's disease; and (5) hyperkalemia. Because all atrial impulses are conducted to the ventricles, there are no adverse hemodynamic effects associated with 1° AV block. First-degree AV block may be considered a warning sign and alerts medical personnel to observe for partial or complete obstruction of impulse transmission to the ventricles, as in 2° and 3° AV block. The intervention for 1° AV block is directed toward removal of the predisposing factor.

There are three types of *2° AV block* (incomplete heart block) in which some, but not all, impulses from the SA node are transmitted to the ventricles. Figure 44-17J represents one form of 2° AV block known as the *Wenckebach type* (Mobitz I). In the Wenckebach form of 2° AV block, conduction of SA node impulses through the AV node is *gradually impeded* until one SA node impulse is completely blocked from entering the ventricles. Thus the primary EKG characteristic of the Wenckebach phenomenon is progressive prolongation of the P–R interval in a cycle of successive beats until one P wave is not followed by a QRS complex. The cycle then begins again. The atrial rate exceeds the ventricular rate, and the ventricular rhythm is irregular. The underlying basic mechanism is either sinus rhythm, bradycardia, or tachycardia.

The electrophysiologic mechanism associated with the Wenckebach phenomenon is increasing refractoriness of the AV node with each successive beat until one atrial impulse cannot be conducted to the ventricles because of absolute refractoriness. The factors that are responsible for this phenomenon are the same as for 1° AV block but to a greater degree, especially ischemia secondary to right coronary artery atherosclerosis. The hemodynamic effects of the Wenckebach phenomenon depend on the frequency with which SA node impulses are blocked from transmission to the ventricles. With infrequent block of atrial impulses, there is little if any effect on the cardiac output and no intervention will be initiated other than increased observation for progression of the process. Conversely, if atrial impulses are frequently not conducted to the ventricles, the diminished ventricular rate will contribute to a decreased cardiac output and concomitant symptoms of decreased tissue perfusion. The Wenckebach type of 2° AV block may be transient, especially if associated with an inferior wall myocardial infarction and therefore resulting from the ischemic process. If the patient is symptomatic, however, the most dependable intervention is insertion of a transvenous pacemaker to increase the ventricular rate and as a prophylactic measure. If for some reason pacemaker insertion is not possible immediately, atropine may be administered to try to improve conduction through the AV node.

The *advanced type* is the most severe form of 2° AV block in which half or more of the SA node impulses are blocked from transmission to the ventricles (Figure 44-17K). On EKG this is characterized by at least two P waves for each QRS complex. The atrial rate thus exceeds the ventricular rate by a factor of 2 or more. The ventricular rhythm is regular if the conduction ratio of SA node impulses to the ventricles is constant, and irregular if the conduction ratio varies. The underlying mechanism is still either sinus rhythm, bradycardia, or tachycardia. The electrophysiologic mechanism associated with advanced 2° AV block is increased refractoriness of the AV node resulting from ischemia or drug toxicity; or ischemia, degeneration, or fibrosis of the bundle branch system. The resultant slow ventricular rate commonly results in a decreased cardiac output and symptoms of decreased tissue perfusion. The most dependable intervention is insertion of a temporary or permanent cardiac pacemaker.

Third-degree AV (complete) block is the most serious form of heart block, in which no SA node or atrial impulses are transmitted to the ventricles because of block at the AV node or bundle branches bilaterally (Figure 44-17L). The underlying basic mechanism of the heart is either SA node in origin or atrial, such as atrial flutter of fibrillation. If the SA node is pacemaker of the heart, what is noted on the EKG are P waves, which are totally unrelated to the QRS complexes as characterized by totally inconsistent P–R intervals. As a result of the complete block of the SA node or atrial impulses, ventricular depolarization is controlled by a subsidiary pacemaker in the junctional tissue or His–Purkinje system. If the junctional tissue assumes the function of cardiac pacemaker for the ventricles, the QRS complexes will be of normal duration and will tend to occur regularly at a rate of 40 to 70 times per minute (junctional rhythm). On the other hand, if the pacemaking function is assumed by ventricular cells, the QRS complexes will be wide and bizarre, as with PVCs, and will tend to occur irregularly at a rate of 20 to 40 times per minute (ventricular rhythm). The atrial rate will exceed the ventricular rate, and the cardiac rhythm will be regular or irregular, depending on the site of the subsidiary pacemaker.

The electrophysiologic mechanism and factors that predispose to complete heart block are as previously mentioned for all heart blocks, but to the severest degree. The hemodynamic effects of complete heart block are dependent on the rate and site of the subsidiary pacemaker. If the junctional tissue assumes the pacemaker function and depolarizes at a sufficient rate, the patient may be asymptomatic. No intervention may be initiated in this instance, especially if the underlying cause is identified as potentially reversible, as with ischemia secondary to right coronary artery occlusion or drug toxicity. Until the condition has stablized, the patient is likely to develop syncope if the junctional pacemaker slows down or if the ventricular pacemaker assumes control.

To decrease the likelihood of syncopal episodes the nurse must instruct the patient to avoid sudden and rapid movements, and straining at stool. Changes in position, especially from the prone to the upright, should be made slowly. Both to reassure the patient and to protect him or her from injury, the nurse should plan to have someone present when the patient gets out of bed. If the ventricular tissue in the His–Purkinje system assumes the pacemaker function or if the junctional tissue depolarizes at an insufficient rate, the cardiac output can be markedly compromised. The patient may experience all the symptoms of decreased tissue perfusion, including syncope and angina, as well as the potential precipitation of ventricular failure. Futher, if the ventricular pacemaker fails there is no other subsidiary pacemaker and ventricular standstill will ensue. When the patient is symptomatic, intervention is directed toward establishment of a sufficient ventricular rate to ensure an adequate cardiac output. The most dependable therapeutic measure in this instance is insertion of a temporary transvenous cardiac pacemaker. If the situation has not abated in 2 to 3 weeks, a permanent cardiac pacemaker may be implanted.

ARTIFICIAL PACEMAKER. The primary purpose of insertion of an artificial cardiac pacemaker is the control of the heart rate as a means to produce an adequate cardiac output. The mechanism by which this is accomplished is by delivering a stimulus for depolarization *to* the heart from an outside energy source rather than initiation of the stimulus within the heart itself. The components of a pacemaker system are a pulse generator, which initiates the stimulus for depolarization at a predetermined rate and electrical intensity, and a pacing catheter, which delivers the stimulus from the power source to the cardiac muscle.

There are two general types of pacemaker systems, temporary and permanent. The two kinds of temporary systems are the transvenous (endocardial) system and the transpericardial (epicardial) system. Temporary pacemaker systems are employed for emergency therapy, for evaluation of arrhythmias, for stabilization of a patient's physiologic condition prior to permanent pacemaker implantation procedures, to override arrhythmias that are potentially life-threatening, and as a prophylactic factor during implantations of permanent pacemakers done under general anesthesia.

The transvenous endocardial temporary pacemaker is the type currently popularized for medical cardiac patients. With this type a catheter electrode is introduced into the venous system percutaneously. Although the most popular insertion site is the right cephalic vein immediately leading into the right subclavian vein, two other available sites are the right jugular vein and the median basilic vein in the right antecubital fossa. The catheter is threaded through the vein to the right ventricle, where it is positioned at the endocardial surface in a trabeculae contiguous with the septum. Passage and positioning of the catheter are accomplished under fluoroscopy, or by EKG guidance. The latter method is more widely used currently and is accomplished by connecting the distal end of the catheter to the precordial lead of a standard electrocardiograph (Spandau, 1970). The distal end of the catheter is then attached to an external pulse generator set at an average voltage of 1.5 milliamperes and a heart rate of between 50 and 100 beats per minute.

The epicardial temporary pacemaker is the type sometimes employed for surgical cardiac patients postoperatively. During an open-heart surgical procedure, particularly for prosthetic aortic valve insertion, platinum electrodes may be sutured to the ventricular pericardium, and the wires extended through the thoracotomy incision. The wires can then be attached to a pulse generator. This type of pacemaker wire insertion frequently is done prophylactically and the pulse generator is not attached. The nurse must be aware that bare pacemaker wires emerging from the thoracotomy incision constitute a grave electrical hazard for the patient. Even minimal amounts of electrical energy in contact with the catheter electrode terminals can cause the patient to develop ventricular fibrillation. One situation this writer recalls that was potentially hazardous involved bare pacemaker terminals extending from a thoracotomy incision in a male patient who was sitting in bed using an electric shaver. The catheter terminals should be individually insulated in some manner. Taping the electrodes in the fingers of a rubber glove is one approach, and personnel should wear rubber gloves whenever handling the pacemaker catheter. There are many situations that are potential electrical hazards for all patients with or without pacemakers in areas with large amounts of electrical equipment.

Permanent implanted cardiac pacemakers are employed for the long-term management of persistent cardiac arrhythmias and conduction defects. With this type of pacemaker system, a transvenous catheter is introduced via the right cephalic vein; passed to the superior vena cava, right atrium; and positioned on the endocardial surface of the right ventricle. The electrode catheter is attached to a pulse generator, which is placed under the skin beneath the right clavicle in a subcutaneous pocket.

The two kinds of pulse generators employed most commonly with both temporary and permanent pacemaker systems are the fixed-rate (set) and demand (standby) types. The fixed-rate pulse generator stimulates the ventricles at a constant preset rate regardless of the patient's own cardiac rhythm. This type of pulse generator is used when a conduction defect such as complete or advanced 2° AV block is unlikely to be resolved. The problem with fixed-rate systems is that if AV node or bundle branch conduction is re-established, competition can occur between the pacemaker and the patient's natural rhythm. If the pacemaker stimulus should discharge during the vulnerable period of the T wave, ventricular fibrillation may develop. For this reason and others, the demand-type pulse generator, which is noncompetitive, is more universally used. The "ventricular inhibited" type of demand pulse generator senses the interval between two successive QRS complexes and discharges only when the patient's ventricular rate falls below preset limits. The "ventricular trigger" demand pulse generator senses a normal QRS complex and fires during the complex, thus avoiding competition. Both of these demand pulse generators can revert to fixed-rate pacemakers if the patient's own QRS complexes fail to occur. One problem with demand pulse generators is that the sensing circuit increases battery drain more than the fixed-rate type. At present mercury-zinc batteries with a 3 to 4 year life or lithium batteries with a 6 to 12 year life are used to power the units (Furman, 1978). Power generators with radioactive isotopes or rechargeable nickel cadmium batteries also are available.

The nurse has major responsibilities when caring for patients with both temporary and permanently implanted pacemakers. With the insertion of either type of pacemaker, there is a significant amount of patient teaching necessary. Kos and Culbert (1971) describe six areas of content for a teaching program, which include cardiac physiology and pathology, pacemaker functioning, pulse taking, medication taking, dietary requirements, and activities and restrictions. Two very fine patient teaching pamphlets have been made available to assist with the instructional process.[13] It would be advantageous if the teaching could take place prior to the insertion procedure. This may be accomplished with patients who are having permanent pacemakers implanted but may be difficult when temporary transvenous pacemakers are inserted rapidly in response to conduction defects that diminish the cardiac output.

Another major area of responsibility when working with pacemaker patients is assessment of complications. Some of the complications resulting from the presence of a foreign body include (1) pulmonary embolus from a thrombus at the electrode catheter

[13] Pamphlets are available through the local chapter of the American Heart Association and through Medtronic, Inc.

tip; (2) infection, phlebitis, or rejection at the pacemaker wire insertion site or at the site of an implanted pulse generator; (3) cardiac irritability from the electrode catheter resulting in PVCs or focal myocardial injury; (4) stimulation of noncardiac sites, such as the diaphragm, resulting in hiccoughs; the phrenic nerve, resulting in seizures; and the intercostal or pectoral muscles, resulting in muscle twitching or spasm; (5) myocardial perforation resulting from a stiff electrode catheter, resulting in cardiac tamponade; (6) septal perforation because of a stiff catheter; and (7) endocarditis. Most of these complications have to do with the position of the catheter and the type of catheter used; therefore, the nurse must be alert to their possible occurrence. The nurse can, however, give aseptic care to the insertion site, as with any surgical incision to decrease or prevent infection. In some hospitals it is policy to apply a topical antibacterial cream daily to the insertion site and cover the area with sterile dressings.

Complications that can result from malfunction in the pacemaker system are generally due to component failure or changes in the heart. One major malfunction is cessation of or intermittent pacing because of pulse generator failure, electrode catheter displacement, interference from extraneous signals, or development of competitive cardiac rhythms. Figure 44-17M depicts the usual cardiac complex initiated by an artificial cardiac pacemaker. It should be noted that a pacing stimulus (spike) initiates ventricular depolarization (wide, bizarre QRS complex) each time; thus the pacemaker is "capturing" the ventricles 100 per cent of the time. The nurse must be aware of the configuration of paced beats in order to make comparisons with the patient's self-initiated beats, to recognize pacemaker-induced PVCs, and to recognize the possibility of septal perforation. Should a pacemaker cease functioning, the nurse should be prepared to (1) replace the batteries in an external pulse generator or replace the generator; (2) notify the physician if the pacing catheter needs to be repositioned or replaced; (3) increase the milliamperage of the pacing stimulus in external systems according to unit policy; and (4) initiate cardiopulmonary resuscitation. Another malfunction of the pacemaker system is an alteration in the pacing rate, usually because of battery depletion. The nurse will note a change in the rate of the pacing spikes from the preset level. A halo effect can be noted on chest x-ray around depleted batteries in an internal system and means that the batteries need replacement.

There must be long-term follow-up of patients with permanently implanted cardiac pacemakers. The patient may be followed in an outpatient pacemaker clinic or in a private physician's office. The community health nurse may also help with the patient's adaptation to the home environment. The parameters evaluated with follow-up care are the pacemaker rate and per cent of capture, which are best done by an electrocardiogram; pacemaker catheter position, which is done by chest x-ray; and ability of a demand pacemaker to convert to a fixed-rate pacemaker, which is evaluated by placing a magnet over the pulse generator. Some areas of patient teaching may need to be reinforced. The patient can participate in all normal activities, including sexual activities, but should exercise caution to prevent jerky movements on the side of the implanted pulse generator, which might dislodge the electrode catheter. The patient should be aware that certain electrical appliances and equipment may suppress pacemaker function if placed in close proximity to the pulse generator. Examples include electrical surgical–dental instruments, diathermy or electric razors placed over the pulse generator site, or the patient coming in close contact with electric motors, gasoline engines, or microwave ovens. The patient should carry a pacemaker history card at all times and inform any new physicians or dentists that he or she has an implanted pacemaker. Telephone transmission devices have been developed that can relay the pacemaker rate and amplitude of the pacing spike from the patient's home to a computer bank in a large medical center. In the future there could be a nationwide hook-up to facilitate assessment of pacemaker function in the thousands of patients with implanted cardiac pacemakers.

CARDIAC ARREST. Two final arrhythmias associated with acute myocardial infarction are the death-producing arrhythmias, *ventricular fibrillation* (Figure 44-17N) and *ventricular standstill* (Figure 44-17O). Ventricular fibrillation is an unco-ordinated "quivering" of the ventricles, which is initiated by rapid, repetitive, chaotic impulse initiation from ectopic foci in the ventricular myocardium. ON EKG this is represented by chaotic, irregular oscillations or an undulating movement of the baseline. These are fibrillatory waves, and there is no normal P-QRS-T sequence, which indicates the absence of normal atrial and ventricular electrical activity. The electrophysiologic mechanism associated with ventricular fibrillation is increased excitability of an ectopic focus that overrides any other pacemaker focus in the heart. There are multiple factors that predispose to enhanced excitability of a ventricular focus, including (1) hypoxia, as occurs in myocardial ischemia and drowning; (2) electric shock occurring during the vulnerable period of the T wave; (3) trauma to the heart, as with crushed-chest injuries; (4) drug toxicity, especially digitalis; (5) hypothermia; and (6) hypokalemia.

As a result of the rapid, uncoordinated "twitching" of the ventricles, there is no effective contraction of the heart and no cardiac output. No vital organs or tissues are perfused, and intervention must be initiated immediately. In the acute care setting or where appropriate equipment and personnel are available, the patient should be defibrillated immediately with direct current unsynchronized precordial countershock at maximum voltage. The electrophysiologic mechanism underlying defibrillation is the application of electrical stimuli, which will depolarize all cells at the same time, with the expected result of the SA node then assuming the cardiac pacemaker function again. At the time of voltage discharge, no personnel should be in contact with the patient or bed. A second defibrillation attempt may be applied immediately if the first attempt is unsuccessful.

The effectiveness of defibrillation is inversely proportional to the degree of metabolic acidosis present. Thus the more acidotic the patient, the less likely defibrillation will be accomplished. Following two unsuccessful attempts at defibrillation, cardiopulmonary resuscitation should be initiated until sodium bicarbonate has been administered intravenously to combat the acidosis. Lidocaine also may be given intravenously to decrease the excitability of the ectopic focus. Defibrillation attempts are then repeated. If the patient develops ventricular fibrillation in a setting where a defibrillator is not available, resuscitation should be initiated immediately until transport to a medical facility is accomplished or a defibrillator is made available.

The second death-producing arrhythmia, ventricular standstill, is characterized on EKG by the absence of QRS complexes, as the name would imply. The electrophysiologic mechanism associated with ventricular standstill is (1) failure of SA node automaticity in conjunction with failure of subsidiary pacemakers, that is, complete cessation of all cardiac electrical activity; or (2) complete block of SA node or atrial impulses at the AV node with failure of subsidiary pacemakers, in which case there may be some form of P wave evident on the EKG. Among the factors that predispose to ventricular standstill are myocardial anoxia, depression of pacemakers with massive doses of antiarrhythmic drugs, hyperkalemia, and circulatory failure. With absent ventricular depolarization there are no ventricular contractions, which (as was the case with ventricular fibrillation) leads to no cardiac output. The result is absent perfusion of all organs and tissues and the classic symptoms of (1) unconsciousness, (2) absent pulse, (3) absent respirations, and (4) dilated pupils.

CARDIOPULMONARY RESUSCITATION (CPR). When a cardiac arrest is suspected, the nurse must make an immediate assessment of the situation in order to begin cardiopulmonary resuscitation (CPR) as quickly as possible. Although many resources suggest that one has 4 minutes to initiate CPR before cellular death occurs, this is misleading. In some individuals brain damage can occur in 1 to 2 minutes, and it has also been documented that the longer the time before CPR is initiated, the greater the rate of mortality. In the assessment of the symptoms noted above, if the patient is unconscious, he or she will not respond to painful stimuli, to being shook, or to having his or her name called. Absence of breathing is best noted by placing one's ear directly over the patient's nose and mouth while simultaneously observing for thoracic excursions. The carotid pulse is palpated to the side of the "Adam's apple" with the flat portion of the fingertips. An absent pulse at this location is evidence that circulation has ceased.

Much is available in the literature and in prepared audiovisual materials on the subject of *CPR*, the prime purpose of which is to establish circulation of oxygenated blood to the brain and other vital organs before cellular death occurs. All nurses should be certified by the American Heart Association at least in Basic Life Support, the techniques of which include (1) obstructed airway, (2) witnessed and unwitnessed cardiac arrest-one and two rescuers, and (3) infant resuscitation. In addition, some will seek certification in Advanced Life Support. The reader is referred to the training materials of the American Heart Association for specifics of the basic CPR techniques. There is little doubt that many thousands of lives can be salvaged each year if CPR is performed by properly trained individuals. In addition, the professional nurse must be familiar with the Nurse Practice Act and Good Samaritan Law of the state in which he or she practices.

Thromboembolic Phenomenon

Thromboembolic phenomenon is another complication associated with acute myocardial infarction. Thrombi may arise from the arterial or venous system. Because mural thrombi commonly form over the infarcted endocardium of the left ventricle, systemic emboli may complicate myocardial infarction. If loosened, mural thrombi may lodge in the cerebrum, causing a cerebrovascular accident, or in the leg arteries, necessitating an emergency embolectomy. There are conflicting viewpoints among clinicians about the anticoagulation of the patient with an acute myocardial infarction, particularly one that is transmural. Some feel that anticoagulants may promote loosening of the mural thrombus and bleeding into the pericardial sac and thus are contraindicated. Others feel that formation or extension of a mural thrombus must be avoided and employ anticoagulants. The use of anticoagulants should be based on the patient's past history and the experience of the physician. Situations like a recent phlebitis or embolism favor anticoagulation, whereas history of ulcer, bleeding tendencies, or hemorrhage argues against anticoagulation.

A major site for thrombus formation in myocardial infarction and heart failure patients is the leg veins, largely because of the bedrest regimen. Patients are generally kept in bed only as long as absolutely necessary. During the time the patient is confined to bed, the extremities should be put through the normal range of motion at least once per shift when the elastic stockings are removed. Elastic stockings are routinely applied in many hospitals to patients on bedrest to prevent venous pooling. They should be removed and reapplied at least every 8 hours. Active exercises of the legs should be taught to the patient. A footboard should be placed in position to support the patient's feet and extremities in good alignment. *Contrary to popular opinion,* however, *the patient should not be taught to push his or her feet against the footboard.* Lavin (1973) reports that this form of isometric exercise produces vasoconstriction of the peripheral vascular bed and causes a marked rise in the residual blood of the left ventricle, which either evokes or accentuates left ventricular dysfunction. Further, the Valsalva maneuver occurs during isometric exercises, which increases the danger to the patient. Rhythmic exercises such as *climbing* the footboard with the *toes* are preferred in addition to active flexion and extension of the feet and turning in bed at regular intervals.

Another potential site for thrombus formation is the site of indwelling cannulas and catheters. Phlebitis is a common occurrence not only because of the cannula per se but because of the various medications and fluids infused. Daniell (1973) reported that the addition of 1 mg of heparin sodium for every milliliter of intravenous solution was found to reduce the frequency of infusion phlebitis. Unfortunately the results of the study were not subjected to statistical analysis.

Ventricular Aneurysm

Ventricular aneurysm is reported to occur in 3 to 30 per cent of patients with an acute myocardial infarction (Alford, 1973). Aneurysm is most commonly associated with anterior transmural myocardial infarctions and predisposes to thrombus formation, left ventricular failure, and ventricular arrhythmias. Ventricular aneurysm is sometimes suspected from changes in the electrocardiogram, physical examination, or chest x-ray; however, definitive diagnosis is primarily accomplished by left heart catheterization with ventricular angiography. In recent years a greater amount of surgical intervention has been attempted in the form of aneurysmectomy. If a significant amount of left ventricle must be removed, however, there may not be sufficient muscle mass to maintain an adequate stroke volume and cardiac output. Many patients are living today with varying sizes of ventricular aneurysms and will continue as such until they succumb to congestive heart failure or cardiogenic shock.

Ventricular Failure (Congestive Heart Failure (CHF))

Ventricular failure has been called the "final common pathway" of heart disease. In other words, all kinds of heart disease will eventually result in some form of heart failure. One difficulty with any discussion of heart failure is the maze of terminology encountered. There are at least ten terms used to connote heart failure.[14] For purposes of this discussion the generic term *heart failure* will be used to encompass all kinds of failure. Various aspects of heart failure will be discussed with respect to the alterations in the left and right heart, hence the terms *left* and *right ventricular failure.* The term *congestive heart failure* is, and will be, applied to the chronic state of combined left and right ventricular failure.

Common to all kinds of heart failure is the factor that the cardiac output is inadequate to meet the metabolic needs of the body. In other words, even if the volume of blood circulation through the body per minute is "normal," it is still insufficient to meet the needs of cells for substances essential to metabolic processes. The reason that the cardiac output is inadequate to meet cellular needs is usually that the heart has failed as the ultimate power source to pump the blood through the circulatory system.

Although the definitive pathophysiologic mechanism by which the myocardial cells lose their ability to contract forcefully is not yet known, research in the field suggests it may be a physiochemical event associated with multiple abnormalities in cardiac cellular metabolism. The abnormalities implicated thus far are (1) depression of the failing heart's ability to utilize fatty acids as a fuel source for glycolysis; (2) depression of the enzyme adenosine triphosphatase, which liberates ATP for the contractile process; (3) decreased calcium ion release from the sarcoplasmic reticulum for the excitation–contraction

[14] The various terms used are *heart failure, cardiac failure, myocardial failure, left ventricular failure, right ventricular failure, congestive heart failure (CHF), high output failure, low output failure, pump failure,* and *power failure.* Many of these terms are used synonymously without regard to mute semantical differences. The nurse may need to clarify what a term means with the particular physician group with whom he or she works.

coupling mechanism; and (4) depression of norepinephrine synthesis and release by cardiac sympathetic nerves, which normally produces inotropic activity of myofibrils (Spann, 1970).

The loss of contractile ability of the cardiac myofibrils has been explained for years on a mechanical basis as an alteration in Starling's Law of the Heart. It will be recalled that this law states that the force of cardiac contraction is a function of the myofibrils' length at the end of diastole. Within physiologic limits, the longer the muscle fibers are at the end of diastole, the more forceful the systolic contraction. If, however, the fibers are stretched to a critical point beyond their limits of extensibility, the force of contraction is markedly diminished and ineffective. The entire process associated with Starling's Law of the Heart can be demonstrated by the stretch of an ordinary brown rubber band. When the band is stretched and released, the force with which it returns to its original form depends on the degree to which the band was stretched. Within the limits of the band's extensibility, the more it is stretched, the more forcibly it contracts. Consider, however, the band that has been stretched and stretched beyond its limits of extensibility. The result is a rubber band that is capable of only weak contraction and that does not return to its original form. Although this is a somewhat simplified explanation of the loss of cardiac contractility in heart failure, it serves to illustrate the mechanical events associated with cardiac dilatation.

The consequences of failure of the heart as a pump occur in varying degrees because of various adaptive mechanisms that are operant to maintain a sufficient cardiac output during periods of rest and activity. These mechanisms include *tachycardia*, *cardiac dilatation*, and *cardiac hypertrophy*. One way the healthy heart adapts to changes in the demands on it is by an increase in the rate of contraction. When activity is increased, the heart and respiratory rates increase within physiologic limits to provide cells with the necessary ingredients to perform metabolic processes necessary to biochemical energy formation. The heart rate returns to normal upon cessation of the activity within a reasonable period of time. In the failing heart, the heart rate increases, gradually at first, in both rest and activity to provide an adequate cardiac output. Eventually, however, there is a marked or unexpected increase in the heart rate during exercise and, finally, at rest, which is out of proportion to the activity. Although this may help to maintain an adequate cardiac output for a period of time, after a while this mechanism will fail. As the ventricular diastolic filling time decreases because of the increased heart rate, the ventricular stroke volume diminishes. Thus cardiac output further diminishes.

Another way in which the heart adapts to changes in the demands made on it is by altering the force of contraction during systole. Essentially the function of the heart as a pump is satisfactory so long as (1) the ventricles are able to eject as much blood into the systemic and pulmonary circulations as is delivered in diastole without a gain in residual blood at the end of systole, and (2) the cardiac output can meet the needs of the tissues under different degrees of activity. The way in which the normal ventricles accommodate an increased volume of blood in diastole is by an increase in the length of the myofibrils. Thus a stronger contraction results, and there is no residual blood in the ventricles at the end of systole. With disease of the heart, however, an increase in the volume of blood entering the ventricles in diastole causes a *sustained* lengthening in the cardiac muscle fibers, or dilatation. For a time this lengthening of the fibers and associated dilatation of the chambers of the heart may enable the heart to meet the needs of all cells, including its own, without signs of embarrassment. In other words, the heart has a reserve power that enables it to maintain an appropriate balance between the blood entering the chambers in diastole and the amount ejected in systole. As the muscle fibers lengthen and the chambers dilate, the contractions become more forceful, but the cardiac reserve power diminishes. Finally the point is reached when further lengthening of the muscle fibers during diastole reaches a critical point, and contractions become weak. At that point, cardiac reserve power is lost. The heart is no longer able to adapt to an increase in venous return or to increase cardiac output in relation to the requirements of cells, and residual blood remains in the chamber at the end of systole. The individual is no longer able to increase activity above resting levels without manifestations associated with failure of the heart as a pump. Eventually the heart will be unable to meet cellular needs even at rest. In other words, adaptive mechanisms fail sooner or later when a condition exists that makes further adaptation necessary, or if there is a direct injury to the myocardium.

As might be expected, the normal size of an individual's heart is roughly proportional to body size. Physical exercise is necessary for a healthy heart, and the heart responds to "lack of use" by atrophy. Likewise, the heart muscle adapts to an increase in workload by hypertrophy. So it is with the "athletic heart." In well-trained athletes, the resting pulse rates are lower than average, but the stroke volume per beat is greater because of an increase in the muscle fibers; thus the cardiac output is maintained. Should the athlete discontinue athletic activities, the heart will respond to the decreased use by some degree of atrophy.

Dilatation of one or more chambers of the heart is associated with hypertrophy of the myocardium. Authorities are not agreed as to whether hypertrophy precedes dilatation of the heart or dilatation precedes hypertrophy. In either event, the hypertrophied heart is far larger than the healthy heart. Hypertrophy is physiologic inasmuch as it occurs in response to an increased workload, and insofar as it enables the heart to maintain the normal equilibrium between intake of blood in diastole and stroke volume during systole. Like other adaptive mechanisms, however, hypertrophy has certain limitations. One important limitation is that as muscle mass increases, the blood supply does not increase to a comparable degree. In the healthy heart, a capillary is thought to be available to supply each muscle fiber. Even when this ratio is maintained in the hypertrophied heart, the quantity of blood delivered to the tissue is reduced in relation to the muscle mass. A larger fiber receives no more blood than the former smaller fiber. This in itself can be physiologic. If, however, something diminishes the blood supply to the muscle fibers, as occurs with coronary atherosclerosis, then the contractile ability of the heart diminishes and the hypertrophy of the muscle fibers is an inefficient adaptive mechanism.

The causes of heart failure, or the factors that impair the cardiac output, can be summarized in four main categories: (1) impaired functional capacity associated with disease of the myocardium, (2) overloading of the cardiac chambers associated with increased resistance or volume states, (3) interference with cardiac diastolic filling, and (4) changes in the cardiac rate or rhythm. It will be noted that although heart disease associated with the above phenomena can precipitate heart failure, these situations also can occur and exacerbate existing heart failure.

The most common cause of heart failure is decreased functional capacity of myocardial cells associated with coronary atherosclerosis and myocardial infarction. Necrotic cells are incapable of contraction; therefore the more extensive a myocardial infarction, the greater the amount of residual blood that remains in the ventricles, and the greater the decrease in cardiac output. A vicious cycle is thus created, because coronary perfusion is further decreased by the lowered cardiac output, and cells are further deprived of materials essential to metabolism and contractile function. For this reason an inotropic agent such as digitalis must be employed. Because of the process of myocardial infarction occurs primarily in the left ventricle, the specific type of heart failure that occurs initially is left ventricular failure. It then becomes only a matter of time before right ventricular failure ensues, and the individual is in congestive, or combined, heart failure.

Other complications associated with myocardial infarction compound the problem and further promote the development of left ventricular and congestive heart failure. These complications include ventricular and septal aneurysms and papillary muscle dysfunction. With a ventricular aneurysm, blood accumulates in the aneurysmal sac during systole, which further decreases the stroke volume and cardiac output. With a septal aneurysm, blood is forced into the septal sac during systole, which predisposes to septal rupture and the development of an interventricular septal defect. Because blood is shunted through the septal defect to the right ventricle during systole, the left ventricular stroke volume decreases along with the cardiac output. With infarction of the left ventricular papillary muscle(s), the mitral valve cusps become incompetent, that is, mitral insufficiency develops. In systole blood is ejected back into the left atrium through the insufficient mitral valve; thus left ventricular stroke volume and cardiac output diminish.

A number of inflammatory and metabolic disorders affect the myocardium, causing decreased contractility of cells and heart failure. The inflammatory process predisposes to decreased cellular contractility because of the increased deposition of connective tissue. Some of the inflammatory diseases are rheumatic fever, diphtheria, infectious mononucleosis, and the collagen diseases, such as lupus erythematosus and scleroderma. Diphtheritic myocarditis is infrequent in the United States, and can be eliminated by childhood immunization. Various metabolic diseases cause biochemical or biophysical changes that interfere with the utilization of essential ingredients by myocardial cells. Examples of these disorders are thyrotoxicosis, hypothyroidism, and beriberi. Most of the metabolic cardiac diseases can be prevented or cured by early and effective treatment of the precipitating abnormality. Some, such as hypothyroidism (myxedema heart), require therapy, such as thyroid hormone, throughout the individual's lifetime.

Overloading of the cardiac chambers because of increased resistance or volume states within the heart or peripheral arterial circulation can precipitate or exacerbate heart failure. The myocardium may fail because the resistance that it must overcome in moving blood into the circulation is excessive. The site of the resistance may be any place between the outlet of the ventricle and the distal circulation. For example, left ventricular failure may be caused by resistance at the aortic valve (aortic stenosis) or in the peripheral circulation (arterial hypertension). Right ventricular failure may be caused by resistance at the pulmonic valve (pulmonic stenosis) or in the pulmonary circulation (pulmonary hypertension associated with lung disease). It all instances, left ventricular stroke volume and cardiac output diminish with increased residual volume in the ventricles at the completion of systole and cardiac dilatation. Any condition that diminishes the cardiac output decreases coronary perfusion, and a vicious cycle ensues.

The heart can fail because the volume of blood entering the atrial or ventricular chambers is in excess of that which can be expelled. The result is residual blood in the chamber at the conclusion of systole, chamber dilatation, and decreased cardiac output. For example, an increased volume state on the left side of the heart occurs with mitral insufficiency. In addition to left atrial overloading in systole, the left ventricular stroke volume and cardiac output diminish. Similarly, left ventricular volume overloading occurs in diastole with aortic insufficiency. On the right side of the heart, overloading of the right ventricle with subsequent failure can occur with pulmonic insufficiency or an interventricular septal defect. A special problem of cardiac volume overloading occurs with general expansion of the blood volume, particularly in elderly persons. With advancing years, even in the absence of overt cardiac disease, there is a reduction in the myocardial reserve power and with it a decrease in the capacity of the heart to cope with excessive expansion of the extracellular fluid volume. Although the degree to which myocardial reserve is diminished differs among elderly persons, any elderly person who is receiving a blood transfusion or intravenous infusion should be closely observed for evidence indicating that the heart is not tolerating expansion of the blood volume. The pulse and respiratory rates as well as the heart and lung sounds should be assessed for evidence of circulatory and respiratory distress. Should either occur, the rate of fluid flow should be reduced to the minimum required to maintain cannula patency, and the physician should be notified immediately.

Interference with filling of the cardiac chambers during diastole will diminish stroke volume and cardiac output and may precipitate heart failure. Two major factors that interfere with chamber filling are (1) obstruction to blood inflow and (2) insufficient volume of blood in the circulatory system. The most common cause of obstructed blood flow is mitral stenosis. Sometimes the stenosis is so severe that the opening is no larger than a broom straw. Such marked narrowing of the mitral valve seriously limits the quantity of blood that can enter the left ventricle with a subsequent decrease in stroke volume, cardiac output, and coronary perfusion. Constrictive pericarditis and cardiac tamponade can also interfere with the filling of the cardiac chambers because of limiting chamber expansion during diastole. The principle that is operant in this situation is that the ventricular chambers can eject into the arterial and pulmonary circulations during systole only the quantity of blood that is received in diastole.

There must be a sufficient volume of blood in the circulation to provide for an adequate venous return. For the left ventricle to eject sufficient blood into the arterial system, it must receive sufficient blood volume from the right heart via the pulmonary circulation. The right heart volume is dependent on an adequate venous return. Thus the cardiac output is equal to the venous return, and any reduction in the venous return causes a reduced cardiac output. The most common cause of an inadequate venous return is shock of various types. For example, in hypovolemic shock, the venous return may fall as a result of blood volume loss, as in hemorrhage, or of excessive loss of fluid into the tissues, as occurs in burns. In other forms of shock, such as bacteremic or anaphylactoid shock, the volume of blood may be within normal limits, but generalized dilatation of the blood vessels may enlarge the capacity of the vascular system so much that the quantity of blood returned to the heart is insufficient to maintain an adequate cardiac output. If these situations persist, death may result.

The final factors that may precipitate or exacerbate heart failure are disturbances in the rate or rhythm of the heart. Excessively fast or slow heart rates predispose to a decreased functional capacity of the myocardium because of a decreased cardiac output and coronary perfusion. It will be recalled that very rapid ventricular rates decrease the ventricular stroke volume because of a reduction in the time for diastolic chamber filling. Examples of rapid rate arrhythmias include sinus tachycardia, atrial flutter or fibrillation with a rapid ventricular rate, and ventricular tachycardia. Similarly, very slow ventricular rates, such as sinus bradycardia, advanced second-degree heart block, and complete heart block, potentially diminish cardiac output and coronary perfusion. Thus any excessively rapid or slow cardiac arrhythmia should not be allowed to persist because of possible precipitation or exacerbation of heart failure.

It should be noted that in the patient with a seriously reduced cardiac reserve, any condition that makes demands on the heart for increased circulation of blood may precipitate heart failure. Thus an infection, particularly when accompanied by a fever and cough, may precipitate heart failure. Similarly, emotional stress, excessive physical activity, ingestion of excessive amounts of sodium, and development of anemia may do likewise. This list is not exhaustive but shows that any disorder that increases demands on the heart can be responsible for heart failure.

It has been noted that the chronic state of combined left and right ventricular failure is known as "congestive heart failure." It also has been noted that given a period of time, left ventricular failure will cause right ventricular failure, and vice versa. The period of time in which this occurs is indeterminate and depends upon the severity of failure in the original ventricle as well as the rapidity with which it develops. The mechanism by which left ventricular failure results in right ventricular failure is generally as follows: (1) because of residual blood in the left ventricle at the end of systole (beginning of diastole)[15] the left atrium, pulmonary veins, pulmonary capillaries, pulmonary artery, and right ventricle are unable to completely empty; (2) incomplete emptying of these chambers and structures results in residual blood and transmission of a "back-pressure" from the left to the right heart; (3) the right ventricular chamber dilates and eventually loses some of its contractile ability, hence right ventricular failure. The pressure in the right ventricle caused by residual blood also is transmitted back to the right atrium, vena cava, and venous system. The increased volume of blood in all the chambers and structures is what connotes the concept of "congestion." The mechanism by which right ventricular failure leads to left ventricular failure is related to the principle that the stroke volume of the left ventricle is dependent on the amount of blood received from the right heart. If the right ventricle is unable to empty completely in systole because of decreased contractility, the left ventricular stroke volume will be proportionally less. As a result cardiac output, coronary perfusion, and left ventricular contractility are diminished, hence left ventricular failure.

Diagnosis of heart failure is accomplished by assessment of the physical manifestations and certain diagnostic tools. For simplicity, it is advantageous to consider the physical manifestations of left and right ventricular failure separately, recognizing that most patients the nurse will encounter are in the chronic congestive heart failure state. In some instances, particularly after myocardial infarction, the nurse is in the position to detect pure incipient left ventricular failure. The manifestations of either left or right ventricular failure may develop over a period of hours, days, weeks, or months, depending upon the form of the underlying cardiac pathology. Generally the outstanding clinical manifestations of heart failure are due to diminished blood flow to tissues and congestion of fluid in tissues, which significantly limits cellular function. Although all tissues are affected when the heart fails, the effects on the vital organs are the most serious.

The clinical manifestations of left ventricular failure are primarily pulmonary in origin. This is due to the resulting engorgement of the pulmonary capillaries as the blood attempting to leave the pulmonary circulation encounters resistance in the left cardiac chambers from residual blood. With engorgement of the pulmonary capillaries, there is mechanical congestion of the lungs, and an increase in the pulmonary capillary hydrostatic pressure, which causes fluid transudation from the capillaries to the interstitial spaces and perhaps into the alveoli. The pulmonary manifestations noted are dyspnea on exertion and at rest, orthopnea, paroxysmal nocturnal dyspnea, Cheyne-Stokes respirations, and pulmonary edema.

In the early stages of left ventricular failure, one of the most outstanding clinical manifestations is dyspnea. Like pain, dyspnea is a subjective phenomenon. The individual becomes aware of his or her breathing and may describe it as "shortness-of-breath." Initially, the individual may be relatively free of dyspnea at rest and experience it only during physical activity or a period of emotional excitement. Dyspnea may be minimal in the morning hours and gradually increase toward evening. It is usually characterized by rapid, shallow respirations. Apprehension usually accompanies dyspnea, because interference with respiration is perceived as a threat to survival. As the disease process progresses, dyspnea may be present at rest. The mechanisms suggested to explain dyspnea in the heart failure patient are (1) decreased lung compliance because of the mechanical congestion of the lungs, with a decreased vital capacity and decreased effective ventilating surface; (2) increased carbon dioxide and decreased oxygen tension of the arterial blood, which stimulate chemoreceptors and thus the medulla to increase respirations; and (3) decreased cardiac output and thus arterial systolic pressure, which stimulates pressoreceptors and thus the medulla to increase respirations. The dyspnea is made worse by concomitant conditions that reduce the vital capacity or ventilating surface of the lungs, such as pleural effusion, pulmonary emboli, and ascites. Assessment of dyspnea is frequently in terms of its occurrence during exertion, dyspnea on exertion (DOE), and if so, what kind of activity precipitates the dyspnea. That which

[15] Normally the diastolic pressure in the left ventricle at the end of systole is 0 mm Hg, because most of the blood has been ejected. With residual blood in the ventricular chamber, the pressure can rise to 25 to 30 mm Hg. This is known as increased left ventricular "end-diastolic" pressure.

is seen frequently on patient charts is in terms of how many flights of stairs, or how many steps, cause shortness of breath (SOB). It is of even greater importance to note if dyspnea occurs at rest.

Dyspnea that occurs when the individual assumes the recumbent position is known as *orthopnea.* The mechanism that produces orthopnea is related to the increased venous return to the right heart that accompanies recumbency. The competent right ventricle pumps the increased venous blood to the pulmonary capillary bed, but because of the residual blood in the left heart chambers, the blood largely remains in the congested pulmonary circuit. Dyspnea ensues, and rales may be present. Orthopnea can often be relieved by elevating the trunk in relation to the rest of the body. When the individual assumes the upright position, venous return is impeded and more of the blood accumulates in the abdomen and lower extremities, thus lessening the congestion. The abdominal organs are pulled down away from the diaphragm, and the vital capacity increases. Assessment of orthopnea is frequently in terms of how many pillows are required to prevent orthopnea, hence the terms *two-pillow orthopnea* or *three-pillow orthopnea.*

Another form of dyspnea experienced by the patient in left ventricular failure is known as *paroxysmal nocturnal dyspnea* (PND), or "cardiac asthma." PND is respiratory distress that occurs after the individual has been sleeping for 1 to 2 hours. The person is awakened from sleep, may be ashen in color and perspire profusely, and is usually extremely apprehensive. Expiratory wheezes may be present because there is often some bronchial constriction, hence the term *cardiac asthma.* The upright position may cause the attack to abate. The explanation given for PND is that although the individual may fall asleep on one or two pillows, during deep sleep the recumbent position occurs, and blood accumulates in the lungs as with orthopnea. Although the attack of PND may abate, its presence is a sign of overt left ventricular failure, and immediate intervention is required. PND may not abate and instead may herald the onset of pulmonary edema.

Pulmonary edema is the severest form of pulmonary capillary congestion and left ventricular failure whereby there is a transudation of fluid from the capillaries to the interstitial spaces surrounding the alveoli. As the process intensifies, transudation of fluid into the alveoli per se results. This process is associated with hypoxia, hypercapnea, and intense dyspnea. The patient gasps for breath and may rip off an oxygen mask because it is too confining. The individual frequently seeks fresh, outdoor air. This writer recalls three specific patients who exemplify the extreme hunger for fresh air. One man in pulmonary edema walked down three flights of stairs from his apartment to the parking lot to get the "good" air. Another patient was found trying to open a window in the coronary care unit for the outside air. In a third situation, the low rate alarm signaled on a cardiac monitor and the nurses noted a straight line on the oscilloscope indicating ventricular standstill. Upon approaching the patient's bed, they found it empty, and the patient was seen wandering down the hall. The patient's explanation was a need to go outside in order to breathe.

Associated with the intense dyspnea of pulmonary edema is extreme anxiety bordering on the panic stage, cyanosis, diaphoresis, and tachycardia. The individual may experience chest pain, which is due to the stretching of alveoli in the congested lungs, and angina associated with the markedly diminished cardiac output. Cough with frothy pink-tinged sputum often accompanies pulmonary edema. The frothiness of the sputum is due to the mixing of the pulmonary edema fluid with air. The pink-tinged color is due to the escape of erythrocytes into the alveoli from the congested capillaries. Frankly bloody sputum, however, is rarely associated with pulmonary edema, and may indicate pulmonary infarction. The degree of pulmonary edema is frequently so excessive that the patient's noisy, gurgly respirations can be heard without a stethoscope. The amount of pulmonary fluid can also be so excessive that it may pour from the patient's nose and mouth, and the patient literally drowns in his or her own secretions. The need for intervention prior to this point is obvious. *Cheyne-Stokes respirations* usually accompany significant pulmonary congestion in acute left ventricular failure.

In addition to the pulmonary manifestations of left ventricular failure, certain cardiovascular signs may be present. Three kinds of abnormal heart sounds are noted. These are a ventricular gallop (S_3) occurring in early diastole, an atrial gallop (S_4) occurring in late diastole, and a summation gallop (both S_3 and S_1) occurring simultaneously because of tachycardia. Pulsus alternans, one strong beat and one weak beat, may occur. This is attributed to alternating initial ventricular fiber lengths and contractility. The point of maximal impulse (PMI) is usually displaced inferolaterally because of cardiac enlargement.

Other symptoms of left ventricular failure are due to hypoperfusion of cells consequent to the diminished cardiac output. One common symptom seen by physicians in private practice is fatigue, or lack of energy, resulting from decreased perfusion of skeletal muscle cells. Cerebral dysfunction is also noted in varying degrees not only because of hypoperfusion but because of increased blood carbon dioxide levels as well.

The clinical manifestations of right ventricular failure are primarily congestive in origin, that is, associated with tissue edema. In right ventricular failure the venous blood returning to the right side of the heart meets increased resistance in the right ventricle or atrium because of residual blood in those chambers. As a result, the pressure in the venous bed increases. With an increased hydrostatic pressure at the capillary level, fluid transudation occurs into the interstitial spaces, causing tissue edema. Although right ventricular failure is most frequently secondary to left ventricular failure, it may occur secondary to another process. The second most common cause of right ventricular failure is chronic obstructive lung disease. This type of right heart failure is known as cor pulmonale. Whether the right ventricular failure is secondary to left ventricular failure or a primary lung disease, the common manifestations are edema, hepatomegaly, ascites, distended cervical veins, oliguria, gastrointestinal disturbances, pleural effusion, and pericardial effusion.

The classic manifestation of right ventricular failure is *edema.* In the early stages of right ventricular failure, the principal evidence of edema may be a weight gain. A gain of 5 per cent or more of the patient's original weight in a short period of time is significant of fluid retention. One patient this writer recalls gained 16 pounds in a 24-hour period and presented with frank pulmonary edema to a hospital emergency room. Before pitting edema occurs, an individual can be expected to store 10 to 20 pounds (5 to 10 liters) of fluid. Usually by the time an individual has overt dyspnea at rest, 20 to 30 pounds (10 to 15 liters) of fluid have been retained. The edema is usually noted in the dependent parts of the body—the feet, ankles, and pretibial region—hence the term *pedal edema.*

In the earlier stages of right ventricular failure, the patient may experience the swelling in the feet and ankles only in the evening and then find that it subsides during sleep. As the right ventricular failure progresses, the patient notes that the ankles swell during the day and that his or her shoes are tight. After sleep the swelling disappears, because of even distribution in the subcutaneous tissue as well as some transudation of the fluid back into the venous system. With further progression of the process, the edema is continuous. The patient complains of a feeling of "heaviness" in the legs, but not of pain. In the patient confined to bed, the edema may be localized in the sacral region and genitalia, and may be overlooked unless the body parts are closely scrutinized. In patients with hemiplegia, the edema is most conspicuous on the paralyzed side, because of loss of autonomic nervous system control to the vessels. When edema is severe, the skin becomes tightly stretched and shiny in appearance. The tissues are poorly perfused because of the marked tissue congestion and thus are predisposed to decubiti, and cellulitis may result from infection. Special care to the skin with regular turning schedules must be implemented for the patient in bed. The orthopneic patient may be resistant to moving and turning.

Generalized edema of the body (anasarca) may mask a serious state of undernourishment. Edema and undernutrition commonly accompany chronic illness, whatever the cause. When the patient responds to therapy, the true state of nutrition becomes evident. It is not uncommon for these patients to appear to be nothing more than "skin and bones" following the removal of edema fluid. In some patients, improvement of their nutritional status may require intravenous amino acid–protein solutions to increase the plasma osmotic pressure before efforts to relieve the edema are successful.

Hepatomegaly, or congestion of the liver, and mild abdominal discomfort accompany right ventricular failure. As the volume of venous blood in the hepatic sinusoids increases because of the elevated venous pressure in the inferior vena cava and portal veins, liver engorgement occurs, particularly in the vicinity of the central hepatic veins. The arterial blood supply to hepatic cells is diminished and necrosis of hepatic cells can occur. Hepatomegaly may also be accompanied by jaundice. Assessment of the degree of liver engorgement is done in terms of how many finger breadths the liver is below the right costal margin of the ribs. Normally the liver is tucked under the right rib cage, with perhaps only the tip palpable. Therefore the liver, which is three to four finger breadths below the right costal margin (3 to 4 fb.↓RCM), is significantly edematous. If the right ventricular failure is so marked as to be associated with functional tricuspid insufficiency, the liver may pulsate with each ventricular contraction because of venous reflux. Manual pressure over the liver can then cause the cervical neck veins to distend abruptly. This maneuver is known as the hepatojugular reflux (H–J reflux), and is indicative of marked right heart distension. When acute swelling of the liver occurs during rapidly developing right ventricular failure, the liver is apt to be tender from the sudden stretching of the liver capsule. The pain is usually a constant ache but may be severe enough to suggest an acute abdomen or right lower lobe pulmonary infarction. With chronic right ventricular failure, extensive fibrosis of hepatic cells may occur, which is known as cardiac cirrhosis. *Hypoglycemia* may also occur, caused by inadequate storage of glycogen in the liver and increased breakdown of glucose to lactic acid in the presence of hepatic anoxia.

Associated with congestion of the venous system is distention of the cervical (jugular) veins. Pulsations of the neck veins may also be noted with each ventricular contraction if functional tricuspid insufficiency is present. Assessment of *cervical-jugular vein distention* (CVD–JVD) is done with the patient in at least a 45° upright position. This is because distention normally occurs in a recumbent position.

Effusion of fluid from the inferior vena cava and portal veins into the abdominal cavity results in *ascites,* which is usually a later development of right ventricular failure. Ascites usually produces no subjective symptoms other than an increase in the abdominal girth. The individual may note the abdominal distention and experience tightness with the waistband of articles of clothing. Assessment of the ascites is accomplished by daily or weekly measurement of the abdominal girth.

Whereas some degree of oliguria is evident with left ventricular failure caused by diminished renal perfusion, it is more striking in right ventricular failure because renal perfusion is further diminished when the pressure in the venous system is elevated. As the right ventricular failure is treated and subsides, urinary output is noted to increase. *Anorexia, nausea,* and *vomiting* are commonly associated with right ventricular failure. The patient frequently complains of "indigestion." Several mechanisms have been identified to explain these gastrointestinal disturbances. The heart and gastrointestinal tract are both supplied by branches of the vagus nerve. It is felt that reflexes arising in one organ may affect the function of the other through reflex pathways. Congestion of the abdominal viscera also contribute to the gastrointestinal dysfunction. In advanced right ventricular failure, cerebral metabolism may be sufficiently disturbed to cause reflex vomiting. These symptoms could also be related to digitalis toxicity.

In advanced stages of right ventricular failure, fluid may accumulate in the pleura, a condition known as a *pleural effusion* (hydrothorax), and in the pericardial sac, known as a *pericardial effusion* (hydropericardium). The mechanism by which this occurs is uncertain, although explanations thus far center on the transudation of fluid from capillaries because of the elevated venous pressure. The problems associated with these effusions are further exacerbation of dyspnea caused by lung compression and further diminishment of cardiac contractility due to cardiac compression. Rapid intervention in these circumstances may be necessary.

Assessment of the chronic congestive heart failure state thus becomes a recognition that the manifestations of both right and left ventricular failure are present. Whereas the congestion of the circulation is readily recognized, the chronicity of the congestion has not been satisfactorily explained. It appears to be more than just the progression of decreased ventricular contractility. The theory proposed to explain the chronic fluid retention has a hormonal basis, and could be schematically represented as in Figure 44-18.

It will be noted that congestive heart failure is an irreversible process and that the therapies utilized are directed to intervene in the above cycle. The best hopes to date are palliation of the process in the absence of cure. Eventually *intractable heart failure* will occur that is unresponsive to all forms of therapy. It is unclear as to whether intractable heart failure and cardiogenic shock are different clinical entities or the same phenomenon. Both phenomena are a terminal event in the largest percentage of patients.

In practice the nurse will encounter more patients with congestive than with single-chamber failure because of the chronicity of the problem. Patients in congestive heart failure offer few diagnostic problems, whereas early diagnosis of impending single-chamber failure is more difficult. It is also more crucial because a therapeutic regimen must be initiated to protect the heart from further injury. In any type of heart failure, the history and clinical assessment are important. The patient, however, sometimes fails to give the physician all pertinent data. In actual practice, the nurse is an important case finder of congestive and single-chamber failure and must work concertedly with patients to seek early and continued medical care.

A few specific tests will facilitate the assessment process for heart failure. In the case of congestive heart failure, various diagnostic tools may merely confirm the clinical findings. Some, however, may be useful in the early detection of incipient left ventricular failure. The assessment tools that frequently are employed include the chest x-ray; electrocardiogram; venous and/or pulmonary capillary pressure readings; and certain blood analyses.

The importance of the chest x-ray in the early detection of left ventricular failure cannot be overemphasized. From x-ray or fluoroscopy of the heart, data can be obtained about the size and position of the heart and great vessels. Of greater importance, however, is the x-ray's ability to detect the early signs of pulmonary congestion, which will be present long before initial signs of cardiac enlargement. Further, the chest x-ray can detect pulmonary congestion in the earliest stages, that is, congestion of the pulmonary veins, which occurs long before interstitial or alveolar edema. Congestion of the pul-

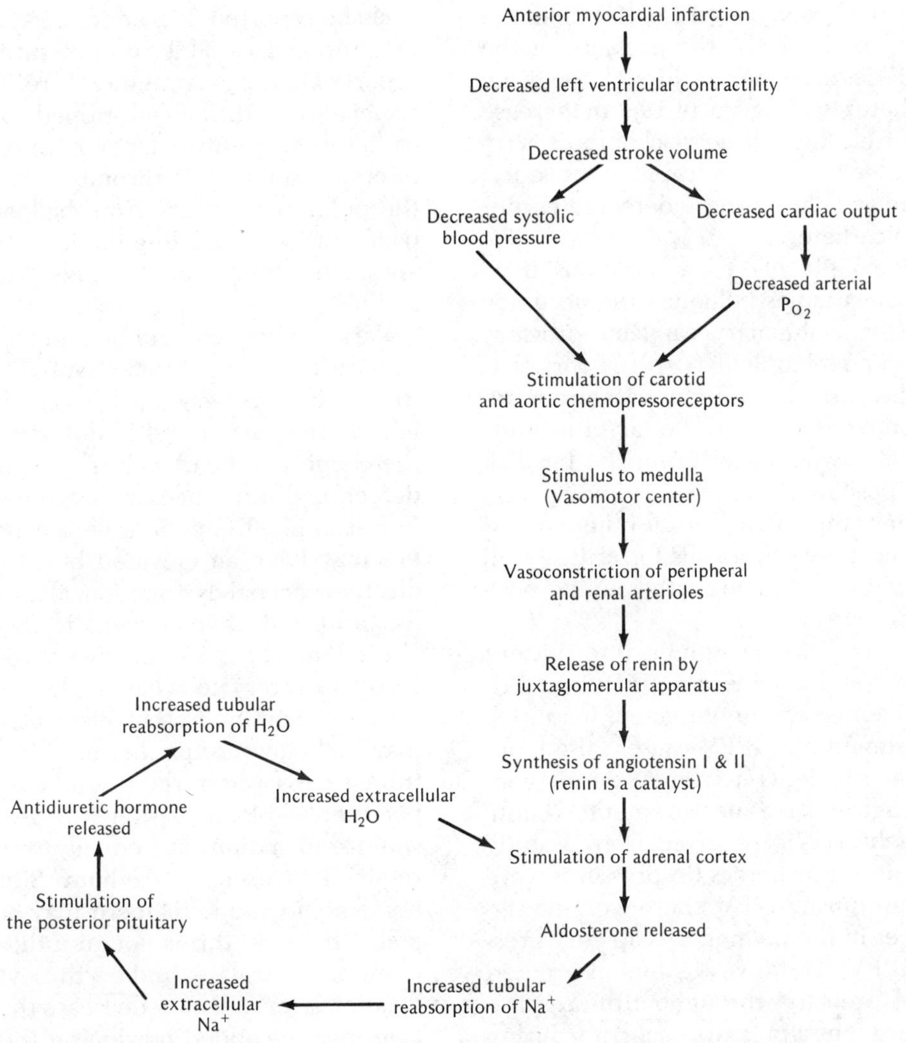

Figure 44-18. Proposed factors leading to chronic fluid retention in congestive heart failure.

monary veins produces no clinical symptoms. It is not until some degree of alveolar edema occurs that rales are even detectable. The advantages of the chest x-ray thus become obvious. It is small wonder that a daily chest x-ray is taken as a routine procedure with select myocardial infarction patients in many coronary care units across the nation.

The electrocardiogram's use in heart failure is related primarily to detection of chamber hypertrophy and arrhythmias associated with heart failure. The electrocardiogram has little use in the early detection of heart failure other than to help to identify cardiac conditions that predispose to heart failure.

For a considerable period of time central venous pressure (CVP) catheters were inserted in patients with myocardial infarction to detect heart failure and to gauge the effectiveness of therapy once initiated. Over the past several years, however, there has been an increasing disenchantment with the CVP as a diagnostic tool. One reason is the many complications associated with the catheters.[16] Perhaps of greater import is the fact that the venous pressure readings are reflective of pressures in the right heart when data about left ventricular function are what is needed. Central venous pressure recordings are therefore of little use in the early detection of left ventricular failure.

The method more commonly employed for early detection of left ventricular failure is introduction of an inflatable balloon-tipped catheter via the left subclavian vein, with subsequent manipulation to the left or right main branch of the pulmonary artery, for measurement of the pulmonary artery and

[16] Complications associated with central venous pressure catheters arise from (1) the insertion process, such as pneumothorax with a subclavian vein insertion site; (2) the presence of a foreign body, such as phlebitis, thromboembolic phenomenon, local and systemic infection, and broken catheter fragments lodged in the heart or lungs; and (3) mechanical problems giving false readings, such as with a blocked or malpositioned catheter.

pulmonary capillary "wedge" pressure. When the balloon is inflated periodically, the pressure in the pulmonary capillaries is measured through the distal lumen of the catheter (see Figure 44-19). An increase in back pressure from the left heart chambers is reflected in an increased pulmonary capillary pressure; thus, left ventricular failure can be detected earlier than with a CVP catheter.

Over the past couple of years, questions have arisen about what variables influence the accuracy of pulmonary artery-pulmonary capillary pressure readings. Woods and Mansfield (1976) report that with regard to the variable *position*, pressure readings in the pulmonary artery can be taken in *non–critically ill* persons without lowering the head of the bed to a flat position. Whereas this finding may raise more questions than it answers, it is hoped that the same or similar answer prevails for critically ill persons who become distressed in the supine position.

Similarly, the effect of concomitant intermittent positive pressure ventilator therapy (IPPV) on PA-PCAP pressure readings was investigated. Inasmuch as it has been assumed that IPPV causes false readings, in most settings patients are removed from ventilators long enough to take measurements. Shinn, Woods, and Huseby (1979) reported from a study of eighteen patients that whereas PA pressures were significantly higher during IPPV, there were no significant differences in the pulmonary capillary pressures on or off IPPV. The investigators also noted fluctuations in PA pressures throughout the respiratory cycle with the highest pressure occurring during peak inspiration. Thus, it is recommended that a mean pressure reading over an entire respiratory

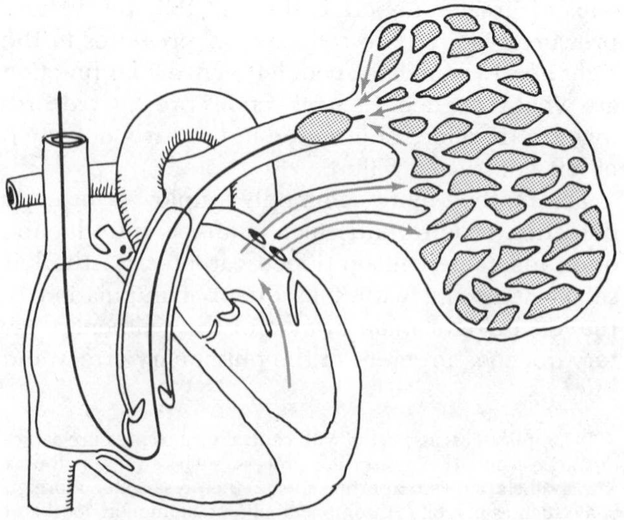

Figure 44-19. Measurement of the pulmonary capillary "wedge" pressure.

cycle be reported. It is anticipated that the influence of additional variables on pressure readings will be reported in the current literature. The complications associated with balloon-tipped pulmonary artery catheters are ventricular arrhythmias, pulmonary infarction, pulmonary thromboembolism, rupture of the pulmonary artery from balloon overdistension, balloon rupture leading to air embolism, infections, and catheter knotting (Nichols, Nichols, & Barbour, 1979).

Various chemical and hematologic analyses of the congestive heart failure patient's blood may be done. Although these blood analyses cannot diagnose heart failure, they are useful in determining the effect of the congestive heart failure on other organs and in detecting disturbances in electrolyte concentrations. For example, the patient with congestive heart failure may have an elevated blood urea nitrogen indicative of renal dysfunction, altered albumin-globulin ratio indicative of hepatic dysfunction, and/or altered blood gases indicative of respiratory involvement. Contrary to what might be anticipated, the serum sodium and other electrolyte concentrations may be below normal because of a dilutional factor from excess water retention. The level of sodium per unit of blood plasma will depend on whether water and sodium are equally retained or water is retained in excess of sodium. Similarly, the blood hemoglobin and hematocrit may be lower than normal. Obviously this is not an indication for replacement of electrolytes and erythrocytes; rather the indication is for means to decrease the water retention. Consider the added burden on the heart should intravenous sodium solutions be given to raise the serum sodium concentrations! Once a significant amount of fluid is removed, the electrolyte and hematologic concentrations will return toward normal levels.

INTERVENTION IN HEART FAILURE. Intervention with the patient in heart failure depends on the degree and suddenness with which the heart fails and the underlying causative cardiac pathology. The therapy is thus dual, directed not only to the failure process but to the predisposing cardiac disease as well. The *primary objective of therapy* in all instances of heart failure is to *increase the capacity of the heart to adapt or respond as efficiently as possible to the demands made on it.* The specific goals to be attained with intervention for the improvement of cardiac efficiency are to (1) increase the strength of cardiac contraction, (2) decrease sodium and water retention, (3) improve tissue oxygenation, (4) decrease the oxygen needs of the heart, and (5) control cardiac arrhythmias. All therapies are usually carried out simultaneously to meet these goals. After the efficiency of the heart has been restored or improved, the reserve power of the heart will need to be evaluated and plans made with the patient and family as to any necessary modifications in living and working habits.

The primary means by which the strength of cardiac contraction is increased is with the use of *digitalis* preparations. Although digitalis has been given to patients for almost 200 years, the precise mechanism by which it achieves the desired effect is still unknown. Two theories purported to explain its effects are (1) the active principle of digitalis in the form of a glycoside interacts in the excitation–contraction coupling mechanism and (2) that digitalis lines the cell membrane extracellularly and delays spontaneous depolarization of cells by slowing the rate of sodium influx and potassium efflux. Regardless of the mechanism by which digitalis preparations act, the effects noted are increased contractility and decreased conductivity of myocardial cells. As a result of the increased contractility, the ventricles empty more completely and the residual blood in the chambers at the end of systole is markedly diminished. This results in a reduction in the size of the heart, which is readily noted on chest x-ray. The increase in stroke volume increases the cardiac output. Consequent to an increased cardiac output, the aortic and carotid pressoreceptors are stimulated, which when relayed to the medulla, result in vagal inhibition of the heart. The ability of digitalis thus to slow the speeding of the failing heart further increases cardiac output, and is of particular value in the patient with atrial fibrillation. As a result of an increased cardiac output, the following clinical effects are noted: (1) decreased heart rate and pulse deficit, (2) increased urinary output, (3) decreased edema formation, (4) decreased cervical vein and liver engorgement, (5) decreased pulmonary congestion and dyspnea, and (6) decreased cyanosis and restlessness.

The particular preparation of digitalis initially employed in the treatment of heart failure depends on the acuity of the patient's clinical state and the physician's personal preference. On rare occasions a therapeutic blood level of digitalis must be achieved rapidly in which case an intravenous preparation may be used. The two most popular intravenous preparations are ouabain and lanatoside C (Cedilanid), primarily because of the rapidity with which a therapeutic effect is noted. Oral preparations will act more slowly, of course, and digoxin has emerged as the most popular preparation. The process by which a therapeutic blood level is reached with digitalis preparations is called digitalization. What this means is that the digitalis preparation that is chosen for use is administered in divided doses until the therapeutic blood level is reached. The initial dosage is the largest, and then the remaining administrations are given at equal time intervals in decreasing increments. Maintenance of the therapeutic blood level is achieved with daily "maintenance" doses. For example, if digoxin were to be used for oral digitalization, the initial dose may be 1 mg to be followed by two 0.5-mg doses at 12-hour intervals, and then two 0.25-mg doses at 12-hour intervals. The daily maintenance dose of 0.25 mg is then implemented. The entire digitalization process thus takes between 24 and 48 hours. The digitalization process is done in this way because digitalis is absorbed by the gastrointestinal tract more rapidly than it is degraded by the liver and excreted from the body by the kidneys. If not administered cautiously, the drug can thus tend to accumulate in the body.

Among the responsibilities of the nurse in the care of patients under digitalis therapy is the administration of the drug at the prescribed times and in the prescribed quantities. The observation of the desired and adverse effects of the drug on the patient is of even greater importance as well as the possible deletion of the dosage on the basis of pertinent observations. There is a very fine line between a dosage that is therapeutic and one that is toxic. A patient may vary from time to time in susceptibility to digitalis. In part this is dependent upon liver and kidney function as influenced by the status of the heart failure. It will be recalled that digitalis is largely degraded by the liver and excreted by the kidneys. Susceptibility to digitalis is also markedly influenced by the level of serum potassium. Hypokalemia and digitalis toxicity are documented to go hand in hand, and it is a rare heart failure patient who is not on diuretics, one of the prime causes of hypokalemia.

Few descriptions of the effects of digitalis have improved on that stated by William Withering who first introduced the drug around the time of the American Revolution. Withering urged that digitalis "be continued until it either acts on the kidneys, the stomach, the pulse, or the bowels; let it be stopped upon the first appearance of any of these effects." In current usage, there is great concern that an epidemic of digitalis toxicity exists in our society. The nurse therefore must be acutely aware of the signs of digitalis intoxication and the mechanisms by which the toxic effects occur. In the past, both in the nursing literature and in practice, great emphasis has been placed on a pulse rate over 60 beats per minute as an absolute criterion for the administration of digitalis preparations. There has been a tendency to neglect other and more significant observations of the pulse relative to developing toxicity.

Digitalis toxicity causes virtually every known cardiac arrhythmia, but generally all fall into the two major categories of the ventricular ectopic rhythms and the AV node conduction defects. The first cardiac manifestation is most frequently the occurrence of premature ventricular contractions commonly in a bigeminal pattern. This is because digitalis, particularly in the presence of hypokalemia, increases the excitability of cells. The PVCs can progress to ventricular tachycardia and ventricular fibrillation. As digitalis accumulates in the body, it also increases the refractoriness of the AV node to atrial impulses. Thus delay at the AV node can progress to complete heart block no matter what the supraventricular mechanism, that is, a patient in atrial fibrillation can develop complete heart block as well as one in normal sinus rhythm. A classic cardiac manifestation of digitalis intoxication is paroxysmal atrial tachycardia with some of the impulses blocked at the AV node.

The nurse must watch for *changes* in the cardiac rate or rhythm, and instruct the patient similarly. Although an electrocardiogram must be taken to identify the specific arrhythmia present, there are certain patterns for which to watch. Guidelines about the pulse that can be used are (1) a change from a regular to an irregular rhythm; (2) a change from an irregular to a regular rhythm; (3) sudden development of a bradycardia or a tachycardia; (4) premature beats which increase in frequency, and (5) runs of tachycardia in an otherwise slow or normal pulse. The reader is referred to an article by Arbeit, Fiedler, Landau, and Rubin (1977) for a detailed presentation on cardiac arrhythmias associated with digitalis toxicity.

Extracardiac symptoms of digitalis toxicity may precede or accompany cardiac manifestations. The first and more common signs of toxicity are gastrointestinal symptoms—anorexia, nausea, and vomiting, developing in that order. By the time vomiting occurs, toxicity is already significant because it indicates that the drug has accumulated to the point that the central nervous system vomiting mechanism has been stimulated. Diarrhea is not common, but when it does occur, the problem of hypokalemia is compounded by additional potassium loss. Even later signs of digitalis toxicity are disturbances in the central nervous system including (1) color visual disturbances such as a yellow-green vision or the presence of white borders around objects, (2) drowsiness that can progress to disorientation and convulsions ("digitalis madness"), and (3) facial neuralgia.

Serum digitalis levels may be utilized in conjunction with the clinical symptoms to verify the presence of digitalis toxicity. Radioimmunoassay methods have been developed to measure the drug content, both free and protein-bound, in the serum. In most patients with clinically apparent toxicity, the serum digitalis level tends to be two to three times higher than normal. It is not uncommon, however, for patients *without* clinical symptoms to have elevated serum digitalis levels. Similarly, there are several factors related to the testing procedure that can render the results invalid and/or unreliable. Thus, there is no single serum digitalis level that can absolutely predict or exclude digitalis toxicity (Kumpuris, Raizner, & Luchi, 1979, p. 713).

Under such seemingly ambiguous circumstances, one might wonder about the real utility of serum digitalis concentrations. It should be noted that the test is used to verify toxicity in the patient with suspicious clinical symptoms. Kumpuris et al. (1979) also cite, as indications for serum digitalis level analyses, (1) suspicion of digitalis toxicity with inability to obtain an adequate or coherent history, (2) absence of the expected digitalis effect despite adequate drug dosage, (3) sudden change in the patient's clinical condition, (4) nonresponse to therapy which exceeds commonly used schedules (p. 714). Interpretation of results relative to other phenomena is the key to the real utility of serum digitalis assays.

The safety of the patient often depends on the accuracy of the nurse's observations on the effects of the digitalis as administered, and on the teaching the nurse does with the patient to recognize and deal with the early signs of toxicity. The patient who takes digitalis will more than likely take it for the remainder of his or her life. As in other situations where the patient and family are responsible for continued treatment, the patient needs to know the what, how, when, and why of the therapy. The patient should know the name of the digitalis preparation used, how much should be taken, when it should be taken, why it is needed, and what signs to watch for that might indicate digitalis toxicity. The patient should notify the physician if any signs of toxicity are present. The patient should be able to take his or her pulse. It should be remembered that the emphasis, however, is not on absolute pulse values but on significant changes in rate and rhythm.

The community health nurse is probably more aware than any other nurse that patients do not comply with medical regimens for a variety of reasons. Such is the case with digitalis administration, and considerable reinforcement of prior patient teaching is required. To illustrate this type of situation, consider this example. A 77-year-old male patient adjusted his dosage of digitalis according to how he felt. When he felt well, he omitted it. When he had a bad day, he took an extra tablet or two. The reasons for the behavior were not explored, but superficially it may relate to the fact that many people judge the state of their health by how they feel. In other words, medicines are to be taken when a person does not feel well. Because the effects of omitting a dose or two of digitalis are not felt immediately, some time may elapse before the patient feels sick. By that time, the patient may be in serious trouble because the heart failure has been exacerbated.

To prevent the possibility of digitalis-induced arrhythmias, particularly in patients receiving diuretics, potassium chloride supplements are frequently administered. In the acute care settings, potassium chloride may be added to the patient's intravenous infusion. In this situation the nurse must initiate actions to ensure that the rate of fluid flow is within established guidelines to prevent death-producing arrhythmias that may result from the too rapid administration of potassium chloride. The infusion site must also be watched for the development of a phlebitis because potassium chloride is very irritating to vessel walls. Potassium chloride supplements are also available for oral administration in liquid form. They often must be administered with food or another liquid as the irritation of the gastric mucosa they produce may create nausea and an unpleasant metallic aftertaste. Enteric-coated potassium chloride tablets are infrequently used these days because of the frequency with which bowel ulceration and strictures have been noted. Patients should be instructed to supplement their diet with foods that are high in potassium. Contrary to popular opinion, orange juice and bananas are not the richest sources of potassium and more can be accomplished with certain meats and poultry, such as veal and chicken, a daily serving of potatoes, raisins, and so on. It would appear that orange juice and bananas are palatable to the largest majority of patients, hence the popularity of these fruit sources. Should digitalis dosage modification and potassium supplementation not prove satisfactory to diminish or abate digitalis toxicity, more aggressive therapy may be initiated with phenytoin (Dilantin), lidocaine, propranolol, or atropine depending on the arrhythmia present. In some instances a temporary transvenous pacemaker may be used to override the underlying arrhythmia until such time as other forms of therapy are effective.

The *second major goal* of intervention with the heart failure process is *to decrease the amount of sodium and water that is retained* in the body and that places an additional workload on the heart. The means by which this can be accomplished is to (1) remove the sodium and water from the body mainly by use of potent diuretics and in rare instances by phlebotomy or dialysis; (2) prevent additional accumulations of sodium and water by restricting the sodium and water intake; and/or (3) contain the excess body water in a localized area by the application of rotating tourniquets.

Diuretics are widely used in the therapy of heart failure to increase the elimination of sodium and water as well as to increase the effectiveness of digitalis on the heart by decreasing the circulating blood volume. It will be recalled that digitalis has a pseudodiuretic effect inasmuch as it improves the circulation to the kidneys and thereby improves urinary output. The diuretics used in the treatment of heart failure are primarily those that interfere with the reabsorption of sodium and water in the renal tubules. In the past the mercurial diuretics were used for this purpose. Today use of the mercurial diuretics is generally limited to patients with massive edema or those who fail to respond to newer diuretics.

The potent diuretics in greatest use are furosemide (Lasix) and ethacrynic acid (Edecrin). Lasix and Edecrin are available in intravenous preparations for use with the heart failure patient in acute distress whereby it is essential to mobilize as much excess fluid as possible from the body in a short period of time. Edecrin produces its desired effect in much the same fashion as Lasix by interfering with the renal tubular reabsorption of sodium. Because of the rapidity with which a profound diuresis is produced with the intravenous agents, potassium depletion can cause serious cardiac arrhythmias. This problem is frequently anticipated, and intravenous potassium chloride given simultaneously. In the less acute situation, oral preparations of Lasix and Diuril are frequently employed. Some physicians will suggest that the patient weigh himself or herself daily and take a prescribed amount of a diuretic if 3 to 5 pounds are gained within a 24-hour period. Such a rapid weight gain is reflective of recent fluid retention. In other situations, the physician will prescribe a daily maintenance dose of a diuretic.

The nurse has the usual responsibilities when administering drugs with a diuretic effect. Both the patient's weight and urinary output should be measured and recorded daily. Particularly pertinent to nurses working with patients in outpatient clinics and in the home is the assessment of patients for signs and symptoms of fluid retention and electrolyte imbalance.

Another means by which excess sodium and water can be removed from the body is by means of a phlebotomy. When a patient has acute pulmonary edema, the blood volume and consequently pulmonary engorgement can be reduced by venesection with the removal of 400 to 500 ml of blood. As may be expected, the patient may require reassurance that the removal of blood is therapeutic in this instance. In some situations the removed blood may be saved, centrifuged, and the packed red blood cells readministered to the patient later should the erythrocyte count indicate this to be necessary. As one might have already surmised, the use of phlebotomy as a therapeutic tool has virtually been eliminated with the current availability of rapid-acting intravenous diuretic agents.

Peritoneal or hemodialysis may also be used as a means to eliminate excessive amounts of sodium and water from the body. (See Chapter 41 for discussion of dialysis.)

In addition to measures utilized to facilitate the excretion of sodium, the prevention of additional accumulation is attempted with the administration of a low-sodium diet. Whereas in prior years the sodium intake was often restricted to 500 to 750 mg per day in acute and nonacute situations, it has generally been recognized that such limitations are too restrictive, promote patient noncompliance, and perhaps are unnecessary in view of the sodium depletion that can occur with the newer more potent diuretics.[17] For these reasons it is not uncommon to see the minimum sodium restricted diet as 1.0 to 1.5 g per day for the majority of heart failure patients. Even in this situation, careful meal planning and food selection are necessary. Once again the nurse can be exceptionally helpful to the patient and responsible family members with hints about food preparation and selection, such as (1) because foods cannot be cooked in salt, the flavor of various foods can be enhanced with a myriad of herbs; (2) baking powders used for bread and cakes are available with a potassium base, as are salt substitutes; (3) label reading is essential in the selection of foods, and anything that contains the words *salt, sodium, monosodium,* or *soda* should be avoided; (4) most preprepared convenience and frozen foods use sodium as a preservative and should be avoided; and (5) the one night-on-the-town restaurant to be avoided is the Chinese restaurant, which uses large amounts of monosodium glutamate in food preparation. If a more severe sodium restriction is necessary, such as 250 to 500 mg per day, then consideration may need to be given to the quantity of sodium used in various medications as a preservative and in the city drinking water.[18] Whatever the sodium restriction, the use of commonly purchased agents for "indigestion" is to be discouraged because of the high sodium concentration.[19]

At one time water intake was markedly restricted for the heart failure patient. Presently the trend is toward moderate or no restriction. In the acute situation, a limitation of 1,200 to 2,000 ml of fluid per 24 hours may be prescribed, which includes all fluids "hidden" in solid foods. For this reason a minimum of 700 to 800 ml per day is required by the dietary staff to provide the patient with well-balanced, nutritious meals. Whatever amount of fluid is left after dietary requirements have been determined should be reasonably distributed over a 24-hour period by the nursing staff.

In addition to removing sodium and water from the body and preventing additional accumulations, it may be necessary to contain the body water in the extremities of the patient with acute pulmonary edema. This is accomplished by the application of rotating tourniquets. The application of three tourniquets high on the extremities will temporarily reduce the volume of circulating blood by approximately 1,500 ml. The containment of the fluid will decrease the volume of blood returning to the pulmonary circulation and thereby minimize the degree of pulmonary congestion and consequent edema formation. Two types of rotating tourniquets can be used, the hand-applied rubber tubing tourniquets and the automatic rotating tourniquet machine, which utilizes blood pressure cuffs. In few instances are the hand-applied tourniquets required these days because of the increased availability of the automatic devices. The disadvantages of the hand-applied tourniquets greatly outweigh the advantages. For example, the rubber tubing is frequently applied too tightly, with the result that the tissues distal to the tourniquet are deprived of arterial blood and become ischemic. Further, the three rubber tourniquets must be rotated every 5 minutes in a rather complicated clockwise fashion, which requires someone to be with the patient at all times for just that purpose. When used correctly, however, the hand-applied rotating tourniquets can have the same therapeutic effect as the automatic rotating tourniquet machine. Although it is seemingly an antiquated procedure, nurses should be familiar with the principles of hand-applied tourniquets should an emergency situation be encountered. The image of a community health nurse packing an automatic rotating tourniquet machine on his or her back seems ludicrous, but some nurses have had to use women's hosiery as hand-applied tourniquets in the home situation.

When the automatic rotating tourniquet machine is used, blood pressure cuffs are usually applied to three extremities and attached to the machine. The arm with the intravenous cannula remains free. The fourth blood pressure cuff should, however, be wrapped around a bath towel and left in the circuit for the entire apparatus to work efficiently. The machine is designed so that when turned on, each cuff

[17] It should be recalled that the average sodium intake in a normal adult is between 5 and 10 g per day.

[18] Information about the sodium content in various medications is available through clinical pharmacies and drug companies. Information about the sodium content in local drinking water usually is available from city and county departments of health.

[19] The sodium content of common antacids are Alka-Seltzer 532 mg per tablet; Bromo-Seltzer, 480 mg per teaspoon; and Rolaids, 53 mg per tablet.

will inflate at 10- to 15-minute intervals until three cuffs are inflated simultaneously. The machine then rotates the pressure in the cuffs every 10 to 15 minutes so that three cuffs are always inflated, including the cuff not on the patient. With this pattern, a cuff is on each extremity 30 to 45 minutes and then is released for 10 to 15 minutes. The machine is also designed to allow control of the pressure within the cuff so that the tourniquet pressure can be adjusted just above the diastolic blood pressure. The pulses in the arteries distal to the tourniquets should be palpated regularly to be sure that arterial blood is gaining access to the extremity. Similarly, the patient's blood pressure should be checked every 1 to 2 hours to determine (1) if the reduction of circulating blood is predisposing to shock and (2) if the pressure in the cuffs needs readjustment.

When the tourniquets are discontinued, they should be removed one at a time at 10- to 15-minute intervals. The simultaneous release of three tourniquets would permit entry of a large amount of fluid back into the circulation, which could readily cause a recurrence of pulmonary congestion. Similarly, the nurse must read the instruction manual with the machine and know what the cuff deflation pattern is should the electrical supply to the machine be interrupted. With some machines, all cuffs will deflate simultaneously should the cord be pulled out of the electrical outlet, whereas others will deflate gradually, one at a time. Following the removal of tourniquets, the patient may demonstrate some transient hyperpnea because of the release of carbon dioxide into the general circulation from the contained venous blood. The duration of rotating tourniquet use with a patient is generally a period of hours in that diuretics and digitalis are usually employed simultaneously, removing fluid from the body and promoting symptomatic relief.

A *third major goal* in the intervention with the heart failure patient is directed toward *improved oxygenation of the tissues.* The previous therapies directed at increasing the efficiency of the heart and eliminating excess fluid from the body will do much to improve tissue perfusion. With the addition of some form of oxygen therapy, the quality of blood circulated to all tissues can be improved. This is of obvious benefit to the heart muscle. In the patient with acute pulmonary edema, the preferred form of oxygen therapy is intermittent positive pressure breathing with a controlled concentration of oxygen. The use of high concentrations of oxygen may be unwise in this situation, as with the chronic obstructive lung disease patient, if the patient is both hypercapnic and hypoxic. The use of the positive pressure breathing apparatus is desirable to force oxygen and edema fluid across the alveolar-capillary membrane. In the less acutely ill patient, oxygen administration by nasal cannula may be used.

In the chronic congestive heart failure patient with pleural effusion or ascites, elimination of the accumulated fluid will promote expansion of the lungs and greater oxygen intake. This may necessitate the performance of a thoracentesis or paracentesis. Unless the state of failure is controlled, however, the fluid will recur.

The *fourth major goal* of therapeutic intervention is to *decrease the oxygen needs of the heart.* This is accomplished primarily by initiating means to promote physical and emotional rest for the patient. The objective toward which rest is directed is to reduce the need for the heart to adapt to varying volumes of venous return. In general the dorsal recumbent position is the most restful for people with a normal cardiovascular system. The dorsal recumbent position has a serious disadvantage, however, for the patient in, or in danger of, heart failure. When the recumbent position is assumed, fluid in tissues below the level of the heart returns to the vessels and increases the blood volume. This, in turn, increases the quantity of blood returned to the heart and with it the need to increase the cardiac output. Should the output of the right ventricle exceed that of the left, the result is pulmonary congestion.

The most advantageous position for the heart failure patient is the semi-Fowler's or Fowler's position. Although it would appear that this position would expend more energy than the recumbent, breathing is facilitated and thus less energy is expended in this act. Further, if the patient's arms are supported by pillows, there is less strain on the shoulder muscles, and the upright position can demand as little energy expenditure as the recumbent position. The primary objective in selecting a position for the patient is what is most comfortable for him or her. Many a heart failure patient will be found sitting up in bed leaning forward to facilitate breathing just as with the chronic obstructive lung disease patient. An overbed table may be placed so that the patient can rest on it while leaning forward.

The congestive heart failure patient may actually be more comfortable sitting in a chair. As mentioned earlier when discussing rest for the myocardial infarction patient, chair rest has many physiologic and psychological advantages but is not a generally accepted practice. In some hospitals the "cardiac bed" is available, which is designed so that the bed can be converted to a chair. The head of the bed becomes the back of the chair, the center becomes the seat, and the foot of the bed is dropped so that the lower legs and feet hang down. A footboard provides support for the feet, and an overbed table and pillows support the arms. The patient's position can then be varied without the need to transfer the patient between bed and chair.

With whatever position is assumed by the patient, the need for turning is present. Most patients on bedrest need to be taught how to turn properly. Human nature leads the patient to take in a breath, hold it, grab onto the side rail, and pull himself or herself over. The patient is thus performing a Valsalva maneuver comparable to straining at stool. It is known that the Valsalva maneuver places an additional burden on the heart and can precipitate or exacerbate heart failure. The patient should be taught to *exhale* and turn over rather than to inhale and turn.

Every effort should be made to increase the patient's level of activity within his or her level of physiologic tolerance. Continued bedrest has other adverse effects on circulatory function. After a few days in the recumbent or semirecumbent position, the capacity to adapt circulation to the erect position is limited. In the healthy person a change from the prone to the upright position is accompanied by peripheral vasoconstriction and a slight rise in blood pressure. These changes protect the brain from an inadequate blood supply as a consequence of the effect of gravity on the blood in vessels below the heart. In the person who has been inactive in bed for a period of time, assumption of the upright position is accompanied by orthostatic hypotension, tachycardia, and possible syncope. The usual explanation for these symptoms is an inadequate cardiac output resulting from an inadequate venous return secondary to lost muscle and venous tone in the legs. Thus for any patient on bedrest, the upright position is assumed gradually, to prevent fainting. First the head of the bed is raised. After the patient has had an opportunity to adapt to this position he or she can shift the legs over the edge of the bed and "dangle." During this time the patient should be encouraged to flex and extend the ankles and swing the legs back and forth. At this time his or her pulse should be checked. If there is a marked tachycardia, this is a sign to go slow. Before finally assisting the patient to his or her feet, the nurse should be sure to have enough help to support the patient should it be needed. After the patient gains balance, he or she should be assisted to walk or be returned to bed. Unnecessary motionless standing should be avoided. Contraction of the muscles of the legs is essential to maintaining the venous return against gravity.

In addition to the wasting of muscle with the accompanying loss of nitrogen, bedrest and inactivity have other adverse effects. Calcium is absorbed from the bones and thereby predisposes to osteoporosis and renal lithiasis. Stasis of blood in the veins combined with chemical changes in the blood predisposes to thrombophlebitis. Gastrointestinal function is impaired. Few if any physiologic and metabolic functions escape adverse effects. Altered psychological functioning as well as mental depression is the rule. (See Chapter 49 for Disuse Syndromes.)

To decrease the oxygen demands of the heart, rest must be both physical and psychological. The anxious patient confined to bed may not only maintain a level of metabolic activity comparable to mild exercise but may also compound this with significant vasoconstriction, tachycardia, and cardiac irritability from circulating epinephrine. During acute pulmonary edema, this situation can be further compounded by the extreme apprehension associated with the inability to breathe. For these reasons morphine sulfate is usually prescribed to allay the apprehension and for its vagal effect. With a decrease in the heart rate, less blood is returned to the pulmonary circulation, and congestion diminishes with a consequent decrease in the degree of dyspnea. Peripheral vasoconstriction is diminished with improved tissue perfusion. After the acuity of the situation has diminished, small dosages of phenobarbital or diazepam (Valium) may be prescribed during the day, with morphine or a sedative prescribed at night to help the patient sleep. The nurse continues to have a major role in anxiety reduction with the heart failure patient.

Other ways to decrease the oxygen demands of the heart are control of energy wasting cardiac arrhythmias, such as atrial fibrillation, and the gastrointestinal symptoms commonly associated with congestive heart failure. An antiemetic agent, such as trimethobenzamide (Tigan), may be ordered for administration when nausea and vomiting require control.

Once the heart failure has been stabilized, the cardiac reserve or functional ability of the patient should be evaluated to determine limitations and strengths. Evaluation may be done in a work classification unit. The degree to which the functional capacity of the heart is impaired in heart failure and other cardiac diseases varies among individuals. Thus a standard therapeutic classification was developed by the Criteria Committee of the New York Heart Association to guide the physician in determining what activities are suited for the patient. Once classified, these therapeutic classes generally indicate what a patient can do, and activities are planned accordingly. The therapeutic classes are the following:

Class A. Patients with cardiac disease whose physical activity need not be restricted.

Class B. Patients with cardiac disease whose ordinary physical activity need not be restricted but who should be advised against severe or competitive physical sports.

Class C. Patients with cardiac disease whose ordinary physical activity should be moderately restricted and whose strenuous efforts should be discontinued.

Class D. Patients with cardiac disease whose ordinary physical activity should be markedly restricted.

Class E. Patients with cardiac disease who should be at complete rest, confined to bed or chair.

Whether or not a person with controlled heart failure will be able to perform a particular job depends on many factors in addition to the amount of energy it requires. These factors include the work experience, emotional state, status in the family, temperament, and dexterity. Many patients neither require nor desire any change in work. Many patients can continue in the same job, with modification in the way in which the work is approached or in the manner in which it is performed.

An example of the latter is the housewife who suffers from heart disease. Considerable work has been done by the American Heart Association to help the housewife with heart disease evaluate her methods of housekeeping and to plan her house and work so that unnecessary work is eliminated and the work she does is performed as easily as possible. In some communities, classes sponsored by the local heart association are taught for housewives. They and their husbands can learn how to evaluate and improve housekeeping methods.

Rehabilitation services are available to patients with heart disease through the Office of Vocational Rehabilitation or the American Heart Association. The first can usually be contacted through the state health department and the latter through the local heart association. At least as important as the rehabilitation of adults is that of children with heart disease. Career planning considering the limitations of the child is important. Emphasis on what the child may do is an essential aspect of helping him or her realize a productive life.

Exactly what each person who has heart disease will be able to do depends on him or her as an individual. The consensus at the present time is that many patients can do something worthwhile. Perhaps the greatest deterrent is fear and misinformation about the effects of exercise on the heart. The first step is to help each patient to develop a healthy and optimistic attitude. Most people in the American society want to be productive and want an opportunity to do something constructive. One of the standards by which they judge their productiveness is that they are economically self-supporting. The stress arising from continued inactivity and dependency may be as great as or greater than that involved in useful work.

Families also need help in interpreting both the patient's limitations and strengths. Nurses can often reinforce the recommendations of the physician and assist the patient and family members to make reasonably realistic plans. This is as important when the family tends to overprotect the patient as when they push him or her too hard. It is difficult to remember when the life of a loved one appears to be threatened "that there is a breadth to life as well as a length. There is no area in a straight line."

Cardiogenic Shock

Cardiogenic shock is a major, potentially lethal complication mainly associated with acute myocardial infarction. Ten to 15 per cent of patients with acute myocardial infarction will develop cardiogenic shock and of that group 80 to 85 per cent will die. Thus cardiogenic shock is the major cause of death in hospitalized acute myocardial infarctions and causes more deaths than cardiac arrhythmias.

The term *low* (cardiac) *output-low perfusion syndrome* perhaps better describes the cardiogenic shock state. It is a clinical syndrome characterized by (1) low systolic blood pressure with a narrow pulse pressure, (2) oliguria-anuria, (3) cold, clammy skin, and (4) confused sensorium. The etiology is unknown, and there is no single accepted therapeutic approach to treatment that helps to explain the high mortality associated with the syndrome. It has not been determined if cardiogenic shock is the end stage of severe heart failure or if they are two separate clinical entities. Data to date suggest that there is a high correlation between patients who develop heart failure and later cardiogenic shock, but in some instances the two processes appear to be mutually exclusive.

Research on the etiology of cardiogenic shock appears to indicate a biochemical origin. One interesting theory purports that as a result of diminished perfusion of the splanchnic circulation, proteolytic enzymes (proteases) are released primarily from the lysosomes of pancreatic cells. These proteases enter the general circulation and act on the plasma proteins to form an entirely new substance in the blood that acts on the weakened myocardium and depresses contractility. The substance is a peptide or glycopeptide and has been named the *myocardial depressant factor* (MDF) (Lefer, 1970, p. 1836). One interesting aspect of the research on MDF is that the process of MDF formation can be blocked by the administration of massive intravenous doses of steroid preparations (Lefer & Verrier, 1970, p. 647).

That the pathophysiologic mechanisms associated with cardiogenic shock are different from those of heart failure is evidenced by the fact that therapies directed toward heart failure are ineffective in the majority of cardiogenic shock patients. The generally accepted aims of therapy for cardiogenic shock are to (1) increase myocardial oxygenation while decreasing oxygen utilization, (2) decrease the metabolic acidosis associated with the shock state, (3) maintain a fuel source for myocardial metabolism, and (4) stimulate the strength of myocardial contraction.

Interventions directed toward increasing myocardial oxygenation are the traditional forms of oxygen therapy plus the experimental use of hyperbaric oxygenation. Oxygen utilization has been decreased by bedrest, analgesics, the control of arrhythmias, and the use of hypothermia. Treatment of metabolic acidosis has been with intravenous sodium bicarbonate solutions. Maintenance of a fuel source is accomplished with intravenous glucose solutions such as a 10 to 20 per cent solution in water to which regular insulin may be added for transport of the glucose across the cell membrane. Digitalis preparations have been used to increase the strength of myocardial contraction. For a period of time, intravenous infusions of glucagon were used to stimulate myocardial strength until warnings were issued that intravenous administrations could cause pulmonary embolism. Dopamine (Intorpin), a sympathomimetic amine, is being used extensively in the treatment of cardiogenic shock with greater positive response in comparison to other vasopressors. Dopamine increases cardiac output primarily by increasing stroke volume. It would appear, however, that there are "dopaminergic" receptors in the renal, mesenteric, and splanchnic beds that dilate in response to dopamine, thus increasing urinary output.

Intravenous administration of corticosteroid preparations such as Solu-Cortef and Solu-Medrol in dosages up to 3,000 to 4,000 mg have been used with some apparent success. Although vasoconstrictor agents such as levarterenol (Levophed) and metaraminol (Aramine) have been used extensively to increase the arterial blood pressure, their worth appears negligible in view of the fact that significant vasoconstriction is already present with the pathophysiologic process of cardiogenic shock.

Among the more vigorous therapies that have been tried with some limited success are circulatory-assist devices, coronary bypass procedures, infarctectomy, and cardiac replacement. The mechanical-assist device that is being used extensively in the treatment of cardiogenic shock is the intra-aortic balloon (IAB). The IAB is introduced into a femoral artery under local anesthesia and threaded retrograde to the descending thoracic aorta. The balloon catheter is positioned between the left subclavian artery and the renal arteries (see Figure 44-20). The balloon-catheter is connected to a console control unit which contains a cardiac monitor and inflation-deflation device. The R-wave of the cardiac complex initiates the inflation of the IAB during cardiac diastole thus increasing coronary and renal artery perfusion. The balloon deflates during systole. The result is an in-

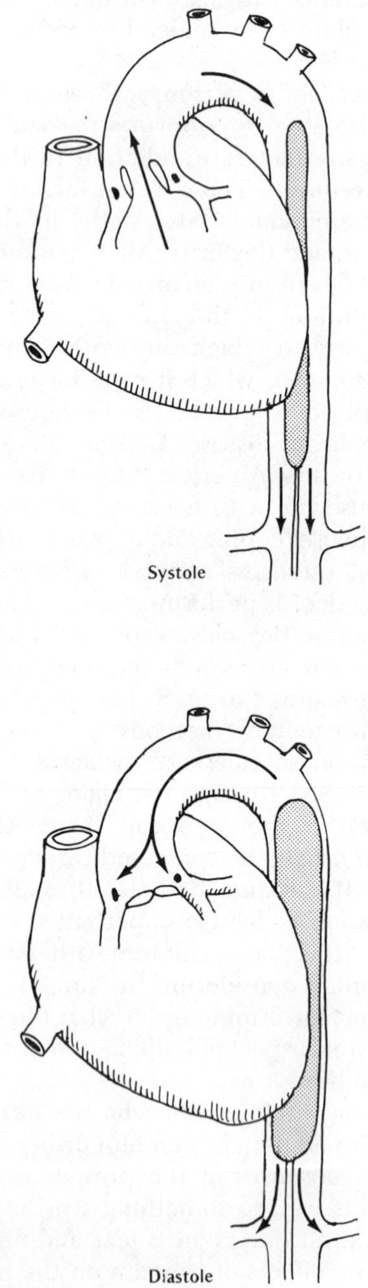

Figure 44-20. The intra-aortic balloon: During systole, the balloon is deflated. During diastole, the balloon is inflated promoting coronary artery perfusion. Note the position of the balloon above the level of the renal arteries and below the left subclavian artery.

creased oxygen supply and decreased oxygen demand with improved oxygenation of ischemic tissue and minimization of myocardial injury-infarction. The care of the patient with an IAB represents a challenge to the nurse.

Summary

In the preceding pages, the consequences of inadequacy or failure of the transport system have been presented with respect to the heart. Emphasis has been placed on the fact that cellular processes, and indeed life itself, cannot be sustained if failure of the transport system occurs. The professional nurse can play a significant role in the prevention of transport failure by application of the assessment-intervention process in all aspects of primary, acute, and long-term care.

References Cited

Adler, J. "Patient Assessment: Abnormalities of the Heartbeat." *Am. J. Nurs.*, **77**:4 (1977), 647–72.

Alexander, J. K., Fred, H. L., Wright, K. E., Turell, D. J., Jackson, R. A., and Jackson, D. "Exercise and Coronary Artery Disease." *Heart and Lung*, **7**:1 (1978), 141–44.

Alford, W. C., Burrus, G. R., Stoney, W. S., and Thomas, C. S., Jr. "The Spectrum of Ventricular Aneurysms." *Heart and Lung*, **2**:2 (1973), 211–17.

Arbeit, S. R., Fiedler, J. P., Landau, T. K., and Rubin, I. L. "Recognizing Digitalis Toxicity." *Am. J. Nurs.*, **77**:12 (1977), 1936–45.

Arlin, M. "Controversies in Nutrition: A Brief Review." *Nurs. Clin. North Am.*, **14**:2 (1979), 199–214.

Baker, K. G., and McCoy, P. L. "Group Sessions as a Method of Reducing Anxiety in Patients with Coronary Artery Disease." *Heart and Lung*, **8**:3 (1979), 525–29.

Barboriak, J. J., and Menahan, L. A. "Alcohol, Lipoproteins, and Coronary Artery Disease." *Heart and Lung*, **8**:4 (1979), 736–40.

Bogdonoff, M. "Psychological Impact of the Coronary Care Unit." in *Advanced Cardiac Nursing*. Philadelphia: Charles Press, 1970.

Brenton, M. *Sex and Your Heart*. New York: Coward-McCann, 1968.

Breu, C., and Dracup, K. "Helping the Spouses of Critically Ill Patients." *Am. J. Nurs.*, **78**:1 (1978), 50–53.

Brown, A. J. "Effect of Family Visits on the Blood Pressure and Heart Rate of Patients in the Coronary-Care Unit." *Heart and Lung*, **5**:2 (1976), 291–96.

Chatham, M. A. "The Effect of Family Involvement on Patients' Manifestations of Postcardiotomy Psychosis." *Heart and Lung*, **7**:6 (1978), 995–99.

Chobin, N., Kangos, J., and Miller, J. "From Project to Ongoing Program." *Am. J. Nurs.* **75**:9 (1975), 1491.

"Clinical Implications of Surgeon General's Report on Smoking and Health." *FDA Drug Bull.* **9**:1 (1979), 4–6.

Cobbs, B. W., Jr. "Clinical Recognition and Medical Management of Rheumatic Heart Disease and Other Acquired Valvular Disease." In *The Heart*, (2nd ed.), Ed. by J. W. Hurst and R. B. Logue. New York: McGraw-Hill, 1970.

Cole, C. M., Levin, E. M., Whitley, J. O., and Young, S. H. "Brief Sexual Counseling During Cardiac Rehabilitation." *Heart and Lung*, **8**:1 (1979), 124–29.

Coodley, E. L. "Prognostic Value of Enzymes in Myocardial Infarction." *JAMA*, **225**, (1973), 595–97.

Daniell, H. W. "Heparin in the Prevention of Infusion Phlebitis." *JAMA*, **226** (1973), 1317–21.

De Pasquale, N. D., and Bruno, M. S. "Prevention of Sudden Cardiac Death." *Heart and Lung*, **2**:6 (1973), 851–56.

DeVillier, B. "Preoperative Teaching of the Cardiovascular Patient." *Heart and Lung*, **2**:4 (1973), 522–25.

Diethrich, E. "Aortocoronary Bypass—Classification and Results." *Heart and Lung*, **4**:3 (1975), 381–89.

Edwards, J. "Protection of the Ischemic Myocardium." Paper presented at the American Heart Association Annual Scientific Sessions. Dallas, Texas, November 1972.

Ehrlick, I. "Patient Selection and Preoperative Evaluation." *Heart and Lung*, **4**:3 (1975), 373–80.

Ellis, R. "Unusual Sensory and Thought Disturbances after Cardiac Surgery." *Am. J. Nurs.*, **72**:11 (1972), 2021–25.

Enos, W. F. "Coronary Disease among United States Soldiers Killed in Action in Korea: Preliminary Report." *JAMA*, **152** (1953), 1090.

The Framingham Heart Study. Public Health Service Publication No. 1515. U.S. Department of Health, Education, and Welfare. Washington, D.C.: U.S. Government Printing Office, 1966.

Fredrickson, S. D., and Levy, R. I. "Familial Hyperlipoproteinemia." In *The Metabolic Basis of Inherited Disease*, 3rd ed. Ed. by J. B. Sanbury, J. B. Wyngaarden, and D. S. Fredrickson. New York: McGraw-Hill, 1972.

Friedberg, C. *Diseases of the Heart*, 3rd ed. Philadelphia: W. B. Saunders Co., 1966.

Friedman, M., and Rosenman, R. H. *Association of Specific Overt Behavior Patterns with Blood and Cardiovascular Findings—Type A Behavior and Your Heart*. Greenwich: Fawcett, 1974.

Furman, S. "Recent Developments in Cardiac Pacing." *Heart and Lung*, **7**:5 (1978), 813–26.

Gentry, W. D., et al. "Anxiety and Urinary Sodium/Potassium as Stress Indicators on Admission to a Coronary-Care Unit." *Heart and Lung*, **2**:6 (1973), 875–77.

Glasser, S. P., Clark, P. I., and Spoto, E. "Heart Rate Response to Fright Stress." *Heart and Lung*, **7**:6 (1978), 1006–09.

Goldstrom, D. "Cardiac Rest: Bed or Chair?" *Am. J. Nurs.*, **72**:10 (1972), 1812–16.

Gordon, E. A. "Use of Energy Costs in Regulating Physical Activity in Chronic Disease." *Arch. Indust. Health*, **16** (1957), 437.

Gotto, A. M., Nichols, B. L., Scott, L. W., Foreyt, J., and Jackson, R. A. "Obesity—Risk Factor No. 1." *Heart and Lung,* **7**:1, (1978), 132–40.

Graboys, T. B. "Clinical Pharmacology of Antiarrhythmic Agents." *Heart and Lung,* **8**:4 (1979), 706–10.

Gronin, S. S. "Helping the Client with Unstable Angina." *Am. J. Nurs.,* **78**:10 (1978), 1677–80.

Harken, D. E. "Postoperative Care Following Heart-Valve Surgery." *Heart and Lung,* **3**:6 (1974), 893–902.

Hellerstein, H. K., and Friedman, E. H. "Sexual Activity and the Post-coronary Patient." *Med. Asp. Hum. Sexual.,* **3**:3 (1969), 70–96.

Higgs, C. "Blood Gases and Myocardial Infarction." *Clin. Sci.,* **35** (1968), 115–22.

Hoffman, M., Donckers, S., and Hauser, M. "The Effect of Nursing Intervention on Stress Factors Perceived by Patients in a Coronary Care Unit." *Heart and Lung,* **7**:5 (1978), 804–9.

Johnston, B. L., Cantwell, J. D., Watt, E. W., and Fletcher, G. F. "Sexual Activity in Exercising Patients after Myocardial Infarction and Revascularization." *Heart and Lung,* **7**:6 (1978), 1026–31.

Julian, D. G. "Angina Pectoris." In *Cecil Textbook of Medicine,* Ed. by P. B. Beeson, W. McDermott, and J. B. Wyngaarden. 15th ed. Philadelphia: W. B. Saunders, 1979.

Killip, T., and Kimball, J. T. "A Survey of the Coronary Care Unit; Concept and Results." In *Acute Myocardial Infarction and Coronary Care Units.* Ed. by C. Friedberg. New York: Grune & Stratton, 1969.

Kumpuris, A. G., Raizner, A. E., and Luchi, R. J. "The Role of Serum Digitalis Levels in Clinical Practice." *Heart and Lung,* (1979), **8**:4 711–15.

Lavin, M. A. "Bed Exercises for Acute Cardiac Patients." *Am. J. Nurs.,* **73**:7 (1973), 1226–28.

Lawson, M. "Progressive Coronary Care." *Heart and Lung,* **1**:2 (1972), 240–52.

Lefer, A. M. "Role of a Myocardial Depressant Factor in the Pathogenesis of Circulatory Shock." *Fed. Proc.,* **29** (1970), 1836–47.

Lefer, A. M., and Verrier, R. "Role of Corticosteroids in the Treatment of Circulatory Collapse States." *Clin. Pharmacol. Ther.,* **11** (1970), 647–56.

Mallison, M. "Updating the Cholesterol Controversy: Verdict—Diet Does Count." *Am. J. Nurs.,* **78**:10 (1978), 1681.

Manley, M. V., and Graber, A. L. "Coronary Prevention in a Community Hospital." *Heart and Lung,* **6**:6 (1977), 1045–49.

McIntosh, H. D., Eknoyan, G., and Jackson, D. "Hypertension—A Potent Risk Factor." *Heart and Lung,* **7**:1 (1978), 137–40.

McIntosh, H. D., Entman, M. L., Evans, R. I., Martin, R. R., and Jackson, D. "Smoking as a Risk Factor." *Heart and Lung,* **7**:1 (1978), 145–52.

McIntosh, H. D., Stamler, J., and Jackson, D. "Introduction to Risk Factors in Coronary Artery Disease." *Heart and Lung,* **7**:1 (1978), 126–31.

Mechner, F. "Patient Assessment: Auscultation of the Heart. Part II (Programmed instruction)." *Am. J. Nurs.,* **77**:2 (1977), 275–98.

———. "Patient Assessment: Examination of the Heart and Great Vessels. Part I (Programmed instruction)." *Am. J. Nurs.,* **76**:11 (1976), 1807–30.

Meltzer, L. "Coronary Care, Electrocardiography, and the Nurse." *Am. J. Nurs.,* **65**:12 (1965), 63–67.

Merkel, R., and Brown, C. "Evaluating Feeding Activities in a CCU." *Am. J. Nurs.,* **70**:11 (1970), 2348–50.

Merrill, S. A., and Froelicher, V. F. "Exercise Testing." *Cardiov. Nurs.,* **13**:6 (1977), 23–28.

Meserko, V. "Preoperative Classes for Cardiac Patients." *Am. J. Nurs.,* **73**:4 (1973), 665–66.

Miller, P., and Shada, E. A. "Preoperative Information and Recovery of Open Heart Surgery Patients." *Heart and Lung,* **7**:3 (1978), 486–93.

Montoya, A., Mullet, J., Piffarre', R., Moran, J.˙M., and Sullivan, H. J. "The Advantages of Open Mitral Commissurotomy for Mitral Stenosis." *Chest.,* **75**:2 (1979), 131–35.

National Institute of Health. *The Dietary Management of Hyperlipoproteinemia: A Handbook for Physicians.* Bethesda, Md.: NIH, 1970, p. 16.

New Label Restrictions and Boxed Warning on Clofibrate." *FDA Drug Bull.,* **9**:3 (1979), 14–15.

Nichols, W. W., Nichols, M. A., and Barbour, H. "Complications Associated with Balloon-Tipped, Flow-Directed Catheters." *Heart and Lung,* **8**:3 (1979), 503–6.

Norris, R. M. "Prognosis in Myocardial Infarction." *Heart and Lung,* **4**:1 (1975), 74–80.

Prebil, K., and Diethrich, E. B. "Cardiac Surgery Using Blood Components without Whole Blood Transfusion." *Heart and Lung,* **3**:5 (1974), 804–7.

Puksta, N. S. "All About Sex . . . After a Coronary." *Am. J. Nurs.,* **77**:4 (1977), 602–5.

Robinson, P. H. "Pericarditis." *Med. Times.,* **107**:1 (1979), 73–78.

Romero, P. E. "Preoperative Teaching for Cardiovascular Surgical Patients." *Cardiovasc. Nurs.,* **14**:6 (1978), 27–32.

Scalzi, C. "Nursing Management of Behavioral Responses Following an Acute Myocardial Infarction." *Heart and Lung,* **2**:1 (1973), 62–69.

Scalzi, C., and Dracup, K. "Sexual Counseling of Coronary Patients." *Heart and Lung,* **7**:5 (1978), 840–45.

Scheer, E. "Enzymatic Changes and Myocardial Infarction: A Nursing Update." *Cardiovasc. Nurs.,* **14**:2 (1978), 5–8.

Schroeder, J. S. "The Prehospital Course of Patients with Chest Pain." *Am. J. Med.,* **64** (1978), 742–48.

Sellers, T. F. "Rheumatic Heart Disease and Other Acquired Valvular Disease." In *The Heart,* 2nd ed. Ed. by J. W. Hurst and R. B. Logue. New York: McGraw-Hill, 1970.

Shinn, J. A., Woods, S. L., and Huseby, J. S. "Effect of Intermittent Positive Pressure Ventilation upon Pulmonary Artery and Pulmonary Capillary Wedge Pressures in Acutely Ill Patients." *Heart and Lung,* **8**:2 (1979), 322–27.

Sokolow, M., and McIlroy, M. B. *Clinical Cardiology,* 2nd ed. Los Altos, Calif.: Lange Medical Publishers, 1979.

Spandau, M. "Insertion of Temporary Cardiac Pacemakers without Fluoroscopy." *Am. J. of Nurs.,* **70**:5 (1970), 1011–13.

Spann, J. F., Jr. "Recent Advances in the Understanding of Congestive Failure (I) and (II)." *Mod. Concepts Cardiovasc. Dis.,* **39**:1 (1970), 73–84.

Stamler, J., Hall, Y., Mojonnier, L., Berkson, D. M., Levinson, M., Lindberg, H. A., Andelman, S. L., Miller, W. A., and Burkey, F. "Coronary Proneness and Approaches to Preventing Heart Attacks." *Am. J. Nurs.,* **66**:8 (1966), 1788–93.

Strong, A. "Caring for Cardiac Catheterization Patients." *Nursing,* **7**:11 (1977), 60–64.

Williams, D. O., Amsterdam, E. A., DeMaria, A. N., Miller, R. R., and Mason, D. T. "Physical Activity in the Rehabilitation of Patients Following Myocardial Infarction. I. Basis of Early Ambulation." *Heart and Lung,* **5**:2 (1976), 317–21.

Winslow, E. H., and MacVaugh, H. III. "Coronary Artery Surgery." *Nurs. Clin. North Am.,* **11**:2 (1976), 371–83.

Woods, S. L., and Mansfield, L. W. "Effect of Body Position upon Pulmonary Artery and Pulmonary Capillary Wedge Pressures in Noncritically Ill Patients." *Heart and Lung,* **5**:1 (1976), 83–89.

General References

Aggressive Nursing Management of Acute Myocardial Infarction. Philadelphia: Charles Press, 1968.

Aranda, J. M., Befeler, B., Castellanos, A., Jr., and Sherif, N. E. "His Bundle Recordings: Their Contribution to the Understanding of Human Electrophysiology." *Heart and Lung,* **5**:6 (1976), 907–18.

Atkinson, A. J., and Nevin, M. J. "Antiarrhythmic Therapy with Procainamide." *Cardiovasc. Nurs.,* **13**:5 (1977), 17–22.

Bjerkelund, C. J. "Anticoagulant Therapy in Myocardial Infarction." *Heart and Lung,* **4**:1 (1975), 61–68.

Bolognini, V. "The Swan-Ganz Pulmonary Artery Catheter: Implications for Nursing." *Heart and Lung,* **3**:6 (1974), 976–81.

Bregman, D. "Management of Patients Undergoing Intraaortic Balloon Pumping." *Heart and Lung,* **3**:6 (1974), 916–28.

Bunke, B. "Respiratory Function after Acute Myocardial Infarction: Implications for Nursing." *Cardiovasc. Nurs.,* **9**:3 (1973), 13–18.

Cassem, N. H., and Hackett, T. P. "Psychological Rehabilitation of Myocardial Infarction Patients in the Acute Phase." *Heart and Lung,* **2**:3 (1973), 382–87.

Chow, R. K. *Cardiosurgical Nursing Care.* New York: Springer, 1976.

Chrzanowski, A. L. "Intra-aortic Balloon Pumping: Concepts and Patient Care." *Nurs. Clin. of North Am.,* **13**:3 (1978), 513–30.

Cogeman, M. M. "Effects of Oxygen on Ischemic Myocardium." *Heart and Lung,* **7**:4 (1978), 635–39.

Cogen, R. "Preventing Complications during Cardiac Catheterization." *Am. J. Nurs.,* **76**:3 (1976), 401–5.

Cohen, N. H., and Lemberg, L. "Cardiac Rehabilitation in the Coronary Care Unit. Part I." *Heart and Lung,* **7**:4 (1978), 667–70.

Cook, R. L. "Psychosocial Responses to Myocardial Infarction." *Heart and Lung,* **8**:1 (1979), 130–35.

DeBusk, R. F. "The Role of Ambulatory Monitoring in Postinfarction Patients." *Heart and Lung,* **4**:4 (1975), 555–61.

Diethrich, E. B. "Pre-infarction Syndrome—Surgical Indications." *Heart and Lung,* **4**:3 (1975), 390–96.

Eckhardt, E. "Intra-aortic Balloon Counterpulsation in Cardiogenic Shock." *Heart and Lung,* **6**:1 (1977), 93–98.

Edwards, M., and Payton, V. "Cardiac Catheterization Techniques and Teaching." *Nurs. Clin. North Am.,* **11**:2 (1976), 271–82.

Elsberry, N. L. "Psychological Response to Open Heart Surgery: A Review." *Nurs. Res.,* **21**:3 (1972), 220–27.

Engel, G. "Emotional Stress and Sudden Death." *Psychol. Today,* **11**:6 (1977), 114 ff.

Foster, S., and Andreoli, K. G. "Behavior Following Acute Myocardial Infarction." *Am. J. Nurs.,* **70**:11 (1970), 2344–48.

Foxworth, G. D. "Rehabilitation for Hospitalized Adults after Open Heart Procedures: The Team Approach." *Heart and Lung,* **7**:5 (1978), 834–39.

Frazee, S., and Nail, L. "New Challenge in Cardiac Nursing: The Intra-aortic Balloon." *Heart and Lung,* **2**:4 (1973), 526–32.

Friedewald, V. E., Jr. "Maximal-Stress, Multiple-Lead Exercise Testing: The Significance of ST-Segment Changes in the Detection of Coronary Arterial Occlusive Disease." *Heart and Lung,* **5**:1 (1976), 91–96.

Friedman, B. "Cardiac Surgery: Skilled Nursing during the Critical Post Operative Period." *Nursing,* **4**:12 (1974), 37–40.

Futral, J. E. "Postoperative Management and Complications of Coronary Artery Bypass Surgery." *Heart and Lung,* **6**:3 (1977), 477–86.

Grace, W. J., and Chadbourn, J. A. "The First Hour in Acute Myocardial Infarction." *Heart and Lung,* **3**:5 (1974), 736–41.

Green, H. L. "Hazards of Electronic Equipment in Critical Care Areas: A Research Approach." *Cardiovasc. Nurs.,* **9**:2 (1973), 7–12.

Griep, A. H., and DePaul, S. "Angina Pectoris." *Am. J. Nurs.,* **65**:6 (1965), 72–75.

Hahn, A., and Dolan, N. "After Coronary Care—Then What?" *Am. J. Nurs.,* **70**:11 (1970), 2350–52.

Hanchett, E. S., and Johnson, R. A. "Early Signs of Congestive Heart Failure." *Am. J. Nurs.,* **68**:7 (1968), 1456–61.

Hansen, M. S., Woods, S. L., and Wills, R. E. "Relative Effectiveness of Nitroglycerin Ointment According to Site of Application." *Heart and Lung,* **8**:4 (1979), 716–20.

Hart, L. K., and Frantz, R. A. "Characteristics of Postoperative Patient Education Programs for Open Heart Surgery Patients in the United States." *Heart and Lung,* **6**:1 (1977), 137–42.

Hathaway, R. "The Swan-Ganz Catheter: A Review." *Nurs. Clin. North Am.,* **13**:3 (1978), 389–407.

Heller, A. F. "Nursing the Patient with an Artificial Pacemaker." *Am. J. Nurs.,* **64**:4 (1964), 87–92.

Henrick, A., and Stephanides, L. "Common Diagnostic Uses of Echocardiography." *Cardiovasc. Nurs.,* **14**:5 (1978), 21–25.

Hirsch, A. T. "Postmyocardial Infarction Syndrome." *Am. J. Nurs.,* **79**:7 (1979), 1240–41.

Hiscoe, S. "The Awesome Decision." *Am. J. Nurs.,* **73**:2 (1973), 291–93.

Horovitz, J. H., and Luterman, A. "Postoperative Monitoring Following Critical Trauma." *Heart and Lung,* **4**:2 (1975), 269–79.

Houser, D. "Ice Water for MI Patients? Why Not?" *Am. J. Nurs.,* **76**:3 (1976), 432–34.

Hudak, C. M., Lohr, T., and Gallo, B. M., eds. *Critical Care Nursing,* 2nd ed. Philadelphia: J. D. Lippincott Co., 1977.

Hunn, V. "Cardiac Pacemakers." *Am. J. Nurs.,* **69**:4 (1969), 749–54.

Jahre, J. A., Grace, W. J., Greenbaum, D. M., and Sarg, M. J. "Medical Approach to the Hypotensive Patient and the Patient in Shock." *Heart and Lung,* **4**:4 (1975), 577–87.

Jillings, C. R. "Phases of Recovery from Open Heart Surgery." *Heart and Lung,* **7**:6 (1978), 987–94.

Johnston, B. L., Cantwell, J. D., and Fletcher, G. F. "Eight Steps to Inpatient Cardiac Rehabilitation: The Team Effort—Methodology and Preliminary Results." *Heart and Lung,* **5**:1 (1976), 97–111.

Kos, B., and Culbert, P. "Teaching Patients about Pacemakers." *Am. J. Nurs.,* **71**:3 (1971), 523–27.

Krone, R. J., Kleiger, R. E., and Oliver, G. C. "Treatment of Chronic Ventricular Arrhythmias." *Heart and Lung,* **6**:1 (1977), 68–78.

Kapoor, A. and Dang, N. S. "Reliance on Physical Signs in Acute Myocardial Infarction and Its Complications." *Heart and Lung,* **7**:6 (1978), 1020–25.

Kessro, B. "Peripheral Arterial Insufficiency Postoperative Nursing Care." *Nurs. Clin. North Am.,* **12**:1 (1977), 143–50.

King, O. M. *Care of the Cardiac Surgical Patient.* St. Louis: C. V. Mosby Co., 1975.

Kleiger, R. E., Martin, T. F., Miller, J. P., and Oliver, G. C. "Mortality of Myocardial Infarction Treated in the Coronary-Care Unit." *Heart and Lung,* **4**:2 (1975), 215–26.

Kleiger, R. E., and Wolff, G. "Indications and Contraindications for Cardioversion of Arrhythmias." *Heart and Lung,* **2**:4 (1973), 552–60.

Kones, R. J., and Benninger, G. W. "Digitalis Therapy after Acute Myocardial Infarction." *Heart and Lung,* **4**:1 (1975), 99–103.

Krone, R. J., and Kleiger, R. E. "Prevention and Treatment of Supraventricular Arrhythmias." *Heart and Lung,* **6**:1 (1977), 79–88.

Lantiegne, K. C., and Avetta, J. M. "A System for Maintaining Invasive Pressure Monitoring." *Heart and Lung,* **7**:4 (1978), 610–21.

Lewis, R. P. "Approach to Sudden Death Outside the Hospital." *Heart and Lung,* **2**:6 (1973), 862–65.

Luchi, R. J., Entman, M. L., Harrison, D. C., and Eknoyan, G. "Use of Cardioactive Drugs in Acute Myocardial Infarction." *Heart and Lung,* **5**:1 (1976), 44–61.

Manwaring, M. "What Patients Need to Know about Pacemakers." *Am. J. Nurs.,* **77**:5 (1977), 825–30.

Marriott, H. J. L., and Vogt, P. "Micturition Angina: A Case Report." *Heart and Lung,* **6**:3 (1977), 510–12.

Maschek, B. J. "Patient Education and the Prevention of Endocarditis." *Nurs. Clin. North Am.,* **11**:2 (1976), 319–27.

Mattea, J., and Mattea, E. "Lidocaine and Procainamide Toxicity during Treatment of Ventricular Arrhythmias." *Am. J. Nurs.,* **76**:9 (1976), 1429–31.

Mayer, G. G., and Kaelin, P. B. "Arrhythmias and Cardiac Output." *Am. J. Nurs.,* **72**:9 (1972), 1597–1600.

Mazzoleni, A. "Electrophysiologic Mechanisms of Sudden Death in Patients with Coronary Artery Disease." *Heart and Lung,* **2**:6 (1973), 841–46.

McAllister, R. G. "The Possible Role of Antiarrhythmic Drugs in the Prevention of Sudden Death." *Heart and Lung,* **2**:6 (1973) 857–60.

McCann, W. J., and Soares, D. M. "The Use of Intra-aortic Balloon Counterpulsation in the Management of Cardiogenic Shock." *Heart and Lung,* **4**:2 (1975), 211–14.

McNeal, G. J. "Tracing Arrhythmias." *Am. J. Nurs.,* **79**:1 (1979), 98–100.

———. "Twenty-four Hour Ambulatory Monitoring." *Nurs. Clin. North Am.,* **13**:3 (1978), 437–48.

Merkel, R., and Sovie, M. D. "Electrocution Hazards with Transvenous Pacemaker Electrodes." *Am. J. Nurs.,* **68**:12 (1968), 2560–63.

Meyer, R. M., and Latz, P. A. "What Open Heart Surgery Patients Want to Know." *Am. J. Nurs.,* **79**:9 (1979), 1558–62.

Moore, S. J. "Pericarditis after Acute Myocardial Infarction: Manifestations and Nursing Implications." *Heart and Lung,* **8**:3 (1979), 551–58.

Naggar, C. Z. "Ultrasound in Medical Diagnosis. Part I. Applications in Cardiology." *Heart and Lung,* **5**:6 (1976), 895–906.

"Nipride (Sodium Nitroprusside)." *Heart and Lung,* **3**:5 (1974), 716.

Palmer, E., and Griffith, E. W. "Effect of Activity during Bedmaking on Heart Rate and Blood Pressure." *Nurs. Res.,* **20**:1 (1971), 17–25.

Pego, R. F., and Luria, M. H. "Left Subclavian Vein Puncture for Insertion of Swan-Ganz Catheters." *Heart and Lung,* **8**:3 (1979), 507–10.

Phibbs, B. *The Cardiac Arrhythmias,* 3rd ed. St. Louis: C. V. Mosby Co., 1978.

Pitorak, E. "Open-ended Care for the Open Heart Patient." *Am. J. Nurs.,* **67**:7 (1967), 1452–57.

Pitorak, E., Hudak, C., Hanusz, P., and O'Gorek, J. *Nurse's Guide to Cardiac Surgery and Nursing Care.* New York: McGraw-Hill, 1969.

Preston, T. A. "The Use of Pacemaking for the Treatment of Acute Arrhythmias." *Heart and Lung,* **6**:2 (1977), 249–55.

Proctor, D., Fletcher, R. D., and Del Negro, A. A. "Temporary Cardiac Pacing." *Nurs. Clin. North Am.,* **13**:3 (1978), 409–22.

Rakocz, M. "The Thoughts and Feelings of Patients in the Waiting Period Prior to Cardiac Surgery: A Descriptive Study." *Heart and Lung,* **6**:2 (1977), 280–87.

Rankin, M. A. "Programmed Instruction as a Patient Teaching Tool: A Study of Myocardial Infarction Patients Receiving Warfarin." *Heart and Lung,* **8**:3 (1979), 511–16.

Rasmussen, S., and Corya, B. C. "The Diagnostic Attributes of Echocardiography in the Patient with Chest Pain or Pulmonary Edema." *Heart and Lung,* **6**:4 (1977), 660–70.

Romhilt, D., and Fowler, N. "Physical Signs in Acute Myocardial Infarction." *Heart and Lung,* **2**:1 (1973), 74–80.

Sandiford, D. M., Shumway, N. E., Stinson, E. B., and Reitz, B. "Cardiac Transplantation: Eight Years Experience." *Heart and Lung,* **5**:4 (1976), 566–70.

Schamroth, L., and Perlman, M. M. "The Electrocardiographic Manifestations of Hypothermia." *Heart and Lung,* **1**:2 (1972), 233–35.

Scher, A. M. "The Electrocardiogram." *Sci. Am.,* **205**:11 (1961), 132–41.

Schroeder, J. S., and Fitzgerald, J. W. "Indications and Techniques for Ambulatory Electrocardiogram Monitoring." *Heart and Lung,* **4**:4 (1975), 540–45.

Schwartz, L. P., and Brenner, Z. R. "Critical Care Transfer: Reducing Patient Stress Through Nursing Interventions." *Heart and Lung,* **8**:3 (1979), 540–46.

Sczekalla, R. M. "Stress Reactions of CCU Patients to Resuscitation Procedures on Other Patients." *Nurs. Res.,* **22**:1 (1973), 65–69.

Shilling, E. "Packmaker Evaluation Clinic." *Am. J. Nurs.,* **73**:10 (1973), 1710–14.

Sivarajan, E. S., Snýdsman, A., Smith, B., Irving, J. B., Mansfield, L. W., and Bruce, R. A. "Low-Level Treadmill Testing of 41 Patients with Acute Myocardial Infarction Prior to Discharge from the Hospital." *Heart and Lung,* **6**:6 (1977), 975–80.

Smith, R. N. Invasive Pressure Monitoring. *Am. J. Nurs.,* **78**:9 (1978), 1514–21.

Spence, M. I., and Lemberg, L. "Cardiac Pacemakers. I. Modalities of Pacing." *Heart and Lung,* **3**:5 (1974), 820–27.

———. "Cardiac Pacemakers. IV. Complications of Pacing." *Heart and Lung,* **4**:2 (1975), 286–95.

Stock, J. P., and Williams, D. O. *Diagnosis and Treatment of Cardiac Arrhythmias,* 3rd ed. London: Butterworth, 1974.

Surawicz, F. "Psychological Aspects of Sudden Death." *Heart and Lung,* **2**:6 (1973), 836–40.

Swan, J. T. "Coronary Bypass." *Am. J. Nurs.,* **75**:12 (1975), 2142–45.

Tanner, G. "Heart Failure in the MI Patient." *Am. J. Nurs.,* **77**:2 (1977), 230–34.

Thatcher, S. K., and Lemberg, L. "Exercise Stress Testing in the Patient with Coronary Artery Disease. Part 1." *Heart and Lung,* **7**:6 (1978), 1062–65.

Thornton, W. E., and Pray, B. J. "Ventricular Arrhythmia and Thioridazine: A Case Report." *Am. J. Nurs.,* **76**:2 (1976), 245–46.

Torrens, P. R., and Hanchett, E. S. "Public Health Nursing and the Congestive Heart Failure Patient." *Cardiovasc. Nurs.,* **3**:4 (1967), 15–18.

Vera, Z., Awan, N. A., Amsterdam, E. A., and Mason, D. T. "Cardiac Pacemakers: Indications and Complications." *Heart and Lung,* **4**:3 (1975), 444–51.

Vinsant, M. O., and Lemberg, L. "Arterial Blood Gases in the Coronary Care Unit. Part I." *Heart and Lung,* **6**:3 (1977), 526–31.

Vismara, L. A., Miller, R. R., DeMaria, A. N., Amsterdam, E. A., Vera, Z., and Mason, D. T. "The Treatment of Ventricular Arrhythmias: Evaluation of Standard Therapy and Recent Advances." *Heart and Lung,* **5**:3 (1976), 485–92.

Weinberg, S. L. "Observations on Ambulatory Electrocardiographic Monitoring in Clinical Practice." *Heart and Lung,* **4**:4 (1975), 546–54.

———. "Quinidine Syncope without Quinidine." *Heart and Lung,* **7**:5 (1978), 779–80.

Westfall, U. E. "Electrical and Mechanical Events in the Cardiac Cycle." *Am. J. Nurs.,* **76**:2 (1976), 231–35.

Whipple, G. H. *Acute Coronary Care.* Boston: Little, Brown, 1972.

Whitman, G. "Intra-aortic Balloon Pumping and Cardiac Mechanics: A Programmed Lesson." *Heart and Lung,* **7**:6 (1978), 1034–50.

Winkle, R. A., and Harrison, D. C. "Beta Blockers in the Treatment of Acute Arrhythmias." *Heart and Lung,* **6**:1 (1977), 62–67.

Winslow, E. H., and Powell, A. H. "Sick Sinus Syndrome." *Am. J. Nurs.,* **76**:8 (1976), 1262–65.

Woods, S. L. "Monitoring Pulmonary Artery Pressures," *Am. J. Nurs.,* **76**:11 (1976), 1765–71.

Young, L. E. "Nursing Interventions with Obese Cardiac Patients." *Nurs. Clin. North Am.,* **13**:3 (1978), 449–56.

Zalis, E., and Conover, M. *Understanding Electrocardiography: Physiologic and Interpretative Concepts,* 2nd ed. St. Louis: C. V. Mosby Co., 1976.

Zeluff, G. W., Pratt, C., and Jackson, D. "Sudden Death—How Can We Prevent It?" *Heart and Lung,* **8**:3 (1979), 568–74.

45

Problems Associated with Shock

We begin with some general considerations. The forces which give meaning to our perceptions of biology are so ramified and interrelated that the boundaries by which we isolate biological entities (cell, organ, organism, species, etc.) are boundaries of our patience, not boundaries on the relations. The more exacting we become, the more smeared these boundaries get. This is one of the most salient features of the biological world. MYERS, 1967

Overview

Shock illustrates more clearly than most disorders the intimate relationship of all parts of the body at all levels of organization. Shock may be initiated by any serious external or internal disorder or agent that impairs the ability to provide cells with required nutrients or interferes with their ability to utilize them. In a way, shock can be the result of a failure of any of the functions discussed in previous chapters. Thus this chapter serves to emphasize and to integrate some of the content presented earlier. As far back as the first extensive studies of shock (Crile, 1899) up to and including studies involving the Vietnam conflict, the understanding of shock has been documented and expanded. Animal experiments have added to the content. Each advance has led to further clarification until our knowledge encompassed all aspects of shock and its treatment.

The term *shock* was first used by a French writer to convey the idea of a violent impression, jolt, commotion, or blow. In 1895, Warren (Warren, 1895) called shock "a momentary pause in the act of death."

Because so much of the body involves itself in the shock syndrome, a definition was needed to include all forms of shock. Many investigators still stress the central role of inadequate tissue perfusion in the chain of events that lead to cellular hypoxia and finally to asphyxia. Wilson (1972) agrees that inadequate tissue perfusion is frequently an early event in hypovolemic and cardiogenic shock, but his findings in septic shock reveal that about two thirds of the patients have normal or high cardiac output. An all-inclusive definition, then, would be inadequate blood flow to vital organs or the inability of the body cell mass to metabolize nutrients normally (MacLean, 1977, p. 67).

Because cellular survival depends on a constant supply of oxygen and nutrients, as well as the removal of products of metabolism, the eventual effects of shock are on cellular metabolism. Whatever the initiating events, and whatever type of shock develops, the diagnosis of shock can usually be made if any two of the following are present (Wilson, 1972):

1. Systolic blood pressure less than 80 mm Hg
2. Urinary output less than 25 ml per hour
3. Metabolic acidosis (low bicarbonate; increased lactic acid)

This chapter was revised by Norma Peters Thomas, R.N., M.S., Visiting Lecturer, College of Nursing, Southeastern Massachusetts University, North Dartmouth, Massachusetts.

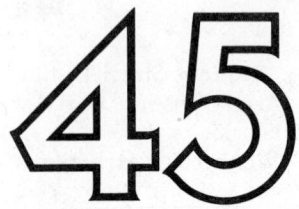

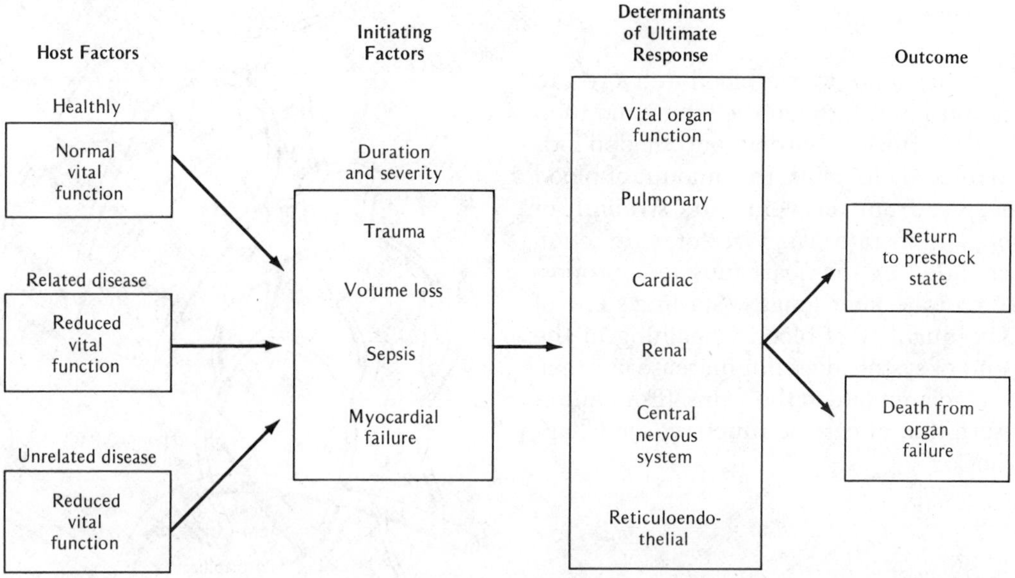

Figure 45-1. The natural history of shock and the factors determining survival. (Used with permission of Grune & Stratton, Inc., from *Prog. Cardiovasc. Dis.*, 1967, Vol. 9, p. 527, by A. P. Thal & J. M. Kinney.)

4. Poor tissue perfusion (cold, clammy skin; low cardiac output)

High-risk shock patients or patients in actual shock require highly sophisticated care. The nurse must understand the current concepts of prevention, cause, nature, effects, and treatment of shock.[1] As we learn to correct one aspect—circulatory and/or renal failure—other crises require further efforts, such as pulmonary failure. Of all forms of shock, the greatest success rate remains in the area of shock due to hemorrhage.

As with any body response to injury, host factors are important in determining the outcome of the treatment of shock. The natural history of shock and the factors determining survival are illustrated in Figure 45-1.

The Cardiovascular System and Shock Mechanisms

As a basis for understanding the pathophysiology of shock and the measures used in treatment, some understanding of the elements involved in tissue perfusion and cell metabolism is essential. The circulatory system is a closed circuit consisting of a pump (the heart), the blood, and a system of tubes or pipes carrying blood to and from the heart and the microcirculation. The components of the tubular system are (1) resistance vessels (arterioles), (2) exchange sites (capillaries), (3) shunts (vessels carrying blood directly from arterioles to venules), and (4) capacitance vessels (veins). Circulation is so regulated that the needs of all tissues are met.

Page (1967) summarizes some of the tasks involved in distributing blood to the tissues in the following:

> The body faces the difficult problem of distributing blood to tissues, each making its own special demands. Blood must be withdrawn from areas not in need of it. For example, the spleen and liver can act as reservoirs from which blood can be safely withdrawn during severe demand. The brain has a special controlling system to insure its supply in preference to less vital areas. To accomplish this constant redistribution of blood requires an elaborate system of sensing devices as well as the means. The complexity of this self-regulating system is almost unbelievable. Not only must it function efficiently, but it must continue to function if some of the control mechanisms are lost. The circulation does not depend on just one vital mechanism.

Four basic components are, therefore, essential to adequate blood circulation:

1. Pump action of the heart
2. Blood volume
3. Arterial resistance
4. Venous bed capacity

[1] This discussion is not intended to meet all the needs of nurses working in shock research units or in intensive-care units equipped with the latest monitoring and supportive devices. The references contain additional information. Because of the intense interest in this field, new papers will be published while this material is being printed.

The Heart as a Pump

The heart applies force to the blood delivered to it by the veins, pushes it through the lungs, and then drives it into the arteries. Cardiac output depends on three interrelated elements: the amount of blood the heart receives from the veins, the strength of its contraction, and its rate. The force of contraction or energy expended by the heart muscle is proportional to the diastolic fiber length (Starling's law of the heart). The quantity of blood remaining in the heart at the end of systole does not increase appreciably nor does it accumulate in the veins. (For a more complete description of cardiac function, see Chapter 44.)

Peripheral Resistance

Essentially, peripheral resistance is determined by the diameter of the blood vessels, particularly the arterioles. When there is no resistance to the flow of blood, the diastolic blood pressure falls to zero. To account for the ability to alter resistance, two types of receptors have been postulated, alpha and beta (Ahlquist, 1948). Alpha receptors in the arterioles respond to stimulation by catecholamines (epinephrine and norepinephrine from the sympathoadrenal system) and sympathomimetic agents by constriction. As the diameter of the arterioles diminishes, the resistance to the flow of blood increases. To overcome this resistance, the heart beats more forcefully, causing the arterial blood pressure to rise. As the blood pressure rises, stretch receptors in the aorta and carotid sinuses are stimulated. They initiate reflexes that can reduce cardiac output and cause the arterioles to dilate. Stimulation of beta receptors results in arteriolar dilatation (especially in skeletal muscles), decreased venous pooling, and an increase in the rate and force of the heartbeat. Through appropriate alterations in peripheral resistance, blood flow to a tissue or an organ can thus be increased or decreased according to the needs of that tissue relative to the rest of the body.

The Capillary Unit

The capillaries are the site of exchange of essential nutrients and cellular wastes between the blood and the tissues. The capillary unit, often called the microcirculation, consists of microscopic arterioles, metarterioles, precapillaries, true capillaries, collecting and distal venules, and small veins (Zweifach, 1959). (See Figure 45-2.)

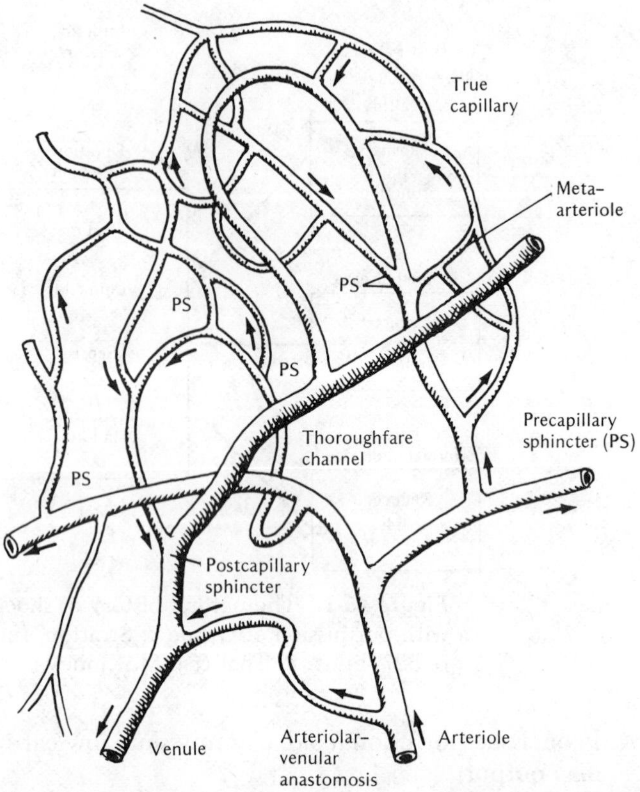

Figure 45-2. Basic scheme of microcirculation. (After an original drawing by Leola Hogan)

The movement of fluid between the capillary bed and the interstitial fluid space is regulated by the filtration pressure within the capillary and the colloid osmotic pressure in the plasma. Filtration pressure increases when the arterioles or precapillary sphincters relax and the venules or postcapillary sphincters constrict; this increased filtration pressure tends to drive fluid from the capillaries into the interstitial space. These vessels appear to be regulated not only by the factors affecting larger vessels, but also by locally produced chemical agents such as tissue metabolites, proteolytic by-products, enzymes, and polypeptides.

In health as well as in shock, blood can be shunted through thoroughfare channels without nourishing or removing materials from the tissues. This mechanism enables the body to shift blood rapidly to the most active and vital cells and organs. Although this ability to shift blood, especially to the heart and brain, may be of temporary advantage, if long-continued it can lead to damage of other important organs such as the kidney, liver, and gastrointestinal tract.

Capacitance Blood Vessels

The capacitance vessels, especially the larger veins, normally hold about 50 to 70 per cent of the blood volume. When veins constrict, the capacity of the vascular system may be greatly reduced. The veins are important in the return of blood to the right atrium. Depending on their degree of constriction they can rapidly return blood to the heart for distribution to the tissues or serve as a reservoir for blood. Unlike in the arteries the pressure within the veins is low. Factors affecting venous pressure are discussed subsequently.

Classification of Shock

In general, classifications of shock are based on either etiology or clinical manifestations. Based on the initiating conditions, shock can be classified as hypovolemic (caused by loss of fluid or blood), cardiogenic (caused by inadequate pumping by the heart), septic or endotoxic (caused by infection), or miscellaneous types (Thal & Wilson, 1965). However, traditional division of shock into such categories as hypovolemic, cardiogenic, or endotoxic is of little practical value, because regardless of the initiating causes, microcirculatory failure is the common factor that leads to death in advanced shock (Ravin & Modell, 1973). Cellular anoxia is indeed the common denominator for all shock states.

Shock Caused by Failure of the Heart as a Pump

Shock caused by the failure of the heart as a pump is characterized by an extremely low cardiac output. Some of the more common causes include myocardial infarction and arrhythmias in which the heart rate is excessively rapid, slow, or irregular. In these disorders, adequate tissue perfusion cannot be maintained because too little blood is forced into the arteries. Cardiogenic shock may also be caused by any disorder interfering with ventricular filling or emptying. Cardiac tamponade caused by excessive fluid or blood in the pericardial sac prevents blood from entering and filling the ventricles. A massive pulmonary embolism obstructs the flow of blood from the right ventricle. Unless the basic disorder is corrected, cardiogenic shock is self-perpetuating and the heart fails to perfuse not only other organs but also its own coronary vessels. Technically, a pump failure occurs.

Shock Caused by a Decrease in Venous Return

Failure of or a significant reduction in venous return to the heart results whenever the intravascular volume of blood fails to adequately fill the vascular capacity. This is usually caused by excessive loss of fluid or blood or decreased vasomotor tone. For a visual appreciation of the pathophysiologic basis of findings in early hypovolemic shock, see Figure 45-3.

Although hemorrhage is the classic example of hypovolemic shock, there are a variety of other causes. These include loss of gastrointestinal fluid from excessive vomiting or diarrhea, from excessive sweating, and through burned surfaces. An uncommon cause of hypovolemic shock is failure to replace the fluid loss from excessive urination. As an example of the latter, Mr. Compo experienced extreme diuresis following the removal of a benign brain tumor from the region of the pituitary gland. Edema and possible damage to the posterior hypophysis resulted in failure to release the antidiuretic hormone. Water lost in his urine was not replaced and as a result his blood volume fell to a point where his circulation could not be maintained. Mr. Compo went into profound shock from which he failed to recover. His life might have been saved had fluid replacement and the administration of ADH followed the observation that his urine output was greatly in excess of his fluid intake.

When the rate of fluid loss is slow, blood volume can be reduced by as much as 10 to 20 per cent without noticeable effects on tissue perfusion. Greater reductions, however, may result in sudden severe cardiovascular insufficiency. As blood volume diminishes, the quantity of blood returned to the heart and cardiac output are also reduced, although usually not by a proportionate amount.

Pooling of Blood

Besides low blood volume, any condition leading to pooling of blood in the capillary or venous circulation can lessen venous return to the heart. Loss of venous tone leads to venous pooling. Loss of arteriolar tone with continued venous constriction leads to capillary pooling. In the latter condition, capillary hydrostatic pressure rises, fluid escapes into the interstitial space, and the blood volume falls. In addition, stasis of blood in the capillary bed favors intravascular clotting that may further interfere with blood flow in the capillaries and venous return.

Hypovolemic Shock: Fundamental Considerations

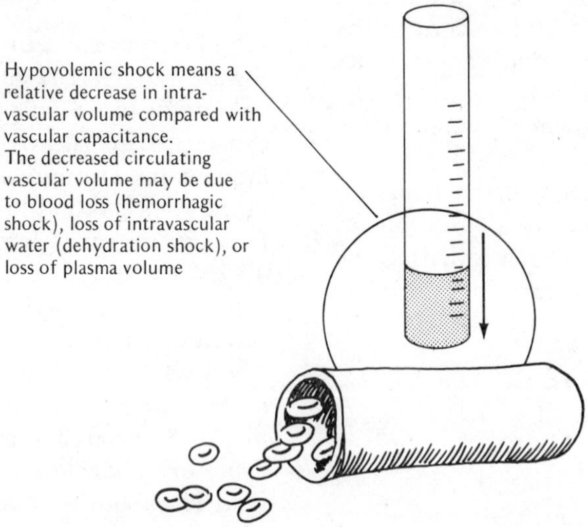

Hypovolemic shock means a relative decrease in intra-vascular volume compared with vascular capacitance.
The decreased circulating vascular volume may be due to blood loss (hemorrhagic shock), loss of intravascular water (dehydration shock), or loss of plasma volume

The Clinical Signs of Hypovolemic Shock, in its Severe Form, Are Easily Recognized

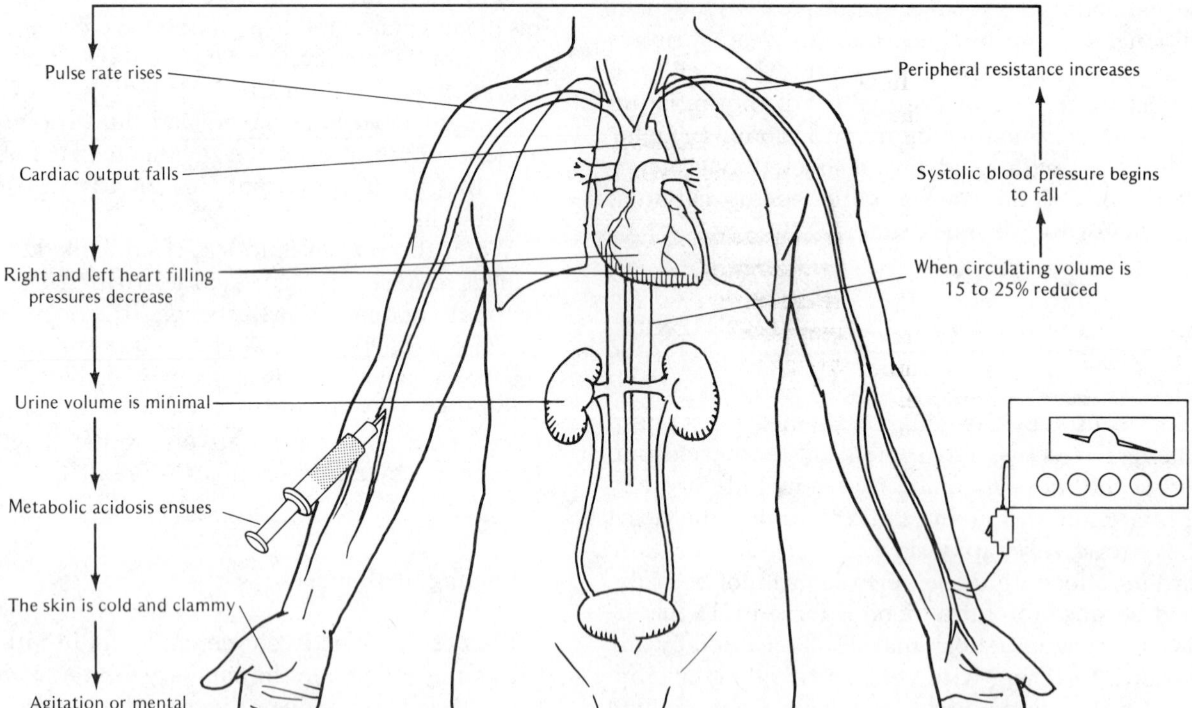

Right and left heart filling pressures decrease

Agitation or mental obtundation apparent

When circulating volume is 15 to 25% reduced

To enhance survival, the diagnosis must be made before blood pressure declines significantly. Close monitoring of patients with a high potential for hypovolemic shock will identify earlier stages.

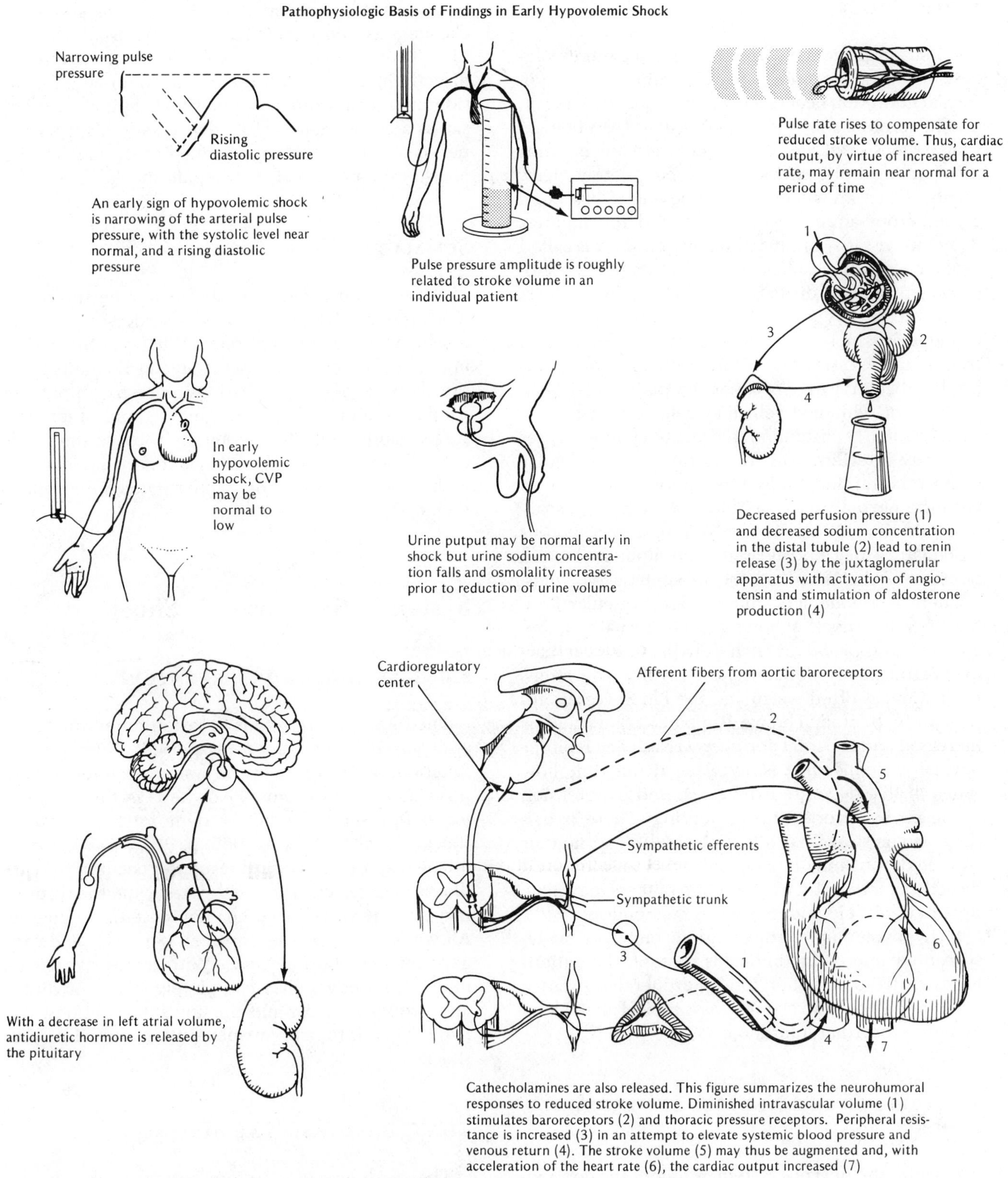
Pathophysiologic Basis of Findings in Early Hypovolemic Shock
Narrowing pulse pressure
Rising diastolic pressure
An early sign of hypovolemic shock is narrowing of the arterial pulse pressure, with the systolic level near normal, and a rising diastolic pressure
Pulse pressure amplitude is roughly related to stroke volume in an individual patient
Pulse rate rises to compensate for reduced stroke volume. Thus, cardiac output, by virtue of increased heart rate, may remain near normal for a period of time
1
2
3
4
In early hypovolemic shock, CVP may be normal to low
Urine putput may be normal early in shock but urine sodium concentration falls and osmolality increases prior to reduction of urine volume
Decreased perfusion pressure (1) and decreased sodium concentration in the distal tubule (2) lead to renin release (3) by the juxtaglomerular apparatus with activation of angiotensin and stimulation of aldosterone production (4)
Cardioregulatory center
Afferent fibers from aortic baroreceptors
2
5
Sympathetic efferents
Sympathetic trunk
3
1
6
4
7
With a decrease in left atrial volume, antidiuretic hormone is released by the pituitary
Cathecholamines are also released. This figure summarizes the neurohumoral responses to reduced stroke volume. Diminished intravascular volume (1) stimulates baroreceptors (2) and thoracic pressure receptors. Peripheral resistance is increased (3) in an attempt to elevate systemic blood pressure and venous return (4). The stroke volume (5) may thus be augmented and, with acceleration of the heart rate (6), the cardiac output increased (7)

Figure 45-3. Pathophysiologic Basis of Findings in Early Hypovolemic Shock. (Used with permission of Hospital Publications, Inc., from Guidelines to evaluation and management of shock. *Hosp. Med.* 15:88–130, Mar. 1979, by C. J. Pepine *et al.*, Fig. 8, pp. 120–21.)

Septic Shock

Clinical experience with hospitalized patients suggests that shock secondary to bacteremia and to myocardial infarction occurs with about equal frequency, but bacteremic shock is more frequent than hemorrhagic shock (McCale, 1973). The exact mechanisms involved in septic shock are not completely clear. Much of the knowledge of septic shock has been gained from animal experiments and the findings do not necessarily apply to human beings. It is called septic because it results from the action of toxic substances produced directly or indirectly by bacteria on blood vessels and other cells. Although these changes are most commonly caused by endotoxin from gram-negative organisms, exotoxin from gram-positive bacteria may occasionally play a role.

Dying or damaged cells may release certain substances such as histamine and proteolytic enzymes that may interfere with the normal cardiovascular activity. Histamine, for example, appears to interfere with the normal reactivity of blood vessels. Vasoactive substances, such as bradykinin, a very potent vasodilator, may be released from alpha-2-globulin fraction of the blood by the proteolytic enzymes.

There is a wide spectrum of cardiovascular findings in septic shock. When sepsis occurs without any complicating problems such as hypovolemia or cardiac insufficiency and does not involve the lungs, the patient is often warm and the blood vessels appear to be dilated. The cardiac output is normal or increased and the total peripheral resistance is either normal or reduced. It is not clear at this time how much of this decreased resistance and hypotension is caused by arteriovenous shunting. There is evidence suggesting that although total blood flow or cardiac output may be adequate, the cells involved directly or indirectly by the septic process may have impaired aerobic and anaerobic metabolism.

If hypovolemia, cardiac insufficiency, or widespread advanced pneumonia is present, the patient tends to have a higher total peripheral resistance and may be cold and clammy, as is typical after blood loss or myocardial infarction.

The Role of the Nervous System in Shock

Because the nervous system regulates the contraction and relaxation of the muscles in the blood vessels, shock may result from the effect on it of injury or drugs. It should be remembered, however, that shock from head trauma is quite rare. Increased intracranial pressure characteristically increases blood pressure until shortly before death. Shock caused by the vasodilator action of the nervous system is classified as neurogenic shock and is usually transitory. The nervous system itself does not have to be directly injured. Fainting, or syncope, may be considered a form of neurogenic shock. Spinal anesthesia, as a consequence of its depressing effect on the nerve supply to the anesthetized area, may also be considered a cause of neurogenic shock.

Summary

As indicated previously, shock may be the result of a large number of unrelated disorders, only a few of which have been mentioned. Whatever the initiating factor, much of the injury in shock results from the damage done to cells by failure to supply the proper amounts of oxygen, glucose, and other substances and failure to adequately remove the products of metabolism. We know, then, that hypoxia is the key mechanism of cellular damage in human shock.

Systemic Responses to Shock

Signs, Symptoms, Intervention

The total body responds to serious injury immediately and effectively for short periods. Normal body functioning continues as the systems call forth their protective mechanisms. "Nowhere is the capacity for self-preservation better demonstrated than in shock" (Thal & Wilson, 1965, p. 9).

The major physiological responses occur in the cardiovascular system, the renal system, and the respiratory system as well as other homeostatic responses. All work together to ensure cell perfusion and oxygenation for short periods. With aggressive treatment, the body rallies completely. Without direct and proper medical and nursing interventions, the body slips into irreversible and eventually fatal shock.

The Cardiovascular System

The cardiovascular system reacts quickly to the menace of shock: pressure receptors in the aorta and carotid artery are stimulated; they in turn stimulate the vasomotor center in the medulla, which activates the sympathetic nervous system to release epinephrine from the adrenal medulla and aldosterone from the adrenal cortex. The increased osmolarity of the blood stimulates the posterior pituitary to secrete the antidiuretic hormone or ADH (see Chapters 15 and 27). These hormones induce vasoconstriction and decrease kidney loss of fluid as well as increasing heart rate and force of contraction. The increase in cardiac output now helps the lessened blood volume to meet cellular oxygenation of tissues. Peripheral vasoconstriction lessens blood flow to nonvital tissues and provides vital organs with needed perfusion. The end result is normal blood flow in the large and vital arteries even though shock is occurring in the nonvital microcirculation. The microcirculation cell mass is much larger than the vital tissue mass so the blood pressure remains near normal.

The informed nurse knows that a decrease in blood pressure is not always an initial sign of early shock because of the above compensatory mechanisms. Reduction of 20 to 25 per cent of blood volume needs to occur before the blood pressure drops significantly (Rich, 1979). A narrowing of the pulse pressure is more common in early shock. Because of pooling of blood in the capillary bed, blood pressure changes are especially important if they occur when the patient has pain or changes in position.

The need for baseline data is exemplified by the elderly woman entering the hospital after a traumatic injury. The admitting nurse reports a "stable" BP of 100/60. The daughter, who has accompanied her mother to the hospital, immediately reports that a normal BP for her mother is 200/100. Clearly, shock is imminent.

Arterial pressure can be measured with the familiar blood pressure cuff attached to a mercury or aneroid manometer. This type of measurement is discouraged in shock, since crucial time can elapse before low volume registers. Many physicians will remove the cuff from the bedside to ensure this method is not used with their patients. Arterial cuff pressure does not reflect the severity of shock and is therefore not sufficiently reliable. In fact, a patient's cuff blood pressure may be within physiological limits and yet his or her tissues may be poorly supplied with blood. The reason for this inadequacy of perfusion is that most arterioles respond to stimulation by the sympathoadrenal system by undergoing powerful vasoconstriction. This response reduces the vascular capacity and brings it into an appropriate relationship with the blood volume. It is useful, inasmuch as the coronary and cerebral vessels are relatively less responsive to the sympathoadrenal system than other blood vessels and they continue to be supplied with blood. It can be detrimental, however, if it is severe and persistent because constriction of the vessels in the extremities, heart, kidneys, and other organs deprives them of an adequate supply of blood.

Venous Pressure

Whereas the arterial blood pressure is a reflection of the state of constriction of the arterioles and the force with which the heart drives blood into the arteries, venous pressure is what remains of that force after the blood passes through the capillaries. Actually, venous pressure is affected by right atrial pressure. With an increase in right atrial pressure, peripheral venous pressure must also rise if blood is to return to the heart. Pressure in peripheral veins also is affected by the distance and relationship of the vein to the right atrium. Hydrostatic pressure is caused by the weight exerted by a fluid against the wall of a tube. The higher the column of fluid, the greater is the pressure against the wall of the tube. When an individual is standing absolutely still, venous pressure is greater in the lower extremities than it is at the right atrium. Although peripheral venous pressure has been measured for many years, it is now known that it does not consistently reflect atrial pressure.

Central Venous Pressure

The pressure of blood in the right atrium, or central venous pressure (CVP), is normally from 0 to 5 cm of water. A CVP of 15 to 20 cm usually indicates that the blood is being returned to the right heart more rapidly than the heart can pump it into the arterial circulation. By continuous monitoring of the central venous pressure, the physician can estimate how the circulating blood volume compares to the pumping action of the heart at any given time. The trend of the response is often more important than the specific level (Cohn, 1970). When a small amount of fluid is administered rapidly and the CVP rises abruptly, this response often indicates that the heart is overloaded. Thal and Wilson (1965) state that the competence of the myocardium in the patient whose CVP is no greater than 10 cm of water can be measured by administering 500 ml of water in 20 minutes. If the CVP rises rapidly, the mycardium is probably loaded to capacity and the fluid intake should be discontinued immediately. If fluids continue to be given, pulmonary edema may result. If, on the other hand, fluids are infused and the arterial pressure increases but the venous pressure does not rise, the patient is probably at least relatively hypovolemic in relation to the competency of the heart.

Pulmonary Artery Pressure

Much has been written about the need for more accuracy in measuring the filling pressure of the left heart. Such measurements become important in patients with cardiopulmonary disease or patients who are at high risk for myocardial infarction.

The Swan-Ganz pulmonary artery wedge pressure (PAWP) flow-guided catheter obtains the pulmonary artery pressure and so reflects the left ventricular filling pressure. Studies reflect discrepancies between the CVP and the PAWP, but current thought still regards CVP as the workhorse of vascular monitoring (Carlson, 1978). In an unstable situation, CVP has first priority since it not only is effective for monitoring right heart performance but also becomes a means of drawing blood samples as well as administering needed medications if necessary.

It is wise to remember that in moderate shock, a CVP catheter is deficient in three ways. It does not indicate the amount of volume needed but measures the competence of the right heart to accept and expel fluids. It takes almost 24 hours for events occurring in the left side of the heart to propagate the lung, right ventricle, right atrium, and superior vena cava. Any pathology in the pulmonary vasculature may produce vascular hypertension (Schumer, 1979). Therefore, PAWP is the choice catheter in moderate to severe shock.

Responses Increasing Blood Volume

In addition to reflexes acting to reduce the capacity of the vascular system, other changes occur that tend to restore the blood volume. As the arterioles constrict, less blood enters the capillaries, thus reducing intracapillary pressure. The quantity of fluid leaving the capillary and entering it from the interstitial space is determined by the balance between (1) the filtration pressure, which the precapillary sphincters (arterioles) and postcapillary sphincters (venules) regulate, and (2) the colloid osmotic pressure of the blood, which is proportional to the concentration of the plasma proteins. Constriction of arterioles and relaxation of venules tend to cause the net filtration pressure to fall below the colloid osmotic pressure of the plasma and result in a tendency of fluid to move from the interstitial space into the capillaries (see Chapter 27).

Renal Responses

The kidney helps to protect the blood volume. Increased secretion of hormones, especially the antidiuretic hormone and aldosterone, promotes the reabsorption of water and sodium by the kidney, thereby aiding in their conservation (see Chapters 15 and 27). Since renal vessels are among the first to constrict in an effort to shift blood to the heart and brain, oliguria is an early sign of shock. The nurse needs to rule out other causes of oliguria by keeping an accurate intake and output, by checking the patency of the urinary catheter, and by obtaining urine specimens for specific gravity. (See Chapter 41 for further discussion of oliguria.)

Thirst occurs because of high sodium levels and because the cellular dehydration dries out mucous membranes. Good and frequent mouth care ensures that the thirst symptom is exactly that and not the result of a caked mouth. Mouth care is exceptionally important, since the gastrointestinal tracts of patients in shock will not usually tolerate oral liquid.

Respiratory Responses

The respiratory system responds primarily to changes in the pH, P_{CO_2} and P_{O_2} of the arterial blood since these levels indicate the amount of O_2 the cells are receiving. Increased CO_2 tension or decreased O_2 tension as well as a decrease in the pH all act to stimulate breathing. The pH is important, since respiratory alkalosis develops as the body compensates for its underlying acidosis with hyperpnea. Both tachycardia and hyperpnea occur to rid the body of its metabolic acidosis. A patient in shock who is not hyperventilating is in trouble (Wilson, 1978b). Accessory muscles are used for respiration. Flaring of the nostrils and restlessness are later signs of respiratory failure.

Nursing interventions rely heavily on coughing and deep breathing several times hourly to prevent atelectasis. Position is changed as often as every 30 minutes in order to prevent fluid accumulation in the lungs.

Current research shows a lack of data to support the Trendelenburg position for the shock patient since this position causes diaphragmatic pressure and severely interferes with respiratory exchange. The supine position along with a clear airway allows maximum heart and brain blood flow. Should more venous return be needed, slight elevation of the legs will accomplish this goal.

Fluid therapy is carefully calculated to decrease the water content of the lungs and still maintain lung tissue perfusion. An important nursing responsibility is that of daily weights for comparison of fluid gains and losses. Weights must be taken on a bed scale; obviously the patient should not be expected to stand.

Other Signs and Symptoms

Since cellular hypoxia is so intrinsic to shock, the body needs to decrease its needs for oxygen. Muscle weakness and fatigue result from the inefficient production of energy by anaerobic rather than aerobic cellular metabolism. Bedrest, a cool environment, and avoidance of any heat which could cause vasodilatation are recommended.

Brain cell hypoxia manifests itself by anxiety, vagueness, restlessness, and a clouded sensorium. Constant reassurance and explanation by the nurse help to reduce patient anxiety. The patient in shock has great emotional anxiety—his or her physical state is no more important than the need for a calm approach by personnel.

Body temperature decreases because of poor circulation and poor metabolism. The skin is usually cool, moist, and pale with blanching at the nail beds. In septic shock, however, the skin can be flushed, dry, and warm. Keeping the skin clean and dry with the least amount of effort by the patient is a major nursing responsibility.

Disseminated vascular coagulation tends to occur in all types of shock, especially septic shock. DIC is a paradox of pooling, clumping, clotting, and bleeding of blood and needs to be recognized and treated early and accurately (see Chapter 42).

Summary of Homeostatic Adjustments in Shock

The body responds to life-threatening situations by initiating reflexes tending to maintain, restore, and/or improve the perfusion of body tissues. Because survival depends on maintenance of function of the heart and brain, the initial response to a diminished cardiac output or fall in arterial blood pressure is to redistribute the circulating blood to maintain adequate blood flow in these organs. By arteriolar and venous constriction, the capacity of the vascular system is reduced, thereby increasing the relative blood volume. Blood volume is also increased by movement of water from the interstitial and cellular spaces into the capillaries. The excretion of salt and water by the kidney is reduced because of the influence of aldosterone and the antidiuretic hormone. The respiratory system attempts to reduce the effects of metabolic acidosis by increased ventilation, thereby producing a compensatory respiratory alkalosis.

Effects of Shock on Specific Organs

Any patient with a serious injury or illness is in danger of developing shock. Shock occurs in all degrees from mild (ischemic) to so-called refractory (stagnant) or irreversible shock. Impending or mild degrees may be compensated for readily by the body's intrinsic homeostatic mechanisms. Depending on circumstances, however, it may progress to a partially compensated and reversible stage and finally to irreversible shock. The term *irreversible* means that the changes in the cells have progressed to the point where present methods of treatment are incapable of reversing the pathophysiologic changes. Sometimes shock develops slowly, and at other times it develops with great rapidity. Whatever the etiologic factor, there appear to be common hemodynamic and metabolic alterations that occur as shock approaches. This "common pathway to irreversibility" is entered upon when blood pressure falls, and catecholamines (epinephrine and norepinephrine) increase. Catecholamines increase peripheral resistance, resulting in diversion of blood from kidneys, bowel, and extremities to the more vital brain and heart. This selective ischemia is necessary for survival, but becomes detrimental if shock is prolonged. Increased peripheral resistance is accompanied by decreased venous return, decreased circulating blood volume, decreased tissue perfusion, and decreased cardiac output, followed in time by anoxia, acidosis, pooling of blood, and cell death (*The Shock Syndrome*, 1969). Unless the patient is rapidly and adequately treated, he or she may go into irreversible shock and die. By means of modern methods of treatment, survival is occasionally possible in some patients who appear to be in irreversible shock.

The heart and Blood Vessels

If shock continues and is severe enough, all tissues eventually suffer. The various parts of the circulatory system deteriorate and a vicious circle may develop. To illustrate, the force of contraction of the myocardium depends on the adequacy of its blood supply. In any condition with a decreased cardiac output, arterial blood pressure falls, leading to decreased systemic blood flow and decreased nutrition of all tissues, including those of the heart. As the nutrition of the heart muscle is further impaired, the force of cardiac contraction becomes increasingly ineffective. With marked tissue ischemia, toxins are believed to be released from the cells. They intensify the condition by (1) increasing capillary permeability, (2) predisposing to intravascular clotting, and (3) depressing the myocardial and vascular responses to catecholamines.[2]

[2] Depression of the myocardium in shock states is currently believed to be due to a myocardial depressant factor (MDF), formed as a consequence of splanchnic ischemia and disruption of intracellular lysosomes that characterize advanced shock (Lefer, 1973).

As systemic blood flow diminishes, stasis of blood develops and the tendency of the blood to clot is increased. Thrombosis within capillaries contributes to the progression of shock and further reduces blood flow. Thus a vicious circle may be initiated with each factor intensifying the severity of the preceding one. Unless the cycle is reversed, death ensues.

With decreased blood volume because of hemorrhage, a similar cycle is initiated. Because of an inadequate blood volume, venous return to the heart is diminished. There is corresponding decrease in cardiac output and a series of events leading to myocardial and tissue ischemia.

The Kidneys

In shock, there is decreased renal perfusion because of constriction of the afferent and efferent arterioles and shunting of the blood away from the glomeruli. This results in reduced renal function and urine volume. The formation of renin by the kidney in response to inadequate blood flow has been described previously. Because of the decrease in blood flow, glomerular filtration diminishes and the kidney loses its ability to regulate electrolyte and acid–base balance. Unfortunately the renal vasoconstriction may continue long after the blood pressure has been restored to normal levels. If the shock progresses, severe oliguria and tubular necrosis may develop. With appropriate therapy and prevention of overloading with fluid, the patient may survive until the kidney repairs itself sufficiently so that normal function returns. This repair takes about 10 to 14 days.

Recognition of impending renal failure even before oliguria appears is essential to the proper treatment of the patient. Among the changes in the urine indicating that the patient is in nonoliguric renal failure are (1) reduced specific gravity and osmolality of the urine, (2) reduced creatinine clearance, and (3) a rise in sodium urine concentration relative to the amount in the serum. Examination of the blood may reveal a progressive rise in urea nitrogen, creatinine, and potassium that will be especially rapid if there is associated tissue damage or infection.

The Intestinal Mucosa

The combination of decreased cardiac output and vasoconstriction also limits blood flow to the intestine. As a result of inadequate perfusion, the capillary endothelium in the intestinal mucosa is damaged, and edema, hemorrhage, and congestion of the intestinal wall may occur. The most serious effect of these changes is the reduced effectiveness of the intestinal mucosa as a barrier between the bacteria and toxins in the intestinal lumen and the blood stream (Jacobson, 1968).

The Reticuloendothelial System

All structures and systems deprived of their blood supply tend to function poorly. In shock, the function of the reticuloendothelial system is depressed. As a consequence, the ability of the body to detoxify harmful agents may be greatly reduced (see Unit V).

The Lungs

Not only may the lungs suffer direct structural and functional changes in shock, but their function may also be impaired because of pulmonary edema secondary to heart failure. The reason for these changes are not well understood. Moreover, unlike the heart and kidney, there is as yet no good, practical way to maintain life while lung function is being restored. Some of the possible causes of lung damage include left heart failure, circulating toxins such as histamine and bradykinin, and constriction of the small pulmonary veins. There is increasing evidence that humoral agents are primarily responsible (Tracing Clues, 1971).

Recently much attention has been directed toward surfactant, a lipoprotein whose main property is the ability to reduce surface tension within the alveoli. If surfactant is destroyed or produced in inadequate quantities, as may occur with shock, anoxia, and trauma, surface tension rises in the alveoli and atelectasis results.

Simeone (1966) and others have wondered whether trauma alone can destroy the integrity of the alveolocapillary membrane and promote the development of congestive atelectasis. Can hypoxia such as that associated with atelectasis affect the integrity of this layer and promote further and more intense atelectasis? Do certain aspects of therapy aggravate these problems?

Structural Changes in the Lung

Certain lung areas become atelectatic because of inadequate perfusion. This is an acute respiratory distress syndrome. The drug of choice in shock patients is O_2, even in those who exhibit no signs of respiratory failure. Forty per cent oxygen by mask at a flow of 8 L/minute is recommended. Mechanical ventilation may be needed for patients with a low P_{O_2} who are dyspneic.

Pulmonary edema commonly results from various trauma and can cause acute respiratory failure and death. It is well to remember that most forms of respiratory failure start with edema. Simple edema is easily removed by the pulmonary lymph system. When edema is severe due to increased pulmonary capillary permeability, the increase in lung water leads to a stiff lung and poor oxygen transport (wet lung) (Wilson, 1978a). The onset of pulmonary edema with decreased cardiac output requires placement of the Swan-Ganz catheter to measure pulmonary artery pressure.

Martin et al. (1968) report that in 100 patients who underwent autopsy following death from shock and/or trauma, the lungs were more frequently involved than any other organ. The lesions included pulmonary edema, congestion, bronchopneumonia, pleural effusions, and pulmonary emboli.

Cell Damage

As discussed in Chapter 29, cellular functions and survival depend on the release of energy from the glucose molecule. Energy is released in the mitochondria by a series of minute steps. The first steps that involve the conversion of glucose to pyruvic acid can take place under anaerobic conditions. Each glucose molecule forms two molecules of pyruvic acid, hydrogen, and a small amount of a high-energy phosphate molecule, adenosine triphosphate (ATP). For the steps in glucose metabolism to continue beyond this point, oxygen is required. Under normal circumstances, pyruvic acid is converted to acetic acid and then to acetyl CoA, which enters the Krebs cycle. In the Krebs cycle, the acetyl CoA is broken down into CO_2 and H. The hydrogen is taken up in the electron transport system, and if adequate oxygen is present, the hydrogen and oxygen combine to form water. The completion of this reaction releases a great deal of energy in the form of ATP. If adequate oxygen is not available, the Krebs cycle stops and the pyruvic acid is converted into lactic acid. If oxygen becomes available again, the lactic acid can be converted into pyruvic acid that can then enter the Krebs cycle. As lactic acid accumulates, it causes metabolic acidosis, which can have a further detrimental effect on cell activity.

The Krebs cycle requires oxygen. When there is a shift from aerobic to anaerobic metabolism, the Krebs cycle is seriously impaired. Insufficient ATP is formed to provide energy to maintain vital functions. The permeability of the cell membrane increases with potassium leaving the cell and sodium and water entering. Other functions necessary to life such as the synthesis of protein and enzymes also fail.

Because of a lack of oxygen and the development of acidosis the membranes or borders around the lysosomes, tiny particles within the cell, may be damaged. When the lysosomal membrane breaks down, powerful hydrolytic enzymes that may play a role in intracellular digestion are released. These enzymes can damage or destroy the cell and surrounding tissues. It may be that lysosome-related injury continues even after hypoxia and acidosis are corrected. This may be one reason that a patient may continue to deteriorate despite correction of the hemodynamic aspects of shock. The injured or anoxic cell may also liberate histamine or similar substances that can interfere with cardiovascular response to catecholaminelike drugs.

These enzymes, especially those with proteolytic activity, may also cause the release of certain very powerful vasoactive substances, kinins, from the alpha-2-globulin fraction of the blood. These proteolytic enzymes, or proteases, convert the inactive precursors, kininogens, into the very active and very powerful kinins. The best known of these kinins is bradykinin, which is the most potent vasodilator known. Other vasoactive substances are the polypeptides angiotensin II and the more recently identified kallidin II (Thal, et al., 1971).

One of the most significant contributions the nurse makes to the care of ill patients is observing them for evidence indicating whether or not they are progressing satisfactorily. All patients who experience traumatic injury, extensive surgery, myocardial infarction, pancreatitis, or other serious illness should be observed for any indications that shock is developing. This observation should be continued until such time as it is *known* that the patient is in a stable state. It is possible for a patient to be treated for shock and to appear to be making a satisfactory recovery only to go later into an even more severe stage of shock. The importance of informed observation cannot be overemphasized because shock must be treated early and vigorously if the patient is to survive.

Because shock involves the entire individual, signs and symptoms reflect changes in function of organs as they respond to altered blood volume, myocardial contraction, and/or vascular tone. Early signs and symptoms result from the activation of the sympathoadrenal system, which may correct or compensate for hypovolemia or other hemodynamic derangements. Early signs and symptoms serve as warning signals that something is wrong. These signs and symptoms usually reflect (1) the response of the sympathoadrenal system; (2) diminished perfusion of blood to the nervous system, heart, kidney, skin, lungs, gastrointestinal tract, and other organs; (3) the primary injury or illness.

Nervous System

Many of the signs and symptoms relating to the nervous system are caused by activation of the sympathoadrenal system. The resultant hyperventilation, anxiety, agitation, apprehension, and restlessness may precede the development of other signs of shock. When they occur, the possibility that the patient is in early shock should be considered, and their presence should be promptly reported to the physician. Not infrequently, restlessness is interpreted as indicating that the patient is in pain when in fact he or she is suffering from hypoxia, which can produce a very similar picture. Eventually, as blood flow to the brain fails, the patient becomes more confused and finally may become comatose. The combination of signs and symptoms which occur together in the high-risk shock patient is important in forming a total picture.

Arterial and Venous Tone

Blood pressure depends on the interrelationship of blood volume, the force of myocardial contraction, and the degree of arterial and venous constriction. Arterial blood pressure tends to rise if there is an increase in cardiac output, blood volume, or vasoconstriction. The reverse is also true; that is, the arterial blood pressure tends to fall if there is a drop in cardiac output, blood volume, or if vasodilatation occurs. The pulse pressure should be noted. As cardiac output decreases, there is generally a corresponding fall in pulse pressure and increased difficulty in breathing.

The state of constriction of the peripheral blood vessels is also reflected by the skin. With peripheral vasoconstriction, the skin is cool and moist. With peripheral stasis it is mottled or cyanotic in persons with little melanin in their skin; in persons with heavily pigmented skin, peripheral stasis gives the appearance of patches of varying color, or of a grayish color. The mucous membranes tend to be pale and dry. Nail beds are cyanotic and, when pressed, refill slowly. Although neck and peripheral veins may be distended in cardiac failure, in other forms of shock they are likely to be collapsed. Although these changes are characteristic of most types of shock, in many patients with sepsis there is a normal or increased cardiac output and the skin is warm, dry, and pink in fair-skinned people; the skin of those who are more heavily pigmented may appear even darker than usual, with occasionally a velvety and/or shiny appearance.

Cardiac Function

The quality of the pulse and its fullness, rate, and rhythm should be noted. A thready pulse is often noted and usually indicates a low cardiac output. The patient is frequently being monitored continuously for the rate and rhythm of the heart. (See Chapter 44 for discussion of common irregularities of rate and rhythm.)

Kidney Function

When the arterial blood pressure or cardiac output is low, blood is shunted away from the kidney, resulting in a decreased glomerular filtration rate of the fluid. Sodium and water reabsorption in the tubules increases, and urine output falls. Measurement of the output of urine is of great importance. A urine output of 25 ml or more per hour is usually a satisfactory minimum. To measure urine output accurately and continuously an indwelling catheter is inserted. Efforts should be made to improve the hemodynamic status of the patient to maintain adequate urine flow. To a certain extent, the kidney is the "window of the viscera." That is, if there is adequate urine (without the use of a diuretic), one can generally assume that the kidney is adequately perfused. If the kidney is adequately perfused, one can usually assume that the other organs are also well perfused. If the urine volume is low and the specific gravity is high, it can usually be assumed that the patient is hypovolemic, has impaired cardiac output, and/or reduced perfusion of the kidney.

Summary

All seriously ill and injured patients require regular and careful observation. In the patient in shock, pulse rate, arterial blood pressure, and central venous pressure may need to be checked every 15 minutes or continuously. At the time these measurements are made, the general condition of the patient should also be noted. Slowing of the pulse, widening of the pulse pressure, and an increase in urine output are usually indices that the patient is improving. EKG monitoring with a cardioscope is also indicated in most critically ill patients.

Tests to Estimate Degree of Cellular Hypoxia

To estimate the degree of cellular hypoxia and the extent to which respiratory mechanisms are effective in compensating for metabolic derangements, arterial pH, blood lactic acid, P_{CO_2}, and standard blood bicarbonate levels may be determined. Venous carbon dioxide content and the carbon dioxide-combining power give only an approximate estimate of the degree of metabolic acidosis. A more accurate estimate of the degree of hypoxia is the arterial lactate. This test is, however, generally limited to research laboratories. Other tests such as the blood hematocrit, cardiac output, and blood volume can also be employed. The hematocrit is easily performed and is useful in determining the need for red cells or the extent of hemoconcentration in disorders such as burns.

Even in the absence of highly sophisticated methods of determining such factors as cardiac output, degree of vasoconstriction, and blood lactic acid, a knowledgeable nurse can detect evidence that shock is developing or becoming progressively worse. The sophisticated tests often confirm what has been discerned by clinical observation. Clinical information is too often collected in a random fashion, varying in quality, and it cannot be retrieved readily. To provide a better definition of shock, standardized methods are necessary for collecting clinical data so they may be interrelated with hemodynamic and biochemical information. Clinical examination of the patient in shock is essential, but it reveals only a part of the complex picture to be analyzed (Thal et al., 1971).

Treatment of Shock

The fundamental objective in shock is to maintain and/or restore cellular metabolism. To achieve this objective, the cells must be provided with adequate amounts of oxygen and glucose and be able to utilize them. The prevention and treatment of shock therefore require attention to the following: (1) identification and correction of the cause of the shock; (2) adequate respiratory function; (3) adequate circulatory function, blood volume, cardiac pumping action, and vascular tone; and (4) correction of any condition that impairs cellular metabolism, such as acid–base and electrolyte abnormalities, and failure of specific organs (Ravine & Modell, 1973).

Maintenance of Respiratory Function

The importance of deficient ventilation and oxygenation in the etiology of shock cannot be overemphasized. An adequate supply of oxygen and the removal of carbon dioxide are essential to biochemical homeostasis. The first step in treatment of shock is to be certain that the airway is open and functioning. In severe respiratory failure, the patient may need ventilatory support from a respirator. An endotracheal tube may be inserted or a tracheostomy performed and a cuffed tracheostomy tube inserted. Because high concentrations of oxygen are known to damage the lung, the physician prescribes the lowest concentration that will maintain a P_{O_2} of 60 mm Hg or higher. The patient must be protected from danger of alkalosis as a consequence of hyperventilation with hand or machine respirators (Thompson, 1973). (See Chapter 40 for causes and treatment of failure of ventilation.)

Maintenance of Adequate Blood Volume

Despite a loss of as much as 25 to 35 per cent in the blood volume, if it is not too rapid there may be only a moderate drop in blood pressure. With a loss of 50 per cent or more, the shock is very severe or lethal. When a patient is hypotensive as a result of hypovolemia, blood pressure may rise rapidly when as little as 500 to 700 ml of fluid are administered.

Fluid Replacement

When enough fluid is lost to affect venous return, then sufficient fluid must be introduced to produce an adequate *cardiac output.* The basic guide to fluid therapy in shock is the concept of "titration" coupled with repeated measurements (Thal et al., 1971). The best gauge for measuring the adequacy of fluid replacement is the response of the central venous pressure or the pulmonary artery pressure to the administered fluid. In general, if a patient is hypovolemic, he or she will have a low central venous pressure, but more important, the central venous pressure rises slowly or not at all as fluid and/or blood is given to the patient. The reverse is true of patients in whom the cardiovascular system is already handling as much fluid as it can. A less accurate index of blood volume is the degree of filling of the neck veins. When fluid is added rapidly and the central venous pressure rises, the neck veins, which are normally collapsed, distend. This response usually indicates that the heart is handling about as much fluid as it can. More fluid may precipitate heart failure. When the central venous pressure fails to rise and the veins remain collapsed, hypovolemia still exists and fluid may continue to be administered.

Even when the fluid deficit appears to be corrected, the patient requires continued observation until such time as it is certain that he or she is in a stable state. The survival of the patient depends on the consistency and accuracy of the observations that are made. As stressed throughout, appropriate actions must be taken if the observations are to benefit the patient.

The kind and amount of fluid used in the treatment of shock depend on the nature and quantity of fluid lost, the urgency of the situation, and the type of fluid available. In general, fluids used in replacement are of three types: blood and plasma, plasma expanders, and electrolyte solutions. In emergency situations, electrolyte solutions such as Ringer's lactate or saline with bicarbonate may be used to expand blood volume, because only a fraction of the erythrocytes is required to carry oxygen. Care must be taken to prevent "wet lung" from excessive infusion of Ringer's lactate, because waterlogged tissues cannot be perfused.

Blood

A rapid loss of as many as 500 ml of blood can usually occur without significant evidence of hypovolemia. In some individuals as many as 1,000 ml may be lost with only mild signs. When more than 1 liter of blood is lost there are usually clinical signs and hemodynamic changes. If bleeding has stopped, fluids that expand the plasma volume will often be adequate to restore homeostasis. When bleeding continues, blood must be used in replacement. Because of the dangers inherent in blood transfusion, it should not be used if another fluid can satisfactorily increase blood volume and maintain adequate oxygen-carrying capacity. Bank blood always presents the danger of hemolysis from mismatched blood and/or serum hepatitis.[3]

[3] The mortality rate associated with blood transfusion is comparable to that of appendicitis. (See Chapters 42 & 52 for discussion of the hazards of transfusion.)

Plasma Expanders

In disorders such as acute pancreatitis, burns, and peritonitis in which the loss of plasma is excessive, fluids containing molecules large enough to be retained in the blood vessels are essential. Plasma, dextran of high or low molecular weight, or electrolyte solutions containing albumin may be used. Dextran of high molecular weight, 72,000 or more, is useful because it tends to remain in the blood. It has a disadvantage, however, because it induces cell aggregation, an already undesirable tendency in slow-moving blood in shock.

Low molecular dextran (40,000) is less effective as a direct plasma expander than the high molecular form. It acts mainly to prevent or hinder cell aggregation and to lessen the viscosity of the blood. As a result, it may improve the circulation of blood and prevent sludging of the red cells.

Before dextran is administered, blood should be taken for blood grouping and cross matching. Dextran should be administered slowly and the patient should have his or her central venous pressure continuously monitored (Gladish et al., 1967).

Electrolyte Solutions

Loss of volume requires whole blood, ideally, but type and cross-matching take valuable time; therefore, use of balanced solutions can maintain needed tissue perfusion. Normal saline, Ringer's lactate and Ringer's bicarbonate solution can be used if appropriate. It would seem safest to use Ringer's bicarbonate, since a poorly perfused liver might be unable to metabolize lactate into CO_2 and water. The unmetabolized lactate is then excreted by the kidney along with sodium chloride and potassium to further alter the acid–base balance (Schumer, 1979). These electrolyte solutions are useful in expanding the extracellular fluid volume. They also have the advantage of reducing viscosity and preventing sludging and aggregation of erythrocytes.

Solutions containing sodium are often contraindicated in cardiac disorders (Lowrey et al., 1971).

Support of the Heart

Some estimate of the condition of the heart can be made by monitoring the EKG and noting the character of the pulse.

Any arrhythmia should be converted because it tends to reduce cardiac efficiency. Quinidine and procaine amide may be used to treat various arrhythmias but it should be remembered that they also tend to reduce myocardial contractility. Digitalis is often very useful in shock because it improves the strength of the failing heart and may reduce the heart rate to more normal values. Isoproterenol (Isuprel) is a sympathomimetic amine that acts primarily on the beta receptors. It increases the strength and rate of cardiac contraction and lowers peripheral vascular resistance, especially in certain muscles.

Regulation of the Size of the Vascular Chamber

Until recently, emphasis has been on maintaining the level of the arterial pressure within so-called normal limits, the belief being that arterial blood pressure is a good index of tissue perfusion. With additional knowledge, however, it is now known that other factors are of equal or even greater importance. In the treatment of shock, the physician must try to evaluate the state of each part of the circulatory system. When in the opinion of the physician the degree of vasoconstriction is insufficient to maintain blood flow, especially to the heart and brain, the physician may prescribe any one of a number of vasopressor agents. Perhaps the most frequently used are metaraminol (Aramine) and norepinephrine (Levophed). Maintenance of adequate arterial pressure is especially important in older patients in whom blood flow through narrowed coronary or cerebral vessels may be pressure-dependent.[4] Both of these drugs can be administered by intravenous infusion and metaraminol can also be injected intramuscularly. However, absorption from the intramuscular site is not reliable enough to be useful in shock.

Norepinephrine is a very powerful vasoconstrictor and care must be taken to prevent it from infiltrating the tissues. If this drug does get outside a vein, it can cause the tissue to slough. It should be injected into large and central veins. The arterial blood pressure of the patient receiving norepinephrine should be under constant surveillance in order to detect undesirable rises in the blood pressure. Moreover, as the patient changes position, the rate of flow may be altered and the patient may receive more or less drug than necessary to produce the desired effect.

There is no place for vasoconstriction therapy in hypovolemic shock since hemodynamically patients are already maximally vasoconstricted (Zamora, 1979). There is some thought that there is no place in the treatment of *any* shock for the vasoconstrictors norepinephrine and metaraminol bitartrate. The resultant overly constricted arterioles increase anaerobic metabolism and so increase acidosis. In order to safely perfuse vital organs until enough fluid has altered the blood volume, dopamine is being used more successfully. Dopamine is a catecholamine which is an immediate precursor in the synthesis of noradrenalin (Kooput et al., 1977). In small doses, a dopamine infusion increases myocardial contractility and cardiac output. It also increases renal blood flow and sodium excretion. But in higher doses dopamine has vasoconstrictive effects caused by alpha-adrenergic stimulation. Blood pressure increases but so does peripheral resistance.

Dopamine is a potent drug. Constant monitoring of blood pressure, pulse, peripheral pulses, color, and temperature of extremities for peripheral ischemia and urinary output are essential. Reduced urine flow in the absence of hypotension is one indicator for decreasing or suspending dosage (Govoni & Hayes, 1978).

Although these drugs may initially be beneficial by maintaining perfusion of the heart or brain, if their use is prolonged they can cause death or irreversible damage in the tissues supplied by the severely constricted vessels. Further, heart failure may be precipitated by a sudden and/or excessive rise in the arterial blood pressure. Therefore vasopressor therapy is used for as short a time as possible. Although vasoconstriction helps to maintain blood flow to the heart and brain in early shock, if prolonged it can result in irreversible injury to the tissues of other organs such as the kidney, lungs, liver, and gastrointestinal tract. If this vasoconstriction is severe and persistent despite the infusing of adequate amounts of fluid or blood, a vasodilating drug may be of value. When vasodilators are used it must be remembered that there is dilatation not only of arterioles but also of the capacitance veins. One to 3 liters of additional fluid or blood may be needed to fill the additional vascular capacity created by the vasodilator drug.

Among the vasodilator drugs in use are phenoxybenzamine (Dibenzyline), phentolamine (Regitine), and chlorpromazine. Phentolamine is useful in patients who remain overconstricted with cold, clammy skin and decreased urinary output after adequate fluid replacement. Phenoxybenzamine is the most powerful (Goodman & Gilman, 1975, p. 534). It blocks the alpha adrenergic receptors in the walls of the blood vessels. Thus the blood vessels do not respond to the naturally produced norepinephrine and peripheral resistance is reduced. It also reduces the response of small blood vessels to agents such as serotonin and histamine. Because phenoxybenzamine does not alter the response of the heart to the catecholamines (epinephrine and norepinephrine), the relative effectiveness of the heart is increased. Although the arterial blood pressure may be lower

[4] See Goodman and Gilman (1975) for a complete discussion of these and other vasoconstrictor drugs.

than normal, tissue perfusion is usually improved. Young patients can usually tolerate vasodilation and low blood pressure quite well, but older patients with sclerotic vessels may not be able to tolerate this hypotension. Under these circumstances a cardiogenic drug used in combination with the vasodilator may be able to maintain or raise the blood pressure by increasing the cardiac output.

Patients who receive vasodilator drugs must be continuously observed for evidence of improvement or of failure of the circulation. Particularly in the patient in hypovolemic shock, a rapid expansion of the vascular capacity without adequate volume to fill the space may lead to a precipitous drop in blood pressure. To protect the patient, central venous pressure must be continuously monitored and the blood volume increased as the vascular chamber enlarges. Because there is some evidence that phenoxybenzamine can cause cardiac damage, it is given slowly.

Maintenance of Renal Function

Measures used to increase blood volume and cardiac output should benefit the kidney as well as other tissues. Correction of metabolic acidosis (discussed subsequently) is essential, because severe metabolic acidosis is injurious to the kidney and other organs. Mannitol, an osmotic diuretic, is a 6-carbon atom sugar. It is filtered in the urine and is neither reabsorbed nor metabolized. It has two uses. By promoting diuresis it helps to prevent the accumulation of hemolyzed cells and other debris in the renal tubules. This action is of most benefit when hypotension is temporary. It is also useful in identifying the patient who has suffered renal damage in shock. The patient whose urine output does not improve after an adequate fluid load of 25 g of mannitol given in 100 to 500 ml of glucose in a 10- to 30-minute period can usually be assumed to have renal damage. Furosemide (Lasix) might also be utilized. If no improvement is noted, dialysis would then be indicated. Generally, if adequate fluid replacement occurs, diuretics are seldom needed (Wilson, 1978b).

An effective method of forcing blood from the nonvital areas of the lower body to the vital heart and brain is use of anti-shock trousers. To see how these trousers counteract bleeding and hypovolemia, refer to Figure 45-4.

Do's and Don'ts for Using M.A.S.T. Effectively

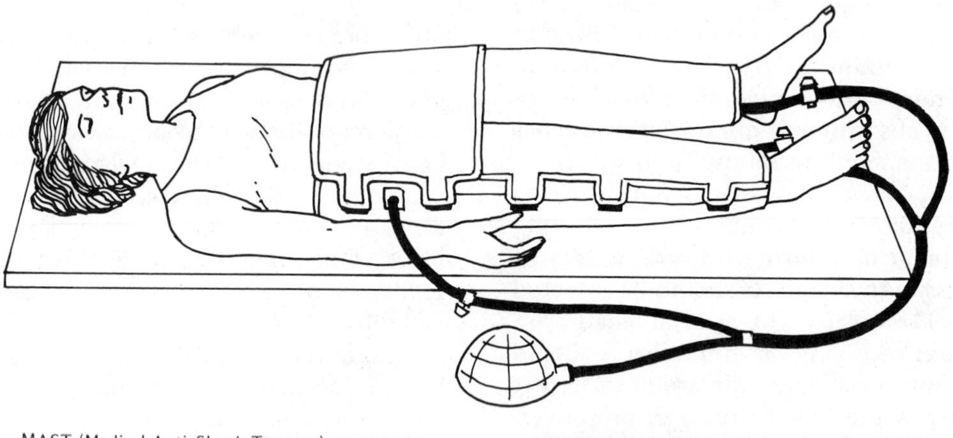

MAST (Medical Anti-Shock Trousers) counteracts bleeding and hypovolemia by slowing or stopping arterial bleeding; by forcing any available blood from the lower body to the heart, brain, and any other vital organ in the upper body; and by preventing return of the available circulating blood volume to the lower extremities.

Do's:

- While patient is wearing MAST: monitor vital signs, blood pressure, apical and radical pulse rate, and respirations; check extremities for pedal pulses, color, warmth, and numbness; and make sure MAST is not too constricting
- Take MAST off only when: a doctor is present; fluids are available for transfusion; and anesthesia and surgical teams are ready for the patient.
- To clean: Wash with warm soap and water; or air dry and store.
- Don't apply MAST if: positions or wounds show or suggest intrathoracic or intracranial major vascular injury; patient has open-extremity bleeding, pulmonary edema, or trauma above the level of MAST application.
- When cleaning, don't autoclave or clean with solvents.

Figure 45-4. Use of Medical Anti-Shock Trousers (M.A.S.T.) to counteract bleeding and hypovolemia. (Used with permission of Intermed Communications, Inc. from Cardiogenic shock: Combatting a high mortality rate, in *Nursing Critically Ill Patients Confidently.* Horsham, Pa.: Nursing Skillbook Series, 1979, by R. R. Rich, Fig. on p. 53.)

Specific Therapeutic Techniques

Adrenal Steroids

Among other drugs used in the treatment of shock are the adrenal steroids. Enthusiasm for their use waxes and wanes. Weissman and Thomas (1962) demonstrated that steroids stabilize the lysosomal membrane and prevent intracellular release of enzymes. They also increase blood volume by increasing sodium retention. Adrenal steroids appear to be of most benefit in patients in septic shock caused by gram-negative organisms.

Hypothermia

Besides measures planned to improve cellular metabolism, reducing the metabolic requirements of cells also should increase the patient's chances for survival. With a 10°C reduction of the body temperature, the needs of cells can usually be reduced by about 50 per cent. In actual practice, the beneficial effects of hypothermia are offset to some extent by the slowing of the heart that accompanies it. In addition, there is an increased possibility of ventricular fibrillation, blood viscosity is increased, and tissue perfusion is impaired. In the patient with a high fever, hypothermia may be helpful in reducing the temperature to a level slightly below normal.

Antibiotics

In almost any type of shock, especially that caused by sepsis, antibiotics are an important adjunct to treatment. As stated earlier, the most frequent cause of septic shock is the gram-negative organisms. Despite the desirability of determining the sensitivity of the causative organisms to antibiotics, there usually is not time. The antibiotic most likely to be selected is the one that, according to the most recent laboratory test, is most likely to attack the offending organism.

Summary

After the patient is in shock, continued observation is required to determine the effectiveness of the corrective measures that have been instituted. It is well to remember that shock is a dynamic, not a static, process. The condition of the patient in shock is usually either improving or deteriorating. Therefore, careful observation accompanied by the prompt reporting of signs and symptoms indicating impending or worsening shock is imperative. Regardless of whether or not the physician has requested that a given patient be observed for evidence of shock, the nurse should nevertheless assume this responsibility with all patients who (1) undergo major surgery or are seriously injured by physical trauma or burning, (2) bleed from a hollow organ or continue to hemorrhage, or (3) have an acute myocardial infarction. This list is suggestive rather than exhaustive. The significant question that the nurse should ask is "Does this patient have a disorder or treatment that is likely to result in failure to perfuse the tissues?" If the answer is yes, the patient should be investigated for signs and symptoms indicating impending or fully developed shock. When they occur, they should be brought to the attention of the physician immediately.

Nursing the Patient in Shock

What are the responsibilities of the nurse in the case of the patient who is in shock or likely to go into shock? The nurse must utilize her or his background knowledge in the following manner:

1. Using clinical data obtained at the bedside, the nurse must assess and evaluate the state of the patient.
2. The nurse must make appropriate nursing interventions in carrying out the treatment prescribed by the physician.
3. The nurse must regulate the environment in relation to the needs of the patient.

Assessment of the Patient

The clinical manifestations of shock are varied and take on importance as they occur together. Each response must be correlated with other responses in order to clarify the total picture. Sensing the patient "just didn't look good" is often the initial step in such a correlation.

The signs and symptoms previously discussed in relation to the pathophysiology of shock provide critical guideposts to the nurse's observation of the shock-prone patient. The central objective of observation is to prevent *irreversible shock,* which is that condition in which blood pressure, peripheral flow, and cardiac output fail to improve despite all measures. Unless shock is aggressively treated within about 3 hours of its onset, it is usually irreversible. Keen observation and prompt reporting by the nurse are critical to the welfare of the patient whose condition places him or her at risk of going into shock.

Although monitoring devices have been made that can collect certain types of information more accurately and reliably than can humans, they cannot and do not replace the knowledgeable nurse and physician. For example, machines can monitor the temperature, pulse, respiration, EKG, EEG, and arterial and venous pressures. They cannot, however, note pink fluid on a dressing, the flaring of nasal alae, or the onset of pain or abdominal distention (Maloney, 1968). Monitoring devices do exactly that; they monitor the patient. Nursing care, fortunately, remains in the hands of nurses.

If they are to be useful, monitoring devices must be properly attached to the patient and in good working order. The significance of whatever information is collected must be interpreted and applied to the patient in an intelligent manner. The rational use of monitoring devices involves recognition of what kinds of information can best be secured by monitors and what their limitations are. Those using monitoring devices must recognize that clinical judgment cannot be replaced by a machine. As an example, Miss Golden is a highly experienced nurse who works in an intensive-care unit. One morning she noted a slight flaring of the nostrils of a patient who had a stab wound in his chest. Had she been less informed and experienced, she might have overlooked the change or discounted its significance. She immediately notified the physician.

Gathering of baseline data is directed toward describing and discovering the cause of the present state. Why are these things happening? Where is this person coming from? Was he or she a high-risk shock patient or is something occurring here and now that is causing these responses?

Nursing Interventions in Carrying Out Medical Prescriptions

As stated previously, one of the critical problems of the patient in shock is the maintenance of adequate respiration. The patient should be moved and turned regularly if at all possible. Because the lung is unevenly perfused and the dependent portions receive the most blood, turning should help to distribute blood to all parts of the lung. Movement also improves ventilation and adds to the patient's comfort. The physician may perform a tracheostomy to reduce the respiratory dead space. A respirator may be prescribed as needed to provide adequate ventilation. Depending on the circumstances, pressure-cycled respirators such as the Bird, or volume-controlled respirators such as the Engström may be necessary in the patient with very high airway resistance or low lung compliance. In cooperative patients with mild ventilatory problems, either the Bird or Bennett is all that is required (Hunsinger et al., 1973).

All these measures improve oxygenation of the blood and the removal of carbon dioxide. Further, they reduce the work of breathing and thus help to reduce demand in relation to supply. As a point of emphasis, none of these measures or devices achieves its purpose unless properly applied and cared for. For example, a tracheotomy does more harm than good unless the airway is kept open, by suctioning, if necessary (see Chapter 40).

Much time and attention must be devoted to the fluid therapy of the patient in shock. Although some intensive-care units are equipped with machines that monitor the infusion of fluids, nurses are responsible for noting the rate of flow and the response of the patient to the solution. Furthermore, they are usually responsible for adjusting the rate of flow in terms of the response of the patient. Because a rapid rise in CVP or PAP indicates a relative hypervolemia (it may or may not be a true hypervolemia) in relation to cardiac competency, the nurse slows the rate of flow of the solution under such circumstances and calls the physician. Continued infusion may cause congestive heart failure or even pulmonary edema.

Medications are usually a constant component of the medical therapy prescribed to treat the patient in shock. Many medications are administered as additives to the intravenous fluids, in which case the nurse must understand their intended physiologic effects and observe closely for their therapeutic or adverse effects. In addition, there are usually a number of medications, such as those prescribed to control pain, restlessness, blood pressure, and so on, for which the nurse must use judgment relative to indications for their administration. Moore and his associates (1969) urge that the nurse avoid excessive administration of p.r.n. medications to the critically ill patient.

Regulating the Environment

Perhaps the most significant nursing function in the care of the patient in shock is the control of the environment of the patient so that demands made on him or her are kept at a minimum. By so doing, the nurse can help to reduce the gap between the need and supply of oxygen and nutrients to the tissues. One of the most critical aspects of environmental modification for the shock patient is the nature and frequency of position change. Until the very recent past, the moment a patient went into shock, he or she was immediately placed in the Trendelenburg position. It was postulated that this position facilitated venous return from the lower portion of the body and improved the circulation to the brain. Recent experimental evidence has demonstrated that this position does not improve cardiac output. At times, circulation through the brain is actually decreased (Simeone, 1966). The decrease in blood flow to the brain in the Trendelenburg position may be caused by the initiation of aortic and carotid sinus reflexes causing constriction of blood vessels supplying the brain. Current thinking is that the patient should be kept flat, or at least on the same plane, with slight elevation of the lower end of the bed, creating a very gradual slope downward to the head, to facilitate drainage of secretions. It is important that the patient be kept moving, to avoid circulatory stasis. Robinson (1972) recommends, on the basis of a study of the effects of positioning on the respiratory needs of acutely ill patients, that critically ill patients who can be turned, be turned 90° every 1 to 2 hours. In-bed activity other than turning should be added and increased just as soon as the patient's vasomotor responses can tolerate positional change without marked hypotensive consequences.

An indispensable corollary to patient positioning and activity is the need of the critically ill patient for planned periods of rest and sleep. The nursing staff should develop, implement, and evaluate a plan with other members of the team to ensure periods of uninterrupted rest for the patient. REM sleep is the stage in which the greatest benefit is derived from sleep; about 90 minutes are required to reach REM sleep, which means that the patient for whom stimulation of some sort is necessary every hour is gradually becoming exhausted. Ensuring some minimal amount of uninterrupted rest for the patient in a critical-care unit is one of the greatest challenges to the skill and judgment of the nurse. Quiet efficiency, competence in giving care, and promptness in attending to the patient's needs can do much to reassure him or her that the personnel are doing what should be done. When the patient is alert and anxious, the nurse should be particularly careful to be unexcited and optimistic so that the patient's anxiety does not increase. One patient reported that the most distressing part of his stay in an intensive-care unit was hearing physicians and nurses talk about him as if he were absent. Furthermore, he was not informed about the purpose of the monitoring equipment or his progress. Attention should be given to maintaining a quiet and calm atmosphere. Visitors should be limited to members of the immediate family. The effect of family members should be evaluated and the length of their visits adjusted to their effect on the patient.

The effects of the flashing lights and the beeps of monitoring and other equipment should also be evaluated. When machines have a disquieting effect on the patient a screen can be placed so that the patient is less aware of them. The nurse, however, must always be able to see the patient and the monitoring equipment.

Attention should be given to the room temperature. At one time a warm room and warm blankets were used. It is now known that warming the patient increases the metabolic rate 7 per cent for each degree (F) of body temperature. If the patient sweats it also increases the loss of body fluids. Currently, a comfortable room temperature is advocated. In a study made on rats, Redding and Mueller (1968) found that, contrary to the belief that 20° to 24°C (68° to 75°F) was the most favorable range to the survival of the animals, those kept at 17° to 20°C (63° to 68°F) actually had the best survival rate. These authors state that the shocked animal is not poikilothermic but is unable to create sufficient energy to maintain core temperature by peripheral vasoconstriction and loss of water by evaporation.

Finally, the nurse is responsible for maintaining strict asepsis to prevent secondary infection of the shock patient. In relation to every aspect of the care of the patient, it is critical that each nurse provide meticulous orientation and reporting to each successive team or shift of nurses who assume responsibility for the care of the shock patient.

Shock Research Units

As in other areas in which active research is being performed, nurses are assisting with medical research in shock. In addition, nurses should be investigating how they can contribute to the prevention of shock and how they can alter or correct the problems before the shock becomes irreversible. Nurses who are employed in shock research units face many problems. Patients brought into the unit are frequently in a moribund condition. New as well as old methods of treatment are utilized and evaluated. Physician and nurse alike may be so occupied with only the shock or their machines that little attention is given to the patient as an individual human being. There are at times so much equipment and so many people in the unit that the nurse has difficulty getting to the bedside of the patient. In some institutions, remote monitoring devices allow the nurse to stay away from the bedside for long periods of time. Some physicians and nurses are questioning the wisdom of this practice.

Summary

Enough is known about the hemodynamic derangements in shock that they can usually be controlled. Much still remains to be learned about the respiratory complications and the metabolic cellular derangements that may result. Much has been learned about shock through experimental work on dogs and other animals, although much of this knowledge does not apply to human beings. To understand and treat shock in humans, tests and treatments must eventually be evaluated on human beings. Each time this is done the physician and the patient or a responsible member of the family must weigh the possible hazards to the patient against the possible benefits. To learn whether a measure is truly effective, human beings may have to be used as controls. Thus one may be denied a treatment while another receives it. This may be a source of stress to the nurse, the patient or family, and the physician. Despite the limitations of current knowledge, under the care of knowledgeable physicians and nurses working as a team, patients are now surviving injuries or illnesses that would have been uniformly lethal only a few years ago.

References Cited

Ahlquist, R. A. "Study of Adrenotropic Receptors." *Am. J. Physiol.*, **153** (June 1948) 596.

Carlson, R. W. "Verge of Death." *Emergency Med.*, **10** (March 1978) 26–31t.

Cohn, J. N. "Monitoring Techniques in Shock." *Am. J. Cardiol.*, **26** (1970) 565–69.

Crile, G. W. *An Experimental Research into Surgical Shock.* Philadelphia: J. B. Lippincott Co., 1889.

Gladish, et al. "Shock: Recognition and Treatment." *Postgrad. Med.*, (July 1967) 42–49.

Goodman, L., and Gilman A., eds. *The Pharmacological Basis of Therapeutics,* 5th ed. New York: Macmillan Publishers Co., 1975.

Govoni, L. E., and Hayes, J. E. *Drugs and Nursing Implications,* 3rd ed. New York: Appleton-Century-Crofts, 1978.

Hunsinger, D. et al. *Respiratory Technology: A Procedure Manual.* Reston, Va.: Reston Publishing Company, 1973.

Jacobson, E. "A Physiological Approach to Shock." *N. Engl. J. Med.*, **278** (April 11, 1968), 836.

Kooput, R. et al. "A Review of the Surgical Treatment of Complications of Myocardial Infarction." *Heart and Lung,* **6** (May–June 1977), 487–92.

Lefer, A. "Role of a Myocardial Depressant Factor in Shock States." *Mod. Concepts Cardiovasc. Dis.*, **12** (Dec. 1973), 59–64.

Lowrey, B. et al. "Electrolyte Solutions in Resuscitation in Human Hemorrhagic Shock." *Surg. Gynecol. Obstet.*, **133** (Aug. 1971), 273–84.

MacLean, L. D. "Shock: Causes and Management of Circulatory Collapse," in *Davis-Christopher Textbook of Surgery,* 11th ed., Ed. by D. C. Sabiston, Jr. Philadelphia: W. B. Saunders Co., 1977, pp. 65–94.

Maloney, J. "The Trouble with Patient Monitoring." *Ann. Surg.*, **168** (Oct. 1968), 605–14.

Martin, A. M. et al. "Pathologic Anatomy of the Lungs Following Shock and Trauma." *J. Trauma,* **8** (Sept. 1968), 687–99.

McCabe, W. "Gram-Negative Bactermia." *Dis.-a-Month* (Dec. 1973).

Moore, F. et al. *Post-Traumatic Pulmonary Insufficiency.* Philadelphia: W. B. Saunders Co., 1969, pp. 184–85.

Myers, J. "On Limitations of Theories of Biology." *Perspec. Biol. Med.*, **10** (Winter 1967), 238.

Page, I. "The Mosaic Theory of Arterial Hypertension—Its Interpretation." *Perspect. Biol. Med.*, **10** (Spring 1967), 327.

Ravin, M., and Modell, J. *Introduction to Life Support.* Boston: Little, Brown, 1973.

Redding, M., and Mueller, C. "Effects of Ambient Temperature upon Responses to Hypovolemic Insult in the Unanesthetized, Unrestrained Albino Rat." *Surgery,* **64** (July 1968), 110–16.

Rich, R. R. "Cardiogenic Shock: Combatting Its High Mortality." In *Nursing Critically Ill Patients Confidently.* Horsham, Pa.: Intermed Communication, 1979.

Robinson, J. "A Study of the Relationship between Positional Change and Respiratory Status in Seriously Ill Adults." Detroit, Mich.: Wayne State University College of Nursing, 1972. Unpublished clinical nursing problem study submitted in partial fulfillment of requirements for the M.S. degree.

Schumer, W. "Hypovolemic Shock," *JAMA*, **241** (Feb. 9, 1979), 615–1b.

The Shock Syndrome. Kalamazoo, Mich.: The Upjohn Company, 1969.

Simeone, F. A. "The Treatment of Shock." *Am. J. Nurs.*, **66** (June 1966), 1290.

Thal, A. et al. *Shock: A Physiological Basis for Treatment.* Chicago: Year Book Medical Publishers, 1971.

Thal, A., and Wilson, R. "Shock." *Curr. Probl. Surg.* (Sept. 1965).

Thompson, G. E. "How to Avoid the Pitfalls in Treating Shock." *Consultant,* **13** (Sept. 1973), 33–35.

"Tracing Clues in Shock Killer—Pulmonary Insufficiency." *Med. World News,* **12** (July 23, 1971), 20–21.

Warren, J. C. *Surgical Pathology and Therapeutics.* Philadelphia: W. B. Saunders Co., 1895, p. 279.

Weissman, C. and Thomas, L. "Studies of Lysosomes: I. Effects of Endotoxin Tolerance, Entotoxin Tolerance, and Cortisone on Release of Acid Hydrolases from a Granular Fraction of Rabbit Liver," *J. Exp. Med.*, **116** (Oct. 1962) 433.

Wilson, R. F. "Acute Respiratory Failure and How to Manage it." *Consultant,* **18:5** (May 1978, a), 25.

Wilson, R. F. "Diagnosis and Treatment of Shock." *Consultant,* **18** (Dec. 1978, b), 109t.

Wilson, R. F. "Diagnosis, Pathophysiology, Monitoring and Treatment of Shock." In *Critical Care Symposium*. Detroit, Mich.: Wayne State University Department of Surgery and the Detroit Surgical Society, 1972.

Zamora, B. O. "Management of Hemorrhagic Shock." *Hosp. Med.*, **15** (July 1979), 6–29.

Zweifach, B. "The Microcirculation of the Blood." *Sci. Am.*, **200** (Jan. 1959), 54.

General References

Alho, A. et al. "Catecholamines in Shock." *Ann. Clin. Res.*, **9**:3 (June 1977), 157–63.

______. "Anaphylaxis and the Community Nurse." *Nurs. Mirror,* **145** (Sept. 8, 1977), 41–42.

Bouwman, D. L. et al. "Effects of Albumin on Serum Protein: Homeostasis after Hypovolemic Shock." *J. Surg. Res.*, **24**:4 (April 1978), 229–34.

Brookman, L. B. et al. "The Early Assessment of Hypovolemia: Postural Vital Signs." *JEN,* **3** (Sept.–Oct. 1977), 43–45.

Carey, L. "Three Questions and Answers about Fluid Therapy in Shock." *Consultant,* **14**:10 (Oct. 1974), 47.

Chrzanowski, A. "Intra-aorta Balloon Pumping; Concepts and Patient Care." *Nurs. Clin. North Am.,* **13** (Sept. 1978), 513–30.

Ciued et al. "Dopamine in Cardiac Failure and Shock." *Br. Med. J.,* **2**:6102 (Dec. 17, 1977), 1563–64.

______. "When a Disaster Happens How Do You Meet Emotional Needs?" *Am. J. Nurs.,* **77** (March 1977), 454.

Feustel, D. "Autonomic Hyperreflexia." *Am. J. Nurs.,* **76** (Jan. 1976), 228–30.

Franco, L. M. "Acute Disseminated Intravascular Coagulation." *Cardiovasc. Nurs.,* **15** (Sept.–Oct. 1979).

Graff, C. "Warning: Don't Jump to Conclusions When a Patient's in Shock." *RN,* **42** (Aug. 1979), 28–8.

Hastings, P. R. et al. "Antacid Titration in the Prevention of Acute Gastrointestinal Bleeding." *N. Engl. J. MED.,* **298** (May 11, 1978), 1041–44.

Hayward, R. P. "Emergency Care of the Cardiac Patient." *Nurs. Mirror,* **144** (April 14, 1977), 45–49.

Kones, R. J. "Rational Therapy in Cardiogenic Shock." *Hosp. Formulary* (Jan. 1977).

Lasser, R. P. et al. "Cardiogenic Shock in the Coronary Care Unit." *Am. J. Cardiol.,* **41**:3 (March 1978), 613.

Pepine, C. J. et al. "Guidelines to Evaluation and Management of Shock." *Hosp. Med.,* **15** (March 1979), 88–130.

Robinson, J. "Septic Shock in Cardiopulmonary Patients." *Hosp. Med.,* **15** (Oct. 1979), 19–28.

Rosenthal, S. "The Treatment of Shock." *J. Trauma,* **19**:11 Suppl. (Nov. 1979), 875–76.

Shires, G. I. "Pathophysiology and Fluid Replacement in Hypovolemic Shock." *Ann. Clin. Res.,* **9**:3 (June 1977), 144–50.

Tharp, G. D. "Shock: The Overall Mechanisms." *Am. J. Nurs.,* **74** (Dec. 1974), 2208.

Thompson, M. A. *Shock Syndrome.* Reading, Mass.: Addison-Wesley, 1978.

Tinker, J. "Intensive Care—4 Shock." *Nurs. Times,* **74**:10 (March 9, 1978), 406–8.

Webb, G. E. "Hypertension and Hypotension in the Recovery Room." *J AORN,* **26** (Sept. 1977), 546t.

Wilson, R. F. et al. "Pathophysiology, Diagnosis and Treatment of Shock." *JEN,* **3** (Sept.–Oct. 1977), 11–25.

46

Problems with Nutrition

Somewhere—the place it matters not—somewhere
I saw a child, hungry and thin of face—
Eyes in whose pools life's joys no longer stirred,
Lips that were dead to laughter's eager kiss,
Yet parted fiercely to a crust of bread.

Prayer for Children [*1944*]
FRANCIS JOSEPH,
CARDINAL SEPPLAN

Taken from *Bartlett's Familiar Quotations* Thirteenth and Centennial Edition p. 953a Little, Brown and Company, Boston, 1955.

The Role of the Nurse in Meeting the Need of Individuals for Food

In general, the physician prescribes a diet designed to meet the individual requirements of the patient for food. The dietary prescription is based on knowledge of the nutritional state of the individual as well as the modifications imposed by the nature of the illness. To illustrate, Mrs. Smith, aged 65, has a diagnosis of diabetes mellitus and obesity. The dietary prescription written by her physician is based on the following knowledge of Mrs. Smith. She is a 65-year-old woman who leads a sedentary life. She is 25 lb. overweight and has diabetes mellitus. A loss of excess weight will probably be accompanied by a lessening in the severity of her diabetes mellitus. The physician prescribes a low-calorie diet approximately meeting her basal needs. The prescription allows an adequate quantity of protein, minerals, and vitamins. By reducing the calories, the carbohydrate and fat are correspondingly restricted. Thereby the physician hopes to lessen the quantity of insulin required by Mrs. Smith. The low-calorie diet will result in gradual loss of weight and some reduction in the severity of her diabetes.

In many hospitals, dietitians translate the dietary prescription into food. They plan the menus and supervise the preparation of food. Like the physician, they depend to a considerable extent on the nursing staff to relay problems encountered by the patient that interfere with his or her ability to eat or to enjoy food. Dietitians also counsel the patient who will continue to modify food intake after leaving the hospital. In public health agencies dietitians may act as consultants to nurses, as well as instructors to patients and their families.

The responsibilities of the nurse in meeting the nutritional needs of patients are many and varied. The extent of these responsibilities differs somewhat in different hospitals and health agencies. In the small community hospitals nurses frequently perform many of the functions of dietitians. No matter how highly organized the food service is, however,

Revised by Gloria J. Smokvina, R.N., Ph.D., Associate Professor of Nursing, Purdue University Calumet; Hammond, Indiana.

the nurse has a significant contribution to make in meeting the nutritional needs of patients. The nurse's objectives are to help the patient to understand why food is essential to health, and to help him or her select, accept, and follow the diet indicated by assessment of his or her nutritional status and/or as prescribed by the physician. To achieve these objectives, the nurse has the following responsibilities:

1. To assist in the collection of data about the food pattern of the patient, likes and dislikes, and the methods and facilities available for food preparation
2. To obtain the diet prescription, if one has not been provided
3. To plan so that the patient receives food suited to his or her needs and, inasmuch as is possible, desires
4. To prepare an environment conducive to eating
5. To prepare the patient so that he or she is in a comfortable position and in condition to eat
6. To prepare the patient for what to expect, if the diet is different from his or her usual food pattern and to explain the reasons for modification in the diet
7. To observe and report the appetite and food preferences of each patient
8. To observe and report the adequacy of the food intake of the patient
9. To observe the patient's attitude toward food
10. To feed or supervise the feeding of patients who are unable to feed themselves
11. To give appropriate emotional support to those who must be fed or must learn to feed themselves or whose food habits require modification
12. To give appropriate assistance to those who need some help
13. To instruct the patient and family and to answer questions about the diet
14. To identify those patients who will require some assistance in obtaining or preparing a suitable diet after dismissal from the hospital
15. To communicate with the patient, family, the physician, and the dietitian in such a way that the needs of the patient are met and the lines of communication are kept open
16. To assist the patient and/or members of the family in meal planning, budgeting, buying, and preparing a nutritious diet
17. To provide assistance to patients and/or members of the family in the home to
    a. Make the required adjustments at home,
    b. Provide assistance to the patient who requires a therapeutic diet, but does not require hospitalization
    c. Assist the patient to modify usual food pattern so that basic and special needs are met
18. To feed the patient by an abnormal route and to aid the patient and/or members of the family in learning how to perform the necessary procedures.[1]

Factors to Consider in Examining a Person for Nutritional Disorders

Studies of Nutritional Status

Examination for the effect of disease on the nutritional status of the individual includes weighing the patient, measuring skin-fold thickness, and observing for signs of rapid loss of weight and dehydration. Changes in the skin, fissuring of the lips, a sore mouth, bleeding gums, and changes in the color of the tongue may also be indicative of nutritional problems. Determinations on the blood levels of specific nutrients or their metabolites and on urinary excretions of metabolites indicate abnormalities in metabolism that result from dietary inadequacy or from interference with nutrition caused by some pathological state. For example, the hemoglobin level, erythrocyte count, and hematocrit provide evidence for or against iron-deficiency anemia. But in a seriously dehydrated patient the levels might appear normal; thus the laboratory determinations would be misleading if the physical examination did not make note of the state of dehydration. Low total protein and serum albumin levels give evidence of protein deficiency that has, in most instances, persisted over a long period of time inasmuch as general tissue depletion has taken place before the blood levels were lowered. Urinary excretions may indicate tissue depletion of some vitamins, or may indicate inability to complete certain metabolic sequences.

Assisting with Diagnosis

Although the making of the medical diagnosis is a primary function of the physician, the nurse assists in a number of ways. One of the most valuable contributions a nurse can make is accurately to observe, report, and record observations. The nurse uses the senses of hearing, touch, sight, and smell to gain information about the patient and the effects of his

[1] Some of these functions may be referred to others.

or her disease and therapy. "Nearness to the patient" is extremely important, for most disorders usually involve a strong emotional component (G.I. Series, 1975). One of the significant aspects of observation is an alertness to changes in the behavior of the patient and to any conditions in the environment that appear to be related. For example, Mrs. Smathers vomits within 15 to 20 minutes from the time she receives morphine sulfate. Mrs. Cletus, who has had a gastric resection, suffers an attack of severe pain during each of her husband's infrequent visits. Mr. Brave, following a gastric resection vomited bright red blood. Each of the preceding has implications for the diagnosis and treatment of the respective individuals. Mrs. Smathers probably has an intolerance to morphine, and another drug should be substituted for it. Unless the nurse makes the connection between the time the drug is administered and the time vomiting occurs, Mrs. Smathers may continue to be made uncomfortable. Unless the observation is made about the time Mrs. Cletus's pain occurs, the emotional factors in her illness may be missed. Finally, unless the nurse knows how much blood Mr. Brave has vomited, the survival of the patient may be threatened.

In addition to collecting information through observation of the patient, the nurse assists in diagnosis by preparing the patient for examination, by performing certain parts of some diagnostic tests, and by collecting secretions or excretions from the alimentary canal. Examinations for disease of the alimentary canal are of three types. The canal or some part of it is directly or indirectly visualized, the contents are collected for examination, or determinations are made of the effects of the disorder on the nutritional status of the individual.

The details for the preparation of patients for different diagnostic tests vary from one institution or physician to another. A few generalizations will, however, be made that should be helpful. The different types of tests will be defined or described and the conditions necessary to their performance suggested.

The direct observation of the lining mucosa of an organ is known as *endoscopy.* The term for a particular endoscopic examination is formed by joining the combining form for the organ with the suffix *scopy:* thus *esophagoscopy, gastroscopy, duodenoscopy, colonoscopy,* or *proctoscopy.* Direct visualization of the mucosa is limited to the organs that are accessible from the natural orifices, the mouth and the anus. An exception is a peritoneoscopic examination. A small incision is made in the abdominal wall to gain entrance into the peritoneal cavity. In addition to providing a means for the examination of the appearance of the mucosa or peritoneum, tissue and secretions can be removed for purposes of examination. New fiberoptic scopes allow for direct visualization, photography, biopsy, excision, and/or fulguration of lesions. As with the passage of any instrument, perforation, bleeding, and infection are potential complications.

X-ray is utilized in fluoroscopy and in making shadow photographs of all organs of the alimentary canal from the esophagus to the anus. In both procedures a contrast medium is introduced into the organ to be studied. In fluoroscopy the progress or movement of the contrast medium through the canal can be followed. As the roentgen rays pass through the body, they are projected onto a fluorescent screen. X-rays are shadow photographs that provide a permanent record.

Noninvasive techniques such as scanning procedures using radioactive substances are useful in detecting organ abnormalities. Ultrasound is sometimes employed to detect abdominal masses, whereas echography, reflected ultrasound imaging, is useful in detecting biliary stones (see Chapter 11, discussion of radiation).

Arteriography with the injection of a dye is employed to detect tumors and sites of blockage. In addition, radioimmunoassay is useful in measuring serum concentrations of alpha-fetoprotein, a cancer-related protein. Carcinogenic embryonic antigen serum levels are frequently elevated in patients with cancer of the colon with liver metastasis.

Secretions from the upper and midportions of the alimentary canal can be removed for examination. Secretions are examined for the concentration of normal constituents and for substances not normally present in the secretion. The capacity of the glands of the stomach to respond to food or other secretory agents can be determined. Both secretions and excretions are examined for blood, pus, and microorganisms. Feces are also examined for parasites and ova.

Preparation of the Alimentary Canal for Examination

The preparation of the patient for examination of the alimentary canal depends on the nature of the test to be performed. In general, food and fluid are withheld in preparation for examinations of the upper and middle alimentary canal and previous to roentgen examination of the large bowel. Food or fluids in the stomach or intestine interfere with the performance of the examination by getting in the way of the instrument or by occupying space. In studies made on gastric juice, the physician is interested in determining the concentration of hydrochloric acid before and sometimes after the acid-secreting glands are stimulated. Therefore gastric juice is tested for acid while the patient is in the fasting state. The patient may then be given a test meal consisting of dry toast or arrowroot cookies and weak tea or water, and the test repeated. Secretion of gastric juice can be further increased by the ingestion of ethyl alcohol or the subcutaneous injection of histamine. Because histamine dilates arterioles and capillaries, susceptible patients may experience a marked drop in blood pressure. It is well for the patient who is to receive histamine to be in bed. If the fall in blood pressure is marked, it may be necessary to place the patient in a supine position. Other effects of histamine include intense headache, shortness of breath, vomiting, and diarrhea. Gastric analysis no longer occupies the position of importance that it once did in the diagnosis of disease of the stomach and intestine.

In endoscopic examinations of the upper alimentary canal, food and fluid should be withheld, because the swallowing reflex is depressed when the pharynx is anesthetized before the tube is passed. Should the patient vomit, he or she is in danger of aspirating food or fluid into the airway. Care of the patient during and following endoscopic examination of the esophagus is similar to that following bronchoscopic examination.

In preparation of the large intestine for examination by x-ray or endoscopy, the bowel is emptied. A clear liquid diet is prescribed prior to the procedure. An irritant or saline cathartic such as castor oil or magnesium citrate may be taken followed with enemas on the evening before and morning of the procedure. When enemas "until clear" are prescribed they should be conscientiously performed, as either feces or gas interferes with the filling of the bowel with the contrast medium and thereby distorts the resulting shadow.

Following roentgen examination of the gastrointestinal tract, particularly after colon x rays, the barium sulfate introduced into the bowel as a contrast medium should be evacuated. The patient may be instructed to take, or be given, an enema to wash out the barium remaining at the end of the procedure. Mineral oil may also be taken daily until all the barium is evacuated. For unless the barium is evacuated, it may form a hard mass in the bowel because the water is absorbed.

Summary

During the period when the patient is undergoing diagnosis, the nurse makes a number of valuable contributions. Through conscientious and informed observations, the nurse collects information about the patient and his or her reactions to the disease, to diagnostic procedures, and to therapy. The nurse helps to prepare the patient both physically and psychologically for the different diagnostic procedures and cares for the patient when and after the examinations are performed. One point that bears emphasis is that many of the methods utilized in the examination of the alimentary canal are unpleasant. They require that meals be withheld and the contents of the canal be removed by catharsis, enema, and stomach tube. In the performance of some examinations a tube may be introduced into the mouth or the anus. Although the patient knows that the various procedures are necessary, he or she still feels miserable. In all probability the patient is anxious about the outcome of the various examinations and may, with or without reason, fear the presence of cancer. Insofar as is possible, the patient should be protected from preventable sources of distress. He or she should be prepared for what to expect and what can be done for self-help. Attention to personal hygiene and to serving meals promptly after a test is completed may not seem to be crucial to the onlooker but can do much to remove controllable sources of irritation.

Determinants of Effects of Disease or Injury of the Alimentary Canal

Any disorder interfering with the capacity to ingest, digest, or absorb one or more nutrients will interfere with the nutritional status of the affected individual. Other effects will depend on the nature of the disorder and the organ or organs affected. As has been repeatedly emphasized, the gastrointestinal tract is sensitive to the general condition or status of the body as a whole. Disorders in other parts of the body are frequently accompanied by one or more disturbances in the gastrointestinal function.

The structures forming the gastrointestinal system are subject to the same types of disorders as other body parts. Disturbances in gastrointestinal functioning may result from messages sent by the mental apparatus, from direct injury to cells, or from a response to injury or threat of injury. Because the system is a muscular structure, under control of the autonomic nervous system, disorders of motility and secretion are frequent.

As is true of all cells, blood supply is necessary to survival. The rich blood supply of the mucosa, the relationship of the veins draining the alimentary canal and the portal circulation to the liver, and the fact that any bleeding into the lumen of the gut is not opposed by a rapid rise in tissue fluid pressure mean that life-threatening hemorrhages are a frequent problem.[2] Massive bleeding into the lumen of the alimentary canal usually initiates the vomiting or defecation reflex, and blood is evacuated in vomitus or from the rectum. Bleeding into the lumen of the alimentary canal is not always massive. Small quantities may be lost at one time or continue to be lost over an extended period of time causing a microcytic anemia.

Blood supply to a portion of the alimentary canal may be cut off by arterial or venous thrombosis, by twisting of the small intestine, or by incarceration of a viscus or the mesentery by a ring through which one or more body structures normally pass. For example, the mesentery of the intestine may slip through the inguinal or femoral ring. Neither the mesentery nor the intestine normally passes through either of these rings, and protrusion into one of them is known as an inguinal or femoral hernia.[3] Should the contents be trapped, the venous return is impeded and swelling occurs. Unless the incarcerated tissue or organ is removed from the hernial sac, the intertissue pressure will be raised sufficiently to prevent blood from entering the area, and tissue necrosis will occur.[4]

Epithelial and other types of cells in the mucosa of glands along the alimentary canal can and do undergo neoplastic change. Neoplasms can be either benign or malignant. For some unexplained reason, neoplasms rarely are found in the small intestine. Neoplasms in the alimentary canal cause harmful effects by obstructing the lumen of the gut and thereby preventing the normal passage of food. Pedunculated neoplasms may twist on their pedicles and cause symptoms associated with the necrosis. In the small intestine they may act as a focus predisposing to the twisting or volvulus of the intestine. The neoplasm may undergo necrosis and predispose to bleeding from ulcerations formed at its surface. Specific effects of any neoplasm will depend on its nature and location in the alimentary canal. Neoplasms are discussed in detail in Chapter 39.

The lining mucosa is exposed to a variety of mechanical, chemical, and living agents of extrinsic origin, as well as to the digestive juices. Cells may be sensitive to ordinarily harmless substances; that is, they are or become allergic. Depending on the nature of the etiology and the extent of the injury, the mucosa may be acutely or chronically inflamed, infected, or ulcerated. If there is sufficient tissue destruction, scar tissue may be formed in the process of healing. Depending on its location and extent, the scar tissue, as it matures and contracts, can reduce the size of the lumen of the gut or block a duct opening into it.

To illustrate the above, Mr. Brave has a peptic ulcer in the proximal portion of his duodenum. Ulceration is due to an imbalance between the capacity of the mucous membrane lining his duodenum to resist digestion and the action of the digestive ferments. In the healing of the ulcer, scar tissue was formed, and as it matured, it contracted. Because the area of ulceration was small and not close to the opening of the ampulla of Vater,[5] healing took place without causing obstruction.

The wall forming the alimentary canal acts as a barrier protecting the internal from the external environment. In health, the internal environment is protected not only from unusable or partly digested nutrients, but from the entrance of digestive enzymes and large numbers of microorganisms. When, as a result of surgery, trauma, or disease, the wall of the alimentary canal is penetrated, its contents escape into the surrounding cavity.

Esophageal Perforation

When the esophagus is perforated, secretions and food can enter the trachea or mediastinum depending on the level of the lesion. Either is serious. The effects of food and fluids entering the trachea have been discussed in Chapter 26. In the mediastinum, the esophagus is near the heart, aorta, lungs, vagus nerves, thoracic duct, vertebral column, and diaphragm. Food escaping into the mediastinum carries bacteria with it. Either food or bacteria can be responsible for abscess formation. Because of its location and poor blood supply, lesions of the esophagus are difficult to treat. For example, Mrs. Bird swallowed a large fish bone. It became lodged in and perforated her esophagus, resulting in secretions and microorganisms gaining access to the mediastinum. A mediastinal abscess was formed as a result. Because of the possibility of perforating the wall of the esophagus, a person should neither manipulate nor

[2] In solid tissues, bleeding raises the intertissue pressure, which opposes further bleeding.

[3] A *hernia* is the protrusion of the contents of a body cavity through a defect in the wall of the cavity. When the protrusion occurs near the surface of the body, it can be felt as a bulge.

[4] When herniated tissue can be returned to its proper cavity, the hernia is said to be reducible. When it cannot be removed, it is irreducible or incarcerated, and when the venous return is obstructed and swelling takes place, it is said to be strangulated.

[5] The duct formed by the union of the common bile duct from the liver and the duct of Wirsung from the pancreas.

allow anyone except a physician to attempt to remove an object caught in the esophagus. Should a chicken or fish bone or other object become lodged in the esophagus, no time should be lost in seeking assistance from a physician. No other person should be allowed to try to remove it.

Peritoneal Perforation

Penetration of structures below the diaphragm allows the contents of the stomach or intestine to escape into the peritoneal cavity. Depending on the site of perforation, digestive juices and bacteria gain access to the peritoneal cavity. Certain anatomical features increase the hazard to the patient. They include (1) the large continuous surface of the peritoneum; (2) the aid given to the distribution of the contents entering the peritoneal space by respiratory, abdominal, and intestinal movements; and (3) the inhibition of phagocytosis and the enhancement of bacterial growth provided by the intestinal contents.

Despite its liabilities, the peritoneum is well adapted to defending itself provided that contamination is not too great or prolonged. As in other areas, the basic defense mechanism is inflammation. A second defense mechanism is the ability to form fibrous adhesions. They cause the mesentery and omentum to adhere together, aiding in the localization of the infection.

When leakage is small, the body may be able to wall off the area and prevent the dissemination of the contents of the alimentary canal throughout the peritoneal cavity. At the time Mr. Brave had a recurrence of his ulcer, it penetrated through the wall of the duodenum and into the peritoneum. He did not have generalized peritonitis, however, because his body was able to wall off the area. Mary Alice Todd had acute appendicitis with the formation of an appendiceal abscess. The inflammatory process around the diseased appendix was sufficient to wall off the leakage from it and to prevent generalized peritonitis.

When, however, a viscus is suddenly perforated and a large quantity of stomach or intestinal content enters or continues to gain entrance to the peritoneal cavity, the protective and reparative powers of the peritoneum may be overcome, resulting in generalized peritonitis. Even with a fairly large opening, the peritoneum is able to defend itself against most bacteria for a few hours. Thereafter, its defensive capacity fails rapidly. Prompt closure of an opening between the digestive tube and the peritoneal cavity is therefore of the greatest importance.

Peritonitis

Peritonitis is frequently secondary to perforation of the alimentary tract, or leakage from the liver, biliary tract, or pancreas. Disease or injury of the alimentary tract, in which perforation of viscus occurs, includes stab and gunshot wounds in the abdomen, perforated peptic ulcers, ruptured appendices or diverticuli, postoperative leakage, and strangulating obstruction of the intestine. One of the hazards in cholelithiasis (gallstones) is that a stone can act as a ball valve, allowing bile to enter the gallbladder, but not to escape. As the wall of the gallbladder distends, its blood supply lessens and predisposes the wall to necrosis and gangrene. With necrosis of its wall, bile escapes into the peritoneal cavity and causes peritonitis.

The manifestations of peritonitis are caused by (1) the responses of the peritoneum, (2) the systemic responses to injury, and (3) sepsis. In generalized peritonitis, from 4 to 12 liters of inflammatory exudate may be formed. Because of its large "weeping" surface, the situation of the patient is similar to that of one who has been burned.

When contents of the alimentary canal escape into the peritoneal cavity, the patient usually experiences abdominal pain. This pain is usually severe and may be either generalized or localized. The patient also presents signs and symptoms of increased sympathoadrenal activity: pallor, sweating, an anxious expression, and rapid pulse and respiration. He or she will eventually have signs and symptoms of sepsis; fever and rapid pulse and respirations. The alimentary tract responds first by vomiting. Eventually gastrointestinal activity is depressed, absorption ceases, and the abdomen becomes distended. The abdominal wall is tender and rigid, and splinting of the diaphragm results in shallow, grunting respirations. Leukocytosis indicates a general response to the injury. Patients who fail to develop leukocytosis generally have a poor prognosis.

Nursing Care

The responsibilities of the nurse differ somewhat with the causes of peritonitis. Individuals who have an acute gastrointestinal disorder or what is commonly referred to as "stomach flu" should avoid ingesting food or fluid during the attack. They should *not* take either a laxative or an enema. When a patient who has a peptic ulcer experiences sudden, severe pain, the physician should be notified immediately. Time should not be wasted on the hypothesis that, given time, the pain will disappear. No fluid, food, or drugs should be administered orally. When there is any doubt about the cause of abdominal pain, or when pain continues for more than a few hours, a physician should be consulted.

Should the pain be caused by perforation of the alimentary tract and the physician decide that the opening is to be closed surgically, the operation is usually performed as soon as possible. The care of the patient following closure is similar to that of any patient having abdominal surgery. Whether or not surgical closure is effected, the prevention of gastrointestinal distention is important. To prevent distention, a long tube is introduced by way of the nose, pharynx, esophagus, and stomach into the small intestine. Suction is applied to establish and maintain decompression. Because the patient is unable to take fluids and foods orally, fluids must be administered parenterally to maintain and correct fluid and electrolyte balance and to provide calories and amino acids. Whole blood may be administered to restore blood proteins. Antibiotics and sulfonamides are usually prescribed to combat bacterial infection.

Pain should be prevented, without unduly depressing the patient. Small doses of morphine or one of the morphine substitutes may be used for this purpose. Morphine has the particular advantage of decreasing the segmenting contractions of the small intestines.

Care directed toward making and keeping the patient comfortable is very important. Because the patient with peritonitis is very ill, he or she should be allowed to be sick. The patient's needs should be anticipated and the responsibility for care assumed by the attendants. He or she should be placed in a comfortable position. Some physicians recommend that the head of the bed be elevated and the patient placed in a semi-Fowler's position. The patient should be moved and turned regularly to prevent respiratory and circulatory complications. The position should also facilitate drainage of pus to the outside when drains are present. The environment should be quiet and nonstimulating. Talking should be limited to that required for care. Personal care, such as mouth hygiene and bathing, should be performed by the nurse. The patient should be protected from unnecessary exertion. As the patient recovers, activity should be increased.

From the preceding general background discussion, it should be clear that no serious disorder in the structure or function of any part of the digestive system is without its effects on the functioning of the entire system or on the body as a whole. It is easier, however, and the presentation is likely to be clearer, if the function or functions of each organ and the effects of alterations in function are presented separately. Discussions will be related primarily to the effects of disturbances in functions of the various organs and the implications of these to nursing. Specific diseases are outlined at the end of this chapter in Table 46-3.

Alterations in the Ability to Ingest Food and Fluids

Inability to Masticate

Lack of teeth is the most common cause of failure to chew food adequately, but teeth that are painful and carious (decayed) also interfere with chewing. Painful lesions of the gums, tongue, or buccal mucosa interfere with the chewing and mixing of food. Inability to open or close the jaws will obviously make chewing difficult, if not impossible. As the result of rheumatoid arthritis, Mr. Gerald has an ankylosis (stiffness or fixation) of the mandibular joints. He can separate his teeth only about 2 cm, which makes it difficult to be introduced for food into his mouth and for him to grind it. He is given soft and liquid foods. Mr. Elmer fractured his mandible in an automobile accident and his jaw has been wired. All food and fluids have to be introduced into his mouth through a tube.

Patients who cannot properly masticate their food should be served food in a liquid or semisolid form. The nurse has a responsibility for determining whether or not the patient needs to have the consistency of some or all food altered in order to eat it. For example, some people with poor natural teeth or dentures can eat most foods but cannot eat meat unless it is tenderized or ground.

In addition to the grinding surface provided by the teeth, the act of chewing requires the power or energy to open the jaws and to close them with force on the food. Power is provided by the muscles of mastication. In disorders such as myasthenia gravis[6]—great muscle weakness—the patient may quickly tire if required to masticate an ordinary diet. To conserve energy and maintain food intake, the food may have to be ground or be soft.

Mouth Care

Because the teeth are essential to proper mastication of food, their care is important. According to

[6] Myasthenia gravis is a disorder in which there is a defect in transmission of impulses at the myoneural junction. The patient experiences weakness. For some reason, many patients with this disorder have difficulty in breathing and swallowing before other muscle function is seriously impaired.

some dentists, the baby should be taught to brush his or her teeth when the first tooth appears. Regular dental care, as well as good nutrition, is important in the care of teeth. The salivary glands are the site of the common infectious disease mumps. Debilitated patients, in whom oral intake is restricted, are susceptible to an infection of the parotid gland, called surgical parotitis. Its prevention is based on an adequate fluid intake, cleanliness of the mouth, and stimulation of the flow of saliva. An adequate intake of fluid makes an important contribution to keeping the mouth clean and moist. In sick and debilitated patients this requires time, planning, and attention of nursing personnel, and it should not be left to chance. Mouth care, including the brushing of the teeth, should be performed at least every 4 hours. Stimulation of the flow of saliva is essential. Measures such as chewing gum and sucking on lemon or orange slices or lemon sour balls are all useful in encouraging salivation.

Dysphagia, Pain, and Heartburn

Difficulty in swallowing is known as dysphagia. Its effects depend on its cause and the degree to which the passageway is obstructed. The person with dysphagia may be unable to swallow either food or fluids or may be able to swallow foods of one consistency, for example, solids, and not be able to swallow those of another, possibly liquids. The patient may also have periods of dysphagia with little or no difficulty in between them. Accurate descriptions of the type and timing of the difficulty in swallowing experienced by the patient are very important in establishing the cause of dysphagia. When an individual is unable to swallow any food or fluid, evidences of dehydration and starvation appear very quickly.

The following anatomic and physiologic features of the pharynx and esophagus, as related to swallowing, influence the nature of the disorders to which the esophagus is prone. (1) The act of swallowing is regulated by the nervous system. (2) The pharynx and esophagus constitute a tube connecting the mouth and stomach. The tube can become obstructed by scars or neoplasms, and it can be perforated by foreign bodies. (3) The tube, being lined with mucous membranes, is subject to the growth of benign or malignant neoplasms. (4) The esophagus passes through the mediastinum; any neoplasms or abscesses of the mediastinal structures may obstruct the esophagus. Perforation of the esophagus allows the esophageal contents to leak into the mediastinum, a most serious event, as the mediastinum is bounded by the pleurae and pericardium. (5) The esophagus is drained by the azygos veins, which serve as an alternate route when the portal vein is obstructed. They are poorly supported by connective and epithelial tissue. In cirrhosis of the liver the blood flow through the portal vein is impeded and seeks alternate routes; one route is the azygos veins. With elevation in venous pressure, the veins dilate, developing varices. As the walls become thin, they are increasingly susceptible to rupture and bleeding. Unlike the situation in solid tissues, the bleeding is not opposed by rising interstitial fluid pressure. Blood is vomited and also evacuated in the feces. (6) The esophagus is incompletely protected by the cardiac sphincter from the effects of gastric juice. Features (1) to (4) may make swallowing difficult because of functional or mechanical obstruction.

Dysphagia may be of reflex or functional origin or may be caused by an obstruction in the pharynx or esophagus. Reflex disturbances are usually responsible for interference with the second stage of swallowing, while obstructing lesions are more likely to be responsible for dysphagia in the third stage.

The factors causing a disturbance in reflex activity in dysphagia are similar to those that cause disorders in reflexes in any part of the body. Dysphagia can conceivably arise from disordered function in any part of the reflex arc—receptors, centers in the central nervous system, or effector nerves or cells.

The swallowing centers in the brain can be stimulated or inhibited, with the result that swallowing or the coordination of the various activities involved in swallowing fails. Inhibition of or failure to transmit impulses over some part of the reflex arc may also be responsible for failure in swallowing.

Functional Dysphagia

As so other centers regulating bodily functions, the swallowing center receives messages from the higher centers in the brain, including the cerebral cortex. Dysphagia may therefore be a manifestation of emotional disturbance. Frequently the patient says that he or she cannot swallow because there is a lump in the throat that the patient believes is caused by a neoplasm. Despite a thorough examination of the esophagus and the information that the esophagus is healthy, the patient states that he or she knows there is a tumor even though it cannot be seen.

Although it is sometimes difficult to demonstrate, the interference with swallowing may be a spasm at some point of the esophagus. Mrs. Clifford is a good example of a patient who is starving because she believes that she has an invisible tumor. She is a lonely widow whose husband died after a long and trying illness. Her children are married and live at a distance. For Mrs. Clifford, life holds little promise.

She suffers from marked dysphagia. As far as can be demonstrated by fluoroscopy, esophagoscopy, and studies of cells taken from the mucosa, her esophagus is free from any evidence of neoplasia or other structural disease. Despite evidence to the contrary, Mrs. Clifford believes that she has cancer. When she tries to swallow, she says, there is a lump in her throat that prevents it.

Mrs. Clifford's food intake is limited almost entirely to small quantities of milk. She has lost so much weight that her skin hangs loosely. As is characteristic in starvation, she lacks energy. The preparation of adequate meals requires more effort than she can muster. Although Mrs. Clifford's illness was precipitated by the loss of her husband, she is now physically ill from a lack of food. Unless her food intake is increased in quantity and quality very soon, irreversible changes will take place in her cells and she will die from the direct effects of starvation. Attention must therefore be given to improving the nutritional status of Mrs. Clifford, if she is to survive. There are no easy answers to the problem of bringing about an increase in food intake in patients such as Mrs. Clifford. In the instance of Mrs. Clifford, a close relative spent some weeks with her. The relative planned the meals around what Mrs. Clifford could and would eat. Progress in the beginning was slow, but as Mrs. Clifford made an effort to eat, she gained strength and her general outlook improved. More food did not cure her basic problems, but it did contribute to her capacity to cope with them. The maintenance of food intake is of no less importance in the patient whose dysphagia is caused by an emotional problem than it is in the patient who has an organic lesion.

Lesions in the Cranial Cavity

In addition to dysphagia caused by disturbances in function, lesions within the cranial cavity interfere with the function of the swallowing centers in the brainstem. Lesions are of two general types: those that lessen the blood supply to the area and those that result in inflammation. Inflammation, by causing swelling also diminishes the blood supply. The blood supply to the swallowing center may be lessened by an obstruction of a blood vessel by a thrombus or an embolus. Intracranial pressure may be raised by neoplasms, particularly those obstructing the free flow of cerebrospinal fluid, and by edema of the brain resulting from the response of the brain tissue to injury. Usually the difficulty with swallowing is manifested as a failure to coordinate swallowing with breathing, so that the patient is in danger of aspirating saliva and secretions from the nasal and pharyngeal cavities, as well as food and fluids. Disturbances in the regulation of swallowing can originate from injury to peripheral nerves supplying the muscles involved in swallowing. Finally, failure of transmission of nerve impulses from a nerve to a muscle will cause dysphagia.

Because the patient cannot manage his or her own secretions, they must be removed by gravity and suctioning. Oral fluids, food, and drugs must be withheld until the patient is able to swallow. The objective is to protect the patient from aspiration of foreign material into the airway. The patient with myasthenia can swallow normally until he or she becomes fatigued; therefore, measures should be taken to limit fatigue.

Obstructive Lesions

In the esophagus itself, dysphagia can be caused by a variety of disorders that obstruct the lumen and block the passage of food and/or fluid. Among the causes of obstruction of the esophagus are neoplasms, malignant and benign, inflammatory strictures, congenital defects, hiatus hernia,[7] foreign bodies, achalasia, and extrinsic pressure. The most frequent causes of mechanical obstruction of the esophagus are neoplasms and strictures caused by the formation of scar tissue. All obstructing lesions have a common effect. They interfere with the ability of the individual to ingest enough food to meet nutritional needs. Patients with one of the above disorders are often in poor nutritional condition when admitted to the hospital. As a matter of fact, they are all too often in a state of near starvation. They are usually treated surgically after the diagnosis is made and the gross nutritional, water, and electrolyte deficiencies and anemia are corrected. Because the route of approach to the esophagus is through the thorax, attention must be paid to reestablishing and maintaining the expansion of the lungs during the immediate postoperative period.

Observation of Patients

Careful and accurate observation of the patient who is dysphagic is important. What, if anything, is the patient able to swallow? Are there any circumstances that affect the ability of the patient to swallow? If the patient regurgitates, what are the characteristics of the emesis? For example, does the regurgitated material contain digested or undigested food particles? Does it contain blood? Does the pa-

[7] A hiatus is a gap or opening in the diaphragm. In hiatus hernia, contents of the abdominal cavity escape through the hiatus into the thoracic cavity. A lay term for hiatus hernia is *upside-down stomach*.

tient complain of pain or other sensations before, during, or after swallowing? When are the symptoms intensified or relieved? The patient may be aware of the point where food is delayed as it passes through the esophagus. When the patient complains of pain or discomfort, where is it located and what is its general character?

Pain

Other symptoms associated with alterations in the function or structure of the esophagus include pain and heartburn. Painful sensations accompany the ingestion of irritating substances such as dilute hydrochloric acid. Regurgitation of the acid chyme from the stomach into the esophagus also causes pain and may cause ulcerations. Spasm or distention of the esophagus, particularly when associated with ulceration of the esophagus, is a cause of pain. When the pain-evoking stimulus is continuously present, the pain is burning in character. When the stimulus is applied intermittently, it is likely to be gripping and intense.

Heartburn

Heartburn, or pyrosis, is a condition experienced by most persons at some time in their lives. Despite its name, heartburn has no relation to the heart or to its function. It is characterized by a burning sensation over the precordium or beneath the sternum and is accompanied by the regurgitation into the esophagus or mouth of the acid gastric juice. Heartburn is one of the discomforts of pregnancy. In persons with hiatus hernia or cardioesophagcal hernia, foods such as cake, sweet rolls, and orange juice induce heartburn. The mechanism for this disorder is not known, though a recent animal study suggests that large meals may be implicated. Large meals appeared to abolish the increases in sphincter pressure observed after eating. As a result, it follows that this would make one more prone to acid reflux and subsequent heartburn. (ACS, 1977).

Uses of Tube Feedings, Elemental Diet, and Intravenous Hyperalimentation

Tube Feeding

Another problem created by the inability to swallow is the maintenance of the fluid intake and the nutritional status of the patient. If the individual is unable to swallow, but a tube can be passed through the esophagus, a nasogastric tube may be introduced into the stomach. Food or fluids may be introduced into the tube at regular intervals or continuously. The latter method requires some means of keeping the food cold to prevent the multiplication of bacteria that cause food poisoning. When a tube cannot be passed through the esophagus, a tube may be placed directly into the stomach by way of an incision in the abdominal wall and stomach (gastrostomy) or jejunum (jejunostomy). Following either a gastrostomy or a jejunostomy, food and fluid are introduced by the tube into the stomach or the jejunum.

For food to be introduced through a tube, it must be in a liquid state. Tube feedings prepared from the foods of a normal diet are preferred to formula feedings because they are generally more appealing to the patient, and they are less likely to produce diarrhea. Any foods that make up a nutritionally adequate normal diet may be blended with liquid in a high-speed blender and strained several times to remove fiber that is likely to clog the tube. For convenience, infant foods including strained meats, vegetables, fruits, and fruit juices, as well as milk, eggs, and cereals, are used because they are low in fiber. Because of the frequency of eggs being contaminated with Salmonella, it is advisable to cook the eggs with milk in the form of a soft, thin custard.

Some patients prechew food before placing it in the tube. Though the spitting of food into a funnel after it is chewed may appear unesthetic or even revolting to the onlooker, one should make an effort to concentrate on the benefit the patient receives from this practice. The patient should be protected from onlookers and embarrassment by adequate screening. Unless the patient plans to chew the food before it is placed in the tube, it should be liquefied. When the patient is physically able and emotionally ready to feed himself or herself, he or she should be taught to perform the procedure. The nurse should be certain that the food served to the patient has been properly liquefied. For weeks Mr. Good, who had developed an esophageal fistula following a laryngectomy and radical neck resection, was repeatedly served lumpy wheat cereal for breakfast. The lumps were large enough to obstruct the feeding tube and they could have been removed easily by straining the cereal. Because of the nature of his surgery. Mr. Good was not able to chew the cereal before introducing it into the tube. Quite understandably Mr. Good interpreted the lumps to mean that the hospital personnel were persecuting him.

Elemental Diet

The elemental diet is a chemically defined, bulk-free diet composed of elemental or semielemental nutrient compounds (Young et al., 1975). It represents a step between parenteral hyperalimentation and oral or tube feedings of normal diets. The elemental diet differs from standard tube feedings in that it contains amino acids, oligopeptides, simple sugars, and a variable fat, mineral, and vitamin content. The osmolarity is highly variable with all preparations being hyperosmolar, and therefore requiring additional water to prevent dehydration. For individuals with a known or suspected lactose intolerance, or for those patients who develop nausea, vomiting, diarrhea, or distention postoperatively, a lactose-free preparation such as Ensure may be tried.

The elemental diet is indicated for patients who are unable to tolerate conventional foods. The diet is completely absorbed in the upper small intestine and provides minimal residue in the lower intestine. The advantages of elemental feeding are that it provides a means of maintaining positive nitrogen balance without exposing the patient to all the risks associated with parenteral nutrition. In addition, it avoids nutrients that may be unacceptable to a diseased gastrointestinal tract. Some conditions for which elemental diet are recommended are preoperative bowel preparation, postoperative colonic and rectal surgery, gastrointestinal fistulas, inflammatory bowel disease, short bowel syndrome, pancreatitis, food allergies, and other conditions that induce catabolic states (Bury, 1976). The major complications of elemental feedings are nausea, vomiting, diarrhea, aspiration hyperglycemia, nonketotic hyperosmolar coma, fluid and electrolyte imbalance, and hypoprothrombinemias. These complications may be prevented or attenuated by slow administration, elevating the head of the bed, monitoring blood glucose and electrolytes, reducing the carbohydrate load, and administering vitamin K.

Intravenous Hyperalimentation

Intravenous hyperalimentation or total parenteral nutrition (TPN) is the intravenous infusion of nutrients above the basal requirements of a patient to meet anabolic needs. Any condition that results in prolonged interference with a patient's ability to ingest, digest, or absorb food, or that creates excessive metabolic demands that cannot be met by other nutritional means, may necessitate TNP. It is used as an adjunct in the treatment of intrinsic inflammatory bowel disease; in catabolic states such as cancer; in intractable, excessive diarrhea; and also by some patients prior to and following major abdominal surgery or surgical resection of the bowel.

The composition of the hyperalimentation solution should vary according to the specific organ impairment and disease being treated. The solution generally contains 20 to 30 per cent glucose for its nitrogen-sparing effect, 5 per cent protein hydrolysate or crystalline amino acids, and 5 per cent solute of vitamins, minerals, and trace elements. Because of its hypertonicity, hyperalimentation fluid is infused into the superior vena cava or the innominate veins via the subclavian or jugular veins. These veins are used because their diameter is large enough to allow blood dilution of the infusing fluid.

Fat emulsions are beginning to be used, since 10 to 20 per cent fractionated soybean oils have been made commercially available. The advantages of the fat emulsion are that it provides twice the caloric value of glucose, is an isotonic fluid which does not exert an osmotic pressure, and it can be administered with other nutrients (amino acids and carbohydrates) into a peripheral vein (Fischer, 1976). When fat emulsions are used, fat-soluble vitamins are given weekly.

Although the optimal amounts of nonessential amino acids are not known, the utilization of the amino acids is improved if all the common nonessential amino acids are included (Wretlind, 1972). Synthetic amino acids mixtures are available, but their use is associated with hyperchloremic acidosis. The hyperchloremic acidosis due to the crystalline amino acid solution may be avoided by giving sodium and potassium requirements as the acetate salt. To achieve a positive nitrogen balance it may be necessary to infuse between 80 and 160 g of protein equivalent per 24 hours. For every 1,000 calories infused it will be necessary to add 40 to 50 mEq of sodium and 30 to 40 mEq of potassium (Fischer, 1976).

A minimum requirement of 100 g of carbohydrate daily is necessary for nourishment of the brain, for prevention of excessive sodium and water loss, and for its anabolic effects. Glucose is used except with patients who are under stress. They receive fructose, which can be utilized without insulin. This concentration of glucose in the hyperalimentation fluid demands an increased secretion of insulin from the pancreas. Administering a graduated amount of glucose gives the body a chance to adapt, but it may be necessary to give exogenous insulin to allow the carbohydrate to be metabolized fully.

The hyperalimentation solution is an excellent growth medium and therefore should be mixed by a pharmacist or nurse using a closed system such as a laminar flow filtered air hood to prevent contamination. The solution is used within 24 hours of its preparation or it is discarded. Electrolytes are added immediately before they are used.

Possible complications that may occur with hyperalimentation are septicemia, sensitivity to peptides, hemothorax, atrial or ventricular irritability, air embolism, hyperglycemia, brachial plexus injury, cardiac overload, dehydration, phlebitis, electrolyte imbalance, hyperosmolar coma, acalculous cholecystitis, and hyperglycemia on discontinuing the infusion, due to insulin rebound.

Nursing Care

Caring for patients who are receiving this type of feeding requires careful observation and a thorough knowledge of the principles of asepsis. The dressings over the intravenous site are changed every 24 or 48 hours under strictly aseptic conditions and the patient is observed for any signs of the onset of an infection. Any elevation in body temperature must be given immediate attention. Urine glucose and acetone are monitored frequently to check the body's utilization of the available carbohydrate. The rate of flow of the solution must be kept constant to avoid radical shifts in the nutrients available to the body. Daily weights should be taken to ensure that the patient's weight is not shifting rapidly because of fluid gain or loss. To avoid exposing the intravenous line to unnecessary sources of clots, the nurse should ensure that the line is not used to administer anything else. An additional intravenous should be used for the administration of medications or blood if they are indicated.

It requires skill and careful planning to replace the nutrients lost to the body by the loss of an ability taken for granted; the ability to ingest food.

Alterations in the Ability to Digest Food and Absorb Nutrients

The Stomach and Proximal Duodenum

Because the stomach and the adjacent portion of the duodenum perform common function and are the site of several frequent disruptions and serious diseases, they will be discussed as a unit. The most frequent disruptions are anorexia, nausea, and vomiting. The diseases are peptic ulcer, gastric carcinoma, and hypertrophic pyloric stenosis. Inflammation of the stomach, or gastritis, is not uncommon. Knowledge of the physiology of the stomach and duodenum is essential to understanding the disorders of this region. (See Table 46-3 at the end of this chapter.)

Vomiting

Possible Effects

Vomiting is a commonly occurring condition. The vomiting reflex can be initiated by a wide variety of intrinsic and extrinsic factors. Frequently more than one element is involved in a patient who is vomiting or who continues to vomit. The prevention and treatment of vomiting depend on its cause and how long it continues. Although vomiting removes irritating materials from the gastrointestinal tract, it also removes water and electrolytes and interferes with the ingestion of food. In a well-nourished person who vomits for a brief period of time, the latter effects are of little moment. Some emotionally disturbed persons who vomit do not lose weight because they actually vomit very little food. In the patient who is debilitated or who continues to vomit not for a few hours but for days, vomiting may result in dehydration, metabolic alkalosis, and serious loss of weight. It may also contribute to the problem of maintaining or improving the nutritional state of the individual. In patients who have had surgery, vomiting may place strain on the site of the incision by increasing pressure within the abdominal, ocular, and cranial cavities. Vomiting after surgery on the eye predisposes to intraocular bleeding. If vomiting occurs in a patient who had undergone surgery on the eyes, it should be brought to the attention of the physician immediately. Orders for antiemetic drugs should be carried out faithfully.

Treatment

Treatment of the patient who is vomiting is based on its cause and effects. If vomiting is associated with acute appendicitis or diabetic acidosis, the obvious treatment is to remove the inflamed appendix or restore glucose metabolism, and to correct the disturbances in water and electrolyte balance. When treatment is directed toward the control of vomiting, procedures are selected that relieve vomiting by (1) removing irritating substances from the stomach, (2) relieving or preventing distention of the stomach, (3) diminishing the sensitivity of the chemoreceptor trigger zone, (4) discontinuing the administration of drugs stimulating the chemoreceptor trigger zone, (5) correcting metabolic disorders in which circulating "toxins" activate the chemoreceptor trigger zone, and (6) correcting imbalances and deficits in water and electrolytes.

When the stomach is distended because of failure to empty, nasogastric suction is usually prescribed. The advantages of this method of emptying the stomach are that distention can be prevented, and repeated and prolonged vomiting can be controlled. (See Chapter 51 for discussion of the nurse's responsibilities for nasogastric suction.)

A number of antiemetic drugs act by raising the threshold of the chemoreceptor trigger zone to stimulation. The first found to be effective was chlorpromazine (Thorazine) most effective phenothiazine is prochlorperazine (Compazine). A more recent drug, benzquinamide hydrochloride (Emete-con), has proven useful in the treatment of nausea and vomiting associated with anesthesia and surgery. Other drugs include dimenhydrinate (Dramamine), trimethobenzamide (Tigan), promethazine (Phenergan) and the barbiturates. Some of these drugs are useful not only in the treatment of vomiting, but also in its prevention in motion sickness.

Physical and chemical agents used in the treatment of disease may induce vomiting. Therapy with x-ray or radioactive isotopes, particularly when applied to the upper abdomen, frequently causes some degree of nausea and vomiting. Usually treatment with radioactive substances is continued, despite the presence of vomiting. Some drugs such as digitalis cause nausea and vomiting when toxic dosages have been reached. When it has been established that vomiting is due to the toxic effects of a drug, it may be discontinued temporarily or permanently or its dosage reduced. Other drugs such as morphine and meperidine (Demerol) induce vomiting in susceptible persons. When nausea and vomiting regularly follow the administration of a drug and diminish in severity as time elapses after it is given, idiosyncrasy to the drug should be suspected. The discontinuance of the drug is usually all that is required to correct the nausea and vomiting.

Nursing the Person

In addition to the treatment prescribed by the physician, the nurse can do much to lessen the discomfort of the patient who is vomiting. There are few more disagreeable or unpleasant symptoms than nausea and vomiting. For many persons, the presence of a kindly and solicitous person makes vomiting more bearable.

The nurse or other person attending the patient may experience nausea while assisting the patient and may find it difficult to stay with him or her. The nurse can suppress the vomiting reflex by swallowing and by concentrating on what can and should be done to assist the patient. Should simple measures be ineffective, the nurse should discuss the problem with the instructor, supervisor, or physician.

During vomiting, nursing care of the patient should be based on two objectives: (1) to prevent the aspiration of vomitus and (2) to increase the comfort of the patient. To lessen the possibility of aspiration during emesis, if at all possible the patient should be turned to one side and the head should be flexed at the neck. Factors predisposing to nausea and vomiting in susceptible patients should be identified and controlled. Insofar as possible, pain should be prevented or kept under control. The room should be well ventilated. Strong odors—dressings, emesis, perfumes—should be eliminated from the environment. The emesis basin should be emptied and washed immediately after use. Because there is a psychic element in vomiting, the suggestion is usually made to keep the basin within easy reach, but out of sight. If, however, the patient is more relaxed when the basin is where it can be seen, this factor should be taken into consideration. After vomiting, the patient should have an opportunity to rinse out his or her mouth. Soiled bed linen should be changed. Becuase moving predisposes to an attack of nausea and vomiting, necessary changes in position should be made slowly. Sometimes the vomiting reflex can be supressed by deep breathing and by initiation of the swallowing reflex. Not infrequently the gastrointestinal tract must be placed at rest for a period of time before oral fluids are tolerated. If the condition of the patient allows, carbonated beverages such as ginger ale or soda may be tolerated when other fluids are not. In children popsicles are frequently tolerated when all else fails. Either cold or hot fluids are generally better tolerated than tepid ones. A combination of measures is sometimes necessary to control vomiting. The patient should be encouraged in the belief that something can be and is being done to control the vomiting.

The following case illustrates the value of simple measures in the control of vomiting triggered by anesthesia and prolonged by metabolic and emotional factors. Alexandra Berry, who was attending college far from home, fell and fractured the radius of her left arm. The fracture site was placed in a splint immediately, but several hours elapsed before Miss Berry was admitted to the hospital and the fracture reduced under thiopental sodium (Pentothal Sodium) anesthesia. As soon as Miss Berry regained consciousness, she was discharged to the college dormitory. For the next 24 hours, she continued to vomit. Since psychic factors were undoubtedly important, the dormitory nurse cleared the room of anxious friends. She also removed the bucket being used as an emesis basin. She obtained a large bottle of chilled ginger ale and encouraged Alexandra to sip it slowly. Each time Alexandra retched, the nurse encouraged her to swallow and breathe deeply. After an hour or so, Alexandra was able to rest comfortably without vomiting. The nurse bathed Alexandra, changed her bed, aired the room, and suggested firmly that the measures that she had instituted would cure her. They did.

Although vomiting was probably induced by the effect of the anesthetic on the chemoreceptor trigger zone, psychic factors were undoubtedly important in its continuance. Miss Berry had a frightening experience, she was far from the comforting presence of her family, and she was treated by a strange physician. Furthermore, with the loss of fluid and failure to ingest food, some degree of electrolyte imbalance presumably increased the activity of the chemoreceptor trigger zone. Factors contributing to the control of vomiting included deep breathing, swallowing, and the drinking of ginger ale. The ginger ale provided fluid required to correct dehydration, and it provided a ready supply of glucose. With the correction of glucose starvation, the rate of mobilization of fat is depressed and the degree of metabolic acidosis is lessened. The probability also exists that Miss Berry responded in a positive way to the presence of an individual who was in control of the situation and who appeared to be convinced that the vomiting could and would disappear. Of course, not all patients are as easily helped as was Alexandra. The specific measures utilized in the therapy of vomiting depend on its cause and its effects.

Among the pertinent observations are the nature of the onset and the circumstances surrounding vomiting. Has the patient been apparently well and then become suddenly ill or has he or she been unwell for a period of time? How long has the patient been vomiting? Is vomiting preceded by nausea? What other signs and symptoms does the patient have? When does the patient vomit in relation to food intake or to the ingestion or injection of drugs? The emesis should be observed for amount, odor, general appearance, and presence of blood. Fresh blood is bright red, while flecks of partly digested blood give the vomitus a coffee ground appearance. In addition to the making of pertinent observations, they should be accurately recorded. Whether or not they are immediately drawn to the attention of the physician will depend on the extent to which prompt action is required. When in doubt, the nurse should notify the physician.

The Dumping Syndrome

Gastric incontinence that follows bypass or destruction of the pyloroantral pump due to gastrectomy, gastroenterostomy, antrectomy, pyloroplasty, or vagotomy may result in the *dumping syndrome*. The patient will experience symptoms because the contents are rapidly "dumped" into the jejunum, shortly after a meal, particularly one containing large amounts of carbohydrate or, in some individuals, lactose. The ability to regulate the rate at which chyme enters the intestine is impaired, with the result that the intestine is dilated by a large volume of concentrated material. The concentrated material in the intestine may in turn cause a contraction of blood volume. In addition, the release of excessive vasoactive hormones from the small intestine may also occur. All of these may operate together in producing the postcibal vasomotor symptoms associated with the dumping syndrome. However, none of the proposed theories completely explains the dumping syndrome in a satisfactory way.

The symptoms frequently experienced are weakness, profuse perspiration, nausea, dizziness, flushing, epigastric fullness, and palpitation. Two to 3 hours after eating, hypoglycemia may occur. The sequence of hypoglycemia is as follows: The rapid entry of a large amount of carbohydrate into the circulation causes a marked, but transient, hyperglycemia. Insulin is secreted in excess of the quantity required to restore the level of glucose in the blood to physiological limits, resulting in hypoglycemia.

A high-protein, high-fat, low-carbohydrate diet given in small, frequent feedings helps to control the symptoms. Meat, fish, poultry, eggs, cheese, and fats are liberally used. Complex carbohydrates such as those in cereals, breads, and vegetables are gradually added, but sugars and sweetened foods are rigorously avoided. Liquids are taken between, but not with, meals. Some patients lie down after eating, whereas others eat in a reclining or semireclining position. Sedatives or antispasmodic drugs may be prescribed. In the postgastrectomy adult, milk should be avoided due to the limited capacity of the jejunum to hydrolyze lactose, rendering a state of lactose intolerance (Condon et al., 1969).

Although the manifestations accompanying the dumping syndrome are frightening and unpleasant, they usually disappear with time. The patient should therefore be reassured that the disorder is not dangerous and that in time he or she will recover. For the American who judges the success of therapy by the immediacy of results, the waiting period may well be a trying one. Today with more conservative surgery being performed in larger university centers, dumping is reported in only 0.4 to 7 per cent of patients (Sawyers, 1978). Proximal gastric vagotomy without drainage preserves gastric emptying and the normal release of duodenal hormones.

Ulceration

Benign ulcers in areas exposed to acid-pepsin are categorized as peptic ulcers. All ulcers in the gut have some similarities. They can be shallow or deep, hypertrophied or proliferating, benign or malignant. They differ in fundamental respects such as etiology, natural history, prognosis, and treatment. (See Table 46-3 at the end of the chapter for details.)

Causes

Ulceration results from an imbalance between the digesting action of gastric juice and the capacity of the gastric and duodenal mucosa to resist digestion. In effect, the digesting action of the gastric juice may be increased, or the resistance of the mucosa lining the stomach and duodenum decreased, or both. Continuous or intermittent hypersecretion of hydrochloric acid is believed to be responsible for the increase in the digesting action of the gastric juice. Hypersecretion can be the result of (1) overstimulation of the secretory mechanisms, (2) failure of the mechanisms inhibiting secretion, or (3) failure of the mechanisms for neutralizing hydrochloric acid. Failure to regenerate epithelium at a rapid rate, failure to secrete an adequate quantity of mucus, and a poor blood supply can all reduce resistance of the mucosa. Ulcerogenic drugs such as aspirin, corticosteroids, phenylbutazone, indomethacin, sympathetic blockers such as reserpine and certain antiobiotics are capable of inducing gastric mucosal irritation, stimulation, or areas of ischemia (Menguy, 1978). Although ulcers in the duodenum are always benign, ulcers in the stomach can be either benign or malignant. Malignant neoplasms in the stomach may eventually ulcerate. Although peptic ulcers are usually chronic, they may also be acute.

Acute ulcers are of two types: Cushing's and Curling's. The acute ulcer of Cushing is found in disorders of the nervous system, particularly in disorders involving the anterior hypothalamus. It is frequently associated with serious brain injury and is thought to be mediated by vagal stimulation resulting in hyperacidity.

Curling's ulcer was first described by Curling, who noted the formation of ulcer of the stomach and duodenum in patients who had been burned. More recently, the formation of acute gastric and duodenal ulcers has been reported in patients who have experienced various types of trauma. Because some degree of stress is involved, these ulcerations and their associated signs and symptoms are frequently referred to as "the stress ulcer syndrome." (See Chapter 52 for discussion of cause, mechanisms, and treatment of stress ulcers.)

Patients who are predisposed by disease or injury to acute ulcer formation should be observed for symptoms and signs indicating ulcer development. Any type of pain or discomfort in the upper abdomen should be brought to be attention of the physician. Onset may be ushered in with hemorrhage or perforation. Either is an emergency and should be treated as such; that is, the physician should be notified immediately. Fluids and food should be withheld until the physician indicates that they can be safely given. The patient should be kept quiet and as comfortable as the situation permits.

Duodenal Ulcer

To summarize some aspects of duodenal ulcer, including methods of treatment, Mrs. Carrie Maple, a 43-year-old charwoman, will be presented. Five years previous to her present admission to the hospital, Mrs. Maple had undergone a subtotal thyroidectomy for the treatment of hyperthyroidism. Shortly thereafter, she experienced pain in the epigastric region about 1½ to 2 hours after eating. X-ray examination of her stomach and duodenum revealed an ulcer in her duodenum. She was treated by diet and an aluminum hydroxide antacid. She responded well and treatment was discontinued after 3 months. Mrs. Maple continued to be well until 2 days prior to her admission to the hospital, when she noted that her stools were tarry. The following day she had lower abdominal pain radiating to her upper abdomen and several loose, tarry stools.

At the time of her admission she was feeling weak and dizzy. Her hemoglobin was 7.8 g per 100 ml of blood and her erythrocyte count was 2.37 million cells per cubic millimeter of blood. Both the hemoglobin level and the erythrocyte count were reduced to approximately half of normal, indicating serious blood loss. Although her hematocrit was 28 per cent (the normal is about 42 per cent), her blood pressure was 142/88, indicating that the blood volume had been maintained despite the loss of blood. (See Chapters 44, 45, and 52.) She required 2,000 ml of blood to raise her hemoglobin to 13.4 g.

In many respects, the history presented by Mrs. Maple is characteristic of the patient with duodenal ulcer.

As stated previously, duodenal ulcer occurs where there is an imbalance between the digesting action of gastric juice and the capacity of the mucosa in the stomach and duodenum to resist digestion. Exactly why ulceration occurs is not known. Authorities agree that certain factors are predisposing. One is that hypersecretion of acid must have a role in ulcer formation. Not all patients, however, can be shown to have hyperchlorhydria, as there is some overlapping between the level of secretion in patients with ulcer and the upper limits of normal secretion.

In duodenal ulcer, secretion of hydrochloric acid is increased as are the number of parietal cells. Some investigators have found an increase in the secretion of gastrin. A number of other hypotheses have been suggested and found wanting. Why any of these conditions occurs is not known. What is known is that ulcers heal and remain controlled providing that acid secretion can be neutralized or reduced by one third to one half by medical or surgical means.

The possibility that duodenal ulcer may have a genetic basis stems from the observation that it occurs more frequently among persons of blood group O than among other groups. It is also associated with the nonsecretion by the stomach of ABH substances. Both of these are hereditary traits that are inherited independently of each other, but their effect is additive. The person who belongs to blood group O and who secretes the ABH substances is less likely to develop duodenal ulcer than the person who inherits both traits. Although these observations have been made, proof is lacking that there is an hereditary factor predisposing to duodenal ulcer. Mrs. Maple had type A blood and was Rh positive. No determination was made of the secretion of ABH substances in her gastric juice or saliva. As far as she knew, no one in her family had ever had an ulcer or bleeding into the alimentary canal. There was no evidence suggesting that heredity directly contributed to her development of a duodenal ulcer.

Despite disagreement about the mechanisms involved, direct observation of the stomach indicates that it responds to different stimuli by hypersecretion and engorgement. The first to report this effect was Beaumont. He made direct observations on the lining of the stomach of Alexis St. Martin who had a gastric fistula. The later work of Wolf and Wolff (1947) further supported and extended the concept that the stomach responds to many forms of stimuli by secretion. Prolonged emotional disturbance associated with anxiety, guilt, resentment, anger, or hostility has been demonstrated to evoke vascular engorgement accompanied by increased secretion and motility of the stomach.

A number of elements including genetic predisposition, emotional stress, sex, and age, as well as other factors may combine to upset the balance between resistance to digestion and the digesting action of acid-pepsin. Duodenal ulcer is probably caused by the interaction of multiple factors.

It will be remembered that the onset of ulcer symptoms in Mrs. Maple followed thyroidectomy to correct hyperthyroidism. As with peptic ulcer, the onset of hyperthyroidism may be coincident with a period of emotional stress. As a shy, retiring person, Mrs. Maple did not conform to the stereotype of the "ulcer personality" of the hard-driving, anxious-to-succeed, "wants what he wants when he wants it" person. She gave some evidence of being depressed, because she was found crying on several occasions. She may have felt angry but turned her anger against herself.

Mrs. Maple's ulcer illustrated an almost textbook picture of the behavior and manifestations of duodenal ulcer. Five years prior to her present attack, she had had pain and nausea, appearing 1½ to 2 hours after eating. The pain responded to treatment with hourly feedings on the hour alternated with hourly doses of an aluminum hydroxide antacid taken on the half hour. As a result of this schedule, she ingested either food or medication each half-hour. *Pain, food, relief* is the most common manifestation.

Despite the fact that normally the gastric mucosa does not produce the sensation of pain, pain is the most frequent symptom associated with peptic ulcer. The two main hypotheses advanced for it are that (1) hydrochloric acid irritates the exposed sensory nerve endings in the edges and base of the ulcer, and (2) pain results from increased motility or spasm of the muscle at the ulcer site. The second view is favored because pain occurs in the absence of an increase of hydrochloric acid.

Although Mrs. Maple did not remember the exact nature or location of the pain associated with her first ulcer, the pain of uncomplicated ulcer is almost always located in the epigastrium and is limited to a small localized area. When an ulcer is located on the posterior wall of the duodenum, the pain sometimes is referred to the back. Pain is steady, and it may be described as gnawing, or it may be dull, aching, or burning.

Three characteristic features of the pain, its chronicity, periodicity, and relationship to the ingestion of food, are considered to be pathognomonic of the disease. Although not true of Mrs. Maple, patients not infrequently have periodic attacks of pain for 5 or 6 years before seeking medical attention, and ulcers may have been present for as many as 40 or 50 years. Recurrences are common, even among patients who continue under medical supervision, and are often triggered by a situation associated with an increase in stress. Sources of stress may include a traumatic injury or a frustrating situation at the office.

During her first attack, the pain experienced by Mrs. Maple demonstrated the characteristic relationship to the ingestion of food inasmuch as it occurred from 1½ to 2 hours after meals. Most patients have pain from 1 to 3 hours after eating and secure relief by the ingestion of food or antacids.

At the time of Mrs. Maple's current admission to the hospital, she had one of the complications associated with peptic ulcer—hemorrhage. At the time of her admission, the priority objective in her care was to stop the bleeding and to restore the elements lost as a result of hemorrhage. (See Chapters 41, 42, 45, and 52 for details.)

The most common complication of ulcers is intractability, or the failure to heal with treatment. New drug therapies, particularly histamine H_2 receptor antagonists such as cimetidine, make possible the control of many so-called intractable ulcers (Zollinger, 1978). Total gastrectomy is greatly reduced, and when surgery is indicated more conservative procedures such as proximal gastric vagotomy without drainage are being performed. Conservative procedures are associated with fewer undesirable effects.

Two other relatively frequent complications, penetration of the duodenal wall (perforation) and obstruction of the pylorus, have been discussed previously. Obstruction may be caused by edema, inflammation, muscle spasm, or the contraction of scar tissue. Unless there are frequent recurrences of the ulcer with the formation of scar tissue in healing, obstruction is likely to be temporary.

Gastric Ulcers

Gastric ulcers and duodenal ulcers may be two different diseases. The reasons this is believed to be so are that

1. Duodenal ulcers occur more frequently in men, whereas gastric ulcers occur in men and women with equal frequency.
2. Patients with gastric ulcers have a high incidence of gastric cancer whereas patients with duodenal ulcers do not.
3. Gastric secretion is elevated in patients with duodenal ulcers but is normal in patients with gastric ulcers.
4. Duodenal ulcer development is more frequently associated with emotional stress than is gastric ulcer development (Yager & Weiner, 1971).

It has been postulated that gastric ulcers are an autoimmune disease or are caused by a reflux of bile. The detergent action of bile acids on the antral epithelium is regarded as a common initiator of tissue damage. This is compounded by the back-diffusion of hydrochloric acid into the gastric wall, which results in chronic gastritis.

As knowledge of the natural history of duodenal ulcer has increased, two problems have become evident. The disease has a tendency to undergo spontaneous remission as well as spontaneous recurrence. Further symptoms tend to be relieved long before the ulcer heals.

Based on the observation that duodenal ulceration does not occur in the absence of hydrochloric acid, medical and/or surgical treatment is instituted to reduce its secretion or to neutralize it. The treatment employed for acid peptic disease is diet, antacids, H_2 receptor antagonists, and, in the head-injured patient, anticholinergics. Attention should be given to psychic, emotional, or social factors producing life stress. Surgical therapy may also be utilized to bring about a similar effect. Proximal gastric vagotomy without drainage has been used in all situations requiring surgical treatment and is considered appropriate in cases intractable to medical therapy. Mrs. Maple was treated successfully by medical means.

DIET. Diet and antacids are usually prescribed in relation to each other in order to secure and maintain the continuous neutralization of the gastric juice. Physicians vary in the emphasis they place on the traditional bland diet. Some physicians prescribe half-hourly feedings of milk and antacid during the phase of acute ulcer activity. Mrs. Maple was allowed clear liquids and milk for the first 2 days of her hospitalization. She was given 3 oz of milk every 2 hours and 1 oz of Maalox—a creamy white, colloidal suspension of magnesium and aluminum hydroxides. By the third day of her hospitalization there was no longer any evidence that Mrs. Maple was bleeding, and the physician prescribed a bland diet with six feedings for her. The bland diet is a transitional diet between milk feedings and an ordinary house diet.

The underlying principles for dietary management in duodenal ulcer are these: (1) A nutritionally adequate diet, often with emphasis on protein, iron, and ascorbic acid, is essential so that the nutrients required for rapid healing of the ulcer are readily available. Many patients, in fact, have some degree of undernutrition because they have consumed inadequate and restricted diets, either prescribed or self-imposed. (2) Regularity of meals requires particular emphasis inasmuch as many patients have eaten hastily at irregular intervals or have skipped meals. Five or six small meals including a light meal at bedtime are recommended. Frequent meals dilute the stomach contents and have some effect on the neutralization of acid. Some protein food, for example, whole or skim milk, should be included in each of the feedings. Although protein foods stimulate acid secretion, they also have a buffering effect that more than balances the acid production. (3) Food selection should be based on individual tolerances. The results of short- and long-term studies indicate that restriction of the diet to bland foods does little to alter the course of the disease. However, the American Dietetic Association lists black pepper, chili powder, caffeine, coffee, tea, cocoa, and alcohol as irritating to the gastric mucosa (Position Paper, ADA, 1971). These foods should be avoided, at least in the early stages of treating an ulcer.

Some clinicians have also questioned the advisability of prolonged use of milk–cream feedings inasmuch as the high saturated fat content of these regimens may predispose to atherosclerosis and coronary thrombosis. (See also "Lipid Metabolism," p. 1001). In addition, the protein in milk is thought to stimulate more gastric secretion than it absorbs unless repeated doses of it are given (Piper, 1969).

ANTACIDS. Antacids are effective in preventing as well as in relieving ulcer pain. Although soluble antacids such as sodium bicarbonate and calcium carbonate neutralize acid most effectively, they cause systemic alkalosis in some patients. As a consequence nonabsorbable antacids such as aluminum hydroxide gel or magnesium trisilicate are prescribed. Aluminum gels have a tendency to be constipating and magnesium salts to cause diarrhea. Therefore magnesium and aluminum oxides are frequently combined. Large quantities of milk and antacids can produce the milk-alkali syndrome.

Different brands of antacids vary in their buffering capacity, in their effectiveness in individuals, and in their sodium content. Mylanta II exhibits the largest capacity for buffering (Samborsky, 1978). Antacids if taken in a fasting state are less effective than if taken 1 hour postprandially. They may be prescribed as frequently as every hour to provide symptomatic relief in acid peptic disease.

Nothing should be ingested that stimulates the secretion of acid without neutralizing it or that directly irritates the gastric mucosa. For example, alcohol is a potent stimulator of gastric secretion, but it does not neutralize the acid after it is secreted. Neither should the patient be given, or take, a drug that directly irritates the gastric mucosa, such as the salicylates. The most frequently used form of this drug is acetylsalicylic acid, or aspirin. The daily or very frequent ingestion of aspirin appears to predispose to hemorrhage from the stomach. Mrs. Maple was given codeine, 32 mg, when she complained of headache. A patient with a diagnosis of peptic ulcer should be instructed *not* to take either aspirin or drugs containing it or other salicylates without a specific prescription from a physician who knows that the patient has an ulcer.

Because there is evidence that smoking decreases acid neutralization by reducing pancreatic biliary HCO_3 secretion in the duodenum and increases duodenogastric reflux, physicians generally discourage smoking. In fact, some physicians feel so strongly about smoking that they refuse to treat patients who do not cooperate. (See Chapters 39 and 43 for a discussion of some of the aspects of discontinuing smoking.)

ANTICHOLINERGICS. Because hydrochloric acid is one of the essential factors in ulcer formation, an ideal drug would appear to be one that depresses its secretion. Such a drug would, in effect, produce a chemical vagotomy. There are a number of drugs available that do block the action of acetylcholine on smooth-muscle and gland cells. Because stimulation of the vagus nerve results in the release of acetylcholine and increases gastric secretion and motility, the effect of the anticholinergics or cholinergic-blocking agents is to decrease secretion and motility. The use of these agents is greatly diminished today due to the undesirable effects of a therapeutic dose. In essence, the therapeutic dose is frequently the toxic dose.

HISTAMINE H_2-RECEPTOR ANTAGONIST. A new field of drug therapy has gained wide acceptance in the management of peptic ulcer in the United States. The drug is a histamine H_2-receptor antagonist known as cimetidine. It is known that histamine stimulates gastric secretion and that it has two known receptors, H_1 and H_2. It is thought that the H_2 receptor is specific for gastric acid secretion. A histamine H_2-receptor antagonist blocks the effect of histamine and thereby reduces the secretion of gastric acid. The precise mechanism of action is unknown. What is known is that cimetidine substantially reduces the volume and secretion of acid in a resting state and following stimulation by food, histamine, pentagastrin, insulin, and caffeine (Clayman, 1977).

H_2 receptors exist in other parts of the body such as the heart, blood vessels, brain, and leukocytes, but no major side effects of blockade have been detected. In England cimetidine is used and found effective in treating both gastric and duodenal ulcers. In the United States its use is not approved for gastric ulceration or erosion, or for reflux esophagitis.

John Chambers suffered with recurrent duodenal ulcers. He was placed on cimetidine 300 mg at mealtime and bedtime. Eight hours following the administration of the drug his pain subsided and he felt much better since his aggravation was gone. Since John's ulcer was recurrent, he was placed on maintenance therapy and will be monitored for side effects. The most common side effects are: reversible gynecomastia; diarrhea; muscle pain; rash; elevated serum transaminase, alkaline phosphatase, and creatinine levels. The effects of long-term therapy are not yet known.

PSYCHIC FACTORS. One of the most important aspects in the care of the patient with a peptic ulcer is attention to the psychic factors in the illness. As indicated previously, gastric secretion, motility, and blood supply to the gastric mucosa are all responsive to a wide variety of stimuli in the environment. Some patients respond positively, that is, their ulcers heal, when they are removed from a stressful environment. For example, Mr. George fits the stereotype of the patient with a peptic ulcer. He was a tense, hard-driving executive. He smoked cigarettes excessively, and, although he never became intoxicated, he consumed several cocktails in the course of most days. He often took work home at night, and his weekends were spent playing golf with business associates. When his ulcer symptoms finally became so severe that he could no longer ignore them, he consulted a physician and the diagnosis of peptic ulcer was confirmed. Mr. George and his physician decided that, instead of being admitted to a hospital, he should take a long-planned hunting trip with his wife. Plans were made for the trip. Mr. George agreed to eliminate smoking and the drinking of alcoholic beverages. He also took a bottle of Mylanta

II, a liquid antacid, with him. Most of all, he planned to relax and enjoy himself. Within a few days of his arrival at the hunting lodge his symptoms had disappeared. At the time of his return to his physician 1 month later, his ulcer was found to be healed and he was free from symptoms.

For some patients, hospitalization is therapeutic because it provides a setting in which the patient can be dependent without feeling guilty about wanting to be dependent. A hospital is a place where one can be looked after. The patient can feel comfortable in allowing others to assume responsibility for his or her care. For this patient, the healing of the ulcer is favored by an atmosphere in which dependency is allowed and encouraged. He or she not only wants, but needs, to have needs anticipated and met. The patient wants and needs to be freed from responsibility for a time. If the patient is undemanding, his or her need for dependence may be overlooked. Mrs. Maple, who was shy and quiet, was such a patient. One statement that she made to the nurse indicated that she had the desire to be dependent. She said, "I'm so glad to have a nurse who does things for me. At home, Joe always makes me decide how the money is to be spent and when to discipline the children. I wish that he would take more responsibility."

At the other extreme is the patient who is unable to allow others to assume responsibility for his or her care and overtly overreacts at the slightest frustration. For example, Mr. Johns watches a clock to be sure that he gets his medication at the exact time it is scheduled. As the hour approaches, his muscles become tense and he becomes more and more angry. Should the nurse be 2 minutes late, he becomes highly distraught. The nurse knows that she cannot possibly distribute medications to thirty patients at the same time and that a reasonable interval before or after the hour is acceptable. Because the patient attacks an approved practice and the nurse herself feels attacked, she too may feel angry. If she can recognize that the behavior of the patient is his usual way of reacting in frustrating situations and that she just happens to be the person who is present, then she may be able to avoid personalizing his remarks and to remain objective. She will be better able to develop a plan to increase the confidence of the patient that he will, in fact, receive the care he requires. Instead of responding with anger, she may try to administer Mr. Johns' medication at the scheduled hour. When the medication is one that can be safely left at the bedside of the patient, this possibility may be discussed with the physician and, with his approval, the drug may be left with the patient. Patients in some hospitals are encouraged to assume responsibility for their own medications. After the nurse has established a trusting relationship with the patient, problems such as the above tend to be less acute.

Because of the importance of psychic stimuli in promoting gastric secretion and motility, drugs are also prescribed to decrease the responsiveness of the individual. Any one of a number of tranquilizing agents may be prescribed for the patient. The desired effect is to lessen the response of the individual to stimuli. These drugs modify the cephalic phase of gastric secretion; that is, they lessen secretion in response to sight, smell, or taste of food. Because of a decrease in the cephalic phase, the gastric phase of secretion may also be less intense.

The indications for and the effects of surgical therapy in the treatment of peptic ulcer have been discussed previously. Should bleeding recur, or perforation, obstruction, or intractability to medical treatment, surgery may be considered in the treatment of Mrs. Maple.

To summarize briefly, at the time of the admission of Mrs. Maple to the hospital, she was suffering from the effects of blood loss. Because an adequate volume of blood is essential to maintaining tissue nutrition, the restoration of the lost blood was the objective receiving priority. As soon as bleeding stopped and the blood that had been lost was replaced, attention was then directed toward treating her ulcer. Because an ulcer is a local manifestation of a constitutional disease, attention to Mrs. Maple as a person was as important as treating her ulcer. The fundamental objective of care was to reduce the effect of acid-pepsin in gastric juice on the lining of the duodenum. Because the stomach responds to a wide variety of stimuli by increased secretion and motility, treatment was planned to decrease Mrs. Maple's responsiveness to environmental stimuli as well as to neutralize gastric acidity.

Because peptic ulcer is a chronic disease characterized by periodic recurrences, Mrs. Maple should know that the ulcer may be reactivated at a later time. She should be advised to see her physician immediately should she develop pain or nausea. Delay not only increases the difficulty in healing the ulcer, but predisposes to complications. Inasmuch as she is able, Mrs. Maple should try to avoid situations that are upsetting to her. Possibly, Mr. Maple could be encouraged to assume more responsibility for family matters. The nurse should discuss the problem with Mr. or Mrs. Maple and with the physician to determine if a referral to social service or to some other agency, such as Family Services Society, would be helpful. As in other chronic illnesses, one of the important factors in the control of peptic ulcers is the strengths and resources of the patient and family.

The Middle Alimentary Canal

Disturbances in the motility, secretion, or absorption in the midportion of the alimentary canal impair nutrition and hydration by decreasing the length of time that nutrients and water remain in the intestine or by interfering with their absorption. The middle part of the alimentary canal is subject to many of the same types of disorders as other parts of the gut. It can be obstructed by neoplasms, twisting (volvulus), scar tissue, incarceration in a hernial ring, or motor failure. Its blood supply can be cut off by twisting, by incarceration, or by thrombosis of the mesenteric artery. Inflammation occurs as the result of the effects of unknown and microbial agents. As in other areas, diverticula occur. Digestion and absorption may be impaired because of failure of delivery of digestive enzymes and bile salts. Fistulae may allow intestinal contents to escape before they can be digested and absorbed. Important disorders are summarized in Table 46-3 at the end of this chapter.

Malabsorption

The effects of ischemia of tissues and of perforation of the intestine have previously been considered. In malabsorption there is a failure to digest or to absorb one or more nutrients. The effects depend on the cause and degree of failure, the suddenness of onset, and which nutrients are not absorbed. For example, in the absence of pancreatic enzymes, fat is not digested. It is evacuated in the stool, which is large, bulky, and foul-smelling. The patient usually loses weight because fat is an important source of calories. The absence of bile salts interferes with the digestion of fats and the absorption of fats and fat-soluble vitamins. Inability to absorb vitamin K means that prothrombin will not be adequately formed and the tendency to bleed is increased. Briefly, as a consequence of failure to digest and absorb food, (1) nonabsorbed food appears in the stool; (2) secondary deficiencies caused by failure of absorption of nutrients develop; and (3) symptoms relating to gastrointestinal function such as diarrhea, anorexia, and nausea occur.[8]

[8] For a list of disorders characterized by malabsorption, see Thomas R. Hendrix and Theodore M. Bayless: "Malabsorption," in *The Principles and Practice of Medicine*, 18th ed., A. McGehee Harvey et al. eds. (New York: Appleton-Century-Crofts, 1972), p. 747.

The Lower Alimentary Canal

Functions and Disease

Although the surgical removal of the entire large intestine is possible, it is attended by considerable risk. A part of all of the large intestine can be bypassed by anastomosing two sections or by bringing a portion of it through the abdominal wall. Complete or partial resection or bypassing of the large intestine, with or without the formation of an artificial anus after the individual has adjusted to the change, is compatible with a full and active life. Although the large intestine completes the absorption of water and stores and evacuates the residue left from the digestion of food, these functions can be accomplished by the remaining portion or by the distal end of the ileum.

The large intestine is the site of a number of important diseases, including cancer, chronic ulcerative colitis, diverticulitis, and hemorrhoids. Abscesses and fissures in the region of the external anal region are not uncommon. The above disorders are summarized in Table 46-3.

Two common effects of disease or disturbances on the function of the large intestine include diarrhea and constipation. Lesions, such as benign and malignant neoplasms or strictures formed in the process of healing, that narrow the lumen of the intestine will in time prevent the passage of the contents through the large intestine, that is, block or obstruct it.

Diarrhea and Constipation

Diarrhea and constipation are terms used to indicate alterations in the normal pattern of defecation. Because of the wide range in bowel habits among healthy individuals, these terms are difficult to define precisely. For the purpose of this discussion, *diarrhea* is defined as *the passage of several unformed stools as a result of the rapid movement of the fecal contents through the large intestine.* By way of contrast, constipation is associated with delay in the passage of feces. Because the feces remain in the intestine for an unduly long period of time, water is absorbed and they are hard and dry. Defecation may be accompanied by discomfort. Both diarrhea and constipation are relatively common, and either can be caused by a disturbance in the regulatory mechanisms controlling the functioning of the large bowel or by mechanical interference with the progress of its contents. Inflammatory disorders of the large intestine are more likely to cause diarrhea than constipation.

Acute disturbances in the function of the digestive system are second only to acute respiratory disease as a cause of morbidity. Any acute disorder increasing the activity of one part of the alimentary canal is likely to affect the function of other parts. An affected individual is likely to experience both vomiting and diarrhea. Like vomiting, diarrhea is one of the defense mechanisms utilized by the gastrointestinal tract to rid itself of harmful agents. In diarrhea, the segmenting contractions of the intestine, a kneading nonpropelling activity, are decreased.

As defined earlier, diarrhea is a condition in which a number of unformed stools are defecated. Diarrhea can result from any condition in which the segmenting contractions become hypoactive, allowing the feces to be moved along the gastrointestinal tract very rapidly. As in other reflex activity, stimuli may act on receptors in the lining of the alimentary canal or be of central origin. Simply, diarrhea can be caused by injury of the lining of the intestine or excessive secretion of water and electrolytes in the intestines stimulated by bacterial toxins, or it may be of nervous origin. See Table 46-1 for causes.

Two examples of diarrhea of neurogenic origin follow. One is Joan Book, who usually has diarrhea just preceding an examination. She calls her condition "nervous diarrhea." Jean Servus is the second example. When Jean consulted her physician because she had had repeated attacks of diarrhea over the past few months, no evidence of an organic lesion was found to account for her difficulty. After some discussion, Jean remembered that her episodes of diarrhea began following a violent quarrel with her father. The problem had not been resolved and she felt that her father was continuing to harass her. Each time Jean and her father had an argument, Jean had an episode of diarrhea. After she understood the relationship of her feelings to diarrhea, it became less troublesome.

Although diarrhea of neurogenic origin is not uncommon, the usual cause is some agent irritating the intestinal mucosa. Irritants can be of endogenous or exogenous origin. Microorganisms are among the more frequent causative agents of acute diarrhea. In the United States infection is most frequently caused by a virus, a Salmonella or the *Endamoeba*

TABLE 46-1 *Causes of Diarrhea*

Psychogenic and/or Neurogenic Innervation

1. Vagal (generalized hypermotility of entire alimentary tract)
   a. Stomach
   b. Small intestine
   c. Ascending colon
   d. Transverse colon
   } Treatment: surgical { a. Vagotomy; b. Gastrectomy
2. Sacral (diarrhea alternates with constipation; irritable colon, mucous colitis)
   a. Descending colon

Classification of Diarrhea

1. Inflammatory
   a. Regional enteritis: distal portion of small intestine
   b. Ulcerative colitis: distal portion of descending colon
2. Irritative
   a. Mechanical: small intestine, transverse and descending colon
      (1) Fecal impaction
      (2) Foreign body
      (3) Neoplasm
      (4) Intussusception
      (5) Extraluminal compression
      (6) Angulation
   b. Chemical: descending colon
      (1) Poisons
      (2) Cathartics
   c. Bacterial: small intestine, descending colon
      (1) Salmonellae
      (2) Shigella
      (3) Staphylococci
      (4) Streptococci
      (5) *B. coli*
      (6) Clostridia et al.
   d. Parasitic: descending colon
      (1) Amebiasis
      (2) Trichinosis
      (3) Ascariasis
3. Malabsorption: small intestine
   a. Tropical sprue
   b. Symptomatic sprue
   c. Celiac disease (adult celiac disease)
   d. Nontropical sprue
   e. Whipple's disease
4. Osmotic: small intestine and descending colon
   a. Saline cathartics
5. Endocrine
   a. Thyroid
      (1) Hyperthyroidism
   b. Adrenals
      (1) Adrenocortical insufficiency
   c. Liver
      (1) Secreting carcinoid tumors (serotonin)
6. Dietary: descending colon
   a. Food intolerance
   b. Vitamin deficiencies
7. Allergic: descending colon
   a. Drug sensitivity
   b. Food sensitivity

histolytica. The nature of each of these is summarized at the end of this chapter. Diarrhea, as well as nausea and vomiting, is frequently associated with the onset of acute diseases of the gastrointestinal tract.

Whenever a person experiences repeated attacks of diarrhea, he or she should be examined by the physician because they may be associated with a serious disorder that may respond if treated early. Furthermore, when diarrhea continues, important nutrients and fluids are lost from the body. In severe diarrhea there is probably always some impairment in absorption. In disorders in which absorption is markedly reduced, large quantities of fat and protein may be lost. For example, in sprue, failure to absorb fat and protein results in large, bulky, foamy feces with a foul odor. Maintenance of even a minimal nutritional status may be difficult.

In obstructive lesions of the large intestine, diarrhea alternates with constipation. As the lumen of the bowel is reduced in size, liquid feces are moved past the site of the obstruction and evacuated. During periods when the feces accumulate behind the obstruction, constipation occurs. The most serious cause of this type of diarrhea is cancer. Fecal impactions can, however, be responsible for the same combination of symptoms. Diarrhea is a manifestation in a number of generalized disorders, such as hyperthyroidism, lymphosarcoma, and tuberculosis. It, too, can be of allergic origin. Radiation therapy of pelvic and abdominal organs predisposes to diarrhea.

From the preceding, the logical conclusion is that diarrhea occurs frequently and is associated with a variety of disorders. The effects of diarrhea depend on its cause and severity as well as how long it persists and the age and state of health of the individual who has it. Age is a significant factor, because diarrhea in a young infant can soon cause a serious depletion of electrolytes, water, and nutrients. Unless the disorder is promptly corrected, the life of the child can be threatened. A bout of diarrhea in a youth or adult is likely to cause some feeling of unfitness, but need not be a source of alarm unless it is very severe or continues for more than a few hours.

Although few persons escape or fail to recover from an occasional episode of diarrhea, excessive or prolonged diarrhea leads to the loss of water and nutrients from the body and predisposes to malnutrition. Undernutrition may be worsened by the fact that anorexia, nausea, and vomiting discourage the intake of food. When cramping accompanies diarrhea, the individual may be afraid to eat. Loss of nutrients may be exaggerated when diarrhea is caused by failure to digest or absorb food, or when there is a large outpouring of mucus into the alimentary canal. Erosion of blood vessels accompanied by bleeding is a frequent observation in patients whose diarrhea is due to an ulcerating lesion or lesions. In chronic or severe diarrhea, nutrition is always affected to some extent by failure to ingest food and by loss of nutrients, mucus, and blood.

Nurse's Responsibilities in Caring for Persons with Diarrhea

In the assessment of the patient with diarrhea it is useful to keep in mind the most common causes as summarized in Table 46-1. An accurate data base may be obtained by the nurse or physician who will in turn try to determine the nature of the cause of diarrhea and what, if any, effect it has on the nutritional status of the individual.

The plan of therapy is dependent on the cause of diarrhea and the general status of the individual. The single most important means of therapy for diarrhea is fluid and electrolyte replacement (Donta, 1975). Fluids are replaced by ingesting small to increasingly larger amounts of liquids high in sodium and potassium such as gatorade, broths, soups, and juices as tolerated. Antiobiotics are indicated in staphylococcal enterocolitis, amebiasis, and severe shigella or salmonella diarrhea. The use of opiates is not recommended in the treatment of toxin-producing enteropathogens and may be harmful. Kaolin and pectin are frequently prescribed for their absorbent qualities to give some consistency to the stool.

It should be remembered that most cases of diarrhea are of viral origin, are self-limiting, and require only palliative therapy. The usual therapy consists of (1) putting the bowel at rest for a period of time by restricting intake; (2) fluid and electrolyte replacement by mouth or intravenously; and (3) general rest. Drugs such as Lomotil if given are used cautiously for they may mask the intensity of the disease. When the patient is known to harbor or is suspected to harbor agents that are transmissible to others, the nurse has the responsibility for planning and enforcing suitable procedures to protect herself or himself and others.

OBSERVATIONS. One important way in which information is collected is by observation of the feces. Pertinent observations include color, odor, consistency—formed, liquid, frothy—number and frequency, and the presence of foreign matter such as blood, mucus, pus, and worms. What symptoms accompany defecation; that is, does the patient have cramping, urgency, pain, or tenesmus on defecation? Tenesmus is the term for the sharp, unpleasant contractions in the lower-left quadrant associated with straining during defecation. Following defecation, the patient feels only partly relieved. The nurse is more helpful by describing the sensations as they are related in the patient's own words than by naming them. Does the patient have abdominal or other pain? Where is it located? Under what conditions are the symptoms of the patient worsened? Improved? For example, is defecation initiated by eating or activity? Is the patient relieved following defecation, or does he or she feel as if the bowels were only partly evacuated? Observations of vital signs are of particular significance when diarrhea is associated with infection or hemorrhage. The nursing of the patient who suffers from a disorder accompanied by chronic diarrhea taxes the patience and ingenuity of any nurse.

To illustrate the problems of the patient with chronic diarrhea, Mrs. Reddy is presented. Mrs. John Reddy, who is 24 years of age, has a diagnosis of chronic ulcerative colitis. A year ago, shortly after her marriage to a promising young businessman, she suffered an attack of diarrhea with pus, blood, and fibrin in the stool. At the time of her admission to Special Hospital, she looked and felt sick. She presented evidence of a poor nutritional state because she had lost 20 lb, her hemoglobin was reduced to 6 g, and her blood proteins were 5.2 g per 100 ml. Each day she passed from ten to twenty rectal discharges of blood, mucus, and pus. With each defecation, she experienced intestinal cramping and straining. Despite frequent defecations, she was not relieved by defecation. The area around the anus was inflamed and sore. When she tried to eat, cramping was intensified. She was aware of the disagreeable odor of her stools. Because of the urgency associated with defecation, Mrs. Reddy was not always able to get on the bedpan in time, and the bed was soiled. Because she was chronically ill and many aspects of her illness were unpleasant, if not repugnant, to others, Mrs. Reddy worried about her marriage and the reaction of her husband to her illness. Quite understandably, she was anxious and depressed.

THE NURSING CARE PLAN. In making a nursing care plan for Mrs. Reddy, her nurse established two objectives. The *first* was to increase her comfort and the *second* to try to improve her nutritional status. To accomplish the first objective, the nurse planned to wash, dry, and powder the anal region after each defecation. To protect the bed from soiling, an absorbent pad of the type used in disposable diapers was placed under Mrs. Reddy's buttocks. It was changed each time it was soiled. The bedpan was washed after every use. To help minimize odor, the room was aired after each defecation. Because the outside temperature was cold, a screen was placed in front of the window and an extra blanket was spread over Mrs. Reddy to prevent chilling. After each defecation, Mrs. Reddy was provided with an opportunity to wash her hands. For the first few days, the nurse gave care to Mrs. Reddy; that is, she allowed her to be sick and dependent. She made few demands on her, accepting her as a very sick woman whose behavior could be explained by her illness and who needed a high quality of nursing care.

The objectives of medical therapy are (1) to improve the general well-being of the patient, (2) to induce a remission of the disease, and (3) to eliminate histological evidence of the disease. For the first 3 days Mrs. Reddy was in the hospital, fluids containing multivitamins were administered by intravenous infusion and she was given 1,000 ml of whole blood. To decrease intestinal peristalsis, her physician prescribed Lomotil every 6 hours. In addition salicylazosulfapyridine, a combination of sulfonamide and salicylic acid, was given orally. For 2 weeks, she was given 50 ml of water containing 20 mg of prednisolone rectally, each evening and, each day prednisolone 0.60 mg was given orally. Because of her improved condition, a soft, high-protein diet was prescribed to be started on her fourth day in the hospital. Before Mrs. Reddy's food arrived, she was prepared for the meal by having an opportunity to brush her teeth and wash her face and hands and was assisted to a comfortable position. The room was aired and a clean bedpan was conveniently placed, but covered. Mrs. Reddy had been encouraged to choose what she wanted for breakfast. She asked for a white wheat cereal and toast. The suggestion was made that she eat slowly and drink only a minimum of fluid during her meal. Fluids were encouraged between meals. Iced fluids are generally avoided because they tend to stimulate peristalsis. When Mrs. Reddy complained of a cramping sensation, the suggestion was made that she contract her buttocks and pull them together and try to contract the anus. By practicing this maneuver, she was sometimes able to prevent defecation.

As her nutritional and general status improved, Mrs. Reddy widened her selection of foods. To occupy her time and attention, and to promote relaxation, her physician prescribed occupational therapy. The occupational therapist suggested she make pot holders on a "Weave It" frame. By using different colored strands, she could design varying patterns. The motions are repetitive and relaxing. The product is useful and can be sold or given to relatives and friends. To encourage relaxation, her nurse planned regular rest periods for her. She tried to control conditions in her external environment, so that Mrs. Reddy was protected from unnecessary stimulation or irritation. Because any kind of stress, including infection, aggravates the disorder, people with colds were banned from her environment.

In addition to medical therapy, surgical procedures are sometimes indicated. To provide rest and allow the diseased portion of the bowel to heal, an ileostomy may be performed. Because there is a tendency for islands of healthy tissue that are surrounded by areas of disease and cicatrization (scarring) to undergo polyp formation and malignant degeneration, resection of the diseased bowel may be required.

Whatever form of therapy is instituted, the patient with chronic ulcerative colitis is sick. Minimizing the disagreeable effects of the disease includes the control of odors, protection of the skin, and control of conditions in the environment tending to stimulate peristalsis. Because of the nature of the disease, nutrition is a problem. One of the major problems in nursing the patient is to improve the intake of food. Unless food intake is improved, recovery is doubtful.

Constipation

In constipation, in contrast to diarrhea, evacuation of feces is delayed, and when they are finally evacuated, feces are frequently hard and dry. Because of the great variability among people, constipation is difficult to define exactly. Many people, though by no means all, defecate once daily. Probably the most frequent cause of constipation is neglect to respond to the normal defecation reflex. Because of failure to respond, the reflex itself becomes less powerful and constipation results. Constipation can also be the result of a disease process or of agents used in the treatment of disease. It can occur in degenerative diseases of the central nervous system, in severe psychoses, in hypothyroidism, in metabolic disturbances, with lesions of the gut, and with the use of such drugs as the ganglionic blocking agents and morphine.

The treatment of simple constipation is primarily education. A regular and convenient time should be selected for defecation. For most people, the defecation reflex is most active after meals, particularly after breakfast. In a family of six or eight with only one bathroom, obviously it will not be available to all members of the family immediately after breakfast. The time selected should be one when the individual can be comfortably relaxed. The individual should be encouraged to "obey" the urge to defecate when it does occur. A diet containing a reasonable amount of fluid, and bulk, and regular exercise, especially before breakfast, are other useful measures in the prevention and treatment of constipation.

For the elderly patient who is poorly motivated or who has a disease that makes change difficult or impossible, the correction of constipation by changing habits of living may not be possible or practical. Measures such as bulky laxatives and oil-retention or other types of enemas may be the most reasonable solutions to the problem. In elderly patients and in those who have neurological disorders affecting bowel function, observation of the regularity of defecation as well as the size and consistency of feces is important to the prevention and early detection of fecal impactions. Sick and debilitated individuals, especially if elderly, and persons with lesions in the nervous system that interfere with the regulation of bowel function are especially predisposed to impaction. Size of the stool is significant because the patient may pass a small amount of feces while retaining and accumulating feces in the lower bowel. Water is absorbed from the fecal material remaining in the bowel, increasing the difficulty with which it is evacuated. In patients who are predisposed to fecal impactions, measures such as bulk-producing cathartics and oil-retention enemas may be successful in the prevention of their formation. After an impaction is formed, it usually has to be broken up manually and removed. Impactions should not occur if the patient is observed and appropriate actions are taken when there is evidence that feces are being retained. Prevention is to be preferred to cure.

Causes and Effects of Obstruction

Any disorder interfering with the forward movement of the contents of the alimentary canal is called an obstruction. As indicated previously, an obstruction in the esophagus interferes with the ability to ingest food. An obstruction of the outlet of the stomach delays or prevents chyme from entering the duodenum. Either the small or large intestine may be the site of an obstruction. For the most part, the discussion of obstruction that follows will be related to blocking of the intestine, large or small. Whatever the nature of obstruction or its site or location, however, it interferes with the accomplishment of the function of the alimentary canal. Three primary types of disturbances predispose to obstruction. They are mechanical blocking of the lumen, reduced or absent peristalsis, and impaired circulation caused by the occlusion of the blood supply. Mechanical blocking may have its origin in abnormalities within the wall of the alimentary canal or outside it. Neoplasms, unreduced volvulus, and incarcerated hernias are a few of many causes of mechanical obstruction.

Neurogenic Obstruction

Absent peristalsis is usually caused by some disturbance in the function of the autonomic nervous system associated with surgical or other trauma. As a result of reflex inhibition of the gastrointestinal tract, the stomach may be acutely dilated by retained secretions and swallowed air. Complete cessation of motor activity of the small intestine produces a functional obstruction and is referred to as paralytic or adynamic ileus. Impairment of the circulation may be caused by a thrombosis of the mesenteric artery, or by distention of the inactive intestine.

In both the neurogenic and the vascular types of obstruction, the lumen of the bowel is open. The effect is that of obstruction, however, because the affected parts of the bowel do not propel its contents forward. As a result of the obstruction the intestine and stomach are distended by gas and fluids. The gas is presumed to have its origin in the air that is swallowed. As the pressure within the bowel increases, absorption decreases. When the pressure within the intestine equals the diastolic blood pressure, absorption ceases. The effect of distention on the circulation of blood to the wall of the intestine is similar to that of pressure on any tissue. First the venous outflow from the tissue is impaired. This leads to a slowing of the blood flow through the tissue and the development of edema. If the condition is allowed to continue, arterial blood flow is impaired and finally ceases. Because of the failure in the flow of blood to the tissue, tissue necrosis occurs. Death of a portion of the alimentary tract may lead to perforation of the viscus and to the death of the individual.

Obstruction in the gastrointestinal tract also leads to shock. One of the factors in the development of shock is that distention of the stomach and intestine is a powerful stimulus to secretion. Secretion combined with a failure of absorption leads to the trapping of a large volume of fluid within the gastrointestinal tract and to a reduction in the blood volume. Therefore, when obstruction is allowed to progress, shock eventually develops. As the stomach and/or bowel distends, the increase in their volume has an adverse effect on respiratory and circulatory function. Increased intraabdominal pressure reduces vital capacity by interfering with the depression of the diaphragm. It also interferes with the return flow of blood from the lower extremities by direct pressure on the veins.

Decompression

Before definitive treatment can be instituted, the stomach and/or intestine must be deflated by the removal of gas and fluid. Decompression is accomplished by the introduction into the stomach or intestine of a tube to which suction is applied. The principles on which decompression therapy is based are described in Chapter 51. As the bowel is decompressed, the blood supply to the wall improves. Because of the improvement of the nutrition of the wall, functional disorders such as adynamic ileus tend to correct themsleves. Structural lesions usually require some form of surgical therapy to remove or relieve the effects of obstruction. One of the important responsibilities of the nurse in the care of the patient who has a gastric or intestinal obstruction is to maintain the suctioning apparatus in good working order. Because respiratory and circulatory functions are impaired, attention must be given to nursing measures that support these functions.

Herniation—Types and Effects

The alimentary canal is subject to two general types of herniation. In the first type the mucosa prolapses through the muscle wall forming a sac or pouch known as a diverticulum. Multiple diverticula are known as diverticulosis. The two most common sites for the formation of diverticula are the colon and the esophagus. As may the appendix, the diverticula may become filled with food or feces and become inflamed or perforated. Inflammation of a diverticulum is known as diverticulitis.

In the other types of herniation, the mesentery or one or more of the organs escape through a ring through which body structures pass. Common types of hernias involving the alimentary canal include esophageal hiatus hernia and inguinal, femoral, umbilical, and postoperative ventral hernia. The name indicates the ring through which the organ prolapses. Thus in an esophageal hiatus hernia, contents of the abdominal cavity protrude through the gap in the diaphragm into the thoracic cavity. Most types of hernia predispose the patient to two dangers, obstruction of the alimentary canal and necrosis of the trapped tissues.

Summary

Understanding of the effects of disease on some portion of the alimentary canal requires knowledge of the following:

1. The structure and function of each part.
2. The mechanisms regulating each part, so that it performs its function in coordination with that of other parts of the alimentary canal.
3. The mechanisms for regulating the function of the alimentary canal so that the nutritional needs of the individual are met.

Disease may be caused by disorders in the regulation of function or by alteration in the structure of the alimentary canal. The manifestations of disease of the alimentary canal result from the effect of injuring agents (in a broad sense) on the structure and function, from failure of the canal to defend the integrity of its lining, and from interference with the intake of food and water. Furthermore, most of the wall of the alimentary canal is richly supplied with blood. Disorders in which the lining membrane is damaged predispose to bleeding. Thrombosis of arteries or veins supplying any part of the alimentary canal predisposes to tissue necrosis. Esophageal and hemorrhoidal veins have the tendency under certain circumstances to dilate and become tortuous, that is, to form varicosities. Although rupture of varices may occur in either location, those in the esophagus are more likely to be the site of serious hemorrhage. Varicosities of hemorrhoidal veins (hemorrhoids) may become thrombosed and painfully inflamed.

The Liver and Biliary Tract

In the preceding sections, disorders in function of the alimentary canal have been discussed. Disorders in function of the liver and pancreas have a direct effect upon nutritional status, for although these two glands are external to the alimentary canal their secretions empty into the duodenum and have a significant role in digestion.

The Liver

The liver is not only the largest, but it is the most complex organ in the body. The liver has four main systems—blood vessels, reticuloendothelial Kupffer's cells, parenchymal cells, and the biliary channels. All these systems are so intimately related that any considerable or continuing pathology in one inevitably leads to disturbances in others. Injury can be the result of direct extension of a pathologic process or the response of the tissues to injury. In the adult, the vascular system of the liver stores and filters blood. Kupffer's cells—a specialized type of reticuloendothelial cells—in the lining of the venous channels of the liver play an important role in defense because they phagocytize potentially harmful agents circulating through the liver. Parenchymal cells secrete bile and play an essential role in the intermediary metabolism of most nutrients. The biliary channels store, concentrate, and conduct bile from the liver to the alimentary canal.

In the study of the liver, one is impressed with the interrelatedness of body functions and structure. For example, the most frequent cause of vascular congestion in the liver is congestive heart failure resulting from the failure of the right side of the heart as a pump (see Chapter 44). In right-sided heart failure, stasis of blood in the right atrium impedes the flow of blood from the inferior vena cava with the result that the blood pressure rises in the inferior vena cava. As the blood pressure rises in the inferior vena cava, pressure is transmitted to the hepatic veins and blood accumulates in the liver, causing the liver to swell and to enlarge. Because the capsule surrounding the liver offers resistance to swelling, pressure within the liver rises. As in any other tissue in which venous congestion occurs, blood supply to the tissue is impeded by failure to remove blood at about the same rate as it enters.

The liver receives over 25 per cent of the cardiac output. Approximately three fourths of the blood delivered to the liver is venous blood and is carried by the portal system. The other one quarter is arterial blood conveyed by the hepatic artery. Because such a high proportion of the blood circulated to the liver is venous blood, oxygen supply, under the most favorable circumstances, tends to be marginal. Any disorder decreasing the blood supply through the liver therefore predisposes to some degree of hypoxia. In addition to causing a deficient supply of oxygen to liver cells, congestion in the liver elevates the blood pressure in the veins forming the portal system. Because fluids move in the direction of least resistance, the elevation of blood pressure within the portal system is reflected by congestion of the wall of the stomach, esophagus, and duodenum. In the esophagus, elevated venous pressure predisposes to esophageal varices. In the stomach and duodenum, elevated portal pressure predisposes to peptic ulcer.

In the liver itself, swelling interferes with parenchymal cell function and may, when severe, obstruct ducts of the biliary canal. Jaundice caused by a failure to remove bile pigments is a frequent sign in severe right-sided heart failure.

Evaluation of Bile Ducts and Gallbladder

The patency of the bile ducts and the capacity of the gallbladder to store and concentrate bile are evaluated by x-ray following the administration of an iodinated organic compound. The usual method for the administration of the dye is by mouth, but it may be given by intravenous injection. Dye may also be injected directly into biliary canals in patients having a T tube or at the time of surgery involving the biliary tract. After absorption of the dye into the blood, it is removed by the liver and secreted into the bile. When the substance is administered orally to a healthy person, sufficient dye will have been excreted into the biliary canals to render them opaque to x-ray in about 12 hours. The success of the examination depends on (1) normal motility and absorbing powers of the alimentary canal, (2) normal liver function, (3) patent biliary channels, (4) an empty gallbladder at the time the test is initiated, and (5) a gallbladder capable of concentrating and storing bile. To make sure that the gallbladder has been emptied before the dye is administered, the patient may be given a fatty meal the morning and noon before the tablets are administered. The evening that the dye is given, the patient has a liquid low-fat meal. Following the initial x-rays, the capacity of the gallbladder to empty can be checked by the ingestion of a fatty meal. Throughout the period of the examination, foods and fluids are limited to those indicated in the directions for the examination. Stimulation of gastric motility and foods stimulating the flow of bile into the alimentary canal are to be avoided after the dye is administered and until the first x-rays have been taken, because they will prevent the dye from being concentrated in the gallbladder.

Approximately 15 per cent of patients with gallstones have concomitant choledocholithiasis, stones in the common bile duct (Way & Sleisenger, 1978, p. 1313). This incidence increases with age. The stones may originate in the gallbladder or, in special circumstances, in the common bile duct itself. When jaundice is present one must search for the obstructing lesion. Numerous invasive and noninvasive tests for the evaluation of bile duct obstruction exist. Tests advocated are intravenous cholangiogram, ultrasound, various cholangiography techniques, liver function tests, scans, and biopsy. A complete preoperative delineation of the scope of the problem is not usually necessary and is expensive.

Secretion of Bile Salts

One of the earliest effects of injury of liver cells is a decrease in the secretion of bile salts. Obstruction of the common hepatic or the common bile duct can prevent bile salts from reaching the intestine. One of the most distressing effects observed in patients with lesions associated with obstruction of the biliary tract is pruritus. It is believed to be caused by excessive amounts of bile salts in the blood. Mr. Pine, who was admitted with a diagnosis of cancer of the head of the pancreas obstructing the common bile duct, had deep scratches over every part of his body that he could reach. To minimize itching he was given tepid baths to which starch was added and lotion was applied to his skin. Room temperature was regulated so that it did not exceed 68°F because heat increases the intensity of itching. To lessen the damage to his skin from scratching, his nails were cut short. If obstruction is incomplete, cholestyramine, an anion exchange resin, may be prescribed to prevent the reabsorption of bile salts from the intestine. It takes 4 to 6 days to be effective.

In the absence of bile salts, a large part of the ingested fat is lost in the stool in the form of soaps. The stool is pale and frothy in appearance. Fat-soluble vitamins A, D, E, and K are also lost in the stool. Because vitamins A and D are stored in sufficient quantities to last for some time, evidence of vitamin A or D deficiency does not usually occur unless the deficiency continues for months. In contrast, absence of bile salts for more than a few days leads to deficiency in vitamin K. Vitamin K acts as a catalyst in the formation of prothrombin. In its absence, whether because of a vitamin K deficiency or the administration of one of its antagonists such as bishydroxycoumarin, the blood fails to clot in the usual period of time. Before the discovery of vitamin K, the surgical treatment of the patient with a common bile duct obstruction was difficult because of the tendency of the patient to bleed. Even small breaks in a blood vessel resulted in bleeding that was difficult to control.

GALLSTONES. Although cholesterol is nearly insoluble in water, it is kept in solution in the bile by bile salts, fatty acids, and lecithin. In some persons, cholesterol and/or bilirubin and calcium carbonate precipitate and form stones (cholelithiasis). Although one constitutent may predominate, even so-called pure stones contain varying proportions of other constituents. For example, a "pure" cholesterol stone is about 98 per cent cholesterol, the other 2 per cent being pigment and calcium carbonate.

Cholesterol stones are common in the Western world, whereas pigment stones are common in parts of Africa and the Far East. Calcium carbonate stones are uncommon in humans but are common in cattle. About 50 per cent of gallstones contain sufficient calcium carbonate to be opaque to x-ray. Stones with little or no calcium can be detected by x-ray only with the use of contrast media. Cholesterol stones are cream-colored, but pigment stones are dark in color.

Etiology. Cholesterol stones are thought to result from the secretion of bile supersaturated with cholesterol. Inflammation or the retention of bile in the gallbladder may be contributing factors (Redinger & Small, 1972).

The incidence of cholelithiasis is higher among women than among men. It has been estimated that about 20 million people in the United States have gallstones and that approximately 300,000 operations are performed yearly for this disease and its complications (Way & Sleisenger, 1978, p. 1294).

Women who have had several children appear to be more susceptible to cholelithiasis than nonparous women. The incidence of cholelithiasis is high among persons having hemolytic jaundice, a condition in which red blood cells are destroyed at an excessive rate. Obesity and diabetes mellitus appear to predispose to gallstones, as do infections of the gallbladder, one notable example being typhoid fever.

The number of stones found in the gallbladder of any one person varies from 1 to more than 200. They vary in shape and size. Single stones are likely to be smooth and round or oval in shape, whereas multiple stones are likely to be small and faceted and variable in size and shape.

Signs and symptoms: Highly variable signs and symptoms accompany cholelithiasis. About half of the patients have no signs or symptoms referable to the biliary tract but have so-called silent cholelithiasis. In those who have stones containing sufficient calcium carbonate, their presence may be demonstrated by an x-ray over the area. Stones may be identified during abdominal surgery or after death during postmortem examination. Signs and symptoms vary from belching and bloating to periodic attacks of biliary colic. Biliary colic is characterized by attacks of pain in the right upper abdomen accompanied by nausea, vomiting, and difficulty in taking a deep breath. The attacks are believed to be caused by muscle spasm initiated by a stone passing through the common duct. Attacks may be precipitated by a fatty meal, but they may also occur during the night when the stomach is presumably empty.

Mrs. Helmer's case is illustrative of the patient who is assumed to be predisposed to cholelithiasis. She is 40 years of age, about 20 lb overweight, and has four daughters. Although gallstones do develop at any age, they are uncommon before the age of 30. Mrs. Helmer was among the 50 per cent of the persons who have cholelithiasis with symptoms. About 2 o'clock one night, she awakened with excruciating pain in her right upper abdomen. It extended through to the region just under the central side of the right scapula. Her pain was so severe that she arose and walked the floor, bending forward with her arms folded firmly across her chest. Although the room was cool, beads of perspiration stood out on her forehead. She complained of nausea, and her breathing was shallow. Because of the severity of her pain, Mr. Helmer called the family physician, who came and gave Mrs. Helmer 15 mg (gr ¼) of morphine sulfate and suggested that she come into his office as soon as possible for diagnostic tests and probably surgery. In the meantime, Mrs. Helmer was told to avoid greasy, fatty, or fried foods and those having strong odor when cooked such as cabbage, turnips, and kale.

The pain was relieved by the morphine and Mrs. Helmer went to sleep. When she awakened in the morning, she had some residual soreness in the affected area, but she felt much better. Although some patients have frequent attacks, Mrs. Helmer continued to feel well for several months. She found that if she avoided fatty foods and cabbage, she was free from symptoms. Being comfortable, busy, and human, she did not make an appointment to see her physician.

Possible complications: Because Mrs. Helmer's gallbladder contained many small stones—over 100 were found in her gallbladder at the time of cholecystectomy—she might have had biliary colic at any time. By delaying treatment Mrs. Helmer was exposing herself to the danger of several serious complications. They include acute and chronic cholecystitis, choledocholithiasis, cholangitis, fistula from the biliary tract to surrounding organs, biliary cirrhosis, carcinoma of the gallbladder, and gallstone ileus. She did develop choledocholithiasis—a stone was lodged in the common duct, causing obstruction. On examination in the laboratory her gallbladder was found to be acutely inflamed.

About a year after the attack described above Mrs. Helmer experienced several acute bouts of pain. None was as severe as the first and she could usually relate an attack to a dietary indiscretion. Her final attack was not quite as severe as the first, but instead of disappearing, her symptoms persisted. She could no longer avoid facing the fact that she was ill and she sought admission to the hospital for diagnosis and treatment. At the time of admission, she had pain in the right upper quadrant, nausea and vomiting, a temperature of 38.3°C (101°F), and leukocytosis. She looked and felt sick. Although chills may precede a rise in temperature, she had none. Careful inspection of the sclera of her eyes revealed some icterus. The level of bilirubin in her blood was 2 mg per 100 ml of blood plasma. The normal range is 0.1 to 1.2 mg per 100 ml. Even in the absence of stones in the common duct a transient icterus can occur. Jaundice is probably caused by edema, spasm, or inflammation of ducts draining the liver.

Although the history and clinical picture pointed toward choledocholithiasis, a few days were required before Mrs. Helmer was ready for surgery. In addition to the diagnostic procedures cited above, she had an x-ray of the abdomen. No preparation was required for it. Her urine was examined for, and, as expected, contained, bilirubin. Urine containing bilirubin is dark in color and forms large bubbles when shaken. Feces were pale or clay-colored.

Treatment and nursing care: Because Mrs. Helmer had fever and had been vomiting, she was somewhat dehydrated. She was given fluids containing glucose in physiological saline solution to correct the loss of water, chlorides, and calories. Because her biliary tract was obstructed and she had not been eating for several days, she was given multivitamins plus vitamin K in the intravenous infusion each day. Nursing of Mrs. Helmer during the period of diagnosis and preparation for surgery was directed toward providing comfort and emotional support and preventing complications as well as carrying out the aspects of diagnosis and treatment usually delegated to the nurse. Mrs. Helmer was a very sick woman who was fighting for survival and she behaved as sick people are likely to do. She regressed to a childlike state. Her tone of voice was whining. She complained repeatedly about how miserable she felt when she had to wait for care even briefly. She was petulant and irritable. She required and was provided with the same kind of care that any acutely ill person needs. She was given mouth care, was bathed, and had her back rubbed. The external environment was regulated to her for quiet and comfort. Because she was a member of a large family and had many friends, she required protection from too many visitors and from those who stayed too long. To prevent respiratory and circulatory complications, she was moved and turned and her extremities were passively exercised. Instructions were limited to preparing her for what was to be done at the time and to answering her questions. The nurse assumed full responsibility for the nursing care of Mrs. Helmer. The nurse anticipated her needs and she limited the demands made on Mrs. Helmer for adapting to her environment, including other people.

Although any change in the condition of a patient should be noted and recorded, observations of particular significance in the instance of Mrs. Helmer include increasing jaundice, color of stools and urine, and abdominal pain.

At some time in the future the treatment of cholesterol gallstones with chenodeoxycholic acid (CDC) may be available for select patients. The treatment involves daily dosage of CDC, which converts bile from a supersaturated to an undersaturated state with respect to cholesterol (Iser et al., 1975). This biliary change dissolves the cholesterol stone. The safety and efficacy of this treatment are being evaluated in clinical trials sponsored by the National Institutes of Health. The rate of stone dissolution is slow and may take from 6 to 24 months. Therefore, its greatest value is prophylactic in the asymptomatic person with cholesterol gallstones.

Failure of the Liver

ETIOLOGY. In addition to disorders involving the vascular system of the liver and the biliary canals, the liver parenchyma may fail. Because of the large reserve of liver parenchyma, evidence of failure of the metabolic and excretory functions is a relatively late manifestation in liver disease. Approximately 80 per cent of the liver can be destroyed before signs of liver failure appear. The liver is further protected by the great regenerative power of its cells. For example, in acute infectious hepatitis, areas of necrosis regenerate leaving no evidence of previous disease.

As stated previously, the most frequent cause of vascular congestion is failure of the right side of the heart as a pump. Parenchymatous cells can be injured by a wide variety of agents. Hepatotoxic agents range from the poisonous mushroom, *Amanita phalloides,* to a host of man-made chemicals (Zimmerman, 1968). Among the latter are chlorinated hydrocarbons used as solvents and chloroform, a general anesthetic; inorganic phosphorus, arsenic, and drugs such as sulfonamides, antithyroid agents, and tetracycline. Alcoholic cirrhosis was once thought to be caused primarily by the resulting malnutrition because it is well known that alcoholics eat poorly. However, fatty livers also occur in well-nourished alcoholics. Moreover, alcohol increases the susceptibility of the liver to other toxic agents. The livers of some individuals also appear to be sensitive to agents not harmful to most persons.

Liver function, as well as the fact that the portal blood passes through the liver before entering the systemic circulation, exposes the liver to higher concentrations of pathogenic agents than other tissues. Some chemicals are concentrated 10- to 100-fold by the liver (Zimmerman, 1968, p. 140). In addition to parenchymal injury from hepatotoxic agents, parenchymal damage can also result from disease or obstruction of the biliary tract.

Three principal factors probably account for similar morphological effects of different etiologic agents. With the exception of hypoxia and certain specific poisons such as carbon tetrachloride and carbon trichloride (chloroform), etiologic agents are poorly defined. In some patients a number of factors may be interacting to cause injury. Second, the number of ways in which liver cells can respond to injury is limited. Third, by the time the effects of disease of the liver are manifested, the defensive reactions of the liver tend to obscure the original injury. According to Faloon (1976), if one remembers the central role of the liver in the biochemistry and physiology of the body, the multiplicity of signs and symptoms of liver dysfunction is understandable. The person with liver disease may not only be jaundiced but also have a decreased prothrombin time, hypoglycemia, abnormal globulin fractions, deficiency in bile acids, and sodium and potassium metabolic disorders.

To illustrate, Mrs. Clarence, aged 42, had a diagnosis of advanced portal cirrhosis of the liver. For the last 10 years she had consumed increasing quantities of alcohol. For 3 or 4 months preceding her admission to the hospital, she had been drinking heavily and eating very little food. The only food that she ingested consistently was an 8-oz. glass of orange juice on arising. Biopsy of her liver demonstrated necrosis of the parenchyma of her liver and extensive fibrosis. What factor or factors were responsible for the injury of Mrs. Clarence's liver? Was it caused by the alcohol or poisons contained in it or was it caused by lack of important nutrients such as protein and the B vitamins? Probably all these factors played a part.

Liver Function Tests

A great variety of tests have been used to determine abnormalities in the physiology and anatomy of the liver. Understanding of the nature and effects of liver disease has been greatly increased by a number of developments: (1) liver biopsy, (2) electron microscopy, (3) improved biochemical techniques, (4) knowledge of the role of intracellular and serum enzymes, (5) ability to study circulatory patterns, and (6) radioisotope scans.

Commonly prescribed tests with their purposes and hazards are summarized. Directions for the performance of each test are not included because they vary in detail from one institution to another. The most important hazards to the patient are included, however, because some tests are accompanied by serious risks. Even when an untoward reaction is likely to occur only once in 1,000 patients, every patient should be treated as if he or she were that one.

BILIRUBIN—DIAGNOSTIC SIGNIFICANCE. Bilirubin, already referred to in the discussion of cholelithiasis, is a product of the degradation of heme, the pigmented portion of hemoglobin. It is discussed in greater detail in Chapter 42.

The level and type of bilirubin or its products found in the blood, feces, or urine have several uses in diagnosis. As products of the breakdown of hemoglobin, they can be used as a measure of the rate of blood destruction. As excretion products, they can be used as a measure of liver function or of the patency of the biliary tract. In some instances, the site of failure may be indicated by the form in which the substance occurs. For example, bilirubin levels in the blood rise (1) when the rate of blood destruction is excessive and the rate of formation is more rapid than the liver can excrete, (2) when certain types of injury to liver cells prevent its excretion, and (3) when the flow of bile from the liver to the intestine is blocked. With elevated bilirubin levels the skin, mucous membranes, and sclera of the eyes become a greenish yellow or jaundiced. The degree of jaundice is affected by the extent to which the bilirubin is elevated.

As it passes through the liver, the bilirubin molecule is conjugated with glucuronic acid to form bilirubin glucuronide, a water-soluble compound. Unconjugated bilirubin is not soluble in water. The van den Bergh reaction is based on the differences in the solubility of the free and conjugated forms. In the test, a color reagent is added to the blood. In obstructive jaundice an immediate change in color, known as the *direct* reaction, takes place; the concentration of bilirubin glucuronide is high. In hemolytic jaundice no color change occurs until the solubility of bilirubin is increased by adding alcohol; this is known as the *indirect* reaction and indicates a high level of unconjugated bilirubin. In inflammatory disorders such as hepatitis, the reaction may be intermediate.

Urine and stool examinations also help to distinguish between obstructive and hemolytic jaundice. In obstructive jaundice, bilirubin glucuronide is excreted in the urine. In hemolytic jaundice the urinary bilirubin is negative. In obstructive jaundice bilirubin does not enter the duodenum and the stool is clay-colored. In hemolytic jaundice bilirubin is secreted into the intestine and the color of the stool is normal.

BROMSULPHALEIN EXCRETION. The ability of the liver to remove a substance from the circulation and to excrete it can be measured by injecting a dye and measuring the rate at which it disappears from the blood. The Bromsulphalein (BSP) excretion test is the most widely used. In normal persons, 10 to 15 per cent of the dye is removed per minute. Less than 5 per cent of the dye should remain in the blood at the end of 45 minutes following injection. The greater the retention of Bromsulphalein, the greater the liver injury is. An occasional patient is hypersensitive to Bromsulphalein. This test should never be performed without appropriate preparation for this possibility.

TURBIDITY-FLOCCULATION TESTS. Two tests, or variations of them, are widely used to determine whether active parenchymal disease exists. These are the cephalin–cholesterol flocculation test and the thymol turbidity test. Blood serum is treated with the appropriate reagent and allowed to stand for a period of time. In the absence of disease no turbidity or flocculation takes place. In the presence of parenchymal disease a marked turbidity or flocculation, depending on the test used, appears. The flocculation is shown by most patients with acute viral hepatitis and is often positive before bilirubin levels are elevated and before jaundice appears. A negative test does not exclude hepatitis, however, inasmuch as up to one fifth of patients may give negative results. A high proportion of patients with cirrhosis shows a positive test, as do those with inflammation of the biliary tract. On the other hand, patients with biliary obstruction of short duration show normal values.

SERUM ENZYMES. Elevation of the level of two

types of enzymes is useful in the diagnosis of liver or biliary tract disease. The tests are based on the principle that enzymes are released into the circulation following injury to a tissue. The tests are not specific for liver or biliary tract disease and are useful only in association with other findings.

Transaminase enzymes—serum glutamic oxaloacetic transaminase (SGOT) and serum glutamic pyruvic transaminase (SGPT)—are found in high concentrations in the liver, heart, and skeletal muscle cells. When there are over 500 units of either enzyme in the blood, the patient is presumed to have liver damage, other conditions having been ruled out.

Serum alkaline phosphatase, another enzyme, is synthesized by the liver, bone, intestines, kidney, and placenta. The level of this enzyme is often elevated in conditions in which new bone is formed and in biliary tract obstruction.

Radiologic Methods

A liver scan is based on the same general principle as the scan of any organ. The organ takes up and concentrates a chemical that can be made radioactive or labeled with a radioactive substance. In the case of the liver, radio-tagged rose bengal, technetium sulfate, gold colloid, or gallium titrate may be used. From the liver scan, the size, shape, and location of the liver can be determined as well as the location of abnormal tissue.

Selective angiography provides for visualization of portal, hepatic, and pancreatic circulation. With this technique it is possible to view portal collateral circulation and to detect tumor masses. Portal pressure may be measured percutaneously or by catheterization of the hepatic or umbilical-portal veins. Portal measurements are elevated in cirrhosis. To demonstrate the patency of splenic and portal collaterals a splenoaortogram may be done. The major dangers of all angiography are: hemorrhage, thromboembolic risk, infection, and dye reaction.

Endoscopy can provide for direct visualization of esophageal varices secondary to portal hypertension. Duodenoscopy may be used for retrograde cholangiography which allows visualization of the biliary ductules. A transhepatic cholangiogram may be helpful in distinguishing hepatic and posthepatic jaundice. This is done by percutaneous puncture and injection of dye into a bile duct. It is a blind procedure and the major hazards are hemorrhage and bile leakage.

Some Gastrointestinal Manifestations of Liver Disease

The signs and symptoms accompanying diseases of the liver depend on a number of factors such as the acuteness or chronicity of the disorder, the extent to which liver function is impaired, and the nature of the response of the liver to injury. Unless cirrhosis of the liver develops, the patient is not likely to develop ascites. Serious disease of the liver affects to a greater or lesser degree the functioning of all parts of the body.

As might well be expected, disorders of gastrointestinal function frequently accompany liver disease. Many of the gastrointestinal manifestations are caused by disorders in motility and are nonspecific, inasmuch as they are commonly seen in illness. They include anorexia, nausea, vomiting, flatulence, diarrhea, constipation, and cramping.

Anorexia is frequently observed in patients with a diagnosis of liver disease. This is of special significance in the nursing of the patient because one of the keystones in the therapy is a nutritious diet. To be of value, food must be eaten. When a patient is severely anorexic, he or she will usually require considerable attention and support to overcome the disinclination to eat. For example, Mr. Clarence, who has acute infectious hepatitis, is anorexic to the point that the thought of food causes a feeling of revulsion. His physician has explained to him that anorexia is a cardinal manifestation in acute hepatitis, but that he will recover more rapidly if he can force himself to eat. Thiamine 10 mg may be given daily to counteract the anorexia. If hemorrhagic tendencies are evident, vitamin K should be given daily. The diet should be high in calories with good quality proteins and carbohydrate rather than fat. The patient should be expected to be a "fussy" or "finicky" eater, even if he or she eats everything when well. The patient should know why eating is important and should be given whatever encouragement and assistance is required. Food preferences should be taken into account in the selection of meals.

Large meals may only serve to increase the anorexia and nausea. It is better to serve three small meals and to use interval feedings of a liquid formula. A variety of milk beverages reinforced with protein can be offered; they may be taken slowly over a period of time and may be well tolerated. If adequate nourishment cannot be given by mouth, tube feeding may be necessary as the main source of nutrition or as a supplement to the small meals eaten.

If the patient becomes exhausted before completion of eating, he or she should be fed. Sometimes the relationship of the family or friends is such that the patient will eat when fed by them. The tray should be checked at the end of the meal, and the quantity of food not eaten should be recorded. If the patient will accept a substitute at a later time, this should be provided. One of the important functions of the nurse is to keep the lines of communication open between the patient, dietitian, and physician.

In disorders of the liver and biliary tract, digestion of food usually proceeds normally unless bile is prevented from reaching the alimentary canal. When bile does not reach the duodenum, the usual cause is biliary tract obstruction.

Changes in gastrointestinal function can also be caused by organic changes associated with liver disease. In portal cirrhosis, the alimentary canal may be congested as a consequence of portal hypertension.

CHANGES IN BLOOD CONSTITUENTS. Disease of the liver is accompanied by changes in a number of blood constituents resulting from the response of the organism to infectious agents or to cellular necrosis. In infectious hepatitis, neutrophils are frequently decreased and monocytes increased, probably caused by a response of mesenchymal tissues to the infectious agent and not by the involvement of the liver per se.

Blood proteins: The liver synthesizes the blood proteins, including the serum albumin, which is especially important in maintaining the osmotic pressure; the fibrinogen, which is essential for blood clotting; and the globulins, which are involved in the immune processes. In serious liver disease the serum albumin level may be less than half the normal value. One effect of this decrease is the tendency of the tissues to hold fluid. By contrast the serum globulin level is increased, and the total serum protein (albumin + globulin) level may appear to be normal. The ratio of albumin to globulin is often less than 1:1, as compared with a normal ratio of 2:1 or 2.5:1.

Anemia: Many patients with disease of the liver have anemia, the type depending on the factors contributing to its incidence. Mrs. Helmer, for example, whose biliary tract was obstructed, developed hypoprothrombinemia from failure to absorb vitamin K. She had a microcytic hypochromic anemia; that is, her red cells were small in size and pale in color. Patients with repeated bleeding from esophageal varices may also have a microcytic anemia. Mrs. Clarence had a macrocytic anemia. Her red cells, though decreased in number, were larger than normal size. Normocytic and macrocytic anemias are common in the patient with cirrhosis of the liver. This type of anemia may be the result of increased blood destruction, or folacin (folic acid) deficiency, or some unknown factor.

Hemorrhagic tendency: An increased tendency to bleed is a frequent finding in patients with disease of the liver. Failure to absorb vitamin K is a common cause. It is also thought that the liver, in some instances, is unable to utilize vitamin K to form prothrombin. Some patients who have a tendency to bleed have normal prothrombin levels; increased permeability of the capillaries or the lack of some other clotting factors may be at fault. Patients with disorders of the liver or biliary tract should be carefully observed for any evidence of hemorrhage. When bleeding occurs, the physician should be apprised of this fact.

Spider telangiectases: A phenomenon associated with cirrhosis of the liver is spider telangiectases. These are small, dilated blood vessels resembling a spider in form. They may be observed in the skin in various parts of the body.

Therapy

Diet and rest are the basic considerations in the therapy of patients with disease of the liver. At least 1 g of protein per kilogram of body weight should be included; somewhat more liberal intake (90 to 120 g) is beneficial to many patients.[9] The protein should be of good quality so that a complete assortment of amino acids is continuously available for maximum regeneration of liver tissue and for replacement of tissue and blood proteins. Sufficient calories from carbohydrates and fats should be provided so that protein can be used for tissue synthesis rather than for energy. The improvement in the level of serum albumin is sometimes exceedingly slow. Yet a nutritionally adequate diet improves the general sense of well-being, restores protein tissues of the body, and may reduce the tendency to edema.

The choice of food depends on the patient's preferences, provided that they are in accord with a nutritionally adequate diet. The restrictions in fat and the omission of spicy foods or strongly flavored vegetables are no longer considered to be necessary. Obviously, intolerance of particular foods should be respected, just as discretion should be used in menu planning. For example, many fried foods, very fatty meats, and rich pastries could produce discomfort, but butter, margarine, cream, ice cream, salad dressing, or an occasional piece of pastry might be enjoyed.

When anemia is present, the type and cause must be determined before satisfactory therapy can be instituted. Supplementary iron salts are prescribed for iron-deficiency anemia because the diet will seldom furnish more than 15 mg of iron per day; this is far too low to be of therapeutic value. Folic acid is often prescribed for macrocytic anemia, especially in alcoholic hepatitis.

In addition to a nutritious diet, the other form of treatment used in the therapy of patients with disease of the liver is rest. Currently the subject of

[9] See page 997 for discussion of exceptions to liberal protein diet.

the extent to which rest should be prescribed is highly controversial. Some, but not all, physicians advocate complete bedrest until the serum bilirubin is reduced to 3 mg or less per 100 ml. Bedrest is thought to shorten the length of illness. Everything should be done to promote relaxation of the patient. All activities that can be done by someone else should be performed for the patient, and the physical, emotional, and social climate should be regulated so that rest is encouraged.

Although the physician prescribes the therapeutic regimen for the patient with a disease of the liver, much of the responsibility for carrying it out is borne by the nurse. Whether the food served to the patient is eaten frequently depends on the patience and the persistence of a nurse who appreciates the importance of a nutritious diet to the recovery of the patient. Whether the patient is provided with an environment in which rest is possible also depends on a nurse who understands the importance of rest to recovery and who acts in accordance with her or his understanding.

EDEMA. As the severity of disease of the liver increases, the patient retains sodium and water. Retained water may be distributed over the body as generalized edema or be concentrated to some extent in body cavities, particularly in the abdominal cavity as ascites and in the pleural cavity as hydrothorax. A number of mechanisms are usually implicated in the development of edema in liver disease. Not all are involved in every patient. Some authorities state that failure to inactivate aldosterone leads to increased retention of sodium and water by the kidney; others state that this failure is doubtful.

Another factor predisposing to edema formation is a decrease in the synthesis of albumin, which is the most important blood protein in the maintenance of the colloid osmotic pressure of the blood. A significant fall in the concentration of serum albumin therefore decreases the water-holding power of the blood.

In the liver itself, two changes may occur that increase the likelihood of the development of ascites. In cirrhosis of the liver, contraction of the liver by scar tissue leads to portal hypertension and to an elevation of the hydrostatic pressure of the blood in the portal capillaries. With increased capillary permeability, albumin and fluid escape into tissues and serous cavities and increase the water-holding power of the tissue and serous fluids.

Treatment of edema: The treatment of edema in the patient with disease of the liver is similar to that for patients with healthy livers but who are edematous because of cardiovascular or renal disorders. To be sure, the edema associated with liver disease sometimes responds slowly to conservative measures and often reforms rapidly.

Restriction of sodium and an adequate to liberal intake of protein are important aspects of diet therapy in edema. Sodium restriction must usually be severe, ranging from no more than 200 to 500 mg daily. Not only must all foods be prepared without salt or other sodium compounds, but the amounts of meat, fish, poultry, eggs, and milk are carefully controlled because these foods are naturally high in sodium. Low-sodium milk is often substituted for regular milk. The sodium-restricted diet is probably one of the most difficult regimens for patients to accept, but by ingenuity in the use of spices and herbs, much can be done to improve the flavor of foods. The patient needs to know why it is important to omit salt and any foods that contain other sodium compounds. In addition, medications that contain sodium should be avoided.

An occasional patient receiving a severely restricted sodium diet may show signs of sodium depletion, including abdominal pain, muscle cramping, weakness, lethargy, confusion, and convulsions. This is especially true in patients who have cirrhosis and chronic renal disease. When any of these signs are detected, the physician should be notified.

The importance of protein for albumin synthesis has been pointed out in a preceding discussion. At a 500-mg sodium level of restriction, it is possible to include about 70 g of protein using regular milk and unsalted meats; when the sodium restriction is lower, low-sodium milk must be used to ensure an adequate intake of protein.

Diuretics may also be employed as adjunct therapy. The nurse should be observant of the diuretic effect. Too brisk diuresis should be avoided. The electrolytes should be monitored closely as should evidence of hepatic encephalopathy (coma).

PARACENTESIS. When ascites or hydrothorax becomes so great that either interferes with the function of the alimentary canal or with breathing, fluid may be withdrawn from the peritoneal or thoracic cavity. Removal of fluid from either cavity involves intrusion in the internal environment, and both procedures should therefore be performed under sterile conditions. The general precautions to be taken when the pleural cavity is entered are discussed in Chapter 40.

Paracentesis (removal of fluid from the peritoneal cavity) is usually performed in the room of the patient or in the treatment room. The nurse has two general responsibilities. One is to prepare the patient and to support and comfort him or her during the procedure and the other is to assist the physician. The latter is also a service to the patient, inasmuch as assistance given by the nurse to the physician facilitates the care provided for the patient. The patient should be so prepared that he or she knows what to expect. Emphasis should be placed on the fact that as the result of the removal of fluid, breathing will be easier, movement will be freer, and eating better. To prevent puncturing of the bladder during the procedure, the urinary bladder should be emptied by the patient or by catheterization before the procedure is attempted. If the paracentesis is performed on the patient in bed, he or she should be brought to the side of the bed and supported in a sitting position. If able, the patient may sit in a chair or with the feet over the edge of the bed. In whatever position the patient is placed, the back should be adequately supported. The skin should be shaved if necessary and thoroughly cleansed.

To lessen the danger of puncturing the colon, the cannula is introduced at the midline and below the umbilicus. After the cannula has been introduced into the peritoneal cavity, tubing is attached to it and the ascitic fluid is drained into a pail or a bottle. Although either is a satisfactory receptacle, the physician may wish to collect the fluid under sterile conditions for purposes of examination or for infusing it into the patient.

After the procedure is completed, the skin at the site of puncture may require a stitch or two to close the incision. A small dressing may be all that is required. When it becomes wet, it should be replaced. The clothing of the patient and bedding should also be checked at the same time and changed as often as necessary. When ascites develops rapidly and the patient requires repeated paracenteses, the problem of keeping him or her dry may be considerable.

During the performance of paracentesis, fluid is withdrawn slowly to prevent syncope resulting from a too rapid reduction in intra-abdominal pressure. At the completion of the procedure an abdominal binder may be applied until the patient has adjusted to the decrease in intra-abdominal pressure.

Throughout the procedure the patient should be apprised of what is expected, of what is being done, and of his or her general progress. For example, when cleansing the skin, the nurse should tell the patient what she or he is doing. When a solution that evaporates rapidly is placed on the skin, the patient should be prepared for the fact that it will be cold. As the physician injects the anesthetic into skin, or introduces the cannula into the peritoneal cavity, the patient should be informed of what is happening. After the peritoneal cavity has been entered and the fluid has started to flow, the patient should be informed. Whether the patient is undergoing paracentesis for the first or the hundredth time, he or she should be included as a participating member of the team. Attention should be given to the physical status of the patient. The pulse, respiration, and color should be noted and any undue change reported to the physician.

Other Signs of Serious Liver Disease

In patients with serious disease of the liver, changes in the mental status, from mild confusion, disorientation, and irrational behavior to stupor and deep coma may appear. Hyperventilation and flapping tremor may also occur. In hyperventilation the depth of respiration is increased, but not the rate. In fact, the rate of respiration may be slower than normal. Not all patients with severe liver disease develop coma, nor do those who become comatose necessarily present the milder signs before developing coma.[10]

Although the reasons for the development of mental changes have not been completely identified, two mechanisms appear to be involved. They are the accumulation of metabolities, probably of a nitrogenous nature, in the internal environment of cells and an abnormal sensitivity of cerebral cells to changes in their fluid environment. Among the nitrogenous substances, ammonia and ammonia-bearing compounds are implicated. Hepatic coma can be precipitated in susceptible patients by orally administered ammonia compounds as well as by certain bacterial metabolites containing methionine. In the healthy liver, substances absorbed from the intestine, such as ammonia, are detoxified before they reach the general circulation. Ammonia is converted to urea. In severe liver disease, the liver cells are assumed to be unable to convert ammonia and other potentially harmful nitrogenous materials to harmless ones. Another possibility is that blood containing these substances does not pass through the liver before it enters the general circulation. Blood flow may be detoured around the liver by naturally occurring or surgical shunts.

Coma can be precipitated in susceptible patients by agents increasing the load of nitrogenous substances or by sodium-excreting diuretics. Thus a high-protein diet predisposes to coma because of the increased production of ammonia by the deamination of the amino acids. When there is impending coma, a protein-free diet or a very low-protein diet (20 to 30 g) is usually prescribed. The calorie intake should be maintained as high as practical by fruit juices reinforced with glucose in order to minimize tissue breakdown. The catabolism of tissues is a

[10] In stupor, the patient can be, but is not easily, aroused. In coma he or she cannot be aroused.

source of ammonia through the breakdown of the constituent amino acids. Even 500 to 600 kcalories per day can be quite effective in keeping tissue breakdown to a minimum.

Ammonium drugs such as ammonium chloride increase the load of nitrogenous substances to be excreted. Carbonic anhydrase inhibitors such as acetazolamide (Diamox) also increase the possibility of coma by increasing the excretion of the sodium ion. Because these agents are also of value in the therapy of the patient with liver disease, the physician may prescribe one or more for a given patient. The nurse should be alert to and promptly report any changes in the patient's mental alertness and status. Nursing of the comatose patient is discussed in Chapter 36.

Nutritional Problems Related to Metabolism

Enzyme Disorders

Inborn Errors of Metabolism

Disorders of metabolism result from the inability of the cell to synthesize a specific enzyme. The capacity to synthesize enzymes depends on the genetic inheritance of the individual. A single gene is involved in a single metabolic reaction. A defective gene may be inherited as a mendelian recessive or dominant. When inherited as a recessive trait, the defect is evident only in individuals inheriting the same trait from both parents. In the absence of the necessary enzyme, a metabolic process is stopped at the point where the missing enzyme acts.

Numerous enzyme-deficiency diseases are now recognized, including such widely known conditions as phenylketonuria, galactose disease, maple syrup urine disease, and leucine-induced hypoglycemia. The metabolic errors produce marked changes in the infant shortly after birth, mental retardation being particularly severe. In some of the diseases it is possible to prevent the severe abnormalities by the early institution of a diet that is carefully regulated to limit or omit the nutrient that cannot be adequately metabolized.

In phenylketonuria, the enzyme that is essential for the conversion of phenylalanine to tyrosine is missing. As a consequence the central nervous system fails to develop and severe mental retardation results. The early detection of the abnormality means that a low-phenylalanine diet can be initiated, thereby making possible essentially normal development of the infant. Galactose disease, resulting from the inability to convert galactose to glucose, likewise leads to severe mental retardation and other abnormalities. It is amenable to treatment, the omission of all sources of milk being essential. Some success has been achieved with the use of very expensive synthetic formulas restricted in isoleucine, leucine, and valine in the treatment of maple syrup urine disease. No treatment has currently been developed for a number of metabolic errors. Similarly, it is now suggested that children be tested at birth, at school age, and at adolescence for familial type II hyperlipoproteinemia. The presence of this condition is known to be important in the genesis of hypercholesterolemia. Susceptible individuals can be detected at birth and treated with a low-cholesterol diet (Schubert, 1973).

Enzyme Inhibitors

The action of enzymes may be inhibited by the action of heavy metals and by certain drugs. One way that mercury is believed to produce toxicity is by inhibiting enzyme reactions. Chemicals such as cyanide are highly toxic because they inhibit enzyme systems catalyzing oxidation-reduction reactions. Death occurs in a matter of minutes following the ingestion or inhalation of cyanide.

The actions of many drugs depend on their ability to depress enzymatic activity. Barbiturates may depress the nervous system by depressing specific enzymes. Acetazolamide (Diamox) induces diuresis by interfering with the ability of the enzyme carbonic anhydrase to catalyze the reaction enabling the kidney to excrete an increased volume of sodium ion in the urine. Sulfonamides are effective in the control of certain bacteria because they depress the enzyme system, enabling them to synthesize folic acid from paraaminobenzoic acid.

Disorder in Carbohydrate Metabolism—Alterations in Blood Glucose

Hypoglycemia

Despite the effectiveness of regulatory mechanisms in keeping the level of glucose in the blood within physiologic limits in most people, they sometimes fail. Depending on the nature of the failure, the level of glucose in the blood falls outside physiologic limits. When the concentration of glucose in the blood falls below 70 mg per 100 ml, the condition is known as hypoglycemia.

Causes

Theoretically, hypoglycemia could result from a failure in the supply of glucose. In diseases of the liver in which its capacity to store glycogen is below physiologic limits, hypoglycemia is at times a problem. Hypoglycemia may also result from failure of the mechanisms for adding glucose to the blood. As a consequence, hypoglycemia is associated with adrenal insufficiency. Probably the most frequent cause of hypoglycemia of a severe degree is overactivity of the mechanism for lowering the level of glucose in the blood, that is, an oversupply of insulin. The insulin may be of endogenous or exogenous origin. If the supply of insulin is excessive, the level of glucose in the blood falls below 70 mg per 100 ml of blood. The effects of lowering the level of glucose in the blood will depend on the suddenness and the extent to which it falls below normal limits.

Signs and Symptoms

Most of the manifestations of hypoglycemia result from failure to supply sufficient glucose to the cells of the nervous system. Glucose is the only fuel from which it can derive energy. Early symptoms and signs in hypoglycemia result from increased autonomic activity. Hunger, often marked, sweating, increased pulse rate, restlessness, irritability, and headache occur early. The patient who is experiencing hypoglycemia for the first time may say, "I feel funny," or "I feel peculiar." Changes in the usual behavior of a patient who is receiving insulin are frequently the result of hypoglycemia. For example, Steven Anderson, who had been a model patient, suddenly became very amorous. Mary Sema was found sitting upright in bed, her eyes fixed and her arms rigidly extended in front of her. Mild-mannered Mr. Boas became violent when treatment of hypoglycemia was delayed until blood could be drawn for glucose analysis. Mr. Johns was admitted to the hospital in coma. Buddy Reiman, aged 12, developed nocturnal enuresis (bed wetting). Each of the above patients was suffering from the effects of hypoglycemia. In each instance, treatment with a readily available form of glucose restored the patient to his or her usual mode of behavior. With the exception of Mr. Johns, glucose was administered by mouth in the form of fruit juice. Moments after an intravenous solution of glucose was begun, Mr. Johns regained consciousness and was demanding to know why he was in the hospital.

Treatment

Because of the possibility of permanent damage to the brain, patients who receive insulin in the treatment of diabetes mellitus should learn to recognize early symptoms and signs of hypoglycemia and how to treat it. Modified insulins create a problem, inasmuch as hypoglycemia may develop without causing warning signs. Persons under insulin therapy should also be taught that exercise improves the utilization of glucose and that hypoglycemia is more likely to develop when unusual amounts of exercise are taken. They should be subject to regular observation when they are hospitalized. Should they develop signs or symptoms indicating hypoglycemia, it should be treated promptly. Usually 100 ml of orange or other fruit juice provide sufficient glucose to correct the condition. Observation should be continued with patients receiving long-acting insulin who experience hypoglycemia. Because of the possibility of recurrence of hypoglycemia in persons receiving long-acting insulin, milk and crackers may be used in treatment because they provide a more sustained source of glucose than do fruit juices or sugar.

Excessive secretion of insulin associated with hyperplasia or an adenoma of islet cells may also be responsible for hypoglycemia. Adenomas are believed to be of infrequent occurrence. Cure is effected by surgical removal. Functional hypoglycemia is a common occurrence. It is usually associated with anxiety and increased nervous tension. Symptoms such as weakness, faintness, tachycardia, and headache follow a meal. The ingestion of carbohydrate alleviates the symptoms temporarily but because carbohydrates act to stimulate the secretion of insulin, a vicious circle, or positive feedback, is initiated.[11] Most patients respond well to a high-protein, high-fat, and low-carbohydrate diet. They should be instructed to avoid the ingestion of highly concentrated carbohydrates because they stimulate the secretion of insulin.

Hyperglycemia

In contrast to hypoglycemia, hyperglycemia is a condition in which the level of glucose in the blood rises above 110 to 120 mg per 100 ml of blood. It can result from the excessive ingestion of glucose, from overproduction of glucose within the organism, or from inadequacy or failure of the mechanism for the removal of glucose from the blood. More than one mechanism may be involved. The condition in which hyperglycemia follows the excessive ingestion of concentrated carbohydrates is known as alimentary glycosuria. The term *alimentary* refers to the fact that glucose is absorbed from the alimentary canal. The presence of glycosuria indicates that the renal threshold for glucose has been exceeded with the result that glucose appears in the urine. Therapy is obvious: Avoid eating excessive quantities of car-

[11] In a positive feedback, a change in one direction intensifies the tendency to change in the same direction.

bohydrate, especially in the form of sugars, at a given meal.

Overactivity of one or more of the mechanisms for the endogenous formation of glucose follows the administration of epinephrine, and this results in an elevated blood glucose. It can also be expected to rise as a part of the reaction of the individual to stressful situations. Many patients have some elevation in blood glucose following a coronary occlusion or major surgery. Because epinephrine stimulates the liver to convert glycogen to glucose, the elevation of the blood sugar depends on glycogen being present in the liver.

Hyperglycemia of sufficient degree to cause glycosuria may also occur in persons with hyperfunctioning adrenal cortices. It is also a finding in acromegaly, a disorder associated with hyperexcretion of the growth hormone by the anterior hypophysis. In these conditions the failure in the homeostasis of glucose is thought to be the result of the overproduction of glucose by the organism. The possibility also exists that some of these hormones also antagonize the action of insulin or interfere with its secretion.

A third source of hyperglycemia derives from a failure of the mechanisms for the removal of glucose from the blood. Although the mechanism that immediately comes to mind relates to the action of insulin, failure of the liver to store glucose is also a cause of hyperglycemia. In serious liver disease, hyperglycemia after a meal, followed by a sharp drop in blood glucose to hypoglycemia levels, is a common finding.

The second source of failure to remove glucose from the blood at a normal rate is a deficiency in the supply of insulin, ineffective insulin, or a decrease in the number of receptor sites for insulin. Whatever the cause, hyperglycemia occurs when the supply of insulin is insufficient or ineffective in removing glucose from the blood. All degrees of failure are possible. In some individuals sufficient insulin is secreted to maintain the level of glucose within physiologic limits provided the ingestion of glucose is moderate or there is no increase in the activity of mechanisms for increasing the production of glucose. In others the deficiency of insulin may be so great that only by restricting the intake of carbohydrate and the administration of exogenous insulin can the blood sugar be maintained within normal limits most of the time. The disease resulting from a failure of the mechanism to remove glucose from the blood at a normal rate is diabetes mellitus (see Chapter 47).

Glucose Tolerance Test

Individuals who are unable to adapt normally to a heavy load of glucose can be identified by a glucose tolerance test. The details for performance of this test differ from one physician or agency to another. In all instances the purpose of the test is to determine the adequacy of the mechanism of the patient for removing glucose from the blood, thereby restoring homeostasis.

For 2 to 3 days preceding the test the patient should eat a diet that provides 250 to 300 g of carbohydrate. The nurse has a responsibility to make sure that the patient understands the instructions and to encourage him or her to eat the food served while in the hospital. On the day of the test, fasting specimens of blood and urine to be used as controls are obtained before the glucose is administered. The patient is then given a weighed amount of glucose (usually 100 g for an adult) dissolved in water and flavored with citric acid or lemon juice. Blood samples and specimens of urine are obtained ½, 1, 2, and 3 hours later.

The results obtained in individuals with normal and abnormal glucose-tolerance curves differ in several respects. The individual who has a normal capacity to respond to an increased supply of glucose has a sharp, but limited, rise in the concentration of glucose in the blood plasma. The maximum elevation should not exceed 150 mg per 100 ml of blood plasma. There is a sharp rise in one-half hour, with little rise thereafter. By the second hour the concentration of glucose in the blood has returned to normal.

The individual with an inadequate capacity to remove glucose from the blood responds to overloading with glucose differently. The fasting blood sugar is higher than normal. The rise in the blood sugar following the ingestion of glucose is higher, and the return to the pretest level is delayed. This type of curve is observed in the patient in the early phases of diabetes as well as in those whose diabetes mellitus is known.

Several modifications of the glucose tolerance test have been developed. In one of these the test dose of glucose is divided into two parts. The second half is given one-half hour after the first. In the person who has a normal adaptive capacity, the level of glucose in the blood does not rise after the second dose of glucose. In the person whose adaptive capacity has been impaired, the level of glucose in the blood continues to rise. When hyperinsulinism is suspected, blood and urine samples may also be collected at 4, 5, and 6 hours after the ingestion of glucose. In patients who produce too much insulin the blood sugar drops to hypoglycemic levels.

The early detection of diabetes mellitus is often accomplished by performing two glucose tolerance tests. Eight hours and again 2 hours before the second test 50 mg of cortisone are administered orally.

The cortisone intensifies the strain on the mechanisms for removing glucose from the blood. In persons with an inadequate insulin reserve, the blood glucose curve obtained during the second test resembles that found in diabetes mellitus. Persons who respond positively to this test are encouraged to follow a regimen to decrease the likelihood of developing diabetes mellitus, that is, to avoid gaining weight.

For example, Mrs. Hale, aged 27, has stress or stage II diabetes mellitus. Both her parents are diabetics. When Mrs. Hale is well and eats moderately and exercises actively and regularly, her fasting blood sugar is within normal limits. When she overeats, has a cold, or is pregnant, her blood glucose tends to rise. She sees her physician regularly and eats moderately. She tries to adjust her food intake so that she maintains her ideal weight. In contrast Mrs. Hale's sister Clara's response to glucose-tolerance tests indicates that her capacity to adapt to glucose is within normal limits. Present-day knowledge is insufficient to be sure that Clara will never develop diabetes. Because the ideal weight favors health and longevity, Clara has been advised to avoid obesity and to exercise regularly. She has also been assured that she does not have diabetes.

Abnormalities of Lipid Metabolism

Obesity, underweight, and diabetes mellitus are widely recognized abnormalities of fat metabolism discussed at other points in this text. A great deal of evidence has accumulated over the last decade to implicate the diet in the elevation of blood cholesterol and other blood lipids and in the incidence of atherosclerosis. (See also Chapter 43.) Blood cholesterol levels are increased when diets are high in saturated fats and low in polyunsaturated fats and by diets high in cholesterol. Animal fat enhances cholesterol absorption whereas plant sterols depress its absorption from the intestines. Mattson et al. found that the average American diet tended to increase serum cholesterol by as much as 40 mg per 100 ml (Mattson et al., 1972). The Inter-Society Commission recommends that Americans (1) ingest sufficient calories to achieve and maintain optimal weight; (2) achieve a cholesterol intake of less than 300 mg per day; (3) reduce total fat to less than 35 per cent of total calories and saturated fat to less than 10 per cent of total calories, with up to 10 per cent as polyunsaturated fat and 10 per cent as monounsaturated fat (Stamler et al., 1970). These diet changes mean that more poultry and fish are eaten and less meat, skim milk is used in place of whole milk, vegetable oils are used instead of solid fats, and eggs, organ meats, and shellfish are restricted.

Inadequate or Disordered Protein Metabolism

Effects of a Lack of Protein

The effects of protein deficiency are described in this chapter under the heading "Undernutrition" (p. 1003–08). Because protein foods are generally good sources of the B-complex vitamins and iron, the signs of deficiency are those of multiple nutrient lacks. Loss of weight, strength, and ability to respond to infection and stress are frequent but nonspecific indicators of deficiency. Anemia is often present because of the lack of both protein and iron for the synthesis of hemoglobin. The colloid osmotic pressure of the blood is gradually reduced as the level of serum albumin falls. Fatty livers have been noted in severe protein undernutrition.

Protein deficiency occurs in many serious illnesses because of inability to ingest protein or because of excessive losses. The deficit is aggravated by the fact that there is an increase in the rate of tissue breakdown for the first few days after a severe injury or a surgical procedure. Proteins may be lost in excessive amounts into the urine, from draining wounds such as burned surfaces, and in accumulations of serous fluids such as ascites. Chronic abscesses, decubiti, or osteomyelitis may be accompanied by an excessive loss of protein. Continued bedrest, even in the healthy, is accompanied by loss of protein for the first 3 or 4 days—then the loss of protein tapers off and the nitrogen balance is restored. Loss of protein from the body is therefore one of the undesirable effects of bedrest. Loss of protein-containing fluid represents a loss not only of protein but of minerals, vitamins, water, and other substances from the body. The effects on the organism will depend in part on the suddenness with which the losses occur, the conditions that are responsible, and the length of time that they persist. Sudden large losses of fluid into serous cavities may, by reducing blood volume, lead to shock. Smaller losses over a period of time lead to malnutrition with a loss of weight, strength, and ability to respond to stress. Resistance of tissue to pressure is less in the undernourished than in the well-nourished. When decubiti form, they resist treatment unless and until protein and other nutritional deficiences are corrected. Recovery depends on the restoration of nutritive elements.

Negative Nitrogen Balance

The underlying reasons for a negative nitrogen balance are many, including (1) insufficient intake of protein in terms of quality or quantity or both, (2) insufficient calorie intake so that dietary protein and body tissues are being used to meet the energy needs, (3) defect in absorption of amino acids from the digestive tract because of enzyme deficiencies or diseases of malabsorption, (4) inability to metabolize one or more amino acids because of genetic defect, and (5) excessive losses of protein in exudates of burns and draining wounds or in the urine because of renal damage.

Problems of Dietary Adequacy of Minerals and Vitamins

Of the fifteen or so mineral elements required by the body, special attention is needed for calcium, iron, iodine, and fluorine. When the allowances for protein and for these elements are met, the needs for other mineral elements will be fully realized.

Calcium can be supplied in the diet in the form of additives as chalk or bone flour or it can be ingested in such foods as milk, cheese, molasses, cauliflower, rhubarb, beans, and egg yolk. The amount of calcium ingested is dependent on the total amount of calcium present in the diet. However, it has been found that where the milk intake is low, the diet is often deficient in calcium (Kon, 1972). Perhaps the best argument that can be made for adequate calcium intake throughout life is on the basis of insurance of normal bone structure. Teenaged girls often drink too little milk in the mistaken notion that it is fattening. Their actual calcium needs are high to meet the requirements for bone growth and maturation. When the demands of pregnancy are superimposed on these already high needs, the young mother-to-be is quite likely to be in negative balance. Osteoporosis, a bone disease affecting large numbers of older people, especially women, has a complex etiology, but it seems clear that those who drink little milk throughout life are more susceptible than those who are milk drinkers. Sometimes the ill effects of low calcium intake become evident in the failure of bones to heal following fracture, particularly in older persons. Before instructing a patient on the necessity of milk in the diet, the nurse should determine the patient's tolerance of milk. An intolerance to milk is common in noncaucasian adults. This intolerance is caused by a decrease in the activity of the enzyme lactase after weaning.

The most serious dietary problem with respect to the mineral elements is that of iron. Infants, young children, adolescent girls, and pregnant women are especially vulnerable to iron-deficiency anemia. To correct this problem, the recommended allowance for iron is 18 mg for girls and women and 10 mg for men (*Recommended Daily Dietary Allowances*, 1974). A good diet based on suggested intakes from each of the four food groups will supply about 6 to 7 mg of iron per 1,000 kcal. Thus the man experiences no difficulty in obtaining the recommended allowance. Not so for women! Most women require about 1,800 to 2,400 kcal daily, and even good diets would therefore supply only about two thirds of the recommended iron allowance. In nutrition education, emphasis must be placed on rich sources of iron including the organ meats, especially liver, enriched and whole grain breads and cereals, some dark green leafy vegetables, meats, egg yolk, legumes, dried fruits, and molasses. The contribution made by these foods, of course, depends on the frequency with which they are consumed as well as the amounts used. According to Höglund, iron absorption is facilitated by the presence of ascorbic acid and is retarded by a full meal. Accordingly, exogenous iron should be administered prior to meals and if possible with ascorbic acid (Höglund, 1970).

Iodine deficiency is most common in the parts of the world far from the sea. During the history of the world, soil has been leached of iodine and iodine washed into the streams and thence into the seas and oceans. Soil in the great plains, such as the center of the United States, and in mountainous regions, such as the Andean Altiplano or the Swiss Alps, is deficient in iodine. In these areas evidence of iodine deficiency has been common. Conditions increasing the need for thyroxine intensify the deficiency. Pregnancy, adolescence, or infections may be associated with enlargement of the thyroid gland in iodine-deficient areas. Prevention of iodine deficiency is achieved by the use of iodized salt.

When added to water in the amount of 1 part per million of water, fluorine has been demonstrated to reduce the rate of dental caries. Excessive concentrations of fluorine cause mottling of the enamel of the teeth. Despite convincing evidence of the value of fluorides in the prevention of dental caries, there has been organized resistance to the introduction of fluoride into drinking water. Some of the opponents claim the fluorine increases the incidence of heart disease in the areas where it is used. Objective analysis of the statistics indicates the falsity of this belief. Other persons object on the basis that fluorine is of value only to the young and that cities should not use tax funds to support a procedure that benefits only a part of the population. Still others object on religious grounds. Some even object on the ground that it violates the right of the individual to choose what he or she will or will not ingest. A review of the history of chlorination of water indicates a similar story.

A nutrition survey conducted in ten states from 1968 to 1970 found individuals suffering from severe deficiencies of vitamin A and vitamin C in this country (Shaefer, 1970). These dietary inadequacies stem primarily form failure to supply sufficient amounts of fruits and vegetables in the diet. The rules for dietary planning to ensure sufficient intake are relatively simple: (1) some dark green or deep yellow vegetable or deep yellow fruit at least every other day to supply ample carotene, the precursor of vitamin A; and (2) some citrus fruit or other good source of vitamin C, such as tomato juice, raw cabbage or dark green leafy vegetable, broccoli, or cantaloupe.

Malnutrition

The term *malnutrition* as used here refers to the condition in which essential nutrients in the tissues are not present in the necessary amounts. The nutrients may be present in either deficient, imbalanced, or excessive amounts.

Malnutrition may be the result of improper intake, improper digestion, absorption, or excretion of nutrients, or improper metabolic use of these nutrients. It is worldwide in scope and differs only in the degree of severity among people living in the affluent and poor nations.

Undernutrition

Undernutrition is a generalized state of deficiency in which a deficient caloric supply is accompanied by insufficient proteins, minerals, and vitamins. Manifestations of specific deficiency diseases may become evident when lack of one nutrient predominates. For example, in beriberi, thiamine is the principal nutrient lacking, and in pellagra the primary deficiency is niacin. However, in each of these conditions the body is supplied with inadequate quantities of most, if not all, nutrients, and some signs characteristic of multiple deficiency are also present.

Undernutrition may be the result of (1) insufficient food being available or ingested, (2) a severe disease of the digestive tract that prevents the absorption of nutrients, as in malabsorption or cancer of the esophagus, (3) a severe and lengthy systemic infection or metabolic disease that interferes with normal metabolism and reduces appetite (Davidson & Passmore, 1969).

Causes of Undernutrition in the United States

Undernutrition is a manifestation of poverty. The poor wherever they live are the most susceptible. Studies over the past decade have demonstrated that the more serious undernutrition plagues the American poor, especially minority ethnic groups, Indians living on reservations, migrant workers, and the aged (Quimby, 1975). Small children and pregnant and nursing mothers are also plagued with severe undernutrition (Eckholm & Record, 1976). The decline in breast-feeding and the increase in the use of high-cost milk substitutes and glass-jar weaning foods has caused a natural resource (human milk) to be ignored while needlessly increasing the cost of feeding infants.

People who lack knowledge or motivation or who are superstitious are also susceptible to undernutrition. Commerciogenic undernutrition is becoming prevalent, both in the United States and in developing countries. In the United States today, 50 per cent of available foods are highly processed. Although there are conflicting reports, it has been reported that many frozen foods are lacking in folate. Also, snack foods that supply primarily calories and little or no protein or vitamins are very widely used.

Other Factors Contributing to Undernutrition

Undernutrition is frequently brought about by some pathologic condition that interferes with adequate food intake, digestion, absorption, or metabolism. The nutritional problems associated with many pathologic conditions have already been discussed in this and other chapters of the text. (See Table 46-3 at the end of this chapter.) Unless careful adjustment is made in the diet, one can expect some degree of undernutrition when one or more of the following conditions exist.

Infections and parasitic infectations accentuate the effects of inadequate diet. The calorie and nutrient requirements are increased because of fever and losses through the gastrointestinal tract.

Anorexia is frequently associated with organic disease as well as psychological disturbances. In the latter, extreme emaciation sometimes results. Acute illness in the well-nourished and the temporary loss of appetite are not likely to be serious. In the chronically ill patient, or in those who are undernourished at the onset of illness, anorexia is of more serious import.

Increased nutritional requirements are imposed by fever, burns, hyperthyroidism, severe anemia, and advanced neoplastic disease. Effects of illness, such as restlessness, dyspnea, or orthopnea, intensify the need of the patient for food.

The degree to which the basal metabolic rate is elevated in the orthopneic patient is illustrated by Mrs. Thims. She had a basal metabolic rate of + 100 per cent. Unless there is a corresponding increase in food ingested, weight loss accompanies any condition in which tissue requirements are increased. In some disorders, such as congestive heart failure, retention of salt and water may mask the loss of body substance. Upon the removal of the edema fluid the patient is found to be emaciated. Sometimes the state of nutrition of the edematous patient is so poor that he or she does not respond to the usual measures to eliminate the edema until nutrition is improved.

In some disorders, the total quantity of food required by the patient may be increased, not by an increase in the requirement of cells, but by excessive losses of nutrients from the body. For example, some disorders of the alimentary tract are accompanied by loss of nutrients. Patients who have large burns or draining wounds or abscesses may lose enormous quantities of nutrients. Large quantities of protein may be lost through abnormally permeable glomeruli in the kidney. In uncontrolled diabetes mellitus, weight loss results from the loss of glucose in the urine. Inasmuch as protein and fats are mobilized for energy and to form glucose, they are also lost. Whatever the cause of the loss, the extent and type of nutrient lost must be estimated and every effort made to restore the balance between supply and demand. The nurse contributes to the estimation of the extent of tissue requirements by making pertinent observations.

Improvement of Nutrition in the United States

Efforts to improve the level of nutrition in the United States need to focus on (1) improving the general level of income and (2) improving the general education of people so that their ability to select a nutritious diet is improved. More specifically, nutrition education must become an integral and important part of the curriculum for every child in the elementary and secondary schools of our nation so that he or she can learn in early life to make wise food choices. Particular attention to the education of mothers and mothers-to-be can be expected to yield good results. Because of the rapid changes in the food products available in today's market, people need continuing information on the products that they buy—their nutritive contributions, comparative costs, methods of preparation, and so on.

Signs and Symptoms

Undernourished infants and children gain weight slowly, remain short in stature, and show delayed maturation of the skeletal structures. Undernourished children have lowered resistance to infection and generally suffer more severe illnesses as protein deficiency interferes with antibody formation. Studies indicate that the malnourished infant will demonstrate a depressed intellectual level later in life. In addition, there are intergenerational effects of this malnutrition. A woman who had poor nutrition and poor health as a child has a significantly higher risk of having a child with a neurointegrative abnormality and a depressed intellect. The younger the child, the more severe are the effects of undernutrition. As the deficiency progresses the child is less able to digest foods, presumably because of a decreased output of digestive enzymes. The serum albumin level gradually falls and the serum globulin level rises, indicating some interference with liver function. Also, if the starvation is severe, ulceration and hemorrhagic lesions of the stomach and colon that interfere with absorption may occur. The skin becomes dry and pigmented, and the hair pigment also changes with grayish or reddish streaking. In severe undernutrition the fluid and electrolyte imbalance may be so serious as to threaten the life of the child.

Adults who are moderately undernourished show few signs except loss of weight. As undernutrition proceeds they will do less and less work unless forced to do it. They become much more susceptible to infections and convalesce more slowly from any illness. The pregnant woman is especially vulnerable, and undernutrition increases the possibility of spontaneous abortions, stillbirths, and premature births. By repeated pregnancies, the poor condition of the mother and the fetus is further aggravated.

As undernutrition progresses in the adult numerous changes take place in body tissues: lowered basal metabolic rate in accord with lowered cell mass and reduced cell activity; changes in hair, skin, and mucous membranes, including dry, pigmented skin, glossitis, and stomatitis; reduction in gastrointestinal enzymes, intestinal ulceration, abdominal distention, diarrhea; neurologic changes such as polyneuritis; lowered serum albumin sometimes accompanied by edema; fatty liver; macrocytic or microcytic anemia; and many other changes.

Treatment

Correction of the undernutrition is effected through an increase in the intake of calories and protein. Easy as this may appear to be to those who have a problem with overweight, the correction of caloric and protein undernutrition may take weeks and months of effort. It often requires (1) a fundamental change in attitudes of the individual and/or family, (2) a building up of the tolerance of the gastrointestinal tract for food, (3) more money to buy food, as well as (4) the patience, understanding, and cooperation of the various members of the health team to achieve success. The reasons for undernutrition vary from one person to another. Therefore, inasmuch as is possible, each person must be treated as an individual.

When undernutrition is extreme, little is gained by suddenly initiating a high-protein, high-calorie diet; in fact, force feeding may be dangerous. Neither the digestive tract nor the cardiovascular system is able to cope with the additional demands posed by large amounts of food. The patient's appetite, during severe undernutrition, often appears to be easily satisfied, and this appears to be, in fact, a protective mechanism. The management of patients with severe undernutrition is therefore complex and requires attention to fluid and electrolyte balance, control of any existing diarrhea, and gradual replacement of nutrients. Initially, small meals of nutritionally balanced foods are given. When the tolerance to small quantities of food is well established, gradual additions are made to the diet.

Examples of Undernutrition

The following individuals illustrate some of the problems that contribute to caloric undernutrition. Some questions that might be considered here are the following: What is the presenting problem (or problems) in each of the four individuals? What are the possible outcomes? Suggest appropriate ways in which a nurse might contribute to the solution of each. In which of the patients presented below is the prognosis favorable, if appropriate action is taken in time?

Sharon, aged 15, had been a plump baby and child and had always eaten well. At the close of the school year she decided to lose weight so that she would be more nearly like her friends in appearance. Because her previous attempts had been unsatisfactory, she felt that her situation was desperate. With the exception of a glass of skim milk and a piece of fruit, three times per day, she refused to eat. Her parents became frantic. The less she ate, the more they scolded and the greater was Sharon's determination to stick to her diet and to lose weight rapidly.

Mrs. Ross, aged 75, lives across town from Sharon. She lives alone in a one-room apartment. Although she has a modest income, her meals consist of health bread and tea. She says other foods disagree with her and that her food intake is adequate. She supports her position by stating that printed on the wrapper covering of the bread is a statement that this bread contains all of the elements required for health. Mrs. Ross has never been fat. She is weak and tired, but after all, as she says, she is an old woman. Her family and friends are gone. She lived during the period when family life was the most intense at any time in American history. When she was a child and until her children left home and her husband died, meals were a social event. The entire family gathered round an abundantly supplied table to eat and enjoy each other's company. Now all that is gone and Mrs. Ross has little incentive to eat.

Mary Alice, aged 17, has arthritis. She was hospitalized for rehabilitation, during which time she made considerable progress. After her return home, she soon returned to almost full-time bedrest. She says that she is too weak and tired to get out of bed. A 3-day food-intake study revealed that her caloric intake was only about 800 calories. Among a number of possible factors contributing to the situation, the easiest to identify and correct is the fact that Mary Alice's mother is a poor cook.

Many of the elements that contribute to problems that arise in the chronically malnourished patient are well illustrated by Mrs. Muncie. As is often true, Mrs. Muncie's malnourished state did not arise suddenly nor was it the result of a single cause. At the time of her admission to the hospital Mrs. Muncie presented an emaciated appearance. Her skin was tightly drawn over her slight frame. She had a large infected decubitus ulcer over her sacrum. Although she had not felt well for some years, she had been able to care for a five-room flat, prepare meals for herself and her husband, and be active in church work. Her present illness had its onset about a week previous to her admission for an episode of diarrhea. Her husband had cared for her at home, because he wanted her to die in peace. A neighbor finally persuaded him to have her admitted to the hospital.

Some of the factors contributing to Mrs. Muncie's chronically malnourished state were revealed by her personal history. She was the thirteenth child born to sharecropper parents in Mississippi. She had completed about the fourth grade in school. Her diet throughout her lifetime was that which she ate as a child. She and her husband had moved to Big City 25 years ago. Insufficient income to cover expenses had been a constant problem. At the time of her admission to the hospital, her husband's wages as a janitor were only $270 a month, but he did have sufficient hospital insurance to cover Mrs. Muncie's hospital expenses. Only by the most careful management were they able to meet all of their obligations. Because her appetite was poor and her husband left early in the morning, she usually ate only two meals a day. The first consisted of either tea or coffee and toast and soup or orange juice. The second meal, which she shared with her husband, usually consisted of a vegetable, preferably greens cooked with fat pork, and cornbread or hot biscuits. Mrs. Muncie had worn dentures since she was 25 years of age.

When she was between the ages of 13 and 25, her father pulled her teeth, one by one, because they were painful. When asked about her weight, she said that she had always been "skinny." Based on her dietary history, Mrs. Muncie's nutrient intake was probably always marginal. Significant factors in her background include poverty, a low educational level, loss of her teeth at an early age, and customs in food selection and preparation that tended to restrict her intake of protein and calories as well as other important nutrients.

An appropriate question at this point is, "How is it that Mrs. Muncie managed to live for more than 60 years on a diet of cooked vegetables, cornbread, and fat pork?" Adults show considerable resistance to food deprivation. In the presence of an inadequate supply of nutrients, cells adapt by decreasing their rate of metabolism. Stores of fat and protein are mobilized and utilized for energy. The only evidence that food intake is less than that required may be loss of weight or a weight that is less than normal. Although the individual is able to do heavy work, he or she rests at every opportunity. During the period in which the individual is able to adapt the metabolic rate of cells to the limited food intake, the malnourished state is said to be compensated. The person may survive in this state for a long period of time. When some condition develops, such as an infection, that places added stress on the individual, adaptation fails and evidence of uncompensated undernutrition appears.

Mrs. Muncie indicated that she had been underweight most of her life when she said "I've always been skinny." Until she had a nephrectomy 6 years ago, she had always been reasonably well. Since that time she had been in her words "poorly." Her present illness was ushered in by an episode of diarrhea. Although she attributed this to some cabbage that she had eaten, diarrhea is frequently the first evidence that chronic undernutrition has entered the uncompensated phase. When she entered the hospital a week later, she was also found to have pyelonephritis in her remaining kidney. As stated previously, an infection is frequently the stress that upsets the unstable balance in chronic undernutrition. Soon after the onset of her illness a decubitus ulcer formed at the base of her spine. It was infected. After compensation failed, Mrs. Muncie was no longer able to protect her tissues from the effects of pressure. Resistance to infection was also impaired.

On physical examination, Mrs. Muncie presented many signs and symptoms of chronic undernutrition. Despite the fact that she was 5 ft 5 in. tall, she weighed only 88 lb. The desirable weight for a woman of small frame and 65 in. tall is from 111 to 119 lb. She did not give the appearance of having lost weight recently. In older individuals, rapid losses of weight are usually accompanied by wrinkling of the skin and loose folds of skin over areas where subcutaneous fat is stored. As the skin ages, it loses its elasticity, and with the loss of elasticity, the ability to adapt the skin to the size of the underlying tissue is diminished. After 50 years of age or so, the skin of the person who loses weight rapidly is likely to be too large for the frame. The severely undernourished person tends to retain water. Although this is more likely to occur in children than in adults, the absence of wrinkling of Mrs. Muncie's skin may have been caused in part by water retention.

Among the other signs and symptoms of chronic undernutrition presented by Mrs. Muncie were wasting of tissues including her muscles; edema; dry, scaling skin; numbness and tingling of her toes; hyperesthesia of feet and legs; weakness and pallor; glossitis (sore tongue); diarrhea; poor wound healing; and anorexia.

Her laboratory findings, which are summarized in Table 46-2, were consistent with a state of chronic undernutrition.

It will be noted that her total blood proteins are within the lower limits of normal, but that the albumin-globulin ratio is reversed. This indicates that albumin is being broken down or lost from the body more rapidly than it can be replaced. Multiple factors probably account for the deficit of albumin. Lack of sufficient intake of protein to provide the amino acids required to replace albumin lost from the body, loss of albumin in the exudate from the decubitus ulcer, and possibly in the diarrheal fluid, utilization of serum albumin to provide energy, and possibly inability of the liver to synthesize albumin—all probably contribute to the reversal of the albumin-globulin ratio. This condition also occurs when large quantities of albumin are lost in the urine. Loss of albumin by this route was not a factor in the instance of Mrs. Muncie. The relatively high serum globulin level accounts for the total protein level being within the normal range, and indicates the response to the prevailing infection. Some degree of dehydration may have also contributed to maintaining the level of protein within normal limits. The blood urea nitrogen elevation may be caused by protein catabolism. The lowering of her carbon dioxide-combining power is consistent with acidosis. It will be noted that her serum sodium is slightly decreased; this indicates some loss of cations. Acid-base balance is discussed fully in Chapters 27 and 41. Acidosis is common in starvation. As might be expected, Mrs. Muncie's hemoglobin is low. Associated with this is a low hematocrit. Anemia is a common occurrence in menstruating women who are undernourished. Although Mrs. Muncie is well past the menopause,

Table 46-2 *Laboratory Values of an Undernourished Patient*

Laboratory Test	Finding—Mrs. Muncie	Normal Range
Blood protein—total	6.6 g/100 ml	6.5–8.3
Serum albumin	1.82	3.5–5.5
Beta globulin	2.51	0.52–1.01
Gamma globulin	2.25	0.61–1.39
Blood urea nitrogen	35 mg/100 ml	10–20
Electrolytes		
Sodium	120 mEq/liter	125–147
Potassium	4.8 mEq/liter	3.5–5.5
Carbon dioxide	26.1 volumes per cent	50–70
Hemoglobin	8.1 g/100 ml	12–16
Hematocrit	31 per cent	36–47
Urine		
Albumin	Negative	Negative

she had been undernourished for much, if not all, of her life.

After Mrs. Muncie was admitted to the hospital, three interrelated problems required immediate attention. The first and central problem was to improve her nutritional status. The second and third were to heal the decubitus ulcer and to eliminate the infection in her kidney—the pyelonephritis. In the early part of her hospitalization, these problems required urgent attention. Others were secondary. To correct her undernutrition, a plioform nasogastric tube was introduced into her stomach. The formula was made by liquefying natural foods in a blender. It contained 1,500 kcal per liter. Other commercially available elemental diets may have been used and given by gavage or orally. The formula was administered slowly with sufficient amounts of water to prevent diarrhea. The tolerance of the digestive tube for food is diminished in undernutrition. Therefore, the ingestion of more than usual amounts of food is likely to aggravate or induce diarrhea in addition to other problems. The diet was supplemented with other essential nutrients as needed.

In addition to efforts to improve her nutritive state, measures were instituted to hasten the healing of her decubitus ulcer. She was placed on a Stryker frame that was turned every 2 hours day and night. Attention was paid to all sites of pressure in order to prevent further tissue breakdown. Warm saline compresses were applied to the ducubitus twice daily for an hour, followed by exposure of the area to a heat lamp for one-half hour. Every effort was made to keep the area clean and dry. Plastic surgery was considered, but not performed because of her poor nutritive state.

Mrs. Muncie's progress was slow. During the first 3 weeks of therapy she gained only 2 lb in weight but she had gained enough strength so that she was able to walk with assistance. She was encouraged to walk because ambulation improves morale and appetite as well as the normal functioning of the alimentary canal. To increase her food intake, her request for a soft diet was granted. Because she tired when eating, she was given assistance at mealtime.

Mrs. Muncie had some assets not available to all patients. She had a devoted husband. She had a strong religious faith. Her husband, who had an excellent work record, was assisted by his employer in establishing that he was 65 years of age and therefore eligible for social security. He planned to retire so that he could care for his wife at home. As soon as the decubitus ulcer was healed, Mrs. Muncie was to be discharged home under the supervision of the outpatient clinic and a visiting nurse. Efforts were made to instruct the husband and wife in selection of food that would meet at least minimum nutritional requirements. Because of their age, limited education and money, and a lifetime of habits, the outlook for marked improvement was poor.

There were also other problems in the care of Mrs. Muncie. The purpose, however, of introducing her case here was to present some of the problems that cause and result from chronic undernutrition. Mrs. Muncie was not from a far-off land, but lived in a large city in the United States. The factors in her condition are those that underlie undernutrition over the world—poverty and illiteracy perhaps being the most fundamental. She did not have a so-called deficiency disease, such as arises when one nutrient is lacking in the dietary. Rather she suffered to a greater or lesser extent from a lack of all nutrients, calories, proteins, vitamins, and minerals.

Had Mrs. Muncie's state been discovered before decompensation occurred, her illness might have been prevented. This would have taken an increase in the ingestion of all nutrients. For each pound gained, an intake of 3,500 calories in excess of those utilized is required. In persons whose food habits and patterns are set, an increase in food intake is often difficult to achieve. It takes time and patience. The individual needs to understand and accept that increase in the intake of food is necessary to health and well-being and to want to improve his or her food habits.

Obesity

Although the incidence of obesity is high among Americans, obesity is neither confined to Americans nor a new problem. It is found among the wealthy, sedentary individuals in all parts of the world. Art objects uncovered in the ruins of ancient civilizations attest to its antiquity. The Venus of Willendorf is a limestone statuette named for the Austrian village in which it was discovered, and the figure is indistinguishable from the present-day fat woman. The Venus of Willendorf, however, is the figure of a Stone Age woman and antedates the development of agriculture by 10,000 years. The group in which the Venus of Willendorf lived were hunters. They probably gorged themselves when food was plentiful, as after a successful hunt, and fasted or starved when food was scarce. In fact, the fatty deposits stood them in good stead during the periods of scarcity.

Considering so many factors affecting energy balance, one must marvel at the homeostatic mechanisms by which many people are able to maintain desirable weight throughout life. Yet, a substantial proportion of the population, perhaps 10 to 20 per cent of all schoolchildren, and 35 to 50 per cent of all adults, experiences overweight and obesity to some degree (Eckholm & Record, 1976). Food in the United States is so plentiful and attractive in its many forms that overeating can easily become a habit. Many people lead sedentary lives at work and in leisure so that they can ill afford the calorie-rich foods so widely available for meals and snacks.

Too many people lack knowledge concerning calorie and nutrient values of foods and often do not realize that even small intakes beyond daily energy needs lead, in time, to gross obesity. This growing public health problem requires a careful study of the many reasons obesity may occur and of ways by which it may be prevented or treated. How is the determination of obesity made?

Definition

Obesity is an excessive accumulation of fatty or adipose tissue. It involves two factors: (1) individual genetic susceptibility and (2) a gross imbalance between food intake and energy expenditure. Ninety-five per cent of all obesity is overconsumptive, probably due to environmental factors. Mayer (1976), in examining the food consumption and energy expenditure of Americans, found that the population is taller and heavier (fatter) despite the slowly decreasing overall food intake. Clearly physical activity diminished more rapidly than caloric intake.

Height-weight tables have long been used to determine the degree of overweight and obesity. Because it is generally agreed that it is undesirable to gain weight throughout life, weight considered to be normal for height and body frame at age 22 years is accepted as desirable throughout life. A weight increase of 10 per cent over the desirable level is usually defined as overweight, and an excess of 20 per cent or more is designated as obesity. Those individuals who are grossly obese are detected visually, but for people who are moderately overweight the height-weight tables do not provide an accurate guide for body fatness. Jim Johnson is a college athlete who weighs 20 lb more than tables indicate he should. He has a well-developed musculature and no evidence of thick folds of fatty subcutaneous tissue; he is not obese. Sally Brown is within 5 lb of her desirable weight but leads a very inactive life. She has moderately thick folds of fatty tissue around the abdomen. She is slightly obese, although the tables do not so indicate.

The normal fat content of the body increases steadily from infancy, girls becoming fatter than boys by the early school years. The percentage of body fat increases throughout life as lean tissue decreases, even though weight remains stationary. The occasional exceptions are those individuals who remain vigorously active throughtout life. At all ages women have a higher percentage of body fat than do males. The thickness of subcutaneous tissue is a more reliable indicator of the degree of fatness than are height-weight tables. Clinicians often make a rough estimation by simply pinching up a fold of skin. By using calipers, the exact thickness of the tissue may be determined at selected points such as the triceps and subscapular skinfolds and compared with normal standards for fatness. Screening the triceps is easiest to measure and a reliable index of total body fatness. Standard tables are not available. However, it must be remembered that clinical judgment may still overrule the dictates of a chart. For in practice it may be more desirable to keep a diabetic patient lean and a tuberculous patient fat (Burton, 1976).

Effects on Health

Hazards of Obesity

Obesity is of concern primarily because it has an adverse effect on health and life expectancy. Adipose tissue places a double burden on the individual. Excess tissue has to be carried as a weight on the individual. Mrs. Albert carries a 55-lb weight with her everywhere she goes, upstairs and down as well as on a level. Obese tissue also has to be supported with nutrients. Each pound of adipose tissue contains 0.7 mile or more of capillaries through which blood circulates.

Diabetes mellitus in adults is highly associated with obesity. It is now believed that obesity is not a cause of diabetes but that it is an early manifestation of the metabolic defect that in later life leads to the typical symptoms of diabetes. Gout and diseases of the liver and gallbladder are also found more frequently in the obese. With a positive energy balance, fatty components in the blood rise and predispose the individual to atherosclerosis and coronary disease. Those individuals who have arthritis or osteoporosis find that the burden of fat to be carried around is an additional handicap.

Although a moderate degree of overweight (10 to 20 per cent) is not always regarded as harmful, statistics indicate that the mortality rate goes up as the weight rises above the desirable level. According to Cowhig, a man who is 20 per cent overweight increases his chances of dying before retirement by one third whereas a man who is 30 per cent overweight is as likely to have a coronary as a man with an abnormal heart pattern (Cowhig, 1972). The adverse effects of obesity are the greatest in males in the years before 40. Excess cardiovascular mortality accounts for a high percentage of the excess mortality among overweight men. A 12-year epidemiologic study, the Framingham study, found that obesity increased the workload of the heart, resulting in an increased risk of sudden death, but not of myocardial infarction (Kannel, 1967).

Causes of Obesity

In the final analysis obesity results when the energy intake is in excess of the body's expenditure of energy. There are, however, many causes for this imbalance.

Overeating

Excessive ingestion of food has been the most frequently cited cause of obesity. Overeating may be related to the cultural pattern or may be an expression of some psychological disorder. Great importance is attached to food in social situations, the food industries entice the consumer with attractive advertising for calorie-rich foods, and eating snacks has become a way of life in America. The dietary patterns of some families predominate in calorie-rich foods. Unfortunately, overemphasis on excessive eating as a cause of obesity has led many health workers to adopt an unjustified moralistic stand against the individual.

Psychological Factors in Overeating

Because the nervous system participates in the regulation of eating, overeating frequently has a psychological basis. In some persons overeating accomplishes two psychological purposes or gains. The first is a primary gain. Food is used to substitute for gratification in life situations. Eating relieves unpleasant feelings—loneliness, frustration, guilt, depression, insecurity, or anxiety. As an example, everyone is acquainted with someone who eats when bored or who makes additional trips to the refrigerator when preparing for an important examination. This is frequently called reactive obesity and may be a compensating factor in adjustment to life, thereby preventing a more serious disturbance.

Secondary psychological gains involve the use of eating not for its direct effect on relieving unpleasant feelings, but to bring about desired changes in interpersonal relationships. It may be used offensively to control or gain attention of others. For example, a youngster overeats because by so doing he pleases his mother. Overeating may be a defensive maneuver utilized by the individual to protect himself or herself from contact with others. For example, Dorothy, aged 15, is 50 lb overweight. She is a shy, anxious girl who fears rejection by her peers. She uses her obesity as a reason for avoiding others. In effect, a thick layer of fat serves to insulate her from people in her environment. Developmental obesity involves the entire growing personality. Experiments indicate that obese individuals may be relatively insensitive to internal hunger satiety clues and thus may lack one of the regulatory devices for eating (Itallie & Campbell, 1972). This may have either a physiologic or psychological basis.

Despite the large amount of information available on the dangers of obesity, excess weight is not necessarily considered undesirable by everyone. Obesity continues to be more prevalent among women of the lower socioeconomic level than among women of any other socioeconomic level (Eckholm & Record, 1976, p. 34). This may be because it is considered a sign that they are financially able to be obese. Loss of weight for such an individual would require reeducation and insight.

Inactivity

One of the most neglected factors in the incidence of obesity is relative inactivity rather than excessive eating of food. In the American culture, machines have largely replaced human beings in the performance of manual labor. In fact, the machine has greatly reduced physical activity in all aspects of the life of human beings. The farmer not only uses a tractor to cultivate fields, but both the farmer and his or her city cousin use a machine to mow their lawns. When a man plays golf, he rides a motorized cart because it speeds his game and is easier. When a person needs something from the corner store, he or she rides in a car. Even children ride to school or to the park. Elevators make it unnecessary to walk from one floor to another. The home is equipped with labor-saving devices from vacuum cleaners to electric beaters and dishwashers. Many recreational activities are for the spectator rather than the participant. Because machines have reduced the need for physical exercise, control of caloric intake combined with regular exercise is necessary for control of weight.

People of middle age and older continue to eat about as much throughout their lives as they did in their youth. Mrs. Simon, age 45, is a good example. Despite lessening activity, she eats about as much as she did when her children were young and she was very active. She has gained 10 lb over the last 8 to 10 years and complains of her thickening waist. Her weight gain is probably caused by failure to adjust her food intake to her diminishing energy requirements.

Endocrine Imbalance

Aberrations of the hormonal control of energy metabolism are responsible for only a small percentage of obese individuals. Hypothyroidism is the best known of these. The lessened secretion of thyroxine reduces the basal metalobic rate, sometimes as much as 30 to 40 per cent, so that the required number of calories to maintain the resting metabolism is reduced. These individuals are likely to be inactive, thereby further decreasing the energy expenditure. Consequently, obesity is likely unless the calorie intake is maintained at levels considerably below the expected normal.

Adrenocortical hyperfunction may lead to a condition known as Cushing's syndrome or moonface obesity. A lesion of the pituitary results in Fröhlich's syndrome, a type of obesity occasionally seen in children. These obesities are characterized by abnormal fat deposits in certain regions of the body.

Heredity

Mr. Johns says, "I'm fat. My father and mother were fat, as were their mothers and fathers." Perhaps heredity is used too often by people as an explanation of their obesity. Frequently the explanation for obesity in several members of a family lies in a cultural pattern dictating the hearty eating of many rich foods. This is not always the case, however. This may be caused by infant feeding practices or by a genetic predisposition to obesity.

The endomorphic (soft, round) individual must continuously control his or her diet and increase activity to control weight, whereas the ectomorphic (lean, wiry) individual is able to follow the dictates of appetite without fear of growing fat. Inasmuch as these body types are inherited, the tendency to obesity may likewise be said to have a genetic origin. The point most worthy of emphasis is that early recognition of body types in children could result in the initiation of effective measures relating to food intake and activity so that obesity could be prevented in these highly prone individuals.

Metabolic Obesity

Marked obesity is frequently accompanied by other clinical or subclinical disorders. These include hypertension, hyperglycemia, hyperlipidemia, hyperuricemia, hyperbilirubinemia, and often as elevated hemoglobin and hematocrit. Most and in some cases all of these disorders disappear when a satisfactory weight loss is achieved. This phenomenon has caused speculation that obesity may be caused by or accompanied by other metabolic abnormalities.

It has been demonstrated that an elevated level of insulin is present in the obese and that the insulin level returns to normal when weight is lost. In addition, in the obese there is a resistance to the usual activity of insulin due to a decrease in the number of receptors available. In the diabetic, as the obesity decreases the receptors become more insulin-sensitive, thereby decreasing the need for insulin supplementation.

Prevention of Obesity

Fifty to 85 per cent of obese children remain obese in later years. Presumably this is caused by a proliferation of fat cells early in life resulting from either an inordinate intake of food during a critical period of development or a genetic predisposition to hypercellularity. The number of fat cells is fixed after adolescence. Fat cells can increase in size in adults, however. Because chronic obesity is especially resistant to treatment, particular emphasis should be given to its prevention in childhood and adolescence. Infant-feeding practices may need to be modified so that the mother does not force the last bit of formula or other food; the fat baby is not necessarily the healthiest baby. Preschool children need to have sufficient diversion by various activities so that they do not become unduly preoccupied with eating. Throughout the school years the child and adolescent should have opportunity to learn about the nutrient and caloric values of food, to know something of food selection for daily meals, and to understand the role of food in weight control. In some instances attention must be given to cultural patterns that encourage excessive food intake through emphasis on calorie-rich foods with great values being attached to eating. The programs of physical education should aim toward physical fitness throughout life by encouraging activities that can be continued into the later years. Friedman (1975) pleads for preventive programs. The family lives together, eats together, and exercises together; thus what is needed is a primary prevention program developed for the entire family and not one particular member who is singled out.

Adults in their 20s and 30s need to be aware of the ease with which they may gain 5 to 10 lb in a year, and that these gains are often the results of small daily excesses of food or of gradual decreases in daily activity. Watching one's weight, engaging in physical activity, and taking prompt steps to correct small gains will eliminate the problems of later obesity.

Treatment of Obesity

The treatment of obesity would appear to be a relatively simple matter, namely, to reduce the energy intake below that of the body's expenditure. Yet in actual practice, obesity is difficult to treat, and the failures are many. Those who have become obese in middle age are most likely to succeed, whereas those who have been obese since childhood or adolescence are seldom successful.

The satisfactory treatment of obesity should meet the following aims: (1) weight loss to a level desirable for the individual, (2) the maintenance of good nutrition throughout the period of weight loss, and (3) lifetime modification of food habits so that the desirable weight is maintained.

To achieve the desired goals, professional guidance is essential throughout. A thorough evaluation of each individual must be made by the therapist to determine the causes of the obesity, the factors that may be useful in bringing about motivation, and whether any psychological factors would contradict the imposition of a weight-losing regimen.

Unless the obese individual has developed sound reasons for weight loss and is determined to follow a prescribed regimen, any efforts by the therapist are doomed to failure. Among the more common reasons are pride in personal appearance, improved health status, avoidance of jibes of family, friends, and business associates, and desire to improve health or to avoid one of the chronic disorders associated with obesity. Sometimes the obese person finds that, to obtain a particular job, he or she must lose weight. The nurse can sometimes assist the patient in expressing why he or she wishes to reduce and to support efforts to continue.

As an example, Mrs. Albert, aged 35, was 55 lb overweight. Her mother had diabetes mellitus, and Mrs. Albert's glucose tolerance curve was indicative of stress diabetes. On this basis, the physician recommended that she lose her excess weight over the next year. To encourage her, her husband offered to buy her a new wardrobe when she reached the desired weight. Both Mr. Albert and the physician frequently complimented her on her improved appearance.

Overeating can be a defense against feelings that are unacceptable to the patient. This possibility should be considered before treatment is begun. For example, one group of obese patients was found to accept treatment more completely when other major medical and emotional problems were first taken care of so the patients could concentrate on the obesity (Shumway & Powers, 1973).

Calorie Level of the Diet

The caloric intake generally prescribed permits a weight loss of 1 to 2 lb per week. Because the loss of 1 lb of adipose tissue is equal to roughly 3,500 kcal, it is apparent that the loss of 1 lb per week would necessitate reducing the daily diet by 500 kcal below the maintenance level. Thus the man who ordinarily needs 2,800 kcal per day would lose 2 lb in a week if he reduced his intake to 1,800 kcal per day. The 65-year-old woman who needs 1,700 kcal per day would lose 1 lb in a week if her diet furnished 1,200 kcal per day.

Extremely low-calorie diets (300 to 900 kcal) are sometimes prescribed because the rapid weight loss that results gives encouragement to the patient. Nutritionally, such diets are inadequate in minerals and vitamins and they may also provide less protein than is desirable. Diets containing less than 1,000 kcal are seldom warranted except for bed patients in a hospital. Not infrequently such diets lead to weakness, dizziness, and, for those with coronary insufficiency, to an increase in anginal attacks. In older persons, too rapid loss of weight may lead to loose, flabby skin, scrawny necks, and sunken cheeks, thus attracting adverse comments from relatives and friends.

Attempts are being made to produce weight loss in the obese through the use of a low-carbohydrate diet. The principle behind the treatment is to attempt to remove glucose, the stimulus for the elevated insulin level found in the obese. The controlled insulin level reduces lipid storage and consequently the obese individual loses weight. A diet of 50 g of carbohydrate per day is claimed to be palatable and to cause weight reduction.

Nutritive Adequacy

The nutritive requirements of the obese, except for energy from food, are the same as those of the nonobese person. Although a protein intake of 55 to 65 g is satisfactory for adults, many people find that a somewhat higher level of protein (80 to 90 g) results in a more satisfying diet. When foods are chosen from the Meal Exchange Lists,[12] including milk, vegetables, meats, and breads and cereals, the mineral and vitamin intakes are likely to be adequate for diets of 1,000 kcal or more. If lower caloric levels are prescribed, mineral and vitamin supplements must be added.

Food Values

The patient must have a thorough knowledge of food values if he or she is expected to follow a diet and to maintain desirable weight throughout life. The Meal Exchange Lists furnish a good starting point for becoming familiar with food values because the calorie and other nutritive values of foods within each list are similar. The initial restriction of food choices to these lists also helps to ensure adequate intakes of all nutrients.

Various methods of food preparation illustrate further how readily the calorie value may be increased. For example, one egg—raw, soft or hard-cooked, or poached—furnished 80 kcal. But when the egg is fried in 1 tsp of fat about 45 kcal have been added. When the egg is beaten with 1 tbsp of cream and cooked as an omelet with 2 tsp of butter, the calorie value has been increased to 175. Cream, butter and other fats, sugar, and flour are ingredients that rapidly increase the calorie content.

The obese individual should recognize that relatively small daily intakes of food in excess of calorie needs are additive in terms of body weight. An average daily excess of 50 kcal amounts to 18,250 kcal in a year or the deposition of about 5 lb of fat. But 50 kcal represent a very small amount of food: 1 tablespoon of heavy cream, or 3 level teaspoons of sugar, or ⅓ cup of whole milk, or 4 ounces of carbonated beverage, or ½ cup of orange juice, or 1½ teaspoons of butter, and so on.

Exercise

Activity has not been sufficiently emphasized as a means of controlling weight because many people have felt that too much exercise was required to lose a small amount of weight and that exercise had the tendency to increase the appetite. An individual who learns that he or she must walk 36 miles to utilize the calories of 1 lb of fat tends to become discouraged. Yet, over the period of 1 year, a walk of 1 mile per day will result in the loss, or in the prevention of gain, of 10 lb. This may be stated in another way: reducing the daily intake by 500 kcal below the body's needs will result in a 4-lb weight loss in 1 month. If the activity is also increased by a daily 1-mile walk, the increased output each day of 100 to 125 kcal will result in the loss of almost an additional 1 lb each month.

Moderate exercise such as walking on a daily basis is preferred to occasional vigorous exercise. Moderate exercise does not increase the appetite, but intense physical activity sometimes does. Even though 18 holes of golf may utilize 800 to 1,000 kcal, the expenditure is nullified if the nineteenth hole includes considerable quantities of beverages and food. In addition to its effect on weight loss, exercise increases muscle tone and improves the physical and mental well-being. The amount of exercise recommended must be adjusted to each individual's health status; a sudden and marked change in exercise patterns is ill advised for older persons.

Variations in Weight Loss

The actual weight loss may vary widely from that calculated. Norma Sims has conscientiously followed her 1,200-kcal diet but has lost no weight in 2 weeks. The nurse reassures her by telling her that it is not uncommon for tissues temporarily to hold water and that she will soon begin to lose weight if she continues to adhere to her diet. Many women experience fluid retention prior to onset of the menstrual period, and this should also be kept in mind. Of course, if there is continued failure to lose weight, the therapist will need to determine whether the prescribed calorie level was appropriate and whether the patient is, in fact, rigorously controlling portion sizes and methods of preparation.

Variations in activity from week to week will also affect the degree of weight loss. Mrs. Thomas, 60 years old, follows her prescribed diet and takes a walk every afternoon. Several weeks of cold weather and icy walks have kept her indoors, and she finds that she is not losing much weight.

Psychological Support

Losing weight is a day-to-day endeavor in which the results become apparent only with the persistent attention to diet and activity. The patient must be given confidence in his or her ability to control food intake. He or she needs the continuing support of the family. Scolding the patient or chastizing the patient rarely produces positive results. The patient

[12] Available from The American Dietetic Association, Chicago.

should be treated in a nonthreatening manner that takes into consideration his or her individuality.

Aldrich, a psychiatrist (1963), indicates that obesity should be viewed as any other addiction. He recommends that it be studied from the point of view of impulses, controls, and consequences. Obesity is a consequence of failure to control the impulse to eat. According to this concept of obesity, the problem faced by the patient and by those who are working with him or her is to help the patient to learn to control the quantity of food eaten. Emphasis is on the patient exercising the control rather than the control being external. For example, Mrs. Leslie, who is chronically obese, sees her physician about every 6 weeks. For the 2 weeks preceding her visit to her physician she literally starves herself. After her visit, she exercises little control over what she eats. Her control is from the physician. Mrs. Leslie wishes to please him or to avoid being scolded. She blames her employer and husband for tempting her with food.

As a consequence of her behavior, Mrs. Leslie feels ashamed. "I should lose weight, I'm a sight." She also rationalizes, "How can I lose weight when you make pie and sweet rolls and leave them out where I can see them?" and "Ben won't eat broiled, roasted, or boiled meat. It has to be fried." Many obese people react in a similar manner. They need help in identifying their own responsibility in controlling their weight.

Drugs in Weight Reduction

Appetite depressants, as well as agents purported to suppress the appetite, come and go. Drugs suppressing the appetite center in the brain usually cause nausea as well as anorexia. Drugs such as amphetamine phosphate and related compounds depress the appetite by inducing a sense of well-being. Because some drugs have dangerous side effects, they should not be taken by persons who are not under medical supervision.

Metabolic stimulants, including hormones, have been tried in weight-reduction regimens. Because the thyroid hormone stimulates metabolism, it has been used to increase weight loss. In the euthyroid individual, the ingestion of exogenous thyroid hormone decreases the secretion of the thyroid gland. When excessive dosages of thyroid are ingested, symptoms of thyroid toxicity appear.

Group Therapy

Some people are better able to achieve weight loss when they ally themselves with a group such as TOPS (Take Off Pounds Sensibly) or Fattys Anonymous. In such groups individuals are able to talk over their problems with others and to compare methods for coping with them. Group meetings provide opportunity for information on dietary control, methods of food preparation, how to resist overeating, the value of exercise, and so on.

Any individual who joins a group should be advised initially by a physician that it is safe to undertake weight loss. Preferably, the person will have had some individual counseling regarding diet prior to joining the group. So that members of a group do not fall prey to misinformation or faddism, it is advisable that a nurse, nutritionist, or physician be available for consultation and guidance.

Surgical Treatment

Surgical treatment is available for individuals who weigh 300 lb or more and who have been unsuccessful in their attempts to lose weight. The purpose of the surgery, the small intestinal bypass, is to reduce the area of absorption in the intestines so that a lowered caloric intake results. A surgical communication is made between the small intestine and the colon in such a way as to balance the area of absorption and the nonfunctional area. After the surgery there is an increased thickness in the remaining bowel and spontaneous recovery of amino acid absorption. However, fat is poorly absorbed and diarrhea is present to some degree for a lifetime (Weismann, 1973). Other possible complications include osteoporosis, a bowel infarction or intussusception, magnesium depletion, cirrhosis, or pulmonary emboli. Anyone undergoing this surgery needs to be aware of the constant necessity of replacing fluids and electrolytes. Gastric stapling has also been tried recently, the intent being to reduce the size of the stomach and thereby reduce the quantity of food ingested. The benefits of either of these surgical procedures are weighed against possible complications before being performed. They are drastic means and are considered as a last resort by many physicians.

Other Measures

The obese individual will welcome any preparation in the attempt to lose weight. Numerous fad diets and preparations ranging from the high-protein Stillman diet to bulk-producing substances, which presumably curb hunger by filling the stomach. Liquid protein diets recently popularized are liquid-based protein hydrolysates of which there are at least fifty brand names. Prolonged use of these diets has been implicated in fifty-eight deaths reported as occurring during the latter half of 1977 and 1978 (*Morbidity and Mortality Weekly Report*, 1978). It is advised that prolonged use of liquid protein diets be limited to research settings.

TABLE 46-3. ***A Survery of Some Disorders of Nutrition and Conditions Involving the Alimentary Tract and Related Structures***

Diagnostic Category	Etiologic Factors	Incubation Period and Nature of Onset	Part of Gastrointestinal Tract and/or Associated Structures Involved	Severity of Illness and Course; Signs and Symptoms	Effect on Adequacy of Nutrition	Major Medical and/or Surgical Treatment
Psychogenic and/or Neurogenic						
Achalasia (cardiospasm)	Physiologic obstruction. Emotional disturbances may precipitate. Supersensitivity to gastrin (augments strength of lower esophageal sphincter).	Dysphagia of the kind in which there is a delay of ingested food entering the stomach.	Esophagus: tortuous, elongated, lower end fails to relax with each peristaltic wave. There is esophageal dilation of varying degree except at distal end, which is undilated. Substernal pain, intermittent dysphagia, regurgitation.	Chronic condition. Progression of dysphagia inconsistent. Regurgitation in recumbent position. Nocturnal wakefulness caused by excessive cough. Pulmonary complications may occur if food is aspirated into the tracheobronchial tree. Esophageal carcinoma, sometimes develops because of prolonged irritation.	Initially satisfactory; then malnutrition caused by insufficient food intake. Weight loss.	Bougienage. If not curative, hydrostatic or pneumatic forceful dilatation is done. Cardioesophagomyotomy if the above methods fail.
Irritable colon	Excessive irritants (laxatives, foods, enemas), or emotional disturbance, or both.	Distention and fullness induced to ingestion of food or liquid, to severe cramplike abdominal pain. Sudden or gradual onset lasting for hours to years depending on duration of the emotional disturbance.	Colon; often palpable and tender. Normal rectum and sigmoid on proctoscopy. Small intestine and colon irritability noted on barium enema.	Defecation or passage of flatus may afford temporary relief or initiate more cramps and tenesmus. Nausea, belching, rumbling, gurgling in abdomen, burning tongue with a brassy taste.	Usually well nourished but occasionally varying degrees of malnutrition are seen.	Relief of anxiety about organic disease. Deeper psychotherapy if needed. Education of patient in relation to diet and fluids, in obtaining and maintaining satisfactory bowel habits.
			Diffuse spasm of lower third of esophagus.	Excessive flatus.		

			Hypermotility of the stomach.	Other physical symptoms related to psychogenesis of disease.		Avoidance of fecal impaction during initial therapy. If constipated, increase the residue in the diet.
				Patient usually wants bowel movement daily and takes laxative or enema to achieve this.		Rest and exercise determined on individual basis.
				Absence of organic disease.		Antispasmodics.
Diverticulum (one) Diverticulosis (many) (An outpouching or herniation of the mucosa through a defect in the muscularis.)	In general, weakness of the muscular wall of the alimentary canal caused by congenital defect. Possibly deficiency of roughage in diet. (A high-residue diet may prevent formation of high-pressure segments.) Excessive psychophysiologic stimulation of colon caused by tension.	Depends on site, size, and presence or absence of inflammation.	Common sites: esophagus, duodenum, and colon. May occur anywhere along the alimentary canal. In the presence of diverticulitis, signs and symptoms of acute inflammation. Effects intensified by peritonitis or mediastinitis.	May be symptomless, acute, chronic, or recurring. Perforation results in mediastinitis or peritonitis, depending on location. Symptoms of mechanical obstruction are present. Occasionally, symptoms of the genitourinary tract are present. Fistula formation and hemorrhage may complicate course of illness.	Depends on site and effects.	Maintenance of ideal body weight. High-residue diet. Avoidance of constipation and bowel irritants. Occasional use of antispasmodics and sedatives.
Diverticulosis		Diverticula are present for years before producing symptoms and then symptoms are correlated with the size of the diverticula and the distortion of the esophageal lumen.	Esophagus.	May be few if any symptoms or minor difficulty in swallowing. Prominent complaint is regurgitation of undigested food particles on assuming the horizontal position.	Weight loss. Malnutrition in later stages caused by failure of food to enter the digestive tract.	Surgical treatment when symptoms occur.

(Continued)

TABLE 46-3 (*Continued*)

Diagnostic Category	Etiologic Factors	Incubation Period and Nature of Onset	Part of Gastro-intestinal Tract and/or Associated Structures Involved	Severity of Illness and Course; Signs and Symptoms	Effect on Adequacy of Nutrition	Major Medical and/or Surgical Treatment
		Two thirds of persons living to 85 years of age in the Western world have them.		Gurgling noises in the neck, nocturnal choking and weight loss may occur. Pulmonary complications occur as a result of aspiration into the trachea.		
	See above.		Colon. See general comments.	See above.	None usually.	
Diverticulitis	Perforation of diverticulum followed by peridiverticular inflammation. Less frequently inflammation of mucosa.	Localized pain and tenderness lower left abdomen.	Most frequently sigmoid colon.	Bowel movements loose and frequent or absent. Occult blood in stool. Fever. Signs of peritoneal irritation.	Depends on extent of involvement.	High-residue diet. Parenteral antibiotics. Anticholinergics. Surgical resection for recurrent attacks.
Meckel's	Persistence of omphalomesenteric duct. Outpouching of serosa and mucosa at point where nutrient artery perforates muscularis layer.	Lower abdominal pain worsened by defecation.	Large intestine. Ileum.	May parallel signs and symptoms of acute appendicitis when inflamed. May cause volvulus, intussusception, or strangulation. Signs of peritoneal irritation. Muscle spasm. Fever. Guarding.	Malabsorption syndrome.	Surgical removal if necessary. Bedrest. Heat to tender abdominal area. Antibiotic therapy. Very soft diet during acute phase; then diet avoiding nuts, seeds, and fibrous foods. Oil enemas.

Ulcerations						
Chronic nonspecific ulcerative colitis	No known single cause. Relationship between emotional stress and onset and exacerbations.	Diarrhea, abdominal pain, blood, pus, fibrin in stools, or excreted as pure exudate.	Rectum and/or colon, ileum: inflammatory reaction involving mucosa and submucosa.	Anemia, weight loss, anorexia, malaise.	Malnutrition. Avitaminosis. Hypoproteinemia. Anemia.	Correction of nutrition and electrolyte loss. Vitamin and iron supplements. Discourage bacterial invasion: antimicrobial therapy. Bedrest.
Acute ulcerative colitis	Possible causes: Bacteria Allergy Autoimmune reaction Ischemia caused by pressure Psychic factors	Diarrhea, toxicity, fever, abdominal pain, distention, tenesmus, spasm, contraction. Constipation rather than diarrhea may be present.	Rectum and rectosigmoid: intensely red, edematous mucous membrane; tissue friable. Ileocecal valve to anus: as above. Colon: engorged, hyperactive. Covered with thick, opalescent, tenacious mucus, high in lysozyme concentration; increased friability of mucous membrane; eventual ulceration and submucosal bleeding. Rectum: see above.	Exacerbations and remissions. Little systemic sign of active inflammation. Course varies with patient. May have local reaction and involvement. May develop carcinoma (3–5% do). May have hyperimmune response.		Control diarrhea by opiates initially and later by sedation and antispasmodics. Psychological support. Parenteral feedings. Elemental feedings. Adrenocortical steroids. Sulfonamide drugs. Surgery may be necessary. All the above apply to both forms of the disease.
Acute ulcerative proctitis			Inflammatory reaction of the rectum with the mucosa being friable and edematous.	Bloody exudate on stool with no systemic manifestation. Rectal urgency if upper rectum involved.		

(Continued)

TABLE 46-3 (*Continued*)

Diagnostic Category	Etiologic Factors	Incubation Period and Nature of Onset	Part of Gastrointestinal Tract and/or Associated Structures Involved	Severity of Illness and Course; Signs and Symptoms	Effect on Adequacy of Nutrition	Major Medical and/or Surgical Treatment
Peptic ulcer						
Duodenal	Unknown—imbalance between digesting action of contents of the stomach and resistance of stomach and duodenum to digestion—see discussion.	Right epigastric pain. High midline pain usually 1 to 3 hours after eating. Nocturnal pain between 2:00 A.M. and 4:00 A.M.	First portion of duodenum: progressively a crater develops in which there is coagulation necrosis at base with infiltration and accumulation of acute and chronic inflammatory cells.	Characterized by exacerbation and remissions. Exacerbations occur most frequently in autumn and spring in temperate climates. Increased muscular activity intitiates pain. May perforate. Pain relieved by eating or alkali.	Protein, iron, and ascorbic acid deficiency with long dietary restriction.	Hospitalization for therapy if possible. Reduction of volume, acidity, and peptic content of gastric juices. Histamine H_2 receptor antagonists. Diet as tolerated. Frequent small volume feedings. Avoid specific secretagogues.
Gastric	Unknown. May be induced by adrenal steroid therapy; adrenergic blocking drugs (tolazine hydrochloride, hydralazine, and hexamethonium). Possibly autoimmune disease or caused by bile reflux.	Left epigastric pain. Pain usually one to several hours after eating, often not relieved or even aggravated by ingestion of food. History of 6 to 7 years of attacks. Exacerbations occur frequently in spring and fall.	Stomach: usually in prepyloric area of lesser curvature. Crater develops and area around becomes hyperemic, edematous, and infiltrated.	Vomiting when obstruction occurs. Anemia. Constipation. Chronic disease may lead to perforation. Frequently fails to respond to medical treatment and recurs.	Anorexia and weight loss frequent. Malnutrition may occur if fear of eating is present or with prolonged vomiting.	Antacids. Parasympatholytics. Sedatives and tranquilizers. Therapy individualized because of role of stress (emotional and physical) in exacerbations. Surgery may be indicated. Rest. Diet as tolerated with frequent small feedings.

Vascular						
Varices Esophageal	1. Increased pressure in veins of portal system—cirrhosis. 2. Thrombosis of portal and/or splenic vein (uncommon).	Hematemesis following local injury to the vessels or sudden elevation of portal pressure. Pressure is increased by straining at defecation, vomiting following a large meal or forceful exertion.	Esophagus: veins are distended and tortuous.	Chronic illness Blood loss. Weight loss.	If etiology is cirrhosis, there is usually generalized malnutrition.	Symptomatic therapy of clinical picture presented. Possible surgery—various shunts, ligation of varices. Low-fiber diet.
Mechanical Obstruction Neoplasia—benign or malignant neoplasms may occur at any level of the alimentary canal. Occurrence in the small intestine is rare. See Chapter 39.						

(Continued)

TABLE 46-3 (*Continued*)

Diagnostic Category	Etiologic Factors	Incubation Period and Nature of Onset	Part of Gastro-intestinal Tract and/or Associated Structures Involved	Severity of Illness and Course; Signs and Symptoms	Effect on Adequacy of Nutrition	Major Medical and/or Surgical Treatment
Hemorrhoids (dilation of either the internal or external hemorrhoidal plexus or both).	Predisposing factors—constipation, motionless standing, pregnancy, hereditary weakness of the wall of the hemorrhoidal vein. May be found in patients with cancer in the rectum or sigmoid colon.	May be present with few symptoms, or may be highly acute, depending on the type of hemorrhoids, the degree of involvement, and complications.	Hemorrhoidal veins in anal canal.	When infected, strangulated, thrombosed, and prolapsed through the anus, symptoms may be exceedingly acute. Severe pain is common. Although bleeding is usually minimal, the loss of large quantities of blood does occur. Tenesmus accompanies strangulation, thromboses, and usually prolapse. Itching follows bowel activity.	None unless continued or excessive loss of blood.	Surgical removal—aftercare is very important. Operated area must be kept clean and strictures prevented from forming. Immediately after operation an ice bag may be placed over the dressing to lessen pain. Sitz baths are started about 24 hours after surgery. Mineral oil to keep stool soft. In the treatment of acutely infected and thrombosed hemorrhoids: Sitz baths, stool softeners, keep area clean.
Choledocholithiasis	Calculi in common duct.	Varies from no symptoms to acute attacks of colic with an unusual degree of nausea and vomiting.	Extra- and intrahepatic biliary passages may become dilated and edematous.	Jaundice may or may not be present. If present, its severity dependent on extent of obstruction. If persistent may lead to distention of the gallbladder.		Viatmin K when jaundice present. Surgical removal of stones.

Hernia (protrusion of the contents of the peritoneal cavity through a defect in the wall).	Developmental defects—trauma, aging, infection, surgery.	Depends on location. Some hernias can be seen and felt as a bulge in the affected area.	Depends on location and whether or not strangulation occurs. With gangrene of the intestine, peritonitis occurs. Locations include Inguinal (direct or indirect) Femoral Umbilical Ventral Postoperative incisions Hiatus or diaphragmatic hernia.	May be few symptoms or signs until hernia becomes incarcerated (irreducible), and intestinal obstruction and strangulation occur. If allowed to continue, bowel becomes gangrenous and peritonitis occurs.	Depends on location.	Surgical repair, preferably before complications develop.
Hiatus hernia		Gradual onset resulting in substernal or epigastric pressure precipitated by eating. Belching. Hot sensations in the back of the throat. Symptoms increase in severity when in recumbent position and are relieved when in the upright position. Sudden respiratory distress follows trauma and has rapid onset.	Stomach and esophagus. Stomach herniates into thorax, leads to esophagitis after regurgitation of gastric contents, continues for a long time. Hyperemia of gastric mucosa, caused by compression of venous drainage, renders it easily susceptible to trauma.	Chronic illness that may be quiescent or lead to development of respiratory embarrassment, cardiac irregularities. Bleeding, slow but persistent.	When acute episode of esophagitis interferes with food ingestion, there is an inadequate quality of nutrition. Anemia, microcytic type.	Avoid excessive filling of herniated pouch: diet is based on small meals, bland foods; restriction of sweets, coffee, alcohol. No food for 3 hours prior to retiring. Antacids. Sleep with head of bed elevated. Surgical treatment depends on the severity of symptoms.

(Continued)

TABLE 46-3 (*Continued*)

Diagnostic Category	Etiologic Factors	Incubation Period and Nature of Onset	Part of Gastrointestinal Tract and/or Associated Structures Involved	Severity of Illness and Course; Signs and Symptoms	Effect on Adequacy of Nutrition	Major Medical and/or Surgical Treatment
Parasites						
Cestodes (tapeworms)	*Diphyllobothrium latum.* *Taenia solium.* *Taenia saginata* *Hymenolepisnana.* Sparganosis. Echinococciasis.	Asymptomatic.		Transient abdominal discomfort; diarrhea, hunger, anemia. Infrequently severe cramping, vomiting, weakness, loss of weight. Usually seeks medical attention because part of parasite is passed per anus.	Malnutrition. Avitaminosis. Weight loss. Anemia. Protein and vitamin deficiency.	Anthelmintics. High-protein, high-calorie diet. Iron therapy.
Hookworm disease	*Necator americanus* (New World). *Ancylostoma duodenale* (Old World).	Have been known to survive 5 years in intestine. "Ground itch" or lesions on feet at point of entry.	Larvae penetrate skin, enter circulation, go to lungs, enter aliveoli, ascend respiratory tree, enter pharynx, and are swallowed. In intestine they mature and adults attach themselves to intestine, sucking about 0.5 ml of blood daily. Primarily in jejunum.	Severity depends on the number of worms and the nutritional status of the host and his or her age. Epigastric pain. Abdominal tenderness. Sometimes nausea, vomiting, and diarrhea because intestine is attacked. Anemia, dyspnea, palpitation, lassitude, tachycardia, constipation may be manifested as infestation progresses.	Anemia. Generalized malnutrition. Poor diet influences course unfavorably.	High-protein, high-calorie diet. Iron therapy. Anthelmintics.

Ascariasis	*Ascaris lumbricoides*	Temperature elevation 4–5 days after ingestion of eggs.	Early transient pulmonary state followed by larval migration and intestinal infestation.	Physical and mental retardation may result from severe chronic infections. Cough and hemoptysis during pulmonary migration. Passage of worm via rectum, epigastric pain, abdominal distention, tenderness, vomiting, and constipation may occur during intestinal infestation.		Symptomatic during pulmonary state, then use chemotherapy.
Amebiasis	*Endamoeba histolytica* as motile trophozoite and nonmotile cyst in the colon.	Chronic: intermittent diarrhea, foul-smelling; abdominal cramping; mild fever. Acute: high fever, severe abdominal cramps, bloody diarrhea, tenesmus, diffuse abdominal tenderness.	Ileum: cyst wall disintegrates and 8 trophozoites result; these pass to colon, attack mucosa, and divide by binary fission; amebic ulceration; cecum, ascending colon, rectum, appendix, terminal ileum.	Vague intestinal symptoms; symptoms of appendicitis, gallbladder disease, peptic ulcer. Dysentery or diarrhea. May eventually enter circulation and infest liver. May infest lung from site in liver. May cause granuloma that encroaches on lumen.	Dehydration. Electrolyte imbalance. Weight loss.	Acute: replace fluid, electrolyte, and blood losses; bed rest; relief of pain and tenesmus; specific chemotherapy. Chronic: specific drug therapy. Hepatic or pulmonary: chloroquine and terramycin are given concomitantly.
Enterobiasis	*Enterobius vermicularis*	Perianal pruritus most troublesome at night. Lower abdominal pain.	Cecum and colon: adults attach themselves to mucosa. Ingested.	May give rise to granulomatous peritonitis in women.		Communal treatment. Piperazine citrate.

(Continued)

Table 46-3 (*Continued*)

Diagnostic Category	Etiologic Factors	Incubation Period and Nature of Onset	Part of Gastrointestinal Tract and/or Associated Structures Involved	Severity of Illness and Course; Signs and Symptoms	Effect on Adequacy of Nutrition	Major Medical and/or Surgical Treatment
Trichinosis	*Trichinella spiralis*	Complaints vary with the severity of infestation and range from mild to severe. Diarrhea characterizes development of adults in the intestine 24 hours after ingestion.	Encysted larvae are ingested and parasites are liberated in duodenum and jejunum. There the parasites anchor themselves to mucosa and extract oxygen and liquid food. Nervous system and heart are frequently involved.	Myositis and systemic reaction when larvae migrate and infest skeletal muscle on seventh day after ingestion; may last up to 6 weeks. Edema, usually periorbital, conjunctivitis, nausea, vomiting, diarrhea, abdominal cramps, and fever within 2–7 days. Mortality rate in epidemics is 5%.	Hypoproteinemia. Dehydration.	Symptomatic therapy. Relief of pain. Maintain adequate fluid and caloric intake. Rest; if necessary, sedation. ACTH and adrenal steroids in severe cases. Anthelmintics.
Bacillary dysentery	*Shigella*	1–6 days; median 48 hours. Colicky abdominal pain followed by profuse diarrhea, fever, tenesmus, chills, nausea, vomiting, headache. Onset sudden and severe in children.	Sigmoid and rectum: acute inflammation leading to coagulation necrosis and ulceration. Mild case: mucosa is strawberry red tint and with diffuse inflammation and hyperemia, bleeding when traumatized.	Passage of pus and mucus. Fever. Nausea. Vomiting. Headache. Malaise. Spontaneous recovery in 2–7 days. 3–6 weeks in severe cases.	Dehydration. Depletion of electrolytes.	Symptomatic. Isolation. Ampicillin. Fluid replacement. Bland diet.

Deficiencies						
Scurvy	Deficiency of ascorbic acid.	Weakness, fatigue, aching in muscles, joints, bones after 90 days of depletion. Hair follicles become prominent after 120 days of deprivation; perifollicular hemorrhage after 165 days. Peak incidence in infants at 8 months with tenderness and swelling of lower extremities.	Skeleton in children: periosteum and costal cartilages separate from bone shaft. A dense, calcified cartilaginous matrix forms in the cartilage shaft junction. Generalized hemorrhages in adults.	Aching muscles, joints, bones. Swollen, painful lower extremities. Swollen gums with hemorrhage; eventual loss of teeth. Rapid improvement with therapy.	Anemia is often an associated finding.	Ascorbic acid.
Pellagra	Niacin deficiency. Low-protein diet with tryptophan deficiency will accelerate the progress; tryptophan is precursor for niacin. Contributing factors are gastrointestinal disease, liver disease, alcoholism.	Follows several months of low intake of niacin, protein, and B-complex vitamins.	Skin: erythema, vesical formation, rough and scaly. Alimentary tract: glossitis, inflammation of the esophagus, ulcer formation in the colon. Nervous system: vertigo, headache, paresthesia, anesthesia, diminished tendon reflexes, coarse tremors, mental disturbances. Degeneration of peripheral nerves, nerve roots, and spinal cord tracts; atrophy of cerebral neurons.	Dermatitis, anorexia, glossitis, lassitude, stomatitis, diarrhea. Later leads to dementia. Symptoms begin to disappear after 24 hours of therapy; almost absent after 3–4 days, except for polyneuritis.	Anorexia. Weight loss. Anemia.	Niacin. High-protein, high-calorie, soft diet. Water and electrolyte replacement. Bedrest. Symptomatic therapy.

(Continued)

TABLE 46-3 (*Continued*)

Diagnostic Category	Etiologic Factors	Incubation Period and Nature of Onset	Part of Gastrointestinal Tract and/or Associated Structures Involved	Severity of Illness and Course; Signs and Symptoms	Effect on Adequacy of Nutrition	Major Medical and/or Surgical Treatment
Beriberi	Thiamine deficiency. Protein, calorie, and multiple B-complex deficiencies coexist. Prevalent in Far East, especially in prisons, asylums, in infants, pregnant and lactating women, and alcoholics. Rare in United States.	Insidious onset. Fatigue, muscle weakness, pain, and atrophy in neurologic form.	Myelin degeneration of peripheral nerves with loss of exoplasm. In alcoholics, bilateral hemorrhagic foci in the mammillary bodies, hypothalamic nuclei, and midline structures. Optic nerve damage and spinal cord lesions. Heart dilatation and occasional hypertrophy of the right ventricle.	Loss of reflexes. Paresthesias and anesthesias. Symptoms progress until patient is bedridden. Dry form: peripheral neuritis. Wet form: edema, muscle cramps. Cardiac form: palpitation, precordial pain, dyspnea, tachycardia, edema, increased pulse and venous pressure.	Weight loss. Anorexia. Multiple deficiencies of B-complex and iron.	Thiamine. High-protein, high-calorie diet.
Undernutrition	Calorie deficiency. Protein deficiency. Associated lack of vitamins and minerals. Endemic undernutrition results from inadequate food supply, poverty, ignorance. Infections, gastrointestinal parasites accelerate effects. Infants, young children, pregnant and lactating women are vulnerable.	Weight loss is initial sign in adults. Other signs only after months of severe deprivation or when aggravated by disease. Infants weaned to low-protein diet show rapid deterioration in growth, development.	Reduced production of digestive enzymes; reduced liver function. Affects growth and mental development of infants and young children.	Children: failure to gain, short stature, retarded mental development. Edema or severe dehydration. Fatty liver, low serum albumin, anemia. Changes in skin and hair pigment. Adults: course usually determined by associated disease.		Gradual addition of nutritionally balanced meals; milk for infants. Elemental diet.

Inflammatory						
Glossitis	Secondary to chronic malabsorption.		Tongue becomes hyperemic. Small ulcers sometimes occur.		Anorexia because swallowing is painful.	Correct underlying disorder.
Stomatitis, catarrhal	Poor oral hygiene. Excessive use of tobacco or alcohol. Associated with debilitated persons. Uremia.		Mouth. Mucous membranes erythematous; increased exudate.			As above.
Aphthous ulcer	Unknown.		Vesicle develops, ruptures, and leaves ulcer.			No treatment; heals spontaneously.
Ulceromembranous	*Bacillus fusiformis.* *Borrelia vincentii.*	Painful, irregular-shaped ulcer covered with whitish gray membrane.	Oral and pharyngeal membranes, particularly gingival tissue. Inflammation and induration surround ulcerations.	Moderate fever, enlargement of submaxilliary lymph nodes.	Temporarily modifies diet.	Penicillin. Dental hygienic measures to eradicate ulcerations.
Parotitis	Hemolytic streptococcus through ducts, blood stream, lymphatics, or extension from adjacent structures.	Enlargement of salivary glands associated with pain and swelling.	Acute inflammation of salivary gland; usually parotid but may be any salivary gland. Blockage of Stensen's duct by a calculus.	Leukocytosis; rapid pulse; trismus; pressure on gland usually produces purulent discharge from duct; fever and chills.	Temporarily modifies diet.	Antimicrobial agents. Therapeutic doses of irradiation are used if antimicrobials fail. Removal of obstruction and local heat application. Surgical drainage if conservative measures fail.
Regional enteritis	Granulomatous response of submucosa to unknown agent(s).		Duodenum: usually leads to stenosis. Upper jejunum: usually leads to stenosis.		Impairment of absorption of amino acids, fats, fat-soluble vitamins, folic acid, iron.	Asulfidine. Antidiarrheal drugs.

(Continued)

TABLE 46-3 (*Continued*)

Diagnostic Category	Etiologic Factors	Incubation Period and Nature of Onset	Part of Gastrointestinal Tract and/or Associated Structures Involved	Severity of Illness and Course; Signs and Symptoms	Effect on Adequacy of Nutrition	Major Medical and/or Surgical Treatment
		Acute right lower quadrant pain and tenderness; disturbance in bowel motility.	Terminal ileum: encroachment of lumen, scarring of muscle, slow spread to other areas of intestine; beefy red appearance. Usually leads to ulceration. Nonstenotic. Fistula forms.	Acute stage can lead to perforation and generalized peritonitis. In nonacute onset, history of intermittent chronic diarrhea, fever, weight loss, crampy pain or distention, anemia. Two thirds develop chronic enteritis. Eventual obstruction of lumen.	"Malabsorption syndrome." Undernutrition.	Surgery: end-to-side ileotransverse colostomy. Provide mental and physical rest. Chemotherapeutics and antibiotics to treat purulent complications. Corticosteroids to convert a subacute obstructing lesion into a nonstenotic one. Diet: high-calorie, high-protein (2 g per kg of ideal body weight per day), low in seasoning and cold fluids and residue. Therapeutic vitamins. Fluid and electrolyte balance restoration.
Sprue	Nontropical: adult form of celiac disease. Primary form involves defect of intestinal epithelium. Secondary form exists in wide range of malabsorption states.	Insidious onset. Diarrhea: 2–3 (or more) mushy, light-colored, foul-smelling stools associated with explosive flatus. Intermittent constipation.	Jejunum: villi become short and blunt, width of crypts of Lieberkühn increases; microvilli become sparse, blunted, and fused. Distortion of columnar cells of the epithelium. Plasma cells of the lamina propria become infiltrated. Mitochondria are enlarged and vacuolated.	Chronic disease. Severe fatigue. Moderate to severe weight loss. Nausea and vomiting and abdominal pain may occur. Nocturnal diuresis. Clinical manifestations of malnutrition. Eventually fractures of bones and tetany. Anemia.	Malnutrition results from inability of food products (properly prepared for absorption) to pass through the mucosa. Vitamin A, C, D, B_{12}, K deficiencies. Deficiencies in electrolytes, potassium and calcium. Hypoproteinemia. Progressively reserves of iron,	Gluten-free diet (do not eat food containing wheat, barley, rye gluten). Takes about 6 months to evaluate this therapy. In presence of nutritional deficiencies, corrective therapy instituted. In presence of malnutrition, adrenocortical hormone therapy initially with diet therapy. Tetany

folic acid, and B_{12} are depleted. Malabsorption of fats and fat-soluble nutrients. Lowered serum cholesterol and phospholipids, copper, prothrombin.	treated with 10% calcium gluconate IV. Electrolyte therapy: potassium chloride, 2–3 g daily. Hemorrhagic complications treated with menadione intramuscularly, 10 mg daily. Antibiotic therapy when sprue is secondary to diverticula, infection, blind loops, and intestinal strictures. Recognize secondary causes of sprue and institute therapy. Postgastrectomy: small, frequent feedings; addition of pancreatin to diet. Androgens for anabolic effect: antibiotics.

(Continued)

TABLE 46-3 (*Continued*)

Diagnostic Category	Etiologic Factors	Incubation Period and Nature of Onset	Part of Gastrointestinal Tract and/or Associated Structures Involved	Severity of Illness and Course; Signs and Symptoms	Effect on Adequacy of Nutrition	Major Medical and/or Surgical Treatment
Hepatitis	Filtrable virus A (infectious hepatitis).	15–50 days. Abrupt onset with high temperature, GI symptoms, and nonspecific constitutional symptoms lasting a few days to 2 weeks.	Liver: cellular damage ranges from swollen or shrunken cells with disintegrating nucleus to massive central necrosis of every lobule of the liver. Kupffer cells are often swollen; edema and cellular infiltration of portal and periportal areas; biliary stasis.	Preicteric stage: fever, anorexia, fatigue predominate. Nausea, vomiting, chilly sensations, indigestion, abdominal pain, headache, pain on eye movement, and arthralgia may occur. Enlarged lymph nodes are common. Icteric stage: jaundice, increases rapidly reaching a maximum in 10–14 days; few days in which anorexia, lassitude, and nausea are striking; right upper abdominal pain. This stage may last a few days to a few weeks, depending on severity. Sudden reappearance of appetite plus sense of well-being indicates beginning of recovery period. Jaundice clears in 4–6 weeks.	Undernutrition as a result of anorexia.	Bedrest. Isolate. Blood and stools considered infectious until fever and jaundice subside. High-protein, high-calorie diet except in massive hepatic necrosis. Parenteral feedings if nausea, vomiting, or anorexia is present. Immune serum globulin may be given prophylactically to those exposed to type A hepatitis.
	Filtrable virus B (serum hepatitis).	60–160 days. Insidious onset with minimal symptoms and little if any fever.				
	Filtrable virus C (non A–B hepatitis).	Occurs in persons following multiple blood transfusions (at least 15).				

Cholecystitis Acute	Biliary calculi, or the action on the wall of the gallbladder caused by a stone. Bacterial infection. Chemical irritants in the bile. Bile supersaturated with cholesterol.	Upper abdominal pain, gradual or acute, associated with biliary colic. Fever.	Gallbladder is distended; serosa is injected; wall is tense and swollen; mucosa is congested. Frequently small amounts of fibrinopurulent exudate.	Becomes chronic but with severe upper abdominal distress. Fever and chills usually. Nausea and vomiting. Mass sometimes palpable.		Removal of calculi after subsidence of acute phase. Symptomatic therapy. Restoration of fluid and electrolyte balance. Low-fat diet. Water-soluble form of vitamins K, A, D, and E. Choledochal exploration. Cholecystectomy.
Chronic	Biliary calculi.	Distinct attacks occurring days to years apart with abrupt onset of abdominal pain, fever, intermittent mild jaundice and digestive complaints.	Chronic inflammatory gallbladder with degenerative changes.	May lead to persistent gallbladder distention as with acute, but having chronic form of jaundice.		Cholecystectomy for cholelithiasis. Medically with antispasmodics, antacids, laxatives, and sedatives. Moderately low-fat diet. Drug dissolution of cholesterol stones.
	Unknown.			Belching, bloating, and epigastric distress after meals. Variety of digestive and systemic complaints. Symptoms aggravated by ingestion of fats. Insomnia.		

(Continued)

TABLE 46-3 (*Continued*)

Diagnostic Category	Etiologic Factors	Incubation Period and Nature of Onset	Part of Gastrointestinal Tract and/or Associated Structures Involved	Severity of Illness and Course; Signs and Symptoms	Effect on Adequacy of Nutrition	Major Medical and/or Surgical Treatment
Cirrhosis	Malnutrition. Alcoholism. Hepatitis.	Insidious onset, with nonspecific complaints of anorexia, weakness, and unusual fatigability.	Liver enlarges and is pale initially; then fibrosis in portal areas and around central veins. Lobular structure becomes distorted with regeneration.	Anorexia, weight loss, eventually (1) hepatocellular failure, manifested by ascites, edema, jaundice, pleural effusion, alteration in serum electrolytes, spider nevi, palmar erythema, gynecomastia; testicular atrophy, loss of axillary and pubic hair, bleeding tendency; (2) portal hypertension manifested by splenomegaly, esophageal varices (with or without massive hemorrhage), visible venous collateral circulation over abdomen, rectal hemorrhoids; and eventually may have (3) hepatic coma; rapid fluctuation of mental and neurologic signs, flapping tremor, and occasionally fetor hepaticus.	Malnutrition in terms of essential nutrients although caloric intake may be adequate or even high. Anemia.	Normal to high-protein, high-calorie diet. Prohibition of alcohol (where it is etiologic factor). Supplemental water-soluble vitamins. Regulation of salt and water balance. Prompt control of hemorrhage and replacement of blood loss. Rest. Antimicrobial therapy in presence of infection. Prednisone. Diuretics. Sodium-restricted diet if ascites present. Paracentesis and/or thoracentesis if needed. Surgery is sometimes used: portacaval shunt. Coma: (1) restriction of protein intake, but calories supplied from fats and carbohydrates; (2) correction of deficiencies in fluids and electrolytes; (3) neomycin; (4) ad-

						ministration intravenously of L-arginine monohydrochloride (25 g in 500 ml water); frequency depends on response of blood ammonia.
Pancreatitis, acute	Obstruction to outflow of pancreatic juices by gallstones in common duct. Direct injury of acinar tissue by toxins, ischemia, inflammation, or trauma. Cancer of ampulla of Vater. Secondary pancreatic edema. Epithelial metaplasia in duct. Alcoholism. Peptic ulcer. Trauma. Steroids. An occasional complication of pregnancy and mumps.	Sudden moderate or severe and prolonged upper abdominal pain and vomiting.	Destruction of parenchyma of pancreas and ductal obstruction. Varying: edema of head of pancreas to patchy or diffuse necrosis of gland. Extensive fibrosis.	Loss of weight although excessive amounts of food are ingested; leading to obstipation; vomiting, distention, and ileus may occur. Tetany may develop. Leads to destructive process in pancreas and fibrotic contracture may cause compression of common duct, producing jaundice. Repeated attacks result in chronic pancreatitis. This, if it progresses sufficiently, may result in calcification of pancreas and diabetes mellitus and steatorrhea.	Incomplete hydrolysis of starches, fats, and proteins and hence incomplete absorption. Marked malnutrition. Avitaminosis. Hypocalcemia.	NPO. Aspiration of gastric contents. Anticholinergic drugs. Analgesics (opiates sparingly and in small doses). Antibiotics. Restoration of fluid and electrolyte balance.
Appendicitis	Obstruction caused by fecalith or stricture. Ulceration. Diffuse phlegmon. Infection.	Acute periumbilical or epigastric pain, followed by anorexia, nausea, and vomiting.	Appendix: inflammatory response to cause.	Anorexia, nausea, vomiting progressing, fever, high leukocyte count. Perforation of the appendix and ensuing peritonitis.	Loss of fluid and electrolytes caused by vomiting. Inadequate nutrient intake because of nausea, anorexia, and vomiting.	Surgical removal of appendix. Correction of dehydration and electrolyte imbalance. Restoration of physiologic function (in absence of peritonitis).

Summary

Survival, growth, productivity, and health all depend on a continuous supply of food. In some areas of the world the amount of food available is insufficient to support the population at much more than a survival level. The reasons for the inadequate food supply include poor soil or unfavorable climate and lack of transportation or food preservation facilities. In the United States malnutrition exists where the supply of food is adequate to feed all. Malnutrition results in stunted growth, mental retardation, and an increased susceptibility to disease. Treatment requires a change in food habits.

Obesity, an excessive accumulation of fatty tissue, is a major public health problem that increases the incidence of chronic diseases and the mortality rate. Although it results from an excess of calorie intake over the energy expenditure, multiple causes are involved. Cultural dietary patterns, ignorance of food values, overeating as a compensation for emotional problems and to meet life stresses, and relative inactivity are the principal factors leading to obesity. Those who have endomorphic body types are more prone to obesity than those of ectomorphic body types. Hormonal imbalance rarely accounts for obesity, and errors of metabolism of fat or carbohydrate have not been firmly established as causes of obesity. The prevention of obesity with emphasis on nutrition education and physical activity during the school years is likely to be much more rewarding than attempts to treat obesity. Successful treatment of obesity requires the extended and sympathetic guidance of the physician, nurse, or nutritionist; the sustained motivation of the patient; adequate counseling regarding control of the diet; and emphasis on a program of physical activity.

For short periods of time, diets inadequate in one or more nutrients may be ingested without causing serious harm. More or less permanent modifications in the diet must meet basic nutritional requirements if malnutrition is to be avoided. In general, diets are modified to (1) accommodate to a disturbance in the structure or function of the gastrointestinal tract, (2) correct the effect of an excess or deficit of essential nutrients, and (3) accommodate to a defect in the capacity to utilize one or more nutrients.

The table on the preceding pages summarized selected characteristics of some common nutritional disorders: diagnostic category; etiologic factors; nature of onset; structure or region involved; symptoms and severity of the course of the illness; effect on nutrition; and major medical and/or surgical treatment.

References Cited

A C S Clinical Congress News. **28** (Oct. 19, 1977), 3.

Aldrich, C. K. "Mechanisms and Management of Obesity." *Med. Clin. North Am.*, **47** (Jan. 1963), 77.

Burton, B. T. *Human Nutrition,* 3rd ed., New York: McGraw-Hill, 1976.

Bury, K. D. "Elemental Diets." In *Total Parenteral Nutrition.* Ed. by J. E. Fischer. Boston: Little, Brown, 1976, pp. 395–411.

Clayman, C. B. "Evaluation of Cimitidine (Tagamet) an Antagonist of Hydrochloric Acid Secretion." *JAMA,* **238** (1977), 1289–90.

Condon, J. R. et al. "Lactose Malabsorption and Postgastrectomy Milk Intolerance, Dumping and Diarrhea." *Gut,* **10** (1969), 311.

Cowhig, J. "Is There More to Obesity Than Food?" *New Scientist,* **55** (July 6, 1972), 31–33.

Davidson, S., and Passmore, R. *Human Nutrition and Dietetics,* 4th ed. London: E. and S. Livingston Ltd., 1969.

Donta, S. T. "Changing Concepts of Infectious Diarrheas." *Geriatrics* (March 1975), p.123.

Eckholm, E., and Record, F. *The Two Faces of Malnutrition.* Washington, D.C.: Worldwatch Paper 9, Library of Congress, Dec. 1976.

Faloon, W. "Hepatic Disorders." In *Pathophysiology,* 2nd ed. Ed. by E. D. Frohlich. Philadephia: J. B. Lippincott Co., 1976, p. 531.

Fischer, J. E. *Total Parenteral Nutrition.* Boston: Little, Brown, 1976.

Friedman, G. M. "Atherosclerosis and the Pediatrician." In *Childhood Obesity.* Ed. by M. Winick. New York: John Wiley & Sons, 1975, p. 118.

G. I. Series. Physical Examination of the Abdomen. Richmond, Va.: A. H. Robins Co., 1975.

Höglund, S. "Deficiency and Absorption of Iron in Man." *Acta Med. Scand.,* **518** 1 Suppl. (1970).

Iser, J. H. et al. "Chenodeoxycholic Acid Treatment of Gallstones." *N. Engl. J. Med.,* **293** (1975), 378.

Kannel, W. B. "The Coronary Profile: 12 Year Follow-up in the Framingham Study." *J. Occup. Med.,* **9** (Dec. 1967), 611–19.

Kon, S. K. *Milk and Milk Products in Human Nutrition.* New York: Food and Agriculture Organization, United Nations, 1972.

Mattson, F. H. et al. "Effect of Dietary Cholesterol on Serum Cholesterol in Man." *Am. J. Clin. Nutr.,* **25** (June 1972), 589–94.

Mayer, J. "The Bitter Truth about Sugar." *N. Y. Times Mag.* (June 20, 1976).

Menguy, R. "Gastric Mucosal Injury from Common Drugs." *Postgrad. Med.,* **63** (April 1978), 82–86.

Morbidity and Mortality Weekly Report. Atlanta, Ga.: U.S. Department of Health, Education, and Welfare, Center for Disease Control, July 7, 1978.

Piper, D. W. "Milk in the Treatment of Gastric Disease." *Am. J. Clin. Nutr.,* **22** (Feb. 1969), 191–95.

Position Paper of the American Dietetic Association on Bland Diet in the Treatment of Chronic Duodenal Ulcer Disease. *J. Am. Diet. Assoc.,* **59** (Sept. 1971), 244.

Quimby, F. H. *Hunger and Malnutrition in the United States: How Much?* Washington, D.C.: Congressional Research Service, Library of Congress, May 1, 1975.

Recommended Daily Dietary Allowances. Washington, D.C.: Food and Nutrition Board, National Academy of Sciences, National Research Council, 1974.

Redinger, R. N., and Small, D. M. "Bile Composition, Bile Salt Metabolism and Gallstones." *Arch. Intern. Med.*, **130** (Oct. 1972), 618–30.

Samborsky, V. "Drug Therapy for Peptic Ulcer." *Am. J. Nurs.*, **78** (Dec. 1978), 2064–70.

Sawyers, J. L. "Proximal Gastric Vagotomy without Drainage." *Postgrad. Med.*, **63** (April 1978), 115–21.

Schubert, W. K. "Fat Nutrition and Diet in Childhood." *Am. J. Cardiol.*, **31** (May 1973), 581–87.

Shaefer, A. E. "Findings and Implications of the National Nutrition Survey." In *Dimensions of Nutrition.* Ed. by J. DuPont. Boulder, Colo.: Colorado Associated University Press, 1970, pp. 243–61.

Shumway, S., and Powers, M. "The Group Way to Weight Loss." *Am. J. Nurs.*, **73** (Feb. 1973), 269–72.

Stamler, J. et al. "Primary Prevention of the Atherosclerotic Diseases." *Circulation*, **42** (Dec. 1970), A55–95.

Van Itallie, T. B., and Campbell, R. G. "Multidisciplinary Approach to the Problem of Obesity." *J. Am. Diet. Assoc.*, **61** (Oct. 1972), 385–90.

Way, L. W., and Sleisenger, M. H. "Choledocholithiasis, Cholangitis, and Biliary Obstruction." In M. H. Sleisenger et al., eds. *Gastrointestinal Disease Pathophysiology, Diagnosis, Management*, 2nd ed. Philadelphia: W. B. Saunders Co., 1978, p. 1313.

Way, L. W., and Sleisenger, M. H. "Cholelithiasis and Chronic Cholecystitis." In *Gastrointestinal Disease Pathophysiology, Diagnosis, Management*, 2nd ed. Ed. by M. H. Sleisenger et al. Philadelphia: W. B. Saunders Co., 1978, p. 1294.

Weismann, R. E. "Surgical Palliation of Massive and Severe Obesity." *Am. J. Surg.*, **125** (April 1973), 437–46.

Wolf, S., and Wolff, H. G. *Human Gastric Function*, 2nd ed. New York: Oxford University Press, 1947.

Wretlind, A. "Complete Intravenous Nutrition." *Nutr. Metab.*, **14** 1–57, Supplement (1972).

Yager, J., and Weiner, H. "Observations in Man with Remarks on Pathogenesis." *Adv. Psychosom. Med.*, **6** (1971), 40–87.

Young, E. A. et al. "Comparative Nutritional Analysis of Chemically Defined Diet." *Gastroenterology*, **69** (1975), 1138.

Zimmerman, H. J. "The Spectrum of Hepatotoxicity." *Perspect. Biol. Med.*, **12** (Autumn 1968), 135–39.

Zollinger, R. M. "Peptic Ulcer Disease." *Postgrad. Med.*, **63** (April 1978), 81.

General References

Alimentary Canal—General

Curtis, C. "Colonoscopy: The Nurse's Role." *Am. J. Nurs.*, **75** (March 1975), 430.

Howie, J. G. "Diseases of the Alimentary System. View from General Practice." *Br. Med. J.*, **1** (Jan. 1977), 159.

Mendeloff, A. In T. Almy (moderator), "Panel 1: Prevalence and Significance of Digestive Disease." *Gastroenterology*, **68** (May 1975), 1351.

Schuster, M. M. "Biofeedback Treatment of Gastrointestinal Disorders." *Med. Clin. North Am.*, **61** (July 1977), 907.

Upper Alimentary Canal

Alp, M. H. et al. "Personality Pattern and Emotional Stress in the Genesis of Gastric Ulcer." *Gut*, **11** (1970), 773.

Friedman, G. D. et al. "Cigarettes, Alcohol, Coffee and Peptic Ulcer." *N. Engl. J. Med.*, **290** (1974), 469.

Henn, R. M. et al. "Inhitition of Gastric Acid Secretion by Climitidine in Patients with Duodenal Ulcer." *N. Engl. J. Med.*, **293** (1975), 371.

Hunt, T. K. "Injury and Repair in Acute Gastroduodenal Ulceration." *Am. J. Surg.*, **125** (1973), 12.

Mirsky, I. A. "Physiologic, Psychologic, and Social Determinants in the Etiology of Duodenal Ulcer." *Am. J. Dig. Dis.*, **3** (1958), 285.

Wilson, D. E. et al. "Effects of an Orally Administered Prostaglandin Analogue (16, 16-dimethyl Prostaglandin E_2) on Human Gastric Secretion." *Gastroenterology*, **69** (1975), 607.

Wormsley, K. G. "The Pathophysiology of Duodenal Ulceration." *Gut*, **15** (1974), 59.

Alimentary Canal—Surgery

Cody, H. S. et al. "Choice of Operation for Acute Gastric Mucosal Hemorrhage. A Report of 36 Cases and Review of Literature." *Am. J. Surg.*, **134** (Sept. 1977), 322.

Durham, N. "Look Out for the Complications of Abdominal Surgery." *Nurs. '75*, **5** (Feb. 1975), 24.

Esselstyn, C. B., Jr. "Surgical Management of Actively Bleeding Duodenal Ulcer." *Surg. Clin. North Am.*, **56** (Dec. 1976), 1387.

Fikei, E., and Cassella, R. "Jejunoileal Bypass for Massive Obesity." *Ann. Surg.*, **79** (1974), 460.

Greenstein, A. J. et al. "Reoperation and Recurrence in Crohn's Colitis and Ileocolitis." *N. Engl. J. Med.*, **293** (Oct. 2, 1975), 685.

MacGregor, I. L. et al. "Gastric Emptying of Solid Food in Normal Man and after Subtotal Gastrectomy and Truncal Vagotomy with Pyloroplasty." *Gastroenterology*, **72** (Feb. 1977), 206.

Mersheimer, W. L. et al. "A Critical Analysis of 51 Patients with Jejunoileal Bypass." *Surg. Gynecol. Obstet.*, **145** (Dec. 1977), 847.

Sawyers, J. L. "Proximal Gastric Vagotomy without Drainage." *Postgrad. Med.*, **63** (April 1978), 115.

Elemental Diet and Total Parenteral Nutrition

Fazio, V. et al. "Parenteral Nutrition as Primary or Adjunctive Treatment." *Dis. Colon Rectum,* **19** (1976), 574.

Herlihy, P. et al. "Total Parenteral Nutrition." *J. Am. Dietet. A.,* **70** (March 1977), 279.

Jeejeebhoy, K. et al. "Total Parenteral Nutrition at Home: Studies Surviving 4 Months to 5 Years." *Gastroenterology,* **71** (1976), 943.

Layden, T. et al. "Reversal of Growth Arrest in Adolescents with Crohn's Disease after Parenteral Alimentation." *Gastroenterology,* **70** (1976), 1017.

Ricour, C. et al. "Continuous Enteral Feeding in Children. Technique and Indications in 170 Cases from 1969 to 1975." *Arch. Fr. Pediatr.,* **34** (Feb. 1977), 154.

Vogel, C. et al. "Intravenous Hyperalimentation in the Treatment of Inflammatory Disease of the Bowel." *Arch. Surg.,* **108** (1974), 460.

Middle and Lower Alimentary Canal—Disorders

Aston, S. J., and Machlfeder, H. I. "Intussception in the Adult." *Am. Surg.,* **41** (Sept. 1975), 576.

Bertholf, C. B. "Protocol: Acute Diarrhea." *Nurse Practitioner,* **3** (May–June 1978), 17.

Best, W. R. et al. "Development of Crohn's Disease Activity Index." *Gastroenterology,* **70** (March 1971), 439.

Buhac, I., and Balint, J. "Diarrhea and Constipation." *Am. Fam. Physician,* **12** (Nov. 1975), 149.

Burkitt, D. P. et al. "Effect of Dietary Fiber on Stools and Transit Time and Its Role in the Causation of Disease." *Lancet,* **2** (Dec. 30, 1972), 1408.

John, G. I. "Symptomatic Treatment of Acute Self-Limiting Diarrhea in Adults." *Practitioner,* **219** (Sept. 1977), 396.

Painter, N. S., and Burkitt, D. "Diverticular Disease of the Colon, a 20th Century Problem." A. Smith, Ed. *Clin. Gastroenterol.,* **4** (Jan. 1975), 3.

Phillips, S. F. "Diarrhea, Pathogenesis, and Diagnostic Techniques." *Postgrad. Med.,* **57** (Jan. 1975), 65.

Liver and Biliary Tract—Disorders

Baranowski, K. et al. "Viral Hepatitis." *Nurs. '76,* **5** (May 1976), 31.

Bartrum, R. J., Jr., et al. "Ultrasonic and Radiographic Cholecystography." *New Eng. J. Med.,* **296** (March 1977), 538.

Gerolami, A., and Sarles, H. "Letter: B-sitosterol and Chenodeoxycholic Acid in the Treatment of Cholesterol Gallstones." *Lancet,* **2** (Oct. 1975), 721.

Hawkins, I. F. et al. "Radiologic Approach to Obstructive Jaundice and Pancreatic Disease." *Med. Clin. North Am.* (1975), 121.

Hoofnagle, J. H. et al. "Transmission of Non-A, Non-B Hepatitis." *Ann. Int. Med.,* **87** (July 1977), 14.

Krugman, S. "Hepatitis: Current Status of Etiology and Prevention." *Hosp. Prac.,* **10** (Nov. 1975), 39.

Loeb, P. M. et al. "Endoscopic Pancreatocholangiography in the Diagnosis of Biliary Tract Disease." *Surg. Clin. North Am.,* **53** (1973), 1007.

Porta, E. A. "Nutrition and Diseases of the Liver and Gallbladder." *Prog. Food Nutr. Sci.,* **1** (May 1975), 289.

Shahinpour, N. "The Adult Patient with Bleeding Esophageal Varices." *Nurs. Clin. North Am.,* **12** (June 1977), 331.

Toouli, J. et al. "Gallstone Dissolution in Man Using Cholic Acid and Lecithin." *Lancet,* **2** (Dec. 1975), 1124.

The Liver and Biliary Tract—Pancreas

Belinsky, I. "Fiberoptic Advances: Visualizing the Pancreatic and Biliary Ducts." *Am. J. Nurs.,* **76** (June 1976), 936.

Johnson, R. M. et al. "Treatment of Acute Pancreatitis: In Search of a Rationale." *Proc. Instit. Med. Chicago,* **29** (1973), 268.

Olsen, H. "Pancreatitis: A Prospective Clinical Evaluation of 100 Cases and Review of the Literature." *Am. J. Dig. Dis.,* **19** (1977), 1007.

47

Problems Associated with Diabetes Mellitus

Leonard Thompson was a 14-year-old boy in the wards of Toronto General Hospital whose diabetes had been slowly progressing since December 1919. By January 1922 he was very weak and not expected to live much longer. On 11th January he was given the first injection of pancreatic extract. There was a transient 25 per cent fall in blood glucose, but no discernible clinical benefit. Daily injections were given between January 23rd and February 4th with obvious improvement. Urine glucose fell, acetone bodies disappeared from the urine, '. . . the boy became brighter, more active, looked better and said he felt stronger' (Banting et al, 1922). When administration of extract was discontinued all the symptoms and findings recurred. In other patients, RQ was found to rise '. . . confirming the increased utilization of carbohydrate.'

TATTERSALL

Ed. Robert Tattersall; "Evolution of Insulin Treatment"
Clinics in Endocrinology 6:2:485 (July) 1977.

Overview

In the not too distant past one of the critical tests of the skill of a nurse was the ability to meet the needs of a patient with an acute infectious disease such as typhoid fever or pneumonia. When the patient recovered, the nurse could rightly take credit for having made an important contribution. As infectious diseases have been brought under control, the incidence of chronic illness has risen so that they now account for a significant portion of morbidity and mortality. The challenges presented by patients who are chronically ill are no less great than they are with patients with acute infectious diseases. Chronically ill patients often have a wider range of problems and need a greater variety of services than are needed to meet the needs of the acutely ill. Restoration of the patient to optimum status and prevention of progress of the illness often demands the continued efforts of the patient, family, nurse, physician, and other health and welfare personnel as well as the members of the community. With patients in whom progress toward recovery is slow and in whom control or prevention of the progression of disease is the goal rather than complete recovery, the nurse may not be able to see immediate results of her or his efforts. Instead of a relatively brief and intense relationship in which the patient is dependent on the nurse, the nurse often has a more or less prolonged relationship. This relationship with the patient changes from time to time, from dependence to independence to interdependence. To meet the needs of the patient, the nurse should be able to identify clues indicating the type of relationship best suited to the needs of the patient at a given time and to adapt her or his behavior accordingly. The nurse must also be able to accept failure of the pa-

This chapter was revised by Kathlene F. Monahan, Associate Professor of Nursing, Wayne State University College of Nursing, Detroit, Michigan.

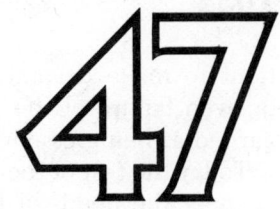

tient to make dramatic progress toward recovery or even failure of the patient to accept what is regarded as being essential to his or her welfare.

Today the test of the skill of the nurse is the ability to meet the needs of the chronically ill patient. If a single disease were to be selected as the modern-day test of nursing knowledge and skill, diabetes mellitus would undoubtedly receive many votes. There are many reasons that this is true. Diabetes mellitus has a relatively high incidence. It affects all age groups. Its complications are many and serious. There are, however, effective means for its detection, diagnosis, and treatment. With modern methods of therapy, persons with diabetes mellitus can live almost as long as those who do not have diabetes. Even more important, they can have full and useful lives with few restrictions on their activities. Persons with diabetes mellitus have been Rhodes scholars, mountain climbers, hockey players, television stars and statesmen. They marry, bear and rear children, and can lead successful, vigorous, productive, lives—a far cry from the predictable fate of the diabetic before the era of insulin therapy. Then the diabetic could only look forward to an early death. This was described so well by Leon Uris (1976, p. 343) in *Trinity:*

> Diabetes the doctor told him [Thomas]. The laboratory tests were conclusively grim. The condition was apparently terminal, for no known medicine could change the chemical balance that was destroying his body. Thomas had contracted the disease at least a year ago and it was a miracle the man had not already fallen into a lethal coma.

Health programs, as they relate to diabetes mellitus, have two general objectives. The first is to prevent or, if this is not possible, to delay the onset of the disease. The second is to maintain the health and vigor of the individual throughout life. In the achievement of these objectives the nurse has three general responsibilities. The first is to aid in the detection of persons who are predisposed to or in the early stages of diabetes mellitus. The second is to participate in the education of the patient, family, and the community in the management of diabetes mellitus. The third is to meet the needs of the sick person for nursing. Frequently the nurse performs all these functions simultaneously.

Historical Review

Diabetes mellitus is not a modern disease and its actual cause is unknown. There is evidence that it is one of the oldest diseases known. The first recorded reference to diabetes mellitus is believed to be in the Papyrus Ebers, which dates back to about 1500 B.C. (Major, 1955, p. 235). The term *diabetes* was introduced by a Roman physician, Aretaeus (A.D. 81–138). His was the first written description of the clinical manifestations of diabetes. He described it as a melting of the flesh and limbs. Considering the state of knowledge of the time, his description is surprisingly accurate.

Diabetic urine was described in the fifth century by Susruta as "honey urine." Some 1,200 years later, Thomas Willis (died 1673) reported that the urine from a patient with diabetes mellitus tasted sweet.

In 1775 Dobson identified the material in urine as sugar. Almost a century later the first reasonably accurate determinations of the quantity of glucose in the blood were made by Claude Bernard. He also discovered glycogen as well as the function of the liver in its storage. In 1869 Langerhans described the islet cells in the pancreas that now bear his name. About 20 years later Von Mehring and Minkowski demonstrated that diabetes mellitus was induced in a dog by pancreatectomy. In 1921 Banting and Best isolated insulin from the islet cells in the pancreas, and in 1922 they made insulin available for patients. Because insulin usually corrects the disturbance in carbohydrate metabolism, scientists believed that the nature of diabetes mellitus was understood. This belief was shaken in 1930 when Houssay (1942) reported that the severity of diabetes mellitus following pancreatectomy in the dog could be ameliorated by the removal of the anterior pituitary gland. Later Long and Lukens (1936) demonstrated that the same effect can be produced in the cat by adrenalectomy.

After more than 10 years of study (1945–1955) Sanger and his associates (1960) finally clarified the structure of the insulin molecule. It is a polypeptide consisting of two chains joined by three —S—S— (disulfide) bridges. They were able to demonstrate the sequence of amino acids in the molecule, as well as the fact that the sequence of amino acids differs somewhat in different species. Complete synthesis of insulin was achieved by Katsoyannis in 1966. Economical production of a synthetic insulin has not yet been achieved. From the patient's point of view the introduction of oral hypoglycemic agents in the late 1950s was a historical landmark.

In 1960 Yalow and Berson (1960) described an immunoassay method of measuring insulin. This procedure provided a sensitive and precise test for insulin that is relatively easy to perform. Equally or more important, information gained from the use of this procedure led to the challenging of many of the accepted "facts" about the nature of diabetes and its control. In 1967, Steiner and Oyer identified a single-chain precursor molecule—proinsulin. Proinsulin is converted to insulin and the C-peptide in the pancreatic beta cells.

The fact that diabetes mellitus may be present despite normal or even elevated immunoreactive insulin and/or insulinlike substances in the blood, led scientists to question whether the primary defect was a lack of insulin secretion.

Current research is directed toward investigation of hormone receptor sites on the plasma membranes of target body cells. The cell receptors act first to recognize specific hormones and then combine with it (the hormone) to form a hormone-receptor complex. This complex activates the cell. The biological effect of the hormone is a function of the hormone-receptor complex. The receptors for insulin and glucagon have been identified (Hormone Receptors, 1976, p. 211). The identification of these receptors has provided a major tool for study of the basic causes of diabetes. The concentration of receptors and receptor affinity for the hormone determines the ability of insulin to activate cellular events. The majority of maturity-onset diabetics appear to produce normal quantities of insulin, but a normal amount of the hormone produces a subnormal hormonal effect. This is defined as insulin resistance. The mechanisms of insulin resistance may operate before, at, or beyond the level of hormone receptor interaction, for example, circulating anti-insulin antibodies, genetic defects at the receptor sites, or decrease in the number of insulin receptor sites (Flier et al., 1979; Bar & Roth, 1977; Beck-Nielson, 1978). For the juvenile-onset type of diabetes (approximately 10 per cent of diabetics), evidence continues to support the theory that the basic defect is lack of insulin secretion (Sherwin & Felig, 1978).

The study of the chemistry and mechanisms of insulin has been voluminous. As a result there have been tremendous strides in the development of purer forms of insulin. These studies have resulted in increased knowledge about beta-cell secretory function. The term *knowledge explosion* is truly applicable to diabetes mellitus.

In 1974 the United States Congress passed the National Diabetes Mellitus Research and Education Act (Public Law 93–354). This act established a National Commission on Diabetes and charged it with formulating a long-range plan to combat diabetes. The development of the long-range plan to deal with diabetes followed a 9-month study by the commission. This comprehensive report examined the magnitude of the disease, its causes, consequences, and resources, and provides a solid base for further study, research, and governmental action. The establishment of the national commission and its findings in the landmark report clearly illustrate the human and social significance of diabetes mellitus.

The Nature and Causes of Diabetes Mellitus

Definition

Diabetes mellitus is not easy to define. The more that is learned about diabetes, the more difficult it becomes to define. Some authorities now believe it is not a discrete entity, but a complex syndrome. The oldest definition of diabetes mellitus is based on the observation that certain persons have a disorder characterized by the excretion of an abnormally large volume of urine or polyuria. The term *diabetes,* which is derived from the Greek and means "to pass through a siphon," was therefore applied to this condition. Mellitus—*mel* is Latin for "honey"—was added in the eighteenth century by Willis.

Based on the current state of knowledge diabetes mellitus is defined as a chronic genetically determined disorder of metabolism in which there is (1) a relative or absolute lack of insulin characterized by disturbed metabolism of glucose, fat, and protein and (2) accelerated atherosclerosis and microangiopathic vascular disease and neuropathy. The early symptoms and signs are usually related to the metabolic defects, whereas the late ones are complications resulting from the vascular disease.

Classification by Etiologic Factors

Over time various classifications of clinical diabetes have been suggested. A common classification is I. primary or genetic diabetes: *(a)* ketosis-prone type, *(b)* ketosis-resistant type; II. secondary diabetes: *(a)* destruction by disease or surgical excision of pancreatic tissue, *(b)* insulin antagonism produced by endocrine disease, excess secretion of growth hormone, hydrocortisone, aldosterone, catecholamines, thyroxine, or glucagon; *(c)* insulin antagonism from iatrogenic administration of drugs, for example, glucocorticoids, thiazide diuretics, oral contraceptives; *(d)* central nervous system disease.

Types of Primary or Genetic Diabetes Mellitus

There are two types of primary or genetic diabetes mellitus: (1) growth-onset (juvenile), (2) maturity-onset (adult diabetes mellitus).

Growth-Onset, Juvenile

Although it may occur later, the juvenile-onset type usually develops before age 15. It is characterized by an absolute insulin deficiency and by a rapid onset with rapid progression to coma. In the early stage of the disease the patient has an increase in insulin like activity substances in the plasma and the islet cells undergo hyperplasia and hypertrophy. After about 3 months of treatment about one third of the patients undergo a remission. Their insulin requirement diminishes and they respond well to sulfonylurea and/or phenethylbiguanide. Within 3 months to a year, they have a relapse and return to a diabetic state. They are then dependent, as are those who do not have a remission, on insulin for the control of their diabetes for the rest of their lives.

The terminology juvenile diabetes may imply it develops only before the age of 15. It may occur at any age and refers to the degree of insulin deficiency and adiposity. The juvenile diabetic is severely insulin-deficient and generally slender. Synonyms include ketosis-prone diabetes, insulin-dependent diabetes (IDD); and insulin-deficient diabetes.

Maturity-Onset

Although maturity-onset diabetes may develop in children, its usually develops after the age of 35 or 40 years. Among its characteristic features are (1) absence of ketosis, (2) excess adiposity, (3) delayed release of insulin after ingestion of glucose, (4) absence of symptoms, and (5) frequent vascular complications. Synonyms are ketosis-resistant diabetes, adult-onset diabetes, insulin-independent diabetes (IID), and lipoplethoric diabetes.

Classification by Therapeutic Requirements

Diabetes mellitus may also be classified according to the therapeutic requirements of the patient. Thus Underdahl (1967) places patients in four groups: A, B, C, and D. About 50 per cent of the patients have mild diabetes and are in group A. They can be controlled by diet. About 25 per cent of patients have moderate diabetes and are in group B. They require oral hypoglycemic agents plus diet to control their diabetes. Another 20 per cent have severe diabetes. They require insulin as well as diet to control their diabetes. Finally, about 2 to 10 per cent of the diabetics have what is variously called brittle, unstable, or labile diabetes. Diabetes in patients in group D is extremely difficult to control because they have a syndrome of excessive insulin sensitivity and ketosis proneness. Despite rigid adherence to the therapeutic regimen, these patients fluctuate between hyper- and hypoglycemia. Most patients with the maturity-onset type of diabetes are in either group A or group B.

Those with the growth-onset type of diabetes are in either group C or group D. The onset of the disease is sudden and is manifested by polyuria, polyphagia, polydipsia, ketoacidosis, and coma. The patient with the growth-onset type of diabetes mellitus is very sensitive to exogenous insulin. Early in the course of the disease his or her response to insulin is erratic. After 2 or 3 months of treatment, about one third of the patients undergo a remission. Their insulin requirement diminishes and they respond well to a sulfonylurea and/or phenethylbiguanide. Within a few months to a year, these patients have a relapse and require insulin to control their diabetes.

Classification by Natural History

Diabetes mellitus may also be classified according to its natural history. The actual or potential biochemical disturbances of diabetes mellitus are viewed on a continuum from a prediabetic state to an overt manifestation state. This type of classification system permits assessment of the severity of the problem and provides guidelines for treatment for the various stages (Table 47-1).

The earliest stage is prediabetes, which is defined as the period of time from birth until a genetically predisposed person has an impaired tolerance for glucose. This state may be very short or very long, as overt diabetes mellitus develops at all ages from very young babies to those 80 years of age. In fact, it may never develop. Prediabetes is suspected in individuals who have close relatives who are diabetic, such as two diabetic parents or a diabetic identical twin. Therapy in this state is prophylatic. For example, the person is encouraged to maintain normal weight. The significance of the postulated prediabetic state lies in the potential for identification of such individuals and application of preventative measures. Needless to say, this is a fertile area for research.

Stage II is termed the stress type. It is sometimes called subclinical or suspected diabetes. It is characterized by the appearance of hyperglycemia induced by stress. The stressors may be infections, trauma, fever, myocardial infarctions, iatrogenic drugs, pregnancy, and so on. When the stress is controlled, the

TABLE 47-1 *Stages in the Natural History of Diabetes Mellitus*

Stage	Fasting Blood Sugar	Glucose Tolerance Tests	Ketones	Insulin
I Prediabetes	Normal	Normal	0	Apparently normal
II Stress type (subclinical)	Normal Abnormal under stress	Normal	0 or +	Probably decreased
III Chemical type (Latent)	Normal	Abnormal	0	Decreased
IV Overt type	Increased	Abnormal	0 or +	Decreased

Adapted from Danowski, T. S. (1976).

individual may return to the prediabetic state with normal blood glucose. During the stress stage, the person may require hypoglycemic therapy.

Stage III is chemical or latent diabetes. In this stage there is mild glucose intolerance. The fasting blood sugar levels are normal. The postprandial and glucose tolerance tests are abnormal. The person maintains insulin secretory ability and is able to handle carbohydrates. It tends to progress to the next stage and it appears most often in overweight adults.

In the fourth stage, or overt diabetes, the individual has fasting hyperglycemia (high blood glucose) and glycosuria (glucose in the urine). He or she may be ketosis-prone or ketosis-resistant (Fajans, 1971).

As implied earlier, diabetes may progress rapidly or slowly. Tolerance for glucose may improve as well as deteriorate. Fluctuations are particularly common among those with mild forms of the disease. Regression even from the overt form of the disease also occurs. Fajans states that instances of overt ketotic diabetes regressing to the prediabetic stage have been reported.

Stage III and stage IV diabetes treatment options include diet management. If this approach is inadequate, hypoglycemic therapy is added to the treatment program.

Although the disease often appears suddenly in children, diabetes is sometimes identified in the latent or chemical stage of the disease. These children have the nonprogressive course characteristic of the maturity-onset type. Like adults, they are identified by a glucose tolerance test.

The various stages of diabetes have been presented in this section. The classification terms for diabetes have been undergoing change. The nurse may also find such terms as *florid diabetes*—this describes the state characterized by hyperglycemia whenever the blood glucose is measured (Whitehouse, 1978).

EPIDEMIOLOGY

The nurse is always concerned about the epidemiology of disease. Understanding the distribution and dynamics (epidemiology) of a disease serves as a basis for meeting objectives of disease detection and for education of patient, family, and community. Because diabetes and other chronic diseases are not reportable, they are not subjected to the type of surveillance used for communicable diseases. As surveys and techniques of detection and diagnosis improve, reporting will increase and it may be possible to identify and to improve preventive measures. In 1900, diabetes mellitus ranked twenty-seventh as a cause of death; presently it ranks in sixth place.

The prevalence (that is, the total number of persons with diabetes mellitus at a specific time) is not known with absolute certainty. According to the 1975 National Health Interview Survey, a rate of 20.4 per 1,000 population or an estimated 4.8 million persons in the United States reported diagnosed diabetes. Between 1965 and 1975, the prevalence of diabetes increased by 50 per cent in the United States. There is some question if there is a true increase in the frequency. The data may represent an increase in recognition due to increased use of automated blood chemistry laboratory techniques. Diabetes mellitus occurs in all age groups and in both sexes. The prevalence rate increases with age, from 1.3/1,000 (1 in 77) for persons under 17 years of age to 78.5/1,000 (1 in 12) in persons over the age of 65. Diabetes is reported more frequently in females (2.4 per cent) than in males (1.6 per cent).

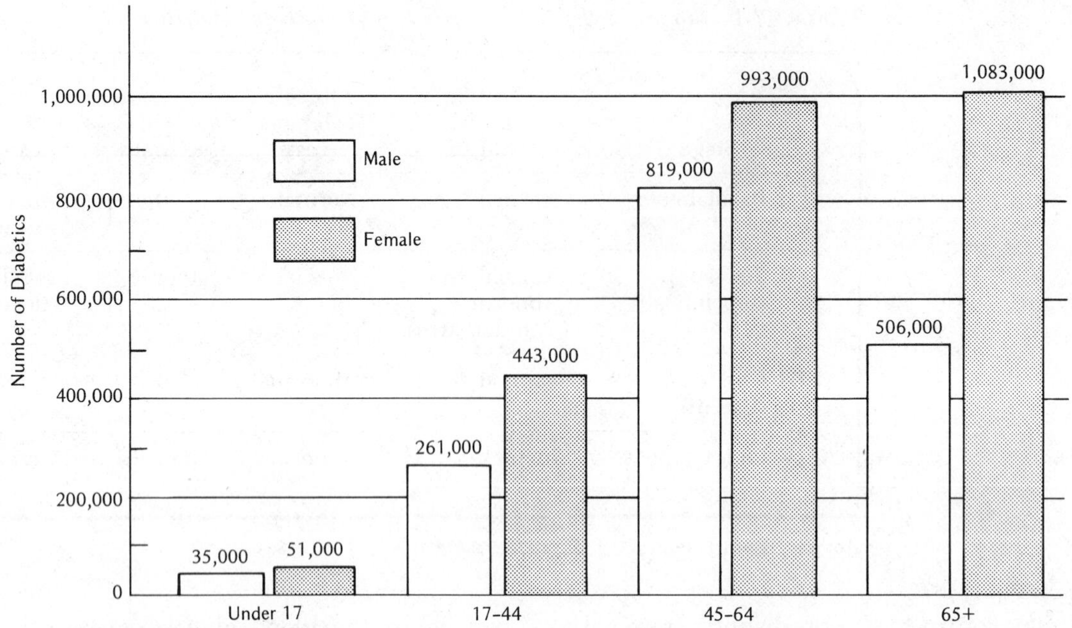

Figure 47-1. Reported number of diabetics by age and sex, 1973
Source: 1973 Health Interview Survey data, National Center for Health Statistics.

Females have a prevalence rate of 24.1/1,000. This is a 50 per cent increase from 1965 data when it was 16.1/1,000. The prevalence rate for males is 16.3/1,000. The most dramatic changes in prevalence of reported diabetes is the increase of diabetes in nonwhites under the age of 45. This group has a percentage change of 150 per cent. Figure 47-1 shows the reported prevalence by age and sex. Nonwhites are 20 per cent more likely than whites to have diabetes.

Incidence is the frequency of new cases of a disease developed during a specified time period. Data concerning the annual incidence of diabetes shows that 325,000 persons reported they have been diagnosed as diabetic in the previous 12 months in 1965. In 1973, 612,000 persons reported a diagnosis of diabetes in the previous 12 months.

Table 47-2 shows the relationship of family income and incidence and prevalence of diabetes mellitus. There is a marked inverse relationship. This relationship appeared in every age group except in the age group under 17 years (*Diabetes Data*, 1978).

Despite the widely held belief that the prevalence of diabetes mellitus is increasing, this may not be true. In 1963, 17 years after the first Oxford study, 65.7 per cent of the residents aged 34 to 55 years who lived in Oxford during the first study were restudied. The percentage of diabetics was found to be the same in the second as in the first study (O'Sullivan, 1969).

In the 1930s and 1940s there was marked improvement in the life expectancy of diabetics. Since that time, there has been little improvement. This may be due to the fact that diabetes patients are living long enough to develop the more dangerous concomitants (Kessler, 1971). The factors contributing to the great improvement in the life expectancy of persons in the 1930s and 1940s include (1) greater understanding of the nature of normal as well as abnormal energy metabolism, (2) more appreciation of the value of diet in the control of hyperglycemia, (3) the discovery of insulin and its use in therapy, (4) the recognition that the control of diabetes mellitus is the responsibility of the patient and family, and (5) the development of educational programs to prepare the patient to assume this responsibility. Reasons for failure to prevent the concomitants of diabetes is one of the problems being studied intensively today.

TABLE 47-2 ***Annual Incidence and Prevalence Rates (per 1,000) of Diabetes by Reported Family Income—United States, 1973***

Reported Family Income	Incidence	Prevalence
Total	3.0	20.4
Less than $5,000	4.5	40.2
$5,000–9,999	3.4	20.0
$10,000 or more	2.2	13.7

Source: Computed from 1973 Health Interview Survey data, National Center for Health Statistics.

Group Differences

The fact that diabetes mellitus appears to be more common among certain groups of people than others merits some comment. The incidence is higher among those who live in urban areas than those who live in rural areas. This is probably caused by the fact that persons living in urban areas are frequently more sedentary than those living in rural areas. It is recognized that exercise decreases the demand for insulin. The possibility also exists that persons living in urban areas have more adequate and better quality medical care available, and a higher *apparent* incidence of diabetes may be shown.

Most authorities emphasize that the incidence of diabetes mellitus is higher among Jews than among non-Jews. Joslin attributes this finding to the high incidence of obesity among Jewish people Joslin (1959). Cohen (1961) challenges the belief that the incidence is higher among Jews than non-Jews. He suggests that it is based on data collected in clinics patronized by a disproportionate number of Jewish people. In the study of the incidence of diabetes mellitus in Israel, Cohen found the incidence to be similar to that of people living in other countries. He also discovered that the Yemenites and Kurds, who traditionally have a very low incidence of diabetes mellitus, became diabetic at about the same rate as other Israelis when they adopted Western habits—food as well as habits of living and working.

Etiologic Factors

Current evidence supports the belief that the basic defect in diabetes mellitus is an inability to secrete sufficient insulin to meet metabolic demands. This failure may be partial or complete. In the maturity-onset type of diabetes, there is often a delayed release of endogenous insulin in relation to a glucose challenge. Some diabetics secrete sufficient insulin to maintain the homeostasis of glucose under most circumstances. In diabetics who secrete some insulin, homeostasis fails when the demand for insulin exceeds its supply or a condition exists that is characterized by a diminished responsiveness to insulin.

Numerous factors appear to be important in the development of diabetes mellitus. Some are amenable to preventive measures and others are not. The nurse can utilize such knowledge as a disease detector and in other situations can design and implement nursing actions to delay or to prevent progression from the nondiabetic state to the diabetic state. The etiologic factors most frequently indicated as predisposing to the diabetic state are age, sex, body weight, heredity, and hormonal factors.

Age

It has been known for over 50 years that the ability to adapt to glucose diminishes with aging. As a result some authorities question whether the same standards should be used for the glucose tolerance test in older persons as for young and middle-aged adults. Despite a large number of studies of the effect of aging on glucose tolerance test performance in different age groups, there is as yet no definitive answer to this question. In summarizing these studies Andres (1971) states that whatever the population studied, on the average there is a progressive decline in performance decade by decade of life on the commonly used diagnostic tests for diabetes. Tolerance is decreased more 1 hour after the ingestion of glucose than 2 hours after. This result is subject to two interpretations. One is that with aging there is a general adaptive decline that affects most of the population. The other interpretation is that a decline in glucose tolerance indicates the development of true diabetes. These are significant distinctions as they determine whether aging individuals with some decrease in glucose tolerance should be treated as normal or diabetic.

Sex

Diabetes is more common in women than in men in the United States and Europe. Black women outnumber black men. High parity (over six children), an obstetric history of stillborns, and/or delivery of large infants all seem to increase the likelihood of a woman developing diabetes after the age of 45 or 50. Other studies relate the increased prevalence to obesity factors and do not attribute it to diabetogenic effects of pregnancy.

Body Weight

There is a close relationship between obesity and maturity-onset diabetes. It is well recognized, but poorly understood. "Heredity loads the cannon, but obesity and certain other stress pull the trigger" (Marble et al., 1971, p. 23).

The incidence of diabetes in obese individuals is substantially greater than in the general population. Depending on the source of the statistics, from 60 to 80 per cent of persons with the maturity-type diabetes are obese at the onset of the disease. Glucose intolerance is significantly higher among the obese than in those who are of normal weight. The enlarged adipose tissue depots and enlarged adipose cells appear to be insulin-resistant. There appears to be a decrease in the concentration of insulin receptors of target cells in the obese.

The beta cells respond to the increased glucose load by releasing insulin, but the adipose tissue's relative resistance retards or prevents passage of the hormone into the cell. This accounts not only for the high relationship between diabetes and obesity, but also for the difficulties encountered in treating the obese diabetic.

As implied earlier with weight loss, the demand for insulin decreases and glucose tolerance improves. Children differ from adults inasmuch as obesity is not a factor in the development of diabetes mellitus. The onset in children frequently occurs during periods of increased linear growth. Obesity plus a family history increases the likelihood of developing diabetes.

Heredity

The relationship of heredity to diabetes mellitus has been observed since at least the seventh century A.D. Despite evidence that heredity is a factor in diabetes mellitus, it cannot be demonstrated in all persons. Statistics from different clinics indicate that from 20 to 50 per cent of diabetic individuals have a positive family history for diabetes. Despite evidence that heredity is important in the development of diabetes, its genetic basis remains controversial.

Countless enzymes, hormones, and receptors each coded by a single gene are involved in metabolic homeostasis. Since genes are polymorphic and since the impact of environmental stressors varies from person to person, the complexity of the study of the genetics of diabetes mellitus is enormous (Goldstein & Podolsky, 1978). Some authorities believe that diabetes is inherited as an autosomal recessive trait, but not all agree. Inheritance of diabetes mellitus among experimental animals is by a variety of patterns—autosomal recessive, dominant, and multifactorial traits.

There is evidence that the diabetes mellitus syndrome may be a heterogenous group of disorders that share glucose intolerance. Heterogenicity implies that different genetic defects and/or environmental factors may result in diabetes. This would help to explain the reason for such findings as that (1) only about 50 per cent of offspring of diabetic parents develop diabetes mellitus, (2) different types of diabetes mellitus (juvenile- and maturity-onset diabetes), and (3) different manifestations in different ethnic groups (Rimoin, 1971; Zonana & Rimoin, 1976).

Genetic studies have supported a definite association between the HLA B-8 antigen and juvenile-, but not maturity-onset, diabetes (Zonana & Rimoin, 1976, p. 604). Autoimmune phenomena have also been found in juvenile diabetics. Clear genetic differences have been indicated between the two forms of diabetes.

An interesting view of the hereditary nature of diabetes is presented by Neel (1962), who suggests that in prehistoric times the diabetic gene enhanced human being's chances for survival. The diabetic tends to have accelerated growth in childhood, early menarche, large babies, and later a tendency toward obesity. Thus the diabetic woman was able to reproduce during her short life span, and obesity protected her against famine.

Hormonal Factors

A deficiency in the supply of available insulin in relation to the quantity required to prevent hyperglycemia is conceded to be the principal endocrine factor in diabetes mellitus. The possibility exists that disturbances in the functioning of other endocrine glands may in some instances play a significant role in its genesis. To date, proof is lacking that abnormal function of glands such as the adrenal cortex or anterior pituitary causes diabetes mellitus unless the reserve capacity of the beta cells is inadequate. The hormones secreted by the adrenal cortex or anterior pituitary may precipitate diabetes mellitus in persons who have a preexisting tendency to diabetes mellitus. Evidence to support a possible relationship of other hormones to the development of diabetes mellitus is derived from animal experiments and the observation that persons with acromegaly, Cushing's syndrome, and hyperthyroidism sometimes manifest hyperglycemia and glycosuria.

Some persons under treatment with adrenocortical hormones or adrenocorticotropin also develop hyperglycemia, and this is sometimes called steroid diabetes. This drug-induced diabetes may occur as soon as 3 days within initiation of treatment and usually disappears in nondiabetic-prone individuals with cessation of treatment.

Because of their capacity to provoke hyperglycemia and glycosuria in persons who are predisposed to diabetes mellitus, hydrocortisone and cortisone may be employed to identify persons who are in the latent (prediabetic) stage of the disease. This test is called the cortisone—glucose tolerance test.

A recent observation of the effect of altering hormonal balance on glucose tolerance is that about 15 per cent of women who are taking combined estrogen-progestogen oral contraceptives develop chemical diabetes (Oakley et al., 1973).

The progestins do not affect the metabolism of carbohydrate. However, the synthetic estrogen mestranol used in five preparations (Enovid, Ovulen, Ortho-Novum, Norinyl, and C-Quen) "impairs glucose metabolism to some extent in the majority of normal women, and even more so in those with potential or actual diabetes" (Ellenberg & Rifkin, 1970, p. 465). Diabetic and prediabetic women should take oral contraceptives with mestranol only on the advice and under the supervision of a physician.

Oral diuretic agents can also produce a chemical diabetes. The impaired carbohydrate metabolism may be the result of depletion of total body potassium by the thiazides. Urine of individuals on thiazide therapy should be checked regularly for sugar. Known diabetics on such therapy may require increased dosage of hypoglycemic agents.

The mechanisms of action by which hormones other than insulin predispose to the development of diabetes mellitus have not been proved. Several hypotheses have been proposed: (1) The hormone or hormones act in some manner to decrease the secretion of insulin; (2) the hormone or hormones antagonize, inhibit, or block the peripheral action of insulin; and (3) the hormone or hormones act indirectly by producing conditions that increase the demand for insulin.

In permanent diabetes the growth hormone can be shown to elevate the blood sugar. It impairs glucose tolerance and responsiveness to insulin. Its mechanism of action is not known. The adrenal steroids promote the formation of glucose (gluconeogenesis) by the liver and may decrease its peripheral utilization.

Somatostatin (somatotropin release-inhibiting factor) in addition to its inhibition of secretion of the growth hormone, inhibits secretion of other hormones. When it is injected into the blood stream, insulin, glucagon, and the growth hormones disappear. Blood glucose will fall in spite of the inhibition of insulin. These effects are brief and will last 30 minutes after discontinuing the infusion. It appears to act directly on the alpha and beta cells of the pancreas to inhibit secretion of glucagon and insulin. There exists increasing evidence that excess of the growth hormone and hyperglycemia may accelerate the development of the chronic complications of diabetes. The potential use of somatostatin in the treatment of diabetes is yet to be determined (Gerich, 1977; Rizza & Gerich, 1978).

The mechanisms of action by which hormones other than insulin predispose to the development of diabetes mellitus have not been proved. Several hypotheses have been proposed: (1) the hormone or hormones act in some manner to decrease the secretion of insulin; (2) the hormone or hormones antagonize, inhibit, or block the peripheral action of insulin; and (3) the hormone or hormones act indirectly by producing conditions that increase the demand for insulin.

Precipitating Factors

Any disorder that alters carbohydrate metabolism can induce diabetes mellitus; for example, pancreatectomy, malignant neoplasms of the pancreas, chronic pancreatitis, or hepatic cirrhosis all can induce diabetes. It also occurs in a high percentage of patients who have hemochromatosis, a disorder of iron metabolism characterized by the deposit of iron in the pancreas and other tissues. Deposits in the skin lead to the characteristic coloring that gives the disorder its name, bronze diabetes. The deposits of iron in the tissues lead to irritation and fibrosis. With destruction of the beta cells in the pancreas, diabetes mellitus ensues. Diabetes commonly accompanies Cushing's disease, a disorder in which there is an increase in the secretion of adrenocortical steroids.

Permanent diabetes mellitus in animals can be induced in a number of ways: (1) the removal of nine tenths or more of the pancreas, (2) the destruction of the beta cells in the islands of Langerhans by a chemical such as alloxan, (3) the prolonged administration of crude extracts of the anterior pituitary gland or of purified growth hormone, and (4) the prolonged parenteral administration of glucose.

The last two experimental conditions appear to have a common element: they increase the demand for insulin by causing a persistent elevation in the blood sugar. Because the secretion of insulin is believed to be regulated by the level of glucose in the blood, a continued elevation in blood glucose places a strain on the beta cells in the pancreas. Eventually insulin-secreting cells are exhausted. After animals treated with the growth hormone or prolonged administration of parenteral glucose die, their beta cells in the pancreas are usually found to have undergone degeneration. At autopsy, some, but not all, diabetics are found to have experienced destruction of the beta or islet cells.

Summary

To recapitulate, the manifestations of diabetes mellitus result from a relative or absolute lack of insulin. Some of the possible causes for this deficiency have been suggested. Heredity, obesity, and age appear to be associated with the development of diabetes mellitus.

Among other factors that may contribute to the diabetic state are anti-insulin antibodies, other hormones, and resistance of the peripheral tissues to insulin. Although insulin antibodies have been identified, they are found only in patients who have taken insulin. Among the hormones that antagonize the effect of insulin are the glucocorticoids, the growth hormone, epinephrine, and glucagon. What the role of each of these factors is in the genesis of diabetes mellitus is still in some doubt. The combination of optimum age, obesity, and hereditary tendency may be sufficient to induce diabetes mellitus. The tendency to develop the disease may be further increased by such factors as dietary excesses and too little exercise.

Organic Metabolism and Energy Balance

The concepts of organic metabolism and energy balance were discussed in Chapter 29 but will be briefly reviewed here. Metabolism requires a continuous supply of nutrients to maintain cell structure and function (Vander et al., 1975, p. 62). Metabolism is a highly integrated process in which all classes of molecules, carbohydrates, lipids, and proteins, can be used if necessary to provide energy for the cell through ATP (adenosine triphosphate) synthesis. Each class of molecule can, to a large extent, provide the raw materials to synthesize members of other classes (Vander et al., 1975, p. 89). The human body's remarkable ability to convert one type of molecule to another provides a mechanism whereby a continuous supply of energy can be stored, liberated, and utilized. Human beings therefore do not have to eat continuously to have an adequate nutrient supply.

Glucose is the major energy source for body cells and the only energy source for the central nervous system and red blood cells. Carbohydrates and lipids are constantly being broken down and resynthesized. The same is true of protein.

During the absorptive state (which lasts approximately 4 hours after a meal) the main source of energy is glucose from the readily available exogenous food supply. The nutrients enter the blood directly from the gastrointestinal tract. During the post absorptive state, carbohydrate is synthesized in the body from endogenous sources. This energy metabolism can be seen as a process whereby the energy stored in food is converted to a form that can be stored for future use and/or gradually liberated by a series of stepwise chemical reactions for use in cells.

Certain facts about glucose should be kept in mind. Only 350 to 400 g of glucose, including glycogen, are present in the body at any time. It is readily converted to fat and thus contributes to the reserve energy supply. It may furnish carbon atoms for certain amino acids. Glucose is the most likely precursor of pentose (a 5-carbon atom sugar) of the nucleic acids, DNA and RNA. Further, it is a major source of glycerol, which is required for the esterification of fatty acids in adipose tissue.

Because glucose is not chemically a very active substance, glucose must be converted to the chemically active glucose-6-phosphate before it can be used at body temperature. This reaction requires the presence of the enzyme hexokinase and is the first step in the utilization of glucose, regardless of whether the glucose is converted to glycogen, utilized as energy, or converted to fat and stored. The entrance of significant quantities of glucose into the cell also requires a transport mechanism. After glucose enters the cell and is converted to glucose-6-phosphate, the cell is protected against too much energy at one time by the stepwise release of energy. Furthermore, different pathways are available in the utilization of glucose and many chemical reactions in the utilization of glucose are reversible. Not only is energy liberated and utilized, but it is fixed as chemically useful energy and stored in the form of high-energy bonds such as the high-energy phosphate bonds.

A number of conditions must be met for energy metabolism to proceed normally. In the first place appropriate metabolites in the proper form must be present. Some of these are supplied from exogenous as well as endogenous sources, and they must enter the cell at an appropriate rate, neither too slowly, nor too rapidly. For example, at least 100 g of glucose must be metabolized daily to prevent the utilization of fat at an excessively rapid rate. Most of this glucose comes from outside sources as the quantity of glycogen (a storage form of glucose) stored in the liver is sufficient to supply the glucose needed for about 4 hours. Glucose can also be obtained from muscle glycogen storage. By the process of glycolysis it is broken down into pyruvate and lactate circulated via the blood to the liver, and there is synthesized into glucose. Some chemical reactions depend on the presence of certain metabolites that are formed during metabolism to provide the energy required for the reaction. For example, for glucose to be transferred into cells and converted into glucose-6-phosphate, high-energy adenosine triphosphate is required. In some chemical reactions a metabolite necessary to initiate the reaction is released or regenerated at the end of the reaction so that it is again available. For example, acetyl CoA and oxaloacetic acid combine at the beginning of the Krebs cycle to form citric acid. Oxaloacetic acid is regenerated at the end of the reaction.

In addition to the availability of appropriate metabolites at varying stages of metabolism, enzymes and coenzymes are required to catalyze the various chemical reactions involved in the release or storage of energy. Some of these are synthesized by the cells, whereas others, such as thiamine, must be ingested in the diet.

Maintenance of Plasma Glucose Concentration

The maintenance of adequate plasma glucose levels is crucial. Brain survival is dependent upon this maintenance. The first source of glucose is absorption from the intestinal tract. This source lasts for approximately 4 hours after a meal. The second source is glycogenolysis and the third is gluconeogenesis.

Glycogenolysis

The glucogen stores, particularly in the liver, can be rapidly converted to glucose. The process by which the liver converts glycogen to glucose and secretes it into the hepatic vein is known as glycogenolysis. This is a rapid reaction occurring in a matter of minutes. The rapid conversion of glycogen to glucose is adapted to protect the individual in emergency situations against a drop in blood glucose. The process is regulated by epinephrine and glucagon. The total quantity of glycogen in the liver is limited. A normal liver contains 60 to 100 g of glucose; at 4 kcal/g, this provides 240 to 400 kcal, and would provide the body's total caloric needs for about 2½ to 4 hours. Glycogen cannot be expected to protect the level of glucose in the blood for more than a brief period of time.

Gluconeogenesis

The liver glycogen stores will only maintain blood glucose levels for a few hours, and the third line of defense, gluconeogenesis, maintains plasma glucose levels by forming glucose from nonglucose precursors (pyruvate, lactate, glycerol, and amino acids). This formation is called gluconeogenesis. If a person fasts for 24 hours, the hepatic synthesis can account for 180 g of glucose.

Gluconeogenesis differs from glycogenolysis in two respects. Rather than being a rapid and brief source of glucose to the blood, it is a slow and sustained reaction. It protects the level of glucose in the blood in disorders in which the supply of glucose is deficient or loss is excessive. Thus the level of glucose in the blood is maintained in starvation, despite a failure in the supply from exogenous sources. It is also maintained in disorders of the kidney in which excessive quantities of glucose are lost in the urine. Gluconeogenesis occurs in the liver and kidney. Ordinarily the kidney accounts for less than 10 per cent of the glucose production. In periods of prolonged starvation it may account for 45 per cent (Brobeck, 1973, sect. 7, p. 133).

Whereas the rate of glycogenolysis is regulated by epinephrine and glucagon, the rate of gluconeogenesis is regulated by glucagon and the adrenal glucocorticoids (cortisol of hydrocortisone). Gluconeogenesis is regulated by the level of substrates (plasma lactate, pyruvate, amino acid, and glycerol) in the blood. For example, increased exercise and activity of the sympathetic nervous system increases lactate production and this results in replenishment of glycogen stores in the liver and muscle (Brobeck, 1973, sect. 7, p. 138).

In addition to protecting the level of glucose in the blood by making more glucose available to the blood, reduction in the utilization of glucose by peripheral tissues may also be a factor in the maintenance of the blood glucose. In starvation, tissues adapt in such a manner that they utilize less glucose than when the glucose supply is adequate. One factor in adaptation to starvation is a drop in total metabolism. On the basis of tissue culture experiments it is postulated that the muscles of starving animals utilize relatively more fatty acids than glucose.

Similar to other aspects of glucose metabolism, hormones are believed to regulate the processes involved in blocking the peripheral use of glucose. These hormones, which are often called insulin antagonists, are the growth hormone (anterior pituitary) and the adrenal glucocorticoids. The nature of the action of these hormones in blocking peripheral glucose oxidation is not known.

One factor that may possibly contribute to the elevation of glucose in the blood is an increase in the rate of destruction of insulin. A number of tissues, especially the liver, have been demonstrated to inactivate insulin. The insulin-destroying mechanism in the liver has been referred to as insulinase, but the nature of the system has not been firmly established. Another factor influencing the level of glucose in the blood is the state of hydration of the individual. When water loss exceeds the loss of solute, solute levels rise. Thus the levels of glucose and electrolytes are increased in states of dehydration.

In the nondiabetic person, the factors tending to elevate the level of glucose in the blood are promptly counteracted by factors tending to lower it. The reverse is also true. As long as the rates at which glucose enters and leaves the blood are equal, the concentration of glucose in the blood is maintained within physiologic limits. Any disturbance that interferes with the mechanisms for elevating or lowering the blood glucose may, depending on the direction of change, lead to hyper- or hypoglycemia. As an example, if the mechanisms for lowering blood glucose are ineffective and/or those for elevating it are hyperactive, hyperglycemia will result. Both of these factors are likely to be involved in diabetes mellitus. Despite the practice of discussing diabetes as if it were simply a disorder of glucose metabolism, it is not. Its pathophysiology involves all facets of metabolism.

Mechanisms for Elevating the Level of Glucose in the Blood

In the regulation of the level of glucose in the blood, certain cells recognize the need of the organism for glucose. When this need is sufficiently great, it is translated into the sensation hunger. Hunger motivates the individual to search for, find, and ingest food. There are three sources or routes by which glucose enters into the blood. The usual route of entry is absorption from the alimentary canal. A second route of entry is the secretion of glucose by the liver. In time of need, the liver can maintain the level of glucose in the blood within normal limits, despite the absence of food intake. Although the liver is able to do this in the absence of hormonal factors, the rate at which glucose is secreted into the hepatic vein by the liver is modified by hormones. A third and less common route is by parenteral injection as by intravenous infusion. Parenteral injection is usually reserved for patients who are unable to ingest food into or absorb it from the alimentary tract.

The supply of exogenous glucose leads to increased plasma glucose levels. This results in an increase in insulin secretion and decrease in the secretion of epinephrine, glucagon, and growth hormone. Conversely, during the fasting state, plasma glucose is decreased. This results in decreased insulin secretion and an increase in secretion of epinephrine, glucagon, and growth hormone.

Mechanisms for Lowering the Level of Glucose in the Blood

The normal response to satiety is to cease ingesting food or to decrease the supply of exogenous glucose. After absorption, glucose is distributed through the body water, thereby reducing its concentration in any compartment, including that of the blood. A third mechanism for lowering the blood glucose is exercise. Exactly how exercise affects the level of glucose in the blood is not well known. It is valuable in the treatment of diabetes mellitus as working muscle oxidizes glucose independently of insulin.

Insulin Release

Although a number of hormones are involved in elevating the level of glucose in the blood, the only hormone known to lower the blood glucose is insulin. The regulation of the release of insulin is highly complex. Among the factors that are believed to increase its release are (1) a rise in the level of glucose as well as the rate at which it rises in the blood; (2) a substance secreted by the jejunum, triggered by the absorption of glucose; (3) stimulation of the vagus nerve; (4) glucagon; and (5) amino acids. Glucose placed in the jejunum causes a greater rise in insulin release than the same quantity given by infusion. This fact may be of some importance when glucose is given by intravenous infusion for the purpose of supplying calories. Presumably less glucose will be lost in the urine when the rate of administration is slow to moderate than when it is rapid.

Release of insulin in response to glucose is biphasic. In phase I preformed stored insulin is rapidly released in response to glucose, amino acids, and other stimuli. In phase II insulin composed of preformed insulin, newly synthesized insulin, and proinsulin is secreted in response to glucose only. Further, measurable amounts of insulin are found in the plasma at all times. The quantity varies with the level of glucose. In other words, there is a feedback relationship between the level of glucose in the blood and the secretion of insulin (Sherwin & Felig, 1978, p. 696).

In addition to the biphasic release of insulin, there is also a diurnal variation in its release. The diurnal (that is morning and evening) response of normal subjects to glucose loading was studied by Carroll and Nestel. They found a decrease in glucose tolerance and a delay in release of plasma insulin in the evening when compared with the morning response. In fact, if accepted diabetic diagnostic criteria were used, the normal subjects would be classified as mild diabetics (Carroll & Nestel, 1973).

In another study glucose tolerance tests were carried out on 122 male volunteers aged 40 and over. In those with fasting blood sugar levels above 110 mg/100 ml the degree of diurnal variation was least in those with the highest morning blood sugars. They also tended to have lower evening fasting blood glucose levels. In 40 controls, those with blood glucose below 110 mg/100 ml, subjects' evening glucose tolerance tests showed significantly higher postglucose blood sugar levels (Jarrett & Keen, 1970).

Another interesting observation is that the diurnal variation was significantly and inversely related to the degree of obesity: the morning test might be normal and there could be considerable hyperglycemia in evening. As the abnormality increases, there is difficulty in correcting the hyperglycemia during the night. Loss of diurnal variation and evening hyperglycemia may be the first stage in glucose intolerance.

Mode of Action of Insulin

Despite considerable knowledge of the effects of insulin, how it produces these effects at the molecular level is not known. It is generally agreed that insulin is the storage or anabolic hormone and is involved in the metabolism not only of glucose but of protein and fat. Krahl (1972) lists the major biological phenomena stimulated by insulin as the (1) transport of glucose, ions, and amino acids across cell membranes; (2) formation of glycogen; (3) conversion of glucose to triglycerides; (4) synthesis of nucleic acid; and (5) synthesis of protein.

Three types of cells are the target sites for the metabolic actions of insulin, the liver, adipose tissue, and muscle. These cells require insulin for the transfer of glucose through the cell membrane. Levine (1971) suggests that a protein receptor on the cell membrane may be the site of the primary action of insulin. He postulates that as a result of the combination of insulin and its receptor, changes occur in the membrane that facilitate glucose, potassium, and amino acid transport. Further, a chemical signal of unknown composition is released. This signal triggers reactions in the interior of the cell that result in a speeding up of anabolic reactions, that is, synthesis of glycogen and fat, incorporation of amino acids in protein, and the increased formation of nucleic acids.

In insulin deficiency, that is, the diabetic state, there is a drastic reduction in the entry of glucose into insulin-sensitive muscle and fat cells. Whereas insulin promotes the storage and maintenance of glycogen, in its absence glycogen is broken down to glucose. With a deficit of intracellular glucose, free fatty acids are released from the triglycerides in fat cells. The fatty acids are used for fuel and give rise to ketone bodies.

A further response to the lack of glucose in cells is an increase in the production of a number of "glucose-elevating" hormones. Among them are the growth hormone, epinephrine, glucagon, ACTH, and cortisol, with the apparent effect of increased mobilization of fatty acids and gluconeogenesis. In addition the growth hormone and cortisol increase the body's resistance to administered insulin (*Diabetes Mellitus*, 1973, p. 27). All of these changes have the effect of raising the blood glucose and providing fuel for cells. Inasmuch as cells are provided with fuel, the effect is adaptive. In many respects, however, the events accompanying an insulin deficit are maladaptive.

Pathophysiology

The basic pathologic process in diabetes mellitus is that the cells are starving. They are starving in an extracellular pool of glucose. The exogenous supply of glucose is there, but because of varying degrees of insulin deficiency the glucose has no transport mechanism for entry into the cell. The body's indicators show that the cells need glucose, and it activates mechanisms to provide this vital energy fuel. The mechanism's activities are the same ones discussed under glucose metabolism. It decreases use of glucose by peripheral tissues, it mobilizes fat stores, and it intensifies the breakdown of protein. These mechanisms of the body would be adaptive *if* the exogenous glucose stores were really depleted, as they would be in true starvation. Some authorities refer to the diabetic situation as "relative starvation."

Effect on Carbohydrate Metabolism

The sequence of events resulting from the effects of a lack of insulin on carbohydrate metabolism is diagrammed in Figure 47-2.

Effect on Fat Metabolism

The deficiency of insulin and diminution in the use of glucose have important effects on the capacity of the individual to synthesize, store, and maintain storage depots of fat. With a lack of insulin and failure to utilize normal amounts of glucose, large quantities of fat are mobilized from fat stores and are poured into the blood in the form of fatty acids.

The liver is inundated with fat, most of which it metabolizes only to the acetyl CoA stage. (Ordinarily, acetyl CoA would enter the Krebs cycle by uniting with oxalacetate, but this is deficient.) The two carbon atom fragments unite to form acetoacetic acid (diacetic acid and beta-hydroxybutyric acid), and an accumulation of these acids in the blood results in metabolic acidosis, one of the characteristic features of which is Kussmaul breathing (deep and rapid breathing). In addition, as the production of ketoacids exceeds the capacity of the kidney to reabsorb them, they are excreted in the urine, and in the process of excretion they take cations such as sodium and potassium with them. Because electro-

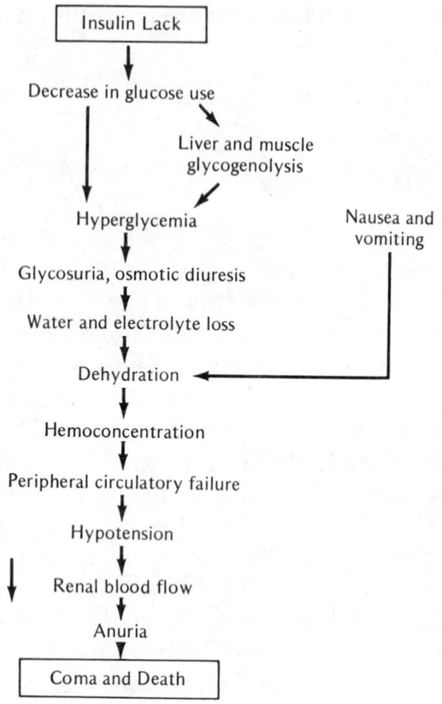

Figure 47-2. The effect of insulin lack on carbohydrate metabolism. (Reproduced with permission from Tepperman, J.: *Metabolic and Endocrine Physiology,* 3rd edition. Copyright © 1973 by Year Book Medical Publishers, Inc., Chicago.)

lytes are osmotically active, they also require water for their excretion. With the loss of sodium ions, the total quantity of sodium in the body is diminished, and with the decrease the water-holding power of extracellular fluid is also reduced. With a loss of sodium, the total volume of water in the extracellular

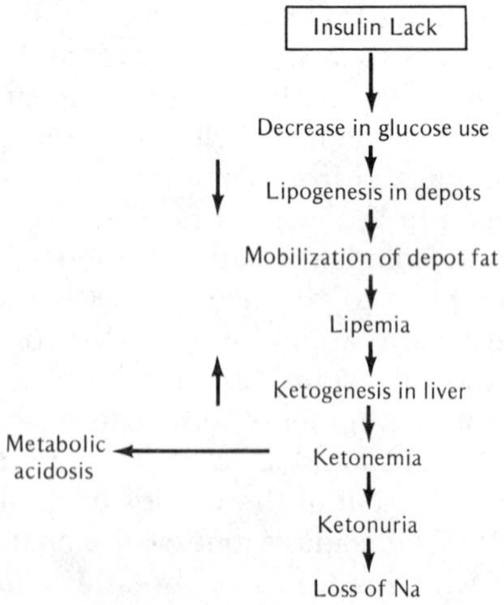

Figure 47-3. The effect of insulin lack on fat metabolism. (Reproduced with permission from Tepperman, J.: *Metabolic and Endocrine Physiology,* 3rd edition. Copyright © 1973 Year Book Medical Publishers, Inc., Chicago.)

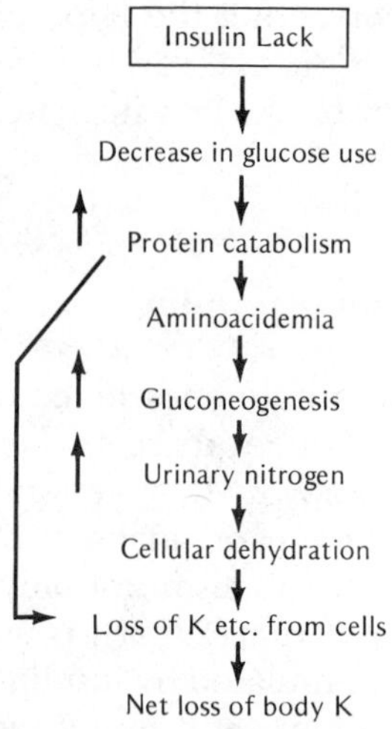

Figure 47-4. The effect of insulin lack on protein metabolism. (Reproduced with permission from Tepperman, J.: *Metabolic and Endocrine Physiology,* 3rd edition. Copyright © 1973 by Year Book Medical Publishers, Inc., Chicago.)

fluid falls. Blood volume drops and predisposes to peripheral circulatory failure. The effects of a deficiency of insulin on fat metabolism are summarized in Figure 47-3.

Effect on Protein Metabolism

Not only does a lack of insulin impair the use of glucose and fat, but it also affects protein metabolism (Figure 47–4). With a deficiency in the supply of insulin, protein synthesis, especially in muscles, is lessened and protein catabolism exceeds protein anabolism. The amino acids released are deaminated in the liver, the NH_2 fragment is removed, and the carbon-containing residues are converted to glucose or fatty acid. Protein catabolism results in a loss of nitrogen and potassium from the body and thereby contributes to hypovolemia and its associated effects.

Effects on Body Fluids, Electrolytes, and Acid-Base Balance

Intake of food and fluids is interfered with by anorexia, nausea, and vomiting. This triad, along with the glycosuria and ketonuria, depletes body fluid and electrolytes.

Loss of glucose in the urine has several undesirable effects. First, it is wasteful, and unless food intake is increased in proportion to loss, it will be associated with a loss in body weight and strength. Second, glucose is osmotically active. It holds water in the urine and thereby causes polyuria. With polyuria, not only water but electrolytes such as potassium and sodium are lost. Thirst and an increase in fluid intake prevent dehydration, unless and until the individual develops nausea and vomiting. With dehydration, the blood becomes concentrated and blood volume falls; blood pressure drops and circulation to the tissues fails. As circulation to the tissues fails, generalized tissue anoxia causes a shift to anaerobic metabolism. Lactic acid appears in increasing concentrations in the blood and reflects an elevation of the hydrogen ions in the cell. Unless the condition is corrected by improving the supply of oxygen to the cells, death from heart failure ensues.

The increase in ketone bodies, inorganic phosphates, and other proton donors results in an increase in hydrogen ions. The loss of sodium decreases the cation pool for neutralization. The kidneys attempt to balance the situation by excreting more hydrogen ions. The ventilatory buffer system responds by tachypnea. The breath of the acidotic patient will have a "fruity" odor as the acetone bodies are excreted by the lungs. When the ventilatory and renal regulators are no longer able to compensate for the metabolic acidosis, Kussmaul breathing appears, usually at serum total CO_2 levels of about 10

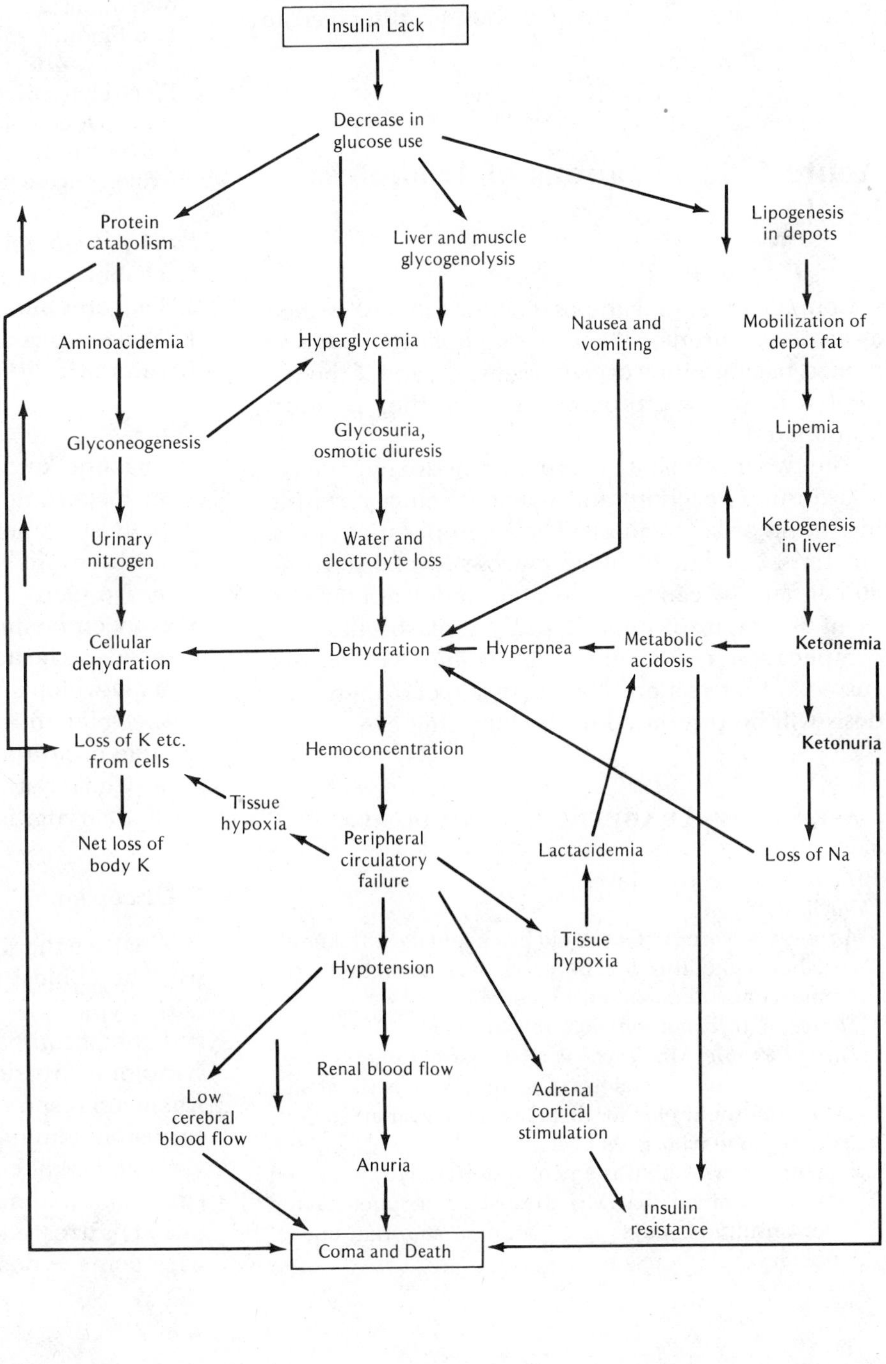

Figure 47-5. Composite summary of the pathophysiology of diabetic acidosis. Note particularly connections among the three general areas of metabolism. (Reproduced with permission from Tepperman, J.: *Metabolic and Endocrine Physiology,* 3rd edition. Copyright © 1973 Year Book Medical Publishers, Inc., Chicago.)

mEq/liter. The tachypnea and deep breathing produce a secondary respiratory alkalosis, which increases loss of CO_2 from the body, decreases P_{CO_2}, diminishes H_2CO_2 formation, and thereby decreases the hydrogen ion concentration.

From the foregoing discussion, it should be obvious that insulin influences the manner in which carbohydrate, fat, and protein are metabolized. Adequate supplies of insulin facilitate the use of glucose and favor synthesis and storage of fat. Inadequate insulin is accompanied by impaired use of glucose, mobilization of fatty acids, in some instances triglycerides, and amino acids. As a consequence, nutrition of the cells is reduced, water and electrolytes are lost, and, unless these deficits are corrected, circulation to the tissues is threatened. A composite summary of the pathophysiology of diabetic acidosis is displayed in Figure 47-5.

Acute Complications of Diabetes Mellitus

Complications of diabetes mellitus can be classified as acute or chronic. The acute complications are so named because they are emergencies; and if the patient is to survive, prompt intensive therapy must be initiated.

The two major acute complications are hypoglycemia (insulin reaction) and hyperglycemia resulting in acidosis or ketoacidosis. These complications present the two ends of blood glucose level spectrum, and either one can result in coma and death if treatment is not instituted. Hypoglycemia occurs as a complication of diabetes control and will be discussed in that section. The discussion of diabetic acidosis will be presented in the following case.

Case Study: Diabetic Ketoacidosis

Patient: Mrs. Beatrice Joyce
Data Base

Admission Note: A 60-year-old black female with known diabetes mellitus for 14 years, was brought to the emergency department by her son.

Source of Information: Son, reliable.

Patient Profile: Mrs. Joyce is a 60-year-old unemployed widow, who lives alone. Diagnosed diabetic at age 46. Treatment plan for diabetes: lente insulin, 20 units daily, 1,800 caloric ADA diet.

Present Illness: Client is a poor historian. However, son has ascertained that Mrs. Beatrice J. stopped taking her insulin 4 days ago "because she ran out of needles." Level of consciousness has become increasingly obtund. She has become progressively disoriented. Increased thirst and urination; vomiting, amount and frequency unknown. No report of any urine tests. No insulin for the last 4 days. Thin black female also appears to be acutely ill.

Significant Physical Examination Findings

Temp. 97; pulse 98; resp. 24; BP 110/70.

Level of consciousness: Lethargic, responds slowly to verbal stimuli.

Skin: Good turgor.

EENT: Eyeballs slightly soft, tongue and lips dry, throat injected.

Resp: Kussmaul respirations. Fruity odor to breath. Lungs clear to palpation and auscultation.

Cardiac: Normal sinus rhythm.

GI: Abnormal tenderness—right upper quandrant. No distention.

Lab Findings: Blood glucose—870 mg%, ph 7.04, P_{O_2}—126, P_{CO_2}—16.

Electrolytes: Na 125 mEq/L; K 6.0 mEq/L Cl 92 mEq/L; CO_2 combining power 5.0 mEq/L Hg 12.6g, HCT 5.3%; WBC 29,300

Urine: glucose 4+, ketones 3+

Patient Problem List:

1. Diabetes ketoacidosis
2. Diabetes mellitus, ketosis-prone (juvenile type)
3. Noncompliance with therapeutic regimen
4. Intercurrent infection

Plan:

1. Diabetic ketoacidosis
   a. Restore normal CHO metabolism
   b. Restore normal fluid and electrolyte balance
2. Diabetes mellitus, ketosis-prone
   a. No plan
3. Noncompliance with therapeutic plan
   a. Identify etiology of noncompliance
   b. Develop specific plan to increase compliance
   c. Defer to #1 corrected
4. Rule out intercurrent infection
   a. Cholecystitis
   b. Pharyngitis

Discussion

What are the signs and symptoms of diabetic acidosis? The clinical picture presented by Mrs. Joyce is fairly typical. The effects were caused by acidosis and the accompanying dehydration. The signs and symptoms are slow onset, florid face, soft eyeballs, Kussmaul respirations, acetone (fruity) breath, tachycardia, abdominal pain, nausea, vomiting, dry skin, variable loss of consciousness, and dehydration. The laboratory findings were also consistent. Hyperglycemia if untreated will progress to ketosis → acidosis → coma → death. (Refer to Figure 47-5.)

Is There a Difference between Ketoacidosis and Diabetic Coma?

Diabetic acidosis and coma refer to the situation where there is "a major loss of carbohydrate tolerance. Such cases may be subdivided in accord with the serum total CO_2 content at the time of admission. Cases with values above 20 mEq per liter are classified as ketonuria. Those with a serum total CO_2 content between 20 and 10 mEq per liter are termed ketoacidosis, and those with values lower than 10 are termed acidosis, coma" (Ellenberg & Rifkin, 1970, p. 674). The patient may or may not be comatose with CO_2 less than 10 mEq per liter. Blood glucose levels in ketoacidosis usually exceed 300 mg, but they may be lower. The level of consciousness does not correlate with blood glucose level. Mrs. Joyce's laboratory findings, blood glucose 870 mg per cent and CO_2 combining power 5.0 mEq per liter, would support a diagnosis of ketoacidosis. If she had been comatose, the diagnosis would have been acidosis, coma.

Nonketotic Hyperosmolar Coma

The diabetic is not immune to other types of coma. Hyperosmolar nonketotic coma (NKHO) in the diabetic has been increasingly recognized. The life-threatening hyperosmolarity is seen more often in the maturity-onset diabetic and in persons over the age of 60. Usually the person has been classified as a mild diabetic and has been treated by diet and/or oral hypoglycemic agents. The chief characteristics include hyperglycemia, heavy glycosuria, and minimal or no ketonuria or ketonemia. The CO_2 content is normal. Physical examination will demonstrate severe dehydration, absence of Kussmaul-type respirations, and no odor of acetone on the breath. The blood glucose is usually between 600 and 2,000 mg. The patient has a severe water deficit in addition to losses of potassium and sodium. Treatment consists of fluid and electrolyte replacement. Insulin therapy must also be instituted. Insulin dosages are calculated in the same manner as for diabetic ketoacidosis. However, in most instances the amount of insulin required to treat NKHO is thought to be less than for ketotic patients, as these patients have greater insulin sensitivity. The nurse must be especially alert to evidence of hypoglycemia as the patient can easily become hypoglycemic. A diabetic coma sheet should be used to monitor the treatment (Bonar, 1977; Guthrie & Guthrie, 1977).

Causes of Diabetic Acidosis

The causes of the major loss of carbohydrate tolerance can include any of the following: newly diagnosed or initial presentation, ignorance, neglect of therapy, intercurrent diseases or infection. Identification of the etiology except for intercurrent disease or infection does not take priority during the acute stage of illness.

Mrs. J. omitted her insulin for 4 days, her throat is injected, and her white count is elevated. Omission of insulin and intercurrent infection appear to be etiological factors. As indicated in her therapeutic plan, identification of etiology of noncompliance will be deferred until the patient is in a more stable state.

Numerous studies have shown that most cases of ketoacidosis are precipitated by infections (56 to 67 per cent), other precipitating factors include myocardial infarctions, cerebrovascular accidents, and trauma. In all these conditions there is an increase in circulating glucagon and cortisol, and/or catecholamines (Alberti & Nattrass, 1978, p. 800).

Why Does the Patient Have GI Symptoms?

Nausea, vomiting, gastric stasis, ileus, and abdominal pain may be present in severe ketoacidosis. There is no clear reason for this. Some authorities attribute it to potassium and magnesium deficiency (Alberti & Nattrass, 1978, p. 801). In the process of ruling out intercurrent infections, it may be necessary to consider an acute abdomen.

Why Wasn't Mrs. J's Temperature Elevated?

Mrs. J's temperature of 96°F and a white count of 29,300 seem to be incompatible. Mild hypothermia or inappropriate normothermia appear to be the rule in diabetic ketoacidosis. This finding is attributed to the peripheral vasodilation of the acidemia (Alberti & Nattrass, 1978, p. 801). The leukocytosis correlates with the degree of ketosis not with the infection. This is found whether there is an infection present or not. The two major signs of infection, fever and high white count, are not helpful in ruling out an intercurrent infection.

Sequelae of Insulin Deficiency

The chain of events resulting in the state of diabetic ketoacidosis are illustrated in Figure 47-5. To summarize: insulin deficiency → hyperglycemia → fatty acid mobilization → ketone body accumulation → deficits in water and electrolytes.

Goal in the Treatment of Diabetic Ketoacidosis

The goal of the health team is to reestablish carbohydrate tolerance as evidenced by the absence of the signs and symptoms of diabetic acidosis. The members of the health team work collaboratively to achieve this goal. The response of the patient to therapy and often whether or not he or she recovers depend on the promptness with which therapy is initiated. Depending on the situation, the nurse may be called on to prepare, administer, and supervise the therapeutic regimen prescribed by the physician. In addition, the nurse is responsible for observing the patient and his or her reaction to therapy. The nurse may be required to modify the therapy in relation to its effects on the patient and report to the physician only when the patient fails to respond in the desired manner to the prescribed therapeutic regimen.

Re-establishment of Carbohydrate Tolerance

Efforts to correct the carbohydrate metabolism and to restore fluid and electrolyte balance are carried out simultaneously. Imbalance in one affects the other, and one cannot be corrected without correcting the other. However, to facilitate discussion they will be presented separately. Details of the fluid replacement and insulin therapy were not stipulated in this case presentation because every patient is an individual, and the details of the treatment required by each patient will differ. In addition, the treatment modalities will depend on individual physician preference, the degree and duration of coma, and the surface area of the patient. It was felt it would be more beneficial to the reader if general guidelines for controlling the insulin dosage and fluid replacement were presented.

Restoration of Carbohydrate Metabolism

The carbohydrate metabolism is restored by providing Mrs. Joyce with a supply of rapid-acting unmodified insulin. Some authorities recommend insulin dosages ranging from 20 to 100 units. Others suggest the initial dose should be one tenth of the blood glucose level, one half administered intravenously and one half subcutaneously. For example, Mrs. Joyce's blood glucose was 870 mg. Therefore she would receive 45 units intravenously and 45 units subcutaneously. Other authorities suggest the following for the initial insulin therapy: if the blood sugar is less than 600 mg and the patient is in coma, give 80 to 100 units; if the patient is not in coma, give 25 to 50 units. If the blood sugar is over 1,000 mg, 320 to 400 units may be ordered. Mrs. Joyce was not in coma and she received 25 units intravenously and 25 units intramuscularly.

Following the initial insulin dose, the insulin requirements are guided by hourly or bihourly blood glucose levels. When the blood glucose is 300 mg or less, the insulin requirements are determined by the results of serial urine glucose and acetone tests. The physician will order a certain quantity of unmodified insulin based on the number of pluses found in the urine for glucose and additional amounts if ketone bodies are present. A typical order might be: Give 5 units of unmodified insulin for each plus in the urine for glucose and if the urine is moderately or mildly positive for acetone. If the urine acetone is strongly positive, give 10 units for each plus in the urine glucose. Insulin orders for children are approximately one half those for adults. The mortality rates for severe diabetic ketoacidosis range from 5 to 15 per cent in specialized centers to 20 to 30 per cent in less specialized centers. In the elderly, the mortality rate may be 50 per cent or more. Alberti & Nattrass, 1978, p. 199).

There has been a trend since 1973 toward low-dose insulin regimens. These regimens involve continuous intravenous (4 to 6 units per hour) insulin and/or intermittent intramuscular administration of small doses of insulin. A bolus of intravenous insulin will probably disappear from the circulation in approximately 40 minutes. The continuous intravenous infusion provides for maintenance of circulating insulin levels.

In addition to insulin therapy, Mrs. Joyce was placed on bedrest as soon as she was admitted. Reduction in activity reduces metabolism and thereby decreases the catabolism of fat and protein.

Disruption of the Fluid, Electrolyte, and Acid–Base Balance

Mrs. Joyce lost water by three avenues: hyperventilation, vomiting, and urination. Within limits the kidney can compensate for the loss of water by other routes by concentrating urine.

Two factors prevented Mrs. Joyce's kidney from conserving water. Her renal threshold for sugar was exceeded, so that water was excreted passively due to increased osmolality of the glomerular filtrate. Second, the kidney plays an important role in the maintenance of acid–base balance by conserving or eliminating excess anions or cations. Elimination of either anions or cations requires water. In acidosis, cations are required to excrete the anions of the ketoacids. The mechanisms by which the kidney conserves cations, other than the hydrogen ions, also fail. (See Chapter 41). Acidosis therefore contributes to the depletion of water and electrolytes. With the loss of water the hematocrit increases and the blood volume decreases. These changes, if severe and continued, predispose to failure of the cardiovascular system.

To accommodate the increase in anions of the ketoacids, the concentration of bicarbonate anions is lowered by hyperventilation (Kussmaul breathing; see Chapter 41), and sodium cations are made available to maintain electroneutrality. One result is a reduction in the carbon dioxide content as well as in the carbon dioxide—combining power of the blood plasma. The latter is the result of the sodium ion being unavailable to combine with the bicarbonate ion. On admission the carbon dioxide content of Mrs. Joyce's blood has been lowered to 5.0 mEq per liter. The normal range is from 21 to 30 mEq per liter.

Restoration of the Fluid, Electrolyte, and Acid–Base Balance

Initially intravenous isotonic saline (1,000 ml) is started. The rate of administration should depend on the patient's cardiovascular status (previous myocardial infarctions, congestive heart failure, and so on) and current level of tissue perfusion. If the patient's CO_2-combining power is less than 10 mEq per liter or the blood ph is below 7, solutions containing sodium bicarbonate are administered to correct the base deficit. The quantity of fluids given may vary from 2,000 to 5,000 ml in a 24-hour period.

When the patient's serum glucose levels start to decrease, glucose solutions are started. This may seem contradictory to give glucose when levels are above normal. However, the patient must be provided with a readily available source of carbohydrate as the glycogen storage has been depleted.

Electrolyte deficits are identified by laboratory tests and EKG findings, and replacements are ordered accordingly. The patient should be closely observed for signs of electrolyte deficiency. For example, hypokalemia is likely to occur approximately 4 to 6 hours after initiation of treatment. Potassium may be added to the fluids if the urine output is greater than 50 ml per hour.

If the patient is vomiting following admission, gastric intubation and lavage may be ordered to guard against aspiration pneumonia. Oral intake may be resumed, if other indicators show it would be safe after approximately 6 to 12 hours. Indicators for resumption of oral intake are cessation of overbreathing and an acceptable state of consciousness. The diet progresses from clear liquids to a full diet.

Some of the Special Dangers Associated with the Insulin and Fluid Therapy

The ketoacidotic patient is in a most precarious situation and the assessment and monitoring of the patient's response to the therapeutic interventions are imperative. In addition to those already discussed, some other dangers will be cited.

Insulin resistance usually accompanies acidosis and is probably a contributing factor to its development. As the acidosis is corrected, the patient becomes less resistant to insulin and the patient is predisposed to hypoglycemia. This is most likely to occur 12 to 24 hours after initiation of therapy. About 20 per cent of the patients will develop this, and if not corrected it may cause death.

Any patient who receives a large volume of fluid by intravenous infusion should be carefully observed. Patients may be anuric at the time of admission or may develop anuria later. Observation of the urine output, including quantity and frequency of voiding, is highly important. As hypovolemia is corrected, urine output should increase. In general, the capacity of the patient to tolerate a large volume of fluid depends on the severity of the hypovolemia, the general health status, and adequacy of the cardiovascular and renal systems. Any patient receiving a large volume of fluid should have the rate of infusion and its general effects closely observed. Depending on the circumstances and available facilities, the patients central venous pressure may be monitored.

A complication that develops infrequently, but is disastrous when it does, is cerebral edema or spinal fluid acidosis. They respond to insulin and fluids with a drop in blood glucose, and then relapse without evidence of recurring acidosis. The pathogenesis of this syndrome is not understood. It is believed to be the result of too-rapid lowering of the blood sugar with a shift of water into the brain or the result of rapid and excessive administration of sodium bicarbonate solutions, along with insufficient potassium. This complication is treated by infusions of 0.20 per cent mannitol and dexamethasone (Shuman, 1976; Winegrad & Clements, 1971).

Consequences of the Patients Failure to Respond to the Insulin and Fluid Therapy

Eventually, if the acidosis continues, the cardiovascular system fails. The pulse becomes weak and thready, and the blood pressure falls; anuria develops, and the patient dies. When adequate therapy is instituted early enough, recovery is the rule (see Figure 47-4).

Other Factors to Consider in Providing Care for the Patient in Ketoacidosis

Although all persons who care for the patient have a responsibility for the safety of the patient, much of the burden for his or her protection falls on the nurse. During the period when the patient is less than normally responsive, he or she must be protected from falling and from the effects of pressure. It is essential that the patient be under intelligent and continuous observation. Mrs. Joyce was less alert than usual, but she was not stuporous. Drowsiness followed by stupor, coma, and death can be expected unless the acidosis is corrected. Until the patient is fully recovered, he or she should not be held responsible for his or her own safety. Side rails should be kept raised on the bed. Insofar as possible, patients should be moved and turned regularly unless they are so restless that this is unnecessary. Some patients in acidosis are restless and thrash. When the patient is restless precautions must be taken to prevent falling or injury from unprotected side rails. Protection from overheating and chilling must be provided. Extra heat should not be applied to patients in a state of shock as heat increases vasodilatation and intensifies the failure of the circulation.

Because the recovery of the patient depends on the restoration of homeostasis, the related factors have been emphasized. Although physiological homeostasis is given priority, this does not mean that the patient as a human being should be neglected. Care should be taken to avoid making unwarranted statements or talking about other patients in the presence of the patient. Conversation should include the patient but should not make unnecessary demands on him or her. The patient should be addressed by name, be informed about the care being given, and the progress being made. Attention should be paid to physical comfort. Until the survival of the patient is assured, attention is, however, directed toward three principal objectives: to restore normal carbohydrate metabolism as promptly as possible, to replace the water and electrolyte balance, and to protect the patient from injury. If the recovery of the patient is to be ensured, time is of the essence. Consequently, when a patient is admitted, therapy should be started promptly.

During the acute phase the nurse will need to address the psychological needs of the family members. It is essential that they be kept informed regarding the treatment plan and the patient's progress, and the nurse must be sure this is carried out.

The treatment plan for the patient in diabetic ketoacidosis has been identified and presented. The collaborative efforts of the health team are essential to ensure the patient's recovery. It is obvious that careful monitoring of the therapy is a key ingredient. Drug and fluid and electrolyte administration is guided by laboratory data. A diabetic flow sheet is recommended for every patient. Such data need to be readily available and will facilitate patient care.

Patient Problem No. 3 Noncompliance with Therapeutic Regimen

The plan for this problem was to (1) identify the etiology of noncompliance and (2) develop a specific plan to increase compliance. This problem is not easy to resolve. It will require careful assessment and will obviously be individualized. Mrs. Joyce's son reported on her admission that she had not taken insulin for 4 days because "she had run out of needles." Why had a diabetic of 14 years permitted this to happen? Was it financial problems? No resources for getting to a store? The nurse explored this with Mrs. J. The patient said she had told her son this, but the real reason was a friend had been able to stop taking insulin and was getting along fine. So Mrs. J. decided if her friend could do it she could, too. The nurse was able to ascertain that the friend was obese and had been able to stop taking insulin when her weight was within normal limits. From this assessment the nurse developed a teaching plan to help Mrs. Joyce, a juvenile-type diabetic, to understand why this would not work for her. The nurse also identified that Mrs. Joyce had limited knowledge of appropriate actions to take when she had diarrhea or vomiting or any indications of an infection. The teaching plan included measures to correct this. Mrs. Joyce's family was included in the teaching program. Along with the patient, they developed a plan for closer supervision of Mrs. Joyce. Hopefully, there will be no recurrence.

The factors that contribute to noncompliance can be identified in the assessment process, and obviously the plan will be dependent on the etiology. If the reason is inadequate finances, then the plan will need to involve measures to resolve the problem, including the assistance of a social worker.

Case Summary

By the evening of the day Mrs. Joyce was admitted to the hospital, her hypovolemia had been corrected. Although several days elapsed before her blood glucose became relatively stable, ketonemia had been largely corrected. She was able to eat the food prescribed for her. Following the correction of the DKA, the abdominal pain subsided. However, gallbladder studies were done and they were negative. No infection was identified. Mrs. Joyce was hospitalized for 6 days and was discharged from the hospital on lente insulin 25 units daily and 2,000 kcal ADA diet. She was scheduled to return to the outpatient department in 2 weeks.

Chronic Complications of Diabetes: The Diabetic Syndrome

Several abnormalities occur with such frequency in diabetes mellitus that some authorities refer to them as concomitants of the disease, that is, they are part of the disease. Major concomitants are large-vessel disease and small-vessel disease. Manifestations of these concomitants are evident in the eyes, mouth, nervous system, vascular system, skin, and kidneys. As they occur so frequently, the nurse must be alert for evidence of their presence whenever assessing and/or caring for a diabetic patient. In addition, knowledge of the concomitants and the measures to prevent or retard them is basic in any educational program for the diabetic.

Vascular Lesions: Diabetic Microangiopathy

The vascular lesion believed to be characteristic of diabetes is an abnormality of the capillary basement membrane. Some believe that it results from an inherited trait directly or indirectly related to the diabetic gene. This disorder is not a complication, but a part of the disease. It probably affects in varying degrees the capillary beds throughout the body, as it has been reported in many different types of tissues. Some go so far as to say that small vessel disease initiates diabetes mellitus. Others relate the disorder to the length of time an individual has been diabetic. In one study less than one third of insulin-dependent diabetics who had been diabetic 4 years or less had significant thickening of the basement membrane, whereas it was present in 100 per cent of those who had the disease for 20 years or more (Williamson et al., 1971; Oakley et al., 1978). The angiopathy is known to be universally distributed in the body. Retinopathy, nephropathy, and possibly the neuropathy occurring in diabetes are associated with a thickening of the capillary basement membrane.

Large-Vessel Disease

Atherosclerosis occurs in the diabetic at an earlier age than it does in the nondiabetic. The hyperlipemia and hypercholesterolemia that accompany diabetes may be predisposing factors. Among the arteries particularly prone to atherosclerosis are those supplying the brain, heart, lower extremities, and kidneys. Recent studies implicate diabetes mellitus as a factor in early coronary artery disease. About 20 per cent of all patients with coronary heart disease have associated hyperglycemia. Twenty-five per cent of known diabetics are under treatment for heart disease (*Report of National Commission on Diabetes,* 1975, p. 35).

With the increase in the life expectancy of patients with diabetes mellitus, chronic disorders involving the vascular and nervous systems and the kidney have become increasingly important. Studies indicate that a high percentage of persons who develop diabetes in childhood and live into adult life develop vascular concomitants.

Vascular concomitants also are frequent among persons who are middle-aged or older at the time of onset. They occur earlier and to a more severe degree in diabetics than in nondiabetics. They are more rapidly progressive in young persons who have long-standing diabetes that has been inadequately treated. More than 50 per cent of the deaths in patients who have had diabetes for more than 15 years are caused by vascular lesions. All types of arteriosclerosis occur alone or in combination. The arteries most commonly involved are those supplying the lower extremities, the heart muscle (coronary arteries), the brain, the eye, and the kidney.

Vascular disorders are important because they have a high incidence among persons with diabetes. After they are established, they tend to be progressive. They differ from acute complications as they do not cause the diabetes to become more severe. Authorities do not agree about the value of maintaining the level of blood glucose within physiologic limits in preventing vascular lesions. Some authorities are questioning whether the present criteria for diabetic control are adequate. The suggestion has been made that periods of *mild* hypoglycemia might be of benefit to the patient.

Renal Complications

Complications involving the kidney are very common among persons with long-standing diabetes mellitus. Renal complications include those resulting from nephrosclerosis, intercapillary glomerulosclerosis, and pyelonephritis. All these conditions can and do occur in nondiabetics. They are, however, likely to be more severe and more rapidly progressive in diabetics than in nondiabetics. When they are progressive, they lead to a loss of renal function and with it to azotemia (the accumulation of the waste of protein metabolism in the blood).

Of the renal disorders the one that is most common in diabetes mellitus is pyelonephritis, but the one that is the most characteristic is intercapillary glomerulosclerosis or Kimmelstiel-Wilson's disease. This disorder is frequent and its incidence is rising. Although its diagnosis requires renal biopsy, it is presumed to be present when edema, hypertension, azotemia, and proteinuria are present. In the diabetic other pathology frequently associated with intercapillary sclerosis is diabetic retinopathy and anemia. Although intercapillary sclerosis may remain stable for long periods of time, after severe edema and albuminuria occur the life expectancy of the patient can be measured only in months. Kidney failure is now the cause for about half the deaths in long-term juvenile diabetes and about 6 per cent of the deaths in the older, stable, diabetic (*Diabetes Data,* 1978).

Neuropathies

The neuropathies of chronic diabetic syndrome can affect any or all of the peripheral pathways, motor or sensory, somatic or automatic. Common manifestations are leg pains, muscle weakness, alterations in gastrointestinal mobility, neurogenic bladder (difficulty in emptying due to poor muscle tone), impotence, and postural hypotension. A common sign found on physical examination is absence of ankle jerk reflex. Patients with peripheral neuritis often suffer numbness, tingling, and pain that is sometimes very severe.

Frequency rates on neuropathy are extremely variable because of lack of consistent measurements among investigators. The signs and symptoms are usually intermittent, may vary in intensity, and increase, diminish, or vanish. They occur in relation to uncontrolled diabetes or may be the presenting symptom preceding diagnosis (Bonar, 1977, p. 225).

Peripheral Vascular Disease

The neuropathies plus the angiopathy account for the high incidence of peripheral vascular disease in the diabetic. The principal clinical manifestations are ischemic lesions of the foot and intermittent claudication. The protective mechanism of sensation is diminished or lost and the individual has decreased perceptual ability for superficial or deep pain. In addition, there is loss of temperature sensation. This makes the diabetic a prime candidate for painless trauma of the lower extremities. The trauma may result from mechanical, chemical, or thermal injury. The pathogenesis of diabetic foot lesions is displayed in Figure 47-6.

Eye Complications

Complications arising from the effects of diabetes on the various structures of the eyes are risks faced by the diabetic. Blindness is twenty-five times more common in diabetics than in nondiabetics, and approximately 5,000 diabetics become blind each year (*Diabetes Data,* 1978). Diabetes is the most important known systemic condition causing blindness.

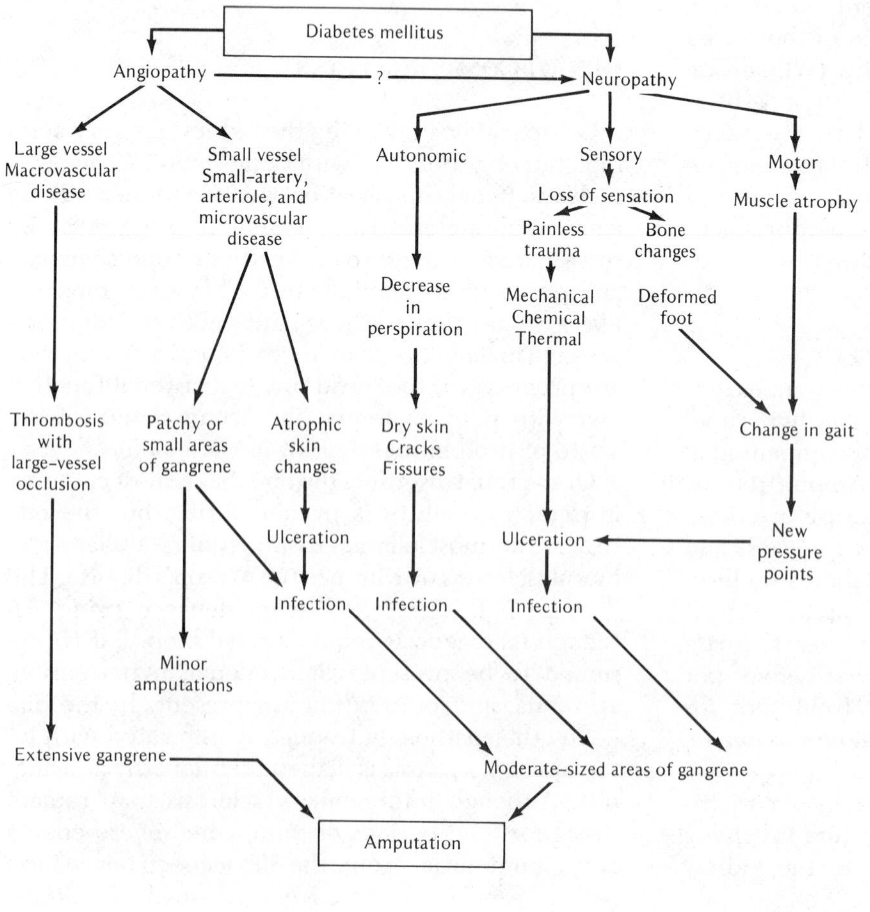

Figure 47-6. Pathogenesis of diabetic foot lesions. (From Levin, Marvin E.: Medical evaluation and treatment. In Levin, Marvin E., and O'Neal, Lawrence W., editors: *The Diabetic Foot,* 2nd ed., St. Louis, 1977, The C. V. Mosby Co.)

Ophthalmalogical disorders can include refractory errors, cataracts, glaucoma, and, the most serious, retinopathy. The macro- and microangiopathies, osmotic variations with resultant edema, excessive sorbitol formations, hemorrhages, and exudates contribute to the eye complications of the diabetic and can lead to blindness. Methods of treatment for severe diabetic retinopathy are laser photocoagulation and pituitary ablation.

Although the type of cataract occurring most frequently in diabetic patients does not differ from the ordinary senile cataract, it does occur somewhat more frequently among diabetics than among nondiabetics. The problems of the patient are those of any individual who is losing or threatened with loss of vision. Yearly ophthalmologic examinations are a must for the diabetic patient. A number of therapies have been demonstrated to retard the rate of vision loss, and regular periodic assessment will help to identify patients in early stages of complications. Some refractive changes in the diabetic are temporary, and with control of the disease there will be improvement. Therefore it is recommended that changes in eyeglass prescriptions be delayed until an appropriate treatment regimen has been implemented.

Infection

Despite the frequency with which the onset of diabetes is coincident with an infection, infection is believed to act as a precipitating rather than an etiological factor. In other words, infection acts as a nonspecific stress. The changes that occur during the infection serve to intensify the disorder so that the clinical manifestations become evident. Changes increasing the insulin requirement, during infection, include an increase in the secretion of adrenocortical steroids and an increase in the rate of metabolism as a result of fever. Fever also predisposes to dehydration and acidosis, which also tends to aggravate the diabetic state.

The poorly controlled diabetic is more threatened by infections than is the nondiabetic. The host mechanisms of the diabetic may be altered. For example, the vascular insufficiency that may accompany diabetes can result in decreased blood flow to the affected tissues. This can lead to retardation of granulocyte mobilization and adverse effects on phagocytic function. In addition there may be proliferation of anaerobic organisms because of the decrease in oxygen tension of poorly perfused tissues (Ellenberg & Rifkin, 1970, pp. 735–38).

Moniliasis, a Candida infection, can occur as a vaginitis or vulvovaginitis. This results in a pruritus vulvae and has been correlated with glycosuria.

Diabetics appear to have increased susceptibility to tuberculosis. For this reason it is imperative that baseline and annual skin testing measures should be instituted for all diabetics. The consequences of infection in the diabetic patient *cannot* be underestimated. Infection has an adverse effect on diabetes mellitus, and diabetes mellitus increases the difficulty of curing certain types of infections.

Among the infections of the skin are furuncles (boils) and carbuncles (multiple boils adjacent to each other). In health, the skin serves as a storehouse for glycogen. In uncontrolled diabetes, the glycogen in the skin is depleted and the glucose content of the skin rises with the hyperglycemia. When diabetes is poorly controlled, the skin is predisposed to infections by the *Staphylococcus aureus.* There is also evidence that function of the polymorphonuclear leukocytes is impaired. Two requirements, that is, control of diabetes and cleanliness of the skin and clothing, are important to the prevention of skin complications. The diabetic with dry skin appears to be more susceptible to skin infections.

Urinary tract infections are observed in the diabetic. Increased frequency of catheterization, nephropathy, and neurogenic bladder have been identified as predisposing factors.

Infections of the lower extremity account for a large number of infections requiring hospitalization.

Summary

This section has presented the chronic complications of diabetes mellitus. The complications can develop in almost every organ of the body. Their increasing incidence is related to the fact that diabetics as well as nondiabetics have an improved life expectancy. All these disorders occur earlier and are more rapidly progressive in the diabetic than in the nondiabetic. The nurse must be alert to them and assess and monitor the diabetic patient for them.

Onset, Diagnosis, and Clinical Manifestations

Comparison of the Onset in the Adult and Child

In the young, the onset of diabetes mellitus is likely to be rapid and acute, whereas in the middle-aged, obese adult, it is often slow. Among the latter, diabetes may be present for some time before the individual becomes aware of its manifestations. One estimate is that the middle-aged, obese adult is diabetic for about as many years before the disease is discovered as he or she survives after the diagnosis is made. Often, though not invariably, onset is precipitated by some physical or emotional stress.

Diagnosis frequently follows the discovery of glucose in the urine on a routine physical examination, or in association with an infection, or after a person seeks medical attention for the diagnosis and treatment of a related or unrelated disorder.

Diagnosis of Diabetes Mellitus

Diabetes mellitus is diagnosed by the presence of its clinical manifestations, presence of glycosuria, and hyperglycemia.

Clinical Manifestations

The classical triad of diabetes is polyuria, polydipsia, and polyphagia (increased urine output, increased thirst, and increased appetite). Additional related signs include undue fatigue, weight loss, dryness of the mouth, sensory disturbances of the lower extremities, blurred vision, impotence in the male, and menstrual irregularity and pruritus vulvae in the female.

Testing

The finding of glucose in the urine is presumptive but not conclusive evidence that a person has diabetes mellitus as glycosuria can be present in a person who is nondiabetic. Glycosuria occurring after the excessive ingestion of carbohydrates is known as alimentary glycosuria. The person who has this form of glycosuria may well be prediabetic. Glycosuria also occurs in persons who have a low renal threshold for glucose. The most frequent cause, however, is diabetes mellitus.

The point at which sugar will start to spill into the urine is called the renal threshold. Sugar will start to spill into the urine when the blood glucose exceeds 160 mg. If there is a high renal threshold, quite common in the elderly diabetic, glucose may not start to spill until the blood sugar level is 250 mg (Ellenberg & Rifkin, 1970, p. 487).

Substances for testing for glycosuria fall into two major categories. In the first group are the copper reduction tests: Clinitest and Benedict tests. The presence of reducing substances in the urine (melituria) can also be associated with lactation (lactose lactosuria) and rare "metabolic errors" (pentosuria, fructosuria, and so on). The reduction tests will give a false-positive reaction for glucose in the preceding conditions. In the second group are the specific enzyme glucose-oxidase tests, Testape and Clinistix. Clinistix will indicate only the presence or absence of glucose, whereas Testape will estimate the actual amount. Because they test only for glucose and are more convenient, they are the preferred tests. The nurse should compare the corresponding readings of Clinitest and Testape. The corresponding readings for 1+ through 3+ indicate different concentrations of glucose. For example a 1+ Testape finding represents a 0.1 per cent glucose concentration and a 1+ Clinitest represents a 0.5 per cent glucose concentration. Whatever test is used, the directions must be carefully followed. A false-negative reaction can be obtained if the Testape is dropped in the urine and not exposed to the air. Certain drugs will inhibit the glucose-oxidase tests and give false-negative readings. A common offender is ascorbic acid in dosages of 300 to 1,000 mg. (Ascorbic acid is frequently used as a buffering agent for many of the antibiotics.) One other comment must be made about the enzyme tests. They are sometimes difficult to read because of the poor color differentiation in the 3+ to 4+ range. For the diabetic with visual difficulties it may be almost impossible.

Not only is urine testing for glucose helpful in case finding, but it is also used as a guide in patient management. Therefore the nurse must assume responsibility for patient education in this area.

Blood Tests for Hyperglycemia

Confirmation of hyperglycemia can be ascertained by a variety of applications of the blood glucose test. A fasting hyperglycemia at or above 125 mg or a postprandial hyperglycemia over 160 mg are usually pathognomonic without any further testing. If the blood glucose levels fall below those levels, and diabetes mellitus is suspected, further study is indicated. Oral or intravenous glucose tolerance tests can be used to confirm the diagnosis. Specific details of these tests are discussed in Chapter 46.

Role of the Nurse in Prevention and Diagnosis

Nurses have numerous opportunities to assist in the identification of persons who either have diabetes or are potential diabetics. Review of the etiologic factors gives the nurse clues as to the target populations. In addition she or he, regardless of the field of practice, must always be alert to the signs and symptoms of diabetes. Any individual with symptoms suggesting diabetes mellitus should be encouraged to seek medical attention.

The suspicion of the school nurse should be aroused when a child develops polyuria and polydipsia. The public health nurse who visits in the home should be alert to the possibility of diabetes in family members. Recently a visiting nurse who was making a call to a mother with a new baby inquired about other members of the family. She learned that 5-year-old Suzie was unusually irritable, that she was constantly "passing water," and that she drank large amounts of water and was constantly hungry. The nurse obtained and tested a sample of urine. When she found that it was highly positive for glucose and acetone, she informed the mother that the child should see a physician as soon as possible. An appointment was made with the family physician, who examined Suzie and confirmed the fact that she had diabetes mellitus.

Some patients are discovered to have diabetes after they are admitted to the hospital. Most hospitals have a rule that before a patient can undergo any type of surgical procedure, the urine must be checked for glucose. In two instances known to the author, a nurse noted on the morning of surgery that the urine of a patient had not been checked for sugar. When the urine was tested, it was found to contain glucose. In both instances surgery was delayed until the patient's diabetes was brought under control.

The nurse can also assist in community screening programs. These programs are usually sponsored by the American Diabetes Association through its local branches and the county medical society. Each fall these groups sponsor a Diabetic Detection Week. During the week materials are made available through local pharmacies so that individuals can test their urine for glucose. An educational program is carried on at the same time to encourage individuals to avail themselves of this opportunity. The program is publicized by the various communication media. Persons found to have glycosuria are referred to their physicians for diagnosis and, if needed, treatment.

In addition to opportunities for the nurse to participate in programs for the identification of persons who have diabetes mellitus, nurses have a role in the prevention of the disease. Because of the frequency with which diabetes in the middle-aged person is associated with obesity, individuals are encouraged to avoid overweight by diet and exercise. The preventive aspects related to genetic counseling are less clear. Persons with diabetes or persons with families in which there is a known history of diabetes should be acquainted with the risks involved when planning marriage.

Psychological Aspects

Fink (1967) has proposed a model of the processes of adaptation to stressful situations. He proposes that psychological phases follow a sequential pattern as follows:

Stage 1. Shock; in this phase the person's cognitive structure is characterized by disorganization. There is inability to plan or to reason.
Stage 2. Defensive retreat, characterized by denial.
Stage 3. Acknowledgment, giving up the past, and starting to face reality.
Stage 4. Adaptation, acceptance of the modification in health. Planning to care for self and to prevent complications.

When a person learns that he or she has diabetes mellitus, even when its presence was suspected, he or she experiences disbelief and then grief. The sequence described by Fink can be observed. The progression through the sequential phases varies with each individual. Unfortunately some patients never progress to the fourth stage. The degree of shock will depend on the individual and what the diagnosis and treatment mean to him or her. Any preexisting problem can be expected to be intensified. The patient and family can be expected to react to knowledge of the diagnosis as they do to other crisis situations in life. Authorities frequently emphasize the advantages of diabetes over other chronic disorders. In time the patient may come to a similar conclusion, but at the time the diagnosis is established he or she is thinking of what has been lost and not of other more serious possibilities. The patient compares diabetes with health and prefers health. The nurse can usually be of more help to the patient if she or he can help in identifying and expressing feelings rather than telling the patient how lucky he or she is.

At the time the patient learns that diabetes is incurable, he or she should learn that it is controllable. Whether or not it is kept under control depends to a large extent on the patient and family. In the past, physicians have tended to assume the primary responsibility for the regulation of diabetes. The trend is toward placing the responsibility for control on the patient and family. Physicians and nurses are available and willing to help the patient assume this responsibility. Furthermore, the measures that are required are for his or her well-being. The patient learns to control the disease because this is the way to good health. He or she does not take insulin or other medication and regulate food intake to please the physician or the nurse or someone else but to promote health. The basic treatment in diabetes is done by the patient and it is done every day. The control of diabetes mellitus is a way of life, but it should not be all of life.

When diabetes is diagnosed in a young child, the parents are the ones who experience the negative feelings. Their child is less than perfect. If the disease is to be controlled, the child must have special care and attention. Questions arise. Will other children in the family develop the disease? Is the fact that the child is ill the result of something the parent did or did not do? Try, however, to imagine the feelings of an 8-year-old boy or a 13-year-old girl who learns that he or she has diabetes. Are they likely to be consoled by the fact that they do not have leukemia? When diabetes is diagnosed in the middle-aged, they may be well aware of the complications. They resent the fact that they may have to alter their life style. For the elderly, it may be viewed as the end of their independence.

In addition to the fact of diabetes itself, negative emotions are usually engendered by the measures required in treatment. Although children of 5 or younger learn to inject their own insulin, older adults find this procedure particularly frightening. Men and women who are employed may be concerned about whether they will be able to continue in their current jobs. Those who are not yet gainfully employed face the possibility that diabetes will limit their choice of vocation as well as their chances of getting and holding a position. Will others know and if they do will the diabetic be accepted? Will he or she be able to do what friends do? Will he or she be able to marry and to have children? Boys who have dreamed of being athletes find their ambitions threatened. Restrictions real and imagined are likely to appear to be insurmountable to the patient and to the family as well.

A danger common to any patient with a disease requiring long-term therapy is that when feeling well the person decides that he or she is cured and discontinues the regimen. Or when the person finally realizes that he or she is not going to get well in the usual interpretation of the term, he or she may decide to try some quick cure such as a special food or a cure-all. The person may also deny having diabetes or that anything can be done to change its course. Deviations from the prescribed regimen will result in a loss of, at best, the control of the diabetes mellitus and, at worst, life. The diabetic does not move smoothly through the four stages described by Fink. He or she may have progressed to stage 4 and slip back to stage 2. Mrs. Joyce, a diabetic of 14 years, is an example of this.

Although much has been accomplished to reduce the cost of insulin, diet, and medical supervision, diabetes mellitus does place an economic burden on families whose incomes are limited. For this reason, patients with diabetes mellitus may be declared medically indigent at a higher level of income than nondiabetics. Enough problems have been raised to suggest that the psychosocial problems arising in relation to a diagnosis of diabetes mellitus are many and highly individualized.

During the period immediately following diagnosis the patient and family require psychological support. This should start with the patient's admission to the office of the physician, to the clinic, or to the hospital. The type and amount of support will vary with each individual. Both the patient and family have a right to expect professional personnel to try to understand their feelings and to accept their behavior as having meaning. An important objective in the care of the patient should be to provide a climate in which he or she feels accepted and therefore free to express feelings and be supported in the attempts to accept the diagnosis and what it entails. The nurse should try to convey to the patient that, while understanding or trying to understand his or her feelings, the patient will be able to learn to do what must be done and will be provided with the necessary assistance.

A second period of stress for the patient occurs at the awareness of the fact that he or she is developing one or more of the chronic manifestations of diabetes.

A patient recently cared for by this writer had been a diabetic for over 30 years. She, despite careful compliance with prescribed therapy, had developed numerous diabetic complications. She had had surgery for cataracts, bilateral transmetatarsal amputations, hypophysectomy for diabetic retinopathy. In addition she had a neurogenic bladder. She reported, "It wasn't too bad when I was younger, but now I can see myself dying by parts."

Control of Diabetes Mellitus

Successful management of diabetes mellitus depends on the intelligent cooperation of the patient and family. Unlike recovery from an acute infectious disease, recovery from diabetes does not follow a period of acute illness. Diabetes mellitus is permanent. Remissions can and do occur, but even these patients should not think of themselves as cured.

The days and weeks that immediately follow the diagnosis of diabetes mellitus are important in the life of the patient. During this time the patient learns what it means to be diabetic and how the disease can be managed. The general objectives of therapy include (1) to individualize the regimen so that the patient can live as full and useful a life as is possible within the limitations of the disorder, (2) to correct the underlying metabolic abnormalities in order to restore homeostasis, (3) to attain and maintain ideal body weight, (4) to delay the progression of chronic complications, and (5) to prevent acute complications of the disease. Diabetes is not easily controlled. Its management requires a knowledgeable patient and knowledgeable health personnel.

The fundamental methods used in the treatment are diet, insulin or hypoglycemic agents, exercise, and education. The continued management and control of diabetes mellitus depend on the patient. Education as to the nature and behavior of the disease is required so that the patient understands the reasons for what he or she must do and develops the skills required for it.

Diet

The keystone for management of the diabetic is dietary control. In most respects the goals of the diet for the diabetic patient are similar to those for the nondiabetic. They are to provide

1. Sufficient calories to establish and maintain body weight. The number will vary with the age, sex, body size, activity, and growth and development requirements.
2. An adequate intake of all nutrients, including minerals and vitamins.
3. Modifications in amounts and types of foods as required in the control of complications of diabetes and other diseases.
4. Meal spacing so that absorption coincides with peak levels of insulin in the blood and protects from hypoglycemia during the night. For patients on intermediate-acting insulin, food is usually distributed in five meals—three main meals with a small meal about 4 P.M. and another at bedtime. For the patient who is taking insulin, it is essential that a regular meal schedule be observed.
5. Integration of exercise and diet with medications.

Most diabetic diets contain 50 to 60 per cent carbohydrates with 10 to 15 per cent in the form of disaccharides and monosaccharides. Fats should comprise no more than 35 per cent of the total calories. The remaining calories are protein (Arky, 1978, p. 658). Patients are encouraged to select unsaturated fats as recommended by the American Heart Association. Concentrated sweets and refined sugars should be avoided.

In the preinsulin era the only therapy available was restriction of the carbohydrate intake. The present trend is toward more liberalization of the diet. The chance of developing diabetes mellitus doubles for every 20 per cent of excessive weight. Correction of obesity by simple caloric restriction is one of the most effective measures for control of the noninsulin-dependent diabetic.

An advantage of metabolic control of diabetes is that the ideal weight is more likely to be maintained and less insulin is required. In the achievement of the objective to plan the diet in terms of the individual pattern of living of the patient, the nurse, wherever employed, is in a particularly advantageous position to be helpful. The nurse should obtain information about the economic status of the patient, what foods are available as well as their cost, his or her religion, national origin, social status, occupation, idiosyncrasies, misconceptions and beliefs about food, facilities for preparing food, and where and with whom he or she eats. Unless the family diet is inadequate, the family food pattern is used as a base. One of the objectives is to disrupt the family as little as possible. The diet of the patient is kept as nearly like the rest of the family's as possible. The visiting nurse can often be of great service to the person who prepares the meals for the person with diabetes. For the most part special foods are not required. Water-packed canned fruits and vegetables are now available at most grocery stores. They can be substituted for fresh fruits and vegetables when these are not available or are expensive. Frozen vegetables are available in variety. Patients should be taught to read labels of canned or frozen food products to identify if they are packed with sugar. If they are, the contents can be rinsed with water.

The patient and the person who prepares the meals should learn to identify the carbohydrate, protein, and fat content of foods. They should know why the carbohydrate content is restricted. When a patient is in ketosis, the carbohydrate content may be restricted to 100 g per day.

Whether patients are taught to weigh, measure, or approximate the size of servings depends on the patient. Patients may be more comfortable when they weigh their food, whereas others may reject the idea entirely. The patient and the person who prepares the food should be well acquainted with food exchange lists and know how to use them.

The physician makes the decision as to the number of calories and distribution of carbohydrate, protein, and fat in the patient's diet. This prescription is translated by the dietitian into terms of food and methods of preparation. The usual method is to use diabetic exchange lists. These exchange lists categorize foods into groups as follows:

List 1. Milk exchanges—contains 12 g carbohydrate, 8 g protein, and trace fat. Calories 80.
List 2. Vegetables—Contains 5 g carbohydrate and 2 g protein. Calories 25.
List 3. Fruit—Contains 10 g carbohydrate. Calories 40.
List 4. Bread—Contains 15 g carbohydrate and 2 g protein. Calories 68.
List 5. Meat, lean—Contains 7 g protein; 3 g fat. Calories 55.
List 6. Fat—Contains 5 g fat. Calories 45.

The dietitian will designate how many portions from each of the lists the patient is permitted to eat for each meal and snack. Those foods selected from lists must be measured initially in the instruction of all new diabetics, to give them the basis for judging amounts. As indicated previously, some individuals may require continual measurement of foods, whereas others may do well with estimation of portions. The dietary treatment should not encumber the patient's life. Greater patient compliance with the dietary regimen can be achieved if the preillness dietary habits of the patient are carefully assessed. Using this as a baseline, proposed modifications can be adapted for the individual patient. Unless the patient receives detailed instruction and the diet is planned to take into account usual food pattern, he or she is quite likely to disregard the diet prescription or to unnecessarily restrict food intake.

MEDICATION

In many patients, diabetes cannot be controlled by dietary measures. When the patient's hyperglycemia cannot be controlled by diet, either insulin or oral hypoglycemic agents are administered.

Insulin

Treatment with exogenous insulin is indicated in the following situations: diabetic ketoacidosis, juvenile diabetes, diabetes developing before the age of 40, unstable diabetes, oral hypoglycemic failure, diet therapy failures, and during stress of pregnancy, infections, major surgery. For the ketosis-prone individual and the unstable adult an exogenous insulin supply is always required. For the others it may be an intermittent requirement (Bonar, 1977, p. 62) that is required during periods of stress.

In the nondiabetic, insulin is released in response to food intake. The beta cells have the ability to release approximately 40 units daily, and there are another 200 units stored for emergency. The diabetic does not have an endogenous supply, and an exogenous form is provided.

Various types of insulin preparations have been developed. These are summarized in Table 47-3. They fall into three general categories: fast-acting (regular and semilente), intermediate (NPH and lente), and long-acting (PZI and ultra lente). The actions of each preparation vary as to time of onset, duration of action, and peak activity time. Hypoglycemic reactions are most likely to occur at time of peak action.

Regular insulin is the only form given intravenously, and it has a clear appearance. The other insulin preparations have a turbid appearance. Each type of insulin comes in three concentrations; U-40, U-80, and U-100. This refers to the concentration of insulin per millileter. U-40 has 40 units per ml, U-

TABLE 47-3 *Time of Action of Various Insulin Preparations*

Type	Preparation	Time of Onset (hours)	Duration of Action (hours)	Peak Activity (hours)
Fast-acting	Crystalline zinc insulin (regular)	1/2–1	8	2–4
	Semilente	1/2–1	14	2–4
Intermediate-acting	Isophane insulin injection (NPH)	2	20–30	6–12
	Lente	2	24–28	6–12
Long-acting	Protamine zinc injection (PZI)	6–8	36+	14–24
	Ultralente	7	36+	18–24

80 has 80 units per ml, and U-100 has 100 units per ml. Syringes are specially calibrated for each concentration. Eventually, the only concentration available will be the U-100 strength. This will decrease confusion and cut down on errors.

In 1971, single peak insulin (SPI) became available. This refers to chromatographic analysis of its purity. SPI is 99 per cent insulinlike; it has 75 per cent pure insulin and 25 per cent desamino insulin. Single-component insulin (SCI) is 99 per cent insulin. Its production is more costly and studies have not shown it to be superior to SPI (Galloway & Bressler, 1978; Bonar, 1977).

Unmodified or regular insulin was the first type to be available. As shown in Table 47-3, it is promptly absorbed after subcutaneous injection and its effect begins within 30 minutes. It reaches its peak action in 2 to 4 hours and its duration is approximately 6 hours. It is obvious the patient would require three or four injections daily if this were the only insulin preparation available. Because it acts quickly, it is used in the treatment of diabetic acidosis. It is also used to supplement the effect of the types of insulin with prolonged actions.

Modified insulins differ from regular insulin in that something is added to make the insulin relatively insoluble and thereby delay the rate at which it is absorbed with the result that the period over which the insulin acts is prolonged. These modifications decreased the need for repeated injections of regular insulin. Protamine zinc insulin, the first of the modified insulins to be developed, has a prolonged action. It was developed by Hagedorn of Denmark, who added a basic protein, protamine—a substance obtained from the sperm of a certain fish—to insulin. Protamine precipitates with insulin and delays the rate at which it is absorbed as the protamine must be broken down before the insulin is released. Because of its prolonged action, hyperglycemia in patients requiring more than 40 units of insulin is difficult to control with protamine zinc insulin. Although the period of maximum action is from 12 to 24 hours, action may continue for from 48 to 72 hours. There is therefore an overlapping of dosages, making it difficult to secure a uniform depression of the blood glucose. Hypoglycemic reactions are frequent.

A more nearly physiologic effect can be achieved by administering part of the insulin dosage as unmodified and part as protamine zinc insulin, either as two separate injections or by mixing the two and giving one injection. The success of this method depends on the ability of the patient to assume responsibility for measuring and mixing the two types of insulin. A commercially prepared mixture of protamine zinc insulin and regular insulin is available.

Following the introduction of protamine zinc insulin, other modifications were introduced that more nearly meet all the following criteria. They require only one injection, have a sufficiently rapid onset of action, and are absorbed over an appropriate period of time. The three most successful preparations are isophane or NPH insulin,[1] globin zinc insulin, and lente insulin. Isophane insulin is a modified protamine zinc insulin. It behaves essentially like a mixture of two parts regular to one part protamine insulin. As the two types are mixed, the problems in administration are simplified. The essential difference between globin and isophane insulin is that globin rather than protamine is used to prolong the period of absorption.

The lente insulins are the newest preparations. They differ from other slow-acting insulins in that they do not contain a foreign protein. They are made by precipitating insulin with zinc and then resuspending it in an acetate buffer solution. By altering the conditions under which the preparations are made, particles of different sizes can be made. Ultra lente contains particles of large size and has the duration of action of over 30 hours; its duration of action is similar to that of protamine zinc insulin. Lente insulin contains particles of small size. Insulin is released more rapidly from small than from large particles, and duration of the action of lente insulin is approximately 24 hours. Semilente insulin is composed of amorphous particles, and the duration of its action is from 12 to 18 hours. The two preparations of insulin in most common use today are isophane and lente insulin. The types of insulin along with the time of onset and duration of action are summarized in Table 47-3.

The objective of insulin therapy is to enable the individual to utilize sufficient food to meet nutritional needs and, within limits, the desire for food. For many patients this objective can be achieved by a single injection of protamine zinc insulin or one of the intermediate-acting insulins, either alone or in combination with crystalline insulin. The ideal preparation of insulin would be one in which the insulin is released in response to hyperglycemia. At this time there is no such preparation. A reasonably good approximation can, however, be achieved in many patients. This is done by planning the distribution of carbohydrate in the diet of the patient and his or her pattern of exercise in relation to the duration of action of the type of insulin used. Because individuals differ from each other and the same individual differs from time to time, the details of the therapeutic plan will be different for each person. Persons who require less than 40 units of insulin

[1] NPH—Neutral Protamine Hagedorn. It was developed in Hagedorn's laboratories.

per day often do very well on a single injection of protamine zinc insulin. Those who require more than 40 units of protamine zinc insulin to control their diabetes usually respond better to one of the intermediate insulins either singly or in combination with crystalline insulin. If the patient requires more than 60 to 70 units of intermediate insulin per day, better control may be achieved by split-insulin dosage. This means approximately two thirds is given in the morning and one third in the evening.

The last few years has seen the development in research centers of other approaches for maintaining normoglycemia control. For example (1) pancreatic or beta-cell transplants. These have the disadvantage of problems with immunosupression, frequent infections, and availability of donors. (2) Development of artificial pancreas or portable insulin pumps. These sophisticated technological systems will probably be used more to identify if maintenance of normal blood sugar will prevent or retard development of chronic complications. The majority of diabetics will probably continue to use insulin injections (Irsigler & Kritz, 1979).

Adverse Reactions

Insulin therapy can produce adverse reactions. The most serious is the hypoglycemic reaction. Hypersensitivity reactions may also occur.

HYPOGLYCEMIA. Hypoglycemia, the state of blood glucose levels below 50 mg (below 30 mg in the full-term newborn infant in the first 48 hours) is most threatening to the brain. Deprivation of glucose to the brain results in utilization of its 2-g reserve and irreparable damage to the neurons of the cerebral cortex (Plum & Posner, 1966, p. 106–25).

Although not all patients experience it, hypoglycemia is an ever-present possibility in the patient who takes insulin or one or more oral hypoglycemic agents. Situations that predispose to hypoglycemia, or, as it is commonly called, insulin reaction, include a delay in or omission of a meal, an increase in the amount of exercise taken, an improvement in the patient's glucose tolerance, an error in the measurement of insulin, resulting in excess dosage.

Signs and symptoms associated with hypoglycemia are caused by its effect on the nervous system. According to Sussman et al. (1963), hypoglycemia affects the nervous system in the following order: (1) parasympathetic nervous system, (2) cerebral effects, (3) sympathoadrenal system, and (4) hypoglycemic coma. Parasympathetic effects include hunger, nausea, and bradycardia. Cerebral effects include yawning, lethargy, lassitude, and the inability to carry out a conversation or to count. Some patients may be confused, disoriented, and aphasic or may make inappropriate remarks or develop acute catatonic or manic states. Thus a patient who is receiving insulin should be suspected of developing hypoglycemia when there is a change in mood or personality.

The symptoms most likely to be noted by the patient are those caused by increased sympathoadrenal activity. They include nervousness or anxiety, sweating, and tachycardia. The patient may describe the state by saying that he or she feels funny or peculiar.

The patient who is taking regular insulin is usually aware of being hypoglycemic. He or she can, therefore, protect himself or herself from a severe reaction. In contrast, the patient who is taking intermediate or long-acting insulin may have difficulty recognizing the warning signs, as they may be less obvious. Generally, intermediate and long-acting insulins lower the blood glucose more gradually than rapidly acting insulin. If the patient happens to be driving an automobile, or is in a position involving danger, the possible consequences are obvious. Hypoglycemic reactions are most likely to occur at the time of peak insulin action (see Table 47-3).

During a period in which a patient is recovering from an acute illness or the diabetes is being brought under control, nurses should be alert to the possibility that the tolerance of the patient for glucose is likely to be improving and hypoglycemia may occur. Changes in the behavior of the patient should be interpreted in this light.

Although the urine may provide information about the level of glucose in the blood, the results may also be misleading. When urine accumulated in the bladder over a period of time is tested, it can contain glucose despite the presence of hypoglycemia at the time. For example, Mr. Rugge, a known diabetic, was admitted to the emergency room of City Hospital in an unconscious state. A catheterized specimen of urine was examined for glucose and produced a maximum color change: it was 4+ for glucose. He was transferred to an inpatient ward, where another sample of urine was obtained and tested for glucose. This time glucose was absent. Mr. Rugge was given 10 g of glucose by intravenous infusion. In a matter of seconds, consciousness returned, and in less time than it takes to tell, he was sitting up in bed demanding, "What happened? Why am I here? I'm hungry. Can't somebody get me something to eat?" Prompt and effective treatment of hypoglycemia quickly restores the individual to well-being. Untreated and severe, it may cause irreparable damage to the brain.

PREVENTION OF HYPOGLYCEMIA. Application of knowledge of the duration of the action of each of the various insulins enables the physician, nurse, or patient to predict when hyperglycemia and hypoglycemia are most likely to occur (see Table 47-3).

The physician prescribes the distribution of carbohydrate in the diet of the patient in relation to the type of insulin used.

Patients should be instructed to maintain an inflexible meal schedule insofar as possible. The distribution of carbohydrate through the day should take into account the time of maximum action of the type of insulin the patient is using. When a meal is delayed, 5 to 10 g of glucose should be taken. This glucose can be subtracted from the next meal. Exercise should be regular rather than sporadic, and when it is increased, the patient may take 5 to 10 g of glucose to prevent hypoglycemia.

To protect patients who are receiving protamine zinc insulin from nocturnal hypoglycemia, some of the carbohydrate from the evening meal is saved for a lunch at bedtime. Milk and crackers or toast and butter are satisfactory. Patients taking intermediate-acting insulin are frequently advised to save some of the carbohydrate from their lunch as a mid- or late-afternoon snack. By distribution of the intake of carbohydrate over the time when insulin absorption is at its height, the patient is protected from attacks of hypoglycemia. The importance of the mid-afternoon and prebedtime lunch should be emphasized to the patient. A hypoglycemic reaction may not be too serious when the person is in the protected environment of home, but a sudden loss of consciousness when out in public can endanger his or her life. If the patient is driving a car, not only the person's life but the lives of others are in danger. Some physicians recommend that patients who are planning to drive a car in the later afternoon take 5 to 10 g of glucose before starting out. One-fourth to one-half glass of orange juice or a Life Saver or two contain enough glucose to protect the patient from hypoglycemia. As pointed out earlier, the patient requires less insulin when the diabetes is under control than when he or she is hyperglycemic. During periods when control is being established, the patient should therefore be observed for signs of hypoglycemia. He or she should also be asked to report any changes in the way he or she feels. The patient should learn the common manifestations of hypoglycemia. The prevention of hypoglycemia is preferable to its cure.

There should be no delay in treatment. If the patient can swallow, a readily absorbable carbohydrate feeding can be given. If this is impossible, glucagon is given by the parenteral route. If the patient fails to respond, 10 to 20 g of glucose are administered intravenously. In some hospitals the method to be used in the treatment of hypoglycemia is included in the standing orders. In others individual physicians leave a prescription or ask to be called. Whatever the practice, there should be no unnecessary delay in instituting effective therapy. Furthermore, should the nurse be in a position where there is some doubt as to whether the patient is hypoglycemic or acidotic, and the physician is not readily available, the nurse should treat the patient for hypoglycemia. Delay in its correction can result in harm to the patient—"the longer hypoglycemia lasts, the more it is likely to produce irreversible neuronal loss" (Plum & Posner, 1966, p. 134). Five or 10 g of glucose will not affect the course of acidosis appreciably.

ALLERGIC REACTIONS. Local or systemic reactions may occur in individuals receiving insulin therapy. They are more likely to occur during the initial treatment. Local reactions may occur at the site of injection. Local allergic reactions are common when patients are taking protamine zinc insulin and are unusual when other types of insulin are used. The reaction is manifested by redness, swelling, itching, and discomfort at the site of injection. The first symptoms appear in from 2 to 12 hours after the injection and reach their height in from 18 to 24 hours. In from 3 to 4 weeks this type of reaction subsides. Fortunately, patients rarely are allergic to the protein of insulin itself. When they are, they are more likely to be allergic to beef or sheep insulins than to pork insulin. This type of allergic reaction is usually controlled by changing to insulin from a different species. In a few instances, a desensitization procedure may be required.

Disorders of the subcutaneous tissue may occur as a result of insulin treatment. They are insulin-induced hypertrophy and insulin lipodystrophy. In the former, there is thickening and lump formation at the injection site. In the latter, there is a decrease or absence of fat tissue resulting in concave depressions of the skin. Insulin injections into the hypertrophic areas can cause absorption delays and account for instability in diabetic control. Children of both sexes and adult females seem to be predisposed to this condition. The cause is not known. The rotation of the sites of injection is encouraged to prevent either hypertrophy or atrophy of adipose tissue. Fat atrophy is also less likely to occur if insulin is administered at room temperature. These disorders are considered to be benign, that is, self-limiting in time. However, they can be distressing to the patient, because they are disfiguring.

PRESBYOPIA. A considerable number of persons whose diabetes is rapidly brought under control with insulin develop a temporary presbyopia, a condition in which the individual can see at a distance but has difficulty in accommodating to near vision. Particularly to the young patient, presbyopia may be quite disturbing. He or she should be reassured that the condition will clear up in from 3 to 4 weeks and delay having the eyes examined for glasses as any prescription obtained during this period will not be suitable later.

Oral Hypoglycemic Agents

About 20 years ago it was discovered that certain chemical compounds administered orally had a hypoglycemic effect. Of the most widely used were the sulfonylurea preparations and the biguanide preparations. The sulfonylureas apparently act by stimulating the operative beta cells to release insulin. Four preparations are available at the present time. They have varying rates of absorption and peak concentrations. These rates determine the frequency of administration and dosage. See Table 47-4. Sulfonylurea drugs can be potentiated by interactions with other drugs, such as coumadin, dilantin, high doses of salicylates, and MAO inhibitors. When taking other drugs, the patient's drug dosage may need to be decreased to prevent hypoglycemia.

The mode of action of the biguanide preparations is unknown. They appear to increase glucose uptake in peripheral tissues and increase sensitivity to insulin. They are used in combination with the sulfonylurea compounds. Only one preparation, phenformin, was used in the United States. However, it was banned in 1977 because of the dangerous side effect, lactic acidosis. Approximately 3,000 patients continue to use the drug. Physicians are able to obtain it if investigatory new drug (IND) applications are filed with the Federal Food and Drug Administration (Kolata, 1979). Much controversy has occurred as a result of the University Group Diabetes Program (UGDP) study. Questions concerning the validity have been debated and the controversy continues. It is now believed that so much uncertainty prevails regarding the action taken, that it needs to be reconsidered.

Investigations have shown the oral hypoglycemic agents to be indicated only for the maturity-onset, nonketotic type of diabetes, blood sugar controllable on less than 40 units of insulin, and only if the individual is less than 20 per cent overweight. The use of these agents should not be substituted for dietary control or reduction of obesity.

Because these agents can be taken orally and the patient does not have to be subjected to daily injections, the oral hypoglycemic agents are probably here to stay. Diabetic patients on the oral agents must receive preparation to live with the disease. They need to understand the disease and how to care for themselves.

Patients receiving oral hypoglycemic agents should know that the drug (1) is effective in many older diabetics but rarely in the young, (2) is not a form of insulin, (3) does not act like insulin, (4) is not effective during infections or other forms of stress, as insulin is required at these times, and (5) can cause hypoglycemia. In some patients the favorable effect of the sulfonylureas lasts only from 4 to 6 months. Other measures—diet and exercise—are still important and should not be neglected. The only real change in the regimen of the patient is that he or she can take the drug by mouth rather than taking insulin by subcutaneous injection. When, as is not at all uncommon, the patient is taking several drugs, some system should be devised to help to remember which of these drugs controls blood sugar and when and how to take each drug.

Exercise

Exercise is known to be an important adjunct in the treatment of the diabetic. It decreases insulin requirements and lowers the blood glucose of diabetic patients. The pathophysiologic mechanisms for this are not fully understood. It has been proposed that insulin receptors become more sensitive to insulin and transport is thereby facilitated (Vranic et al., 1979).

Table 47-4 *Oral Hypoglycemia Agents*

Drug	Proprietary Name	Duration of Action	Frequency of Administration
Sulfonylureas			
Tolbutamide	Orinase	6–12 hr	Bid or tid
Acetohexamide	Dymelor	12–24 hr	Daily or bid
Tolazamide	Tolinase	6–18 hr	Daily or bid
Chlorpropanide	Diabinese	24–36 hr	Daily
Biguanides			
Phenformin	DBI or Metrol	4–6 hr	Daily or bid
Phenformin TD (Time-dispersal)	DIB-TD	12–14 hr	Daily or bid

The patient with diabetes is encouraged to exercise regularly. The type, amount, and degree of activity should be about the same from day to day. Sudden increases, particularly in the patient who is taking insulin, are to be avoided. The beneficial effect of exercise sometimes creates problems for the patient who has been hospitalized. Hospital space and policy often make it difficult for the patient to duplicate the amount of exercise taken outside the hospital. After discharge, he or she may have a series of hypoglycemic attacks. To prevent this, some physicians encourage patients who are able to leave the hospital for an afternoon, or several afternoons, to try to duplicate their usual activity. When patients must for some reason exercise more than is usual, they should protect themselves by taking 5 to 10 g of glucose (1 to 2 lumps of sugar).

The short-term and chronic effects of exercise are the subjects of intensive study. The impact of exercise on diabetics with microangiopathy is also being studied. There is concern that delivery of oxygen to working muscles may be particularly hazardous if the patient already has a compromised blood supply to a vital organ. Exercise programs need to be individually adjusted to the general health and physical training of the patient. It is contraindicated if the patient is in ketoacidosis.

General Care

Skin Care

The diabetic patient should be the cleanest person "on the block." Personal cleanliness, as well as clean clothing, is very important. Diabetic patients are more susceptible to "athlete's foot" and to pyogenic infections of the skin than nondiabetics. Cleanliness reduces the number of bacteria and other microorganisms on the skin. The removal of the secretions from between the toes and from the skin makes conditions less favorable for the growth and multiplication of bacteria.

Instruction must be practical. This means that it should be adapted to the situation of the patient, including customs, habits, and living conditions. For example, although a daily bath is frequently recommended as a desirable practice, some modifications are often necessary. For the patient with very dry skin frequent bathing intensifies the dryness and predisposes to itching. A patient living in a cold-water flat or in a farmhouse where water has to be carried in and out and where only one room is heated may find the effort and lack of privacy great obstacles to seriously considering a daily bath. Habits and customs also differ from one group to another. The elderly person who has always bathed once or twice a week is not likely to take kindly to the suggestion of a daily bath. When frequent bathing is rejected or is impractical, the nurse should stress the daily washing of the feet, the neck, and the pubic region.

Foot Care

In the diabetic patient the care of the feet cannot be overemphasized. Arteriosclerosis develops earlier and progresses more rapidly than it does in the nondiabetic. An injury to the toes that would pass unnoticed in the nondiabetic can, if neglected, lead to gangrene of the toe, foot, and leg. The feet of the diabetic patient require special care. Cleanliness, protection of the feet, well-fitting shoes, daily inspection for blisters, cuts, scratches, avoidance of temperature extremes, avoidance of chemicals for removal of corns or calluses, proper cutting of nails, and prompt treatment of injuries when they occur are imperative. Nurses caring for diabetic patients cannot exercise too much care in the protection of the patient's feet from injury.

One of the most important causes of injury to the lower extremities is heat. Diabetics are remarkably sensitive to heat and may be burned by hot-water bottles, electric pads, and hot moist packs. Therefore heat in any of these forms should not be applied below the knees. If moist dressings are applied, they should be just warm (37.8 to 40.6°C, 100 to 105°F). (See Chapter 43 for detailed instruction.)

Other

The diabetic patient should be taught to treat minor infections such as a common cold or an acute gastrointestinal infection by going to bed. He or she should avoid the use of sweetened cough mixtures and other agents that are sometimes taken during acute respiratory infections. The patient should test urine at 3-hour intervals during the day and at 6-hour intervals during the night. Because any infection in the diabetic patient is an emergency, he or she should contact the nurse or physician and follow their advice.

The diabetic should also receive instructions as to frequency of physician or clinic visits. The diabetic patient should receive yearly physical examinations. Just because the patient is a diabetic he or she is not immune to other diseases and careful surveillance is important.

Education—Overview

The goal of diabetic education programs is for the diabetic patient to assume responsibility for managing his or her own disease. The patient is assisted to achieve this goal by (1) understanding the nature of the disease, (2) understanding how diabetes affects life style, (3) developing the knowledge and skills to carry out diet, exercise, and medication prescriptions, (4) developing knowledge and understanding of the common complications and how to recognize, prevent, and treat them.

If the patient is going to be assisted in self-care, it is necessary to provide the knowledge that will help in understanding the nature of the disease. This assists the individual in knowing what is happening to him or her and why compliance with the prescribed treatments is essential. In addition, it can serve as a basis of identification of problems and their possible solutions. Knowledge to a limited degree serves as motivation for patients to follow therapeutic regimens.

The patient must receive information that will lead to understanding and compliance with the diet prescription. This means information will be needed about the type of diet, exchange lists, selection, spacing, and frequency of meals. In addition, data regarding the avoidance of excesses will be needed. The patient will need to understand the exercise prescription—that the diet and medication are balanced for expected type and amount of exercise. If there is any modification in any part of the treatment triad (diet, exercise, or medication), he or she should have instructions on how to handle the situation.

The diabetic needs to know the following about medication prescription: the type of insulin or hypoglycemic agent, the prescribed amount, frequency of dose, mode and technique of administration, signs and symptoms of untoward reactions, and what to do if they occur. In addition, the diabetic must receive instruction in personal hygiene. The above identified areas form the nucleus for diabetic instruction programs. The instruction must be developed and carried out based on assessment of the individual patient. The assessment will dictate how rapidly and how detailed the educational program will be. It is important to remember that not everything can be learned at the first exposure. The program should plan for progression, reinforcement, and periodic evaluation. Diabetes is a chronic disease and educational programs cannot be a "one-shot deal."

The period during which the severity of diabetes is being evaluated and regulation is effected should be utilized to prepare the patient and the members of the family to assume the responsibility for controlling the diabetes. During this period the patient should learn what he or she needs to know to understand the nature of the disease and to develop the skills needed to maintain control. He or she requires practice in a supportive environment until skill and confidence in the ability to carry out the necessary procedures are developed. The patient should receive the maximum rather than the minimum of instruction. To accomplish this, teaching should begin as soon as the diagnosis is established. The objective should be for the patient to be the master of diabetes mellitus rather than for it to be the master. The reward of mastery is a more nearly normal life. The instruction of every diabetic patient must be planned. The plan for the patient's instruction must suit the individual patient and situation if it is to work. However, whether the instruction of the diabetic patient is given by a special instructor or is shared by a number of people, each person should know what his or her responsibilities are and every provision should be made to see that these functions are accomplished.

For the nurse to provide the patient with the assistance needed, she or he should have a body of knowledge and have developed skills in teaching as well as in the performance of the necessary procedures. Some hospitals have well-organized plans for the instruction of patients with diabetes mellitus. In these programs nurses are usually responsible for certain aspects of the instruction of the patient. The nurse must therefore be familiar with the total program. In hospitals and other agencies that do not have an organized instructional plan, the nurse should discuss the content of the plan for teaching with the patient's physician so that the patient is protected from conflicting instructions.

In addition to making the most of the patient's interest in learning and being sure that he or she knows what is to be learned, the teaching should provide for thoughtful and understanding learning. Time should be taken to learn what the patient already knows or thinks he or she knows as well as wants to know about diabetes. In the opinion of the author, there is a tendency to overestimate what persons who have had diabetes for some time know about their disease and its control. Although the average patient may not benefit from knowing the chemical reactions involved in the testing of urine, patients are much more likely to test urine regularly if they understand why they test it and if they know how to use the results. Sometimes the physician may ask the patient to keep a record of the results of urine testing. The patient should know that the information will help guide the physician in regulating the diabetes. As in other learning, the program should provide for sufficient repetition to make certain that the patient has had sufficient knowledge and practice to have confidence for self-care. Some of the factors that influence the amount of practice that a given patient needs are the ability of the patient to learn, interest in learning, and self-confidence. A great deal of encouragement is sometimes necessary. Emphasis should be on accomplishment rather than on failure.

As in other types of learning, the situation should provide the patient with an opportunity to perform procedures as nearly as possible as they will be carried out at home. Practice periods should be distributed over a period of time rather than be limited to a single intensive session. Unless the instruction of the diabetic patient is carefully planned, this factor in learning is likely to be disregarded. Instruction may include little more than a hasty demonstration and inadequate practice. The patient is then dismissed with the vain hope that he or she has mastered a set of complicated instructions and will be able to manage the diabetes. The worried patient goes home hoping for the best. Often, as a result of failure to appreciate the importance of the control of diabetes plus a lack of confidence in the ability to care for himself or herself, the patient lapses into old habits and sooner or later is readmitted to the hospital where the same procedure is repeated. Both group and individual instruction are arranged. More recently, some of the content has been programmed and placed on a teaching machine. Each method has its advantages and disadvantages. One of the advantages of group instruction is that the patient may be encouraged by learning that other people's problems are not unlike his or her own. Patients may have an opportunity to share experiences and solutions to problems. Individual instruction allows for modification of the plan for the needs and problems of the patient. Programmed instruction permits the patient to progress in learning at his or her own rate. Theoretically, the patient does not progress until each step is mastered. This form of instruction also ensures that each patient receives a minimum of instruction. A well-planned program should cover all aspects required by the patient.

Whether patients are taught in groups or individually, instruction should be carefully planned and adapted to the needs of each individual patient. A variety of factors may interfere with the ability of the patient to learn. Sometimes a patient is of low intellectual level. Other factors are more frequently responsible, however. The fact that the patient is adjusting to a new and anxiety-provoking diagnosis may decrease learning capacity for the time being because the patient is unable to give attention to learning. His or her ability to learn may be lessened because he or she is not feeling well. Frequently the time in the hospital is too short to master the necessary knowledge and skill. As soon as the patient begins to feel well, he or she is discharged. The ability or willingness to reveal significant factors in the home and work situation may be lacking. Most, though by no means all, patients are motivated to learn. Other patients may have the motivation but because of educational or physical handicaps be unable to develop the required knowledge and skills needed to control their disease. Some patients do not see well enough to measure insulin and to carry out the details of the procedure unless they have a special type of syringe that is available for the use of blind patients. When the patient is unable for one reason or another to learn, members of the family or a neighbor may be enlisted to give the necessary assistance.

Insulin—Equipment and Administration

The patient must know the type of insulin, concentration (U-80, U-100), and the prescribed dosage. It is essential that the appropriate syringe be used for the insulin concentration prescribed. Diabetic patients on insulin may use either disposable or reusable syringes. The former are used one time only and then discarded. Patients find them highly desirable because they do not require sterilization. Although minimal, cost may be considered a disadvantage. If reusable syringes and needles are used they should be sterilized by boiling before each injection. Boiling is simplified by placing the separated barrel and plunger of the syringe and the needle in a metal strainer. The strainer is placed in a saucepan of cold water and boiled for 5 minutes. When the syringe is removed from the water, care should be taken not to contaminate any part of the needle or syringe that comes in contact with the insulin or is introduced into the patient. When the syringe and needle are kept in alcohol, the alcohol container should be emptied, washed, and boiled at the time the syringe is sterilized. Before the syringe is filled with insulin, alcohol should be removed from the barrel by moving the plunger in and out of the barrel a number of times. The skin over the site of injection should be clean, and just before the injection is made, it should be cleansed with alcohol.

The hour at which the patient takes the insulin will depend on the type of insulin, the severity of the diabetes, when blood sugar is highest, and the practices of the physician. The most common time is 20 to 30 minutes before breakfast for patients receiving one injection a day. Modified insulins containing a precipitate should be gently rotated until the sediment is thoroughly mixed with the clear solution. Vigorous shaking should be avoided to prevent bubble formation.

Insulin, though usually called a protein, is a polypeptide and is digested in the alimentary canal. It must therefore be administered parenterally. The usual method is by subcutaneous injection into loose subcutaneous tissues. Because daily, or more frequent, injections are required over the lifetime of the individual, care should be taken to rotate the sites, so that one area is not used more often than once each month. When a patient injects his or her own insulin, the anterior aspects of the thigh and the abdomen are usually the most convenient sites. For those patients who have automatic syringes, the lateral aspect of the upper arm may also be used.

Patients should be taught that because insulin is a protein, it is advisable to keep it in a cool place but that it should not be allowed to freeze. The bottle in current use need not be kept in the refrigerator. When traveling it should not be kept in the glove compartment or the trunk. It should be protected from temperature extremes. Patients with diabetes mellitus must be taught the signs and symptoms of hypoglycemia and hyperglycemia. In addition they need to know what to do if the signs and symptoms occur.

The patient with diabetes mellitus should carry some form of identification that includes not only personal data but the fact that he or she is diabetic, insulin dosage, and the name of the physician. Carrying a card is of greatest importance to those who are taking insulin or who are subject to ketosis. A number of types of identification tags and cards are available.

Urine Testing

Although the concentration of glucose in the blood of a fasting person provides accurate information about the adequacy of control of diabetes mellitus, the frequency with which the test is performed is limited by the fact that blood must be withdrawn before it can be examined. Under most circumstances, the quantity of glucose in the urine provides a reasonably accurate estimate of the degree to which the homeostasis of glucose is being achieved. Because urine is easily obtained and glucose and acetone are excreted in the urine when the renal threshold is exceeded, and the qualitative test for glucose and acetone are relatively simple, urine is widely used to evaluate the control of diabetes mellitus. Depending on the severity of the diabetes and whether or not the patient takes insulin, as well as the views of the physician, the patient may be instructed to test urine as frequently as four times a day or as infrequently as once or twice a month. For most individuals who work, two testings a day are a practical maximum. During a period in which diabetes mellitus is under regulation or is changing, more frequent testing may be desired to dtermine when hyperglycemia and/or hypoglycemia occurs.

Whereas blood to be tested for glucose is usually taken when the patient is fasting, no simple statement applies to the kinds of samples of urine examined for glucose. All urine may be saved for 24 hours so that the total quantity of glucose excreted per day can be determined. Each and every voiding may be checked as a means of evaluating fluctuations in the blood glucose. The patient may be instructed to void at specific times of the day and the urine is added to previous voidings and mixed. A sample of the mixture is then tested for sugar and acetone. In another method the patient voids and discards the voiding unless a 24-hour specimen is being collected, when the urine is added to previous voidings. The patient drinks a glass or two of water and then 1 hour later collects a sample of urine (a fresh specimen) for testing. Because the urine is secreted over a known and relatively short period of time, it more accurately reflects the level of glucose in the blood at the time of testing than is likely to be true of the other methods. Whatever method is used, however, the patient should be instructed in its use. He or she should have practice not only in performing the method used at home but in evaluating the results. If the patient is to adjust the insulin dosage in relation to the quantity of glucose in urine, he or she should also be given explicit written as well as verbal instructions and should practice adjusting insulin dosage while still being instructed.

The tests for glucose and for ketone bodies are useful in evaluating the success of the control of diabetes mellitus. The patient should be instructed to seek medical attention immediately when the quantity of glucose in the urine increase over 1+ or 2+ as well as when ketone bodies appear in the urine. An experienced and intelligent diabetic patient may be able to evaluate why glucose appears in the urine and to make the appropriate adjustment. When these adjustments are not successful, he or she should see the physician.

Teaching is More than Telling

A not unimportant, but frequently little appreciated, part of teaching the patient is the teaching given by the nurse in the care and supervision of the patient. The nurse is in a favorable position to encourage the patient to express and examine feelings about diabetes mellitus, to learn personal misconceptions and doubts, and to answer or obtain answers to questions. Some instruction the nurse gives directly as instruction. Other teaching is done by example, for if the nurse carries out and supervises care conscientiously she or he does much to impress the patient with its importance. For example, if the nurse collects the urine specimens promptly and correctly, the patient will be impressed with the importance of regular and frequent testing of the urine. If the nurse uses care in washing feet and dries them well with a soft cloth, the patient is more certain to follow the example set. If the nurse insists that the patient who starts barefooted for the bathroom stop and put on slippers, she or he is not only emphasizing what the patient has been taught but is giving actual practice in it. The patient who is provided with a footstool and encouraged to elevate his or her feet is learning by doing.

Throughout the discussion of the needs of the patient with diabetes mellitus, emphasis has been placed on the importance of preparing the patient for self-management so that the diabetes is kept under control. Diet, exercise, and, when necessary, insulin or an insulin substitute are the principal measures used in the control of diabetes mellitus. Education is an essential aspect of therapy.

Because the patient and family must eventually assume the responsibility for the management of the diabetes mellitus, the nurse must not do for patients what they are able to do for themselves. The nurse should, however, interpret her or his actions so that the patient understands the reason for encouraging him or her in self-care. Recognition should also be given to progress made by the patient. The nurse must exercise a high degree of judgment in making the decision that the patient is or is not ready to assume more responsibility. In some instances, the patient is unable to assume full responsibility for care and a member of the family must be taught to assist. Insofar as the patient is able to participate, he or she should be included in any instruction. Whenever possible, one or more members of the family should also be included in the instructional plan, as family members can be helpful to the patient.

Even when instructions given in the physician's office or in the hospital are well planned and carried out, the patient and/or family still may have some problems. When a visiting nurse service or public health nurse is available in the community, the patient can be helped to make the adjustment to full responsibility by visits from a nurse. Even when a patient is well taught in the hospital, problems are likely to arise in adjustment at home or to the work situation. In addition to the usual sources of stress in hospitalized patients, he or she is adapting to diabetes and all that is entailed in its control.

The need for ongoing education programs and continuing evaluation of their effectiveness is emphasized by the following studies of patient's compliance with therapy. Two studies of diabetic patients at home indicate that they make many errors in the management of their disease. In the first, made by Watkins and her associates (1967), the patients were rated on the management of insulin, urine tests, diet, foot care, and disease control. In every category from 20 to 80 per cent of the patients made errors. As an example, of sixty patients, forty-eight had unacceptable practices in administration of insulin and thirty-one made errors in dosage. Furthermore, the longer they had the disease, the more insulin errors they made. Those who knew more about diabetes managed better but their disease was more poorly controlled. Only one patient demonstrated acceptable practice in all areas.

In the second study, Leifson (1969) found that patients made numerous errors in testing urine. Eighty-six per cent timed them improperly, 19 per cent used outdated test material, and 67 per cent stored the material improperly.

Both of these studies indicate the need for further study of the kind of help patients need if they are to manage their diabetes. Very likely the kind of assistance patients require changes over time. As an example, as vision fails old methods for measuring insulin may be inadequate. These studies also raise some other questions, such as why should patients who know more about diabetes be in poorer control? Certainly more information is needed if people with chronic conditions are to live productive and healthy lives. The National Commission on Diabetes has identified the lack of educational programs for diabetes. The two studies cited are just an example. Other studies have found that professional health team members have a "significant lack of knowledge of basic concepts of diabetes and its management" (Etzwiler, 1978, p. 858).

Throughout this text, attention has been given to the problem of enlisting the patient's help in restoring and maintaining his or her own health.

Mendelsohn (1968) challenges some of the current ideas about mass education in public health. To emphasize the point that mass communication efforts of the past have failed despite the expenditure of large sums of money, he cites the ever-rising number of traffic accidents. For educational efforts to be successful, he states (p. 133) that the program must take into account the following:

1. Simple exposure is not enough; interest is a prerequisite.
2. Humans are complex actor-reactors. They function in dynamic situations that they define for themselves in different ways.
3. Facts are not enough. Time must be spent in altering socially derived perceptions and in helping

the patient develop insight into the actual health threat.

4. Two variables are involved in any health threat: perceived susceptibility (it can or cannot happen to me) and perceived severity.

Tolstoy, in *The Death of Ivan Ilyich* (1963), defined the latter when he had Ivan Ilych say "Is it or is it not serious?" He did not care what the diagnosis was. He wanted to know what the implications were.

Although Mendelsohn makes other useful points, one more will be cited. He says that people do not want the facts, nor do they know what to do with them. They must be told what to do in an interesting, explicit, dramatic, and exact manner.

In the practice of nursing, nurses want to help patients with long-term illnesses live as comfortably and usefully as they can. To accomplish this objective we must learn

1. What kinds of help the patient who is newly diagnosed needs and how this help can best be given.
2. What kinds of continuing help and supervision the patient needs and how this help can best be given.

Unanswered Questions

When insulin was discovered in 1922, it was thought diabetes would no longer be a major problem. The concomitants of the disease, the diabetic syndrome, were unknown. Much of what was accepted as certain is now uncertain. The questions to be answered are increasing rather than decreasing. Among the unanswered questions are the following: (1) What is the nature of the cause of diabetes? (2) Who is diabetic? (3) How and where does insulin act? (4) How are different tissues affected by insulin? (5) Do the abnormalities in glucose tolerance occurring among the aged indicate diabetes mellitus or are they a "normal" part of aging? (6) Do some diabetic patients maintain glucose metabolism by utilizing noninsulin-dependent metabolic pathways? (7) Is the level of glucose in the blood the best way of measuring the degree of control of diabetes or are there better methods? (8) Does vascular damage precede the development of diabetes? (9) How can the vascular and neurologic concomitants of diabetes be prevented? (10) What are the long-range effects of the various degrees of carbohydrate restrictions? (11) What kind of program is needed to assist the patient and family to learn to cope with diabetes mellitus? (12) What kind of follow-up is required if the patient is to manage his or her disease properly? The last two questions are of particular importance if nurses are to provide maximum assistance to patients.

Summary

The nurse has major responsibilities in the care of the diabetic patient. She or he must provide instruction, guidance, and understanding for the control and management of the condition. The nurse must be prepared to provide nursing care for the patient if acute or chronic complications should occur. Last but not least, the nurse must recognize that the diabetic is not exempt from other diseases. She or he must be prepared to evaluate the impact of a concurrent illness on the diabetes and the impact of the diabetes on the concurrent illness. The sick diabetic has all the problems of any person who is ill and they are compounded by the diabetic state. The special needs of the diabetic must be recognized and met. The nurse who assists in the care of the diabetic patient has the satisfaction of knowing that the quality of life of the diabetic can be improved by intelligent nursing care.

References Cited

Alberti, K. G. M. M., and Nattrass, M. "Severe Diabetic Ketoacidosis." *Med. Clin. North Am.*, **62**:4 (1978), 799–814.

Andres, R. "Aging and Diabetes." *Med. Clin. North Am.*, **55** (1971), 835–46.

Arky, R. A. "Current Principles of Dietary Therapy of Diabetes Mellitus." *Med. Clin. North Am.*, **62** (1978), 655–62.

Bar, R. S. S., and Roth, J. "Insulin Receptor Status in Disease States of Man." *Arch. Inter. Med.*, **137** (1977), 474–80.

Beck-Nielsen, H. "The Pathogenic Role of an Insulin-Receptor Defect in Diabetes Mellitus of the Obese." *Diabetes*, **27** (1978), 1175–81.

Bonar, J. *Diabetes: A Clinical Guide.* Flushing, N.Y.: Medical Exam Publishing Co., 1977.

Brobeck, J. R. *Best & Taylor's Physiological Basis of Medical Practice*, 9th ed. Baltimore: Williams & Wilkins Co., 1973.

Carroll, K. F., and Nestel. "Diurnal Variation in Glucose Tolerance and Insulin Secretion in Man." *Diabetes*, **22** (1973), 333–37.

Cohen, A. M. "Prevalence of Diabetes among Different Ethnic Jewish Groups in Israel." *Metabolism*, **10** (1961), 50–58.

Danowski, T. S. "The Diagnosis of Maturity-Onset Diabetes Mellitus." In *Diagnosis and Treatment of Maturity-Onset Diabetes Mellitus.* Symposium presented at Department of Continuing Education in Health Sciences, University of California, Los Angeles, 1976.

Diabetes Data, Compiled 1977. U.S. Department of Health, Education, and Welfare. DHEW Publication No. (NIH) 78–1468. Washington, D.C.: U.S. Government Printing Office, 1978.

Diabetes Mellitus, 7th ed. Indianapolis, Ind.: Lilly Research Laboratories, 1973, p. 27.

Ellenberg, M., and Rifkin, H. *Diabetes Mellitus: Theory and Practice.* New York: McGraw-Hill, 1970.

Etzwiler, D. D. "Education of the Patient with Diabetes." *Med. Clin. North Am.,* **62** (1978), 857–65.

Fajans, S. S. "Classification and Natural History of Genetic Diabetes Mellitus." In *Diabetes Mellitus: Diagnosis and Treatment,* Vol. 3. Ed. by S. S. Fajans and K. E. Sussman. New York: American Diabetes Association, 1971.

Fink, S. L. "Crisis and Motivation: A Theoretical Model." *Arch. Phys. Med. Rehab.* (1967), 592–97.

Flier, J. S., Kahn, C. R., and Roth, J. "Receptors, Antireceptor Antibodies and Mechanisms of Insulin Resistance." *N. Engl. J. Med.,* **300** (1979), 413–19.

Galloway, J. A., and Bressler, R. "Insulin Treatment in Diabetes." *Med. Clin. North Am.,* **62** (1978), 663–80.

Gerich, J. E. "Somatostatin." *Arch. Inter. Med.,* **137** (1977), 659–65.

Goldstein, S., and Podolsky, S. "The Genetics of Diabetes Mellitus." *Med. Clin. North Am.,* **62:4** (1978), 639–54.

Guthrie, D. W., and Guthrie, R. A. *Nursing Management of Diabetes Mellitus.* St. Louis: C. V. Mosby Co., 1977.

"Hormone Receptors: New Clues to the Cause of Diabetes." *Science,* **193** (1976), 220–22.

Houssay, B. A. "Advancement of Knowledge of the Role of the Hypophysis in Carbohydrate Metabolism during the Last Twenty-Five Years." *Endocrinology,* **30** (1942), 884–90.

Irsigler, K., and Kritz, H. "Long Term Continuous Intravenous Insulin Therapy with a Portable Insulin Dosage-Regulating Apparatus." *Diabetes,* **28** (1979), 196–203.

Jarrett, R. J., and Keen, H. "Further Observations on Diurnal Variation in Oral Glucose Tolerance." *Br. Med. J.,* **4** (1970), 334–37.

Joslin, E. P. et al. *Treatment of Diabetes Mellitus,* 10th ed. Philadelphia: Lea & Febiger, 1959.

Kessler, I. J. "Mortality Experience of Diabetic Patients." *Am. J. Med.,* **51** (1971), 724.

Kolata, G. B. "The Phenformin Ban: Is the Drug an Imminent Hazard?" *Science,* **203** (1979), 1094–96.

Krahl, M. E. "Insulin Action at the Molecular Level, Facts and Speculations." *Diabetes,* **21:** Suppl. 2 (1972), 695–702.

Leifson, J. "Glycosuria Tests Performed by Diabetics at Home." *Pub. Health Rep.,* **84** (1969) 32.

Levin, M. E., and O'Neal, L. W. *The Diabetic Foot,* 2nd ed. St. Louis: C. V. Mosby Co., 1977.

Levine, R. "New Horizons in Our Knowledge." *Am. Geriatric Soc.,* **19** (1971) 903.

Long, C. N., and Lukens, F. D. W. "The Effects of Adrenalectomy and Hypophysectomy upon Experimental Diabetes in the Cat." *J. Exper. Med.,* **63** (1936) 465–90.

Major, R. H. *Classic Descriptions of Disease,* 3rd ed. Springfield, Ill.: Charles C Thomas, 1955.

Marble, A. et al. *Joslin's Diabetes Mellitus,* 11th ed. Philadelphia: Lea & Febiger, 1971.

Mendelsohn, H. "Which Shall Be: Mass Education or Mass Persuasion for Health?" *Am. J. Pub. Health,* **58** (1968) 131–37.

Neel, J. V. "Diabetes Mellitus: A 'Thrifty' Genotype Rendered Detrimental by 'Progress?' " *Am. J. Human Gen.,* **14** (1962) 353.

Oakley, N. W. et al., "Diurnal Variations in Oral Glucose Tolerance: Insulin and Growth Hormone Changes with Special Reference to Women Taking Oral Contraceptives." *Diabetologia,* **9** (1973) 235–38.

Oakley, W. G., Pyke, D. A., and Taylor, K. W. *Diabetes and Its Management,* 3rd ed. London: Blackwell Scientific Publications, 1978.

O'Sullivan, J. B. "Population Retested for Diabetes after 17 Years: New Prevalence Study." *Diabetologia,* **5:4** (1969), 211–14.

Plum, F., and Posner, J. *Diagnosis of Stupor and Coma.* Philadelphia: F. A. Daivs Co., 1966, pp. 106–25.

Report of National Commission Diabetes. DHEW Publication No. (NIH) 76–1022. **3:2** (1975)

Rimoin, D. L. "Inheritance of Diabetes Mellitus." *Med. Clin. North Am.,* **55** (1971) 807–19.

Rizza, R. A., and Gerich, J. E. "Somatostatin and Diabetes." *Med. Clin. North Am.,* **62** (1978) 734–46.

Sanger, F. "Chemistry of Insulin." *Br. Med. Bull.,* **16:3** (1960) 183–88.

Sherwin, R., and Felig, P. "Pathophysiology of Diabetes Mellitus." *Med. Clin. North Am.,* **62:4** (1978) 695–711.

Shuman, C. R. "Acute Complications of Maturity-Onset Diabetes Mellitus." In *Diagnosis and Treatment of Maturity-Onset Diabetes Mellitus.* Symposium presented by the Department of Continuing Education in Health Sciences, University of California, Los Angeles, 1976.

Sussman, K. E. et al. "Failure of Warning in Insulin Induced Hypoglycemia." *Diabetes,* **12** (1963) 39.

Tepperman, J. *Metabolic and Endocrine Physiology,* 3rd ed. Chicago: Year Book Medical Publishers, 1973.

Tolstoy, L. "The Death of Ivan Ilyich." In *Six Short Masterpieces by Tolstoy.* New York: Dell Publishing Co., 1963.

Underdahl, L. O. "Classification of Diabetes Mellitus According to Therapeutic Requirements." In *Diabetes Mellitus: Diagnosis and Treatment,* Vol. 2. Ed. by G. S. Hamwi and T. S. Danowski. New York: American Diabetes Association, 1967.

Uris, L. *Trinity.* Garden City, N.Y.: Doubleday, 1976.

Vander, A., Sherman, J., and Luciano, D. S. *Human Physiology—The Mechanisms of Body Function,* 2nd ed. New York: McGraw-Hill, 1975.

Vranic, M., Horvath, S., and Wahren, J. "Exercise and Diabetes: An Overview." *Diabetes,* **28** (1979), 107–10.

Watkins, J. D., and Williams, T. F. et al. "A Study of Diabetic Patients at Home." *Am. J. Pub. Health,* **57** (1967), 452–59.

Whitehouse, F. W. "The Diagnosis of Diabetes." *Med. Clin. North Am.,* **62:4** (1978) 627–37.

Williamson, J. R., Vogler, N. J., and Kilo, C. "Microvascular Disease in Diabetes." *Med. Clin. North Am.,* **55** (1971), 847–61.

Williamson, J. R., and Kilo, C. "Basement Membrane Thickening and Diabetic Microangiopathy." *Diabetes,* **25** (1976) 925–27.

Winegrad, A. I., and Clements, R. S. "Diabetes Ketoacidosis." *Med. Clin. North Am.*, **55** (1971) 908–9.

Yalow, R. S., and Berson, S. A. "Immunoassay of Endogenous Plasma Insulin in Man."*J. Clin. Invest.*, **39** (1960) 1157–75.

Zonana, J., and Rimoin, D. L. "Current Concepts in Genetics." *N. Engl. J. Med.*, **295** (1976), 603–5.

General References

Alberti, K. G. M. M. "Low Dose Insulin in the Treatment of Diabetic Ketoacidosis." *Arch. Intern. Med.*, **137** (1977), 1367.

Backsheider, J. E. "Self-Care Requirements, Self-Care Capabilities, and Nursing Systems in the Diabetic Nurse Management Clinic." *Am. J. Pub. Health*, **64** (1974), 1138–46.

Berger, M., Berchtold, P., Cuppers, H. J., and Drost, H. "Metabolic and Hormonal Effects of Muscular Exercise in Juvenile Type Diabetes." *Diabetologia*, **13** (1977) 355–65.

Bowen, R., Rich, R., and Schlotfeldt, R. M. "Effects of Organized Instruction for Patients with the Diagnosis of Diabetes Mellitus." *Nurs. Res.*, **10** (1961), 151–59.

Braverman, I. M. "Cutaneous Manifestations of Diabetes Mellitus." *Med. Clin. North Am.*, **55** (1971), 1019–29.

Colwell, J. A., and Halushka, P. V. "Platelet Function and Diabetes Mellitus." *Med. Clin. North Am.*, **62** (1978) 753–66.

Diabetes Care. Bimonthly publication, clinical journal, American Diabetes Association.

Ellenberg, M., "Diabetic Neuropathy: Clinical Aspects." *Metabolism*, **25** (1976), 1627–55.

"Employment of Diabetics. Special Report." *Diabetes*, **21** (1972), 834.

Fajans, S. S., ed. *Diabetes Mellitus.* DHEW Publication No. NIH 76–854. Washington, D.C.: U.S. Government Printing Office, 1976.

Felig, P. "Body Fuel Metabolism and Diabetes Mellitus in Pregnancy." *Med. Clin. North Am.*, **61** (1977), 43–67.

Felig, P., Wahren, J., Sherwin, R., and Palaiologos, G. "Amino Acid and Protein Metabolism in Diabetes Mellitus." *Arch. Inter. Med.*, **137** (1977), 507–13.

Forland, M., Thomas, V., and Shelokov, A. "Urinary Tract Infections in Patients with Diabetes Mellitus." *JAMA*, **238** (1977) 1924–26.

Fusaro, R., and Goetz, F. "Common Cutaneous Manifestations and Problems of Diabetics." *Postgrad. Med.*, **49** (1971) 84–90.

Garber, R. "The Use of a Standardized Teaching Program in Diabetes Education." *Nurs. Clin. North Am.*, **12** (1977), 375–91.

Goodman, L. S., and Gilman, A. *The Pharmacological Basis of Therapeutics*, 5th ed. New York: Macmillan Publishing Co., 1975.

Hoffman, W. H., O'Neill, P., Khoury, C., and Bernstein, S. S. "Service and Education for the Insulin-Dependent Child." *Diabetes Care*, **1** (1978) 285–88.

Horvath, S. M. "Review of Energetics and Blood Flow in Exercise." *Diabetes*, **28**: Suppl. T (1979), 33–38.

Howard, R. B., and Herbold, N. H. *Nutrition in Clinical Care.* New York: McGraw-Hill, 1978.

Kane, W. "Diabetic-Foot Problems." *Minn. Med.*, **56** (1973) 369–73.

Kaufman, M. "A Food Preference Questionnaire for Counseling Patients with Diabetes." *Am. Dietet. Assoc.*, **49** (1966) 31–37.

Keithley, J. K. "Proper Nutritional Assessment Can Prevent Hospital Malnutrition." *Nursing '79*, **9** (1979) 68–72.

Keyes, M. "The Somogyi Phenomenon in Insulin-Dependent Diabetes." *Nurs. Clin. North Am.*, **12** (1977), 439–45.

Kolata, G. B. "Blood Sugar and the Complications of Diabetes." *Science*, **203** (1979) 1098–99.

Krall, L. P., ed. *The Joslin Diabetes Manual*, 11th ed. Philadelphia: Lea & Febiger, 1979.

Krall, L. P., and Chabot, V. A. "Oral Hypoglycemic Agent Uptake." *Med. Clin. North Am.*, **62** (1978), 681–94.

Kyllo, C. J., and Nuttall, F. Q. "Prevalence of Diabetes Mellitus in School-Age Children in Minnesota." *Diabetes*, **27** (1978), 57–60.

L'Esperance, F. A. "Diabetic Retinopathy." *Med. Clin. North Am.*, **62** (1978) 767–86.

Levin, L. S. "Patient Education and Self-Care: How Do They Differ?" *Nurs. Outlook*, **26** (1978) 170–75.

"Long-Range Plan to Combat Diabetes." *Diabetic Forecast*, **28**: Supp. 1 (1975).

Lowery, B. J., and DuCette, J. P. "Disease-Related Learning and Disease Control in Diabetes as a Function of Locus of Control." *Nurs. Res.*, **26** (1976), 358–62.

Managing Diabetes Properly. Nursing skill book. Horsham, Pa.: Intermed Communications, 1977.

Marston, M. V. "Compliance with Medical Regimens: A Review of the Literatures." *Nurs. Res.*, **19** (1970), 312–23.

McCarthy, J. A. "Somogyl Effect: Managing Blood Glucose Rebound." *Nursing '79*, **9** (1979), 38–41.

McGarry, J. D., and Foster, D. W. "Hormonal Control of Ketogenesis." *Arch. Intern. Med.*, **137** (1977), 495–501.

Micossi, P., Pontiroli, A. E., and Baron, S. H. "Aspirin Stimulates Insulin and Glucagon Secretion and Increases Glucose Tolerance in Normal and Diabetic Subjects." *Diabetes*, **27** (1978), 1196–1204.

Miller, L. V., Coldstein, J., and Nicolaisen. "Evaluation of Patients' Knowledge of Diabetes Self-Care." *Diabetes Care*, **1** (1978), 275–80.

Myers, S. A. "Diabetes Management by the Patient and a Nurse Practitioner." *Nurs. Clin. North Am.*, **12** (1977), 415–26.

Newsholme, E. A. "The Control of Fuel Utilization by Muscles during Exercise and Starvation." *Diabetes*, **28**: Supp. T (1979), 1–7.

Notkins, A. L. "The Causes of Diabetes." *Sci. Amer.*, **241** (Nov. 1979), 62–73.

Power, L., Bakker, D., and Cooper, M. *Diabetes Outpa-*

tient Care through Physician Assistants. Springfield, Ill.: Charles C Thomas, 1973.

Raskin, P., and Unger, R. H. "Glucagon and Diabetes." *Med. Clin. North Am.,* **62** (1978), 713–22.

Renshaw, D. C. "Impotence in Diabetes." *Dis. Nerv. Sys.,* **36** (1975), 369–71.

Sackett, D. L., and Haynes, R. B. *Compliance with Therapeutic Regimens.* Baltimore, Md.: Johns Hopkins University Press, 1976.

Sanders, K., Mills, J., Martin, F. I. R., and DelHorne, D. J. "Emotional Attitudes in Adult Insulin-Dependent Diabetics." *J. Psychosomatic Res.,* **19** (1975), 241–43.

Schumann, D. "Refining Urine Test Tactics." *Managing Diabetes Properly.* Horsham, Pa.: Intermediate Communications, 1977.

Shagon, B. P. "Diabetes in the Elderly Patient." *Med. Clin. North Am.,* **60** (1976) 1191–1208.

Spiro, R. G. "Investigations into the Biochemical Basis of Diabetic Basement-Membrane Alterations." *Diabetes,* **25** (1976), 909–13.

Steinke, J. "Management of Diabetes in the Surgical Patient." *Med. Clin. North Am.,* **55** (1971), 939–45.

Suren, J. V. "Education of the Culturally and Educationally Deprived Diabetic." *Nurs. Clin. North Am.,* **12** (1977), 427–37.

"Symposium on Sex and Diabetes." *Diabetes Care* **2**:1 (1979).

Thompson, R. G. "The Management of Diabetes Mellitus in the Adolescent." *Med. Clin. North Am.,* **59** (1975), 1349–1157.

Vincent, P. "Factors Influencing Patient Noncompliance: A Theoretical Approach." *Nurs. Res.,* **20** (1971) 509–16.

Vranic, M., and Kawamori, R. "Essential Roles of Insulin and Glucagon in Regulating Glucose Fluxes during Exercise in Dogs." *Diabetes,* **28**: Supp. T (1979), 45–52.

Weisenfeld, S. "Absorption of Insulin to Infusion Bottles and Tubing." *Diabetes,* **70** (1968), 766–70.

West, K. M. "Diet Therapy of Diabetes: An Analysis of Failure." *Ann. Inter. Med.,* **79** (1973), 425–34.

"When a Pregnant Woman is Diabetic." *Am. J. Nurs.,* **79** (1979), 448–60.

White, P. "What It Means to Be Female and Diabetic." *Diabetic Forecast,* **28** (1975).

Willer, B., and Miller, G. H. "Client Involvement in Goal Setting and Its Relationship to Therapeutic Outcome." *J. Clin. Psychol.,* **32** (1976), 687–89.

Williams, S. R. *Essentials of Nutrition and Diet Therapy,* 2nd ed. St. Louis: C. V. Mosby Co., 1978.

Wishner, W. J., and O'Brien, M. D. "Diabetes and the Family." *Med. Clin. North Am.,* **62** (1978), 849–56.

Zifferblatt, S. M., and Wilbur, C. S. "Dietary Counseling: Some Realistic Expectations and Guidelines." *J. Am. Dietet. Assoc.,* **70** (1977), 591–95.

48

Mr. Allen, A Patient Who Was Burned

The worst possible casualty which can happen and still leave a victim surviving is a major burn. The pain, suffering, disfigurement and potential rejection by society are inestimable.

KELLEHER, 1980

The energy crunch has seen a resurgence of the back-to-basics school. Increased use of wood stoves, do-it yourself repair work, and car upkeep all contribute to energy saving but with the potential of accidental trauma. Burn trauma will affect over 2 million Americans yearly in the 1980s.

The Patient

On the evening of April 4, 14-year-old Dennie Allen and his 15-year-old friend, Jim Knight, were in the basement of Dennie's home filling the gasoline tank of his new mini bike. During the procedure, some of the gasoline was spilled. When the stream of gasoline reached the furnace, an explosion occurred. Dennie ran up the stairway calling for help. When he reached the top of the stairway, he noticed that Jim was not behind him. He ran back into the basement to help his friend, with the result that he was badly burned. Fortunately, the nearby general hospital had excellent facilities for both emergency and burn treatment, and within a half-hour Dennie and Jim were receiving emergency treatment.

Burn shock is essentially the same as any other shock with its underlying fluid dislocations. Burn shock is slow to develop and so burned patients are usually quite alert for 20 minutes to several hours and can give a reliable account of what happened.

In some burn centers, current thought centers on the patient being the primary decision maker in choosing between a full therapeutic regimen or ordinary care (Imbus & Zawacki, 1977). The patient's status is assessed by the burn team and chances of survival are realistically estimated. Those patients whose burned areas are of a nature that has no precedent for survival are allowed to choose between aggressive care and ordinary care. In such a setting, supportive nursing care of the highest caliber is essential.

Dennie was awake and alert throughout his treatment in the emergency room, which lasted until 9:30 P.M. During this period, he was given meperidine HCl (Demerol) for his pain; two intravenous catheters were inserted to (1) administer fluids and (2) continuously monitor central venous pressure; and an indwelling urinary catheter was inserted to monitor renal function.

As soon as treatment was initiated, both Dennie and Jim were admitted to a surgical unit. During

This case is based upon the experience of a burned patient followed and described by Marie Ray. At the time, Miss Ray was Assistant Professor of Nursing, College of Nursing, Wayne State University, Detroit, Michigan, and a Clinical Specialist for surgical patients in the general hospital to which Mr. Allen was admitted.

This chapter was revised by Norma Peters Thomas, R.N., M.S., Visiting Lecturer, College of Nursing, Southeastern Massachusetts University, North Dartmouth, Massachusetts.

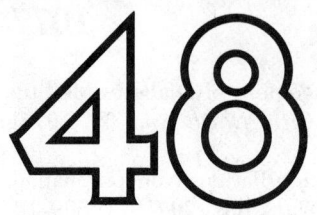

the night Dennie had a nasogastric tube inserted and was subsequently transferred to the burn unit. It has been well established that successful burn treatment is related to the availability of special burn facilities (Are Our Burn Facilities Insufficient, 1973).

Any significant burn should be treated at a burn center. A burn center is a collection of interested people (Stahl, 1977). In 1978, the American Burn Association compiled a list of burn care treatment centers. Dennie was fortunate this general hospital had such a special burn unit.

The Extent of Burn Injury

Mr. Dennie Allen had sustained second- (partial thickness) and third-degree (full thickness) burns over about 40 per cent of his body. Figure 48-1 demonstrates the affected areas: face, head, hands, abdomen, legs, and thighs. Although it does not show in Figure 48-1, he also had blisters of the palate, which made swallowing painful for several days after injury. Because he had facial burns, tracheal burns were considered to be a possibility, and a tracheostomy was considered but was determined to be unnecessary as he showed no evidence of respiratory distress. Estimates of body surface burned vary with age-related differences in body surface. Figure 48-2 presents a guide to burn estimation that provides for age-related differences; Mr. Allen's burns are indicated.

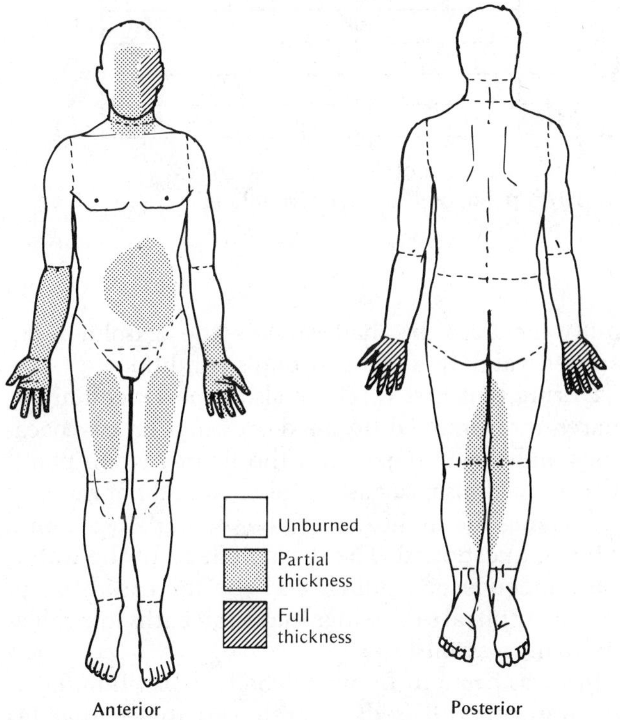

Figure 48-1. Distribution of burns of Mr. Allen's body surface

Physical examination on admission revealed a slender, well-nourished black male adolescent weighing 120 lb (55 kg), about 5 ft, 6 in tall, with generalized edema, especially of his face and hands; second- and third-degree burns of face; blisters of the palate; eyelids swollen closed, and difficulty manipulating his mouth; second-degree burns of anterior neck and lower thorax; third-degree burns of left abdomen; second- and third-degree burns of right forearm with blister formation; third-degree burns of both hands; and second- or third-degree burns of anterior and medial aspects of both thighs.

The following history was obtained from Dennie and his family during the first few weeks of hospitalization.

Age: 14 years (11–21–57).
Marital status: Single.
Father: Living and well, employed for 25 years at an auto plant. Sometimes worked two jobs. Visited seldom because of working two jobs.
Mother: Living and well; housewife.
Siblings: Five (two married siblings).
Occupation: Unemployed student, grade 9A—Junior High School.
Health insurance: CHA (Community Health Association).
Living accommodations: Single home, all family living in home, except married siblings.
Significant persons: Mother, father, friend (Jim Knight).
Religion: Baptist.
Medical history: Free of significant illness. Allergic to procaine penicillin procainamide, possibly all of "caine" family. Previously reacted with polyarthritis and pericarditis. (No record of why he had received penicillin.)
Personal habits: Enjoyed sports (basketball), television, and socializing with friends. No smoking, drinking, or drugs. Expressed wish to be a lawyer in the future.

Table 48-1 (see end of chapter) summarizes and emphasizes the pathophysiologic changes that occurred in Mr. Allen because of his burns and specifies the medical therapy instituted and the nursing care required. Because little reference is made in the table to Mr. Allen's behavior, it is necessary to present here a brief description of his psychological response to his injury and subsequent hospitalization. Mr. Allen was admitted to the special burn unit the afternoon after his arrival at general hospital, and remained in that unit throughout the period of hospitalization to which most of this discussion relates.

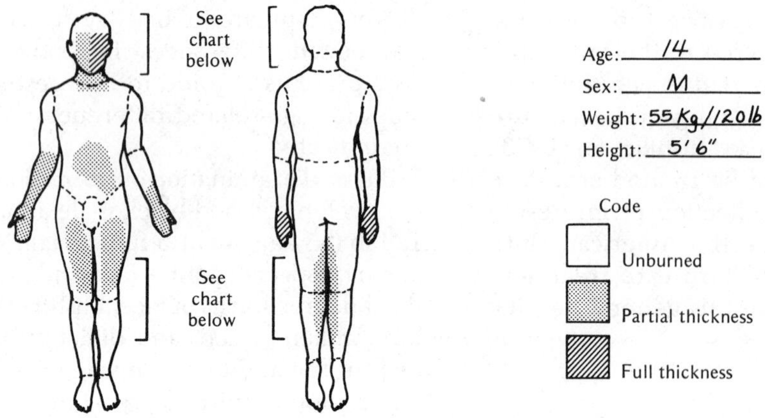

Area	Inf.	1–4	5–9	10–14	15	Adult	Part	Full	Total	Donor Areas
Head	19	17	13	11	9	7		11		
Neck	2	2	2	2	2	2	2			
Ant. trunk	13	13	13	13	13	13				
Post. trunk	13	13	13	13	13	13				
R. buttock	2½	2½	2½	2½	2½	2½				
L. buttock	2½	2½	2½	2½	2½	2½				
Genitalia	1	1	1	1	1	1				
R.U. arm	4	4	4	4	4	4				
L.U. arm	4	4	4	4	4	4				
R.L. arm	3	3	3	3	3	3	3			
L.L. arm	3	3	3	3	3	3				
R. hand	2½	2½	2½	2½	2½	2½		2½		
L. hand	2½	2½	2½	2½	2½	2½		2½		
R. thigh	5½	6½	8	8½	9	9½	8½			
L. thigh	5½	6½	8	8½	9	9½	8½			
R. leg	5	5	5½	6	6½	7	6			
L. leg	5	5	5½	6	6½	7	6			
R. foot	3½	3½	3½	3½	3½	3½				
L. foot	3½	3½	3½	3½	3½	3½				
					TOTAL		34	16		

Figure 48-2. Burn estimate diagram. (Adapted with permission of The C. V. Mosby Co. from *Nursing Care of the Patient with Burns,* 1976, p. 56, by Florence Greenhouse Jacoby.)

Psychological Responses of the Patient, His Family, and the Staff

During the first postburn week, Mr. Allen exhibited an egocentricity and constriction of interest that was graphically illustrative of regressive adaptation; as mentioned previously, he never lost consciousness, and during this first week his overwhelming concern was, "What does my face look like?" He also asked repeatedly about the condition of Jim, who had been admitted to another unit with burns of one arm and both legs. Repeatedly, he was told that his friend was doing well. Nevertheless he continued to ask and requested to see Jim. Dennie felt guilty because he had spilled the gasoline. He wanted validation of his friend's condition.

During that first week he also experienced nightmares and removed his head dressings on two occasions and threw objects on the floor. At one point, he removed his nasogastric tube. He did not remember having the nightmares. The use of daily tubbing is being questioned. The drying effects of the water, the incidence of chilling, and the increased use of wet silver nitrate dressings make tub baths less valuable than previously.

Jim was brought by wheelchair to visit him. Dennie was very pleased and relieved to see that his friend was indeed well.

However, even though the nurse had described

Dennie's facial burns to Jim in preparation for the visit, Jim would not look directly at Dennie and said very little. Dennie's trust and confidence in the ability of others to see through his appearance to the person within was constantly being challenged. Whenever he met someone for the first time, his eyes were riveted on the newcomer's face to detect any hint of revulsion or rejection.

A burn patient suffers physiological stresses plus gross psychological insult (Psychic Survival, 1978). A major burn with its airways, tubes, IVs, bandaging, and restrictions exemplifies sensory deprivation in its purest form. The patient elects to meet the trauma in an adaptive or maladaptive manner. Whatever the patient does, he or she needs great inner resources. It is the scarring damage to self-esteem and the reminder when looking in other people's eyes, that he or she is different, perhaps even repulsive, that is harder to bear than the physical pain. It's no picnic out there—society is cruel (Kelleher, 1980).

Jim visited two or three times a week, until his own discharge from the hospital. Gradually he had become more talkative and less reticent with Dennie. After Jim's first visit, Dennie became more concerned about himself, the extent of his facial burns and the burns of his hands. He expressed his concern by asking, "How bad are my burns?" "Am I going to heal?" At this point, the explanation of daily baths, débridement, and application of $AgNO_3$ (silver nitrate cream) was given. He continued to ask all of the staff and his family the same questions about his hands and face for some time. During the fifth week of his hospitalization, Mr. Allen experienced a great deal of anxiety prior to going to the operating room (OR). He was taken to the OR six times for débridement, pig skin application, and split thickness graft application. Upon interview, it was found that he feared being alone in pain after each débridement and grafting. The pain was greatest during his baths and after each trip to the OR. His mother or a staff member would sit with him after each surgical procedure. Also, his pain medication was given as liberally as ordered.

His mother and grandmother were constant visitors, and both were very helpful, especially during explanations of care, such as the part that bathing and silver nitrate play in the healing process of burns, or the part that protein plays in the healing process. They would validate the explanations by nodding their heads and using the same explanation during subsequent questioning by the patient. All of this family had difficulty assisting Dennie to tolerate his pain. They often came to the nurses' station requesting pain medication and became upset when his medication was not due.

The family is most supportive to the patient by having realistic expectations. The nursing staff's attitude is highly contagious and highly visible. Their unquestioning support is vital.

By the fifth week, Mr. Allen had begun to develop contractures and scarring of his eyelids, mouth, hands, and legs. Physical therapy had been involved with him from the beginning of hospitalization. Active and passive exercises had been instituted, along with night splints for both hands. The problem of contractures and scarring continued throughout the remaining days of his hospitalization and after discharge.

As was mentioned earlier, the Physical Medicine and Rehabilitation (PM & R) Department was involved with the care of the patient early in his hospitalization. The therapists ordered and applied splints for both arm and hands. The splints were applied nightly and removed during the day so that he might use his hands to feed and help care for himself. Burn gloves were used instead of hand dressings. $AgNO_3$ cream is placed inside of a soft material glove and the glove is placed over the burned hands. With this technique, the patient may use his hands. Also the PM & R Department prescribed exercises. The patient carried out the exercises while in the tub and every 2 hours during the day. His mother assisted him with his exercises a great deal of the time. In searching for a solution to the problem of scarring and contractures, one of the PM & R therapists found that at the Shriners' Burn Institute in Galveston, Texas, hypertrophic scar formation was being prevented by the application of constant pressure to the healing areas. The pressure can be applied by splints, bandages, and tight-fitting stretch fabric garments. To be effective in reducing scarring, the bandages or garments must be worn 24 hours a day. If removed, the bandages should be replaced within 1 hour. As long as the scar remains hyperemic and firm, the pressure should be continued. The following explanation has been offered for the effectiveness of constant pressure in reducing scarring (Making the Least of Burn Scars, 1972).

> Fibroblasts initiate a contraction in the early healing wound that results, first, in the buckling of collagen, and, later, in the formation of nodules. As the disoriented collagen develops intermolecular cross-linking, the scar becomes stable and resistant. . . . The application of pressure, then, tends to elongate the fibroblasts and to keep the collagen in its normal parallel pattern as it stabilizes.

Even mature collagen can be remodeled by prolonged external force. Dennis Allen wore Ace bandages over his extremities, hands, and trunk continuously except for bathing times; however, the ace bandages were difficult to manage. His mother and older brother were taught how to bathe him and wrap the bandages.

Mr. Dennis Allen was discharged using ace bandages, and returned to the PM & R Clinic for therapy once a week. Soon after discharge, he was measured by the Jobst Company and a complete body suit—including a face mask (similar to a ski mask)—was made.[1] When pressure is applied to healing tissue, hypertrophic scarring can be greatly reduced. The completely healed skin is fairly smooth and flexible. The Jobst garment applies constant pressure for a long time. It is a specially designed elastic woven material that provides tridimensional control with normal movement.

Family and staff feared that the experience of seeing himself in the body suit the first time would be traumatic to Dennie. The day finally came when he was confronted with the completed body suit. After working for some time to get the suit on, he stood before the mirror for a while, then suddenly jumped into a Jose Greco pose and stamped his heels against the floor. Everyone breathed a sigh of relief; he had accepted the suit and hood. Dennie had one bad incident when he visited the corner store in his neighborhood with some friends. A young man teased him about his "Captain Marvel" suit and asked him to take off his "mask." Dennie explained the reason for and purpose of the mask, but his doubting tormentor proceeded to pull off the mask. After having seen that he had indeed been burned, and what the scars looked like, his playmates no longer viewed him as a marvel.

He has returned to school, and continues to be seen in PM & R Clinic. He has ahead of him a long series of plastic surgery procedures to release contractures and improve facial scars.

Acceptance of the Role of a Sick Person

In most respects, Mr. Allen fulfilled the role of a patient that is expected in our culture. When he became ill, he was provided with, and accepted, medical treatment. He surrendered his independence and decision-making prerogatives to medical and paramedical personnel. Although he was very ill, he cooperated by making progress toward recovery. As he improved physically, he accepted the care that was necessary. He expressed his appreciation to those who cared for him and followed the instructions (orders) of the professional staff explicitly and without question. As his condition improved, his behavior began to deviate from that expected of the person in the sick role, that is, despite his verbal assertions that he desired to regain independence and mobility, he frequently whined during treatments and the onset of activity, was easily discouraged and would allow others to do for him things that he had previously been able to manage slowly by himself, and made many requests of personnel. The high tolerance of nurses for deviant behavior of persons in the sick role because of severe burns seems to be a common phenomenon. Davitz and Pendleton found that nurses inferred the greatest degree of suffering in patients who had been burned and consequently might be expected to empathize more with burned patients than with patients having other illnesses (Davitz & Pendleton, 1969). The approval that was accorded Mr. Allen by those responsible for his care may have been caused in part by the fact that his family also behaved as relatives are expected to behave in our culture. His father, mother, grandmother, and brother all served as a strong stabilizing force in helping to maintain Mr. Allen's psychological equilibrium throughout the severe physiologic and psychological stress to which he had been subjected. The general tenor of verbal and written comments of nursing staff throughout Mr. Allen's hospitalization suggests their acceptance, empathy, and high tolerance for his prolonged dependency.

The patient must learn to live with what he or she has, and must be allowed to recognize and mourn his or her losses—included in that mourning are the demands, the complaints, and the uncooperativeness. The staff cannot allow itself the privilege of rejection of what is actually normal behavior in the psychic survival of the burn patient (Psychic Survival, 1978).

Physiologic Responses

Table 48-1 describes the cellular, neuroendocrine, cardiovascular, renal, pulmonary, and metabolic responses to severe burn injury. Coagulation problems also are increased in a burn injury. The coagulation process is disturbed, thromboplastin is released, fibrinogen is then released by injured platelets, and venous stasis occurs along with intravasular clump-

[1] Pictures of stretch fabric garments and wrappings that may be applied to burn wounds in various parts of the body to control scarring can be seen in B. A. Wills et al., "Positioning and Splinting the Burned Patient," *Heart & Lung*, 2 (Sept.–Oct., 1973), 696–706.

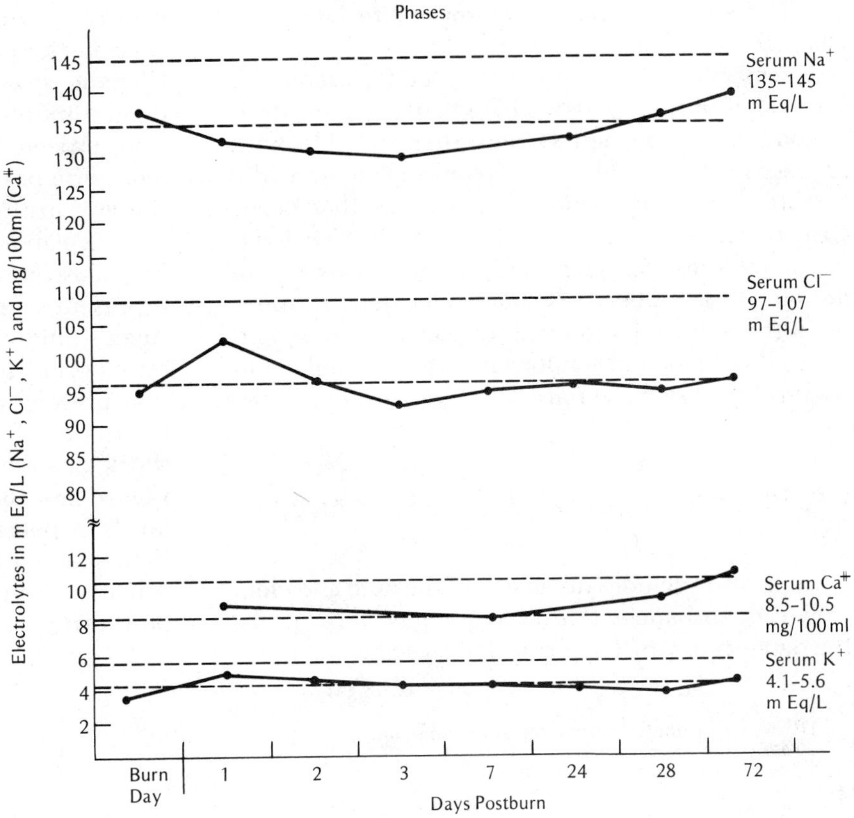

Figure 48-3. Serum levels of potassium, calcium, chloride, and sodium for 72 days post-burn for Mr. Allen.

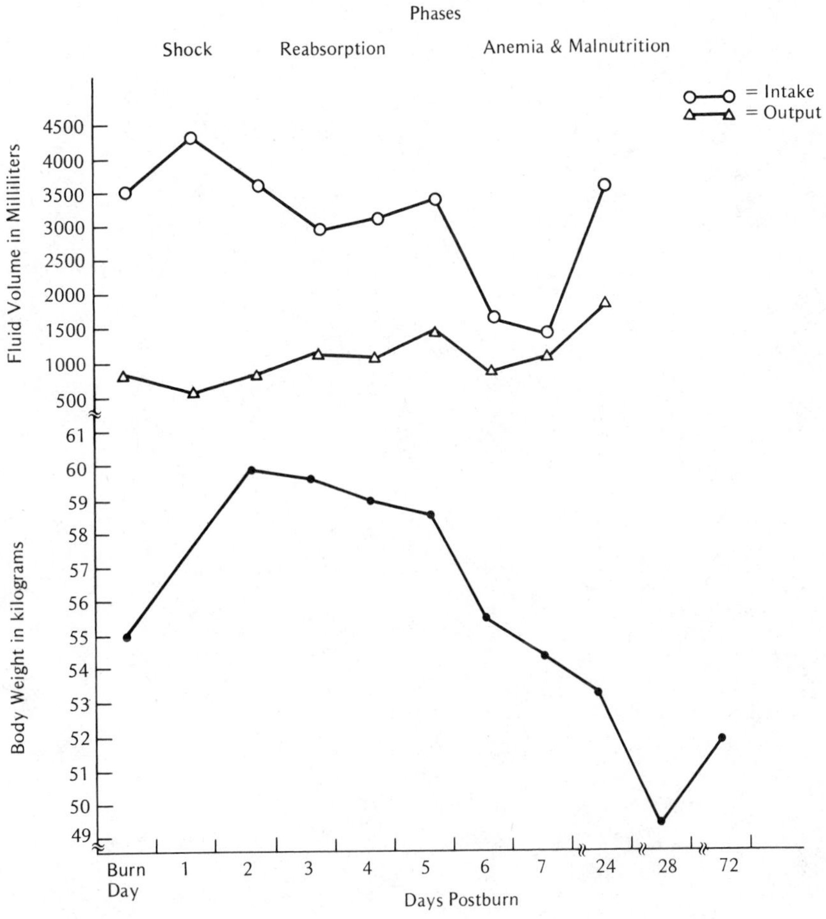

Figure 48-4. Fluid intake, urinary output, and body weight recordings for 72 days post-burn for Mr. Allen.

ing. The entire process may progress to DIC[2] (see Chapter 42) (Busby, 1979).

As expected by formulas developed for predicting survival of burned patients based on age and extent of body surface burned, Dennis Allen was able, with aggressive treatment, to overcome all of the life-threatening injuries and complications that occur with thermal burns (Artz, et al., 1979). The long-term problems of physical and psychological rehabilitation persist. Their resolution will depend more upon the determination and courage of Dennis, and upon the love and understanding of family and friends than upon the miracles of modern medicine.

Fluid and Electrolyte Disturbances

Table 48-1 includes discussion of the fluid and electrolyte disturbances that accompany severe burns; the dangers to which a person is exposed when there is disruption of the integrity of the skin and alterations in the defense mechanisms of the respiratory tract; hazards to a person's convalescence from prolonged immobilization; and alterations in metabolism, especially of proteins, in the immediate and long-term postburn period. In each case the medical therapy instituted for Mr. Allen is presented, and there is elaboration of actions indicated for the nurse. Two illustrations have been developed to graphically represent some of the most significant aspects of Mr. Allen's fluid and electrolyte status during the postburn period, to assist the reader in applying information presented in Table 48-1 to the condition and treatment of Mr. Allen during the phases of burn shock, reabsorption, and anemia and malnutrition. Figure 48-3 presents a summary of selected serum levels of potassium, calcium, chloride, and sodium; Figure 48-4 presents a summary of his fluid intake, urinary output, and body weights during the same postburn period.

[2] DIC = disseminated intravascular coagulation.

TABLE 48-1 ***Physiologic Changes, Medical Prescription, and Nursing Intervention***

Changes	Medical Prescriptions	Nursing Intervention
General Description of Physiologic Events that Follow Severe Thermal Trauma		
The end results of the complex, interrelated consequences of thermal trauma are a reduction in plasma and extracellular volume, the development of acidosis, swelling of erythrocytes, elevated hematocrit, microcirculatory stasis, decreased cardiac output, circulatory failure with fall in blood pressure, and decreasing renal blood flow. Medical therapy is aimed at averting, modifying, or correcting these abnormal physiologic conditions. Sequence of events is generally as follows: 1. Heat injures cells. 2. Injured cells lose K^+ (as well as Mg^{2+} and PO_4^{2-}) and acquire Na^+. 3. Intracellular enzymes such as proteases, thromboplastin, and various "toxic factors" are released or produced. ATP is converted to ADP and ultimately to inorganic PO_4^{2-} and adenine nucleotides. Histamine is released and its production increased. Damaged cells are anoxic. Tissue perfusion is depressed by blockage of the microcirculation secondary to erythrocyte aggregation by platelet adhesion enhanced by ADP and by formation of microthrombi. Blood viscosity is also increased by these factors plus released tissue thromboplastin and hypercoagulability of the blood. Microcirculatory stasis develops locally and at a distance from the site of trauma, leading to cellular anoxia and resultant metabolic acidosis. Acidosis reduces renal blood flow. If the elevated P_{CO_2} of respiratory acidosis is superimposed on the reduced bicarbonate concentration of metabolic acidosis, intracellular pH can become dangerously low, leading to rapid and sudden death. 4. The acquisition of Na^+ by injured cells reduces the tonicity of the extracellular fluid; this, together with the increasing H^+ concentration of cells, causes uninjured cells to imbibe water. The intracellular gain in water from hypotonic extracellular fluid has been demonstrated to result in decrease in plasma volume without prior "plasma loss."	Three requirements of an effective burn regimen: 1. Replacement of Na^+ and water gained by the injured tissues. 2. Neutralization of an increased H^+ concentration (metabolic acidosis) and restoration of both bicarbonate and P_{CO_2} to normal. 3. Reduction in the viscosity and hypercoagulability of the blood (Busby, 1979).	Acquire operational knowledge of the physiologic events that follow severe thermal trauma. Observe for: *Dehydration* Thirst Dry mucosa Decreased turgor of intact skin Decreased salivation Weight loss Decreased urine output Elevated temperature Elevated hematocrit Increased pulse Increased specific gravity of urine Soft tongue *Hyponatremia* Muscle weakness or cramps Apathy Tremors Anorexia Decreased turgor of intact skin Increased pulse Decreased blood pressure and pulse pressure Orthostatic hypotension *Hypokalemia* Anorexia Nausea and vomiting Abdominal distention Paralytic ileus Muscle weakness Absent or weak deep tendon reflexes Depressed sensorium

(Continued)

TABLE 48-1 *(Continued)*

Changes	Medical Prescriptions	Nursing Intervention
5. Plasma constituents, some ions, and some protein molecules accumulate in zones of injury; their transport, via the lymphatics, is greatly increased. Edema represents the influx into the zones of injury of Na^+ and water in isotonic proportions like extracellular fluid; thus the total "loss" of Na^+ in the edema fluid, plus that exchanged for cellular K^+, exceeds the "loss" of edema water into injured tissues. Reduction not only in plasma volume but also in "functioning" extracellular volume follows. The fact is that plasmapheresis (massive removal of plasma protein without salt and water) does not cause shock; plasma protein levels of 1.0 g/100 ml or lower may prevail with no signs of shock. In marked contrast, removal of Na^+ promptly leads to shock and circulatory collapse. Edema formation is mediated in part by bradykinin produced by the tissue proteases. If blisters are formed, some plasma proteins may be contained therein. Thinking is divided as to treatment of blisters. Some say leave them alone as they provide a sterile dressing. Others may break the blisters and apply antibiotic ointment to reduce the possibility of infection. Some plasma proteins accumulate in the edema fluid at the site of injury, with cell proteins entering the circulation, but specific "plasma loss" is a minor fraction of the total fluid shift. Actually, the plasma protein concentration is supranormal (8.0–8.5 g/100 ml) soon after the burn, before fluid therapy, caused by Na^+ depletion, reflecting the movement of water out of the plasma (Pruitt, April 1979). 6. A consequence of reduction in extracellular fluid volume is augmentation of aldosterone activity, resulting in Na^+ retention and cellular K^+ loss manifested by urine low in Na^+ but high in K^+. In addition, Cl^- excretion, especially after infusion of NaCl, is relatively suppressed. The resulting metabolic acidosis inhibits the normal vasomotor response to catecholamines, which are produced in supernormal amounts and appear in the urine with bradykinin. Angiotensin II may also be produced, or activated, in small but sufficient amounts to cause intense renal vasoconstriction and stimulate the extrarenal response of increased aldosterone secretion. These factors, as well as metabolic acidosis, all contribute to a decreased renal blood flow. The metabolic acidosis arises from several sources. Following tissue destruction produced by thermal trauma, PO_4^{2-} and other intracellular acidic anions are released. These, together with lactic acid and other acids, which accumulate		*Metabolic acidosis* Depressed level of consciousness, some degree of disorientation General malaise Dull headache Abdominal pain Nausea and vomiting Kussmaul respirations Elevated P_{CO_2} Decreased blood pH

during intervals of impaired circulation and tissue anoxia, flow into the blood. They cause metabolic acidosis characterized by reduction in plasma HCO_3^-. The blood pH will fall until hyperpnea can ventilate the CO_2 produced, and decrease the P_{CO_2} below normal, to restore the 20:1 ratio of bicarbonate/carbonic acid.

7. Frequently the free egress of CO_2 is impeded by actual damage to the airways or by edema of face, nose, and especially the neck, and the P_{CO_2} becomes elevated above normal. If P_{CO_2} remains elevated despite assisted ventilation, a normal pH can be obtained only by compensated elevation in bicarbonate. There is a limit to the buffering capacity of the elevated plasma bicarbonate and hence mechanical ventilatory aids and perhaps tracheostomy may be necessary (Monafo, 1971).

Mr. Allen's Admission to Emergency Hospital:

Mr. A was considered to be critically burned according to the starred items in the following criteria:

1. Critical burns.
   *a. Burns complicated by respiratory tract injury.
   b. Partial-thickness burns of more than 30% of body surface.
   *c. Full-thickness burns of *face, hands,* feet, genitalia, or *more than 10% of body surface.*
   d. Burns complicated by fractures or major soft-tissue injury.
   e. Electrical burns.
2. Moderate burns.
   a. Partial-thickness burns of 15 to 30% of body surface.
   b. Full-thickness burns less than 10% of body surface, provided the hands, face, or genitalia are not involved.
3. Minor burns.
   a. Partial-thickness of less than 15% of body surface.
   b. Full-thickness of less than 2% of body surface (Artz et al., 1979).

Intensive supportive care is needed at this time. Intramuscular or subcutaneous narcotics in the first hour postburn are anathema: you'll just need to ventilate the patient once IVs are begun and circulation picks up that storehouse of narcotic that was given and didn't go anywhere because of venous stasis. Remember that major burns do not have much pain because of deadened nerve endings.

(Continued)

TABLE 48-1 *(Continued)*

Changes	Medical Prescriptions	Nursing Intervention
Extent of Mr. A's burn was estimated as shown in Figure 48-2. The initial estimate of the type and amount of fluids to be administered to Mr. A in the first 48 hours was calculated by the Brooke formula, according to the severity of the burn: 1. 0.5 ml of colloid per kg of body weight for each 1% of body surface burned. 2. 1.5 ml of electrolyte (crystalloid) solution per kg of body weight for each 1% of body surface burned. 3. 2,000 ml of glucose in water (Artz et al., 1979).	Intravenous fluids for the first 24 hours: 5,000 ml Colloid: Albumin Crystalloid: Ringer's Lactate Water: 5% dextrose in water	If using the rule of nines, remember that the palm of your hand is 1% of your body surface. In clear, unexcited, low tones explain to Mr. A—whether or not he asks or seems frightened—that he will have 1. Two tubes into his shoulder veins by which to feed him for a while. 2. A tube into his bladder to be sure of how his kidneys are working. 3. Medication to ease the pain and help him relax.
When the skin is burned, cells are damaged, there is an increase in capillary permeability, and plasma seeps very rapidly into and out of the burn area. This plasma, the fluid portion of blood, contains crystalloids or electrolytes and colloids, that is, albumin and globulin. Even though protein in the plasma is leaking out, it remains questionable whether it should be replaced with serum albumin or plasmanate. The serum albumin from both of these replacements appears to leak out into the tissue and may actually hold fluid in the pulmonary area. Therefore, in the first 24-hour period it's safer to treat with protein free IVs and give albumin in the second 24-hour period when the body system has tightened up (Stahl, 1977). The burned patient has lost integrity of the semipermeable membrane. Use of plasma or whole blood or colloids is probably wasteful since they will only seep into the extracellular space and be lost. However, by using Ringer's lactate, which closely resembles extracellular fluid, we can perfuse the body until the integrity of the semipermeable membrane has been restored. This usually happens 18 to 24 hours after the burn (Gillespie, 1979). There is no formula that can replace careful medical and nursing supervision on an individualized basis.		Set up two independent intravenous injection setups with prescribed solutions, placing one on each side of Mr. A. Prepare a central venous pressure (CVP) set to attach to one of the conduit systems. Set up a male catheterization tray for physician, or if he is occupied with crucial tasks, obtain a qualified male attendant. Insert a rectal probe and attach it to the battery-powered box, which registers continuous temperatures. Take either pedal, femoral, carotid, or supraclavicular pulses, because of the location of Mr. A's burns. When taking CVP readings, have the bed flat. Connect indwelling urinary catheter to sterile drainage set and a sterile, stable, calibrated collecting reservoir. A urinometer that operates automatically every hour is ideal. First urine may be chocolate brown or red due to hemoglobin pigment released into plasm by destroyed red blood cells.
Fluid and Electrolytes Clinical shock is a preventable syndrome, provided adequate therapy can be instituted soon after injury. Patients with burns exceeding 10–15% of body surface receive the fluid equivalent of approximately 10% of body weight, or 100 ml/kg. This is given initially at the rate of at least 500 ml hourly, and more slowly subsequently depending on the status of the patient. A patient weighing 60 kg would thus receive at least 6,000 ml of fluid in the first 24 hours. Of this, slightly more than half would be given in the first 12 hours (Stahl, 1977).	Foley to urinometer: Measure and record every hour. Vital signs ever hour. Central venous pressure every 2 hours.	The easiest way to monitor fluid replacement is by monitoring renal function on a 24-hour flow sheet. Be sure connecting drainage tubing is free of any obstruction that will interfere with free gravity flow and that collecting reservoir is protected against being turned over or broken (e.g., if a bottle is used, suspend from bed frame). Be sure measurement is done in a receptacle with calibrations of at least as fine as 5 ml.

Mr. A arrived at General Hospital one-half hour after he was burned. To ensure that he would receive uninterrupted fluid and electrolyte therapy essential to the early management of his burns, two percutaneous intracatheters were inserted, one in each of his subclavian veins. Because changes in body fluids are reflected by changes in body weight, it is of the utmost importance to monitor the patient's weight frequently, regardless of the severity of illness. Replacement therapy of burn patients cannot be undertaken blindly. The guidelines available from measurements of body weight, blood pH, urine output, and serum and urine electrolytes are of proved value in preventing the patient from being drowned with fluid (Stahl, 1977). Mr. A was watched closely for signs of renal failure, which fortunately never developed; the lowest urine volume he exhibited during the shock phase was 530 ml/24 hours on the first postburn day. There are many possible and interrelated causes of renal failure in the burn patient, but the major one is low plasma volume. Others include pigment load from intravascular hemolysis and muscle necrosis, toxins, endotoxemia, and preexisting renal disease (Sevitt, 1979). Close observation of the pattern of CVP readings must accompany notation of hourly urine outputs, as they are intimately related. Pulmonary edema with normal CVP is possible but rare. The upper limit of safety varies with the individual patient; 20 cm of water is high (measured from a point 4 cm below the anterior chest wall at the sternal angle) and 30 cm of water is very high. Patients with valvular cardiac disease and invasive gram-negative sepsis appear to tolerate and require a higher CVP than others. Rate of rise is a better guide than absolute level. If an aliquot of 200 ml of plasma given in 30 min causes the venous pressure to increase by 5 cm of water, its absolute value being greater than 10 cm of water, there is probably no immediate need for further volume replacement (Sevitt, 1979). Remember that the CVP does not tell when too much fluid is taxing the heart. As an indicator of left heart performance a PAWP is necessary (See Chapter 45). As the physicians in the emergency room were establishing access for intravenous replacement, they were simultaneously evaluating his respiratory status. They made the decision not to perform a tracheostomy, despite his face and neck burns, but to watch him closely for any signs of obstruction. At no time did Mr. A require either intubation or a tracheostomy, except for purposes of administering anesthesia later in his postburn course when grafting procedures were performed in the operating room, after the third burn day.	Weigh stat. and q.d.	Unless otherwise instructed, volumes of less than 30 ml or greater than 50 ml/hour should be reported stat. to the physician. Measure and record specific gravity every hour or as often as cumulative hourly volumes enable the urinometer to float. A concentration in excess of 1.020–1.030 may indicate progressive hemoconcentration and should be reported. Note character of the urine for: Deepening amber color Pink tinge (blood ?) Casts, sediment (albumin or cells ?) Odor

(Continued)

TABLE 48-1 *(Continued)*

Changes	Medical Prescriptions	Nursing Intervention
Pulmonary Complications Burn treatment, especially in burn centers, is quite sophisticated as well as successful. Aggressive fluid therapy and correct usage of topical and systemic antibiotics ensure survival of most patients in the early stages of burn injury. More and more patients, however, survive only to develop pulmonary complications. Despite the term, respiratory burn, there is little evidence to support the existence of thermal coagulation necrosis of the tracheobronchial tree as a clinical or pathological entity in the absence of steam or readily combustible vapors or gases. Reflex closure of the glottis, the cooling effect of the upper airway, and the poor heat-carrying capacity of air all account for the protection of the respiratory tree. Even though the respiratory tract is not burned, the smoke and toxic gases that are incomplete products of combustion are potent chemical irritants to the respiratory mucosa. Mucosal and submucosal swelling results in obstruction of varying degrees. Bronchial wheezing and rales can be heard. These symptoms, however, can appear anywhere from 2 to 3 days to 2 to 3 weeks postburn. Facial burns of any degree should suggest the possibility of pulmonary involvement. A burned lung will not show on admission x-ray. Schall et al. have shown that a Xenon Lung Scan used in a variety of other pulmonary diseases may prove to be an early warning system in burned lung (Scan for a Scorched Lung, 1979). Early treatment of pulmonary complications is imperative. Unlike pneumonia, the acute respiratory distress syndrome involves the development of pulmonary exudate and loss of surfactant activity, which impairs gas exchange and reduces pulmonary compliance (Pulmonary Burns, 1977). Postmortem pathological findings in the respiratory tree seem to be related to prolonged positive pressure ventilatory assistance with oxygen. Major trauma and shock have been shown to cause decreases in surfactant, with resultant atelectasis causing alterations in diffusion and perfusion. (See Chapter 45.) If there is doubt as to involvement of the pulmonary tract, fall in P_{O_2} or a rise in P_{CO_2} will indicate the need for improving ventilation. In contrast, a falling plasma bicarbonate concentration will indicate need for additional sodium bicarbonate solution rather than the balanced electrolyte solution with which fluid replacement therapy is begun (Morton, 1979).	Cough, deep breathe frequently. Chest x-ray two times per week.	Observe for signs of pulmonary edema: Increased restlessness Cyanosis of toenail beds, feet, conjunctival sac Increase in moist, labored respirations Complaints of feeling of chest constriction, desire to sit up Marked increase in pulse Alteration (possible decrease) in blood pressure Increased CVP Hemoptysis On admission, observe for: Singed nasal hairs Clean inside as well as outside of nose. Blackened rim of nares, especially when adjacent skin is not burned Rapid, noisy respirations—as wind passing over a dry reed Dry, wracking cough Cyanosis of unburned skin and toenail beds[3] Rales Black particles and/or blood in sputum Know location and operation of: Oxygen equipment Respirators Laryngoscope Endotracheal tubes Tracheostomy set Aspirator Measure and record the circumference of the neck q.4.h. (Mr. A's increased 1 in. the first 24 hours; despite this, he was able to breathe adequately unassisted and without tracheostomy.) Stimulate cough reflex with tip of suction catheter, which should not be passed into the trachea below the larynx or into the bronchi but only to the point of stimulating the patient to cough. Use scrupulous surgical aseptic technique in handling the suction catheter. Asceptic technique in everything. Foley catheter, IVs, cut downs, N/G tubes.

Impaired respiratory mechanics and obstruction of the upper airway are the two most critical indications for tracheostomy and/or ventilation. Otherwise, even in the presence of facial and neck burns, singed nasal hairs, and a history of smoke inhalation, the decision for tracheostomy should be deferred (Pruitt, April 1979).

Patients with smoke inhalation may demonstrate immediate or delayed hoarseness or begin expectorating sooty mucus. Humidification is strongly recommended, preferably with ultrasonic nebulizers, which provide very fine water particles less than 5 μ in diameter, which can reach the lower bronchial tree. The hyperventilation of burned patients can quickly desiccate the tracheobronchial mucosa (Pruitt, April 1979).

Deep breathing and coughing should be encouraged frequently. Occasionally, instillation of saline through a percutaneous tracheal catheter effectively stimulates the cough reflex. Direct suctioning down the tracheobronchial tree produces considerable trauma and irritation of an already inflamed mucosa. Whether through the nasal route or directly through the tracheostomy, suctioning should be performed *gently*. The most important part of the endotracheal aspiration is the stimulation of the cough reflex. As the patient brings the secretions up high in the trachea, they should then be gently aspirated. Vigorous and deep probing of stiff catheters down the tracheobronchial tree is to be condemned (Jacoby, 1976).

Progressive activity, especially ambulation when burned surfaces do not include the feet, should begin even during the early postburn period as one of the best means of preventing pulmonary complications.

Enthusiasm for the use of intermittent positive pressure breathing must be tempered with caution, as these devices are potential sources of infection (Jacoby, 1976).

The simple act of washing hands is the one most effective means of combating infection.

Instruct Mr. A to deep breathe and cough (starred items were not feasible with Mr. A because of the location of his burns):

*1. Inspire against pressure of nurse's hands on anterolateral surface of thorax.
*2. Expire forcibly, with assistance of nurse's hands, to compress thorax as completely as possible.
3. After a sequence of exchanges, cough at the onset of the expiratory phase.
4. Have tissue over Mr. A's nose and mouth before he coughs.
5. Instruct, demonstrate, and supervise him in the use of blow bottles.

Help Mr. A learn how, and how much, to move himself in bed. (More details in relation to mobility problems).

Because Mr. A had no involvement of his feet, he was helped to stand and shift his weight from one foot to the other by the fourth postburn day.

(Continued)

TABLE 48-1 *(Continued)*

Changes	Medical Prescriptions	Nursing Intervention
Skin and Vascular Problems Although age and general physical condition prior to the thermal injury influence mortality in major burns, the ultimate determining factor in survival is the burn wound itself. Both the depth and extent of the burn are critical. The characteristic pathological lesion caused by thermal injury is coagulation necrosis. Before healing can be complete, this necrotic tissue must be sloughed and replaced by skin. If only a portion of the thickness of skin is involved, then regeneration of skin can take place from remaining epidermal elements. If the full thickness of skin is destroyed, healing of the wound will require the use of skin grafts. As indicated previously, Mr. A had full-thickness burns of over 10% of his body surface. Prior to the final healing of the burn wound, the effects of thermal injury on the skin covering of the patient are major factors influencing ultimate survival. The chemical and physical alterations in the skin render this organ incapable of serving its function in the overall body homeostasis. The vapor barrier capacity of the skin, which preserves the aqueous milieu of the body, is an important quality of normal skin. The keratinized superficial skin layers and the lipids within the skin normally prevent the escape of large volumes of water. A superficial second-degree burn may destroy the keratinized surface and permit increased water vaporization. Full-thickness coagulation necrosis of the skin destroys not only the keratin but also the lipid-containing portions of the skin. The dry, full-thickness burn has practically no vapor barrier. Although to visual inspection it appears otherwise, evaporation through a dry eschar is much greater than water loss from an equal surface of wet, blistered skin. Not until full, mature epithelium, regrown or grafted, covers the wound does water vaporization return to essentially normal levels (Jouglard, et al., 1979).		Nurses must assume function of skin: By adherence to strict asepsis in every detail of nursing care, they protect the patient from infection. By regulation of the environment, they prevent loss of bodily fluids and heat. By having a nonjudgmental attitude and giving 100% support, nurses are a key factor in the patient's adjustment to cosmetic changes and decreased sensations.
Traditionally, eschar is allowed to slough off wounds at its own pace over several weeks. Now, a laser scapel and enzymes have been used for excision of dead skin, which is then replaced with a graft within a few days of the original injury (Consensus for Treatment, 1979). The laser method reduces blood loss and tissue destruction. With a large portion of the body surface burned, loss of water vapor may result in rapid dehydration of a patient. The peak period of vapor loss is between 5 and 10 days postburn. After this time, there is a gradual reduction of water loss, but evaporation continues to be greatly increased until coverage of the		Conserve heat loss, and thus energy expenditure, by creating and maintaining environmental temperature and humidity at a level that will allow Mr. A, at rest, to be in a state of thermal neutrality: 1. Collaborate with physicians, hospital engineers and architects, nursing and hospital supervisory personnel, and equipment sales representatives to develop means by which to gain more precise control over environmental temperature and humidity.

burn wound itself by skin is obtained. Because 1 sq m of full-thickness burn can lose up to 3,000 ml of water per hour, an adult with a 50% full-thickness burn can lose over 6 liters of water per day. With each liter of water requiring 560 calories for evaporation, the caloric expense of such a burn may be up to 4,000 calories for evaporation of water alone.

[The total number of calories per hour liberated by an individual is divided by total body surface area, which, for the average adult, is 1.73 sq m. This means that the basal metabolic rate is 48.3 calories/sq m/hour, or approximately 1965 calories in 24 hours (48.3 calories × 1.73 sq m × 24 hours (Guyton, 1971).] Considering that Mr. A had a 10% full-thickness burn, its caloric expense was substantially more than that required by his body surface in the unburned state. Such an enormous expenditure of energy accompanying heat loss usually results in a marked drop in body temperature, resulting in a relative hypothermia. Further energy in the form of muscular activity is then required to maintain the body temperature at anything approaching a normal thermal response. When heat loss exceeds heat production, an absolute hypothermia exists. Clinical data suggest that manipulation of the ambient temperature and water vapor pressure by more precise methods might actually permit the achievement of thermal neutrality in the burned patient (Stahl, 1977).

The flow of blood through vessels of the local area is related to the vascular alterations from the coagulative thermal injury to the burn tissue. The degree of thrombosis of the blood supply in the wound is in proportion to the intensity and duration of the heat applied. Where the heat injury has been intense, a blood coagulum without fibrin develops in the vessels. In addition, agglutination of red blood cells forms overt thrombi. Within 24 hours, the devitalized tissue at the site of the burn injury shows marked edema, without subcutaneous cellular infiltration. The obstructed circulation around a third-degree burn prevents access of blood-borne inflammatory elements to the site of injury, which is responsible for the minimal inflammatory response in the burn wound, even in the presence of infection of the devitalized tissue (Munster, 1970). After 1 week, granulation tissue begins to develop and brings with it a new blood supply but is not an effective barrier to infection for 3 weeks (Jouglard et al., 1979). In the absence of infection, the period of avascularity of the partial-thickness burn usually lasts only 24–48 hours, though circulation may be decreased for longer periods. Preservation of the deep epithelial elements from destruction by infection or ischemia prevents the conversion of second-degree burns to third-degree burns.

2. Try to maintain a temperature of 75–80°F and a humidity of 40–70%, being guided to alterations by the response of Mr. A in terms of his report of what feels comfortable, results of frequent measurements of his body temperature, and any objective evidence of shivering (Price & Wood, 1968).
3. Initiate, request, or offer to participate in multidisciplinary research on the effects of control of environmental temperature and humidity on the duration of the catabolic phase in the postburn period.
4. The Apollo cover is a canopylike transparent conductive metal that covers the body and by means of radiant heat, consistently keeps the patient's environmental temperature at optimum level for increased wound healing and decreased heat loss.

(Continued)

TABLE 48-1 *(Continued)*

Changes	Medical Prescriptions	Nursing Intervention
One of the most frequent sites of infection is related to the need of the burned patient for intravenous fluids, while the vascular system is ideally suited to the proliferation of microorganisms that may enter via any route. Approximately one fourth of patients who have had a cutdown develop some complication, ranging from mild cellulitis around the cutdown site to frank suppurative thrombophlebitis with septicemia. Although the saphenous venous system is the most common area for suppurative thrombophlebitis, sepsis has occurred from infected veins in the upper extremities as well as the external jugular system (Pruitt, May 1979). Mr. A showed no evidence of suppurative thrombophlebitis. Both subclavian intracatheters were removed by the seventh postburn day, which was considerably longer, on a continuous basis, than the recommended 72 hours.	Intracatheter 1: Discontinue on postburn day 4. Intracatheter 2: Discontinue on postburn day 7.	Observe for signs and symptoms of (suppurative) thrombophlebitis: 1. Tender vein with a red streak. 2. Pus coming from cutdown site. 3. Abscesses along the course of the vein. 4. Complaint of burning or pain along vein when intracatheter is irrigated to keep it patent. (This is probably the most sensitive and earliest symptom of inflammation of the vein.)[4]
Management of the Burn Wound Occlusive dressings are no longer recommended for major burns. Patients are frequently febrile and have little control over their temperature-regulating mechanism, and occlusive dressings interfere with heat loss. Dressings must be changed at least every 2 to 3 days, requiring general anesthetic, which interrupts the patient's oral intake. In addition, the absence of physical therapy, febrile courses, lack of daily inspection of the burn wound, and the requirement of using an operating room all weigh against occlusive dressings as the primary mode of therapy for large areas of burn (Shuck & Moncrief, 1969). For a short period postburn, the surface of the wound is generally sterile. Within 48 hours, however, bacteria appear to contaminate the surface of the wound and then colonize the depths of the eschar. The source of the contaminating bacteria is not generally agreed on. Studies of the numberous phage types of *Pseudomonas aeruginosa* that may involve the wounds of different patients on the same ward strongly suggest that this microorganism may constitute a part of a given patient's normal flora prior to injury. Thus the role of self-contamination in the pathogenesis of burn wound colonization is presently under serious consideration. Failure to prevent bacterial colonization of wounds under the most aseptic ward precautions may well lie in the problem of self-contamination of wounds by the patient's own cutaneous or fecal flora (Artz et al., 1979). The presence of bacteria within the hair follicles may prevent their detection on swab cultures of the skin surface (Artz et al., 1979).		The burn patient and his or her environment must be as sterile as possible to eliminate any reservoirs of infection. Validate with the attending physician whether or not strict medical asepsis, including gown, gloves, and masks, are required before going to the enormous preparation of such a unit. It may be that careful hand washing, careful assignment of the smallest possible number of persons to render care to the patient, and use of pHisoHex for all general hygiene will suffice. Reverse isolation to protect the patient from other patients, staff, visitors, and environment can also be used. Check with attending physician as to whether or not the patient should be shaved. If so, carry out the procedure with sterile technique and pHisoHex solution.

All hair should be shaved from the burned area and from adjacent sites of unburned skin and shaved frequently throughout the hospital course to prevent crusting and its attendant proliferating of microorganisms (Shuck & Moncrief, 1969).

Pseudomonas aeruginosa has been recognized with increasing frequency as the most prevalent colonizer and deadly invader of the burn wound. Staphylococci and certainly streptococci no longer occupy the positions of importance that they formerly held in relation to the establishment of fatal infection (Artz et al., 1979).

Any successful, objective treatment of patients with extensive burns must provide for effective wound bacteriostasis, until epithelialization is complete, impede the leak of water vapor through the wound, and permit closure of it with skin or a satisfactory substitute at the earliest possible moment (Monafo, 1971).

The ideal topical antiseptic should meet several criteria:

1. Effective clinical bacteriostasis.
2. Nonabsorbability, and therefore lack of systemic toxicity.
3. Absence of direct histotoxicity or of potent allergenicity.

One-half per cent aqueous silver nitrate solution reasonably satisfies these criteria, both hypothetically and clinically (Monafo, 1971).

Because of the disadvantages of the patient's being constantly wet, and the subsequent added heat and energy loss, silver nitrate cream or ointment base has been developed that has retained all the advantages of the active ingredient, silver nitrate, and has eliminated much of the discomfort for the patient and tediousness of application for the nursing staff of continuous wet dressings. The silver nitrate cream applied to Mr. A was in hydrophilic ointment, which contains the following ingredients:

Stearyl alcohol,	250 g
Methylparaben,	0.25 g
Prophylparaben,	0.15 g
Polyoxyl-40 stearate,	50 g
Propylene glycol,	120 g
Water	330 g[5]

Gentamycin q.8.h.
Erythromycin q.6.h.

Garamycin (Gentamycin) is an aminoglycosides drug which is an active agent for a wide variety of gram-negative bacteria. Aminoglycosides are excreted in large amounts by burn patients and so the body has low levels of aminoglycosides. The recommended dose of garamycin for use in burn patients is, therefore, substantially higher than the dose used in other disorders (The Underuse of Amphotericin, 1977).

Ointments, beside limiting infection are a good cover since only cornified epithelial cells are adapted to the desiccating effects of air. When there are no cornified cells, air hurts, so covering area with ointment allows patient to be more comfortable and less in need of analgesics.

Realize that nothing applied topically truly sterilizes the skin wound. What does happen is that bacteria decrease in number when topical antibacterials are applied. This decreased number of bacteria cannot be handled by the body's defense mechanisms. In this way, efforts can proceed to convert an open dirty wound to a closed clean wound (Artz et al., 1979). Meanwhile, the body copes since it is the degree of infection and not the presence of infection that wears away at our defenses. Again, absolute sterile technique cannot be overemphasized.

Dressings must be kept wet so that reepithelization will take place, but remember to keep the patient dry to prevent chilling. Expect difficulty in inspecting skin that is discolored black from $AgNO_3$.

(Continued)

TABLE 48-1 *(Continued)*

Changes	Medical Prescriptions	Nursing Intervention
Silver has practically no allergenic potential and a low systemic toxicity. Because of the minimum absorption of silver that occurs through burn wounds, argyria has not been observed in any patient treated in this way. The silver salts of the biologically important anions (chloride, carbonate, proteinate) are highly insoluble. This is the reason that no significant absorption of silver occurs through wounds. Application of silver nitrate to open burns results in the precipitation of silver salts on the wound. A brown or blue-black keratinous crust of these salts forms over newly healed or epithelializing surfaces and on eschar as well. Because of the insolubility of these silver salts, and because of the hypotonicity of silver nitrate, the dressing causes the leaching from the wounds of significant amounts of the serum minerals and possibly of the water-soluble vitamins and other substances. This loss into the dressing continues until the wounds are epithelialized and, for Na^+ and Cl^-, is a constant function of the surface area of open wound (Monafo, 1971).		
Burn wounds are avascular, so you need topical agents to control the number of organisms. Mafenide cream (Sulfamylon) actively penetrates through the eschar into unburned tissue. It is, however, painful for a time after application, it is drying, and it cannot be used under a closed dressing. Furthermore, it is a synthetic topical sulfonamide and needs to be used with caution in patients with renal dysfunction. In burn shock, a major buffer of the body, the renal tubule, is impaired. Most buffering will therefore be done by the pulmonary system through its compensating mechanisms of tachypnea or hyperpnea. The resulting increase in respiratory exchange must be closely monitored while the patient is on Sulfamylon.		
Many agents are used to protect the patient from infection. These antibacterials could help increase the incidence of fungal infections. Amphotericin is a potent drug used to treat Candidiasis. Risks to the patient are high—sometimes you buy a life with a partial loss of hearing (The Underuse of Amphotericin, 1977). The patient or family must have an explanation of the risks involved in order to give informed consent for use of the drug.	Second postburn day: Apply 0.5% $AgNO_3$ cream dressings every day to all burned areas and to donor sites. Third postburn day: Tub bath q.d. for débridement before daily dressings.	Prepare dressings for application before taking Mr. A to tub room. Have tub room as steamy and warm as possible before removing old dressings to prevent chills. Gently remove top loose layers of old dressings. With adequate numbers of assistants, help Mr. A into tub. Let him sit quietly until relaxed.
Salt is added to the tub bath to lessen the osmotic gradient and thus to decrease the loss of electrolytes and minimize subsequent dehydration.	Add 1½ lb of NaCl to bath water. Use Epigard (trade name) for $AgNO_3$ dressings.	Keep water running slowly while Mr. A is in the tub to help maintain temperature of the water. Place snorkel over his nose and mouth, submerge total head.

Epigard is one result of efforts to find a new "artificial skin" to appy to third-degree burns as a substitute for homo- and heterografts. It can be used to apply antimicrobial agents. Its advantages are (1) better adherence and conformity to wound than previous synthetic skins, (2) meshlike surface for phagocyte-bacterial interaction, (3) acceleration of new skin growth, (4) imperviousness to bacteria, (5) it is nonantigenic, (6) shelf-stable, and (7) relatively inexpensive (Plastic Sandwich Sheet, 1972).		Gently remove old dressings with help of bath water. Weigh Mr. A when he gets out of the tub and before applying new dressings.
Burke and Yannas have developed a semiartificial skin, a semisynthetic material of skin graft made from cow collagen with a polysaccharide base. It appears to be a satisfactory skin replacement that reacts in a positive manner; it infiltrates living tissue when placed on a wound and induces growth of fibroblasts and blood vessels without inflammation. Experiments thus far have been restricted to guinea pigs but it is soon to be used as graft material as well as a matrix for normal human epithelial growth (Consensus for Treatment, 1979).		Apply dressings to wound, placing them properly the first time, to avoid rubbing dressing across burn surface. Topical agents are only as good as the person applying them. Wrap dressings with Kling, flannel, or stockinette. Remove and treat dressings gently to avoid disrupting granulation tissue.
In patients with burns of more than 20% in extent, there are frequently clinically significant deficits of Na^+, Cl^-, and K^+ and less frequently of Ca^{2+} and Mg^{2+}. Deficits can be induced by the dressing within as little as 6 hours but is most likely to occur within the first few weeks following injury. By this time the patient is usually on oral intake, and so dietary supplement of NaCl, K, and Ca must be adequate and regulated according to the serum and urine concentrations of these minerals and the absence or presence of the clinical signs of their deficits (Monafo, 1971).		Observe for: Hyponatremia Hypochloremia Hypokalemia Hypocalcemia: Tetany Trousseau's sign Chvostek's sign Paresthesias Muscle spasm (especially of facial muscles) Mood changes
As can be seen in Figure 48-3, Mr. A experienced a mild electrolyte imbalance. Topical 0.5% silver nitrate is not an escharotic and will not injure regenerating epithelium or other normal tissue. In a series of more than 140 patients treated with topical silver nitrate, not once did a full-thickness wound result at any of the donor sites subsequent to the cutting of split-thickness skin grafts; all donor sites were continuously covered with the silver nitrate dressing. Donor sites treated like this healed regularly within 10 to 12 days so that the recutting of more skin from them was then routinely possible (Monafo, 1971).	NaCl tablets Ca gluconate tablets KCl liquid Vitamin C tablets Multivitamin tablets Vitamin A caps	Give vitamin and mineral supplements with feedings or meals to minimize the amount of water required to be taken by Mr. A.
Penicillin and oxacillin are given routinely throughout convalescence as a precaution against streptococcal and staphylococcal lymphangitis (Monafo, 1971). Because Mr. A had an allergy to penicillin, other antimicrobials were used.	Decadron q.8.h. × 4 days Tetracycline q.6.h. Check temperature q.4.h. If temperature is over 101°F, get blood culture. Then give Tylenol p.r.n.	Observe for sensitivity: Fever with chills Angioedema Decreased blood pressure Increased pulse

(Continued)

TABLE 48-1 *(Continued)*

Changes	Medical Prescriptions	Nursing Intervention
Homograft skin is placed over the granulating surface for no more than 4–5 days, because its removal becomes progressively difficult. If left longer, at the time of removal bleeding and the retention of dermal homograft remnants in the granulating surface are troublesome (Jacoby, 1976).	Twenty-first postburn day: Start surgical débridement and grafting	Be aware that steroids can delay healing because steroids are antiinflammatory and inflammation is part of the process of healing.
Hemografts serve many functions in the treatment of the burn wound.	Psychiatric consultation	
Their use tends to clean up untidy wounds, because débridement is effected with each homograft change. They provide a vapor barrier for the granulating surface with resultant decrease in water evaporation and exudation. They also serve as an excellent test of the granulating surface for its acceptability to autograft, which is especially important in large burns in which donor sites are limited and autograft failure can be disastrous. In massive burns, where donor sites must be used more than once, the homograft will preserve granulation tissue until donor sites can be reharvested. After homograft has been applied, the wound becomes immediately and dramatically free of pain (Artz et al., 1979). However, débridement continues to be painful. Mr. A was acutely anxious throughout this series of treatments in the operating room.	Valium and Compazine Demerol after tub bath and return from operating room.	
On admission, Mr. A had suffered extensive destruction of his body's first barrier of defense against invasion of microorganisms, and he was covered with charred clothing. He was therefore subject to infection by anaerobic microbes, especially *Clostridium tetani.*	Tetanus toxoid, 0.5 ml s.c., stat.	Explain that the injection is to protect him against infection. Because this induces active immunity, observe for signs and symptoms of anaphylaxis. (See Chapter 24.)
"Burn wound sepsis" is a pathological entity characterized by the presence of greater than 10^5 organisms per gram of tissue with demonstrable invasion of adjacent unburned tissues (Artz et al., 1979). Development of burn wound sepsis creates a condition that facilitates invasion of the blood stream by colonizing microorganisms. The onset of septicemia may be insidious or acute. A blood culture in any burned patient whose rectal temperature is 103°F or higher is indicated.		Observe for septicemia: Paralytic ileus Increased bleeding tendency Mild jaundice Elevated body temperature Increased pulse Decreased blood pressure Decreased urine output Confusion, disorientation
Before leaving discussion of changes in the skin of a burned patient, it is necessary to point out one of the enormous advantages of using topical antiseptics in the treatment of the burn wound; there is absolutely none of the previously characteristic foul smell that promptly identified the presence of a burned patient on any hospital unit. This improvement alone has made the illness and its prolonged treatment more bearable for patients and has helped nursing personnel attack the many nursing problems of the burned patient with greater zeal.		

Urinary Bladder In a 2-year study of 88 autopsies on fatally burned individuals at the U.S. Army Surgical Research Unit, 62% were found to have bacteriuria, and 100% of these either still had the indwelling catheter in place or had recently had it removed (Artz et al., 1979).	Remove Foley catheter, but continue to measure and record urinary output (third postburn day).	Give scrupulous attention to perineal care, especially around the urethral orifice, while an indwelling catheter is in place. Urge the physician to endorse removal of the catheter as soon as evidence of Mr. A's fluid status and ability to take oral fluids warrants.
Chondritis of the Ear The pathogenesis of chondritis of the ear in burned patients remains a mystery. The complication usually develops late, during the second and fifth week postburn. Depth of burn is no indication of the ultimate course. *Pseudomonas* and *Staphylococcus aureus* are the most frequently cultured organisms from this site, but there are instances of sterile culture and frank necrosis. The incidence is unaffected by the use of topical antiseptic treatment. The patient complains of severe pain, and swelling and redness of the ear become apparent. Spontaneous rupture with drainage of purulent material may occur directly through healed second-degree burn or in areas of complete skin loss. Drainage and total removal of necrotic cartilage are required. When destruction is extensive, it may be necessary to remove all of the cartilage. The end result is a markedly deformed ear (Pruitt, May 1979). Mr. A's left ear began to drain green purulent exudate in the sixth week, but débridement and grafting preserved the ear.		Prepare Mr. A's family and visitors for the changes in his appearance before they go in to visit him, to prevent their shock from being an additional burden on Mr. A's already overstressed psychological status. Be very supportive of the family and provide an environment in which verbal expression of their fears and feelings is perfectly acceptable.
Eye The problem of burns around the eyes involves primarily the periorbital tissues, especially the lids. Appropriate care involves prevention of secondary injury to the eye from infection or exposure. During the early course of face burns, it is important to irrigate the eyes several times a day with normal saline solution to wash out exudate and debris. After irrigation, an antibiotic ophthalmic ointment or solution should be instilled three or four times a day.	Neosporin ophthalmic gtts both eyes t.i.d.	
If conjunctiva is exposed because of contraction of eyelids, inflammation and corneal ulceration may develop rapidly. Exposure of the cornea while the patient is sleeping and intractable conjunctivitis are indications for early release of eyelid contractures (by means of tarsorrhaphy) (Pruitt, May 1979).		Ask physician if he would approve frequent administration of methyl cellulose eye gtts., to prevent further drying and deterioration of the cornea until such time as the eyelid contractures are released.

(Continued)

TABLE 48-1 *(Continued)*

Changes	Medical Prescriptions	Nursing Intervention
Musculoskeletal System		
One of the most formidable obstacles to maintaining or restoring mobility in the burned patient is the patient's fear of pain or fear of moving a burned extremity because of anticipation of pain. If the patient learns early that the limbs can be moved without causing extreme discomfort, he or she is better able to cooperate with subsequent efforts. After even a few days or a week of absolute immobility following acute burn trauma, the patient will be extremely fearful of and resistant to any passive or active motion (Artz et al., 1979). Throughout the period covered by this report of Mr. A's injury and hospitalization, his reponses to efforts to move him either passively or actively were consistent with the preceding description; every success in getting him to move either a single joint or his whole body was accomplished only with painstaking persistence, patience, and endless time and reassurance. It is a testimony to his nursing care that within the first 2 weeks postburn Mr. A was able to hold his own glass by cupping both covered hands around the container; was able to get in and out of bed by himself, though it required from 15 to 20 minutes for each operation; and was able to ambulate around the ward unassisted.	Encourage ambulation (on fourth postburn day). Range-of-motion exercises with dressing changes while in bathtub.	Remember that it's much easier to prevent deformities than it is to correct them. Get patient involved in his own care. Do what he can no matter how long it takes him to do it: brush teeth, comb hair, eat, and so on.
It is significant to note that the extent to which he was willing to make the effort required to accomplish the preceding activities on his own depended largely on who was encouraging or pushing him. It seems evident that, with the severely burned patient perhaps more than with any other type of patient, the nurse must reinforce the will to live and to try by caring enough to continually harass the patient. Perhaps this persistent caring is the best means the patient has of knowing that, despite disfigurement and relative helplessness, he or she is still worthy of being a person with a future.		Alternate flat and elevated headrest to prevent hip flexion deformity. Apply $AgNO_3$ cream directly to burned surfaces of hands, and then apply white cotton gloves to increase possible range of motion in the hand. Apply forearm splints during extended rest periods of the day and at h.s. Teach and remind to do exercises of the facial muscles.
The goals of physical therapy are relatively simple: 1. Prevention of contracture. 2. Maintenance of joint motion. 3. Maintenance of muscle tone. Accomplishment of the goals of physical therapy is through the recognized measures of positioning and of active, passive, resistive, and iosmetric exercise. In positioning, special attention is given to all major joints: ankles, knees, hips, shoulders, elbows, wrists and hands (Artz et al., 1979). Ankles are supported at 90° of dorsiflexion. Knees are straight but not hyperextended.		Position, turn, and exercise him to provide optimum exposure of all burned areas, redistribution of pressure, and immobilization of arms and head: 1. Head must be in neutral position with sandbags placed to prevent rotation (to protect grafts on neck) when Mr. A is on his back. 2. Do not address Mr. A until you are standing directly in his vision. Place bed so he can see those entering his room without having to turn his head.

Hips are in neutral rotation and symmetrically abducted to 10 to 15°.

Shoulders are abducted at least 60° and are alternately externally and internally rotated.

Elbows are flexed no more than 30 to 40°.

Wrists are supported in slight extension.

At the metacarpophalangeal joints, fingers are allowed to drop into flexion, and the thumb into an abducted and slightly flexed position.

In burns of the neck, the head is positioned so that there is slight extension of the neck but no more than that amount that will allow the patient to close his or her mouth easily (Artz et al., 1979).

In each case, the position chosen or prescribed is the one that facilitates the most useful position for subsequent movement of the body.

The amount of active motion possible in the burned extremity is determined by whether or not joints are bridged by unburned skin and by whether or not grafts have been applied within the past 48–72 hours (Artz et al., 1979).

Because of the primary role of the hand in our ability to be self-sufficient, one of the most serious threats to mobility is the development of interphalangeal joint stiffness. This stiffness is not caused by the burn itself, but happens during the period of systemic treatment of the burned patient and results from immobilization, edema, contraction, and fibrous-protein synthesis as the wound begins to heal (Peacock, 1969). Muscle atrophy progresses relentlessly in the catabolic phase following a severe burn; although this cannot be prevented, a degree of muscle tone and muscle awareness can be retained. In the catabolic phase, which in most patients roughly corresponds to that period preceding skin coverage or wound closure or the formation of healthy granulating surfaces, no measures, dietary or otherwise, will bring the patient into nitrogen equilibrium. The nitrogen loss through exudate, but principally through the urine, far exceeds any realistic dietary intake (Artz et al., 1979).

Evidence does not support the assumption that the routine programmed exercise of the severely burned patient impedes skeletal demineralization. Immobility is only one of the causes of bony atrophy in severe burns, and considered alongside protein deficit and hyperadrenalism, it could easily be the least important. It is, however, one factor that can be controlled to some extent from the outset. It is safe to assume that exercise affects favorably the degree of local atrophy in burned extremities, whereas its effect on generalized demineralization is probably negligible (Artz et al., 1979).

3. Teach, supervise, and encourage:
   Quadriceps setting exercises.
   Gluteal setting exercises.
   Flexion extension exercises of legs and feet.
   Wiggling toes and pressing on footboard. (See Chapter 51.)
4. Keep elbow joint as nearly straight as possible, support arms (under elbow to produce extension) with rolled towels, bath blankets, or small pillows to elevate hands just above shoulder (to promote venous return and decrease edema of wrapped hands) when Mr. A is on his back.
5. As soon as facial burns have granulated, Mr. A should be encouraged to chew gum and blow up balloons.

(Continued)

TABLE 48-1 *(Continued)*

Changes	Medical Prescriptions	Nursing Intervention
Protein Metabolism Proteins are the basic components of cellular protoplasm, composed of carbon, hydrogen, oxygen, nitrogen, and often sulfur. With complete hydrolysis, proteins yield various crystalline amino acids, which may be 1. Synthesized into protein. 2. Metabolized to H_2O and CO_2 for energy production. 3. Converted to glucose or fat. Of the 23 known amino acids, 10 are essential in the diet because they cannot be synthesized in the body; foods containing these are called complete proteins. Incomplete protein can be synthesized from products of glucose and fat metabolism and also occurs in vegetable proteins. Amino acids absorbed in the intestine go directly to the liver via the portal vein, where some are stored and others are sent on to body tissues. In the absence of food, protein will be deprived of its nitrogen and converted into glucose to keep up the blood sugar level and to provide the glucose essential to the burning of the body fat for fuel. As much as 58% of protein, by weight, may thus be turned to glucose to be burned along with fat for fuel, or serve as the sole source of fuel when body fat is exhausted. The nitrogen output of the fasting man is thus raised because he uses protein for fuel as well as for building purposes. To minimize this extravagant use of protein in a patient unable to ingest (or digest) food by the oral route, carbohydrate should be given to supply the glucose necessary to provide energy and spare protein. The normal adult is in nitrogen equilibrium; intake equals excretion, and the total quantity of protein stores remains essentially stable. Positive nitrogen balance implies that the rate of anabolism exceeds the rate of catabolism. Negative nitrogen balance exists when catabolism exceeds anabolism. Burn injuries are the greatest stimulation to the catabolic process (Bartlett et al., 1977). The weight loss, negative nitrogen balance, and progressive weakness can be a prelude to impaired healing, poor ventilation, sepsis, and death.		Encourage complete proteins: Milk Eggs Cheese and cottage cheese Fish Fowl Liver, kidneys Veal Pork Lamb Lean meat Encourage proportional intake of incomplete proteins: Legumes three to four servings per day Cereals Cereal products: whole wheat bread, crackers Encourage low alkaline ash juices (to minimize renal calculus formation while increasing vitamin, mineral, and fluid intake): Cranberry juice Raspberry juice Plum juice Assess Mr. A's tolerance for, and encourage: Cream soups Eggnogs, flavored if necessary Meat stock broth Identify Mr. A's favorite drinks: Fruit juices Milk Milk shakes Refrain from forcing more than Mr. A takes willingly to avoid his developing a strong aversion to food early in his convalescence. Allow 10 to 15 minutes for offering liquids, as his willingness to drink may be in direct proportion to the relation and encouragement of nurse's attitude. Observe closely for: 1. Eructation. 2. Nausea. 3. Abdominal distention. 4. Complaints of cramps, abdominal pain. Discontinue feedings if any of the preceding signs or symptoms develop, and report to physician immediately.

An adult ingesting a normal diet excretes from 10–15 g of urinary nitrogen per day; the same adult, following an extensive burn, may excrete as much as 30 g of urinary nitrogen per day. During the first few days postburn, increased excretion of urinary nitrogen is not evident because of impaired renal function. High excretion becomes evident within 3 to 5 days postburn, reaching a maximum in the first and second postburn week. Magnitude of urinary nitrogen loss varies with the following factors: 1. There is rough correlation between the severity of the burn and the amount of nitrogen excreted; the more extensive the burn, the larger the nitrogen excretion. 2. Preburn body weight is positively correlated with nitrogen excretion. 3. Men generally excrete more than women. 4. Usually, increased nitrogen excretion does not occur in patients malnourished before injury. The metabolic demands of a big burn are tremendous. It is the most severe long-term traumatic episode that the human organism can survive (Stahl, 1977). Burned patients are usually unable to accept an adequate oral diet during the early postburn period. The gastrointestinal tract is used when possible—alimentation is used otherwise. Starvation, with its disproportionate lean tissue destruction, leads to hypoproteinemia very early. The nitrogen excretion from major thermal injury can approach 40 g/day. Starvation in the uninjured individual is compensated by a decrease in resting metabolism, but the burned patient has a tremendous increase in metabolic activity as reflected by oxygen utilization. The metabolic expenditure during the first postburn week is 200% of normal. In addition, in the burned patient, total metabolic expenditure cannot be lowered, and as catabolism proceeds, there are decreased stores for energy conversion. As open or infected wounds produce exudation, further protein loss occurs. Two to 3 g of protein for each percentage of burn is the average loss per 24 hour, and as much as 7–8 g of protein for each percentage of body surface burned can be lost from a burn wound in 1 day (Shuck & Moncrief, 1969).	Xylocaine viscous p.r.n.	Apply topical Xylocaine rinse to mouth a few minutes before feeding Mr. A, until blisters of palate heal.
A loss of 30 g of tissue protein represents an accompanying loss of approximately 1 g of total protein per 100 ml of serum; thus early wound closure is of paramount importance. In this same postburn period, a low nitrogen intake contributes further to the negative nitrogen balance.		Weigh dressings when dry, before applying them to Mr. A, and again when they are removed, as a basis for estimating the loss of protein via wound exudate.

(Continued)

TABLE 48-1 *(Continued)*

Changes	Medical Prescriptions	Nursing Intervention
In the early postburn period, Mr. A was in negative nitrogen balance (excessive catabolism) because of imbalance created by excessive losses in wound exudate and increased excretion of urinary nitrogen, mostly as urea, resulting from hydrolysis of proteins for energy and extensive destruction of tissue protein by burn injury. When amino acids are burned for fuel, they are deprived of their nitrogen and reduced to compounds containing only carbon-hydrogen-oxygen, which burn like sugar and fat. The nitrogen, being of no use as fuel, is converted into a relatively harmless soluble substance, urea, and excreted in the urine.		
An energetic nutritional regimen of a high-protein, high-caloric diet, instituted 7 to 10 days after burning, may reduce substantially the duration of negative nitrogen balance. Unless special efforts are made to achieve ingestion of such a diet, negative nitrogen balance can be expected to last more than a month. The well-treated burned patient returns to nitrogen equilibrium, or more likely to positive balance, after a month.	4,000-calorie high-protein, high-vitamin, soft (bland) diet, in frequent small feedings (fifth postburn day).	Observe frequency and consistency of bowel movements. (Mr. A was consistently confronted with the added problem of constipation.) Ask physician for p.r.n. enema order and prevent impaction.
Increased energy requirements during the catabolic phase pose serious nutritional problems. Intravenous hyperalimentation providing up to 8,000 kcal per day has resulted in weight stabilization and wound healing in burned patients. (See Chapter 46 for nursing implications of intravenous hyperalimentation.)		
In a high-calorie, high-protein diet, the ratio of calories to nitrogen in the intake is important because protein synthesis will not occur in the absence of adequate caloric intake. The calorie/nitrogen ratio is the ratio of nonprotein calories to protein nitrogen in the diet. 1 g of carbohydrate equals 4 kcal. 1 g of fat equals 9 kcal. 1 g of protein equals 4 kcal.		
About 40–50% of the chemical energy of carbohydrate and fat, and 80–85% of the chemical energy of protein, is converted to heat in the process of metabolism. A lack of caloric intake from the first two food sources will result in gradual combustion of body tissue. The burned patient loses weight as he or she loses muscle mass and fat. The depletion syndrome includes low levels of total body protein, potassium, magnesium, sulfate, and other intracellular ions. Water and extracellular salts tend to remain in excess until the patient approaches nitrogen equilibrium.		

B-complex vitamins, especially thiamine, are essential to the enzyme systems responsible for facilitating use of glucose by the cell. Ascorbic acid is essential for growth, cell activity, maintenance of strength of blood vessels, and formation of supporting tissues. Plasma ascorbic acid concentration is low after severe burns; ascorbic acid is one of the precursors of the adrenocortical steroids and thus is depleted during the body's response to stress. This, in combination with increased tissue demands for vitamin C for healing the extensive areas of injury, requires administration of large doses of ascorbic acid. Anemia develops rapidly in severely burned patients who survive the initial period of shock. Amount of destruction of red blood cells (RBCs) following thermal injury is variable and in general is a significant problem only with deep burns. An additional factor that would have prolonged the catabolic phase of Mr. A's postburn period is the development of a Curling's ulcer. Mr. A did not develop this complication. The incidence of gastroduodenal ulceration on one series of 88 patients who were fatally burned at the Brooke Army Medical Center was 47% (Artz et al., 1979). (See Chapter 52 for discussion of "stress ulcers.")	Multivitamins ii p.o. q.d. Ascorbic acid, 500 mg p.o. t.i.d.	Encourage foods rich in vitamin C. Ask family to contribute some of the following if not available in quantity from the kitchen: Citrus fruits Melons Berries Tomatoes Raw vegetables Encourage foods high in iron: Beans Soybeans Green leafy vegetables: Kale Turnips Lean meats: liver Dried fruits: Prunes Apricots Observe for: Coffee-ground emesis Hematemesis Poor food tolerance Melena Abdominal distention Epigastric pain Ileus

Mr. A withstood the onslaught of every one of the insults to which the severely burned patient is subject. A large burn assaults the patient in three overlapping ways: hypovolemic shock, followed by sepsis and starvation, succeeded in turn by a period of limited function and nutritional inadequacy. The response to volume depletion, though doubtless subtle and complex, is at least well enough understood for treatment to be effective. Current understanding of the endocrine and metabolic response to starvation and sepsis in the second phase serves less well as a guide to treatment, and it is here that the majority of patients are lost. Mr. A won his battle for survival, but the struggle to improve the quality of his life goes on.

[3] Cyanosis in the black patient is detected best on the soles of feet, palms of hands, nail beds, and mucosa as ashen gray.

[4] Lucy M. Brand, a nurse now in independent practise, made this observation based on her 10 years of experience in caring for the acutely ill surgical patient, including burned patients.

[5] Contents according to Emergency Hospital Pharmacy.

References Cited

"Are Our Burn Facilities Insufficient for the Job?" *Med. World News,* **14** (Nov. 9, 1973), 65–67.

Artz, C. P. et al. *Burns—A Team Approach.* Philadelphia: W. B. Saunders Co., 1979.

Bartlett, R. H. et al. "Nutritional Therapy Based on Positive Caloric Balance in Burn Patients." *Arch. Surg.,* **112** (Aug. 1977), 974–80.

Busby, H. C. "Nursing Management of the Acute Burn Patient and Nursing Management of Optimal Burn Recovery." *J. Contin. Educ. Nurs.,* **10** (July–Aug. 1979), 16–30.

"Consensus for Treatment of the Sickest Patients You'll Ever See." *JAMA,* **241** (Jan. 26, 1979), 345–48.

Davitz, J., and Pendleton, S. H. "Nurses' Inferences of Suffering." *Nurs. Res.,* **18** (March–April 1969), 100–7.

Gillespie, R. W. "The Burn at First." *Emer. Med.,* **11** (May 15, 1979), 186–87+.

Guyton, A. C. *Textbook of Medical Physiology,* 4th ed. Philadelphia: W. B. Saunders Co., 1971, p. 829.

Imbus, S. H., and Zawacki, B. E. "Autonomy for Burned Patients when Survival Is Unprecedented." *N. Engl. J. Med.,* **297** (Aug. 11, 1977), 308–11.

Jacoby, F. G. *Nursing Care of the Patient with Burns,* 2nd ed. St. Louis: C. V. Mosby Co., 1976.

Jouglard, J. P. et al. "Severity and Prognosis after Early Excisions from One to Twenty Percent of the Body Surface Area." *Scand. J. Plast. Reconstr. Surg.,* **13**:1 (1979), 121–25.

Kelleher, R. E. *The Standard-Times* (New Bedford, Mass.), Feb. 22, 1980.

"Making the Least of Burn Scars." *Emer. Med.,* **4** (March 1972), 25.

Monafo, W. W. *The Treatment of Burns.* St. Louis: Warren H. Grun, 1971.

Morton, J. H. "Fluid Replacement in Patients with Large Area, Full and Partial Thickness Burns." *Arch. Surg.,* **114**:3 (March 1979), 247–52.

Munster, A. M. "Alterations of the Host Defense Mechanisms in Burns." *Surg. Clin. North Am.,* **50** (1970), 1217.

Peacock, E. "Burned Hands: And How to Heal Them." *Consultant,* **9** (March–April 1969), 18–20.

"Plastic Sandwich Sheet for Burn Therapy." *Med. World News,* **13** (Oct. 27, 1972), 19.

Price, W. R., and Wood, M. "Operating Room Care of Burned Patients Treated with Silver Nitrate." *Am. J. Nurs.,* **68** (Aug. 1968), 1705–07.

Pruitt, B. A. *The Burn Patient: I Initial Care.* Chicago, London: Yearbook Medical Publishers, April 1979.

______. *The Burn Patient: II Later Care and Complications of Thermal Injury.* Chicago, London: Yearbook Medical Publishers, May 1979.

"Psychic Survival after the Burn.," *Emer. Med.* (Jan. 1978), 197–200.

"Pulmonary Burns: Delayed Disaster." *Emer. Med.* (Oct. 1977), 163–65.

"Scan for a Scorched Lung." *Emer. Med.,* **11** (June 15, 1979), 87–88.

Schuck, J. M., and Moncrief, J. A. "The Management of Burns: General Considerations and Sulfamylon Method." *Curr. Probl. Surg.* (Feb. 1969).

Sevitt, S. "A Review of the Complications of Burns, Their Origin and Importance for Illness and Death." *J. Trauma,* **19**:5 (May 1979), 358–69.

Stahl, W. "The Superficial Burn and Beyond." *Emer. Med.* (Nov. 1977), 113–22.

"The Underuse of Amphotericin." *Emer. Med.* (Sept. 1977), 126–29.

Willis, B. A. et al. "Positioning and Splinting the Burned Patient." *Heart and Lung,* **2** (Sept.–Oct. 1973), 696–706.

General References

Alawneh, I. "Acute Non-Calculous Cholecystitis in Burns." *Br. J. Surg.,* **65**:4 (April 1978), 243–45.

Baxter, D. R. "Problems and Complications of Burn Shock Resuscitation." *Surg. Clin. No. Am.,* **58**:6 (Dec. 1978), 1313–22.

Clark, A. M. "The Treatment of Burns in Children." *Aust. Fam. Physician,* **7**:4 (April 1978), 371–77.

Drucek, C. et al. "Hemodynamic Analysis of Septic Shock in Thermal Injury: Treatment with Dopamine." *Am. Surg.,* **44**:7 (July 1978), 424–27.

"The Eccentricities of Gentamicin." *Emer. Med.* (Sept. 1977), 122–26.

Edlich, R. F. et al. "Emergency Department Treatment, TRIAGE, and Transfer Protocols for the Burn Patient." *JACEP,* **7**:4 (April 1978), 152–58.

Emig. E., and Lloyd, J. "How to Get Burned Children Home Sooner." *RN,* (July 1977), 37–39.

Govoni, L., and Hayes, J. *Drugs and Nursing Implications.* New York: Appleton-Century-Crofts, 1978.

Isler, C. "Save Victims of Lightening." *RN* (Aug. 1976), 37–39.

Jacoby, F. G. *Nursing Care of the Patient with Burns.* St. Louis: C. V. Mosby Co., 1972.

Konigoua, R. et al. "Clinical Forms of Endotoxemia in Burns." *Scand. J. Plast. Reconstr. Surg.,* **13**:1 (1979), 612.

Leavitt, M. "Andy Was a Fighter—In More Ways than One." *Nursing '79,* **9** (April 1979), 64–66.

Linn, B. S. et al. "Evaluation of Burn Care in Florida." *N. Engl. J. Med.,* **296** (Feb. 10, 1977), 311–15.

Marvin, J. A. "Burn Nursing as a Specialty." *Heart and Lung,* **8** (Sept.–Oct. 1979), 913–17.

Rubin, A. B. "Black Skin." *RN* (March 1979), 31–35.

Schuck, J., and Wachtel, T. "Burned But Not Too Badly." *Emer. Med.* (Aug. 1977), 24–30.

"Where Burns Get Special Care." *Emer. Med.* (Nov. 15, 1979), 153–70.

49

Problems Associated with Disuse Syndromes—Including the Integument

Iron rusts from disuse,
stagnant water loses its purity,
and in cold weather becomes frozen:
even so does inaction sap the vigors
the mind.
LEONARDO DA VINCI, Notebooks—(c. 1500)

Disuse Syndromes—The Consequence of Prolonged Bedrest and Inactivity

In 1947, Dr. R. A. Asher, a British physician, warned of the dangers of going to bed. He describes what an overdose of bedrest can do: "Look at a patient lying long in bed. What a pathetic picture he makes! The blood clotting in his veins, the lime draining from his bones, the scybala sticking up in his colon, the flesh rotting from his seat, the urine leaking from his distended bladder, and the spirit evaporating from his soul" (Asher, 1947). In reviewing Dr. Asher's statement sentence by sentence, we find that just about every body system has been included with a rather dramatic, almost laughable, description of the serious consequences of prolonged bedrest and inactivity. Many of the problems encountered with patients who have long-term problems are a result of disuse syndromes. Disuse problems are the most common and serious complication of chronic illness. It is important to realize that often the primary disability is greatly overshadowed by the unanticipated effects of disuse. Each leads to further inactivity and thereby aggravation and extension of disease. The chronically ill patient with weakness, pressure sores, contractures, osteoporosis, and incontinence is too common a sight.

This chapter was contributed by Rita H. O'Neill, R.N., M.S., Associate Professor of Nursing, College of Nursing, Southeastern Massachusetts University, North Dartmouth, Massachusetts.

CAUSES OF SECONDARY DISABILITY

Secondary disabilities are those that result from inactivity or from contraindicated or injurious activities. Disabilities caused by inactivity are termed *disuse syndromes.* Those disabilities caused by contraindicated or injurious activities are termed *misuse syndromes.* Both types of secondary disability are preventable. Disability from immobilization or secondary disability is a preventable health problem (Olson, 1967). The belief that reduction or elimination of disability caused by disuse is dependent on nursing care is the basis for the following discussion of the disuse syndromes. This requires awareness of the specific secondary disabilities that may arise in different conditions and the application of specific preventive nursing measures. Obviously, such preventive practice must begin immediately in the care of all disabled patients; otherwise a disproportionate amount of effort is expended in dealing with secondary disabilities, many of which cannot be reversed.

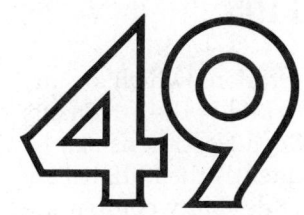

Knowledge of the physiologic and psychologic alterations which result from confinement, whether to bed or the astronauts' couch, is advancing rapidly. Such alterations can be drastic in their effects. Frequently the initial disease state is negligible as a cause of disability compared with the deteriorative effects of disuse. For example, the expected disability of uncomplicated hemiplegia is paralysis of the extremities and the lower face on one side of the body. If a hemiplegic is neglected and does not start a rehabilitation program, in all likelihood, in the course of weeks he or she will develop such complicating disorders as bed sores, urinary tract infection, painful and contracted joints, constipation and bowel impaction, and urinary incontinence.

Causes of Disuse Syndromes in Illness

In illness, disuse may be due to a number of causes. The principal ones are

1. *Loss of sensation.* Normally, change of position is stimulated by discomfort. Any person who has loss of sensory stimuli may maintain the same position for too long a time with resulting damage.
2. *Pain.* Painful disorders of the joints and surrounding soft tissue lead to protective limitation of motion and produce local disuse effects. The person with rheumatoid arthritis may limit motion of the involved joints for too long, which may cause damage.
3. *Immobilization as a result of braces and/or casts.* The immobilized part(s) may suffer disuse.
4. *Paralysis.*
5. *Joint Stiffness.*
6. *Enforced rest,* in bed or chair, during illness or convalescence.
7. *Mental disorders* that cause immobilization.

Effects on Motor Function

Motion is necessary for the maintenance of the structural stability and metabolism of the musculoskeletal system and requires both basic tonicity and intermittent workload of the skeletal muscles.

Atrophy of Skeletal Muscles

If a muscle or a muscle group is not used for exercise at fairly regular intervals, the muscle mass diminishes in volume. This can be seen, for example, in the shrinkage of a limb after application of a cast. Muscle strength as well as size is diminished. The greatest disuse occurs in denervated muscle, muscle that has lost its nerve supply. Muscle fibers that have not contracted for sometime gradually diminish in size, and the proportion of muscle fibers and connective tissue change so that there is more and more fibrous tissue and less and less muscle mass. Muscle atrophy generally adds to weakness and therefore adds to the individual's overall disuse. This establishes a vicious cycle which leads to physical and psychological deterioration.

Contracture of Joints

A contracture is a limitation of the range of motion caused by shortening of soft tissue structure around a joint. Contractures occur when muscles do not have the activity necessary to maintain the integrity of their function, that is, the full range of shortening and lengthening of its fibers. As a disuse phenomenon this disability occurs whenever a joint is not moved frequently through its range of motion. Contractures may also occur with muscle imbalances in which one muscle is weak and its antagonist is stronger, or spastic, or both.

Clinically, limitation of range of motion due to contractures is detected when one attempts to move a joint passively through its full range. There is either a sensation of resistance that blocks further movement without any special discomfort to the patient, or there is pain and active resistance by the patient. In a true contracture, there is limitation of movement even when the patient is anesthetized.

The most common and disabling contractures are *hip flexion* contractures, *knee flexion* contractures, and contractures of the *shoulder.* Knee and hip flexion contractures develop commonly in the patient who is confined to a chair or wheelchair or spends most of the time in a Fowler's position in bed. In these positions, full extension of the hips and knees never occurs. Knee and hip flexion contractures also result from spastic paraplegia. In this case, the spasticity of the flexor muscles maintains the patient's knees and hips in a flexed position. Pain or paralysis around the shoulder girdle predisposes to contractures. If severe, it is called "frozen shoulder." Plantar flexion contractures of the feet and toes may arise from pressure of tight bed clothes and also from a combination of paralysis and the pull of the powerful gastrocnemius muscle.

Whatever the predisposing cause of the contracture, the fibers of the involved muscle shorten and atrophy, resulting in a limited range of motion of the joint. Such a process may initially produce a reversible contracture than can be overcome by exercise and stretching, but eventually it will involve tendons, ligaments, and the joint capsule and become irreversible, requiring surgical intervention or prolonged mechanical stretching for its release.

Prevention of Contractures

The prevention of contractures is much easier than their treatment. The following nursing measures are of great value in the prevention of contractures:

Positioning
Maintain body joints in their most functional anatomical position. Give special attention to the prevention of hip and knee flexion contractures which may be caused by improper placement of pillows or from gatched beds that keep hips and knees continuously flexed. A bed board and a firm mattress are helpful in maintaining correct body positioning. A foot board can be helpful in preventing plantar flexion (foot drop). Be sure the foot board is used properly. It should be placed firmly against the patient's feet to hold them at right angle with the legs. It should not be placed at a distance where stretching to reach it will create the plantar flexion position of foot drop.

Mobilization
Frequent and scheduled change of patient position and range of motion of all joints should be carried out. This definite and specific schedule must be included in the nursing care plan and cannot be left to chance. "Change position frequently" is not a specific enough directive. The intervals and the specific positions must be specified. Whenever possible, the patient should assume some of the responsibility for checking his or her position and for performing range of motion exercises. Teaching that encourages participation of the patient and family can be vital in the prevention of contractures.

Osteoporosis

Osteoporosis is a wasting of bone characterized by simultaneous loss of bone matrix and minerals. The vital matrix of bone is fundamental to its growth and carries calcium which gives bone its solidity. Throughout life, the matrix and the calcium are constantly being built up and broken down by opposing cell forces in a dynamic state of equilibrium. This activity depends upon the stress and strain of mobility and weight bearing for proper functioning. Nurses should be aware that decalcification takes place during immobility regardless of the quantity of calcium intake.

Osteoporosis occurs also as a primary disorder in hyperparathyroidism and Cushing's disease and after menopause. This condition is recognized in x-ray by diminished density or opacity of bone. Osteoporosis is disabling for the following reasons: (1) it may cause pain; (2) it leads to fractures; and (3) it leads to excessive excretion of calcium, which may produce formation of stones in the urinary tract.

Osteoporosis, as a result of disuse, can be prevented or decreased by the maintenance of weight bearing and muscle movement and the avoidance of complete immobility. A daily program of muscle activities against resistance should be planned. Having the patient stand or walk between parallel bars will provide weight bearing and normal stress on the bone. If the patient is unable to stand, placing him or her in a weight-bearing position on a tilt table or oscillating bed will accomplish weight bearing and stress on bones.

Effects on Elimination

Urinary Elimination

The human renal and urinary excretory system is designed to function optimally when one is in the erect position. What happens to the function when one is ill, supine, and allowed to remain immobile?

When a human being is in the erect position, urine flows out of the renal pelvis and into the ureter in accordance with the laws of gravity. There is only a small portion of the renal pelvis where stasis of urine might occur. The anatomy of the kidney is such that in the erect position the hilus of the kidney emerges from the medial aspect. But when a person is in the supine position, the hilus of the kidney is uppermost and all the urine formed must be excreted into the ureter against gravity. Peristaltic contraction may not be of continuous and sufficient strength to overcome this resistance, and the renal pelvis may fill completely before the urine is expressed into the ureter. If a supine position is maintained for even a few days, urinary stasis occurs. Any particle contained in the urine may settle into the calyces and become the nucleus for formation of a renal calculus or the focus for infection. Many disuse factors may contribute to stone formation including the following:

1. Increased calcium excretion through the kidney (hypercalciuria) because of demineralization of bone

2. Stagnation of urine in the kidney pelvis or bladder because of supine position and/or inadequate change of position
3. Urinary tract infections that are common in the severely disabled, especially in those who have residual urine
4. Alkaline urine due to diet or infection which favors precipitation of calcium salts

Urinary complications are of constant concern to the disabled. Disuse osteoporosis brings about abnormal calcium deposits. Oliguria, retention, or stasis of urine also precipitate stone formation and infection. Chills, temperature elevation, decrease of urinary output, or hematuria may be the first signs of urinary complications.

Because most urinary bacteria thrive in an alkaline medium, attempts must be made to maintain an acidic medium. The patient should be encouraged to drink fruit juices that assist in maintaining the acidity of urine. Such fruits are cranberries, plums, and prunes. The most important single measure will be adequate fluid intake. At least 3,000 ml daily is recommended, provided cardiovascular and/or circulatory complications are not present.

The length of time for training the bladder varies greatly. The incontinent male may wear an external urinary collecting device that will be attached to his leg. Incontinence creates a greater problem for the female patient, since there are no successful female collection devices. Some patients are never able to achieve bladder training and will need permanent indwelling catheters, intermittent catheterization, or cystostomies. Intermittent catheterization has proven to be a highly effective way to eliminate the need for an indwelling Foley catheter. The technique embraces the concept of intermittent introduction of a urethral catheter to provide drainage to the bladder, thus preventing distention and eliminating a residual medium in which bacteria may grow. Further, it eliminates the chronic presence of a foreign body that incites an inflammatory action and allows bacterial invasion. Depending upon the disability, the patient or a family member may be taught intermittent catheterization.

There has been a great deal of debate with regard to the infection rate and the training of those doing the catheterization. Studies have shown no great variation in incidence depending on who does the catheterization, the physician only, patients only, or others. In learning to manage urinary elimination the patient has much to learn from the nurse, whether it be the technique of self-catheterization or the total management of an indwelling catheter or cystostomy. Watching for sufficient output is as important as providing the appropriate amount and kind of fluid to ingest. Knowing only how to irrigate the catheter is not enough; as stated before, the patient must know the total management of equipment.

Bowel Elimination

Constipation is a problem that confronts all immobilized patients. The process of bowel elimination depends upon the integration of smooth and skeletal muscle activity and complicated visceral reflex patterns. Immobility may interfere with these mechanisms and because of diminished expulsive power, the loss of defecation reflex, or both, may cause constipation. The primary muscles involved in the elimination process are the abdominals, the diaphragm, and levator ani. These muscles are necessary to increase intraabdominal pressure preliminary to the act of defecation and for the expulsion of fecal mass. Muscle atrophy and loss of tone occur in the immobilized, the debilitated, or the malnourished. Also, lack of exercise brings about a generalized weakness of muscles which may interfere with the mechanical expulsion mechanism. Thus, the patient is unable to assist with the elimination process, and retention or incomplete evacuation of fecal material results.

The usual hospital treatment for constipation is use of laxatives and/or enemas. This will never suffice as a desirable program for a disabled person. Repeated enemas decrease normal bowel tone and, in the instance of the paralyzed patient, the highest degree of peristalsis possible must be maintained. Enemas should be used only as a beginning step in initiating a bowel program; they should never be considered a total solution to evacuation for the disabled person.

Each person has a definite pattern of elimination. It is learned and established early in childhood. Therefore, the patient's habits prior to disability should be determined and incorporated into the plan. The nurse should also consider the time of day most convenient for evacuation after the patient returns home. Generally, the time chosen will be early morning or evening. Mass peristalsis occurs most often following meals and is believed to be strongest following breakfast. To establish regularity, the patient should be taught to eat breakfast, respond to the signal for defecation, and allow at least 10 to 15 minutes for this process. If feasible, the patient should be permitted to use the lavatory or, for the totally immobilized patient, the environment can be modified to provide privacy and make it possible to assume a position that best promotes evacuation. Gentle, digital stimulation to the anal sphincter may be helpful in activating evacuation for some patients.

Regulating bowel function is accomplished by using stool softeners, prune juice, and suppositories in addition to adequate food and fluid intake. Determining the amount needed and the program for each patient is usually done by the trial and error method. It is generally accepted that evacuation twice a week in sufficient amounts and consistency is compatible with healthy body function. The nurse will usually strive for at least an every-other-day pattern.

Dietary regimen must be individualized. It is important to learn which foods have a natural laxative effect for the person and provide these foods in the necessary amounts. Prune juice is usually considered the most effective laxative. Adequate fluids and fruit juices are encouraged to stimulate reflex activity, and to assure enough water in the feces. The diet must contain sufficient amounts of bulk and cellulose. This poses a problem for the edentulous patient and for the nurse and dietician who plan his or her diet. The abuse and misuse of laxatives and enemas may lead to an interruption of normal colonic mobility patterns and to cathartic habituation.

Even with a well-planned bowel program, *fecal impaction* may develop especially in the aged or in patients with neurologic diseases. Fecal impactions develop from prolonged retention of feces in the rectum or colon. When the fecal material remains in the bowel, water is continually withdrawn from it, and the material becomes increasingly more dry and hard. Excessive hardening of the stool can also be caused by medication or diet. The bulk of the stool may become so great that the person has a continuous desire to defecate. The rectal muscles contract but, due to the hardened consistency of the stool, it cannot be molded for expulsion. The older person may have a relaxation of the rectal musculature. When the rectum is distended with stool, the patient may have no desire to defecate due to the blunting or the loss of the defecation reflex. The earliest symptom of an impaction is the frequent passage of liquid material around the impacted stool. Often this situation is erroneously treated as diarrhea, thus increasing the magnitude of the patient's problems. An impaction should be dislodged and removed by gentle digital action. Some authorities recommend that this be followed by an oil retention enema and soap suds or saline enemas. It may be necessary to repeat this treatment for several days until normal patterns are reestablished.

Functional bowel programs are not achieved quickly. During the period before the schedule is achieved bowel movements can occur at any time, thereby causing embarrassment and discouraging the patient. Psychological trauma caused by evacuation during meals, during visiting hours, or at occupational or physical therapy is obvious. Through continued efforts, patience, and support to the patient, a workable bowel program will evolve. The patient does need a definite program for the rest of his or her life, and only by working toward evacuation at a specific hour can this function be controlled: there is no reason to delay its establishment. Optimism is in order, as a plan can be achieved in time. The value to the patient of once again "controlling" evacuation of feces is immeasurable.

Effects on Peripheral Circulation—Localized Areas of Ischemia

PRESSURE SORES

Skin breakdown is always a matter of grave concern to the disabled person. Breaks in the skin due to prolonged pressure, particularly over bony prominences, are referred to as *bedsores, decubitus ulcers,* or *pressure sores.* A pressure sore is defined as an area of necrosis caused by excessive and prolonged pressure.

Despite the frequency of pressure sores and their costs to the patient and society, comparatively little research has been done to determine their causes and how they can be effectively prevented and treated. It is generally agreed that the dominant ischemic agent in producing decubiti is *pressure* over bony prominences, and that immobilization, undernutrition, and lack of sensory nerve supply are major predisposing factors. All these factors lead to a decrease in the quantity and quality of blood delivered to the affected tissues. Other contributing factors include age, sex, temperature of affected tissues, edema, continence or incontinence of urine and feces, sepsis, and adrenal steroids.

The most successful treatment of bedsores is their prevention. The significance of prevention is emphasized by the cost of curing a decubitus ulcer. In 1967, Bliss and McLaren estimated the cost to range from $2,000 to $10,000. In 1977—just 10 years later—the cost of treatment of decubiti for a single patient was estimated at $15,000 or more (Sather et al., 1977). Seventy per cent of all patients developing decubiti do so within the first 2 weeks after admission. Therefore, the first step in prevention is the systematic and prompt identification of susceptible patients followed by the institution of preventive measures.

To facilitate the identification of susceptible patients, several authors have developed guides or rating scales (Bliss & McLaren, 1967; Verhonick, 1961;

Williams, 1973; Gosnell, 1973; and Gruis & Innes, 1976). There is general agreement that the major areas to be observed are skin integrity, mental status, continence, mobility, activity, and nutritional status. Figure 49-1 presents a skin integrity assessment tool which can be used to estimate a patient's risk for pressure sores.

Pressure: The Ischemic Agent

Whether the patient sits or lies, the weight of his or her body is borne by tissues covering bony prominences. The skin and subcutaneous tissue are compressed between the bony prominences and the mattress or chair seat. When the patient lies on the back the points of greatest compression are the shoulders, sacrum, and heels. Weight may also be borne by the back of the head of babies and patients who do not use a pillow. In patients who sit, the weight of the trunk and head is borne by the ischial tuberosities. The patient lying on the side bears weight on the hip, knees, ankle, and shoulder. In the absence of a pillow, the weight of the head may be concentrated on the ear. *Approximately 7 pounds of pressure per square inch of surface on the tissue is sufficient to shut off the blood supply.* In some patients tissue necrosis may occur in as little as 30 minutes.

Shearing Pressure

Patients in a sitting position, be it in a bed or chair, are susceptible to a second type of pressure, shearing pressure. As the patient slides down in the bed or chair, the skin and subcutaneous tissues lag behind the bony prominences, which move in a forward direction until the sacrum bears the weight of the body. As the bone passes over the tissue, it damages or even destroys small blood vessels. When patients are pulled up in bed without being lifted, the shear-

Name: ______________________
Disease: ______________________
Sex: ______________________

Directions: For each of the 9 variables which present an ordinal scale, *circle* the number of the word or phrase which best summarizes your observations related to that characteristic. *Add* the patient's risk score.
A score of 7 or more on the 5 boxed variables places the patient at risk for pressure scores (Exton-Smith, 1967).

Age:
0 under 25
1 25 to 35
2 35 to 45
3 45 to 55
4 over 55

Weight:
0 Normal weight
1 Under weight
2 Malnourished
3 Over weight
4 Obese

General infection process
1 Absent
2 Present
(Specify kind and location)

Skin integrity:
1 Intact
2 Broken

General condition:
0 Good
1 Fair
2 Poor
3 Bad

Mental status:
0 Alert
1 Confused
2 Apathetic
3 Stuporous

Activity:
0 Ambulant
1 Walking with help
2 Chairfast
3 In bed all day

Mobility:
0 Full
1 Slightly limited
2 Very limited
3 Immobile

Incontinence:
0 None
1 Occasional
2 Usually of urine
3 Usually of urine and feces

State of nutrition (lab finding)
Hb. __________
T.P. __________
Alb __________
Glb __________
Hct __________

Figure 49-1. Skin integrity assessment tool to determine patients who are at risk for pressure sores. (Rowhanieh Rowhani developed this guide as a graduate student in Medical-Surgical Nursing, in partial fulfillment of requirements for the Master of Science in Nursing degree from Wayne State University College of Nursing, Detroit, Michigan, 1971.)

ing force is applied in the opposite direction. The injury to the tissues may be further increased by incorrect massage.

Major Predisposing Factors

Skin Integrity

The skin of a patient predisposed to decubiti should be carefully inspected the first time the patient is seen and regularly thereafter. The state of the skin should be accurately described so that data are available for future comparisons. An observation guide will help to ensure that pertinent observations are made. Such information as the following is essential: skin intact or broken, excoriated, or a necrotic area, or indurated, or swollen. Any abnormalities should be measured so that changes in size can be determined. Skin color, especially over pressure areas, should be described and compared to that of surrounding skin. If there are color changes, the length of time the skin takes to return to that of the surrounding skin should be noted and recorded. The longer that it takes the skin to return to its prepressure color, the greater the degree of ischemia.

Changes in the color of skin over an area of pressure are caused by the amount and oxygenation of blood in the tissues underlying the skin surface. At the point of greatest pressure, sufficient to obstruct the flow of blood to the area, skin color will be a lighter hue than that of surrounding skin which is receiving unimpaired blood supply; when pressure is relieved and blood pools or rushes to the area to nourish the ischemic tissue, the skin color will be a darker hue than that of surrounding skin. In patients whose skin has little or no pigment, the blanching of ischemia will appear white, and the reactive hyperemia will appear as some shade of red. In patients whose skin is heavily pigmented, the blanching of ischemia will appear as a lighter hue of the color of the surrounding skin, and the reactive hyperemia will appear as a darker hue of the color of the surrounding skin (Mitchell, 1979). Gruis and Innes (1976) have observed that reactive hyperemia may last from a few seconds to an hour.

Other pertinent observations include skin tone, presence or absence of sensation, and skin creases where the patient lies on the bed. Skin creasing is a normal phenomenon. Careful regular inspection of the skin followed by recording of observations provides a basis for evaluating the effectiveness of preventive measures. Changes in care can then be based on this information.

Intact skin is a vital defense against the entrance of microorganisms as well as the loss of body constituents. The size of a break in the skin is not the only index of its seriousness. A sore a millimeter across, infected by virulent organisms, may lead to a fatal septicemia. Conversely, a large, craterlike sore several inches across and extending through the subcutaneous tissues may be walled off, but leak large quantities of protein and other constituents in body fluid.

Ischemia is the first stage in the formation of a pressure sore. This is noticed by a *blanching* of the skin. At this point strict measures to prevent formation of the pressure sore should be instituted at once. The second stage is termed *hyperemia*. The area will be red, raised, and warm to the touch. Cell destruction and hemorrhage have already occurred. This is the time when most pressure sores are observed, and measures are instituted to prevent further damage. Unfortunately, cell destruction occurs at this stage. It is extremely difficult to halt the progress of a pressure sore in a paralyzed person, no matter how elaborate the measures that are instituted. The final stage is a *break in the skin*. No matter how small the area, it is now a pressure sore.

The most common site of pressure sores are the anatomical areas over bony prominences: the sacrum, iliac crests, ischial tuberosities, greater femoral trochanters, and heels. Whatever the location, true pressure sores undergo a characteristic clinical evolution. The skin first becomes red and may develop a large blister. The discolored area darkens gradually and becomes dark and hard. Over a period of weeks, the necrotic tissue is sloughed off gradually, leaving a deep ulcer. Though the development of the ulcer may take several weeks because of the delay in sloughing of dead tissue, a pressure ulcer frequently is caused by one period of continued pressure. The damage may occur following as little as an hour of immobility and pressure.

Mental Status

The mental status of the patient should be evaluated because the confused, very sick, apathetic, stuporous, or comatose patient is unable to protect pressure areas from injury. As examples, the confused patient may resist efforts to mobilize him or her. Restraints may cause further immobilization. If the patient resists the restraints or is excessively active, the skin may be further damaged by friction.

RESTRAINTS. The simplest and least disrupting type of restraint to keep a patient from falling or getting out of bed is bed rails, but when greater protection is needed it may be necessary to apply restraints to any or all of the following areas: chest, waist, hands, wrists, and ankles. Because these usually are also areas prone to developing pressure sores, it is imperative to observe the following safety precautions (Kukuk, 1976):

1. If restraints are being applied in an agency, be sure to follow agency policies and guidelines for restraints.
2. Explain to the patient and family why restraints are necessary.
3. Use two people to apply restraints, to minimize patient discomfort and maximize effectiveness of restraints.
4. Be sure restraints do not pinch or bind the patient beyond the absolute minimum limitation of motion required for safety.
5. Restrain the patient in a natural, comfortable position. If possible, position the patient so he or she can see the immediate environment.
6. Check on the patient and change the position frequently, preferably several times an hour. If possible, have a family member or friend stay with him or her.

ABILITY TO EAT. The nutritional status of the very sick, apathetic, or stuporous patient may be impaired by the inability to eat, a limited food intake, or refusal to eat. The very sick, apathetic, or stuporous patient, as well as the unconscious patient, suffers most from immobility and lack of food and fluids.

Continence or Incontinence

Despite the belief that incontinence of urine and feces predisposes to decubiti, experimental evidence does not support this belief (Bliss & McLaren, 1967; Gosnell, 1973; Williams, 1973). If incontinent patients continue to move about, they do not develop decubiti. Further, some of the worst pressure sores occur on the heels, one of the driest areas of the body.

Immobilization

One of the factors causing pressure on vulnerable tissues is immobilization. The healthy person changes position with great frequency. Even at night he or she may change it many times. As a result of debility, serious illness, or the application of restraints to keep a confused or disoriented patient in bed, the patient may not be able to move about. Deeply unconscious patients may not move at all. Further, interference with movement is not limited to the patient who is bedfast, for patients who are placed in chairs may not move all day.

Nutritional Status

Pressure ulcers are more likely to occur in malnourished persons who are in negative nitrogen balance. Once the patient regains a positive nitrogen balance, and there is more nitrogen intake then output, there will usually be improvement in regeneration and growth of the tissues. Negative nitrogen balance may be expected as a response to injury. A greater amount of nitrogen is excreted than can be ingested. Because of protein loss caused by tissue breakdown, protein-sparing agents are sometimes given. Although it is not possible to reverse negative nitrogen balance in the period immediately following injury by a high dietary intake of protein, the patient must be encouraged to eat foods containing sufficient protein, vitamins, and minerals. After the catabolic phase is completed, protein foods are essential to an adequate anabolic response. Vitamins B and C (ascorbic acid) are also essential to wound healing.

One of the common methods of estimating the nutritional state of an individual is noting the degree to which his or her weight compares to normal and whether or not the patient appears to have lost weight recently as evidenced by loose skin. Some estimate can also be made by asking a person what he or she usually eats, as well as by observing what is or is not eaten. Among the nutrients required to maintain the integrity of the skin are ascorbic acid and protein. Particularly among the elderly, insufficient protein intake is common. Elderly persons limit their food intake for economic and social reasons, as well as because they have little desire to eat meat and other high protein foods. Debilitated patients are also likely to have had a deficient food intake. They may lack the necessary appetite to eat and tire easily.

Lack of Nerve Supply

None of the reported studies were concerned with a lack of sensory nerve supply per se. However, difficulty in maintaining the integrity of the skin of hemiplegics and paraplegics is well known. Among the predisposing factors are immobility and inactivity. It is possible that the loss of nerve supply impairs the ability to adapt the blood flow to tissue needs. During the first weeks following a traumatic injury that results in paraplegia, a marked catabolic response may aggravate the tendency toward tissue breakdown. Probable elements predisposing to decubiti: loss of sensation plus immobility plus diminished blood supply plus catabolism plus (?) factors equals decubiti.

Other Contributing Factors

Age, Sex, and Adrenal Steroids

In a study of geriatric patients Bliss et al. (1967) found that the incidence of decubiti increased as age exceeded 65 years. Immobility and poor nutrition combined with the loss of subcutaneous fat were likely factors. This assumption is supported by Williams (1973), who found that the incidence of decubiti was higher among the thin than among the obese. Williams also found a higher incidence among men than women (six to one) with the two youngest males (23 and 26) developing decubiti. Although she suggests that this finding may be due to the small sample studied, and it may be, there is a possible explanation. Males between the ages of 15 and 25 (approximately) have a more severe catabolic response to injury than do older or younger males and females of all ages. After a serious injury, tissue breakdown may proceed at such a rapid rate that decubiti are difficult to prevent (see Unit V). Corticosteroids predispose to decubiti probably for the same reason (protein catabolism).

Pressure, Temperature, Humidity

Verhonick et al. (1972) studied by thermography the relationships among pressure, temperature, and humidity of sites predisposed to decubiti. One of the findings is that the longer pressure is applied to a pressure-sensitive area, the longer it takes for it to return to normal temperature.

Preventive Measures

Prevention is the best treatment for a pressure sore. All areas of possible skin breakdown must be inspected frequently. During each position change, the skin should be inspected for areas of tenderness, edema, coldness, or redness. Meticulous skin care should be given and a dry wrinkle-free bed provided. A regular toilet schedule on a 24-hour basis, time-tailored for each individual patient, will reduce the incontinence that contributes to skin breakdown.

For the paralyzed bed patient, turning is as essential to skin integrity as breathing is for life. All four sides are to be utilized. Maintenance of skin integrity is almost completely the responsibility of the nursing staff. There should be no reason for the physician to write orders on these patients to be turned. Although pressure sores will occur in some instances in spite of diligent nursing care, most occur as a direct result of improper care.

To test the effectiveness of a variety of methods used in the prevention of bedsores, Bliss and McLaren (1967) studied a number of them. They report that measures such as massage, soap and water, witch hazel. pHisoHex, and silicone are ineffective. Among the devices found to be of limited value were sheepskin, nylon pads, and sponge rubber mattresses.

Regular turning every 2 hours was not successful or practical with geriatric patients, as 50 per cent of these patients developed trunk sores. Some patients were confused and uncooperative and some, such as patients in congestive heart failure, could

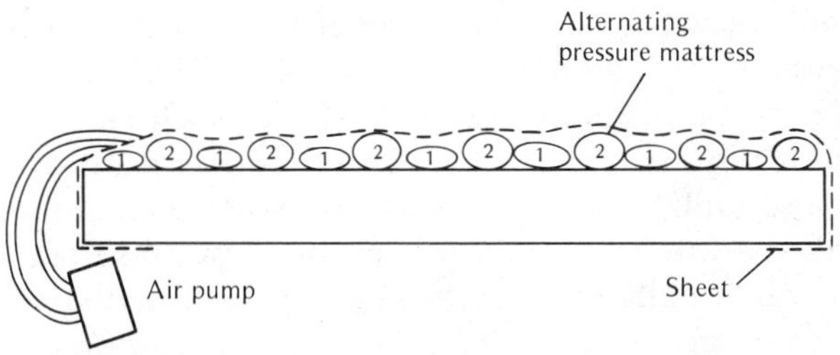

Figure 49-2. Diagram of a large-cell ripple mattress showing transverse cells. An alternating-pressure mattress is a plastic (or sometimes rubber) air mattress, rather like a beach mattress, but connected to a motorized air pump that causes different parts of it to be alternately blown up and let down underneath the patient. All the cells labeled 1 are connected to the motor by one set of tubes and all those labeled 2 by another. Once every five minutes the 1 cells inflate while the 2 cells deflate; then the 2 cells inflate while the 1 cells deflate. The body thus rests first on the row of 1 cells and then on the row of 2 cells, so that the points of support, and therefore of pressure, are constantly being changed.

not or would not move. Regular turning was successful with patients with cord injuries where patients were positioned on pillows and there was a regular turning team.

Two types of mattresses were found to be successful. The first is a mattress that molds itself to the shape of the body, such as an air or water mattress. The second is a large-cell alternating-pressure mattress.[1] This mattress consists of alternating plastic or rubber tubes or cells. The cells are arranged so that they lie either transverse or parallel to the length of the bed. The air cells are connected to a pump which causes alternate cells to inflate and deflate. (See Figure 49-2, in which the cells are transverse to the bed.) Bliss et al. (1967, p. 382) reported that during the test period no patient placed on a mattress with transverse cells developed decubiti on either trunk or heels. They also found that the mattress with the cells parallel to the length of the bed was highly effective in preventing trunk sores. It was ineffective in preventing heel sores as the type of mattress used was not long enough to protect the heels. Mattresses are available that do protect the heels.

When an alternating pressure mattress is used, only one sheet is used to cover it, and it is tucked in loosely. The effectiveness of the mattress is progressively reduced by each additional layer of linen. The sheet should be free of wrinkles and crumbs. To encourage the patient to move, the top bed covering should be loose. Wrist and ankle restraints are to be avoided. When they are used, they should be

[1] There is also a small-cell mattress.

removed at frequent and regular intervals and the patient moved. Whatever type of mattress is used, it must be properly placed on the bed. The mattress itself requires protection. The effectiveness of mattresses inflated by air or water depends on maintaining the integrity of the covering. A pin inserted to attach a light cord or tubing can ruin a mattress. The pump must also be kept working properly.

Another pressure-distributing device is the flotation bed. There are a number of types. One consists of a plastic tank which fits on a standard hospital bed frame. It is filled with water and covered with a heavy sheet of plastic. In another, a plastic bag of water is placed in the tank. In both types the linen is placed on the bed in the usual way. Because the patient "floats" on water, weight is evenly distributed rather than being concentrated on bony prominences (Noonan & Noonan, 1968). A new type of flotation bed is the air bed.

Another flotation device is a square pad filled with a gel the consistency of human fat; one example of this is the Stryker Flotation Pad. The pad is large enough to protect the sacrum of bed patients and the ischial tuberosities of sitting patients. It can be moved from the bed to chair as the patient moves from one to the other. To prepare the bed for the flotation pad, a sponge-rubber mattress with a 16-inch square hole in the center and covered by a fitted sheet is placed on the mattress. The pad is placed in the hole. Like a water or air mattress the flotation pad accommodates itself to the contours of the part of the body resting on it. Just as with other pressure-relieving devices, the skin of the patient should be checked regularly to determine its condition. No matter how effective such aids are, their ultimate success depends on the competence of the professional staff utilizing them.

Positioning

When a patient is in bed, pressure can also be minimized by keeping the patient as flat as possible. A triangular-shaped pad is available to elevate the legs just enough to reduce pressure on the heels, or a thin pillow can be placed under the legs, just raising the heels from the bed. Care should be taken to prevent a ridge from pressing the tissue proximal to the heel. Provided the support extends far enough up the lower leg, preferably to the popliteal space, the broad surface on which the legs rest tends to distribute the weight.

A turning frame such as the Stryker or Foster frame is used particularly for a patient with neurological injuries to prevent and treat bedsores as well as to immobilize him or her. The patient must be turned regularly and frequently enough to prevent prolonged pressure.

Diet

In addition to the preceding, attention should be given to the patient's intake of food, with particular attention to protein—meat, eggs, fish, cheese, milk—and ascorbic acid—orange juice, green leafy vegetables—and other fruits and vegetables.

When the skin breaks down, the first line of defense of the body is disrupted, and bacteria have a portal of entry. The situation may be further aggravated by the loss of tissue nutrients in serous or bloody drainage from the area.

Devices that reduce the incidence of bedsores are those preventing the continued concentration of pressure on tissue and distributing the weight of the body over a wide area. A variety of pads and mattresses have been designed to accomplish these objectives. Success in the prevention of decubiti depends on the identification of susceptible patients and the proper use of appropriate measures to limit and relieve pressure. (See Figure 49-3 for a pictorial summary of the major pathogenetic factors in bedsores).

Treatment

If a pressure sore does develop, treatment will be ordered by the physician. There are probably as many treatments as there are physicians. Except for general agreement that the area should be kept clean, there are any number of variations in treatment. If infection is present, antibiotics will usually be given. A sterile dressing will usually be placed over the pressure sore. When the pressure sore penetrates the subcutaneous fat, plastic surgery is usually necessary. A full-thickness skin graft will be performed.

The search for special devices or mattresses to help prevent pressure ulcers has continued for years. However, none of the current devices replace a meticulous turning schedule and vigilant personal care. Alternating pressure mattresses are used and there are a variety of useful seat chairs that have been developed for wheelchair use. Water beds of various kinds have also been developed. Doughnuts or rubber rings are not to be used, as they only transfer and increase pressure to surrounding areas. As soon as possible, the patient should become involved in daily observation of the skin. To examine all his or her body surface, a long-handled mirror should be used. The patient should be taught how to shift weight to relieve pressure in both wheelchair and bed; he or she should do wheelchair push-ups every 20 minutes.

As stated earlier, the best treatment is *prevention.* The first step is in identifying patients who are likely to develop decubiti and in instituting preventive

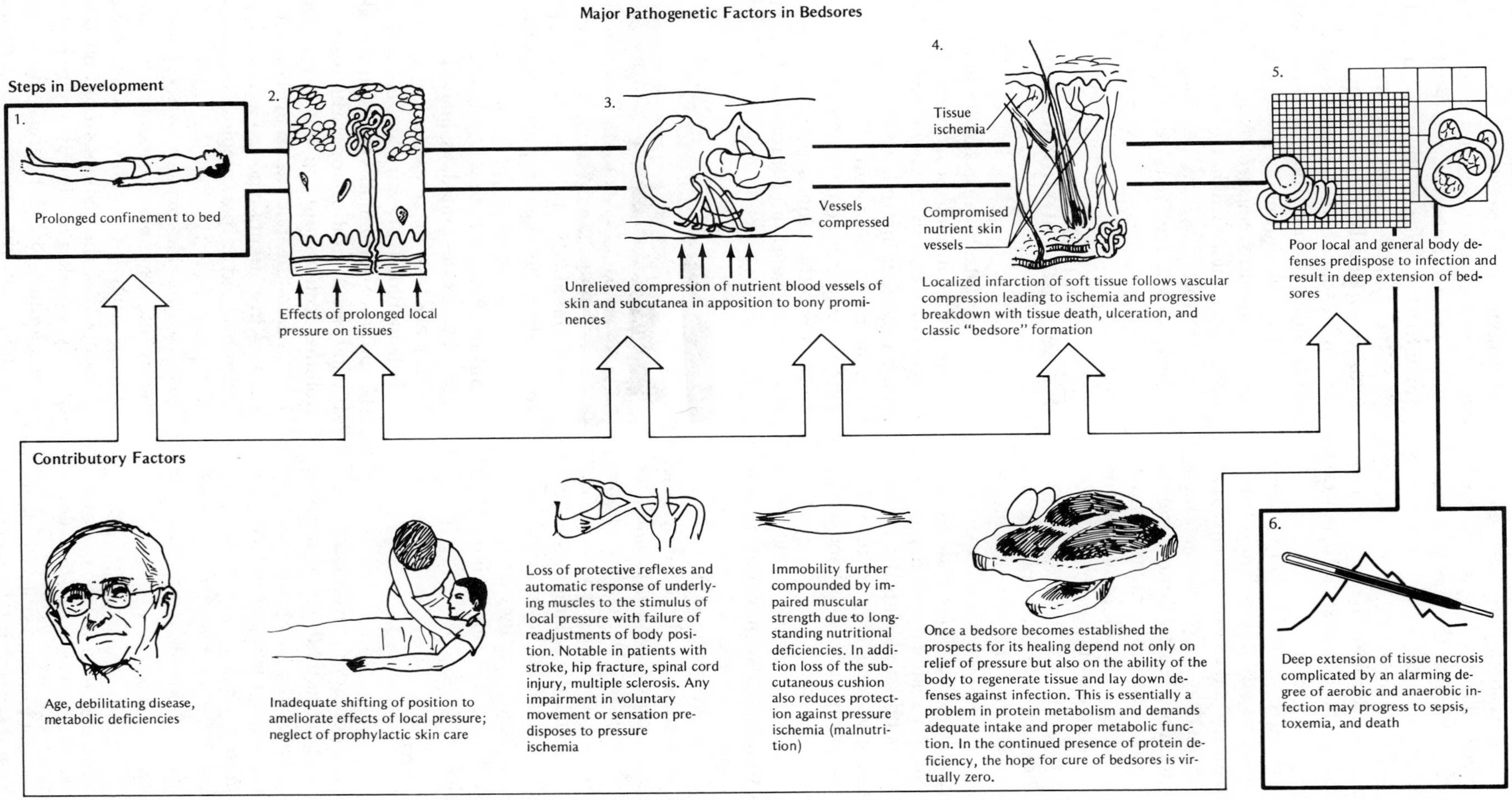
Major Pathogenetic Factors in Bedsores
Steps in Development
1.
Prolonged confinement to bed
2.
Effects of prolonged local pressure on tissues
3.
Vessels compressed
Unrelieved compression of nutrient blood vessels of skin and subcutanea in apposition to bony prominences
4.
Tissue ischemia
Compromised nutrient skin vessels
Localized infarction of soft tissue follows vascular compression leading to ischemia and progressive breakdown with tissue death, ulceration, and classic "bedsore" formation
5.
Poor local and general body defenses predispose to infection and result in deep extension of bedsores
Contributory Factors
Age, debilitating disease, metabolic deficiencies
Inadequate shifting of position to ameliorate effects of local pressure; neglect of prophylactic skin care
Loss of protective reflexes and automatic response of underlying muscles to the stimulus of local pressure with failure of readjustments of body position. Notable in patients with stroke, hip fracture, spinal cord injury, multiple sclerosis. Any impairment in voluntary movement or sensation predisposes to pressure ischemia
Immobility further compounded by impaired muscular strength due to longstanding nutritional deficiencies. In addition loss of the subcutaneous cushion also reduces protection against pressure ischemia (malnutrition)
Once a bedsore becomes established the prospects for its healing depend not only on relief of pressure but also on the ability of the body to regenerate tissue and lay down defenses against infection. This is essentially a problem in protein metabolism and demands adequate intake and proper metabolic function. In the continued presence of protein deficiency, the hope for cure of bedsores is virtually zero.
6.
Deep extension of tissue necrosis complicated by an alarming degree of aerobic and anaerobic infection may progress to sepsis, toxemia, and death

Figure 49-3. Major pathogenetic factors in bedsores. (Adapted with permission of Hospital Publications, Inc., from Bedsores, *Hosp. Med.* 13:83–103, May 1977, pp. 84–85, by S. E. Moolten.)

measures. Susceptible areas should be observed for reddening around a blackened area. The initial break in the skin may be no more than the size of a common pinhead. Generally the area is painful and the pain is similar to that accompanying blistering of the heel. In patients with edema of the sacrum and buttocks, large areas can be denuded in a matter of a few hours.

The difficulty in curing bedsores is emphasized by the number of measures advocated. They range from the use of comb honey and raw or refined sugar to coating the area with a drug. The same measures as are used in prevention are basic: (1) mobilization of the patient, (2) measures to minimize pressure on susceptible and affected areas, (3) providing the patient with an adequate intake of protein and ascorbic acid, (4) treating the wound aseptically as well as keeping it clean and dry[2] (5) bladder training and the use of an external condom if the patient is incontinent, (6) prevention of tissue edema, (7) exposure of the wound to air and ultraviolet light, (8) debriding the wound surgically or by packing it with dry gauze, and (9) cleansing the wound by placing the patient in a tub of water. Large wounds may require skin grafting. As implied earlier, measures utilized in the treatment of decubiti are legion.

Psychological trauma caused by the formation of a pressure sore can be great. This new body insult is but another cause for increased dependence on others. Pressure sores are always unsightly and are often draining and foul smelling. Frequently, the pressure sore progresses to the point of prohibiting any activity other than bedrest. The patient can no longer be in a wheelchair; all therapies must be accomplished from bed. Again the rehabilitation program is at a standstill and cannot be resumed until the pressure sore heals. This delay may be for a period of months, and during this time other disuse problems may develop.

Summary

Prevention and to a considerable extent the therapy of decubiti are the responsibilities of nursing. Success depends on identifying those who are susceptible and instituting appropriate preventive measures. Important considerations in the preventive management of bedsores are summarized in Figure 49-4). Many of the same measures are as useful in treatment as in prevention. They include pressure relief, mobilization, and improvement in or maintenance of good nutrition. Candidates for decubiti include the very old, the thin, the immobile and inactive, the confused and unconscious, the seriously injured, especially young males, the paralyzed and the undernourished. The first step in prevention is the identification of those who are susceptible. The second is the initiation of appropriate preventive and therapeutic measures. Nurses also have a responsibility to explore further questions such as (1) Who is susceptible? (2) How can they be identified? (3) Which preventive measures are effective? (4) Why?

[2] Dextranomer Debrisan is a promising new substance for helping to keep the wound clean and dry. It is a sterile insoluble powder contained in tiny beads, and consisting of a three-dimensional network of cross-linked dextran macromolecules. The powder absorbs four times its weight in water, and also absorbs the products of collagen and tissue breakdown, and of contaminating bacteria (DiMascio, 1979).

Effects on Cardiovascular Function

The heart itself works harder in the resting supine position than in the resting erect position. The physiologic effects on the heart of bedrest as a treatment for myocardial infarction has received much attention in recent literature. Three major changes in cardiovascular system function that have been identified are orthostatic hypotension, increased workload of the heart, and thrombus formation.

Orthostatic Hypotension

Orthostatic hypotension is defined as the rapid fall of blood pressure when a recumbent patient is placed in an upright position. It indicates a deterioration of the ability of the autonomic nervous system to equalize the blood supply when the person who has been recumbent for a long period attempts to stand up. Nurses are aware that when patients first get up after several days in bed, they may suffer from weakness, dizziness, and may even faint.

Fall of blood pressure in this case is caused by dilatation of the blood vessels in the abdomen and the lower extremities under the weight of the blood volume accumulating in the lower portions of the body when the patient is upright. It is especially marked in patients who have had a lumbar sympathectomy and in paraplegics and/or quadriplegics. The patient faints when the blood supply is inadequate to provide oxygen to the brain. There is a failure of vasomotor responses to compensate for change from a recumbent to an upright position.

Seeing that the patient's position is changed frequently will alter the intravascular pressure and provide stimulus to the neural reflexes of the vessels and help prevent hypotension. Probably the most effective measure is changing the patient's position

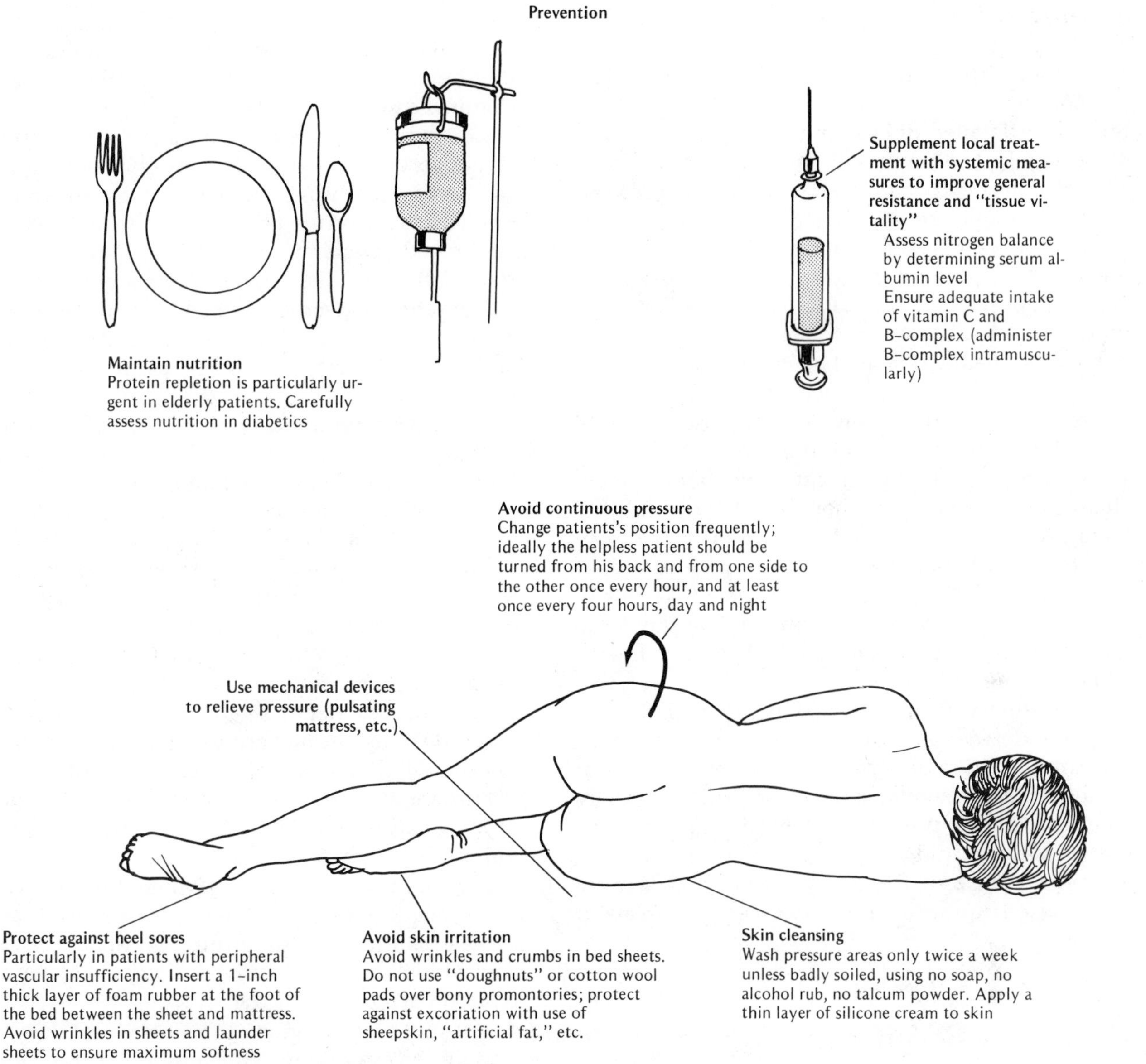
Prevention
Maintain nutrition
Protein repletion is particularly urgent in elderly patients. Carefully assess nutrition in diabetics
Supplement local treatment with systemic measures to improve general resistance and "tissue vitality"
Assess nitrogen balance by determining serum albumin level
Ensure adequate intake of vitamin C and B-complex (administer B-complex intramuscularly)
Avoid continuous pressure
Change patients's position frequently; ideally the helpless patient should be turned from his back and from one side to the other once every hour, and at least once every four hours, day and night
Use mechanical devices to relieve pressure (pulsating mattress, etc.)
Protect against heel sores
Particularly in patients with peripheral vascular insufficiency. Insert a 1-inch thick layer of foam rubber at the foot of the bed between the sheet and mattress. Avoid wrinkles in sheets and launder sheets to ensure maximum softness
Avoid skin irritation
Avoid wrinkles and crumbs in bed sheets. Do not use "doughnuts" or cotton wool pads over bony promontories; protect against excoriation with use of sheepskin, "artificial fat," etc.
Skin cleansing
Wash pressure areas only twice a week unless badly soiled, using no soap, no alcohol rub, no talcum powder. Apply a thin layer of silicone cream to skin

Figure 49-4. Important considerations in the preventive management of bedsores. (Adapted with permission of Hospital Publications, Inc., from Bedsores, *Hosp. Med.* 13:83–103, May 1977, p. 100, by S. E. Moolten.)

from horizontal to vertical. This can be achieved by elevating the head of the bed or, when permissible, sitting the patient in a chair. For the immobile patient, the use of tilt tables to gradually achieve a vertical position may be helpful. The Circle Electric Bed also provides an opportunity to change from horizontal to vertical position without getting the patient out of bed. When getting the patient out of bed after any prolonged period of bedrest, the nurse should ensure the safety of the patient by changing his or her position in stages, closely monitoring the pulse, blood pressure, and subjective symptoms at each stage of position change. See Chapter 50 for further discussion of causes of, and exercises to prevent, orthostatic hypotension.

Thrombus Formation

It is believed that immobility predisposes to thrombus formation by contributing to venous stasis, hypercoagulability of the blood, and external pressure against the veins. Venous stasis in the legs results from the lack of muscular contraction which ordinarily promotes venous return. Dehydration, which often accompanies immobility, is considered as a factor in hypercoagulability of the blood. External pressure on the blood vessels is a common problem familiar to nurses. The lateral recumbent position, which is the most frequently used position, may also result in both circulatory stasis and damage to the intima of the blood vessels due to pressure. When the intima is damaged, a layer of platelets is laid down over the damaged area, and this plaque may be the basis for a clot. These problems in turn may result in a pulmonary embolism which can be fatal. See Chapter 41 for detailed discussion of thrombi.

These effects of immobility on the cardiovascular system indicate that no patient should be allowed to remain immobile any longer than absolutely necessary. Even when bedrest must be imposed, nursing measures can prevent the hazards of immobility. Exercises to prevent loss of muscle tone and to promote muscular pressure on veins to assist the return flow of blood to the heart should be included in the nursing care plan. These might include active and passive range of joint motion exercises, isometric exercises, and self-care to the maximum permitted.

Patients need to be taught how to move and change position in bed without building up intrathoracic pressure. An overbed frame and trapeze can be provided, if necessary, and the patient taught to use it properly. To prevent dangers inherent in repeated Valsalva maneuvers, the patient should be told to exhale rather than hold his or her breath while moving in bed.

Preventing constipation and positioning the patient for defecation in a well-supported sitting or squatting position also will reduce the workload of the heart. Anticoagulants are used prophylactically when prolonged immobilization will be necessary postoperatively and when patients are on bedrest for more than 2 or 3 days. And finally, as activity is permitted, it must be graduated carefully to avoid fatigue.

Effects on Respiratory Function

Respiration as a physiologic process is the gaseous exchange between an organism and its environment. Oxygen is absorbed and carbon dioxide is eliminated. The purpose of the respiratory movement is to renew the air in the alveoli, to ventilate, to move air in and out (See Chapter 26). Changes in normal physiologic function of the respiratory system during short periods of immobility may at first be compensatory or adaptive as the body strives to preserve homeostasis. Respirations become slower and less deep to compensate for the lessened demand when a patient is immobile and/or confined to bed. This leads to decreased respiratory movement, decreased movement of secretions, and disturbed oxygen-carbon dioxide balance (Olson, 1967, p. 783). The etiological factors involved in deficient respiration are (1) habitual poor posture; (2) inadequate or asymmetric motion of the ribcage due to weakness and paralysis of muscles; (3) pathologic changes in the thoracic viscera (such as from asthma, emphysema, and tuberculosis); (4) weakness or paralysis of the diaphragm; and (5) weakness or paralysis of the abdominal muscles.

The normal movement of secretions out of the tracheobronchial tree is decreased whenever one of the normal cleansing mechanisms, such as coughing or changes in posture or position, is made ineffective. Prolonged immobility causes stasis and pooling of secretions. The maintenance of a patent airway may be threatened. Secretions may become thick and tenacious due to poor fluid intake and dehydration, and this will further interfere with the movement of secretions. The immobilized patient may contract bronchitis or hypostatic pneumonia. The collection of stagnant secretions in the dependent parts of the lungs also provide an excellent medium for bacterial growth within the body, especially for pneumococcal, pseudomonal, staphylococcal, and streptococcal organisms. Drugs such as anesthetics, narcotics, and sedatives may also contribute to respiratory complications by decreasing the rate and depth of lung expansion and ventilation and by depressing the cough center.

If there is a decrease in respiratory movement and a decrease in movement of secretions, there is limited diffusion of oxygen and carbon dioxide. The disturbance in the exchange will alter the normal oxygen–carbon dioxide balance, with a continuous buildup of carbon dioxide because it cannot adequately be expired and development of hypoxia because adequate oxygen cannot be inspired. If this process continues without intervention, respiratory acidosis will develop. (See also Chapter 41 for acid–base imbalance.)

Many of the activities the nurse performs daily pertain to respiration. While observing the patient's respiratory rate, the nurse makes many important observations in regard to the quality of the respirations. Are they deep or shallow? Moist or dry? Easy or labored? Is the patient using neck muscles or abdominal muscles? Are there any signs which would indicate hypoxia such as restlessness or forgetfulness? Another nursing activity is to help the patient routinely cough, turn, and breathe deeply. The nurse must be able to teach the patient how to breathe deeply using abdominal muscles, diaphragm, and intercostals to facilitate deep inhalation and prolonged expiration and must encourage him or her to do breathing exercises regularly. Patients, as well as nurses, must understand how beneficial it is to chest and lung expansion for the patient to turn off of the back or side, stretch out, and sit up straight at regular and frequent intervals; also it should be understood how coughing secretions up and out facilitates adequate oxygen–carbon dioxide exchange. If the patient is unable to cough effectively, it may be necessary to use chest percussion and tapping to help loosen secretions and postural drainage to remove them from the tracheobronchial tree. (See Chapter 40 for description of these techniques.)

References Cited

Asher, R. A. "The Danger of Going to Bed." *Br. Med. J.* (1947), 967.

Bliss, M. R., and McLaren, R. "Preventing Pressure Sores in Geriatric Patients. Part 1." *Nurs. Mirror,* **123** (Jan. 27, 1967), 381.

———. Part 2. *Nurs. Mirror,* **123** (Feb. 10, 1967), 434.

Bliss, M. R. et al. "Preventing Pressure Sores in Hospital: Controlled Trial of a Large-Celled Ripple Mattress." *Br. Med. J.,* **1** (Feb. 18, 1967), 394.

DiMascio, S. "Debrisan for Decubitus Ulcers." *Am. J. Nurs.,* **79** (April 1979), 684–85.

Exton-Smith, A. N. cited in *Nurs. Times,* Aug. 4, 1967, p. 1033.

Gosnell, D. J. "An Assessment Tool to Identify Pressure Sores." *Nurs. Res.,* **22** (Jan.–Feb. 1973), 55–59.

Gruis, M. L., and Innes, B. "Assessment: Essential to Prevent Pressure Sores." *Am. J. Nurs.,* **76** (Nov. 1976), 1762–64.

Kukuk, H. M. "Safety Precautions: Protecting Your Patients & Yourself." *Nursing 76,* **6** (June 1976), 49–52.

Mitchell, A. C. "Black Skin: An Historical, Psychological and Health Care Perspective. *J. Cont. Ed. in Nurs.,* **10** (1979), 28–33.

Moolten, S. E. "Bedsores." *Hosp. Med.,* **13** (May 1977), 83–103.

Noonan, J., and Noonan, L. "Two Burned Patients on Flotation Therapy." *Am. J. Nurs.,* **68** (Feb. 1968), 319.

Olson, E. V. "The Hazards of Immobility." *Am. J. Nurs.,* **67** (April 1967), 780–96.

Sather, M. R. el al. "Pressure Sores and the Spinal Cord Injury Patient." *Drug Intelligence Clin. Pharm.,* **11** (March 1977), 154–168.

Verhonick, P. J. "Decubitus Ulcer Observations Measured Objectively." *Nurs. Res.,* **10** (Fall 1961), 211–14.

——— et al. "Thermography in the Study of Decubitus Ulcers." *Nurs. Res.,* **21** (May–June 1972), 233–37.

Williams, A. "A Study of Factors Contributing to Skin Breakdown." *Nurs. Res.,* **22** (May–June 1973), 238–43.

General References

Disuse Syndromes & Mobility Problems

Anderson, H. C. *Newton's Geriatric Nursing,* 5th ed. St. Louis: C. V. Mosby Co., 1971.

Belger, A. J., and Greene, E. H. *Winter's Protective Body Mechanics.* New York: Springer Publishing Co., 1973.

Bonner, Charles, ed. *The Team Approach to Hemiplegia.* Springfield, Ill.: Charles C Thomas, 1969.

Browse, N. *The Physiology and Pathology of Bed Rest.* Springfield, Ill.: Charles C Thomas, 1965.

Brunnstrom, S. *Clinical Kinesiology,* 3rd ed. Philadelphia: F. A. Davis Co., 1972.

Carini Esta, and Owens, Guy. *Neurological and Neurosurgical Nursing.* St. Louis: C. V. Mosby Co., 1973.

Cohen, Lillian. *Communication Problems after Stroke.* Minneapolis: Sister Kenny Institute, 1971.

Downey, John A., and Darling, Robert C., ed. *Physiological Basis of Rehabilitation.* Philadelphia: W. B. Saunders Co., 1971.

Ehlrich, George, ed. *Total Management of the Arthritic Patient.* Philadelphia: J. B. Lippincott Co., 1973.

Elden, H. R., ed. *Biophysical Properties of the Skin.* New York: John Wiley & Sons, 1971.

Ford, J. R. *Physical Management for the Quadriplegic Patient.* Philadelphia: F. A. Davis Co., 1975.

Garret, J. S., and Levine, E. S. *Rehabilitation Practices with the Physically Disabled.* New York: Columbia University Press, 1973.

Harmon, Vera, and Steele, Shirley. *Nursing Care of the Skin.* New York: Appleton-Century Crofts, 1975.

Hutchinson, E. C., and Acheson, E. J. *Strokes: Natural History, Pathology and Surgical Treatment.* London: W. B. Saunders Co., 1975.

Krusen, F. H., Kottke, F. J., and Ellwood, P. M. *Handbook of Physical Medicine and Rehabilitation,* 2nd ed. Philadelphia: W. B. Saunders Co., 1971.

Larson, Carroll, and Gould, Marjorie. *Orthopedic Nursing.* St. Louis: C. V. Mosby Co., 1974.

Lawton, E. *Activities of Daily Living for Physical Rehabilitation.* New York: McGraw-Hill, 1963.

Leutennegger, Ralph R. *Patient Care and Rehabilitation of Communication Impaired Adults.* Springfield, Ill.: Charles C Thomas, 1975.

Licht, Sidney, ed. *Stroke and Its Rehabilitation.* Baltimore: Waverly Press, 1975.

May, Elizabeth Edkhardt, Wayonner, Neva, and Hotte, Eleanor. *Independent Living for the Handicapped and the Elderly.* Boston: Houghton, Mifflin Co., 1974.

Miller, M., and Sachs, M. *About Bedsores.* Philadelphia: J. B. Lippincott Co., 1974.

Mooney, T. O., Cole, T. M., and Chilgren, R. A. *Sexual Options for Paraplegics and Quadriplegics.* Boston: Little, Brown, 1975.

O'Brien, Mary, and Pallett, Phyllis. *Total Care of the Stroke Patient.* Boston: Little, Brown, 1978.

Rosebury, T. *Life on Man.* New York: Viking Press, 1969.

Steinberg, F. A., ed. *Cowdry's the Care of the Geriatric Patient,* 5th ed. St. Louis: C. V. Mosby Co., 1976.

Winter, C. *Nursing Care of Patients with Urologic Diseases,* 3rd ed. St. Louis: C. V. Mosby Co., 1975.

General Rehabilitation

Alshuler, A. et al. "Even Children Can Learn to Do Self Catherization." *Am. J. Nurs.,* **77** (Jan. 1977), 97–101.

Flynn, R. J. et al. "Normative Sex Behavior and the Person

with a Disability." *J. Rehabil.*, **43** (Nov.–Dec. 1977), 34–38.

Glass, D. D. et al. "Sexual Adjustment in the Handicapped." *J. Rehabil.*, **44** (Jan.–March 1978), 43–47.

Smith, J. et al. "Sexuality and the Severely Disabled Person." *Am. J. Nurs.*, **75** (Dec. 1975), 2194–97.

Amputations

Kegel, B. et al. "Functional Capabilities of Lower Extremity Amputees." *Arch. Phys. Med. Rehabil.*, **59** (March 1978), 109–20.

Kerstein, M. D. "The Air Prosthesis for Amputees." *RN*, **39** (July, 1976), 42–43.

Martin, Nancy. "Rehabilitation of the Upper Extremity Amputee." *Nurs. Outlook*, **18** (Feb. 1970), 50–51.

Reinstein, L. et al. "Sexual Adjustment after Lower Extremity Amputation." *Arch. Phys. Med. Rehabil.*, **59** (Nov. 1978), 501–4.

Reyes, R. L. et al. "Elderly Patients with Lower Extremity Amputations." *Arch. Phys. Med. Rehabil.*, **58** (March 1977), 116–23.

Shoenfeld, Y. et al. "Orthostatic Hypotension in Amputees and Subjects with Spinal Cord Injuries." *Arch. Phys. Med. Rehabil.*, **59** (March 1971), 138–41.

Solomon, G. et al. "A Burning Issue: Phantom Limb Pain and Psychological Preparation of the Patient for Amputation." *Arch. Surg.*, **113** (Feb. 1978), 185–86.

Cerebral Palsy

Flechsig, L. "Living with Cerebral Palsy." *Am. J. Nurs.*, **78** (July 1978), 1212–13.

Hawley, D. et al. "Reducing Muscle Spasms in a Child with Cerebral Palsy." *Am. J. Nurs.*, **78** (July 1978), 1214–15.

Hitchcock, R. R. "Stereotactic Surgery for Cerebral Palsy." *Nurs. Times*, **74** (Dec. 1978), 2064–65.

Scherzer, A. I. et al. "Physical Therapy as a Determinant of Change in the Cerebral Palsied Infant." *Pediatrics*, **58** (July 1976), 47–52.

Immobility Disuse Syndromes

Asher, R. A. J. "Dangers of Going to Bed." *British Med. J.*, **2** (1947), 967.

Brower, Phyllis, and Hecks, Dorothy. "Maintaining Muscle Function in Patients on Bed Rest." *Am. J. Nurs.*, **72** (July 1972), 1250–53.

Carnevali, Doris, and Bruechner, Susan. "Immobilization—Reassessment of a Concept." *Am. J. Nurs.*, **70** (July 1970), 1502.

Downs, Florence. "Bed Rest and Sensory Disturbances." *Am. J. Nurs.*, **74** (March 1974), 434–38.

Gaul, A. L. et al. "Hyperbaric Oxygen Therapy." *Am. J. Nurs.*, **72** (May 1972), 892–96.

Gibson, C. J. et al. "Urinary Output and Incidence of Acute URI in Patients with Indwelling Bladder Catheters." *Arch. Phys. Med. Rehabil.*, **59** (Jan. 1975), 17–20.

Gordon, Janet E. "Circolectric Beds." *Nursing '77*, **7** (Feb. 1977), 42–46.

Kelly, Mary M. "Exercise for Bedfast Patients." *Am. J. Nurs.*, **66** (March 1966), 2209–12.

Kuhn, Hannah et al. "Intermittent Catherization as a Rehabilitative Nursing Service." *Arch. Phys. Med. Rehabil.*, **55** (Oct. 1974), 439–43.

Lapides, Jack et al. "Follow-up on Unsterile Intermittent Self Catherization." *J. Urol.*, **111** (1974), 184–87.

Olson, Edith V. et al. "The Hazards of Immobility." *Am. J. Nurs.*, **67** (April 1967), 780–97.

Rubin, C. F. et al. "Auditing the Decubitus Ulcer Problem." *Am. J. Nurs.*, **1974** (Oct. 1974), 1820–26.

Multiple Sclerosis

Hornby, A. "Multiple Sclerosis: The MS Sufferer in the Community." *Nurs. Times*, 74 (May 1978), 130–31.

McNairn, N. "About Multiple Sclerosis." *Can. Nurse*, **74** (July–Aug. 1978), 35–43.

"Multiple Sclerosis: Home Study Unit for Continuing Education in Nursing." *Am. J. Nurs.*, **80** (Feb. 1980), 273–302.

Pulton, T. W. "Multiple Sclerosis: A Social-Psychological Perspectice." *Phys. Ther.*, **57** (Feb. 1977), 170–73.

Schnertzer, L. "Rehabilitation of Patients with Multiple Sclerosis." *Arch. Phys. Med. Rehabil.*, **59** (Sept. 1978), 430–37.

Parkinson's Disease

Davis, J. C. "Team Management of Parkinson's Disease." *Am. J. Occup. Ther.*, **31** (May–June 1977), 300–8.

Erb, Elizabeth. "Improving Speech in Parkinson's Disease." *Am. J. Nurs.*, **73** (Nov. 1973), 1910–14.

Fischback, F. T. "Easing Adjustment to Parkinson's Disease." *Am. J. Nurs.*, **78** (Jan. 1978), 66–69.

Geden, C. E. "Rehabilitation of a Patient with Parkinson's Disease." *Nurs. Times*, **73** (Sept. 1977), 1470.

Rheumatoid Arthritis

Attenborough, C. G. "Total Knee Replacement." *Nurs. Times*, **73** (Sept. 1977), 1514–17.

Ehrlich, G. E. "Arthritis Management: Treating Rheumatoid Arthritis with Behavioral and Clinical Strategy." *Nurs. Dig.*, **4** (Nov–Dec. 1976), 24–28.

Meyers, M. H. et al. "Total Hip Replacement—A Team Effort." *Am. J. Nurs.*, **78** (Sept. 1978), 1485–88.

Wright, V. "Rheumatoid Arthritis: Conservative Managements." *Nurs. Times,* **73** (Dec. 1977), 1878–81.

Skin Breakdown

Agris, J., and Spira, M. "Pressure Ulcers: Prevention and Treatment." *Clin. Symposia* (1979), **31**:5.

Cameron, G. "Pressure Sores: What to Do When Prevention Fails." *Nursing, 79,* **9** (Jan. 1979), 42–47.

Michelsen, D. "How to Give a Good Back Rub." *Am. J. Nurs.,* **78** (July 1978), 1197–99.

Spinal Cord Injury

Bactol, G. "Psychological Needs of the Spinal Cord Injured Person." *J. Neurosurg. Nurs.,* **10** (Dec. 1978), 171–75.

Beckman, A. H. et al. "Sexual Adjustment of Spinal Cord Injured Veterans Living in the Community." *Arch. Phys. Med. Rehabil.,* **59** (Jan. 1978), 29–33.

Hodges, L. C. et al. "Human Sexuality and the Spinal Cord Injured: Role of the Clinical Nurse Specialist." *J. Neurosurg. Nurs.,* **10** (Sept. 1978), 125–29.

Larrabee, J. H. "The Person with a Spinal Cord Injury." *Am. J. Nurs.,* **77** (Aug. 1977), 1330–36.

Lawsen, N. C. "Significant Events in the Rehabilitation Process: The Spinal Cord Patient's Point of View." *Arch. Phys. Med. Rehabil.,* **59** (Dec. 1978), 573–79.

Perkash, I. "Intermittent Catherization Failure and an Approach to Bladder Rehabilitation in Spinal cord Injury Patients." *Arch. Phys. Med. Rehabil.,* **59** (Jan. 1978), 9–17.

Sperling, Keith. "Intermittent Catherization to Obtain Catheter Free Bladder Function in Spinal Cord Injury." *Arch. Phys. Med. Rehab.,* **59** (Jan. 1978), 4–8.

Stroke

Anderson, T. P. et al. "Quality of Care for Completed Stroke without Rehabilitation: Evaluation by Assessing Patient Outcome." *Arch. Phys. Med. Rehabil.,* **60** (March 1979), 103–7.

Belt, Linda. "Working with Dysphasic Patients." *Am. J. Nurs.,* **74** (July 1974), 1320–23.

Dzau, Ruth, and Boehme, Anita. "Stroke Rehabilitation: A Family Team Education Program." *Arch. Phys. Med. Rehab.,* **59** (May 1978), 236–39.

Feldman, J. L., and Shultz, M. E. "Rehabilitation after Stroke." *Cardiovasc. Nurs.,* **11** (March–April 1975), 29–32.

Fox, Madeleine J. "Patients with Receptive Aphasia: They Really Don't Understand." *Am. J. Nurs.,* **76** (Oct. 1976), 1596–1600.

Granger, Carl V. et al. "Stroke Rehabilitation: Analyses of Repeated Barthel Index Measures." *Arch. Phys. Med. Rehab.,* **60** (Jan. 1979), 4–7.

Kavchak-Keyes, M. A. "Comeback from Disaster: Helping the Stroke Patient Learn to Help Himself." *Nursing '79,* **9** (Jan. 1979), 32–35.

Lynn, P. A. et al. "Research in Rehabilitation of Stroke Patients." *Chest Heart Stroke J.,* **3** (Fall 1978), 25–31.

Orade, Donna, and Waite, Nancy. "Group Psychotherapy with Stroke Patients during the Immediate Recovery Phase." *Am. J. Orthopsych.,* **44** (April 1974), 386–89.

Schwartzonan, S. T. "Anxiety and Depression in the Stroke Patient: A Nursing Challenge." *J. Psychiatr. Nurs.,* **14** (July 1976), 13–17.

Skelly, Madge. "Aphasic Patients Talk Back." *Am. J. Nurs.,* **75** (July 1975), 1140–43.

Strickland, E. "Stroke. . . . How Can You Help?" *Nurs. Times,* **74** (Nov. 1978), 327–29.

Wylie, Charles M. "The Value of Early Rehabilitation in Stroke." *Geriatrics,* **25** (1970), 107.

50

Problems with Mobility

Keep the faculty of effort alive in you by a little gratuitous exercise every day. That is, be systematically ascetic or heroic in little unnecessary points, do every day or two something for no other reason than that you would rather not do it, so that when the hour of dire need draws nigh, it may find you not unnerved and untrained to stand the test.

William James
The Principles of Psychology (1890) Quoted in *Bartlett's Familiar Quotations* Thirteenth and Centennial Edition. By John Bartlett, Boston: Little, Brown and Company. 1955

Care of the Person Who Has Sustained a Cerebral Vascular Accident

Overview of Care

Cerebral vascular disease is the third leading cause of death and disability in the United States and affects half a million Americans yearly. Approximately 2 million people are currently suffering with long-term disabilities resulting from stroke. Some of these disabilities can be reduced or prevented by conscientious application of rehabilitation principles. In other cases a rehabilitation program can assist the patient to live a more comfortable and productive life in spite of deficits that cannot be cured or altered. The first step in developing a rehabilitation plan for the patient with stroke is a complete evaluation of strengths and limitations. Rehabilitation planning should begin with institution of both short- and long-term goals as soon as the stroke is diagnosed. Even though it may not be possible to predict the patient's rehabilitation potential at this early stage of illness, it is imperative that nurses caring for the patient with stroke understand techniques of preventing complications that will retard rehabilitation if the patient does have the potential for it. Complications that have a direct effect on rehabilitation, such as contractures, pressure sores, and bowel and bladder problems have been reviewed in the previous chapter on disuse syndromes.

This chapter was contributed by Rita H. O'Neill, R.N., M.S., Associate Professor of Nursing, College of Nursing, Southeastern Massachusetts University, North Dartmouth, Massachusetts.

Exercise

Only at such time as the physician orders active or passive range of motion for the patient should the indicated exercises begin. The length of time following the disability until range of motion exercises can be started will be determined by the patient's condition. For example, if a cerebrovascular accident has occurred as a result of thrombus or embolus, these activities may be indicated within 48 hours. If, however, the stroke was caused by hemorrhage, the physician may not allow activity for 6 to 8 weeks. When exercises are indicated and ordered, the necessity of their daily occurrence cannot be overemphasized. Talking with the physician about when he or she wishes exercises to begin is always in order.

Alignment

From the time of admission the body should be maintained in good physiologic alignment. This is accomplished by the use of sandbags, pillows, trochanter rolls, foot boards, splints, and slings. Nursing students are urged to observe their own position when supine. The importance of diligent attention may then be more apparent. They will observe that the feet are in plantar flexion and the legs are externally rotated. Not infrequently their arms will be abducted and flexed. Prolonged bedrest may result in flexion deformities that fix the joints abnormally in these positions, thus prohibiting full range of motion. Measures instituted by the nurse are designed to prevent and correct these deformities.

The patient who has had a stroke should have the affected arm supported by a sling when either sitting or walking. If the arm is not supported, subluxation or partial dislocation of that shoulder may ensue. When a sling is used, three considerations are important: first, the wrist must also be supported to prevent wrist drop; second, the weight of the arm in the sling should not exert excess pressure on the cervical vertebrae; last, the extremity should be taken through range of motion and not allowed to become contracted in the sling.

Probable Outcomes

All the preventive nursing measures that are detailed for disuse syndromes will be necessary to prevent further complications. The prognosis for functional recovery following stroke is limited by coexistence of such chronic illnesses as hypertension, cardiac decompensation, obesity, emphysema, and diabetes mellitus. The time that elapses between onset of stroke and the institution of rehabilitation efforts is also important, since in most cases of longstanding untreated disability, the results of even the most intensive therapy are poor (Licht, 1975, pp. 221–25).

Patients who have failed to show any return of motor function within 1 to 2 months after onset of stroke cannot be expected to recover muscle control to any appreciable degree. Unless rehabilitation has been neglected or medical problems have caused delay or interruption of the rehabilitation program, maximum achievement of functional performance generally occurs within 4 to 6 months of the start of therapy (Licht, 1975). Predictor items that have been identified to assist in establishing rehabilitation potential include (1) positive acceptance of the disability on the part of the patient, (2) presence in the home of a spouse or other family member to assist the patient, (3) good bladder control, (4) good visual–motor coordination, (5) early return of muscle tone, (6) early return of tendon jerks, (7) early return of voluntary motion, (8) good strength in muscles of hands and trunk, and (9) skill in feeding (Licht, 1975, pp. 435–71).

No two rehabilitation programs can be the same; each must be tailored to the individual patient's abilities and disabilities. Since a patient with receptive aphasia may not be able to follow many verbal instructions, it will be necessary to use a different approach in teaching an exercise program. When a patient has weakness or paralysis accompanied by a perceptual disorder, he or she will need to use a very different technique for dressing from another patient with the same physical deficit who has no perceptual impairment.

Hemiplegia

Hemiplegia or hemiparesis is easily observable and presents definite indications for specific nursing care. The traditional approach relies heavily on active-assistive exercise programs. In active-assistive exercises the patient is instructed to concentrate on the activity and attempt to perform the movements voluntarily while the nurse or physical therapist carries out the range of motion exercises. Most self-care activities such as bathing, grooming, using the toilet, dressing, and eating are referred to as bilateral activities, because they normally involve the use of two hands. One of the greatest losses for the patient who has suffered a stroke can be the loss of a functional hand or arm. A functional hand requires motor control, intact sensory discrimination, and exquisite coordination to perform intricate movements with skill and speed. Following stroke the upper extremities frequently remain useless, because those qualities that make the difference between a functional and nonfunctional hand are either totally lost or severely impaired. The occupational therapist can teach the patient various techniques for using the involved arm to assist the functional arm in carrying out self-care activities. The most important motor ability of the body is that of opposition of the thumb and fingers to pinch, grasp, or clasp. When this function has been lost, the therapist will explore with the patient alternative methods that may be available for gripping and holding objects. Occasionally adaptive equipment for the hand may be used to improve function and assist in self-care. When the dominant side has been paralyzed, the therapist will initiate a retraining program for the good arm in which the patient is taught to write and use various implements such as keys and flatware. This is necessary because this patient will have had less dexterity of the nondominant hand even before being paralyzed by the stroke. Once the patient begins to progress with use of the unaffected nondominant hand, he or she can be taught to use the affected hand for holding and stabilizing objects to be manipulated with the good hand (Licht, 1975, pp. 347–79).

Whereas the right hemiplegic has aphasic problems, the left hemiplegic is more prone to spatial-perceptual difficulties. Speech may be quite fluent and may mask brain damage. This patient will have difficulty with position sense and body parts sense. Not only are these problems harder to perceive, but left hemiplegics tend to plunge ahead into activities, believing and saying they are capable of activities of which they are not. They will, for example, transfer without locking wheelchair brakes, or attempt to walk without looking to see if their foot is planted firmly on the floor. These patients present a danger to themselves because of their masked brain damage and spatial-perceptual difficulties and must be protected for their own safey. The patient with hemiplegia has an excellent chance of both bowel and bladder control because the reflex is intact and there is partial sensation. Although there will be exceptions, right and left hemiplegics tend to demonstrate some different functional and behavioral changes. These differences can be useful guides for planning nursing care. Right hemiplegia occurs following damage to the left side of the brain. The right hemiplegic is more prone to demonstrate aphasia. Aphasia may be mild, moderate, or severe and it may be expressive or receptive.

The Aphasic Person

A large number of persons suffering from cerebral vascular accident or head trauma experience brain damage in those areas responsible for the comprehension and expression of language. The loss of language functioning is termed *aphasia.* Other problems (hemiplegia, hemianopsia) may also be present. If present, they can compound the communication difficulty. This reduction in language includes understanding things that are heard, seen, or written and the expression of a message whether expressed orally, through gestures, or in written form. Expressive language is that language used to reveal our needs and thinking to other persons. Receptive language is the language each of us uses to understand what others communicate to us. Inner language is that language individuals use to think or talk to themselves. The patient who has had a stroke may have had damage of varying degree to any or all of these three types of language. Therefore, if patients have expressive aphasia, it does not mean that they cannot hear or understand what is said to them or in their presence. This fact must be clearly and completely understood by all persons (staff, visitors, and other patients) coming into contact with patients who are unable to speak. When attempting to communicate, the nurse should talk with such a patient as if he or she does understand. Above all, it should never be forgotten how devastating and frightening it would be to the patient to have others discuss, within his or her hearing, the hopelessness of the condition. The following terms are symptoms of aphasia and may help the nurse describe the patient's aphasic problem.

ANOMIA—difficulty in recalling specific words such as nouns and verbs. The patient knows what they are, but cannot recall their name from memory.

JARGON—the word used to describe utterances by the patient that are unintelligible; the use of nonsense sound combinations instead of words.

TELEGRAPHIC LANGUAGE—the use of only major information words to express ideas, such as "wife, son, visit" instead of "My wife and son came to visit me." The patient omits such words as articles, prepositions, and adjectives.

PERSEVERATION—continues to make a response after that response is no longer appropriate.

APRAXIA—the inability to perform voluntary motor acts. The patient may say a word perfectly one minute when not thinking about it, but be unable to repeat it when asked to do so.

DYSARTHRIA—a motor speech defect of the oral musculature resulting in imprecise articulation of speech sounds. Patient may clearly utter short words or phrases, but speech becomes less intellegible as length and rate of speech increases.

RETENTION PROBLEMS—the impairment of the patient's ability to retain events that were recently performed, heard, or seen.

AUTOMATIC SPEECH—reciting automatic or overheard language units although unable to provide other messages. Such language units include social amenities, rote lists, profanity. Automatic speech can often mislead family and personnel caring for the patient about the patient's true expressive abilities.

If the patient does not demonstrate the ability to communicate verbally, it must be ascertained if he or she understands what is being said. Following the onset of aphasia, one of the earliest and most basic forms of communication is the use of yes and no. Whether or not the patient has a reliable yes/no response must be carefully ascertained. A verbal or physical yes response may be demonstrated, but the patient may respond to any or all questions in this manner. As soon as the patient uses any form of yes/no response he or she should be asked questions that require both yes/no answers, such as, "Are you a man?" "Are you a woman?" "Is the sun shining?" "Is it raining?" The patient may be capable of responding nonverbally to questions that require yes or no answers. When the patient does respond by shaking his or her head or blinking the eyes, he or she should use these nonverbal responses appropriately. However, neither the patient nor those in the environment should be allowed to rely on nonverbal communication if verbal communication is possible.

The patient with aphasia is not mentally ill as a result of the cerebral episode. There may be disorientation or emotional lability. The patient may be unable to inhibit inappropriate or excessive laughter or tears. The threshold for frustration and anger may be lowered. A person who cannot communicate, when he or she desires to do so, becomes very frustrated. In addition, the patient is probably not understanding everything being said. All patients with aphasia have some difficulty processing auditory information. Constant smiling, nodding of the head, and other affirmative behavior in response to questions, comments, or actions may be misleading and does not necessarily mean that the patient understands.

It is extremely important to begin language evaluation and therapy as soon as the patient can focus attention. The primary responsibility of the speech therapist is to evaluate, screen, and treat patient problems in the area of language (verbal and nonverbal), articulation, voice, rhythm, and audiology. Therapy is directed toward restoring the patient, insofar as possible, to his or her previous ability in these areas. The goals of a speech and language program are based on the needs of the individual patient. In general, the speech pathologist begins remediation when the patient has some performing success. The guiding purpose of the program is to help each patient regain as much functional language as possible. For some this may only be the ability to indicate yes or no to questions concerning their needs. The prognosis of recovery of language skills varies with the severity of the language problem, motivation on the part of the patient, adjustment, help from family, and other physical and emotional involvement. The greater the language loss and the less spontaneous recovery that occurs, the poorer the prognosis.

Those involved in caring for the patient with communication problems have an opportunity to assist him or her in avoiding additional frustration and overcoming the problem. The following are some approaches that may be utilized:

1. Do not appear rushed. Give the patient the feeling you have time for him or her. The patient needs more time than most people to express himself or herself and process what is heard. Consequently, feeling rushed will add to frustration and anxiety and result in poorer language performance or possibly in giving up altogether.
2. When speaking to the patient, speak slowly, clearly, and not too loudly. Use brief sentences of only a few words. Speak on a concrete level. Let the patient watch your face as you talk.
3. If the patient does not understand your statement or question the first time it is verbalized, repeat or rephrase it. Use of gestures or objects may aid comprehension for at least a yes/no response.
4. Give the patient every opportunity to communicate in some way.
   a. Soliciting yes/no response to questions.
   b. Using a communication chart, either with pictures or words.
   c. Having a volunteer or family member play simple games with the patient and read to him or her
5. There are some patients who do not appear to respond to any verbal or visual stimuli. Stimulate language in any way possible:
   a. Talk about things you are doing for him or her.
   b. Talk about cards or visitors received.
   c. Discuss new items of general interest.
   d. Require a gestural response and prompt the patient's movement as you request it (as "lift your arm" or "sit up" or "roll over").

When a patient is frustrated, depressed, angry, or lashes out against his or her inability to communicate, never overlook the problem or tell the patient he or she will be communicating "as good as new soon." If a patient has not recovered speech and language spontaneously within the first few weeks of the hospital stay, a long period of speech remediation may be required. Tell the patient you know he or she has difficulty communicating and that everyone wants to help him or her regain as much as possible.

Assessing Functional Levels

Although comprehensive initial patient assessments require a great deal of nursing time, it is time extremely well spent. Obtaining pertinent data early is the only way goal-directed patient programs can begin early. The initial assessment tool will contain all the pertinent general information contained in a general nursing history, but will, in addition, give more attention to self-care activities. By self-care activities we mean those activities of daily living (ADL) that are essential to all people—eating, dressing washing, ambulating, and toileting. In addition to these initial assessment data, rehabilitation patients must be reassessed frequently to determine if short-term goals are being achieved and to aid in setting new and realistic goals with the rehabilitation team and the patient.

One tool that is useful for periodic assessment of self-care activities is the Barthel index. The index has a maximum score of 100 (ten items being scored) for complete functional competence. The ten self-care activities being evaluated are feeding, bathing, personal toilet or grooming, dressing, bowel control, bladder control, toilet transfers, chair/bed transfers, ambulation, and stair climbing. It is suggested that the rehabilitation team use this index to evaluate patients every 2 weeks in order to monitor progress in acquiring functional skills (Granger, 1979). This tool does not include other factors that may influence progress or outcomes such as medical, perceptual, emotional, cognitive, language, or family problems, but it provides a very specific means of determining patient progress in the area of self-care activities which is so vital in the rehabilitation program.

Care of Persons with Spinal Cord Injury

Because of increased numbers of persons injured in automobile and athletic accidents and in crimes of violence, nurses frequently have patients with spinal cord injury to care for during their acute phase on general wards. There are few patients who so promptly and devastatingly reveal poor care as these; but, on the other hand, nurses who can maintain in good shape the bodies and spirits of their patients with pathology in the spinal cord may justifiably feel great satisfaction.

Everything one has learned of the structure and function of the spinal cord and peripheral nervous system can be put to use. Everything one knows of normal development of the personality and the effects of sudden helplessness on it will be invaluable knowledge to the sensitive nurse. If transection is functionally complete, one knows that afferent impulses cannot ascend from below the level of the lesion to the brain or efferent impulses descend to parts below the break in continuity of the cord. There will be paralysis, necessarily, and there will be anesthesia and vasomotor instability of the body beginning a little higher up than the level of the lesion. The patient will be unaware of his or her distended bladder and unable to empty it or the bowel voluntarily. Sooner or later the patient will be aware of inadequacy of sexual function. If the lesion is in the thoracic cord or above, breathing will be affected and the weak chest movements will keep the patient continuously in danger of pneumonia.

The problem of the patient with a severed spinal cord are numerous and complex. Some complications are preventable; some are not. Most do not happen early in the disability and, therefore, are an excellent example of why diligent concern on the part of the nurse must continue.

Spasms

One such complication is spasms. Following the initial spinal cord injury, the patient enters a period known as spinal cord shock. During spinal cord shock the paralysis is flaccid. Spinal shock may last from weeks to months. Eventually, the lower motor neuron, or reflex are, which has not been damaged, begins to function again. Because there is no longer central nervous system control or modulation of the reflex arcs below the level of injury, the paralysis becomes and remains spastic. Involuntary muscular contraction of the lower extremities will be observed. Very little stimulus is needed to set the reflex arc into action. Such things as jarring of the bed, or merely touching of the leg can send the part into spasm. The patient will notice his or her leg "moves" or "jumps." It is not difficult to imagine the meaning of this event to the patient. Whereas the legs have been "dead," they now obviously have "come back to life." The nurse should help the patient understand what is happening.

Spasms vary in severity from person to person. They may present no problem at all and, in fact, may be of physiologic value. On the other hand, they may increase in severity to the point of producing flexion contractures. Spasms may increase to the point of preventing the patient from wearing long leg braces, thereby prohibiting ambulation. When the physiatrist feels that because of spasms no further rehabilitation can be accomplished, a chemical block may be offered to the patient. Accepting or refusing chemical or surgical rhizotomy is a decision that can be made only by the patient. Rhizotomy will result in a permanent flaccid paralysis as it destroys the reflex arc, but it will enable the patient to continue the rehabilitation process. Few patients accept rhizotomy immediately, and some never agree to the procedure. The rehabilitation team can only make apparent why rhizotomy is indicated. The decision belongs to the patient.

Skin Breakdown

Skin breakdown is another matter of grave concern to the paralyzed person. Able bodied persons constantly shift their body weight to relieve and redistribute pressure. This is not possible for the paralyzed person. Because of lack of sensation, they are not aware when they have been in one position too long; and if they were aware, they could not move because of motor paralysis. No matter whether in bed or in wheelchair, it is imperative that body weight be distributed evenly over as wide a surface as possible. Prevention is the best treatment for pressure sores, as discussed in depth with the disuse syndromes.

Bowel and Bladder Problems

Bowel and bladder problems also plague the patient with paraplegia. A regimen must be established for each as soon as possible, or physical and psychological trauma will occur. Bladder sensation and control are lost following complete transection, or cross section, of the spinal cord. Immediately after injury the bladder becomes atonic, or without tone, and remains so throughout the period of spinal shock. When reflexes again affect the detrusor muscle, the bladder will empty itself. The amount of urine the bladder is capable of holding varies. If the bladder can accommodate 250 to 350 ml and then expel this urine, the patient is said to have an automatic or reflex bladder. Initially an indwelling catheter will have been inserted. When attempts are made to "train" the bladder, the catheter may be removed. The patient's intake and output will be accurately measured and recorded. If, after a period of time, the bladder continues to empty itself, with residuals of 60 ml or less, the patient will be catheter free. It is hoped that the bladder will continue to hold and then expel its maximum amount of urine. When reflex bladder is a reality, expulsion of urine will be mainly determined by the amount of fluid the patient drinks. He or she must carefully calculate intake in order to know when to anticipate the expulsion of urine. In upper motor neuron lesions, expulsion of urine by the bladder may be facilitated by tactile stimulation of the areas innervated by the pudendal nerve. In lower motor neuron lesions, exertion of manual pressure over the bladder (Credé method) or straining may be helpful in inducing urination.

The length of time required for training the bladder varies greatly. The male patient may wear an external urinary collecting device that will be attached to his leg. Some patients are never able to achieve a reflex bladder and therefore will need permanent indwelling catheters or cystostomies. Long-term use of an indwelling catheter in the male patient can produce a penile scrotal fistula. The shaft of the penis should be elevated and the penile scrotal junction examined. If a fistula is present, one will observe the catheter through the fistula. This problem can be prevented by taping the catheter to the abdomen whenever the patient is in bed. To avoid some of the problems associated with indwelling catheters, the use of intermittent catheterization is gaining in popularity. Refer to the urinary elimination section of Chapter 49, on disuse syndromes.

Autonomic Hyperreflexia

Following severe spinal cord injury, only isolated cord reflexes, cut off from any inhibiting control from above, remain. Most of these reflexes, if they occur, have nuisance value only. An important exception to the innocuous nature of residual reflexes is *autonomic hyperreflexia* (disturbed or abnormal reflexes), an excessive autonomic response to normal stimuli experienced by a patient with a spinal cord lesion usually above T_6 or T_4 (Feustel, 1976). The genitoanal area is the most sensitive and frequent source of visceral or cutaneous stimuli below the level of cord injury which triggers autonomic hyperreflexia. When caused by a plugged catheter or bladder or urethral obstruction, tremendous backup of urine greatly distends the bladder. The reflexes sent by the distended bladder may be carried to all parts of the cord. This constitutes a medical emergency and must be corrected immediately. Again, the patient does not feel the sensation of a distended bladder so he or she cannot tell the nurse. However, the patient will be extremely anxious and may complain of a severe headache. Blood pressure will be elevated; it is not uncommon to observe a systolic reading of 300.

In the hypertensive crisis which follows *autonomic hyperreflexia*, different impulses ascend in the lateral funiculi to the level of the lesion, which blocks transmission up the spinothalamic tracts and posterior columns. But because the autonomic reflex is mediated through the intact lateral horn cells, reflex arteriolar spasm takes place in the skin and viscera, causing hypertension and profuse sweating below the level of the lesion. Other signs are slow pulse, diaphoresis, pilomotor reflex, and temperature elevation. This complication will most often occur when an indwelling catheter is being utilized, although fecal impaction may also be the cause. See Figure 50–1 for other symptoms of autonomic hyperreflexia.

Hypertension persists because compensatory vasodilation cannot occur below the lesion, due to blockade of efferent impulses to the sympathetic motor preganglionic neurons in the thoracic and lumbar segments. Emergency treatment of autonomic hyperreflexia is to remove the triggering stimulus, which may be a full bladder, or rectum, sudden changes of environmental temperature or air movement, or pressure against the patient's skin.

From the onset of symptoms, the nurse should monitor the patient's blood pressure every 5 min-

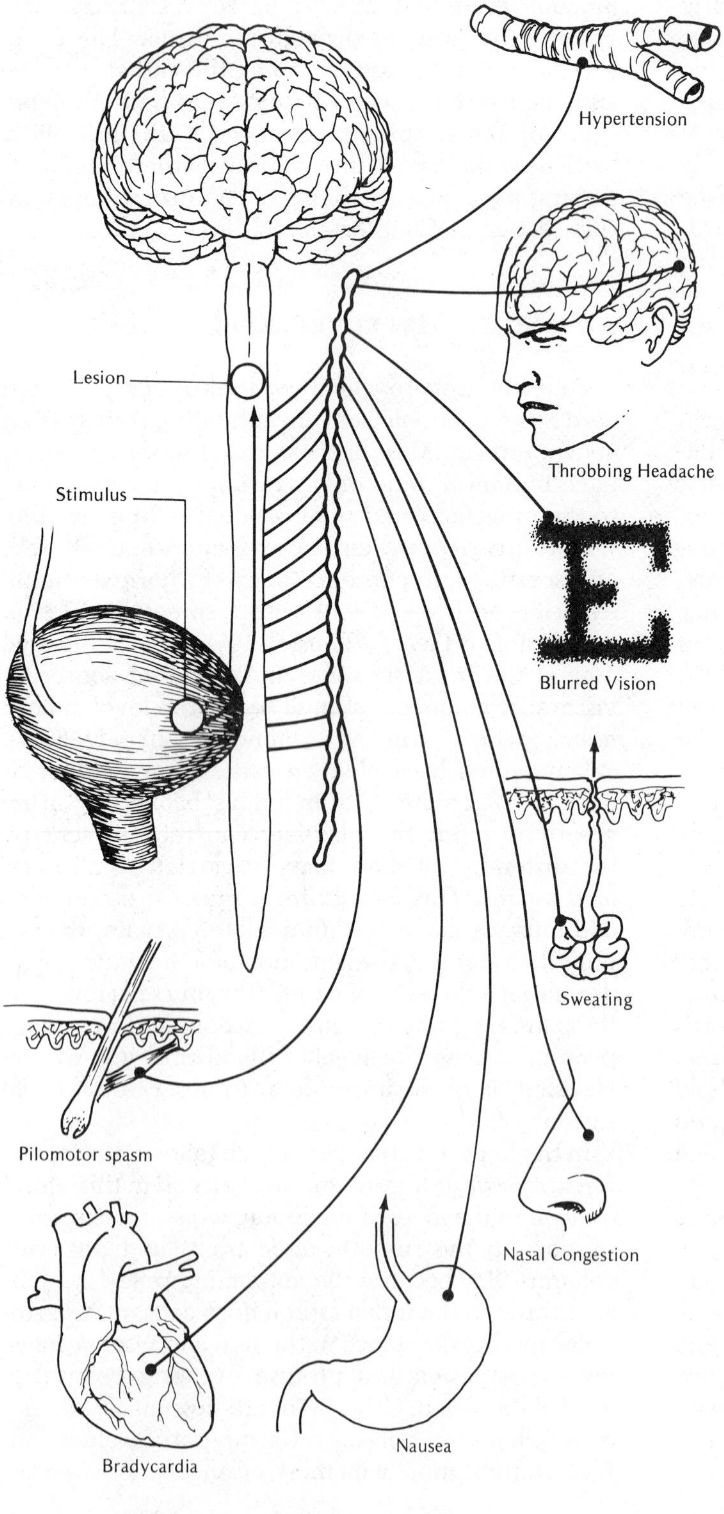

Figure 50-1. The symptoms of autonomic hyperreflexia, a dire threat to some patients with spinal cord injury, are triggered by distention or contraction of the bladder or rectum, stimulation of pain receptors, and stimulation of the skin. Immediate removal of the triggering factor is the essential treatment. (Used with permission of the American Journal of Nursing Company, from Autonomic hyperreflexia. *Am. J. Nurs.* 76:228–230, Feb. 1976, p. 229, by D. Feustel.)

utes; if the triggering stimulus cannot be removed or the blood pressure does not decrease, the physician may have to administer by rapid intravenous injection an alpha-adrenergic blocking agent, such as diazoxide (Hyperstat I.V.) [Feustel, 1976].

Sexuality

Some patients are able to broach the subject of sexuality to the team member with whom they feel most comfortable during their rehabilitation program. Others are not. In order to place sexuality in perspective as one aspect of the total care program, it is wise to indicate to the patient early in the rehabilitation program that sexual counseling is available. This acknowledges that it is not a taboo subject and that staff members are ready to talk about this aspect, and it leaves the timing for such discussion up to the patient. During counseling sessions, less emphasis is placed on orgasm, erection, and ejaculation, and the more crucial elements of the relationship and communication between partners are stressed. Depending upon the level of injury, whether the lesion is complete or incomplete, and the individual characteristics of the patient, alternative sexual practices that satisfy both partners usually can be found. Generally speaking, when a relationship is strong, a couple will be able to experiment with various sexual activities until they find ways that are gratifying and aesthetically pleasing to both partners as well as physiologically possible (Stryker, 1977, pp. 96–97).

Summary Considerations

The helpless patient lies dead weight in gravity position on the bed and quickly begins to develop contractures and foot drop. The muscles, whose nerves are no longer supplied by axons coming from anterior horn cells that are being constantly excited by stimuli coming from above, lose tone and will atrophy. A soft atrophic muscle supports poorly; the veins are not well pumped by vigorous muscle contractions any more, so the circulation is not brisk and the patient's tissues are prepared to break down easily.

If the patient has a badly fractured spinal column, he or she may have to be immobilized. But if the cord is damaged either traumatically or by disease without significant fracture of bone, effective nursing care seems to hinge largely on cleanliness and movement. A good rule for the nurse to have is: "I must see every square inch of this patient's body every day."

There are mattresses that are made in cells and are inflated by circulating fluid so that the pressure is continuously changing under the weight of the motionless body and limbs of the patient. These are excellent, but one may not always have such a mattress and, even with one, there is need for meticulous care.

The patient should be washed with soap and plenty of water daily, rinsed with clear water, and dried by brisk friction with a Turkish towel. This, in itself, exercises the tissues as well as cleans the skin. The clean, dry patient needs a perfectly smooth, dry bed. He or she will not feel the wrinkle or the bread crumb that injures the skin of the buttock. The supports of the flail feet must be kept clean and smooth as well as those pads arranged to prevent hyperextension of the knees. All the movement that can be provided is to the patient's advantage: joints stay mobile; skin and muscle, which is of poor tone, are relieved of pressure; vital capacity remains higher than otherwise; the often cheerless and disheartened person gets a little change of view.

Although drugs for control of urinary tract infections are excellent today, the paralyzed patient is at risk. High fluid intake that provides for a copious output of dilute urine is less likely to become infected and to burn tissues than the meager output of concentrated urine of the dehydrated incontinent. Whatever may be the eventual pattern of bowel and bladder evacuation of the chronic patient with a damaged spinal cord, it is not established at once. The newly incontinent invalid demands great sensitivity on the part of the nurse, and this includes awareness that prevention of fecal impactions is accomplished best through knowing what is taking place from day to day and seeing that this preventable complication does not occur. The fluid fecal seepage that keeps the bed damp and soiled indicates both impaction and inattentive nursing, and will be followed by tissue breakdown.

Skin surfaces that lie on top of one another are not shifted in the paralyzed. Moving the patient tends to separate the skin surfaces, remove pressure, and permit air to bathe them. Often a patient, even one acutely ill, can be moved about a good deal if the nurse understands the advantages of it. A litter provides different pressures on the body from those of a mattress on a bed; a wheelchair has a firm surface, and an upholstered chair a more resilient one. These little changes are helpful and supplement the absolutely essential ones of daily complete bath and toweling repeated at night for back, sacrum, and buttocks at least. Moving, shifting body position, and providing a high water intake are things that can be done to try to prevent renal calculi, which so frequently occur when bones decalcify as a result of continuing immobility. These renal stones compound the danger of stasis in the urinary tract.

A mere "ounce of prevention" is not enough in nursing the patient with spinal cord injury; there are too many issues at stake. Each one of them, the integrity of lungs, skin, urinary tract, and joints, needs its own ounce if the patient is to be accorded even a chance for a "pound of cure."

Care of Persons with Arthritis

The terms *rheumatism* and *rheumatic diseases* embrace a variety of disorders, all of which are characterized by pain and stiffness referable to the musculoskeletal system. *Arthritis* means joint inflammation and includes a number of specific diseases, among them, gout and a group of collagen diseases. The two main types of arthritis, however, are osteoarthritis or, as it is sometimes called, degenerative or hypertrophic arthritis, and rheumatoid arthritis. Arthritis is a major health problem which is responsible for much of the existing chronic illness and crippling of adults. Today, arthritis is the number one crippling disease in the United States. About 13 million Americans suffer from some form of arthritis, and more than 3 million of these people report that the disease limits their ability to carry on customary activity. Arthritis affects more people and causes more crippling than any other chronic disease (USDHEW, 1972). The suffering caused by arthritis is immeasurable. Some arthritis develops in almost everyone who lives long enough.

Osteoarthritis

Most individuals over the age of 50 show some degenerative cartilaginous changes. Osteoarthritis is a degenerative process in the joints, often associated with the normal aging process and resulting from the wearing down of the normal articular cartilage. Enzymatic degradation probably plays some part in the joint deterioration. A high percentage of individuals do not complain of symptoms, although x-ray studies reveal pathological changes. Osteoarthritis is not a systemic disease and most commonly is limited to the weight-bearing joints of the hips, knees, and spine. The joint cartilage gradually becomes thin and may eventually disappear, thus markedly impairing the smooth gliding surface of the involved joint or joints. The process does not cause pain. Pain develops as the process is far advanced and as a consequence of the rubbing together of the rough bony surfaces. Osteoarthritis may occur as a result of chronic trauma to joints, in joints aggravated by continual occupation-related stress as in the typist's fingers, for instance. Obesity may contribute to the increased joint stress and to the development of osteoarthritis.

Heberden's nodes develop in many patients. These bony enlargements of the distal phalangeal joints of the fingers occur most frequently in women, but do not significantly affect hand and finger function. There may be aching in affected joints. In most cases of osteoarthritis there is aching, pain, and stiffness in the involved joints, but not acute inflammation. Degenerative joint disease starts slowly with morning stiffness, especially in damp weather or after a period of heavy activity. Slowly the involved joints are uncomfortable, and finally they are painful when they are exercised. The discomfort yields to bedrest, aspirin, and warmth only to reappear with activity.

In planning nursing care the major objective is to relieve discomfort, preserve joint function and protect the joints from undue stress and trauma. Since osteoarthritis in some form or other affects almost everyone over the age of 50, many patients will be suffering from this condition in addition to their basic diagnosis. Weight reduction may decrease strain on the spine, hips, knees and efforts to improve posture and strengthen muscles may be helpful. Periods of physical activity should be followed by periods of rest. Local application of heat and analgesics may relieve the pain, but because of the chronicity of osteoarthritis, narcotics are not recommended. Acetylsalicylic acid (aspirin) is the most effective medication. Indomethacin (Indocin) or phenylbutazone (Butazolidin) may be used if conservative treatment with salicylates fails. Patients who are unable to tolerate aspirin may tolerate acetoaminophen (Tylenol). Muscle spasm may be relieved with diazepam (Valium), methocarbamol (Robaxin), or meprobamate (Equanil). Systemic corticosteroid therapy is not given for osteoarthritis, but intraarticular injections (such as hydrocortisone acetate) may be helpful in treating selected joints.

A brace may be prescribed to stabilize the spine or the knees and to relieve pain. Therapeutic efforts are aimed largely at reducing strain and pain in the involved joints. Residence in a warm, dry climate is beneficial for some patients. Orthopedic procedures such as total hip replacement and knee replacement may provide dramatic relief for patients with severe osteoarthritis.

Gouty Arthritis

Primary gout is a familial metabolic disorder of purine metabolism which results in abnormal amounts of urates in the body. The basic disorder in gout seems to be an inability to metabolize purines, which are products of the digestion of certain proteins. This inability results in an accumulation of uric acid in the blood stream. Deposits of sodium urate crystals (tophi) occur in the margins of the joints, in the cartilage of the ear, in the kidneys, on the skin, and, rarely, in the heart and other organs. These deposits of crystals then initiate local irritation and an inflammatory response. It is possible to have hyperuricemia without having gout. However, secondary gout can arise as a result of increase of purine metabolism resulting from some blood dyscrasias such as polycythemia and certain leukemias.

The main clinical problem with gout is arthritis. Early in the course of the illness, a recurring acute arthritis occurs which is usually monarticular, that is, involving one joint. Later a chronic, deforming arthritis occurs. About 95 per cent of patients with gout are men over age 30. If gout develops in women, it usually does so after menopause. Gout is characterized clinically by acute periodic episodes of pain, swelling, and inflammation in a joint. The joints of the foot (great toe, instep, or ankle) are most often affected; however, any joint may be involved.

During acute gouty arthritis, the involved joint(s) is usually intensely painful, swollen, and extremely tender. The skin over the joint feels warm and tense and appears dusky red or purple. Other symptoms commonly occur such as headache, tachycardia, fever, malaise, anorexia. The patient may be completely incapacitated. The pain usually is so severe that even the weight of the bedclothes is intolerable. Movement of the joint is out of the question. Spontaneously, in about 2 weeks—or sooner, with treatment—swelling, redness, and pain are gone, and the joint appears to be as good as ever. However, after years of attacks the permanent damage to the joint becomes evident. Attacks become more and more frequent over the years.

Laboratory findings with gout include: (1) elevated WBC and sedimentation rate during acute attacks, (2) elevated blood uric acid (unless uricosuric medications are being taken), and (3) presence of crystals of sodium urate in materials aspirated from a tophus or joint fluid. Early diagnosis and treatment of gout are important. The emphasis of treatment has shifted from the simple treatment of recurrent attacks to permanent supervision and treatment aimed at preventing acute attacks and progressive disability. Progressive renal dysfunction is the greatest threat to life.

Acute attacks may be terminated by administering medications such as (1) colchicine; (2) phenylbutazone (Butazolidin); (3) indomethacin (Indocin); or (4) corticotropin (ACTH). The treatment of acute attacks also includes bedrest (continued for at least 24 hours after acute symptoms subside) and analgesics. Fluids are forced to reduce precipitation of urates in the kidney. Some patients receive added relief from hot or cold compresses.

Although gout cannot be cured in the sense of removing the basic metabolic difficulty of constant or recurrent hyperuricemia, the attacks can be controlled. The regimen must be individualized for each patient and changed from time to time in response to the changes in the course of the disease. Understanding the nature of gout, understanding the importance of taking prescribed medications, and practicing self-discipline will help the patient control the occurrence of acute attacks.

The excess uric acid in the body of a patient with gout is derived from a process of internal biosynthesis; consequently there is not a great deal of emphasis on dietary management. Dietary management was formerly regarded as most important in gout control and rigidly prescribed. However, since the effect of dietary control upon urate levels is relatively small, a much more lenient attitude is now taken. Restriction of the purine content of the diet may be temporarily recommended until the serum urate concentration returns to normal. Foods high in purine include kidneys, sweetbreads, anchovies, sardines, meat broths, and leguminous vegetables, such as beans. Low purine or purine-free foods, usually allowed, include chocolate, coffee, tea, fruit juices, fruit, bread, cereals, eggs, gelatine, milk, sugar, and nonleguminous vegetables. A moderate ingestion of alcohol does not appear to precipitate acute attacks or to be otherwise harmful. However, the patient should avoid foods or alcoholic beverages which precipitate attacks and should practice moderation.

Drug therapy is extremely important in the treatment of acute attacks as well as the control of gout. Daily administrations of colchicine have preventive actions (that is, they reduce frequency of acute attacks) and may be continued indefinitely. Also uricosuric drugs may be given, such as probenecid (Benemid), sulfinpyrazone (Anturane), or salicylates. Uricosuric medications block the tubular reabsorption of filtered urates in the kidney and thus reduce the metabolic pool of urates by increasing uric acid excretion. Salicylates cannot be given with any other uricosuric agents. The patient should be told not to take salicylates, if taking other uricosuric agents, because they antagonize the action of other uricosuric agents (Goodman & Gilman, 1975). Another method of ongoing treatment is the administration of xanthine oxidase inhibitor allopurinol (Zyloprim). This drug inhibits uric acid formation. Fluid intake should be at least 3 liters per day when uricosuric drugs are being taken, and attempts are made to keep the urine alkaline in order to prevent formation of urinary calculi. The patient is taught to test his or her urine (Luckmann & Sorenson, 1974, p. 1235).

Rheumatoid Arthritis

Rheumatoid arthritis is a chronic systemic disease of unknown cause, characterized most prominently by recurrent inflammation involving the synovium or lining of the joints. Constitutional symptoms and joint changes, which may become permanent deformities, are part of the disease. Rheumatoid arthritis is of greatest significance because of the disability it causes. All too frequently the patient and family do not recognize that much can be done to prevent severe deformities. Rheumatoid arthritis is found throughout the world, although some believe it is more common in temperate than in torrid climates. This crippling disease strikes during the most productive years of adulthood. The majority of new cases begin between the ages of 25 and 50, but no age is spared, as rheumatoid arthritis may afflict infants or even the very old. Still's disease is the juvenile form of rheumatoid arthritis. It causes severe crippling if the cervical spine is involved along with the other joints. The systemic effects are usually more severe than those of the adult forms of arthritis.

Theories of Etiology

The etiology of rheumatoid arthritis is unknown. It is probable that arthritis is not caused by a single factor, but that one or more factors trigger the onset. Theories of etiology include the following:

1. Disorder of autoimmunity. The body, for unknown reason, produces abnormal antibodies that are directed against its own tissues. Part of the evidence supporting this theory is the abnormally high levels of certain types of gamma globulins in the blood of patients with rheumatoid arthritis. The characteristic "rheumatoid factor," a complex protein found in the blood of patients with this disease, closely resembles an antibody.
2. Infection. Some researchers believe that rheumatoid arthritis may be due to infection from bacteria, viruses, or myocoplasma, and that the organism, probably a virus, may be the cause of the abnormal "autoimmune" reaction which causes the body to produce antibodies against its own tissue.
3. Faulty adaptation to physical or psychic stress. Psychic stress as a cause of rheumatoid arthritis is associated more often with degenerative joint disease. Studies have proved that illness is more likely to occur when an individual experiences stress. Thus, although the cause-and-effect relationship between illness and stress is often a matter of conjecture in an individual patient, data implicating psychological stress as a causative factor is the onset of many illnesses among groups of people studied indicate the need for concerned attention to the patient's history and present life circumstances when illness strikes.
4. Inherited factors. Children of arthritic parents have a greater tendency to develop the disease than those whose ancestors have no such history. Heredity may be a factor, but the evidence pointing to this theory could be explained also by environmental factors. Perhaps a latent virus infection was passed from the mother to the child.

Manifestations

Since rheumatoid arthritis is a systemic disease, manifestations include lassitude, generalized fatigue, muscular atrophy and weakness, loss of body weight, and in the most severe cases exhaustion. Secondary anemia is frequently associated with rheumatoid arthritis. The sedimentation rate is usually elevated during an acute attack and is followed closely during the course of therapy since it provides an index of disease activity.

An acute attack frequently starts with swelling and stiffness in one or more joints. The stiffness may be especially noticeable when the individual arises in the morning. The involved joints may loosen up as the patient moves about and performs customary activities. These early manifestations may be followed by an acute episode in which joints become enlarged, red, warm, and very painful. Muscular aching, pain, weakness, and fatigability are early complaints. Multiple joints may be involved, especially the knees, ankles, elbows, wrists, and proximal joints of the phalanges.

As the disease progresses, the muscle wasting around affected joints accentuates the appearance of swelling. The proximal finger joints swell the most, and as deformity develops, the fingers deviate toward the ulnar aspect of the hand. Extremities become cold and moist. Patients in this stage of the disease have considerable pain even at rest and especially on motion. Although the supporting muscles are in spasm, the ligaments are lax. Consequently, the affected joints are unstable and move in unnatural directions. Inflammation of the synovial membrane results in roughening of the smooth articular surfaces and pain upon motion. There is narrowing of the joint spaces. In severe cases there is complete joint destruction and partial or complete ankylosis of the involved joints. Formation of excess synovial fluid is stimulated, the joint capsule may become thickened and distended, and the ligaments and joint cartilages are damaged. The joints become enlarged due to thickening of the capsules, accumulation of fluid, and muscle atrophy. Acute attacks may occur periodically and last several weeks or months, followed by remissions.

Without treatment, and sometimes with it, the joint may be destroyed totally. As the synovial space is replaced with bony growth, motion is lost. When the joint becomes immobile, the pain of the inflammation is lessened, but there is still discomfort because of contractures and immobility. One of the aims of treatment is to decrease the inflammation of the joint before it develops into one bone.

Objectives of Care

The primary objective of nursing in the acute stage of rheumatoid arthritis is the prevention of crippling deformities. Other objectives are (1) to maintain joint mobility and muscle power, (2) to promote comfort, (3) to halt the activity of the disease, (4) to help the patient and family adjust to the chronic disability, and (5) to assist the patient to become functionally independent as soon as possible.

Therapy

The patient is placed on a program of rest, physical therapy, and an extended course of treatment with salicylates supplemented by other anti-inflammatory agents. Optimal health conditions should be maintained, since supporting the resistance of the body to the inflammation is one of the few truly therapeutic steps that medicine has to offer. Rest, both systemic and local, is balanced carefully with exercise. The patient should be encouraged to eat an optimum diet, even though he or she may have little appetite. Unless there are other complications such as diabetes or hypertension, this diet need not be modified from that of a normal individual.

Drugs

Drug therapy is not curative, but it helps the patient to feel less pain and in some instances it depresses the inflammatory process. Because of the long-term nature of this disease, the relief of pain with narcotics is avoided. The nurse is responsible for observing reactions to drugs and accurately reporting them. The most widely used drugs are the salicylates; aspirin is the major drug in this group. In early rheumatoid arthritis it seems to reduce inflammation and to afford specific relief of joint pain and stiffness. In chronic rheumatoid arthritis the relief appears less dramatic, but is still present, and probably it is more related to the general analgesic properties of aspirin than to any specific action. The dosage may vary according to the patient's tolerance. Salicylates are usually given to the point of toxicity, that is, the development of tinnitus. The usual dose of aspirin in rheumatoid arthritis is two to four (0.3 g) tablets two to six times a day. Some physicians give the drug until the serum level of salicylates reaches 25 mg per 100 ml. The patient must be carefully observed for side effects such as allergic reaction and gastrointestinal bleeding. Some patients decrease the dose or omit tablets entirely, and yet control of the symptoms depends on a high sustained blood level of the drug.

Phenylbutazone (Butazolidin) is an anti-inflammatory analgesic and antipyretic drug that may be used on a short-term basis in a dosage of 400 to 600 mg per day. It is poorly tolerated by some patients and should be given with meals. Blood studies should be done frequently to detect possible untoward effects, such as decrease in white blood cell count and bone marrow depression.

Indomethacin (Indocin) is an analgesic anti-inflammatory medication which appears to be more effective in treating rheumatoid arthritis than the salicylates. Its efficiency is believed to be similar to that of phenylbutazone. Numerous untoward effects may occur, such as headaches, nausea, vomiting, anorexia, peptic ulcer, abdominal pain, diarrhea, and mental confusion.

Other medications that may be used in the treatment of rheumatoid arthritis are gold compounds, antimalarials, and adrenocorticosteroids. Immunosuppressive drugs are also being used on an investigational basis, and more anti-inflammatory drugs are being developed.

Rest

It is important to remember that rheumatoid arthritis is not merely a disorder of the joints, but rather a systemic disease. The amount of systemic rest that is necessary varies depending upon the severity of the patient's disease at a given time. With extensive systemic and articular involvement, complete bedrest is indicated. Complete bedrest is anti-inflammatory. As a general rule, the more acute the disease or the greater the number of joints involved, the greater is the benefit of bedrest. With mild rheumatoid arthritis, 2 to 4 hours of rest daily may be adequate. Commonly the prescribed amount of rest is dictated by the patient's condition. Nursing attention must be extensively directed at preventing complications of immobility and disuse, and the student is again referred to the section on disuse syndromes. Providing rest for joints involved with rheumatoid arthritis helps reduce articular inflammation. Weight-bearing joints may be rested by complete bedrest. Splints may also be applied to more completely rest inflammed joints. Splints also relieve pain by relieving muscle spasm and prevent or reduce deformities. Splints must be removed for exercise and other treatments, such as heat applications. To prevent fibrous ankylosis of joints, the joints are periodically exercised; for example, splinted joints may be carried through a full range of motion once or twice daily. With improvement, some patients require splints only at night or perhaps not at all for a while.

Activity

Prescribed amounts of activity help the patient with rheumatoid arthritis to attain and maintain optimum levels of function and independence. Activity also helps the patient to feel more comfortable mentally. Acute inflamed joints are extremely painful when moved. The patient is often reluctant to move because of the pain. Occupational therapy provides an excellent means of encouraging purposeful movement. Encouraging self-care activities also provides purposeful movement. A variety of self-care appliances are available to help the patient with rheumatoid arthritis maintain a maximum level of independence. These include such things as eating utensils with special handles, long-handled "reachers," and specially elevated chairs and toilet seats.

Physical therapy is of great importance in the treatment of rheumatoid arthritis because it prevents and corrects deformities, controls pain, strengthens weakened muscles, and improves function. During exercise, the patient may experience some pain which persists for a short time. This is not unusual; however, pain which lasts for several hours following exercises may indicate that the exercises are excessive and need to be modified. Exercises are the most important single part of the physical therapy program for a patient with rheumatoid arthritis. Rest and therapeutic exercises must always be kept in proper balance. Because fatigue is a common symptom, the patient's tolerance of exercise must be carefully evaluated. Overactivity can inflame affected joints. Exercise should be performed within the limits of pain tolerance.

Surgery

Surgical procedures are gaining increasing importance as part of the rehabilitation of the patient with arthritis. A variety of procedures may be performed to relieve general symptoms, improve function, and correct deformities. Not too many years ago surgery was used only late in the course of arthritis, after severe destruction or deformity had occurred. Preventive surgery is now used during early phases of treatment.

Rheumatoid arthritis is usually best treated by a conservative approach with salicylates, rest, and physical therapy. An important part of a successful rehabilitation program involves teaching the patient about the nature of his or her illness and about the best methods of treatment. Victims of arthritis often tend to try "quack" cures to obtain relief. Patients who do not understand the nature of rheumatoid arthritis are especially vulnerable to claims made by manufacturers of quack remedies. According to the Arthritis Foundation, more than $400 million per year is spent by arthritics on worthless treatments or devices.

Early, active therapy, before the establishment of fibrosis or bony ankylosis, is most successful. Treatment goals include (1) preservation of function, (2) reduction of pain and inflammation, (3) prevention or correction of deformities. It is desirable for the patient with rheumatoid arthritis to be seen by both a rheumatologist and an orthopedic surgeon.

Individually prescribed rehabilitation programs are essential in the treatment of rheumatoid arthritis. Because rheumatoid arthritis is a chronic disorder, the patient will require a long-term rehabilitation plan. The patient will also require long-term medical supervision. Since the patient is the central figure in the rehabilitation program, he or she must be accurately advised about how to help himself or herself. For example, the patient must understand the nature of the illness in order to be responsible for taking medications and carrying out prescribed exercise programs. The patient needs to be familiar with reportable side effects of the medications being taken. These aspects—the importance of medications, exercising, resting—must be emphasized during patient and family education sessions. The patient should also be informed of local assistance programs and organizations that may be helpful. For example, the Arthritis Foundation provides many services such as information services, home living assistance programs, and helpful education booklets. The Arthritis Foundation has also been very active in trying to combat quackery through these public information programs.

A community nurse can help a patient with rheumatoid arthritis plan modifications in activities and home environment to make it easier to perform activities of daily living. The entire rehabilitation team may be involved in helping the person adapt to the chronicity and disabilities of the illness. Although some persons with rheumatoid arthritis find it necessary to change their type of employment, many are able to continue their jobs. Those individuals who need to make job changes may be helped by the State Department of Vocational Rehabilitation if vocational retraining is needed.

Family members need to be included in the rehabilitation program so they can understand the nature of the person's illness and participate in his or her care. Both the patient and family should understand that much disability and deformity can be prevented with vigorous, early therapy and adherence to prescribed treatment programs.

References Cited

Feldman, L. J., and Schultz, M. E. "Rehabilitation after Stroke." *Cardiovasc. Nurs.,* **11** (1975), 29–34.

Feustel, D. "Autonomic Hyperreflexia." *Am. J. Nurs.,* **76** (Feb. 1976), 228–30.

Goodman, L. S., and Gilman, A. *The Pharmacological Basis of Therapeutics,* 5th ed. New York: Macmillan Publishing Co., 1975, p. 865.

Granger, C. V., et al. "Stroke Rehabilitation: Analysis of Repeated Barthel Index Measures." *Arch. Phys. Med. Rehabil.,* **60** (Jan. 1979), 4–7.

Licht, S., (ed.) *Stroke and Its Rehabilitation.* Baltimore: Williams & Wilkins, 1975.

Luckmann, J., and Sorensen, K. *Medical-Surgical Nursing.* Philadelphia: W. B. Saunders Co., 1974.

O'Brien, M. T., and Pallett, P. *Total Care of the Stroke Patient.* Boston: Little, Brown, 1978.

Sivarajan, E. S. et al. "Progressive Ambulation and Treadmill Testing of Patients with Acute Myocardial Infarction during Hospitalization." *Arch. Phys. Med. Rehabil.,* **58** (June 1977), 241–47.

Sperling, K. "Intermittent Catheterization to Obtain Catheter Free Bladder Function in Spinal Cord Injury." *Arch. Phys. Med. Rehabil.,* **59** (Jan. 1978), 4–8.

Stryker, R. *Rehabilitation Aspects of Acute and Chronic Nursing Care,* 2nd ed. Philadelphia. W. B. Saunders Co., 1977.

U.S. Department of Health, Education, and Welfare. *Arthritis Source Book.* Washington, D.C.: U.S. Government Printing Office, 1972.

General References

Boegil, E. H., and Steele, M. S. "Scoliosis." *Am. J. Nurs.,* **68** (Nov. 1968), 2399–403.

De Bush, R. F., et al. "Colonary Care Unit Activities Program: It's Role in Post Infarction Rehabilitation." *J. Chronic Dis.* **24** (1971), 373–81.

Guerrieri, B. O. "Survey of the Knowledge of the Nurse in Direct-Care Services Concerning Proper Bed Positioning of the Patient with Hemiplegia." *Nurs. Res.,* **17** (March–April 1968), 157–59.

Lapides, J. et al. "Follow up on Unsterile Intermittent Self Catheterization." *J. Urol.* (1974), 184–87.

Meadows, S. P. "Subarachnoid Hemorrhage." *Nurs. Mirror,* **132** (June 4, 1971), 19–23.

Meyer, J. S. *TIA's—The Early Warning System of Impending Stroke.* Kansas City, Mo.: Marion Laboratories, Inc., 1971.

Smith, S. W. "Subdural Hematoma in Adults." *Postgrad. Med.,* **42** (Aug. 1967), A59–A64.

Van Horn, G. "Cerebrovascular Disease." *DM* (June 1973).

Webb, P. H. "Neurological Deficit after Carotid Endarterectomy." *Am. J. Nurs.,* **79** (April 1979), 654–58.

51

Problems Associated with Uncomplicated Surgical Treatment

"Notice"

As of today, May 15, 1847, every doctor or student who comes from the dissecting room is required, before entering the maternity wards, TO WASH HIS HANDS thoroughly in a basin of chlorine water which is being placed at the entrance. This order applies to all, without exception.

I. P. SEMMELWEIS, M.D. (THORWALD, 1957)

Overview

However thoughtfully planned and skillfully performed, surgery imposes significant psychological and physiologic stress on the person undergoing operation. The nurse who aspires to being effective in helping patients who are treated surgically will have to synthesize and apply knowledge from all areas discussed in previous chapters, as well as to understand and deal appropriately with the consequences of breaching the skin, as the body's first line of defense against injury; exposing, handling, and cutting such tissues as nerves, capillaries, lymphatics, and viscera,[1] interfering with the body's early warning nervous system (central and autonomic) via anesthetics and analgesics; blood and fluid loss and their replacement; and various intubations and drainages. Surgery is a special mode of medical treatment of disease and injury. This chapter discusses its development and the major requirements of the patient treated surgically.

[1] *Viscera* are the hollow and multilayered walled organs of the digestive, respiratory, urogenital, and endocrine systems as well as the spleen, heart, and great vessels.

History of Surgery

Moore (1959), a contemporary Harvard physician who has contributed extensively to understanding of the metabolic problems of surgical patients, defines *surgery* as that field of medicine that assumes responsibility for the cure of a large segment of human disease that is "largely acute, focal, or traumatic . . . (involving) care of the entire range of injuries and wounds, local infections, benign and malignant tumors, as well as a large fraction of those various pathologic processes and anomalies which are localized in the organs of the body." This concept of modern surgery is a far cry from the surgery performed by the uneducated barber surgeons of the early Middle Ages, whose operations were so frequently followed by complications that the surgeons often cut and ran. The decadence of surgery in about the first 1500 years A.D. has been ascribed to its separation from medicine and neglect of anatomy during that period. This was not characteristic of Egyptian, Greek, and Roman antiquity, from which come some of the earliest records of surgical instruments and procedures. The treatment of disease and injury by surgical methods probably goes back to the beginning of humankind. The earliest records of surgical procedures are primitive tools found in burial grounds. Other early records include writings and drawings on stone tablets and on the walls of caves and houses. Ancient Egyptian papyri describe problems in medicine, surgery, obstetrics and gynecology, and veterinary medicine. A variety of surgical procedures were performed by primitive humans, including the setting of broken bones and the treatment of wounds. Trephining, a procedure in which a hole is made in the skull, was performed by primitive surgeons in many parts of the world. Skulls, eight to ten thousand years old, bearing marks of trephination, have been found in France and other parts of Europe. In the New World, Peru is the site where trephining was practiced most extensively, but it was performed as far north as Alaska. As far back as 4000 B.C., the Egyptians did circumcisions as well as ophthalmic surgery. The Homeric legends refer to regimental surgeons as fighters and physicians (Bettmann, 1956). Histories of other civilizations contain reference to surgical treatment, but much of the early surgery was both cruel and crude. Its use was hampered by inadequate knowledge of effective and humane ways to control pain, hemorrhage, and infection. Some of this surgery was done not for the purpose of removing diseased tissue or of correcting anatomic defects but to allow evil spirits to escape. By modern standards, making an opening in the skull to provide an avenue for the escape of a demon seems strange, but in relation to the knowledge of the time it was logical.

Some of the knowledge essential to the practice of surgery was discovered and then lost, to be reintroduced at a later time. For example, the use of ligatures was known and described by Celsus shortly before the beginning of the Christian era. Since their use by Ambroise Paré (1510–1590), ligatures have been used as the method of choice in hemostasis.

Phases in the Development of Surgery

Much of the knowledge on which modern surgical treatment of disease is based has been acquired in the last 100 to 150 years. Since the early nineteenth century the science of surgery has developed so that an increasing number of surgical procedures can now be performed with reasonable safety and benefit to the patient. Conditions that have plagued humankind since the beginning of time, such as acute appendicitis, cholecystitis, hernia, compound fractures, and even structural defects of the heart, have been brought under control.

Modern surgery has gone through two phases in its development. In the first, the objective was to make surgery safe and humane. In the second, the objective was to make the patient safe for surgery. Both are important to the welfare of the patient. The first phase has its origins in the sciences of anatomy, chemistry, bacteriology, psychology, sociology, and anthropology.

The three elements that are essential to safe and humane surgery are hemostasis, asepsis, and anesthesia. Without an adequate method to control bleeding, the patient may die from hemorrhage. Before the development of the science of bacteriology, patients frequently died from infection. Because anesthesia made possible the prevention of pain, the surgeon can take the necessary time to handle tissues gently and perform the surgical procedures carefully and accurately. Knowledge of anatomy and the factors that influence wound healing was important to the development of surgical methods.

Controlling Bleeding

Because humans have always been faced with bleeding, the methods of stopping the flow of blood were developed early. Methods used to control hemorrhage developed in three stages. As might be anticipated, pressure was the first to be used; the second was the cauterization of wounds; and the third was use of some type of material to tie the ends of blood vessels. One of the most significant contributions to modern surgery was made by Halsted, who correlated surgical technique with wound healing. He emphasized the careful handling of tissue. For hemostasis, he clamped only the blood vessels with as little of the surrounding tissue as possible. He used a fine ligature that was tied just tight enough to approximate the tissues without strangulation. The care taken by the surgeon in making and closing a surgical incision is one of the important factors in recovery of the patient.

As in many other fields of knowledge, the introduction of new methods did not entirely replace the old, but each new procedure increased the ability to control hemorrhage. All these methods are still used today. The causes, effects, and treatment of hemorrhage will be discussed later in Chapter 52.

Modern Asepsis

The modern concept of asepsis is based on two premises, neither of which is really new. One is that the environment contains something that, when it is introduced or it enters into a wound or individual, can cause harm. The other is that something can be done to prevent the harmful agent (spirit or microbe) from entering the body or its harmful influence can be nullified. As an example, some primitive people isolated the sick by placing them outside the village walls or abandoned their houses when someone died in them. Others made loud noises or practiced some kind of ritual to frighten the evil spirit or immobilize it.

Asepsis as it is known today developed in three stages: the first was the stage of isolation and cleanliness; the second was the stage of antiseptic surgery; and the third and present stage is the stage of asepsis. The value of isolation and cleanliness was demonstrated in the 1840s by Semmelweis, a young Hungarian physician who practiced in Vienna.[2] Despite lack of precise knowledge of microorganisms, Semmelweis instituted measures that were successful in the prevention of puerperal fever. These measures were based on the observation that the incidence of puerperal fever was much lower in a ward where the women were delivered by midwives than in a ward where the women were examined by medical students who had come from autopsy rooms where they had handled tissues of women who had died of puerperal fever. Next he instituted techniques to control the factor he believed to be responsible. He insisted that physicians and medical students wash their hands before they examined patients. Despite active opposition to this rule, the lives of many mothers were saved by it. Semmelweis died a depressed and disappointed man; although he had proved over and over the soundness of his ideas, they were not rapidly accepted by his colleagues. As happens even today, there was a considerable lag between the development of knowledge and its acceptance and use in practice.

The work of many men, some who preceded Semmelweis and some who followed him, contributed to the development of modern aseptic surgery. Among those usually mentioned is the seventeenth-century Dutch lens grinder, Leeuwenhoek. He is credited with being the first to see bacteria. It was not until 1850–1865, or nearly 200 years later, that the foundation was laid for antiseptic and, soon thereafter, aseptic surgery. A French chemist, Louis Pasteur, was employed by the wine growers of France to identify the cause of the souring of wine and to devise techniques for preventing it. As a result of his work the theory of spontaneous generation was disproved for all time and the germ theory of disease was established. According to the germ theory, disease is caused by a living agent. After it is introduced into an individual, the agent establishes itself, grows, multiplies, and may cause disease.

Other men, notably Lister and Koch, added to the body of knowledge that contributed to the acceptance of the germ theory. Lister, a physiologist and surgeon, read reports of the studies made by Pasteur on the cause and prevention of the souring of wine. If microorganisms present in the air caused wine to sour, might not microorganisms infect wounds? To remove microorganisms from the air, Lister had the operating room sprayed with a dilute solution of carbolic acid previous to the start of the operation. Following the operation he placed a disinfectant bandage over the incision. He had some success with the latter, for he found that he could prevent the infection of compound fractures, that is, fractures in which the skin is broken and there is direct communication between the broken bone and the external environment. Compound fractures treated in this manner healed as well as simple ones, that is, those in which the skin remained intact. Lister reported his experiments and clinical trials in 1867.

The third stage, or the stage of asepsis, quickly followed the stage of antisepsis. In 1877 Robert Koch published *The Cause of Infection in Wounds.* In what has come to be known as Koch's postulates, he stated the conditions that must be fulfilled for a microorganism to be established as the cause of a disease. The work of Semmelweis, Pasteur, Lister, Koch, and others demonstrated that the pus that was formed in a wound resulted from the introduction of an outside agent and was not an essential part of the healing process. With this knowledge as a basis, methods were developed to prevent microorganisms from gaining access to the wound.

Previous to these discoveries, wounds were so regularly infected that pus was considered an essential aspect of wound healing. The type and quantity of pus present in a wound depended on the infecting microorganism and often provided a clue to the prognosis. Thus abundant, creamy pus with little or no odor was usually associated with recovery and was therefore called laudable pus. A thin, watery, or malodorous pus is characteristic of hemolytic or anaerobic streptococcal infection and implied a poor prognosis. Presently, it is known that any type of infection in a wound delays healing and may threaten the life of the individual.

Despite a large body of knowledge acquired over the last 100 years or so indicating that the external environment contains microorganisms capable of causing disease, wounds continue to be infected. Among the elements contributing to infections are a lack of understanding of existing knowledge and failure to follow prescribed techniques. For example, Miss Smith, a nurse in the operating room, awakens in the morning with a sore throat or a boil on her neck. A heavy operative schedule is planned for the

[2] About the same time Oliver Wendell Holmes published an essay, "On the Contagiousness of Childbed Fever."

day. Should she go to work or should she remain at home? If she goes to work, she may be able to rationalize her behavior by saying, "I'm not very sick. I'll wear a mask. It's on the back of my neck. I'm needed." But she will be demonstrating that she does not know what she, as an operating room nurse, should know or that she does not accept her knowledge as having validity. Other considerations take precedence in influencing her behavior. A classic example of the type of consideration that takes precedence over knowledge in influencing nurses' behavior is the symbolic significance of wedding and engagement rings. It is increasingly common to see nurses in all areas of a hospital, with the possible exception of the operating suite, wearing rings while giving direct patient care. Hemstrup-Hansen (1963) cultured the ringed and nonringed fingers of ten nurses on medical–surgical units just prior to their lunch hour, when the likelihood of recent hand washing was greatest. Nonringed finger cultures grew 2,000 microorganisms, whereas ringed finger cultures grew 66,200 microorganisms. In view of the fact that hands are the most frequent mode of transfer of microorganisms in cross infection, the sentimental attachment to rings constitutes a serious impediment to the effectiveness of hand washing as a measure to control hospital infections.

Among the additional elements contributing to the continued problem of wound infection are susceptibility of the host and the ecological balance between or among microorganisms. It is likely that there are others as well (see also Chapter 38).

Fundamentally, the practice of asepsis depends on two factors:

1. Knowledge of the factors to be controlled and development of suitable techniques
2. The conviction of practitioners that the knowledge is valid and that the techniques are practical and will accomplish their purpose

Semmelweis failed not because his observations or techniques were unsound but because his colleagues refused to accept them as valid, practical, and necessary.

Anesthesia

The third element required, if surgery is to be safe and humane, is some means of preventing pain during the performance of surgery. Prior to the middle of the nineteenth century, surgery was limited to emergency procedures or those absolutely essential to life. Agents that were used to prevent painful sensations were limited to belladonna, hemp, opium, and alcohol. Most of these drugs lessened the patient's perception of pain or memory of it. In some instances the patient was rendered unconscious by a blow on the head. When the condition of the patient was believed to contraindicate the administration of large doses of alcohol or opium, the patient was held or tied and the operation performed with all possible speed. After the introduction of safe and effective anesthetic agents, time and speed were no longer the prime considerations.

Thus the discovery and acceptance of a variety of safe chemical agents have been important to the development of surgery. The chemical discovery of the anesthetic agents preceded their actual use by many years. The first anesthetic, nitrous oxide, was discovered in 1776 by Priestly. In 1799 Sir Humphrey Davy reported that it prevented pain and suggested that it might be used in surgical operations. Although others experimented with nitrous oxide and ether, the first recognized use of anesthesia for a surgical operation did not come about until Morton, in October 1846, successfully anesthetized a patient with ether at the Massachusetts General Hospital.

Today a great variety of anesthetic agents are available. Some are suitable for inducing unconsciousness; others may be used to anesthetize a region of the body or a small area of the skin or mucous membrane. Methods used in their administration are also varied and are related to the state in which the agent occurs. For example, gaseous anesthetics are administered by way of a face mask or through a tube intratracheally. Liquid anesthetics that evaporate rapidly can anesthetize the skin by freezing it. Other liquids produce anesthesia when applied to mucous membrane. Liquids may also be injected into the skin, sensory nerves, and spinal canal and even intravenously. Because of the variety of agents now available, an anesthetic agent can be selected that suits not only the desired method of administration but also the condition of the patient.[3]

Before the discovery of effective and safe anesthetics, speed was one of the essential features in the performance of a surgical procedure. As a consequence, incisions were often crudely made and tissues suffered unnecessary damage.

Dramatic progress in making surgery safe and humane through improvements in hemostasis, asepsis, and anesthesia has led to successful aggressive surgical treatment of persons previously considered poor surgical risks. Among those who successfully undergo major surgery today are such unlikely groups as the

[3] For detailed information about various anesthetic agents, the student is referred to L. S. Goodman and A. Gilman. *The Pharmacological Basis of Therapeutics,* 5th ed. New York: Macmillan Publishing Co., 1975, sects. II and III.

elderly, the massively obese (Braasch, 1971), those with advanced vascular insufficiency and gangrene (Symposium on vascular grafts, 1979), and even persons with classical hemophilia (Croom & Hutchin, 1969). Continual improvements in making surgery safe and humane for the patient have resulted from the explosion of knowledge in the physical and biological sciences and the emergence of a vast and complex biomedical technology that requires a highly specialized and centralized setting for its application to patient care. For example, since the discovery of x-rays by Röntgen in 1895, the ever-expanding requirement for complicated, expensive, and bulky equipment for radiologic studies has contributed to establishing the hospital as the primary locus for medical, and especially surgical, care (Brieger, 1977). As a result, "surgical nursing" has become almost synonymous with "hospital nursing"; this is unfortunate, inasmuch as the pre- and posthospitalization care available to a patient can substantially influence the nature and consequences of events during the episode of hospitalization, and ultimately the effectiveness of surgical treatment.

As biomedical technology evolves and knowledge of psychology, biochemistry, and physiology advances, surgeons are directing their attention to making patients safe for surgery. Knowledge of physiologic and biochemical processes has led to the discovery of methods that can be used to support patients during prolonged surgical procedures. As the relationship between the capacity of the patient to adapt physiologically and psychologically and his or her recovery has come to be appreciated, methods to evaluate patient status and to correct abnormalities have been developed. With greater understanding of the physiological needs of people and the effects of surgery on structure and function, the care of the patient can be better regulated, so that recovery is facilitated.

Elements in the Nursing Care of Patients Treated Surgically

The nurse can contribute to the care of the patient treated surgically from the time he or she seeks, or is directed by the nurse to seek, medical care until the patient has recovered sufficiently to resume normal activities, is entrusted to the care of family or friends, or, as happens infrequently, dies. The nurse shares with the physician the responsibility for helping the patient to understand his or her health problem, and to understand and accept the nature, indications for, and expected consequences of the proposed surgery, as well as to monitor and support psychophysiologic defenses throughout the preoperative, operative, and postoperative periods. In planning the nursing care for all phases of a patient's experience with surgery, the following general factors must be considered:

1. The patient as an individual with rights and responsibilities, with characteristic patterns of stress[4] response and with assets and limitations, all of which may affect or be affected by
   a. The risks to which the patient is exposed before, during, and after surgery.
   b. Problems related to the incision and approach to the organ or tissue.
   c. The functions of the involved organ or region of the body and their effect on functions of other areas of the body.
   d. The disorder under treatment and the effects of therapy.
2. The patient's perception of the nature of his or her disorder, the therapy, and prognosis.

Right of Access and Informed Consent to Surgery

One of the most basic considerations for the nurse related to the first general factor is the right of the individual to have access to surgery whose purpose, procedure, and consequences the patient comprehends and about which he or she or those close to him or her are able to make an informed decision. The primary purpose of Medicare and Medicaid legislation in the 1960s was to increase access of socioeconomically disadvantaged groups to medical care. Through analysis of National Health Interview Survey data, Bombardier and associates (1977) found that between 1963 and 1970 there was a large increase in surgical treatment of the aged, those of lower education levels, and nonwhites in urban areas. Predictably, lower-income groups used surgical procedures that were rated lowest on a necessity scale to a lesser extent than did middle- and upper-income groups.

In the wake of the dramatic increase in elective surgery on Medicare and Medicaid recipients, the Department of Health, Education, and Welfare initiated, in the late 1970s, a Second Opinion Program to encourage Americans to ask the advice of at least

[4] *Stress* can be defined as the stereotyped reaction pattern of the living organism in response to a variety of influences affecting homeostasis. [Lennart Levi: *Stress: Sources, Management & Prevention* (New York: Liveright Publishing Corporation, 1967), p. 167.]

two physicians before undergoing nonemergency surgery such as procedures involving gallbladder; hemorrhoids; ear, nose, and throat; and certain orthopedic procedures (Mitchell, 1979). A second, and even third, opinion is now required by some third-party payers as a prerequisite to payment of the surgeon for services rendered.

The Second Opinion Program is closely related to the broader issue of the right of the individual to give informed consent for treatment. Although much attention has been given to the individual's moral and legal right to submit to surgery and other treatment only after having given an informed consent, much controversy still swirls around the issue of how to ensure that consent has been informed. Grundner (1980) analyzed five representative surgical consent forms for readability, and found that the readability of all five was equivalent to material intended for upper-division undergraduate or graduate students. Grundner drew the implication that thousands of persons may be undergoing surgery each year on the basis of inadequate consent.

In a follow-up study of 200 cancer patients one day after each had signed a consent form for chemotherapy, radiation therapy, or surgery, Cassileth and associates (1980) found that only 60 per cent understood the purpose and nature of the procedure, and only 55 per cent correctly listed even one major risk or complication.

Rennie (1980) attributes the difficulty to "the inevitable and gross inequality between the two parties interested in consent to a medical procedure. One is fit and medically knowledgeable, the other sick and medically ignorant." Rennie (1980) proposes that the issue will be best addressed by physicians accepting education of the patient, through the process of consent, as a worthwhile therapeutic goal. In the role of patient advocate, the nurse is obliged to see that education of the patient to the purpose, nature, and probable outcomes of treatment takes place in a way that promotes maximum understanding and which places before the patient clear alternatives to consider in making the decision.

Psychological Stress

In all phases of the surgical experience, in relation to any of the general factors cited earlier, the patient may experience a disturbing or even disabling degree of anxiety as a result of the stress response. A primary responsibility of the nurse is to prevent, or recognize and minimize, anxiety of patients. For most persons some aspect of even minor surgical therapy is tantamount to a crisis situation. An individual's behavior can be expected to be similar to the behavior in any other highly stressful situation, as discussed in Chapter 19. Although many of the sources of psychological stress are similar to those to which any sick person is likely to be exposed, there are some that are peculiar to, or more likely to occur among, surgical patients. One of the most common sources is the inadvertent insensitivity of personnel to the stress-inducing potential of almost any aspect of the surgical experience and the hospital environment. Because of their familiarity with the risks and other aspects of surgical treatment, physicians and nurses may not be sufficiently aware of the uniqueness of the experience to each patient. Furthermore, their perception of the proposed procedure and its consequences may be quite different from that of the patient. Unless they are aware of the possibility of differences in perceptions and are alert to clues indicating the emotional state of the individual, they may not be as helpful as they should.

As an illustration, 15-year-old Jesse is to have a wart removed from the sole of his foot. Although his physician has tried to reassure him that removal of the wart is a relatively simple procedure, Jesse fears that he will lose his leg or at least his foot. Physicians and nurses know that a removal of this wart is a minor procedure, and they cannot understand why Jesse continues to turn on his light and to make unnecessary demands for service. About 3 o'clock in the morning, when the night nurse was answering his light for the fifteenth time, she said, "Jesse, you are having trouble getting to sleep, aren't you? It's hard to sleep when you are away from home. Would you like me to stay with you for a little while?" She sat quietly beside his bed. In a few minutes Jesse asked, "Are they going to cut my foot off tomorrow?" When the nurse knew what was troubling Jesse, she was able to reassure him by saying, "My goodness, no," and then explained what was planned.

During the period of diagnosis, the patient may be subjected to a variety of procedures some of which are strenuous, embarrassing, and even painful. At the time surgery is performed, the diagnosis may be uncertain or the patient may believe that it is. Even when the diagnosis has been established as something relatively benign, it is not unusual for a patient to fear that he or she may have cancer. The patient may not understand the nature of the procedure to be performed or believe that it will be more extensive than it is actually planned to be. Uncertainty about the diagnosis and required treatment can be the source of severe stress. Jesse was under psychological stress because he did not understand the extent of the planned surgical procedure.

Another example is Mrs. Thomas, who had a small lump in her breast. Although her physician tried to assure her that the tumor was almost certainly benign, Mrs Thomas was sure that it was malignant and that she would have a radical mastectomy. Previous to the removal of the tumor for examination, she was in a state of near-panic. During the period of recovery from the anesthetic, she wept and referred over and over to loss of her breast. Not until she was fully recovered from the anesthetic could she be assured that her breast had not been removed.

Among other sources of concern to some patients are the anesthetic, its effect, and its effectiveness in preventing pain, as well as the possibility that they may behave in an embarrassing manner. Mr. Thome wonders whether he will be awake or asleep during the operation. He has heard that people sometimes reveal secrets or say foolish or embarrassing things as they go to sleep. The man in the room next to him was awake while he was operated on, but he is not sure that he would like that either. Is it really possible to prevent pain when one is awake? How does one lie awake and allow someone to cut into one's abdomen? If he is awake, will the time of the operation pass quickly or will it be endless and seem to go on and on? Will he have pain after the operation?

In some types of surgery, organs having special meaning to the patient may have to be removed. Although any organ can have some special significance to a given individual, certain ones are more likely to have special meaning than others. Because the heart is essential to survival, surgical procedures on the heart are especially likely to be associated with anxiety and fear of death. Surgery on the organs of reproduction may affect the individual's self-concept, so that he or she feels less of a man or woman. In the American culture, the breast is a symbol of femininity. A woman may therefore feel less a woman after losing a breast. When a surgical procedure either temporarily or permanently prevents a husband and wife from having sexual relations, it may affect the stability of the marriage or the individual may fear that it will. When the loss of a part of the body necessitates changes in the way of life of the patient or in his or her role at work or in the family, the patient usually experiences some degree of anxiety.

Another source of anxiety is the risk to which the patient exposes himself or herself by undergoing surgical therapy. The nurse should be aware of the fact that every operation, no matter how minor, is accompanied by some risk. The risk may be slight or it may be great. When a new procedure or an exceptionally hazardous one is performed, the patient may be aware of the nature of the risk. The patient may also know that if surgery fails, chances for living are negligible. Some of the preceding continue to be sources of anxiety during the period of recovery following the operation. Attention is given to provide the patient with sufficient care of good quality to assure him or her that needs will be met. Possibly too little consideration is given to the effects of what the patient regards as too much care. For example, during the period when Mr. Norman was being prepared for, and immediately following, the introduction of an aortic prosthesis (artificial aortic valve), he received more attention than he had possibly experienced over his entire life span. The effect was not to assure him but to frighten him, for he said, "Who am I to receive all this care? No one has ever cared this much about me before. Why should they do so at this time? I must be terribly sick, or people would continue to ignore me as they have in the past." Following the immediate postoperative period, Mr. Norman became deeply depressed. Although some depression is common, Mr. Norman was unusually depressed. During an interview with a psychiatrist, he expressed his feelings. The nurse who cared for him before and immediately after the operation remembered that he had made a similar comment to her but she had not recognized its significance. Possibly, if he had had an opportunity to express his feelings previous to surgical therapy his depression would have been less severe.

Measures to Minimize the Patient's Anxiety?

One of the most reassuring things about modern surgical treatment is the proportion of patients who benefit from it. Exclusive of obstetric deliveries, it is estimated that some 11 million to 12 million people undergo surgery in the United States each year. The extent to which surgery has been made safe for the patient is demonstrated by the fact that over 99.5 per cent of those operated upon survive the surgery (Rothenberg, 1965).

The nurse should know the mortality and complication rates of the type of surgery proposed for the patient. It is *not* appropriate for the nurse to *initiate* discussion of the mortality and morbidity associated with a particular operation, but it is essential that the nurse's response to a patient's questions, or follow-up of the physician's explanations, be informed and based in reality. Especially when the patient's reluctance to consent to surgery is due to fear of death, he or she is entitled to the most complete and recent information available to help in the decision of whether the possible benefits are worth taking the known risks. However, great care should be taken to avoid creating anxiety in patients who do not wish to have extensive information about the proposed operation. Recent emphasis on the legal right of the patient to give informed consent to surgical procedures can prompt physicians and nurses to give more information than the patient wants, needs, or can interpret, with the result that the anxiety of the patient is needlessly intensified. As with every other patient problem, assessment of the individual must precede appropriate action.

Although fear of death continues to be a major source of anxiety, especially in the preoperative period, there are many other relatively mundane concerns that may be anxiety provoking unless the patient is helped to formulate and get answers to questions. On the basis of many years of experience as a surgeon, Rothenberg (1965) had identified questions most frequently asked by patients about prospective surgery.

What caused my disease? Will the operation cure me?
Is this operation necessary? What will happen if I don't have the operation?
How long will I be hospitalized?
How much will the operation and hospitalization cost? How can I pay for it?
Will I be awake during the operation?
Will there be complications from the operation? Will I be able to eat? Will I have pain, or nausea and vomiting?
Do I need special nurses after surgery? Can my family and/or friends stay with me?
Will there be a big scar? Where? When can the stitches come out?
How soon after the operation may I:
  Shower? Take a tub bath?
  Drive or ride in a car?
  Do light and heavy lifting?
  Climb stairs?
  Take walks? How far?
  Return to work?
  Resume marital relations?
  Resume hobbies and preferred recreation?
Will I have to take medication after leaving the hospital? What will it cost? How/where will I fill prescriptions?

Creating a climate in which the patient is encouraged to raise such questions is a necessary first step to minimize psychological stress. Additional areas about which information should be provided to the patient and those concerned about him or her include hospital routines, the recovery room, and postoperative procedures. The patient wants to be assured that those who are responsible for care are competent and will be available when he or she needs them. Although some of the preceding are the responsibility of the surgeon, nurses are frequently faced with questions that the patient asks for information and reassurance. Even when the surgeon provides the patient with a detailed explanation, the patient may be so overwhelmed and confused by the fact that surgery is necessary that he or she comprehends very little of what is told. In addition, the patient may stand in awe of the surgeon and hesitate to ask questions. Later, after having had an opportunity to think about the situation, the patient may have questions that should be answered. The nurse has an obligation to secure answers to the questions the patient is asking. Whether the nurse answers the questions personally or refers them to the physician and how she or he answers those that are not referred depends on the nature of the questions and the nurse's own competence.

When the patient has questions that the nurse cannot or is not permitted to answer, she or he can still be helpful to the patient. The nurse can express interest in the patient by listening and, if required, initiating action. Someone who is willing and able to listen may be all the patient wants or needs. The nurse can also help the patient to clarify questions and can encourage him or her to ask the surgeon for information. The nurse can also determine the urgency of the need of the patient to have questions answered. Miss Elder had been in the hospital for some weeks for the treatment of a fractured hip. The fracture was treated by open reduction, following which Miss Elder was encased in a double spica cast. About a week previous to the incident related here, she had been told that she might go home on the following Tuesday and all the arrangements had been made. The day before she planned to leave the hospital, the surgeon made a window in the cast in order to examine and dress the wound. After the required equipment was delivered to the room, the surgeon explained what he was going to do. Because Miss Elder was unprepared for the procedure, she heard nothing. Although her wound was healing nicely, she quickly concluded that it was not healing and that she would not be discharged from the hospital. She was so upset that she could not ask the surgeon for an explanation. Shortly after the surgeon left, a nurse found Miss Elder in tears. Although the nurse knew that Miss Elder was to be discharged as planned, she was sure that reassurance of the patient depended on direct word from her physician. She immediately called him and he assured her that Miss Elder was to be discharged the following day. This information was relayed to Miss Elder so that she could relax and complete her plans for leaving the hospital.

In some hospitals the problem of what patients can be told about the nature of their illness, why surgery is needed, and what can be expected during all phases of illness is met by the preparation of two types of manuals that the patient may be given to read and the nursing staff given to use as a guide in answering questions. One type includes essential information about the nature of a particular disease and its therapy, or its content may deal primarily with the surgical aspects of therapy. For example, one manual might cover the disease diabetes mellitus and its treatment. Another might be prepared for the use of the patient having a colostomy or thoracic surgery. These manuals emphasize what the patient needs to know to help himself or herself recover and give answers to frequently asked questions. They are usually prepared by a committee of physicians and nurses.

A second type of manual provides information about hospital routines such as admission procedures, visiting hours, and special facilities such as the recovery room. The guide may also include suggestions about how the patient and visitors can help to facilitate the recovery of the patient as well as what they can expect from the hospital personnel. It may be given to the patient before admission by the physician or at the time of admission. Any material preparing the patient for what to expect and for what is expected of him or her should be helpful. In addition to well-prepared written explanations, the patient needs oral instruction as to what to expect.

Efforts to structure patient expectations as a means of reducing anxiety and distress should include information on the *sensations* likely to accompany a procedure or event. Too often preparatory instruction is limited to the structural elements of diagnostic and therapeutic procedures, such as descriptions of equipment, positions to be assumed, personnel to be involved, timing and duration of the event. Rarely does preparation include description of the various sensations that may accompany the event. Discovering the sensory component of surgical procedures is a fertile field for nursing research. Johnson (1972) found that in preparing patients for gastroscopy, information that reduced the discrepancy between expectations about sensations and patients' actual experience during the procedure resulted in less distress, as measured by motor behavior, vital signs, and amount of Valium[5] required during the procedure. Description included such sensations as the needle stick during administration of IV medication, followed by drowsiness; the changes in lighting of the examining room during the procedure; and the sensation of fullness similar to that after eating a large meal when air is pumped into the stomach.

Admission to the hospital is accompanied by emotional stress and, at the time, the patient is likely to be more or less confused. Some attention should be given to the family of the patient. Relatives should know the time the patient is expected to be taken to the operating room and whether or not he or she is expected to return to the room immediately after the operation or will be cared for in a recovery room or an intensive-care unit. For example, a patient may remain in a recovery room only until consciousness is regained and major physiologic derangements have been corrected, or may stay in an intensive-care unit for 24 to 48 or more hours. Whatever the practice is, the patient and family should be prepared for what to expect. They should know that the recovery room or intensive-care unit is a service provided for the welfare of the patient.

[5] Trade name for diazepam, N.F., a central nervous system depressant used for relief of mild to moderate symptoms of anxiety, including preoperative apprehension.

Summary

The psychological status of the patient is an important factor in the patient's capacity to withstand the stress imposed by surgery. How the patient regards the surgical procedure that is to be performed, as well as its possible effects, influences chances for survival and for recovery. The nurse may be helpful to the patient and to the family by providing a climate in which the patient feels free to express feelings and in which he or she feels accepted and esteemed as an individual human being. The nurse can also be helpful to the patient by relaying any concerns to the physician, so that the physician can more accurately assess the psychological status of the patient and plan to correct misconceptions and misinformation. Only when fears are examined can they be put into their true perspective and confined. Measures to prevent or minimize psychological stress of the patient or family will be equally applicable in any phase of the surgical experience. Attention will now be directed to the physiologic status of the patient treated surgically. It must be emphasized that mind and body always respond or function as a unit and that, because of the connecting links of the hypothalamus and hypophysis, emotional responses inevitably have a somatic component, and many physiologic responses have an emotional component. Separation of these two domains of behavior here is purely for the purpose of clarity in presentation.

The Preoperative Period

A patient who is in physiologic homeostasis and is emotionally prepared for surgery tolerates surgical intervention well. The purpose of all activities in the preoperative period is to optimize those conditions necessary to emotional and physiologic homeostasis, thereby increasing the likelihood that the patient will react appropriately to, and correct derangements caused by, surgical trauma and its consequences (Polk, 1977).

The preoperative period may be defined as the period of time beginning with the moment it is recognized that surgery is needed and ending when the patient arrives in the operating room. During this period the nature of the patient's illness is determined and a therapeutic plan is made. For example, Mr. Thome has had symptoms of indigestion periodically for the last 6 months. For the most part, his symptoms have been mild and he has been able to explain them to his satisfaction and secure relief by taking antacids. One morning he awakened feeling nauseated and with a pain in his upper abdomen. He reviewed what he had eaten during the last 24 hours to determine what might be responsible for his symptoms. He took two anti-indigestion pills. Instead of the pills relieving his feeling, however, the symptoms increased and he began to feel frightened. His wife suggested that she call a doctor, who determined that he needed surgery. Mr. Thome had entered the preoperative period, which did not end until he was transferred to the operating room, where he expected to have a partial gastrectomy for the removal of a portion of his stomach.

During the early preoperative period the nurse may act as a case finder and a health educator by encouraging the patient who is in the "Is it or isn't it?" stage to seek medical attention. Delay in the treatment of some disorders increases the danger of serious complications and may lessen chances for recovery. As an illustration, acute appendicitis, when operated on early, is accompanied by only a small risk. The death rate following appendectomy is less than 0.3 per cent when the operation can be performed before perforation. The complication rate after perforation has been shown in at least one study to be seven times that of the preperforation rate (Allen, 1965).

At the time Mrs. Thome called the family physician, Mr. Thome entered the phase of diagnosis. He still had moments of "Is it or isn't it?" He also felt relief that at last he was under medical care, but his relief was mixed with anxiety about the nature of the cause of his symptoms and the treatment that would be required. At this time Mr. Thome was subjected to a series of investigations directed toward answering two questions: What was the nature and extent of his illness? What was his physiologic and psychological status? Answers to the first question determined whether or not surgery was indicated in his treatment and the type of procedure that would be of benefit to him. Answers to the second question provided information about any abnormalities that required correction before he was operated on and his capacity to adapt to surgical therapy.

Any disorder that reduces the capacity of the individual to adapt and to maintain homeostatic conditions increases the risk of surgery. Among the many disorders increasing risk are shock; hemorrhage; disorders in water and electrolyte balance; acidosis and alkalosis; anemia; pulmonary, cardiac, and renal disorders; undernutrition; hypoproteinemia; obesity; adrenal insufficiency; alcoholism; hyperthyroidism; diabetes mellitus; disease of the liver; and psychic and emotional disturbances. All these disorders lessen, in some manner, the capacity of the individual to maintain homeostasis. Some, such as disturbances in water and electrolyte balance, indicate impairment of one or more homeostatic conditions. When the life of the patient is not immediately threatened, surgical treatment is usually delayed until the physiologic and psychological condition of the patient is improved as nearly as possible to the optimum condition. In the investigation of the patient, the surgeon is interested in uncovering any condition that will either make the development of a complication more likely or reduce the capacity of the person to adapt to stress.

Most of the disorders that increase surgical risk have been discussed in previous chapters. The following comments will be limited to relating those disorders to surgical risk. To make the patient safe for surgery, preoperative evaluation and preparation must consider the age; the nutritional, pulmonary, and cardiovascular status of the patient; and the patient's neurologic, renal, hepatic, and gastrointestinal function. All are interrelated in determining the capacity of the patient to tolerate additional stress and to respond favorably to surgery.

Age

Because there is a relationship between age and the capacity of the individual to maintain physiologic homeostasis under stress, the age of the patient has some bearing on the risks to which he or she is exposed during surgical therapy. Very young children tolerate the trauma of surgery remarkably well and recover quickly. They are, however, easily upset, and they are particularly sensitive to chilling, exposure, and rough handling. Gius (1966) states that the loss of an ounce of blood by an infant may be equivalent to the loss of a pint of blood by an adult. The infant should therefore be closely observed for evidence of blood loss, because seemingly small losses represent a relatively large part of the blood volume. He or she must also be protected from conditions in the environment predisposing to chilling. These include a low environmental temperature, drafts, and wet clothing. With proper care, an infant survives surgical therapy very well.

At the other end of the life span, the elderly patient has generally been believed to tolerate surgical therapy poorly. Although modern surgical management has greatly reduced the hazards of surgery to the elderly patient, some surgeons have known for many years that old age, by itself, is not a contraindication to surgical therapy. One surgeon who is frequently quoted on this point is Sir James Paget (1954). He wrote

> Years, indeed, taken alone are a very fallacious mode of reckoning age: it is not the time but the quantity of a man's past life that we have to reckon. . . . The old people that are thin and dry and tough, clear-voiced and bright-eyed, with good stomachs and strong wills, muscular and active, are not bad; they bear all but the largest operations very well. But very bad are they, who, looking somewhat like these, are feeble and soft-skinned, with little pulses, bad appetites, and weak digestive powers; so that they cannot in an emergency be well nourished.

Moyer (1965) in a summary of a review of the literature on the influence of age on operative mortality, concludes that (1) the operative mortality is higher among the aged in disorders accompanied by pus formation or other complications such as perforation of a viscus, (2) the operative mortality rate is the same for all groups in disorders that are seldom accompanied by complications, and (3) the death rate from burns is higher among the aged than among younger persons.

In more general terms, the elderly person's capacity to respond to the stress of a single surgical procedure of short duration is satisfactory, but he or she is less able to tolerate prolonged stress and multiple stresses than are younger persons. The elderly person is less able to tolerate disorders accompanied by prolonged physiological disturbances. Because the elderly person has less reserve than the younger person the old person's capacity to maintain and to restore homeostasis in the presence of continued strain is less than that of a younger person. He or she is more likely to have one or more chronic diseases that decrease reserve or place a burden on the capacity to adapt. When the strain placed on the adaptive capacity is within his or her reserve, the older person responds favorably. As in the care of the very young, attention should be given to preventing unnecessary demands on the adaptive capacity of the elderly person.

When planning and implementing the nursing care of the elderly patient, the nurse should be mindful of the fact that as people age, their renal, cardiovascular, and pulmonary reserves diminish. As a consequence, these structures are less able to cope with conditions placing stress on their functional capacity, and they are more likely to be sites of complication than they are in young persons. Among the elderly, the exact chronological age of the patient is of less significance than outlook and physiological status. A hopeful, optimistic attitude combined with a good nutritional status and reasonable cardiovascular, renal, and pulmonary reserve makes an elderly person quite safe for surgery. Even with such traumatic surgery as resection of abdominal aortic aneurysms, a study of a series of 152 patients over 74 years of age found that once a patient had been operated on successfully, his or her life expectancy tended to parallel that of the normal population for that age group (Beven, 1970).

Nutritional Status

Among the important factors significant to the nutritional status of the surgical patient are blood volume, hemoglobin and plasma proteins; water and electrolytes; vitamins, especially B and C; and body weight. Blood volume may be considered normal, or adequate, when tests of organ function reveal no abnormality attributable to inadequate perfusion. Hematocrit levels below 35 per cent may be restored to normal by administering packed cells or, if accompanied by hemoglobin levels below 9 to 10 g per 100 ml, may be treated by transfusion of whole blood. It is generally agreed that any deficit for which a single unit (500 ml) of whole blood would be adequate replacement should be treated by other means, because of the present hazards of whole blood transfusion. Many surgeons believe that suspensions of packed red cells are superior to whole blood transfusion in the correction of preoperative anemia. Williams (1969) found in correcting preoperative anemia in patients over 60 years of age who had compensated heart disease that blood volume expansion was almost entirely caused by red cells, and was greater 24 hours after packed cells than after whole blood transfusion.

Nutritional elements most important to wound healing are protein and vitamins B and C, which, being water-soluble, are not stored and are therefore quickly exhausted. Whenever the patient is taking nothing by mouth, even for 2 to 3 days, the minimum daily requirement of vitamins B and C must be provided, usually in intravenous feedings. Undernutrition, with or without hypoproteinemia, significantly increases the risk factor because of the catabolic response to surgical trauma, which uses amino acids as an energy source via gluconeogenesis. Except in a crisis, surgery will be delayed until the patient's nutritional status is improved by some form of hyperalimentation,[6] which may be administered orally, by nasogastric or gastrostomy tube feedings, or intravenously.

Of the patients who are treated surgically, some are more likely to be undernourished than others. Chronically ill and aged persons are more likely to be malnourished than are previously healthy children and adults. Persons who have disturbances in the functioning of the alimentary tract are predisposed to malnutrition. These disturbances result from failure to either ingest, absorb, or retain food in the alimentary canal long enough for it to be digested and absorbed. The patient who has had a chronic loss of protein-containing body fluids, including blood, is likely to suffer from hypoproteinemia. One often neglected aspect relating to nutrition is the effect of diagnostic examinations that require the withholding of food and purging. For example, examinations of the alimentary canal are usually preceded by withholding of food and fluids, sometimes for an extended period of time. This may create serious problems in the already dehydrated and undernourished patient. Unless contraindicated, food and fluids should be served at the completion of a diagnostic test. Between-meal and bedtime snacks can be added to increase the patient's intake. If the patient is losing excessive amounts of fluid or is not taking in proper amounts of food or liquids, the physician should be notified so that he or she may order supplemental feedings of intravenous fluids. All these measures require a thoughtful concern for the welfare of the patient and appropriate planning. All the measures suggested in Chapters 29 and 46 may be required to improve the nutritional status of the patient sufficiently to make him or her safe for surgery.

Some disorders that are associated with undernutrition are also responsible for the loss of water and electrolytes. In addition to insufficient water and/or electrolytes, water may accumulate in body cavities or in the interstitial spaces in the form of edema. Measures required to correct water and electrolyte balance *must* be taken prior to surgery. (See Chapter 41 for problems of fluid and electrolyte balance.)

Excessively obese patients should be placed on a weight-reduction regimen and whenever possible surgery delayed until the patient reaches a satisfactory weight. Obesity burdens the patient with a number of handicaps. Because fat has a poor blood supply, these patients are more susceptible to infection. Fat is more difficult to approximate than other tissues. Large amounts of fat also increase the difficulty of exposing organs in the abdominal cavity and may reduce the pulmonary vital capacity by pressure on the diaphragm. Although obese patients present difficult technical problems, a 5-year study of 400 obese and nonobese patients undergoing cholecystectomy demonstrated that obesity per se was not associated with a higher postoperative morbidity or mortality rate (Manax & Pemberton, 1971).

Pulmonary Status

Significant pulmonary complications occur in 20 to 40 per cent of patients following abdominal or thoracic operations, making pulmonary complications the largest single cause of morbidity and mortality in the postoperative period. Respiratory failure is a major cause in 25 per cent of postoperative deaths and a major contributory factor in another 25 per cent (Schwartz, 1979, p. 499). The high incidence is due to the large number of factors that can produce a pattern of shallow monotonous tidal ventilation without intermittent deep breaths (sighing respirations), which soon leads to alveolar collapse, followed by atelectasis, tachypnea, hypoxia, fever, and pneumonitis. Instructing and exercising the patient in deep breathing and coughing preoperatively are critical measures to help prevent alveolar collapse and the events that follow. The ideal prophylactic respiratory maneuver is one in which high alveolar inflating pressure is exerted for a long period of time, using the inhaled volume rather than the peak airway pressure as the critical measurement. See Chapter 40 for management of pulmonary complications.

The aggressiveness with which measures are instituted to prevent pulmonary complications is guided by assessment of risk factors exhibited by the patient. Table 51-1 summarizes risk factors for pulmonary complications of surgery. Additional factors associated with a high incidence of pulmonary complications are oral infections, unconsciousness, and prolonged bedrest.

In the preoperative period, all patients must have an x-ray examination of the chest as an essential part of the assessment of the status of the respiratory system. It is useful in detecting tuberculosis and emphysema as well as many other disorders of the lung that may not be found during a routine history and physical examination. Depending upon the disorder and condition of the patient, pulmonary function tests discussed in Chapter 26 may be performed.

In addition to initiating deep-breathing exercises, preoperative measures to prevent pulmonary complications should include insisting that the patient

[6] *Hyperalimentation* is the administration of sufficient nutrients above basal requirements to achieve tissue synthesis, positive nitrogen balance, and anabolism. See Chapter 46 for detailed discussion.

TABLE 51-1 *Risk Factors for Postoperative Pulmonary Complications*

Variable	This Factor	Is a Greater Risk than (>)	This Factor
Age	Elderly	>	Youth and early adulthood
Sex	Men	>	Women
Type of anesthesia	Inhalation	>	Spinal or local
Duration of anesthesia	Deep and long	>	Short and light
Smoking	Smokers	>	Nonsmokers
Site of incision	Upper abdomen	>	Lower abdomen

stop smoking for at least 3 weeks prior to elective procedures, treating chronic bronchitis with specific antibiotics, improving nutrition and general muscular strength, and postoperatively resuming early activity and ambulation, and avoiding fluid overload (Bartlett et al., 1973).

Cardiovascular Status

In the evaluation of the cardiovascular system, the condition and reserve capacity of the heart and blood vessels are investigated. When there is evidence of pathology, the physician then tries to estimate the adequacy of the cardiac reserve; this helps to determine if the patient will be able to tolerate the strain of surgery. Contrary to popular opinion, the patient may have considerable cardiovascular pathology and the heart may still be able to tolerate certain surgical procedures with little or no difficulty.

In the evaluation of the state of the blood vessels, two factors are reviewed. One is the capacity of the body to adapt the diameter of the blood vessels to the changing needs of the organism. The other is the adequacy of the blood supply to the tissues that will be operated on. The level of the blood pressure of the patient provides information about the first factor. In a patient with a blood pressure below 90 systolic or above 120 diastolic, the capacity to adapt to the stress of surgery is likely to be inadequate or greatly diminished. The patient with an excessively low systolic blood pressure may be suffering from a variety of fluid and electrolyte problems, cardiovascular disease, or adrenal insufficiency. The patient with the high diastolic pressure is especially likely to develop or already have significant impairment of renal function. Because healing is dependent on the adequacy of the blood supply, an estimation of the capacity of the heart and blood vessels to deliver sufficient blood to the tissues is essential. Pallor and coldness of extremities and blanching on pressure with slow return of color are indications that the amount of blood being delivered to the tissue is greatly reduced.

The capacity of the circulatory system to deliver adequate amounts of oxygen, glucose, and other metabolic necessities to the tissue depends not only on the competence of the heart as a pump and the adaptability and patency of the blood vessels but on the quantity and quality of the blood. After an acute hemorrhage both the quality and quantity of the blood may be diminished. With long-standing nutritional deficiencies or chronic loss of blood, the quality of blood may be poor. The most commonly used measures of the quantity of blood in relation to the size of the vascular system are blood pressure, pulse, and central venous pressure. Blood volume determinations may also be of value. The quality of the blood in relation to its red cell content may be measured by either the hematocrit or the hemoglobin content, or both. A reduction of either indicates a decrease in the oxygen-carrying capacity of the blood. Because the adequacy of the oxygen-carrying power of the blood and the blood volume both directly affect the chances of the patient for survival, surgery is seldom scheduled until arrangements have been made to replace needed blood. If the surgical procedure is one entailing a large loss of blood, additional blood may be required to replace that which is lost at the time of the operation. Cardiac and cerebrovascular complications are minimized by avoiding hypovolemia, which is accompanied consistently by hypotension, and subsequently by hypoxemia.

Hemostatic risk must be assessed preoperatively. In a 6-year study of hemostatic risk in surgical patients at San Francisco General Hospital, abnormal bleeding problems were found in 1 per cent of preoperative patients (Davis, 1969). Identification of hemostatic risk is based on findings from (1) the history of effects on the patient of trauma such as tonsillectomy, dental extractions, nose bleeds (epistaxis), heavy menstrual flow (menorrhagia), and bruising (ecchymosis) disproportionate to trauma; (2) physical examination; (3) complete blood count (CBC), including estimate of platelets; (4) time tests for thromboplastin and prothrombin; and (5) the tourniquet test for capillary fragility. Problems and management of impaired function of the transportation system are discussed in Chapters 42, 43, and 44 and in the chapter on shock (Chapter 45).

Neurologic Function

A thorough neurologic assessment of the patient is necessary prior to any major surgical procedure, because (1) anesthetics and analgesics act directly to depress the nervous system, (2) functions of all body systems are regulated and integrated totally or in part by the neuroendocrine system, and (3) both the psychological and physical components of pain, which is an almost universal consequence of any surgical procedure, are phenomena of the nervous system. Comprehensive evaluation of neural regulation of body responses is discussed in Unit IV. Unless there is evidence of primary or secondary neurologic impairment, preoperative evaluation is usually limited to physical examination findings of the cranial nerves; motor, sensory, and reflex responses of upper and lower extremities; and cerebellar responses.

Renal Function

In any condition in which the body is placed under increased physiologic stress, the capacity of the kidney to function is of great significance. It functions in homeostasis to eliminate or conserve water and electrolytes and it eliminates the wastes of protein metabolism. In the absence of evidence to indicate that the kidney reserve is limited or that the kidney is diseased, the urine is tested for sugar, acetone, and albumin. The presence of sugar and acetone in the urine are not tests of kidney function but they are important because they may indicate that the patient has diabetes mellitus. Albumin in the urine usually indicates the presence of kidney disease or some condition that limits its blood flow. In a woman, albuminuria may not be significant unless the urine specimen is obtained by catheter. To estimate the adequacy of kidney function, the level of the creatinine, urea, or nonprotein nitrogen in the blood is determined. Other tests of kidney function include the capacity of the kidney to concentrate phenolsulfonphthalein in the urine or to increase its specific gravity when water is withheld.

Evaluation of renal function is important not only because it influences operative risk but because it affects the capacity of the patient to handle the parenteral fluid and electrolytes administered during the postoperative period. Although output should be compared with intake in all patients, these measurements are especially important in patients with renal disease. The kidney normally produces 35 g of solute in 24 hours. Urine concentration to a specific gravity of only 1.010 requires 1,500 ml to excrete 35 g of solute. It is therefore advisable to maintain a 24-hour urine output of at least 2,000 ml. A diseased kidney requires more fluid volume to clear the daily metabolic products than does the normal kidney. With appropriate hydration, renal complications of major surgical procedures have become relatively uncommon (Polk, 1977, p. 128). The nurse should take the responsibility for checking specific gravity, as well as volume output, of urine, whenever the patient's history and circumstances indicate the need for a measure of urine concentration. Use of the urinometer is a simple procedure for which the nurse does not require a directive from the physician.

Digestive System

Hepatic Function

The nutritional status of the patient and his or her ability to control bleeding and repair tissue are largely dependent upon critical metabolic functions of the liver. Maintenance of blood glucose levels depends upon glycogenesis, glycogenolysis, and gluconeogenesis; maintenance of plasma proteins depends upon synthesis of essentially all the body's albumin and fibrinogen, and over half the globulins; control of potentially harmful blood ammonia levels depends upon formation of urea from ammonia, with urea being excreted in the urine; the oxygen-carrying capacity of red cells depends upon the liver's storage of iron as ferritin, for the formation of hemoglobin; and blood clotting depends upon formation of prothrombin and factors VII, IX, and X. An additional contribution of the liver to the welfare of the surgical patient is that many of the central nervous system depressant drugs administered throughout the surgical experience must be detoxified in the liver. If preoperative medical evaluation reveals abnormalities in such areas as plasma proteins, blood sugar, or blood clotting, additional liver function tests may be required. If the patient has a defective blood-clotting mechanism or excessive blood loss is anticipated during the operative procedure, vitamin K may be administered preoperatively to facilitate formation of prothrombin and the three blood-clotting factors by the liver.

Stomach and Small Intestine

The nurse plays a major role in the preoperative preparation of the gastrointestinal tract, which usually requires several days preceding major abdominal operations. Regardless of whether the gastrointestinal tract is directly involved, preparation of the patient for surgery often includes emptying this tract. Food and fluids are withheld and the lower bowel is emptied by the administration of one or more enemas. Preparation for colon surgery may involve several enemas and laxatives for 3 or more days. Intravenous fluids may also have to be given to elderly patients, especially if there is any evidence of dehydration or hypovolemia.

In the past, to make sure that the stomach was empty at the time of surgery, food and fluids were withheld from midnight until the surgery was performed the following day. Many surgeons have modified this procedure to correspond to the time it takes the stomach to empty, for prolonged abstinence from food and fluids is of no general value and increases the likelihood of dehydration. Unless there is an obstruction, food usually remains in the stomach 6 hours or less. Liquids leave the stomach even quicker. In fact, liquids may pass immediately from the esophagus to the duodenum. To make sure that the stomach is empty, food intake is restricted for at least 8 to 10 hours, and fluids are prohibited for 4 or more hours before surgery. The nervous adult or older child may have food sit in his stomach for many hours. This is less likely to occur in infants and children, and fluids should be restricted in the latter as little as possible. An empty stomach is important, because it reduces the likelihood of the patient's vomiting and aspirating gastric juice into the lung; when gastric juice is inhaled, it produces a very serious type of pneumonitis. However, dehydration of the patient is not necessary to prevent aspiration.

In preparation for many major abdominal operations such as gastric surgery, a nasogastric tube may be used to empty the stomach. When the patient has an obstruction of the intestinal tract, decompression of the bowel may be necessary before he or she can be operated on with safety. The cause and effects of obstruction of the alimentary canal are presented in Chapter 46. Gastric or intestinal intubation with suction often is employed during the preoperative as well as the postoperative phase of surgery to reduce vomiting and gastric or intestinal dilatation.

Decompression is accomplished by the introduction into the stomach or intestine of a tube to which suction is applied. Removal of fluids and gas from the stomach can be accomplished by a single-lumen Levin tube. Removal of the contents from the jejunum or ileum requires a long intestinal tube with either a single or double lumen. A bag or balloon is often added to the end of the tube to facilitate its movement after it enters the duodenum. When a single-lumen tube is used, a bag filled with mercury is attached to the tip before it is inserted. When a double-lumen tube is used, one lumen opens into a balloon that is distended with water, air, or mercury; the other lumen provides for the removal of fluid and gas. Either type of tube is passed through a nostril, the pharynx, and the esophagus into the stomach. After the short tube (Levin) reaches the stomach, it is taped to the face. No tube should be taped to the nose and above the eye, because when the tube is taped in this position it presses on the underside of the nostril and may cause pressure necrosis. It should be anchored in the position that it takes naturally. (See Figure 51-1.)

The long tube is passed from the stomach through the pylorus and into the duodenum. The passage of the tube through the pylorus may be facilitated by having the patient lie on his or her right side. After the tube enters the duodenum, the physician inflates the balloon; peristalsis, if present, may carry the balloon and tube through the intestine. To hasten the movement of the tube toward the site of the obstruction, the physician may leave an order for the nurse to advance the tube a specific distance

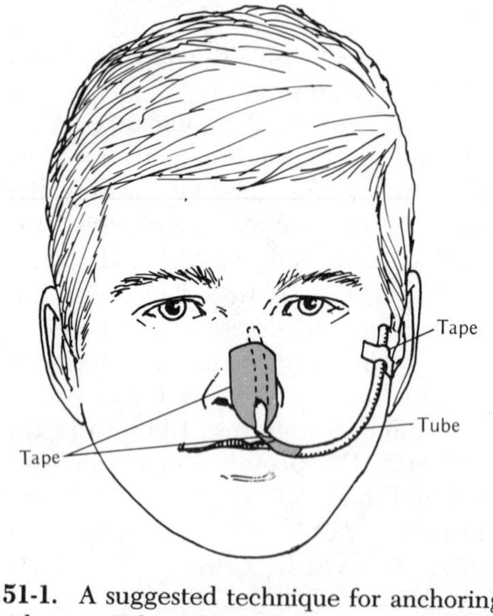

Figure 51-1. A suggested technique for anchoring nasal tubes with tape. When this technique is used, adherence of the tape to the nose must be checked frequently. Perspiration and skin oils cause the tape to loosen. The tape is split half its length, and the split ends are wrapped securely in opposite directions around the tube after the broad end has been taped to the nose. The free end of the tube can then be taped over the zygomatic arch or secured to the clothing of the patient to prevent pulling on the tube.

at regular intervals of time. If able, the patient can assist in this by swallowing as the tube is pushed forward. The act of swallowing also helps to suppress the gag reflex. During the procedure the physician can check the location of the tube by x-ray or by fluoroscopic examination. When the tube reaches the desired site, it is then taped in the manner previously described.

After either the short or long tube has reached the stomach, suction is applied. There are a number of methods for producing suction. The method that is selected depends on the wishes of the physician and the equipment provided by the hospital.[7] Whatever method is utilized to secure suction, the force should be gentle, usually not in excess of 1.5 lb of negative pressure. When excessive suction is applied, the mucosa lining the intestine or stomach may be sucked into the opening in the tube, damaging the mucosa and occluding the tube. The injury to the mucosa is similar to that induced in the mucosal lining of the trachea and bronchi by excessive suction. To secure suction, the system must be airtight and the device should be checked at intervals to be sure that it is working. However, because secretion is not constant, fluid does not flow continuously from the tube. Should there be doubt as to whether or not the system is operating, the tube leading to the stomach can be irrigated with a small amount of saline. If fluid returns when the apparatus is connected, then it is operating satisfactorily. Frequent irrigations of the tube or the use of large amounts of water should be avoided, as water and electrolytes required by the body are removed in the process. However, gastrointestinal secretions contain solid particles that may accumulate and obstruct the tube. The tube should therefore be irrigated at regular intervals and frequently enough to keep it patent. Occasionally when a tube is irrigated, the fluid runs in, but an obstruction to its return acts as a ball valve. In this event the fluid introduced into the stomach contributes to further distention of the stomach. Sometimes the obstruction of the tube can be eliminated by changing the position of the patient or the tube. If this does not relieve the obstruction, the physician should be notified. To prevent the loss of fluids and electrolytes, some surgeons prescribe the use of air to check the patency of the tube. Smaller amounts of air can be introduced, and thus distention avoided. If one places a stethoscope just below the xiphoid process and listens, the muffled "woosh" that accompanies the passage of air through a patent gastric tube will be heard. The amount of air required varies with the length and diameter of the tube; with a Levin tube, for example, 15 to 25 cc are usually adequate.

When the outlet of the stomach is obstructed, a large tube with multiple openings may be required to remove the food particles and other debris that accumulate. Cleansing of the stomach may be furthered by pouring water or saline into the tube and then sucking out the fluid. The procedure is repeated until the solution that returns is clear. Because of the size of the tube, it is passed through the mouth and is removed at the completion of the procedure.

Many patients regard gastrointestinal intubation as one of the most disagreeable aspects of the entire hospital or operative experience. Mrs. Repeat illustrates this point very well. Two years ago, she had abdominal surgery. She says, "The thing that I dread the most is having all those tubes. Worst of all is that tube they put into my stomach." When gastric intubation is a part of a patient's preoperative preparation, he or she should be helped to understand how intubation contributes to recovery. The patient should also understand how the tube is passed and what he or she can do to help and what will be done to assist. The patient should know that the tube will be lubricated to make it pass more easily, and should also know that swallowing as the tube is passed will help and that he or she will be reminded to swallow at the appropriate times. The patient who has had the symptoms of obstruction may welcome the relief that the introduction of the tube brings.

Although the physician may pass the tube, it is increasingly common practice that the nurse be taught and expected to pass short nasogastric tubes. Before doing this, the nurse should prepare by studying the anatomy of the area and becoming acquainted with the possible difficulties that may be encountered. In addition to preparing the patient for what to expect and for what is expected of him or her, the nurse also prepares the patient physically. The patient may be in either the recumbent or the sitting position. In either event, the head should be hyperextended until the tube is in the esophagus. The head may then be flexed in order to facilitate swallowing of water. Because the patient is likely to gag and may vomit, and because secretions are increased, a supply of paper tissues and an emesis basin should be within easy reach. The required equipment and supplies should be at hand and in working order before the procedure is started. Thorough lubrication of the tube makes for ease in passing it. If oil is used, any excess should be removed to decrease the danger of aspiration of oil into the lungs. Because of this possibility, some physicians prefer to use glycerine or a water-soluble substance to lubri-

[7] For students who wish an extensive review of intubation and drainage of the alimentary canal, see V. Henderson and G. Nite. *Principles and Practice of Nursing*, 6th ed. New York: Macmillan Publishing Co., 1978, Chap. 23, pp. 1212–57.

cate the tube. As the tube is passed the patient should be reminded at appropriate intervals to swallow. Some patients find swallowing easier if they are allowed sips of water as the tube is passed. Patients should be kept appraised of the success of their efforts and they should know when the tube reaches the stomach. The nurse can check the placement of the tube in the stomach by (1) aspirating stomach contents by syringe attached to the lumen of the tube, or (2) using a syringe to quickly introduce 20 to 25 cc of air, while simultaneously listening with a stethoscope just below the xiphoid process for the "woosh" of air passing through the tube into the stomach. Any prolonged coughing or labored or crowing respirations may indicate that the tip of the tube has entered the larynx; the tube should be withdrawn slightly, the patient instructed to swallow, and then the tube quickly advanced while the glottis is closed. The nurse should be mindful of the fact that it is difficult to pass a tube through the upper alimentary canal without the cooperation of the patient who is conscious. The patient should know what his or her role is and be helped to carry it out.

The mouth of the patient with gastric or intestinal decompression requires the same or more care than that of a patient who is not taking food and fluid by mouth. The patient should have an opportunity to brush his or her teeth and rinse the mouth with mouthwash three or four times a day. Mouthwash, if not overused, is refreshing. Too frequent rinsing of the mouth contributes to dehydration by loss of saliva. The flow of saliva may be stimulated by encouraging the patient to chew gum or to suck lemon or orange slices or sour lemon balls. The saliva helps to keep the mouth moist and clean. It also washes out the ducts leading from the parotid gland and decreases the possibility of surgical parotitis. Free drainage from any gland is essential to its health. Blocking of the duct from a gland favors the development of infection in the gland. After the mouth has been cleansed, the tongue and other mucosa may be coated with a milk of magnesia substrate. If the patient is unable to perform his or her own oral hygiene, a half-strength solution of hydrogen peroxide (3 per cent) should be applied to all surfaces of the tongue, teeth, mucosa, and palate every 4 hours. The foam is promptly removed and the mouth should be rinsed with water (Passos & Brand, 1966).

When the tube is left in place for some days, the throat may be irritated by it. The patient may be allowed sips of water or anesthetic troches to relieve the soreness. When the patient is allowed water, attention should be given to limiting the amount of water taken to that prescribed by the physician. Any water that is taken returns through the tube, bringing with it electrolytes that are secreted into the stomach. The relief that the patient obtains is therefore at the expense of the body's electrolytes. Some surgeons remove the tube after 2 or 3 days and allow the patient to have a period of rest. The tube is then reinserted 12 or 18 hours later if the patient continues to require it. After the tube has been removed, the nurse should observe the patient for signs and symptoms that indicate that the gastrointestinal tract is not functioning. These include distention, a feeling of fullness, nausea, or vomiting. The sensation of fullness is often the earliest symptom to indicate that the stomach is not emptying properly and along with any other symptoms should be reported promptly. To detect developing distention the abdomen may be measured with a tape. One way to test the function of the alimentary canal without removing the tube is by clamping it for a period of time. When the tube is clamped, the patient should be checked for the symptoms listed. Later the tube is unclamped, and the amount of fluid escaping from the tube is measured. Any accumulation of fluid indicates that gastrointestinal function has not yet been restored.

Because the nostril through which the tube is passed may be irritated by the tube, it may be passed through the opposite nostril when it has to be reintroduced. However, sometimes structural abnormalities make it difficult if not impossible to use the other nostril. Tubes in the nose and pharynx stimulate increased local secretions which may be aspirated or interfere with ventilation. This must be seriously considered in patients with any pulmonary difficulty or complications.

As long as the tube is in place, the nurse should observe the amount and character of fluid that is returned through it. Any abnormality of color or odor is important. Because the effectiveness of the procedure depends on the equipment being in working order, the nurse must check at regular intervals to make sure that the system is airtight and operating.

As peristalsis resumes or the obstruction is relieved, the surgeon removes the tube or clamps it. The removal of a tube from the stomach is relatively simple. The removal of the long tube is more complicated. If the tube has passed the ileocecal valve, the surgeon may cut the tube and allow it to progress through the gastrointestinal tract, as the forcible return of the tube and balloon through the valve may damage it. The tube should not be released at the nose until it has been secured below. Otherwise a laparotomy may be required to retrieve the tube. The patient may need to be reassured that the tube will progress through the alimentary canal just as the normal contents do. When the tube is returned through the mouth, the physician pulls gently and allows the intestine time to release its attachment to the tube.

When removing either a short or a long tube through the nose or mouth, care should be taken to pinch or clamp the tube to prevent gastric or intestinal contents from running out of the tube as it is withdrawn; otherwise, as the tip passes the larynx, there is danger of the patient aspirating the gastric or intestinal liquid.

When gastrointestinal fluids and electrolytes are removed by suction, the oral fluid intake of the patient is restricted and fluids must be administered by intravenous infusion. To have a basis for determining the adequacy of the fluid intake of the patient, the urine output and the other fluids should be measured accurately as long as the gastric or intestinal tube is in place.

Colon and Rectum

In addition to the preparation of the upper alimentary canal for surgery, the colon and rectum are often emptied by the administration of one or more enemas. The reason generally advanced is that this practice lessens the possibility of soiling the peritoneal cavity if the bowel is entered during surgery; there also may be less difficulty with constipation postoperatively. Not all surgeons agree with the routine practice of giving an enema in the preoperative preparation of patients. However, when the intestine itself is the site of surgery, it is cleansed to lessen the likelihood of spillage of fecal contents into the peritoneal cavity. In surgical procedures involving organs in the pelvic cavity, an empty bowel is essential to the exposure of the operative site and to its protection from injury. When barium studies have been made of the gastrointestinal tract, the barium should be removed by enemas or laxatives, if necessary, in order to prevent it from forming an impaction postoperatively. In some disorders such as acute appendicitis, enemas are contraindicated; the fluid introduced into the intestine can raise the pressure within the intestine and stimulate peristalsis. When the solution contains soap or some other irritating agent, peristalsis is further intensified, and the danger of perforation of the appendix is increased.

In surgery on the large intestine, prevention of contamination of the wound and the peritoneal and pelvic cavities by feces requires that special measures be taken to lessen the volume of feces. Bacteria are responsible for more than half the weight of the dried stool. These organisms are harmless and may even be helpful as long as they remain in the intestine. However, when they escape into the peritoneal or other body cavities, they may cause serious morbidity. By using antibiotics and chemical antiseptics that are not absorbed from the intestine, the bacterial count in the intestine can be greatly reduced. Most surgeons agree that the danger of developing superinfections as a result of intestinal antisepsis has been overemphasized. Mechanical cleansing of the colon does not reduce the colonic flora to the desired low level necessary for careful elective operations on the colon and rectum. A period of 3 days of combined mechanical cleansing and antibiotic therapy is necessary to achieve optimum results (Cohn & Nance, 1977).

Administration of enemas that are both effective in cleansing the large bowel and minimally upsetting to the patient requires considerable nursing skill. Hogstel (1977) reported a recent case in which a patient was awarded damages for injury caused by an enema that was not given in a safe manner, according to established procedure. Hogstel's review of basic principles highlights the importance of the reclining position to the effectiveness of a cleansing enema. Cleansing enemas should be administered to the patient lying either on the left side, with right leg flexed on the trunk, or if this is not possible, in the dorsal recumbent position. Fluid should be introduced slowly, to allow maximum volume to reach the ascending colon before the patient expels the liquid. The common practice of routinely delegating cleansing enemas to nursing assistants is to be condemned, unless the nurse has direct evidence that the assistant has both the skill and judgment to perform the procedure effectively. *Cleansing enemas should never be given to the patient while he or she is standing, or sitting on the toilet or commode.*

Preparation of the Skin

The first line of defense of the body against injuring or invading agents is a healthy and intact skin. Each of the functions of the skin makes an important contribution to the patient's response to, and recovery from, surgery. These functions include (1) protection against chemical, thermal, mechanical, and biological injury; (2) control of body temperature; (3) control of water balance; (4) housing for the sensors that facilitate communication with the external environment; and (5) facilitation of motion by providing a pliable covering to the body. The operative incision disrupts the skin and subjects the patient to mechanical and biological injury. Attention to the skin in the preoperative period is directed primarily toward minimizing biological injury, that is, infection.

A complex and fascinating community of microorganisms maintains itself on our skin, with the densest populations found on the face and neck, and in the axilla and groin, as well as on the sole of the foot and between the toes. The trunk and upper arms have much sparser microbial populations (Marples, 1969). Among the most numerous bacterial residents of the skin are two that frequently cause surgical infections: staphylococci and streptococci. In the healthy intact skin, protection against staphylococci is provided by the dryness of the keratin layer; defense against streptococci is provided by (1) bactericidal and fungicidal fatty acids in sebaceous secretions and (2) lysozyme, which hydrolyzes the acetyl-amino polysaccharide constituent of the bacterial membrane (Robson et al., 1973).

Despite differences in details or routines, the objective toward which the preparation of the skin is directed is to reduce the number of microorganisms on it to a minimum and at the same time protect it from injury. The skin must be thoroughly cleansed but not broken or damaged in the process. In some hospitals, patients who are able to do it are asked to shower or take a tub bath, and those who are not able to are given a bed bath. In other hospitals, only those patients whose skins can be seen to be dirty are bathed. When showering or bathing is part of the preoperative preparation, the patient should understand that this requirement is not a reflection on his or her standard of cleanliness or hygiene. When a sudsing agent containing a germicide is employed, the germicide must have time to act. With an agent containing hexachloraphene, the suds should be left on the skin for at least 5 to 10 minutes.

Whether or not the entire body is showered or bathed, the region surrounding the site of the surgery should undergo special cleansing to remove microorganisms and materials that may harbor microorganisms. When cationic surface-active agents such as benzalkonium chloride solution (Zephiran Chloride) are employed in preparation of the skin, soap should not be used as the lathering agent previous to the operation. Because soap is anionic (Harvey, 1975) it antagonizes the action of the cationic agents.

The practice of removing hair as part of the preoperative skin preparation is falling into disrepute. Present evidence on wound infection rates following various methods of preoperative skin preparation argues against shaving, as razor trauma provides a portal of entry for exogenous organisms, "with the injured tissue serving as a substrate for bacterial growth" (Robeson et al., 1973, p. 30). In a study of 406 patients to determine the influence of the method of hair removal on the risk of postoperative wound infection, the infection rate was 5.6 per cent after razor preparation, 0.6 per cent after depilatory, and 0.6 per cent after no preparation. The longer the time interval between shaving the skin and surgery, the higher the infection rate: 3.1 per cent when done just prior to the operation; 7.1 percent when done up to 24 hours prior to surgery; and 20 per cent when done over 24 hours before surgery (Reynolds & Seropian, 1971). Because of the weight of evidence, the shaving of hair, if there is to be any, and final cleansing of the operative area are now frequently done in the operating room, just prior to surgery. Obviously, when the surgical incision is to be in a surface area with a heavy growth of hair, the hair must be cut close to the skin and/or shaved. The size of the area to be shaved depends upon the nature of the proposed surgical procedure and the directions of the surgeon. Pubic hair should be shaved only when necessary. The discomfort suffered by the patient as the hair grows outweighs the advantage of its removal. For this reason some surgeons do not require the pubic hair to be shaved preceding a dilatation of the cervix and curettage of the uterus. Eyebrows should not be removed.

Preparation of the scalp for a surgical incision also requires some modification of the ordinary procedure. Before the hair can be cut and the scalp shaved, a permit from the patient or a responsible member of the family is usually required. As a rule, arrangements are made to have a barber cut the hair and shave the scalp. The removal of the hair is a source of considerable psychological stress. Members of the family, such as the spouse or mother, may also be understandably distressed. For a considerable number of persons, their hair is truly their crowning glory. Before the hair is removed, the nurse should make sure that the patient is not facing a mirror and that a head scarf or cap is ready to cover the head as soon as it is shaved. Some hospitals provide wigs for patients. The hair should be placed in a paper bag and given to a relative. A patient who has long hair may want to have a headpiece made from it. Headpieces and fancy caps are now available to disguise the head and should be used whenever possible.

Because of the serious nature of bone infections, some orthopedic surgeons order that the skin be specially prepared. The skin is shaved and then washed with a detergent and covered with sterile towels; this washing may be repeated twice daily for several days. Particular attention should be given to preventing nicks in the skin. The towels should be anchored so that they stay in place and the equipment and materials used should be sterile. Close attention should be paid to all principles involved in the maintenance of asepsis.

Altered Control of Body Temperature

The surgical patient is at risk of hypothermia from the time the preanesthetic medication is administered until after the effects of anesthesia have dissipated. Many of the preanesthetic medications, as well as anesthetics, depress central heat-regulating mechanisms, with the result that heat production mechanisms are depressed; as the person's body is necessarily exposed for skin preparation and incision, and as tissues are irrigated during the operation, heat loss is increased. (See Chapter 20, Thermal Responses.) Ozuna and Foster (1979) recommend that during the perioperative period the individual be protected from inadvertent hypothermia by:

1. Raising the temperature of the surrounding environment with radiant heat
2. Using warm irrigating solutions
3. Warming inhaled gases, such as O_2 by nasal cannula or catheter
4. Increasing the insulation around the person's body with warm cotton blankets
5. Frequent pre- and postoperative monitoring of body temperature

Rest and Activity

In addition to the identification and treatment of risk factors in the preoperative period, preventive care requires that the patient maintain a balance of rest and activity. If the patient has no disorder that confines him or her to bed, the physician's directive may be "up ad lib." or "ambulatory," or there may be no activity order specified. It is a nursing responsibility to ensure that patients who are hospitalized for preoperative preparation have a rest and ambulation schedule that promotes readiness for surgery.

Patients who remain at home during the period are less likely to be able to remain in bed. Although the patient was once kept in bed because it was thought that rest conserved strength, studies indicate that bedrest results in a loss of strength as well as of proteins and other nutrients. Exercise within the limits tolerated by the patient improves psychological as well as the physiologic status. When the patient feels unwell, he or she may have to be encouraged to be up and about; on the other hand, the patient who feels reasonably well may require some protection from overactivity. The patient should have the help that is needed to get out of bed and to walk. To make certain that the patient does ambulate, there should be a plan to ensure it. Because most people eat better when they are out of bed, the plan may include getting the patient into the chair for meals. Depending on how the patient feels, he or she may have a rest period followed by a bath and then another rest period followed by a walk down the hall. When in bed, the patient should be encouraged to do deep-breathing exercises and to flex and extend the feet and legs. (See Chapter 52 for discussion of preambulation exercises to prevent orthostatic hypotension in the postoperative period.) By alternating periods of activity with rest, the patient builds up strength and is at the same time protected from overactivity.

Sedation Before Surgery

To ensure that the patient sleeps well and to reduce apprehension, the surgeon usually prescribes a sedative for the patient the night preceding and the morning of surgery. The specific drug selected varies with the surgeon but is often one of the barbiturates such as pentobarbital (Nembutal), 0.05 to 0.1 g, or secobarbital (Seconal), 0.1 to 0.2 g. Occasionally this has to be repeated later in the night. When the patient has been prepared for sleep, he or she should know whether or not the nurse expects to visit during the night. Nothing can be more frightening to a person who sleeps in a room alone at home than to go to sleep and to be awakened by someone opening the door and coming into the room. For example, Miss Tee was admitted to the hospital in the late afternoon for diagnostic surgery the following day. About 9 o'clock in the evening she was given secobarbital (Seconal), 0.2 g, and prepared to sleep. The door to her room was closed. At midnight an aide opened the door and entered the room to remove the water glass. Miss Tee awakened frightened, and, needless to say, she had difficulty returning to sleep.

The morning of surgery the same drug that was administered the preceding night may be repeated. In addition, morphine, 8 to 15 mg, or meperidine hydrochloride (Demerol), 50 to 100 mg, may be administered an hour before the operation is scheduled. Currently there appears to be disagreement among physicians about the necessity and desirability of using either morphine or meperidine hydrochloride preoperatively. Some surgeons are of the opinion that they serve no useful purpose because, previous to the operation, patients do not have pain and the barbiturates are at least as effective as morphine in relieving preoperative apprehension. In addition, these drugs may have some undesirable effects. In some patients they cause nausea and vomiting. They can also depress respiration, the cough reflex, and the activity of cilia in the tracheobronchial tree because they can increase the tone of the tracheobronchial musculature. In humans they can be harmful in the patient who is asthmatic. All these effects decrease the capacity of the patient to cleanse the tracheobronchial tree and aerate the lung. The influence of morphine on mechanisms for cleansing the tracheobronchial tree is particularly undesirable in patients having thoracic and upper abdominal surgery. Drugs such as promethazine hydrochloride (Phenergan), an antihistaminic, which relieves preoperative apprehension, may be administered alone or as a potentiator for smaller dosages of a narcotic, barbiturate, or other CNS depressant.

Certain disorders or circumstances alter or increase the patient's response to morphine. For example, the patient with hypothyroidism often becomes stuporous and suffers respiratory depression following relatively small doses of morphine. Infants and children can usually tolerate morphine quite well if the dosage is adjusted to their body weight. In contrast, there is evidence that elderly persons may be extremely sensitive. Because morphine depresses the respiratory center and increases the cerebrospinal fluid pressure, it is contraindicated in patients who are undergoing brain surgery or who have had surgery on the brain; in such patients it is contraindicated after, as well as before, the operation.

To further reduce anxiety of the patient toward surgery and to counteract the tendency toward increased tracheobronchial secretions, atropine sulfate or scopolamine hydrobromide is frequently prescribed to be administered to the patient about 1 hour before the operation is scheduled. When the tranquilizing effects are desired, scopolamine is more likely to be selected than atropine because of its increased tendency to cause drowsiness, amnesia, euphoria, and fatigue. Occasionally it produces excitement, talkativeness, restlessness, and even delirium and hallucinations. The patient who is given scopolamine when in pain is more likely to respond with excitement than if given it when free of pain. The nurse should anticipate this possibility when a patient who is in pain is given scopolamine. The more important action of both atropine and scopolamine is the depression of the effector cells of organs enervated by postganglionic cholinergic fibers with a resultant decrease in secretions in the tracheobronchial tree. Because one of the actions of these drugs is dilation of the pupil, these anticholinergic drugs are contraindicated in patients who have glaucoma.

Responsibilities of the Nurse on the Day of Surgery

Whatever the nature or extent of surgery proposed for a patient, there are certain routine provisions that must be made for comfort and safety before he or she goes to the operating room on the day of surgery. *Before the patient's preoperative medication is prepared,* the nurse should

1. *Ascertain whether or not the permit for the patient to undergo the contemplated surgery has been signed by the patient or a representative.* Practice varies as to whether the nurse or the physician secures the signature of the patient. Whoever is responsible for obtaining the signed operative permit should explain the nature of the operation and its risks prior to the signing of the permit. This should generally be done the day prior to surgery.
2. *Have the patient take a complete bath, if able, or bathe him or her.* Following the bath, the patient is dressed in hospital pajamas, a cap is applied to cover the hair, and all polish is removed from finger- and toenails to facilitate observation for early signs of impaired tissue perfusion. All jewelry should be removed, and a wedding band secured.
3. *Check for, remove, and store dentures and ensure that the patient has a clean mouth.* Because of the danger of aspiration into the airway of dentures or removable bridges, they should be removed before the patient is transferred to the operating room. Occasionally a patient has very strong feelings about having others see him or her without teeth. In rare instances, when the psychological stress created by removing dental prostheses is very great, the nurse should explore the possibility of the patient keeping them in place until in the operating room. They can then be removed and returned to the patient's room or ward. Care should be taken to prevent the loss of dentures. Their loss or damage subjects the patient to inconvenience and psychological stress and may be an added expense to the hospital and patient.
4. *Ensure that the patient is wearing a proper identification label.* If the patient does not already wear some form of identification such as an identification bracelet, an identification tag should be prepared and attached to him or her before being transferred to the operating room. On it should be the full name, hospital number, the name of the surgeon, and any other pertinent information.
5. *Identify from the patient, when possible, the relatives or friends who will be present, or awaiting information, during the operation.* If those persons important to the patient are present, all can be oriented to the place, time, and sources of progress reports on the patient. Those in attendance on the patient should be guided to the waiting area and informed by the nurse when the patient has arrived in the operating suite.

Just before the preoperative medication is administered, the nurse should

6. *Take the patient's blood pressure, temperature, pulse, and respiration.*
7. *Have the patient void.* To prevent distention and possible injury to the urinary bladder during the operative period, the urinary bladder should be emptied just before the patient is transferred to the operating room. To facilitate exposure of pelvic organs and to reduce the possibility of injury to the bladder during surgical procedures in the pelvic cavity, an indwelling catheter is usually introduced prior to surgery in this region. Although the nurse on the unit may be responsible for preoperative insertion of an indwelling catheter, it is increasingly common for the catheter to be inserted in the operating room, under surgical aseptic conditions, to minimize the danger of infection.

After the patient receives preoperative medication, he or she should not be disturbed again until being transported to the operating suite. When recording vital signs and administration of the preoperative medication, the nurse should

8. *Check the completeness of the patient's chart,* to include
   a. Morning temperature, pulse, and respiration.
   b. Results of the hematocrit or hemoglobin, urinalysis, and type and cross match for possible transfusion.
   c. Drugs that were administered preoperatively.
   d. Any significant observation that relates to the patient's emotional or physiologic status.

Should any of the preceding be found to be abnormal, the abnormality should be drawn to the attention of the physician.

Although the practice varies from hospital to hospital, the patient may be transported to the operating room in the bed, on a cart, or in a wheelchair. Even if an orderly is responsible, when possible, the nurse should accompany the patient. In some hospitals relatives are encouraged to accompany the patient as far as the entrance of the operating suite. Throughout the entire preoperative period every effort should be made to convey to the patient and family that (1) the welfare of the patient is the prime consideration in his or her care, and (2) all persons who participate in care are competent and trustworthy.

Summary

In the preoperative preparation of the patient, the care of the patient is planned and organized to meet the following objectives: (1) to prepare the patient psychologically, (2) to prepare him or her physically, and (3) to prepare the patient physiologically for the operative experience. The time available to accomplish each of these may vary from 1 day to several weeks or months. Unless emergency surgery is contemplated, the patient who is in the hospital for only a short period of time receives much of the preliminary preparation for the operation in the physician's office and/or clinic. The way in which nurses in the office or clinic treat the patient and his or her problems contributes to the patient's preparation for the hospital experience. Courtesy and thoughtfulness on the part of everyone from the doorman to the nursing personnel contribute to the patient's feeling of being welcome and that everyone is interested in his or her welfare.

The Operative Period

The operative period begins the moment the patient is anesthetized and ends when the last stitch or dressing is in place. This period will be discussed in terms of the general purposes for which surgery is performed, functions and responsibilities of members of the surgical team, and special considerations for the safety of the patient related to anesthesia, position on the operating table, and maintenance of asepsis.

Purposes of Surgery

To obtain tissue for examination. One of the purposes for which surgery is performed is to observe the gross or microscopic structure of an organ or tissue. When tissue is removed for the purpose of microscopic examination, the procedure is called a biopsy. The word *biopsy* comes from the Greek. *Bio* is derived from *bios,* which means "life." *Opsy* comes from *opsis,* which means "sight" or "vision." The term *biopsy* means not only the taking of tissue but also its microscopic examination. Biopsy is useful in confirming diagnosis, estimating prognosis, and following the course of disease and the effectiveness of treatment. To illustrate, Mrs. Stubby has a lump in her breast. The surgeon removes the lump and the pathologist examines it microscopically. He reports to the surgeon that the tumor is benign or that it is malignant. Should it be malignant, the surgeon removes the breast and surrounding lymph nodes. From the examination of the breast tissue and the lymph nodes, the nature of the neoplasm can be determined and the extent to which it has spread can be estimated. If the lesion is benign, Mrs. Stubby's prognosis is excellent and she should make a complete recovery. Should the lesion be malignant, both the nature and extent of spread will be important in predicting her chances for recovery.

Tissue may be removed for study by various methods. The method used depends on the nature and location of the lesion. In the instance of Mrs. Thomas, her breast tumor was removed by surgical excision. A patient with a tentative diagnosis of myelogenous leukemia has bone marrow removed from the sternum by means of a punch. A punch is a hollow instrument similar in appearance to a large needle; it is introduced into, and removes, a piece of tissue. Tissue may also be obtained by aspiration, a method useful when the lesion contains fluid or when fluid is formed in a serous cavity. Tissue may be procured by a number of other methods, which include (1) curettage, or the scraping of the surface of a lesion; (2) dragging of a sponge over the surface of tissue, usually a mucous membrane; (3) irrigation or washing of a serous cavity; and (4) examination of cells in sputum or other secretions. The last, which is known as the Papanicolaou technique, is based on the fact that cells are shed into secretions (see Chapter 39).

After the surgeon removed the tumor from Mrs. Thomas, it was sent to the pathological laboratory for examination. The pathologist examined its gross appearance and then he gave it to a technician who prepared slices of tissue from the tumor for examination by two methods. One is called a frozen section and the other a paraffin or permanent section. Each has its advantages and disadvantages. In this instance the surgeon wished to have an immediate report and a frozen section was made at once. Later another portion or the rest of the tumor was placed in paraffin after it had been fixed in a suitable preservative. Although the latter method is more accurate, either method can be utilized with good results by experts. When the results obtained by frozen section indicate that the patient requires additional surgery, it can be instituted without delay.

To establish diagnosis by visualization of internal structures. Besides biopsy, exploratory surgery with or without the removal of tissue may be performed for the purpose of establishing diagnosis. At times, despite the best efforts of the physician and the use of modern diagnostic devices, a diagnosis cannot be confirmed or rejected, nor can the extent of a disease process be known for sure. For example, Mr. James has bronchogenic carcinoma. His surgeon is not certain whether the tumor can be cured with resection. One way of determining this is to examine the mediastinum through a small incision in the neck. If the procedure, called a mediastinoscopy, shows that there are no involved lymph nodes in the mediastinum, then the chances of the surgeon curing the patient are greatly increased. Mrs. Smith has had periodic attacks of severe pain in her abdomen. Despite inconclusive evidence as to its cause, the surgeon operates and finds the source of her pain, which is corrected.

To cure disease. In addition to its use in the diagnosis of disease, surgery is performed to effect a cure by the removal of diseased tissue or a diseased organ. Organs such as the kidney or lung may be removed provided the other organ of the pair is healthy. Some organs such as the stomach or large intestine may be removed in part or in entirety. The resection of most or all of the stomach is often followed by some impairment in nutrition and/or health. A tumor may be removed with or without the removal of surrounding tissue. Cure can sometimes be effected by the drainage of an abscess that is well walled off. Following the removal of the contents of the abscess, the surrounding tissues are then able to complete the process of repair.

During surgery the normal functional relationships or normal continuity of structures may be disrupted following the removal of an organ or a part of the organ. For example, when Mr. Brave had the distal two thirds of his stomach removed following repeated hemorrhage from a peptic ulcer in the duodenum, a new connection between the remaining portion of the stomach and the intestine was required. Following fractures in which the ends of the bone are displaced, surgery may be required to restore and maintain the normal alignment of the bones. In the treatment of hernia, the contents that have escaped from a body cavity are replaced and the opening through which they escaped closed. Deformities resulting from failures in development or from disease may be corrected. One of the major triumphs of modern surgery is that, in the abnormal heart, openings may be closed, valves opened or reconstructed, and blood vessels rerouted so that the effects of deformities are overcome.

To repair structures disrupted by trauma. Advances in surgery have consistently been associated with violence in the life of humankind, from the time of earliest recorded medical history. Modern surgery is no exception; World War II and more recent warfare in Southeast Asia have led to improved understanding and management of massive trauma. In addition, the high rate of automobile accidents and the increasing number of violent crimes in our society result in unbelievably complex traumatic injury to the victims. The interest and success of surgeons in meeting these new challenges have led to the emergence of new specialties in emergency and critical-care medicine.

To relieve symptoms. Surgery may also be performed to relieve symptoms, even when there is no expectation that the patient can or will be cured. Operations that are performed to relieve symptoms and to increase the comfort of the patient without any definite attempt at cure are said to be palliative. Palliative surgery is of several types. Infected and necrotic tissue may be removed in order to lessen odors and to relieve pain, detours may be established around obstructing neoplasms, pressure on vital structures may be relieved, and pain may be eliminated. For example, in advanced cancer of the breast in which ulceration of the skin and superficial tissues has occurred, the breast may be removed, not because the removal of the breast is expected to cure the patient, but to relieve the pain and remove the infection that accompanies ulceration.

In conditions accompanied by obstruction of any tubular structure such as the intestines, bile ducts, ureters, or bladder, surgery may be performed so that the contents of the tube are rerouted around the obstruction. For example, in cancer of the head of the pancreas, the expanding neoplasm may obstruct the common bile duct. The obstruction can be relieved by connecting the gallbladder or a portion of the common duct to the duodenum or jejunum. In cancer of the urinary bladder, the ureters may be transplanted into the ileum or sigmoid colon or opened onto the abdominal wall. A colostomy may be performed to relieve an obstruction of the transverse, descending, or sigmoid colon or rectum. A gastroenterostomy, a new opening between the stomach and jejunum, may be made to relieve the symptoms accompanying the blocking of the pyloric end of the stomach. Many of these same procedures are also used in the treatment of disease in which the outcome is expected to be curative. Any treatment whose primary objective is to relieve symptoms rather than produce a cure is palliative.

Expanding lesions in the cranial cavity or spinal canal can cause symptoms by pressing on the brain, spinal cord, or nerve tissue and by increasing intracranial pressure. Relief of symptoms can sometimes be secured by removing a portion of the skull or part of a vertebra. In the latter instance, the lamina and the spinous process of the vertebra are most likely to be removed.

Under certain circumstances the nerve supply of an organ or part may be interrupted to relieve muscle spasm or pain. In some patients whose spinal cords have been transected, muscle spasms may be severe. By cutting the motor nerve root to the involved muscles, a spastic paralysis is converted into a flaccid, or limp, one. In patients with severe and intractable pain, such as that associated with trigeminal neuralgia, sensory nerve fibers may be cut or destroyed by injection of certain chemicals, such as alcohol, into or around the nerve. Occasionally a patient suffering from advanced cancer may have severe pain that is not relieved by the usual methods. The surgeon may then cut the lateral spinothalamic tract in the spinal cord; the fibers in this tract carry pain impulses from the affected part to higher centers. When any tissue is deprived of its sensory nerve supply, it loses one of its most important defense mechanisms; therefore the involved area should be inspected regularly for redness, pallor, and other evidence of impending tissue injury, and measures should be instituted to protect the area from damage. For example, the eye of a patient who has had the ophthalmic branch of the trigeminal nerve interrupted is deprived of its sensory nerve supply. He or she should be taught to protect the eye from dust and other foreign bodies and to inspect it regularly for redness, especially after being out of doors or in a dusty area. The patient who has a transection of the sensory pathways in the spinal cord should be instructed to change position regularly and to keep the bed and clothing free from crumbs and wrinkles. He or she should also inspect the involved areas regularly. When the patient is unable to do these things, they should be done for him or her. Unless these points receive special attention, a decubitus ulcer may develop, especially over bony prominences. (See Chapter 49 for a more complete discussion of the prevention and management of decubitus ulcer.)

As indicated, when the patient arrives in the operating room, the surgical procedure that has been planned can be expected to accomplish one or more purposes. It may establish the nature and extent of the illness or how well the patient is responding to therapy. It may effect cure or relieve symptoms.

The Surgical Team

During the operative period the needs of the patient are met by a team of individuals each of whom has a well-defined role and tasks and on whom other members of the team depend. The objectives of the surgical team during the operative phase are (1) to achieve the purpose of the surgical therapy, (2) to keep the patient safe during the operative procedure, and (3) to keep the surgery safe for the patient. Each of these objectives is important. Failure to achieve any one of them may result in injury or death to the patient. Some members of the team are removed from direct contact with the patient, but every member acts in behalf of the patient. The broad spectrum of knowledge and skills required for successful performance of the more sophisticated operative procedures makes the management of today's surgical service analogous to running a massive conglomerate corporation. Surgical team members who participate directly or indirectly in the care of the patient during the operative period may include biomedical engineers, physiologists, electronic technicians, photographers, television technicians, in addition to the more traditional members of the team—the surgeon, the anesthetist, and the nurse. Discussion will focus briefly on the functions of only the traditional members of the surgical team.

The Surgeon

The surgeon is the leader of the team, but certain circumstances may make it necessary for him or her to temporarily relinquish the leadership role. Throughout the operative phase the surgeon gives attention to the prevention of serious physiologic disturbances. He or she ties blood vessels before or immediately after cutting them. The surgeon may reduce excessive loss of fluid by covering exposed organs with moist towels. Organs and tissues are handled gently. The surgeon estimates blood loss, or when procedures are long and there is the possibility of considerable loss of blood, the sponges are weighed. He or she takes time to identify structures so that the blood supply to the tissues in the area is maintained and injury to important structures is prevented. He or she also attends to the nature of the response of the patient and modifies the surgical procedure according to the reaction of the patient. During the operative phase, the complications that are most troublesome and frequent are those of hemorrhage, shock, and hypoxia. Because these complications may also be problems in the postoperative phase, they will be discussed later. During the operative phase of surgical therapy, the purposes of the operation are, hopefully, accomplished, and the dangers to which the patient is exposed are controlled. Many of the problems encountered by the patient during the postoperative phase depend on the care and attention the patient received during the operation or in earlier phases of treatment.

The Anesthetist

A second member of the surgical team is the anesthetist. In the late nineteenth century, nurses were trained as anesthetists, and many years passed before physician anesthetists appeared in this country. Because of rapid advances in biomedical technology related to surgical treatment, as well as the use of increasingly potent anesthetic agents, a sound foundation in medicine became mandatory throughout the entire perioperative period. Brunner and Eckenhoff (1977, p. 217) make the following strong statement about the responsibility of the anesthesiologist:

> Ideally, all patients should be evaluated preoperatively by an anesthesiologist. This is not possible at present because of an acute shortage of physician anesthetists. Of necessity, therefore, a surgeon or internist sometimes assumes responsibility for preanesthetic evaluation and preparation. Because these physicians lack extensive experience with the physiologic changes that occur during anesthesia and with the pharmacologic idiosyncracies of the anesthetized patient, this must be regarded as a temporary necessity that is less than ideal. If a physician anesthetist is available and fails to assume his responsibility in this respect, he is not giving his patients the care due them and he risks being considered a technician rather than a physician.

During the operative procedure the anesthetist has several important responsibilities. One is to induce a sufficient degree of anesthesia to prevent the patient from having pain, and another is to secure the degree of relaxation necessary to the performance of the operation. The anesthetist is also concerned with the observation and maintenance of the physiologic status of the patient. He or she pays particular attention to maintaining

1. A clear or patent airway. In addition to the usual problems encountered in the maintenance of an open airway, the patient must be protected from aspirating secretions from the gastrointestinal tract. The danger of aspiration is increased in patients who have emergency surgery, because time may not be sufficient to have the stomach emptied properly.
2. Adequate breathing and exchange of gases (oxygen and carbon dioxide) in the lungs.
3. The systemic circulation.

Throughout the entire operative period the anesthetist is charged with the responsibility of observing the general condition of the patient and reporting the results of this observation to the surgeon. He or she observes and records the pulse, respiration, and blood pressure of the patient at regular intervals. When the surgery is associated with a large loss of blood, the anesthetist may also monitor the central venous pressure, especially in poor-risk patients. Should an abnormality occur, he or she calls this to the attention of the surgeon so that appropriate measures can be taken.

The Nurse

The third member of the surgical team is the nurse and nursing assistants. The nurse has two general responsibilities. One is to anticipate and meet the needs of the surgeon for instruments and supplies during the operative procedure. The other is the general management of the operating room so that all those who are participating in the surgical procedure have what they need and the safety of the patient is protected. Obviously, these two functions require two nurses. The first nurse is usually called a scrub, or instrument, nurse because she or he scrubs the hands and arms before donning a sterile gown and gloves; the second is called the circulating nurse. Although the activities of the nurse who handles instruments may appear to be the more difficult and responsible role, it is not. The circulating nurse has multiple responsibilities, as she or he must anticipate and plan to meet the needs of each member of the operating team; be alert to threats to the patient's safety; watch for breaks in technique or for conditions that, if allowed to continue, will lead to a loss of asepsis; save and count discarded sponges and instruments; control the number and behavior of visitors in the operating room; and remind the surgeon and others that the patient is awake when this reminder is necessary. In general this nurse manages the environment of the patient, so that the progress of the procedure is furthered and the safety of the patient is protected. Few activities of the circulating nurse are glamorous or exciting. Yet the smooth running of the operating room depends on having a circulating nurse who has initiative and intelligence and who exercises sound judgment.[8] All members of the team are important. Each member of the team contributes to the success of the surgical procedure.

Anesthesia

Before the operative procedure is begun, the patient is anesthetized. The type of anesthetic used and the method by which it is administered will depend on the type and length of the procedure to be performed, the condition of the patient, his or her preferences, the equipment available, the skill and the training of the anesthetist, and the preference of the surgeon. Intelligent observation and safe care of the patient in the immediate postoperative period, as well as during the operation, require that the nurse know the type, action, and hazards of the anesthetic used. All types of anesthesia may be classified as either *regional* or *general,* and both types interfere with normal neural function.

Regional anesthesia is a reversible blockade of pain receptors and conduction fibers in an area determined by the anatomic site of application. The sensorium remains clear, and the patient continues to be able to see, hear, taste, and smell. The patient who has been given a regional anesthetic is likely to be drowsy from the preoperative medication, but he or she is awake and able to sense all but touch and pain in the area of anesthesia. Operating room personnel should keep uppermost in their minds the fact that the patient is awake and constantly remind each other of this fact. Conversation other than that directed to the patient should be avoided. The patient should be greeted by the surgeon or told that the surgeon will arrive shortly. He or she should be apprised of what to expect and protected from physical harm. Because the patient is drowsy, he or she should not be left alone on a cart in a corridor or in the operating room.

Regional anesthesia may be produced by such physical agents as cold and pressure, as well as by anesthetic drugs. Spinal anesthesia, one type of regional anesthesia frequently used in major surgery, requires injection of the local anesthetic into the cerebrospinal fluid via an intervertebral space in the lumbosacral area (Brunner & Eckenhoff, 1977, pp. 202–04). Many patients are reluctant to have spinal anesthesia, fearing nerve damage with pain or loss of function. Current evidence indicates that the hazards of neurologic complications following spinal anesthesia are minimal because of improved technique and drugs. A study of over 10,000 patients to whom spinal anesthesia was administered revealed no major CNS problem, and minor problems consisted of complaint of backache by 2.7 per cent of patients and complaint of positional headache by 3.5 per cent of patients (Black et al., 1969).

General anesthesia is a reversible state of insensibility with loss of consciousness, produced by a variety of chemical agents that act on the brain. Although there are now nearly 20 general anesthetic agents available for clinical use, nitrous oxide alone or in combination with other drugs is chosen for most of the general anesthesias administered (Brunner & Eckenhoff, 1977, p. 209). Because of the high incidence of pulmonary complications following major surgery under general anesthesia, much attention is given to selecting the anesthetic expected to pro-

[8] For basic references on the humane and technological nursing care of the patient during the operative period, see the following citations in the General References at the end of the chapter: Rhodes et al., 1978; and LeMaitre & Finnegan, 1980.

duce the best possible relaxation with the least compromise of ventilation. Diethyl ether (ether) is a highly volatile liquid with a pungent, flammable vapor capable of producing all depths of surgical anesthesia to respiratory arrest. Like other flammable anesthetics, its use is now markedly restricted in the United States, but it is still widely used in emerging countries (Brunner & Eckenhoff, 1977, p. 211).

The prime concern of the nurse with general anesthesia is related to the first 6 to 8 hours of the immediate postoperative period, when the patient passes through the same stages of general anesthesia that he or she did in induction, except that the order is reversed. Therefore discussion of the stages of anesthesia is presented in the order in which the nurse observes them in the postoperative patient.

In the induction of the anesthetic, the concentration of the anesthetic gas or mixture of gases is higher in the alveoli than it is in the blood. Therefore the gas moves from the alveoli into the blood at a more rapid rate than it moves out of the blood into the alveoli. When the desired level of anesthesia is reached, the amount of gas inhaled by the patient is adjusted so that the amount entering the blood equals that leaving the blood. At the termination of the operation or at some suitable point previous to it, the administration of the anesthetic gas is terminated. In the period of recovery, the process is reversed. As the patient inhales air or oxygen, the concentration of the anesthetic gas in the alveoli is diluted and, as a consequence, its partial pressure is reduced. With the reduction in the partial pressure of the gas in the alveoli, the gas in the blood escapes into the alveoli, where it is mixed with inspired air and exhaled. This process continues until all the gas is removed from the body.

The degree of general anesthesia may be divided into four stages. During stage IV respiratory paralysis of central origin occurs. This depth of anesthesia is seldom seen except in the operating room when large amounts of anesthesia may be used. Death occurs unless ventilation is maintained by the anesthesiologist.

Stage III is known as the stage of surgical anesthesia. The patient is unconscious and reflexes are depressed or paralyzed. This stage is divided into four planes, according to the degree to which reflexes are depressed or paralyzed, with plane 1 being the lightest and plane 4 the deepest. Most surgical procedures are carried out in plane 2.

As the patient eliminates the anesthetic, he or she goes into the second stage of anesthesia or the stage of excitement or delirium. This stage, as the name implies, is accompanied by a number of hazards to the patient. Although the patient becomes unconscious in stage II, there is great variability in the degree of excitement manifested by patients as they pass through this stage. Some remain relatively quiet, whereas others may be so disturbed that they are difficult to control. As a result of the use of modern drugs and anesthetics, the length of the stage of excitement has been shortened and decreased in severity. The nurse should, however, be alert to the possibility of the patient's becoming excited. She or he should take appropriate steps to decrease the likelihood of the patient becoming excited and to protect him or her from injury if this occurs. Bedside rails should be raised, and someone should be in constant attendance on the patient. The environment of the patient should be regulated so that all sources of stimulation such as noise, drafts, and loud talking are eliminated. The patient should be handled gently. In the past, efforts were sometimes made to increase the rate at which the patient regained consciousness by stimulation, shouting, or shaking. Because the rate of the recovery of the patient depends on the rate at which the anesthetic agent is eliminated, these procedures cannot be counted on to be very effective, and they may be harmful. In addition to increasing the likelihood of the patient's becoming excited during stage II, the capacity of the patient to adapt the functioning of the cardiovascular system to rapid changes in position is reduced and as a result blood pressure may fall.

During stage I, the patient is drowsy. He or she can be awakened and will respond to questions, but then lapses back into sleep. The patient may waken and complain of pain and in a moment or two return to sleep. At this time the nurse must assess the need of the patient for a pain-relieving medication, by estimating the severity of the pain experienced by the patient and the extent of recovery from the anesthetic and preanesthetic medications. Questions the nurse should be able to answer before administering an analgesic medication include the following: Has the patient recovered sufficiently from the effects of the anesthetic to require a pain-relieving medication? Is the respiratory status of the patient such that it is safe to administer a drug that depresses respiration? What evidence indicates that the patient does or does not require an analgesic? The objective is neither to give nor to withhold medication; too great delay in the administration of an analgesic can cause as much harm to the patient as administering one too soon. The objective should be to minimize the pain experienced by the patient and at the same time protect him or her from the hazards of overmedication. One of the most sensitive indicators that the patient in stage I is experiencing pain is restlessness; it should be emphasized that restlessness may also be caused by hypoxia. The administration of a narcotic to a hypoxic patient will cause further respiratory depression and may result in death.

During the operation, cardiac arrhythmias are a hazard for which all team members, and especially the anesthetist, must be on the alert. A frequent cause of arrhythmias is an abnormal serum potassium level, either hypo- or hyperkalemia. Surgery on the heart or great vessels requiring cardiopulmonary bypass (a pump oxygenator to shunt cardiopulmonary circulation around the operative site) exposes the patient to the hazard of hemodilution, with significant hypokalemia and arrhythmia, especially if the patient received preoperative diuretics. Potassium chloride infusions administered during cardiopulmonary bypass and in the immediate postoperative period may prevent or quickly correct hypokalemia (Fujikura et al., 1972).

Another one of the parameters that is usually monitored continuously by the anesthetist is the patient's temperature. Hyperpyrexia as an idiosyncratic response to general anesthesia is always sudden and often fatal, requiring prompt detection for the treatment to be effective (Hamelberg, 1969).

The periods of induction and of recovery from anesthesia are the most critical in the entire operative experience. Gius (1966, p. 314) compares the induction and recovery from anesthesia to the takeoff and landing of an aircraft. In both situations human and mechanical failures occur. Many of the hazards to the patient and the circumstances contributing to accidents are known and should therefore be preventable. The principal complications during the period of anesthesia are circulatory collapse, cardiac arrest, respiratory complications, and injury or death caused by fire and explosions. During the period in which the patient recovers from the effects of the anesthetic, the problems in his or her care continue to be (1) the maintenance of a clear airway, (2) the prevention of the aspiration of saliva and gastric secretions, and (3) the maintenance of cardiovascular stability. The nurse shares in the responsibility for the care of the patient during both the operative and postoperative periods, but the extent of her or his responsibility is usually greater during the period of recovery. Nowhere, however, are the identification and control of unsafe acts more important than in the care of the patient who is in one of the stages of anesthesia.

Positioning for Operation

A major factor in minimizing tissue trauma during the operation is positioning the patient in such a way that visualization of the operation field is optimized. The combined effect of muscle relaxation in the patient from preoperative medication and/or anesthesia and the great versatility of operating tables in the surface angles that can be achieved can result in very extreme and unnatural positions of the patient throughout the operation. After arriving in the operating room, the patient is transferred from the cart or bed to the operating room table. (The patient may or may not have been previously anesthetized.) The position in which he or she is placed on the table after being anesthetized depends on the organs to be exposed during the operation. Pressure over bony prominences with compression of underlying tissues and hyperextension of muscles sometimes contribute to discomfort in the postoperative period. To prevent movement and/or falling during the period of surgery, the patient is strapped to the table. The straps should be well padded and loose enough to allow adequate circulation to the extremities. The elbow should be padded, especially on the inner or medial side, to prevent ulnar nerve palsy. Care should be taken not to let the arms of the anesthetized patient dangle over the side of the table. The table should be well padded. These points are of particular importance during a lengthy operation.

Surgical Asepsis

Dramatic reduction in postoperative infection as a cause of morbidity and mortality has resulted in part from development and rigorous application of measures to control transmission of microorganisms from the environment to the wound in the operating room. In view of the fact that complete sterilization even in the operating room remains a virtual impossibility, progress in control of postoperative infection is also partly the result of support of the patient's resistance by judicious use of antibiotics. In a study of the propriety of administration of antiobiotics to 300 consecutive surgical patients in three university-affiliated teaching hospitals, Gardner and associates (1979) found that nonuse was usually appropriate. However, there was a high incidence of inappropriate use of antibiotics. Errors in use, in order of frequency, included the following:

1. Misjudgments in attempted prophylaxis of operative wound infection, such as failure to use preoperative administration or use in clean operations without implanted foreign bodies
2. Attempted treatment of undefined and undiagnosed fever.

As indicated in Chapter 10, measures to prevent or control any infection must be based upon information about (1) the reservoirs of sources of microorganisms, (2) the vehicles by which they are spread, (3) the resistance of the microorganisms to environmental conditions including their susceptibility to physical and chemical agents, (4) the conditions favoring the spread and growth of the microorganism, and (5) susceptibility of persons exposed to the microorganisms.

The reservoirs or sources of microorganisms may be animals or contaminated objects or materials, but they are usually people who are carriers of, or are infected by, the offending organism. When the reservoir is people, organisms come not only from body orifices, but also from the body surface; the unique way in which the human body serves as a source of airborne contamination is by the convection currents produced by the heat of the body acting as the carrier of microorganisms. The nose and throat of hospital personnel are a major source of virulent organisms, especially staphylococci. In the general population, only 15 per cent to 20 per cent of people are nasal carriers of virulent staphylococci; among hospital personnel, single nasal culture will reveal about 40 per cent as carriers, and repeated nasal cultures raise the proportion of nasal carriers identified to 80 per cent (Postlethwait, 1977). This high carrier rate among hospital personnel not only increases the probability of wound contamination during surgery, but also is related to the increased infection rate among patients whose preoperative hospitalization is prolonged. One study found a postoperative infection rate of 6 per cent in patients hospitalized 2 days or less before operation, whereas the rate was 14.7 per cent in patients hospitalized for 3 weeks or more before operation. It has been well documented that the number of bacteria in the air and indirectly in the wound is related to the activity and number of personnel in the operating room. Measures to control this source include isolation of the operating suite from all other hospital traffic; provision of separate viewing rooms for those not involved in performing the operation but who have a legitimate reason for observing the operation; the rigorous monitoring by the circulating nurse of all persons entering the operating room; and the use of air conditioning that delivers air under positive pressure with a complete change and filtering of air every 5 to 10 minutes.

Not only are other persons possible sources of microorganisms, but the skin and mucous membrane of the patient may be. In one study that cultured patients' wounds before closure to identify possible sources within the operating room of organisms recovered, the nose or skin of the patient was the source in 50 per cent of the cases, whereas the hands of the scrub team were the source in only 6 per cent, and the nose and throat of the scrub team the source in 14 per cent of the cases (Postlethwait, 1977, p. 326).

Vehicles for the transmission of microorganisms from the reservoir to the wound include the hands, air, instruments, linens, sutures, and any other material coming in contact with the wound. In the practice of asepsis, attention is given to preventing contact between any reservoir and the patient and to ridding vehicles of any microorganism. The methods employed depend on the character of the object to be disinfected and the susceptibility of the microorganism to destruction.

Because the incision through the skin or mucous membrane provides a portal of entry for microorganisms into the underlying tissues, measures are instituted to prevent the introduction of bacteria into the incision. The site of the incision is thoroughly cleansed. When time permits, cleansing procedures may be initiated some time before the patient is transferred to the operating room. Although transient bacteria on the skin surface can be killed with appropriate solutions, the resident bacteria around hair follicles and in sebaceous glands cannot be destroyed. The wound must be protected from resident bacteria by sterile draping and final preparation for the incision in the operating room. Many surgeons now apply an adherent plastic sheet over the operative area and then make the incision through it, thus providing a tight seal between the open wound and resident bacteria on the surrounding intact skin. Draping of the patient is completed prior to the skin incision, preferably with waterproof materials that minimize bacterial penetration. Synthetic and paper materials are now available that allow little or no bacterial penetration when wet.

To isolate members of the surgical team from the wound, they remove clothing worn in the other areas of the hospital or on the street and don special clothing. The hair is covered with a cap or turban and the mouth and nose are covered with a mask. The purpose of the mask is to prevent the spread of microorganisms from the nasal and pharyngeal mucosa to the wound of the patient. The duration of protection from face masks varies with such factors as the fit of the mask to the face, the amount of talking by the wearer, and, most important, the filtering efficiency of the mask. Efficiency ranges from a low of 15 per cent for one of the gauze masks to a high of 99.7 per cent for one of the fiberglass masks (Postelthwait, 1977, p. 329). Even when masks are properly constructed and worn, they do not trap all the microorganisms carried by the droplets of moisture during talking. Because masks are only partly effective, all but the most necessary conversation in the operating room should be discouraged.

After the thorough scrubbing of the hands and

arms, a sterile gown is donned and rubber gloves are placed on the hands. The gown and gloves act as a barrier between the member of the surgical team and the wound. Before gloves were introduced, various chemicals were utilized to reduce the number of microorganisms on the hands. Semmelweis dealt with the problem by insisting that persons examining patients wash their hands in a solution containing chlorine. Lister introduced the use of carbolic acid, or phenol. Interestingly, rubber gloves were introduced by Dr. William Halsted, who had them made to protect the hands of a nurse who assisted him. She had developed a mercury dermatitis that made working in the operating room impossible. Because he valued her services, he had a pair of rubber gloves made for her. Later, other members of his operating team wore them, first to protect their hands and then later to protect the wound.

In addition to the preceding, all materials and instruments coming in contact with the wound are sterilized before they are used in the operative procedure. A variety of physical and chemical agents are now available for this purpose. They can be selected not only on the basis of being effective against organisms in either the vegetative or spore state but according to the type of material to be sterilized.

Susceptibility of the patient to organisms lodged in the wound during operation is minimized by judicious use of antibiotics. Although discernible evidence of wound infection may develop only after 24 hours or more, the ultimate presence or degree of infection is determined by events within the critical 2 or 3 hours following contamination. Therefore antibiotics must be administered before, at the time of, or within 3 hours after bacterial implantation if infection is to be prevented or altered (Postlethwait, 1977, p. 329). Probability of infection is greater in emergency than elective operations, and is greater in prolonged operations than in short ones. Also the presence of factors previously identified as classifying the patient as high risk for surgery (see discussion of the preoperative period) tend to be associated with greater susceptibility to infection.

Maintenance of asepsis is one of the important elements in making surgery safe for the patient. Each and every member of the surgical team is responsible not only for his or her own conduct but for that of other team members. Thus the nurse reminds the surgeon that he or she is in danger of, or has, contaminated the gloves, gown, a drape, or an instrument. The surgeon likewise reminds the nurse. Every team member is asepsis-conscious and acts to protect the safety of the patient. Although prophylactic use of antibiotics has made a dramatic contribution to making surgery safe for the patient, antibiotics cannot be used as a substitute for maintenance of sterile technique, application of basic surgical principles, and judgment in selection and timing of surgical procedures.

Summary

Throughout the operative period, the patient is totally dependent upon others for safety and welfare. Depending upon the anesthetic agent and the preoperative medication, he or she may be sufficiently awake during the operation to talk with the surgical team or may be unconscious. In either case the patient should be protected from the insult of depersonalization, and his or her person and body treated at all times with deftness and respect. Whatever the purposes of the operation, the patient must be protected from the hazards of the anesthesia, from unsafe acts on the part of all members of the surgical team, and from the hazards of infection, shock, and hemorrhage, to which surgery predisposes him or her.

The Postoperative Period

The postoperative period begins the moment the surgeon completes the last stitch and continues until the metabolic and tissue changes resulting from the surgical procedure have returned to normal. This may require several days, weeks, or months. One of the major goals during this period is to anticipate, prevent, and, if necessary, treat postoperative complications. When this goal is accomplished, the patient has the greatest chance for optimal recovery. Whether or not complications are prevented frequently depends on the quality of nursing that the patient receives. Many nurses enjoy the care of patients in the postoperative phase of surgery because the results of their efforts are immediately evident. The patient fulfills the expectations of the nurse by getting well promptly. Changes indicating progress toward recovery can be seen from one day to the next and are sources of satisfaction. There are some disappointments, because not all patients get well and some develop complications.

To anticipate and prevent complications, the nurse requires knowledge of (1) the effects of anesthesia on the capacity of the patient to function, (2) the site of the incision and its effects on function, (3) the organ and tissue operated on and the general nature of the surgical procedure, and (4) knowledge of the manner in which the body responds, locally and generally, to trauma. This knowledge will influence (1) the preparations that are made for the patient in the immediate postoperative phase, (2) how he or she is transported from one area to another, (3) the care the patient receives in the period that follows the completion of the operative procedure until ambulating, and (4) the care given until the patient is fully rehabilitated. The psychological and physiologic status of the patient are not only important in the preparation of the patient for the operation and in assessing his or her ability to withstand the actual procedure, but they influence the patient's recovery from the operation. Age predisposes the patient to, or protects him or her from, certain hazards. Personal habits, such as smoking, make the patient more vulnerable to certain complications, particularly those involving the tracheobronchial tree. The ability to accept any changes in appearance or function that may result from the surgrey influences the timing and content of instruction in preparation for discharge, and ultimately may determine if, or how well, the patient resumes the usual life style.

In the following chapter the postoperative period is considered to consist of three phases: (1) the early postoperative phase, extending from completion of the operation through the time when catabolism still exceeds anabolism (usually completed by the fourth postoperative day); (2) the turning-point phase, when function of critical systems return to normal, anabolism at least balances catabolism, and the patient begins to feel better (usually occurs during the third or seventh postoperative days); and (3) the recovery phase, when muscle strength returns, followed by gain in depleted stores of body fat. (See Unit V for discussion and summary of phases and events in the response to injury.) These phases are not discrete, but overlapping, and problems attributed to one phase can develop in any phase because of unique factors in the operation and in the conditions of postoperative care, and because of unique responses of individual patients. However, there are a few generalizations to guide the care of the patient until he or she reaches the phase of recovery: (1) the periods of induction and recovery from anesthesia are the most critical of the operative experience,[9] (2) the patient can be expected to have some disruption or depression of defense mechanisms, (3) the patient's capacity to adapt physiologically or psychologically is lessened, (4) the functions of organs and systems may be stimulated or depressed, (5) disturbance in one function can be the cause of disturbances in others, and (6) therapeutic measures may have adverse effects.

[9] For discussion of recovery room nursing as a specialty, see Drain & Shipley (1979) in General References at the end of this chapter.

The following chapter will present the nature, causes, and management of problems common to the early postoperative and turning-point phases, followed by measures recommended to prevent problems and promote recovery.

References Cited

Allen, J. G. "Appendicitis and the Acute Abdomen." In *Surgery: Principles and Practice,* 3rd ed. Ed. by C. A. Moyer et al. Philadelphia: J. B. Lippincott Co., 1965, p. 968.

Bartlett, R. H. et al. "Respiratory Maneuvers to Prevent Postoperative Pulmonary Complications." *JAMA,* **224** (May 14, 1973), 1017–21.

Bettmann, O. L. *A Pictorial History of Medicine.* Springfield, Ill.: Charles C. Thomas, 1956, p. 15.

Beven, E. G. et al. "Aneurysectomy in the Aged?" *Surgery,* **67** (Jan. 1970), 34–39.

Black, M. H. et al. "Neurologic Complications Following Spinal Anesthesia with Lidocaine." *Anesthesiology,* **30** (March 1969), 284–89.

Bombardier, C. et al. "Socioeconomic Factors Affecting the Utilization of Surgical Operations." *N. Engl. J. Med.,* **297** (Sept. 29, 1977), 699–705.

Braasch, J. W. "The Surgical Treatment of Obesity." *Surg. Clin. North Am.,* **51** (June 1971), 667–73.

Brieger, G. H. "The Development of Surgery: Historical Aspects Important in the Origin and Development of Modern Surgical Science." In *Davis-Christopher Textbook of Surgery,* 11th ed. Ed. by D. C. Sabiston, Jr. Philadelphia: W. B. Saunders Co., 1977, p. 20.

Brunner, E. A., and Eckenhoff, J. E. "Anesthesia." In *Davis-Christopher Textbook of Surgery,* 11th ed. Ed. by D. C. Sabiston, Jr. Philadelphia: W. B. Saunders Co., 1977, pp. 200–24.

Cassileth, B. R. et al. "Informed Consent—Why Are Its Goals Imperfectly Realized?" *N. Engl. J. Med.,* **302** (April 17, 1980), 896–900.

Cohn, I., Jr., and Nance, F. C. "Intestinal Antisepsis and Peritonitis from Perforation." In *Davis-Christopher Textbook of Surgery,* 11th ed. Ed. by D. C. Sabiston, Jr. Philadelphia: W. B. Saunders Co., 1977, p. 1087.

Croom, R. D., III, and Hutchin, P. "Surgical Management of the Patient with Classical Hemophilia." *Surg. Gynecol. Obstet.,* **128** (April 1969), 793–800.

Davis, C. "Hemostatic Risk." *Am. J. Surg.,* **118** (Oct. 1969), 609–11.

Fujikura, I. et al. "Transient Hypopotassemia and ECG Changes Following Hemodilution Perfusion." *Arch. Surg.,* **104** (May 1972), 640–43.

Gardner, F. T. et al. "Further Definition of Antibiotic Use and Abuse in the Surgical Setting." *Arch. Surg.,* **114** (Aug. 1979), 883–86.

Gius, J. A. *Fundamentals of General Surgery,* 3rd ed. Chicago: Year Book Medical Publishers, 1966, p. 272.

Grundner, T. M. "On the Readability of Surgical Consent Forms." *N. Engl. J. Med.*, **302** (April 17, 1980), 900–2.

Hamelberg, W. E. et al. "Sudden Hyperpyrexia during General Anesthesia." *Surgery*, **66** (Nov. 1969), 850–55.

Harvey, S. C. "Antiseptics and Disinfectants; Fungicides; Ectoparasiticides." In *Pharmacological Basis of Therapeutics*, 5th ed. Ed. by L. S. Goodman and A. Gilman, New York: Macmillan Publishing Co., 1975, p. 1001.

Hemstrup-Hansen, R. "Do Nursing Personnel Aid in the Spreading of Hospital Infection by Wearing Rings on Duty?" Report of a Nursing Problem Study completed in partial fulfillment of the requirements for the graduate course sequence in Medical-Surgical Nursing. Detroit, Mich.: Wayne State University College of Nursing, 1963, unpublished oral report.

Henderson, V., and Nite, G. "Intubation of the Alimentary Tract for Feeding, Medication, and Drainage." In *Principles and Practice of Nursing*, 6th ed. New York: Macmillan Publishing Co., 1978, Chap. 23, pp. 1212–57.

Hogstel, M. "How to Give a Safe and Successful Cleansing Enema." *Am. J. Nurs.*, **77** (May 1977), 816–17.

Johnson, J. E. "Effects of Structuring Patients' Expectations on Their Reactions to Threatening Events." *Nurs. Res.*, **21** (Nov.–Dec. 1972), 499–504.

Manax, W. G., and Pemberton, L. B. "Relationship of Obesity to Postoperative Complications after Cholecystectomy." *Am. J. Surg.* **121** (Jan. 1971), 87–90.

Marples, M. J. "Life on the Human Skin." *Sci. Am.*, **220** (Jan. 1969), 108–15.

Mitchell, M. "Program Helps Patient Get Second Medical Opinion before Surgery." *New Bedford Standard-Times* (Aug. 6, 1979), 7.

Moore, F. D. *Metabolic Care of the Surgical Patient.* Philadelphia: W. B. Saunders Co., 1959, p. vii.

Moyer, C. A. "The Assessment of Operative Risk." In *Surgery: Principles and Practice*, 3rd ed. Ed. by C. A. Moyers et al. Philadelphia: J. B. Lippincott Co., 1965, pp. 220–22.

Ozuna, J. M., and Foster, C. "Hypothermia and the Surgical Patient." *Am. J. Nurs.*, **79** (April 1979), 646–48.

Paget, Sir J. *Clinical Lectures and Essays.* London: Longmans, Green & Co., Ltd., 1877, quoted in U. H. Eversole. "The Anesthetic Management of the Elderly Patient." *Surg. Clin. North Am.*, **34** (June 1954), 622.

Passos, J. Y., and Brand, L. M. "Effects of Agents Used for Oral Hygiene." *Nurs. Res.*, **15** (Summer 1966), 196–202.

Polk, H. C., Jr. "Principles of Preoperative Preparation of the Surgical Patient." In *Davis-Christopher Textbook of Surgery*, 11th ed. Ed. by D. C. Sabiston, Jr. Philadelphia: W. B. Saunders Co., 1977, pp. 119–30.

Postlethwait, R. W. "Principles of Operative Surgery: Antisepsis, Technique, Sutures, and Drains." In *Davis-Christopher Textbook of Surgery*, 11th ed. Ed. by D. C. Sabiston, Jr. Philadelphia: W. B. Saunders Co., 1977, p. 325.

Rennie, D. "Informed Consent by Well-Nigh Abject Adults." *N. Engl. J. Med.*, **302** (April 17, 1980), 917–18.

Reynolds, B. M., and Seropian, R. "Wound Infections after Preoperative Depilatory Versus Razor Preparation." *Am. J. Surg.*, **121** (March 1971), 251–54.

Robson, M. C. et al. "Biology of Surgical Infections." *Curr. Probl. Surg.* (March 1973), 7.

Rothenberg, R. E. *Understanding Surgery.* New York: Pocket Books, 1965, p. 1.

Schwartz, S. I. et al., eds. *Principles of Surgery*, 3rd ed. New York: McGraw-Hill, 1979.

"Symposium on Vascular Grafts: Current State of the Art." *Arch. Surg.*, **114** (June 1979), 665–702.

Thorwald, J. *The Century of the Surgeon.* New York: Pantheon Books, 1957, p. 234.

Williams, R. D. "Whole Blood Versus Packed Red Cells for Preoperative Transfusions." *Surg. Gynecol. Obstet*, **128** (May 1969), 1047–50.

General References

Bell, J. "Just Another Patient with Gallstones? Don't You Believe It." *Nursing 79*, **9** (Oct. 1979), 27–33.

Brand, T. C., and Tolins, S. H. *The Nursing Student's Guide to Surgery.* Boston: Little, Brown, 1979.

Condon, R. E., and Nyhus, L. M. *Manual of Surgical Therapeutics*, 4th ed. Boston: Little, Brown, 1978.

Daniel, R. K. "Microsurgery: Through the Looking Glass." *N. Engl. J. Med.*, **300** (May 31, 1979), 1251–57.

Del Guercio, L. R. M. "Physiologic Monitoring of the Surgical Patient." In *Principles of Surgery*, 3rd ed. Ed. by S. I. Schwartz et al., New York: McGraw-Hill, 1979, pp. 525–45.

Drain, C. B., and Shipley, S. B. *The Recovery Room.* Philadelphia: W. B. Saunders Co., 1979.

Finn, K. "How's Your Post-op Ambulation Technique?" *RN*, **42** (Sept. 1979), 69–72.

King, E. M. et al. *Illustrated Manual of Nursing Techniques.* Philadelphia: J. B. Lippincott Co., 1977.

LeMaitre, G. D., and Finnegan, J. A. *The Patient in Surgery: A Guide for Nurses*, 4th ed. Philadelphia: W. B. Saunders Co., 1980.

Love-Mignogna, S. "Taping and Splinting: Seven Common Problems . . . and How to Avoid Them." *Nursing, 80*, **10** (April 1980), 88–92.

Madden, J. W. "Wound Healing: Biologic and Clinical Features." In *Davis-Christopher Textbook of Surgery*, 11th ed. Ed. by D. C. Sabiston, Jr. Philadelphia: W. B. Saunders Co., 1977, pp. 271–94.

Marcinek, M. B. "Stress in the Surgical Patient." *Am. J. Nurs.*, **77** (Nov. 1977), 1809–11.

Meredith, S. "Those Formidable External Fixation Devices." *RN*, **42** (Dec. 1979), 18–24.

Moore, F. D., "Homeostasis: Bodily Changes in Trauma and Surgery—The Responses to Injury in Man as the Basis for Clinical Management. In *Davis-Christopher Textbook of Surgery*, 11th ed Ed. by D. C. Sabiston, Jr. Philadelphia: W. B. Saunders Co., 1977, pp. 27–64.

Peacock, E. E. "Wound Healing and Wound Care." In *Principles of Surgery*, 3rd ed. Ed. by S. I. Schwartz et al. New York: McGraw-Hill, 1979, pp. 303–24.

Rhodes, M. J. et al. *Alexander's Care of the Patient in Surgery,* 6th ed. St. Louis: C. V. Mosby Co., 1978.

Sabiston, D. C., Jr., ed. *Davis-Christopher Textbook of Surgery,* 11th ed. Philadelphia: W. B. Saunders Co., 1977.

Schweiger, J. L. et al. "Oral Assessment: How to Do It." *Am. J. Nurs.,* **80** (April 1980), 654–57.

Thompson, J. E., and Garrett, W. V. "Peripheral-Arterial Surgery." *N. Engl. J. Med.,* **302** (Feb. 28, 1980), 491–503.

Welch, C. E., and Malt, R. A. "Abdominal Surgery." Part I. *N. Engl. J. Med.,* **300** (March 22, 1979), 648–53. Part II. *N. Engl. J. Med.,* **300** (March 29, 1979), 705–12.

Williamson, R. C., and Chir, M. "Intestinal Adaptation. Part I. Structural, Functional and Cytokinetic Changes." *N. Engl. J. Med.,* **298** (June 22, 1978), 1393–1402. "Part II. Mechanisms of Control." *N. Engl. J. Med.,* **298** (June 29, 1978), 1444–50.

52

Prevention and Management of Postoperative Problems

Surgeons must be very careful
When they take the knife
Underneath their fine incisions
Stirs the Culprit—Life!
EMILY DICKINSON, 1859
Barlett's Familiar Quot. p. 734

Overview

PERSONNEL TRAINING AND SURGICAL SURVIVAL

Training and experience of health care providers are important to the outcomes of all health services rendered, but in the prevention and management of postoperative problems, the training and experience of all personnel are critical factors to successful outcomes. Luft and his associates (1979) examined mortality rates for twelve surgical procedures of varying complexity performed in 1,498 hospitals, and found there was a relationship between a hospital's surgical volume and its surgical mortality. For four of the twelve operations, death rates were 25 to 41 per cent lower in hospitals in which 200 or more of the operations were done annually than in hospitals with lower volumes. Although some procedures such as cholecystectomy showed no relation between volume and mortality, Luft and his associates propose that the data support the value of early regionalization for certain operations such as open-heart surgery, major vascular surgery, and total hip replacement.

TECHNOLOGY AND THE SURGICAL NURSE

When the nurse's practice involves assisting people in the perioperative period,[1] a major factor influencing care is the intensive and ever-changing technology associated with medical diagnosis and surgical treatment. Developments such as microsurgery (Daniel, 1979) have made surgical correction possible for conditions such as incipient stroke (Fein, 1978) and severed nerves, for which medical management was previously the only alternative.

Monitoring

A major component in care of the surgical patient which has increased in complexity as a result of biomedical technology is physiologic monitoring. Physiologic monitoring methods have been classified as follows (Del Guercio, 1979, p. 531):

[1] The *perioperative period* is the time surrounding a surgical procedure, from presentation to the individual of the need for surgery through that time when the person and those with whom he or she shares life can resume unaided control of the activities of daily living.

1. Analysis of samples of tissue, blood, respiratory gases, urine, cerebrospinal fluid, or other body fluids.
2. Techniques which use intrinsic energy sources within the body, such as EKG, EEG, thermogram.
3. Methods which direct extrinsic energy probes at or into the body, with analysis of the emerging energy, such as ultrasound.

The nurse is involved in all three methods to some extent. Initially, the nurse must ensure that the person to be monitored, and those close to him or her, understand what to expect and what is expected of the person. Simultaneously, the nurse may assist with or be solely responsible for collection of samples, or for setting up and/or attaching monitoring devices. Frequently it is the nurse who makes, records, reports, and acts on serial observations of the patient's physiologic status.

Physiologic monitoring is a major responsibility in care of the postoperative patient. To *monitor* is to observe, record, or detect an operation or condition with instruments that have no effect on the operation or condition. This definition highlights a basic problem of all patient monitoring; the measuring systems tend to change the measurements. The ideal monitoring system should be noninvasive and unobtrusive, neither of which is characteristic of most physiologic monitoring techniques. In addition, the use of invasive and obtrusive monitoring systems have not been proven to be life-saving. Only in the coronary care unit can it be statistically documented that lives are saved by electrocardiographic monitoring for early detection of arrhythmia (Del Guercio, 1979, p. 525).

The problem of monitoring the surgical patient is highly complex because there is no known single physiologic variable which can be used to warn of impending disaster. The many systems available to assess cardiorespiratory function and oxygen transport are used primarily when it is obvious the patient is in serious trouble. These systems are generally invasive and are used to assess the response of a desperately ill person to specific modes of therapy. Even then, monitoring devices are not a substitute for observation.

> [T]he most sophisticated and advanced electronic system can never substitute for close surveillance by an experienced and qualified health professional. Monitors in surgery are worthwhile only if they provide physiologic information about the patient which cannot be detected by the five senses of a physician or nurse. In addition, the transducers, signal processors, or readout devices should not so encumber the patient as to interfere with essential nursing care. (Del Guercio, 1979, p. 525)

Traumatic Injury and Postoperative Problems

Elective surgery threatens homeostasis, but because it is performed under controlled circumstances, it is considered controlled trauma (Marcinek, 1977). The incidence of postoperative problems following the controlled trauma of elective surgery is usually low, when the person has been carefully prepared during the preoperative period to minimize the effect of any existent risk factors. However, the probability of postoperative problems increases dramatically when surgery is necessitated by traumatic injury.

The increasing incidence of traumatic injury makes a major contribution to the growing number of Americans receiving surgical treatment, as well as to the growing number receiving critical care during the often complicated postoperative period. Oakes (1979) describes trauma as the twentieth-century epidemic, attributable to the interaction of three social phenomena: industrialization, urbanization, and affluence.

Nurses working with the severely injured function in an environment that is constantly demanding mentally and physically.

> By the very nature of multisystem disruptions resulting from severe injuries, trauma nurses are expected to comprehend extensive scientific data and to synthesize care in life-threatening emergencies. Daily, these care givers are confronted by uncharted areas of pathophysiology and telescoping crises situations. Magnifying the already stressful environment, they require of themselves an epitome of practice that is unparalleled in other critical care specialties. (Oakes, 1979, p. 921)

This chapter discusses the prevention and mangement of common postoperative problems. Although these problems are frequently encountered in critical care nursing, the student is cautioned that knowledge and skill must be substantially expanded to support safe and effective nursing of the critically ill postoperative trauma victim. Trauma nursing is fast becoming a field of advanced specialization in nursing.

High-Cost Hospital Patients

An analysis in 1976 of the cost characteristics of over 2,000 hospital patients revealed that 13 per cent of the highest cost patients consumed as many resources as the remaining 87 per cent, that repeated hospitalizations for the same disease were more characteristic of the high-cost patients, and that unexpected complications during treatment were five times more frequent in the high-cost group

(Zook & Moore, 1980). Since only one person in ten in the United States enters a hospital in any given year, results of the 1976 cost-analysis study suggest that as few as 1.3 per cent of the population consumes over half the hospital resources used in any given year. Many of these patients are treated surgically either for the medical problem that necessitates hospitalization or for treatment of subsequent complications or both.

The nurse is responsible not only for being competent to assist with management of surgical complications of these high-cost heavy users of hospital services, but also for helping to find ways to reduce the probability of readmission and for developing alternative systems of care which respond more effectively and economically to the needs of people with chronic conditions.

For those persons undergoing surgery whose preoperative status and/or proposed surgery indicate a strong likelihood of postoperative problems, it is imperative that the nurse understand the probable causes, manifestations, and management of those postoperative problems.

Causes, Manifestations, and Management of Postoperative Problems

Some of the causes and manifestations of postoperative problems common to major surgical operations are summarized in Table 52-1, and for each problem that is fully explored elsewhere, the chapter is indicated. Especially in the early postoperative period, management is directed toward prevention and early detection of those problems.

TABLE 52-1 *Some Causes and Evidence of Postoperative Problems Common to All Major Operations*

Problem*	Some Common Causes	Possible Nursing Observations
A. Acute respiratory insufficiency (see Chapter 40)	Prolonged effects of anesthesia Tracheal or bronchial obstruction Sedation Pain Chronic lung disease Retained secretions with atelectasis Pneumonitis Pulmonary edema 2° to left heart failure Pulmonary embolism Bronchospasm	Dyspnea Tachypnea Stertorous respirations ↑ Heart rate Cardiac arrhythmias Pallor, cyanosis of skin and mucous membranes Anxiety and restlessness ↓ P_{O_2} ↑ P_{CO_2}
B. Shock (see Chapter 45)	Hemorrhage from unligated artery or vein Vasodilatation caused by anesthesia Abnormal coagulation Unreplaced losses during operation	↓ Arterial blood pressure Low central venous pressure Weak or thready pulse Rapid heart rate Oliguria (<30 ml/hr) or anuria Pallor of skin and mucous membranes Anxiety and restlessness
C. Acid–base imbalance (see Chapter 41)	Incomplete correction of preoperative deficit or excess of water or electrolytes Cause or effect of many uncorrected postoperative problems (see also Chapter 41)	The following laboratory findings may be depressed, normal, or elevated, depending on (1) cause of the imbalance and (2) whether the imbalance is compensated or uncompensated: P_{CO_2} Standard bicarbonate Chloride Sodium Potassium Urinary pH

(Continued)

TABLE 52-1 *(Continued)*

Problem*	Some Common Causes	Possible Nursing Observations
1. *Acidosis* = pH < 7.36† a. Respiratory	Unrelieved acute respiratory insufficiency (see Causes of A) Obesity	See Observations for acute respiratory insufficiency Low pH High P_{CO_2} Chronic productive cough Polycythemia Weakness, dull headache
b. Metabolic	Acid gain acidosis 2° to: Anesthesia Fever and infection Shock Lactic acidosis Thyrotoxicosis Starvation Diabetic acidosis Violent exercise and convulsions Intake of excessive acids 2° to oral or parenteral administration of acids or salts containing Cl ions, and poisoning by ingestion of boric acid, salicylic acid, methanol, or ethylene glycol Retention of metabolic acids 2° to renal disease Loss of base 2° to diarrhea, small bowel, or biliary fistula	$CO_2 < 18$ mEq/L ($<$40 vol %) Weakness or general malaise Dull headache Nausea and vomiting Abdominal pain Deep respirations characteristic of air hunger (Kussmaul breathing) Flushed face Full, bounding pulse
2. *Alkalosis* = pH > 7.44† a. Respiratory	Hyperventilation *Primary* Anxiety CNS lesions Intracranial surgery Alcoholic intoxication Anemia Fever General anesthesia with assisted respiration CHF Intoxication from salicylates, paraldehyde, sulfonamides Thyrotoxicosis High altitude Vigorous exercise *Secondary* Compensatory response to metabolic acidosis	Low P_{CO_2} Dizziness, light-headedness Paresthesia around the mouth Numbness and tingling of fingers and toes Sweating Palpitation Tinnitus and tremulousness Dyspnea and air hunger Feeling of fear, panic, unreality Precordial chest pain Epigastric or lower abdominal pain, with nausea, vomiting, diarrhea Tetany
b. Metabolic	Excessive oral or parenteral intake of base, e.g., $NaHCO_3$ or other alkaline salts Loss of HCl because of vomiting, gastric suction, diarrhea, excessive use of diuretics	Largely dependent on causative disorder Anorexia Nausea, vomiting Drowsiness, confusion, coma Tetany

TABLE 52-1 *(Continued)*

Problem*	Some Common Causes	Possible Nursing Observations
	Loss of K ions because of diarrhea, vomiting, cirrhosis of liver, high renal output failure Prolonged hypercalcemia	
D. Oliguria (see Chapters 27 and 41)	Hypovolemia ↓ Cardiac output Severe hypoxia with metabolic acidosis Renal failure 2° to: §‡ Acute tubular necrosis Blood incompatibilities	<30 ml/hour of urine Specific gravity <1.010/>1.030 ↑ or ↓ central venous pressure Blood urea nitrogen (BUN) > 26 mg % Serum K^+ > 4 mEq/L Serum creatinine > 1.3 mg %
E. Disturbances in mental status (see Units IV and VI)	Excessive depressant effects of anesthesia Cerebral hypoxia 2° to: Respiratory insufficiency Shock Acid–base and/or electrolyte imbalance Intracranial hemorrhage, embolism, thrombosis Hypoglycemia Septicemia Functional brain disorder	Failure to awaken promptly from anesthesia Abnormalities of: Facial expression Cough, gag, swallow reflexes Limb reflexes Pupil size and reflexes Posture Neuromuscular irritability Responses to verbal, tactile, and painful stimuli
F. Jaundice (see Chapter 46)	Hemolysis Leakage of bile into peritoneal cavity Mechanical obstruction of common bile duct Severe sepsis Pulmonary embolism Liver disease 2° to: toxicity of anesthesia or drugs Serum hepatitis Liver hypoxia	Elevated serum bilirubin Elevated serum transaminase Yellow sclera Yellow tinge to skin Dark urine
G. Disturbances in alimentary tract function (see Chapter 46)	Depressant effect of anesthesia Intraperitoneal sepsis Acute gastric dilatation Paralytic ileus Mechanical obstruction Fecal impaction Bacterial overgrowth because of broad-spectrum antibiotics "Stress ulcer syndrome"	Prolonged: Anorexia Nausea and/or vomiting Distention with gas pains Absence of bowel sounds Fecal incontinence Diarrhea
H. Hiccough	Gastric dilatation Irritation of diaphragm Metabolic disorders affecting the brain	Intermittent noise produced by diaphragmatic spasm accompanied by sudden inhalation of air and closure of the glottis

(Continued)

TABLE 52-1 *(Continued)*

Problem*	Some Common Causes	Possible Nursing Observations
I. Infection (see Chapters 10 and 38, and Unit V)	Hypostatic pneumonia Abscesses Urinary tract infection Septicemia Wound infection Infection around tubes, drains, catheters Parotitis Phlebitis	Fever (>100° F) Leukocytosis ↑ Heart rate Swelling, warmth, erythema, drainage—with infection near periphery of body Pain and tenderness
J. Defective wound healing (see Chapter 25)	Infection Hematoma or fluid accumulation Excessive tension on sutures 2° to: Inadequate closure technique Excessive coughing, vomiting, straining, distention Previous irradiation Metabolic derangements	Failure of wound edges to seal within 2 to 3 days Appearance of serosanguinous fluid between skin sutures

* Problems are based on those identified by James D. Hardy: Surgical complications, in *Davis-Christopher Textbook of Surgery,* 11th ed. Ed. by David C. Sabiston. Philadelphia: W. B. Saunders Co., 1977, pp. 424–42.

† Emanuel Goldberger: *A Primer of Water, Electrolye and Acid-Base Syndromes,* 5th ed. Philadelphia: Lea & Febiger, 1975, p. 166.

‡ Arthur C. Guyton: *Textbook of Medical Physiology,* 5th ed. Philadelphia: W. B. Saunders Co., 1976, pp. 504–12.

Recovery from the Anesthetic

The principal complications during the first 6 to 8 hours after the operation, when the patient is recovering from anesthesia, are obstruction of the airway, shock, and hemorrhage. Among the more important objectives of care during this period are to maintain a clear airway, to prevent aspiration of vomitus, to maintain tissue perfusion (and thus blood pressure), and to prevent injury from falling or restless thrashing about. Depending on the type of anesthesia used and the stage of anesthesia the patient is in, he or she may be deeply unconscious or fully awake. Unless or until the patient is responding in the postanesthesia period, his or her problems and care will be similar to those of any unconscious patient.

When the operation is completed, the patient is transferred out of the operating room to recover fully from anesthesia elsewhere. When the surgical procedure or the patient's postoperative status qualify him or her for admission to one of the various special care units such as pulmonary intensive-care unit (ICU), general surgical ICU, or cardiovascular surgical ICU, he or she may be transferred directly to the appropriate ICU to recover from anesthesia, in order to minimize the stress of an additional move. Occasionally a patient who has had a regional anesthetic and a short and uneventful operative period may be transferred directly to his or her own room. But the most common practice, especially following general anesthesia, is to transfer the patient to the recovery, or postanesthesia, room. To prevent obstruction of the tracheobronchial tree and aspiration of gastric secretions and saliva while the patient is being transported from one area to another, all personnel should be constantly on the alert for any signs of altered or interrupted respiration indicating obstruction of the airway. The patient should be accompanied by a professional person capable of instituting remedial or resuscitative measures in the event that respiratory insufficiency or arrest develops in transit. The recovery room has the advantage of having a trained and experienced staff who know what to expect in the postoperative period and how to prevent and treat conditions predisposing to complications. The recovery room is also specially equipped to meet any emergencies that may arise. It should be located in or adjacent to the operating suite so that equipment from the operating room is readily available. Physicians are also more accessible should their services be required.

When the patient arrives in the recovery area, he or she may be fully awake or in any one of the various stages of anesthesia described previously. If unconscious, the patient may have an oropharyngeal airway in place. It should not be removed until the swallowing reflexes of the patient return and the patient tries to remove it. The oropharyngeal airway should not be confused with an endotracheal tube. As may be deducted from its name, an endotracheal tube is placed in the trachea and its primary purpose is to administer an inhalation anesthetic. It should only be removed after the patient is awake and can ventilate adequately. Some physicians and anesthetists measure the patient's tidal volume before removing the endotracheal tube. Patients who have had chest surgery are often placed on a respirator for a few hours or even days before the endotracheal tube is removed. The endotracheal tube should always be removed by a physician because it may have to be reinserted if the patient does not breathe adequately without it. A laryngoscope should be available in case the tube has to be reinserted.

In order to maintain a clear airway, equipment is available to remove secretions from the mouth and pharynx as they appear. The patient should be observed for signs that may indicate some airway obstruction, such as noisy respirations and/or labored breathing. The movements of the chest as well as the use of the accessory muscles of respiration should be observed and abnormalities reported. Cyanosis is a relatively late sign of oxygen deficiency or hypoxia, as it depends on the presence of 5 g or more of reduced (unoxygenated) hemoglobin in the capillary blood. Thus cyanosis may not become evident in an anemic patient until just prior to death. If evidence of obstruction is ignored until the patient becomes cyanotic, the patient's condition has been allowed to deteriorate to an unacceptable degree. Treatment should be promptly instituted to prevent and to relieve obstruction and to lessen the possibility of a serious degree of hypoxia. (See Chapters 26 and 40 to review the effects of a lack of oxygen to the brain and other tissues.)

Should the unconscious patient develop signs indicating any respiratory obstruction, the nurse should check the tongue to make certain that it is not responsible. In prolonged unconsciousness, obstruction can be caused by the lodging of a foreign body transversely in the oral pharynx. One source of foreign bodies is crusting, which frequently develops on the hard palate of patients who breathe through their mouths. This crust may subsequently become dislodged and cause obstruction. Conscientious mouth care and an adequate fluid intake can prevent this complication. The condition of not only the anterior but of the posterior part of the mouth should be regularly determined. Movement of the patient from side to side may promote coughing and expulsion of a mucus plug from the tracheobroncial tree. In the patient who has had head and neck surgery, including thyroidectomy, the area around the incision should be checked for signs of hemorrhage. When the obstruction cannot be relieved by procedures within the province of nursing, the physician should be notified immediately so that the cause of the obstruction can be determined and the appropriate remedy initiated. The therapy prescribed by the physician will be determined by the factors contributing to the hypoxia and the severity of the hypoxia. Every patient who has received general anesthesia is a possible candidate for supplementary oxygen therapy, with the need indicated by a P_{O_2} below 65 mm/Hg. Simple techniques such as administering oxygen via nasal cannula or face mask may suffice, or more aggressive measures such as administration of respiratory stimulants and/or ventilatory assistance with pressure or volume cycle respirators may be required to raise the P_{O_2} (Drain & Shipley, 1979). In addition to being able to recognize manifestations of hypoxia, the nurse must be skillful in use of equipment and preparation of drugs used to treat hypoxia.

When laryngospasm is responsible for obstruction of the airway, action must be taken promptly to relieve it or the patient will die from the effects of hypoxia. The nurse can recognize this condition by the characteristic crowing sound occurring during respiration. The sound is caused by the movement of air through the narrow space between the vocal folds, which are tightly adducted because of laryngeal muscle spasm. The patient appears to be struggling to breathe, especially during inspiration, and uses accessory muscles of respiration. Although the simplest method used to treat laryngospasm is to administer oxygen under pressure by way of a tight-fitting mask placed over the face, laryngospasm can also be relieved by the introduction of an endotracheal tube by a physician. A nurse must *never* attempt this procedure. The administration of oxygen under pressure is usually successful. Enough oxygen gets by the adducted vocal folds to reduce the degree of hypoxia sufficiently to cause the folds to relax. When the proper equipment is not readily available, a tracheostomy may have to be performed to establish an open airway. Other indications for tracheostomy such as pressure on the trachea and excessive secretions, as well as the care of the patient with a tracheostomy, are discussed in Chapter 40.

The patient should be turned at regular intervals from side to side. As soon as he or she responds, the patient should be encouraged to perform deep-breathing exercises and to cough at hourly intervals or until the lungs have been cleared of any secretions. An upright position increases the effectiveness of coughing and the vital capacity. Slight pressure over the incision by the nurse may reduce the pain of coughing or make the patient feel more secure about the incision. When the condition of the patient permits, some surgeons direct that the patient be placed in the sitting or standing position to cough and to do breathing exercises. Although either position increases the effectiveness of mechanisms for cleansing the tracheobronchial tree, the patient who has so recently experienced a major operation may become very anxious when the suggestion is made to sit up or get out of bed. He or she should therefore be given appropriate psychological and physical support.

Positioning of the patient during postanesthesia recovery has critical consequences for maintaining both a patent airway and a stable blood pressure. During the first 6 to 8 hours after surgery, the patient's cardiovascular system does not adapt well to rapid changes in position. Even when blood pressure is stable at the completion of the surgical procedure, movement or jarring of the patient is likely to cause it to fall. Care should be taken to handle the patient slowly and gently and to avoid bumping the cart or bed.

To prevent obstruction of the respiratory tract by secretions and aspiration of saliva and gastric juice, the patient should be placed in a position favoring drainage. Although some surgeons recommend that the unconscious patient be transported on his or her side, this is seldom done except with children or if the patient is vomiting. The patient may be transported with the head and shoulders slightly lower than the legs and buttocks. Excessive lowering of the head, however, increases the pressure of the viscera on the diaphragm, reduces ventilation, increases intrathoracic pressure, and may actually decrease blood flow to the brain by initiating reflex constriction of the carotid arteries. The head should be turned to one side, in order to keep the posterior portion of the tongue and soft tissues from blocking the glottis. This position not only favors the drainage of fluid from the tracheobronchial tree and the mouth, but it also reduces stasis of blood in the lower extremities. Return of fluid and blood to the general circulation is important for maintaining cardiac output. During the period that the patient is unconscious and well relaxed by the anesthetic, an oropharyngeal airway placed in the mouth may be helpful in keeping the tongue and soft tissues from falling back into the pharynx. In the event that the airway becomes obstructed, the mandible should be raised and moved forward. If the mouth can be opened, the tongue can be grasped with a gauze square and pulled forward so that the obstruction of the airway is relieved.

Until the patient regains consciousness, the head should be lowered slightly and/or turned to the side unless there is some reason contraindicating it. The child who has had a tonsillectomy under general anesthesia is usually placed face down. Because blood and saliva will drain from the mouth by gravity, aspiration of these materials into the tracheobronchial tree is avoided and the extent to which the patient is bleeding can be determined. The patient having intracranial or head and neck surgery is not placed in the head-down position. No matter where a part is located, if it is placed in a dependent position, gravity decreases venous return from it and increases the chance of swelling and bleeding. The position of the patient may also be modified by the presence of other disorders. The obese or emphysemic patient should be placed in a sitting position to facilitate breathing. The patient with a spinal anesthetic should usually be kept relatively flat in bed. Because spinal anesthesia lessens the ability to adjust the diameter of the blood vessels to position changes, it predisposes to severe postural hypotension (the blood pressure falls when the individual rises to sit or stand). A less dangerous effect is headache (spinal headache), which is thought to be caused by a reduction in the pressure of the cerebrospinal fluid. To prevent either or both of these complications, the patient is usually kept in the supine or recumbent position for a longer time than the patient having a general anesthetic.

When placing the patient on the side, the nurse should keep two points in mind. One is that the weight of the body should not be allowed to rest on the dependent arm. The other is that the weight of the body should be distributed so that the body holds itself on the side. To prevent pressure on the arm, the body may be turned on the side with the lower arm parallel to the side. The arm on the dependent side is then pulled through so that it lies posterior to the trunk. The nurse then stands behind the patient and places one hand under the iliac crest and the other under the trochanter of the femur and pulls the body toward herself or himself. The upper leg and thigh may be flexed at the knee and be carried forward over the dependent leg. The side-lying position not only facilitates the drainage of secretions, but it helps to maintain the tongue and soft tissues forward so that they do not block the pharynx or larynx. (See Figure 52-1 for illustration of each of the positions discussed.)

Until the patient is fully recovered from anesthesia and the cardiovascular pulmonary status has stabilized, the nurse should check frequently on all the

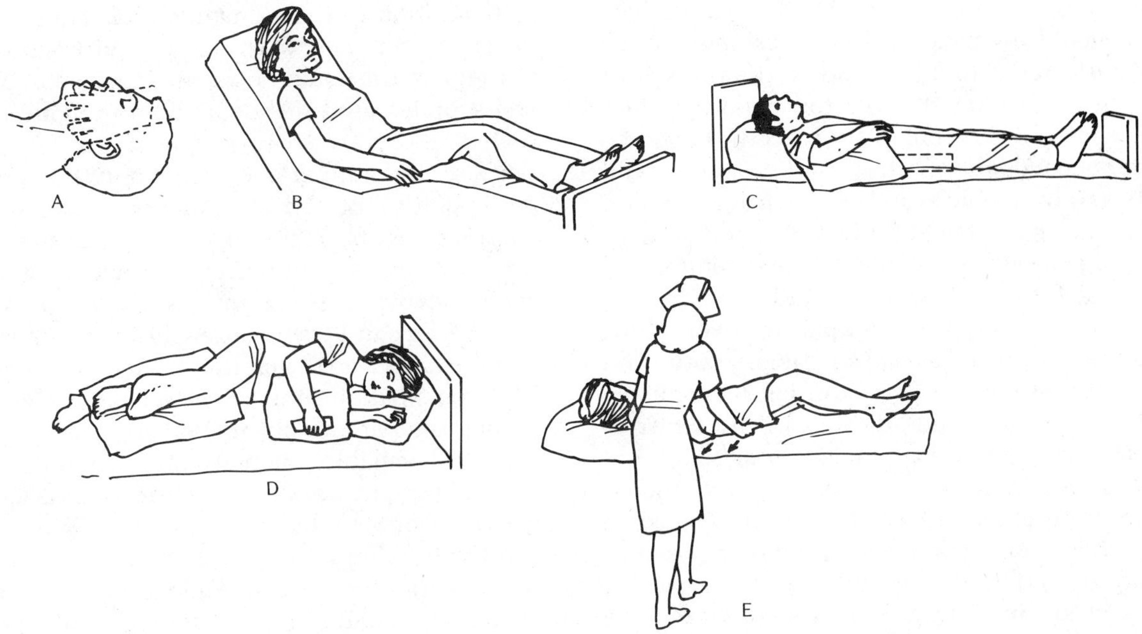

Figure 52-1. Positioning of the patient during postanesthesia recovery. (After an original drawing by Leola Hogan.)
A. Mandible raised.
B. Sitting position.
C. Supine—spinal anesthetic.
D. Side lying.
E. Turning patient to the side-lying position. To prevent pressure on the arm, the body may be turned on the side with the *lower* arm parallel to the side. The arm on the *dependent* side is then pulled through so that it lies *posterior* to the trunk. The nurse then stands behind the patient and places one hand under the iliac crest and the other under the trochanter of the femur and pulls his body toward herself. The upper leg and thigh may be flexed at the knee and be carried forward over the dependent leg.

vital signs. These include the pulse and blood pressure, and central venous and arterial pressures when appropriate manometers are in place, as well as the depth, rhythm or pattern, and rate of respiration. Unless the vital signs of the patient are being recorded by continuous electronic monitoring equipment, the nurse should check them every 5 minutes for the first hour, then every 15 minutes for the next 3 to 4 hours, and then hourly until they are stable. This frequency should be viewed as a guide, not a rule; judgment based on all available data and the progressive pattern of the patient's vital signs should be the basis upon which the nurse either increases or decreases the frequency of monitoring vital signs.

Frequent measurements of central venous pressure enables one to evaluate how well the heart is handling the volume of blood in the cardiovascular system. The response to a fluid load rather than the absolute level gives the most accurate information (Fisher, 1979). When evaluation is made of the condition of a patient, all evidence should be taken into consideration. The fact that the blood pressure of a patient is within the range expected for the patient should not cause the nurse to discount other evidence that the patient is in trouble. As a matter of fact, accumulation of carbon dioxide may cause the blood pressure to be higher than it would be otherwise.

Preparations to Receive the Patient from the Operating or Recovery Room

Assuming that the patient recovers from the anesthesia without respiratory or cardiovascular complications, he or she will usually be returned to the room on the day of surgery. Preparations for the care of the patient following surgery should be begun as soon as he or she is transferred to the operating room. The bed or frame on which the patient is to be placed should be secured and prepared. In preparing the bed three criteria should be met. First, the bed should be made so that the patient can be easily transferred into it. In general, the transfer of the patient is facilitated if the top bedding is not tucked in at the foot but placed neatly folded to one side. Second, the mattress and pillows should be protected from emesis and drainage as necessary. For example, for a patient having a general anesthetic or a procedure involving the gastrointestinal tract or the head and neck, the pillow under the head should be protected by a plastic cover. However, the patient who has had a local anesthetic and the drainage of an abscess of the leg is not likely to stain the pillow under the head. The mattress and pillow under the leg are in danger of being contaminated by drainage from the leg and should therefore be protected. Last, there should be some consideration of any special equipment or positions that may be required. To illustrate, if the patient is expected to have a general anesthetic, or to have the eyes bandaged following eye surgery, or is elderly, side rails should be placed on the bed to remind the patient of where the edges of the bed are and to reduce the chance of falling out. A patient having surgery on his or her back may be placed on a frame so that turning from face to back is facilitated. If the patient is to be encased in a cast, a board may be placed under the mattress to provide a firm support for the cast. Although most hospitals are now equipped with beds having Gatch frames to elevate the head of the bed, few have the type that facilitate elevation of the foot of the bed.[2] The necessity for elevating the foot of the bed should be anticipated when the patient goes directly from the operating room to his or her room following a prolonged and difficult operation or when there is any other reason for anticipating that the patient may be unconscious or in shock. Some surgeons prefer to have their patients in a slight Trendelenburg position to facilitate drainage of secretions from the airway and to prevent the aspiration of vomitus or other liquids.

In the past the warming of the bed was considered to be essential. Although warming of the bed probably does no harm, unless the room and bed are cold, it probably is unnecessary. If hot-water bottles or other heating devices are used, they should be removed before the patient is transferred to the bed to prevent burns and/or overheating. Overheating may cause sweating and may contribute to the dehydration of the patient. The aim should be to maintain the temperature of the room so that the patient is comfortable.

[2] Some carts or stretchers used in recovery rooms are adjustable and a patient can be placed in almost any position desired.

In addition to the preparation of the bed, equipment and supplies that will be required in the care of the patient should be assembled. The equipment and supplies used will depend on the kind of anesthetic used and the nature of the surgical procedure. Because the number-one problem in the immediate postoperative period for patients having a general anesthetic is the maintenance of adequate ventilation and the prevention of obstruction of the tracheobronchial tree, provisions should be made to remove oral and tracheobronchial secretions and to prevent saliva and vomitus from being aspirated. With some patients this can be accomplished by positioning the patient, but suction apparatus should always be available. Suction apparatus must also be available and in working order for patients who have gastric or other tubes.

A tracheostomy tray should be placed at the bedside of patients who have undergone head and neck surgery, including thyroidectomy, in anticipation of the possibility of acute obstruction of the airway. Other equipment should be obtained and prepared as required. This might include equipment for administering oxygen, drainage or irrigation sets, and solutions. Because practice varies, no attempt will be made to list all the types of equipment or supplies that may be required in the care of the patient; however, whatever is necessary should be obtained and tested to make certain that it is in working order before the patient is returned to the room.

Although the danger of airway obstruction is greatest during postanesthesia recovery, other pulmonary complications continue to be a danger throughout the postoperative period, with the operative site being a more important determinant of the incidence of pulmonary complications than either the anesthetic agent or its route of administration (Polk, 1977). Maintenance of ventilation is critically important to both the prevention and treatment of other postoperative complications. Any development that alters the metabolic rate, fluid and electrolyte balance, transportation system, or renal function of the patient can affect, or be affected by, the pulmonary status. Two of the most common postoperative problems that may require assisted ventilation are shock and hemorrhage, with their inevitable effect on renal function and acid–base balance. The reader is referred elsewhere for detailed discussion of acid–base balance (Chapter 41) and shock (Chapter 45), but hemorrhage and its management are presented in detail as surgical problems.

Shock

A relatively frequent complication occurring during the operation and early postoperative phase of surgery is shock. In serious states of shock, life may be threatened unless the disorder is treated promptly and effectively. As defined elsewhere, shock is an abnormal physiologic state characterized by inadequate cellular metabolism. This may be caused by poor tissue perfusion or other factors. Postoperatively it is often caused by a serious discrepancy between the capacity of the blood vessels and the circulating blood volume. Any disorder resulting in a marked increase in the capacity of the blood vessels or noticeably decreasing the volume of circulating blood can cause shock. One effect of the disparity between blood volume and the capacity of the blood vessels is a fall in the blood pressure. The consequence, in terms of cells, is failure to deliver enough oxygen and other substances to maintain adequate metabolism.

In a closed system such as the vascular system, the pressure of the fluid within the system above simply hydrostatic pressure is maintained by three factors: (1) an effective pumping mechanism, (2) fluid to pump, and (3) appropriate resistance in the pipes or vessels. Although any abnormalities of one of these factors may be involved in development of shock in the surgical patient, the last two are probably the most frequent. In the patient who is treated surgically or who suffers serious physical trauma or is burned, fluid volume is decreased by loss of blood and the loss of body fluids. Dehydration may be an initiating or sustaining factor in shock because it contributes to a reduction in circulating blood volume. Shock caused by the reduction in the circulating blood volume is classified as hypovolemia, and in the surgical patient a frequent cause of hypovolemia is hemorrhage.

Hemorrhage, Hemostasis, and Replacement

Causes and Consequences of Hemorrhage

Hemorrhage, which is a very profuse flow of blood, is one of the most common causes of hypovolemic shock, and is a very real possibility in all phases of any surgical operation. In the instance of Mr. Brave, bleeding from an eroded blood vessel located in a peptic ulcer caused him to seek medical attention. Mrs. Smith lost approximately 3 pints of blood during the removal of her uterus (hysterectomy), and Sunny Day bled profusely from the tonsillar fossa in her pharynx after tonsillectomy. Johnny Hopper suffered an open or compound fracture (a break in a bone in which one or more fragments protrude through the skin) when he fell from a tree. In all these patients the primary factor causing hemorrhage was a disruption in the continuity of one or more blood vessels.

Although physical injuries are usually responsible for breaks in the continuity of blood vessels, the condition of the wall of the blood vessel influences its ability to withstand trauma or chemical destruction. Examples of disorders weakening the walls of blood vessels include arterial aneurysms or venous varicosities. In an arterial aneurysm, the wall bulges as a result of disease or structural defect. As it bulges, the wall thins and becomes less resistant to the pressure of the arterial blood. Furthermore, the tension against the wall of a vessel increases with its diameter (Laplace's law). Sooner or later it is likely to rupture and result in arterial hemorrhage. When varicosities—elongated, tortuous, thin-walled veins—are located in the esophagus, food passing over may cause erosion of the already thin wall and cause serious hemorrhage. In addition to localized areas of weakness in the walls of blood vessels, deficiency of vitamin C is accompanied by a generalized fragility in the walls of capillaries.

The upper gastrointestinal tract is frequently the site of hemorrhage in an extensively burned patient or one whose operation was necessitated or characterized by massive trauma, or whose postoperative course is complicated by sepsis, shock, or other causes of systemic hypovolemia. Because this bleeding was believed to be due to excessive adrenocortical response to stress, it has been widely referred to as the "stress ulcer syndrome." However, in a study of over 2,000 combat injuries in Vietnam, Strempple and his associates (1973) found, that among the 3 per cent who developed gastrointestinal bleeding, there was no increase in urinary steroid excretion following trauma, thus casting doubt on the role of the adrenals in initiating mucosal erosion. Based on the finding of multiple areas of focal necrosis throughout the gastrointestinal tract, they suggest use of the term *acute gastrointestinal focal necrosis syndrome (AGFNS),* which implies no etiologic mechanism. Their concept of the pathogenesis of this type of gastrointestinal bleeding is presented in Figure 52-2. The common precursor appears to be systemic hypovolemia, with mucosal erosion following release of vasoactive amines and excessive back diffusion of H^+ ions. The nurse should observe gastric and intestinal drainage closely for signs of fresh or old blood, and note the pattern of vital signs for any indication of blood loss. Antacid therapy has proved to be an important prophylactic measure to protect against mucosal erosion resulting from back diffusion of H^+ ions (Silen, 1980). While the patient is NPO, the antacid can be administered via the nasogastric tube.

Following injury to a blood vessel, the body re-

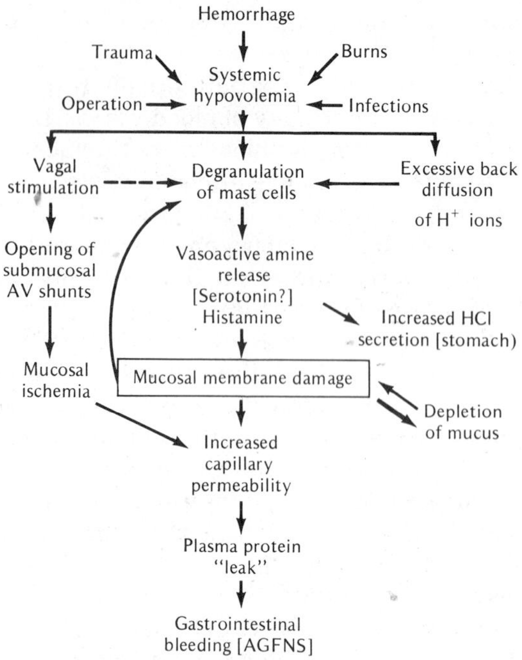

Figure 52-2. Conceptual model of the pathogenesis of the "stress ulcer syndrome." (From The stress ulcer syndrome, by J. F. Stremple *et al.* in *Current Problems in Surgery,* April 1973. Copyright © 1973 by Year Book Medical Publishers. Fig. 29, p. 52. Used by permission.)

sponds to protect itself from an excessive loss of blood. Among these responses are the self-sealing mechanism, the elevation of interstitial fluid pressure created by the escaping blood, and the immobilization of the injured area by muscle spasm. In the self-sealing mechanism, the muscle in the cut end of the blood vessel contracts and thereby reduces the diameter of the lumen. Muscle contraction occurs whether the blood vessel is large or small and may be sufficient to control bleeding, even from large arteries. Sealing of the remaining lumen is accomplished by the formation of a blood clot within the terminal portion of the cut end of the blood vessel.

Platelets play a critical role in the self-sealing mechanism. When the endothelial lining of a blood vessel is intact, platelets do not adhere to the surface. However, breaks in the continuity of blood vessels expose the subendothelium, of which *collagen* is a constituent. It is to the collagen that platelets adhere. Breaks in large blood vessels are plugged by an aggregation of large numbers of platelets (Zucker, 1980).

The second process at work in hemostasis is the result of *tissue factor* liberated by the cut blood vessel. The exposure of the blood to tissue factor sets in motion a complex series of reactions whereby the plasma protein prothrombin is converted into thrombin; the thrombin in turn converts fibrinogen into fibrin. The fibrin formed at the site of the injury supports and reinforces the platelets in the hemostatic plug, and it also solidifies blood that remains in the wound channel (Zucker, 1980, p. 89). As the clot matures, it, too, contracts and forms a tight plug in the end of the blood vessel. The self-sealing mechanism is usually successful in limiting blood loss from small wounds and from areas where the surface tissue has been removed, as in an abrasion or burn.

When a large area of tissue has been denuded or for some other reason the self-sealing mechanism is ineffective, sufficient blood may be lost to form a soft clot over the site of bleeding. The clot, instead of contracting and sealing the underlying blood vessels, remains soft and the vessels behind it continue to bleed. Before blood loss can be checked, the soft clot must be removed.

To illustrate, after the surgical removal of the tonsils, the surgeon dries the denuded area by gently patting the surface with a sponge. He or she continues this process until the cut ends of the blood vessels have constricted and the blood has clotted within them. Should bleeding recur, a clot forms external to cut ends of the blood vessels and bleeding continues underneath it. One theory advanced to explain continued bleeding is that the blood clot probably releases fibrolysin, which prevents clotting in the ends of the blood vessels. Control of bleeding usually requires that the soft blood clot be removed and that the area again be dried. Pressure is often applied to control bleeding until the self-sealing mechanism becomes effective.

Following prostatectomy, bleeding from the lining of the bladder usually occurs. Because of its anatomy, pressure over the bleeding sites is difficult, if not impossible, to apply. Continued bleeding is usually the result of a soft clot adhering to the lining of the bladder and interfering with the formation of clots within the disrupted blood vessels. Bleeding can usually be prevented or stopped by the removal of blood and clots from the bladder by irrigation. When irrigation of the bladder is prescribed following prostatectomy, sufficient fluid should be introduced to remove blood and blood clots, and the procedure should be performed frequently enough to prevent clot formation within the bladder lumen.

Besides the self-sealing mechanism, blood loss into a closed space is opposed by the rise of tissue pressure caused by blood accumulating in the space. As tissue fluid pressure rises, it exerts pressure against the wall of the bleeding vessel. Blood flow ceases when the interstitial pressure exceeds the blood pressure. Conversely, bleeding into a body cavity where blood can escape is more likely to be severe because the blood is removed from the cavity. Thus bleeding from the nose or into the alimentary canal or other hollow organs is more likely to be profuse. Muscle spasm in an affected part contributes to immobilization and may also increase the pressure exerted against the exterior of the involved blood vessels. All these factors may combine to lessen the quantity of blood lost.

Hemorrhage has one effect: It lessens circulation of blood by decreasing blood volume. When a large quantity of blood is lost quickly, the blood pressure falls. As much as 10 to 20 per cent of the blood volume can be lost without any appreciable effect on the blood pressure, especially if it is lost slowly. A rapid loss of 30 per cent or more is usually associated with a considerable drop in blood pressure. As stated, if the fall in blood pressure is not too great, it may help to produce hemostasis by reducing blood flow through the severed blood vessels. The effect of the decrease in the blood volume is counteracted by (1) the constriction of blood vessels, thereby reducing the size of the vascular bed; (2) constriction of the arterioles, which increases peripheral resistance; and (3) transfer of fluid from the interstitial and cellular spaces to the blood. All these mechanisms help to maintain perfusion of the heart and brain by reducing the disparity between the size of the vascular bed and the blood volume.

In addition to a decrease in the volume of circulating blood, hemorrhage causes a reduction in the oxygen-carrying capacity of the blood caused by a loss of erythrocytes and hemoglobin. Serious as the loss of hemoglobin is, it is not of as much immediate importance in acute hemorrhage as it is later on in chronic blood loss. The effects of the loss of hemoglobin are discussed in Chapter 42.

When arteries are disrupted, a third problem is created because the tissues supplied by the artery are partly or completely deprived of their blood supply. For example, in an accident with an electric saw, Jim Green's lower leg was severed, so that only about one fourth of the tissue remained intact. Whether or not his foot can be saved will depend in part on whether the arterial blood supply is sufficient or, if not, whether it can be reestablished. Interestingly, it is often the integrity of the veins that is more crucial. Lack of adequate venous drainage may result in severe congestion and death of the involved organ or limb.

Signs and Symptoms of Hemorrhage

In hemorrhage, the site of bleeding determines whether escaping blood increases pressure within an organ or tissue or flows to the outside. In tissues or organs where the escaping blood is trapped, such as in the cranial or spinal cavity, the signs and symptoms may be caused primarily by increased pressure on the brain or cord or by the irritation of the brain or nerves by the blood. Although some blood is lost, the quantity is not sufficient to affect the blood volume.

When bleeding is in an organ or tissue from which it can escape to the outside, blood as well as the consequences of a reduction in blood volume can be observed. Blood escaping from an artery is bright red and comes in spurts; blood from a vein generally has a dusky hue and flows steadily; and capillary bleeding is characterized by seepage.

When the rate and volume of blood loss from the intravascular compartment are sufficient to produce evidence of hypovolemia and hypoxia, the nurse may observe a weak rapid pulse; rapid respirations, at first deep then increasingly shallow; an early slight rise in blood pressure (especially diastolic, because of reflex arteriolar constriction) followed by a gradual fall; and cool, moist skin. The patient may complain of faintness or dizziness, apprehension, thirst, feeling cold, and frequently of pain when escaping blood accumulates, causing pressure and nerve irritation.

Hemostasis

In instances in which bleeding is not self-limiting, therapy of hemorrhage is directed toward two objectives. The first is to stop the hemorrhage. The second depends on the extent of blood loss and the effects of the accumulation of blood on involved structures. When the loss of blood is sufficient to affect the blood volume, a second objective is to replace the blood volume. Blood replacement will be discussed in the next section.

When blood has accumulated in a tissue or organ in sufficient quantity to impair its function, then an objective is to remove the blood or to relieve the pressure created by it. Before bleeding can be treated, it must be detected. Any patient who is predisposed to hemorrhage by the nature of his or her illness or treatment should be under an intelligent program of surveillance. Dressings should be inspected regularly for evidence of fresh blood. Like other fluids, blood runs downhill; parts inferior to the dressing should be inspected. Fluids drained or discharged from affected organs should be examined for blood. When the incision or injury is in an organ or tissue from which blood cannot escape, the patient should be observed for signs and symptoms indicating pressure on the organ or surrounding tissues.

Although bleeding may occur in any incision, it is most likely to take place in large wounds, in those in which the operated surface is exposed, and in highly vascular areas. Internal bleeding may also result from the failure of a ligature to hold a large artery severed during the operative procedure; large amounts of blood can be lost in a very short period of time. Traumatic injuries are a frequent cause of hemorrhage, and certain blood dyscrasias are associated with a tendency to bleed. Formerly operations on patients with obstructions in the biliary tract were likely to be associated with hemorrhage because of failure to absorb vitamin K. Now, many of these patients can be prepared so that they are not subject to any special hazard.

In some surgical procedures the tendency of the patient to bleed can be controlled by appropriate care. As previously indicated, patients having intracranial and head and neck surgery are usually placed in a position with the head and back up. In patients who have surgery on an extremity, the limb is elevated to improve the venous return and to lessen the tendency to bleed into the wound. Occasionally, a special tourniquet is applied to a limb so that surgery can be performed distally in a bloodless field. This may be done safely for up to 1 or 1½ hours at a time. The extremity is also immobilized until the danger of hemorrhage has decreased. As discussed earlier following prostatectomy, bleeding from the bladder is controlled by bladder irrigation. In the control of bleeding from any organ, the location of the structure and the nature of its functions have to be considered. In general, measures are used to immobilize the part, overcome the force of the blood pressure, or support or assist the self-sealing mechanism.

One of the most common methods (perhaps the oldest) of controlling hemorrhage, particularly in the emergency situation, is the application of *pressure.* The points at which bleeding may most easily be stopped by applying pressure are those where large blood vessels overlie bony prominences. The vessels that meet this criterion include the temporal, facial, carotid, brachial, and femoral arteries. Pressure should be applied with the cleanest available material. Although tourniquets have long been used to control bleeding from an extremity, they often do more harm than good. Their use is not advocated. If a tourniquet is applied, it should be tight enough to prevent blood from entering the affected limb and it should be left in place until the patient is examined by a surgeon. If the tourniquet is not tight enough to occlude the arterial flow but does occlude venous return, blood loss distal to the tourniquet will be greater than without any tourniquet at all. The patient should be treated as soon as possible to protect the tissue that is deprived of its blood supply. A properly applied tourniquet should be left in place only 1 or 2 hours; if prolonged, this method of hemostasis in itself may cause severe tissue injury.

Hemorrhage from an accessible organ or cavity such as the uterus or the nares may sometimes be controlled by packing the organ with sterile gauze. The gauze is usually left in place until the self-sealing mechanism controls bleeding. Occasionally, bleeding is renewed after the packing is removed, and the packing may have to be replaced. Patients should always be observed following the removal of packing for evidence of recurrent hemorrhage.

Although the application of pressure is frequently life-saving when utilized to control bleeding from a large artery or vein, large vessels often must be ligated before hemorrhage is actually checked. Otherwise the bleeding starts again as soon as the pressure is removed. The self-sealing mechanism is usually successful in curbing blood loss from small vessels. Pressure applied over an area in which there is bleeding from small vessels may be of value until the self-sealing mechanism is effective in controlling bleeding.

Another old, but probably newer, method of controlling the loss of blood is *cauterization* of the wound. In its earliest use, cauterization was not the carefully confined and controlled application of heat to a limited area of tissue that it is today. One old method of cauterizing tissue was to pour boiling oil into the wound. Styptics, astringents, or a hot iron were also used. Although the techniques used in cauterizing wounds have changed and cautery is less frequently utilized than it once was, it still has its uses. Many surgeons now use electric cautery with fine tips to control bleeding during surgery. Not only is it useful in controlling hemorrhage, but it may also be employed to destroy tissue. For example, it is used in brain surgery to both destroy tissue and prevent bleeding. Cautery is often employed to open colostomies; in this procedure a loop of the colon is brought above the surface of the skin and allowed to remain closed until the second or third day after the initial surgical procedure. This procedure is not painful because the tissues of the intestine do not have nerve endings that are sensitive to heat. The patient may be frightened, however, because he or she does not believe that it will not hurt. To lessen the fear, the patient's eyes should be covered with a small towel and he or she should be informed about the successful progress of the procedure. Through the use of heat enough tissue is destroyed to provide an opening into the intestine, and the blood vessels in the affected tissue are sealed.

Although pressure and cauterization are of value in hemostasis, neither method provides an adequate means of controlling the loss of blood during a major operative procedure. It was not until materials were available that could be used to tie the ends of blood vessels that the prevention of blood loss during surgery became a practical reality. Early materials to be used in tying off blood vessels were silk or linen thread. As noted earlier, *ligatures* have been known for centuries, but their regular use is of relatively modern origin. Today the surgeon has the choice of many materials, some of which are absorbable and some of which are not. During an operative procedure the surgeon also has instruments, hemostats, that can be used to close the ends of vessels before they are severed or to grasp them after they are cut.

Additional techniques that have been used to reestablish continuity of blood vessels include the use of extreme cold (cryosurgery) and laser beams (*l*ight *a*mplification by *s*timulated *e*mission of *r*adiation) (Polanyi, 1976). Another technique used in Vietnam for temporary control of intraperitoneal and lower-extremity hemorrhage secondary to massive trauma is the application of the "G-suit," which contains inflatable rubber bladders used to protect pilots from the consequences of blood pooling in the extremities under dive pressures that exceed the pressure of gravity. The counterpressure against the body surface acts as a sort of body tourniquet (Cutler & Daggett, 1971).

Summary

A variety of methods are available to prevent and to limit the loss of blood. The method selected depends on a variety of factors. Among them are the urgency of the situation, the rate at which blood is being lost, the extent to which blood volume has already been diminished, the site of bleeding, as well as the facilities at hand. As in shock, the safety of the patient depends on the rapidity with which hemorrhage is detected and appropriate measures are instituted.

In addition to stopping the bleeding, treatment should restore blood volume if it has been significantly decreased. When the loss of blood is within the limits to which the patient is able to adapt, no special measures may be required, but when the loss of blood seriously threatens the blood volume, measures such as intravenous fluids, plasma, volume expanders, and blood transfusion may be required.

Blood Replacement

Although attempts have been made to transfuse blood for at least 400 years, the ability to transfuse blood with reasonable safety to the patient is an accomplishment of the twentieth century. In some of the early experiments, blood taken from one dog was successfully transfused into another. Transfusion of human blood from one person to another was less successful and at least half of the recipients died. Because of the frequency with which death occurred, laws were passed prohibiting blood transfusions in England, France, and Italy. Before blood can be safely transferred from one person to another, three factors must be considered: (1) the blood groups and the Rh-Hr system, (2) calcium and blood clotting, and (3) diseases transmitted by blood.

The Basis for Blood Grouping

In 1900 Landsteiner made an observation that was to serve as the basis for the discovery of why at least one half of those who were transfused with the blood of another died. He noted that when the red blood cells of one person were exposed to the serum of another, they sometimes clumped or agglutinated. During the next 2 years Landsteiner and his associates investigated this phenomenon more fully. From these studies they learned that all human beings could be placed in one of four blood groups. The blood group to which any individual belongs is determined by the presence or absence of one or both of two antigens or isoagglutinogens in the erythrocytes. Landsteiner called these antigens A and B. Persons whose erythrocytes contain neither antigen A nor antigen B were classified as belonging to blood group O, the most common blood group among Caucasians, as 40 to 45 per cent of the population have type O blood. Those who have isoagglutinogen A in their erythrocytes belong to blood group A; this is the next most frequent type, as about 40 per cent of the population belong to group A. Those who have isoagglutinogen B in their erythrocytes belong to group B; about 10 per cent of the population are in group B. About 4 per cent of the population have both isoagglutinogen A and B in their erythrocytes and are in group AB.

Agglutination depends on the presence in the serum of an antibody, agglutinin, that reacts with the antigen in the erythrocyte. The agglutinin reacting with isoagglutinogen A is named anti-A and the one reacting with B is called anti-B. The blood serum of a person does not contain the agglutinin that reacts with the isoagglutinogen in his or her red cells. Thus type A blood contains anti-B but not anti-A agglutinin. Persons in blood group O do not have either antigen A or B in their red cells, but they do have both anti-A and anti-B in their serum. Persons in blood group AB have antigens A and B in their erythrocytes, but they do not have either agglutinin in their serum. Because the blood of the donor is diluted as it enters the blood of the recipient, there is relatively less concern about the effect of the antibodies in donor serum on the red blood cells of the recipient. Some authorities question the dilution factor as an explanation of why the donor's isoagglutinins do not agglutinate the erythrocytes of the recipient. Whatever the reason, the antibodies in the donor's serum do not usually adversely affect the recipient's red cells. Because erythrocytes of group

O blood do not contain either antigen, they can be transfused into persons with other types of blood. For this reason a person with group O blood is said to be a universal donor; theoretically his or her blood can be transfused into all other individuals. Although group O blood can often be transfused into persons of other blood groups without causing a reaction, it can cause a reaction, especially if there is a high titer of anti-A and anti-B in the serum of the donor. When the titer of antibody is high, the agglutinin in the blood serum of the donor can react with the isoagglutinogen of the recipient to produce hemolysis of the erythrocytes of the recipient. Persons with group O blood must be transfused with group O blood. Despite their ability to give to other groups, they can take only from their own group.

Because antibodies are absent from the serum of persons with group AB blood, they can theoretically receive blood from persons of all blood groups, and, therefore, these persons are known as universal recipients. They can give blood only to persons with type AB blood. Because not all persons react as expected on receiving blood, cross matching is an essential part of the preparation for blood transfusion. In cross matching, the erythrocytes of the donor are exposed to the serum of the recipient and the erythrocytes of the recipient are exposed to the serum of the donor.

As Landsteiner and his associates studied the factors influencing the agglutination of erythrocytes, they learned that there were more antigens and isoagglutinogens than A and B. Perhaps the most important of these other isoagglutinogens are those belonging to the Rh-Hr system. Six cell characteristics have been identified with this system. These factors have two sets of names, the American and the British. They are Rho, rh', rh", Hro, hr', hr". The corresponding British nomenclature is D, C, E, d, c, c_1. The red cells of each person contain at least one member of each of the three groups of antigens. In some persons the red cells contain four, five, or six of them. The number of possible combinations is therefore great. In general, if the patient's red cells have D antigens, he or she is considered to be Rh positive. More recently, however, the presence of both C and E has also been considered to be Rh positive. As a consequence, more exact Rh typing and matching is being done, especially in potential mothers.

Rh–Hr antigens differ from A and B antigens in that the antibody that acts against them is not normally found in the blood serum. It is formed when an Rh-negative person is given Rh-positive blood. This happens under two circumstances. In one, a person who is Rh-negative is transfused with Rh-positive blood. Although there is no obvious reaction, the individual reacts by producing antibodies in the blood serum against the Rh factor. Should this person receive a transfusion of Rh-positive blood at a later date, a serious reaction occurs. In the second situation an Rh-negative woman who is pregnant with an Rh-positive child is sensitized to the Rh factor. Usually nothing obvious occurs during the first pregnancy, and often during the second pregnancy, to indicate that the woman is becoming sensitized to the Rh factor. In many instances a number of normal children can be borne before the mother becomes sensitized to the Rh factor. Apparently, the sensitization comes about because the red cells of the Rh-positive baby escape through the placenta and stimulate the production of anti-Rh antibodies in the mother. These antibodies pass from the mother through the placenta into the blood of the baby, causing hemolysis of the red cells of the baby. The condition in the baby is known as erythroblastosis fetalis. If these babies are born alive, they may still suffer severe brain damage from the high levels of bilirubin that can develop in the fetus because of the hemolysis. If the condition is not too severe, their lives may be saved and brain damage prevented by an exchange transfusion in which the blood of the baby is removed and replaced by Rh-negative blood.

Many different agglutinins have been discovered since recognition of the ABO and Rh factors and have been referred to as Kell, Duffy, Kidd, and others. In 1926 an especially interesting type of agglutinin was described by Landsteiner and Levine (1926). This agglutinin in the blood plasma of an individual coagulates the erythrocytes when the temperature of the blood plasma is reduced below normal body temperature. Because the activity of the agglutinins depends on temperature, they are called cold agglutinins. Cold agglutinins are present more frequently in the blood of Negro donors than in Caucasians. They are also frequent in persons who have cirrhosis of the liver, severe anemia, hemolytic anemia, and many other chronic diseases. Cold agglutinins were not of much significance when blood was administered soon after it was drawn. It has assumed more importance now that blood is stored under refrigeration in blood banks. When patients are known to have cold agglutinins, blood is warmed before it is administered. After the blood is warmed, its temperature may be maintained at 37°C (98°F) by passing the tubing through a blood warmer. Some commercial blood warmers are now available and are used in many of our larger operating rooms, especially if there may be a need for massive transfusions. Because blood proteins can be altered or denatured by heat, care should be taken not to overheat the blood. Any mixing of the blood should be gentle, as hemolysis of red cells is increased by mechanical stress. Because of the increased possibility that the blood plasma of the patient with chronic illness may contain cold agglutinins, when being transfused with cold blood he or she should be observed carefully and frequently for symptoms indicating hemolysis of cells. Hemolysis may result from the action of cold agglutinins in the serum of the donor on the red cells of the recipient or from the action of cold agglutinins in the serum of the recipient on the red cells of the donor.

Besides the antigens and antibody systems just presented, there are other rare antigens that may be present in erythrocytes. In certain diseases, such as hemolytic anemia, the red cells of the person become sensitized to an antibody in his or her own serum. The cells of these patients, as well as those of persons who are Rh-negative and who have been sensitized to the Rh factor, react with Coombs's serum. Coombs's serum is prepared from the serum of rabbits exposed to human globulin. The rabbit serum then contains antibodies that will react with any human antibodies that are globulins. If the human red blood cells have any antibodies attached to them, the antihuman globulin will cause the red cells to agglutinate. Because Coombs's serum reacts only with the red blood cells that are sensitized in the living organism, and have antibodies (globulin) attached to their red blood cells, the test is useful in determining the presence of hemolyzing antibodies in the blood serum of the patient. One of the important uses of the Coombs's test is in determining the presence of antibodies against the Rh factor in a person with Rh-negative blood. When the test is performed by treating blood cells from the individual with Coombs's serum, it is called a direct Coombs's test. In the indirect Coombs's test known cells are exposed to the patient's serum in order to identify antibodies in the patient's serum.

Second in importance to the discovery of blood groups was that sodium citrate was safe in certain circumstances and could be used to prevent the clotting of blood. The citrate ion combines with the calcium ion. Ionized calcium is necessary for the clotting of the blood. Before this discovery, blood had to be transferred immediately from one person to another, usually by direct transfusion. When sodium citrate is added to blood, it prevents blood clotting and simplifies the transfer of the blood from the donor to the recipient. A more recent innovation, the development of methods for the refrigeration and storage of blood, has made even greater delay possible. Because the life span of erythrocytes is from 100 to 120 days, the oxygen-carrying capacity of blood continues for some time. However, blood that is 3 weeks old or older is considered to be too old. Progress is being made in preserving the viability and oxygen carrying capability of RBCs which have been frozen and stored at −80°C for up to 10 years. However, the process is expensive and not widely available (Chaplin, 1978). White blood cells and platelets die within a few hours after blood is drawn. Therefore, when their action is desired, the blood must be freshly drawn. Freshly drawn blood can be used to restore any of the elements of the blood. Stored blood is satisfactory for restoring the blood volume, erythrocytes, and the blood proteins, but it is of no value in the replacement of platelets or leukocytes.

Blood and Blood Components

Supply and Demand

Increases in the number of elective surgical procedures on high-risk patients, the number of dramatic and aggressive procedures requiring large volumes of intraoperative blood, the incidence of accidents requiring surgical treatment with replacement therapy, and the persistence of warfare have increased the demand for blood and its components during the past decade. It has been estimated that the nation's need for blood would be met if 7 per cent of the eligible population contributed each year (Allen, 1971), but that is not the case. At present, only 3 to 4 per cent of eligible donors contribute (Isler, 1973). Where, then, does the necessary blood come from and how is it obtained? Because too few people donate their blood, more and more has to be purchased. In addition to the cost and the possibility of the price rising greatly, blood that is purchased from a commercial agency is much less reliable than donated blood; people who sell their blood are more likely to misrepresent their medical histories. Blood-borne diseases for which there is no ready method of identification include hepatitis and malaria. The protection of the patient depends on the honesty of the potential donor in admitting he or she has had either or both of these diseases.

Blood is obtained by two types of agencies; one is voluntary and the other commercial. Voluntary agencies include the Red Cross, hospital blood banks, and community blood banks. Commercial blood banks, located in large cities, collect, process, and distribute blood for the purpose of making a profit. They depend on paid donors for blood, and the risk that the blood will carry organisms of one or more of the blood-borne diseases is therefore greater. Some authorities feel that the only way to reduce the increasing incidence of post-transfusional hepatitis is to devise a strong federally licensed blood program to provide quality blood. Nursing has begun to speak out against the existence of commercial blood banks, spurred by the increasing incidence of hepatitis in nurses who work with transfusion therapy (Commercial Blood Banks, 1979). But unless individual citizens are ultimately to be conscripted as donors, the power of persuasion and motivation will continue to be the most influential factor in continuing efforts to maintain a supply equal to our growing need for blood. Multiple factors, mostly psychological and cultural, account for the failure of people to donate blood in proportion to the need and their capacity to give. In some communities two or more agencies may work cooperatively or vie with each other to collect blood from willing and available donors. The Red Cross is the largest single agency collecting blood, but it does not have centers in some communities and does not completely fill the need in others.

Many persons who have not donated blood hesitate to do so because they fear the consequences to themselves or the unpleasantness of the procedure. There are altruistic and selfish reasons for donating blood. There is no more personal way of helping one's fellow human being than by donating blood. Many voluntary agencies encourage individuals to donate blood by promising that should they or a member of their families need blood within a specified period of time, it will be available. In terms of safety, a healthy person who is between the ages of 18 and 59 can give blood every 8 to 10 weeks for an indefinite period of time without his or her health being threatened.[3]

Giving blood is not a status-giving activity. In factories, proportionately more blood is donated by the workers on the assembly line than by union stewards or office personnel, and the executive class gives least of all. Because blood for transfusion is essential to save lives, nurses have a responsibility to help to interpret to the public why it is needed and why the donation of blood is safe and is a source of satisfaction to the donor.

Therapeutic Uses of Blood

The uses of blood transfusion, whatever the nature of the patient's illness, can be summarized as follows:

1. To restore blood volume
2. To restore red blood cells
3. To provide platelets or other factors important in clotting
4. To provide protein and/or other nutritive elements

Of the preceding, the first two are the most common purposes of blood transfusion. The need for either may arise out of conditions that are treated medically or surgically. In addition, blood transfusion makes certain forms of treatment possible. Many surgical procedures could not be performed today were it not for the availability of human blood and the ability to transfuse it safely. Many patients undergoing prolonged surgical procedures require from 2 to 10 pints or more of blood to maintain an adequate blood volume and oxygen-carrying capacity. The more extended the operation and the greater the loss of blood, the more blood is needed. Some surgical procedures could not be started without blood. Although the newer types of pumps used in heart surgery require little or no blood for priming, a large quantity of blood may be used before the procedure is completed. As much as 500 to 700 ml of blood are required to prime an artificial kidney. Some treatments such as total-body irradiation could not be performed were it not for the ability to replace the cellular elements of the blood. In the seriously undernourished patient, blood is sometimes administered for its nutritive value. For example, each pint of blood contains approximately 35 g of protein in the form of plasma protein. Cellular elements are further sources of protein and other nutrients.

Additional information about blood and blood components—including indications for their use, modes of action, storage conditions, and resulting therapeutic life span, and side effects—is summarized in Table 52-2.

Hazards of Administration

Despite the frequency with which blood and its components are transfused, transfusions are always attended by the possibility of a serious complication. The dangers may result from (1) transmission of blood-borne diseases, (2) transfusion of incompatible or contaminated blood, and (3) too rapid infusion of blood into the individual. Under appropriate circumstances all of the above can be life threatening. The incidence of morbidity and mortality associated with transfusion is of great concern. In the United States alone some 3,000 persons die each year as a consequence of transfusion. Serum hepatitis, the major cause of death, kills 12 per cent of the victims, followed in frequency by hemolytic transfusion reactions. (Baker & Nyhus, 1970). Reports of the inci-

[3] The Red Cross has a well-organized plan for blood donors. They accept as a donor any healthy adult 18 through 60 years of age who weighs at least 110 lb. Those under 21 years of age must have written consent of a parent or guardian, unless they are married. Unmarried minors may be donors without written consent of a parent or guardian if they are living away from home and are self-supporting or if they are members of the armed services. Donors are allowed to give whole blood every 8 weeks but not more than five times in a calendar year. With the advent of plasmaphoresis, a process through which plasma is removed and cells returned to the donor, eligible donors may be allowed to contribute more frequently.

TABLE 52-2 *Blood Products and Uses**

	Indication(s)	Action(s)	Storage	How Long Usable	Side Effect(s)
Whole Blood and Cellular Products					
Whole blood	Acute hemorrhage (loss of more than 1 liter), hypovolemic shock; should be given only for the above indications	Restores blood volume, raises hematocrit level (oxygen-carrying capacity of the blood)	At 4°C with ACD or CPD†	21 days	Hives, chills, temperature elevation, shortness of breath, back pain; congestive heart failure; shock, if serious anaphylactic reaction
Red blood cells, packed	Acute anemia with hypoxia, aplastic anemia, some chronic anemias, bone marrow failure from malignancy	Elevates hematocrit, O_2-carrying capacity	At 4°C with ACD or CPD†	21 days in original container; 24 hours if container is opened	Same as above (RBC antigenicity same)
Red blood cells, frozen	As above; preferable for pre- or post-transplant patients (to prevent sensitization); or for patients sensitized by previous transfusions	As above	At −65°C to −95°C with glycerol added	Two years (24 hours after thawing)	Less likely to cause WBC antigenic reaction because RBC thawed, washed, antigens removed before administration
White blood cells (leukocytes)	Used experimentally in severe leukopenia with infection or threatened infection, research	Raises leukocyte level	Not stored	Given as soon as collected	Elevated temperature; may develop graft-vs.-host disease
Platelet concentrate (not used in idiopathic thrombocytopenic purpura [ITP] nor in disseminated intravascular coagulation)	Severe platelet deficiency (thrombocytopenia), bleeding in thrombocytopenic patients (as acute leukemia) if count below 10,000 platelets per cu mm blood	Raises platelet count, produces hemostasis in bleeding patient by aiding clot formation	Incubator at room temperature, continuous rotation	48 hours	Patient may develop antibodies and destroy platelets in subsequent transfusions; fever, chills, hives not uncommon

(Continued)

TABLE 52-2 *(Continued)*

	Indication(s)	Action(s)	Storage	How Long Usable	Side Effect(s)
Single-Donor Plasma					
Fresh plasma	Clotting deficiency when concentrates are not available or clotting factor deficiency has not been fully diagnosed, shock	Elevates low clotting-factor level; in shock, expands blood volume	Not stored	Given within 6 hours of collection	Rare; congestive heart failure
Plasma removed from whole blood up to 5 days after 21-day expiration date	Shock due to loss of plasma, burns, peritoneal injury, hemorrhage; while awaiting blood cross-matching	Expands blood volume	At 15°C to 30°C	3 years	Rare; as above
Fresh-frozen plasma	Clotting factor deficiency when specific concentrate unavailable or exact factor deficiency undiagnosed, shock	Produces hemostasis in bleeding patient, raises level of deficient clotting factor	At −18°C to −30°C, at −30°C or lower with ACD or CPD†	6 months, thawed just before use; 12 months with ACD or CPD†	Rare; as above
Other Plasma Products					
Cryoprecipitate‡ (contains factor VIII [AHG] concentrate)	Hemophilia patient during bleeding or at start of bleeding episode, preparation for surgery, preventively	Elevates low factor VIII level; prevents, controls bleeding in hemophilia patient	−18°C or below	12 months	Rare
Superconcentrate of factor VIII (AHG), lyophilized commercially prepared	As above	As above	Refrigerated	Manufacturer's dating period§	Rare
Factors II, VII, IX, X complex	Special clotting-factor deficiencies	Elevates low clotting-factor level, stops bleeding, allows surgery	5°C	As above	Hepatitis (from these plasma derivatives)
Fibrinogen (factor I)	Bleeding fibrinogen deficiency	Replaces lacking fibrinogen	5°C	5 years	As above

Albumin 5%, 25%	Used interchangeably in shock due to hemorrhage, trauma, infection, surgery, burns; prevention, treatment of cerebral edema	Restores blood volume, protein	At 2°C to 10°C At room temperature no warmer than 37°C	5 years 3 years	No hepatitis risk (products are heat-treated)
Plasma protein fraction (PPF)	As above	As above	Refrigerated At room temperature no warmer than 30°C	5 years 3 years	As above
Some Immunoglobulins‖					
Immune serum globulin	Agammaglobulinemia or hypogammaglobulinemia	Raises gamma globulin levels, produces passive temporary immunity to infectious hepatitis, poliomyelitis, similar infections	5°C	3 years	Rare
Tetanus immune globulin	Nonimmunized patient at risk of tetanus	Provides temporary immunity	5°C	1 year	Rare
Pertussis§ immune globulin	Exposure to pertussis, clinical symptoms of pertussis	Provides temporary immunity, combats the disease	5°C	3 years from date placed in solution	Rare
Mumps immune globulin	Exposure to mumps, clinical symptoms of mumps	Provides temporary immunity, combats the disease	5°C	Same as above	Rare
Measles immune globulin	Exposure to measles, modification of measles	Provides temporary immunity	5°C	3 years	Rare

* From "Blood: The Age of Components," by Charlotte Isler in RN magazine for June 1973. Copyright © 1973 by Medical Economics Company, Oradell, N.J. 07649. Used with permission.

† Acid citrate dextrose or citrate phosphate dextrose.

‡ Cold-insoluble part of plasma left after thawing of fresh frozen plasma.

§ Follow manufacturer's instructions.

‖ All immune serum globulins are given IM. The specific immunoglobulins are made commercially from gamma globulin of persons hyperimmunized to certain bacterial or viral diseases.

dence of nonfatal reaction to transfused substances vary between 2 and 10 per cent of all recipients. *Immediate reactions* are those that occur during, immediately after, or up to 96 hours after transfusion. Immediate reactions result primarily from transfusion of incompatible or contaminated blood and too rapid infusion. *Delayed reactions* may develop from 10 to 120 days after the last transfusion and result primarily from disease transmission and sensitization to previous transfusion (Baker & Nyhus, 1970). The danger of immediate and delayed reactions is present in every blood transfusion. The fact that the incidence of reactions is as low as it is serves as a tribute to the care that is taken from the moment the blood is taken from a donor until it is infused into a recipient.

Procedures for Safe Administration

To make sure that the patient receives properly matched blood, hospitals have rules regulating the collection and labeling of blood, the removal of blood from the blood bank, and the identification of the patient who is to receive the blood. All of these regulations are for the purpose of protecting patients from receiving mismatched blood. They should be meticulously followed.

All labels for blood taken from a patient for typing and cross matching should include the full name of the patient, diagnosis, the name of the physician, and the hospital or clinic number. This information should be printed or written legibly. The possibility always exists that two patients with identical names and diagnoses may be present in the hospital at the same time. An added precaution to the complete labeling of all slips is to have the slips made at the bedside at the time the blood is drawn. In some hospitals only the physician is allowed to remove blood from the blood bank. As a further precaution, only one unit may be removed at a time. Blood taken from the blood bank should be labeled with the names of the patient and the donor, the date the blood was drawn, the blood group, and the hospital where the blood is to be administered. The safety of the patient depends on all persons paying strict attention to details, so that unsafe acts are prevented.

Infusions of blood are frequently administered by a "double setup." One tube is attached to the bottle of blood and another to a bottle of physiological saline or glucose in water solution. The two tubes join leading to the patient by means of a Y tube. The flow of blood or fluid into the patient can be regulated by opening or closing the tubing leading from one or the other of the bottles, or by regulating the level at which each bottle is hanging. If glucose is to follow a transfusion, the tubing should first be rinsed with saline to prevent blood clotting.

Because of the possibility of reactions and the need for prompt action to prevent or minimize disability or death as a consequence of reactions, any person receiving a transfusion must be under close surveillance of a nurse or physician.

Causes of a Transfusion Reaction

Transmission of Disease

Of the diseases that may be transmitted through blood transfusions, those that are of the greatest concern are syphilis, malaria, and homologous serum jaundice (serum hepatitis). Persons who have syphilis can be identified by one of a number of serologic tests. Each of these tests is named after the man who originated it (Kline, Kahn, and Hinton). These tests depend on the presence of an antibodylike substance (sometimes called reagin) in the blood serum. It appears in the patient's blood serum soon after the onset of the disease. Those who have a history of having had malaria or who have been in a malarious area within a 2-month period are not used as blood donors.

Although persons having a history of jaundice are not used as blood donors, a person can have hepatitis without apparent jaundice and thus be unaware that he or she can transfer hepatitis virus when his or her blood is transfused into a recipient. In the United States, hepatitis is probably the most common disease to be transmitted by transfusion. Because of the possibility of serum hepatitis, some physicians avoid the administration of blood unless it is absolutely essential. It was hoped that use of frozen RBCs would prevent posttransfusion hepatitis, but Alter and his associates (1978) found that hepatitis is transmitted in frozen blood. Serum hepatitis may develop up to 120 days after transfusion and is associated with a high mortality and morbidity rate. For example, 4 months ago Mrs. Seven was delivered by cesarean section of a 6-lb baby boy. She required a blood transfusion. Two months after delivery she became ill. Because she was acutely ill and jaundiced, she was admitted to the hospital for diagnosis. Although her progress was satisfactory, she had to spend 6 weeks in the hospital. Until there are methods of identifying carriers of the virus that produces jaundice, this condition will remain one of the major risks that occur with the transfusion of blood.

Because blood is pooled in the preparation of plasma, plasma is more likely to be contaminated with the virus of hepatitis than is whole blood. Storage of plasma at room temperature for 6 months usually removes any risk that hepatitis will be transmitted by the plasma.

Infusion of Incompatible Blood and Platelets

A second danger is the infusion of incompatible blood, which results in the agglutination and hemolysis of the erythrocytes of the donor by isoagglutinins in the blood plasma of the recipient. Should the blood plasma of the donor have a high titer of isoagglutinins, the erythrocytes of the recipient can also be agglutinated. Such cells tend to be hemolyzed more readily than normal. Signs and symptoms are caused by the blocking of blood vessels by agglutinated cells or hemolysis of cells. Oliguria or anuria may be caused by a blocking of the renal tubules by hematin that is released on hemolysis of red cells and/or reduced blood flow through the kidney.

Because platelets are harder to match than red blood cells, there is a high incidence, in persons receiving multiple transfusions, of developing antibodies against the foreign platelets if they are not of the same type as the recipients'. Immunosuppression may be required if the person's need for platelets is persistent (Zucker, 1980, pp. 96–99). See Chapter 24 for discussion of homotransplantation and immunosuppression.

Allergic and Febrile Response

These two frequent types of reaction to transfusion are thought to be variations of the same problem, caused by unidentified antigens from the donor or the transfusion equipment reacting with recipient antibodies. Persons who have had an allergic reaction to previous transfusion have a 60 to 65 per cent chance of having another allergic reaction with subsequent transfusions, and should be watched even more closely than usual (Baker & Nyhus, 1970, p. 669).

Rate and Volume of Infusion

Too much blood or blood given too rapidly may cause heart failure, which may be severe enough to produce pulmonary edema. Judgment as to the rate at which blood is to be administered is the responsibility of the physician. At times, when a large volume of blood has been lost in a short period of time, the life of the patient may depend on blood volume being restored rapidly. Almost continuous monitoring of the central venous pressure is vital in such patients. In other instances, blood must be administered slowly to protect the circulation from overload. Occasionally, when danger of overload is especially great, most of the plasma is removed and only the packed red blood cells are transfused.

An exchange volume of 5 liters within 12 hours or less may cause some of the following alterations that accompany massive transfusion: (1) acidosis, resulting partly from the acidifying action of acid citrate dextrose (ACD) solution used for blood storage; (2) hypothermia, induced by infusion of large amounts of blood at refrigerator temperature;[4] (3) citrate overload, which induces deficits in ionized calcium, possibly resulting in congestive heart failure, with increased central venous pressure, slowed heart rate, and arrhythmia; (4) hyperkalemia, resulting from the leaching of potassium from red cells after 3 or more days of blood storage; and (5) dilutional coagulation defects, related to decrease in platelets and factors V and VII.

Responsibility of the Nurse in Transfusion Therapy

The nurse's responsibility for transfusion therapy begins during the preoperative period, when she or he gathers baseline assessment data about the circulatory status of the patient. This information, combined with knowledge of the proposed surgical procedure and the patient's actual blood loss, will allow the nurse to anticipate if and when transfusion is likely. The nurse should be certain that the patient is typed and cross-matched and has had a hemoglobin determination, with reports in the record, before he or she is transported to the operating room to undergo *any* surgical procedure. It is *mandatory* that all personnel involved in any aspect of transfusion therapy know the institutional policies and procedures for obtaining, monitoring, and reporting the effects of transfusable substances, as the resulting consistency and efficiency of action may be life-saving for the patient.

Table 52-3 summarizes information about the incidence, evidence, and management of the three most common types of immediate transfusion reaction. No reference is made in the table to the equally important observation and nursing management of the patient related to the fact that he or she is receiving a transfusion, regardless of whether or not a reaction develops. Especially when the transfusion is whole blood, both patient and visitors tend to associate "blood" with "life" and to assume that the patient's condition is critical. The nurse must provide opportunity for fears to the expressed and for questions to be asked and answered as fully and diplomatically as possible, and the nurse must convey by frequent presence and touch that she or he understands and respects their fears and can be relied upon to guide the patient through this often disturbing treatment. Frequently, in the process of starting or chang-

[4] Thirty-three calories of heat are required to warm 1,000 ml of blood from 4°C refrigerator temperature to 37°C. In the seriously ill patient, this increase in metabolic rate may result in tissue hypoxia, and the direct effect of cold on the myocardium may result in ventricular fibrillation.

TABLE 52-3 ***Incidence, Evidence, and Management of Three Most Common Types of Immediate Transfusion Reaction***

Type of Reaction	Incidence*	Nursing Observations	Management
Allergic	45%	*Common* Fever as high as 103°F Chills Itching Erythema Urticaria Nausea/vomiting *Rare* Headache Dyspnea Stridor Wheezing	1. Stop the transfusion, notify physician to assess cause. 2. IV administration of antihistamines. 3. Occasionally, administration of epinephrine or steroids. 4. Measures to reduce fever. (See Chapter 37.) 5. Send *stat.* urine specimen for analysis; continue to measure and observe urine output. 6. Send remaining blood to blood bank to analyze for incompatibility and bacterial contamination; attach report of reaction. 7. Have fresh sample of recipient blood drawn and send to blood bank (or laboratory) for analysis.
Febrile	43.7%	Sudden onset of fever, or chills and fever	Same as for allergic reaction
Hemolytic	10.2%	Chills and fever, early in transfusion	Measures 1, 5, 6, and 7 above.
		Sensation of burning of the face Tachycardia Nausea and vomiting Pain in chest, flank, or back Dyspnea Apprehension, feeling of impending doom Severe hypotension, or shock Spontaneous unexpected diffuse bleeding Icterus Hemoglobinuria and/or anuria	8. IV administration of osmotic diuretic in a water load of dextrose or Ringer's lactate, often with $NaHCO_3$ and hydrocortisone. 9. IV administration of vasopressors for hypotension. (See Chapter 41 for treatment of renal failure.)

* Incidence of reactions is based upon results of a 7-year study of 131,614 units of blood and various blood components infused into 47,909 recipients. One hundred per cent of observed reactions developed in 5.19 per cent of patients transfused. (Robert J. Baker and Lloyd M. Nyhus: "Diagnosis and treatment of immediate transfusion reaction." *Surg. Gynecol. Obstet.*, **130:** 665–72 (April 1970) 665.

ing a transfusion, blood splashes on the bedding or the patient. One of the most effective measures to convey respect and concern for the patient's comfort is to wash and change the linen promptly; the sight of one's own blood replacement all over the bedding is a most disconcerting reminder of one's tenuous hold on life. Also, patients tend to hold themselves rigid while being transfused. Care should be taken to move and reposition them frequently.

In addition to making the patient physically and psychologically as comfortable as possible during transfusion, it is the nurse's responsibility to make the observations that would yield the signs and symptoms elaborated in Table 52-3. Should any of those signs and symptoms occur, blood flow should be terminated and the physician notified immediately to assess the patient. As indicated under "Nursing Observations," one of the earliest and most sensitive indicators of reaction is an elevated temperature. Therefore it is advisable to monitor this parameter before and at intervals during a transfusion.[5]

Summary

By virtue of the nature of surgical treatment, the patient almost always loses some blood. The signifi-

[5] See the continuing education feature on Blood Therapy in the *American Journal of Nursing,* May 1979, for an excellent presentation of nursing involvement in all aspects of blood therapy.

cance of the bleeding, in terms of its threat to the survival of the patient, depends on the degree to which the circulation to the cells is maintained. Although shock can and does exist in the absence of blood loss, hemorrhage increases the ease with which a patient may go into shock from any cause. Effective nursing care of the patient treated surgically requires that the nurse have (1) a working knowledge of the causes, manifestations, and management of shock and hemorrhage and (2) an understanding of and skill in applying appropriate nursing measures related to hemostasis and transfusion therapy.

Surgery and Renal Function

The critical importance of the kidney in maintaining the composition and distribution of body fluids is documented in Chapter 27, and its participation in body defenses against and responses to injury is described in Unit V. All surgical procedures inflict some degree of injury on the body; consequently, the monitoring and maintaining of renal function are always important considerations in care of the surgical patient.

In the period immediately following surgery, or a traumatic injury, the formation of urine by the kidney is depressed. Oliguria is generally believed to be caused by an increase in the production of the antidiuretic hormone (ADH) by the posterior pituitary gland. Accompanying the retention of water is sodium retention, which may be the result of an increase in the production of the adrenocortical steroids. Because of this tendency to retain salt and water after injury (surgery), the urine output of the patient is likely to be decreased below normal levels for periods varying from 12 hours to several days, depending upon extent of response and nature of concurrent fluid replacement and diuretic administration. Following routine abdominal procedures, patients will usually have a decrease in glomerular filtration rate (GFR) of 20 to 30 per cent on the first postoperative day, which returns to preoperative values over a 4-day period (Stahl & Stone, 1970). This oliguria may be prevented to a certain extent by infusion of adequate amounts of fluid before, during, and after surgery. Following a period of oliguria, the patient may have a period of diuresis. In patients who have been in severe shock for an extended period of time, oliguria or even anuria may continue for days or even weeks. Unless the fluid intake of the patient with renal failure is balanced against the fluid output, he or she may die from overloading with water. Because of the possibility of continued suppression of urine following surgery, the accurate measurement and recording of the urine output and the fluid intake for the first days following surgery are of great importance. Measurement of the specific gravity and/or osmolality of the urine is also important. Small quantities of urine with a high specific gravity are usually indicative of dehydration, hypovolemia, and/or poor renal perfusion. If the specific gravity is low, the diagnosis is more difficult and the oliguria may be at least partially related to renal disease or failure. Acute renal failure in general surgical patients is most often due to hypotension and sepsis. Occasionally acute renal failure is preceded by high urine output in some patients who respond to massive trauma and sepsis with an obligatory water loss followed by circulatory collapse and renal failure if fluid replacement is not adquate (Gupta et al., 1971).

Urinary Retention

In addition to the possibility of oliguria or anuria, a considerable number of patients experience retention of urine; that is, they are unable to void during the early postoperative period. Retention of urine can be a troublesome condition. Regardless of the cause of urinary retention, its early detection is indispensable to prevent overdistention and possible subsequent injury to the bladder. Early detection requires that the nurse use objective, as well as subjective, evidence. In the immediate postoperative period it is essential to know the surgical procedure performed, how long it lasted, at what time it was completed; estimated blood loss and total fluid replacement; any medications received during or after surgery that might affect renal or bladder function; composition and absorption rate of current infusions; and composition, route, and volume of any fluid intake other than intravenous infusions since surgery. This information is evaluated in relation to the timing, volume, and character of all urine output since surgery; urine that drained from an indwelling catheter in place during surgery should be considered. If *total intake* is greatly in excess of *total output* since the operative period, and the patient has no significant fluid deficit to make up as a result of the operation , is not sweating profusely, and shows no signs of circulatory overloading, there is a distinct possibility of urinary retention. Although the postoperative adult patient whose bladder contains more than a few hundred milliliters of urine often complains of discomfort, urgency, or frequency, there are many individuals who do not experience or report these symptoms when they have a full bladder. Therefore it is imperative that the nurse educate her or his fingers to detect by palpation the feel of a full bladder against the abdominal wall, directly above the symphysis pubis bone. As soon as the patient is returned from the operating suite, initial observations should include palpation for the bladder, to obtain a baseline with which to compare subsequent palpations. Finally, frequent voiding of small amounts of urine may be indicative of retention with overflow.

The consequences of unrelieved distention of the urinary bladder are due to the resultant overstretching of the mucosa, which predisposes to breaks in its continuity and diminished blood supply to the wall of the bladder. Both disorders predispose to infection of the urinary bladder. This applies especially to patients who are catheterized for retention with overflow. The overstretching of the muscle wall may also delay the return of normal function. Also, sustained distention of the bladder predisposes to the reflux of urine into the ureters, with the possibility of distention and infection of the ureters and even of the kidney itself.

Many circumstances can lead to the relatively common problem of urinary retention: obstructions in the bladder or urethra, primary neurologic disease, acute illness with secondary impairment of neurologic function, and frequently as a complication of childbirth. But probably the most frequent cause of retention is surgery. With surgery in the region of the bladder, such as gynecologic surgery, or in operations on the large bowel or rectum, the mechanical trauma of the procedure frequently results in temporary depression of the patient's ability to empty the bladder.

Another cause of urinary retention is that some patients cannot void in bed. The position is abnormal and psychological conditioning against it may be very strong. In surgical patients the frequency of urinary retention has been reduced by early ambulation. Patients not yet allowed to ambulate may be assisted to stand beside the bed (for men) or to use a beside commode. Before considering whether to obtain medical permission for the patient to be out of bed to void, the nurse must carefully evaluate the possible hazards from such factors as location and status of the incision, drainage tubes, dressings, infusions, and the probability of severe orthostatic hypotension, which will subject the patient to the danger of falling. (See discussion of orthostatic hypotension later in this chapter.)

Whether the patient is in bed, on a bedside commode, or in the bathroom, there are a number of nursing measures to help the patient to induce voiding. Because tenseness of the patient aggravates the problem, the approach to the patient should be relaxed and the patient protected from anxiety-provoking situations. A screen around the bed or in front of the door will help to shield the patient from unexpected visitors. A warm bedpan is a necessity. Relaxation is sometimes encouraged by placing the feet of the patient in warm water. Suggestion sometimes works. Water is allowed to run from the tap, or warm water is poured over the vulva of a woman. When the bladder is not overly full, the patient may be urged to try to void and, if not able, to try at a later time. One thing to be avoided is to encourage the patient to try too hard, as he or she then becomes overly tense and is unable to relax the sphincters in the urethra. Sometimes gentle manual pressure at the rim of the symphysis pubis, over the fundus of the bladder, will assist in starting the stream of urine.

Catheterization for the Treatment of Urinary Retention

When other measures are ineffective in encouraging the patient to void, or the nature of the surgical procedure is such that the bladder should not be allowed to become distended, catheterization may become necessary. When catheterization is required, it must be prescribed by the physician, who makes the decision about whether the patient is to be catheterized when the bladder is full, at regular intervals, or whether an indwelling catheter be inserted. Two objectives should guide the nurse in preparations for, and performance of, catheterization. The first is to remove urine from the bladder. The second is no less important than the first and is more difficult to achieve—to prevent infection of the urinary tract. The two types of procedures most commonly associated with bacteremia are catheterization of the urinary bladder and intravenous infusion (Smith, 1979). Both types of procedures are frequently performed in care of the surgical patient.

To prevent infection as a consequence of catheterization, all equipment and materials should be sterile, the procedure itself should be clean, and trauma to urethra and bladder avoided. The danger of trauma to the bladder and urethra by the catheter can be lessened by using the smallest possible catheter, lubricating it well, and encouraging the patient to relax. The lubricant lessens friction by preventing the catheter from coming in direct contact with the wall of the urethra. Relaxation can usually be achieved by asking the patient to take a deep breath at the moment the catheter is introduced. The patient should have been prepared for what to expect and should be adequately covered, so that his or her modesty pattern is observed. Should an obstruction to the passage of the catheter be encountered, the catheter should not be forced. It will usually slip into the bladder if the pressure on the catheter is reduced and the patient is asked to take a deep breath. When the catheter is in place, it must be held there, as the pressure of the urine in the bladder is likely to carry it out. Should the catheter escape from the urethra, another sterile catheter must be introduced.

To minimize the number of microorganisms introduced into the bladder, a number of precautions should be taken. The catheter should be sterile and well lubricated with sterile, and possibly antibacterial, lubricant. Cleansing of the area around the urethral meatus should be done with a bacteriostatic agent, applied with sterile cotton balls or sponges held either with a sterile forcep or hemostat, or in a sterile gloved hand. Whatever technique and equipment are used, thorough hand washing must precede the entire procedure. Most hospitals are now using prepackaged sterile disposable catheterization sets, in which all materials, except possibly the cleansing solution, are included. Directions for use are always provided and should be carefully read.

To expose the meatus adequately, the female patient should be in the recumbent position, with the knees flexed and the legs separated. A good light placed to illuminate the area is essential. Unless the patient is in a position that permits adequate exposure of the meatus, the nurse cannot see what she or he is doing, the catheter is likely to be contaminated before it is introduced, and urethral trauma is more difficult to prevent. If the catheter becomes contaminated before it is introduced, another sterile catheter should be obtained.

Unnecessary discomfort to the patient should be prevented. In patients who have surgery on the perineum, exposure of the meatus may be painful. This discomfort can be minimized by preparing the patient for what to expect and by assuring the patient that every effort will be made to handle the tissues with gentleness. When the patient to be catheterized is a male, the female nurse should still provide the same instruction and precautions for him as she does for a female patient. In relation to the procedure itself, she is responsible for setting up the equipment and obtaining a physician, a nurse, or a qualified male attendant to catheterize the patient. Catheterization can usually be performed with a minimum of distress to the patient. Time must be taken to prepare the patient for what to expect and for what he or she can do to assist the nurse. Another precaution is that urine should not be drained off too fast from a greatly distended bladder. Regardless of how long it takes to drain the urine, the nurse must *remain with the patient* to observe closely the patient's response, and to prevent the catheter from being expelled by the pressure of the remaining urine in the bladder.

Care of an Indwelling Catheter

When an indwelling catheter is left in place, attention should be given to the maintenance of continuous free drainage. The tubing should be free of kinks, twists, or bends, and from pressure of resting body parts. It should be arranged so that the urine flows downhill into the drainage bottle. A sterile closed drainage system with an antiseptic added to the collecting container should be used. Disposable collecting systems are available and are safer and more convenient than glass bottles. A rigid portable collecting container should be used for ambulatory patients. The tubing leading from the bladder should be below the level of the bladder but above the level of the urine. At no time should the collecting reservoir be elevated to the level of the bladder, even when the patient is ambulating; this precaution will prevent backflow into the bladder. Irrigation may be necessary to maintain patency of the catheter or, as previously mentioned, to remove soft clots from the bladder to prevent bleeding. One way to irrigate the catheter that eliminates the possibility of introducing microorganisms is to make sure that the patient has a fluid intake sufficient to produce a urine flow rate of at least 50 ml per hour, thus preventing the upward migration of motile bacteria in the collection tubing. Because cranberry juice helps to keep the urine acid, it may be offered to patients who find it acceptable; acid urine inhibits bacterial growth. The physician may prescribe that the catheter be either irrigated at regular intervals to ensure its patency or irrigated as necessary to clear obstructing sediment or clots. The procedure must be carried out according to strict surgical aseptic principles. Because the probability of infection increases each time the closed drainage system is opened, provision for closed-system irrigation may be made by using a setup that incorporates a reservoir of sterile irrigating solution attached by a Y connecting tube to the drainage system, at the indwelling catheter.

Several recently reported studies on hospital infections all indicate that the most frequent site of infection is the urinary tract, accounting for more than one third of all hospital infections (Eickhoff, 1972). The present character of hospital infections suggests that the cause may be due primarily to factors that adversely affect host defense mechanisms. This is especially true of surgical patients, many of whom undergo complex and prolonged procedures when their defenses are so compromised that surgery would not even have been attempted in earlier decades. These high-risk patients frequently require indwelling urethral catheters to facilitate continuous accurate monitoring of renal function because of the increased possibility of prolonged postoperative oliguria or anuria. The catheter acts as a foreign body predisposing to infection by mechanical means. In addition, it provides a three-lane highway by which bacteria may travel to the bladder (Cleland et al, 1971): (1) bacteria can be pushed in by the catheter when it is first introduced into the bladder; (2) bacteria can move up the lumen of the catheter; and (3) bacteria can move up the space between the urethral wall and the catheter (periurethral route). Meticulous care in performing catheterization, as described previously, substantially blocks the first lane. Use of the second lane can be minimized by a fluid intake adequate to ensure continuous secretion of acid urine and by careful handling of the collection system to prevent reflux of urine into the bladder, as described previously. Nursing measures aimed at preventing contamination of the bladder from the third periurethral route consist of washing around the meatus and the proximal few inches of the visible catheter to remove mucoid secretions and exudate with a bacteriostatic agent such as hexachlorophene (pHisoHex)[6] soap solution, followed by conscientious washing and drying of the entire perineal area, in both men and women, with special attention to the perianal area, to be repeated at least twice daily. Whatever materials and technique are used, perineal care should be considered primarily as a means to prevent gross soiling and contamination of a patient's urinary catheter, and to promote the hygiene and comfort of the patient. In an experimental study of 184 female patients to determine the effectiveness of four types of perineal care in preventing bacteriuria after insertion of an indwelling catheter, Cleland and others (1971, p. 318) found that none of the four types of perineal care was any more effective in preventing bacteriuria than the patient's own efforts to administer self-care. Two factors that were of great concern were that none of the available closed-drainage-system products was mechanically dependable or properly used by patients or staff and that personnel with the least preparation cared for the drainage systems. Both of these factors must be addressed by responsible nursing leadership, in view of the fact that other controlled studies (Eickhoff, 1972, p. 33) have demonstrated that careful management of closed drainage from urinary tract catheters can effect a substantial reduction in urinary tract infection and subsequent gram-negative sepsis. Systemic broad-spectrum bactericidal agents such as kanamycin sulfate (Kantrex), acetyl sulfisoxazole (Gantrisin) and various nitrofurantoin (Furadantin) preparations are beneficial in preventing and treating bacteriuria, alone or in combination with acidifying agents such as methenamine mandelate (Mandelamine).

Prolonged presence of an indwelling catheter may affect muscle tone and competence of the internal sphincter to the point that restoration of normal voiding is difficult following removal of the catheter. After the catheter is removed, the quantity of each voiding should be measured accurately so that retention with overflow is detected should it occur.

[6] Hexachlorophene preparations are restricted to use with physician's prescription as the result of current FDA recommendations. Check with your hospital formulary or local pharmacist.

Summary

Urinary tract infection is a possibility in any patient who is subject to repeated catheterization or in whom the bladder is allowed to become overdistended or in whom urine is retained. Preventive measures include an adequate intake of fluids and prevention of overdistention of the bladder with urine. When catheterization is necessary, attention should be given to defend the drainage system's three portals of entry: the urethra and urethral meatus, the connection between the catheter and the tubing, and the end of the drainage tube. Trauma to the urethra and bladder should also be avoided. Drug therapy, although necessary and effective in controlling urinary tract infection, should not be considered a substitute for cleanliness and maintenance of effective drainage.

Surgery and Gastrointestinal Function

Usual Responses to General Anesthesia and Surgical Trauma

The gastrointestinal system is affected as greatly as the respiratory and cardiovascular–renal systems by events in the operative period. As emphasized earlier, the gastrointestinal tract is very sensitive to the state of health of an individual. Furthermore, the sympathoadrenal system, which is activated by the physical and psychological stress of surgery, depresses the activity of the alimentary canal. Some disturbance in the functioning of the alimentary canal is therefore to be expected in patients who have been anesthetized and have undergone surgical treatment. The effects are usually manifested as anorexia, nausea, and vomiting. These effects may persist for several hours or days. Because of the inactivity of the alimentary canal, bowel sounds are usually absent for at least several hours after general anesthesia.

In patients who have surgery on the gastrointestinal tract, function returns more slowly. It usually takes 2 or 3 days for the patient to be able to tolerate fluids and for the normal bowel sounds to appear. All the preceding effects are normal accompaniments of surgical treatment and do not constitute complications unless they are prolonged or unusually severe. To prevent overdistention of the bowel and to increase the comfort of the patient whose gastrointestinal functioning is expected to be slow in returning, nasogastric suction may be instituted. Because the responsibilities of the nurse in the care of the patient treated with nasogastric suction were discussed earlier in the chapter, they will not be repeated here. It is noteworthy that a group of surgeons (Hoshal et al., 1971) is sufficiently concerned about the complications of respiratory insufficiency, aspiration, infection, and nasopharyngeal inflammation that often attend use of nasogastric tubes that they have developed a "tubeless decompression" that relies on the presence of gastric and intestinal motility and postural mechanical drainage to keep the stomach decompressed postoperatively. An experimental study to test the effectiveness of tubeless decompression found fewer complications, earlier ambulation, less patient discomfort, and an average hospital stay 3 days shorter than for patients who had the conventional nasogastric tube in place for five postoperative days.

When nasogastric suction is used, and has been discontinued, the nurse observes for such symptoms as a feeling of fullness and nausea, which suggests that the gastrointestinal tract of the patient is not ready to tolerate fluids. As indicated earlier, developing abdominal distention can be detected early by measuring the abdomen with a tape measure.

When the bowel sounds are returning, but before water is tolerated, other fluids, such as ginger ale or a similar carbonated beverage, may be tried. Some patients find tea more acceptable than water or coffee. Dry crackers or toast may be better tolerated than fluids. Sitting the patient upright is sometimes helpful in preventing vomiting. Simple nursing procedures such as providing the patient with mouthwash after he or she vomits and emptying and washing the emesis basin promptly help to increase the comfort of the patient. Because suggestion sometimes plays a part in the continuance of vomiting, the emesis basin, although placed within easy reach, should be out of sight. When vomiting continues and there does not appear to be an organic basis for it, the physician may order a drug such as dimenhydrinate, U.S.P. (Dramamine), or chlorpromazine (Thorazine). Just as the character and amount of fluid removed in gastric suction should be observed and recorded, the characteristics of emesis such as odor, color, consistency, and the type or description of solid particles should be noted and recorded. Choking or a paroxysm of coughing during or after vomiting indicates the possibility of aspiration of vomitus. Evidence of aspiration should be reported to the physician. The circumstances under which the patient vomits are sometimes significant and should be observed. Should vomiting continue longer than is expected, a search should be made for its cause.

Because nausea and vomiting are frequent accompaniments of disease, by themselves these symptoms mean little more than that the patient is sick. Nausea and vomiting in the postsurgical patient can be caused by a great variety of disorders. These disorders may include idiosyncrasy to drugs, emotions, pain, shock, uremia, disturbances in water and electrolytes or acid-base balance. If the nausea and vomiting are persistent, it is more likely to be of serious surgical significance and is often associated with a physiological or mechanical obstruction somewhere along the alimentary canal.

Perhaps the simplest cause of vomiting in the postoperative patient is idiosyncrasy to a drug. An observant nurse may note that the vomiting occurred after the administration of a drug, such as morphine or meperidine hydrochloride. It is most severe soon after the drug is administered and recedes as the time for the next dose approaches.

Discomfort from gas pains following major surgery or trauma is not uncommon. Gas pains differ from vomiting in that they indicate that gastrointestinal function is returning but that its activity is not yet coordinated. Since the introduction of nasogastric suction and early ambulation, few patients have severe gas pains. When a patient does have severe gas pains, the insertion of a rectal tube or a small enema may provide relief. Both must be prescribed by the physician. The patient should be encouraged to be active and to walk. Because analgesic drugs such as morphine reduce the activity of the alimentary canal, they favor the development of gas pains. They should therefore be administered only as required to prevent pain in the postoperative patient.

Gastrointestinal Complications

Although disturbances in gastrointestinal function are more likely to be prolonged when a surgical procedure involves the gastrointestinal tract, peritoneum, or abdominal organs, they may follow any operative procedure. The three most serious gastrointestinal complications are acute gastric dilatation, paralytic ileus, and mechanical obstruction of the intestine. Both acute gastric dilatation and paralytic ileus may result from inadequate or abnormal peristalsis and/or abnormal swallowing of air. Obstruction may result from functional failure, or it may be the consequence of organic changes involving the wall of the digestive tube. Obstruction may occur soon after surgery or years later. Functional disturbances along the gastrointestinal tract tend to be self-perpetuating; that is, they act like a positive feedback system. As the motility of the digestive tube decreases, secretions and air accumulate, causing distention. Distension further inhibits motility. With the distention of the wall of the stomach or intestine, the wall thins and lessens the capacity of blood vessels to deliver blood. A vicious circle ensues: decreased motility → distention → thinning → decreased blood supply → decreased motility. When functional disturbances are accompanied by vomiting or the need for continued suction, they may also lead to hypovolemia and serious disturbances in water and electrolytes unless appropriate quantities of fluids and electrolytes are given intravenously.

Symptoms indicating that the function of the gastrointestinal tract is not returning as expected include (1) nausea and vomiting more than 12 to 24 hours after surgery (this may persist longer in patients having surgery on the gastrointestinal tract or in those with peritonitis), (2) distention of the abdomen, (3) pain in the abdomen (gas pain), (4) absent bowel sounds, and (5) evidence of obstruction on x-ray. High-pitched, tinkling bowel sounds often indicate a mechanical obstruction of the bowel. Postoperatively, this is usually caused by a poorly functioning anastomosis, adhesions, or a hernia.

Acute Gastric Dilatation

In the patient who develops an acute gastric dilatation, prodromal symptoms may include a feeling of fullness, hiccoughs, and retching. Overflow vomiting may also occur. The patient vomits small amounts of dark-colored, foul-smelling fluid. Gastric dilatation may develop rapidly and present a picture of acute shock. Unless the stomach is emptied and kept empty until function returns, death is a possibility. The nurse assists in the prevention of acute gastric dilatation by maintaining the function of the gastric suction apparatus and by regulating the amount of fluid that the patient ingests orally until the capacity of the gastrointestinal tract to tolerate fluids has been tested. The nurse also helps to prevent the gastric dilatation from becoming serious by reporting early signs and symptoms indicating that gastrointestinal function has not been reestablished.

Adynamic Ileus

Gastrointestinal activity is often greatly reduced or even paralyzed (ileus) after surgery, especially if the stomach, intestines, or colon was involved. Failure to keep this inactive bowel decompressed may result in distention of the abdomen with increased stress on the abdominal incision or impairment of respiration. The bowel that is extremely distended also tends to remain paralyzed for longer periods of time.

In adynamic ileus the motor activity of the gastrointestinal tract is not strong or coordinated enough to maintain normal peristalsis. As a result the normal bowel sounds do not return as expected. Loops of small and large intestine fill with gas, but neither gas nor feces are passed by rectum. Gastric suction and the insertion of a rectal tube may relieve the symptoms. When distention is not relieved by gastric suction, a long tube may be necessary to decompress the more distal small bowel. Efforts have been made to relieve paralytic ileus by administering alpha-sympatholytic drugs that have an alpha-adrenergic receptor blocking effect, intended to relieve the peristaltic reflex from the inhibitory effect of catecholamines. These drugs, in combination with the more traditional parasympathomimetics, such as neostigmine, have been reported effective in restoring peristalsis in patients suffering from paralytic ileus. An enema given when peristalsis is resumed seems to enhance the effects of the drugs (Petri et al., 1971).

Mechanical Obstruction

Prior to any attempt to relieve paralytic ileus with medication, it is imperative, and often difficult, to distinguish ileus from mechanical obstruction. As stated previously, the usual causes of postoperative mechanical obstruction are a poorly functioning anastomosis, adhesions, or a hernia. Early diagnosis and treatment of intestinal obstruction with fluids, decompression, and surgery are essential to patient survival (Stahlgren & Morris, 1977; Literte, 1977).

Fecal impaction may cause mechanical obstruction, although it does not usually cause difficulty during the first hours after surgery. Fecal impaction may result when barium is introduced into the alimentary canal and incompletely removed prior to surgery. As the water is absorbed from the barium, it forms a hard mass similar to a plaster cast. Barium impactions can usually be prevented by the removal of the barium within 1 to 2 days after the x-ray examination is completed. This can be accomplished by the administration of a mild laxative and/or cleansing enemas. Both of these must be prescribed by the physician. Identification of the need for such a prescription is a responsibility of the nurse. She or he should also be alert to signs and symptoms indicating that a barium impaction has been formed. Should the enema fail to remove the barium, this should be reported and recorded. Aged patients may also develop fecal impactions either following surgery or in the course of an illness. Symptoms that suggest the presence of an impaction include painful defecation, a feeling of fullness in the rectum, pain in the rectum, and constipation or a diarrhealike stool. A rectal examination reveals a hard mass that may have to be broken up before it can be passed.

To lessen the possibility of fecal impactions, some surgeons prescribe mineral oil for the patient the day before surgery and for a few days after gastrointestinal function is resumed. Some surgeons also prescribe an enema for the patient on the second or third day postsurgery or after there is evidence that gastrointestinal activity has resumed. Others do not believe that enemas are necessary. When enemas are given, the extent of their effectiveness should be reported. Especially in elderly patients, not only should the fact that feces were evacuated be noted but also the size of the stool should be described. Symptoms indicating the possible development of a fecal impaction should be reported and recorded.

Peritonitis

Although peritonitis is more appropriately considered with infections, the nurse's observation for and assistance with prevention of peritonitis is guided by knowing that peritonitis is caused by injuries or lesions of the gastrointestinal tract, as well as of the biliary system, pancreas, and genitourinary tract (Hau, 1979). Causes, manifestations, and management of peritonitis are detailed in Chapter 46.

Nutritional Status

As soon as the gastrointestinal tract begins to function normally, as evidenced by the presence of bowel sounds, absence of abdominal distention, and/or the passage of feces or gas per rectum, fluids and food may be ordered by the surgeon. The length of time that oral food and fluids are withheld varies with the nature of the surgical procedure, the type of anesthetic used, and the response of the patient. Usually patients having operations on the alimentary canal are not able to tolerate food as early as those having surgery on other parts of the body. When fluids are first administered, the volume may be restricted to 15 to 30 ml per hour and increased gradually to fluids as desired. Fluids should be discontinued and the physician notified if the patient vomits, becomes distended, or complains of a feeling of fullness. (See Chapter 46.)

When a patient was reasonably healthy before surgery, the appetite can be expected to return within a few days. Except in those patients who have special requirements, patients are returned to a full diet as soon as they are able to tolerate it. Patients having surgery on the stomach usually require some reduction in the volume of food eaten at one time. The consistency may also be modified by reducing the amount of roughage contained in it. The objectives are to prevent distention of the stomach with strain on the sutures and to meet the nutritional requirements of the patient. Thus the patient is fed four to six small meals each day. Foods having a high cellulose content, such as cabbage and cucumbers, are eliminated. All patients require an adequate intake of protein and vitamin C.

Operations on the gastrointestinal tract, particularly on the small bowel, pose grave postoperative nutritional problems of glucose, nitrogen, potassium, and fluid balance. For as long as 3 weeks after the operation, patients who undergo extensive small bowel resection may experience severe diarrhea. Provided the terminal ileum and ileocecal valve are retained, good nutrition can be maintained by hyperalimentation following resection of up to 70 per cent of the small bowel. In the absence of the cecum and ileocecal valve, nutrition may be impaired with resection of even 50 to 60 per cent of the small bowel (Shires & Canizoro, 1979). An added burden of the postoperative nutritional requirements of at least 20 per cent of patients having small bowel resection is the development of such wound complications as infection, fistulas, dehiscence, and cellulitis (Storer, 1979). As indicated in the discussion of nutritional problems in Chapter 46, hyperalimentation feedings may be administered orally, by nasogastric or gastrostomy tube, or parenterally.

Parenteral hyperalimentation was pioneered in 1966 by Dr. Stanley Dudrick in an attempt to deal with postoperative malnutrition as a cause of death following otherwise successful operations. It has been estimated that at least 10 per cent of all hospital deaths are attributable to malnutrition and another 30 per cent are due in part to insufficient nourishment. In 1978, Dr. Dudrick estimated that only 5 to 10 percent of hospitals actually used parenteral hyperalimentation regularly, despite widespread awareness of the technique (Life Jacket, 1978). However, as prepared solutions and improved techniques are developing to control the infection and circulatory complications, use of intravenous hyperalimentation is becoming more widespread. As frequently happens when a new medical modality is introduced into hospital practice, it has been followed by a new technical specialist role for the nurse—"hyperalimentation nurse." Nursing responsibilities in caring for a person receiving intravenous hyperalimentation are discussed in detail in Chapter 46.

Whatever the route of administration, hyperalimentation predisposes the patient to infection, fluid shift because of the "pulling" effect of the hyperosmolar feeding solution, and irregularities of fecal elimination.

Gastrointestinal problems following major surgery under general anesthesia, especially following bowel surgery, are among the most distressing events with which the patient must cope throughout the surgical experience. Within 2 or 3 days after surgery, just about the time incisional pain subsides and becomes bearable, gas pains from gastric and intestinal dilatation commence, accompanied occasionally by nausea and vomiting. In addition to the pain of abdominal distention, the patient is frequently subjected to the indignity of rectal tubes and the cramping discomfort of enemas. If the patient is unfortunate enough to suffer diarrhea, or has fecal diversion from a colostomy, ileostomy, or fistula, he or she must bear the added stress of frequent and often liquid and odorous stools and the hazard of excoriated skin at the portal of exit. Meeting the challenges presented by disturbances in gastrointestinal function during the postoperative period requires great skill, knowledge, patience, creativity, and caring from the nurse. It is ironic, and perhaps prophetic of the role confusion currently experienced by many nurses, that so many of the functions and procedures nurses have delegated to less prepared assistants relate to assisting the patient with these functions.

Other Serious Postoperative Problems

Many serious complications or problems that challenge effective management of the surgical patient occur after the immediate postoperative period. Among these are intravascular clotting, infection, wound disruption, pain, fever, hiccough, and distorted self-concept.

Intravascular Clotting

Two problems that result from intravascular clotting are venous thrombosis and pulmonary embolism. Pulmonary emboli usually result from venous thrombi that break off and block a portion of the pulmonary artery bed. Like complications occurring after surgical procedure, thromboembolic phenomena are not unique to the postsurgical patient. They may develop in any patient in whom the nature of the disorder or some other factor favors intravascular clotting. The capacity of the blood to clot under appropriate circumstances is a valuable defense against the loss of blood. In health, the factors causing the blood to clot are controlled so that its fluid state is maintained. Although the reasons for the formation of blood clots within blood vessels are not well understood, three factors are believed to contribute to the possibility: (1) a roughening of the vascular endothelium lining the blood vessel by a microorganism or a chemical or physical agent, (2) a stasis or slowing of blood flow, and (3) changes in the composition of the blood that increase its tendency to coagulate.

Venous Thrombosis

In health, damage to platelets and other elements in the blood is minimized by the smoothness of the vascular edothelium. Further protection is offered by the probability that a single layer of negatively charged molecules of protein repels negatively charged platelets and prevents the platelets from coming in contact with the vascular endothelium. Incident to surgery, as well as to disease, the vascular endothelium can be injured by microorganisms, trauma, or chemical agents with the result that it becomes roughened. The roughened surface increases the likelihood of thrombocytes being broken down. When the wall of a thrombocyte is ruptured, it releases thromboplastin, which, in the presence of calcium ions, reacts with prothrombin to form thrombin. Thrombin then interacts with the blood protein, fibrinogen, to form fibrin. The fibrin forms a network of long, sticky threads or strands that entraps, in a manner similar to sticky flypaper, platelets (thrombocytes) and red cells and forms a blood clot.

The second factor favoring the formation of blood clots in blood vessels is stasis, or slowing of the flow of blood. Inactivity combined with the supine or sitting position favors stasis in the veins of the legs. With a normal rate of blood flow, cells are concentrated in the center of the blood vessel and are separated from the intima by a layer of plasma. As the rate of blood flow slows, cells tend to leave the center core and move toward the periphery, where they come in contact with the intima. Thus stasis of blood is believed to increase the likelihood of venous thrombosis in patients who are predisposed to it by other factors.

One aspect of the response to surgical or other trauma and to disease is an increase in the tendency of the blood to clot. Inasmuch as this response contributes to the effectiveness of the self-sealing mechanism, it is homeostatic. Like other homeostatic mechanisms, it can also be the source of problems. A number of changes in the blood contribute to its increased tendency to clot. Thrombocytes increase in number and become sticky. Instead of repelling each other, they tend to adhere one to another. Leukocytosis also occurs. When dehydration is allowed to develop, all the solid elements, including platelets and fibrinogen, increase in proportion to plasma and further increase the tendency of the blood to clot. In the absence of an adequate clotting mechanism, the individual faces the possibility of hemorrhage. When it is too active or clotting occurs in inappropriate sites, the clotting mechanism is also a source of danger to the individual.

As stated previously, knowledge of why intravascular clotting occurs following surgery or trauma is incomplete. But among the many factors believed to predispose to thromboembolic phenomena are advanced age of the patient, the volume and duration of intravenous infusions, hypotension, inflammation and infection, intimal injury, the foreign body effect of intravascular catheters, and deficient endogenous fibrinolytic activity. Although blood clots may form in any vein, deep veins in the lower extremities are most commonly affected. Something, perhaps a roughening of the endothelial lining of the vein, causes blood platelets to accumulate in that area. They release thromboplastin, which initiates the process of blood clotting. After a clot is formed, it continues to grow, provided the clot does not obstruct the flow of blood. The continued growth of the clot depends on blood flowing over it to provide the materials from which the clot is formed. Growth usually ceases when the clot reaches a site where the vein in which it is formed joins another vein. The rate of blood flow is increased at the point where two vessels unite; the thromboplastin in the blood from the vein containing the thrombus is diluted and its clotting effect is reduced. Clots formed in the deep veins in the calf of the leg may propagate into the femoral and iliac veins.

As the clot forms, the fibrinogen within the clot is converted into fibrin. If there are thrombocytes in the clot, the fibrin threads within the clot fold and pull the clot together, resulting in clot retraction. The clot is also invaded by macrophages that digest the red blood cells and release their hemoglobin into the body fluids. Later, fibroblasts enter and organize the clot, so that within a few weeks it becomes a firm, fibrous mass. After a period of months, all that may remain of the thrombus is a small fibrous band.

Although the factors responsible for intravascular clotting are not entirely clear, stasis seems to play a major role. Two of the benefits of early ambulation after surgery are the improvement in venous return from the legs and the reduction of thromboembolic complications. Many authorities disagree about the relationship of phlebothrombosis and thrombophlebitis. Some believe that these two conditions are phases of the same condition. Others state that they are two different conditions. Be that as it may, the predominating feature in phlebothrombosis is the formation of a blood clot. In thrombophlebitis the predominating characteristic is inflammation of the wall of the vein, which may extend to the surrounding tissue and involve lymphatic channels as well. In phlebothrombosis, the problem is to prevent the detachment of a portion of the clot. The floating clot, or embolus, in a vein is dangerous because it can block the flow of blood through the pulmonary arteries or its branches.

Pulmonary Emboli

Clots originating in the leg veins reach the right atrium and ventricle of the heart by way of the inferior vena cava. From the right ventricle, the embolus enters the pulmonary circulation via a pulmonary artery. It continues to move forward until it obstructs an artery through which it cannot pass. If the clot is large enough to obstruct more than half of the pulmonary circulation, the patient may die without warning or go into a severe shocklike state. Smaller clots move into the pulmonary circulation until they reach arteries too narrow for them to pass. They then obstruct the flow of blood to the area supplied by the occluded artery. This tissue, deprived of its blood supply, may die or become infarcted.

The symptoms and signs that accompany small emboli vary. The patient may have pain in the chest similar to the pain of pleurisy and described by the patient as a "catch in the chest" when he or she breathes. Hemoptysis (blood in the sputum) occurs in only a small percentage of patients. When there is hemoptysis, the sputum is brick red at first, but later it becomes dark red or brownish black. Small clots may also be expectorated. Although the patient usually has some fever, it rarely exceeds 101.4°F and lasts only 4 or 5 days. Most patients with pulmonary emboli may have only a relatively sudden onset of dyspnea. Any patient who suddenly becomes short of breath, especially 10 to 14 days after surgery, should be considered to have a pulmonary embolus until proved otherwise. Findings from a study of surgical patients followed throughout the postoperative period by fluoroscopic lung scan demonstrated that changes compatible with pulmonary embolus can be detected prior to development of symptoms in the patient. Presymptomatic diagnosis and treatment can reduce mortality from this serious complication. (Allgood et al., 1970).

Phlebothrombosis—Signs and Symptoms

Although patients with phlebothrombosis may have little in the way of signs or symptoms to indicate the presence of a clot, they may have a slight increase in temperature over normal levels. In some patients the temperature remains slightly elevated longer than is usual and there may be a small elevation in the leukocyte count. One of the most common symptoms is leg pain, usually in the calf. Should the patient mention the pain, he or she is likely to ascribe it to wearing slippers with heels that are lower than those to which he or she is accustomed. The patient may suffer only mild symptoms and go on to complete recovery or may develop a severe from of thrombophlebitis or a pulmonary embolism. Only about half of the patients with pulmonary emboli have leg symptoms at the time of embolus.

Unlike phlebothrombosis, a massive embolus is not likey to be formed in thrombophlebitis. Thrombophlebitis is more likely to be followed by disturbances in venous drainage with the development of incompetent venous valves and chronic stasis of blood in the feet or legs.

Thrombophlebitis—Signs and Symptoms

In the patient who has a thrombophlebitis, symptoms may range from mild to exceedingly severe. At the site of the thrombus, the cardinal signs of inflammation may be marked. The concern of the surgeon in the care of the patient is the prevention of the changes that may lead to chronically dilated leg veins with insufficient valves.

As with other complications, prevention is preferred to cure. Authorities, however, do not agree as to the value of the various methods that are employed in prevention. With few exceptions, the following are stressed: early ambulation, leg exercises while the patient is in bed, avoidance of pressure against the leg and thigh by a pillow or knee roll, maintenance of sufficient fluid intake to prevent dehydration, and prevention of hypotension.

Therapy

For the patient who is predisposed to intravascular clotting or who has already developed phlebothrombosis or thrombophlebitis, the physician will usually prescribe heparin therapy concurrently with an oral anticoagulant such as bishydroxycoumarin or one of its substitutes, to be administered for at least 7 to 10 days (Coon & Willis, 1972). The action of heparin in preventing coagulation of the blood involves at least four interrelated effects: (1) It acts as antiprothrombin to prevent the conversion of prothrombin to thrombin. (2) It antagonizes the action of thromboplastin, by a mechanism not fully understood. (3) It prevents the conversion of fibrinogen to fibrin. (4) It prevents the agglutination or clumping of platelets. Bishydroxycoumarin produces its effect by inhibiting the synthesis of prothrombin. Because heparin interferes with the action of substances already present in the blood, its action is prompt. Because bishydroxycoumarin inhibits the synthesis of prothrombin, its maximum effect does not occur for from 2 to 4 days and its action continues for some days after it has been discontinued. There is little or no question about the effectiveness of heparin when it is given properly; the bishydroxycoumarin-like substances, on the other hand, have had conflicting reports on their ability to prevent or retard clotting. In patients in whom the anticoagulant effect is immediately required, heparin may be administered by intravenous or deep intramuscular injection until the bishydroxycoumarin has had an opportunity to be effective. Bishydroxycoumarin is almost always administered orally. All patients who are being treated with anticoagulant therapy should be observed for evidence of bleeding. Should it occur, the condition should be reported immediately. The physician may discontinue the drug or decrease the daily dosage. To reduce the danger of hemorrhage in the patient who is receiving bishydroxycoumarin or one of its substitutes, the prothrombin time is initially checked either daily or every other day. The objective is to keep it between 25 and 15 per cent of normal.

Bedrest with elevation of the affected leg is usually prescribed for the patient with thrombophlebitis. Although elevation of the leg is a simple procedure, its effectiveness in promoting venous return and the comfort of the patient depend on its being properly done. Because water runs downhill, distal parts should be higher than proximal parts. Support of the leg should extend along its entire length. Pillows should be placed so that they form a firm base under both the leg and thigh, and after they are in place, the muscles of the leg and thigh should appear to be relaxed. The pillows should look as if they were supporting the leg rather than the leg the pillows. Moreover, pillows have a way of becoming disarranged. Any position, no matter how comfortable at the beginning, becomes tiring. The obvious conclusion is that the nurse should check the patient regularly. He or she should have an opportunity to change position and to have the supporting pillows rearranged, so that they continue to be supporting.

The physician may prescribe heat to be applied locally to the area. When warm, moist packs are used, they should be kept warm and some method should be employed to keep the bed dry. Chilling increases vasospasm and aggravates the condition.

Treatment of Pulmonary Embolism

Should the patient develop signs and symptoms indicating the possibility of a pulmonary embolism, the physician should be notified immediately. The development of a pulmonary embolism, especially a large one, is a frightening event for the patient, the family, and those responsible for his or her care. An embolism may occur during the sleep or it may be associated with some ordinary activity such as getting out of bed or using the bedpan. Should the patient be out of bed at the onset of symptoms, he or she should be returned to bed and supported in a comfortable position. If short of breath, the patient is likely to be more comfortable in a sitting than in a supine position. If at all possible, someone should remain with the patient until he or she is comfortable and the acute symptoms are relieved.

In addition to anticoagulant therapy, the patient is placed on absolute bedrest and oxygen therapy is usually prescribed. Drugs to relive the apprehension of the patient and to relax smooth muscle spasm may also be ordered. These include morphine, atropine, and papaverine. When conservative medical treatment by anticoagulants and rest is ineffective, pulmonary embolism may be treated surgically with partial or complete interruption of the inferior vena cava, either by applying a serrated clip, performing a compelete ligation, or insertion of a balloon catheter that is left in place only until a solid thrombosis of the vena cava occurs, after which the balloon is deflated and withdrawn (Sabiston, 1977). An umbrella-shaped filter has also been introduced for surgical treatment of pulmonary embolism (Doyle, 1980). Despite the exotic surgical alternatives, anticoagulant therapy remains the treatment of choice for those who can tolerate it.

Infections

Perhaps the most nearly unique aspect of the surgical patient is the incision that is made to approach the organ to be operated upon. As emphasized earlier in this chapter, the incision disrupts one of the individual's most important defenses against infection. All patients who have surgery run a certain risk of developing an infection in the wound or operative site, as well as in other parts of the body into or through which instruments, drains, and tubes of various types are inserted for visualization, aspiration, drainage, or instillation. Application of principles of asepsis throughout a patient's hospitalization has been instrumental in reducing infection caused by external environmental bacteria. In fact, some authorities (Robson et all, 1973) believe that the present incidence of infection in the surgical patient is rarely due to bacterial invasion from the external environment, but is most often due to "a quantitative disturbance of the normal balance, allowing invasion by bacteria for which man himself is the primary reservoir." Lowering of systemic or local host resistance as a result of operative or traumatic wounding may alter the balance sufficiently to resut in infection. A major objective in care of the surgical patient is to prevent infection by maintaining the balance in favor of the host, through support of his or her defenses and through the control of environmental bacteria by asepsis, antisepsis, and antibacterial agents.

A critical factor in strengthening patient resistance to infection is a proper state of nutrition. Not only does starvation with inadequate proteins and vitamins hinder wound healing and increase the chance of infection, but obesity also predisposes to wound infection. Adipose tissue is more vulnerable to infection than many other tissues because it has relatively poor blood supply and is difficult to approximate properly.

Other systemic alterations that lower the level of resistance of the patient to infection include (Robson et al., 1973, pp. 10–13):

1. Age. In old age, there is a decrease in antibody production. In the newborn, there is decreased phagocytosis.
2. Blood glucose level. Gram-negative infections thrive with levels below 110 mg %, whereas gram-positive infections thrive with levels above 130 mg %.
3. Deficit or excess of adrenocorticosteroids.
4. Decreased tissue perfusion and shock.
5. Malignancy, when in the terminal stages or when treated by chemotherapy.
6. Irradiation, which decreases white blood cells and impairs local blood supply by producing local fibrosis.
7. Burn injury, which destroys local cellular defenses.

Of particular relevance to the surgical patient are local wound factors that decrease resistance to infection: (1) necrotic tissue; (2) decreased local wound perfusion; (3) presence of a foreign body, such as a catheter, drain, or sutures; (4) hematoma; and (5) dead space.

Classification of organisms as pathogens or nonpathogens is no longer meaningful. *Pathogencity* is a measure of an organism's ability to injure host tissue, and may be defined as "any organism that arrives with the capacity to survive in a host, whose multiplication results in injury, which in turn elicits an active response from that host" (Robson et al., 1973, p. 20). Research reports indicate that there seems to be a critical number of bacteria that can be handled by the host before clinical infection develops, within the range 10^5 or 10^6 organisms, that is, about a million organisms per gram of tissue or milligram of biological fluid. In fact, *sepsis* has been defined as organisms greater than 10^5 per gram of tissue (Robson et al., 1973, pp. 16–17). The number of organisms required to produce clinical infection appears to vary little with the type of organism.

The following factors may be involved in postoperative wound infections. They are listed in the order of their significance as causative factors (Smith, 1979):

1. Recovery of organisms from wound washings
2. Nature of the operation

3. Duration of the operation
4. Age of the patient
5. Presence of drains
6. Anemia

Pyogenic bacteria, which cause primary postoperative wound sepsis, originate most frequently from the skin of the patient and of the operating team and from the gastrointestinal tract of the patient undergoing bowel surgery (Smith, 1979).

The nurse contributes most to prevention and control of postoperative infection by meticulous execution of medical and surgical asepsis to prevent cross-contamination, and by scrupulous and regular attention to the cleanliness of the patient's skin, to mucous membrances, and to oral hygiene and by removal of secretions and crusts from any tubes, where they enter natural or man-made orifices of the body. In addition, the nurse contributes to the management of infection by administering, and observing for response to, medications, especially antibiotics. The incidence of adverse drug reactions among postoperative patients has been reported as high as 10 to 15 per cent with antibiotics causing the majority of adverse reactions (Marcoux & Peters, 1969). The patient receiving antibiotics must be observed closely for allergic or anaphylactic reactions. At the first sign of rash, itching, elevated temperature, changes in respiration or pulse and blood pressure, or other signs of toxicity pertinent to specific drugs, the physician should be notified and the next dose of the antibiotic withheld pending medical evaluation of the patient's condition. The process of wound healing and further consideration of inflammatory and immunologic responses are presented in Chapter 24 and 25.

Wound Disruption

When the surgical patient has a satisfactory response to injury, the operative wound will begin to increase in strength immediately after suturing and will continue to gain strength at a relatively rapid and constant rate for over 4 months, and at a slower rate for over a year. Wound healing following uncomplicated surgery is often sufficiently established within 7 days to allow removal of the sutures. Four efficient stages of wound healing are described and illustrated by Schumann (1980), as presented in Figure 52-3.

Wounds rarely regain either the strength or elasticity of normal tissues. The rank order of some important tissues according to their rate of strength gain are (1) skin—fasters; (2) muscle and fascia—moderate or middle rate; and (3) tendons—slowest (Madden, 1977). The nature and sequence of overlapping events in the repair process are shown in Figure 52-4.

The nurse needs to know when to anticipate removal of sutures and how to plan with the patient for safe resumption of activity. This information is determined in large part by the rate of strength gain and ultimate strength of the wound.

Any factors that impair the process of wound healing will increase the likelihood of wound disruption. Disruption of the wound is one of the serious sequelae of impaired wound healing. Separation of the wound may occur at any time following the closure of the incision. It may occur immediately after the wound is closed and before the patient has been transferred from the operating room or at some later time. A common time is about the seventh day. The degree to which the wound separates varies. When the skin as well as the underlying tissue separates and the contents of the abdominal cavity extrude, the condition is known as evisceration. Although disruption of any wound may occur, the most common site is in midline abdominal incisions.

Although wound disruption is possible in any patient, certain conditions in the various phases of surgery predispose to it. In the preoperative phase, obesity, undernutrition, particularly of protein and vitamin C (ascorbic acid); conditions associated with metabolic disorders, such as diabetes mellitus, Cushing's syndrome, and uremia, and advanced cancer or liver disease appear to predispose to impaired wound healing. Weight reduction, when a patient is obese, and attention to the nutritional staus of patients during the preoperative period are important preventive measures. During the operative phase, many of the activities of the surgeon are directed toward making and closing the incision in such a manner that wound healing is favored or, conversely, is protected from disruption. Thus attention is given to the site and direction of the incision. Wound healing is a consideration of the selection of sutures and in the suturing technique. Careful hemostasis and the maintenance of asepsis are also important. With the exception of asepsis, all the preceding preventive measures are mainly the responsibility of the surgeon.

During the postoperative phase a variety of conditions predispose to separation of an abdmoninal incision. Perhaps the most frequent cause is some disorder that places strain on the incision by increasing intra-abdominal pressure. Thus separation of the wound is associated with abdominal distention, retching, unrelieved coughing, sneezing, hiccoughs, or uncontrollable motor activity. When any of these disorders exist, attention should be directed toward their relief. The nurse has a responsibility to report any of the disorders to the physician and to carry

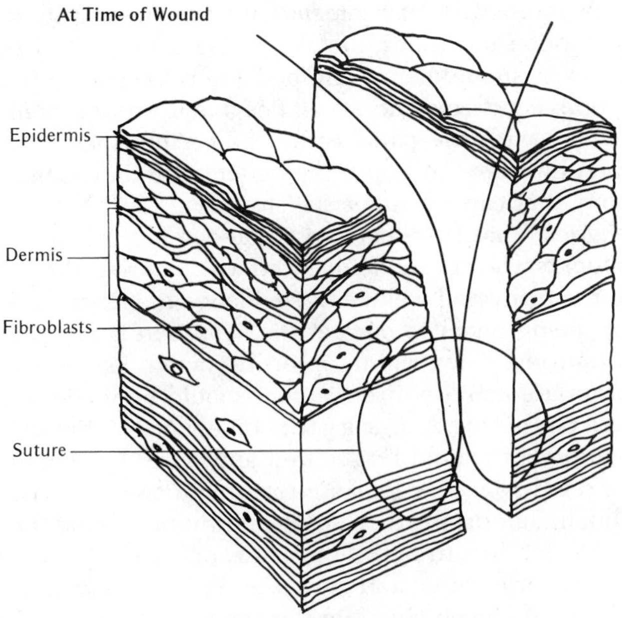

Once the surgeon's knife makes an incision, blood from ruptured vessels fills the gap, as does cellular debris from epidermal and subdermal layers. Within an hour, the blood begins to clot. Glue-like fibrins in the clot, aided by sutures, bind the wound edges together. Meanwhile, fibroblasts close in to surround the wound.

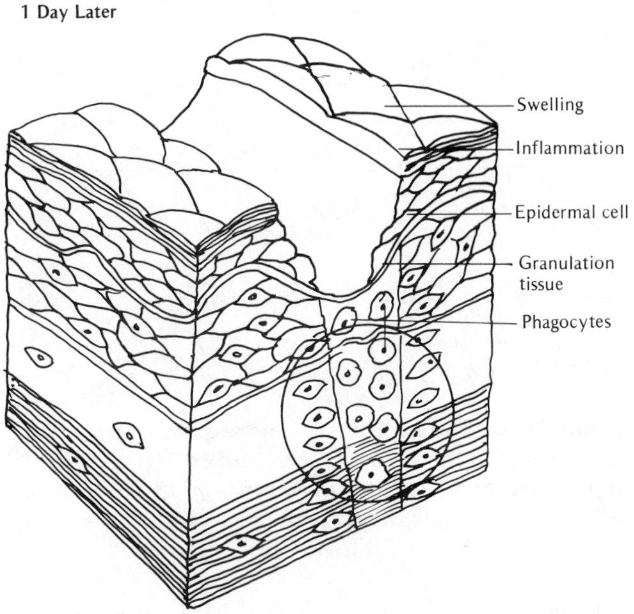

After the clot has set, the wound edges swell and become inflamed. White blood cells (specifically, phagocytes) from surrounding vessels move into the clot to ingest bacteria and cellular debris, thereby gradually deomlishing the clot. By the end of the first day, epidermal cells and granulation tissue have begun to push into space formerly occupied by the clot.

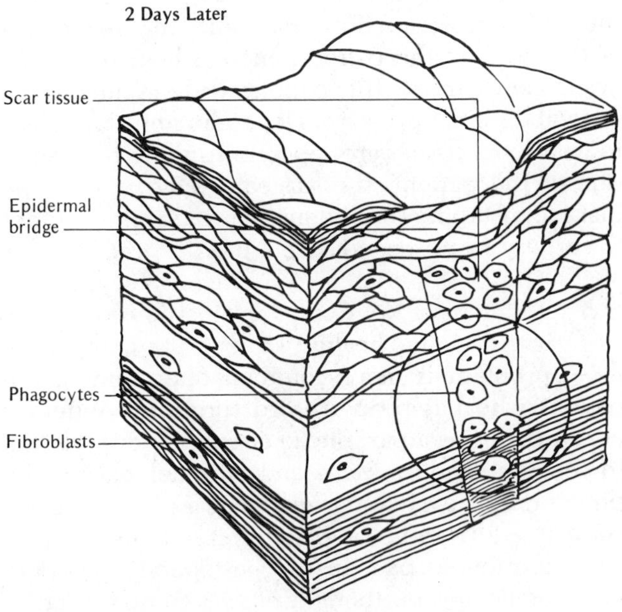

About 2 days after the incision, epidermal cells have bridged the wound. (In a large open wound, not shown here, the epidermal bridge may form under a scab, which will later be cast off.) While the phagocytes continue their cleanup, collagen-producing fibroblasts have entered the wound and begun reconstructing dermal tissue. A scar, in other words, is beginning to form.

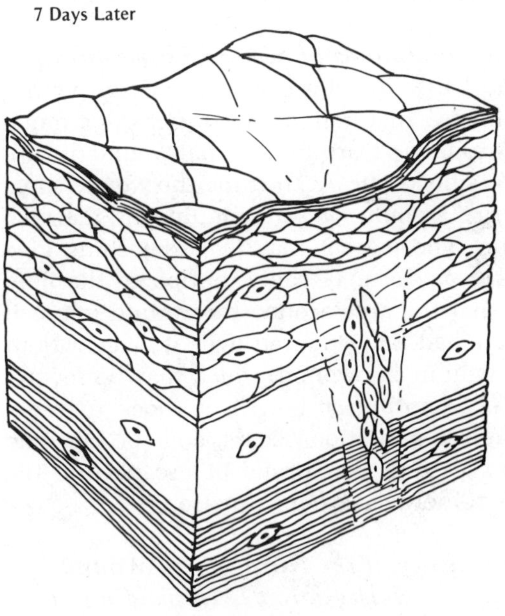

If the wound is in an area of low tension, by the seventh day the sutures will have been removed. Meanwhile, the epidermis has restored itself, and the scar tissue has grown more compact. At this point, the fibroblasts are at their most numerous and active. Along with their collagen building comes replacement of other damaged connective tissue, including lymphatics, blood vessels, and supporting stromal matrixes. This rebuilding process continues during the succeeding weeks until (assuming the healing goes well) all functions have returned to near normal and the scar has paled significantly.

Figure 52-3. Wound healing in four efficient stages. (From "How to Help Wound Healing in Your Abdominal Surgery Patient." *Nurs. 80,* **10** (Apr. 1980), 34–40, by D. Schumann, p. 36.)

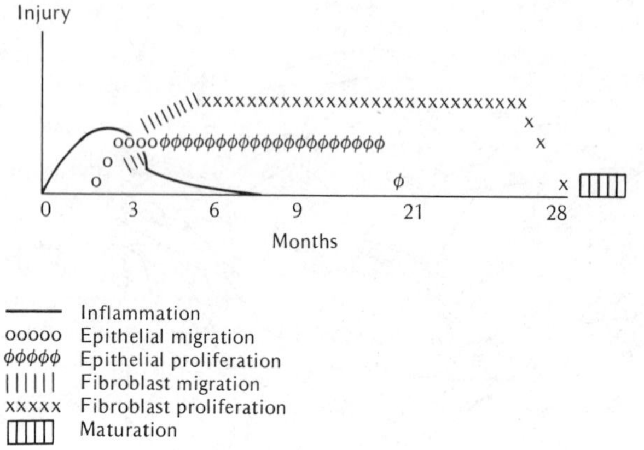

Figure 52-4. The nature and time sequence of overlapping events in the repair process. (From "The Nature of Wound Healing." *Nurs. Clin. North Am.* **14** (Dec. 1979), 667–82, Fig. 1, p. 668, by P. Bruno.)

out measures for their relief. Should the surgeon believe that the patient is seriously predisposed to wound disruption or that separation of the wound is imminent, he or she may use special "retention sutures" that encompass all layers of the abdomen for 1 to 2 inches on either side of the incision and apply a binder to the abdomen of the patient.

Signs and Symptoms of Wound Disruption

Staining of the dressing over the incision with a serosanguineous material, which looks very much like cherry soda, is a warning sign that wound disruption will possibly occur. At the time the wound separates a large amount of serosanguineous material may escape. The patient may feel something give or burst. He or she may call attention to the fluid by saying that the area around the wound felt as if warm water had been poured over it. The patient may have pain in the wound, which may be severe. In addition, vomiting and signs of shock may develop. When evisceration occurs, coils of intestine may protrude from the wound or escape into the bed, an extremely hazardous situation

Responsibilities of the Nurse When Wound Dehiscence or Evisceration Is Impending or Has Occurred

When there is evidence that wound dishiscence or evisceration is impending or has occurred, the physician should be immediately notified. At best, these sequelae to impaired wound healing are extremely serious. As little time as possible should be lost between the event and the initiation of treatment. The patient should be instructed to lie quietly on his or her back in a horizontal position. If coils of intestine can be seen, they should be covered with sterile towels or other sterile materials, which are kept moist with physiologic saline. Because wound disruption predisposes to shock, the patient's blood pressure should be determined and pulse and respirations counted. When at all possible, a nurse should remain with the patient until he or she is seen by the physician. To assure the patient that all is being done that can be, he or she should be told that the physician has been notified and is coming. For most patients who are suddenly faced with a serious threat to their physical well-being, evidence that measures are being taken to correct the condition is in itself reassuring. They rightly interpret action as the appropriate activity. Preparations should be made for the physician. A nasogastric tube and suctioning equipment should be secured and the tube should be ready to insert. Because retching increases intra-abdominal pressure, a local anesthetic should be ready for use to anesthetize the pharynx. A mask and a sterile gown and gloves, as well as sterile towels, should be obtained for the surgeon. Sterile saline should be warmed and available. If intravenous fluids are not running they should be made available for starting by the physician. When the surgeon arrives, he or she will decide on the place and type of therapy. When the condition of the patient permits, most surgeons prefer to have the patient transferred to the operating room for treatment. In the process of transferring the patient, enough help should be available to move the patient without increasing intra-abdominal pressure. Depending on the extent to which the tissues are separated and on the condition of the patient, the surgeons may support the incision by taping the abdomen or return the patient to surgery for a secondary closure.

Pain

No problem is more common than pain to the patient who has been treated surgically. Whether or not pain was a part of the circumstances that led to seeking medical care, and whether or not the preoperative evaluation and preparation were accompanied by pain, the patient often fears and usually experiences pain in the postoperative period. Pain should not be thought of as a complication of surgery in the same sense that hemorrhage, shock, and wound dehiscence are complications. Rather, pain should be considered an inevitable consequence of the mechanical trauma of manipulating and cutting tissue, of pressure resulting from transudation fluid that accumulates with inflammation at the site of injury, of pressure resulting from accumulation of gases within the gastrointestinal tract prior to resumption of peristalsis, and of psychic stress associated with such factors as fear of death or threats to the self-concept of the patient. A primary responsibility of the nurse in the postoperative period is to help the patient manage that pain normally associated with his or her particular operation in such a way that psychophysiologic complications are prevented and recovery is promoted. The management of ordinary postoperative pain is elaborated in the following section on preventive nursing measures.

When there is a discrepancy between the pain normally associated with a particular operation and the pain experienced by a patient who has undergone that operation, extraordinary pain may indicate development of a major postoperative complication and/or an exceptionally high level of anxiety.

Distorted Self-Concept

In the discussion of the preoperative phase of surgical therapy, some mention was made of the psychological aspects of surgery as a threat to the survival of the individual. Many aspects of surgical therapy can provoke anxiety. This anxiety may be further augmented by the disease, or what the person perceives to be the disease, that makes surgery necessary. Many aspects of the total surgical experience threaten the self-concept of the individual. During the operative phase of treatment, the patient loses complete control over what happens. He or she is utterly dependent on the surgeon, the anesthetist, and the assistants to the surgeon. The patient faces, and then experiences, pain and fear of pain. Throughout the entire experience, from the day the patient becomes aware that he or she is ill until convalescence has been completed, the unknown plays a part in his or her reactions. Was surgery necessary? Was it successful? Was the cause of the illness cancer? Was it all removed? Has the physician told the truth?

The surgical treatment of disease frequently threatens one's self-concept, by actual fact or by the perception of the individual. These are the persons who, though they make a full physiologic recovery, have some change in their anatomy that threatens their self-concept. Full psychological recovery depends on their accepting the change in themselves as necessary and for their welfare. This involves a change in self-concept without a prolonged period of depression or other evidence of failure to accept reality.

Types of surgery that place the greatest strain on the adaptive capacity of the individual are those involving the loss of a part of the body (1) that is obvious to others, such as an eye or an extremity; (2) in which the patient has an emotional investment; or (3) that involves an obvious change in function, such as with a colostomy, ileostomy, or cystostomy. The patient can and should be expected to experience some grief and anger. He or she may also feel a certain degree of shame or guilt. The reader is referred to Chapter 31 for a more complete discussion of this very important psychosocial aspect of care of the surgical patient.

Fever

A symptom that may also be of great importance during the recovery of the patient is fever. For the first 2 or 3 days postoperatively a slight elevation of temperature and of leukocyte count may be expected because of the tissue damage. A marked increase in body temperature during the first 24 to 72 hours, however, frequently indicates a developing atelectasis. Later elevations may be caused by thrombophlebitis or an infection in the operative site, urinary tract, or other foci identified in the previous section on infections. In addition to serving as a sign of major postoperative complications, the hyperthermia itself can cause tissue damage. Nursing objectives related to fever for care of the postoperative patient include (1) monitoring body temperature as frequently as other vital signs in the immediate postoperative period, and regularly thereafter, to ensure early detection of elevation;[7] (2) instituting measures (such as turning, deep breathing, and coughing) designed to prevent complications associated with fever; and (3) in the presence of fever, instituting measures to increase heat loss by increasing radiation, convection, conduction, and evaporation.

Measures to increase heat loss are included in Chapters 20 and 37. For the surgical patient, factors of special importance include ensuring that (1) fluid intake closely approaches *total* fluid losses or output from urine, stool, sweating, insensible loss via lungs, and drainage from tubes or wounds; (2) light and absorbent clothing and bedding are used to cover the patient; (3) moist clothing and bedding of the diaphoresing patient are changed promptly; (4) the patient receives at least a partial bath, with special attention to trunk and extremities, several times a day during the febrile period; (5) there is good circulation of air in the patient's room, without exposure to drafts; and (6) humidity of air in the patient's room is as low as engineering features of the hospital will allow. When these conservative measures are insufficient to keep the patient's temperature elevation within safe limits, the nurse may administer or apply

[7] Until the patient has passed the turning-point stage, body temperature should be checked at least once a day, at a time when the patient's normal temperature would be expected to be at its highest. Research on circadian rhythms indicates that temperature, which varies about 1 or 2°F each 24 hours, tends to reach the high point in the afternoon and evening. [Gay Gaer Luce: *Biological Rhythms in Human and Animal Physiology* (New York: Dover Publications, Inc., 1971), p. 44.]

measures prescribed by the physician, such as antipyretic drugs, alcohol sponges, or other forms of total body cooling.

Hiccough

Hicough (singultus) is an annoying, though not usually dangerous, symptom. It results from a paroxysmal and intermittent contraction of the diaphragm. It may be the result of chemical or mechanical irritation of the peritoneum or pleura that invests the diaphragm. Hiccoughs will often respond to simple measures—a drink of water, something that startles the person, a cough, a change in position. Other procedures that may be prescribed by the physician include rebreathing air in a paper bag, cabon dioxide inhalation, gastric lavage or suction, and sedatives. In extreme cases in which hiccoughs are prolonged and do not respond to other treatments, crushing the phrenic nerve may be required. Severe and continuous hiccoughing is exhausting because it interferes with rest and the ingestion of food and fluid.

Measures Recommended to Prevent Complications and Promote Recovery

Control of Pain

The nature, assessment, and management of pain are discussed in detail in Chapter 36, because both the physical and psychological components of the pain experience constitute neurologic phenomena. However, the prevalence of postoperative pain as an abstacle to active participation by the patient in activities designed to prevent postoperative complications warrants additional comment at this time.

To fulfill the role in the prevention and relief of pain, the nurse must be able (1) to care for the patient so that preventable pain is avoided; (2) to evaluate the nature and cause of pain, as a basis for instituting appropriate measures; (3) To evaluate the effectiveness of measures used to relieve pain; (4) to inspire confidence in the patient that the nurses can be trusted to anticipate and meet his or her needs; and (5) to continue to offer comfort and support to the patient whose pain persists despite the use of all conceivable measures to relieve pain.

The best treatment of pain is the removal of its cause. Because the mechanisms of pain perception involve both peripheral and central processes, the cause of postoperative pain will usually have both a peripheral and central component. Afferent impulses produced by the injuring agent flow into the central nervous system, where they are given meaning by the emotional state of the individual based upon past and present experience. This makes pain an *experience* rather than a sensory modality in a strict neurologic sense, and psychological events play an essential role in determining the quality and quantity of its ultimate perception (Duthie & Hoaglund, 1979). Apprehension, with the resulting tension, is likely to be increased when a patient fears that he or she is going to be hurt. The tension resulting from fear and anxiety can be expected to increase the degree of pain suffered by the patient. When the patient knows that those who are responsible for care will be gentle, that they will not allow him or her to suffer unnecessarily, and that when pain is unavoidable he or she will be warned to allow for preparation, the patient is less likely to be unnecessarily apprehensive, and consequently is less likely to experience intensified pain. Johnson's (1972) research on the reduction of distress experienced by patients during threatening events uses measures directed at the central processes of the pain experience, by providing the patient with accurate information on the sensory component of the forthcoming event.

Peripheral pain processes are activated by all the types of agents that injure tissues: mechanical, chemical, thermal, and biological. (See Unit III for the nature and effects of injurious agents.) In the postoperative period the most common types of pain that result from injury are (Duthie & Hoaglund, 1979, p. 1810)

1. *Local pain,* felt at the site of injury in superficial structures.
2. *Diffuse pain,* felt throughout a regional or segmental area involving deep-lying tissue.
3. *Radicular pain,* characterized by radiation from the center to the periphery; often associated with paresthesia and tenderness along the nerve root; frequently accompanied by sensory loss, depression of area reflexes, and muscle paresis or paralysis.
4. *Referred pain,* occurring with injury to deep structures and resulting from misplaced pain projection caused by cortical misrepresentation.

Physical nursing measures, associated with explanation and positive suggestion of benefit, contribute significantly to relief of peripheral pain caused by (1) torsion or pulling; (2) pressure; and (3) ischemia.

Torsion or Pulling

The most effective way to prevent or relieve pain caused by torsion or pulling is to maintain body structures in anatomic alignment. Support should be provided as needed to achieve positions that will eliminate strain on parts. Parts particularly subjected to strain in the postsurgical patient include extremities used as sites for intravenous infusion; head, neck, and shoulders; hips, knees, and feet; and the lumbosacral area of the back. Basic to securing good alignment and to preventing strain on muscles is a firm mattress. When a patient is heavy, a board under the mattress may be required to achieve a firm surface. In some institutions a nurse may place a board under the mattress when it is required; in others a prescription from a physician must be secured. In the prevention of strain, the body and any of its parts should be moved as a unit. In moving the torso, the patient can assist by trying to keep his or her spine straight and stiff. The movements of all who participate in the turning should be synchronized so that everyone moves together. Counting "one, two, three, go" is helpful. Devices such as pillows, sand bags, and molds or splints, casts, braces, and corsets may also be useful in supporting or immobilizing a part subjected to strain.

To move an extremity, the part should be supported so that strain is minimized and unnatural movements are avoided. Both hands may be used, supporting the part on the palms of the hands, or the extremity can be supported by placing the hand and arm under its length. Pressure should be avoided over painful areas. Here again, movement may be made less painful by the use of a splint, brace, cast, or even a pillow to support the painful part while it is moved.

Deep breathing and coughing, which are so critical to prevention of postoperative pulmonary complications, are painful to the patient with a thoracic or abdominal incision. Incisional discomfort can be decreased by applying the hands on each side of the incision and moving the skin and underlying structures toward the incision line, or by placing the hands or a firm pillow directly over the incisional area to provide reinforcing resistance to the vibration of coughing. Whether the nurse or the patient provides the support depends on the location of the incision and the wishes and the capability of the patient. In patients who cough in excess of that required to maintain the patency of the tracheobronchial tree, a binder may be required to provide continuing support for the incision.

A special case of pain caused by torsion or pulling results from muscle spasm, a common occurrence with orthopedic injury. Relief of muscle spasm is best accomplished by applying traction to the bone into which the spastic muscle inserts. When the patient is in traction, the nurse ensures that the torso and extremities of the patient remain in anatomic alignment; that the ropes and pulleys are intact and running freely; that weights are *suspended* and not caught on bed or frame or resting on the floor; and that all body surfaces in contact with traction equipment are protected against injury from pressure and friction.

When immobility of the trunk or thigh is required, or movement is accompanied by excessive pain, the desired result may be attained by placing the patient on a Foster, Stryker, or Bradford frame or on a Circo-Lectric bed. They also facilitate the giving of patient care.

Another frequent cause of pain caused by pulling in the surgical patient is tension on tubes. Whether the portal of entry of a tube is a natural or manmade body orifice, care must be taken to secure tubes as close to the portal of entry as possible, to prevent slack from catching on clothing, equipment, or adjacent body parts as the patient moves about. Whenever possible, a system should be used which secures the tube on opposite sides for maximum stability. Figure 52-5 illustrates two methods for securing tubes to prevent pulling. Occasionally the purpose of a tube is to apply traction to some internal tissue, such as bleeding esophageal varices. In that event the tube should not be secured by any means at the portal of entry.

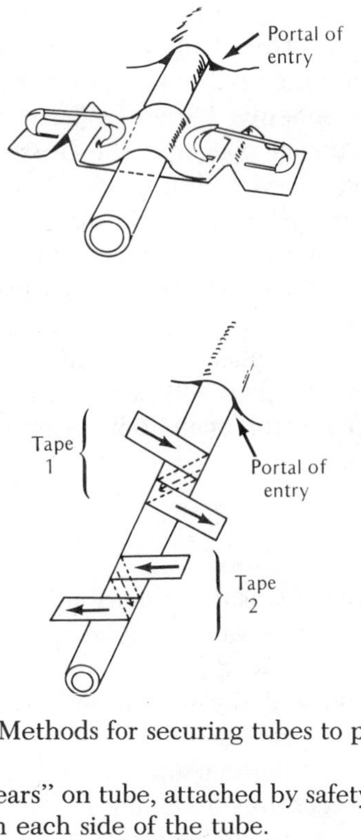

Figure 52-5. Methods for securing tubes to prevent pulling on tissue.

A. Taped "ears" on tube, attached by safety pins to the flap of tape on each side of the tube.

B. A length of tape extending from skin attachment on one side of tube, around its circumference, then reattached to side of origin. Repeat application of tape in opposite direction.

Pressure

Pressure as a cause of pain may originate in the external and/or the internal environment of the patient. Measures to protect the patient against pressure originating in the external environment are discussed with the prevention and treatment of decubitus ulcers in Chapter 49. A common cause of pressure originating in the internal environment is edema, or swelling. Swelling, particularly in tissue surrounded by a bony wall or encased in a circular bandage or cast, is painful and may be dangerous. The most effective treatment for this is to reduce the swelling by utilizing the force of gravity to remove the excess fluid. Mrs. Erie offers a good example. She was admitted for the reduction of a fractured tibia, which was followed by the application of a cast. Several hours after the cast was applied, she called and asked to have something for her pain. Her toes on the affected side were slightly swollen. Instead of getting Mrs. Erie an analgesic, the nurse elevated her leg on pillows and told Mrs. Erie that, as soon as the swelling was relieved, her pain would disappear. An hour or so later Mrs. Erie said that she was free of pain and was able to eat breakfast. If the toes were cold or cyanotic, the cast should immediately be cut or bivalved by a physician.

Ischemia

Any factor that produces mechanical obstruction to the flow of arterial blood to an area can result in local anemia, or ischemia, and part of the tissue response to ischemia is pain. When ischemic pain is due to external pressure, the nurse may relieve the pain by relieving the pressure and exercising the painful part or placing it in a dependent position to allow gravity to assist in increasing arterial blood flow. When there is no apparent external cause for ischemic pain, it may signal development of a serious postoperative complication, in which case the nurse should report the pain and associated manifestations to the physician for evaluation prior to taking any other action.

Analgesics

The nursing measures described earlier may be effective in preventing or relieving superficial or local pain experienced by the patient in the postoperative period, but the severe deep pain associated especially with prolonged and extensive thoracic, orthopedic, or abdominal operations, or with minor operative procedures involving nerves, requires analgesic medication. Failure to relieve severe deep pain may cause failure of homeostatic defense mechanisms, foretold by weakness, hypotension, pallor, sweating, bradycardia, and nausea and vomiting. The selection of the medication and the interval at which it is given is the prerogative of the physician. The nurse administers the medication within the framework of the prescription of the physician. When the physician prescribes the medication at stated intervals, the drug must be given at the times prescribed unless the patient develops signs of depression of the respiratory or nervous system or other toxic effects. When the prescription left by the physician permits the nurse to use discretion, then she or he may give the drug as often as required. Usually the prescription or the policy of the agency sets some limits on the maximum frequency with which a drug can be administered. This is usually every 3 to 4 hours. Generally, the patient gets more benefit from the drug if the pain is not allowed to become too severe. There is some evidence to support the observation that patients who can count on having their pain relieved promptly suffer less pain than those who cannot. Dickman (1959) made a study to determine the effect of knowing or not knowing on the quantity of drug required by postoperative patients for comfort. Patients who knew that they could have a pain-relieving medication required less medication than those who did not know. Most patients tolerate painful or unpleasant procedures better if they have their medication before the procedure is performed.

During the first 48 hours after surgery, most patients benefit from receiving analgesic medication at least once during the period of the day when they are subjected to greatest activity, such as bathing, blood tests, ambulation, visitors; at least once during the evening, when environmental stimulation decreases and fatigue intensifies pain; and at least twice during the night, when fears are greatest and distractions least available. Except in unusual circumstances the patient in the immediate postoperative period who is receiving intelligent nursing care should not have to ask for pain medication. Although the patient should not be required to ask for pain medication before having pain evaluated and treated, when the patient says he or she has pain the complaint should be taken seriously and every effort made to determine the cause. Too often nurses and physicians stereotype patients' responses to pain in a way that impairs their ability to seek and evaluate subtle evidence to explain pain, with occasional tragic consequences for the patient. Mr. Big was such a patient. He was a handsome, trim, and muscular 28-year-old man who had emergency abdominal surgery for a ruptured appendix. He had had no previous illnesses or operations, and for the first 3 or 4 days following surgery his pain medication seemed adequate to control his pain. By the fifth postoperative day, his requests for pain medication were becoming as frequent as every 2 or 3 hours, and the staff began to suspect either addiction or attention-seeking as the cause. Physical findings were not significant, and it was not until the tenth postoperative day that the surgeon finally performed an exploratory laparotomy. To everyone's dismay, Mr. Big had developed an extensive mesenteric thrombosis, with resultant gangrene of the small bowel. He died 2 days after his second operation, from overwhelming sepsis and irreversible shock. During the postoperative course, or during any other period associated with a painful disorder, increases in complaints of pain are more often traceable to physical causes than to addiction; assuming addiction to medication as a *first* hunch is analogous to expecting to see zebras rather than horses at the first sound of hoofbeats.

On the basis of close observation as a guide to judicious use of analgesic medication and appropriate use of the nursing measures described above, the nurse should be able to help the patient achieve sufficient comfort and activity to prevent many complications and to promote prompt recovery.

Exercise and Rest

All postoperative patients have some degree of anxiety about coughing, deep breathing, and ambulating, because of concern about bursting their stitches and an instinctive avoidance of those activities which increase incisional pain. Finn (1979) suggests the following precautions to protect the incision and promote mobilization:

1. Thorough explanation of wound closure, to dispel the common misconception that skin sutures are holding the wound together.
2. Pain medication about 20 minutes prior to coughing or getting out of bed.
3. Demonstration of and assistance with splinting the incision in association with deep breathing and coughing techniques.
4. Rest period after coughing and ambulation.
5. Two persons to assist the patient with the first venture out of bed, using basic techniques for transfer and moving which maximize and support the patient's participation.

Control of pain promotes optimal exercise and rest, and optimal exercise and rest facilitate the control of pain. The sympathoadrenal medullary response of the patient to surgical trauma is intensified and prolonged by bedrest and can be minimized in degree and shortened in length by the early mobilization of the surgical patient. Following surgery, the patient undergoes metabolic changes similar to that of the general response to injury. It is more pronounced in the young healthy individual than it is in the debilitated and elderly and it is intensified by bedrest. In the early stages, it is characterized by increased catabolism of protein and a negative nitrogen balance.

Among the positive effects of exercise following surgery is the reduction in the loss of nitrogen. It has long been known that simple bedrest leads to a loss of nitrogen and a depression in the appetite (Coller & DeWeese, 1949). It also leads to a loss of muscle tone and to muscle weakness. Excessive rest results not only in nitrogen loss from muscles but also calcium loss from bones. In active healthy young persons, especially young men, who are suddenly and completely inactivated, loss of calcium may be so great that it forms kidney stones. This tendency can be counteracted to a certain extent by exercise and a high fluid intake. Return to physiologic functioning of the respiratory circulatory, gastrointestinal, and nervous systems is earlier in patients who exercise.

For the purpose of this discussion exercise following surgery will be considered under three headings: (1) mobilization or exercise of the patient in bed, (2) mobilization or exercise of the patient out of bed, and (3) exercises for the restoration of specific functions. All types of exercise have a common goal, the restoration of function. The effects of exercise can be summarized as a law of nature: parts, especially muscles, develop in proportion to the stresses and strains placed on them.

Exercise in Bed

Many of the exercises performed in bed have been previously presented in other chapters. Mobilization and exercise are essential for patients who for some reason cannot get out of bed. These exercises are essential for the protection of respiratory, circulatory, and joint function and to prevent the loss of muscle strength and tone. Depending on the condition of the patient, exercise can be passive, that is, performed by the nurse, or it can be active, that is, performed by the patient. Exercise can also be assistive, with the nurse helping the patient to exercise.

For patients who are confined to bed for more than a day or two, a variety of simple devices are available to increase the mobility of the patient as well as enable him or her to assist with his or her own care. One such device is the overhead swing, or "monkey bar," which, when used, strengthens the arm muscles, enables the patient to move about in bed, and allows the patient to assist with care. A rope or sheet tied to the foot of the bed may be used by the patient to pull himself or herself into a sitting position. The arms and shoulders may be strengthened by the patient placing hands palms down on the bed and raising the buttocks from the bed. This exercise is useful in the preparation of the patient for crutch walking.

Exercise should be an integral part of the care of virtually all patients. When a patient is treated by bedrest, the nurse should include range of motion exercises as part of the morning and evening care. When the patient is able, he or she may perform these exercises alone. As the term *range of motion* implies, extremities are moved at the joints within the limits of the usual range of motion for the patient. One precaution should be observed in the performance of these exercises: the nurse should never force a part beyond the point at which it moves freely or causes pain. This is especially important after any trauma at or near a joint.

Although exercise out of bed is more beneficial, exercise in bed can also be beneficial and has its indications. Exercise improves the psychological status and morale of the patient. To the extent that exercise is accompanied by relaxation of the patient, it lessens pain, and, as a consequence, less postoperative medication is required. Mrs. Hammer illustrates the latter point. During a recent pregnancy Mrs. Hammer was found to have a marked elevation of her blood pressure. At the time of delivery, she went into hypovolemic shock as a result of severe hemorrhage. Despite reasonably prompt replacement of blood loss, she became anuric and remained so for about 10 days. After this time her urine output began to increase but her renal function was still very poor, as evidenced by the low fixed specific gravity of her urine and the rising blood levels of potassium and urea. When potassium and urea levels rose to a critical level, peritoneal dialysis was initiated and Mrs. Hammer was instructed to lie still. What the physician meant was that Mrs. Hammer should not toss about or get out of bed. What Mrs. Hammer perceived was that she must not move a muscle. In fact, she was so fearful and held herself to rigidly that she developed muscle soreness that persisted for a week.

Because Mrs. Hammer was being "specialed" by a physician, she was given little attention by a nurse. When a nurse finally asked her how she felt, she said, "Awful. Nobody does anything for me, no one even talks to me." The nurse gave Mrs. Hammer a bath and, as she did, she put her extremities through their normal range of motion. She showed Mrs. Hammer how she could wiggle her toes and exercise her arms and legs without disturbing the tubing. Except for giving directions and instructions, the nurse did not talk very much. When she had completed Mrs. Hammer's care, she asked her how she felt. At this time Mrs. Hammer said, "Oh, so much better. I had just about given up." Although there were other factors in Mrs. Hammer's improvement, exercise was one.

Exercise Out of Bed

The earliness with which surgical patients are ambulated varies with the surgeon, the surgical procedure, and the patient. Leithauser (1951), who was one of the more vigorous proponents of early ambulation, advocated that patients be ambulated as soon as they had recovered from the depressing effects of the anesthetic. The only exceptions were patients who were in shock, experiencing severe uncontrolled hemorrhage, or in thyroid crisis. Some surgeons add sepsis to this list of exceptions because exercise can promote the spread of an infection.

When early ambulation was first introduced, patients, nurses, and physicians were fearful that harm might come to the patient. They had been indoctrinated with the belief that bedrest was necessary to the healing of the wound and that exertion by the patient was dangerous. Patients who entered the hospital expecting to have good rest were surprised and somewhat frightened because they were forced to get out of bed and walk. Today patients are mentally better prepared to ambulate. They know that the neighbor across the street was out of bed a few hours after he returned from the operating room. Despite previous warning, however, the patient who gets out of bed for the first time after undergoing a major surgical procedure is frequently frightened and anxious.

A frequent and justifiable cause for apprehension when the patient first gets out of bed in the immediate postoperative period is the development of *orthostatic hypotension,* or drop in blood pressure caused by failure of vasomotor responses to compensate for change from a recumbent to an upright position. The normal compensatory response of blood pressure to change from a recumbent to a standing position is illustrated in Figure 52-6. In normal individuals compensation usually is complete within 30 seconds. Factors that interfere with the mechanisms of normal vasomotor compensation with position change are numerous. Those that are present or that may develop in the operative and postoperative periods include spinal anesthesia; injury to nervous and circulatory systems; interference with blood supply to lower extremities; injury to lower extremities; confinement to the recumbent position for 24 hours or longer; and drugs that depress sympathetic nervous system, dilate blood vessels, or reduce blood volume. When getting the patient out of bed following surgery, or after any prolonged period of bedrest, the nurse should ensure safety of the patient by changing his or her position in stages, closely monitoring the

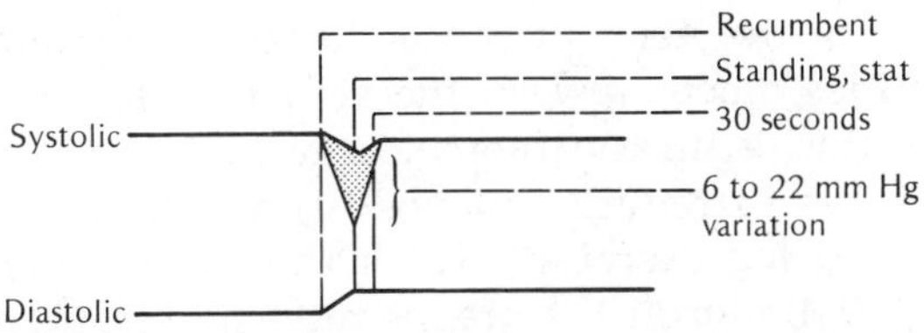

Figure 52-6. Normal compensatory response of blood pressure to change from a recumbent to an upright position. (From *Effects of Preambulation Exercises on Postoperative General Surgery Patients Experiencing Postural Hypotension* by Madeline L. Bluemle. Detroit: Wayne State University Master's Thesis, 1972, p. 94. Used by permission.)

pulse, blood pressure, and subjective symptoms at each stage of position change.

In an experimental study to test the effectiveness of preambulation exercises in reducing symptoms of patients who had experienced postural hypotension on the first postoperative ambulation, Bluemle (1972) found the following simple rhythmic leg exercises significantly reduced subsequent symptoms. Exercises were performed in bed prior to ambulation, according to the following instructions.

1. Lie flat in bed.
2. Flex one knee, keeping the foot on the bed.
3. Straighten the lower leg as far as possible.
4. Bring the lower leg down to the flexed knee position.
5. Straighten the leg.
6. Repeat with the other leg.
7. Repeat with each leg, alternately, six times.
8. If unable to do unaided, assistance will be given as needed.

The five positions of each leg are illustrated in Figure 52-7.

In addition to taking measures to help the patient equilibrate the circulatory status with position change, the nurse who is assisting a patient out of bed must be sure there is enough competent assistance available to assure the patient that he or she will not be allowed to fall. The patient should also be assured that the wound will not suffer from the activity. When a patient is large or heavy, a male nurse or orderly can make a real contribution to the actual physical safety and confidence of the patient. In the process of getting out of bed, the patient should be allowed sufficient time to adjust to each change in position.

Preparatory to getting the patient out of bed, the bed should be lowered. Then the patient turns on the side and, as he or she starts to sit up, swings the feet over the edge of the bed. By the time the patient is in the upright position, the feet are over the edge of the bed. At this point the patient may wish to rest with hands on the edge of the bed or on the shoulders of a nurse standing in front of him or her. Then the patient should be assisted to the standing position. In those hospitals where the height of the bed is fixed, the simplest way to get the patient out of bed is to let him or her slide off the edge of the bed until the feet touch the floor. The patient should be supported and encouraged to cough, so that secretions are eliminated from the tracheobron-

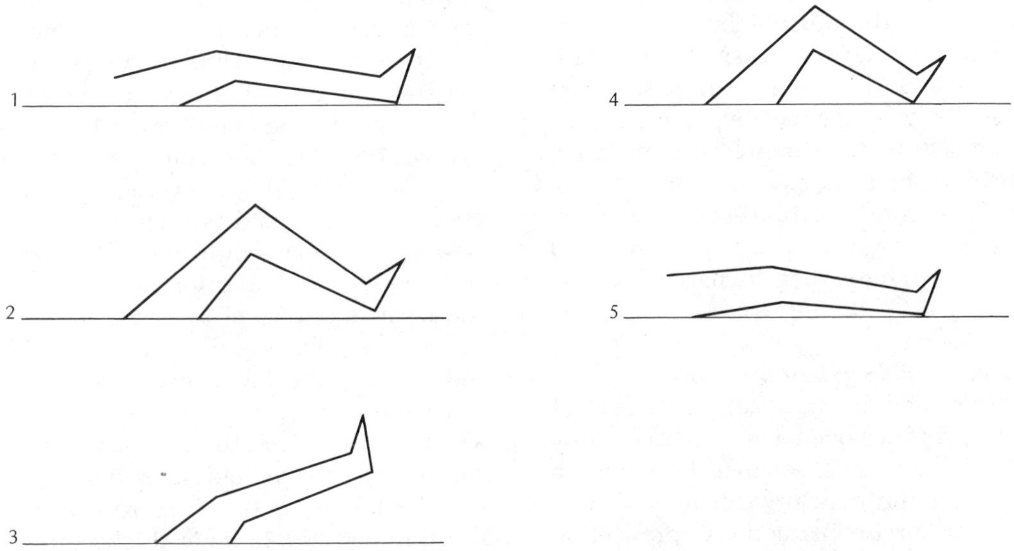

Figure 52-7. Preambulation leg exercises. (From *Effects of Preambulation Exercises on Postoperative General Surgery Patients Experiencing Postural Hypotension* by Madeline L. Bluemle. Detroit: Wayne State University Master's Thesis, 1972, p. 94. Used by permission.)

chial tree. He or she should then be encouraged to walk to the foot of the bed and return to the center of the bed and be assisted back into bed. If the patient is short and the bed is high he or she may step on a stool 6 to 8 inches high before getting into bed. After a period of rest, the patient is again encouraged to get up and walk. With each successive period out of bed, strength and courage usually improve.

Following chest surgery, ambulation offers some difficulties but these are not insurmountable. If the patient has chest drainage tubes, attention should be given to preventing tension on them. If the bottles are moved, they should be kept below the point where the tubes enter the thorax so that fluid will not be sucked back into the pleural cavity. Suction is discontinued and tubes are clamped only when prescribed by the physician. Ambulation of the patient receiving intravenous fluids can be accomplished if the arm with the needle is stabilized. When the needle is introduced into a vein over a joint, the joint must be immobilized with a splint. Attention should be given to the prevention of any tension on the tubing. In patients with indwelling catheters, the catheter should either be attached to a leg bag or the regular collecting reservoir carried with the patient, being sure it is held below the level of the bladder.

The term *to ambulate* means "to walk," not to get up and sit in a chair. Patients should be discouraged from sitting in a chair. They should either be walking or in bed, because in the sitting position the dependent position of the legs and the weight of the body on the thighs interferes with venous return from the legs. Venous stasis predisposes to the development of thrombophlebitis, which, in turn, may lead to pulmonary embolism. Venous stasis in the legs of some elderly patients may be so severe that, if they sit for a long time, hypotension may develop. The benefits to the patient from ambulation include less pain in the operative site, earlier disappearance of pain, a protein-sparing action, reduction in certain postoperative sequelae, improvement of the patient's morale, and earlier discharge from the hospital.

Exercise to Restore Specific Functions

Exercises performed by the patient to protect *pulmonary function* have been described previously in Chapter 51 and in some detail in Chapters 26 and 40. The benefits of preoperative deep breathing, coughing, and leg exercise instruction in preventing postoperative pulmonary complications have been well documented (Risser, 1980). Those same exercises also aid in promoting *circulation.* With inspiration the pressure within the thoracic cavity falls. Blood in the veins of the abdomen, head, and extremities moves toward the area with lower pressure, that is, in the thoracic cavity. Circulation in the lower extremities may be further stimulated by foot and leg exercises, which should be taught to the patient during the preoperative period. Contraction of the muscles of the feet and legs squeeze on the deep veins in the legs and push the blood toward the heart. The valves in the veins support the column of blood so that it can move only in the direction of the heart. Inactivity allows blood to stagnate or pool in these veins. This venous stasis tends to occur in anyone who sits quietly for an extended period of time. Examples include the person who takes a long bus ride and the elderly person who sits in a chair from morning until night without moving. Stasis of blood in leg veins also occurs during the operative and early postoperative phases of surgery. This is particularly marked in spinal anesthesia which causes complete paralysis of the muscles of the legs for up to several hours. Because of the tendency for blood to pool in the lower extremities during anesthesia, some surgeons wrap the lower extremities from toes to the knee or to the groin with elastic bandages.

Unless there is a specific contraindication, patients undergoing surgical procedures should perform foot and leg exercises regularly. These exercises consist of dorsiflexion alternating with hyperextension of the feet. The knee and the thigh should also be flexed and then extended. The movements of the leg and thigh are often referred to as bicycle exercises, because the movements are similar to those used in riding a bicycle. Although foot and leg exercises are more beneficial when the patient is able to perform them alone, they may also be performed by the nurse as passive exercises. Until the patient is up and walking, they should be initiated at 1- or 2-hour intervals, depending on the condition of the patient and the prescription of the surgeon. As with the deep-breathing exercises, most patients require some reminding, encouragement, and assistance.

Many physicians discourage the use of pillows or rests under the knees for two reasons. One is that the localized areas of pressure where the legs rest against the pillows tend to interfere with the venous return from the lower extremities and predispose to venous stasis and thrombosis. Pillows or knee rests also tend to reduce the mobility of the patient, because they help to hold the patient up in bed. Without the pillow or the knee rest, the patient slides down in bed. When he or she becomes uncomfortable, the patient boosts himself or herself up in bed to increase comfort and in the process stimulates circulation, respiration, and muscle activity.

Exercise may be prescribed to protect or restore

function of a specific structure or part. For example, the loss of muscle tone in an extremity can be reduced by the performance of muscle-setting exercises. To prevent the loss of strength in a leg encased in a cast the physician sometimes prescribes special exercises that require contraction of the quadriceps muscles. The nurse can practice performing this exercise on herself or himself as preparation for teaching patients. As the quadriceps muscles shorten, the kneecap can be felt to move. Before encouraging a patient to exercise a muscle or muscles in an extremity that has had surgery, the nurse should consult with the physician about when the exercises may be started.

Following a radical mastectomy, exercise of the arm and shoulder on the affected arm may be prescribed by the physician to maintain joint motion and muscle tone in the area. Surgeons' opinions differ as to the time exercises should be started. When the resection has been extensive, closure of the wound may be difficult and proper healing of the wound may depend on immobilization and rest of the area. The nurse should always consult with the surgeon before initiating any exercises that may affect the operated area. Specific exercises that are used are described in Chapter 39.

When patients are treated by physical therapy, the nurse should know what the purpose of the therapy is and how she or he can assist the work of the therapist. Although this discussion has been related to the needs of the postsurgical patient, it is also important in the care of any bedfast patient, regardless of the diagnosis or treatment. The proper amount and kind of exercise are important factors in restoring any patient to health. Whether the exercise is performed in bed or out of bed, it improves the psychological as well as the physiologic status of the patient. Although a program of exercise is begun in the early postoperative period, it continues to be important in all phases.

Rest

Although exercise is important in the care of the patient, adequate rest must also be emphasized. Despite Leithauser's contention that patients will not overexert themselves, some patients do require protection from overactivity. As the patient begins to recover, he or she may feel farther along in convalescence than he or she actually is. The patient should be encouraged to exercise to moderation and stop before becoming fatigued.

Another source of exhaustion of patients is the number of procedures performed on them. Frail or seriously ill patients are sometimes exhausted by the continuous activity, especially in intensive-care units. Mr. Watts had open-heart surgery and his diseased aortic valve was replaced with a prosthesis. For the first 3 days postoperatively, he was in borderline shock. On his first postoperative day, he was to be turned from side to side, to do deep-breathing exercises, and to cough each hour. All the preceding are required to prevent postoperative atelectasis and to promote the re-expansion of the lung. However, because Mr. Watts was frail and unable to cooperate well, each maneuver took the better part of an hour. At one point when his care had just been completed and he was prepared to rest, the surgeon and his assistants came in. The patient was then raised to a sitting position and moved so that his chest could be examined. Shortly after the physicians departed, the patient vomited without any warning and soiled the bed with emesis. The bed required changing, further depriving Mr. Watts of rest. His nurse felt that there was another requirement—that is, some planning between the surgeon and the nurse so that the visit of the physician could be substituted for one of his exercise periods. The nurse has the responsibility for taking initiative to protect the patient from too rigorous exercise and to make sure that he gets needed rest. This lack of needed rest may be expecially important after heart surgery or any extended stay in an intensive-care unit. A study of rest and activity patterns of patients in an intensive-care unit following open heart surgery found that all patients were deprived of sleep during their first six postoperative nights, and none received enough uninterrupted sleep during the other 16 hours of each day to have made up for the sleep loss (McFadden & Giblin, 1971). Severe psychosis of depression may result in 1 or 2 days if the patient is awakened every 15 to 60 minutes and is not allowed adequate sleep or rest.

Tubes

Of the many aspects of surgical treatment viewed by the patient with apprehension, distaste, or even fear, there is probably no single aspect any more distressing to most patients than the indignity and discomfort associated with the myriad of tubes used in their care. The most frequent question asked by an intubated patient is, "When can the tube come out?" No effort will be made here to describe all the tubes that may be encountered by the nurse in caring for the surgical patient, because their number is legion and daily the ingenuity of surgeons adds to the list. However, regardless of whether or not the nurse has ever previously encountered a particular tube in nursing practice, there are a number of questions she or he can ask related to *any* tube that will assist in planning and providing safe and effective care to the patient.

1. How much and what kind of discomfort for the patient is associated with this tube? Are there any physical or psychological measures that can alleviate that discomfort?
2. Where is the portal of entry of the tube? In many instances the portal of entry is under a dressing and is not visible. Does the tube enter through a natural body orifice of one created by accidental or surgical trauma? Intact skin and mucous membranes of natural orifices provide some added protection against infection and against the effects of pressure and irritation of the tube on surrounding tissue.
3. Where is the "working end" of the tube? Does it enter a clean or sterile cavity? Tubes inserted into the gastrointestinal tract are in an organ considered to be clean, and can be handled according to principles of medical asepsis, whereas tubes inserted, for example, into the pleural space or peritoneal cavity are considered to be in a sterile cavity and must be handled according to principles of surgical asepsis.
4. What is the purpose of the tube? Is it in place to drain fluid and/or air from a particular area, or does it serve as a means to introduce fluid, medication, or gases into the patient?
5. Does the tube have to be advanced or withdrawn periodically? Or is it to remain fixed? How is it, or how should it be, secured to prevent accidental dislodgment?
6. Does the presence of the tube prohibit moving or ambulation of the patient? If not, what precautions or preparations are necessary to ensure continuing effective operation of the system while mobilizing the patient?
7. Is there a reservoir attached to the tube? Is the reservoir collecting material *from* the patient, and if so, what are the expected quality and amount, and how do the expected characteristics compare with what is present? Is the reservoir providing material for instillation or infusion via the tube *into* the patient? If so, what is the *exact* nature of the material, what are its purpose and action, and what responsibilities does the nurse have for administration of the material to the patient?
8. When was the tube inserted? How long has it been in place? When and under what circumstances will it be removed? Will accidental removal constitute a life-threatening crisis for the patient? If so, from whom will the nurse need immediate assistance? Where and how can that person be contacted promptly?
9. What are the institutional practices and procedures governing (a) the responsibility of the nurse relating to insertion, maintenance of function, and removal of the tube; (b) the reporting and recording of the function and status of the tube and its effect on the patient; and (c) the care and final disposition of equipment after the tube is removed from the patient?

The nurse who is competent in caring for the patient treated surgically provides immeasurable comfort and assistance to the patient in preventing postoperative complications, by careful observation and appropriate care of tubes used in the surgical treatment.

Summary

In the last century surgical therapy has become a reality; diseases in all parts of the body are now treated by surgical methods. In its development, surgery was first made safe for the patient by the development of techniques of hemostasis, asepsis, anesthesia, and increased skill in incising and treating tissues. More recently, advances in knowledge have made it possible to give proper attention to making the patient safe for surgery. As a result, most patients are restored to health and vitality after surgery with a minimum of discomfort and disability. This is true of patients in all age groups and even those who have extensive surgery. Some of the complications that may delay recovery or cause death have been indicated.

Despite numerous possibilities for difficulty in the postoperative period, most patients have what is called an uneventful recovery. In those who do develop a complication, signs and symptoms are usually detected early so that procedures are promptly instituted to correct the problem. Much of the credit for the reduction in operative morbidity and mortality can be given to the application of knowledge of physiology, microbiology, and psychology to the care of the patient in all phases of the operative experience. Credit must also be given to nurses who carry out, or assist patients in carrying out, procedures to protect and support bodily processes. Because of the amount of time nurses spend with patients, they also are in a position to observe and report early signs and symptoms that indicate a complication is developing. Despite the united efforts of the patient, nurse, and physician, complications do occur. Many of the possibilities have been indicated in the preceding discussion. Surgery places stress on physiologic and psychological functioning. Even in minor surgery, the combination of the effects of an anesthetic and a surgical procedure many result in depression or disorganization of function. If continued, some disturbances in function are self-perpetuating or lead to more serious changes that are difficult to correct.

Complications that develop in the postoperative period can be summarized as having their origin in (1) abnormal function of one or more systems—respiratory, gastrointestinal, urinary, or cardiovascular; (2) stress that exceeds the adaptive capacity of the individual—shock, hemorrhage, psychological disturbances; (3) failure to heal the wound; and (4) sepsis—wound infection or infection of other structures such as the urinary bladder, leg veins, peritoneum, or lungs.

Pulmonary complications associated with surgery have been identified, especially those believed to originate in obstruction of portions of the tracheobronchial tree by accumulated secretions, inadequate coughing or ventilation, or aspiration of salivary and/or gastric secretions. Prevention of these problems by preoperative evaluation and preparation and by maintenance of adequate ventilation during and after surgery has been discussed here and in Chapter 40.

During the postoperative period the objective in the care of the patient is to enable him or her to return to optimal physiological and psychological functioning as rapidly and safely as possible. The surgical procedures, including the incision, the anesthetic, the pain-relieving medications, and excessive bedrest, combine to depress and to disorganize bodily functions. An important part of the patient's care is to anticipate, protect, and maintain the functions that are disrupted. To do this effectively requires some understanding of physiology and how function can be maintained until the patient can carry it on independently. In assessing the needs of the patient in the postoperative period, the nurse should try to determine the functions with which he or she requires assistance. Individual factors, such as age and personal habits, that may influence the prognosis of the patient should be given consideration. For example, the elderly patient usually has a lowered capacity for responding to stress. His or her respiratory reserve decreases with age and he or she is more susceptible to respiratory complications than earlier in life. The patient who has chronic bronchitis as a consequence of heavy smoking over a period of years is especially predisposed to respiratory complications. In addition, the chronic cough renders the patient more liable to wound disruption. Both these patients, then, require more than the usual attention toward keeping the tracheobronchial tree clear of secretions.

Only a small part of the patient's convalescence is spent in the hospital. As soon as the requirements of the patient can be met at home, he or she is likely to be discharged form the hospital. Plans for the discharge of the patient should include instruction in those aspects of care that require some modification of the daily patterns of living. The patient should know when to visit the physician, how much rest and exercise he or she should take, any modifications of the diet that are required, and when return to work can be anticipated. Even when the patient has made what is called an uneventful recovery, the nurse should ask the question, will this patient and family be able to meet his or her needs after leaving the hospital? If the answer is yes, as it will be in many instances, then nothing more needs to be done. If the answer is no, then the next question is, what kind of help does the patient or family require? And then, what are the resources in the community that can be utilized to provide the help the patient and family require? What steps should be taken to secure continuing care for the patient?

References Cited

Allen, J. G. "Commercial Blood in Our National Blood Program." *Arch. Surg.*, **102** (Feb. 1971), 122–26.

Allgood, R. J. et al. "Prospective Analysis of Pulmonary Embolism in the Postoperative Patient." *Surgery*, **68** (July 1970), 116–22.

Alter, H. J. et al. "Transmission of Hepatitis B Virus Infection by Transfusion of Frozen-Deglycerolized Red Blood Cells." *N. Engl. J. Med.*, **298** (March 23, 1978), 637–42.

Baker, R. J., and Nyhus, L. M. "Diagnosis and Treatment of Immediate Transfusion Reaction." *Surg. Gynecol. Obstet.*, **130** (April 1970), 665–72, 665.

"Blood Therapy: A Home-Study Feature Approved for ANA Continuing Education Contact Hours." *Am. J. Nurs.*, **79** (May 1979), 925–48.

Bluemle, M. L. *Effects of Pre-Ambulation Exercises on Postoperative General Surgery Patients Experiencing Postural Hypotension.* Detroit: Wayne State University, Master's thesis, 1972, pp. 65–66.

Bruno, P. "The Nature of Wound Healing." *Nurs. Clin. North Am.*, **14** (Dec. 1979), 667–82.

Chaplin, H., Jr. "Frozen Blood." *N. Engl. J. Med.*, **298** (March 23, 1978), 679–80.

Cleland, V. et al. "Prevention of Bacteriuria in Female Patients with Indwelling Catheters." *Nurs. Res.*, **20** (July–Aug. 1971), 310.

Coller, F. A., and DeWeese, M. S. "Preoperative and Postoperative Care." *JAMA*, **141** (Nov. 5, 1949), 644.

"Commercial Blood Banks Threat to Nurses." *Mass. Nurse*, **48**:8 (Aug. 1979), 1.

Committee on Guidelines of the Society of Critical Care Medicine. "Guidelines for Organization of Critical Care Units." *JAMA*, **222** (Dec. 18, 1972), 1532–35.

Coon, W. W., and Willis, P. W., III. "Thromboembolic Complications during Anticoagulant Therapy." *Arch. Surg.*, **105** (Aug. 1972), 209–12.

Cutler, B. S., and Daggett, W. M. "Application of the 'G-suit' to the Control of Hemorrhage in Massive Trauma." *Ann. Surg.*, **173** (April 1971), 511–14.

Daniel, R. K. "Microsurgery: Through the Looking Glass." *N. Engl. J. Med.*, **300** (May 31, 1979), 1251–57.

Del Guercio, L. R. M. "Physiologic Monitoring of the Surgical Patient," in *Principles of Surgery*, 3rd ed., Ed. by I. Schwartz. New York: McGraw-Hill, 1979, pp. 525–45.

Dickman, H. M. "A Pilot Study of Pain in the Postoperative Patient." Detroit: Wayne State University, unpublished Master's essay, 1959.

Doyle, J. "The Intracaval Filter: New Nursing Challenge." *RN*, **43** (May 1980), 38–42.

Drain, C. B., and Shipley, S. B. *The Recovery Room*. Philadelphia: W. B. Saunders Co., 1979, Chap. 15, "General Recovery Room Care."

Duthie, R. B., and Hoaglund, F. T. "Manifestations of Musculoskeletal Disorders." In *Principles of Surgery*, 3rd ed. Ed. by S. I. Schwartz. New York: McGraw-Hill, 1979, p. 1809.

Eickhoff, T. C. "Hospital Infections." *Dis.-a-Month* (Sept. 1972), 7–8.

Fein, J. M. "Microvascular Surgery for Stroke." *Sci. Am.*, **238** (April 1978), 58–67.

Finn, K. "How's Your Post-op Ambulation Technique?" *RN*, **42** (Sept. 1979), 69–72.

Fisher, R. E. "Measuring Central Venous Pressure: How to Do It Accurately . . . and Safely." *Nursing 79*, **9** (Oct. 1979), 74–78.

Gupta, S. L. et al. "Renal Insufficiency after Trauma and Sepsis." *Arch. Surg.*, **103** (Aug. 1971), 175–83.

Hau, T. "Secondary Bacterial Peritonitis: The Biologic Basis of Treatment." *Curr. Probs. Surg.*, **16**:10 (Oct. 1979).

Hoshal, V. L. et al. "Gastric Decompression Following Vagotomy and Drainage Procedures." *Arch. Surg.*, **102** (April 1971), 248–50.

Isler, C. "Blood: The Age of Components." *RN*, **36** (June 1973), 31–41, 34.

Johnson, J. E. "Effects of Structuring Patients' Expectations on Their Reactions to Threatening Events." *Nurs. Res.*, **21** (Nov.–Dec. 1972), 499–504.

Landsteiner, K., and Levine, P. "On the Cold Agglutinins in Human Serum." *J. Immunol.*, **12** (Dec. 1926), 441.

Leithauser, D. J. et al. "Prevention of Embolic Complications from Venous Thrombosis after Surgery." *JAMA*, **147** (Sept. 22, 1951), 301.

"Life Jacket: It Saves People Who Cannot Eat." *Time* (Oct. 9, 1978), 104.

Literte, J. W. "Nursing Care of Patients with Intestinal Obstruction." *Am. J. Nurs.*, **77** (June 1977), 1003–06.

Luft, H. S. et al. "Should Operations Be Regionalized? The Empirical Relation between Surgical Volume and Mortality." *N. Engl. J. Med.*, **301** (Dec. 20, 1979), 1364–69.

Madden, J. W. "Wound Healing: Biologic and Clinical Features." In *Davis-Christopher Textbook of Surgery*, 11th ed. Ed. by D. C. Sabiston et al. Philadelphia: W. B. Saunders Co., 1977, p. 280.

Marcinek, M. B. "Stress in the Surgical Patient." *Am. J. Nurs.*, **77** (Nov. 1977), 1809–11.

Marcoux, J. P., and Peters, G. A. "Some Adverse Drug Reactions Common in the Postoperative Period." *Surg. Clin. North Am.*, **49** (Oct. 1969), 1123–36.

McFadden, E. H., and Giblin, E. C. "Sleep Deprivation in Patients Having Open-Heart Surgery." *Nurs. Res.*, **20** (May–June 1971), 249–54.

Oakes, A. R. "Trauma: Twentieth Century Epidemic." *Heart and Lung*, **8** (Sept.–Oct. 1979), 918–22.

Petri, G. et al. "Sympatholytic Treatment of 'Paralytic' Ileus." *Surgery*, **70** (Sept. 1971), 359–67.

Polanyi, T. G. "The Physics of Lasers for Surgery." *Gynescope*, 17 (1976).

Polk, H. C., Jr. "Principles of Preoperative Preparation of the Surgical Patient." In *Davis-Christopher Textbook of Surgery*, 11th ed. Ed. by D. C. Sabiston, Jr. Philadelphia: W. B. Saunders Co., 1977, p. 127.

Risser, N. L. "Preoperative and Postoperative Care to Prevent Pulmonary Complications." *Heart and Lung*, **9** (Jan.–Feb. 1980), 57–67.

Robson, M. C. et al. "Biology of Surgical Infections." *Curr. Probl. Surg.*, (March 1973), 3–4.

Sabiston, D. C., Jr. "Pulmonary Embolism." In *Davis-Christopher Textbook of Surgery*, 11th ed. Ed. by D. C. Sabiston, Jr. Philadelphia: W. B. Saunders Co., 1977, pp. 1849–55.

Schumann, D. "How to Help Wound Healing in Your Abdominal Surgery Patient." *Nursing 80*, **10** (April 1980), 34–40, 36.

Shires, G. T., and Canizaro, P. C. "Fluid, Electrolytes, and Nutritional Management of the Surgical Patient." In *Principles of Surgery*, 3rd ed. Ed. by S. I. Schwartz et al. New York: McGraw-Hill, 1979, pp. 65–97, 92–93.

Silen, W. "The Prevention and Management of Stress Ulcers." *Hosp. Prac.*, **15** (March 1980), 93–100.

Smith, G. "Primary Postoperative Wound Infection Due to Staphylococcus Pyogenes." *Curr. Probs. Surg.*, **16**:7 (July 1979).

Stahl, W. M., and Stone, A. M. "Prophylactic Diuresis with Ethacrynic Acid for Prevention of Postoperative Renal Failure." *Ann. Surg.*, **172** (Sept. 1970), 361–69.

Stahlgren, L. H., and Morris, N. W. "Intestinal Obstruction." *Am. J. Nurs.*, **77** (June 1977), 999–1002.

Storer, E. H. "Small Intestine." In *Principles of Surgery*, 3rd ed. Ed. by S. I. Schwartz et al. New York: McGraw-Hill, 1979, pp. 1169–90.

Stremple, J. F. et al. "The Stress Ulcer Syndrome." *Curr. Probl. Surg.* (April 1973).

Zook, C. J., and Moore, F. D. "High-Cost Users of Medical Care." *N. Engl. J. Med.*, **302** (May 1, 1980), 996–1002.

Zucker, M. B. "The Functioning of Blood Platelets." *Sci. Am.*, **242** (June 1980), 86–103.

General References

Akiyama, H. "Surgery for Carcinoma of the Esophagus." *Curr. Probs. Surg.*, **17**:2 (Feb. 1980).

Berry, E. C., and Kohn, M. L. *Introduction to Operating Room Technique,* 4th ed. New York: McGraw-Hill, 1972.

Boyd, D. R. et al. "Trauma Registry: New Computer Method for Multifactorial Evaluation of a Major Health Problem." *JAMA,* **223** (Jan. 22, 1973), 422–28.

Del Bueno, D. J. "Recognizing Fat Embolism in Patients." *RN,* **36** (Jan. 1973), 48–55.

Burnett, W., and McCaffrey, J. "Surgical Procedures in the Elderly." *Surg. Gynecol. Obstet.,* **134** (Feb. 1972), 221–26.

Brazier, M. A. B. *The Neurophysiological Background for Anesthesia.* Springfield, Ill.: Charles C Thomas, 1972.

Browse, N. L. *The Physiology and Pathology of Bed Rest.* Springfield, Ill.: Charles C Thomas, 1965.

Bunker, J. P. *The Anesthesiologist and the Surgeon: Partners in the Operating Room.* Boston: Little, Brown, 1972.

Cohen, S., and Stack, M. "How to Work with Chest Tubes: Programmed Instruction." *Am. J. Nurs.,* **80** (April 1980), 685–712.

Committee on Pre- and Postoperative Care, American College of Surgeons. *Manual of Preoperative and Postoperative Care,* 2nd ed. Philadelphia: W. B. Saunders Co., 1971.

Franklin, B. *A Dissertation on Liberty and Necessity, Pleasure and Pain* (reproduced from the 1st ed.) New York: Facsimile Text Society, 1930.

Frawley, T. F. "Axioms on Metabolic Considerations in Postsurgical Patients." *Hosp. Med.,* **6** (Jan. 1970), 107–21.

Gius, J. A. *Fundamentals of Surgery.* Chicago: Year Book Medical Publishers, 1972.

"Giving Medication Through a Nasogastric Tube." *Nursing '80,* **10** (May 1980), 71–73.

Hardy, J. D. *Critical Surgical Illness.* Philadelphia: W. B. Saunders Co., 1971.

Henderson, V., and Nite, G. "Application of Surgical Dressings." In *Principles and Practice of Nursing,* 6th ed. New York: Macmillan Publishing Co., 1978, pp. 1431–48, Chap. 33.

Kintzel, K. C. *Advanced Concepts in Clinical Nursing,* 2nd ed. New York: J. B. Lippincott Co., 1977.

Leithauser, D. J. *Early Ambulation.* Springfield, Ill.: Charles C Thomas, 1946.

Lewin, I. et al. "Physical Class and Physiological Status in the Prediction of Operative Mortality in the Aged Sick." *Ann. Surg.,* **174** (Aug. 1971), 217–31.

Mackenzie, R. *Risk.* New York: Viking Press, 1970.

Marshall, H. R. *Pain, Pleasure, and Anesthetics.* New York: Macmillan Publishing Co., 1894.

Maurer, J. "Providing Optimal Oral Health." *Nurs. Clin. North Am.,* **12** (Dec. 1977), 669–85.

Moore, F. D. *Transplant: The Give and Take of Tissue Transplantation,* 2nd ed. New York: Simon & Shuster, 1972.

Ranson, J. H. C. "Acute Pancreatitis." *Curr. Prob. Surg.,* **16**:11 (Nov. 1979).

Saltzstein, E. C. "Ambulatory Surgical Unit: Alternative to Hospitalization." *Arch. Surg.,* **108** (Feb. 1974), 143–46.

"Symposium on Bioinstrumentation for Nurses." *Nurs. Clin. North Am.,* **13** (Dec. 1978), 559–640.

"Symposium on Current Surgical Nursing." *Nurs. Clin. North Am.,* **8** (March 1973), 107–98.

"Symposium on Orthopedic Nursing." *Nurs. Clin. North Am.,* **11** (Dec. 1976), 639–730.

"Symposium on Trauma." *Nurs. Clin. North Am.,* **13** (June 1978), 175–265.

Tichener, J. L., and Levine, M. *Surgery As a Human Experience.* New York: Oxford University Press, 1960.

Van Way, C. et al. "An Assessment of the Role of Parenteral Alimentation in Management of Surgical Patients." *Ann. Surg.,* **177** (Jan. 1973), 103–111.

Zuidema, G. D. et al. *The Management of Trauma,* 3rd ed. Philadelphia: W. B. Saunders Co., 1979.

Preoperative Preparation

Graham, L. E., and Myers, E. "Evaluation of Anxiety and Fear in Adult Surgical Patients." *Nurs. Res.,* **20** (March–April 1971), 113–22.

Lindeman, C. A. "Influencing Recovery through Preoperative Teaching." *Heart and Lung,* **2** (July–Aug. 1973), 515–21.

Schmitt, F. E., and Woolridge, P. J. "Psychological Preparation of Surgical Patients." *Nurs. Res.,* **22** (March–April 1973), 108–16.

Winslow, E. H., and Fuhs, M. F. "Preoperative Assessment for Postoperative Evaluation." *Am. J. Nurs.,* **73** (Aug. 1973), 1372–74.

Cardiovascular Pulmonary Function

Blacher, R. S. "The Hidden Psychosis of Open-Heart Surgery." *JAMA,* **222** (Oct. 16, 1972), 305–8.

Clagett, G. P., and Salzman, E. W. "Current Concepts: Prevention of Venous Thromboembolism in Surgical Patients." *N. Engl. J. Med.,* **290** (Jan. 10, 1974), 93–96.

Collart, M. E., and Brenneman, J. K. "Preventing Postoperative Atelectasis." *Am. J. Nurs.,* **71** (Oct. 1971), 1982–87.

Fonkalsrud, E. W. et al. "Prophylaxis against Postinfusion Phlebitis." *Surg. Gynecol. Obstet.,* **133** (Aug. 1971), 253–56.

Lecky, J. H., and Ominsky, A. J. "Postoperative Respiratory Management." *Chest,* **62** (Aug. Suppl. 1972), 50–54.

Lum, L. G. et al. "Splenectomy in the Management of the Thrombocytopenia of the Wiskott-Aldrich Syndrome." *N. Engl. J. Med.,* **302** (April 17, 1980), 892–96.

Malt, R. A. "Control of Massive Upper Gastrointestinal Hemorrhage." *N. Engl. J. Med.,* **286** (May 11, 1972), 1043–46.

Ratnoff, O. D. "A New Property of an Old Remedy: Fibrinolysis and Aspirin." *N. Engl. J. Med.,* **296** (March 10, 1977), 566–67.

Rob, C. G. "A History of Arterial Surgery." *Arch. Surg.*, **105** (Dec. 1972), 821–23.
Roche, J. K., and Stengle, J. M. "Open-Heart Surgery and the Demand for Blood." *JAMA*, **225** (Sept. 17, 1973), 1516–21.
Scarloto, M. "Blood Transfusions Today: What You Should Know and Do." *Nursing '78*, **8** (Feb. 1978), 68–72.
Skillman, J. et al. "Cardiorespiratory, Metabolic and Endocrine Changes after Hemorrhage in Man." *Ann. Surg.*, **174** (Dec. 1971), 911–22.

Urinary System Function

Bergstrom, N. I. "Ice Applications to Induce Voiding." *Am. J. Nurs.*, **69** (Feb. 1969), 283–85.
Fass, R. J. et al. "Urinary Tract Infection: Practical Aspects of Diagnosis and Treatment." *JAMA*, **225** (Sept. 17, 1973), 1509–13.
Tank, E. S. et al. "Urinary Tract Complications of Anorectal Surgery." *Am. J. Surg.*, **123** (Jan. 1972), 118–22.

Other Problems

Robach, S. A., and Nicoloff, D. M. "High Output Enterocutaneous Fistulas of the Small Bowel." *Am. J. Surg.*, **123** (March 1972), 317–22.
Stephenson, C. A. "Stress in Critically Ill Patients." *Am. J. Nurs.* **77** (Nov. 1977), 1806–09.
"Symposium on Impressions of Pain: A Nursing Diagnosis." *Nurs. Clin. North Am.*, **12** (Dec. 1977), 609–68.
"Symposium on Wound Healing." *Nurs. Clin. North Am.*, **14** (Dec. 1979), 665–778.
Trimpi, H. D. et al. "Guide to the Management of Rectal Abscesses." *Hosp. Med.*, **12** (Sept. 1976), 79–88.
Wang, S. M. S., and Wilson, S. E. "Subphrenic Abscess: The New Epidemiology." *Arch. Surg.*, **112** (Aug. 1977), 934–36.

APPENDIX A

Critical Requirements for Safe-Effective Nursing Practice

In 1971 the Council of State Boards of Nursing of the American Nurses' Association authorized a study to examine the validity of the State Board Test Pool Examination (SBTPE). A research steering committee was formed by the Council of State Boards to oversee the implementation of the study by the National League for Nursing. A research advisory committee, appointed by the Steering Committee and composed of clinical nurses and test construction specialists, assisted in overall guidance and direction of the NLN staff. As part of this study of the SBTPE, the project on *Critical Requirements for Safe-Effective Nursing Practice* was contracted by the NLN to the American Institutes for Research (AIR).

The scope of AIR's contract was to provide a data base for use in the development of tests to validate the SBTPE licensing examination. The research staff of AIR collected approximately 14,000 critical incidents of nursing behavior from 2,795 nurses at all levels of experience and responsibility in five clinical specialties: Medical-Surgical, Maternal-Newborn, Pediatrics, Community Health, and Psychiatric Nursing. Participants from 67 health care agencies in all four geographic regions of the country contributed incidents to this project.

Although the data collection plans were to collect 2,000 incidents from nurses in each of the five clinical specialties, the enthusiasm of the participants resulted in considerably more incidents in two of the specialties: Medical-Surgical, 4,084, and Community Health, 3,211.

Because of budget and time restrictions, a decision was made by the NLN project management that 2,000 incidents from each clinical specialty would be classified and analyzed. All of the pediatric, psychiatric, and maternal-newborn incidents were analyzed, and a representative sample of 2,000 incidents was selected from the other two specialties, so that every institution and respondent was covered. The total number of incidents analyzed was approximately 11,150.

The critical incidents were inductively classified to derive the classification scheme reflected in the following pages, which include an overall summary and the complete category structure of Critical Requirements for Safe-Effective Nursing Practice, as well as detailed descriptions and analyses of all the categories.

The final report of the project is contained in Council of State Boards of Nursing. *Examining the Validity of the State Board Test Pool Examination for Registered Nurse Licensure.* Kansas City, Mo.: American Nurses' Association, 1979.

Complete Category Structure of Critical Requirements for Safe-Effective Nursing Practice*

I. Exercises Professional Prerogatives Based on Clinical Judgment
   A. Adapts Care to Individual Patient Needs
      1. Adapts rules or policies when flexibility will benefit patient
      2. Adapts standing orders, routines, or usual procedures to accommodate individual patient differences
      3. Designs safe inventive device, method or improvisation for patient care

* Subcategory behaviors in *italics* are *negative behaviors* from critical incidents for which there were no positive counterparts stated by respondents.

4. Makes environmental change to facilitate care of the patient

B. Fulfills Responsibility to Patient and Others Despite Difficulty
1. Persists in providing thorough care despite discouraging prognosis or results
2. Accepts (does not shirk) full responsibility for assigned patients
3. Adjusts for staffing deficiencies by optimizing work schedules and patient priority assignments
4. Volunteers to help beyond assigned responsibility
5. Provides for health care needs of individuals who are not assigned patients

C. Challenges Inappropriate Orders and Decisions by Medical and Other Professional Staff
1. Questions appropriateness of orders for medication or treatment
2. Questions decision not to take needed action or to discontinue needed treatment
3. Questions incomplete investigation when diagnosis is in doubt
4. Refuses to implement inappropriate order
5. Seeks another authority when order is in doubt and there is resistance to changing it
6. Intervenes to prevent harm to patient or violation of patient's rights by medical or other professional staff

D. Acts as Patient Advocate in Obtaining Appropriate Medical, Psychiatric, or Other Help
1. Obtains medical or nursing consultation, assistance or orders
2. Arranges for home nursing services
3. Refers patient or family to special disease center or other health programs
4. Uses community resources to help patient resolve nonmedical problems
5. Persists in obtaining help patient needs
6. Acts as patient's spokesman; supports patient against unwarranted opposition, obstructiveness, neglect, or possible physical harm
7. Provides or arranges transportation to and from agency, or arranges more accessible care

E. Recognizes Own Limitations and Errors
1. Refrains from initiating or implementing care which violates the limits of licensure or authority
2. Recognizes need for instruction or assistance in unfamiliar situations
3. Obtains assistance when situation requires additional help, more skilled personnel, or greater resources
4. Recognizes, corrects, and reports own errors

F. Analyzes and Adjusts Own or Staff Reactions in Order to Maintain Therapeutic Relationship with Patient
1. Recognizes own inability to deal with patient or situation and obtains substitute
2. Avoids allowing frustration, anger, impatience, or irritation with patient to be communicated to patient in nontherapeutic or punitive manner
3. Avoids letting prejudice or moral judgments interfere with patient care
4. Avoids showing favoritism, becoming overinvolved in patient's problem, or overly attached to patient
5. Assesses impact of her or his action on patient and family, to avoid hurting feelings; making suggestive remarks; conveying disgust, threats, blame; or denying the patient's dignity
6. Overcomes own uneasiness, discomfort, or fear in order to give effective care
7. Encourages and participates in staff's exploration of feelings generated by patient care problems

II. Promotes Patient's Ability to Cope with Immediate, Long-Range, or Potential Health-Related Change

A. Provides Health Care Instruction or Information to Patient, Family, or Significant Others
1. Teaches and promotes preventive health care
2. Teaches and helps patient work with normal body processes during labor
3. Gives initial and continuing instruction on management of condition, including treatment devices
4. Gives instruction in the use of medications or home remedies
5. Ensures that instruction is understood
6. Delays teaching until patient is emotionally or physically able to accept it

B. Encourages Patient or Family to Make Own Decision About Accepting Care or Adhering to Treatment Regimen
1. Respects and evaluates patient's right to refuse care

2. Recognizes when patient's misperception of treatment prevents him or her from making realistic decision to seek, accept, or to refuse it
3. Obtains patient's informed consent for procedure
4. Gains patient's cooperation by explaining what is to be done, why it is necessary, and what patient must do
5. Initially considers patient's preference, comfort, or need for assistance and gradually helps patient move toward achieving prescribed care
6. Asks other staff or "significant others" to encourage patient to accept care
7. Persists in persuading patient or family to seek, accept, or not to discontinue needed care

C. Helps Patient Recognize and Deal with Psychological Stress
1. Helps patient deal with feelings associated with body image or self-concept
2. Provides factual, reality-oriented information to help patient or family deal with real or imagined fears and anxieties
3. Facilitates patient's exploration and expression of feelings
4. Uses confrontation appropriately, as a method of helping patient recognize and control behavior
5. Uses self as source of reassurance by presence, touch, or words which convey understanding and encouragement
6. Arranges sedation or analgesia before painful or anxiety-inducing procedure
7. Uses supportive, therapeutic measures other than sedatives or restraints to help patient manage anxiety or stress
8. Aids patient in adjustment to hospital, new setting, aftercare facility, or home
9. Supports dying patient and family in death process

D. Avoids Creating or Increasing Anxiety or Stress
1. Provides means by which patient can signal for help and shows patient how to signal
2. Provides means of communication for patient who cannot express himself or herself or who is sensorily deprived
3. Uses discretion in disclosing guarded or alarming information
4. Refrains from and stops others from discussing potentially anxiety-provoking subjects without considering that patient or family may be able to hear and understand
5. Refrains from giving excessive details, misinformation, or confusing answers to patient's questions
6. Recognizes when care may be perceived as physical, sexual, or environmental threat and takes needed action

E. Conveys and Invites Acceptance, Respect, and Trust
1. Gives credence to and follows up on patient's or family's complaint or criticism
2. Keeps promises or appointments made, without undue delay
3. Is honest with patient or family and avoids pretense of feelings, placation, or raising of false hopes
4. Fulfills patient's need to be spoken to, responded to, or accepted
5. Respects patient's need for privacy and protection of modesty
6. Allows patient to gain or maintain own self-esteem and standards of aesthetics and grooming
7. Respects cultural, religious, and other differences which affect patient's care
8. Maintains confidentiality of patient information
9. Shows concern for patient verbally and by doing little "extra" things for him or her

F. Facilitates Interaction of Family or Significant Others with Patient
1. Facilitates parent-newborn interaction
2. Arranges for patient contact with family member or significant other
3. Alleviates family's concern about patient's care, condition, or treatment
4. Helps patient and family recognize and deal with their feelings about each other and develop a trusting relationship
5. Encourages family or significant other to get concurrent counseling or therapy
6. Keeps family or others from interfering in nurse-patient communication or from disrupting the therapeutic environment
7. Gives reassurance and support to family member giving complex and demanding care to patient

G. Stimulates, Remotivates Patient or Enables Him or Her to Achieve Self-Care and Independence
1. Provides sensory and social stimulation

to raise patient's level of consciousness or increase development
2. Employs reality orientation techniques and structuring of activities
3. Encourages patient to make social contact with others and to participate in activities
4. Supports and encourages steps toward independence
5. Correctly assesses and periodically reassesses patient's ability to assume care of daily health needs
6. Helps patient perceive need for and deal with termination of treatment or dependency relationship
7. Helps patient assume responsibility and accountability for his or her own behavior

III. Helps Maintain Patient Comfort and Normal Body Functions
A. Keeps Patient Clean and Comfortable
1. Gives complete hygiene care to helpless patient
2. Frequently changes incontinent patient, colostomy patient, or patient with drainage
3. Makes patient as comfortable as possible during treatment or procedure

B. Helps Patient Maintain or Regain Normal Body Functions
1. Helps patient maintain appropriate food and fluid intake
2. Helps patient maintain normal bowel functions
3. Helps patient maintain or regain normal bladder function
4. Helps patient maintain normal body temperature

IV. Takes Precautionary and Preventive Measures in Giving Patient Care
A. Prevents Infection
1. Uses aseptic technique in treating wounds, lesions, ostomies, decubiti, etc.
2. Avoids contaminating equipment or using contaminated materials on patient
3. Institutes and observes isolation technique
4. Correctly uses reverse isolation
5. Washes hands between patients
6. Prevents moisture in patient's lesions
7. Checks contacts of patient with communicable disease to ascertain immunity status or presence of symptoms

B. Protects Skin and Mucous Membranes from Injurious Substances or Agents
1. Gives thorough skin care
2. Minimizes contact of skin with injurious or irritating substances
3. Periodically deflates or avoids overinflation of inflatable internal devices to prevent pressure and tissue damage
4. ______4. *Applies dressing, tape, or treatment device too tightly, causing circulatory impairment or tissue damage*

C. Uses Positioning or Exercise to Prevent Injury or the Complications of Immobility
1. Adjusts patient's extremities to prevent strain, nerve damage, footdrop, injury
2. Uses turning or passive and active exercise to prevent complications (e.g., pneumonia, decubiti, venous stasis, etc.)
3. Positions patient's body to permit drainage or prevent aspiration or suffocation
4. Positions patient to ensure effectiveness and safety of treatment
5. Maintains body alignment in moving immobile patient
6. Maintains ordered or optimum position to prevent injury to operative site or to actual or potential fracture site
7. Avoids changing position of patient too quickly or traumatically

D. Avoids Using Potentially Injurious Technique in Administering Care and Managing Intrusive Treatments
1. Selects correct, suitable, properly fitting or functioning equipment to be used on patient
2. Inserts or removes intrusive devices without causing pain, discomfort, or injury
3. Selects correct line, tube, or wire from multiple lines for connection of equipment, insertion or withdrawal of substances (tube feedings, parenteral infusion, irrigations, suctioning, etc.)
4. Uses safe techniques in introduction of fluid into the patient's body
5. Uses safe technique in the withdrawal or drainage of fluids from patient's body
6. Uses safe technique in the administration of respiratory treatment
7. Checks to see that automatic equipment is on correct and safe setting
8. Refills, replaces, calibrates, or repairs equipment attached to patient's body
9. Avoids disruption of treatment process or harm to patient by inadvertent disconnection of equipment
10. Gives undivided attention to treat-

ment or care requiring continuous presence and attention

11. ______11. *Inadvertently cuts or injures patient while giving care*
12. Applies and maintains traction correctly

E. Protects Patient from Falls or Other Contact Injuries
1. Uses side rails or crib net; closes isolette door
2. Uses adequate restraints, applied correctly
3. Uses padding, helmets, or other protective devices to prevent patient from self-injury
4. Locks brakes or hinges on furniture or movable equipment
5. Assists patient during ambulation
6. Avoids leaving patient unattended or unobserved when there is danger of falling
7. Obtains help or uses safe body mechanics in moving, transporting, or ambulating heavy or helpless patient
8. Correctly and safely uses wheelchair, stretcher, or appropriate vehicle to transport patient
9. Avoids leaving patient in high or elevated position so patient cannot reach floor
10. Intervenes physically to prevent patient from falling or to soften the fall
11. Ensures that infant is handled carefully to prevent dropping or bumping

F. Maintains Surveillance of Patient's Activities
1. Maintains close observation of potentially dangerous patient activity (smoking, dangerous games, unsupervised shopping by addict)
2. Arranges close supervision or system of checks to prevent wandering, unauthorized absence, seduction, or deceitful behavior
3. Ensures that patient is escorted by hospital personnel when leaving unit or hospital, or when engaged in off-unit activities
4. Avoids delay in searching for missing patient
5. Physically intervenes when violence of one or several patients threatens safety of other patients (including sexual assaults)
6. Removes self from area or does not turn back on patient when patient becomes assaultive or sexually aggressive

G. Reduces or Removes Environmental Hazards
1. Prevents burns from heat lamps, warm soaks, other heating and treatment devices
2. Shields parts of patient's body from x-ray, phototherapy, or other irradiation
3. Searches for and removes, or does not leave potentially dangerous objects or substances in patient's environment
4. Restricts smoking, flowers, or strong perfume in room when it is detrimental to patient(s)
5. Observes safety regulations in the use of electrical equipment
6. Adjusts, repairs, replaces malfunctioning or broken equipment or furniture
7. Does accurate sponge count in surgery
8. ______8. *Mislays keys; leaves potentially dangerous rooms, cupboards, doors, or windows unlocked*
9. ______9. *Fills tub above safety level when bathing patient*
10. Does not allow water to remain on floor

V. Checks, Compares, Verifies, Monitors, and Follows-Up Medication and Treatment Processes

A. Checks Correctness, Condition, and Safety of Medication Being Prepared
1. Compares medication card, reminder list, etc. with Kardex or chart
2. Verifies that medication labels and instructions agree with patient's orders
3. Checks expiration time and condition of medication
4. Considers compatibility, potency, and stability of medications
5. Prepares and verifies correct dosage
6. If interrupted, repeats each medication preparation step to prevent error

B. Ensures that Correct Medication or Care Is Given to the Right Patient and that Patient Takes or Receives It
1. Checks that care being administered is intended for that patient
2. Places or replaces correct identifying bracelet on patient
3. Accurately and completely labels all substances to be administered
4. Checks that patient ingests oral medication
5. Ensures that medication she or he does

not personally administer is administered correctly

C. Adheres to Schedule in Giving Medication, Treatment, or Test
   1. ______1. *Gave medication, treatment, or test late or missed it entirely*
   2. ______2. *Gave medication, treatment, or care sooner than scheduled or too often*
   3. Reschedules medication administration times to cover patient's absence from unit or to compensate for medication error

D. Administers Medication by Correct Route, Rate, or Mode
   1. ______1. *Gave medication by a different route than route ordered*
   2. ______2. *Gave medication rapidly by IV push instead of properly diluting it in IV solution*
   3. ______3. *Used wrong orifice or site to administer medication*
   4. ______4. *Failed to give facilitating or buffering substance with medication*
   5. ______5. *Gave too large an amount of liquid in subcutaneous or intramuscular injection*

E. Checks Patient's Readiness for Medication, Treatment, Surgery, or Other Care
   1. Checks patient for allergies
   2. Checks patient for other contraindications before administering care; withholds or discontinues contraindicated care
   3. Obtains and checks data on which dosage is predicated
   4. Observes dietary, fluid, or medication restrictions before surgery, treatment, or test
   5. Safely prepares patient for surgery, delivery, or other intrustive procedure

F. Checks to Ensure that Tests or Measurements Are Done Correctly
   1. Schedules, prepares for, and performs test or measurement correctly
   2. Ensures that specimen is collected correctly and delivered to laboratory
   3. Labels and dates specimens and requisitions correctly

G. Monitors Ongoing Infusions and Inhalations
   1. Checks, regulates, and maintains rate of flow of parenteral infusions
   2. Prevents or detects infiltration of IV, tissue damage, or phlebitis
   3. Regulates volume, rate, or duration of oxygen or other inhalations

H. Checks for and Interprets Effects of Medication, Treatment, or Care and Takes Corrective Action If Necessary
   1. Observes for signs of effectiveness of medication or treatment and, if ineffective, gives additional or alternative care
   2. Checks for, interprets, and correctly treats adverse reaction to medication, treatment, or care
   3. Watches for symptoms resulting from wrong medication or formula, and institutes care to compensate for the error
   4. Observes and evaluates patient for postoperative or postpartum complications

VI. Interprets Symptom Complex and Intervenes Appropriately

A. Checks Patient's Condition or Status
   1. Makes periodic checks as ordered or necessary
   2. Increases frequency of checks, measurement, observations, or visits when need is indicated by patient's condition or situation
   3. Continuously checks, observes, or stays with patient whose condition or treatment requires close monitoring
   4. Avoids superficial or incomplete checking
   5. Checks that patient's condition is satisfactory or that orders are completed before discharge

B. Remains Objective, Further Investigates, or Verifies Patient's Complaint or Problem
   1. Queries patient and family to ascertain cause or extent of problem
   2. Verifies observation or hunch by obtaining or performing tests or measurements
   3. Repeats test or asks for confirmation of unusual findings
   4. Rechecks condition or situation personally instead of relying on assessment or reports of others
   5. Avoids discounting patient's or family's perception or report of problem

C. Uses Alarms and Signals on Automatic Equipment as Adjunct to Personal Assessment
   1. ______1. *Fails to place, replace, or keep patient on monitor when indicated*

2. ______2. *Fails to set warning device or alarms on monitors or other equipment*
3. Avoids relying too heavily on monitor; checks patient personally
4. Responds immediately and correctly to alarm or signal or lack of alarm

D. Observes and Correctly Assesses Signs of Anxiety or Behavioral Stress
1. Recognizes when changes in patient's mental or behavioral status has physiological basis
2. Recognizes that patient's behavior necessitates psychiatric assessment or treatment
3. Recognizes signs of escalation or loss of control; sets and enforces limits
4. Recognizes when agitated, violent, confused, assaultive, or sexually abusive patient should be restrained, secluded, or medicated
5. Maintains continuing assessment of patient in restraints, seclusion, or under sedation
6. Assesses patient's behavior as potentially suicidal, self-destructive, self-abusive, assaultive, or homicidal and takes appropriate action
7. Recognizes when patient's attention-seeking behavior should not be reinforced and when intervention is indicated
8. Assesses patient's readiness for off-unit privileges or weekend passes, etc., and withholds if contraindicated

E. Observes and Correctly Assesses Physical Signs, Symptoms, or Findings and Intervenes Appropriately
1. Notes signs, symptoms, or abnormal results and associates symptom complex with probable cause
2. Observes, correctly assesses minimal, early, or atypical signs and takes appropriate action
3. Makes the correct *differential* assessment of cause of patient's condition
4. Assesses patient's state of consciousness as being subject to sudden change and takes precautions to prevent injury

F. Correctly Assesses Severity or Priority of Patient's Condition and Gives or Obtains Necessary Care
1. Assesses patient's condition as requiring immediate attention and gives or arranges for it
2. Recognizes that patient's acute condition requires treatment on acute unit and arranges for appropriate care
3. Assesses vigorousness and frequency of care required and intervenes appropriately
4. Correctly assesses the patient's need for prn medication or treatment

VII. Responds to Emergencies

A. Anticipates Need for Crisis Care
1. Prepares equipment, supplies, medication, and environment for management of actual or anticipated crisis
2. Alerts staff to be prepared for potential crisis (delivery of neonate in distress, administration of potentially dangerous medication)

B. Takes Instant, Correct Action in Emergency Situations
1. Restores or enhances breathing (suctions, provides clear airway, gives O_2, etc.)
2. Initiates cardiopulmonary resuscitation and defibrillation procedures
3. Immediately relieves condition that interferes with successful resuscitation (fluid in peritoneal cavity from dialysis, etc.)
4. Stops bleeding
5. Recognizes onset of shock, checks for cause, and takes immediate action
6. Initiates measures to counteract poisoning, drug overdose, or anaphylaxis
7. Prevents cerebral air embolism or pneumothorax when tubes are inadvertently disconnected
8. Prevents entry of foreign substances or objects into the system (broken needles, endotube, etc.)
9. Covers eviscerated organs or opened incision with moist dressings and arranges for immediate surgery or repair
10. Delivers infant safely, and with safety to mother, in precipitous delivery situation
11. Treats sudden maternal or fetal distress by appropriate supportive measures and prepares for immediate delivery if necessary
12. Gives appropriate first-aid burn care
13. Physically restrains patient from imminent suicide attempt

C. Maintains Calm and Efficient Approach Under Pressure
1. ______1. *Panicked, was unable to act,*

or acted ineffectively in emergency situation

2. Avoids alarming patient in giving infant emergency care
3. Summons help in quickest, safest, most efficient manner
4. Postpones management activities, paper work, or deferrable patient care in order to give emergency care
5. Adjusts pace or sequence of care to cope with crisis
6. Ensures that patient is attended or protected during crisis
7. Decides relative efficiency of transporting patient to source of help or vice versa
8. Quickly locates most accessible source of emergency medication or equipment

D. Assumes Leadership Role in Crisis Situation

1. Directs others, works with team, and uses all available resources in giving crisis care
2. Manages environment, personnel, and patients in fire or other disaster
3. Extends usual R.N. role to give emergency treatment or medication without order or to obtain immediate test data on which to base emergency care

VIII. Obtains, Records, and Exchanges Information in Behalf of the Patient

A. Checks Data Sources for Orders and Other Information about Patient

1. Checks and rechecks patient's orders before giving care
2. ______2. *Makes error or omission in reading or interpreting doctor's order on chart or Kardex*
3. Checks chart for information about patient's history, condition, and previous care given
4. Searches previous record for similar symptoms or relevant data

B. Interviews, Obtains, and Validates Information from Patient and Family

1. Obtains historical or other facts that contribute to understanding of patient's problem
2. Detects need to verify authenticity of information obtained
3. Provides therapeutic support, avoids threatening approach
4. Uses good interview technique
5. ______5. *Fails to listen to what patient really is saying and to respond to patient's obvious anxiety*

C. Transcribes or Records Information on Chart, Kardex, or Other Information System

1. ______1. *Fails to transcribe order*
2. ______2. *Makes transcription or transposition error*
3. Checks transcription of orders and corrects errors
4. Charts that care was given
5. Charts observation of patient's symptoms and status or test results
6. ______6. *Charts inaccurately*
7. ______7. *Falsifies records (charts care as having been given when it was not)*

D. Exchanges Information with Nursing Staff and Other Departments

1. Obtains information about patient or assignment from nursing staff before giving care
2. Gives complete, accurate shift or other report of patient's status, condition, and treatment given, to members of nursing team
3. Notifies other staff of particulars of special treatment, care, plan, restrictions, or change (posts signs, uses special notes, flags information, etc.)
4. Reports significant change to team leader or supervisor and asks for direction and guidance
5. Relays patient request to team member responsible for that care measure
6. Maintains two-way communication with other departments about patient appointments, discharge, diet, laboratory results, supplies, etc.

E. Exchange Information with Medical Staff

1. Obtains clarification of ambiguous written or verbal order
2. Obtains verification of STAT or verbal order
3. Informs doctor of significant change, symptom, reaction, laboratory result, etc., and asks for order
4. Informs or reminds doctor of relevant facts, etc., and offers suggestions in diagnosis and management of patient's care
5. ______5. *Gives doctor insufficient or incorrect information in reporting patient's symptoms*

IX. Utilizes Patient Care Planning
   A. Develops, Uses, and Follows up on Patient Care Plan
      1. Plans care in accordance with patient condition, needs, limitations, etc.
      2. Revises care plan in light of changes in patient condition or needs
      3. Anticipates or makes certain patient has correct medication or equipment he or she will need and appropriate directions for taking medication
      4. Develops strategy for management of contingencies; devises alternative plan
      5. Follows up to ensure that patient is carrying out plan
   B. Utilizes or Coordinates Other Health Care Personnel in Patient Care Planning
      1. Includes doctor, other staff, or other agencies in the planning conference
      2. Communicates changes in patient care plan to other departments, services, or agencies
      3. Ensures that there is staff consistency and continuity in implementing the care plan
   C. Involves Patient, Family, or Significant Other in Planning Care
      1. Determines ability of patient, family, or significant other to provide needed care
      2. Encourages and helps patient and family to participate in planning and therapeutic activities; fully informs patient and family of care plan

X. Teaches, Supervises, and Acts as Resource Person for Staff
   A. Teaches Correct Principles, Procedures, and Techniques of Patient Care
      1. Demonstrates and explains new or unfamiliar procedures and methods to new staff or when asked for help by other staff
      2. Notes and corrects errors or omissions of care and explains principles and procedures of correct care, stressing importance
      3. Teaches importance of adapting care or asking for assistance when routine care is contraindicated by patient's condition
   B. Supervises and Checks the Work of Staff for Whom She or He Is Responsible
      1. Makes effective and realistic personnel assignments
      2. Checks correctness and adequacy of patient care plan and of patient care given by team member

Summary: Overall Composite of Analysis Section of Category Descriptions

A. KNOWLEDGES
   1. Knowledge about the patient
   2. Knowledge of patient's orders, treatment regimen, or nursing care plan
   3. Knowledge of language, symbols, and terminology necessary to interpret orders and patient data, and to be used in charting and transcription of information
   4. Knowledge of ward situation, including patient census and staffing
   5. Awareness of type of information required about the patient and his or her problem
   6. Sources of information
   7. Knowledge of chart and record formats so search for information will be systematic
   8. Knowledge of resources and lines of authority
   9. Knowledge of pharmacology
   10. Knowledge of anatomy, physiology, body processes, and the interrelation of body systems
   11. Knowledge of the effects of body position, pressure, and prolonged inactivity on body systems and of methods of intervention to prevent complications
   12. Knowledge of physical and emotional needs of patient and/or family
   13. Knowledge of principles and techniques in administration of medication or treatment
   14. Knowledge of techniques and underlying principles of common nursing interventions
   15. Knowledge of tests as a basis for assessment
   16. Recognition of the need to investigate or verify patient's complaint
   17. Knowledge of correct procedure for taking vital signs and other measures and for performing certain common tests, such as urine sugar and acetone determination
   18. Knowledge of signs and symptoms and their implications
   19. Knowledge of signs of stress, stress behavior, and factors that induce stress
   20. Knowledge of therapeutic measures to relieve stress and anxiety
   21. Knowledge of ways to help patient achieve self-care and independence
   22. Knowledge of emergency procedures and resources

23. Knowledge of equipment and how it functions
24. Knowledge of safety factors
25. Knowledge of the need for and the techniques of communication
26. Information needed to supervise and interact with staff
27. Knowledge needed to teach staff and patients
28. Knowledge of agency policies and procedures and their underlying rationale
29. Awareness of roles and functions of medical support staff
30. Awareness of team concepts
31. Awareness of self-limitations
32. Awareness of priority of patient care over administrative duties
33. Awareness of legal responsibilities, nurse licensure, and limits of authority
34. Knowledge of record-keeping procedures

B. Abilities

35. Observation and assessment skills
36. Investigative and analytical skills
37. Problem-solving ability
38. Ability to doubt or question orders or care administered by others
39. Ability to attend to and take verbal orders
40. Ability to read and understand medical orders and patient-care information
41. Ability to use correct interviewing and counseling technique
42. Ability to analyze and adjust own feelings
43. Ability to use interpersonal skills
44. Ability to alleviate stress
45. Ability to gain patient acceptance and cooperation
46. Ability to promote self-care and independence
47. Ability to develop a patient care plan and follow it
48. Ability to organize time and to set priorities
49. Ability to remember to perform necessary care or activities
50. Ability to create or adapt equipment and methods to solve specific problems
51. Ability to perform common nursing interventions
52. Ability to correctly and safely use equipment and intrusive or externally applied devices on patient
53. Ability to recognize unsafe situations and to intervene correctly to prevent or minimize harm to patient
54. Ability to correctly and safely apply emergency interventions
55. Ability to record and report information
56. Teaching skills
57. Ability to direct others and to fully use available resources
58. Ability to recognize own limitations and to obtain help, approval, or orders
59. Ability to recognize when an error has occurred, her or his own or others

C. Affect

60. Acceptance of responsibility
61. Awareness of professional responsibilities and limitations
62. Self-awareness and self-control
63. Self-confidence and courage of convictions
64. Willingness to accept help or criticism or to seek opportunities for learning
65. Concern for patient and family
66. Tact, sensitivity to feelings of others
67. Respect for patient's rights
68. Willingness to relinquish patient's dependence and to find satisfaction in patient's independence
69. Willingness to work cooperatively with others and to give help if needed
70. Commitment to importance of specific aspects of nursing care
71. Honesty
72. Adaptability and flexibility
73. Deliberateness and decisiveness in taking action
74. Sense of urgency in a crisis situation
75. Risk-taking
76. Caution
77. Objectivity and tolerance
78. Resistance to unthinkingly following rote procedure
79. Attention to detail
80. Concentration and resistance to distraction
81. Sense of vigilance
82. Thoroughness and conscientiousness
83. Persistence

D. Motor Skills

84. Skill in administering intramuscular injections
85. Skill in inserting intravenous needle
86. Skill in drawing blood samples from patient's vein
87. Skill in using protective devices without injury to patient (e.g., tongue blades)
88. Speed and dexterity in readying emergency equipment or applying life-saving interventions
89. Adeptness, deftness, gentleness, and sureness of motion in giving vigorous first aid or in using intrusive or potentially traumatic procedures

APPENDIX B

Guide for Assessing the Needs of the Patient

1. Personal information
   - 1.1 General impression
   - 1.2 Patient's and family's perception of the illness and how he or she should be treated
   - 1.3 Apparent degree of illness
     - 1.31 Acutely ill, seriously ill, critically ill, improving, convalescent, failing to improve
   - 1.4 Cerebral activity[1]
     - 1.41 Mental status[2]
       - 1.411 Oriented
       - 1.412 Disoriented
     - 1.42 Level of consciousness[2]
       - 1.421 Fully conscious
       - 1.422 Inattentive
       - 1.423 Drowsy
       - 1.424 Confused
       - 1.425 Stuporous
       - 1.426 Comatose
   - 1.5 Previous experience with illness in hospital ____
     Previous experience with illness at home ____
   - 1.6 Age __________ Sex __________
   - 1.7 Drugs
     - 1.71 Drugs used
     - 1.72 Drug sensitivities
   - 1.8 Problems with communication ____
     - 1.81 Language ____
       - 1.811 Does not speak English ____
         Speaks ____
       - 1.812 Inability to speak ____
       - 1.813 Impediment in speech ____
       - 1.814 Hearing impairment ____
       - 1.815 Other ____
     - 1.82 Manner in which patient communicates satisfaction or dissatisfaction ____
     - 1.83 How does he or she seem to relate to others? ____
   - 1.9 Cultural differences that may affect patient's attitudes, food preferences, expectations, modesty pattern, time orientation, or customary sleeping garments ____
   - 1.10 Religion ____
     - 1.101 Does patient wish to see minister, priest, rabbi? ____
     - 1.102 Religious practices with which he or she desires assistance ____
   - 1.11 Education and intellectual level
     - 1.111 Level of schooling ____
     - 1.112 Interest in learning ____
     - 1.113 Hobbies and recreational interests ____
     - 1.114 What does the patient like to talk about? ____
     - 1.115 Prejudices ____
     - 1.116 Aspirations ____
   - 1.12 Role and place in family ____

[1] Although the following characteristics of cerebral activity might appropriately be included under the "Physical and Physiologic Status" heading of this guide, they are elaborated here because of their importance to the nurse in assessing the priority of needs of the patient.

[2] For definition of these terms, the reader is referred to glossaries of neurologic and psychiatric terms.

1.121 Position in family ____
1.122 Position in community ____
1.123 Apparent self-image. How does he or she answer the questions Where am I? What am I? Who am I? ____
1.124 How does the family appear to regard patient? ____
1.125 Is there anything in the family relationship that may have an effect on the patient? ____
1.1251 Favorable ____
1.1252 Unfavorable ____
1.126 Is there a relative or friend who may be helpful in meeting the patient's needs? ____
1.127 If he or she has no family, what resources are available as a substitute? ____
1.128 Who is the head of the family? ____
1.13 Residence
1.131 Place of birth ____
1.132 Present residence ____
1.133 Travel (especially overseas—recent or in the past) ____

2. Social and economic status
2.1 Occupation and position ____
2.2 Insurance
2.21 Hospital ____
2.22 Medical ____
2.23 Income ____
2.3 Adequacy of income to meet needs ____
2.4 Adequacy of housing ____

3. Emotional status[3]
3.1 Apprehensive ____
3.2 Anxious ____
3.3 Agitated ____
3.4 Restless ____
3.5 Irritable ____
3.6 Shy, timid ____
3.7 Withdrawn ____
3.8 Depressed ____
3.9 Discouraged ____
3.10 Happy ____
3.11 Demanding ____

[3] These terms are intended to assist the nurse in identifying the nature of the emotional needs of the patient, to enable her or him to formulate the most effective plan or approach possible. Their purpose is not to label or categorize the patient but rather to help the nurse better understand and describe patients' behavior as a necessary first step to assisting them in coping with their illness.

4. Patient's expectations
4.1 How does the patient view his role as a sick person? ____
4.2 What does he or she expect of those administering care? ____
4.21 Nurses ____
4.22 Doctors ____
4.23 Others ____
4.3 How does he or she expect the family to behave? ____
4.4 How does he or she think the illness should be treated? ____
4.5 What does the patient want to know and do? ____

5. Previous experience and background that may be factors in patient reactions and expectations
5.1 Previous hospitalizations ____
5.2 Previous care by nurses ____
5.3 Life experiences ____

6. Personal habits (which of these is the patient able to perform alone, with which does he or she require assistance, which must be performed for him or her?)
6.1 Mouth care
6.11 Dentures ____
6.12 Brushing teeth ____
6.2 Bathing
6.21 Modifications ____
6.3 Hair (clean, dirty, tangled, matted) ____
6.31 Shampoo ____
6.32 Combing ____
6.33 Wig or hairpiece ____
6.4 Nails (clean, dirty, long, short) ____
6.5 Beard ____
6.6 Bowel or defecation habits
6.61 Usual time ____
6.62 Time of last defecation ____
6.63 Abnormalities ____
6.631 Constipation ____
6.632 Diarrhea ____
6.633 Incontinence ____
6.64 Dependent drainage ____
6.641 Colostomy ____
6.642 Ileostomy ____
6.643 Fistula ____
6.644 Draining wound ____
6.7 Sleep and resting habits
6.71 Rest periods ____
6.72 Sleep ____
6.721 Usual time for retiring ____
6.722 Usual hour for arising ____
6.723 Any assistance or modifications that

the patient requires to get adequate sleep ____

- 6.8 Food habits and patterns
  - 6.81 Likes, dislikes, preferences ____
  - 6.82 Timing of meals when at home ____
  - 6.83 Any ideas about food that may have a bearing on patient's food intake ____

7. Exercise
   - 7.1 Active or sedentary habits ____
   - 7.2 Usual forms of exercise ____
   - 7.3 Limits of exercise ____
     - 7.31 Paralysis ____
     - 7.32 Weakness ____
     - 7.33 Prosthesis ____
8. With what daily activities of living does the patient require help?
   - 8.1 Eating ____
   - 8.2 Bathing ____
   - 8.3 Dressing ____
   - 8.4 Getting out of bed ____
   - 8.5 Walking ____
   - 8.6 Bathroom ____
   - 8.7 Uses crutches, braces, wheelchair, walker, etc. ____
9. Physical and physiologic status
   - 9.1 Height ________ Weight ________ (lean, normal, overweight)
   - 9.2 Vital signs:
     Temperature ____
     Pulse ____
     Respiration ____
   - 9.3 Blood pressure ____
   - 9.4 Condition of skin
     - 9.401 Intact ____
     - 9.402 Breaks or wounds ____
     - 9.403 Dry ____
     - 9.404 Moist ____
     - 9.405 Wrinkled ____
     - 9.406 Tense ____
     - 9.407 Bruised ____
     - 9.408 Rash ____
     - 9.409 Flushed ____
     - 9.410 Pale ____
     - 9.411 Jaundiced ____
     - 9.412 Ulcers or sores ____
     - 9.413 Edematous areas ____
   - 9.5 Teeth
     - 9.51 Own teeth ____
     - 9.52 Edentulous ____
     - 9.53 Dentures ____
   - 9.6 Vision
     - 9.61 Good ____
     - 9.62 Defective ____
     - 9.63 Blind ____
     - 9.64 Prosthesis ____
   - 9.7 Eyes
     - 9.71 Conjunctiva ____
     - 9.72 Lids ____
   - 9.8 Hearing
     - 9.81 Good ____
     - 9.82 Impaired ____
   - 9.9 Body alignment ____
   - 9.10 Position ____
   - 9.11 General sensation ____
     - 9.111 Sensory deficit ____
     - 9.112 Inability to detect changes in temperature ____
10. Needs with which the patient requires assistance
    - 10.1 Maintenance of oxygen supply ____
      - 10.11 Clear airway ____
      - 10.12 Assistance with breathing ____
      - 10.13 Additional supply of oxygen ____
        - 10.131 Mask or catheter in proper position ____
        - 10.132 Mask comfortable ____
        - 10.133 Tent tucked in ____
      - 10.14 Evidence of general oxygen deficit ____
      - 10.15 Difficulty in breathing ____
      - 10.16 Signs or symptoms indicating deficit of oxygen ____
    - 10.2 Maintenance of water balance
      - 10.21 Intake ____
      - 10.22 Output ____
      - 10.23 Weight ____
      - 10.24 Condition of skin and mucous membranes ____
      - 10.25 Thirst ____
    - 10.3 Nutritional needs ____
      - 10.31 Interference with capacity to eat ____
        - 10.311 Anorexia, nausea, vomiting ____
      - 10.32 Condition preventing absorption of food ____
        - 10.321 Diarrhea ____
    - 10.4 Capacity to maintain excretory function ____
      - 10.41 Urine
        - 10.411 Voids ____
        - 10.412 Indwelling catheter ____
        - 10.413 Color, odor, appearance of urine ____
      - 10.42 Bowel ____
    - 10.5 Special observation of urine
      - 10.51 Glucose ____
      - 10.52 Acetone ____
      - 10.53 Specific gravity ____

- 10.54 Color ____
- 10.55 Odor ____
- 10.56 Filter ____

11. Capacity to maintain motor function
    - 11.1 Difficulty in swallowing ____
    - 11.2 Difficulty in walking ____
    - 11.3 Difficulty with grasping ____
    - 11.4 Motor incoordination ____
    - 11.5 Motor instability ____
    - 11.6 Motor weakness ____
    - ____
12. Ability to maintain appropriate position and body alignment ____
13. Therapeutic measures and devices
    - 13.1 Blood transfusions ____
    - 13.2 Indwelling catheter ____
    - 13.3 Cast ____
    - 13.4 Nasogastric or gastric suction ____
    - 13.5 Surgical procedure ____
    - 13.6 Barron pump ____
    - 13.7 Tracheostomy ____
    - 13.8 Other ____
14. Signs and symptoms associated with a disease state
    - 14.1 Pain ____
    - 14.2 Fever ____
    - 14.3 Abdominal distention ____
15. Medical diagnosis ____
16. Condition of physical environment
    - 16.1 Equipment used in the care of the patient ____
    - 16.2 Furnishings ____
    - 16.3 Floors—clean and dry ____
    - 16.4 Room temperature and ventilation ____
    - 16.5 Lights ____
17. Safety precautions
    - 17.1 Side rails ____
    - 17.2 Low bed ____
    - 17.3 Other ____
18. What instruction does patient require?
19. What problems does he or she have in accepting the goals that are possible for him or her?
20. What aspects of the medical care plan have a bearing on the patient's needs for nursing?
    - 20.1 Diagnostic measures
    - 20.2 Therapy
21. Which aspects of the patient's care require assistance from members of other disciplines?
22. What care and service is the patient likely to require following discharge from the hospital? Need for continuing care?

APPENDIX C

Assessment of Spiritual Concerns

Spiritual Concerns

Etiology

Challenged belief system
Separation from religious-cultural ties
Anticipated role change
Concerned about relationship with God
Unresolved feelings about the concept of death
Search for more meaning or purpose in existence
Disrupted religious practices

Defining Characteristics

Investigates various beliefs
Verbalizes inner conflict about beliefs
Questions credibility of religious cultural system
Discouraged
Mild anxiety
Bewildered
Anticipatory grief
Questions meaning of own existence
Concern about relationship with God/diety
Unable to participate in usual religious practices, such as daily prayers, communion, meditation, worship services
Attempts to substitute simplified rituals for usual worship
Unable to obtain specific foods required by faith/belief system

Spiritual Despair

Etiology

Self-disintegration
Lack of will to live
Lost belief in self
Lost belief in treatment
Lost belief in value system and/or God

Defining Characteristics

Hopelessness
Sense of meaninglessness
Loss of spiritual belief
Death wish (escapism)
Sense of exhaustion
Sense of abandonment
Sees no meaning in suffering
Requires extreme effort to function
Withdrawal
Severe depression
Loss of affect
Refusal or passive acceptance of therapy
Refusal to communicate with loved ones
Discontinued religious participation

Spiritual Distress

Etiology

Separation from religious-cultural ties
Challenged belief and value system

Sense of meaninglessness/purposelessness
Remoteness from God
Disrupted Spiritual Trust
Moral-ethical nature of therapy
Sense of guilt/shame
Intense suffering
Unresolved feelings about death
Anger toward God

DEFINING CHARACTERISTICS *COMMON TO ALL ETIOLOGIES:*

(One of the following *must* be present):
Struggling with meaning in life/death
Seeks spiritual assistance
Disturbance in concepts/perception of God or belief system
Disturbance in sleep/rest pattern
Moderate to severe anxiety
Crying
Varying degrees of grieving
Depression
Preoccupation
Psychosomatic manifestations
Degrees of anger
Degrees of guilt

DEFINING CHARACTERISTICS *RELATED TO SPECIFIC ETIOLOGIES:*

Separation from Religious-Cultural Ties

Loneliness
Sense of powerlessness
Doubts
Credibility of religious-cultural system

Challenged Belief and Value System

Ambivalent about own and others belief systems
Difficulty in receiving assistance

Sense of Meaninglessness/Purposelessness

Cynicism
Considers suicide
Questions meaning in suffering
Feelings of uselessness
Withdrawal
Apathy
Self-destructive behavior
Sexual activity disturbance

Remoteness from God

Lacks a feeling of unity with God
Sense of spiritual emptiness
Gains little satisfaction in prayer
Verbalizes that God seems very distant
Verbalizes a desire to feel close to God

Disrupted Spiritual Trust

Doubts compassion of superior being
Worries about loss of trust
Ambivalence
Resentment
Feelings of alienation

Moral-Ethical Nature of Therapy

Sense of powerlessness (trapped feeling)
Ambivalence in decisions
Questions or refuses therapeutic regimen
Agrees to morally/ethically unacceptable therapy
Frantic seeking of advice or support for decision-making

Sense of Guilt/Shame

Wish to undo, redo, relive the past
Expressions of shame, regret, sinfulness, guilt
Bitterness, recrimination
Inability to forgive self or receive forgiveness
Views illness as punishment from God
Doubts acceptance by God
Self-belittling
Projection of blame
Self-destructive behavior
Sexual activity disturbance

Intense Suffering

Questions meaning of suffering
Fear of ability to endure suffering
Ambivalence toward God
Questions credibility of God/belief system
Expresses that suffering is necessary
Reparation
Self-focus as demonstrated by withdrawal, irritability, restlessness/agitation, self-pity, or fatigue

Unresolved Feelings about Death

Fears (of darkness, being alone, going to sleep, etc.)
Concern about life after death
Disturbing dreams

"Gallows" humor
Demanding behavior
Avoidance/preoccupation with subject of death

Anger Toward God

Feels resentment/hostility/alienation
Perceives illness as punishment from God
Reluctance to participate in spiritual rituals
Rebelliousness
Displacement of anger toward religious representative

Rating of Independent Nursing Involved in Treating the Health Problem

Degrees of Independent Nursing Therapy

Assessment is high
Intervention is medium to high with interdependence with other disciplines in various areas

Etiologies for Future Consideration

Religious Immaturity

Defining characteristics:
Unclear differentiation regarding beliefs/values ("I believe what I was taught")
Feels no freedom of religious choice
Persistent indecision about spiritual beliefs
Motivated by self-gratification
Verbalizes little about religious meaning in relation to health/illness
No verbalization of feelings, acts, and experiences related to belief system
Excessive verbalization about spiritual relation to health/illness
Lack of integration. Behavior incongruent with stated belief
Evidence of magical thinking
Uses religious themes to manipulate people
Dabbling in a variety of religious experiences
Inability to make commitment, closed to growth

Distorted View of Basic Religious Tenets

Defining characteristics:
Guilt
Sees illness as punishment
Inadequate substitution of rituals

Unresolved Hostility toward a Particular Church, Religion, Religious Representative

Defining characteristics:
Anger
Cynicism
Outburst
Refusal to accept visitation by religious representative

APPENDIX D

Summary of Some of the Responses to Injury

Phase I	Neuro-endocrine	Psychological	Circulatory	Metabolism	Water and Electrolytes	Blood
A. Onset		Shock Anxiety, fear Guilt, shame Frustration Denial Aggression: ill-tempered, irascible Passivity: pitiable, complains, obsequious Elation: neurotic level of function Indecisiveness, vacillation $\downarrow$				
B. Injury 2–4 days patient looks and feels sick	sympatho-adreno-medullary response (1–12 hr) $\uparrow$ Norepinephrine $\uparrow$ Epinephrine	Surrender, abdication of responsibility Listless, sleeps, "regressive integration" Egocentricity Constriction of interests or lack of interest Emotional dependency, with ambivalence toward those on whom dependent	Tachycardia $\uparrow$ Cardiac output $\uparrow$ Systolic blood pressure Vasoconstriction $\uparrow$ Diastolic blood pressure Splenic contraction to maintain blood volume $\uparrow$ Blood volume	$\uparrow$Hepatic glycogenolysis, hyperglycemia	Water loss from lungs, skin sweating	$\uparrow$ Platelets and fibrinogen $\downarrow$ Prothrombin time Results in acceleration of blood clotting $\uparrow$ Sedimentation rate (varies with blood content of fibrinogen)

Respiration	Alimentary Canal	Other	Wound	Needs of the Patient
↑ Rate and depth Bronchial dilation ↑ Oxygen consumption As a result of anesthesia, drugs, unconsciousness, immobility, and other effects of illness, increased secretion into and interference with mechanisms for clearing the	Peristalsis decreased or absent for 12–48 hr No appetite	Skin: ↑ sweating (cholinergic) Immobilization and splinting of wound with pain Resistance to movement, tries to find a comfortable position Hypothermia first 12 hr or so, then fever should not be over 100°F for 24–48 hr, and then re-	Lag or inflammatory phase Strength of wound is low Exudation of fluid into the wound—contains leukocytes and antibodies; exudate also contains protein, mucopolysaccharides, and ascorbic acid from which collagen fibers are formed	The specific regimen for each patient is prescribed by the physician Oral food and fluids are withheld until peristalsis is restored; encourage deep breathing, coughing, and turning, exercises of the extremities, and ambulation; patient requires assistance and support; protect from unnecessary stimulation, provide for periods of rest and quiet, use analgesics and other measures to prevent unnecessary pain; the nurse should assume responsibility for the care of the dependent patient; observe vital signs, urinary output in relation to intake, and if intake is exceeding output to an unexplained degree, report observation to the physician Note time, onset, degree of elevation of fever; should it be over 37.7°C (100°F) or continue at or above this level longer than

(Continued)

Phase I	Neuroendocrine	Psychological	Circulatory	Metabolism	Water and Electrolytes	Blood
Catabolism exceeds anabolism	Adenohypophysis (anterior pituitary) ↓ ACTH Adrenocortical response ↑ Glucocorticoids ↑ Cortisol (peak 6 hr)	Hypochondriasis		↓ Adrenal cholesterol and ascorbic acid ↑ Gluconeogenesis ↓ Cellular glucose utilization ↑ Protein catabolism ↓ Protein synthesis Negative nitrogen balance Nitrogen excretion in urine increased; may lose 7–15 g per day in ordinary soft-tissue injury ↑ Fat mobilization (from fat depots) ↑ 17-hydroxycorticosteroid excretion		Leukocytosis Lymphocytes and eosinophils diminish in number Hyperglycemia

Phase II	Neuroendocrine	Psychological	Circulatory	Metabolism	Water and Electrolytes	Blood
		Defensive retreat				
	↑ Adrenal androgens (slight)			↑ 17-ketosteroid excretion in urine		
	↑ Aldosterone			↑ 11-oxysteroid excretion		
	Neurohypophysis ↓ ↑ ADH			Rapid weight loss	Sodium retention Potassium excretion Water retention resulting in oliguria for approximately 12 hr after injury	

Respiration	Alimentary Canal	Other	Wound	Needs of the Patient
tracheobronchial tree predispose to obstruction of the airway		turn to normal	During this time tissue debris and foreign materials are removed; this phase may be prolonged by the accumulation of blood, pus, or any other material in the wound that must be removed before wound healing can take place	usual 24–48 hr, this indicates that an infection may be developing; for example, incipient infection is often characterized by a marked rise in body temperature to 38.3°C (101°F) or higher All abdominal and chest wounds should be supported when the patient coughs; excessive and ineffective coughing should be avoided as it may lead to the disruption of an abdominal wound

Respiration	Alimentary Canal	Other	Wound	Needs of the Patient
		↓ Gonad secretion, amenorrhea, ↓ libido		

(Continued)

Phase II	Neuro-endocrine	Psychological	Circulatory	Metabolism	Water and Electrolytes	Blood
					Diuresis may begin in 1–2 days Diuresis of water and salt	
Turning point 3–7 days	Adreno-medullary signs past	Ambition with weakness	Normotension	↓ 17-hydroxy-corticosteroid excretion	Potassium excretion	Eosinophils and other
Patient begins to look and feel better	Adrenocortical secretion returns to normal	"I feel better today" Interested in surroundings, grooming and visitors	Normal cardiac output	↓ Nitrogen excretion Wound begins to acquire tensile strength (stitches out)	Body water still slightly high	leukocytes normal

Phase III	Neuro-endocrine	Psychological	Circulatory	Metabolism	Water and Electrolytes	Blood
Muscular strength returns 2–5 weeks	Normal	Acknowledgment Reintegration of personality Relinquishes: dependence egocentricity provincial reactions rebellion against dependency Wants to go home Ambulation no longer painful Ambition with increasing strength ↑	Normal	Positive nitrogen balance Weight gain Anabolism exceeds catabolism Resynthesis of muscle tissue	Normal	Normal

Respiration	Alimentary Canal	Other	Wound	Needs of the Patient
Normal	Bowel sounds return Appetite improves	Temperature returns to normal	Chemical and morphological changes occur in the wound leading to the formation of scar tissue and the healing of wound	During this period the patient may feel better than he or she actually is; patient should be protected from overactivity and overstimulation; food intake should be encouraged; high-quality proteins and food containing ascorbic acid are of particular importance The patient should be encouraged to be up and walking

Respiration	Alimentary Canal	Other	Wound	Needs of the Patient
Normal	Absorption capacity returns	Needs adequate diet and exercise May attempt premature overwork	Wound broader, raised red scar, tensile integrity established and function of soft tissues resumed	Patient should not return to work involving heavy muscular exercise until this phase has been completed Normal strength returns Adequate intake of protein and calories; may need 2,000–3,000 calories per day; severely burned patients may need more; patients leaving the hospital during the seventh to tenth day may need to be instructed to eat well; without an adequate intake of food convalescence may be delayed

(Continued)

Phase IV	Neuro-endocrine	Psychological	Circulatory	Metabolism	Water and Electrolytes	Blood
		↓ Adaptation and change				
Fat gain several months	Normal	Returns to work	Normal	Positive nitrogen balance, carbon and energy balance Normal strength	Normal	Normal

Respiration	Alimentary Canal	Other	Wound	Needs to the Patient
Normal	Normal	Looks underweight, at beginning Clothes fit loosely May tend to overeat Normal sexual function returns	During this time the wound loses its convex and reddened appearance; it becomes a concave, thin white line	The patient is able to return to ordinary occupation The patient's food intake should exceed his or her energy output until desired weight is regained; when this has been accomplished, food intake should be balanced with energy output so that obesity is avoided

This table has been synthesized from the cited and general references of Unit V on the relationship of psychological, physiological, and wound responses during the four phases of recovery from surgical injury. Needs of the patient for which the nurse has major responsibility during each phase are specified.

INDEX

D

F

J

K

L

O

Q

R

T

U